OXFORD TEXTBOOK OF
SPORTS
MEDICINE

OXFORD MEDICAL PUBLICATIONS

EDITORS

MARK HARRIES
Consultant Physician
Northwick Park Hospital
and
Clinical Director
British Olympic Medical Centre

CLYDE WILLIAMS
Professor of Sports Science
Loughborough University

WILLIAM D. STANISH
Professor of Surgery
Dalhousie University
Halifax, Nova Scotia
Canada

LYLE J. MICHELI
Director
Division of Sports Medicine
Children's Hospital
Boston, MA
USA

OXFORD TEXTBOOK OF
SPORTS
MEDICINE

SECOND EDITION

Edited by

Mark Harries
Clyde Williams
William D. Stanish
and Lyle J. Micheli

Oxford   New York   Tokyo
OXFORD UNIVERSITY PRESS
1998

Oxford University Press, Great Clarendon Street, Oxford OX2 6DP

Oxford   New York
Athens   Auckland   Bangkok   Bogota   Bombay
Buenos Aires   Calcutta   Cape Town   Dar es Salaam
Delhi   Florence   Hong Kong   Istanbul   Karachi
Kuala Lumpur   Madras   Madrid   Melbourne
Mexico City   Nairobi   Paris   Singapore
Taipei   Tokyo   Toronto   Warsaw

and associated companies in
Berlin Ibadan

Oxford is a trade mark of Oxford University Press

Published in the United States
by Oxford University Press, Inc., New York

First edition (hardback) published 1994; paperback published 1995
Second edition published 1998

A catalogue record for this book is available from the British Library

Library of Congress Cataloging in Publication Data
(Data applied for)

ISBN 0 19 262717 1

Typeset by Interactive Sciences Ltd.
Printed in Great Britian by Butler and Tanner Ltd., Frome

Preface to the first edition

We are all encouraged to take exercise as one contribution to a healthy life-style. However, participation in exercise and sport carries with it the risk of injury. Injuries occurring in the course of recreational activity are treated in exactly the same way as those sustained in the work-place or during the daily round of domestic activities. Why then sports medicine?

Sports medicine has evolved over the last 50 years from a core activity of treating injuries to one which now uses a multidisciplinary approach to the care of those injured whilst participating in sport. The rationale for this approach (and the legitimate claim on the title 'sports medicine') is that those who look after the injured are professionally obliged to offer advice on how injuries can be both treated and avoided.

Practitioners in all branches of sports medicine must now be well informed about those activities which have the potential to lead to injury. Understanding the physical and physiological demands that heavy and sustained activity places on participants in sport, whatever their age, requires a special knowledge of the adaptive responses to exercise.

In writing the *Oxford Textbook of Sports Medicine* we have included sections on environmental sciences as well as aspects of basic physiology, psychology, and biomechanics. While coverage is comprehensive, we have not included highly specialized subjects such as the fine details of surgical procedures. Each chapter offers the experience and perspective of its author in a way which informs; often the approach challenges the basis on which cherished beliefs have been built. We have tried above all to produce a concise reference work that will support all those involved in the broad spectrum of sports medicine.

To our authors we offer our thanks and trust that despite all, we have managed to remain friends. Our thanks also go to the staff of Oxford University Press for their help and guidance.

Preface to the second edition

The first edition of this textbook was published in 1994 and received many highly appreciative and constructive reviews. These, together with helpful comments from colleagues, have encouraged us to produce a second edition to keep pace with the fast moving and changing specialty of sports medicine. To this end, our loyal authors have updated and rewritten all existing chapters and we have commissioned new contributions on overtraining, eating disorders, nutrition and ergogenic aids, and making weight for sports participation. A new section containing chapters on the female athlete and exercise in pregnancy has been incorporated. The organization of the book into sports science and clinical aspects is judged to be particularly successful and has been retained. Topicality, as in the previous edition, has been deemed of utmost importance: authoritative chapters on issues such as drug abuse and gender verification are included.

Our grateful thanks go to all our authors and colleagues for their help, comments, and encouragement. We must particularly acknowledge the contribution of John Sutton who died unexpectedly during the preparation of this edition. He will be greatly missed as a scientist, a member of the organizing committee of the millennium Olympic Games, and not least by his family, friends, and colleagues. Much of his contribution to the first edition has been retained here and has been admirably updated by Martin Thompson.

Finally, we thank our secretaries for their sterling work and unfailing support, and our friends and publishers Oxford University Press.

March 1998

Mark Harries
Clyde Williams
William D. Stanish
Lyle J. Micheli

Contents

Introduction—Man as an athlete

1 Sports science

2 Sport and the environment

3 Medical aspects of exercise and sport

* It is with regret that we must report the death of John Sutton during the preparation of this edition.

List of contributors

PER-OLOF ÅSTRAND
Professor Emeritus, Physiolology, Karolinska Institute,
Stockholm, Sweden
Introduction—Man as an athlete

ROALD BAHR
Professor of Sports Medicine, Norwegian University of Sport
and Physical Education, Oslo, Norway
1.2.5 Eating disorders in athletes

MARIO M. BERKOWITZ
Orthopedic Surgery Resident, Long Island Jewish Medical
Center, New York, USA
4.3.3 Injuries of the rotator cuff

DARREN W. BOOTH
Consultant Physiotherapist, Department of Athletics, Acadia
University, Wolfville, Nova Scotia, Canada
6.5. Athletes with a disability

MARK K. BOWEN
Fellow and Junior Attending Orthopedic Surgeon,
Sportsmedicine and Shoulder Service, The Hospital for
Special Surgery, New York, USA
4.3.3 Injuries of the rotator cuff

OWEN H. BRADY
Senior Registrar, St Vincent's Hospital, Dublin, Ireland
4.2.3 Acute injuries of the meniscus

JEAN-LOUIS BRIARD
Chirurgie Orthopédique et Réparatrice, Traumatologie
Clinique du Cèdre, Bois-Guillaume, France
4.2.5 Fractures and dislocations

ROBERT M. BROCK
Sports Medicine Orthopaedic Surgeon, North York General
Hospital, North York, Ontario, Canada
*7.2 Emergencies of the musculoskeletal system in sport: 'the fallen
athlete' (Rodin)*

RICHARD BUDGETT
Director of Medical Services, British Olympic Association and
British Olympic Medical Centre, Northwick Park Hospital,
Harrow, Middlesex, UK
3.6 The overtraining syndrome

LINDA CASTELL
Senior Research Associate, Cellular Nutrition Research Group,
University Department of Biochemistry, Oxford, UK
3.6 The overtraining syndrome

GUGLIELMO CERULLO
Orthopaedic Surgeon and Sports Medicine Doctor, Clinica
Valle Giulia, Rome, Italy
5.2 Stress fractures

CATHERINE M. COADY
Department of Orthopaedic Surgery, Dalhousie University,
Nova Scotia, Canada
4.3.4 Injuries of the acromioclavicular joint

DAVID A. COWAN
Professor of Pharmaceutical Toxicology and Director, Drug
Control Centre, King's College London, UK
3.4 Drug abuse

JAY S. COX
Professor of Orthopedic Surgery, Pennsylvania State
University, University Park, USA
4.3.4 Injuries of the acromioclavicular joint

SANDRA L. CURWIN
Associate Professor and Director of Physical Therapy, Husson
College, Bangor, Maine, USA
4.4.4 The aetiology and treatment of tendinitis

FOSCO DE PAULIS
Director of Computed Tomography Service and Radiology,
Santa Maria di Collemaggio Hospital, L'Aquila, Italy
5.2 Stress fractures

WAYNE DERMAN
Associate Professor of Sport Science and Sports Medicine,
University of Cape Town Medical School, South Africa
5.5 Overuse injuries of the foot and ankle

MICHAEL J. DUNBAR
Senior Resident in Orthopaedic Surgery, Dalhousie University,
Halifax, Nova Scotia, Canada
5.3 Chronic exertional compartment syndrome

DAVID ELLIOTT
Honorary Professor of Occupational Medicine, Robens
Institute of Health and Safety, University of Surrey, UK
2.1 The underwater environment

MALCOLM A. FERGUSON-SMITH
Professor of Pathology, Cambridge University and Honorary
Consultant in Medical Genetics, Addenbrooke's Hospital,
Cambridge, UK
3.5 Gender verification and the place of XY females in sport

MIKAEL FOGELHOLM
Senior Researcher, The UKK Institute, Tampere, Finland
1.2.3 Making weight for sports participation

PETER A. FRICKER
Professor of Sports Medicine and Director of Medical
Services, Australian Institute of Sport, Canberra, Australia
4.4.1 Acute and overuse ankle injuries

JANE H. GIBSON
Consultant Rheumatologist, Fife Rheumatic Diseases Unit,
Cameron Hospital, Fife, UK
3.8 Exercise and the skeleton

J. ROBERT GIFFIN
Chief Resident, Division of Orthopaedic Surgery, University of
Western Ontario, London, Canada
4.2.5 Fractures and dislocations

F. ST C. GOLDEN
Consultant in Applied Physiology, Robens Institute, University
of Surrey, Guildford, UK
2.2 Immersion in cold water: effects on performance and safety

G. F. GOUBRAN
Consultant Oral and Maxillo-Facial Surgeon, Charing Cross,
Ealing, Royal Free, and Clementine Churchill Hospitals, and
Honorary Consultant, Royal Masonic Hospital, London, UK
7.3 Maxillofacial injuries in sport

BASIL J. S. GROGONO
Orthopaedic Surgeon, Dalhousie University, Halifax, Nova
Scotia, Canada
6.5 Athletes with a disability

A. B. GROSSMAN
Professor of Neuroendocrinology, St Bartholomew's Hospital,
London, UK
3.7 The endocrinology of exercise

LEW HARDY
Professor of Health and Human Performance, University
College of North Wales, Bangor, Gwynedd, UK
1.4 Sport psychology

MARK HARRIES
Consultant Physician, Northwick Park and St Mark's Hospital,
and Honorary Clinical Director, British Olympic Medical
Centre, Harrow, Middlesex, UK
3.2 The lung in sport

JAN HENRIKSSON
Professor of Physiology, Karolinska Institute, Stockholm,
Sweden
*1.1.3 Adaptations in skeletal muscle in response to endurance
training*

ROBERT C. HICKNER
Assistant Professor, School of Health and Human Performance
and School of Medicine, East Carolina University, Greenville,
North Carolina, USA
*1.1.3 Adaptations in skeletal muscle in response to endurance
training*

TREVOR A. HOWLETT
Consultant Physician and Endocrinologist, Leicester Royal
Infirmary, UK
3.7 The endocrinology of exercise

BRIAN J. HURSON
Consultant Orthopaedic Surgeon, Department of
Orthopaedics, St Vincent's Hospital, Dublin, Ireland
4.2.3 Acute injuries of the meniscus

J. C. HYNDMAN
Professor of Surgery, Dalhousie University, Halifax, Nova
Scotia, Canada
6.2 The growing athlete

PAUL J. JENKINS
Lecturer in Endocrinology, St Bartholomew's and The Royal
London Medical School, Queen Mary and Westfield College,
London, UK
3.7 The endocrinology of exercise

ROBERT J. JOHNSON
McClure Professor of Orthopedics and Academic Vice-
Chairman, Department of Orthopedics and Rehabilitation,
University of Vermont, Burlington, USA
4.2.1 Acute knee injuries: an overview

GRAHAM JONES
Director, Applied Psychology Research Unit, Lane 4
Management Group Ltd., Maidenhead, Berkshire, UK
1.4 Sport psychology

PETER R. M. JONES
Professor of Human Functional Anatomy, Department of
Human Sciences, University of Loughborough, Leicestershire,
UK
1.5 Anthropometry and the assessment of body composition

HENRYK K. A. LAKOMY
Lecturer, Loughborough University, Leicestershire, UK
1.3.2 Strength and power

CONSTANCE M. LEBRUN
Director of Primary Care Sport Medicine, Fowler-Kennedy
Sport Medicine Clinic, University of Western Ontario,
London, Canada
6.3.1 The female athlete

D. ROBERTSON LLOYD-SMITH
Clinical Assistant Professor, Allan McGavin Sports Medicine Centre, University of British Columbia, Vancouver, Canada
4.4.1 Acute and overuse ankle injuries

TERRY R. MALONE
Director and Associate Professor of Physical Therapy, University of Kentucky, Lexington, USA
4.3.5 Shoulder rehabilitation: principles and clinical specifics

BARRY J. MARON
Director, Minneapolis Heart Institute Foundation, Cardiovascular Research Division, Minneapolis, Minnesota, USA
3.1 Cardiac adaptations to exercise training

R. J. MAUGHAN
Professor of Human Physiology, University Medical School, Aberdeen, UK
1.2.2 Fluid and electrolyte loss and replacement in exercise

ANGUS M. McBRYDE
Professor and Chairman, Department of Orthopedic Surgery, Medical University of South Carolina, Charleston, USA
4.4.2 The acute ankle sprain

GARY R. McGILLIVARY
Assistant Professor, Department of Orthopedics and Co-Medical Director of Hand Therapy, Loma Linda University, California, USA
7.7 Injuries to the wrist and carpus

DARRELL MENARD
Health Promotion Coordinator, Directorate of Health Protection and Promotion, National Defence Headquarters, Ottawa, Ontario, Canada
6.4 The ageing athlete

LYLE J. MICHELI
Director, Division of Sports Medicine, Children's Hospital, and Associate Clinical Professor of Orthopedic Surgery, Harvard Medical School, Boston, Massachusetts, USA
5.6 Overuse injuries of the spine
6.1 Introduction: considerations for unique groups

JAMES S. MILLEDGE
Consultant Physician, Hertfordshire, UK
2.3 Altitude

JEFFREY MINKOFF
Minkoff Orthopedic Associates, New York, USA
4.2.4 The patella: its afflictions in relation to athletics

CRAIG M. MINTZER
Staff Orthopedic Surgeon, Jewett Orthopedic Clinic, Orlando, Florida, USA
5.6 Overuse injuries of the spine

MICHELLE F. MOTTOLA
Associate Professor of Anatomy and Kinesiology and Director of R. Samuel McLaughlin Foundation—Exercise and Pregnancy Laboratory, University of Western Ontario, London, Canada
6.3.2 Exercise and pregnancy—What do I tell my pregnant patient?

MICHAEL F. MURPHY
Associate Professor, Emergency Medicine and Anaesthesia, Dalhousie University, Halifax, Nova Scotia, Canada
7.4 Cardiopulmonary and abdominal emergencies in sports medicine

E. A. NEWSHOLME
Emeritus Professor in Biochemistry, University of Oxford, UK
3.6 The overtraining syndrome

BENNO M. NIGG
Professor, Faculty of Physical Education, University of Calgary, Alberta, Canada
1.3.1 Biomechanics as applied to sports

T. D. NOAKES
Liberty Life Professor of Exercise and Sports Science, Department of Physiology, University of Cape Town, South Africa
5.5 Overuse injuries of the foot and ankle

N. G. NORGAN
Senior Lecturer, Department of Human Sciences, University of Loughborough, Leicestershire, UK
1.5 Anthropometry and the assessment of body composition

BARRY W. OAKES
Associate Professor, Department of Anatomy, Monash University, Australia
4.4.3 Tendon/ligament basic science

CHRIS OSINGA
Resident, Department of Orthopaedic Surgery, Dalhousie University, Halifax, Nova Scotia, Canada
7.5 Spine injuries

GEOFFREY PASVOL
Professor in Infection and Tropical Medicine, Northwick Park Hospital, Harrow, Middlesex, UK
3.3 Infections in sports medicine

ANTONIO PELLICCIA
Professor of Pathophysiology in Sports Medicine, Institute of Sports Science, Department of Medicine, Italian National Olympic Committe, Rome, Italy
3.1 Cardiac adaptations to exercise training

JEFFREY T. POTTS
Fellow, Department of Physiology, University of Texas
Southwestern Medical Center, Dallas, USA
1.1.2 Cardiovascular responses to exercise and training

GIANCARLO PUDDU
Orthopaedic Surgeon, Clinica Valle Giulia, Rome, Italy
5.2 Stress fractures

PETER B. RAVEN
Professor and Chair, Physiology Department, University of
North Texas Health Sciences Center, Fort Worth, USA
1.1.2 Cardiovascular responses to exercise and training

JONATHAN REEVE
MRC External Scientific Staff and Consultant Physician,
Department of Medicine, University of Cambridge, UK
3.8 Exercise and the skeleton

DAVID C. REID
Professor of Orthopaedic Surgery, Adjunct Professor of
Rehabilitation Medicine, and Honorary Professor of Physical
Education, University of Alberta, Edmonton, Canada
7.5 Spine injuries

THOMAS REILLY
Professor of Sports Science, School of Human Sciences,
Liverpool John Moore's University, UK
2.5 Circadian rhythms

PER A. F. H. RENSTRÖM
Professor, Section of Sports Medicine, Department of
Orthopaedics, Karolinska Hospital, Stockholm, Sweden
5.1 An introduction to chronic overuse injuries
7.8 Pain about the groin, hip, and pelvis

HARALD P. ROOS
Department of Orthopaedics, University Hospital, Lund,
Sweden
7.8 Pain about the groin, hip, and pelvis

R. MITCHELL RUBINOVICH
Attending Orthopedic Surgeon, Alice Hyde Hospital, Malone,
New York, USA
4.3.2 Glenohumeral instability

KENT SAHLIN
Associate Professor of Physiology, Department of Physiology
and Pharmacology, Karolinska Institute and Department of
Human Biology, University College of Physical Education and
Sports, Stockholm, Sweden
*1.1.4 Anaerobic metabolism, acid-base balance, and muscle fatigue
    during high intensity exercise*

WIM H. M. SARIS
Professor of Nutrition, Nutrition Research Centre NUTRIM,
University of Maastricht, The Netherlands
1.2.3 Making weight for sports participation

MICHAEL L. SCHWARTZ
Associate Professor, Department of Surgery (Neurosurgery),
University of Toronto, Ontario, Canada
7.6 Head injuries in athletics

M. P. SCHWELLNUS
Professor of Sports Medicine, University of Cape Town
Medical School, South Africa
5.5 Overuse injuries of the foot and ankle

ALBERTO SELVANETTI
Sports Medicine Doctor, Clinica Valle Giulia, Rome, Italy
5.2 Stress fractures

SUSAN M. SHIRREFFS
Research Fellow, University Medical School, Aberdeen, UK
1.2.2 Fluid and electrolyte loss and replacement in exercise

BARRY G. SIMONSON
Minkoff Associates, New York, USA
4.2.4 The patella: its afflictions in relation to athletics

WILLIAM D. STANISH
Professor of Surgery, Dalhousie University, and Director,
Orthopaedic and Sport Medicine Clinic of Nova Scotia,
Halifax, Canada
4.1 Introduction: acute sports injuries
4.2.2 Knee ligament sprains—acute and chronic
4.3.1 Introduction: shoulder injuries in athletics
5.3 Chronic exertional compartment syndrome
5.4 Overuse injuries of the knee
7.1 Introduction: special considerations in sports injuries

JORUNN SUNDGOT-BORGEN
Associate Professor of Exercise and Health, Norwegian
University of Sport and Physical Education, Oslo, Norway
1.2.5 Eating disorders in athletes

JOHN R. SUTTON*
Professor of Medicine and Head, Department of Biological
Science, Faculty of Health Science, University of Sydney,
Australia
*2.4 Physiological and clinical consequences of exercise in heat and
    humidity*

CHARLES H. TATOR
Professor and Chair of Neurosurgery, University of Toronto
and Program Director, Toronto Hospital Neuroscience Centre,
Ontario, Canada
7.6 Head injuries in athletics

J. E. TAUNTON
Professor and Co-Director, Allan McGavin Sports Medicine
Centre, University of British Columbia, Vancouver, Canada
4.4.1 Acute and overuse ankle injuries

* It is with regret that we must report the death of John Sutton during the preparation of this
edition.

MARTIN W. THOMPSON
Associate Professor and Head—School of Exercise and Sport Science, Faculty of Health Sciences, University of Sydney, Australia
2.4 Physiological and clinical consequences of exercise in heat and humidity

M. J. TIPTON
Reader in Human and Applied Physiology, University of Surrey/Institute of Naval Medicine, Gosport, Hampshire, UK
2.2 Immersion in cold water: effects on performance and safety

ANDREW H. TURTEL
Team Orthopedist; New Jersey Nets National Basketball Association (NBA), Private Practice, New York City, USA
4.2.4 The patella: its afflictions in relation to athletics

NANCY E. VINCENT
Orthopaedic Surgery and Sports Medicine Consultant, Lethbridge, Alberta, Canada
5.3 Chronic exertional compartment syndrome

SUSAN A. WARD
Professor of Sport Science and Head of Sport and Exercise Science Research Centre, School of Applied Science, South Bank University, London, UK
1.1.1 Respiratory responses of athletes to exercise

RUSSELL F. WARREN
Surgeon-in-Chief and Professor in Surgery, Sportsmedicine and Shoulder Service, The Hospital for Special Surgery, New York, USA
4.3.3 Injuries of the rotator cuff

BRIAN J. WHIPP
Professor of Physiology, St George's Hospital Medical School, London, UK
1.1.1 Respiratory responses of athletes to exercise

CLYDE WILLIAMS
Professor of Sports Science, Loughborough University, Leicestershire, UK
1.2.1 Diet and sports performance

MELVIN H. WILLIAMS
Professor and Eminent Scholar, Old Dominion University, Norfolk, Virginia, USA
1.2.4 Nutritional ergogenic aids/supplements and exercise performance

ROBERT M. WOOD
Resident in Orthopaedic Surgery, University of Alberta, Edmonton, Canada
5.4 Overuse injuries of the knee

PLATES

Plates for Chapter 3.3 Infections in sports medicine

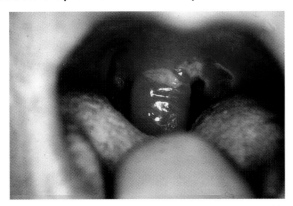

Plate 1   Pharyngitis due to the β-haemolytic streptococcus with ulceration of the uvula.

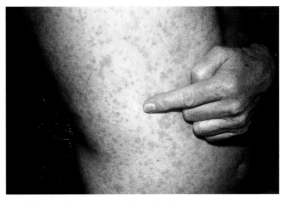

Plate 2   Pharyngitis due to the Epstein–Barr virus showing a pale membrane.

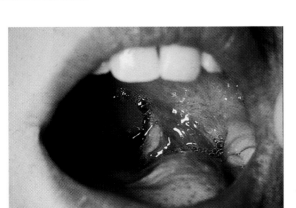

Plate 3   Petechiae between the hard and soft palate suggestive of infectious mononucleosis.

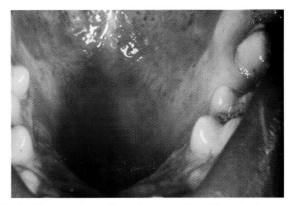

Plate 4   The maculopapular rash seen in about 5 per cent of cases of infectious mononucleosis.

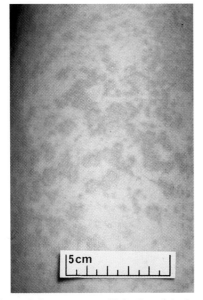

Plate 5   β-Haemolytic streptococcal infection of the leg with tracking lymphangitis and inguinal lymphadenopathy.

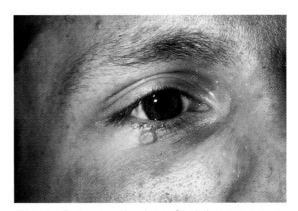

Plate 6   Bullous impetigo due to *Staphylococcus aureus*.

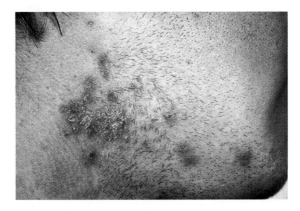

Plate 7   Raised pearly-pink umbilical lesions of molluscum contagiosum.

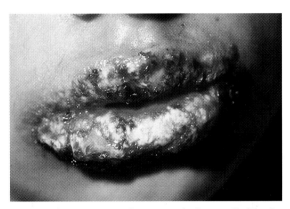

Plate 8 Ulcerated lips in a patient systemically unwell with primary herpes simplex virus infection.

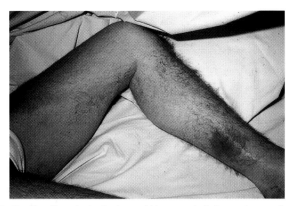

Plate 9 Small vesicular lesions of Herpes gladiatorum in a rugby player.

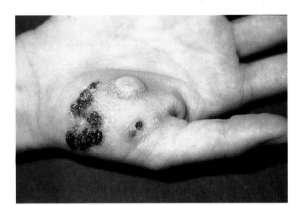

Plate 10 Tinea unguium after 3 weeks' antifungal treatment.

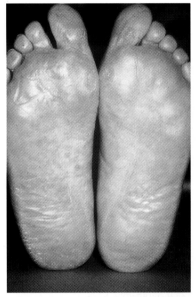

Plate 11 Raised lesions of tinea corpotis.

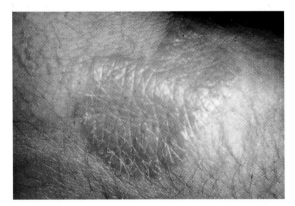

Plate 12 Severe involvement of the feet in tinea pedis.

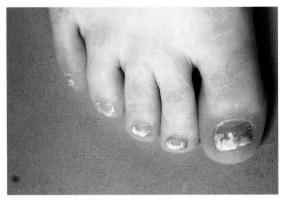

Plate 13 Hypopigmentation due to pityriasis (tinea) versicolor.

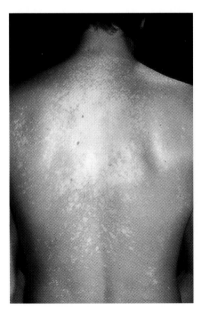

Plate 14 Maculopapular rash seen in an acute HIV seroconversion illness.

Plates for Chapter 7.3 Maxillofacial injuries in sport

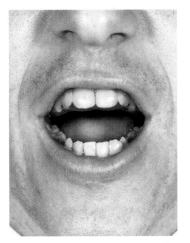 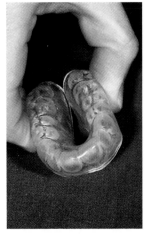

Plate 1 Custom-made, vacuum-formed, soft-bite guard made from a 4-mm thick thermoplastic sheet.

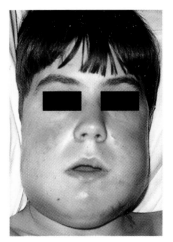

Plate 2 Facial swelling following a bilateral fracture of the condyles.

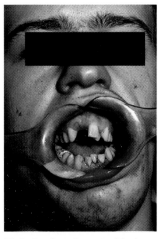

Plate 3 Anterior open bite in a patient with bilateral condylar fracture.

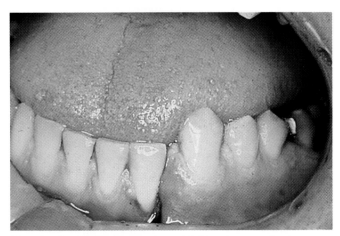

Plate 4 Mandibular parasymphyseal fracture between the lower canine and lateral incisor.

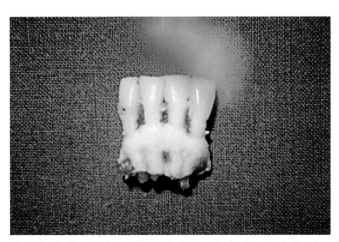

Plate 5 A dissected mandibular dentoalveolar fracture including the four lower incisors.

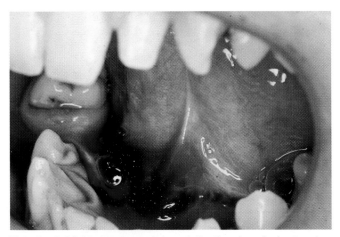

Plate 6 Sublingual ecchymosis is an indicative sign of a fractured mandible.

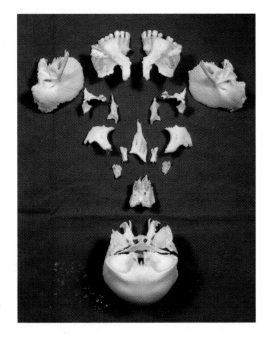

Plate 7 Components of the middle and upper third of the facial skeleton.

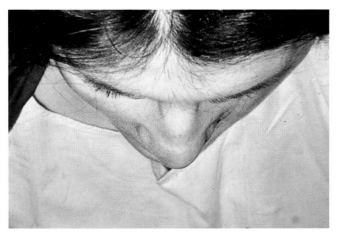

Plate 8 Flattening of the cheek following fracture of the left zygomatic complex.

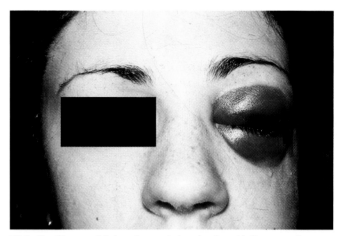

Plate 9 Circumorbital ecchymosis in a fractured left zygomatic complex.

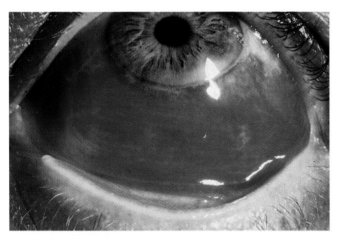

Plate 10 Subconjunctival ecchymosis.

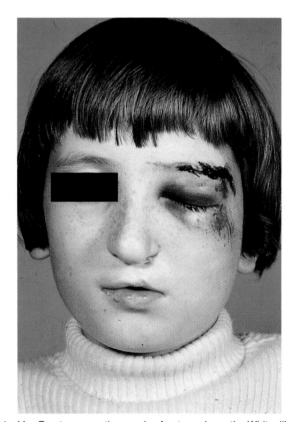

Plate 11 Frontozygomatic complex fracture above the Whitnall's tubercle. Note the drop of the level of the left eye.

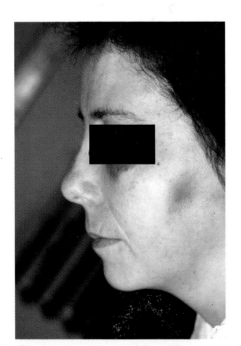

Plate 12 Circular depression 'dimple' overlying a zygomatic arch.

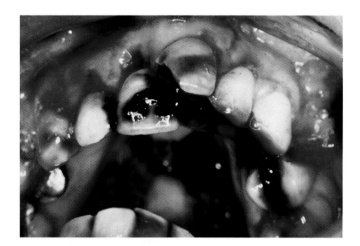

Plate 13 Dentoalveolar fracture of the upper right central and lateral incisors. Note the derangement of occlusion and the dried blood on the palate.

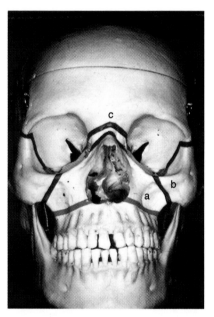
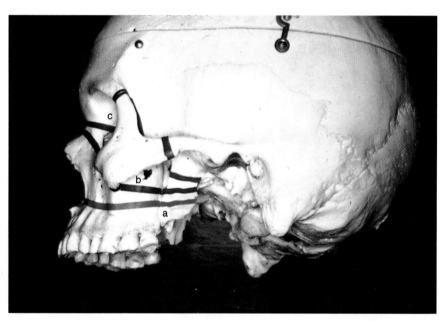

Plate 14 Le Fort lines of the fractures of the middle third of the facial skeleton. (a) Le Fort 1 (red). (b) Le Fort 2 (blue). (c) Le Fort 3 (green). (Skull front and lateral views side by side.)

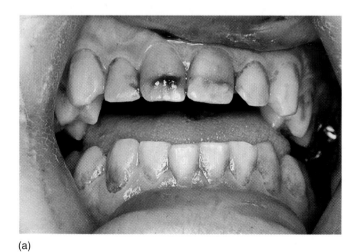
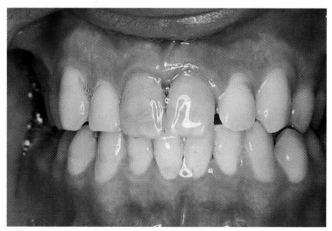

(a)

(b)

Plate 15 (a) Occlusion in Le Fort fracture before treatment. (b) Same patient after treatment.

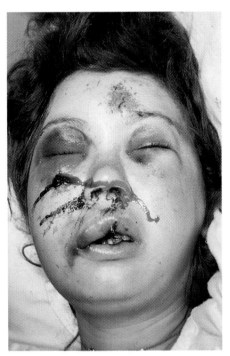

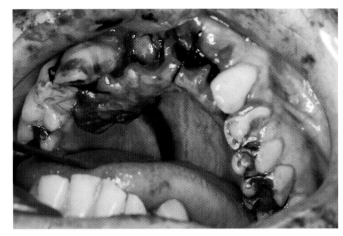

Plate 17   Split palate, missing incisors, and sheared teeth in a Le Fort 2 fracture.

Plate 16   Le Fort 3 fracture. Note the bilateral circumorbital ecchymosis, ballooned face, flattened nasal bridge, and bloodstained CSF rhinorrhoea from the left nostril.

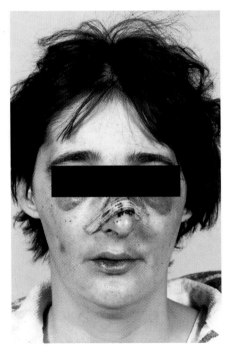

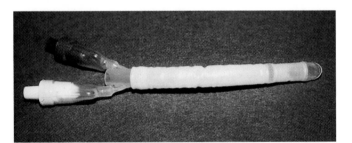

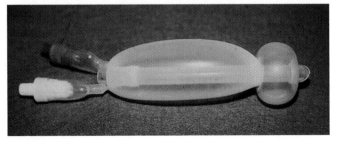

Plate 18   Laterally deviated fractured nasal complex. (Note the bilateral circumorbital ecchymosis.)

Plate 19   Epitek nasal catheters.

Introduction

Introduction—Man as an athlete*

Per-Olof Åstrand

The purpose of this introductory chapter on man as an athlete is to put the textbook in a broad historical perspective for readers.

A brief sketch of our evolutionary history is presented to remind us that it has taken a long time to become the way we are. The history of competitive sports is summarized, with special emphasis on the ancient and modern Olympic games, and then the reasons for the improvement in world records during this century are discussed with examples mainly from track and field events.

Our biological heritage

According to the natural sciences it is believed that our solar system was created some 4600 million years ago.[1] Evidently, the atmosphere surrounding our planet at that time did not contain oxygen. This was a prerequisite for the evolution of life from non-living organic matter. Without atmospheric oxygen there was no high altitude ozone, and hence ultraviolet radiation from the sun reached the surface of the Earth. This radiation then provided the energy for the photosynthesis of organic compounds from such molecules as water, carbon dioxide, and ammonia. The process that enabled living organisms to capture solar energy for the synthesis of organic molecules (e.g. glucose) can be clearly traced in fossils that are about 3500 million years old. Similarly, the familiar anaerobic fermentation (i.e. glycolysis) is probably the oldest energy-extracting pathway found in life on Earth.

The ancient organisms split the water molecule by photosynthesis, gradually releasing free oxygen into the atmosphere. It may have taken some 2000 million years to create an atmosphere in which one out of every five molecules was oxygen. As oxygen became toxic for many of the original oxygen producers, new metabolic patterns (i.e. aerobic energy yield) were developed that utilized oxygen as a hydrogen acceptor.

A new milestone in the biological evolution was reached approximately 1500 million years ago when the unicellular organism with a nucleus, the eukaryote, was developed.[2] The energy-absorbing and energy-yielding processes typical of our cell activities today, such as the ATP–ADP system, are merely copies of events that occurred thousands of millions of years ago. ATP has been described as the energy currency of life because it is used as the principal energy source for all biological processes. The body has a surprisingly small store of ATP, for example the ATP stores in muscles are so small that they are used up as a result of only a few contractions of muscle.

If we had to carry around our daily requirement for ATP, as an energy store, then it would add about 50 to 100 per cent to our body weight. The energy-producing systems of the body are, however, designed to deliver ATP as and when it is required, that is above and beyond the ATP requirements for simply sustaining life of a resting person. The aerobic metabolism of the fuel stores of fat and carbohydrate is increased when we need additional ATP and when the rate of ATP use is greater than aerobic metabolism can sustain then we call on anaerobic degradation of glycogen, a process which is several thousand million years old.

Thus, over thousands of millions of years of evolution, a unicellular living organism was created. By some sort of trial and error, the fundamental biological principles for maintaining life were developed and they are still in efficient operation. A comprehensive textbook of biochemistry written some 1500 million years ago would no doubt still be up to date in its treatment of the functions of the cell.

The evolution was now ready for the next major step—the creation of larger animals. That stage probably began 700 million years ago.[3] In this evolution of larger animals, the individual cell retained its original size (i.e. the same size as the unicellular organism living more than 1000 million years ago), but more cells were grouped together to increase the size of the organism.

As an inevitable consequence of grouping thousands of millions of some 200 different types of cells together in one organism (the human being), the individual cell lost its intimate contact with the external environment. This problem was solved by bathing each cell in water (i.e. the interstitial fluid). Like the amoeba, each cell in our body (with some exceptions) is surrounded by fluid, the composition of which is basically very similar to that of the ancient oceans. The organism brought the sea water with it, so to speak, in a bag made of skin.

In the course of the diversification of the multicellular organisms, which occurred over the last 700 million years, new types of organisms appeared and dispersions took place within already established groups. It should be noted that the history of the mammals covers the last 220 million years, if not more. The first primates (the order including man) can be traced back some 60 to 70 million years to a period when the dinosaurs still dominated the scene. With the extinction of the dinosaurs, there was a mammalian dispersion into vacant niches. Another evolutionary explosion occurred, with a dispersion of flowering plants, insects, fishes, birds, and mammals.

---

* Parts of this chapter have been published earlier (Åstrand P-O, Rodahl K. *Textbook of work physiology.* New York: McGraw-Hill, 1986; ch.1).

What then are the mechanisms that underlie the origin of species and the evolutionary relationships among them (i.e. darwinism)? Lewin[4] has summarized the current views held by different researchers in this field. According to the modern ideas, evolution is a consequence of the gradual accumulation of genetic differences due to point mutations and rearrangements in the chromosomes. The direction of an evolutionary change is determined by natural selection, promoting the variants that are best fitted to their environment. However, the fact remains that fossils do not generally document a smooth transition from old morphologies to new ones. This was also discussed by Darwin. For millions of years species remain unchanged in the fossil record, suddenly to be replaced by something that is substantially different but clearly related.[4]

Because the accumulation of small genetic changes cannot exclusively explain the development of new species, a new theory called punctuated equilibrium has been advanced. According to this, individual species may remain virtually unchanged for long periods of time. They are then suddenly punctuated by abrupt events in the environment and a new species arises from the original stock. It is conceivable, however, that future fossil records may fill many of the gaps and provide some of the missing links. It may have been only 5 million or as many as 20 million years ago that the family tree of primates developed a branch, the hominids, which finally resulted in *Homo sapiens sapiens*, the only surviving hominid. Not until about 4 million years ago do the African fossils reveal the presence of the hominid genus *Australopithecus*. The pelvis permitted an upright posture and bipedal gait with the arms free. There are archaeological records of tools, pebble choppers, and small stones that are probably more than 3 million years old.[5] Tool-making was thus established before there was a marked brain expansion in the hominid stock. Although a few varieties have been identified, the *Australopithecus* was a relatively homogeneous genus that survived for more than 2 million years. The next well-identified member of our family tree may have been the first true man. *Homo habilis* existed from 2.3 to 1.5 million years ago. He was replaced by *Homo erectus*, who had a modern pelvis and moved with a striding gait. They lived as hunters and food gatherers and had a wide geographical range. The body height was probably 150 to 160 cm. They made use of fire, as evidenced by a hominid occupation site 1.4 million years old.

The general public is probably most familiar with the Neanderthal man (*Homo sapiens neanderthalensis*) who, from archaeological findings, appears to have been well established some 200 000 years ago.[6] Neanderthal men were skilled hunters of large and small game, forming bands similar to those of more recent hunting people, and were probably linked into tribal groupings, or at least groups with a common language. They formed a human population complex extending from Gibraltar across Europe into East Asia. The Neanderthal population was as homogeneous as the human population of today. On average, the brain encased in the Neanderthal skull was slightly larger than the brain of modern man. Although Neanderthal men had the same postural abilities, manual dexterity, and range and character of movement as modern man, they had more massive limb bones and a larger muscular mass and power. The departure of the Neanderthal population occurred some 35 000 years ago. When they disappeared from the scene anatomically, modern man, *Homo sapiens sapiens*, was already in existence.

There are different opinions concerning '. . . the latest phase in human origins—the emergence of people like you and me, our species *Homo sapiens*, with its widespread varieties of physique and color'.[6] One hypothesis is that modern humans evolved in Africa and then spread throughout the world, developing racial features in the process. Modern humans and Neanderthal man could be distinct lines that diverged from a common ancestor more than 200 000 years ago in Africa and Europe, respectively. At a later stage they spread and in some parts of the world they shared the environment.

An alternative hypothesis is a 'gene-flow' model with a genetic contribution varying from region to region, with the rate of intermixture gradually increasing as modern man evolved. Stringer[6] points out that in the gene-flow model, racial features preceded the appearance of modern man, whereas the African model reverses the order. He supports the African model with dispersal of early modern humans from Africa within the past 100 000 years. However, the dating of our origin as modern man is controversial.

A human being living 50 000 years ago probably had the same potential for physical and intellectual performance, playing a piano or constructing a computer, as anyone living today. Therefore, from all indications, *Homo sapiens sapiens* has remained biologically unchanged for at least 50 000 years. By 30 000 years ago, modern man had spread to nearly all parts of the world. It was not until some 10 000 years ago that the transition from a roaming hunter and food gatherer to a stationary farmer began.

To illustrate the evolutionary time-scale, let us compare the 4600 million years our planet has existed with a 460-km journey (Fig. 1). Life began after the first 100 km of the trip had been covered. Another 200 km was required before the unicellular organism with a nucleus was born. Multicellular animals were living when we arrived at the 400-km mark. Evolutionary radiation of the mammalian stock began somewhere around the 453-km mark. The first hominid appeared approximately 6 km later. *Australopithecus*, joined the journey 200 to 400 m from the end, and Neanderthal man disappeared about 3.5 m from the finish line. The cultivation of land and keeping of livestock occurred 1 m from our present position. A 100-year-old person today has merely covered a distance of 10 mm of the 460-km journey.

The purpose of this brief summary has been to present an outline of our genetic background. Many structures and functions are common to different species in the animal kingdom. For instance, there appears to be no fundamental difference in structure, chemistry, or function between the neurones and synapses in man and those in a squid, a snail, or a leech.[7] Therefore we can learn a great deal from studying different species. It is remarkable that all living organisms have a genetic code based on the same principles. For instance, data indicate that man and the chimpanzee share more than 99 per cent of their genetic material.[8] However, minimal genetic changes can affect major morphological modifications. Consequently, we should be careful when extrapolating findings from one species to another, because over millions of years many species undergo minor or major modifications in their physical and other characteristics. In general, evolution is a very conservative process. For instance, all vertebrates, including the hominids, have backbones of a similar design. This supports the hypothesis that backbones have evolved only once, that is all vertebrates share a common ancestor with a backbone. At an early stage the human embryo will start to develop gills but these are replaced with lungs.

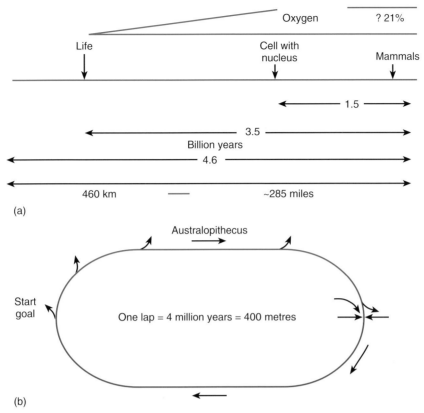

Fig. 1 (a) The 4.6-billion-year history is illustrated as proportional to a journey of 460 km (285 miles). After some 300 km (186 miles) we find an eukaryote—a cell with a nucleus. A textbook dealing with the structure and metabolism of that cell would not need much updating to describe the basic histochemistry of our cells. (b) The history of the hominids, starting with *Australopithecus*, covers the last 400 m (see text) and farming and agriculture started 399 m into this period (10 000 years ago). *Homo sapiens neanderthalensis* died out at 3.5 m (35 000 years ago). The twentieth century covers the last 10 mm.

In general, vertebrate locomotion is genetically programmed. Fish can swim and birds can walk as soon as they hatch. Many species of mammals are well developed at birth. Thus, some are able to walk or run as soon as they are born, and some of these are able to attain a speed of 35 km/h when they are only a few days old. Evidently, survival may depend on their ability to get away. In the case of man, who is utterly helpless at birth and entirely dependent on parental care, it may be advantageous not to be able to move very far from their parents until a reasonable level of maturity has been attained.

The evolutionary process continues, and mammalian history has seen a wave of extinctions, which has been particularly severe for large mammals including the hominids. Extinctions are a measure of the success of evolution in adapting organisms, because particular adaptations provide entry into a relatively empty niche. In the balance between existence and extinction, the odds are not favourable. It has been estimated that 2000 million species have appeared on Earth during the last 700 million years, but the number of multicellular species now living is only a few million (i.e. only 0.1 to 0.2 per cent have survived).

The cortex of the human brain mirrors man's evolutionary success. Just as the proportions of the human hand, with its large opposable and muscular thumb, reflect successful adaptation for life in trees and later for the use of tools, so does the anatomy of the human brain reflect a successful adaptation for manual and intellectual skills.

In the same way as upright walking and tool-making were the unique adaptations of the earlier phases of human evolution, the physiological capacity for speech was the biological basis for the later stages. Indeed, it is by language that human social systems are mediated. Speech is the form of behaviour that differentiates man from other animals. The use of language to transfer knowledge and experience from one generation to the next has enabled man, biologically unchanged for tens of thousands of years, to accelerate progress. In addition, language has enabled humans to apply their endowed intellectual resources in a technical revolution leading to entirely new and complex tools, weapons, shelters, boats, wheeled locomotion, exploratory voyages, and the attainment of the impossible—space travel. Nevertheless, in the midst of these splendid achievements, there are those who wonder whether the evolution of the human brain has gone too far. Although its ability to conceive, invent, create, and construct is astonishing, it remains to be seen whether or not it has retained or developed equally well its capacity for ethical conduct or responsible application of its endowed potential. When our ancestors roamed around in small bands, any destructive consequence of their activity was quite limited. However, because of social developments and technical innovations, basically the same brain is now capable of self-destruction.

Like all higher animals, man is basically designed for mobility. Consequently, our locomotive apparatus and service organs constitute the main part of our total body mass. The shape and dimensions of the human skeleton and musculature are such that the human body cannot compete with a gazelle in speed or an elephant in sturdiness, but it is indeed outstanding in diversity. The basic instrument of mobility is the muscle. It is a very old tissue. The earliest animal fossils were the burrowers living some 700 million years ago. By muscle force, these animals could dig into the sea-bed. They retained the metabolic pathways developed when the air had no oxygen (i.e. the anaerobic energy yield). The pyruvic acid formed in our muscles under anaerobic conditions is now removed by the formation of lactate. One old-fashioned alternative could have been the transformation of the pyruvate into ethyl alcohol. There may be those who now regret that the skeletal muscles did not select this alternative route. Had this occurred, producing pyruvate by exercising to exhaustion or running uphill might have been a very popular endeavour!

The skeletal muscle is unique in that it can vary its metabolic rate to a greater degree than any other tissue. In fact, active skeletal muscles may increase their oxidative processes to more than 50 times the resting level. Such an enormous variation in metabolic rate must necessarily create serious problems for the muscle cell, because as the consumption of fuel and oxygen increases 50-fold, the rate of removal of heat, carbon dioxide, water, and waste products must be dramatically increased. To maintain the chemical and physical equilibrium of the cell, there must be an enormous increase in the exchange of molecules between intracellular and extracellular fluid (i.e. fresh fluid must continuously flush the exercising cell). When muscles are thrown into vigorous activity, the ability to maintain the internal equilibria necessary to continue the exercise is entirely dependent on those organs that service the muscle's circulation. Food intake, digestion and handling of substrates, endocrine system, kidney function, and water balance are also very much affected by variation in metabolic rate.

Almost 100 per cent of the biological existence of our species has been dominated by outdoor activity. Hunting and foraging for food and other necessities have been conditions of human life for millions of years. We are adapted to that style of life. This applies to our emotional, social, and intellectual skills. After a brief spell in an agrarian culture, we have ended up in an urbanized, highly technological society. There is obviously no way to revert to our natural way of life, which was not without its problems. With insight into our biological heritage, however, we may yet be able to modify our current lifestyle. Understanding of the function of the body at rest, as well as during exercise under various conditions, is important as a basis for an optimization of our existence.

Children are definitely spontaneously physically active. Unfortunately, in our modern society, we discourage this activity by furnishing houses and apartments to fit parents' needs, keeping children indoors in schools and doing homework for many hours, creating heavily overpopulated 'concrete deserts', and producing television programmes to capture their attention. Children should keep quiet and stay clean and neat! Vigorous physical activity is asocial behaviour in too many circumstances. From the time of puberty, human nature has an inclination toward physical laziness. There is no appetite centre for physical activity.

Some years ago, the present author visited the Bushmen of the Kalahari Desert, probably the last remaining Stone Age people. They followed the lifestyle of the true hunters and food gatherers. Gathering sufficient food meant trudging long distances, for the men in their hunting efforts, and for the women and children in their collection of berries, melons, roots, and various plants. The sequence of walking, stopping, and squatting to dig, and walking again, is physically demanding. When the women gather enough and return home, they still have to collect and carry firewood for the cooking and the night fire. Most of the year, the game and food plants are not found in any abundance. To get enough to eat, the Bushmen have to exercise for hours almost every day. The driving factor for the habitual physical activity is hunger and thirst, not a particular love for exercise. I never saw an adult Bushman out jogging, but the walking was fast! The Bushmen are well trained with emphasis on endurance.

History of sports

For obvious reasons we do not know anything about athletic activities during the Stone Age. People probably liked games and plays, and they sang and danced. There is definite evidence in sculptures, reliefs, and paintings some 5000 years old that Egyptians exercised. The hieroglyphic sign for swimming dates from the same period.

It is not until the Olympic Games began that the history of organized athletic activities can be revealed. While the origin of the Olympic Games is not known exactly, there is a historical record of the ancient games beginning in Olympia in the western Peloponnese, Greece, in 776 BC. Thereafter they were held at 4-year intervals for more than 1100 years. There are various traditional explanations of the origin of the games. One attributes the festival to Heracles, the most famous Greek hero. In art and literature he is represented as an enormously strong man of moderate height, a huge eater and drinker, very amorous, and generally kind but with occasional outbursts of brutal rage. This great fighter and hunter is famous for the Twelve Labours, or *Dodekathlos*, which include the capture of the lion of Nemea, the cleansing of the stables of Augeas in Elis, the capture of the Cretan Bull, and seizing the cattle of Geryon. Another myth tells us that there was a chariot race between Pelops and King Oenomaus who used to challenge the suitors of his daughter Hippodamia. Pelops successfully persuaded Oenomaus' servant to remove the wheel spindle pins; the chariot crashed and the King was killed. Unfair play is not a modern phenomenon in sport! Pelops married Hippodamia and became King of Pisa. He conquered Olympia where, for the glory of Zeus, he arranged competitions.

The earlier Olympic programmes consisted almost exclusively of exercises of the Spartan type, testing endurance and strength with a special view to war. Later, more and more events were added: chariot races and horse races, wrestling and boxing, and the pentathlon including long jumping, quoit (discus) throwing, javelin throwing, running, and wrestling. Winners became national heros: musicians sang their praise and sculptures preserved their strength and beauty in marble. From 444 BC poets, writers, philosophers, and orators also competed. As late as in London 1948 artists competed.

Olympia became an expression of the Greek ideas that the body of man has a glory as well as his intellect and spirit, that the body and mind should alike be disciplined, and that it is by the harmonious discipline of both that men best honour Zeus. Nobles and peasants met on equal terms. It should be noted that women were not allowed as competitors or, except for the priestesses of Demeter, as spectators.[9] There are written reports still available from the ancient Games but reports on 'records' are very scarce. The winner in long jump in 668 BC apparently jumped 7.05 m. In 516 BC Milo picked up a 4-year-old heifer at Olympia and, after carrying it around the altar in triumph, he killed it and ate it all in 1 day—a real olympic performance! In 724 BC a runner was tripped up by his scarf tangling around his feet and was killed. This event was the basis for a law wherein athletes in the future were to compete naked. An early example of preventive medicine in sports!

In AD 393 the Games were closed and after that no runners placed their feet in the hollows of the starting line in the stadium of Olympia—except for tourists.

Baron Pierre de Coubertin took the initiative to revive the Olympic Games for athletes of all countries of the world, regardless of national rivalries, jealousies, and differences of all kinds, and with all considerations of politics, race, religion, wealth, and social status eliminated. At an enthusiastic conference at the Sorbonne, Paris, in 1894, it was decided that the games of the First Olympiad of the modern cycle should take place in Athens in 1896. However, we know too well that at times the high ideals expressed by Pierre de Coubertin have been neglected.

Modern athletics

Many modern sports have their origins in games played with and without balls and equipment enjoyed during the Middle Ages and later. Preparation for hunting, war, and defence made training of archery, javelin throwing, fencing, shooting, boxing, and wrestling necessary for survival. During the Middle Ages the knights' tournaments were frequently a life-and-death struggle.

Historians claim that Great Britain was the cradle of modern, organized sports and competitions. At the beginning of the nineteenth century, sports were introduced in schools, and in the middle of that century, championships were arranged at colleges and universities and competitions took place between them, for example the famous Boat Race between Oxford and Cambridge. In 1880 the British Amateur Athletic Association was founded. As mentioned above, a few years later Baron Pierre de Coubertin launched the flagship of sports, the Olympic Games.

Why are sports records improving?*

Several factors, which vary in importance depending on the characteristics of the sport, must be considered.

The following factors will be discussed in detail:

- selection from a larger and healthier population

- better training methods and preparation

- improved techniques

- improved materials

- psychological aspects

- scientific support

- doping

- physiological aspects

* Parts of these section have been published earlier (Åstrand P-O, Borgström A. Why are sports records improving? In: Strauss R, ed. *Drugs and performance in sports*. Philadelphia: WB Saunders, 1987; 147–63).

Examples chosen mainly from track and field events will be used in this discussion. Figures 2 to 7 illustrate the development of world records in several sports from the beginning of this century, when systematic documentation of the world's best performances started. For obvious reasons, one can trace the effects of the two World Wars in the statistics: there is a hiatus in progress during, and for some years after, the wars.

Selection from a larger and healthier population

More and more individuals, particularly women, are attracted by sports activities. Increasing numbers of nations are represented in the sports arena. As preventive and curative health measures become more successful throughout developing countries, millions of teenagers should have a chance to enjoy sports. These factors make it more likely that individuals with talent for a particular sport will be noticed by the experts.

Better training methods and preparation

Training volume has increased and training methods have improved dramatically. Today, top athletes are not 'true amateurs' as in the days when the Olympic oath included the statement that athletes did not compete for improvement of their economic status. Certainly, top athletes have always managed to make money in their sport, but today this is permissible and can involve large sums. In other words, athletes can now devote more time to training and can train year round in an optimal climate.

In the ancient Games an olive crown was awarded to the winner and he became a hero. In the eary modern Olympic Games, practical prizes, such as an umbrella, were awarded. A tragic case is the North American Indian, James Thorpe, who won the decathlon event in Stockholm in 1912. He was disqualified because he had received a few United States dollars when playing basketball. However, in 1980 his family received retrospectively the gold medal.

Improved techniques

In some events, changes in the rules have made developments in techniques possible. In the early rules for the high jump, it was stated that when passing the cross-bar: (i) the jumper's buttocks should be on a lower level than his or her head and (ii) the feet should precede the head. In 1936 the rules were changed and the only restriction was that the take-off should be accomplished from one foot. Until then the scissors style had dominated. However, the 'western roll,' originally introduced by Horine in 1910, had given H.M. Osborne the gold medal in the 1924 Olympic Games, although the judges had great problems in deciding whether or not his jumping style conformed to the rules. Probably this and other similar incidents made it necessary to change the rules. Dick Fosbury's victory with his 'flop style' in the 1968 Olympic Games provided a spectacular introduction of today's dominant technique.

Covering the circle for the shot put, discus, and hammer throwing with rubber material or concrete facilitated the development of new techniques.

In cross-country skiing, the skating technique was actually introduced long before in the orienteering event on skis, because in this event the skiers had to use lanes and roads that were often icy. However, not until the Olympics in 1976, when the American skier William Kock applied this technique and won the silver medal in the 30-km event, did it become launched more officially.

When the breast stroke in swimming was modified to increase speed, a new event was born—the butterfly. Both styles are energetically expensive, and so it is realistic that the longest distance swum in competition is 200 m. Some techniques have been prohibited for safety reasons, namely climbing on the pole in pole vault and turning a somersault in the long jump. In Spain the technique in a traditional sport was adopted for the javelin throwing. The thrower initiates the throw with fast rotations, and the back part of the javelin is prepared with soap to reduce the friction against the palm when the javelin glides out of the hand. For evident reasons, this 'soap style' is forbidden.

Improved materials

Technological innovations have played an important role in the performance explosion in many events. The introduction of artificial surfaces on tracks improved conditions and, most importantly, maintained consistant lane quality throughout a competition. Previously, the inner lane of track deteriorated as it became worn by large numbers of feet. The Pan American Games in 1967 were the first major event to be held on an artificial surface. The modern materials on the thrower's circle also provided long-lasting and equal conditions for all competitors. When starting blocks were permitted, the start in sprint events became faster.

The introduction of the fibreglass pole improved world records in pole vault in the 1960s. This is well illustrated in Fig. 2. Such a pole was first introduced during the latter part of the 1950s, and an American, Alburley Dooley, was a pioneer in the development of a technique that efficiently utilized the elastic properties of the pole. Without a foam rubber mat, the landing after the high jump and pole vault would be hazardous. In fact, without this equipment the 'flop style' and fibreglass pole would be too dangerous to use.

The aerodynamic properties of the javelin and discus have been improved. The long throws, as illustrated in Fig. 3, can be a threat to spectators. Also, it is often difficult to judge whether or not the javelin hits the ground with its point first. In 1986 a rule was passed which introduced a new javelin model with different aerodynamic characteristics from those of the traditional model. It is estimated that Hohn's world record (104.80 m) is equivalent to a throw of approximately 85 m with the new model. The length–reducing effect is less pronounced with shorter throws. An 'old' 90-m mark would now be comparable with approximately 78 m, and 60 m is comparable with 59 m. There is an effect similar to that of the badminton shuttlecock. In addition, there is a much better chance of the javelin landing correctly on its point. The introduction of rules and equipment which reduce the performance as evaluated in metres is unique to javelin throwing.

Psychological aspects

Good performance depends on expectation, which in part determines tactics. With a world record of 3 min 30 s (3:30) in the 1500-m run, the goal may be to run it in 3:29, but not in 3:20! In some events there are no barriers, that is the limits are unknown. A

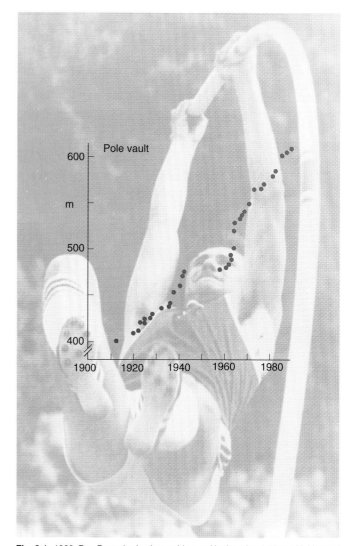

Fig. 2 In 1960, Don Bragg broke the world record by jumping 4.80 m with his steel pole. In 1961, the first record using a fibreglass pole was set (4.83 m), and 2 years later John Pennel jumped 5.20 m. The fibreglass pole effectively stores some of the athlete's energy developed during the run and, with good technique, that energy can be utilized at exactly the right moment. During the last 20 years, this catapult pole has changed very little in quality. Therefore the continual improvement in records must be due to better skill and power of the record breakers. Without the development of foam rubber mats on which to land, jumping with fibreglass poles would be dangerous. The photograph shows Sergei Bubka (of the former USSR) setting a new record by jumping 5.88 m in the Saint-Denis Stadium 1984 (Dagens Nyheter, Pressens Bild AB). Now his record is 6.15 m (1994).

perfect example is Bob Beamon's 8.90-m aerial trip in the long jump in 1968. That jump improved the world record by 55 cm (Fig. 4)! At that time the world record in high jump was 2.28 m. Who would have dreamed of putting the cross-bar up to 2.4 m, which would have resulted in a similar improvement in the record?

From a psychological viewpoint, it is often a handicap to run in front of the pack for most of a 1500-m race. This drawback has, at least partly, a physiological background. Even if there is no wind, the speed of the runner causes significant air resistance. Running behind another competitor in a 'shielded' position can save 4 to 6 per cent of the energy cost.[10] From both a psychological and a physiological aspect, a steady speed throughout the race up to the final spurt usually gives the best time.

Scientific support

It is difficult to prove to what extent medical science has helped athletes in their pursuit of new records. Often the athletes have been one step ahead, applying trial and error methods, followed by the physiologists whose studies have revealed mechanisms that can explain why a particular regimen can enhance performance. However, basic research from the 1930s and 1940s, confirmed in more recent studies, has proved that diet and fluid balance can affect physical performance decisively. As early as 1939, Christensen and Hansen[11] reported that a carbohydrate-rich diet improved endurance in heavy exercise and that training could have a glycogen-saving effect that enhances aerobic capacity (see Chapter 1.2.1). Scientific data supported the belief in

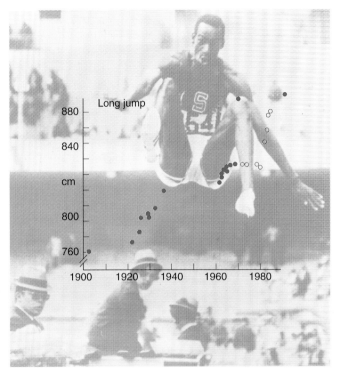

Fig. 4 Bob Beamon's meteoric jump, sending him 8.90 m from the take-off point in the 1968 Olympic Games in Mexico City, was spectacular. 'No other world track and field record excels the previous best performance by a comparable margin ... Beamon's feat outshines all others. It is unlikely that the 8.90-m record will ever be beaten' (Ernst Jokl). The open circles denote the best results achieved during the years following 1968. Carl Lewis gradually came closer. However, it was Mike Powell who broke the record with a jump of 8.95 m in 1991. The photograph shows Bob Beamon (of the United States) in his 8.90-m jump in the 1968 Olympic Games in Mexico City (Pressens Bild AB).

the beneficial effects of a warm-up before high-intensity exercise.

Unfortunately, many athletes are injured during training and competition. Physicians and physical therapists try, often successfully, to enable the athlete to return to the arena as quickly as possible. Methods for treatment and rehabilitation are examined critically; if successful, they are then available for everyone.

Doping

It is a tragedy that so many athletes, coaches, and physicians break the rules by using illegal substances in their attempt to improve performance and so win competitions and set new world records (see Chapter 3.4). It is only in some sports that the substances on the International Olympic Committee (**IOC**) list of prohibited substances may improve performance beyond what the athlete can expect to achieve as a result of training, skill acquisition and an 'in depth' knowledge of their sport. Nevertheless, many coaches and athletes are only too ready to adopt, without question, new concepts which are claimed to improve performance. There are some procedures which clearly improve the physiological function of athletes and so, in theory, they should improve their performances. One such illegal procedure is blood doping because it increases an athlete's capacity for oxygen transport. In sports in which success depends largely on the athlete's ability to sustain a high rate of oxygen consumption to support a fast race pace, such as in middle- and

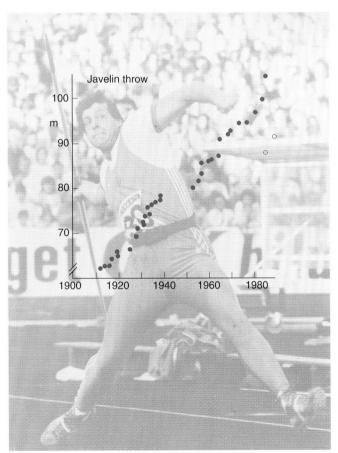

Fig. 3 In 1932 Matti Järvinen of Finland, holder of the world record in javelin throwing, predicted that one day someone would throw the javelin farther than 100 m. His record at that time did not exceed 75 m. In 1984 Uwe Hohn (of the former DDR) achieved a throw of 104.80 m. There has been a dramatic development of the aerodynamic characteristics of the javelin over the years, with Frank Held (of the United States) as a pioneer. He broke the world record in 1953 and again in 1955. Held threw a specially designed javelin some 4 m further than was possible with traditional equipment, but this design was not approved by the authorities. One problem is to combine the javelin's aerodynamic ability to 'float' on the air with a landing on its tip in accordance with the rules. A javelin throw is more effective if the body is bent into an extreme 'bow' before the throw. Stretched muscles can develop more force than muscles at a shorter initial length. The javelin throw is anatomically very demanding, and most throwers suffer from orthopaedic problems, particularly in the elbow, at least once during their careers. The champion discus thrower Adolfo Consolini (of Italy) is reported to have achieved a throw of 114 m using the forbidden 'soap style' (see text). The photograph shows Uwe Hohn throwing the javelin 104.80 m (Pressens Bild AB).

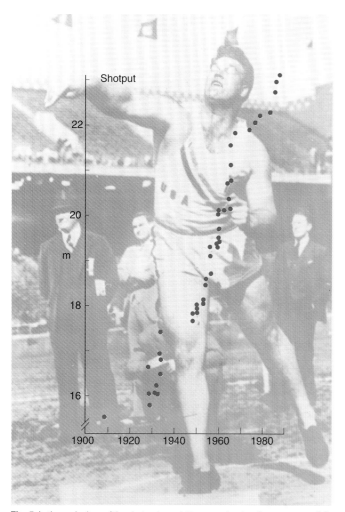

Fig. 5 In the early days of the shot put event, it was predominantly a one-arm affair. Jack Torrance put the shot up on his finger tips and could thereby add extra power from the wrist. He reached a 'phenomenal' 17.40 m in 1934, a result that survived attacks until 1948 (with the Second World War as a restriction in between). Parry O'Brien, in particular, introduced a new technique starting in a low position with the back facing the direction of throw. The strength of leg and trunk muscles became more important, and it was logical that more strength training was included in preparation for the competitive season. O'Brien dominated the scene from 1953 until his last record noted in 1959. At the beginning of the 1950s the cinders in the ring were replaced by concrete, which facilitated the introduction of new techniques. In the mid-1970s some shot putters launched a rotation to initiate the put. As mentioned in the text, up to the mid-1980s there was a trend toward stagnation in the breaking of records despite the growing popularity of the use of anabolic steroids. The photograph shows Jack Torrance (of the United States) (Pressens Bild AB).

long-distance walking, running, swimming, or cycling races, blood doping provides a clear advantage. However, this procedure will not, for example, make an Olympic champion out of even a very good recreational endurance athlete because all the other ingredients for success must also be in place before the full benefit of blood doping can be realized.

It is interesting that the world record in shot put only increased from 21.78 m in the mid-1960s to 22.02 m in 1982 (in 1997 it stands at 23.12 m) (Fig. 5). During that period the intake of anabolic steroids increased dramatically and probably involved many world-class shot putters. It is tempting to conclude that the intake or injection of such hormones has not contributed significantly to the world record statistics in shot put.

There are some grey zones. According to the IOC anti-doping regulations, the administration to, or use by, a competing athlete of any agent with the sole object of increasing artificially the performance during the competition, is deemed to be doping. What about the so-called 'bicarbonate loading', ingestion of sodium bicarbonate before an 800-m race, or creatine supplementation before sprinting events? These substances are, so far, not on the doping list but apparently they can enhance performance[12],[13] and in an artificial way (see Chapter 1.2.4).

Physiological aspects

Are the athletes of today superior in their physiological potential as compared with their predecessors? A high maximal oxygen uptake (V_{O_2}max; aerobic power) is essential for success in sports utilizing large muscle groups in all-out efforts for several minutes or longer. In activities in which the body weight is carried, this aerobic power is related to body weight, that is oxygen uptake in ml/kg per min. However, in such exercises as rowing and swimming, oxygen uptake is expressed in litres of oxygen per min. (In comparative biology, oxygen uptake expressed in $ml\ min^{-1}\ kg^{-0.75}$ is an important parameter.) In 1937, Robinson et al.[14] reported that Don Lash, who held the world record for the 2-mile race (3.22 km), attained a maximal oxygen uptake of 81.5 ml/kg per min when running on a treadmill. Today, competitors have similar values but they run much faster (Lash's record was 8 min 58.4 s; in 1997 the best time recorded is 7 min 58.6 s). This fact is intriguing. Evidently, modern training principles allow the athlete to exercise at or closer to maximal aerobic power for longer periods of time. Another reason for improved performance is a higher power and capacity of the anaerobic metabolic pathways (see below).

Better shoes and tracks cannot explain the superiority of modern athletes. Ron Clark's time of 27 min 39.4 s for 10 000 m on a cinder track in 1965 is not far from Henry Rono's 27 min 22.5 s on an artificial surface in 1978. For the 100-m distance, Jim Hines' time of 10.03 s on a cinder track at sea-level is not significantly slower than his time of 9.95 s when running on an artificial surface, the same year, but at high altitude, which favours the sprinter because air resistance is reduced. The better results recorded for distance races that demand the ability to sustain a high rate of oxygen consumption cannot be explained by better tracks or running surfaces in general (Fig. 6).

There is a personal limit for maximal oxygen uptake. For example, a Swedish cross-country skier who in 1955 had just qualified for the national team had at that time a maximal oxygen uptake of 5.48 litre/min. In 1963 it was about the same (5.60 litre/min), but he had trained almost daily during the intervening 8 years and had successfully participated in two Olympic Games and two world championships, winning several gold medals. In repeated tests during 1955 another skier never exceeded 5.88 litre/min in maximal oxygen uptake. He trained intensively and competed successfully until 1964, winning a gold medal in the 50-km race in that year's Olympic Games. There are just two examples from longitudinal studies of top athletes in running disciplines. There are indications that running times improve despite little change in the maximal aerobic power. Training can improve running economy and the ability to run faster before a continuous accumulation of lactate sets in.[10]

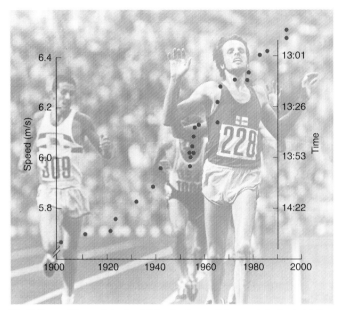

Fig. 6 The world records for the 5000-m track event follow a relatively straight line from 1920 onward. The introduction of an artificial track surface did not noticeably improve the records. An extrapolation to the world record for the year 2000 is tempting. The photograph shows Lasse Virén (of Finland) winning the 5000-m race at the 1972 Olympic Games in Munich (Pressens Bild AB).

No methods are available for an exact measurement of an individual's maximal anaerobic power and capacity. Therefore we do not know whether today's athletes have better anaerobic metabolism to support the contractile machinery of exercising muscles than did earlier generations. An increase in blood lactate concentration reflects a breakdown of glycogen in muscle. However, one cannot calculate from blood concentration how much lactate is produced. It is interesting to note that this lactate concentration is usually higher if measured after an important competition than after an all-out test in the laboratory. Apparently, the tolerance for high lactate values and low pH can be modified by psychological factors. It is remarkable that the pH in the arterial blood can fall below 7.0 after repeated 1-min maximal runs (see Chapter 1.1.4). A comparison of peak blood lactate concentrations after maximal physical performance in the laboratory or in connection with competition in top athletes does not indicate any differences over the last 30 years.

There is a continual increase in body height (H) in most developed countries. If a proportional increase in all dimensions is assumed, maximal strength, related to the surface area of the muscles, should be proportional to H^2 and maximal work and torque, should be proportional to H^3. The mean height of the participants in the decathlon in the 1960 Olympic Games in Rome was 184 cm. Approximately 30 years earlier the average height was 176 cm. These heights compare as the ratio 1.045:1, their muscle strength as 1.09:1, and work or torque as 1.14:1. Therefore, owing to different dimensions, the 4.5 per cent taller decathlete can be expected to be 9 per cent stronger and to have the capacity to do 14 per cent more work than the shorter competitor. These advantages are particularly evident in such events as throwing the javelin and discus and putting the shot. If these data are extrapolated to the development of world records in the shot put, similar changes in body dimensions alone could explain a gain from 16 m in 1930 to

approximately 18 m in 1960. However, in that year the shot was put 20 m. No doubt, in sports in which body size influences the results, from a democratic point of view the competitors should be classified according to weight as in boxing, wrestling, and weightlifting. Such classifications would, however, be unrealistic in track and field events.

Sexual dimorphism

Pierre de Coubertin was adamantly opposed to competitive sports for women. His Games were intended to emulate the male hedonistic ideals of Ancient Greece and the manly ethos of sports in Victorian public schools. However, in the Olympic Games of 1900 women competed in golf and tennis, and in 1912 swimming was included in the programme, but track and field events were not introduced until the Amsterdam Games in 1928 and consisted of the 100 m, 400-m relay, and 800 m races, high jump, and discus throwing. Earlier, women's Olympic Games had been suggested and, actually, the First Women's International Championships in track and field events was held in Paris in 1922. American female physical educators strongly opposed female elite competitions. In 1928 many women collapsed after the 800-m race and it was not reintroduced into the programme until 1960. In 1984 women ran the marathon and in the 1988 Olympics they also ran the 10 000 m.

An interesting statement made by a woman from the University of Illinois in 1928 was: 'Women can never hope successfully to compete in the men's world of athletics, and that when they do, they not only endanger their health but at the end become akward, ugly, and in every way unattractive'.

World records for women and men are compared in Table 1. In swimming, the highest speeds attained by women are, on average, 90.4 per cent of those reached by men. In track events women's performances are at the same ratio with top speeds at the 89.3 per cent level. In speed skating, women reach 91.0 per cent of men's world record speeds. In bicycling the figure is 83.8 per cent; perhaps a number of women with talent for bicycling have not yet discovered this discipline.

The large difference between women and men in world records in track and field events is noticed in the high jump, with the women's cross-bar reaching 85.3 per cent of the men's 2.45 m, and the long jump, in which the best woman jumped 84.0 per cent of Mike Powell's 8.95 m.

In sports testing strength (bench press, squat, deadlift) the weight handled by women is on average 70.3 per cent of the men's world record, (range 58.6 to 81.4 per cent in weight classes 52 to 82.5 kg).

It is interesting to follow the development of results for women and men over the years. In 1950 the highest speed during the 100-m race for women was 88.7 per cent of the best male performance (93.8 per cent in 1995). In 1950 in the 800-m race the highest speed for women was 80.2 per cent. Few women competed over longer distances, even though the 800-m race appeared in the Olympic Games as early as 1928. In high jump, the women's record was 81 per cent of the men's best result in 1950, 83 per cent in 1960, 84 per cent in 1970, and, as mentioned, close to 85 per cent in 1997. In long jump the figures are 77 per cent, 78 per cent, 77 per cent, and 84 per cent, respectively. The women's records have gradually

Table 1 Women's world records compared with those of men (valid September 1997)

Track and field		Swimming		Speed skating		Cycling	
Event	%	Event	%	Event	%	Event	%
100 m	93.8	50 m	89.0	500 m	90.9	1 h	83.8
200 m	90.5	100 m	89.3	1000 m	90.4		
400 m	87.6	200 m	91.3	1500 m	91.0		
800 m	89.8	400 m	91.8	3000 m	92.2		
1500 m	90.0	800 m	93.9	5000 m	90.6		
5000 m	86.7	1500 m	91.8				
10 000 m	84.7	*Breaststroke*					
Marathon	89.9	50 m	92.2				
4 x 100 m	90.4	100 m	90.4				
4 x 400 m	89.3	200 m	89.9				
High jump	85.3	*Butterfly*					
Long jump	84.0	50 m	87.0				
		100 m	90.2				
		200 m	91.5				
		Backstroke					
		50 m	86.7				
		100 m	89.5				
		200 m	92.1				

The data are taken from a selection of records valid 15 September 1997. The women's times (speeds) are given as a percentage of the men's records (= 100%). A similar calculation is performed for the jumping events.

crept closer to the men's levels. There are speculations, which have gained worldwide interest in the mass media, that women will eventually catch up to the men's world records, sooner in the marathon than in other events.[15] Whipp and Ward[15] extrapolate from world record progression, expressed as mean running velocity versus historical time, for women and men respectively and conclude that women may overtake men in the marathon by the year 2000 and in the 200-m sprint by the year 2050. If that were to happen it would be tempting for a female marathon runner to masquerade as a man and race in the men's event in the next century. Whipp and Ward ignore the fact that there are basic, genetically fixed differences that are decisive for physical performance demanding muscular strength and high aerobic power even when related to body mass. Women cannot compensate by 'natural means' for their lower haemoglobin concentration and this is reflected by a lower maximal aerobic power. There are no physiological data indicating that women have a particularly high potential for long-distance events such as the marathon race.

World records in swimming as compared with running

Swimming appears to be the discipline that has the world record for breaking world records. During the 1972 Olympic Games in Munich the swimming competitors produced 30 world records in 29 events. There are claims that swimming is still a developing discipline. Figure 7 illustrates the advances in 200-m freestyle swimming and 800-m running since the turn of the century. The reason for selecting these events is that the present world records are not far from each other with regard to the times involved. Records in running can survive for years, but in swimming the records have been broken frequently since 1950. One factor to consider is that the per-

centage increase in the number of pools over the years exceeds the number of new running tracks. Specific training of muscular strength and flexibility may improve swimming performance more than running ability. Many countries are handicapped because swimming cannot be recommended as a recreational sport where waters are polluted and can cause serious diseases (e.g. bilharzia (schistosomiasis) in tropical areas).

Altitude training

Is training at high altitude beneficial for the oxygen transport system? The reason for bringing up this question here is that a study of the improvement of world records can enlighten the discussion. Acclimatization too is essential in the preparation for optimal performance in events demanding high aerobic power if the competition takes place at high altitude. The 1968 Olympic Games in Mexico City were not the first challenge forcing athletes to face new environmental conditions. In the 1960 Olympic Games in Squaw Valley the athletes had to gasp at an altitude of approximately 2000 m (6600 feet).

It is a common belief that training at high altitude will also enhance the performance at lower altitudes. The history of world records does not support this hypothesis. In the years 1966 and 1967, and particularly in 1968, the cream of the world's athletes spent long periods of time in Mexico City or at similar altitudes. Many scientific studies were conducted on these athletes. However, few world records in middle- and long-distance running were broken in those years. Nor were there any spectacular records in swimming. New records would be expected at sea-level if a sojourn at high altitude elicited an additional improvement of maximal aerobic power and endurance. In fact, in 1968, when certainly all Olympic candidates were extremely well prepared, there were no new world records in middle- and long-distance running.

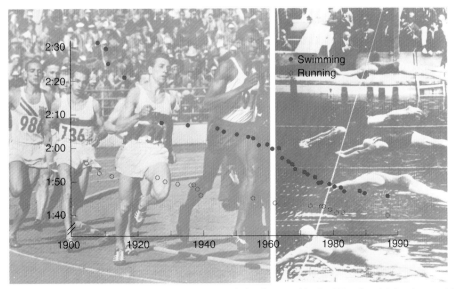

Fig. 7 The development of world records in swimming and running is shown. Swimming speed for the 200-m freestyle has improved 27 per cent since the 1920s, whereas running 800 m has improved only 12 per cent. The left-hand photograph shows Arthur Wint (of Jamaica) leading in the 800-m final at the 1952 Olympic Games in Helsinki, no. 986 is Ulzheimer (of Germany), no.736 Steines (of Germany), and no. 986 Whitfield (of the United States), the winner (UPI Photo; Pressens Bild AB). One of the swimmers is Johnny Weissmüller, winner of five gold medals in the 1924 and 1928 Olympic Games, better known for his movie role as Tarzan.

The beneficial effect of acclimatization is an increase in haemoglobin concentration. The problem is that at high altitude it is inevitable that peak intensity during training in endurance events cannot reach the same level as at sea-level. In Finland they have launched a 'high altitude house', located at sea-level, but by diluting the normal room air with nitrogen one can simulate conditions equivalent to oxygen pressures at 2000 to 3000-m altitudes. Athletes spend some 15 h/day for weeks indoors and they can go outdoors and train at sea-level conditions. An ideal quality of life for an athlete?

The record

Eric Segal[16] writes:

But without any question, the most famous barrier in sports history was the four minute mile. And yet I seriously wonder if it would have acquired such mystique if the first man to break it had not been that eloquent obsessive, Roger Bannister. Anyone who reads his aufobiography cannot help but sense what an all-consuming fixation it was for him to run merely two seconds faster than he ever had before. After all, Glenn Cunningham, that great miler of the 1930s, claimed that he had often run better than four minutes in practice sessions, but it had never seemed important to do so officially in a race. He had just wanted to win. Not Bannister. To him, breaking four minutes for the mile would be extending the 'ultimate' in human capability. Indeed, as a doctor Bannister believed that the effort required would be so enormous that the runner would expend his entire oxygen reserve a few yards before the finish and have to complete the race as a semiconscious reflex action. He planned his race according to his own theories. The rest is history. The photos of Bannister after his epoch-making run on May 6, 1954, show a totally exhausted man who by hint of courage and scientific preparation systematically depleted himself of all his resources to surpass all previous limits. His face shows that his body had not an ounce in reserve. He could not have done an instant better. The ultimate time for the mile had to be 3:59.4. This was, I repeat, May 6, 1954. And yet on August 7 of the same year, Bannister ran 3:58.8 without collapsing. Paradoxically, running a mile even faster proved to be less exhausting. Because once he had surpassed the four-minute

'limit,' there was no magic in 3:58. Nor did there appear to be in 3:50. Values are what they are, Hamlet tells us, 'because thinking makes it so.' On July 18, 1979, the London Daily Express wrote the following: 'Coe came up to the final straight looking almost relaxed, hardly gasping ... what a fantastic contrast to the complete exhaustion of ... Sir Roger Bannister'. The limits are, of course, purely mental. Sebastian Coe was so relaxed in Oslo because he did not consider 3:49 any kind of ultimate. And when he finally begins to think in these terms, some mad idealist will appear in track shoes and prove him wrong. There are simply no absolute limits.

Swedes like to remember the comments of two runners who broke many world records in middle-distance running in the 1940s, Gunder Hägg and Arne Andersson: first of all, 1 mile is not a Swedish distance; second, the goal is to win, not to make spectacular times.

Conclusion

Many factors have contributed to improvements in sports world records. The complexities of the disciplines are decisive for the quantitative impact of the various factors. Probably the basic endowment of the human being has been the most stable factor. Changes in training methods, tactics, techniques, rules, equipment, material, economy, and an increase in the number of people engaged in sports have all contributed to the improvements. It will probably be many years before we can write the final history of all world records—records that will never be surpassed.

A retardation in the curves can be seen in some events but not in others. As mentioned previously, in the javelin event it will be very difficult to beat Hohn's record owing to equipment modifications. In certain disciplines not discussed here one can, with great confidence, say that 'this record can never be improved'. One such discipline is shooting. With all bullets awarded 10 points, present rules do not permit a better achievement.

It should be emphasized that sports that cannot be evaluated by world records also are very popular with participants and spectators: racket sports, American football, boxing, cricket, soccer, gymnastics, skiing, golf, alpine and cross-country skiing, just to mention a few. Beating a world record is not an essential stimulus for action and spectators' interest.

References

1. Dickerson RE. Chemical evolution and the origin of life. *Scientific American* 1978; **239(3)**: 62–78.

2. Vidal G. The oldest eukaryotic cell. *Scientific American* 1984; **250(2)**: 32–41.

3. Valentine JW. The evolution of multicellular plants and animals. *Scientific American* 1978; **239(3)**: 104–17.

4. Lewin R. Evolutionary theory under fire. *Science* 1980; **210**: 883–7.

5. Lewin R. Ethiopian stone tools are world's oldest. *Science* 1981; **211**: 806–7.

6. Stringer CB. The emergence of modern humans. *Scientific American* 1990; **264(6)**: 68–74.

7. Kandel ER. Small systems of neurons. *Scientific American* 1979; **239(3)**: 67–76.

8. Washburn SL. The evolution of man. *Scientific American* 1978; **239(3)**: 146–54.

9. *Encyclopaedia Britannia*. London: William Benton, 1963.

10. Åstrand P-O, Rodahl K. *Textbook of work physiology*. New York: McGraw-Hill, 1986: Ch. 14, 651.

11. Christensen EH, Hansen O Arbeitsfähigkeit und Ehrnärung. *Skandinavischen Archiv für Physiologie* 1939; **81**: 160–71.

12. Balson PD, Ekblom B, Söderlund K, Sjödin B, Hultman E. Creatine supplementation and dynamic high-intensity intermittent exercise. *Scandinavian Journal of Medicine and Science in Sports* 1993; **3**: 143–9.

13. Linderman J, Fahey TD. Sodium bicarbonate ingestion and exercise performance. *Sports medicine* 1991; **11(2)**: 71–7.

14. Robinson S, Edwards HT, Dill DB. New records in human power. *Nature* 1937; **85**: 409–10.

15. Whipp BJ, Ward SA. Will women soon outrun men? *Nature* 1992; **355**: 25.

16. Segal E. Reflections on the right to one's own limit. In: Pabst U, ed. *Baden-Baden report: the limits in sports. 11th Olympic Congress 1981*. Munich: Nationales Olympisches Komitee für Deutschland, 1980.

1

Sports science

1.1 Physiology

1.1.1 Respiratory responses of athletes to exercise

Brian J. Whipp and Susan A. Ward

Introduction

The appropriateness of the ventilatory response to dynamic muscular exercise is best considered with respect to the degree of arterial blood-gas homeostasis it achieves for moderate exercise and by the degree of compensatory hyperventilation at work rates that engender a metabolic acidosis. These responses, however, comprise only one part of an integrated system, with external pulmonary and internal tissue gas exchange components which are linked via the circulation. The system components operate as a coupled unit during exercise: mechanically coupled anatomically and control coupled physiologically.

In highly trained athletes, the pulmonary demands of high intensity exercise can lead to the effective limits of the convective fluid flow being approached or even exceeded: that is, air through the airways and blood through the pulmonary capillary bed. Furthermore, these high ventilatory demands can require a level of respiratory muscle power that is so great that a large fraction of the total increase of cardiac output can be required by the respiratory muscles. In addition to diverting blood flow from the muscles generating the external work, this can also exceed the ability of the respiratory muscles to provide ventilation wholly aerobically; respiratory muscle fatigue being the potential consequence.

The assessment of the athlete's respiratory system performance during exercise is therefore not straightforward; however, it should address three interrelated issues:

- To what extent are the 'requirements' met? The major requirements are for arterial P_{O_2}, P_{CO_2} and pH regulation. These variables need to be determined directly or, when this is not possible, reliable and valid estimators should be used.

- What is the 'cost' of meeting these requirements? This necessitates an assessment of: (i) how much ventilation (and its pattern) is utilized to meet the requirements, and (ii) the amount of respiratory muscle work involved—along with its oxygen and blood flow cost.

- To what extent is the system 'constrained' or 'limited'? This requires estimation of whether the effective limits of the system are achieved or approached; for example, with respect to limiting airflow, volume change, and gas exchange

efficiency. Flow-volume and tidal volume-inspiratory capacity considerations, the maximum voluntary ventilation, and the maximum sustained ventilatory capacity provide useful frames of reference for mechanical reserve, and the alveolar–arterial P_{O_2} difference provides an important index of gas exchange efficiency.

The ventilatory requirements during exercise

Ventilatory response characteristics

The ventilatory demands of muscular exercise vary with respect to its 'intensity'. It is important, therefore, to determine the intensity domain of a particular work rate in order to establish whether the ventilatory response is appropriate. Although there is no generally agreed upon procedure for normalizing work intensity, we believe that two widely used procedures fail to meet the demands of critical scrutiny in this regard, at least with respect to the respiratory system: the 'met' increment and the 'percentage' of maximal oxygen uptake (%$\dot{V}_{O_2}$max).

The onset of the metabolic (lactic) acidaemia of exercise does not occur at a common 'met' increment in different individuals. Consequently, different subjects at the same 'met' level can have markedly different degrees of metabolic acidaemia. Similarly, there is a wide variation in the percentage of $\dot{V}_{O_2}$max at which the metabolic acidosis becomes evident. In normal individuals, this can range from 40 to 80 per cent of $\dot{V}_{O_2}$max,[1] tending to be greater the fitter the subject, but with a large variability at any particular level.

For these reasons, it is preferable to utilize the measured or estimated degree of metabolic acidaemia as the index of exercise intensity. The range of work rates within which there is not a sustained metabolic acidaemia may be considered to be of moderate intensity: in the athlete, this range is substantial. Work rates at which blood lactate concentration and [H$^+$] are elevated, but eventually stabilize or even decrease as the exercise continues, are of heavy intensity. For those higher work rates at which blood lactate concentration and [H$^+$] are not only elevated but increase inexorably throughout the test, the work rate is of severe intensity.

For moderate constant-load exercise, oxygen uptake ($\dot{V}_{O_2}$) increases mono-exponentially following a short delay, reflecting the vascular transit time between the 'exercising' muscle and the lungs. This response has a time constant (τ) that typically ranges from 20 to 40 s, such that a steady state is attained within about 3 min.[2-6] However as $\tau\dot{V}_{O_2}$ appears to be shorter in athletes,[7] the time to steady state is also reduced. As a consequence of the high tissue CO_2 capacitance, CO_2 output ($\dot{V}_{CO_2}$) takes longer to reach a steady state, resulting in a longer τ.[2-6] The time constant for ventilation ($\dot{V}_E$) is longer still, and consequently a steady state is normally not attained until 4 to 5 min.[2-6,8] The lack of a metabolic acidosis and the attainment of steady states in $\dot{V}O_2$, $\dot{V}CO_2$ and $\dot{V}_E$ allows exercise in this intensity domain to be sustained for long periods with relative ease.

During heavy exercise, $\dot{V}_E$ is further stressed both by the metabolic acidosis *per se* and the gas-exchange consequences of the acidosis. In response to constant-load exercise within this domain, blood lactate concentration and arterial pH (pH_a) eventually stabilize,[9-11] as do the circulating levels of adrenaline and noradrenaline.[11] $\dot{V}O_2$, $\dot{V}CO_2$ and $\dot{V}_E$ also attain new steady-state levels. However, relative to moderate exercise, the $\dot{V}O_2$ response develops far more slowly, such that its time constant is prolonged. This delays the attainment of a steady state. Furthermore, at these work rates a further, acidosis-related component of $\dot{V}O_2$ is superimposed upon this initial response, adding to the steady-state O_2 cost—and hence ventilatory cost—of the exercise.[12,13]

In contrast, in the severe intensity domain, both $\dot{V}O_2$ and lactate concentration continue to increase throughout the work until $\dot{V}O_2max$ and the limit of exercise tolerance are attained.[10,11] Likewise, pH_a continues to fall,[10,11] but at a rate that depends on the degree of respiratory compensation. In this domain, the duration for which a given work rate may be sustained has been shown to be hyperbolically related to the work rate.[11,14,15]

As there is no systematic metabolic (or respiratory) acid–base derangement in the steady state of moderate exercise, pH_a is regulated as a result of ventilation changing in proportion to $\dot{V}CO_2$; i.e. through regulation of arterial PCO_2 (PCO_2a). This is implicit in the Henderson–Hasselbalch equation:

$$pH_a = pK' + \log \frac{[HCO_3^-]_a}{\alpha PCO_2a} \qquad (1)$$

where α is the solubility coefficient for CO_2 in plasma and is equal to 0.03 mmol/mmHg at 37 °C; pK', which is related to the first 'apparent' ionization constant of carbonic acid, is equal to 6.1; and $[HCO_3^-]_a$ is the arterial bicarbonate concentration. The influence of PCO_2a and ventilation on the regulated level of PCO_2a can be incorporated into this consideration by means of the 'alveolar air' equation for the 'ideal' lung*[16-18]:

$$\dot{V}_A[BTPS] = \frac{863 \dot{V}CO_2[STPD]}{PCO_2a} \qquad (2)$$

where $\dot{V}CO_2$ (the CO_2 production rate) is expressd at standard temperature and pressure, dry (STPD), and the alveolar ventilation ($\dot{V}_A$) is expressed at body temperature, ambient pressure, saturated with water vapour (BTPS). Substituting for PCO_2a in equation (1) yields:

$$pH_a = pK' + \log \left\{ \frac{[HCO_3^-]_a}{25.6} \cdot \frac{\dot{V}_A}{\dot{V}CO_2} \right\} \qquad (3)$$

where the constant 25.6 is the product of the conversion constant

863 and α. It should be noted that as long as $[HCO_3^-]_a$ is unaltered, pH_a can only be regulated if $\dot{V}_A/\dot{V}CO_2$ is maintained constant; i.e. a proportional increase of $\dot{V}_A$ with $\dot{V}CO_2$ during the work.

However, it is the *total* ventilation ($\dot{V}_E$) that needs to be controlled, and the extent to which this is translated into alveolar ventilation is dictated by the physiological dead space fraction of the breath (V_D/V_T):

$$\dot{V}_A = \dot{V}_E(1 - V_D/V_T) \qquad (4)$$

Therefore, substituting for $\dot{V}_A$ in equation (3), we obtain:

$$pH_a = pK' + \log \left\{ \left[\frac{[HCO_3^-]_a}{25.8} \right] \cdot \left[\frac{\dot{V}_E}{\dot{V}CO_2} \right] \cdot [(1 - V_D/V_T)] \right\} \qquad (5)$$

This integration of the Henderson–Hasslebalch and alveolar air equations allows pH regulation relative to the demand for CO_2 clearance to be considered in terms of three distinct components:

(1)　the acid-base 'set point' component, $[HCO_3^-]_a$;

(2)　the respiratory 'control' component, $\dot{V}_E/\dot{V}CO_2$; and

(3)　the ventilatory 'efficiency' component, $(1 - V_D/V_T)$.

The metabolic acidosis of heavy and severe exercise leads to additional drive to $\dot{V}_E$. In normal subjects, this is thought to derive predominantly from the metabolic acidaemia;[19,20] however other influences also contribute, such as increased levels of circulating catecholamines, further-increased levels of circulating potassium ions and adenosine, sufficiently high body temperature, and in some subjects anxiety, pain, and apprehension.[4,21-23] In the highly fit subjects who develop arterial hypoxaemia at these work rates[24] there is presumably an additional drive via peripheral chemoreception. As a result, $\dot{V}_E$ increases at a greater rate than $\dot{V}CO_2$, causing PCO_2a to fall. It is the magnitude of this compensatory reduction in PCO_2a that constrains the fall of pH_a.

These considerations underscore the importance of establishing the transitional work rate between the moderate and heavy intensities of exercise. This has been termed the 'lactate threshold' (θ_L), and represents the highest $\dot{V}O_2$ that can be attained without a sustained lactic acidosis.[25-28] Likewise, it is also important to identify the work rate that separates the heavy and severe intensity domains. This has been termed the 'fatigue threshold'* (θ_F)[11] or 'critical power':[14] it appears to correspond to the highest work rate (supra-θ_L) that can be sustained without blood lactate concentration, $[H^+]$ and $\dot{V}O_2$ continuing to increase throughout the work bout.[10,11]

However, an important caveat to this consideration of the ventilatory determinants of PCO_2a or pH_a regulation is the recognition that the control studies under laboratory conditions may not be appropriate for consideration of actual athletic performance.

Estimation of functional parameters

We consider here the techniques that identify the parameters which partition the intensity domains of exercise.

---

* The 'ideal' lung is characterized by diffusion equilibrium between alveolar gas and pulmonary end-capillary blood, regional matching of ventilation to perfusion, and the absence of a right-to-left vascular shunt. Therefore, alveolar PO_2 and PCO_2 equal arterial PO_2 and PCO_2

* The parameter θ_F has been termed the fatigue threshold,[11] not in the sense that there is no fatigue at lower work rates, but that the fatigue will be of a different character from that which results in $\dot{V}O_2max$ being attained.

Table 1 Markers of the lactate threshold

Marker	Comments
Incremental work tests	
1. Blood and muscle [L⁻]/[P⁻]	Best single estimate that [L⁻] increase is probably consequent to anaerobiosis (i.e. corrects for pyruvate-dependent [L⁻] changes). Arterialized capillary blood or arterialized venous blood from high flow to low metabolic rate region (e.g. dorsum of hand) is acceptable. Direct venous samples are inadequate
2. Blood [L⁻] and HCO₃	As [L⁻] and HCO₃] changes are often curvilinear above θ_L, a plot of log [L⁻] or log [HCO₃] vs. $\dot{V}O_2$ or, even better, log [L⁻] or log [HCO₃] vs. log $\dot{V}O_2$ gives linear components intersecting precisely at θ_L
3. Ventilatory response variables	In subjects with normal chemosensitivity and normal pulmonary mechanics, the beginning of a systematic increase in $\dot{V}_E/\dot{V}O_2$ and PO_2et without PCO_2et decreasing provides a valid index of θ_L: R beginning to increase more rapidly and $\dot{V}_E/\dot{V}CO_2$ becoming relatively constant (usually after having decreased) often, but not always, gives added support; breathing frequency also often begins to increase more rapidly
4. V-slope method	When the early kinetic non-linearity and the hyperventilatory region are discarded, a plot of $\dot{V}O_2$ vs. $\dot{V}O_2$ gives two linear components, the intersection of which occurs at θ_L (validated, to date, only for 1 min incremental tests). As this method only relies on the accelerated $\dot{V}CO_2$ above θ_L, it is expected to be valid even when $\dot{V}_E$ does not respond as required in method 3
Constant-load tests	
5. Blood [L⁻] and [HCO₃]	Sustained change is required to know if exercise is supra-θ_L. Several studies are needed to determine the location of θ_L
6. $\Delta \dot{V}O_{2(6-3)}$	For sub-θ_L exercise $\Delta \dot{V}O_{2(6-3)}$ is zero (i.e. steady state as attained after 3 min). When $\Delta \dot{V}O_{2(6-3)}$ is positive, a slow $\dot{V}O_2$ kinetic phase is evident, the magnitude of which correlates well with the increase in blood [L⁻]. Although several tests are needed to determine the location of θ_L, this index is useful for confirming that a particular work rate is or is not greater than θ_L

Lactate threshold

A wide range of techniques have been advocated for estimation of θ_L, and include both direct and indirect estimators (Table 1).[29] While various exercise regimens have been used, the most useful has proved to be the rapid-incremental test, in which the work rate is increased in a continuous ramp profile or by a constant, small increment (e.g. 15–25 W, for healthy subjects) at a regular interval (typically each min or less) until the subject's limit of tolerance is reached.

The lactate threshold is highly task specific. It occurs at a much lower $\dot{V}O_2$ for arm exercise than for leg exercise, and is typically lower for cycle ergometry than for treadmill exercise.

The response profile of blood lactate concentration during incremental exercise is often not the most sensitive estimator for θ_L. The reason is that there may be no clear break-point in the profile that can be identified with sufficient confidence, at least for some investigators. As a component of the blood lactate concentration increase reflects pyruvate-dependent increases, a clearer estimate is provided by the ratio of lactate to pyruvate concentrations.[30] Another approach has been to transform the lactate concentration (or [HCO₃⁻]ₐ) response to a logarithmic function, to linearize its rising phase.[31] The intersection of this phase with the earlier region of shallower slope (i.e. the moderate exercise region) coincides with non-invasive estimators of θ_L (described in detail below).

However, one can forego the necessity for serial blood sampling and even, in many cases, enhance the discriminability of θ_L by utilizing a particular cluster of pulmonary gas-exchange responses. The compensatory hyperventilation for the metabolic acidosis of heavy and severe exercise occurs coincidentally with the increase in lactate concentration and decrease in [HCO₃⁻] in tests for which the work rate is incremented in a quasi-steady-state manner (i.e. increment durations of more than 4 min), that is, $\dot{V}_E$ begins to increase more

rapidly than $\dot{V}CO_2$ (and $\dot{V}O_2$) and PCO_2a is reduced.[26,32] In contrast, when the work-rate incrementation rate is more rapid, the compensatory hyperventilation is strikingly attenuated (Fig. 1). In this situation, there is a range of work rates immediately above θ_L within which $\dot{V}_E$ increases with $\dot{V}CO_2$ in approximately the same proportionality as for moderate exercise. Under these conditions, $\dot{V}CO_2$ has contributions both from metabolic sources and from HCO₃⁻ buffering reactions. Therefore, as PCO_2a does not fall in this region, it has been termed the range of 'isocapnic buffering'.[33] Respiratory compensation for the lactic acidosis (i.e. PCO_2a actually decreasing) only begins for rapid-incremental tests (Fig. 1) at a work rate which is typically about midway between θ_L and $\dot{V}O_2$max.[34]

The phenomenon of isocapnic buffering forms the basis for probably the most widely used techniques for θ_L estimation.[33] Thus, for a rapid-incremental protocol, θ_L is taken as the $\dot{V}O_2$ (not the work rate) at which the alveolar (end-tidal) PO_2 (PO_2et) and the ventilatory equivalent for O_2 ($\dot{V}_E/\dot{V}O_2$) start to rise systematically without a simultaneous fall in the end-tidal PCO_2 (PCO_2et) (Fig. 1).[1,29]

An additional approach, known as the 'V-slope' technique,[35] has arisen out of the recognition that in some individuals the respiratory system may be compromised in its ability to generate the required increases in $\dot{V}_E$ at higher work rates, such as in subjects with insensitive peripheral chemoreceptors or high airways resistance. As a result, if there is no or only a poor additional ventilatory response, it proves difficult, or impossible, to discriminate θ_L according to these criteria.[34]

However, the work rate at which the metabolic acidaemia first becomes evident is also associated with an accelerated rate of CO_2 production.[36] This reflects the additional contribution from HCO₃⁻-mediated buffering of lactic acid.[37] For example, in order to sustain a given ATP production rate under anaerobic conditions

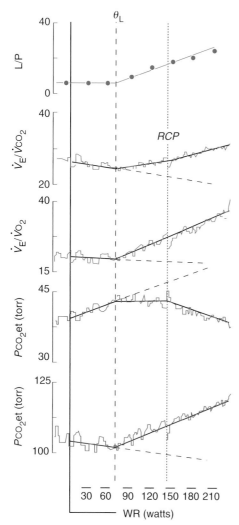

Fig. 1 Responses in a normal subject of the ratio of blood lactate to pyruvate concentration (L/P), ventilatory equivalents for CO_2 and O_2 ($\dot{V}_E/\dot{V}_{CO_2}$, $\dot{V}_E/\dot{V}_{O_2}$) and end-tidal gas tensions (P_{CO_2}et, P_{O_2}et) to an exhausting incremental exercise test (15 W/min), as a function of $\dot{V}_{O_2}$. The full vertical line indicates the start of the test, the broken vertical line indicates the lactate threshold (θ_L), and the dotted vertical line indicates the onset of the respiratory compensation phase (RCP) for the lactic acidosis. It should be noted that θ_L occurs at the work rate where both $\dot{V}_E/\dot{V}_{O_2}$ and P_{O_2}et start to increase, but P_{CO_2}et does not yet fall. Typically, the RCP occurs approximately midway between θ_L and $\dot{V}_{O_2}$max.

relative to aerobic conditions, the glycogen utilization rate must increase more than 12-fold—a major concern, of course, for the marathon runner who runs too fast early in the race. The formation of two lactate molecules from one glucosyl unit of glycogen yields only three ATP molecules, compared with the 37 that result from its complete aerobic catabolism to CO_2 and H_2O. Therefore, the ATP production rate can only be sustained if the glycolytic flux increases by a factor $37/3 = 12.3$. The resulting 24.6 mmol/L lactic acid yield will be predominantly buffered by the HCO_3^- system;[9,38] $[HCO_3^-]_a$ will therefore decrease by about 22 mmol/L (i.e. some 90 per cent of 24.6). This yields an increase of about 22 mmol in CO_2 production. However, 6 mmol of this replaces the CO_2 that would have occurred aerobically for this rate of ATP formation (i.e. as no O_2 is used in the glycogen-to-lactate catabolism, no CO_2 is directly released). The net increase in CO_2 production rate is therefore

22 mmol anaerobic CO_2–6 mmol aerobic CO_2 = 16 mmol net CO_2 yield. This results in an increase in $\dot{V}_{CO_2}$ for these reactions during supra-θ_L exercise by a factor of about 2.5, relative to purely aerobic conditions.

It should be noted that this analysis considers the volume released from the blood compartment with no arterial hypocapnia. It does not consider the changes within the exercising muscle compartment, which has a resting intracellular $[HCO_3^-]$ less than half that of blood, but which interacts with the blood compartment through ion-exchange mechanisms. Interested readers are referred to articles by Wasserman *et al.*[1] and Jones[39] for further consideration of this topic.

Beaver *et al.*[35] proposed that θ_L could be identified from the relationship between $\dot{V}_{CO_2}$ and $\dot{V}_{O_2}$. This relationship, which is characterized by a relatively linear relationship during moderate exercise, is shown by an increased, but still essentially linear, slope within the isocapnic buffering phase. The intersection of these two linear phases has been shown to agree closely with the beginning of the increase in blood lactate concentration and the ratio of lactate to pyruvate concentrations and the decrease in $[HCO_3^-]$ (Fig. 2).[35]

It is important to point out that the resolving power of these

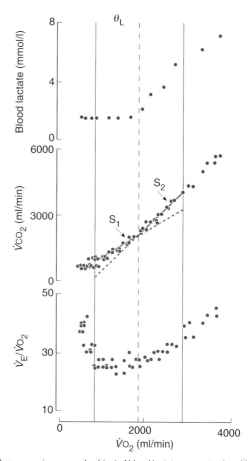

Fig. 2 Responses in a normal subject of blood lactate concentration, $\dot{V}_{CO_2}$, and the ventilatory equivalent for O_2 ($\dot{V}_E/\dot{V}_{O_2}$) to an exhausting incremental test (20 W/min), as a function of $\dot{V}_{O_2}$. The broken vertical line indicates the lactate threshold (θ_L), and the left- and right-hand solid vertical lines demarcate the 'region of interest' for the V-slope analysis.[35] The V-slope parameters, S_1 and S_2, are the slopes of the regressions of the sub-θ_L and supra-θ_L regions of the $\dot{V}_{CO_2}$–$\dot{V}_{O_2}$ relationship, respectively. It should be noted that the intersection of these two regressions coincides with θ_L. (Modified from ref. 13.)

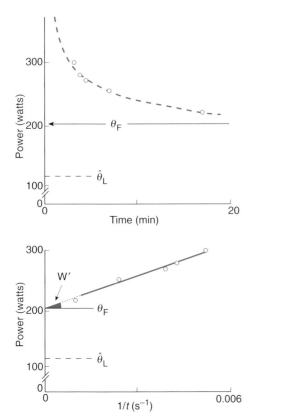

Fig. 3 The upper panel shows the power-duration (P–t) relationship for high intensity exercise. The lower panel shows the determination of parameters W' and θ_F from the linear P–$1/t$ formulation. θ_L is the estimated lactate threshold. (Modified from ref.11.)

non-invasive approaches depends on the rate at which the work rate is increased. The more slowly the work rate is increased the more slowly blood $[HCO_3^-]$ will fall, and therefore the smaller will be the contribution to $\dot{V}CO_2$ from the blood-buffering reactions.[40,41] Rapid-incremental work rates are therefore preferable. However, it should be recognized that the total extra volume yield of CO_2 accruing above θ_L is considerably greater for slow-incremental than for fast-incremental tests, owing to the reduction of PCO_{2a} and the tissue CO_2 stores with which it equilibrates. This is because of the greater compensatory hyperventilation in the slow tests.[42]

Fatigue threshold

The tolerable duration for high intensity exercise decreases hyperbolically as a function of the absolute work rate[11,14,15] (Fig. 3):

$$(P - \theta_F) \cdot t = W' \tag{6}$$

where θ_F corresponds to the lower limit or asymptotic power. However, to date, this relationship has only been validated for exhaustive exercise lasting 30 min or less. Interestingly, W' has the units of work and hence represents a constant amount of work that can be performed above θ_F, regardless of the rate at which it is performed. It may therefore be regarded as an energy store comprised of O_2 stores, a phosphagen pool, and a source related to anaerobic glycolysis and the consequent production and accumulation of lactate.[11,14,15]

The asymptote θ_F (or critical power[14]) has been shown to represent the highest work rate for which a steady state can be

attained in pulmonary gas exchange, blood acid–base status, and blood lactate concentration, given sufficient time.[10,11] θ_F may therefore be regarded as reflecting a rate of energy-pool reconstitution which dictates the maximum power that can be sustained without a continued and progressive anaerobic contribution. Like θ_L, θ_F is high in trained individuals and can be increased by training.[43]

In many subjects, this higher sustainable lactate level occurs at about 4 to 5 mmol/l. This may therefore be the reason that the work rate yielding a 4 mmol/l blood lactate concentration has proved such a useful index of endurance performance. However, the maximal sustainable lactate can be markedly different in different subjects. It is therefore important that training strategies utilize intensity indices that are specific for individual athletes rather than utilizing those which characterize groups of athletes where the group mean value may have a wide dispersion.

θ_F can be readily estimated by transforming the P–t relationship (eqn 6) into its linear formulation:

$$P = (W'/t) + \theta_F \tag{7}$$

where W' and θ_F are the slope and intercept, respectively (Fig. 3). The parameters W' and θ_F are determined from the linear regression of P against $1/t$ from a series of discrete bouts of exhausting supra-θ_L constant-load exercise, preferably performed on different days.[11] Four to five tests typically provide good definition of the relationship, especially if the tolerable duration is spaced relatively evenly on the $1/t$ axis (i.e. not evenly with respect to t).

It is important to emphasize that this relationship is unlikely to provide a precise representation of the actual physiological behaviour at the very extremes of performance, as there are distorting factors such as (i) limitations of muscular (mechanical) force-generation for the very highest power requirements and (ii) constraints resulting from substrate provision, thermoregulatory, or body-fluid requirements for markedly prolonged exercise.[11]

Determinants of ventilatory requirements

Alveolar ventilation

The alveolar air equation described earlier (eqn 2) provides the basic frame of reference for predicting the ventilatory requirement of a particular task. This relationship demonstrates that both $\dot{V}CO_2$ and PCO_{2a} are important in determining the magnitude of the $\dot{V}_A$ requirement for a particular task. The greater the demand for metabolic CO_2 clearance, the greater will be the $\dot{V}_A$ requirement, at a particular 'set-point' for PCO_{2a} regulation. Lowering of the set-point, for example as in a sea-level native sojourning at high altitude or with metabolic acidosis induced hyperventilation, will require a larger increase in $\dot{V}_A$ to effect a given rate of CO_2 clearance.

Furthermore, both $\dot{V}CO_2$ and PCO_{2a} determine the compensatory potential of a particular increment of $\dot{V}_A$. As a result, the greatest stress to potential encroachment on the functional ventilatory limits for the elite athlete results from the combination of high levels of $\dot{V}CO_2$ and low levels of PCO_{2a}; the less fit individual is protected from such limitation by the relatively low achievable levels of metabolic rate.

Total ventilation

Substituting for $\dot{V}_A$ in eqn (2) from eqn (4) provides the total ventilatory requirement for a given work rate:

$$\dot{V}_E = \frac{863 \dot{V}_{CO_2}}{P_{CO_2a}(1 - V_D/V_T)} \qquad (8)$$

It should be noted that eqn (8) does not, on cursory inspection, appear to characterize the linear, isocapnic $\dot{V}_E$–$\dot{V}_{CO_2}$ relationship for steady-state moderate exercise. What makes $\dot{V}_E$ linearly related to $\dot{V}_{CO_2}$ isocapnically under these conditions is that V_D/V_T decreases hyperbolically with respect to $\dot{V}_{CO_2}$.[44]

Equation (8) indicates that the three variables $\dot{V}_{CO_2}$, P_{CO_2a}, and V_D/V_T collectively determine the overall ventilatory requirements for exercise. This can be illustrated with reference to an elite athlete and an untrained individual exercising at their respective θ_L and $\dot{V}_{O_2}$max levels, based upon some reasonable assumptions.

For example, assume the untrained individual to have a steady-state $\dot{V}_{O_2}$ of 2 l/min and the athlete to have a $\dot{V}_{O_2}$ of 5 l/min at θ_L. With the further assumption that carbohydrate is the substrate undergoing oxidation (i.e. respiratory quotient or $RQ = 1.0$), the corresponding requirements for metabolic CO_2 clearance (i.e. $\dot{V}_{CO_2}$) will be also 2.0 l/min for the untrained subject and 5.0 l/min for the athlete. Assume that both have a normal setpoint P_{CO_2a} of 40 mmHg. The $\dot{V}_A$ requirements will be 43 l/min for the untrained subject and 108 l/min for the athlete (i.e. eqn 2). V_D/V_T, however, is likely to be somewhat lower for the athlete owing to the higher work rate at θ_L. Therefore, the untrained individual with a V_D/V_T of 0.15 at θ_L has a $\dot{V}_E$ requirement of some 50 l/min; for the athlete, with a V_D/V_T of 0.1, the requirement is 120 l/min (i.e. eqn 4).

A similar analysis can be applied at maximum exercise, with the assumption that $\dot{V}_{O_2}$max for the untrained subject is 3 l/min, and 7 l/min for the élite athlete. However, while carbohydrate is still likely to be the dominant metabolic substrate ($RQ = 1.0$), R is now dissociated from RQ owing to the additional CO_2 clearance coming from HCO_3^- buffering of lactic acid and the reduction of CO_2 stores resulting from the compensatory hyperventilation. With the reasonable assumption that R at maximum is 1.2 in both subjects,[1] $\dot{V}_{CO_2}$max will be 3.6 l/min for the untrained subject and 8.4 l/min for the athlete. Allowing for a 10 mmHg reduction of P_{CO_2a} at maximum (i.e. $P_{CO_2a} = 30$ mmHg), the $\dot{V}_A$ requirements will be 103 l/min and 241 l/min (eqn 2), respectively, for the untrained individual and the athlete. However, both subjects are now likely to have a similar V_D/V_T at maximum of 0.1, which yields a $\dot{V}_E$ requirement of 114 l/min for the untrained subject, and 267 l/min for the athlete (eqn 4).

This is an enormous ventilatory demand, even for a large athlete. Consequently, if the athlete's $\dot{V}_E$ is mechanically limited at a value less than this, eqns (2) and (4) indicate that P_{CO_2a} would not be appropriately reduced. Therefore, the fall of arterial and muscle pH would be less constrained; more-rapid fatigue would be the consequence. It should be noted also that arterial hypoxaemia would also result, as evidenced by the lower $\dot{V}_E/\dot{V}_{O_2}$.

Some investigators[45,46] have suggested that athletes tend to have low peripheral chemosensitivity to hypoxia (as do their non-athletic relatives). As both hypoxia and H^+ are sensed by the carotid bodies, it is tempting to speculate that they are also insensitive to the exercise-induced metabolic acidaemia. Whether this reduced peripheral chemosensitivity also ameliorates the sensation of shortness of breath in the athlete remains to be determined.

The costs of meeting the ventilatory requirements of exercise

The increased ventilatory requirements for arterial blood-gas and acid–base homeostasis during exercise exact increased mechanical cost, with respect to both work and power, from both the respiratory and cardiac 'pumps'.

Ventilatory costs

The provision of energy at a sufficient rate to support the increased costs incurred by the respiratory muscles during exercise requires increased local vascular perfusion, as well as adequate levels of stored substrates that can be mobilized readily. Without this, respiratory muscle fatigue ensues.

Mechanical costs

The respiratory power (i.e. work rate) generated during the breathing cycle is manifest as the pressure changes which distend the lungs via the chest wall (the elastic component or elastance) and also airflow through the conducting airways (the resistive component or resistance). The third component of the total pulmonary impedance, the accelerative component (or inertance), is often disregarded as it is mostly such a small component of the total. This is because, although the chest wall has a large mass, its acceleration during breathing is low, and although the acceleration of the inspired gas can be high, its mass is low.

During exercise, the respiratory power increases curvilinearly with respect to $\dot{V}_E$, such that a greater increment in power is required to establish a given increase in $\dot{V}_E$ as the work rate increases.[47-52] In moderately fit subjects exercising near maximum, respiratory muscle power has been estimated to be only about 30 per cent of that achieved on a maximal volitional test (i.e. the maximum voluntary ventilation, MVV*).[53] The average in the more recent work of Klas and Dempsey[54] was 40 per cent.

Similarly, the maximum exercise $\dot{V}_E$ is appreciably less than the MVV in such subjects. This difference has been termed the 'breathing reserve' (Fig. 4).[1] As the MVV is largely independent of fitness and training status, a highly fit athlete who is capable of achieving high levels of $\dot{V}_E$ during exercise has a lower breathing reserve than does the less fit subject.

The greater mechanical cost of ventilation at high work rates is predictable on the basis of the increased contributions from turbulence (and even inertia) when air flow is high.[56,57] In addition, there may also be an increased elastic work of breathing, owing to a decreased compliance of the lungs in the tidal range during exercise;[58-61] this effect has been ascribed to the increase in pulmonary blood volume.[61] Other studies, in contrast, have reported no change in compliance,[62,63] or even an increase.[47] However, the progressive increase of end-inspiratory lung volume that occurs as V_T increases during exercise will tend to encroach on the upper, poorly compliant region of the compliance curve;[64] although this effect will be ameliorated by the decrease in end-expiratory lung volume.

It is important to recognize that estimates of the components of respiratory muscle work often fail to take into account several factors that may be important at maximal work rates in élite athletes, i.e. with extremely high levels of $\dot{V}_E$ and high breathing frequencies. For example, there may be considerable distortion of the chest wall

* The $\dot{V}_E$ that may be volitionally attained for periods as short as 15 s.

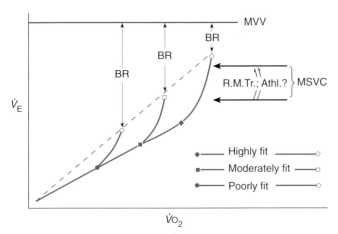

Fig. 4 Schematic representation of the $\dot{V}_E$ response to exhausting incremental exercise as a function of $\dot{V}_{O_2}$ for poorly fit (circles), normal (squares) and highly fit (diamonds) subjects. The $\dot{V}_E$ responses are similar below the lactate threshold (full symbols) regardless of fitness. However, $\dot{V}_E$ at maximum exercise ($\dot{V}_{Emax}$) is progressively higher the greater the maximum $\dot{V}_{O_2}$ (open symbols), and the breathing reserve (BR) therefore becomes reduced (BR = MVV–$\dot{V}_{Emax}$). The MVV is largely independent of fitness and training. However, the maximum sustained ventilatory capacity (MSVC) can be increased by endurance training of the respiratory muscles (R.M.Tr) and is considered to be high in highly fit athletes (Athl.?). (Modified from ref. 55.)

at these high work rates,[65,66] and its inertial contributions to the total impedance may no longer be neglected.[67,68]

Attempts have been made to partition respiratory muscle power to individual muscles of respiration.[69] However, those estimates that are presently available have been obtained during maximal volitional ventilatory manoeuvres; we do not believe that this condition is useful as a mechanical or metabolic analogue of ventilation during muscular exercise.

Metabolic costs

The mechanical costs of ventilation appear to be satisfied, in large part, by the aerobic energy-yielding process in the respiratory muscles. Thus, during exercise, the O_2 consumption of the respiratory muscles ($\dot{V}rm_{O_2}$) increases progressively relative to $\dot{V}_E$. However, the relationship is concave upwards; i.e. a greater increment in $\dot{V}rm_{O_2}$ is required to establish a given increase in $\dot{V}_E$ as work rate increases.[49,54,67,70–77] It is important to point out that estimation of $\dot{V}rm_{O_2}$ in humans is technically quite difficult, owing to its small size relative to whole-body $\dot{V}_{O_2}$.

A further confounding influence is the fact that if $P_{CO_2}a$ is allowed to fall in tests which attempt to mimic the exercise hyperpnoea at rest, then the whole-body $\dot{V}_{O_2}$ is increased by the alkalosis, by about 10 per cent per 10 mmHg reduction in $P_{CO_2}a$.[78] This is large compared with the actual $\dot{V}_{O_2}$ cost of exercise ventilation.

However, while $\dot{V}rm_{O_2}$ is small when $\dot{V}_E$ is at resting levels, it can be a significant factor during near-maximal exercise,[54] especially in highly fit athletes who attain extremely high levels of $\dot{V}_E$. Normal subjects have been reported to attain a $\dot{V}rm_{O_2}$ of some 0.5 l/min for a $\dot{V}_E$ in excess of 120 l/min; i.e. about 14 per cent of the total $\dot{V}_{O_2}$ for a subject with a $\dot{V}_{O_2}$max of 4 l/min. Shephard[76] has reported that, in the $\dot{V}_E$ range of 90 to 130 l/min, $\dot{V}rm_{O_2}$ increases by about 4.4 ml/min per l/min increase of $\dot{V}_E$. In athletes, who attain much higher levels of $\dot{V}_E$ at maximum, $\dot{V}rm_{O_2}$ is presumably even greater.

The vascular perfusion of the respiratory muscles ($\dot{Q}rm$) plays an important supportive role in the generation of $\dot{V}rm_{O_2}$. As arterial O_2 content (Ca_{O_2}) remains essentially stable over the entire work-rate range (however, $P_{O_2}a$, can decrease at high work rates in highly trained athletes,[24] as described below), the increased O_2 delivery to the respiratory muscles necessary to sustain increased levels of $\dot{V}_E$ depends on an appropriate increase in $\dot{Q}rm$.

What is less certain in humans is the exact magnitude of the $\dot{Q}rm$ response during exercise, and how it is partitioned between the contributing muscle groups. Whipp and Pardy[55] have provided an estimate of the $\dot{Q}rm$ response to maximum exercise in moderately fit subjects, using the $\dot{V}rm_{O_2}$ data of Shephard,[76] together with the assumption that the arterio–venous O_2 content difference across the respiratory muscles increases to 15 ml/100 ml at maximum. This yielded a value for $\dot{Q}rm$ at maximum exercise of 3.8 l/min (i.e. $\dot{V}rm_{O_2}$ = 570 ml/min and $\dot{V}_E$ = 130 l/min) or about 15 per cent of a maximal cardiac output of 25 l/min. However, extrapolating to the human respiratory musculature from blood flow measurements in the diaphragm of the dog made by Robertson et al.[79], Bye et al.[80] have suggested that $\dot{Q}rm$ may be as high as 8 l/min and $\dot{V}rm_{O_2}$ in excess of 1 l/min at maximum exercise. Johnson[81] has even argued that the upper limit for sustained operation of the respiratory muscles may be set by the cardiovascular system, through the vascular pressure-flow properties of the respiratory muscles.

These considerations raise the important issue of whether the demands for O_2 utilization by the respiratory muscles during exercise outstrip the ability of vascular supply mechanisms to deliver O_2 at the appropriate rate. Do the respiratory muscles resemble other skeletal muscles in having a demonstrable lactate threshold?

It is known that the duration for which a particular level of $\dot{V}_E$ may be sustained bears an inverse curvilinear relationship to $\dot{V}_E$ during voluntary hyperpnoea. We may infer that such a relationship also holds for the hyperpnoea of muscular exercise.[77,82] However, while this relationship may be qualitatively similar, there may be significant quantitative differences, both with regard to the actual mechanical cost of achieving a given level of $\dot{V}_E$ (i.e. the respiratory muscle recruitment pattern and mechanical efficiencies are likely to be different) and the metabolic cost of the $\dot{V}_E$ which is attained.

The actual response, however, resembles the hyperbolic whole-body power-duration relationship described earlier (Fig. 3) (eqns 6 and 7). Whether the $\dot{V}_E$–duration relationship is also well described by a hyperbolic function and whether it provides a reasonably accurate representation of the relationship that actually occurs during high intensity exercise has not yet been established.

In the context of the $\dot{V}_E$–duration relationship, the MVV constitutes an upper limit for exercise ventilation.* An index of respiratory muscle endurance is provided by the horizontal $\dot{V}_E$ asymptote—the 'maximum sustained ventilatory capacity' (MSVC),[77,83] which may be usefully regarded as the highest level of ventilation which can be sustained for 'long periods'. As a corollary, respiratory muscle fatigue is considered to develop when $\dot{V}_E$ exceeds MSVC.[84,85] In moderately fit individuals, the MSVC lies in the range of 55 to 80 per cent of the MVV;[77,82,86–89] however, in highly fit athletes, it may be as much as 90 per cent of MVV.[90]

---

* This is based on the unlikely assumption that the respiratory muscles operate during the MVV manoeuvre in the same manner as for the spontaneous breathing of exercise (i.e. with respect to recruitment pattern, mechanical cost, and efficiency of contraction) and that there is no exercise-induced bronchodilatation or bronchoconstriction

It is tempting to speculate that the MSVC represents the highest $\dot{V}_E$ that can be sustained without a sustained and progressive metabolic acidosis of the respiratory muscles; i.e. analogous to the fatigue threshold or critical power for whole-body exercise. Furthermore, the actual characterization of the $\dot{V}_E$–duration relationship has not been well described in elite athletes, who are likely to have highly trained respiratory musculature. There is a special paucity of information on athletes such as swimmers and rowers, in whom the demands of the performance impose a mechanical imperative on the pattern of breathing.

Both $\dot{V}rmo_2$ and respiratory muscle endurance increase in normal individuals after specific respiratory muscle endurance training.[77,80] Whether this increased $\dot{V}rmo_2$ was the result of an increased $\dot{Q}rm$, an improved O_2 extraction, or both is not known. Also, it is not known whether the regional 'matching' of $\dot{Q}rm$ to local metabolic rate is optimized to any extent by training strategies.

Perfusion costs

In contrast with the respiratory muscles, cardiac power and cardiac output appear to be essentially linearly related throughout the entire work-rate range.[81]

Cardiac muscle power has been estimated to be about 30 times greater than the respiratory muscle power in normal subjects at rest.[81] However, at maximum exercise, the respiratory muscle power may be as much as three times greater than the cardiac power.[81] In fact, the actual difference at maximum exercise may be more marked than this, as no respiratory compensation for the metabolic acidosis was included in the $\dot{V}_E$ response profile. Respiratory muscle power may therefore have been underestimated both absolutely and relative to the cardiac power at the higher work rates attainable in the athlete (see above).

These observations on the relative costs of ventilatory and cardiac pump function support the contention that although the myocardial O_2 consumption increases with increases in cardiac output, it is likely to be a trivially small component of the total,[81,91] even at the high maximal cardiac outputs that can be achieved by some highly fit athletes.

Constraints and limitations on respiratory system performance

The oxygen transport and utilization system has been characterized as a series of linear conductances representing the convective flow of air into the lung, the diffusional exchange into the pulmonary capillary blood, the convectional flow of oxygen to the contracting muscle units, and the final diffusive flux of oxygen to the mitochondrion to serve as the terminal oxidant in the electron transport chain.

While the role of the muscular and cardiovascular components of this transfer in limiting exercise has been the focus of considerable research (see ref. 92 for a review of the proposed site(s) of limitation and an analysis of the competing arguments), the lung itself has recently been considered a potential site of constraint or limitation in highly trained athletes as a result of the high flow requirements for each of the pulmonary fluids—air and blood.

In the context of the respiratory system, constraint refers to a condition in which the achieved ventilatory response is lower than the required response, owing to the influence of an opposing mechanism, despite the system not being limited from further increases in $\dot{V}_E$; e.g. the presence of applied resistive loads.

In contrast, limitation refers to situations in which the variable is actually prevented from increasing, despite an increased ventilatory requirement. For example, reduced lung recoil and/or increased airways resistance limits the maximum expiratory air-flow attainable during exercise (at a particular lung volume) despite further increases in ventilatory drive; increased elastance (i.e. reduced compliance) in patients with diffuse interstitial fibrosis limits the achievable tidal volume during exercise.

Ventilatory constraints

The operating limit for tidal volume (V_T) in humans ranges from zero to vital capacity. The breathing frequency can range from zero to about 5 to 7 Hz,[93] with the upper limit being set by the rate at which the neuromuscular apparatus can generate rapid alternating movements.[68,93] In moderately fit individuals, however, the ventilatory pump during maximum exercise typically operates at a frequency of no more than 1 Hz and a V_T of only about 50 to 60 per cent of the vital capacity. As the maximum V_T attained during exercise does not increase appreciably as a result of physical training or increased fitness, further increases in $\dot{V}_E$ must be accomplished through breathing frequency.

One source of mechanical constraint of ventilation during exercise arises from the limitations imposed on expiratory airflow by the determinants of the maximum expiratory flow-volume (MEFV) curve (i.e. the expiratory flow-volume that results from a forced volitional manoeuvre). In moderately fit subjects, ventilation at maximum exercise, and the flow profiles with which it is accomplished, appear to fall well below the maxima of the MEFV curve.[60,61,94,95] However, when high levels of $\dot{V}_E$ are attained (as would be the case for the highly fit athlete), these maxima may be encroached upon.[54,95-98] In older athletic subjects, in whom lung recoil is reduced, this can occur at appreciably lower metabolic rates.[98] Consequently the genetic make-up of the athlete, in terms of airway dimensions and lung recoil, can play a decisive role in whether the airflow demands can be met without flow limitation over a part of the expirate. A further complicating factor is that, following prolonged muscular efforts (marathon and ultra marathon events), there are reports of reductions in respiratory muscle strength and endurance, and also the vital capacity.

A second consideration relates to the respiratory muscle work that is expended in sustaining a particular level of $\dot{V}_E$ with a particular V_T–frequency combination. In 1925, Rohrer[56] argued that any particular level of $\dot{V}_E$ would have an associated breathing frequency at which a minimal level of respiratory work would, in theory, be exacted. For example, were a given level of $\dot{V}_E$ to be generated with a high frequency (and therefore a low V_T), this would increase the flow-resistive component of the respiratory work. In contrast, when the same level of $\dot{V}_E$ is accomplished with a large V_T and therefore a very low breathing frequency, this results in an increased contribution from the elastic component of the respiratory work,[75,97] if the lung volume encroaches on the flatter portion of the lung compliance curve.

Ventilatory limitations

Mechanical

Several observations support the view that, in moderately fit indi-viduals, ventilation is neither mechanically limited nor associated with respiratory muscle fatigue during maximal exercise:

(1) such subjects can increase $\dot{V}_E$ substantially above the spontaneous maximal value at maximum exercise by volitional means;

(2) inspiratory muscle fatigue cannot be demonstrated in such subjects at high work rates;[99]

(3) the ratio of maximum exercise $\dot{V}_E$ to MVV is relatively low (i.e. about 60 to 70 per cent);[96,100-102] and

(4) the spontaneous expiratory $F–V$ curve at high work rates does not encroach on the boundaries of the MEFV curve.[60,61,94]

In contrast, evidence of both ventilatory mechanical limitation and inspiratory muscle fatigue may emerge in subjects who are more fit. For example, in subjects with a $\dot{V}_{O2}$max of about 5 to 6 litre/min and a maximum exercise $\dot{V}_E$ of about 110 to 160 litre/min (i.e. some 80 per cent of MVV), Hesser *et al.*[53] reported that the spontaneous expiratory $F–V$ curve impacted on the outer envelope of the MEFV curve during maximal exercise. Similar findings have been reported by Olafsson and Hyatt,[60] Grimby *et al.*,[96] Johnson,[81] and Klas and Dempsey[54] (Fig. 5). It appears, however, that such subjects only generate sufficient pleural pressures to establish the maximum flow.[54,59,96] In contrast, subjects generate appreciably greater (and 'wasteful') pressures during MVV manoeuvres.[54] Furthermore, Bye *et al.*[80] have demonstrated evidence of diaphragmatic fatigue both in terms of electromyographic criteria and also as a result of reduced maximum transdiaphragmatic pressures after exhausting exercise.

However, one should be cautious about using the resting MEFV curve, and even the resting MVV, as the frame of reference for deciding whether there is airflow limitation during exercise. The reasons for this are as follows.

• Locating the spontaneous expiratory $F–V$ curve on the MEFV curve is crucial. It is often assumed that the subject's total lung capacity does not change. It is better to 'trap' an $F–V$ display oscillographically on a particular breath and then have a MEFV manoeuvre performed immediately thereafter, ensuring that the subject really goes to the extremes of thoracic excursion on the manoeuvre.

• Some bronchodilatation can result during exercise from the increased circulating levels of catecholamines—this presumably accounts for the increased MVV that has been reported during exercise.

• In many subjects, the maximum expiratory effort $F–V$ manoeuvre does not yield the optimum maximum expiratory flow $F–V$ curve, although this is more likely to be a factor in older athletes with diminished lung recoil and airways function than in healthy young athletes.

There is also now a consistent body of evidence which demon-strates that, when helium is used to replace nitrogen in the inspirate at high work rates, $\dot{V}_E$ abruptly increases with consequent hypo-

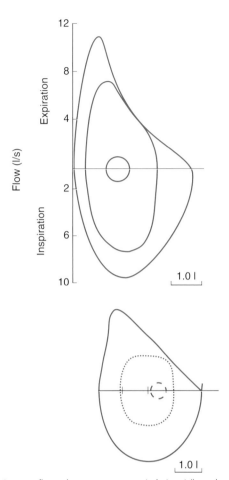

Fig. 5 Spontaneous flow–volume curves generated at rest (inner loop) and max-imal exercise (middle loop) in a fit subject (upper panel) and a normal untrained subject (lower panel) compared with their maximum flow–volume curves (outer loop). See text for discussion. (Modified from ref. 54 and from ref. 93.)

capnia,[103-105] even when care is taken to mask the sudden sensation of cold in the airways associated with helium breathing.[104] As helium is about 39 per cent less dense than nitrogen, it is thought that the turbulent component of airflow resistance is reduced when helium is breathed. It appears, therefore, that there is normally a component of airflow constraint at high work rates. This will pre-sumably be appreciable in elite athletes who attain high levels of $\dot{V}_E$. However, as airway dimensions play an important role in the onset and magnitude of the airflow turbulence, lung structure will also be important.

It should be noted that reduction of the vital capacity and respiratory muscle strength and endurance have only been demon-strated consistently in athletes following prolonged exer-cise.[102,106,107]

Consequently, at high work rates an athlete is confronted with a control dilemma: if $\dot{V}_E$ is increased further to provide respiratory compensation for the metabolic acidosis (i.e. to constrain the pH fall in blood and exercising muscle), the additional $\dot{V}_E$ necessary can be so large (as described above) it is likely to induce ventilatory mech-anical limitation and possibly ventilatory muscle fatigue.[108] How-ever, the absence of this additional $\dot{V}_E$, although tending to protect the subject from pulmonary mechanical limitation, predisposes both to arterial hypoxaemia and also a more precipitous fall in blood and muscle pH which impairs contractile responses[109] and exacerbates intramuscular fatigue.

Metabolic

The respiratory muscles may also reach their metabolic limits during maximum exercise in highly fit athletes. This reflects not only that $\dot{V}_E$ at maximum exercise is high in such subjects, but also that the relationship between $\dot{V}r m_{O_2}$ and $\dot{V}_E$ becomes steeper in this $\dot{V}_E$ range.[49,67,70,71-76,83,110] Thus, a greater component of the systemic O_2 supply is diverted away from the musculature of the exercising limb at high levels of $\dot{V}_E$.

This raises the notion of a theoretical limiting (or maximal) level of $\dot{V}_E$, above which the O_2 requirement of the respiratory muscles becomes sufficiently large that it requires all of the subsequent increase in whole-body $\dot{V}_{O_2}$ to sustain this high rate of ventilation. This has been estimated by several investigators to lie in the range 120 to 160 l/min,[48,67,76] i.e. levels of $\dot{V}_E$ which are not uncommon in elite athletes. Should the energetic requirements of the musculature of the exercising limbs be preferentially met, then the muscles of respiration would be predisposed towards fatigue. Conversely, if the requirements of the respiratory muscles are to be met, the limb muscles would be predisposed to premature fatigue. In reality, the cardiovascular control system presumably treats the respiratory muscles during exercise as for other skeletal muscles with increased flow requirements, partitioning the flow in proportion to the magnitude of the metabolic demands.

Perfusion-related limitation

It is important to understand not only why some athletes do not become hypoxaemic at high work rates, but also why there is not a systematic hyperoxaemia. End-tidal, mean alveolar, and 'ideal' alveolar P_{O_2} increase systematically above θ_L; arterial P_{O_2} does not! Consequently, the alveolar (ideal)–arterial P_{O_2} difference ($[A–a]O_2$) increases further, reaching 20 to 30 mmHg at high work rates.

At sea level, moderately fit individuals maintain arterial P_{O_2} and O_2 saturation at, or close to, resting values even during exhausting work rates.[111-113] As the topographic distribution of $\dot{V}_A$ and $\dot{Q}$ has been shown to improve during upright exercise,[114-116] it has been assumed that the distribution of alveolar ventilation-to-perfusion ($\dot{V}_A/\dot{Q}$) within the lung was also improved and hence that the lung exchanged gas more efficiently during exercise than at rest.

However, this notion has been brought into question, as a result of recent investigations utilizing the multiple inert gas technique of Wagner et al.[117] For example, Gledhill et al.[113] have demonstrated that the mean $\dot{V}_A/\dot{Q}$ for the entire lung increased during steady-state exercise. This must occur, because:

$$\dot{V}_A.(F_{O_2}I - F_{O_2}A) \Leftarrow \dot{V}_{O_2} \Rightarrow \dot{Q}(C_{O_2}a - C_{O_2}\bar{v})$$

and therefore:

$$\frac{\dot{V}_A}{\dot{Q}} = \frac{C_{O_2}a - C_{O_2}\bar{v}}{F_{O_2}I - F_{O_2}A} \quad (9)$$

(For simplicity, we have disregarded the effect of the different inspired and expired tidal volumes which occurs when $R \neq 1$, as it does not materially affect the argument.) $C_{O_2}\bar{v}$ decreases systematically with increasing work rate in this range, whereas $F_{O_2}A$ remains relatively constant; therefore $\dot{V}_A/\dot{Q}$ increases. In contrast, however,

the $\dot{V}_A/\dot{Q}$ dispersion within the lung was reported to be increased and to constitute a major influence on the widening of the $[A–a]O_2$ that is normally seen during moderate and heavy exercise. Likewise, Hammond et al.[118] demonstrated increased $\dot{V}_A/\dot{Q}$ inequality at high work rates (i.e. $\dot{V}_{O_2} > 3$ l/min). However, they argued that this could not entirely account for the widened $[A–a]O_2$. The mechanisms of the gas-exchange 'impairment' implicit in the wider dispersion of $\dot{V}_A/\dot{Q}$ at high work rates remain to be elucidated.

In contrast, at more moderate work rates ($\dot{V}_{O_2}$ less than about 2 litre/min), Derks[119] reported the $\dot{Q}$ distribution to be unchanged (or even narrowed). Furthermore, neither Hammond et al.[118] nor Gale et al.[120] were able to detect statistically significant changes in $\dot{V}_A/\dot{Q}$ dispersion.

The work of Hammond et al.[118] and Dempsey et al.[24] coupled with the earlier work of Johnson et al.,[121] implicates diffusion impairment as a contributor to the widened $[A–a]O_2$, at least for very high work rates. Based upon the demonstration that $P_{O_2}a$ fell at such work rates in highly fit subjects, Dempsey et al.[24] have suggested that a diffusion impairment could arise from a pulmonary capillary transit time that was too short (owing to the high pulmonary blood flow) to allow diffusion equilibrium to be attained throughout the lung. The observations of Hammond et al.[118] cohere with this view. Neither the increased dispersion of $\dot{V}_A/\dot{Q}$ nor the increased post-pulmonary shunt that these investigators demonstrated in highly fit subjects (exercising in 'the steady state' at 300 W) were sufficiently large to entirely account for the widening of the $[A–a]O_2$ at this high work rate.

Whether there is equilibrium of pulmonary end-capillary P_{O_2} with the alveolar P_{O_2} depends both on the rate at which P_{O_2} rises in the capillary bed (i.e. its time constant) and the time available for exchange. As the diffusing capacity for O_2 ($D_{O_2}l$) is a crucial determinant of the time constant, a large $D_{O_2}l$ is vital in preventing arterial hypoxaemia, in addition to a long residence time in the pulmonary capillary bed. (The reader is referred to refs 121 and 122 for a more comprehensive consideration of limitations of diffusive gas exchange during exercise).

Normally, approximately 0.3 s is required for the P_{O_2} (and hence haemoglobin saturation) of the blood traversing the pulmonary capillary bed to increase to its equilibrium with the alveolar gas; this will be longer during exercise, however, especially in trained athletes.[24,81,122]). Therefore, if the flow through the capillary bed is sufficiently great, the blood will leave the gas exchanging region and pass into the pulmonary veins before equilibrium occurs: hypoxaemia is the inevitable consequence.

Whether or not there is sufficient residence time in the pulmonary capillary bed depends both on the capillary volume (V_c) and the pulmonary blood flow ($\dot{Q}$); i.e.

$$T_{tr} = \frac{V_c \text{ (ml)}}{\dot{Q} \text{ (ml/s)}} \quad (10)$$

where T_{tr} is the mean transit time.

Therefore, to prevent critical reductions of the pulmonary capillary residence time, the athlete must recruit capillary volume as the capillary flow increases. However, there is a morphological limit to the capillary dimension.[123]

The relationship between T_{tr} and V_c is presented in Fig. 6. It should be noted, were there to be no increase in the resting V_c of about 80 ml, then the critical transit time of 0.3 s would be achieved at a $\dot{V}O_2$ of only 2 l/min. Doubling the capillary volume to 160 ml would lead to the critical transit time occurring at a $\dot{V}O_2$ of 'only' 5 l/min. At a $\dot{V}O_2$ of 7 l/min, this occurs even if the capillary bed has expanded to 200 ml. The broken line in the left panel reflects the increase in the time necessary for equilibrium as work rate increases.[24,81,122] However, this relationship is presently uncertain at high work rates and hence this line should only be considered an approximation, but one that is notionally important for the mechanism.

It should further be recognized that there is a distribution of both pulmonary capillary length and diameter, and therefore probably a similar distribution of transit time. As transit times longer than the critical do not further increase oxygenation but the shorter ones do reduce it further, then the actual hypoxaemia-inducing effect will begin to be manifest at work rates less than suggested by the mean transit time consideration.

A useful rule of thumb to determine the minimum pulmonary capillary volume (ml) that will maintain the mean transit time at 0.3 s is to multiply the cardiac output (l/min) by 5 (for a mean transit time of 0.6 s, the multiplier is 10) i.e.

$$V_c(T_{tr} \, 0.3) = 5 \times \dot{Q} \qquad \text{or} \qquad V_c(T_{tr} \, 0.6) = 10 \times \dot{Q}$$

The ability of the élite athlete to perform intense exercise without developing arterial hypoxaemia depends critically on such factors, in order to minimize or obviate the development of diffusion impairment[122] which provides additional stress on already taxed mechanisms of tissue energy provision and ventilatory control and which can therefore limit exercise performance. This is supported by the fact that when the hypoxaemia was prevented by increasing the inhaled O_2 fraction to maintain resting levels of PO_2a, exercise tolerance increased significantly.[124]

Consideration of Fig. 7 raises the question of why all subjects exercising at high levels of pulmonary blood flow do not develop arterial hypoxaemia. The answer is likely to reside in the fact that

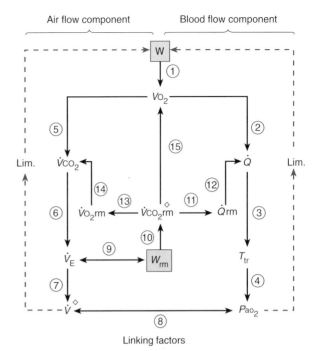

1. Work efficiency
2. Tissue O_2 extraction
3. Pulmonary capillary blood volume
4. Pulmonary capillary transit time dispersion
5. Respiratory exchange ratio (metabolic and buffering components)
6. Arterial pCO_2
7. Pulmonary mechanics; breathing pattern
8. Carotid chemoreceptor stimulation
9. Respiratory muscle mechanical efficiency
10. Respiratory muscle work efficiency
11. Respiratory muscle O_2 extraction
12. Respiratory muscle fractional utilization of $\dot{Q}$
13. Respiratory muscle respiratory quotient
14. Respiratory muscle fractional contribution to $\dot{V}CO_2$
15. Respiratory muscle fractional utilization of $\dot{V}O_2$

Fig. 7 Schematic representation of the stress cascade predisposing to pulmonary limitation (i.e. airflow limitation, respiratory muscle fatigue, and arterial hypoxaemia) during exercise. The full arrows connect the links in the cascade and the broken lines indicate limiting (Lim.) feedback influences on work rate. Full diamonds indicate points at which a large-value potential for the particular variable is crucial to minimize the likelihood of limitation. See text for discussion.

the genetic make-up of some athletes leads to development of a large-volume pulmonary capillary bed. Consequently, it is likely that for future record performances in athletic events, it will no longer be sufficient to be 'élite' in the metabolic and cardiovascular capabilities, but also in terms of pulmonary capabilities.

This is likely to be dominated by hereditary factors, as physical training does not systematically improve these indices of pulmonary function. However, it should be pointed out that this concept is based on studies in adults; i.e. when the lung is mature. Whether these adult dimensions can be improved by training during the period of lung growth remains to be determined.

A further potential concern for the elite athlete is that the high pulmonary vascular pressures during exercise[125] predispose to increased pulmonary interstitial oedema. Whether or not there is net fluid flux ($\dot{J}$) across the alveolar–capillary membrane during exercise will depend upon the difference between the hydrostatic pressure tending to 'push' water out of the vascular bed and the

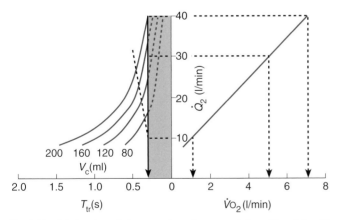

Fig. 6 The right-hand panel shows a schematic representation of the relationship between cardiac output ($\dot{Q}$) and $\dot{V}O_2$. The left-hand panel shows a schematic representation of the relationship between cardiac output ($\dot{Q}$) and the mean pulmonary capillary transit time (T_{tr}), with superimposed isopleths for pulmonary capillary blood volume (V_c). The full vertical line indicates a critical transit time of 0.3 s. The dotted line reflects the increase in the time necessary for diffusion equilibrium at higher work rates. See text for discussion.

osmotic pressure tending to 'pull' it back. These forces may be quantified with respect to the Starling equation; i.e.

$$\mathcal{J} = K(P_c - P_i) - K\sigma(\pi_c - \pi_i) \tag{11}$$

where K is the filtration coefficient, P_c and π_c are, respectively, the vascular hydrostatic and colloid osmotic pressures in the capillary, and P_i and π_i are these pressures in the pulmonary interstitial (i.e. perimicrovascular) space. The term σ is the 'reflection coefficient', which is an index of the degree of the membrane impermeability to protein.

Not surprisingly, perhaps, the behaviour during exercise of many of the variables in the Starling equation is poorly understood. However, while transpulmonary microvascular pressure and the area of the perfused surface both increase during exercise, there is no evidence of impaired capillary permeability.

O'Brodovich and Coates[126] cite three safety mechanisms that prevent pulmonary oedema: (i) increased lung lymph flow, (ii) fluid movement into the interstitial space that will dilute its protein concentration and hence lower its osmotic pressure, and (iii) the low compliance of the interstitial space which will lead to a large increase in perimicrovascular pressure for a small change in volume. Mechanisms (i) and (ii) occur even with mild exercise, and (iii) becomes operative if oedema occurs. Based upon a careful analysis of the available evidence, O'Brodovich and Coates,[126] and also Brower and Permutt,[127] have concluded that these safety mechanisms are adequate in normal humans to prevent the development of pulmonary oedema. Furthermore, the evidence suggesting the development of interstitial oedema during severe exercise is not only indirect, but inconclusive. However, it is important to establish conclusively whether or not this occurs in highly trained athletes, because the presence of such oedema during severe exercise would predispose the athlete to: (i) reduced gas exchange efficiency and hypoxaemia, and (ii) pulmonary 'J'-receptor stimulation with its attendant tachypnoea and possibly increased respiratory sensation and even decreased exercise tolerance through inhibition of spinal motor neurones.[128]

It has been demonstrated that pulmonary artery pressures can increase to values in excess of 40 mmHg in healthy young subjects, with pulmonary wedge pressures of 25 to 30 mmHg.[125] Similarly high pulmonary vascular pressures have been observed in older, but healthy, subjects at appreciably lower levels of cardiac output.[125] This predisposes not only to increased pulmonary interstitial oedema, but also to potential structural damage to the extremely thin alveolar–capillary interface.[129]

The safety mechanisms cited by O'Brodovich and Coates[126] (see above) appear adequate in preventing the development of pulmonary oedema in normal subjects.[126,127] However, whether or not pulmonary interstitial oedema (and even regional alveolar flooding) develops during severe exercise in highly trained athletes needs to be determined conclusively (case reports are suggestive, however). Were such oedema to occur, it would compromise exercise performance in the affected athlete, because of further hypoxaemia and the consequences of 'J'-receptor stimulation (see above).[128]

West and his associates[130] have spearheaded investigations of stress failure of the fine-structured pulmonary capillaries at the high levels of capillary pressure which are associated with high intensity exercise. They demonstrated that, in contrast to sedentary controls, short-term, high intensity muscular exercise in élite cyclists led to significantly increased concentrations of red blood cells, total protein, and leukotriene B4 in broncho-alveolar lavage fluid. They concluded that this was likely to be a consequence of mechanical stress failure rather than being a primary inflammatory response, as they could demonstrate no difference between the exercising control group and the élite cyclists for tumour necrosis factor bioactivity, lipopolysaccharide or interleukin 8. In more recent studies, however, these investigators have been unable to demonstrate increased levels of red blood cells or leukotriene B4 in the broncho-alveolar fluids of such élite cyclists who had exercised for 1 h at 80 per cent of $\dot{V}_{O_2}$max. Therefore, stress-related failure of the pulmonary blood–gas interface in élite athletes, when it occurs, may only result from supramaximal efforts.

Conclusion

As data on the performance of the pulmonary system during competition, or even mock competitive conditions, are sparse, this chapter has focused on the pulmonary consequences of high and sustained metabolic rate. Our considerations are therefore based almost entirely on experiments performed in the laboratory. Space constraints also precluded consideration of the young and maturing athlete, the effects of ageing on pulmonary performance limits, or of environmental stressors.

The influence of preparatory breathing responses for certain events (e.g. the deep inspiration followed by explosive expiration used prior to high power events such as shot-putting, sprinting, and weightlifting) on the subsequent pattern of response is largely unknown, as is the influence of deliberately chosen modifications of the spontaneous breathing control. An example of this is the 'breath-play' method,[131] which has been suggested for athletes. This proposes what is termed 'upside-down' breathing, which demands active expiration with (attempts at) passive inhalation. Clearly, the control of blood-gas and acid–base status during actual competition, especially when it involves such peculiar modifications of normal control, awaits exploration.

What is clear is that pulmonary function is likely to be an important determinant of success in a wide range of athletic performance. Genetics will naturally play a predominant role in determining the extent to which the capacity of the pulmonary system will be sufficient to allow the athlete's full metabolic potential to be expressed; i.e. as shown schematically in Fig. 7. In this figure, we show potential pulmonary limitations to sustaining the required work rate. The solid lines connect the links in the stress cascade which can lead to airflow limitation, respiratory muscle fatigue, and also arterial hypoxaemia. The broken lines demonstrate the limiting feedback on the work rate. The open diamonds represent points at which a large-value potential for the particular variable is crucial for minimizing the likelihood of limitation. It should be noted, in our terminology, that the maximum metabolic rate of the task-performing muscles would be constrained by the pulmonary limitations, i.e. the systemic $\dot{V}_{O_2}$ has the potential to increase further under these conditions.

To what extent training focused on the pulmonary system, especially during the period of lung growth, will be capable of extending the pulmonary limits, or even decrease the rate of their deterioration with age, will probably prove to be a topic of not inconsiderable interest for future record-breaking performances.

References

1. Wasserman K, Hansen JE, Sue DY, Whipp BJ. *Principles of exercise testing and interpretation*. Philadelphia: Lea and Febiger, 1987.

2. Linnarsson D. Dynamics of pulmonary gas exchange and heart rate changes at start and end of exercise. *Acta Physiologica Scandinavica*. 1994; 415(Suppl.): 1–68.

3. Casaburi R, Whipp BJ, Wasserman K, Beaver WL Koyal SN. Ventilatory and gas exchange dynamics in response to sinusoidal work. *Journal of Applied Physiology*, 1977; **42**: 300–11.

4. Whipp BJ. The control of the exercise hyperpnea. In: Horbein T, ed. *The regulation of breathing*, Part II. New York: Marcel Dekker, 1981; 1069–139.

5. Hughson, RL Morrissey M. Delayed kinetics of respiratory gas exchange in the transition from prior exercise. *Journal of Applied Physiology* 1982; **52**: 921–9.

6. Griffiths, TG Henson, LC Whipp, BJ. Influence of inspired oxygen concentration on the dynamics of the exercise hyperpnoea. *Journal of Physiology (London)* 1986; **380**: 387–407.

7. Hagberg, JM Hickson, RC Ehsani, AA Holloszy, JO. Faster adjustment to and from recovery from submaximal exercise in the trained state. *Journal of Applied Physiology*. 1980; **48**: 218–4.

8. Herxheimer, H Kost, R. Das Verhaltnis von Sauerstoffauf-nahme and kohlensaurausscheidung zur Ventilation bei harter Muskelarbeit. *Zeitschrift für klinische Medizin*. 1932; **108**: 240–7.

9. Wasserman, K VanKessel, AL Burton, GC. Interaction of physiological mechanisms during exercise. *Journal of Applied Physiology*. 1967; **22**: 71–85.

10. Roston, WL Whipp, BJ Davis, JA Effros, RM Wasserman, K. Oxygen uptake kinetics and lactate concentration during exercise in man. *American Review of Respiratory Diseases* 1987; **135**:1080–4.

11. Poole, DC Ward, SA Gardner, GW Whipp, BJ. Metabolic and respiratory profile of the upper limit for prolonged exercise in man. *Ergonomics* 1988; **31**: 1265–79.

12. Whipp, BJ. Dynamics of pulmonary gas exchange. *Circulation* 1987; **76**:VI-18–28.

13. Henson, LC Poole, DC Whipp, BJ. Fitness as a determinant of oxygen uptake response to constant-load exercise. *European Journal of Applied Physiology* 1989; **59**: 21–28.

14. Moritani, T Nagata, A deVries, HA. Muro, M. Critical power as a measure of physical work capacity and anaerobic threshold. *Ergonomics* 1981; **24**: 339–50.

15. Hughson, RL, Orok, CJ Staudt, LE. A high velocity treadmill running test to assess endurance running potential. *International Journal of Sports Medicine* 1984; **5**: 23–5.

16. Rahn, H. A concept of mean alveolar air and the ventilation––bloodflow relationships during pulmonary gas exchange. *American Journal of Physiology* 1949; **158**: 21–30.

17. Riley, R.L., and A. Cournand. 'Ideal' alveolar air and the analysis of ventilation–perfusion relationships in the lung. *Journal of Applied Physiology* 1949; **1**: 825–47.

18. Rahn, H., and W.O. Fenn. *A graphical analysis of the respiratory gas exchange. The O2–CO2 diagram*. 1955; Washington, DC: American Physiology Society.

19. Sutton, J Jones, NL Towes, CJ. Growth hormone secretion in acid–base alterations at rest and during exercise. *Clinical Science and Molecular Medicine* 1976; **50**: 241–7.

20. Wasserman, K Whipp, BJ Koyal, SN Cleary, MG. Effect of carotid body resection on ventilatory and acid–base control during exercise. *Journal of Applied Physiology*. 1975; **39**: 354–8.

21. Dejours, P. Control of respiration in muscular exercise. In: Fenn WO, Rahn H. eds. *Handbook of physiology. Respiration*, Vol. 1. Washington DC: American Physiological Society 1964; 631–648.

22. Cunningham, DJC. Integrative aspects of the regulation of breathing; a personal view. In: Widdicombe JG, ed. MTP *International Reviews of Science. Physiology*. Series 1. Vol 2. *Respiration*. Baltimore: University Park Press, 1974; 303–69.

23. Linton, RAF Band, DM. The effect of potassium on carotid chemoreceptor activity and ventilation in the cat. *Respiratory Physiology*. 1985; **59**: 65–70.

24. Dempsey, JA. Hanson, P. Henderson, K. Exercise-induced alveolar hypoxemia in healthy human subjects at sea level. *Journal of Physiology (London)* 1984; **355**: 161–75.

25. Wasserman, K. McIlroy, MB. Detecting the threshold of anaerobic metabolism. *American Journal of Cardiology* 1964; **14**: 844–52.

26. Wasserman, K. Whipp, BJ. Koyal, SN Beaver, WL. Anaerobic threshold and respiratory gas exchange during exercise. *Journal of Applied Physiology* 1973; **35**: 236–43.

27. Reinhard, U. Muller, PH. Schmullingm, R.-M. Determination of anaerobic threshold by the ventilation equivalent in normal individuals. *Respiration* 1979; **38**: 36–42.

28. Stegmann, H Kindermann, W Schnabel, A. Lactate kinetics and individual anaerobic threshhold. *International Journal of Sports Medicine* 1981; **2**: 160–5.

29. Whipp, BJ Ward, SA Wasserman. K. Respiratory markers of the anaerobic threshold. *Advances in Cardiology* 1986; **35**: 47–64.

30. Wasserman, K Beaver, WL Davis, JA Pu, JZ Heber, Whipp, DBJ. Lactate, pyruvate and lactate-to-pyruvate ratio during exercise and recovery. *Journal of Applied Physiology* 1985; **59**: 935–40.

31. Beaver, WL Wasserman, K Whipp, BJ. Improved detection of the lactate threshold during exercise using a log–log transformation. *Journal of Applied Physiology* 1986; **59**: 1936–40.

32. Wasserman, K Whipp, BJ. Exercise physiology in health and disease. *American Review of Respiratory Diseases* 1975; **112**: 219–49.

33. Wasserman, K Whipp, BJ Casaburi, R Beaver, WL Brown, HV. CO₂ flow to the lungs and ventilatory control. In: Dempsey JA, Reed CE, eds. *Muscular exercise and the lung* Madison: University of Wisconsin Press, 1977; 103–35.

34. Whipp, BJ Davis, JA Wasserman, K. Ventilatory control of the 'isocapnic buffering' region in rapidly-incremental exercise. *Respiratory Physiology* 1989; **76**: 357–68.

35. Beaver, WL Wasserman, K Whipp, BJ. A new method for detecting the anaerobic threshold by gas exchange. *Journal of Applied Physiology* 1986; **60**: 2020–27.

36. Douglas, CG. Co-ordination of the respiration and circulation with variations in bodily activity. *Lancet* **ii** 1927; 213–18.

37. Beaver, WL Wasserman, K Whipp, BJ. Bicarbonate buffering of lactic acid generated during exercise. *Journal of Applied Physiology* 1986; **60**: 472–8.

38. Keul, J Doll, E Keppler, D. *Oxidative energy metabolism of human muscle*. Baltimore: University Park Press, 1972.

39. Jones, NL. Acid-base physiology. In: Crystal RG, West JB, eds. *The lung: scientific foundations*. New York: Raven Press, 1991: 1251–65.

40. Whipp, BJ Mahler, M. Dynamics of gas exchange during exercise In: *Pulmonary Gas Exchange*, Vol. II. West, JB, ed. New York: Academic Press, 1980; 33–96.

41. Wasserman, K Beaver, WL Whipp, BJ. Gas exchange theory and the lactic acidosis (anaerobic) threshold. *Circulation* 1990; **81** (Suppl). II: 14–30.

42. Ward, SA Whipp, BJ. Influence of body CO₂ stores on ventilatory-metabolic coupling during exercise. In: Honda Y, Miyamoto Y, Konno K, Widdicombe JG. eds. *Control of breathing and its modeling perspective*. New York: Plenum Press, 1992: 425–31.

43. Poole, D.P., S.A. Ward, and B.J. Whipp. Effect of training on the metabolic and respiratory profile of heavy and severe exercise. *European Journal Applied Physiology* 1990; **59**: 421–9.

44. Whipp, BJ Ward, SA. Ventilatory control dynamics during muscular exercise in man. *International Journal of Sports Medicine* 1980; **1**: 146–59.

45. Weil, JV Swanson, GD. Peripheral chemoreceptors and the control of breathing. In: Whipp BJ, Wasserman K, eds. *Exercise: pulmonary physiology and pathophysiology. Lung Biology in Health and Disease*, Vol. 52. New York: Dekker, 1991: 371–403.

46. Ohyabu, Y Honda, Y. Exercise and ventilatory chemosensitivities. *Annals of Physiology and Anthropology* 1990; **9**: 117–21.

47. McIlroy, MR Marshall, R Christie, RV. The work of breathing in normal subjects. *Clinical Science* 1954; **13**: 127–36.

48. Margaria, RG Milic-Emili, G Petit, JM. Cavagna, G. Mechanical work of breathing during muscular exercise. *Journal of Applied Physiology* 1960; **15**: 354–8.

49. McGregor, M Becklake, MR. The relationship of oxygen cost of breathing to respiratory mechanical work and respiratory force. *Journal of Clinical Investigation* 1961; **40**: 971–80.

50. Milic-Emili, G Petit, JM Deroanne, R. Mechanical work of breathing during exercise in trained and untrained subjects. *Journal of Applied Physiology* 1962; **17**: 43–6.

51. Thoden, JS. *et al.* Ventilatory work during steady-state response to exercise. *Federal Proceedings* 1969; **28**: 1316–21.

52. Holmgren, A. Herzog, P. Astrom, H. Work of breathing during exercise in healthy young men and women. *Scandinavian Journal of Clinical and Laboratory Investigation* 1973; **31**: 165–74.

53. Hesser, CM Linnarsson, D Fagraeus, L. Pulmonary mechanics and work of breathing at maximal ventilation and raised air pressure. *Journal of Applied Physiology* 1981; **50**: 747–53.

54. Klas, JV Dempsey, JA. Voluntary versus reflex regulation of maximal exercise flow:volume loops. *American Review of Respiratory Diseases* 1989; **139**: 150–6.

55. Whipp, BJ Pardy, R. Breathing during exercise. In: Macklem PT, Mead J. eds. *Handbook of physiology. Respiration (pulmonary mechanics)*. Washington, DC: American Physiological Society, 1986: 605–29.

56. Rohrer, F. Physiologie der Atembewegung. In: Bethe ATJ, von Bergmann G, Embden G, Ellinger A eds. *Handbuch der normalen und pathogischen Physiologie*. Berlin: Springer, 1925; 70–127.

57. Otis, AB Fenn, WO Rahn, H. Mechanics of breathing in man. *Journal of Applied Physiology* 1950; **2**: 592–607.

58. Hanson, JS Tabakin, BS Levy, AM Falsetti, HL. Alterations in pulmonary mechanics with airway obstruction during rest and exercise. *Journal of Applied Physiology* 1965; **20**: 664–8.

59. Gilbert, R Auchincloss, JH. Mechanics of breathing in normal subjects during brief, severe exercise. *Journal of Laboratory and Clinical Medicine* 1969; **73**: 439–50.

60. Olafsson, S Hyatt, RE. Ventilatory mechanics and expiratory flow limitation during exercise in normal subjects. *Journal of Clinical Investigation* 1960; **48**: 564–73.

61. Stubbing, DG Pengelly, LD Morse, JLC Jones, NL. Pulmonary mechanics during exercise in normal males. *Journal of Applied Physiology* 1980; **49**: 506–10.

62. Granath, A Horie, E Linderholm, H. Compliance and resistance of the lungs in the sitting and supine positions at rest and during exercise. *Scandinavian Journal of Clinical Laboratory Investigation* 1959; **11**: 226–34.

63. Chiang, ST Steigbigel, NH Lyons, HA. Pulmonary compliance and nonelastic resistance during treadmill exercise. *Journal of Applied Physiology* 1965; **20**: 1194–8.

64. Jones, N.L Killian, KJ Stubbing, DG. The thorax in exercise. In: Roussos CH, Macklem PT, eds. *The thorax. Lung biology in health and disease*, Vol. 29. New York: Dekker, 1988: 627–62.

65. Goldman, MD Grimby, G Mead, J. Mechanical work of breathing derived from rib cage and abdominal V-P partitioning. *Journal of Applied Physiology* 1976; **41**: 752–63.

66. Grimby, G Goldman, M Mead, J. Respiratory muscle action inferred from rib cage and abdominal V-P partitioning. *Journal of Applied Physiology* 1976; **41**: 739–51.

67. Otis, AB. The work of breathing. *Physiological Reviews* 1954; **34**: 449–58.

68. Otis, AB. The work of breathing. In: Fenn WO, Rahn H, eds. *Handbook of physiology. Respiration*, Vol. 1 Washington, DC: American Physiological Society 1964: 463–76.

69. Rochester, DF Farkas, GA Lu, JY. Contractility of the *in situ* human diaphragm: assessment based on dimensional analysis. In: Sieck GC, ed. *Respiratory muscles and their neuromotor control*. New York: Liss, 1987.

70. McKerrow, CB and Otis, AB. Oxygen cost of hyperventilation. *Journal of Applied Physiology* 1956; **9**: 375–9.

71. Campbell, EJM Westlake, EK and Cherniack RM. Simple methods of estimating oxygen consumption and efficiency of the muscles of breathing. *Journal of Applied Physiology* 1957; **11**: 303–8.

72. Bartlett, RG Jr., Brubach, HF Specht, H. Oxygen cost of breathing. *Journal of Applied Physiology* 1958; **12**: 413–24.

73. Cherniack, RM. The oxygen consumption and efficiency of respiratory muscles in health and emphysema. *Journal of Clinical Investigation* 1959; **38**: 494–9.

74. Fritts, HN Filler, J Fishman, AB Cournand, A. The efficiency of ventilation during voluntary hyperpnea. *Journal of Clinical Investigation* 1959; **38**: 1339–48.

75. Milic-Emili, G Petit, JM. Mechanical efficiency of breathing. *Journal of Applied Physiology* 1960; **15**: 359–62.

76. Shephard, RJ. The oxygen cost of breathing during vigorous exercise. *Quarterly Journal of Experimental Physiology* 1966; **51**: 336–50.

77. Leith, DE Bradley, M. Ventilatory muscle strength and endurance training. *Journal of Applied Physiology* 1976; **41**: 508–16.

78. Karetsky, MS. Cain, SM. Factors controlling O_2 uptake. *Chest* **61**: (Suppl.): 48S–49S, 1972.

79. Robertson, CH. Jr., Foster, GH Johnson, Jr RL. The relationship of respiratory failure to the oxygen consumption of, lactate production by, and distribution of blood flow among respiratory muscles during increasing inspiratory resistance. *Journal of Clinical Investigation* 1977; **59**: 31–42.

80. Bye, PTP Esau, SA Walley, KR Macklem, PT Pardy, RL. Ventilatory muscles during exercise in air and oxygen in normal men. *Journal of Applied Physiology* 1984; **56**: 464–71.

81. Johnson, RL. Jr. Heart–lung interactions in the transport of oxygen. In: : Scharf SM, Cassidy SS, eds. *Heart–lung interactions in health and disease. Lung biology in health and disease*, Vol. 42. New York: Dekker, 1989: 5–41.

82. Tenney, SM. Reese, RE. The ability to sustain great breathing efforts. *Respiratory Physiology* 1968; **5**: 187–201.

83. Bradley, ME. Leith, DE. Ventilatory muscle training and the oxygen cost of sustained hyperpnea. *Journal of Applied Physiology* 1978 **45**: 885–92.

84. Belman, MJ. Mittman, C. Ventilatory muscle training improves exercise capacity in chronic obstructive pulmonary disease patients. *American Review of Respiration Diseases* 1980; **121**: 273–80.

85. Bai, TR Rabinovitch, BJ Pardy, RL. Near-maximal voluntary hyperpnea and ventilatory muscle function. *Journal of Applied Physiology* 1984; **57**: 1742–48.

86. Shephard, RJ. The maximum sustained voluntary ventilation in exercise. *Clinical Science* 1967; **32**: 167–76.

87. Freedman, S. Sustained maximum voluntary ventilation. *Respiratory Physiology* 1970; **8**: 230–44.

88. Keens, TG Krastins, IRB Wannamaker, EM Levison, H Crozier, DN Bryan, AC. Ventilatory muscle endurance training in normal subjects and patients with cystic fibrosis. *American Review of Respiratory Diseases* 1977; **116**: 853–60.

89. Peress, L McLean, P Woolf, CR Zamel, N. Ventilatory muscle

training in obstructive lung disease. *Bullétin Européen Physiopathologie Respiratoire* 1979; **15**: 91–2.

90. Folinsbee, LJ Wallace, ES Bedi, JF Horvath, SM. Respiratory patterns and control during unrestrained human running. In: Whipp BJ, Wiberg DM, eds. *Modelling and control of breathing.* New York: Elsevier, 1983; 205–12.

91. Dill, DB Edwards, HT Bauer, PS Levenson, EJ. Physical performance in relation to external temperature. *Arbeitsphysiologie* 1931; **4**: 508–18.

92. Rowell LB (1986) *Human circulation: regulation during physical stress.* New York: Oxford University Press.

93. Otis, AB and Guyatt, AR. The maximal frequency of breathing in man at various tidal volumes. *Respiratory Physiology* 1968; **5**: 118–29.

94. Leaver, DJ and Pride, NB. Flow-volume curves and expiratory pressures during exercise in patients with chronic airway obstruction. *Scandinavian Journal of Respiratory Diseases* 1971; **77** (Suppl.): 23–7.

95. Jensen, JE Lyager, S Pederson, OF. The relationship between maximum ventilation, breathing patterns and mechanical limitation of ventilation. *Journal of Physiology (London)* 1980; **309**: 521–32.

96. Grimby, G Saltin, B Wilhelmsen, L. Pulmonary flow-volume and pressure–volume relationship during submaximal and maximal exercise in young well-trained men. *Bulletin de Physio–Pathologie Respiratoire* 1971; **7**: 157–72.

97. Milic-Emili, G Petit, JM Deroanne, R. The effects of respiratory rate on the mechanical work of breathing during muscular exercise. *Internationale Zeitschrift für Angewandte Physiologie, Einschliessliche Arbeitsphysiologie* 1960; **18**: 330–40.

98. Johnson, BD and Dempsey, JA. Demand vs. capacity in the aging pulmonary system. *Exercise and Sports Science Reviews* 1991; **19**: 171–210.

99. Macklem, P.T. Discussion of 'Inspiratory muscle fatigue as a factor limiting exercise' by A. Grassino, D. Gross, P.T. Macklem, C. Roussos, and G. Zagelbaum. *Bullétin Européen de Physiopathologie Respiratoire* 1979; **15**: 111–5.

100. Pierce, AK Luterman, D Loudermilk, J Blomqvist, G Johnson, Jr. RL. Exercise ventilatory patterns in normal subjects and patients with airway obstruction. *Journal of Applied Physiology* 1968; **25**: 249–54.

101. Brown, HV Wasserman, K Whipp, BJ. Strategies of exercise testing in chronic lung disease. *Bullétin Européen de Physiopathologie Respiratoire* 1977; **13**: 409–23.

102. Bye, PTP Farkas, GA Roussos, C. Respiratory factors limiting exercise. *Annual Review of Physiology* 1983; **45**: 439–51.

103. Nattie, EE and Tenny, SM. The ventilatory response to resistance unloading during muscular exercise. *Respiratory Physiology* 1970; **10**: 249–62.

104. Ward, SA Whipp, BJ Poon, CS. Density-dependent air flow and ventilatory control in exercise. *Respiratory Physiology* 1982; **49**: 267–77.

105. Hussain, SNA Pardy, RL Dempsey, JA. Mechanical impedance as determinant of inspiratory neural drive during exercise. *Journal of Applied Physiology* 1985; **59**: 365–73.

106. Gordon, B Levine, SA Wilmaers, A. Observations on a group of marathon runners. *Archives of Internal Medicine* 1924; **33**: 425.

107. Warren, GL Cureton, KJ Sparling, PB. Does lung function limit performance in a 24-hour ultramarathon? *Respiratory Physiology* 1989; **78**: 253–64.

108. Whipp, BJ and Davis, JA. Does ventilatory mechanics limit maximum exercise? In: Russo, P, Gass G, eds. *Exercise. A Workshop.* Sydney, Australia: Cumberland College, 1979: 20–6.

109. Edwards, RHT. Human muscle function and fatigue. In: Porter R, Whelan J, eds. *Human muscle fatigue* London: Pitman, 1981: 1–34.

110. Pardy, RL Hussain, SNA Macklem, PT. The ventilatory pump in exercise. *Clinics in Chest Medicine* 1984; **5**: 35–49.

111. Hansen, JE Stelter, GP Vogel JA. Arterial pyruvate, lactate, pH, and Pco_2 during work at sea level and high altitude. *Journal of Applied Physiology* 1967; **23**: 523–30.

112. Jones, N.L: Exercise testing in pulmonary evaluation: Rationale, methods, and the normal respiratory response to exercise. *New England Journal of Medicine* 1975; **293**: 541–4.

113. Gledhill, N Froese, AB Dempsey, JA. Ventilation to perfusion distribution during exercise in health. In: Dempsey J, Reed CE, eds *Muscular exercise and the lung* Madison: University of Wisconsin Press, 1977: 325–43.

114. West, BJ and Dollery, CT. Distribution of blood flow and ventilation–perfusion ratio in the lung measured with radioactive CO_2. *Journal of Applied Physiology* 1960; **15**: 405–10.

115. Bryan, AC Bentivoglio, LG Beerel, F MacLeish, H Zidulka, A Bates, DV. Factors affecting regional distribution of ventilation and perfusion in the lung. *Journal of Applied Physiology* 1964; **19**: 395–402.

116. Bake, B Bjure, J Widimsky, J. The effect of sitting and graded exercise on the disrtibution of pulmonary blood flow in healthy subjects studied with the 133-Xenon technique. *Scandinavian Journal of Clinical Laboratory Investigation* 1968; **22**: 99–106.

117. Wagner, PD Saltzman, HA West, JB. Measurement of continuous distributions of ventilation–perfusion ratios: theory. *Journal of Applied Physiology* 1974; **36**: 588–99.

118. Hammond, MD Gale, GE Kapitan, KS Ries, A Wagner, PD. Pulmonary gas exchange in humans during exercise at sea level. *Journal of Applied Physiology* 1986; **60**: 1590–8.

119. Derks, CM. Ventilation–perfusion distribution in young and old volunteers during mild exercise. *Bullétin Européen de Physiopathologie Respiratoire*. 1980; **16**: 145–54.

120. Gale, GE Torre-Bueno, J Moon, R Saltzman, HA Wagner, PD. $\dot{V}_A/Q$ inequality in normal man during exercise at sea level and simulated altitude. *Journal of Applied Physiology* 1985; **58**: 978–88.

121. Johnson, Jr., RL Taylor, HF DeGraff, Jr. AC. Functional significance of a low diffusing capacity for carbon monoxide. *Journal of Clinical Investigation* 1965; **44**: 789–800.

122. Hughes, JMB. Diffusive gas exchange. In: Whipp BJ, Wasserman K, eds. *Exercise: pulmonary physiology and pathophysiology. Lung biology in health and disease*, Vol. 52. New York: Dekker, 1991; 143–71.

123. Weibel, ER. *The pathway for oxygen.* Cambridge, MA: Harvard University Press, 1984.

124. Powers, SK Lawler, J Dempsey, JA Dodd, S Landry, G. Effects of incomplete pulmonary gas exchange on $\dot{V}o_2$max. *Journal of Applied Physiology* 1989; **66**: 2491–5.

125. Reeves, JT Dempsey, JA Grover, RF. Pulmonary circulation during exercise. In: Weir EK, Reeves JT, eds. *Pulmonary vascular physiology and pathophysiology. Lung biology in health and disease*, Vol. 38 New York: Dekker, 1989; 107–133.

126. O'Brodovich, H and Coates G. Lung Water and Solute Movement during exercise. In: Whipp BJ, Wasserman J, eds. *Exercise: pulmonary physiology and pathophysiology. Lung biology in health and disease*, Vol. 52. New York: Dekker, 1991; 253–70.

127. Brower, R. and Permutt S. Exercise and the pulmonary circulation. In: Whipp BJ, Wasserman K, eds. *Exercise: pulmonary physiology and pathophysiology. Lung biology in health and disease*, Vol. 52. New York: Dekker, 1991; 201–20.

128. Paintal, AS. The mechanism of excitation of type-J receptors and the J-reflex. In: Porter R, ed. *Breathing: Hering–Breuer Centenary Symposium.* London: Churchill, 1970; 59.

129. West JB, Mathieu-Costello O. Strength of the pulmonary blood-gas barrier. *Respiratory Physiology* 1992; **88**: 141–8.

130. West JB, Mathieu-Costello O. Stress failure of pulmonary capillaries: role in lung and heart disease. *Lancet* 1992; **340**: 762–7.
131. Jackson, I. *The breathplay approach to whole life fitness.* New York: Doubleday, 1986.

1.1.2 Cardiovascular responses to exercise and training

Peter B. Raven and Jeffrey T. Potts

Introduction

Physical exercise is associated with increases in the rate and depth of breathing to increase ventilation of the lungs, and increases in heart rate and stroke volume to increase cardiac output. These cardio-respiratory adjustments insure adequate delivery of oxygen to the active muscles. Thus, physical exercise involves an interaction among the respiratory, cardiovascular, and cellular energetic systems of working muscles.

The gas transport mechanisms for coupling cellular and pulmonary respiration are schematically illustrated (Fig. 1) using interlocking gears representing the functional interdependence of the major systems involved in oxygen delivery.

The increase in oxygen use by active muscle occurs as a result of an increase in oxygen extraction from blood perfusing active muscle, vasodilation of peripheral vascular beds within active muscle, an

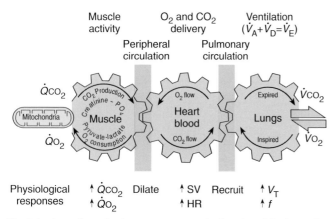

Fig. 1 A scheme illustrating the gas transport mechanisms for cellular (internal) to pulmonary (external) respiration. The gears represent the functional interdependence of the physiological components of the system. The large increase in $\dot{V}_{O_2}$ utilization by the muscles ($\dot{Q}_{O_2}$) is achieved by increased extraction of oxygen from the blood perfusing the muscles, the dilatation of selected peripheral vascular beds, an increase in cardiac output (stroke volume and heart rate), an increase in pulmonary blood flow by recruitment and vasodilatation of pulmonary blood vessels, and finally, an increase in ventilation. Oxygen is taken up ($\dot{V}_{O_2}$max) from the alveoli in proportion to the pulmonary blood flow and degree of $\dot{V}_{O_2}$ desaturation of haemoglobin in the pulmonary blood. In the steady state, $\dot{V}_{O_2}$max = $\dot{V}_{O_2}$. Ventilation (tidal volume, V_t, and breathing frequency, f) increases in relation to newly produced carbon dioxide ($\dot{Q}_{CO_2}$) arriving at the lungs and the drive to achieve arterial carbon dioxide and hydrogen ion homeostasis. (Reproduced with permission from Wasserman *et al. Principles of exercise testing and interpretation.* Philadelphia: Lea & Febiger, 1987.[1])

Table 1 Acute cardiorespiratory responses to dynamic and static exercise

	Dynamic	Static
Cardiac output	++++	+
heart rate	++	+
Stroke volume	++	0
Peripheral resistance	–––	+++
Systolic blood pressure	++	++++
Diastolic blood pressure	0 or –	++++
Mean arterial pressure	0 or +	++++
Left ventricular work	Volume load	Pressure load

+/– represents the relative magnitude of change in each variable from resting value.

increase in cardiac output and vasoconstriction in non-active vascular beds to maintain blood pressure, and an increase in pulmonary blood flow and ventilation.[2] In this review, we advance the hypothesis that regulation of exercise respiratory, cardiovascular, and metabolic function is based on the detection of error signals related to skeletal muscle oxygen demand. Monitoring these error signals leads to appropriate corrections in systemic blood flow and pressure facilitating the transport of oxygen to active skeletal muscle. Furthermore, we postulate that exercise training alters the respiratory, cardiovascular, and metabolic responses to exercise by altering the sensitivity of those mechanisms regulating systemic blood flow and pressure.

During exercise, working muscle utilizes oxygen for the generation of free energy to be stored in ATP and produces carbon dioxide as a byproduct. Therefore, transfer of oxygen and carbon dioxide between the atmosphere and mitochondria requires a highly co-ordinated interaction between cardiovascular and respiratory mechanisms linked to muscle metabolic activity to ensure adequate arterial oxygen content and the appropriate perfusion pressure to couple oxygen delivery and blood flow to the metabolic needs of the working muscle (see Fig. 1).

Physiological responses of static and dynamic exercise

The acute metabolic and haemodynamic responses associated with exercise and training are dependent upon the type of muscle contraction. In general, the type of muscle contraction is either static or dynamic, or some proportional combination of the two. However, the acute cardiovascular responses to exercise and training are quite different to the responses to sustained and habitual use of these types of contractions. The acute cardiorespiratory responses to dynamic and static exercise are summarized in Table 1.

Static muscle contractions

There is no doubt that the blood flow through skeletal muscle during static exercise is impeded by local mechanical compression of the vasculature; however, there is no clear consensus of the critical level of force development required to reduce the circulation through active skeletal muscle. Systematic studies of blood flow through the human forearm at varying levels of tension development during static contraction have shown that at low, non-fatiguing tensions (up to 10 per cent of maximal voluntary contraction) the blood flow increases linearly with tension and reaches a steady state in several minutes.[3,4] During fatiguing tensions (60 to 70 per cent of maximal voluntary contraction), blood flow increases linearly until fatigue is reached, after which the blood flow becomes progressively lower, presumably because of the increasing mechanical impediment to muscle perfusion.[5] In the human forearm, mechanical occlusion occurs at 60 to 70 per cent of maximal voluntary contraction;[3,6] however in other muscle groups, occlusion by mechanical compression may vary between 20 and 70 per cent of maximal voluntary contraction.[7,8] Interestingly, the fall in muscle perfusion during fatiguing static contraction occurs despite a large reflex increase in muscle perfusion pressure elicited by activation of muscle afferent fibres.[3,5,6]

Static isometric muscle contractions produce a sustained increase in heart rate and systolic, diastolic, and mean arterial pressures in direct relation to the force or relative intensity of the contraction. The increase in heart rate is due to vagal withdrawal, while muscle ischaemia due to the static contraction potentiates the blood pressure response.[9,10] Static contractions are also associated with a small increase in left-ventricular end-diastolic pressure and an enhanced contractile state.[11] However, there is relatively little change in cardiac output or total peripheral resistance. Thus, static exercise results primarily in an afterload pressure on the heart.

Cardiovascular adaptations to strength training

Weightlifting and resistance training utilizing sustained isometric contractions and slow muscle contractions of high force output increase muscular strength. The gain in strength is due to both neural factors and muscle hypertrophy. Neural involvement is indicated by an increase in maximal integrated electromyographic activation without a change in force per fibre output or the number of innervated motor units.[12] The increase in muscle hypertrophy is due primarily to an increase in muscle fibre cross-sectional size as a result of increases in the number of myofibrils per fibre, sarcoplasmic volume, total protein, and hypertrophy of connective, tendinous, and ligamentous tissues.[12] The increase in muscle myofibril size actually decreases mitochondrial density. In some cases, muscle hypertrophy can result from an increase in fibre number (hyperplasia) as a result of stimulation of dormant stem cells.[13] Strength training increases intramuscular stores of ATP, creatine phosphate, and glycogen, but produces little change in anaerobic glycolytic and aerobic oxidative enzyme activities. Muscle hypertrophy is generally not as large in women as in men because of lower levels of circulating testosterone.

Cross-sectional studies[14] suggest that strength training increases left ventricular mass without affecting left ventricular volume. This indicates that chronic strength training alters the LaPlace constant (increased wall stress) of the heart, which in some cases may lead to an increase in myocardial oxygen demand similar to that seen in hypertensive individuals with concomitant cardiac hypertrophy. However, strength training has little or no effect on maximal cardiac output, stroke volume, heart rate, and arterial–venous oxygen difference, and, hence, maximal oxygen uptake during dynamic exercise.[15-17]

Dynamic muscle contractions

Dynamic contractions and cellular metabolism

During the onset of dynamic exercise, the heart rate increases due to withdrawal of vagal tone and an increase in sympathetic adrenergic activity.[18,19] The increase in sympathetic activity increases plasma noradrenaline concentration, cardiac contractility, and muscle sympathetic nerve activity.[19] The increase in plasma noradrenaline concentration is due to an increase in spillover from the vascular α-adrenergic receptors which mediate vasoconstriction. The amount of spillover is directly related to the exercise intensity.[20]

The increase in heart rate increases cardiac output, which in turn increases the mean arterial pressure. Vasoconstriction in splanchnic and renal vascular beds redistributes blood to the large central veins, increasing venous return and the central blood volume and thereby providing support for increases in stroke volume and cardiac output.[21] Thus dynamic exercise causes a volume load to the heart.

The accumulation of metabolites as a result of muscle contraction produces local muscle vasodilation.[22] However, the local muscle vasodilation response is not great enough to override the tonic vasoconstrictor tone or totally abolish vasoconstrictor activity.[23] Much speculation exists as to the agent facilitating active muscle vasodilation. Some candidates include levels of muscle carbon dioxide and muscle pH, lactic acid, adenosine, bradykinin, cyclo-oxygenase products of arachidonic acid, and potassium, but no one agent can explain all features of the local vasodilator response to muscle contraction.[24] These substances may function by sensitizing the responses of group III and IV afferents during muscle contraction.[25,26] Whatever the substance(s) and the mechanism(s) it is clear that changes in the chemical milieu of the interstitium of skeletal muscle plays a critical role in activating muscle afferents during muscle contraction. It has been postulated that arterial baroreceptors and muscle chemoreflexes function to regulate sympathetic outflow, and thus muscle perfusion pressure and blood flow.[9] The degree of metabolic vasodilation in active skeletal muscle is opposed by sympathetic vasoconstriction, which has been shown to be under direct control of the carotid baroreceptor reflex.[27] However, in order for the arterial baroreflex to modulate sympathetic outflow, the reflex must be reset to the prevailing level of systemic pressure during exercise. Recently, direct evidence for resetting of the carotid baroreceptor reflex has been reported during dynamic leg exercise.[28,29] Thus, optimal perfusion of active skeletal muscle is achieved by active vasoconstriction to non-active vascular beds which redistributes systemic blood flow to active muscle, and the modulation of metabolic vasodilation in active tissue by the arterial baroreceptor reflex.

Effect of dynamic contractions on central circulatory responses

Oxygen uptake

In the laboratory, oxygen uptake $\dot{V}O_2$ is determined by indirect calorimetry.[30] Under these circumstances, $\dot{V}O_2$ is equal to pulmonary minute ventilation V_E multiplied by the difference in the inspired

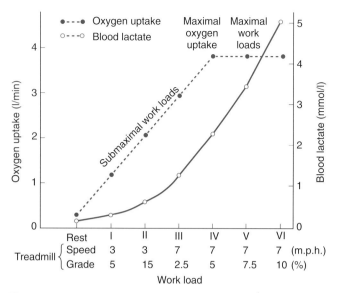

Fig. 2 The objective determination of maximal oxygen uptake $\dot{V}_{O_2}$max on a tread-mill. The plateau of oxygen uptake $\dot{V}_{O_2}$max occurs while the subject continues to perform work at increasing workloads. Note also the exponential increase in plasma lactate concentrations as workload increases beyond 50 per cent $\dot{V}_{O_2}$max. (Reproduced from Mitchell and Blomqvist *New England Journal of Medicine* 1971; **284**: 1018–22, with permission.[15])

and expired oxygen percentages at the mouth as expressed in the following equation:

$$\dot{V}_{O_2} \text{ (l/min)} = V_E \text{ (l/min)} \times \tag{1}$$
$$\text{(inspired fraction of } O_2 - \text{expired fraction of } O_2)$$

Oxygen uptake at rest is approximately 0.25 l/min. Maximum oxygen uptake $\dot{V}_{O_2}$max of a sedentary 70-kg man averages 3.0 l/min (43 ml/kg per min). $\dot{V}_{O_2}$max is determined during graded increases in exercise workload during cycle ergometer or motorized treadmill tests (Fig. 2).[15,31]

$\dot{V}_{O_2}$max is confirmed when additional increases in workload produce no further increase in $\dot{V}_{O_2}$.[15,31] Therefore, $\dot{V}_{O_2}$max is a rate measurement and indicates the maximal level of aerobic power output. Oxygen uptake can also be expressed as cardiac output Q_c multiplied by the systemic oxygen extraction, or the arteriovenous oxygen difference across active tissues, as:

$$\dot{V}_{O_2} \text{ (l/min)} = Q_c \text{ (l/min)} \times \tag{2}$$
$$\text{(arterial } O_2 \text{ content} - \text{venous } O_2 \text{ content)}$$

Therefore, maximal oxygen uptake can also be determined by measuring maximal cardiac output and the arteriovenous oxygen difference. Maximal cardiac output is the product of maximal heart rate and maximal stroke volume, while the maximal arteriovenous oxygen difference depends upon the maximal oxygen content of the arterial blood and minimal oxygen content of the venous blood. The major factors affecting cardiac output are heart rate and stroke volume determinants, which are summarized in Fig. 3.

Cardiac output

Cardiac output Q_c is equal to the heart rate (HR) multiplied by the stroke volume (SV), as indicated by the equation:

$$Q_c = HR \text{ (beats/min)} \times SV \text{ (ml/beat)} \tag{3}$$

At rest, cardiac output approximates 5 to 6 l/min. However, cardiac output increases to 20 to 25 l/min during maximal exercise in a sedentary individual. Cardiac output increases to its maximum as a result of increases in heart rate and stroke volume and the attainment of their respective maxima.[15,21,32] During maximal exercise, arterial haemoglobin saturation and oxygen content remain relatively constant at 97 per cent and 20 ml/dl of blood, respectively. However, venous oxygen content decreases substantially due to an increase in muscle oxygen extraction. During maximal exercise, the arteriovenous oxygen difference increases from 6 ml O_2/dl of blood at rest to 16 ml O_2/dl of blood at maximal exercise.

From eqn 3 above, an example calculation for an individual with a maximal heart rate of 180 beats/min and a maximal stroke volume of 140 ml/beat is:

$$\dot{V}_{O_2}\text{max} = 180 \text{ beats/min} \times 140 \text{ ml/beat} \times 16 \text{ ml/dl} \tag{4}$$
$$= 4.032 \text{ l/min.}$$

Heart rate

Heart rate is the number of ventricular contractions occurring during a period of 1 min. At rest, heart rate is approximately 70 beats/min in a sedentary individual, and is determined by the relative contributions of the parasympathetic and sympathetic nervous systems.[19] Increases in heart rate from a resting value up to an exercise rate of 100 beats/min are primarily a result of the withdrawal of vagal tone and minor increases in sympathetic activity. However, once the heart rate reaches 100 to 110 beats/min, further increases in heart rate occur as a result of an increased sympathetic activity and continual vagal withdrawal up to a heart rate of 150 to 160 beats/min. Above 150 to 160 beats/min only slight adjustments in vagal tone occur as the heart rate increases to the maximum (Fig. 4).[33]

During exercise, heart rate increases in proportion to the workload and oxygen uptake, and reaches 190 to 200 beats/min at $\dot{V}_{O_2}$max.[18,19] Heart rate during submaximal exercise is elevated in individuals in whom stroke volume is reduced owing to a decrease in myocardial contractility as a result of deconditioning or cardiac disease.[15]

Stroke volume

Stroke volume is the amount of blood ejected from the heart with each heart beat and is equal to the difference between the amount of blood in the heart after completion of filling (the end-diastolic vol-

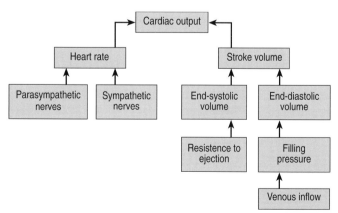

Fig. 3 A schematic block diagram summarizing the major factors determining cardiac output.

ume) and the amount remaining after ejection (the end–systolic volume).[34] At rest, stroke volume is 80 to 90 ml/beat, while during maximal exercise, stroke volume increases to 110 to 115 ml/beat (Fig. 5). As will be discussed in the section on cardiovascular adaptations to dynamic exercise training, alterations in diastolic function of the left ventricle in endurance-trained athletes facilitates enhanced ventricular filling and augmented stroke volume during near-maximal exercise.

The rhythmic muscle contractions of dynamic exercise increase venous return and the intrathoracic and pulmonary capillary blood volumes.[35,36] The increase in these central volumes increases the reserve volume, thus providing for an enhanced preload for the heart. Therefore, increases in stroke volume are achieved by an increase in pulmonary vascular pressure which increases left ventricular filling pressure and end-diastolic volume and by an increase in left ventricular contractility, as indicated by an increase in ejection fraction and decrease in end-systolic volume (Figs 5 and 6).[34]

Myocardial oxygen consumption

During dynamic exercise, increases in heart rate, myocardial contractility, stroke volume, and blood pressure are associated with an increase in myocardial oxygen consumption. The arteriovenous oxygen difference across the heart during exercise is only slightly greater than at rest.[15,37] This indicates that the increase in myocardial oxygen consumption is almost totally dependent upon an increase in coronary blood flow. The large increase in coronary blood flow with exercise suggests that a large vasodilator error signal

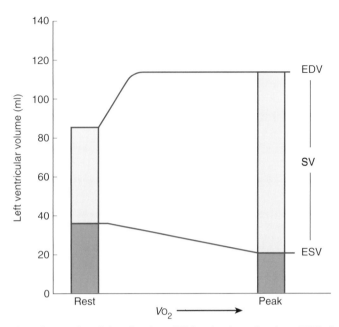

Fig. 5 Changes in end-diastolic volume (EDV) and end-systolic volume (ESV) of the left ventricle during upright bicycle exercise from rest to $\dot{V}_{O_2}$peak. (A modification of the data of Poliner *et al.*[34] and reproduced with permission from *Circulation* 1980; **62**: 528–34. Copyright 1980 American Heart Association.)

overrides the existing tonic vasoconstrictor tone.[38] While myocardial oxygen consumption during exercise is difficult to measure in the human, the product of heart rate and systolic blood pressure (the rate–pressure product) is highly correlated to myocardial oxygen consumption and cardiac work and is used in clinical settings to assess the results of pharmacological, surgical, or exercise therapy.

Systemic arteriovenous oxygen difference

At rest, haemoglobin leaving the lungs for the peripheral vasculature is approximately 97 per cent saturated with oxygen, producing an arterial oxygen content of 20 ml/100 ml of whole blood. As

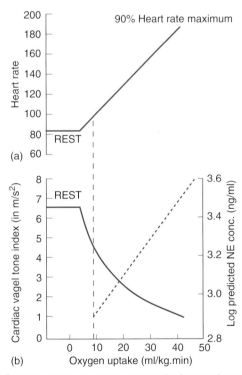

Fig. 4 (a) Changes in heart rate during a progressive increase in workload exercise test to 90 per cent of the maximal heart rate. It should be noted that the initial increase in heart rate from rest to 100 beats/min involves only vagal withdrawal. (b) Between heart rates of 100 beats/min and the maximum heart rate the increase is a result of further vagal withdrawal and increasing sympathetic drive to the heart (log concentration of noradrenaline) with the sympathetic drive predominating at heart rates in excess of 150 beats/min.

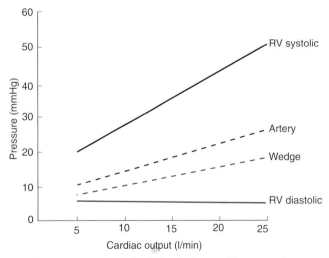

Fig. 6 Changes in right-ventricular (RV) and pulmonary (P) pressures from rest to maximal cardiac outputs during supine exercise. (Adapted from Ekelund and Holmgren,[21] and reproduced with permission from Chapman CB, ed. *Physiology of muscular exercise*. American Heart Association Monograph 15. Copyright American Heart Association 1967.)

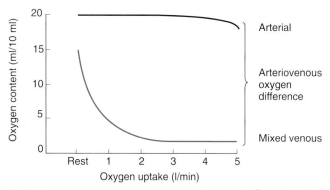

Fig. 7 Change in arteriovenous oxygen content from rest to $\dot{V}_{O_2}$max of 5 l/min. Individuals with high $\dot{V}_{O_2}$max values tend to have some arterial desaturation at maximal capacity; however, they appear to be able to extract more oxygen at the working muscle resulting in mixed venous oxygen contents of 2 to 3.ml O_2/100ml of blood at $\dot{V}_{O_2}$max. (Adapted from ref. 33, and reproduced with permission.)

blood is transported through metabolically active tissues, large pressure gradients occur between the capillary and mitochondria.[36] These pressure gradients for oxygen establish the release of oxygen from haemoglobin and diffusion into the cell. Not all oxygen is released from the haemoglobin as it passes through the peripheral tissue. Varying levels of venous oxyhaemoglobin saturation reflect the amount of oxygen extracted at the tissue level. The difference between systemic arterial and venous oxygen contents is called the arteriovenous oxygen difference and is an indicator of oxygen extraction. During exercise, the increase in the arteriovenous oxygen difference is also solely due to an increase in oxygen extraction by working skeletal muscle (Fig. 7).

Blood volume

The onset of exercise is usually associated with a reduction in plasma volume due to a redistribution of fluids from the vascular to the interstitial space. However, in most cases this shift is the result of movement to an upright exercise body position or to an increase in mean arterial pressure related to exercise intensity.[39] After the initial fluid shift, an equilibrium is reached between vascular fluid influx and efflux resulting in a constant plasma volume. A 'true' decrease in plasma volume usually only occurs as a result of total body dehydration due to prolonged exercise, high sweat rates, and heat stress.[40]

Either the onset of exercise or the decrease in plasma volume stimulates the release of neuroendocrine hormones associated with fluid and electrolyte balance. The release of these hormones, namely arginine vasopressin, atrial natriuretic peptide, and aldosterone, is related to the intensity of the exercise, and during continuous exercise to a decrease in cardiac filling pressure. The increase in the plasma concentration of these hormones and constancy of the plasma volume during continuous exercise suggests an active regulation of the vascular fluid volume for the purpose of maintaining cardiac output and mean arterial pressure.[40]

Vascular resistance and conductance

Mean arterial blood pressure provides the driving force for systemic blood flow, and involves the interplay of cardiac output and peripheral vascular resistance. The major factors determining the mean systemic arterial pressure include the cardiac output and peripheral vascular resistance (Fig. 8). In the laboratory, cardiac output is

determined by the product of heart rate and stroke volume, while total peripheral resistance (TPR) is equal to the ratio of mean arterial pressure (MAP) to cardiac output Qc:

$$\text{TPR (mmHg/l per min)} = \text{MAP (mmHg)}/Q\text{c (l/min)} \qquad (4)$$

Systolic and diastolic blood pressure at rest are normally 120 and 80 mmHg, respectively. However, during maximal exercise, systolic blood pressure increases to between 200 and 240 mmHg, while diastolic pressure changes little or decreases to 60 mmHg resulting in a widening of the pulse pressure and a moderate increase in mean arterial pressure.

During dynamic exercise, local muscle vasodilation produces a decrease in total peripheral resistance. In order to maintain mean arterial pressure and an adequate muscle perfusion pressure, cardiac output increases. During maximal exercise, the increase in cardiac output in relation to the change in mean arterial pressure indicates that the decrease in total peripheral resistance is associated with an increase in vascular conductance. Since skeletal muscle vascular conductance can exceed cardiac pumping capacity, reductions in splanchnic and renal blood flow and vasoconstriction in non-active and exercising muscle occur in order to maintain cardiac output at a level high enough to insure adequate muscle perfusion pressure and muscle blood flow.[9,33,41]

Pulmonary ventilation

Pulmonary ventilation at rest is 10 to 14 l/min, and breathing rate is 10 to 14 breaths/min. However, during maximal exercise, ventilation will increase to 100 to 120 l/min, while respiration rate will increase to 40 to 50 breaths/min.[42] Tidal volume also increases to approximately two-thirds of the forced vital capacity with most of the increase occurring by 50 per cent $\dot{V}_{O_2}$max. At the onset of dynamic exercise, pulmonary ventilation increases due to neurogenic and neurohumoral mechanisms which increases both breathing frequency and tidal volume. Thus ventilation is equal to breathing rate multiplied by the volume of each breath:

$$\dot{V}_\text{e} \text{ (l/min)} = f_\text{b}\text{(breaths/min)} \times V_\text{t} \text{ (l/breath)} \qquad (5)$$

During maximal exercise, arterial lactic acid concentration increases in a curvilinear pattern as a result of an increased energy production via anaerobic glycolysis (Fig. 2). Arterial hydrogen ion concentration is maintained constant up to approximately 50 to 60 per cent of $\dot{V}_{O_2}$max. At this point, called the ventilatory or anaerobic threshold,[1,2] it is proposed that increases in carbon dioxide flow stimulate

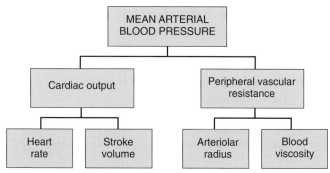

Fig. 8 Physiological factors that effect flow and resistance to produce the resultant mean arterial pressure, i.e. resistance = pressure/flow.

carotid chemoreceptors which further increases pulmonary ventilation (hyperventilation) as a compensatory mechanism to regulate the plasma carbon dioxide partial pressure P_{CO_2}, hydrogen ion concentration $[H^+]$, and arterial pH (see Chapter 3.1). Increases in $[H^+]$ produced with lactate during inadequate oxygen delivery to active muscle increases capillary oxygen partial pressure P_{O_2} and facilitates oxygen diffusion to mitochondria.[2] Muscle chemoreceptors sensitive to the concentration of lactic acid (or other metabolic byproducts) provide another and probably more dominant mechanism contributing to exercise hyperpnoea.[41]

Dynamic exercise produces an increase in venous return as a result of the pumping action of the exercising limbs and diaphragm. The increase in venous return in conjunction with vasodilation of the pulmonary vasculature produces an increase in pulmonary capillary blood volume. The increase in pulmonary capillary blood volume increases lung oxygen diffusion capacity which serves to maintain arterial P_{O_2} and oxyhaemoglobin at nearly 97 per cent saturation. As long as arterial oxyhaemoglobin saturation is maintained, pulmonary ventilation is not normally a limiting factor to $\dot{V}_{O_2}$max. However, it is evidence of hypoxaemia during maximal exercise in athletes who are extremely well trained.

Factors limiting maximal oxygen uptake capacity

There is substantial evidence that in the normal person $\dot{V}_{O_2}$max is the objective measure of the supply of oxygen to the exercising muscle, i.e. it is the maximum capacity to deliver oxygen. However, despite the integrative aspects of the oxygen transport system, it is generally held that cardiac output is the major limiting factor in the achievement of $\dot{V}_{O_2}$max.

Cardiac function

During maximal exercise, arterial P_{O_2} is maintained constant, while skeletal muscle vascular conductance is expanded. This indicates that oxygen delivery is greatly increased. However, the vascular conductance capacity of skeletal muscle is larger than the capacity of the heart to expand cardiac output, and whole-body $\dot{V}_{O_2}$max is produced through engagement of only one-third of the total skeletal muscle mass.[23,33] Thus the limited ability to expand cardiac output in relation to the vascular conductance capacity strongly suggests that cardiac output is the limiting factor to oxygen delivery and $\dot{V}_{O_2}$max. If a larger muscle mass is engaged during exercise, vasoconstriction is thought to occur in the arterioles of the exercising limbs to avoid a reduction in blood pressure (Fig. 9).

If vasoconstriction did not occur, exercise requiring a majority of the muscle mass of the body would require a cardiac output of up to 60 l/min to prevent a drop in blood pressure.[23] However, a major unanswered question is the nature of the signal for the sympathetically mediated vasoconstriction.

Pulmonary function

The lack of dyspnoeic sensations during exhaustive exercise suggests that pulmonary blood gas transport is most efficient. However, during graded exercise there is a progressive widening of the alveolar to arterial P_{O_2} difference due to intraregional variations in the relationship between alveolar ventilation and blood flow distribution in the lungs.[35] The presence of arterial oxygen desaturation during maximal exercise suggests that respiratory function can be a limit-

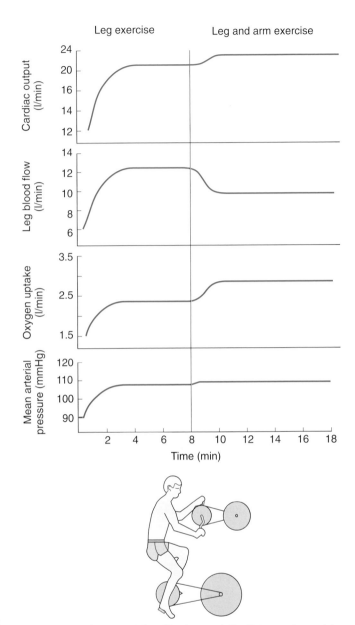

Fig. 9 A schematic representation of the decrease in flow that occurs in exercising legs when additional arm exercises are added. The cardiac output increases to increase flow to exercising arms and the distribution of cardiac output to the legs is reduced as a means of maintaining mean arterial pressure. However, the locus of the error signal necessary to produce and maintain active vasoconstriction in the legs has not been determined. (Modified from the data presented in ref. 33 and reprinted with permission.)

ing factor to $\dot{V}_{O_2}$max. However, as long as pulmonary blood flow and pulmonary capillary blood volume increase during maximal exercise, mean pulmonary capillary transit time appears sufficient to permit alveolar–arterial oxygen equilibration (Fig. 10).[35]

Skeletal muscle oxygen utilization

While many researchers contend that central circulatory factors limit $\dot{V}_{O_2}$max, others[30,36] argue that the major limitation to $\dot{V}_{O_2}$max is the rate at which oxygen is moved by diffusion from haemoglobin in the red cell to the muscle mitochondria. This concept is supported by evidence showing that $\dot{V}_{O_2}$max is reduced by decreases in the oxygen carrying capacity of red cells and muscle ischaemia due

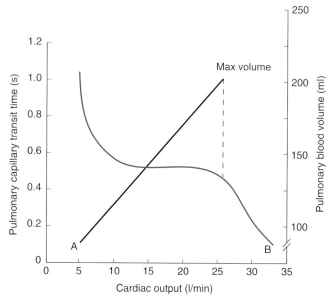

Fig. 10 A schematic outline of progressive increases in pulmonary capillary blood volume (A) in relation to decreases in pulmonary capillary transit time (B) with increasing cardiac output. As can be seen early on in exercise, capillary recruitment increases the capillary blood volume and decreases mean transit time without arterial haemoglobin desaturation. From 15 l/min to 25 to 28 l/min cardiac output, arterial haemoglobin saturation is maintained because of the increasing capillary recruitment, increasing pulmonary capillary volume, and constant transit time. When maximum capillary volume is achieved at cardiac outputs of 25 to 28 l/min, the transit time decreases until it is insufficient to provide complete arterial haemoglobin saturation. (Redrawn from data presented in ref. 33 and reprinted with permission).

to peripheral vascular diseases, and by evidence showing little increase in $\dot{V}O_2$max during the breathing of hyperoxic gases.[43] It is also worth noting that the limitations to $\dot{V}O_2$max will differ depending upon the training status of the individual.

Factors influencing maximal oxygen uptake capacity

Much of the physiological variation in $\dot{V}O_2$max can be attributed to genetics, gender, age, body composition, and habitual level of physical activity.[15]

Genetics and $\dot{V}O_2$max
Evidence supports the concept that genetic factors are associated with individual differences in $\dot{V}O_2$max values and changes in $\dot{V}O_2$max with training.[44] It has also been shown that there is a maternal effect on maximal exercise heart rate, blood lactate, and $\dot{V}O_2$max.[45] Recent evidence[46] suggests that sequence variations in mitochondrial DNA may contribute to individual differences in $\dot{V}O_2$max and its response to training. In addition, the greater cardiorespiratory functional capacity of endurance athletes is usually manifested at an early age prior to extensive training.[47] The selection of endurance sports by some athletes may be related to early success in endurance events due to an already elevated $\dot{V}O_2$max. However, the $\dot{V}O_2$max of endurance athletes is also a result of adaptations in cardiovascular, respiratory, and muscle metabolic structure and function as a result of endurance training.[33] Thus, attainment of world-class status in endurance sports is probably due

to a combination of genetic endowment and participation in a programme of long-term training.

Body composition and $\dot{V}O_2$max
Maximal oxygen uptake expressed relative to body weight (ml/kg per min) enables the comparison of individuals of high and low body weight, and is the most useful way of expressing cardiorespiratory functional capacity. Endurance athletes usually have a lower body weights compared with sedentary individuals. However, while the sedentary individual possesses a greater amount of body fat, the lean body weight of sedentary individuals and endurance athletes are remarkable similar.[48,49] Maximal oxygen uptake can be altered by changes in body composition. Decreases in body fat due to dieting alone, accompanied by little or no change in lean body weight, will increase $\dot{V}O_2$max when $\dot{V}O_2$max is expressed relative to body weight[50], but not in absolute values (i.e l/min).

Gender and $\dot{V}O_2$max
Maximal oxygen uptake is also influenced by gender. $\dot{V}O_2$max expressed in absolute units (l/min) increases linearly with increases in height, weight, and age in both boys and girls. The physical stature and body weight of boys and girls is similar up to puberty making their $\dot{V}O_2$max values nearly equivalent.[32] During and after puberty, males experience an increase in lean muscle mass, while females increase their body fat. As a result, males experience a greater increase in $\dot{V}O_2$max. The magnitude of these changes in certain individuals may contribute to the type of sport they choose to perform. Endurance athletes tend to be individuals of low body weight and body fat, while strength and power athletes tend to be large and muscular. As adults, the $\dot{V}O_2$max of females is about 20 per cent lower than that of males.[31,51] However, this difference is reduced to about 5 per cent when $\dot{V}O_2$max is related to fat-free, lean body mass. The residual small differences in $\dot{V}O_2$max values may be due to the lower haemoglobin concentration of females.[52]

Age and $\dot{V}O_2$max
The maximal oxygen uptake of children and adults expressed in litres per minute is proportional to height and body weight, and increases in a linear pattern with body growth.[32] Cross-sectional studies show that after the age of 20 years there is a decline in $\dot{V}O_2$max ranging from 0.3 to 0.5 ml/kg.min per year.[52-54] The decrease in $\dot{V}O_2$max is also associated with a decrease in maximal exercise heart rate of 0.5 to 1.0 beats/min per year.[54] The age-related decline in $\dot{V}O_2$max appears to be due to a decrease in maximum heart rate, cardiac output, and systemic arteriovenous oxygen difference. However, much of the age-related decline in $\dot{V}O_2$max can be explained by a more sedentary lifestyle and an increase in body fat. The $\dot{V}O_2$max of athletes engaged in endurance training is higher than that of sedentary individuals of similar age, and individuals who maintain a physically active lifestyle have a smaller amount of body fat and a slower rate of decline in aerobic endurance capacity with advancing age.[54]

Physical activity and $\dot{V}O_2$max
Cardiorespiratory functional capacity is most profoundly influenced by the amount of habitual physical activity.[55] Prolonged exposure to bed rest and detraining leads to a decrease in $\dot{V}O_2$max (Fig. 11), while endurance training produces an increase in $\dot{V}O_2$max.[15,31,54,55]

   The rate and magnitude of increases in $\dot{V}O_2$max are related to the age of the individual, level of $\dot{V}O_2$max prior to the commencement of training,[23,54,55] and to the frequency, intensity, and duration of the exercise training programme.[56]

Cardiovascular adaptations to dynamic exercise training

The adaptive responses to habitual endurance exercise occur throughout training.[57-60] The adaptations to endurance exercise occur in both central and peripheral circulatory function and lead to increases in maximal oxygen uptake and muscle oxygen extraction, and an improved ability to sustain submaximal steady-state exercise. The increase in $\dot{V}O_2$max is primarily related to an increase in maximal cardiac output and secondarily to an increase in oxygen extraction across active muscles (Fig. 12).

$\dot{V}O_2$max and training

Cross-sectional studies show that the $\dot{V}O_2$max of endurance-trained athletes is higher than that of sedentary individuals.[61] The $\dot{V}O_2$max of sedentary individuals is usually less than 40 ml/kg per min. The $\dot{V}O_2$max of world-class male endurance athletes can exceed 80 ml/kg per min, while the $\dot{V}O_2$max of local-area champions may vary between 60 and 70 ml/kg per min. There is a strong relationship between training volume, as determined from the product of exercise frequency, duration, and intensity, and $\dot{V}O_2$max capacity.[33,54-56] In the sedentary individual, endurance training can increase $\dot{V}O_2$max by 15 to 30 per cent during the first 2 to 3 months of training. Further increases of up to 40 to 50 per cent can occur over the next 9 to 24 months of training. However, there is little change in $\dot{V}O_2$max after this point. Despite this plateau of $\dot{V}O_2$max and because of continued intracellular metabolic adaptations, performance in endurance events may continue to improve with continued endurance exercise training. The termination of training results in a slow and gradual decline in $\dot{V}O_2$max to pretraining levels

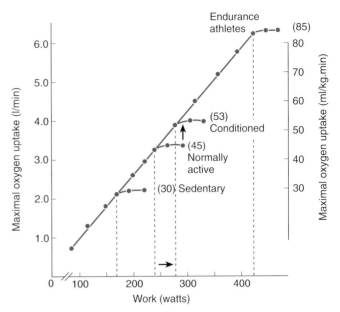

Fig. 12 The range of $\dot{V}O_2$max that exists within a normal healthy adult population. The range includes sedentary individuals with $\dot{V}O_2$max = 30 ml/kg per min, normally active individuals with $\dot{V}O_2$max = 45 ml/kg per min, active people who carry out a 2 to 3-month training programme with $\dot{V}O_2$max = 53 ml/kg per min, and the world-class endurance performer with $\dot{V}O_2$max = 85 ml/kg per min. (Reprinted from ref. 33 with permission.)

over a 6-month period with a more rapid decline in the metabolic energy supply systems of the skeletal muscle (see Chapter 1.1.3).

Submaximal exercise responses

The cardiorespiratory response to submaximal exercise is improved by endurance exercise training. Heart rate for any given absolute level of submaximal power output is reduced, while stroke volume is increased.[31,55] The reduced heart rate is only partially related to a decrease in sympathetic stimulation because the decline in plasma catecholamines is completed by the third week of training, while the decline in resting and submaximal heart rates continues over a longer period of training. Resting heart rates of world-class endurance runners vary from 30 to 40 beats/min and remain in sinus rhythm.[1,36] However, pre- and post-training concentration of plasma catecholamines are similar at any given percentage of $\dot{V}O_2$max. These differences imply that the reduction in heart rate during submaximal exercise is due to other factors such as a decrease in the sensitivity of β_1-receptors on the heart,[62] the increased vagal control of the heart,[63] or an increase in filling volume at any given heart rate as a result of training-induced increases in blood volume.[40]

The cardiac output, arteriovenous oxygen difference, and oxygen uptake for any absolute level of exercise are unchanged by endurance exercise training. As a result, muscle blood flow and blood flow to inactive tissues during submaximal steady-state exercise are not affected by endurance training.

The rate of attainment of the steady-state responses for oxygen uptake, cardiac output, and heart rate occur more rapidly after endurance training.[64,65] The more rapid attainment of a cardiorespiratory steady-state during submaximal exercise after training is possibly a reflection of the increased muscle mitochrondial volume, which increases ATP replenishment and reduces the magnitude of

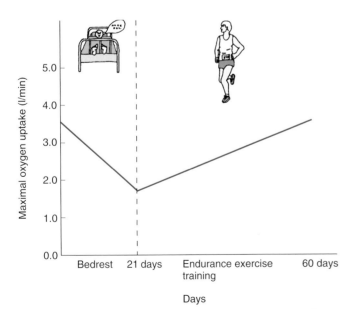

Fig. 11 A representative description of the loss of maximal oxygen uptake $\dot{V}O_2$max with complete bed rest and the prolonged exercise training necessary to achieve the same level of $\dot{V}O_2$max that occurred prior to the bed rest. (Adapted from Saltin et al.[55] and reproduced with permission from *Circulation* 1969; **38** (Suppl.): 1–78. Copyright 1969. American Heart Association.)

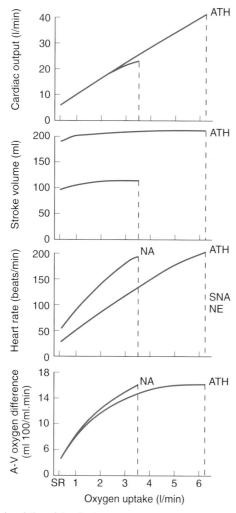

Fig. 13 A description of the circulatory responses to graded exercise in normal active individuals and world-class performers. The large differences in cardiac output range and resting and exercise stroke volumes of the athletes compared with those of the normally active individuals should be noted. In fact, the primary difference in the greater $\dot{V}_{O_2}$max of the athletes is clearly the difference in resting stroke volumes. This difference is maintained throughout exercise to $\dot{V}_{O_2}$max and is evidence of the training-induced increase in pumping capacity of the heart. NA = normally active, ATH = athletes, NE = norepinephrine (noradrenaline), SNA = sympathetic nerve activity. (Adapted from data presented in ref. 33 and reprinted with permission.)

cellular oxygen deficit, and also leads to a more rapid increase in blood flow to active muscle.[2]

Haemodynamic adjustments

Exercise training increases $\dot{V}_{O_2}$max by increasing maximal cardiac output and maximal arteriovenous oxygen difference. Endurance training does not change maximal exercise heart rate. However, maximal stroke volume is increased as a result of an increase in cardiac filling pressure (Fig. 13). The greater preload and cardiac filling pressure of the endurance athlete during exercise is probably caused by several factors: (i) training-induced augmentation in total circulating blood volume probably contributes to the elevation of ventricular filling pressure and is reflected by an increased pulmonary capillary wedge pressure,[66] and (ii) ventricular filling is further augmented during exercise by an increase in the compliance of the left ventricle.[67] Together, these alterations in circulatory blood vol-

ume and the pressure–volume relationship of the left ventricle function to augment ventricular filling and emptying and continue to increase stroke volume even at very high heart rates associated with near maximal exercise. Interestingly, the same alteration in left-ventricular pressure–volume relationships which facilitates stroke volume responses during exercise has also been shown to contribute to syncope and orthostatic intolerance which is consistently observed in athletes.[68]

In contrast to the suggestion by Rowell[33] (Fig. 13), current findings suggests that endurance training augments the exercise stroke volume of the endurance-trained individual. Gledhill *et al.*[67] have reported that stroke volume progressively increased in endurance-trained, but not sedentary, individuals throughout incremental work rates with no plateau. The mechanism mediating this response was thought to reside in the athlete's ability to augment ventricular filling and emptying rates at high heart rates of 140 to 190 beats/min despite a considerable reduction in diastolic filling time (Fig. 14).

These findings imply that ventricular preload and/or left ventricular compliance was considerably enhanced in athletes. This finding has been supported by an earlier study by Levine *et al.*[68], who reported that endurance-trained athletes possess a greater ventricular diastolic chamber compliance and distensibility than non-athletes.

Endurance exercise training does not affect maximal systolic blood pressure. However, maximal diastolic blood pressure is decreased by endurance training, probably as a result of an increased capacity for muscular vasodilation.[69] The increase in vasodilator capacity lowers total peripheral resistance and reduces ventricular after-load. This enables the endurance athlete to generate a higher maximal exercise cardiac output while maintaining a normal mean arterial pressure. The greater vascular conductance of the endurance-trained athlete leads to an increased capacity for muscle oxygen extraction. The increased capacity for muscle oxygen extraction may also be related to an increase in oxygen diffusion capacity due to an increases in muscle vascularity and capillary density. This increase in oxygen diffusion capacity from vessel to respiratory chain enzymes also increases $\dot{V}_{O_2}$max.[23]

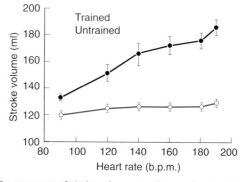

Fig. 14 The responses of stroke volume at each target heart rate during incremental work rates in untrained and endurance-trained individuals. The large differences in stroke volume between sedentary individuals and athletes are probably due to the training-induced increase in myocardial contractility and blood volume. The progressive increase in stroke volume in the endurance-trained individuals with no plateau should be noted. This augmentation in stroke volume, especially at high heart rates of 140 to 190 beats/min, is evidence of a training-induced alteration in diastolic function of the left ventricle. (Adapted from data presented in ref. 67 and reprinted with permission.)

Respiration function

The endurance-trained athlete can produce a higher maximal pulmonary ventilation and breathing rate.[42] However, maximal tidal volume is unchanged by training. The higher pulmonary ventilation of endurance athletes can produce arterial hypoxaemia, thereby limiting $\dot{V}o_2$max.[35] In addition, the endurance athlete can generate higher levels of lactic acid and tolerate a lower pH level, i.e. greater metabolic acidosis. Endurance training shifts the oxygen–haemoglobin dissociation relation such that, at any given level of Po_2, oxygen is released more readily from haemoglobin. The improved oxygen–haemoglobin dissociation may be due to a greater erythrocyte concentration of 2,3-diphosphoglycerate.[31]

Cardiac structure

Endurance exercise training increases cardiac mass and volume.[14] Left atrial and right ventricular dimensions and intraventricular septal and posterior wall thickness are consistently larger in endurance athletes. Endurance athletes have a larger absolute left-ventricular mass and left-ventricular end-diastolic volume even in relation to lean body mass. However, the ratio of left ventricular mass to left-ventricular end-diastolic volume, and ratio of left-ventricular wall thickness to left ventricular chamber radius are unchanged. The parallel increase in left ventricular mass and volume occur to maintain a constant relation between systolic blood pressure and the ratio of left-ventricular wall thickness to ventricle radius.[14,55] Thus wall tension, or stress, is held constant in accordance with LaPlace's law. While the results from humans are equivocal, studies in experimental animals show that chronic physical exercise increases myocardial capillary growth and enlarges extramural vessels.[70] It has been postulated that these changes lead to an increase in myocardial perfusion capacity.[58]

Blood volume and thermoregulation

Chronic endurance training leads to an increase in plasma volume, red cell volume, and hence, total blood volume. Initially, the increase in blood volume is confined to an increase in plasma volume,[9,20] but as training progresses there is a gradual increase in the total number of red blood cells. Haemoglobin concentration is unaffected by training, but because of the increase in the number of red cells, total haemoglobin content is increased. The increase in plasma volume with training is related to the level of sympathetic activity and total body dehydration during the exercise training sessions,[40,71,72] the release and concentration levels of neuroendocrine hormones affecting the renal reabsorption of water and electrolytes,[73] and to the intravascular influx of albumin to maintain plasma colloid oncotic and osmotic pressure.[40,71,72] These alterations in volume-regulating hormones and plasma proteins persist after the training session and it is through these sustained increases that the blood volume changes occur during recovery from the exercise training session. In addition, endurance training increases the renal sensitivity of these hormone responses, producing more efficient reabsorption of water and sodium.[73]

Endurance training increases the capacity to dissipate body heat during exercise.[74] This is accomplished through a reduction in the threshold for sweating at any given level of central thermoregulatory drive, and to an increase in the sensitivity of the central mechanisms. Heat acclimatization alone reduces the threshold for sweating of the sweat glands, but does not appear to change the sensitivity of the central mechanism for heat dissipation. Furthermore, endurance training and heat acclimatization have little effect on cutaneous blood flow. Accordingly, for any given level of heat stress, an equivalent workload is accomplished with a lower cardiovascular strain than occurs before endurance training and heat acclimatization. In addition, endurance exercise training is associated with an increased sensitivity of neuroendocrine hormones responsible for renal reabsorption of water and electrolyte, and an enhanced perception of the need to drink. These changes serve as the basis for the finding that endurance training increases plasma volume and diastolic reserve.[74]

Mechanisms of cardiovascular regulation during static and dynamic exercise

Theory of cardiovascular control during exercise

The primary function of the cardiovascular system is to supply oxygen and energy substrates to tissues of the body and remove metabolic waste products. The matching of cardiovascular and metabolic function during exercise is based on open-loop and closed-loop feedback circuits. The basic pattern of effector activity at the onset of exercise is set by centrally generated somatomotor ('central command') and cardiovascular motor signals (Fig. 15).[9,10,41]

In this model, 'central command' initiates the cardiovascular response and sets the level of sympathetic and parasympathetic autonomic efferent activity of the heart and vascular vessels in parallel with recruitment of the requisite motor units to perform muscular work.[41,75] In addition, this activity is then modulated by mechanosensitive and chemosensitive afferent nerve fibres (unmyelinated type III and IV nerves) in active muscle which sense changes in muscle contractile force, metabolism, and perfusion pressure or flow.[9,10,22,41] Furthermore, afferent input to the brainstem via the nucleus of the solitarius tract from carotid baroreceptors plays an important role in the expression of the cardiovascular response to exercise. Animal experimentation has shown clearly that the blood pressure response to exercise is altered by baroreceptor denervation[76] and recent evidence in humans has shown that the carotid baroreceptor reflex is reset acutely during exercise.[29] Therefore, in addition to the roles played by central command and skeletal muscle afferents in cardiovascular regulation, the arterial baroreceptor reflex also plays an integral role in establishing the level of autonomic activity during exercise.

Adjustment of error signal between oxygen demand and supply

Exercise increases oxygen utilization and hence oxygen demand. The increase in oxygen demand is met by increases in respiratory and cardiovascular functions to provide and maintain oxygen delivery to the active skeletal muscle for the purpose of maintaining energy production. At the onset of exercise, recruitment of muscle fibres and the increase in oxygen utilization by the increased active muscle causes, for a short period of time, a large error signal between oxygen demand and oxygen supply of the active muscle. Since the respiratory, cardiovascular, and muscle metabolic systems

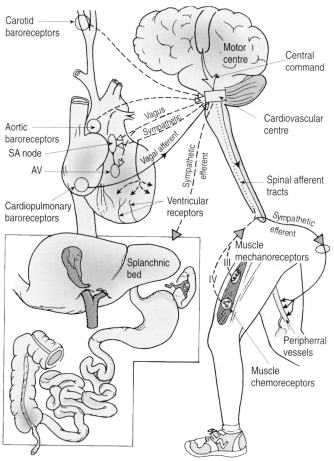

Fig. 15 A schematic description of the neural control of the circulation during exercise. Central command from the cortex establishes the required cardiovascular reference activity at the cardiovascular centre in parallel with the muscle fibre activity (EMG) of the working skeletal muscle in direct proportion to the required force output of the muscle. Muscle mechanoreceptors and muscle metaboreceptors via type III and IV afferent neural fibres provide the cardiovascular centre with information regarding the adequacy of the perfusion of the muscle. The error signal generated at the cardiovascular centre results in increased sympathetic stimulation of cardiac output (heart rate and stroke volume) and regional vasoconstriction. Cardiopulmonary baroreceptors regulate peripheral vasoconstriction reflexly and are thought to monitor and maintain cardiac filling pressure. The arterial baroreflexes appear to act as a brake to increases in blood pressure by counteracting heart rate increases and vasoconstriction mediated via the muscle reflexes. Local venovasospinal reflexes and/or encephalinergic modification of the sympathetic ganglia may play a role in regulating flow through the working muscle.

are partially regulated by negative feedback mechanisms, this error signal (an imbalance between oxygen delivery, fibre activation, and energy metabolism) is detected by peripheral mechano- and chemoreceptors.[9,10] The mechano- and chemoreceptors transmit afferent impulses to the cardiovascular centres in the brain which regulate the dissemination and distribution of efferent signals to target arterioles for the purpose of correcting the error signal. In muscle, the metabolic error signal involves the monitoring of the 'phosphorylation state', which may be linked to muscle blood flow, while in the respiratory system, this involves monitoring the partial pressures of oxygen and carbon dioxide by chemoreceptors. In the cardiovascular system, the error signal is linked to alterations in central and peripheral blood pressure due to variations in cardiac output and total peripheral resistance. The interplay between cardiac output and peripheral resistance forms the basis of feedback from peripheral sensors which monitor blood flow (muscle chemoreceptors) and blood pressure (baroreceptors) in conjunction with 'central command.'

During dynamic exercise, cardiovascular adjustments include a reduction in working muscle vascular resistance, increases in heart rate and cardiac contractility, and an increase in pulmonary ventilation. However, it is not known whether the primary signal is a 'flow error' based on the accumulation of muscle metabolites that activate group III and IV chemosensitive muscle afferents as a result of a mismatch between blood flow and metabolism, or as a 'blood pressure error' that activates arterial baroreflexes and raises blood pressure as a result of a mismatch between cardiac output and vascular conductance.[9,10,41]

The coupling of oxygen demand and oxygen supply during dynamic exercise

The oxygen uptake of an individual with an arterial oxygen content of 20 ml/dl of blood and a total blood volume of 5 l is 1 l/min of oxygen. This indicates that 5 l/min of cardiac output is necessary for effective transport of 1 l/min of oxygen. This ratio of 5 l/min of cardiac output per 1 l/min oxygen uptake is constant from rest to maximal oxygen uptake. In normal individuals, the coupling of cardiac output Q_c and oxygen uptake $\dot{V}o_2$ is unaffected by sex, age, body size, exercise position, and aerobic fitness capacity.

Table 2 Cardiorespiratory responses of a normal man to exercise at maximal oxygen uptake

Condition	Oxygen uptake (l/min)	Oxygen uptake (ml/kg.min)	Cardiac output (l/min)	Heart rate (beats/min)	Stroke volume (ml)	Arteriovenous O₂ difference (ml/100 ml)	Mean arterial pressure (mmHg)
Rest	0.25	3.5	5	70	70	5	100
Maximal exercise	3..0	43.0	25	190	132	16.0	115

The $\dot{V}_{O_2}/\dot{Q}_c$ relationship is also maintained during exposure to high altitude and during anaemia,[15,31] but is disrupted in pathological conditions that hinder the transfer of oxygen from ambient air to the mitochondria.[15,37] Pulmonary disease reduces alveolar diffusion capacity and reduces the oxygen content of the arterial blood. The oxygen content of the blood is also reduced with anaemia, carbon monoxide poisoning, and in genetic conditions altering the oxygen-binding capacity of haemoglobin. Oxygen delivery is reduced in any disease or condition that reduces cardiac output and cardiac function, or reduces venous return.[37] Thus the remarkable aspect of cardiovascular regulation during exercise is the exquisitely sensitive coupling that exists between the metabolic demand for oxygen and the delivery of oxygen to the working muscles by the cardiovascular system.

Oxygen uptake is also limited by defects in cellular metabolism regulating ATP regeneration.[20] Patients with deficiencies in phosphorylase (McArdle's disease) or phosphofructokinase have an impaired ability to utilize intramuscular glycogen as an energy substrate. In these disorders, the coupling of cardiac output with oxygen uptake is disrupted as evidenced by a two- to threefold greater than normal slope of increase in cardiac output in relation to oxygen uptake, and by the reduced arteriovenous oxygen difference at maximal exercise. However, the delivery of bloodborne oxidizable substrates (such as free fatty acids, glucose, or lactate) provides fuel for muscle metabolism, allowing an increase in oxygen uptake during graded exercise and returning the cardiac output to oxygen uptake

relationship to nearly normal.[20] Thus activation of metabolically sensitive muscle afferents by changes in muscle oxidative phosphorylation is linked to the regulation of cardiac output.

Summary

Cardiovascular function plays an integral role in the linking of oxygen supply with oxygen demand.[77,78] During exercise, the cardiovascular system functions to deliver oxygen and energy substrates to metabolically active skeletal muscle. Increases and decreases in blood flow to active and non-active tissues, respectively, occur in response to blood-flow error and blood-pressure error signals. Flow error signals sensed in active muscle and pressure error signals sensed by arterial baroreceptors appear to play a major role in the regulation of cardiac output and distribution of peripheral blood flow. The ATP concentration in active muscle appear to play an important role in setting oxygen demand. The level of oxygen demand in turn establish the appropriate error signals which produce and maintain oxygen delivery. Endurance training increases the capacity to perform exercise. A large portion of the increase in maximal exercise capacity occurs as a result of an increase in oxygen delivery due to an increase in exercise stroke volume, cardiac output, and vasodilatory capacity, while a smaller portion is due to an increased capacity for oxygen extraction by muscle as a result of an increase in muscle mitochondrial volume. Endurance training appears to alter the sensitivity of certain effector tissues to neurohumoral agents, which subsequently alter physiological responses at rest and during exercise.

References

1. Wasserman K, Hansen JE, Sue DY, Whipp BJ. *Principles of exercise testing and interpretation*. Philadelphia: Lea and Febiger, 1987.
2. Wasserman K, Hansen JE, Sue DY. Facilitation of oxygen consumption by lactic acidosis during exercise. *News in Physiological Sciences* 1991; **6**: 29–34.
3. Humphreys PW, Lind AR. The blood flow through active and inactive muscles of the forearm during sustained hand-grip contractions. *Journal of Physiology* (*London*) 1963; **166**: 120–35.
4. Lind AR, McNicol GW. Local and central responses to sustained handgrip contractions during other exercise, both rhythmic and static. *Journal of Physiology* (*London*) 1987; **192**: 575–93.
5. Lind AR. Cardiovascular adjustments to isometric contractions: static effort. In: Shepherd JT, Abboud FM, eds. *Handbook of physiology: the cardiovascular system*, Sec. 2, Vol. III, Part 2. Bethesda, MA: American Physiological Society, 1983: 947–66.
6. Lind AR, Williams CA. The control of blood flow through human forearm muscles following brief contractions. *Journal of Physiology* (*London*) 1979; **288**: 529–547.

Table 3 Cardiorespiratory responses at rest and in response to maximal exercise after endurance exercise training

Variables	Resting	Maximal exercise
Pulmonary oxygen uptake	No change	Increase
Cardiac output	No change	Increase
Heart rate	Decrease	No change
Stroke volume	Increase	Increase
Cardiac contractility	No change	No change
Muscle blood flow	No change	Increase
Splanchnic blood flow	No change	Decrease
Muscle oxygen extraction	No change	Increase
Pulmonary ventilation	No change	No change
Respiration rate	No change	Increase
Respiratory tidal volume	No change	Increase

7. Bonde-Peterson F, Mork AL, Nielson, E. Local muscle blood flow and sustained contractions of human arm and back muscles. *European Journal of Applied Physiology and Occupational Physiology* 1975; **34**: 43–50.

8. Saltin B, Sjogaard G, Gaffney FA, Rowell LB. Potassium, lactate, and water fluxes in human quadriceps muscle during static contraction. *Circulation Research* 1981; **48** (Suppl.1): 18–24.

9. Rowell LB, O'Leary DS. Reflex control of the circulation during exercise: chemoreflexes and mechanoreflexes. *Journal of Applied Physiology* 1990; **69**: 407–18.

10. Rowell LB, Sheriff DD. Are muscle 'chemoreflexes' functionally important? *News in Physiological Sciences* 1988; **3**: 250–3.

11. Mullins CB, Blomqvist CG. Isometric exercise and the cardiac patient. *Texas Medicine* 1973; **69**: 53–8.

12. Fox EL. *Sports physiology.* Philadelphia: W.B. Saunders, 1979: 121–58.

13. Mikesky AE, Giddings CJ, Matthews SW, Gonyea WJ. Changes in muscle fiber, size and composition in response to heavy-resistance exercise. *Medicine and Science in Sports and Exercise* 1991; **23**: 1042–9.

14. Longhurst JC, Kelly AR, Gonyea WJ, Mitchell JH. Left ventricular mass in athletes. *Journal of Applied Physiology* 1980; **48**: 154–62.

15. Mitchell JH, Blomqvist G. Maximal oxygen uptake. *New England Journal of Medicine* 1971; **284**: 1018–22.

16. Smith ML, Graitzer HM, Hudson DL, Raven PB. Baroreflex function in endurance- and static exercise-trained men. *Journal of Applied Physiology* 1988; **64**: 585–91.

17. Smith ML, Raven PB, Cardiorespiratory adaptations to training. In: Blair SN, Painter P, Pate RR, Smith LK, Taylor CB, eds. *Resource manual for guidelines for exercise testing and prescription.* Philadelphia: Lea and Febiger, 1988: 62–5.

18. Clausen JP. Circulatory adjustments to dynamic exercise and effect of physical training in normal subjects and in patients with coronary artery disease. *Progress in Cardiovascular Diseases* 1976; **18**: 459–95.

19. Ekblom B, Kilbom A, Soltysiak J. Physical training, bradycardia, and autonomic nervous system. *Scandinvian Journal of Clinical and Laboratory Investigation* 1973; **32**: 251–6.

20. Lewis SF, Haller RG. Skeletal muscle disorders and associated factors that limit exercise performance. *Exercise and Sport Sciences Reviews* 1989; **17**: 67–113.

21. Ekelund LG, Holmgren A. Central hemodynamics during exercise. In: Chapman CB, ed. *Physiology of muscular exercise*, American Heart Association Monograph No.15. New York: American Heart Association, 1967: I33–43.

22. Mitchell J, Schmilt RF. Cardiovascular reflex control of afferent fibers from skeletal muscle receptors. In: Shepher JT, Abboud FM, eds. *Handbook of physiology: the cardiovascular system*, Part III. Bethesda, MA: American Physiological Society, 1983: 623–58.

23. Saltin B. Physiological adaptation to physical conditioning. Old problems revisited. *Acta Medica Scandinavica* 1986; Suppl. **711**: 11–24.

24. Kaufman MP, Forester HV. Reflexes controlling circulatory, ventilatory, and airway responses to exercise. In: Rowell LB, Shepherd JT, eds. *Handbook of exercise*, Sect. 12, *Integration of motor, circulatory, respiratory, and metabolic control during exercise.* Bethesda, MA: American Physiological Society, 1996.

25. Rotto DM, Schultz HD, Longhurst JC, Kaufman MP. Sensitization of group III muscle afferents to static contraction by products of arachidonic acid metabolism. *Journal of Applied Physiology* 1990; **68**: 861–7.

26. Rotto DM, Kaufman MP. Effects of metabolic products of muscle contraction on the discharge of group III and IV afferents. *Journal of Applied Physiology* 1988; **64**: 2306–13.

27. Strange S, Rowell LB, Christensen NJ, Saltin B. Cardiovascular responses to carotid sinus baroreceptor stimulation during moderate to severe exercise in man. *Acta Physiologica Scandinavica* 1990; **138**: 145–53.

28. Papelier Y, Escourrou P, Gauthier JP, Rowell LB. Carotid baroreflex control of blood pressure and heart rate in men during dynamic exercise. *Journal of Applied Physiology* 1994; **77**: 502–6.

29. Potts JT, Shi XR, Raven PB. Carotid baroreflex responsiveness during dynamic exercise in humans. *American Journal of Physiology* 1993; **265**: H1928–38.

30. Connett RJ, Honig CR, Gayeski TEJ, Brooks GA. Defining hypoxia; a systems view of V_{O_2}, glycolysis, energetics, and intracellular P_{O_2}. *Journal of Applied Physiology* 1990; **68**: 833–42.

31. Snell PG, Mitchell, JH. The role of maximal oxygen uptake in exercise performance. *Clinics in Chest Medicine* 1984; **5**: 51–62.

32. Astrand P-O. *Experimental studies of physical working capacity in relation to sex and age.* Copenhagen: Munksgaard, 1952.

33. Rowell LB. *Human circulation: regulation during physical stress.* New York: Oxford University Press, 1986: 1–416.

34. Poliner LR, Dehmer GJ, Lewis SE, Parkey RW, Blomqvist CG, Willerson JT. Comparison of supine and upright left ventricular performance during rest and exercise on normal subjects. *Circulation* 1980; **62**: 528–34.

35. Dempsey JA. Is the lung built for exercise? *Medicine and Science in Sports and Exercise* 1986; **18**: 143–55.

36. Wagner PD. The determinants of V_{O_2}max. *Annals of Sports Medicine*, 1988; **4**: 196–212.

37. Mitchell J. Exercise training in the treatment of coronary heart disease. *Advances in Internal Medicine* 1975; **20**: 249–71.

38. Stone, HL. Control of the coronary circulation during exercise. *Annual Review of Physiology* 1983; **45**: 213–27.

39. Hagan RD, Diaz FJ, McMurray R, Horvath SM. Plasma volume changes related to posture and exercise. *Proceeding of the Society of Experimental Biology and Medicine* 1980; **165**: 155–60.

40. Convertino VA. Blood volume: it's adaptation to endurance training. *Medicine and Science in Sports and Exercise* 1991; **23**: 1338–48.

41. Mitchell JH. Neural control of the circulation during exercise. *Medicine and Science in Sports and Exercise* 1990; **22**: 141–54.

42. Folinsbee LJ *et al.* Exercise respiratory pattern in elite cyclists and sedentary subjects. *Medicine and Science in Sports and Exercise* 1983; **15**: 503–9.

43. Kaijser L. Limiting factors for aerobic muscle performance: the influence of varying oxygen pressure and temperature. *Acta Physiologica Scandinavica* 1970; Suppl. **346**: 1–96.

44. Klissouras V. Heritability of adaptive variation. *Journal of Applied Physiology* 1971; **31**: 338–44.

45. Lesage R, Simoneau JA, Jobin J, Leblanc J, Bouchard C. Familial resemblance in maximal heart rate, blood lactate, and aerobic power. *Human Heredity* 1985; **35**: 182–9.

46. Dionne FT, Turcotte L, Thibault MC, Boulay MR, Skinner JS, Bouchard C. Mitochondrial DNA sequence polymorphism, V_{O_2}max, and response to endurance training. *Medicine and Science in Sports and Exercise* 1991; **23**: 177–85.

47. Murase Y, Kobayshi K, Kamei S, Matsue H. Longitudinal study of aerobic power in superior athletes. *Medicine and Science in Sports and Exercise* 1981; **13**: 180–4.

48. Hagan RD, Gettman LR. Maximal aerobic power and serum lipoproteins in male distance runners matched to sedentary controls by physical characteristics and body composition. *Journal of Cardiac Rehabilitation* 1983; **3**: 331–7.

49. Upton SJ, Hagan RD, Rosentswieg J, Gettman LR. Comparison of the physiological profiles of middle-aged women distance runners and sedentary women. *Research Quarterly of Exercise and Sport* 1983; **54**: 83–7.

50. Hagan RD, Upton SJ, Whittman J, Wong L. The effects of aerobic conditioning and/or caloric restriction on body composition, maximal aerobic power, and serum lipoprotein fractions in overweight adult men and women. *Medicine and Science in Sports and Exercise* 1986; **18**: 87–94.

51. Drinkwater BL. Physiological responses of women to exercise. *Exercise and Sport Sciences Reviews* 1973; **1**: 126–54.

52. Astrand I. Aerobic work capacity in men and women with special reference to age. *Acta Physiologica Scandinavica* 1960; Suppl. **169**: 49.

53. Hagan RD. The kinematics of aging. In: Nelson CL, Dwyer AP, eds. *The aging musculoskeletal system: physiological and pathological problems.* Collamore Press, 1984: 91–102.

54. Raven PB, Mitchell JH. Effect of aging on the cardiovascular response to dynamic and static exercise. In: Weisfeldt, ML, ed. *The aging heart: its function and response to stress,* Vol. 12. New York: Raven Press, 1980: 269–96.

55. Saltin B, Blomqvist CG, Mitchell JH, Johnson RL, Wildenthal K, Chapman CB. Response to exercise after bed rest and after training. *Circulation* 1969; **38** (Suppl. 7): 1–78.

56. Adams WC, McHenry MM, Bernauer EM. Long-term physiologic adaptations to exercise with special reference to performance and cardiorespiratory function in health and disease. *American Journal of Cardiology* 1974; **33**: 765–75.

57. Saltin B, Henriksson J, Nygaard E, Andersen P. Fiber types and metabolic potentials of skeletal muscles in sedentary man and endurance runners. *Annals of the New York Academy of Sciences* 1977; **301**: 3–29.

58. Scheuer J, Tipton CM. Cardiovascular adaptations to physical training. *Annual Review of Physiology* 1977; **39**: 221–51.

59. Winder WW, Hagberg JM, Hickson RC, Ehsani AA, McLane JA. Time course of sympathoadrenal adaptations to endurance exercise training in man. *Journal of Applied Physiology: Respiratory, Environmental and Exercise Physiology* 1978; **45**: 370–5.

60. Winder WW, Hickson RC, Hagberg JM, Ehsani AA, McLane JA. Training-induced changes in hormonal and metabolic responses to submaximal exercise. *Journal of Applied Physiology: Respiratory, Environmental and Exercise Physiology* 1979; **46**: 766–71.

61. Pollock ML. Submaximal and maximal working capacity of elite distance runners. Part I: Cardiorespiratory aspects. *Annals of the New York Academy of Sciences* 1977; **301**: 310–22.

62. Brundin T, Cernigliaro C. The effect of physical training on the sympathoadrenal response to exercise. *Scandinvaian Journal of Clinical and Laboratory Investigation* 1975; **35**: 525–30.

63. Smith ML, Hudson DL, Graitzer HM, Raven PB. Exercise training bradycardia: the role of autonomic balance. *Medicine and Science in Sports and Exercise* 1989; **21**: 40–4.

64. Hagberg JM, Coyle EF, Carroll JE, Miller JM, Martin WH, Holloczy JO. Faster adjustment to and from recovery from submaximal exercise in the trained state. *Journal of Applied Physiology* 1980; **48**: 218–24.

65. Holloszy JO. Biochemical adaptations to exercise: aerobic metabolism. *Exercise and Sport Sciences Reviews* 1973; **1**: 45–71.

66. Blomqvist CG, Saltin B. Cardiovascular adaptations to physical training. *Annual Review of Physiology* 1983; **45**: 169–89.

67. Gledhill N, Cox D, Jamnik R. Endurance athletes; stroke volume does not plateau: major advantage is diastolic function. *Medicine and Science in Sports and Exercise* 1994; **26**: 1116–21.

68. Levine BD, Lane LD, Buckey JC, Friedman DB, Blomqvist CG. Left ventricular pressure-volume and Frank–Starling relations in endurance athletes: implications for orthostatic tolerance and exercise performance. *Circulation Research* 1991; **84**: 1016–23.

69. Snell PG, Martin WH, Buckey JC, Blomqvist CG. Maximal vascular leg conductance in trained and untrained men. *Journal of Applied Physiology* 1987; **62**: 606–10.

70. Scheuer J. Effects of physical training on myocardial vascularity and perfusion. *Circulation* 1982; **66**: 491–5.

71. Convertino VA, Brock PJ, Keil LC, Bernauer EM, Greenleaf JE. Exercise training- induced hypervolemia: role of plasma albumin, renin, and vasopressin. *Journal of Applied Physiology: Respiratory, Environmental and Exercise Physiology* 1980; **48**: 665–9.

72. Greenleaf JE, Sciaraffa D, Shvartz E, Keil LC, Brock PJ. Exercise training hypotension: implications for plasma volume, renin, and vasopressin. *Journal of Applied Physiology: Respiratory, Environmental and Exercise Physiology* 1981; **51**: 298–305.

73. Wade CE, Freund BJ. Hormonal control of blood volume during and following exercise. In: Gisolfi CV, Lamb DR, eds. *Perspectives in exercise science and sports medicine,* Vol. 3: *Fluid homeostasis during exercise.* Indianapolis: Benchmark Press, 1990: 207–245.

74. Stolwijk JA, Roberts MF, Wenger CB, Nadel ER. Changes in thermoregulatory and cardiovascular function with heat acclimation. In: Nadel ER, ed. *Problems with temperature regulation during exercise.* New York: Academic Press, 1977: 77–90.

75. Melcher A, Donald DE. Maintained ability of carotid baroreflex to regulate arterial pressure during exercise. *American Journal of Physiology* 1981; **241**: H838–49.

76. Smith ML, Hudson DL, Graitzer HM, Raven PB. Blood pressure regulation during cardiac autonomic blockade: effect of fitness. *Journal of Applied Physiology* 1988; **65**: 1789–95.

77. Essen B. Intramuscular substrate utilization during prolonged exercise. *Annals of the New York Academy of Sciences* 1977; **301**: 30–44.

78. Raven PB, Stevens GHJ. Cardiovascular function and prolonged exercise. In: Lamb DR, Murray R, eds. *Perspectives in exercise science and sports medicine,* Vol. 1: *Prolonged exercise.* Indianapolis, IN: Benchmark Press, 1988: 43–74.

1.1.3 Adaptations in skeletal muscle in response to endurance training

Jan Henriksson and Robert C. Hickner*

Introduction

Skeletal muscle cells possess a quite remarkable capacity for adapting to changes in metabolic demand. Endurance training, for instance, induces marked adaptive changes in several structural components and metabolic variables in the engaged skeletal muscles. Different training regimens affect the muscle's content of metabolic enzymes, its sensitivity to hormones, and the composition of the contracting filaments. Other adaptations affect membrane transport processes and the muscular capillary network. The adaptive changes in metabolic enzymes and capillaries are the best-described consequences of endurance training, and both these factors are likely to be important determinants for an individual's physical working capacity. The enhanced muscle glucose transport and insulin sensitivity represents another major effect of exercise and training on muscle metabolism. This chapter is devoted to a

* Jan Henriksson was supported by grants from the Swedish Medical Research Council, the Karolinska Institute, the Research Council of the Swedish Sports Federation, and the National Institutes of Health, USA.

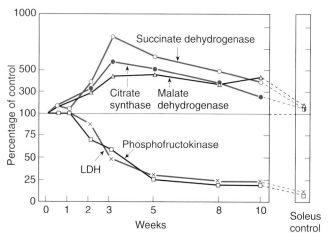

Fig. 1 Enzyme changes induced by chronic electrical muscle stimulation. The rabbit anterior tibial muscle was stimulated at 10 impulses/s, 24 h a day, for 3 days to 10 weeks. The figure depicts changes in three oxidative and two glycolytic enzymes: succinate dehydrogenase, citrate synthase, and malate dehydrogenase are enzymes in the citric acid cycle; LDH and 6-phosphofructokinase are involved in glycolysis. The value for unstimulated control muscles has been set at 100 per cent. To the right, enzyme levels are given for the slow-twitch soleus muscle in unstimulated control rabbits, thus illustrating that, as a result of the chronic stimulation, the originally fast-twitch anterior tibial muscle acquires a clearly higher oxidative enzyme content than a normal slow-twitch muscle. (Reproduced from ref. 7 with permission.)

closer look at the cellular adaptation to endurance training, particularly with regard to changes in the referred variables.

Estimation of the metabolic capacity of skeletal muscle

The muscle-biopsy procedure,[1] whereby small (10–100 mg) muscle pieces are sampled, can be combined with sensitive biochemical techniques to permit the capacity of different metabolic pathways in human muscle to be estimated. Today, biochemical measurements can be performed even at the single-fibre level.[2] The most important metabolic pathways for energy delivery in exercising muscle are glycolysis/glycogenolysis, fatty acid oxidation, the citric acid cycle, and the respiratory chain. The capacity of these pathways is limited mainly by the amount of pathway enzymes contained in the cell. In this context, some enzymes, the rate-limiting or flux-generating ones, are more important than others. Such enzymes have low activity and constitute bottlenecks in the pathways. Theoretically, therefore, an increased concentration of the rate-limiting enzyme with unchanged concentrations of the other pathway enzymes would be sufficient to increase the capacity of the entire metabolic pathway.[3] Generally, however, with a change in the capacity of a metabolic pathway, for example due to training or inactivity, the content of all enzymes, whether rate-limiting or not, changes in the same direction. This can be illustrated by the changes recorded in the anterior tibial muscle of the rabbit in response to chronic electrical stimulation. In this situation there is an almost identical decrease in all glycolytic enzymes, although only one, phosphofructokinase, is considered to be rate-limiting (Figs 1 and 2). The reason for this is not entirely clear, but it may be that relatively constant proportions of the different enzymes in a certain metabolic pathway are necessary in order to maintain the metabolic equilibrium of a cell. Therefore it is possible to obtain a good estimation of the cellular capacity of a

specific metabolic pathway just by measuring the content (maximal activity) of any one of its enzymes. The choice of enzymes for analyses is therefore largely dependent on the simplicity and speed of the available analytical methods. A list of enzymes, the levels of which are commonly used as a measure of the capacity of their respective metabolic pathways, is given below.

Glycolysis: phosphofructokinase, lactate dehydrogenase (**LDH**)

Fatty acid oxidation: 3-hydroxyacyl-CoA dehydrogenase

Citric acid cycle: citrate synthase, succinate dehydrogenase

Respiratory chain: cytochrome *c* oxidase.

The maximal adaptability of skeletal muscle: results of experiments involving chronic electrical stimulation

It is of considerable theoretical interest to know how skeletal muscle adapts to a maximal training stimulus. This knowledge can be used as a frame of reference against which the effects of, for instance, different endurance-training regimens can be compared and evaluated. One way of obtaining such information has been to subject a normally rather inactive muscle, such as the rabbit anterior tibial muscle, to chronic electrical stimulation. This can be done in a way that is essentially painless to the animal. During anaesthesia, a stimulator (of fingertip size) is implanted close to the common peroneal nerve under aseptic conditions so that, when activated, it subjects the anterior tibial muscle to chronic stimulation via the common peroneal nerve. The stimulator is activated non-invasively by means of an electronic flash-gun after the rabbit has been allowed to recover from the operation. When stimulating with a continuous train of pulses at a frequency of 10 Hz, as in most studies, there is a

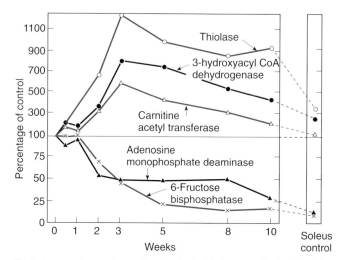

Fig. 2 Enzyme changes induced by chronic electrical muscle stimulation. Thiolase and 3-hydroxyacyl-CoA dehydrogenase represent the fat degradation (fatty acid oxidation) pathway and carnitine acetyl transferase is one of the enzymes required for the transfer of fatty acids from the cytosol into the mitochondria. Adenosine monophosphate (**AMP**) deaminase is related to the enzymes involved in high-energy phosphate transfer, whereas fructose bisphosphatase catalyses the reversal of the 6-phosphofructokinase reaction (Fig. 1) and is therefore required for the regeneration of glycogen from lactate. For further explanations, see the caption to Fig. 1. (Reproduced from ref. 7 with permission.)

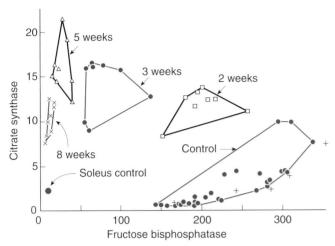

Fig. 3 Enzyme changes in single, skeletal muscle fibres induced by chronic electrical muscle stimulation. The anterior tibial muscle of the rabbit was stimulated as described in the text and the legend to Fig. 1. Single fibres were isolated by microdissection from muscles stimulated for different periods of time (2, 3, 5, and 8 weeks, respectively) as well as from unstimulated control muscles. Citrate synthase is a member of the citric acid cycle, and was therefore used as a measure of the fibre's oxidative capacity, while fructose bisphosphatase catalyses the reversal of the phosphofructokinase reaction in glycolysis and was used as a measure of glycolytic capacity. The average value for fibres in the control slow-twitch soleus muscle is included for reference (for explanation see the legend to Fig. 1). All fibres in a normal unstimulated (control) muscle have a high content of glycolytic enzymes, whereas the content of oxidative enzymes varies 10-fold. The chronic stimulation induces a high oxidative capacity in all fibres, whereas the glycolytic capacity decreases to low levels. Values are in moles (citrate synthase) or millimoles (fructose bisphosphatase) per kilogram dry weight per hour at 20 °C. Each symbol (except soleus control) denotes one individual fibre. (Reproduced from ref. 25 with permission.)

very small amplitude oscillation of the hindpaw, but without any observable effect on the use of the limb in posture control and locomotion or on the general well being of the animal. These investigations have revealed a quite remarkable capacity of skeletal muscle for adaptation to the extreme metabolic demand imposed by the chronic stimulation. This response will therefore be described in some detail in the present chapter before turning to a discussion of the effects of more physiological endurance-training regimens.

The rabbit anterior tibial muscle is a predominantly fast muscle, containing no more than 6 per cent slow-twitch fibres. However, the chronic stimulation programme results in a striking fibre-type transformation so that, after stimulation durations of 5 to 6 weeks or more, the anterior tibial muscle contains only slow-twitch fibres. Simultaneously, the normally very fatiguable anterior tibial muscle becomes highly fatigue-resistant. The increased endurance is probably a result of the pronounced enzyme and microcirculatory adaptation induced by the chronic stimulation, but the fibre-type transformation may also be of major importance in this respect. For a more detailed description of the effects of chronic stimulation on muscles, see the reviews by Salmons and Henriksson,[4] Jolesz and Sreter,[5] and Pette.[6]

Enzyme adaptation

The stimulation-induced enzyme changes are summarized in Figs 1, 2, and 3. Of all enzymes analysed, hexokinase (not shown) displays the most rapid response to chronic stimulation. The main function of this enzyme is to channel (by phosphorylation) glucose,

taken up by muscle, into the muscle cell's glycolytic (or glycogen synthetic) pathway. An increase in hexokinase (which upon chronic stimulation was demonstrable within 1 day, more than doubled in 3 days, and increased 11-fold at its peak) is not normally seen in endurance training, but the observed response illustrates the capacity of skeletal muscle to adapt rapidly to the use of blood glucose as the preferred energy substrate. The absence of an increase in hexokinase in response to endurance training makes sense physiologically, since, with a large trained muscle mass, a high consumption of blood-derived glucose during exercise would rapidly override the capacity of the liver to replenish the consumed blood glucose.

The enzymes of the citric acid cycle and fatty acid β-oxidation are commonly referred to as oxidative enzymes. These enzymes display large increases on stimulation, but the increases occur somewhat later than that of hexokinase. In our investigations[7] maximal changes (6–12-fold) were reached after 2 to 5 weeks. Thereafter, the enzyme concentrations decreased somewhat before stabilizing at a lower level (Figs 1 and 2). It is not known whether this two-phase pattern of change is specific for chronic stimulation or whether it may also occur with certain endurance-training programmes. However, to date there has been no report that this may occur in response to endurance training in man or any other species. It may therefore be speculated that the secondary decline in oxidative enzymes, which is observed with chronic stimulation, is caused by the fibre-type transformation from fast twitch to slow twitch. There is evidence that the latter fibre type is more energy efficient at slow contractions,[8] and this could then at least partly explain why the levels of oxidative enzymes could be kept at slightly less than maximal values after fibre-type transformation had been completed. Contrary to what was observed for the oxidative enzymes, chronic stimulation led to a drastic decrease in the glycolytic enzymes as well as creatine kinase (namely enzymes supplying energy to the muscle during short-term, intense exercise). Following 2 months of continuous stimulation, only 20 per cent of the initial glycolytic enzyme content remained in the anterior tibial muscle. When stimulation was stopped, the levels of enzymes whose activity had increased then declined towards the initial value—at first rapidly and later more slowly—and had returned to normal after 5 to 6 weeks. This was also true of the glycolytic enzymes, which increased when stimulation was stopped, but normalization occurred more rectilinearly with these enzymes.[9] It may be noted that the normally large variation in enzyme content among different fibres in the same muscle, and even between those of the same type, is reduced with chronic stimulation (Fig. 3). However, no corresponding information is available with regard to the effect of endurance training, although some information can be found in Chi et al.[10]

Other adaptations induced by chronic stimulation

There is a doubling of the number of blood capillaries per unit muscle cross-sectional area, thus greatly improving the muscle's blood supply.[11] The time course of this change has not been studied in detail, but preliminary data indicate that it is roughly similar to that of the oxidative enzymes. Concomitant with these changes there is, as mentioned above, a dramatic improvement in the muscle's endurance. In a previous investigation,[9] this variable was measured as an index: the remaining muscle force following a 5-min period of intense muscle stimulation divided by the muscle force exerted during the first few contractions. This index increases from a normal value of 0.5 to 1.0 in muscle that has been continuously stimulated for 6 weeks. Following discontinuation of the chronic stimulation, the fatiguability again increases, with the time needed for normalization (5–6 weeks) being similar to that of the metabolic enzymes and the capillary supply.

An interesting general observation from these chronic stimulation experiments is that the different biochemical and morphological adaptations to chronic stimulation fit into a 'first in, last out' pattern for the response to stimulation and recovery. This means that the earlier the stage at which a parameter changes during the course of stimulation, the later the stage at which it returns to control levels during recovery. (For further information see Brown *et al.*[9]). This may be a general rule governing training adaptations, and implies that a threshold level of muscle activity must be exceeded in order to induce and maintain a specific adaptation.

This summary of what is likely to be the maximal activity-induced adaptability of skeletal muscle might serve as a background to a description of the effect of endurance training on skeletal muscle characteristics. It may be argued that chronic stimulation in the rabbit is quite different from endurance training in man. However, when we sought to reconcile observations from chronic stimulation and endurance training,[4] it was found that results from the two experimental approaches differ only in degree. The properties that change in response to exercise are also those that change at an early stage of stimulation; the properties that are resistant to change under exercise conditions change only after prolonged stimulation. Therefore there is a hierarchy of stability in the properties of skeletal muscle, which is also revealed by the rate at which a parameter returns to control values following cessation of stimulation (see above).

Human skeletal muscle: effects of endurance training

The first observations of the effects of endurance training on metabolic enzymes in skeletal muscle (rat) were made by Russian investigators in the 1950s, but a detailed investigation of these changes was first performed by Holloszy and co-workers.[12] In 1937, Petrén *et al.*[13] had already shown that the capillary network of rat skeletal muscle was influenced by training. The first human studies on muscle metabolic enzymes were published around 1970.[14,15] During the 1970s and 1980s improved methodology allowed more detailed studies both on humans and other species. For the human studies, small muscle-biopsy specimens (20–100 mg) were obtained, usually from the thigh muscle, but also from other muscles like the gastrocnemius, deltoid, and triceps. Different groups of individuals were compared in these studies, for example untrained persons versus athletes in different sports, or, alternatively, a group of previously untrained individuals was studied repeatedly with muscle biopsies taken during a training period. Despite the fact that different parts of the same muscle may often differ with regard to fibre-type composition, capillary density, and enzyme content, the muscle-biopsy technique has proved to be surprisingly useful for these studies. This technique allows relatively small changes to be detected, such as a change in enzyme content or capillary density of 15 to 20 per

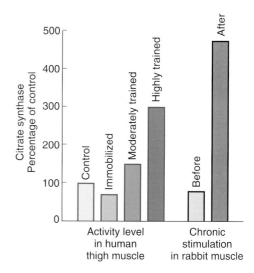

Fig. 4 The influence of the physical fitness level on skeletal muscle oxidative capacity, measured as the content of citrate synthase. Muscle tissue from normal sedentary individuals (controls) is compared to muscle subjected to encasement in plaster after injury (immobilized), or to 2 to 3 months of moderate endurance training, as well as to values recorded in top-class cyclists and long-distance runners (highly trained). As a further comparison, the corresponding values from the rabbit anterior tibial muscle before and after 3 to 5 weeks of chronic electrical stimulation are indicated on the right. (The human data have generously been placed at our disposal by Dr Eva Jansson, Department of Clinical Physiology, Karolinska Hospital, Stockholm; the results regarding chronic stimulation are from ref. 7.)

cent, when a group of five or six subjects is studied with single biopsies before and after training. Generally, however, the biopsy technique is not sensitive enough to allow conclusions to be drawn from the analysis of a single sample. With several samples from the same muscle, the methodological error is markedly reduced.

Enzyme changes

The effects of endurance training on human muscle can be illustrated with the observed difference between endurance athletes and untrained individuals (Fig. 4). With regard to oxidative enzymes (namely enzymes of fatty acid oxidation, the citric acid cycle, and the respiratory chain), the values are approximately threefold higher in the trained thigh muscle of the athletes than in the thigh muscle of untrained individuals. With total inactivity, such as in muscle encased in plaster after an injury, the content of oxidative enzymes decreases to 70 to 75 per cent of the 'untrained level'. It can be speculated that lower levels than this would be incompatible with the survival of the muscle cell. The maximal range of oxidative enzyme content in the human thigh muscle is therefore approximately fourfold, but it can be assumed that a very long training time would be required for an individual to cover this whole range. A comparison with chronically stimulated rabbit muscle (Fig. 4) reveals that muscles of endurance athletes have approximately 40 per cent lower levels of oxidative enzymes than these chronically stimulated muscles. The difference with respect to fat oxidation enzymes is somewhat greater. If possible differences between the rabbit and man are ignored, this result can be taken to indicate that the trained muscles of the best endurance athletes have an oxidative capacity that is 50 to 65 per cent of the theoretically attainable maximal level.

Another important question concerns the magnitude of the

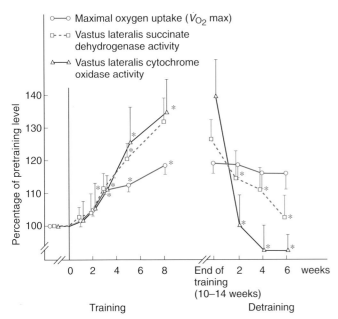

Fig. 5 The effect of endurance training on the content of oxidative enzymes in human skeletal muscle. A group of previously untrained subjects trained for 10 to 14 weeks on bicycle ergometers (40 min/day, 4 days/week; the rate of work corresponded to 80 per cent of the maximal oxygen uptake) and was subsequently studied for 6 weeks after cessation of training. Thigh muscle-biopsy samples were analysed for the oxidative enzymes succinate dehydrogenase (of the citric acid cycle) and cytochrome c oxidase (the last enzyme of the respiratory chain). In addition, the maximal oxygen uptake during cycling was determined using the Douglas bag technique. It is noteworthy that, in the post-training period, the whole-body $\dot{V}_{O_2}$max is maintained significantly longer than the muscle oxidative enzyme content. (Modified from ref. 232.)

enzyme changes that can be attained with a few weeks or months of more moderate endurance-training regimens. Here, information is available from a large number of investigations in which different research groups have studied the effects of 2- to 3-months training on the oxidative enzyme content of leg or arm muscles. These studies have usually involved bouts of 30 to 60 min of exercise at intensities corresponding to 70 to 80 per cent of $\dot{V}_{O_2}$max three to five times per week. With a group of previously untrained individuals, the general finding is an approximately 40 to 50 per cent increase in the content of oxidative enzymes in the trained muscle (Fig. 5). This increase occurs gradually over 6 to 8 weeks of training, with the most rapid change taking place during the first 3 weeks.[16]

The oxidative enzymes are located in the mitochondria. Therefore, their expression is controlled by factors which influence both nuclear and mitochondrial DNA. However, in skeletal muscle there is a tight coupling between the mitochondrial and the nuclear genome, and mitochondrial RNA and DNA are increased to about the same extent as the mitochondrial volume in muscles following training. Therefore, a given mitochondrial volume unit is supplied by a constant proportion of nuclear- and mitochondrially-encoded proteins irrespective of training state.[17] On the other hand, the relative content of different enzymes in mitochondria are likely to change with training. This can be concluded from experiments with chronic electrical stimulation[7] and from studies comparing mitochondria isolated from fast- and slow-twitch skeletal muscle.[18] Regarding the nuclear genome, there is evidence of plasticity in myonuclear number with changes in muscle activity. Therefore,

variations in the amount of available nuclear DNA may be one factor of importance for the adaptability in muscle size and enzyme content in response to chronic changes in neuromuscular activity.[19] Mitochondria reside in two separate locations in skeletal muscle; immediately below the cellular membrane (subsarcolemma) or interspersed among the myofibrils. The functional difference between these two pools of mitochondria has not been well characterized. It has been speculated that the subsarcolemmal mitochondria are involved in supplying energy to different membrane transport processes, whereas the intermyofibrillar mitochondria supply energy for muscle contractions. The recent finding that in trained subjects subsarcolemmal mitochondria amount to 30 per cent of total mitochondria compared to 14 per cent in the untrained[17], would then imply that the relative increase of the energy demand of membrane transport processes with exercise training may be even higher than that of the contracting filaments.

The importance of exercise intensity and duration of training

A question of practical importance is the intensity and duration of training needed to obtain optimal results with respect to enzyme adaptation. For an untrained person, some increase in the muscle content of oxidative enzymes can be obtained by fairly light running (jogging), but the enzyme adaptation becomes much more marked if the training intensity is increased to work rates demanding 70 to 80 per cent of the individual's $\dot{V}_{O_2}$max. In theory, even higher training intensities would result in a further enhancement of the muscle's oxidative capacity, but in practical terms this may not be so since another important factor is the duration of the training bouts. There are no conclusive human data illustrating this interdependency between exercise intensity and duration, but Dudley *et al.*[20] obtained interesting information from a detailed study in rats. These workers subjected rats to training in the form of treadmill running 5 days per week for 2 months at varying speeds and daily training durations (Fig. 6). The rats trained at six different running speeds, demanding approximately 60, 70, 80, 95, 105, and 115 per cent of their maximal oxygen uptake. At the two highest speeds, the exercise was performed intermittently. For each speed, the muscle enzyme adaptation increased with the duration of the daily exercise, but no additional training effect was noted when the daily duration exceeded 60 min. At the two highest speeds, the rats could only tolerate exercise for 30 and 15 min daily, but this was sufficient for training effects to occur that were similar (red vastus, fast-twitch oxidative glycolytic fibres) or much higher (white vastus, fast-twitch glycolytic fibres) than those induced at the highest exercise intensity that could be tolerated for 60 min (corresponding to 95 per cent of the maximal oxygen uptake). However, in the slow-twitch soleus muscle, the enzyme changes at the two highest speeds were clearly decreased. This could indicate that a daily exercise duration of 15 to 30 min was too low to result in maximal enzyme adaptation in this muscle. As might be expected, the initial period of the daily exercise bout gave the highest training effect per unit of training time, with successively smaller effects for the following periods. In a previous study by Fitts *et al.*[21] rats trained 10, 30, 60, or 120 min/day on a motor-driven treadmill and displayed progressively larger increases in the gastrocnemius muscle oxidative capacity with increasing exercise duration. Beyond 120 min there were no further increases. The

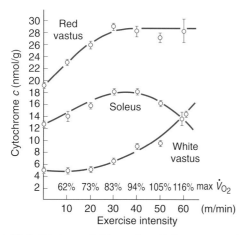

Fig. 6 The effects of endurance training on the oxidative enzyme content of different muscles in the rat. The rats were trained on a treadmill 5 days per week for 2 months at varying running speeds (usually 45 to 60 min daily). The muscle content of cytochrome c, a respiratory chain component, was measured as an indicator of muscle oxidative capacity. The three muscles, representing different fibre types, were red vastus (fast-twitch oxidative glycolytic, type IIa), soleus (slow-twitch, type I), and white vastus (fast-twitch glycolytic, type IIb). The approximate percentage of the rat's maximal oxygen uptake demanded at each speed is indicated. (Reproduced from ref. 20 with permission.)

available data thus indicate that beyond a certain time the law of diminishing returns applies, that is to say less adaptations occur per unit increase in training duration.

Effect of the fibre-type specific recruitment pattern

An interesting observation in Dudley *et al.'s* study[20] was that the training response differed markedly between the fibre types. For a training effect to occur in the fast glycolytic fibres (type IIb), the exercise intensity had to require at least 80 per cent of the rat's $\dot{V}_{O2}$max (Fig. 6). Higher running speeds gave successively better training effects in this fibre type. In contrast, for the fast oxidative glycolytic fibres (IIa), the training effect increased with increasing running speeds up to an intensity (speed) demanding 80 per cent of $\dot{V}_{O2}$max (30 m/min). Higher running speeds did not result in an enhanced training effect. The slow-twitch fibres (type I) responded in yet another fashion. In this fibre type, the training effect increased up to a running speed demanding 80 per cent of the $\dot{V}_{O2}$max. At the two highest speeds, there was a decreased training effect. These fibre-type specific training effects are likely to be explained by the recruitment pattern of different muscles during running. The deep part of the thigh muscle, which was the source of the fast oxidative glycolytic fibres in the cited study, is fully activated during running at 30 m/min; consequently, this training speed results in a maximal-training effect. The superficial part of the thigh muscle, which was the source of the fast glycolytic fibres, has a higher activation threshold. No training effect is therefore seen at low running speeds, but above the activation threshold there is a linear relationship between running speed and training effect. The soleus muscle, which contains almost exclusively slow-twitch (type I) fibres, is fully activated at 30 m/min. Therefore, higher running speeds than this would not be expected to increase the training effect. However, there is no obvious explanation for the finding by Dudley *et al.*[20] that running speeds faster than 30 m/min resulted

in a successively diminished training effect in this muscle but not in the fast-twitch oxidative glycolytic deep vastus muscle.

Fibre-type recruitment in humans

The results of the training studies in laboratory rats clearly illustrate that knowledge of the fibre-type recruitment pattern during exercise is essential when trying to predict the effects of different training regimens. For humans, quite detailed information is available from cycle ergometer exercise at different rates of work. It has been shown that, as in the rat, the slow-twitch (type I) muscle fibres are the first to be activated and are kept activated even at higher exercise intensities. With increasing rates of work there is a recruitment of the fast-twitch motor units, with type IIa followed by type IIb. It is believed that fibres (motor units) of all types are recruited at exercise intensities demanding more than 80 to 85 per cent of the $\dot{V}_{O2}$max. However, very strenuous exercise is probably required to activate maximally all the type IIb motor units in a given muscle (for references, see Saltin and Gollnick[16]).

This fibre-type recruitment pattern probably also applies to other activities, such as running. However, it is possible that the recruitment of high-threshold IIb units is less marked in running than in cycling, especially at high exercise intensities when cycling may involve quite forceful pedalling. Training at an exercise intensity slightly above that resulting in a marked increase in the blood lactate concentration is generally sufficient for a maximal recruitment of the muscle's slow-twitch (type I) fibres. However, there is no evidence that more intense exercise would decrease the training effect in this fibre type as it did in the rat studies referred to above. A maximal training effect on the muscle's IIa and IIb fibres demands higher rates of work—how high may be dependent on the percentage fibre-type composition of the particular muscle. Available evidence indicates that with long exercise durations and the resulting glycogen depletion, there is a time-dependent increase in the recruitment of higher threshold motor units; therefore long-duration exercise would be expected to result in an increased training effect.[16,22,23] It may be concluded that, for a large training effect per unit of training time, it is advisable to use high training intensities. With very heavy exercise, however, the duration of the exercise bouts may be insufficient for an optimal training effect. The rat study by Dudley and colleagues[20] gives some hints about the optimal balance between the intensity and duration of training, but there are still insufficient human data available.

Effect on glycolytic enzymes

The muscle cell's content of glycolytic enzymes is not, or only marginally, affected by endurance-training programmes of 2 to 6 months' duration. The content of glycolytic enzymes is normally low in the skeletal muscles of endurance athletes, but this finding is entirely explained by the large percentage of slow-twitch fibres in their muscles. The content of glycolytic enzymes in this fibre type is normally only half of that in the fast-twitch fibres. The mean glycolytic enzyme level of slow-twitch or fast-twitch muscle fibres in athletes has thus been found to be normal, or even slightly enhanced.[10,24] This finding is in accord with what has been observed during chronic stimulation (see above), when there is a complete fibre-type transformation from fast-twitch glycolytic (type IIb) to slow-twitch (type I) fibres. In this situation the glycolytic enzyme content of the muscle is decreased to 20 per cent of the initial level (Figs 1, 2, and 3), a decrease which reflects the large difference in glycolytic potential between fast-twitch glycolytic and slow-twitch fibres in the rabbit.[25] It therefore seems as if the type of muscle fibre, based on its composition of myofibrillar proteins, is a strong determinant of its glycolytic enzyme content. The same is not true of most of the oxidative enzymes, which change with training and inactivity completely independently of the specific myofibrillar protein isoforms of the fibre.

Effect on the prevalence of different fibre types and on fibre size

When stains for myofibrillar ATPase have been used as the basis for fibre-type classification, most longitudinal studies in humans have failed to demonstrate an interconversion of fibre types (namely fast-twitch to slow-twitch) in response to endurance training. The stable nature of a muscle's fibre-type composition is further illustrated by the results of chronic stimulation studies in rabbits. Although in this situation there is a gradual and complete replacement of fast-twitch by slow-twitch fibres, quite long periods of chronic stimulation are required for this to take place. The fibre-type changes are also the first to revert to normal when stimulation is discontinued.[9] On the basis of these findings, the high percentage of slow-twitch (type I) fibres in endurance athletes and the opposite finding in sprinters have therefore been ascribed to genetic factors.[26] However, endurance training is known to lead to a complete type transformation within the fast-twitch (type II) fibres from type IIb to type IIa.[27,28]

The concept that endurance training does not change the relative occurrence of fast- and slow-twitch fibres has been challenged in recent years. Thus it has been shown, for example, that:

1. Endurance training of long duration leads to the appearance of fibres intermediate between fast- and slow-twitch (Fig. 7).

2. The muscles of the dominant leg in different types of athletes, such as badminton players, contain a significantly increased percentage of slow-twitch fibres (for reference, see Schantz[29]).

3. In several studies of detraining the percentage of fast-twitch muscle fibres increases (for references, see Schantz[29]).

In accord with these results are analyses of the myofibrillar protein isoform pattern within single muscle fibres. Bauman et al.[30] demonstrated the appearance with training of fast-twitch fibres containing a mixed pattern of fast- and slow-myofibrillar protein isoforms. Therefore it is reasonable to conclude that extensive endurance training will result in an enhanced percentage of slow-twitch fibres. The extent to which this might occur still remains to be demonstrated. The reasons why fibre-type transformation was not seen in the early studies are probably that: (1) these studies were too short; and (2) the muscles investigated were postural muscles and therefore relatively trained even in the pretraining state. (For a detailed discussion, see Schantz[29])

It is difficult to predict the effect of endurance training on fibre size, since this depends, to a large extent, upon the fibre size prior to training. However, it is often reported that trained individuals have smaller fibre areas than untrained subjects. The different demands

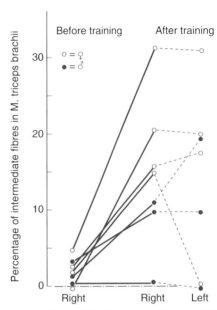

Fig. 7 Increases in myofibrillar ATPase intermediate human skeletal muscle fibres in response to extensive endurance training. Muscle biopsies were obtained from the triceps brachii muscle (upper arm) in seven individuals before and after training and were investigated by means of histochemical fibre-typing (myofibrillar ATPase). The training consisted of skiing with sledges for 500 miles over a period of 36 days. It is believed that the emergence of intermediate fibres reflects ongoing fibre-type transformation from fast to slow twitch. (Reproduced from ref. 233 with permisson.)

placed on the muscle fibre to determine fibre size may be illustrated by a recent training study in humans.[31] In this investigation slow-twitch muscle fibre area decreased with endurance training, increased with strength training, but showed no change when endurance training and strength training were combined.

Effects on capillarization and blood flow

Skeletal muscle capillarization in humans is rapidly enhanced with endurance training. At high, submaximal-exercise intensities two months of training is sufficient to increase the total number of muscle capillaries by 50 per cent (Fig. 8).[32–34] A two- to threefold difference has been found between endurance athletes and untrained individuals with respect to the capillary count per muscle fibre (leg muscles).[16] There is a lack of information about the extent to which capillary neoformation is dependent upon training intensity and duration. However, it is known that less-intense training regimens often result in oxidative enzyme increases without any change in capillarization. In spite of the increased capillarization with training, muscle blood flow at the same absolute workload is reduced in the trained state.[14,35] This could be secondary to an increased transit time of blood through the capillaries (due to the increased capillary density), by which the required amount of oxygen can be supplied at a lower blood flow.

Less is known about vascular function in response to training. There is some evidence from animal studies that physical training may lead to an attenuation of vasoconstrictor responses, possibly mediated via an increased release of endothelium-derived relaxation factor (nitric oxide) (see refs 36, 37). Exercise training was also found to augment flow-dependent dilation in rat skeletal muscle arterioles due to an increased release of both endothelium-derived

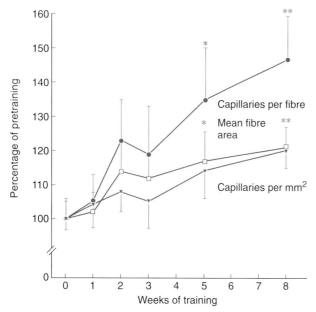

Fig. 8 The effect of 2 months' endurance training (identical with that described in Fig. 5) on capillary formation in the human thigh muscle. Muscle biopsies were histochemically stained for capillaries, which appear as dark spots in a muscle cross-section (amylase–periodic acid–Schiff reagent method). The number of capillaries per fibre was calculated in each muscle cross-section as the number of cross-sected capillaries divided by the number of cross-sected muscle fibres. * (p < 0.05) and ** (p < 0.01) denote significant differences from pretraining values. (Modified from ref. 32.)

nitric oxide and prostaglandins.[38] Peak vasodilator activity during reactive hyperaemia has also been shown to be enhanced with endurance training,[39,40] but the vasodilator response to methacholine chloride (an endothelium-dependent vasodilator) has been reported to be unchanged with exercise training.[41] Green *et al.* have also presented evidence that basal and stimulated activity of the nitric oxide dilator system is identical in the trained and untrained forearm of tennis players.[42]

Effects of training on muscle sensitivity to hormones of the sympathetic nervous system (adrenaline and noradrenaline)

The effects of sympathetic hormones on muscle metabolism are predominantly exerted via adrenergic β-receptors (of the β2 subtype), which are mainly activated by adrenaline. It is unclear whether endurance training is accompanied by an increase in β-receptor density,[43–45] although the existence of this training effect is supported by findings that muscle oxidative capacity normally correlates positively with β-adrenoceptor density.[43,46] This correlation may not be causal, however, since it was found to disappear in the fast-twitch but not in the slow-twitch fibres after treatment with clenbuterol, a selective β2-adrenergic agonist.[47] It may be speculated that the different behaviour of the two fibre types is explained by differences in the specific receptor subtypes in the slow-twitch and fast-twitch muscle fibres. For example, results in the rat suggest that the β3-receptor, which lacks phosphorylation sites involved in receptor desensitization and downregulation, is particularly prominent in the rat slow-twitch soleus muscle (see Torgan *et al.*[47] for references).

When clenbuterol was given to exercise-trained obese Zucker rats, this β2-agonist was found to attenuate the increase in oxidative enzyme (citrate synthase) activity in fast muscle, and also to prevent the training-induced improvement in insulin-stimulated glucose uptake. In addition, clenbuterol-treated groups displayed a 42 per cent decrease in β-adrenoceptor density. These results indicate that clenbuterol administration, possibly through β-adrenoceptor down-regulation, attenuated a cellular reaction essential for the training-induced increase in oxidative enzyme activity and improvement in skeletal muscle insulin sensitivity.[48]

Effect on muscle contractile characteristics

There is some evidence that muscle contractile characteristics may, to some extent, be influenced by training. In the rat, 8–12 weeks of treadmill running resulted in a significant increase in both the unloaded maximal-shortening velocity ($\dot{V}_0$) and the ATPase activity of the slow-twitch type I fibre of the soleus.[49] In humans, slow-twitch fibres from the gastrocnemius muscle were found to be 19 per cent faster ($\dot{V}_0$) when obtained from élite endurance-trained master runners than from sedentary controls.[50] The authors speculate that this adaptation may permit these fibres to maintain a greater level of force production during rapid contractions, thereby reducing the athlete's reliance on the more fatiguable type IIa fibres.[51]

Various isozymes of carbonic anhydrase occur in skeletal muscle, being different in fast- and slow-twitch fibres.[52] There is some evidence that this enzyme may influence both muscle contractility[52] and metabolism,[53] but there is, at present, very little information on its adaptation to training.

Rate of loss of the training-induced adaptation in skeletal muscle oxidative capacity and capillarization following cessation of training

An increase in the oxidative capacity of a muscle, induced by 2 months of endurance training, is lost in 4 to 6 weeks if the training is stopped (Fig. 5). This loss of muscle oxidative enzymes occurs faster than the decrease in muscle capillarization[54] and in the whole-body maximal oxygen uptake that can be attained during bicycling (Fig. 5). The time course of the decrease in muscle oxidative enzyme content following cessation of training agrees well with that observed when chronic stimulation in the rabbit is discontinued (see above). In the latter case, however, the return to pretraining levels of both muscle capillarization and oxidative enzyme content occur simultaneously. There has been only one detailed investigation of the enzyme changes that take place during the detraining of individuals who for several years previously had participated in endurance training (very well trained, although not top, athletes).[10] It was found that the oxidative capacity of the slow-twitch fibres rapidly decreased with detraining to the level found in untrained control subjects. Interestingly, however, the oxidative capacity of the fast-twitch fibres, despite the detraining decrease, maintained an elevated level throughout the 12-week period of detraining studied. One theory put forward was that, because of prolonged endurance training, changes had occurred in the normal impulse pattern of fast motor neurones in the spinal cord. In the latter study, as in Fig. 5, the relative decrease in oxidative enzymes occurred faster than the decline in $\dot{V}O_2$max. In the referred study, however, there was also a significant decrease in $\dot{V}O_2$max after 12 days of detraining (these data are reported in ref. 55). It is possible that these individuals were kept more inactive during the detraining phase compared to the study depicted in Fig. 5.

Possible intracellular signals mediating the enzyme adaptation of training

The enzymes, as well as other protein molecules, have a limited lifespan. They are built up and degraded in a continuous cycle in which the biological half-life of many of the mitochondrial enzymes is about a week and that of the glycolytic enzymes is one to a few days. Accordingly, the cellular content of a certain enzyme is the result of this balance between synthesis and degradation. It has been shown that a change in the rate of synthesis of enzyme proteins is the most important factor in explaining the enzyme changes resulting from chronic stimulation or training.[6,56,57] It is also clear that changes in the rate of protein synthesis with training may be effected via both transcriptional and post-transcriptional regulation. Furthermore, the time courses of the responses of these respective pathways may differ.[58]

At present, one aspect of research is focused on exploring the biochemical mechanisms underlying the altered rate of enzyme synthesis; that is to say, how information that an increased amount of an oxidative enzyme is needed in the muscle cell is transferred to the genes. As an example, the interaction between training and diet for the achieved muscle enzyme adaptation has recently begun to be explored.[59] Suggested mediators for the increase in muscle oxidative capacity include the following:

(1) decreases in the concentration of adenosine triphosphate (ATP) or other high-energy phosphate compounds;

(2) decreases in oxygen tension;

(3) increases in sympathoadrenal stimulation of the muscle cell;

(4) release of substances from the motor nerve; and

(5) calcium-induced diacylglycerol release with the subsequent activation of protein kinase C.

Regarding a decrease in high-energy phosphate compounds as a possible mediator of the training-induced increase in muscle oxidative capacity, this hypothesis is strongly supported by the results of studies where rats were fed a creatine analogue, β-guanidinopropionic acid. This analogue, which results in the depletion of muscle stores of creatine and phosphocreatine, has been found to induce 40–50 per cent increases in markers of muscle oxidative capacity such as cytochrome c concentration and citrate synthase activity. Similar increases were found in markers of skeletal muscle insulin sensitivity, such as the expression of the glucose transporter protein GLUT-4 and hexokinase activity.[60] On the other hand, a reduced oxygen tension seems unlikely to induce an increase in mitochondrial enzyme content, but may influence glycolytic

enzymes. This can be concluded from studies in Quechuan-speaking natives of the Peruvian Andes (>3300 m), where it was reported that hypoxia produced a shift from oxidative to glycolytic metabolism in slow-twitch type I fibres in humans.[61] A reduction in muscle oxidative capacity with residency at high altitude has also been reported in most, but not all, (four out of five) studies performed (see ref. 61). An increased sympathoadrenal stimulation as a stimulus for oxidative enzyme synthesis is supported by the study in the obese Zucker rat mentioned earlier.[48] On the other hand, no changes in cAMP, the β-adrenergic second messenger, has been detected up to 4 h postexercise in rats.[62]

It has also been discussed that the flux through the enzyme reaction may be important, possibly influencing enzyme degradation. Finally, the results of studies on the enzyme 5-aminolaevulinate synthase are of interest in this context. This enzyme is necessary for the synthesis of haem in skeletal muscle. Several components of the respiratory chain are haemoproteins. An interesting observation in training studies is that this enzyme increases much earlier and to a greater extent than the mitochondrial enzymes. It therefore seems that a training-induced increase in the capacity of the mitochondrial respiratory chain demands an increased synthesis of haem.[63]

The availability of advanced genetic techniques as well as improved cell-culture systems has led to a renewed interest in this area of research, and this will probably lead to a better understanding of the mechanisms whereby the skeletal muscle cell adapts to different normal and pathological states.

Muscle glucose uptake and insulin action

Another major effect of exercise and physical training on muscle metabolism is that of an increased glucose uptake. Glucose uptake into the cell occurs by markedly different processes in different tissues. In skeletal muscle and adipocytes, as well as fibroblasts, cellular glucose transport occurs by facilitated diffusion. This process is passive, in the sense that glucose moves from areas of higher concentrations to lower concentrations without requiring energy. The transport involves a mobile carrier molecule which facilitates hexose transport through the membrane. This mechanism results in saturation kinetics of the glucose transport process. The Michaelis constant K_m for the transport of glucose from the outer to the inner surface of the cell membrane (namely the glucose concentration at which the transport rate is half-maximal) is approximately 5 to 10 mmol/l in several tissues including skeletal muscle.[64] Thus the transport rate responds to fluctuations in the blood glucose concentration (more correctly, interstitial glucose concentration), but, in addition, it is regulated by hormones and other extra- and intracellular factors. Specifically, contractile activity and insulin are the two most potent stimulators of skeletal muscle glucose transport.

Glucose is transported into mammalian skeletal muscle by a glucose transporter. The most abundant glucose transporter in mammalian skeletal muscle is the insulin-regulatable glucose transporter, GLUT-4.[65] A second isoform of the glucose transporter (GLUT-1) has also been isolated from skeletal muscle, although the role of this transporter is restricted to basal conditions. Under basal conditions the major portion of the cellular GLUT-4 content is present in an intracellular pool, but upon stimulation (through contraction or insulin) the transporters are translocated to the sarcolemma where they facilitate glucose transport. In order to increase glucose uptake, either the number of transporters in the plasma membrane or the activity of the available transporters must increase. Glucose uptake following a single bout of exercise appears to be enhanced by an increase in both the number of transporters and transporter activity.[66–68]

It is believed that muscle contraction and insulin stimulate glucose uptake through two separate pathways. This belief has been supported by the observations: (1) that the effect of contractile activity and a maximal dose of insulin on glucose transport are additive *in vitro*,[69–72] and possibly even synergistic *in vivo*;[72] and (2) that the time courses of the effects are different.[64] Furthermore, the appearance of GLUT-4 in the plasma membrane of muscle in response to a maximal stimulus of insulin and contraction has also been shown to be additive.[73] This finding agrees well with the recent identification of two separate pools of intracellular GLUT-4, which responded to insulin and exercise, respectively.[74] However, a detailed description of how these two pathways differ cannot be given at present, although this is currently a very active area of research.[75–77]

The term 'insulin sensitivity' is defined as the concentration of insulin required for half-maximal activation of glucose transport; however, it is not always possible to measure glucose transport at maximal insulin concentrations. In such cases, insulin sensitivity is often incorrectly defined as the glucose transport activity at a specific, submaximal insulin concentration. In this case, it would be more correct to state that there is an enhancement of the insulin-mediated glucose uptake at the given submaximal insulin concentration. Insulin responsiveness is said to be improved when an enhanced effect of a maximal insulin stimulus is registered.

Methods of determining insulin-stimulated glucose transport

Glucose tolerance, or the ability of the body to process an ingested glucose load, can easily be measured using the oral glucose tolerance test. In this test, subjects ingest a drink containing 75 to 100 g of glucose. Blood samples are obtained during the following 3 h for the analysis of plasma insulin and glucose. The data are then plotted, with the glucose tolerance being inversely related to the areas under the glucose and insulin curves.

Whole-body insulin sensitivity and responsiveness can be determined using the hyperinsulinaemic–euglycaemic clamp procedure developed by DeFronzo *et al.*[78] During this procedure, insulin is infused via the brachial vein at a low dose (less than $100 \text{ mU/m}^2/$ min), followed by a high dose (more than $2000 \text{ mU/m}^2/\text{min}$), during two consecutive 2-h periods. Blood samples are taken every 5 min to monitor blood glucose levels, and glucose is infused via the brachial vein at rates necessary to keep the blood glucose level constant. Insulin sensitivity and responsiveness are then determined from the amount of glucose infused via the brachial vein during the low- and high-dose stages. As skeletal muscle is the primary site of glucose disposal under these conditions,[79,80] it is generally presumed that skeletal muscle insulin sensitivity or responsiveness is being measured by this technique. Furthermore, several studies indicate that skeletal muscle is the major site of the increased peripheral insulin sensitivity associated with physical training.[81,82] This was recently verified by a study using positron emisson tomography

to directly determine the uptake of [^{18}F]fluoro-2-deoxy-D-glucose in skeletal muscle.[83]

Glucose transport following a single bout of exercise

Following an acute bout of exercise, glucose uptake into skeletal muscle is stimulated. This is partly a direct effect, occurring independently of insulin.[69,70] Recent evidence indicates that the effect is initiated by the increase in cytoplasmic calcium.[84] In addition, however, the sensitivity of the muscle glucose transport process to insulin is also increased.[85–87] Both the direct and insulin-mediated effects of contraction are sustained into the postexercise period. The direct effect seems to be reversed within a few hours,[88] whereas the enhanced insulin sensitivity, as a result of an acute exercise bout (which is not detectable until the direct effect has been partially reversed), lasts longer (usually 1 to 2 days).[70] The rate of reversal varies and seems to depend upon the refilling of glycogen stores (see below). Recently, Cartee and Holloszy[89] obtained evidence that the enhanced insulin sensitivity is indicative of a process which is not limited to insulin, but which may be thought of as a non-specific increase in the susceptibility of glucose transport to stimulation by a variety of agents. There is evidence that the increased insulin action following an acute bout of exercise is, to a large extent, a local effect restricted to the muscle groups that were recruited during the exercise session.[90]

An increase in both transporter number and intrinsic activity has been demonstrated in human muscle following bicycling exercise.[91] The translocation of the transporters was associated with an increase in vesicle-associated membrane protein, suggesting that the translocation of glucose transporters occurs via a mechanism similar to neurotransmitter release.[91] With respect to insulin-mediated effects, the increases following a single bout of exercise result in enhanced insulin action at physiological insulin concentrations[90,92,93] and probably also at maximally stimulating insulin concentrations.[70,72,94]

Glucose transport in response to endurance training

Although, as indicated in the previous discussion, it is a well-established fact that an acute exercise bout leads to an increase in muscle glucose uptake, the question of whether training produces an additional effect has been debated.

Response of glucose transporter protein (GLUT-4)

In their study, Houmard *et al.* found that 13 middle-aged men increased their GLUT-4 content in gastrocnemius muscle almost twofold with 14 weeks of exercise training to the same level as that found in age-matched distance runners.[95] Training studies have since yielded similar results, and furthermore it has been clearly shown that this is an early training adaptation. Thus, if subjects perform exercise training for 2 h daily, GLUT-4 may double in concentration in only 5–7 days.[96,97]

In the rat, the GLUT-4 changes with endurance training are mainly reported to occur in the predominantly red (fibre type I,

IIA) but not in the white (fibre type IIB) muscle groups, thus corresponding to the fibre-type recruitment pattern during training practices (rat). No corresponding information is available in humans (see ref. 95 for references).

In the rat, the content of GLUT-4 in skeletal muscle, as well as the insulin-stimulated glucose uptake, is highly correlated to the proportion of oxidative fibres in the muscle.[98] These results, and the results of denervation studies, demonstrate that glucose uptake and GLUT-4 are regulated in close relation to the oxidative capacity of the muscle and its activity level. The importance of muscle activity is further illustrated by the fact that denervation reduces GLUT-4 more than severe diabetes. The close correlation between GLUT-4 concentration and muscle oxidative capacity may, however, be dissociated under some experimental conditions.[47] Although GLUT-4 is often reduced with stopping training,[99-101] the decreased insulin sensitivity observed with the short-term cessation of muscle training is not always associated with a decrease in GLUT-4 content.[102] These results indicate that oxidative capacity and GLUT-4 protein content do not always change in tandem.[102] Also, endurance training does not result in a persistent increase in skeletal muscle glucose uptake or transport in the rat, despite an increase in GLUT-4 protein content.[103] Furthermore, the GLUT-4 concentration seems to be more decisive for the insulin-stimulated, glucose uptake capacity in fast-twitch than in slow-twitch muscle. This indicates that, in the rat, the limiting factors for the rate of insulin-stimulated glucose uptake may be different in the two fibre types.[47] It may also be, as the authors speculate, that glucose transporters exist in different pools of different sizes in the fast- and slow-twitch fibres and that these pools may or may not be accessible to insulin stimulation.

Changes in other factors which influence glucose transport and insulin action in skeletal muscle

The increase in glucose transporters is accompanied by several other factors which also increase the action of insulin. The glycogen-synthase step is, beside membrane glucose transport, considered to be the most important point of control for glucose uptake into skeletal muscle.[104,105] Several reports indicate that endurance training results in an increase in the activity of glycogen synthase in muscle.[106,107] In addition, hexokinase activity in trained muscle correlates closely with the enhancement of the GLUT-4 content,[108] suggesting that the capacity for glucose transport and phosphorylation are under close coordinate control. Insulin receptor binding and tyrosine kinase activity are unlikely to be affected by training,[109] but there are reports that endurance training leads to an upregulation of proteins in the insulin signalling pathway distal to the insulin receptor, such as the insulin receptor substrate-1 and MAP kinase.[110] Other profound adaptations in skeletal muscles to physical training that may affect muscle glucose handling are enhanced vascularization and oxidative capacity.[111,112] The extent of muscle capillarization may be especially important in this respect, in view of the evidence showing extensive binding of insulin to the vascular endothelium.[113] Recent data obtained from various groups of patients suggest a novel mechanism for insulin resistance: a decrease in the ability of insulin to stimulate blood flow.[114] Since muscle capillarization is increased in aerobically trained individuals,[32] it is possible that the opposite mechanism enhances insulin sensitivity in trained

athletes. However, no clear evidence supporting this view is currently available.[106]

Furthermore, it has been shown, both in rats and humans, that insulin action is related to the fatty acid composition of the skeletal muscle cell membrane. The fibre types differ in the lipid composition of membranes, with the more oxidative muscles containing a higher amount of unsaturated fatty acids. However, in a recent study this factor was found to be unaffected by a 45-day training period in the rat,[115] although it can be beneficially modified by dietary changes.

Contraction-stimulated glucose transport

There is very little information available regarding possible training effects, but Idström et al.[116] and Ivy et al.[117] failed to demonstrate any chronic training effect in the rat on contraction-induced glucose transport in the perfused hindquarter. However, these studies were complicated by the fact that insulin was present in the systems. This problem was avoided in a study by Ploug et al.[94] using the perfused hindquarter, who found an increased contraction-stimulated glucose-transport rate with training, but only in slow-twitch fibres. This effect, which could not be ascribed to an influence of the last training session, was paralleled by signs of an increased abundance of glucose transporter proteins. During submaximal exercise, on the other hand, a recent investigation in humans[118] suggested that endurance training in fact reduces glucose transport. Dela et al.[119] argued that the decreased glucose transport seen in the referred study[118] was due to an increased supply of free fatty acids in the plasma of trained subjects, which would reduce glucose transport.

Thus, when Dela and colleagues performed a study under conditions of a maximal insulin stimulus, which would suppress lipolysis, they found glucose uptake during a superimposed muscular contraction to be increased in the trained as compared to the untrained leg. This may indicate that training increases the potential for an increased glucose uptake during exercise, but that this potential is not fulfilled under normal circumstances. This may be due to high plasma free fatty acid concentrations or to other adaptations which favour fat combustion in the trained state. In agreement with this notion are the results of McConell et al.[120] who found that glucose uptake during a conventional protocol of cycling at 72 per cent $\dot{V}o_2$max is not related to the muscle content of GLUT-4.

Results with respect to insulin-mediated glucose disposal and glucose tolerance

The fact that training can increase insulin-mediated glucose disposal has been demonstrated in a number of studies,[93,94,121,122] but most of this effect is likely to be mediated by short-term effects of the last exercise bouts, which are lost within a few days following the cessation of training (see below). In healthy individuals these changes in insulin action are not usually accompanied by similar changes in glucose tolerance,[123-125] since the plasma insulin level during a glucose tolerance test changes in a reciprocal manner relative to the changes in insulin action (Fig. 9).

In accordance with the notion that the effect of the last exercise bout is the important factor, in a number of studies the enhanced

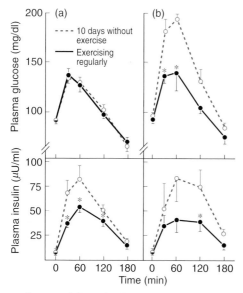

Fig. 9 Plasma glucose and plasma insulin concentrations during an oral glucose-tolerance test where 100 g of glucose was ingested at time zero. (a) Ten master athletes showed no deterioration in glucose tolerance with inactivity. However, the increase in plasma insulin concentration during the glucose-tolerance test indicates that insulin sensitivity was impaired with inactivity. (b) Four master athletes showed deterioration in glucose tolerance in response to 10 days without exercise compared with 16 to 18 h after a usual training session when they were exercising regularly. * Exercising regularly vs. 10 days without exercise, $p < 0.05$ (mean ± SEM). (Reproduced from ref. 126 with permission.)

insulin-mediated glucose disposal in trained individuals has been found to be rapidly lost after the cessation of exercise training.[126,127] King et al.[128] studied nine endurance-trained subjects in the trained state (within 24 h of the last exercise bout) and again after 10 days of physical inactivity using the hyperinsulinaemic–euglycaemic clamp procedure. When the plasma insulin concentration was maintained at approximately 80 mU/ml (high physiological level), the glucose disposal rate averaged 8.7 ± 0.5 mg/kg/min before and 6.7 ± 0.6 mg/kg/min after 10 days of inactivity ($p < 0.001$) (Fig. 10(a)). These results were supported by those of Mikines and co-workers[93,129] (Fig. 10(b)); they observed a reduction of insulin sensitivity in physically trained men 5 days after the cessation of training to levels identical with those observed in untrained individuals, who, in turn, could increase their insulin sensitivity to the same level as that seen in well-trained individuals by performing just one 60-min exercise bout. Nagasawa et al.[127] studied insulin-mediated glucose disposal in rats after 5 weeks of wheel running, as well as 1, 2, 3, 7, and 14 days after the last exercise session, using the hyperinsulinaemic–euglycaemic insulin-clamp technique. They found insulin action to be enhanced in the trained rats compared with sedentary controls; however, the enhanced insulin-mediated glucose disposal was lost 3 days after the cessation of training. On the other hand, Hughes et al. observed an increased insulin sensitivity and GLUT-4 content in the thigh muscle following 12 weeks of training in 18 individuals with reduced glucose tolerance when subjects were studied 96-h postexercise, when they argue that the acute effects of exercise should have waned.[130]

Thus most investigations performed to date indicate that much of the enhanced glucose uptake at submaximal insulin concentrations noted in trained individuals is not a true training-induced

adaptation but merely an effect of the last exercise bout. Although Houmard et al.[102] found no decrease in GLUT-4 content with 14 days of inactivity, glucose transporter (GLUT-4) content has been shown to decrease (20–30 per cent) with 7 to 10 days of inactivity in endurance-trained athletes.[99,101] This decrease has also been found to be associated with reduced insulin sensitivity[101] and oxidative capacity[99,120] with cessation of training.

Results with respect to insulin responsiveness

As discussed previously, endurance training leads to an increased number of glucose transporters in both rat and human muscle due to an increased synthesis of transporter protein. Fibre-type differences may play a role in this process, since Rodnick et al.[131] found an increased transporter number with training in fast-twitch muscle only, with no change in the slow-twitch soleus muscle. It is possible that such fibre-type related differences may explain the variable results which have been noted with respect to the change in insulin responsiveness connected with endurance training. Several studies have, however, shown that endurance training results in an increased insulin responsiveness in skeletal muscle,[93,122,132,133] which seems consistent with the increased muscle content of glucose transporters as indicated above.

Mikines et al.[129] claim that this adaptation is not due to residual

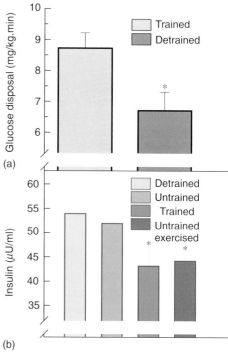

Fig. 10 Effects of exercise and inactivity on insulin sensitivity. (a) Nine well-trained individuals were studied with the hyperinsulinaemic–euglycaemic clamp procedure in the trained exercising state (16 h after the last exercise bout) and again after 10 days of physical inactivity. Insulin sensitivity is estimated from the whole-body glucose disposal rate at a submaximal plasma insulin concentration (78 µU/ml) (mean ± SEM). (From ref. 128) (b) Insulin sensitivity (the insulin concentration eliciting 50 per cent of maximal insulin-mediated glucose disposal) was measured in seven trained individuals in the habitual state 15 h after the last training bout and 5 days after the last training session (detrained). In addition, seven untrained subjects were studied at rest and after 60 min of bicycle exercise at 150 W (mean ± SEM). (Hyperinsulinaemic–euglycaemic clamp experiments from refs 93 and 129.)

effects of the last bouts of exercise. They found insulin responsiveness to be clearly higher (40 per cent) in endurance-trained than in untrained subjects, and that these results were not influenced if the trained subjects had (1) performed one training session or (2) stopped training for 5 days. In untrained subjects, a 1-h exercise session resulted in a 15 per cent increase in insulin responsiveness, but not to the level found in trained subjects. However, in the light of the conflicting data reported by King *et al.*[121,128] the question of whether endurance training actually results in a long-term adaptation with respect to insulin responsiveness must still be left open. These authors found no difference in insulin responsiveness with respect to glucose uptake between 11 endurance-trained individuals in the habitual state 16 h after a normal exercise session and a group of 11 untrained controls. Consistent with these results, there was no change in the insulin responsiveness of the trained subjects following 10 days without exercise. It may, however, be difficult to determine the insulin responsiveness with respect to glucose transport in humans without simultaneously applying a vasodilator. This is because the increase in muscle blood flow at maximal insulin stimulation is inadequate to maintain the interstitial glucose concentration at a normal level. The lowered interstitial glucose concentration will thereby limit the glucose transport into the muscle cell.[134] Compatible with these data are results from Bourey *et al.*[135] and Dela *et al.*[119] showing an increase in glucose disposal when exercise is superimposed on a maximal insulin stimulus.

It may be concluded that endurance training leads to an increased insulin sensitivity, and possibly also responsiveness, in the engaged skeletal muscles. Whether this represents a long-term adaptation or is just the result of consistently performing a single bout of exercise cannot yet be determined. This question may be purely academic, however, and the results demonstrate the importance of regularly performed exercise to protect against the development of insulin resistance, for example with ageing, or to improve insulin action in such pathological states as obesity and non insulin-dependent diabetes mellitus. It may also be noted that not all types of exercise are associated with increased insulin action, as one bout of eccentric exercise has been found to be associated with insulin resistance (see below for discussion).[94,136] However, strength training has been reported to be effective in enhancing whole-body insulin sensitivity.[137-139] An interesting observation was recently made on 19 male marathon runners, who displayed insulin resistance on the morning after a marathon race in spite of marked muscle glycogen depletion. This was termed 'the postmarathon paradox' and was explained by an increased rate of lipid oxidation, which the authors hypothesized to be a protective mechanism in order to spare body glucose following an exhaustive exercise session.[140]

Metabolic significance of the training-induced adaptation in insulin action

Glycogen storage

The main routes of disposal of the glucose taken up by the muscle cell in response to insulin are:

(1) glycogen formation;

(2) oxidation;

(3) lactate formation.

Although the oxidation of glucose increases in response to insulin infusion,[93,129] this increased oxidation does not account for the entire glucose uptake seen in response to insulin. It should also be noted that much of the increase in oxygen consumption in response to insulin is due to increased glycogen synthesis.[90] Lactate formation in response to insulin has been estimated to account for only 10 per cent of the glucose uptake in human skeletal muscle.[90] Therefore it can be concluded that a significant proportion of the glucose uptake in skeletal muscle is directed towards glycogen synthesis.[90,141,142]

Thus a major change associated with the increased insulin action in endurance-trained skeletal muscle is likely to be an increased glycogen storage capacity which allows faster replenishment of muscle glycogen stores following exercise bouts. However, the increased rate of insulin-stimulated glycogen synthesis observed in trained individuals is not great enough to account for the entire increase in glucose uptake due to exercise training.[93,142] It has been shown that the concentration of muscle glycogen is higher in trained than in untrained individuals. The resting glycogen concentration in untrained human muscle has been found to range between 70 and 110 mmol/kg wet weight of muscle,[15,16,143] while that in endurance-trained muscle may range from 140 to over 230 mmol/kg wet weight.[143,144] Particularly convincing evidence that local, and not only dietary, factors are responsible for this difference in storage capacity between trained and untrained muscle comes from studies of one-leg training.[145,146] In these studies it was found that the trained leg possessed from 6 to 60 mmol glucose units/kg wet weight more glycogen than the untrained leg. However, this increased level of glycogen is reduced to that of untrained muscle upon detraining or immobilization.[147] As discussed above, muscle glycogen synthase activity has also been found to be higher in trained than in untrained individuals,[99,129,148,149] and this enzyme can be activated by insulin.[150,151] Skeletal muscle GLUT-4 content has also been shown to correlate with glycogen storage following endurance exercise training.[99] It is therefore likely that the latter adaptation to endurance training is important for rapid glycogen resynthesis following exercise. It is somewhat surprising that no published investigations have actually demonstrated that glycogen resynthesis rates are higher in trained than untrained humans. Data from Blom *et al.*[152] fail to demonstrate a higher muscle glycogen resynthesis rate in the 22 h immediately following running exercise in trained than in untrained subjects, although glycogen supercompensation was seen in the trained but not in the untrained subjects in the subsequent 2 days. It can be speculated that the lack of glycogen supercompensation in the untrained subjects may have been due to muscle damage following such an unaccustomed bout of running. Glycogen supercompensation was indeed demonstrated in untrained subjects in the first muscle glycogen studies performed.[153] In fact, muscle glycogen resynthesis rates have recently been found to be higher in trained than in untrained subjects following cycle ergometry exercise to exhaustion (RC Hickner, SB Racette, C Mier, M Turner, JO Holloszy, unpublished observation). Both the rate of resynthesis over the initial 6 h postexercise and the peak muscle glycogen concentration attained 48 h postexercise were

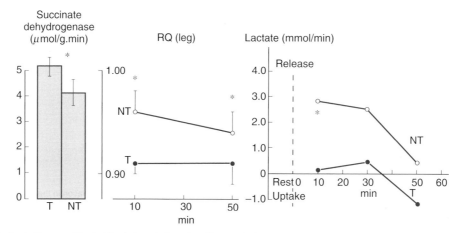

Fig. 11 The metabolic significance of the training-induced adaptation of human skeletal muscle. A group of subjects underwent one-leg endurance training on a bicycle ergometer for 6 weeks. With one well-trained leg (T) (the level of succinate dehydrogenase being 25 per cent higher than in the non-trained leg (NT) (left-hand figure)), the subjects performed two-leg bicycle ergometer exercise at 70 per cent of $\dot{V}o_2$max, in which both legs performed identically. Arterial and venous catheterization made it possible to measure the oxygen uptake $\dot{V}o_2$ and the carbon dioxide production $\dot{V}co_2$ of both legs separately. The $\dot{V}co_2/\dot{V}o_2$ ratio, known as the respiratory quotient (RQ), indicates the relative contributions of carbohydrate and fat to the oxidative metabolism; an RQ of 1.0 indicates oxidation of carbohydrate only and an RQ of 0.7 indicates oxidation of fat only. Thus the middle figure indicates that fat is a more important energy source for the trained leg than for the untrained one. There is a larger formation and release of lactate (right-hand figure) accompanying the greater use of carbohydrates in the untrained leg. In the trained leg, the lactate release is low, and towards the end of the exercise bout there is even a tendency towards an uptake of lactate from the blood ($n = 6$, mean ± SEM). (Modified from ref. 146.)

significantly higher in the trained than in the untrained subjects when they were fed a high-carbohydrate diet over the 48 h post-exercise.

The replenishment of glycogen stores following a bout of exercise is associated with a reversal of the enhanced insulin sensitivity.[154] Gulve et al.[154] found that this reversal was related to glycogen concentration and not to the increased glucose transport into the muscle, but could say nothing about the effectors beyond the level of glucose transport. However, it is unlikely that the reversal of insulin action is solely linked to glycogen replenishment *per se*, since an enhanced glycogen synthesis was found in response to insulin even when the glycogen concentration in the muscle had returned to control levels.[90,141] With regard to muscle insulin responsiveness, Cartee et al.[85] found a complete reversal following an exercise bout even when rats were fed a fat diet after exercise in order to keep the muscle glycogen concentration well below that measured in fasted sedentary rats. The fact that a corresponding reversal was not observed with respect to insulin sensitivity may indicate different controlling mechanisms for insulin sensitivity and responsiveness.

Muscle glycogen concentration and performance

The initial muscle glycogen concentration is important for sustained exercise (longer than 1 h) at work rates above 60 to 80 per cent of $\dot{V}o_2$max. Bergström et al.[155] found that subjects exercising at 75 per cent of $\dot{V}o_2$max could sustain exercise for 114 min when muscle glycogen stores were at concentrations comparable to those found in resting untrained muscle (97 mmol/kg wet weight), but were able to exercise for only 57 min at this intensity when muscle glycogen concentrations were 35 mmol/kg wet weight. When the muscle glycogen level was comparable to that found in endurance-trained individuals (184 mmol/kg wet weight, attained with a 3-day high-carbohydrate diet), subjects were able to exercise for 167 min.

Other authors have confirmed a close association between muscle glycogen depletion and fatigue.[156,157] Glycogen storage in skeletal muscle therefore appears to be one of the major limiting factors in prolonged performance, and accordingly preservation of these stores during exercise is of great importance.

Metabolic significance of the increased oxidative capacity in muscle induced by training

After the cessation of chronic electrical stimulation (see above), the restoration of a normal muscle oxidative enzyme content and capillarization follows a time-course similar to that of the normalization of muscle endurance. This indicates that the adaptations described are of importance for the muscle's capacity to perform prolonged exercise. This can be further illustrated by an investigation in which a group of subjects underwent one-leg endurance training on a cycle ergometer for 6 weeks. With one well-trained leg (the level of the oxidative enzyme succinate dehydrogenase being 25 per cent higher than in the untrained leg), the subjects then performed two-leg endurance exercise at 70 per cent of $\dot{V}o_2$max, in which both legs performed identically. The energy metabolism of the two legs could be analysed and compared by means of arterial and venous catheterization and muscle-biopsy analysis.

As illustrated in Fig. 11, there was a significantly smaller release of lactate from the trained leg than from the untrained one, and a significantly larger percentage of the energy output in the trained leg stemmed from fat combustion. In the following, a large number of studies will be reviewed showing that at the same absolute exercise intensity (and possibly even at the same relative intensity (percentage $\dot{V}o_2$max)), trained individuals rely more than untrained subjects on fat as an energy substrate. This is the case despite the fact that, at a given workrate, the plasma level of free fatty acids is either similar or lower in endurance-trained subjects.

Endurance training and glycogen-depletion rates

Training can result in reduced muscle glycogen utilization during exercise in several ways. The amount of muscle glycogen utilization and lactate formation in the rat plantaris muscle subjected to 3 min of electrical stimulation has been found to be reduced after training.[158] The cause of this decreased muscle glycogen utilization upon initiation of exercise was not clear, but it was accompanied by smaller increases in inorganic phosphate, adenosine monophosphate (AMP), and estimated free ADP concentrations in the trained than in the untrained muscles during the electrically induced contractions. Furthermore, the trained muscles displayed smaller decreases in ATP and phosphocreatine concentrations. The authors concluded that the observed changes were consequences of the adaptive increase in muscle mitochondria (see below and Fig. 12 for hypothetical mechanisms). Furthermore, they suggested that reduced levels of inorganic phosphate in trained muscle might have played a role in the decreased initial burst of glycolysis. The validity of these results was supported by Jansson and Kaijser[159] and Green et al.,[160] who found that training exerts its greatest effect in reducing glycogen degradation early in exercise (Fig. 13).

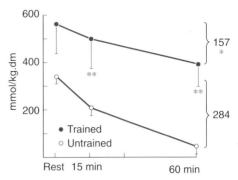

Fig. 13 Muscle glycogen concentration in the quadriceps femoris muscle, vastus lateralis, at rest and during bicycle exercise in untrained (open circles) and trained (filled circles) subjects. All subjects exercised at an identical relative intensity (65 per cent of $\dot{V}O_2$max). Glycogen values are expressed as mmol glucose units/kg dry weight ($n = 5$; mean ± SEM). Statistical comparisons are between untrained and trained subjects: $*p < 0.05$, $**p < 0.01$. (Reproduced from ref. 159 with permission.)

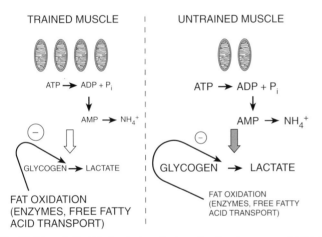

Fig. 12 A hypothetical biochemical mechanism whereby a large concentration of oxidative enzymes (namely citric acid cycle and fat oxidation enzymes and respiratory chain components) in trained muscle would lead to a greater reliance on fat metabolism, a lower rate of lactate formation, and sparing of muscle glycogen during exercise. The increased content of oxidative enzymes in trained skeletal muscle is explained, to a large extent, by a larger mitochondrial volume (volume fraction), indicated schematically with mitochondrial symbols. Suppose that in the untrained muscle there are only half as many enzyme molecules of the citric acid cycle and half as many components of the respiratory chain than in the trained muscle (which is a reasonable assumption (see Fig. 4)). Owing to the lower enzymatic capacity and mitochondrial volume fraction of the untrained muscle, it follows that, at a given rate of work, that is to say at a given rate of oxygen uptake, each mitochondrial unit has to be activated twice as much in the untrained as in the trained muscle. An important component of this activation is the increased level of the degradation products of ATP (for example ADP), which are the result of muscle contractions. These substances must thus be stabilized at a higher concentration in the untrained than in the trained muscle. However, these ATP degradation products are also powerful stimulators of the glycolytic pathway; thus leading to a higher glycolytic rate in untrained muscle, resulting in a greater lactate release and carbohydrate oxidation. The fat oxidation rate is higher in trained muscle mainly due to the higher content of enzymes of fatty acid transport and oxidation. This leads to a more pronounced inhibition of glycolysis in the trained than in the untrained muscle, where the rate of fat oxidation is lower (the glucose–fatty acid cycle.[183]). Together, these factors lead to a sparing of glycogen during exercise in trained skeletal muscle. (Reproduced from ref. 12 with permission.)

Green et al.[160] were also able to show that this effect occurs in both fast- and slow-twitch fibres. Glycogen depletion has been found to be reduced during prolonged exercise in trained individuals compared with untrained individuals working at the same absolute rate (the same rate of oxygen consumption),[21] although the rate of glycogen depletion is likely to be similar if the subjects are exercising at the same relative exercise intensity (same percentage of $\dot{V}O_2$max).[161] Saltin and Karlsson[162] found the latter to be true when the same subjects were studied before and after training; however, Jansson and Kaijser[159] have recently demonstrated reduced glycogen utilization in the muscles of endurance-trained subjects when exercise was performed at the same relative intensity (65 per cent of $\dot{V}O_2$max) (Fig. 13).

The metabolic changes with exercise training occurs rapidly. Training lasting 7 to 10 days (2 h/day) is sufficient to induce a marked reduction of lactate production and glycogen utilization during an acute exercise bout as well as lowering the RQ. Spina et al.[163], as well as Chesley et al.,[164] but not Green,[165] found a mitochondrial adaptation on the same time-scale, which therefore could explain the glycogen-sparing effect that develops early during the course of exercise training.

Lactate formation

It is well documented that endurance-trained individuals have lower blood lactate levels than untrained individuals during exercise both at the same absolute exercise intensity[166-169] and at the same relative exercise intensity (percentage of $\dot{V}O_2$max).[159,161,170] As mentioned above, this metabolic adaptation to training becomes evident quite rapidly. After only 5 to 6 days of cycling for 2 h/day, the increase in muscle lactate during identical exercise intensities is drastically reduced (50 per cent).[171] This is probably attributable to a decreased rate of lactate formation in trained muscles, as indicated by several studies of the arteriovenous difference for lactate.

Thus, while significant lactate disposal occurs in resting skeletal muscle during high-intensity exercise, the lower blood lactate concentrations following endurance training are unlikely to result from an increased lactate removal by resting trained skeletal muscle.[172] Jansson and Kaiser[159] studied trained and untrained individuals exercising at an identical relative intensity and found also in this case that the femoral arteriovenous difference for lactate tended to be higher in the trained than in the untrained individuals at both 15 min and 60 min of exercise. This is in accordance with the one-leg training study shown in Fig. 11. The fact that glycogen depletion occurs at lower rates in trained than in untrained muscle supports the notion of a decreased rate of lactate formation in trained muscle (see the preceding text for references). The enzyme isoforms of lactate dehydrogenase (**LDH**) are also known to shift to favour the LDH_{1-2} (heart) over the LDH_{4-5} (muscle) isoforms following endurance training.[173] This adaptation in favour of the heart isoform increases lactate conversion to pyruvate in aerobically trained skeletal muscle and decreases the conversion of pyruvate to lactate. This may well be a major cause of the reduced glycogen utilization in trained as compared to untrained individuals. The reduction of lactate production with training is also supported by the findings of Favier et al.[174] who observed that after a 3-min electrical stimulation of the gastrocnemius–plantaris–soleus muscle group, the lactate concentration in all muscle fibre types was considerably lower in trained than in untrained animals. Thus, the decreased lactate production with training occurs in all fibre types, although lactate accumulation is related to the type of fibre,[175] with slow-twitch fibres producing less lactate. In addition to the proposed mechanism described in Fig. 12, and the shift in the LDH isoenzyme pattern, the increased capacity of the malate–aspartate shuttle system for the transport of NADH electrons from the cytosol into the mitochondria probably also contributes to the reduced lactate production in response to training.[176] However, these changes, which result in a lower blood lactate concentration after training, are lost upon cessation of training. Costill et al.[177] found that postexercise blood lactate levels increased gradually towards pretraining levels during 4 weeks of detraining. The data given in this section exclude the possibility that the decreased blood lactate concentration during exercise in the trained state is simply due to an increased clearance of lactate as has been suggested previously.[178,179] However, an increased lactate clearance in endurance-trained individuals cannot be ruled out, but further studies are needed to evaluate this possibility.

Utilization of blood-derived glucose

In addition to a decreased utilization of muscle glycogen, the carbohydrate-sparing effect of training also involves a decreased utilization of blood-derived glucose. In the study by Coggan et al.[118] this could account for approximately half the total decrease in carbohydrate oxidation following training during the final 30 min of a 2-h cycle ergometer exercise session at 60 per cent of the pretraining $\dot{V}o_2max$. Similar results were reported by Jansson and Kaijser.[159] They found no change in blood glucose extraction by the legs after 15 min of bicycle exercise at 65 per cent of the $\dot{V}o_2max$, but after 60 min of exercise the blood glucose extraction was considerably lower in the trained subjects, corresponding to only 5 per cent of the total oxidative metabolism vs. 23 per cent for the untrained subjects. This low blood glucose utilization may explain why the trained, unlike the untrained, subjects in this study were able to maintain or even increase their blood glucose concentration throughout the exercise. A lower utilization of blood glucose during exercise in the trained state could explain the reduced liver-glycogen depletion during exercise reported earlier in rats after training.[21,180] Jansson

and Kaijser[159] suggested that the increased blood glucose extraction by the legs of the untrained subjects was secondary to their low muscle glycogen concentration during the later stages of the exercise session. This would be in accord with Essén et al.[181] and Gollnick et al.[182] who demonstrated an inverse relationship between blood glucose extraction and muscle glycogen concentration.

Possible mechanism behind the glycogen-sparing effect

Taken together, the available evidence, including the results of the one-leg training study (Fig. 11), indicates that the lower reliance on carbohydrates in endurance-trained individuals may be explained, to a large extent, by local factors within the trained muscle. These may include a larger utilization of intracellular or extracellular adipose tissue stores (see below), but the high content of mitochondrial oxidative enzymes is also likely to be important in this respect. This assumption is supported by the results of a study in rats in which it could be shown that the amount of glycogen (muscle plus liver) remaining after an endurance-exercise test on a rodent treadmill was directly proportional to the muscle's content of oxidative enzymes.[21] Figure 12 shows a possible biochemical mechanism whereby a large concentration of oxidative enzymes (namely citric acid cycle and fat oxidation enzymes and respiratory chain components) leads to a situation in which a major portion of the energy supply is derived from fat metabolism, with a lower rate of lactate formation and sparing of muscle glycogen during exercise. The training-induced enhancement of muscle capillarization probably contributes to the metabolic adaptation seen in trained muscle. A conceivable mechanism for this effect might involve an augmented muscle supply of oxygen and fatty acids. An additional factor that may contribute to the lower carbohydrate utilization during prolonged exercise in the trained state has been suggested to be increased levels of citrate, which has been implicated as a major inhibitor of phosphofructokinase and therefore glycolysis.[183] However, recent evidence of a lower glucose 6-phosphate concentration after training suggests that the training-induced reduction in carbohydrate utilization results from attenuation of glycolytic flux before the phosphofructokinase step and is not due to citrate-mediated inhibition of phosphofructokinase.[184]

However, increased levels of citrate in combination with other factors, such as inhibition of pyruvate dehydrogenase activity or of cellular glucose uptake, have been considered important in leading to reduced carbohydrate utilization in times of high fatty acid oxidation. This metabolic link between fat and carbohydrate metabolism, which has been termed the glucose–fatty acid cycle (or Randle cycle[183]), has, however, recently been questioned.[185] As pointed out by Green et al.,[186] there may in addition be other adaptive changes, particularly during the early part of training, which lead to a reduction in anaerobic glycolysis and carbohydrate utilization during exercise. These may include the distribution of the workload to more muscles and muscle fibres, thereby lessening the work done by a single muscle fibre. The reduced rate of glucose utilization during exercise after training may also be influenced by endocrine adaptations to exercise training. These include a reduced plasma noradrenaline and adrenaline response to acute exercise as well as a lower glucagon response.

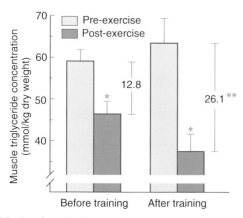

Fig. 14 Utilization of muscle triglyceride during exercise in the untrained and the trained state. Nine previously untrained subjects performed a prolonged bout of bicycle ergometer exercise of the same absolute intensity before and after adapting to a strenuous 12-week endurance-training programme. The exercise test required 64 per cent of the pretraining $\dot{V}o_2$max. Muscle biopsies were obtained from the quadriceps femoris muscle, vastus lateralis. *Pre-exercise versus postexercise, $p < 0.05$; **before training versus after training, $p < 0.01$. (Modified from ref. 169.)

Utilization of free fatty acids

As previously discussed, it is known that, at the same absolute exercise intensity, trained individuals rely more on fat as an energy substrate than do untrained individuals. The source of this increased fat supply has been debated, however, since the plasma levels of free fatty acids are often lower in endurance-trained individuals, probably secondary to a slower rate of free fatty acid release from adipose tissue.[187,188] Furthermore, it has been shown that endurance-exercise training results in decreased plasma free fatty acid turnover and oxidation during submaximal exercise.[188] Hurley et al.[169] studied nine male subjects before and after a 12-week programme of endurance training. When exercising at the same absolute intensity (64 per cent of the pretraining $\dot{V}o_2$max) before and after training, plasma free fatty acid and glycerol concentrations were found to be lower in the trained state than in the untrained state. Despite this, the respiratory exchange ratio was reduced in the trained state, indicating a greater reliance on fat oxidation. Muscle triglyceride utilization was found to be twice as great (12.8 ± 5.5 mmol/kg dry weight compared with 26.1 ± 9.3 mmol/kg dry weight; Fig. 14) and muscle glycogen utilization 41 per cent lower in the trained, as opposed to the untrained state. The increased muscular capacity for free fatty acid oxidation was reflected in the 90 per cent increase in the level of β-hydroxyacyl-CoA dehydrogenase, which was used as a marker for the mitochondrial enzymes involved in free fatty acid oxidation. It was concluded that the greater utilization of fat in the trained compared with the untrained state was fuelled by increased lipolysis of intramuscular triglycerides. This conclusion was supported by Jansson and Kaijser,[159] who concluded that the reduced reliance on carbohydrate metabolism in trained compared with untrained individuals exercising at the same relative exercise intensity would have been covered by intramuscular triglycerides. They based this conclusion on the finding of no difference between trained and untrained individuals in the ratio of plasma free fatty acid extraction to oxygen extraction by the working legs.

Therefore, the notion that the muscle oxidation rate of plasma-derived free fatty acids depends only on the plasma free fatty acid

concentration and blood flow[189,190] still seems undisputed. However, there is still a limited amount of information available in this area. Kiens et al.[191] found no decrease in intramuscular triglycerides during a 2-h bout of one-leg knee extension exercise in either the trained or untrained leg of subjects trained unilaterally on the bicycle ergometer. The authors speculated that this could be attributable to the small increase in sympathoadrenal activity during one-leg, as opposed to two-leg exercise. This sympathoadrenal activation may have been too low to induce intramuscular lipolysis. In this case, it is possible that the observed increased reliance on fat metabolism observed after training was due to an increased uptake of free fatty acids from the blood.

Intramuscular triglyceride concentration

As intramuscular triglycerides appear to be an important factor in the sparing of muscle glycogen, one might expect an increased resting level of intramuscular triglycerides in trained muscle. However, this has not been definitively demonstrated in human muscle. Three studies in which the same subjects were studied before and after training demonstrated an increase in muscle triglycerides of approximately 50 per cent with training.[192–194] Howald et al.[195] reported a significant increase in the volume density of intracellular lipid in fast-twitch, but not in slow-twitch, fibres in an electron micrography study of endurance training. However, Hurley et al.[169] found no significant difference between pre- and post-training muscle triglyceride concentrations in subjects who underwent an intensive 12-week running and cycling training programme. Conflicting results have been found in studies on the rat, where both a decrease[196,197] and no change[198] of muscle triglyceride concentration in response to training have been noted.

Mechanisms involved in increased fat oxidation

If neither the utilization of plasma free fatty acids nor the concentration of intramuscular triglycerides is clearly affected by training, one must conclude that changes responsible for increased fatty acid utilization in the trained state would be related to:

(1) increased lipolysis of existing intramuscular or plasma triglycerides;

(2) increased transport of fatty acids into the mitochondria; and/or

(3) the increased number of mitochondria within the muscle.

The increased mitochondrial density and the increased content of mitochondrial enzymes in aerobically trained muscle are accompanied by increases in the enzymes involved in activation, transfer into the mitochondria, and β-oxidation of fatty acids.[12,16,199] Paulussen and Veerkamp[200] have presented evidence that this adaptation may include increases in the low molecular weight fatty-acid binding proteins, which may play an important role in the intracellular transport and targeting of fatty acids. A change in the activity of regulatory molecules may also be included in this response, as a 36 per cent decrease in malonyl-CoA (an inhibitor of carnitine acyl-transferase I activity) has been noted during 30 min of treadmill exercise in rats.[201] This would lead to an increased oxidation of fatty acids. Whether malonyl-CoA is reduced in trained individuals is not known at present, however. At a given exercise intensity, these adaptations in skeletal muscle would permit the rate of fatty acid oxidation to be higher in the trained than in the untrained muscle, even in the presence of a lower intracellular fatty acid concentration in the trained state. The latter could be secondary to the lower sympathoadrenal activation in the trained state[202] which, unopposed, would lead to decreased lipolysis not only of adipose tissue but also intramuscular triglycerides. Since β-receptor mechanisms regulate skeletal muscle triglyceride hydrolysis,[203] it is possible that an increased β-receptor density may, at least partially, oppose the lower sympathoadrenal activation in the trained state. However, to date, an increased density of β-receptors has been found in response to training only in the rat.[43,44] Martin *et al.*[45] found no increase in β-receptor density in human subjects following 12 weeks of endurance training (however, see the discussion above on the effect of training on muscle sensitivity to hormones). Another potentially more important factor regulating intramuscular triglyceride utilization may be a training-induced increase in hormone-sensitive lipase, the enzyme which hydrolyses intracellular triglycerides into fatty acids.[204] However, no information is currently available on this issue.

Another potential source of free fatty acids for skeletal muscle is the hydrolysis of intravascular triglycerides, catalysed by the enzyme lipoprotein lipase which is located on the intraluminal surface of the capillaries. There has been conflicting evidence, however, as to whether[205,206] or not[207] this enzyme is increased by endurance training. Lipoprotein lipase (LPL) may be activated following a single bout of exercise during some,[208,209] but not all conditions,[208] and it is possible that the resulting variability may mask possible effects of training. In fact, recent studies seem to prove that LPL is increased by endurance training. One study reported an LPL increase by training, but that this increase was considerably blunted by feeding following the last bout of exercise.[210] Unlike skeletal muscle LPL, the lipoprotein lipases of adipose tissue and heart are highly regulated by feeding and are not responsive to endurance training. This difference is illustrated by a study of detraining in athletes, which resulted in a decrease in muscle LPL (through post-translational mechanisms), whereas adipose tissue LPL increased probably yielding a condition favouring adipose tissue lipid storage.[211]

Yki-Järvinen *et al.*[212] recently presented evidence of a feedback mechanism which serves to maintain a certain rate of cellular fatty acid oxidation under conditions of changing inflow of plasma free fatty acids. This mechanism is supposed to involve stimulation of lipoprotein lipase at times of lowered intracellular free fatty acid concentration resulting from either insufficient hormone-sensitive lipase activity or lowered plasma free fatty acid concentrations. Whether such mechanisms are important in explaining the increased fat reliance in endurance-trained muscle remains to be demonstrated.

Amino-acid concentrations in muscle and plasma

In the postabsorptive state, skeletal muscle constitutes the major source of circulating amino acids in the body. Despite this, very little information is available concerning the influence of endurance training on muscle production and the release of individual amino acids. We have found some evidence that trained individuals may

have higher basal amino-acid concentrations in skeletal muscle and plasma than untrained individuals.[213] In this study, we compared seven endurance-trained individuals ($\dot{V}O_2max$ = 59.4 ± 2.5 ml/kg/min) and eight sedentary controls ($\dot{V}O_2max$ = 38.7 ± 1.4 ml/kg/min). It was found that the average amino-acid concentrations in skeletal muscle were higher in the trained group for 8 of 11 measured amino acids, but there was a statistically significant difference only for glutamate (+39 per cent, $p < 0.05$) and taurine (+36 per cent, $p < 0.05$). With respect to the basal plasma amino-acid concentrations, 10 out of the 11 amino acids (all except serine) displayed higher levels in the trained subjects. However, the differences were quite small (16.1 ± 5.5 per cent, mean ± SD) and reached statistical significance only in the case of plasma phenylalanine (15 per cent higher in the trained group, $p < 0.05$). Graham *et al.* found that trained subjects had higher intramuscular concentrations of glutamate, phenylalanine, taurine, and alanine both at rest and during exercise than untrained individuals.[214] In another study,[215] 12 members of a major university track team, who ran an average of 110 km per week, were compared with 13 controls who ran less than 5 km per week. It was found that the trained subjects had significantly higher plasma concentrations of leucine (41 per cent), isoleucine (27 per cent), and tyrosine (23 per cent). Evidently, more research is needed to confirm these findings and to determine the underlying mechanisms responsible for this adaptation.

Exercise-induced muscle damage

Although concentric contractions dominate in most activities involved in exercise and training, the majority of activities also include movements requiring eccentric muscle contractions. It is known that an acute bout of eccentric exercise may result in negative effects on skeletal muscle. It is also known that muscle soreness, lasting from a few days to one week, almost invariably follows eccentric exercise in individuals unaccustomed to such exercise.[216] Such negative effects of eccentric exercise may include a reduction in maximal voluntary force, as well as in maximal twitch and tetanic tension, leading to greater fatiguability.[217,218] Oedema, increased plasma creatine kinase levels,[219] and ultrastructural damage, such as myofibrillar disorganization and Z-band disruption, are also apparent.[220,221] Excretion of 3-methyl-histidine, an indicator of protein degradation within skeletal muscle, has also been found to increase following eccentric exercise. Incidentally, it has been suggested that this apparent increase in protein degradation may be a prerequisite for the exercise-induced hypertrophy of skeletal muscle.[219]

In addition to these effects of eccentric exercise, a failure to replenish glycogen stores following such exercise has been noted in a number of studies.[136,222] It has recently been suggested that this defect may be due to the development of insulin resistance following eccentric exercise. Using the hyperinsulinaemic–euglycaemic clamp technique, Kirwan *et al.*[136] found that insulin-mediated glucose disposal was reduced by about 40 per cent in subjects 2 days following a 30-min bout of downhill running. Ploug *et al.*[94] also observed the development of insulin resistance in the red gastrocnemius and soleus muscles of untrained rats subjected to a single 6-h swimming bout. However, these effects are likely to disappear when the eccentric exercise is performed regularly. Thus prior exposure to the specific eccentric exercise has been found to induce protection against several of these negative effects.[220,223,224]

The mechanism by which this adaptation occurs is not known, but it may be an acute response to eccentric exercise, as indicated in the study by Byrnes et al.[225] These authors have found that a single 30-min bout of downhill running on a 10 per cent decline reduced or eliminated the delayed onset of muscle soreness and the increased circulating creatine kinase levels following a single bout of downhill running performed at any time up to 6 weeks later.

Summary

A proposal has been put forward suggesting how the increased mitochondrial density may mechanistically influence endurance performance.[226,227] It was reasoned that ADP and/or ATP concentrations may be changed from their homeostatic levels less in muscles which contain a higher mitochondrial density, a hypothesis supported by the data of Saltin and Karlsson,[170] Constable et al.,[158] and Dudley et al.[228] This increased proportion of ATP/(ADP plus inorganic phosphate) during exercise in trained muscle would inhibit phosphofructokinase and result in less stimulation of glycogen phosphorylase, thereby slowing glycolysis and the accompanying glycogen depletion and lactate production. In addition, the increased fat oxidation in trained skeletal muscle is likely to have a major role in the sparing of muscle glycogen.[229] Furthermore, Nosek et al.[230] found a strong correlation between inorganic phosphate, $H_2PO_4^-$, and a reduction in contraction force, indicating that a lower increase in inorganic phosphate, and thus $H_2PO_4^-$, with training would result in a smaller decrease in force production of the muscle at the same exercise intensity after aerobic training. The adaptations mentioned above are accompanied by increased capillarization in trained skeletal muscle—which provides a longer mean transit time for oxygen and substrate exchange between blood and tissue—as well as by a possible increase in Na^+–K^+ pump activity with training—this would enhance the reuptake of K^+ and thereby delay fatigue of the contraction process.[231] After several years of endurance training, fibre-type transformations from fast twitch to slow twitch[29] (which would serve to increase the overall muscle oxidative capacity and possibly also reduce energy expenditure[8]) would be expected to raise the endurance capacity of the muscle still further. The increased insulin action in the skeletal muscle of individuals regularly involved in endurance training demonstrates the importance of consistent exercise if insulin action is to be improved in pathological states such as obesity and type II diabetes, as well as protecting against the development of insulin resistance with ageing. However, the training-induced adaptations in skeletal muscle must be considered in the light of adaptations in all other organs and organ systems of the body in order to obtain an accurate picture of how endurance training may influence the metabolic homeostasis of the organism as a whole.

References

1. Bergström J. Muscle electrolytes in man. *Scandinavian Journal of Clinical and Laboratory Investigation* 1962; **68** (Suppl.): 1–110.
2. Lowry OH, Passonneau JV. *A flexible system of enzymatic analysis.* New York: Academic Press, 1972.
3. Newsholme EA, Leech AR, eds. *Biochemistry for the medical sciences.* Chichester: John Wiley and Sons Ltd, 1983: 38–42.
4. Salmons S, Henriksson J. The adaptive response of skeletal muscle to increased use. *Muscle and Nerve* 1981; **4**: 94–105.
5. Jolesz F, Sreter FA. Development, innervation, and activity-pattern induced changes in skeletal muscle. *Annual Review of Physiology* 1981; **43**: 531–52.
6. Pette D. Activity-induced fast to slow transitions in mammalian muscle. *Medicine and Science in Sports and Exercise* 1984; **16**: 517–28.
7. Henriksson J, Chi MM-Y, Hintz CS, et al. Chronic stimulation of mammalian muscle: changes in enzymes of six metabolic pathways. *American Journal of Physiology* 1986; **251**: C614–32.
8. Crow M, Kushmerick MJ. Chemical energetics of slow- and fast-twitch muscles of the mouse. *Journal of General Physiology* 1982; **79**: 147–66.
9. Brown JMC, Henriksson J, Salmons S. Restoration of fast muscle characteristics following cessation of chronic stimulation: physiological, histochemical and metabolic changes during slow-to-fast transformation. *Proceedings of the Royal Society of London* 1989; **235**: 321–46.
10. Chi MM-Y, Hintz CS, Coyle E, et al. Effects of detraining on enzymes of energy metabolism in individual human muscle fibres. *American Journal of Physiology* 1983; **244**: C276–87.
11. Brown MD, Cotter MA, Hudlicka O, Vrbová G. The effects of different patterns of muscle activity on capillary density, mechanical properties and structure of slow and fast rabbit muscles. *Pflügers Archiv* 1976; **361**: 241–50.
12. Holloszy JO, Booth FW. Biochemical adaptations to endurance exercise in muscle. *Annual Review of Physiology* 1976; **38**: 273–91.
13. Petrén T, Sjöstrand T, Sylvén B. Der Einfluss des Trainings auf die Häufigkeit der Capillaren in Herz- und Skeletmuskulatur. *Arbeitsphysiologie* 1937; **9**: 376–86.
14. Varnauskas E, Björntorp P, Fahlén M, Prerovsky I, Stenberg J. Effects of physical training on exercise blood flow and enzymatic activity in skeletal muscle. *Cardiovascular Research* 1970; **4**: 418–22.
15. Gollnick PD, Armstrong RB, Saubert IV CW, Piehl K, Saltin B. Enzyme activity and fiber composition in skeletal muscle of untrained and trained men. *Journal of Applied Physiology* 1972; **33**: 312–19.
16. Saltin B, Gollnick PD. Skeletal muscle adaptability: significance for metabolism and performance. In: Peachy LD, et al., eds. *Handbook of physiology—skeletal muscle.* Bethesda, MD: American Physiological Society, 1983; **19**, 555–631.
17. Puntschart A, Claassen H, Jostarndt K, Hoppeler H, Billeter R. mRNAs enzymes involved in energy metabolism and mtDNA are increased in endurance-trained athletes. *American Journal of Physiology* 1995; **269**: C619–25.
18. Jackman MR, Willis WT. Characteristics of mitochondria isolated from type I and type IIb skeletal muscle. *American Journal of Physiology* 1996; **270**: C673–8.
19. Allen WJ, Mont MA, Talmadge RJ, Rubenstein A, Edgerton VR. Plasticity of myonuclear number in hypertrophied and atrophied mammalian skeletal muscle fibers. *Journal of Applied Physiology* 1995; **78**: 1969–76.
20. Dudley GA, Abraham WM, Terjung RL. Influence of exercise intensity and duration on biochemical adaptations in skeletal muscle. *Journal of Applied Physiology* 1982; **53**: 844–50.
21. Fitts RH, Booth FW, Winder WW, Holloszy JO. Skeletal muscle respiratory capacity, endurance, and glycogen utilization. *American Journal of Physiology* 1975; **228**: 1029–33.
22. Vollestad NK, Vaage O, Hermansen L. Muscle glycogen depletion patterns in type I and subgroups of type II fibres during prolonged severe exercise in man. *Acta Physiologica Scandinavica* 1984; **122**: 433–41.
23. Ball-Burnett M, Green HJ, Houston ME. Energy metabolism in human slow and fast twitch fibres during prolonged cycle exercise. *Journal of Physiology* 1991; **437**: 257–67.

24. Essén-Gustavsson B, Henriksson J. Enzyme levels in pools of microdissected human muscle fibres of identified type. Adaptive response to exercise. *Acta Physiologica Scandinavica* 1984; **120**: 505–15.

25. Chi MM-Y, Hintz CS, Henriksson J, *et al*. Chronic stimulation of mammalian muscle: enzyme changes in individual fibres. *American Journal of Physiology* 1986; **251**: C633–42.

26. Komi PV, Viitasalo JT, Havu M, Thorstensson A, Karlsson J. Physiological and structural performance capacity: effect of heredity. In: Komi PV, ed. *International series of biomechanics*. Baltimore, MD: University Park Press, 1976: 118–23.

27. Andersen P, Henriksson J. Training induced changes in the subgroups of human type II skeletal muscle fibres. *Acta Physiologica Scandinavica* 1977; **99**: 123–5.

28. Jansson E, Kaijser L. Muscle adaptation to extreme endurance training in man. *Acta Physiologica Scandinavica* 1977; **100**: 315–24.

29. Schantz P. Plasticity of human skeletal muscle. *Acta Physiologica Scandinavica* 1986; **128** (Suppl. 558): 1–62.

30. Baumann H, Jäggi M, Soland F, Howald H, Schaub MC. Exercise training induces transitions of myosin isoform subunits within histochemically typed human muscle fibres. *Pflügers Archiv* 1987; **409**: 349–60.

31. Kraemer WJ, Patton JF, Gordon SE, *et al*. Compatibility of high-intensity strength and endurance training on hormonal and skeletal muscle adaptations. *Journal of Applied Physiology* 1995; **78**: 976–89.

32. Andersen P, Henriksson J. Capillary supply of the quadriceps femoris muscle of man: adaptive response to exercise. *Journal of Physiology* 1977; **270**: 677–90.

33. Brodal P, Ingjer F, Hermansen L. Capillary supply of skeletal muscle fibres in untrained and enduranced-trained men. *American Journal of Physiology* 1977; **232**: H705–12.

34. Ingjer F. Effects of endurance training on muscle fibre ATP-ase activity, capillary supply and mitochondrial content in man. *Journal of Physiology (London)* 1979; **294**: 419–22.

35. Grimby G, Häggendal E, Saltin B. Local Xenon-133 clearance from the quadriceps muscle during exercise in man. *Journal of Applied Physiology* 1967; **22**: 305–10.

36. Jansakul C. Effect of swimming on vascular reactivity to phenylephrine and KCl in male rats. *British Journal of Pharmacology* 1995; **115**: 587–94.

37. Negrao CE, Irigoyen MC, Moreira ED, Brum PC, Freire PM, Krieger EM. Effect of exercise training on RSNA, baroreflex control, and blood pressure responsiveness. *American Journal of Physiology* 1993; **265**: R365–70.

38. Koller A, Huang A, Sun D, Kaley G. Exercise training augments flow-dependent dilation in rat skeletal muscle arterioles. Role of endothelial nitric oxide and prostaglandins. *Circulation Research* 1995; **76**: 544–50.

39. Snell PG, Martin WH, Buckey JC, Blomqvist CG. Maximal vascular leg conductance in trained and untrained men. *Journal of Applied Physiology* 1987; **62**: 606–10.

40. Martin WH III, Ogawa T, Kohrt WM, *et al*. Effects of aging, gender, and physical training on peripheral vascular function. *Circulation* 1991; **84**: 654–64.

41. Green DJ, Cable NT, Fox C, Rankin JM, Taylor RR. Modification of forearm resistance vessels by exercise training in young men. *Journal of Applied Physiology* 1994; **77**: 1829–33.

42. Green DJ, Fowler DT, O'Driscoll JG, Blanksby BA, Taylor RR. Endothelium-derived nitric oxide activity in forearm vessels of tennis players. *Journal of Applied Physiology* 1996; **81**: 943–8.

43. Williams RS, Caron MG, Daniel K. Skeletal muscle b-adrenergic receptors: variations due to fiber type and training. *American Journal of Physiology* 1984; **246**: E160–7.

44. Buckenmeyer PJ, Goldfarb AH, Partilla JS, Pineyro MA, Dax

45. EM. Endurance training, not acute exercise, differentially alters b-receptors and cyclase in skeletal fiber types. *American Journal of Physiology* 1990; **258**: E71–7.

45. Martin WH III, Coggan AR, Spina RJ, Saffitz JE. Effects of fiber type and training an b-adrenoceptor density in human skeletal muscle. *American Journal of Physiology* 1989; **257**: E736–42.

46. Plourde G, Rousseau-Migneron S, Nadeau A. Effect of endurance training on b-adrenergic system in three different skeletal muscles. *Journal of Applied Physiology* 1993; **74**: 1641–6.

47. Torgan CE, Etgen GJ Jr, Kang HY, Ivy JL. Fiber type-specific effects of clenbuterol and exercise training on insulin-resistant muscle. *Journal of Applied Physiology* 1995; **79**: 163–7.

48. Torgan CE, Etgen GJ Jr, Brozinick JT Jr, Wilcox RE, Ivy JL. Interaction of aerobic exercise training and clenbuterol: effects on insulin-resistant muscle. *Journal of Applied Physiology* 1993; **75**: 1471–6.

49. Schluter JM, Fitts RH. Shortening velocity and ATPase activity of rat skeletal muscle fibers: effects of endurance exercise training. *American Journal of Physiology* 1994; **266**: C1699–713.

50. Widrick JJ, Trappe SW, Blaser CA, Costill DL, Fitts RH. Isometric force and maximal shortening velocity of single muscle fibers from elite master runners. *American Journal of Physiology* 1996; **271**: C666–75.

51. Widrick JJ, Trappe SW, Costill DL, Fitts RH. Force-velocity and force-power properties of single muscle fibers from elite master runners and sedentary men. *American Journal of Physiology* 1996; **271**: C676–83.

52. Geers C, Wetzel P, Gros G. Is carbonic anhydrase required for contraction of skeletal muscle? *News in Physiological Sciences* 1991; **6**: 78–82.

53. Geers C, Benz K, Gros G. Effects of carbonic anhydrase inhibitors on oxygen consumption and lactate accumulation in skeletal muscle. *Comparative Biochemistry and Physiology* 1995; **112**: 111–17.

54. Schantz P, Henriksson J, Jansson E. Adaptation of human skeletal muscle to endurance training of long duration. *Clinical Physiology* 1983; **3**: 141–51.

55. Coyle EF, Martin WH III, Sinacore DR, Joyner MJ, Hagberg JM, Holloszy JO. Time course of loss of adaptations after stopping prolonged intense endurance training. *Journal of Applied Physiology* 1984; **57**: 1857–64.

56. Booth FW, Holloszy JO. Cytochrome c turnover in rat skeletal muscles. *Journal of Biological Chemistry* 1977; **252**: 416–19.

57. Williams RS, Salmons S, Newsholme EA, Kaufman RE, Mellor J. Regulation of nuclear and mitochondrial expression by contractile activity in skeletal muscle. *Journal of Biological Chemistry* 1986; **261**: 376–80.

58. Neufer PD, Dohm GL. Exercise induces a transient increase in transcription of the GLUT-4 gene in skeletal muscle. *American Journal of Physiology* 1993; **265**: C1597–603.

59. Helge JW, Richter EA, Kiens B. Interaction of training and diet on metabolism and endurance during exercise in man. *Journal of Physiology* 1996; **492**: 293–306.

60. Ren J-M, Semenkovich CF, Holloszy JO. Adaptation of muscle to creatine depletion: effect on GLUT-4 glucose transporter expression. *American Journal of Physiology* 1993; **264**: C146–50.

61. Rosser BWC, Hochachka PW. Metabolic capacity of muscle fibers from high-altitude natives. *European Journal of Applied Physiology* 1993; **67**: 513–17.

62. Sheldon A, Booth FW, Kirby CR. cAMP levels in fast- and slow-twitch skeletal muscle after an acute bout of aerobic exercise. *American Journal of Physiology* 1993; **264**: C1500–4.

63. Town GP, Essig DA. Cytochrome oxidase in muscle of endurance-trained rats: subunit mRNA contents and heme synthesis. *Journal of Applied Physiology* 1993; **74**: 192–6.

64. Wallberg-Henriksson H. Glucose transport into skeletal muscle:

influence of contractile activity, insulin, catecholamines and diabetes mellitus. *Acta Physiologica Scandinavica* 1987; **131** (Suppl. 564): 1–80.

65. Klip A, Paquet MR. Glucose transport and glucose transporters in muscle and their metabolic regulation. *Diabetes Care* 1990; **13**: 228–43.

66. Douen AG, Ramlal T, Klip A, Young DA, Cartee GD, Holloszy JO. Exercise-induced increase in glucose transporters in plasma membranes of rat skeletal muscle. *Endocrinology* 1989; **124**: 449–54.

67. Sternlicht E, Barnard RJ, Grimditch GK. Exercise and insulin stimulate skeletal muscle glucose transport through different mechanisms. *American Journal of Physiology* 1989; **256**: E227–30.

68. Goodyear LJ, Hirshman MF, King PA, Horton ED, Thompson CM, Horton ES. Skeletal muscle plasma membrane glucose transport and glucose transporters after exercise. *Journal of Applied Physiology* 1990; **68**: 193–8.

69. Nesher R, Karl IE, Kipnis DM. Dissociation of effects of insulin and contraction on glucose transport in rat epitrochlearis muscle. *American Journal of Physiology* 1985; **249**: C226–32.

70. Wallberg-Henriksson H, Constable SH, Young DA, Holloszy JO. Glucose transport into rat skeletal muscle: interaction between exercise and insulin. *Journal of Applied Physiology* 1988; **65**: 909–13.

71. Garetto LP, Richter EA, Goodman MN, Ruderman NB. Enhanced muscle glucose metabolism after exercise in the rat: the two phases. *American Journal of Physiology* 1984; **246**: E471–5.

72. Wasserman DH, Geer R, Rice DE, et al. Interaction of exercise and insulin action in humans. *American Journal of Physiology* 1991; **260**: E37–45.

73. Gao J, Ren J, Gulve EA, Holloszy JO. Additive effect of contractions and insulin on GLUT-4 translocation into the sarcolemma. *Journal of Applied Physiology* 1994; **77**: 1597–601.

74. Coderre L, Kandror KV, Vallega G, Pilch PF. Identification and characterization of an exercise-sensitive pool of glucose transporters in skeletal muscle. *Journal of Biological Chemistry* 1995; **270**: 27584–8.

75. Sherman LA, Hirshman MF, Cormont M, Le Marchand-Brustel Y, Goodyear LJ. Differential effects of insulin and exercise on Rab4 distribution in rat skeletal muscle. *Endocrinology* 1996; **137**: 266–73.

76. Lee AD, Hansen PA, Holloszy JO. Wortmannin inhibits insulin-stimulated but not contraction-stimulated glucose transport activity in skeletal muscle. *Federation of European Biochemical Societies* 1995; **361**: 51–4.

77. Brozinick JT Jr, Etgen GJ Jr, Yaspelkis BB III, Ivy JL. The effects of muscle contraction and insulin on glucose-transporter translocation in rat skeletal muscle. *Biochemical Journal* 1994; **297**: 539–45.

78. DeFronzo RA, Tobin JD, Andres R. Glucose clamp technique: a method for quantifying insulin secretion and resistance. *American Journal of Physiology* 1979; **237**: E214–23.

79. DeFronzo RA, Jacot E, Jequier E, Maeder E, Wahren J, Felber JP. The effect of insulin on the disposal of intravenous glucose: results from indirect calorimetry and hepatic femoral venous catheterization. *Diabetes* 1981; **30**: 1000–7.

80. Katz LD, Glickman MG, Rapoport S, Ferrannini E, DeFronzo RA. Splanchnic and peripheral disposal of oral glucose in man. *Diabetes* 1983; **32**: 675–9.

81. Horton ES. Role and management of exercise in diabetes mellitus. *Diabetes Care* 1988; **11**: 201–11.

82. Koivisto VA, Yki-Järvinen H, DeFronzo RA. Physical training and insulin sensitivity. *Diabetes/Metabolism Reviews* 1988; **1**: 445–81.

83. Nuutila P, Knuuti J, Heinonen O, et al. Different alterations in the insulin-stimulated glucose uptake in the athlete's heart and skeletal muscle. *Journal of Clinical Investigation* 1994; **93**: 2267–74.

84. Youn J, Gulve EA, Holloszy JO. Calcium stimulates glucose transport in skeletal muscle by a pathway independent of contraction. *American Journal of Physiology* 1991; **260**: C555–61.

85. Cartee GD, Young DA, Sleeper MD, Zierath J, Wallberg-Henriksson H, Holloszy JO. Prolonged increase in insulin-stimulated glucose transport in muscle after exercise. *American Journal of Physiology* 1989; **256**: E494–9.

86. Richter EA, Garetto LP, Goodman MN, Ruderman NB. Muscle glucose metabolism following exercise in the rat. Increased sensitivity to insulin. *Journal of Clinical Investigation* 1982; **69**: 785–93.

87. Zorzano A, Balon TW, Goodman MN, Ruderman NB. Additive effects of prior exercise and insulin on glucose and AIB uptake by rat muscle. *American Journal of Physiology* 1986; **251**: E21–6.

88. Young DA, Wallberg-Henriksson H, Sleeper MD, Holloszy JO. Reversal of the exercise-induced increase in muscle permeability to glucose. *American Journal of Physiology* 1987; **253**: E331–5.

89. Cartee GD, Holloszy JO. Exercise increases susceptibility of muscle glucose transport to activation by various stimuli. *American Journal of Physiology* 1990; **258**: E390–3.

90. Richter EA, Mikines KJ, Galbo H, Kiens B. Effect of exercise on insulin action in human skeletal muscle. *Journal of Applied Physiology* 1989; **66**: 876–85.

91. Kristiansen S, Hargreaves M, Richter EA. Exercise-induced increase in glucose transport, GLUT-4, and VAMP-2 in plasma membrane from human muscle. *American Journal of Physiology* 1996; **270**: E197–201.

92. Ivy JL, Holloszy JO. Persistent increase in glucose uptake by rat skeletal muscle following exercise. *American Journal of Physiology* 1981; **241**: C200–3.

93. Mikines KJ, Sonne B, Farrell PA, Tronier B, Galbo H. Effect of training on the dose-response relationship for insulin action in men. *Journal of Applied Physiology* 1989; **66**: 695–703.

94. Ploug T, Stallknecht BM, Pedersen O, et al. Effect of endurance training on glucose transport capacity and glucose transporter expression in rat skeletal muscle. *American Journal of Physiology* 1990; **259**: E778–86.

95. Houmard JA, Shinebarger MH, Dolan PL, et al. Exercise training increases GLUT-4 protein concentration in previously sedentary middle-aged men. *American Journal of Physiology* 1993; **264**: E896–901.

96. Gulve EA, Spina RJ. Effect of 7–10 days of cycle ergometer exercise on skeletal muscle GLUT-4 protein content. *Journal of Applied Physiology* 1995; **79**: 1562–6.

97. Phillips SM, Han XX, Green HJ, Bonen A. Increments in skeletal muscle GLUT-1 and GLUT-4 after endurance training in humans. *American Journal of Physiology* 1996; **270**: E456–62.

98. Megeney LA, Neufer PD, Dohm GL, et al. Effects of muscle activity and fiber composition on glucose transport and GLUT-4. *American Journal of Physiology* 1993; **264**: E583–93.

99. McCoy M, Proietto J, Hargreaves M. Skeletal muscle GLUT-4 and postexercise muscle glycogen storage in humans. *Journal of Applied Physiology* 1996; **80**: 411–15.

100. Houmard JA, Tyndall GL, Midyette JB, et al. Effect of reduced training and training cessation on insulin action and muscle GLUT-4. *Journal of Applied Physiology* 1996; **81**: 1162–8.

101. Vukovich MD, Arciero PJ, Kohrt WM, Racette SB, Hansen PA, Holloszy JO. Changes in insulin action and GLUT-4 with 6 days of inactivity in endurance runners. *Journal of Applied Physiology* 1996; **80**: 240–4.

102. Houmard JA, Hortobágyi T, Neufer PD, et al. Training cessation does not alter GLUT-4 protein levels in human skeletal muscle. *Journal of Applied Physiology* 1993; **74**: 776–81.

103. Etgen GJ Jr, Brozinick JT Jr, Kang HY, Ivy JL. Effects of exercise training on skeletal muscle glucose uptake and transport. *American Journal of Physiology* 1993; **264**: C727–33.

104. Yki-Järvinen H, Young AA, Lamkin C, Foley JE. Kinetics of glucose disposal in whole body and across the forearm in man. *Journal of Clinical Investigation* 1987; **79**: 1713–19.

105. Bogardus C, Lillioja S, Stone K, Mott D. Correlation between muscle glycogen synthetase activity and *in vivo* insulin action in man. *Journal of Clinical Investigation* 1984; **73**: 1185–90.

106. Ebeling P, Bourey R, Koranyi L, *et al.* Mechanism of enhanced insulin sensitivity in athletes. Increased blood flow, muscle glucose transport protein (glut-4) concentration, and glycogen synthase activity. *Journal of Clinical Investigation* 1993; **92**: 1623–31.

107. Vestergaard H, Andersen PH, Lund S, Schmitz O, Junker S, Pedersen O. Pre- and posttranslational upregulation of muscle-specific glycogen synthase in athletes. *American Journal of Physiology* 1994; **266**: E92-101.

108. Kong X, Manchester J, Salmons S, Lawrence JC Jr. Glucose transporters in single skeletal muscle fibers. *Journal of Biological Chemistry* 1994; **269**: 12963–7.

109. Dela F, Handberg A, Mikines KJ, Vinten J, Galbo H. GLUT 4 and insulin receptor binding and kinase activity in trained human muscle. *Journal of Physiology* 1993; **469**: 615–24.

110. Kim Y, Inoue T, Nakajima R, *et al.* Effects of endurance training on gene expression of insulin signal transduction pathway. *Biochemical and Biophysical Research Communications* 1995; **210**: 766–73.

111. Henriksson J. Influence of exercise on insulin sensitivity. *Journal of Cardiac Risk* 1995; **2**: 303–9.

112. Bassett DR Jr. Skeletal muscle characteristics: relationships to cardiovascular risk factors. *Medicine and Science in Sports and Exercise* 1994; **26**: 957–66.

113. Holmäng A, Björntorp P, Rippe B. Tissue uptake of insulin and inulin in red and white skeletal muscle *in vivo. American Journal of Physiology* 1992; **263**: H1–7.

114. Laakso M, Edelman SV, Brechtel G, Baron AD. Decreased effect of insulin to stimulate skeletal muscle blood flow in obese man. *Journal of Clinical Investigation* 1990; **85**: 1844–52.

115. Kriketos AD, Pan DA, Sutton JR, *et al.* Relationships between muscle membrane lipids, fiber type, and enzyme activities in sedentary and exercised rats. *American Journal of Physiology* 1995; **269**: R1154–62.

116. Idström JP, Elander A, Soussi B, Scherstén T, Bylund-Fellenius AC. Influence of endurance training on glucose transport and uptake in rat skeletal muscle. *American Journal of Physiology* 1986; **251**: H903–7.

117. Ivy JL, Young JC, McLane JA, Fell RD, Holloszy JO. Exercise training and glucose uptake by skeletal muscle in rats. *Journal of Applied Physiology* 1983; **55**: 1393–6.

118. Coggan AR, Kohrt WM, Spina RJ, Bier DM, Holloszy JO. Endurance training decreases plasma glucose turnover and oxidation during moderate-intensity exercise in men. *Journal of Applied Physiology* 1990; **68**: 990–6.

119. Dela F, Mikines KJ, Sonne B, Galbo H. Effect of training on interaction between insulin and exercise in human muscle. *Journal of Applied Physiology* 1994; **76**: 2386–93.

120. McConell G, McCoy M, Proietto J, Hargreaves M. Skeletal muscle GLUT-4 and glucose uptake during exercise in humans. *Journal of Applied Physiology* 1994; **77**: 1565–8.

121. King DS, Dalsky GP, Staten MA, Clutter WE, Van Houten DR, Holloszy JO. Insulin action and secretion in endurance-trained and untrained humans. *Journal of Applied Physiology* 1987; **63**: 2247–52.

122. Rodnick KJ, Reaven GM, Azhar S, Goodman MN, Mondon CE. Effects of insulin on carbohydrate and protein metabolism in voluntary running rats. *American Journal of Physiology* 1990; **259**: E706–14.

123. Heath GW, Gavin JR III, Hinderliter JM, Hagberg JM, Bloomfield SA, Holloszy JO. Effects of exercise and lack of exercise on glucose tolerance and insulin sensitivity. *Journal of Applied Physiology* 1983; **55**: 512–17.

124. Leblanc J, Nadeau A, Richard D, Tremblay A. Studies on the sparing effect of exercise on insulin requirements in human subjects. *Metabolism* 1981; **30**: 1119–24.

125. Seals DR, Hagberg JM, Allen WK, *et al.* Glucose tolerance in young and older athletes and sedentary men. *Journal of Applied Physiology* 1984; **56**: 1521–5.

126. Rogers MA, King DS, Hagberg JM, Ehsani AA, Holloszy JO. Effect of 10 days of physical inactivity on glucose tolerance in master athletes. *Journal of Applied Physiology* 1990; **68**: 1833–7.

127. Nagasawa J, Sato Y, Ishiko T. Effect of training and detraining on *in vivo* insulin sensitivity. *International Journal of Sports Medicine* 1990; **11**: 107–10.

128. King DS, Dalsky GP, Clutter WE, *et al.* Effects of exercise and lack of exercise on insulin sensitivity and responsiveness. *Journal of Applied Physiology* 1988; **64**: 1942–6.

129. Mikines KJ, Sonne B, Tronier B, Galbo H. Effects of acute exercise and detraining on insulin action in trained men. *Journal of Applied Physiology* 1989; **66**: 704–11.

130. Hughes VA, Fiatarone MA, Fielding RA, *et al.* Exercise increases muscle GLUT-4 levels and insulin action in subjects with impaired glucose tolerance. *American Journal of Physiology* 1993; **264**: E855–62.

131. Rodnick KJ, Holloszy JO, Mondon CE, James DE. Effect of exercise training on insulin-regulatable glucose-transporter protein levels in rat skeletal muscle. *Diabetes* 1990; **39**: 1425–9.

132. James DE, Kraegen EW, Chisholm DJ. Effect of exercise training on *in vivo* insulin action in individual tissues of the rat. *Journal of Clinical Investigation* 1985; **76**: 657–66.

133. Davis TA, Klahr S, Tegtmeyer ED, Osborne DF, Howard TL, Karl IE. Glucose metabolism in epitrochlearis muscle of acutely exercised and trained rats. *American Journal of Physiology* 1986; **250**: E137–43.

134. Holmäng A, Möller M, Andersson O, Lönnroth P. Microdialysis of muscle interstitial glucose in healthy and type II diabetic subjects. *Diabetes* 1996; **45** (Suppl. 2): 255A.

135. Bourey RE, Coggan AR, Kohrt WM, Kirwan JP, King DS, Holloszy JO. Effect of exercise on glucose disposal: response to a maximal insulin stimulus. *Journal of Applied Physiology* 1990; **69**: 1689–94.

136. Kirwan JP, Hickner RC, Yarasheski KE, Kohrt WM, Wiethop BV, Holloszy JO. Eccentric exercise induces transient insulin resistance in healthy individuals. *Journal of Applied Physiology* 1992; **72**: 2197–202.

137. Miller JP, Pratley RE, Goldberg AP, *et al.* Strength training increases insulin action in healthy 50- to 65-yr-old men. *Journal of Applied Physiology* 1994; **77**: 1122–7.

138. Smutok MA, Reece C, Kokkinos PF, *et al.* Effects of exercise training modality on glucose tolerance in men with abnormal glucose regulation. *International Journal of Sports Medicine* 1994; **15**: 283–9.

139. Fluckey JD, Hickey MS, Brambrink JK, Hart KK, Alexander K, Craig BW. Effects of resistance exercise on glucose tolerance in normal and glucose-intolerant subjects. *Journal of Applied Physiology* 1994; **77**: 1087–92.

140. Tuominen JA, Ebeling P, Bourey R, *et al.* Postmarathon paradox: insulin resistance in the face of glycogen depletion. *American Journal of Physiology* 1996; **270**: E336–43.

141. Langfort J, Budohoski L, Newsholme EA. Effect of various types of acute exercise and exercise training on the insulin sensitivity of rat soleus muscle measured *in vitro. Pflügers Archiv* 1988; **412**: 101–5.

142. Kern M, Tapscott EB, Downes DL, Frisell WR, Dohm GL. Insulin resistence induced by high-fat feeding is only partially reversed by exercise training. *Pflügers Archiv* 1990; **417**: 79–83.

143. Hultman E, Nilsson LH. Liver glycogen in man: effect of different diets and muscular exercise. In: Pernow B, Saltin B, eds. *Muscle metabolism during exercise.* New York: Plenum, 1971; 143–51.

144. Costill DL. Carbohydrates for exercise: dietary demands for optimal performance. *International Journal of Sports Medicine* 1988; **9**: 1–18.

145. Saltin B, Nazar DL, Costill DL, *et al.* The nature of the training response: peripheral and central adaptations to one-legged exercise. *Acta Physiologica Scandinavica* 1976; **96**: 289–305.

146. Henriksson J. Training induced adaptation of skeletal muscle and metabolism during submaximal exercise. *Journal of Physiology* 1977; **270**: 661–75.

147. Häggmark, T. A study of morphologic and enzymatic properties of the skeletal muscles after injuries and immobilization in man. Thesis, Karolinska Institutet, 1978.

148. Piehl K, Adolfsson S, Nazar K. Glycogen storage and glycogen synthetase activity in trained and untrained muscle of man. *Acta Physiologica Scandinavica* 1974; **90**: 779–88.

149. Tesch P, Piehl K, Wilson G, Karlsson J. Physiological investigations of Swedish elite canoe competitors. *Medicine and Science in Sports and Exercise* 1976; **8**: 214–18.

150. Bogardus C, Ravussin E, Robbins DC, Wolfe RR, Horton ES, Sims EAH. Effects of physical training and diet therapy on carbohydrate metabolism in patients with glucose intolerance and non-insulin-dependent diabetes mellitus. *Diabetes* 1984; **33**: 311–18.

151. Devlin JT, Horton ES. Effects of prior high-intensity exercise on glucose metabolism in normal and insulin-resistant men. *Diabetes* 1985; **34**: 973–9.

152. Blom PC, Costill DL, Vollestad NK. Exhaustive running: inappropriate as a stimulus of muscle glycogen super-compensation. *Medicine and Science in Sports Exercise* 1987; **19**: 398–403.

153. Bergström J, Hultman E. Muscle glycogen synthesis after exercise: an enhancing factor localized to the muscle cells in man. *Nature* 1966; **210**: 309–10.

154. Gulve EA, Cartee GD, Zierath JR, Corpus VM, Holloszy JO. Reversal of enhanced muscle glucose transport after exercise: roles of insulin and glucose. *American Journal of Physiology* 1990; **259**: E685–91.

155. Bergström J, Hermansen L, Hultman E, Saltin B. Diet, muscle glycogen and physical performance. *Acta Physiologica Scandinavica* 1967; **71**: 140–50.

156. Karlsson J, Saltin B. Diet, muscle glycogen, and endurance performance. *Journal of Applied Physiology* 1971; **31**: 203–6.

157. Sherman WM, Costill DL. The marathon: dietary manipulation to optimize performance. *American Journal of Sports Medicine* 1984; **12**: 44–51.

158. Constable SH, Favier RJ, McLane JA, Fell RD, Chen M, Holloszy JO. Energy metabolism in contracting rat skeletal muscle: adaptation to exercise training. *American Journal of Physiology* 1987; **253**: C316–22.

159. Jansson E, Kaijser L. Substrate utilization and enzymes in skeletal muscle of extremely endurance-trained men. *Journal of Applied Physiology* 1987; **62**: 999–1005.

160. Green HJ, Smith D, Murphy P, Fraser I. Training-induced alterations in muscle glycogen utilization in fibre-specific types during prolonged exercise. *Canadian Journal of Physiology and Pharmacology* 1990; **68**: 1372–6.

161. Hermansen L, Hultman E, Saltin B. Muscle glycogen during prolonged severe exercise. *Acta Physiologica Scandinavica* 1967; **71**: 129–39.

162. Saltin B, Karlsson J. Muscle glycogen utlization during work of different intensities. In: Pernow B, Saltin B, eds. *Muscle metabolism during exercise.* New York: Plenum, 1971: 289–99.

163. Spina RJ, Chi MM-Y, Hopkins MG, Nemeth PM, Lowry OH, Holloszy JO. Mitochondrial enzymes increase in muscle in

164. Chesley A, Heigenhauser GJF, Spriet LL. Regulation of muscle glycogen phosphorylase activity following short-term endurance training. *American Journal of Physiology* 1996; **270**: E328–35.

165. Green HJ, Helyar R, Ball-Burnett M, Kowalchuk N. Metabolic adaptations to training precede changes in muscle mitochondrial capacity. *Journal of Applied Physiology* 1992; **72**: 484–91.

166. Bang O. The lactate content of the blood during and after muscular exercise in man. *Scandinavian Archives of Physiology* 1936; **74** (Suppl. 10): 51–82.

167. Cobb LA, Johnson WP. Hemodynamic relationship of anaerobic metabolism and plasma free fatty acids during prolonged, strenuous exercise in trained and untrained subjects. *Journal of Clinical Investigation* 1963; **42**: 800–10.

168. Ekblom B, Åstrand P-O, Saltin B, Stenberg J, Wallström B. Effect of training on circulatory response to exercise. *Journal of Applied Physiology* 1968; **24**: 518–28.

169. Hurley BF, Nemeth PM, Martin WH III, Hagberg JM, Dalsky GP, Holloszy JO. Muscle triglyceride utilization during exercise: effect of training. *Journal of Applied Physiology* 1986; **60**: 562–7.

170. Saltin B, Karlsson J. Muscle ATP, CP, and lactate during exercise after physical conditioning. In: Pernow B, Saltin B, eds. *Muscle metabolism during exercise.* New York: Plenum, 1971: 395–9.

171. Cadefau J, Green HJ, Cussò R, Ball-Burnett M, Jamieson G. Coupling of muscle phosphorylation potential to glycolysis during work after short-term training. *Journal of Applied Physiology* 1994; **76**: 2586–93.

172. Buckley JD, Scroop GC, Catcheside PG. Lactate disposal in resting trained and untrained forearm skeletal muscle during high intensity leg exercise. *European Journal of Applied Physiology* 1993; **67**: 360–6.

173. Karlsson J, Sjödin B, Thorstensson A, Hultén B, Frith K. LDH isozymes in skeletal muscles of endurance and strength trained athletes. *Acta Physiologica Scandinavica* 1975; **93**: 150–6.

174. Favier RJ, Constable SH, Chen M, Holloszy JO. Endurance exercise training reduces lactate production. *Journal of Applied Physiology* 1986; **61**: 885–9.

175. Stanley WC, Gertz EW, Wisneski JA, Neese RA, Morris DL, Brooks GA. Lactate extraction during net lactate release in legs of humans during exercise. *Journal of Applied Physiology* 1986; **60**: 1116–20.

176. Schantz PG, Sjöberg B, Svedenhag J. Malate-aspartate and alpha-glycerophosphate shuttle enzyme levels in human skeletal muscle: methodological considerations and effect of endurance training. *Acta Physiologica Scandinavica* 1986; **128**: 397–407.

177. Costill DL, Fink WJ, Hargreaves M, Fink DS, Thomas R, Fielding R. Metabolic characteristics of skeletal muscle during detraining from competitive swimming. *College Sports Medicine* 1985; **17**: 339–42.

178. Donovan CM, Pagliassotti MJ. Enhanced efficiency of lactate removal after endurance training. *Journal of Applied Physiology* 1990; **68**: 1053–8.

179. Donovan CM, Brooks GA. Endurance training affects lactate clearance, not lactate production. *American Journal of Physiology* 1983; **244**: E83–92.

180. Baldwin KM, Fitts RH, Booth FW, Winder WW, Holloszy JO. Depletion of muscle and liver glycogen during exercise. Protective effect of training. *Pflügers Archiv* 1975; **354**: 203–12.

181. Essén B, Hagenfeldt L, Kaijser L. Utilization of blood-borne and intramuscular substrates during continuous and intermittent exercise in man. *Journal of Physiology (London)* 1977; **265**: 489–506.

182. Gollnick PD, Pernow B, Essén B, Jansson E, Saltin B. Availability of glycogen and plasma FFA for substrate utilization in leg muscle of man during exercise. *Clinical Physiology (Oxford)* 1981; **1**: 27–42.

response to 7–10 days of cycle exercise. *Journal of Applied Physiology* 1996; **80**: 2250–4.

183. Randle PJ, Kerbey AL, Espinal J. Mechanisms decreasing glucose oxidation in diabetes and starvation: role of lipid fuels and hormones. *Diabetes/Metabolism Reviews* 1988; **4**: 623–38.

184. Coggan AR, Spina RJ, Kohrt WM, Holloszy JO. Effect of prolonged exercise on muscle citrate concentration before and after endurance training in men. *American Journal of Physiology* 1993; **264**: E215–20.

185. Sidossis LS, Wolfe RR. Glucose and insulin-induced inhibition of fatty acid oxidation: the glucose-fatty acid cycle reversed. *American Journal of Physiology* 1996; **270**: E733–8.

186. Green HJ, Jones S, Ball-Burnett ME, Smith D, Livesey J, Farrance BW. Early muscular and metabolic adaptations to prolonged exercise training in humans. *Journal of Applied Physiology* 1991; **70**: 2032–8.

187. Holloszy JO. Metabolic consequences of endurance exercise training. In: Horton ES, Terjung RL, eds. *Exercise, nutrition and energy metabolism.* New York: Macmillan, 1988: 116–31.

188. Martin WH III, Dalsky GP, Hurley BF, *et al.* Effect of endurance training on plasma free fatty acid turnover and oxidation during exercise. *American Journal of Physiology* 1993; **265**: E708–14.

189. Hagenfeldt L. Turnover of individual free fatty acids in man. *Federation Proceedings* 1975; **34**: 2236–40.

190. Groop LC, Bonadonna RC, Delprato S, *et al.* Glucose and free fatty acid metabolism in non-insulin dependent diabetes mellitus. Evidence for multiple sites of insulin resistance. *Journal of Clinical Investigation* 1989; **84**: 205–13.

191. Kiens B, Essén-Gustavsson B, Christensen NJ, Saltin B. Skeletal muscle substrate utilization during submaximal exercise in man: effect of endurance training. *Journal of Physiology (London)* 1993; **469**: 459–78.

192. Morgan TE, Short FA, Cobb LA. Effect of long-term exercise on skeletal muscle lipid composition. *American Journal of Physiology* 1969; **216**: 82–6.

193. Bylund AC, Bjurö T, Cederblad J, *et al.* Physical training in man. Skeletal muscle metabolism in relation to muscle morphology and running ability. *European Journal of Applied Physiology and Occupational Physiology* 1977; **36**: 151–69.

194. Staron RS, Hikida RS, Hagerman FC, Dudley GA, Murray TF. Human skeletal muscle fiber type adaptability to various workloads. *Journal of Histochemistry and Cytochemistry* 1984; **32**: 146–52.

195. Howald H, Hoppeler H, Claassen H, Mathieu O, Straub R. Influences of endurance training on the ultrastructural composition of the different muscle fiber types in humans. *Pflügers Archiv* 1985; **403**: 369–76.

196. Fröberg SO. Effects of training and acute exercise in trained rats. *Metabolism* 1971; **20**: 1044–51.

197. Fröberg SO, Östman I, Sjöstrand NO. Effect of training on esterified fatty acids and carnitine in muscle and on lipolysis in adipose tissue *in vitro. Acta Physiologica Scandinavica* 1972; **86**: 166–74.

198. Górski J, Kiryluk T. The post-exercise recovery of triglycerides in rat tissues. *European Journal of Applied Physiology and Occupational Physiology* 1980; **45**: 33–41.

199. Molé PA, Oscai LB, Holloszy JO. Adaptation of muscle to exercise. Increase in levels of palmityl CoA synthetase, carnitine palmityltransferase, and palmityl CoA dehydrogenase, and in the capacity to oxidize fatty acids. *Journal of Clinical Investigation* 1971; **50**: 2323–30.

200. Paulussen RJA, Veerkamp JH. Intracellular fatty-acid-binding proteins. Characteristics and function. In: Hilderson HJ, ed. *Subcellular biochemistry. Intracellular transfer of lipid molecules.* New York: Plenum Press, 1990; **7**: 175–226.

201. Winder WW, Arogyasami J, Barton RJ, Elayan IM, Vehrs PR. Muscle malonyl-CoA decreases during exercise. *Journal of Applied Physiology* 1989; **67**: 2230–3.

202. Winder WW, Hickson RC, Hagberg JM, Ehsani AA, McLane JA. Training-induced changes in hormonal and metabolic responses to submaximal exercise. *Journal of Applied Physiology* 1979; **46**: 766–71.

203. Stankiewicz-Choroszucha B, Górski J. Effect of beta-adrenergic blockade on intramuscular triglyceride mobilization during exercise. *Experientia* 1978; **34**: 357–8.

204. Oscai LB, Essig DA, Palmer WK. Lipase regulation of muscle triglyceride hydrolysis. *Journal of Applied Physiology* 1990; **69**: 1571–7.

205. Svedenhag J, Lithell H, Juhlin-Dannfelt A, Henriksson J. Increase in skeletal muscle lipoprotein lipase following endurance training in man. *Atherosclerosis* 1983; **49**: 203–7.

206. Nikkilä EA, Taskinen M-R, Rehunen S, Härkönen M. Lipoprotein lipase activity in adipose tissue and skeletal muscle of runners: relation to serum lipoproteins. *Metabolism* 1978; **27**: 1661–71.

207. Stubbe I, Hansson P, Gustafson A, Nilsson-Ehle P. Plasma lipoproteins and lipolytic enzymes activities during endurance training in sedentary men: changes in high-density lipoprotein subfractions and composition. *Metabolism* 1983; **32**: 1120–8.

208. Seip RL, Mair K, Cole TG, Semenkovich CF. Induction of human skeletal muscle lipoprotein lipase gene expression by short term exercise is transient. *American Journal of Physiology* 1997; **272**: E255–61.

209. Lithell H, Cedermark M, Fröberg J, Tesch P, Karlsson J. Increase of lipoprotein–lipase activity in skeletal muscle during heavy exercise—relation to epinephrine excretion. *Metabolism* 1981; **30**: 1130–8.

210. Ong JM, Simsolo RB, Saghizadeh M, Goers JWF, Kern PA. Effects of exercise training and feeding on lipoprotein lipase gene expression in adipose tissue, heart, and skeletal muscle of the rat. *Metabolism* 1995; **44**: 1596–605.

211. Simsolo RB, Ong JM, Kern PA. The regulation of adipose tissue and muscle lipoprotein lipase in runners by detraining. *Journal of Clinical Investigation* 1993; **92**: 2124–30.

212. Yki-Järvinen H, Puhakainen I, Saloranta C, Groop L, Taskinen M-R. Demonstration of a novel feedback mechanism between FFA oxidation from intracellular and intravascular sources. *American Journal of Physiology* 1991; **260**: E680–9.

213. Henriksson J. Effect of exercise on amino acid concentrations in skeletal muscle and plasma. *Journal of Experimental Biology* 1991; **160**: 149–65.

214. Graham TE, Turcotte LP, Kiens B, Richter EA. Training and muscle ammonia and amino acid metabolism in humans during prolonged exercise. *Journal of Applied Physiology* 1995; **78**: 725–35.

215. Einspahr KJ, Tharp G. Influence of endurance training on plasma amino acid concentrations in humans at rest and after intense exercise. *International Journal of Sports Medicine* 1989; **10**: 233–6.

216. Ebbeling CB, Clarkson PM. Exercise-induced muscle damage and adaptation. *Sports Medicine* 1989; **7**: 207–34.

217. Davies CTM, White MJ. Muscle weakness following eccentric work in man. *Pflügers Archiv* 1981; **392**: 168–71.

218. Newham DJ, Jones DA, Edwards RHT. Large delayed plasma creatine kinase changes after stepping exercise. *Muscle and Nerve* 1983; **6**: 380–5.

219. Evans WJ, Cannon JG. The metabolic effects of exercise-induced muscle damage. In: Holloszy JO, ed. *Exercise and sports sciences reviews.* Baltimore, MD: Williams and Wilkins, 1991: 99–125.

220. Friden J, Seger J, Sjöström M, Ekblom B. Adaptive response in human skeletal muscle subjected to prolonged eccentric training. *International Journal of Sports Medicine* 1983; **4**: 177–83.

221. Warhol MJ, Siegel AJ, Evans WJ, Silverman LM. Skeletal muscle injury and repair in marathon runners after competition. *American Journal of Pathology* 1985; **118**: 331–9.

222. Costill DL, Pascoe DD, Fink WJ, Robergs RA, Barr SI, Pearson

D. Impaired muscle glycogen resynthesis after eccentric exercise. *Journal of Applied Physiology* 1990; **69**: 46–50.

223. Hunter JB, Critz JB. Effect of training on plasma enzyme levels in man. *Journal of Applied Physiology* 1971; **31**: 20–3.

224. Schwane JA, Armstrong RB. Effect of training on skeletal muscle injury from downhill running in rats. *Journal of Applied Physiology* 1983; **55**: 969–75.

225. Byrnes WC, Clarkson PM, White JS, Hsieh SS, Frykman PN, Maughan RJ. Delayed onset muscle soreness following repeated bouts of downhill running. *Journal of Applied Physiology* 1985; **59**: 710–15.

226. Holloszy JO. Biochemical adaptations to exercise: aerobic metabolism. In: Wilmore JH, ed. *Exercise and sports sciences reviews*. New York: Academic Press, 1973: 45–71.

227. Booth FW, Thomason DB. Molecular and cellular adaptation of muscle in response to exercise: perspectives of various models. *Physiological Reviews* 1991; **71**: 541–85.

228. Dudley GA, Tullson PC, Terjung RL. Influence of mitochondrial content on the sensitivity of respiratory control. *Journal of Biological Chemistry* 1987; **262**: 9109–14.

229. Holloszy JO, Coyle EF. Adaptations of skeletal muscle to endurance exercise and their metabolic consequences. *Journal of Applied Physiology* 1984; **56**: 831–8.

230. Nosek TM, Fender KY, Godt RE. It is diprotonated inorganic phosphate that depresses force in skinned skeletal muscle fibers. *Science* 1987; **236**: 191–3.

231. Kjeldsen K, Norgaard A, Hau C. Exercise-induced hyperkalaemia can be reduced in human subjects by moderate training without change in skeletal muscle Na, K-ATPase concentration. *European Journal of Clinical Investigation* 1990; **20**: 642–7.

232. Henriksson J, Reitman JS. Time course of changes in human skeletal muscle succinate dehydrogenase and cytochrome oxidase activities and maximal oxygen uptake with physical activity and inactivity. *Acta Physiologica Scandinavica* 1977; **99**: 91–7.

233. Schantz P, Henriksson J. Increases in myofibrillar ATPase intermediate human skeletal muscle fibres in response to endurance training. *Muscle and Nerve* 1983; **6**: 553–6.

1.1.4 Anaerobic metabolism, acid–base balance, and muscle fatigue during high intensity exercise

Kent Sahlin†

Introduction

Exercise is a process in which energy stored as complex chemical compounds is transformed into mechanical energy and heat. The transition from rest to exercise involves a drastic increase in energy demand and the metabolic changes pose a potential threat to whole-body homeostasis.

The immediate energy source in practically all energy-requiring processes is the hydrolysis of ATP to adenosine diphosphate (**ADP**) and inorganic phosphate (P_i). The muscle content of ATP is small and has to be replenished continuously by rephosphorylation of ADP to ATP. This is linked to aerobic and anaerobic metabolic processes by which the chemical energy in fuels is released and partially

† The author's research is supported by grants from the Swedish Medical Research Council (08671) and the Swedish Sports Research Council.

trapped as ATP. The breakdown of ATP to ADP and the rephosphorylation of ADP to ATP constitutes the ATP–ADP cycle by which the energy-consuming processes are linked to the energy-yielding processes (Fig. 1). The energy-yielding processes are limited in the rate and amount of energy that can be formed and these features of energetics are important determinants of exercise performance.

The metabolic processes are associated with changes in the hydrogen ion concentration. The hydrogen ion is unique in its high reactivity and its abundancy in biological fluids. Most of the hydrogen ions are bound and the cellular concentration of the free form is only about 10^{-7} mol/l, corresponding to a pH of 7.0. Despite its low concentration, changes in H^+ have a profound effect on biochemical and physiological processes. It is therefore of fundamental importance that the generation and removal of H^+ are under tight control. The whole-body acid–base balance is maintained by renal excretion of acids/bases and by variation in the respiratory CO_2–elimination. Cellular acid–base balance is maintained by (i) intracellular buffering processes, (ii) feedback control of metabolic pathways and physiological processes, and (iii) transmembrane transport of acids and bases.

Muscle fatigue is a limiting factor on performance in many sports and in many cases it is related to energy deficiency. The focus of the present chapter is on the limitations of the energetic processes in muscle with special emphasis on high-intensity exercise and the acid–base balance.

Exercise-induced changes in acid–base balance

The breakdown of ATP is the immediate source of energy and results in the release of H^+:

$$ATP \rightarrow ADP + P_i + n_1 H^+ + energy \qquad (1)$$

where n_1 is between 0 and 1 and dependent on the intracellular pH. Although the rate of ATP hydrolysis is very high in a contracting muscle, the acid–base disturbance is negligible. This is because the reverse reaction (phosphorylation of ADP) proceeds at a nearly identical rate and consumes an equivalent amount of H^+.

The breakdown of phosphocreatine (**PCr**) can rephosphorylate ADP at a high rate in the absence of oxygen. Therefore, phosphocreatine breakdown is an important energy source during short periods of high-intensity exercise, such as sprints. The breakdown of phosphocreatine is catalysed by the enzyme creatine kinase, which has a high level of activity in skeletal muscle. Creatine kinase catalyses an equilibrium reaction and will thus catalyse both the breakdown and resynthesis of phosphocreatine:

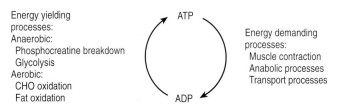

Fig. 1 The ATP–ADP cycle: the link between energy-demanding and energy-yielding processes.

$$PCr + ADP + n_2H^+ \longleftrightarrow ATP + creatine \qquad (2)$$

Combining equations 1 and 2 gives:

$$PCr + (n_2-n_1)H^+ \rightarrow creatine + P_i \qquad (3)$$

Thus the breakdown of phosphocreatine is associated with a removal of protons, the stoichiometry being dependent on the cellular pH.[1] At rest, when intracellular pH is close to 7.0, about 0.4 mol of H^+ are consumed per mol of phosphocreatine utilized, giving a theoretical maximal uptake of protons of about 32 mmol/kg dry wt (PCr = 80 mmol/kg dry wt; pH = 7.0). At the onset of exercise, phosphocreatine breakdown exceeds the formation of lactic acid and the removal of H^+ due to phosphocreatine breakdown is in excess of the released H^+ due to lactic acid formation. Under these conditions, one would expect an increase in pH. An alkaline shift of 0.1 to 0.2 pH units has also been demonstrated during the first seconds of contraction in frog skeletal muscle.[2] Conversely, when phosphocreatine is resynthesized after terminating exercise, the reaction (equation 3) is reversed and H^+ is released. This postexercise proton load explains why the minimum muscle pH is not reached at the end of exercise, when muscle lactate is at its maximum, but after a recovery period of about 1 min.[3]

Exercise-induced acid–base disturbances are normally associated with lactic acidosis. Glucose derived from locally stored glycogen (or from blood glucose) can be degraded to lactate in a series of enzymatic steps called glycolysis:

$$1/2 \text{ Glucose} \longrightarrow \text{Lactate} + H^+ \qquad (4)$$
$$P_i + ADP + n_1H^+ \qquad ATP$$

When the substrate is intramuscular glycogen the energy yield is 50 per cent higher (i.e. 1.5 mol of ATP per mol of lactate). Since lactic acid has a pKa of about 3.7, it is almost completely dissociated under physiological conditions and a stoichiometric release of protons will occur. If the uptake of protons owing to ADP rephosphorylation is included in the balance, the picture becomes more complex.[4] However, since there are no major changes in the ATP or ADP concentration during exercise, the changes in protons owing to ADP rephosphorylation and ATP hydrolysis can be neglected (see above). The metabolism of lactate, either through a reversal of the reaction (equation 4) (which normally occurs in the liver) or through transformation into pyruvate and subsequent oxidation in the mitochondria, will result in a stoichiometric uptake of protons and elimination of the acid load.

Even after a short period of intensive exercise (less than 10 s), production of H^+ via lactic acid exceeds the removal of H^+ by the creatine kinase reaction and pH decreases below the value at rest. The rate of glycolysis may be very high and a large amount of lactic acid can be formed in a short time. If there were no restraints, lactic acid production would kill the organism within a couple of minutes. Powerful brakes on glycolysis have therefore been developed and involve inhibition of key enzymes of glycolysis and muscle fatigue (see below). Lactate has a key position in exercise physiology and the changes in blood and muscle lactate/pH have been thoroughly investigated under a variety of conditions. This interest stems from the close connection between lactate accumulation and muscle fatigue, which was observed by Berzelius as early as 1877 and later substantiated in 1907 by Fletcher and Hopkins[5] and, since then, by numerous other studies. However, the mechanism still remains elusive.

During sustained exercise, the energy demand is met almost exclusively through the formation of ATP by the oxidative processes. The end product of oxidative metabolism is carbon dioxide which, after hydration to carbonic acid, can dissociate into protons and bicarbonate:

$$CO_2 + H_2O \longleftrightarrow H_2CO_3 \longleftrightarrow H^+ + HCO_3^- \qquad (5)$$

Exercise can increase the rate of CO_2 production and thus the proton load by about 20 times. However, normal circulation and respiration will balance the increased CO_2 production through increased elimination of CO_2 via the lungs. Therefore, the hydrogen ion concentration remains normal despite a large increase in the proton load. In fact, the expiration of CO_2 during high-intensity exercise is in excess of the CO_2 formation and constitues one mechanism to counteract lactic acidosis.

The metabolic end-products (CO_2 and H_2O) during steady-state exercise can be handled easily by the organism and the exercise can proceed for a long time without metabolic perturbation. At the onset of exercise and during high-intensity exercise, ATP is also formed through the anaerobic processes: the breakdown of phosphocreatine and glycolysis. The term anaerobic denotes that these processes can regenerate ATP in the absence of oxygen. In contrast to the aerobic processes, the anaerobic processes produce waste products (e.g. H^+ and P_i) that accumulate in the working muscle. Since these waste products impair the contraction process, the anaerobic processes can supply ATP only during short periods of activity and can be regarded as an emergency fuel reserve.

Limitations of the energetic processes

There are two inherent limits on the energetic processes: the maximum rate (power) and the amount of ATP (capacity) that can be produced.[6] The power and the capacity vary drastically between the different energetic processes. The peak values of power and capacity that have been observed in human skeletal muscle during exercise are presented in Fig. 2. Factors such as training status, nutrition, and working muscle mass will modify these values. All energetic processes contribute to energy production during exercise, but the relative contribution of each process varies during different types of exercise. The intensity of the exercise is an important determinant of the extent to which the various energetic processes are recruited. It will influence the relation between aerobic and anaerobic processes and the relation between carbohydrate and fat oxidation. Other factors of importance are the availability of oxygen, training status, availability of fuels, and hormonal changes. The described metabolic processes will set an upper limit to energy production and may thus restrict exercise performance. The sum of the maximal power of the ATP-generating reactions will limit the intensity of the exercise, and the maximal capacity of ATP generation (at a certain exercise intensity) will limit the duration of exercise.

Breakdown of phosphocreatine

The breakdown of phosphocreatine is the energetic process that can sustain the highest rate of ATP production. The maximum rate of

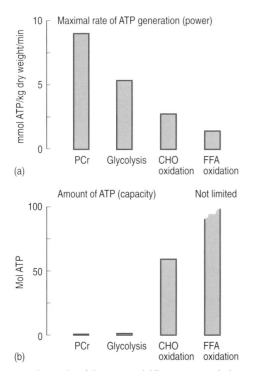

Fig. 2 Power and capacity of the energy-yielding processes in human skeletal muscle. Levels of power are based on observed values during the following conditions: phosphocreatine breakdown, 1.3 s electrical stimulation;[7] glycolysis, 2.6 s electrical stimulation;[7] carbohydrate oxidation (CHO), calculated from O_2 extraction during two-leg cycling, assuming that 72 per cent of $\dot{V}O_2$max (4 litre/min) is utilized by a working muscle mass of 20 kg. Free fatty acid (FFA) oxidation was assumed to be 50 per cent of that of CHO oxidation. Values for capacity have been derived from the muscle content of phosphocreatine, glycogen (80 mmol/kg), maximal muscle lactate accumulation, and a working muscle of 20 kg. The amount of ATP that can be produced from oxidation of FFA is not limited, hence the staple bar is cut off.

phosphocreatine breakdown observed *in vivo* is close to the maximum *in vitro* rate of ATP hydrolysis by the contractile protein.[8] Therefore, it seems plausible that the release of energy during short bursts of activity (e.g. the high jump, shotput, and the start of a 100-m sprint) is not limited by the rate of ATP generation through phosphocreatine breakdown but rather by intrinsic limitations of the contractile proteins or by motor unit recruitment.

The amount of energy that can be produced from phosphocreatine is rather small and is limited by the intramuscular store. The muscle content of phosphocreatine is about 15 per cent higher in fast-twitch fibres than in slow-twitch fibres[9] and thus fast-twitch fibres have a higher capacity for this process. With the maximal rate of phosphocreatine breakdown depicted in Fig. 2, one would expect complete depletion of phosphocreatine in about 10 s. However, the contribution of ATP from other energy sources and decreased energy expenditure owing to fatigue prolong this time. On the basis of thermodynamic considerations, one would expect that the maximum rate of phosphocreatine breakdown would decrease when the phosphocreatine content of the muscle decreases. Availability of phosphocreatine may therefore be a limiting factor on power output even before the muscle content of phosphocreatine is totally depleted. This may explain why the running speed at the end of a 100-m race decreases despite the fact that phosphocreatine is not completely depleted.[10]

Recent studies have demonstrated that the muscle store of total

creatine (phosphocreatine + creatine) can increase by about 10 to 20 per cent with oral creatine supplementation.[11] Evidence has also been presented that creatine supplementation enhances performance during high-intensity intermittent exercise,[12] a type of exercise that occurs frequently in a variety of sports such as soccer, ice hockey, and tennis. These data provide evidence that limitations of the energetic processes may play a major role in performance.

Glycolysis

The degradation of carbohydrate proceeds via glycolysis both during complete oxidation in the mitochondria and when lactate is the end product. In contrast to complete carbohydrate oxidation, in which all of the stored energy is released, incomplete degradation of carbohydrates to lactate exploits only 8 per cent of the stored energy and is therefore an inefficient way of utilizing fuel. Glycolysis can proceed in the absence of oxygen and, owing to the high-level activities of glycolytic enzymes, the energetic power of this process is high. Anaerobic glycolysis (i.e. lactate formation) is an important process for ATP formation when the energetic demand exceeds the oxidative power and under conditions of oxygen deficiency.

The maximum rate of glycolysis (i.e. lactate formation) observed in the human quadriceps femoris muscle after voluntary and electrically induced isometric contraction is 3 to 4 mmol/kg dry wt per second.[7,13] Although most reports demonstrate that lactate formation starts at the very onset of exercise, there appears to be a lag of a couple of seconds before the maximum rate is reached. Lactate is mainly derived from glycogen since the rate of glycogenolysis is much higher than that for glucose uptake. The maximum rate of glycolysis (breakdown of glucose units to pyruvate) is determined by the activities of the enzymes glycogen phosphorylase and phosphofructokinase. The activities of these enzymes are depressed during acidosis and the product of glycolysis (lactic acid) can therefore reduce the rate of glycolysis and the amount of lactic acid accumulation through feedback inhibition. This could be regarded as a safety mechanism, by means of which cellular damage owing to excessive lactic acid accumulation is prevented. Both the power and the capacity of glycolysis (i.e. amount of lactic acid produced) may therefore be limited by product accumulation (i.e. H^+). At the observed maximum rate of glycolysis (3 to 4 mmol/kg dry wt per min), one would expect that saturating muscle lactate levels would be reached after maximal exercise for 30 s. However, because an increased proportion of the energy demand is derived from aerobic processes and because of muscle fatigue (and thus a decreased energy demand) it will take a longer time (about 1 min) before the maximal muscle lactate level is reached.

There is no doubt that glycolysis is an important process for energy production during high-intensity exercise and under anaerobic conditions. This is emphasized by the decreased exercise tolerance in patients with McArdle's disease, in which the patients are deficient in the glycogenolytic enzyme.[14] However, lactate will also be formed during submaximal exercise before the aerobic power is fully exploited. The relative exercise intensity when blood lactate reaches 4 mmol/l or increases above the baseline (lactate threshold) is an important indicator of the local oxidative power and is closely related to endurance during marathon running.[15] The observed relationship is probably explained by an increased rate of glycogen breakdown.

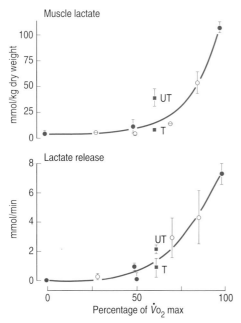

Fig. 3 Muscle lactate and lactate release after cycling for 4 to 15 min at different intensities. Symbols are means ±SE from four to eight subjects in three different studies.○[16,]●[17,]■[18]

Influence of muscle mass

The power of anaerobic energy production appears to be limited either by the activities of creatine kinase and key enzymes in glycolysis or by the activity of myosin ATPase (i.e. the energy demand). The total enzyme activities are proportional to muscle mass and an increased working muscle mass will therefore result in a proportional increase in the maximum anaerobic power and thus exercise intensity. In contrast, the power of aerobic energy production is limited to a significant extent by cardiac output and an increase in muscle mass therefore will not increase aerobic power. The capacity for both carbohydrate oxidation and anaerobic energy production is limited by intrinsic muscular factors such as the amount of glycogen, the amount of phosphocreatine, and the available volume for the distribution of interfering metabolic end-products. Consequently, under both aerobic and anaerobic conditions, a large working muscle mass will be advantageous for the amount of energy, and thus the amount of work, that can be produced. However, an increased muscle mass may not necessarily be an advantage for performance since the energy expenditure may increase owing to the increase in body weight.

Influence of transmembrane lactate flux on acid–base balance

The amount of lactic acid that can accumulate in the muscle cell before impairment of the contraction process is limited. Extrusion of lactic acid into the extracellular fluid provides a mechanism to increase the production of lactate and thus to prolong the duration of exercise. The release of lactate from the working muscle increases with the intensity of the exercise and is related to muscle lactate (Fig. 3). Earlier studies indicated an upper limit of lactate release from the leg during cycling of about 4 to 5 mmol/min.[16] However,

later studies on a smaller working muscle mass (one-leg knee extension) have shown that lactate release can increase up to 20 mmol/min.[19] The higher muscle blood flow and lactate gradient during exercise with a small working muscle mass may explain the high rate of lactate release.

The proportion of produced lactate extruded from the muscle is dependent on the intensity, duration, and nature of the exercise. During high-intensity exercise the release of lactate may range between 17 per cent (maximal cycling at 100 per cent $\dot{V}o_2$max)[17] and 30 per cent (one-leg knee-extension)[19] of the total amount produced. Thus, during high-intensity exercise, most of the produced lactate remains within the muscle despite large increases in blood lactate. In contrast, during prolonged exercise, there is a continuous release of lactate but only a moderate increase in muscle lactate and a major proportion of the lactate is released from the cell.

The transport of lactate is passive (i.e. without expenditure of ATP) and occurs both by free diffusion and facilitated diffusion.[20] Despite the low concentration, there is evidence that free diffusion mainly occurs in the form of undissociated lactic acid. The carrier-mediated process involves a cotransport of lactate and H^+.[20] Carrier-mediated lactate transport has been shown to increase with training and to be related weakly to the percentage of type I fibres.[21] Experiments in humans have shown that the venous–arterial difference for the base deficit (corresponding to the release of H^+) is equal to that of lactate both during exercise and the early recovery period[22] and suggest that the efflux of H^+ is stoichiometric to that of lactate. However, other studies using the one-leg knee extension model indicate that proton release is in excess of lactate release.[23]

During prolonged exercise at a moderate intensity, lactate is released continuously from the working muscle.[24] Despite this large release of lactate from the working muscle, blood lactate and blood pH remain fairly constant and demonstrate that the release of lactate is balanced by an equal rate of uptake by the liver and inactive muscle tissues. The continuous release of lactate from the working muscle should correspond to a large flux of protons into the blood. However, the perturbation of extracellular pH is small and suggests that, in this situation, the transmembrane flux of lactate corresponds to a similar flux of protons.

Changes in muscle and blood pH during exercise

The arterial blood pH at rest is 7.4 and the intramuscular pH is close to 7.0. If the hydrogen ions were in electrochemical equilibrium across the cell membrane one would (owing to the negative potential of the cell interior) expect a much higher concentration of H^+ (corresponding to pH 6.0). The low transmembrane permeability of H^+ and HCO_3^- and the extrusion of H^+ by energy-consuming transport systems ensure that the cellular pH can be maintained far above the value corresponding to the electrochemical equilibrium for H^+.

During high-intensity exercise, lactate accumulates both in muscle and in the blood and the acid–base homeostasis is disturbed. The decrease in pH is attenuated by buffering processes (see below) and by hyperventilation, by which means arterial PCO$_2$ is reduced. After high-intensity exercise the capillary blood pH can decrease to 7.1 or 7.2, or even below 7.0 for short periods of time.[25] Considering that pH values outside the range of 7.0 to 7.8 are regarded as a threat to life, it is clear that exercise is a serious challenge to the organism.

Muscle pH has been measured by different techniques. Using the homogenate technique, muscle pH decreased from about 7.1 at rest to about 6.4 to 6.8 at fatigue. The decrease in pH was linearly related to the increase in muscle lactate (Fig. 4). With the CO_2 technique, where intracellular pH is calculated by the Hendersson–Hasselbach equation, pH at rest in human muscle is 7.0 and the value after cycling to fatigue is 6.4.[27] The intracellular pH can be measured non-invasively by using the nuclear magnetic resonance (**NMR**) technique to monitor the position of the ^{31}P peak of inorganic phosphate. Since the P_i made visible by NMR is located in the cytosol, the measured pH corresponds to that of the cytosol. The intracellular pH obtained at rest using this technique is similar to that measured by other techniques, but during fatigue, values of as low as pH 6 have been reported in the contracting forearm muscle[28] and in the flexor digitorum superficialis muscle.[3] In other studies using NMR,[29] pH decreased during fatigue to a level (pH 6.5 to 6.6) similar to that observed using the homogenate technique.

Buffer capacity

During high-intensity exercise the cellular release of H^+ is mainly due to an accumulation of lactic acid, which can amount to more than 30 mmol/l of muscle water. The change in pH is determined both by the amount of acid or base added and by the cellular buffering capacity ($\beta = \Delta H^+/\Delta pH$). If 30 mmol/l of H^+ ions were added to an unbuffered solution, the pH would decrease to less than 2. However, because of the buffering processes, more than 99 per cent of the released H^+ is bound within the cell and the changes in the free H^+ concentration and pH are diminished. Muscle β can be estimated from the slope of the linear relation between muscle pH and muscle lactate (Fig. 4). From the changes in lactate, pyruvate, and pH during dynamic exercise, β has been estimated to be 73 mmol/l/pH in human muscle.[30] Similar values have been obtained after *in vitro* titration of homogenates from the quadriceps femoris muscle[31] and the gastrocnemius and triceps brachii muscles.[32]

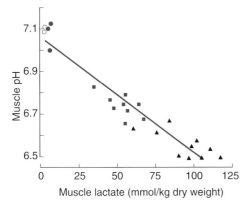

Fig. 4 Relationship between muscle pH (determined by the homogenate technique) and muscle lactate content. Muscle specimens were taken from the quadriceps femoris muscle in man at rest (o) after circulatory occlusion for 10 min(•) and after isometric contraction at 68 per cent of the maximum voluntary contraction force sustained for 25 s (■) or to fatigue (45 s) (▲). Results are from Sahlin *et al.*[26] and are reproduced with the kind permission of the *Biochemical Journal*. $y = -0.00537x + 7.06$; $r = 0.96$.

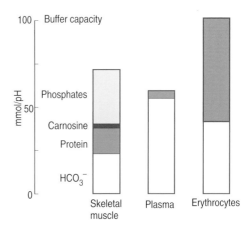

Fig. 5 Buffer capacity of skeletal muscle, plasma, and erythrocytes. The buffering of $HCO_3^- - CO_2$ was calculated as $2.3 \times (HCO_3^-)$ according to Woodbury[33] and assuming an open system (i.e. intact muscle blood flow). In a closed system in which CO_2 is trapped (e.g. in ischaemia), the buffer capacity of $HCO_3^- - CO_2$ is negligible. The buffering by proteins in erythrocytes and plasma is from Woodbury.[33] The composition of buffer capacity in skeletal muscle is from Sahlin.[30]

The magnitude and the composition of β in skeletal muscle are different from those in plasma and erythrocytes (Fig. 5). Phosphate compounds are of major importance for β in skeletal muscle but have a negligible influence on β in erythrocytes and plasma. The CO_2 system is an important buffer system in the blood but it is less important in skeletal muscle. This is explained by the lower pH and thus lower HCO_3^- concentration in muscle. Another effect of the lower intracellular concentration of HCO_3^- is that the change in pH after a change in PCO_2 will be smaller. Consequently, respiratory acid–base disturbances will have a much smaller influence on intracellular pH than on extracellular pH.

Increases in β may improve the exercise capacity during high-intensity exercise since the decrease in pH for a certain increase in lactate will be reduced. After anaerobic training for 8 weeks the buffer capacity increased by 37 per cent (range 12 to 50 per cent, $n = 7$).[34] The increased buffer capacity enabled the subjects to accumulate more lactic acid and the capacity to perform exercise also increased accordingly. Two weeks of high-altitude training increased both the buffer capacity in muscle (by 6 per cent) and the capacity for short-term running.[32] In a cross-sectional study, buffering capacity was found to be higher in trained subjects involved in sports with a high degree of anaerobic energy utilization (ice hockey, football) compared with a control group of untrained subjects.[35] In contrast, no change in β (measured by *in vitro* titration of muscle) was found after 8 weeks of sprint training.[31] Despite the unchanged β, the subjects increased their sprinting capacity and were able to accumulate more lactate in the muscles. The reason for the divergence between studies is not clear.

Effects of acidosis on metabolism

Acidosis and glycolysis

It has been known for a long time that the maximal rate of glycolysis is enhanced during alkalosis and inhibited during acidosis. The main regulatory steps in the metabolic pathway of lactate formation are the activities of glycogen phosphorylase and phosphofructokinase. Both of these enzymes are sensitive to changes in pH and have

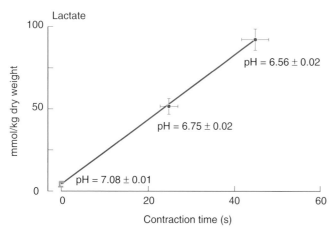

Fig. 6 Muscle lactate during isometric contraction at 68 per cent of maximal voluntary contraction to fatigue. Corresponding values of muscle pH are shown. Results are means ± SE, from ref. 37.

lower activity under acidotic conditions.[36] The rate of glycolysis (measured as the rate of lactate accumulation) has been determined during isometric contraction sustained to fatigue (Fig. 6). Despite a pronounced decrease in muscle pH, the glycolytic rate is maintained. Similar data are available from animal studies (for references, see[38]) and appear to be in conflict with the inhibition of the regulatory enzymes observed *in vitro*. Increases of inorganic phosphate, AMP, ADP, and hexose-phosphates[38] are allosteric activators of phosphofructokinase and are all increased during high-intensity exercise. Similarly, AMP and inosine monophosphate (**IMP**) are allosteric activators of glycogen phosphorylase. Thus acidotic inhibition of glycolysis and glycogenolysis may be counteracted by other metabolic changes and it is clear that a low pH does not necessarily limit the rate of these processes *in vivo*. However, the price for maintaining a high rate of glycolysis at a low pH is increased levels of ADP and AMP, and there is evidence that these changes could be involved in the impairment of the contraction process.

Acidosis and phosphocreatine depletion

The muscle content of phosphocreatine has been shown to be curvilinearly related to muscle lactate.[39] The relationship appeared to be independent of exercise intensity and was suggested to reflect an altered equilibrium state of the creatine kinase reaction induced by increased concentrations of H^+ and ADP (which may be secondary to acidotic inhibition of glycolysis; see above). Thus, during exercise, acidosis may result in phosphocreatine depletion and a decreased maximal rate of ATP generation. A consequence of phosphocreatine depletion is an increase in inorganic phosphorus (equation 3). Acidosis increases both the total P_i concentration in muscle (through displacement of the creatine kinase equilibrium towards phosphocreatine depletion) and increases the proportion of P_i present as $H_2PO_4^-$. Increases in P_i (especially $H_2PO_4^-$) have been implicated as an important factor in fatigue.[28]

Acidosis and aerobic energy production

Although acidosis has certain negative effects on muscle energetics, decrease in tissue pH has a positive effect on muscle oxygenation.

The mechanism is related to a decreased oxygen affinity of haemoglobin (the Bohr effect) and local vasodilation under conditions of acidosis. Tissue acidosis will thus facilitate oxygen uptake and thereby improve aerobic energy production.[40]

The effects of lactic acidosis on the function of isolated mitochondria have been investigated in a number of studies. Acidosis appears to decrease the maximal rate of respiration and the P/O ratio (i.e. the amount of ATP produced per amount of oxygen consumed).[41-43] The observed effects were, however, less pronounced in mitochondria isolated from skeletal muscle[41,44] than in those from other tissues.[41,43] Mitochondria isolated from horse skeletal muscle displayed a decreased maximal rate of respiration to 45 per cent of the control value after high-intensity exercise.[45] Although this occurred in parallel with reductions in pH, other factors may be responsible for this effect. Aerobic energy production is of central importance during dynamic exercise and even small changes in function will influence aerobic performance. Further studies are required to elucidate the influence of acid–base changes on the aerobic processes.

Acid−base changes and exercise performance

During high-intensity exercise, large changes occur in intracellular pH, and lactic acid accumulation is often implicated as a cause of fatigue. An increased hydrogen ion concentration could interfere with the energy supply as discussed above and, secondarily, affect one or several steps in the contraction process. Alternatively, an increased H^+ ion concentration (or associated changes, i.e. increases in $H_2PO_4^-$) may interfere directly with the contractile machinery. *In vitro* experiments with the skinned fibre preparation have shown that increases in P_i and H^+ impair the contraction process.[46,47] It was shown in contracting human muscle that the decline in force was related to the increase in $H_2PO_4^{-28}$, whereas in another study of a patient deficient in myophosphorylase, no correlation was observed between $H_2 PO_4^-$ and the decline in tension.[48] A series of experiments has been performed to investigate the influence of an altered acid–base status on exercise performance. Alkalosis was induced by the administration of bicarbonate and acidosis by the administration of ammonium chloride. During high-intensity exercise of short duration (less than 2 min) there is no detectable influence of prior treatment with these agents on performance.[49,50] However, during exercise of a longer duration and during intermittent exercise, induced alkalosis has been shown to improve performance in some studies.[51-53] Concomitantly, the muscle and blood lactate content during fatigue was augmented.[51,52] The divergent results may be related to the fact that the intracellular pH was affected in some studies but not in others. Extracellular pH is a poor indicator of both the magnitude and the direction of the change in intracellular pH. In fact under certain conditions, such as the administration of ammonium chloride, lactate, or bicarbonate, one may even expect the intracellular pH to change transiently in the opposite direction to that of the extracellular pH. Extracellular alkalosis has been shown to increase postexercise blood lactate.[50-52] It is possible that the improved performance, which was observed after prior treatment with bicarbonate, was related to an increased efflux of lactic acid.

Muscle energetics and fatigue

Our knowledge of the mechanism and the limits of the contraction process has been extended considerably during recent years. However, the mechanism(s) of fatigue is still not fully understood and is a sign of the complexity of the subject. A detailed discussion of fatigue and its mechanisms is beyond the scope of this chapter and the reader is referred to more extensive reviews.[54-56]

The hypothesis that muscle fatigue is caused by failure of the energetic processes to generate ATP at a sufficient rate is classic. The evidence for this hypothesis is that interventions which increase the power (i.e. aerobic training) or capacity (i.e. carbohydrate loading, creatine supplementation, or glucose supplementation) of the energetic processes result in enhanced performance and a delayed onset of fatigue. Similarly, factors that impair the energetic processes (i.e. depletion of muscle glycogen, intracellular acidosis, hypoxic conditions, or reduced muscle blood flow) have a negative influence on performance. It has been argued that since muscle ATP remains practically unchanged during exhaustive exercise, it is unlikely that fatigue is caused by energy deficiency. This line of reasoning may, however, be too simplistic, since temporal and spatial gradients of adenine nucleotides may exist in the contracting muscle. Furthermore, the link between energy deficiency and fatigue may be related to increases in the products of ATP hydrolysis (i.e. ADP, AMP, or P_i) rather than to decreases in ATP *per se*. A small decrease in ATP will cause relatively large increases in ADP and AMP, because of the lower concentrations of these latter compounds. Under a variety of conditions, muscle fatigue is associated with increased catabolism of adenine nucleotides to IMP and ammonia[57] and this supports the hypothesis that muscle fatigue is caused, under many conditions, by energy deficiency.

Concluding remarks

The increased energy demand during exercise is associated with large increases in the rates of the energetic processes and therefore also in the flux of H^+. The increased accumulation of lactic acid causes a decrease in tissue pH, the extent being dependent on the buffer capacity and the efflux of lactic acid. A decrease in the extracellular pH will facilitate tissue O_2 uptake and thus have a positive influence on aerobic energy transduction. However, a decrease in the intracellular pH will interfere with the intracellular energetic processes and decrease the maximal rate of ADP rephosphorylation. Recent studies have shown that, under a variety of conditions, exercise to fatigue results in a breakdown of the adenine nucleotide pool to IMP. This supports the hypothesis that, in many cases, fatigue is related to a mismatch between utilization and generation of ATP. During high-intensity exercise, fatigue is associated in many cases with lactic acid accumulation and acidosis. However, it is clear that, under other conditions, fatigue may occur when the muscle pH is unchanged or even increased. Thus, patients with glycogen phosphorylase deficiency (McArdle's disease) and phosphofructokinase deficiency have low exercise tolerance, although their muscle pH at fatigue is increased. Similarly, during prolonged submaximal exercise, fatigue coincides with glycogen depletion and not with lactate accumulation.

Evidence suggests that, in many cases, the failure of the contraction process is related to energy deficiency and that acidosis is one factor of importance. Therefore, metabolic factors are likely to play an important role in physical performance *in vivo*, but there is no doubt that conditions exist in which fatigue cannot be explained by metabolic changes. Considering the diversity and complexity of exercise, this is to be expected.

References

1. Hultman E, Sahlin K. Acid–base balance during exercise. *Exercise and Sport Sciences Reviews*, 1981; 9: 41–128.
2. Dawson JM, Gadian DG, Wilkie DR. Contraction and recovery of living muscles studied by ^{31}P nuclear magnetic resonance. *Journal of Physiology* 1977; 267: 703–35.
3. Taylor DJ, Bore PJ, Styles P, Gadian DG, Radda GK. Bioenergetics of intact human muscle: a ^{31}P nuclear magnetic resonance study. *Molecular Biology and Medicine* 1983; 1: 77–94.
4. Hochachka PW, Mommsen TP. Protons and anaerobiosis. *Science* 1983; 219: 1392–97.
5. Fletcher WW, Hopkins FG. Lactic acid in mammalian muscle. *Journal of Physiology* (*London*)1907; 35: 247–303.
6. McGilvery RW. The use of fuels for muscular work. In: Poortmans JR, ed. *Metabolic adaptation to prolonged physical exercise*. Basel: Birkhäuser, 1973: 12–30.
7. Hultman E, Sjöholm H. Substrate availability. In: Knuttgen HG, Vogel JA, Poortmans J, eds. *Biochemistry of Exercise*, vol 13. 1983: 63–75.
8. Saltin B, Gollnick PD, Skeletal muscle adaptability: significance for metabolism and performance. In: Peachey LD, Adrian RH, Geiger SR, eds. *Handbook of physiology. Skeletal muscle*. Bethesda: American Physiological Society, 1983: 555–631.
9. Söderlund K, Hultman E. ATP and phosphocreatine changes in single human muscle fibers after intense electrical stimulation. *American Journal of Physiology* 1991; 261: E737–41.
10. Hirvonen J, Rehunen S, Rusko H, Härkönen M. Breakdown of high-energy phosphate compounds and lactate accumulation during short supramaximal exercise. *European Journal of Applied Physiology*. 1987; 56: 253–9.
11. Harris RC, Söderlund K, Hultman E. Elevation of creatine in resting and exercised muscle of normal subjects by creatine supplementation. *Clinical Science* 1992; 83: 367–74.
12. Balsom PD, Ekblom B, Söderlund K, Sjödin B, Hultman E. Creatine supplementation and dynamic high-intensity exercise. *Scandinavian Journal of Medicine and Science in Sports* 1993; 3: 143–9.
13. Ahlborg B *et al.* Muscle metabolism during isometric exercise performed at constant force. *Journal of Applied Physiology* 1972; 33: 224–8.
14. Lewis SF, Haller RG, Cook JD, Nunnally RL. Muscle fatigue in McArdle's disease studied by ^{31}P-NMR: effect of glucose infusion. *Journal of Clinical Investigation* 1985; 76: 556–60.
15. Sjödin B, Svedenhag J. Applied physiology for marathon running. *Sports Medicine* 1985; 2: 83–99.
16. Jorfeldt L, Juhlin-Dannfelt A, Karlsson J. Lactate release in relation to tissue lactate in human skeletal muscle during exercise. *Journal of Applied Physiology* 1978, 44: 350–2.
17. Katz A, Broberg S, Sahlin K, Wahren J. Muscle ammonia and amino acid metabolism during dynamic exercise in man. *Clinical Physiology* 1986, 6: 365–79.
18. Jansson E, Kaijser L. Substrate utilization and enzymes in skeletal muscle of extremely endurance-trained men. *Journal of Applied Physiology* 1987, 62: 999–1005.
19. Saltin B. Anaerobic capacity: past, present and prospective. In: Taylor AW, Gollnick PD, eds. *Biochemistry of exercise VII*. Champaign: Human Kinetics, 1990: 387–412.
20. Juel C. Muscle lactate transport studied in sarcolemmal giant vesicles. *Biochimica et Biophysica Acta* 1991; 1065: 15–20.

21. Pilegaard H, Bangsbo J, Richter EA, Juel C. Lactate transport studied in sarcolemmal giant vesicles from human muscle biopsies: relation to training status. *Journal of Applied Physiology* 1994; **77**: 1858–62.

22. Katz A, Sahlin K, Juhlin-Dannfelt A. Effect of adrenoceptor blockade on H^+ and K^+ flux in exercising man. *Journal of Applied Physiology* 1986; **250**: C834–40.

23. Bangsbo J, Johansen L, Graham T, Saltin B. Lactate and H^+ effluxes from human skeletal muscles during intense, dynamic exercise. *Journal of Physiology* (*London*) 1993; **462**: 115–33.

24. Broberg S, Sahlin K. Adenine nucleotide degradation in human skeletal muscle during prolonged exercise. *Journal of Applied Physiology* 1989; **67**: 116–22.

25. Hermansen L, Osnes JB. Blood and muscle pH after maximal exercise in man. *Journal of Applied Physiology* 1972; **32**: 304–8.

26. Sahlin K, Harris RC, Hultman E. Creatine kinase equilibrium and lactate content compared with muscle pH in tissue samples obtained after isometric exercise. *Biochemical Journal* 1975; **152**: 173–80.

27. Sahlin K, Alvestrand A, Brandt R, Hultman E. Intracellular pH and bicarbonate concentration in human muscle during recovery from exercise. *Journal of Applied Physiology* 1978; **45**: 474–80.

28. Wilson JR, McCully KK, Mancini DM, Boden B, Chance B. Relationship of muscular fatigue to pH and diprotonated P_i in humans: a ^{31}P-NMR study. *Journal of Applied Physiology* 1988; **64**: 33–9.

29. Miller RG, Boska MD, Moussavi RS, Carson PJ, Weiner MW. ^{31}P Nuclear magnetic resonance studies of high energy phosphates and pH in human muscle fatigue. *Journal of Clinical Investigation* 1988; **81**: 1190–6.

30. Sahlin K. Intracellular pH and energy metabolism in skeletal muscle of man. With special reference to exercise. *Acta Physiologica Scandinavica* 1978; Suppl.: 455.

31. Nevill ME, Boobis LH, Brooks S, Williams C. Effect of training on muscle metabolism during treadmill sprinting. *Journal of Applied Physiology* 1989; 67: 2376–82.

32. Mizuno M *et al*. Limb skeletal muscle adaptation in athletes after training at altitude. *Journal of Applied Physiology* 1990; **68**: 496–502.

33. Woodbury W. Regulation of pH. In: Ruch TC, Patton HD, eds. *Physiology and biophysics*. London: Sounder Co., 1965.

34. Sharp RL, Costill DL, Fink WJ, King DS. The effects of eight weeks of bicycle ergometer spring training on buffer capacity. *International Journal of Sports Medicine* 1983, 7: 13–17.

35. Sahlin K, Henriksson J. Buffer capacity and lactate accumulation in skeletal muscle of trained and untrained men. *Acta Physiologica Scandinavica* 1984, **122**: 331–9.

36. Trivedi B, Danforth WH. Effect of pH on the kinetics of frog muscle phosphofructokinase. *Journal of Biological Chemistry* 1966; **241**: 4110–14.

37. Sahlin K, Harris RC, Hultman E. Creatine kinase equilibrium and lactate content compared with muscle pH in tissue samples obtained after isometric exercise. *Biochemical Journal* 1975; **152**: 173–80.

38. Dobson GP, Yamamoto E, Hochachka PW. Phosphofructokinase control in muscle: nature and reversal of pH dependent ATP inhibition. *American Journal of Physiology* 1986; **250**: R71–6.

39. Harris RC, Sahlin K, Hultman E. Phosphagen and lactate contents of m. quadriceps femoris of man after exercise. *Journal of Applied Physiology* 1977; **43**: 852–7.

40. Stringer W, Wasserman K, Casaburi R, Porszasz J, Maehara K, French W. Lactic acidosis as a facilitator of oxyhemoglobin dissociation during exercise. *Journal of Applied Physiolog.* 1994; **76**: 1462–7.

41. Mitchelson KR, Hird FJR. Effect of pH and halothane on muscle and liver mitochondria. *American Journal of Physiology* 1973; **225**: 1393–8.

42. Tobin RB, Macherer CR, Mehlman MA. pH effects on oxidative phosphorylation of rat liver mitochondria. *American Journal of Physiology* 1972; **223**: 83–8.

43. Hillered L, Ernster L, Siesjö BK. Influence of *in vitro* acidosis and hypercapnia on respiratory activity of isolated rat brain mitochondria. *Journal of Cerebral Blood Flow and Metabolism* 1984; **4**: 430–7.

44. Mukherjee A, Wong TM, Templeton G, Buja LM, Willerson JT. Influence of volume dilution, lactate phosphate, and calcium on mitochondrial function. *American Journal of Physiology* 1979; **237**: H224–38.

45. Gollnick PD, Bertocci LA, Kelso TB, Witt EH, Hodgson DR. The effect of high intensity exercise on the respiratory capacity of skeletal muscle. *Pflügers Archiv* 1990; **415**: 407–13.

46. Donaldsson SKB, Hermansen L, Bolles L. Differential, direct effects of H^+ on Ca^{2+} activated force of skinned fibers from the soleus, cardiac and adductor magnus muscles of rabbits. *Pflügers Archiv* 1978; **376**: 55–65.

47. Cooke R, Franks K, Luciani GB, Pate E. The inhibition of rabbit skeletal muscle contraction by hydrogen ions and phosphate. *Journal of Physiology* (*London*) 1988; **395**: 77–97.

48. Cady EB, Jones DA, Lynn J, Newham DJ. Changes in force and intracellular metabolites during fatigue of fatigued human skeletal muscle. *Journal of Physiology* (*London*) 1989; **418**: 311–25.

49. Kindermann W, Keul J, Huber G. Physical exercise after induced alkalosis (bicarbonate or tris-buffer). *European Journal of Physiology* 1977; **37**: 197–204.

50. Katz A, Costill DL, King DS, Hargreaves M, Fink W.J. Maximal exercise tolerance after induced alkalosis. *International Journal of Sports Medicine* 1984; **5**: 107–10.

51. Jones NL, Sutton JR, Taylor R, Toews CJ. Effect of pH on cardiorespiratory and metabolic responses to exercise. *Journal of Applied Physiology* 1977; **43**: 959–64.

52. Sutton JR, Jones NL, Toews CJ. Effect of pH on muscle glycolysis during exercise. *Clinical Science* 1981; **61**: 331–8.

53. Costill DL, Verstappen F, Kuipers H, Janssen E, Fink W. Acid–base balance during repeated bouts of exercise. Influence of $NaHCO_3$. *International Journal of Sports Medicine* 1984; **5**: 228–31.

54. Fitts RH. Cellular mechanisms of muscle fatigue. *Physiological Review.* 1994; **74**: 49–94.

55. Westerblad H, Lee JA, Lännergren J, Allen DG. Cellular mechanisms of fatigue in skeletal muscle. *American Journal of Physiology* 1991; **261**: C195–209.

56. Sargeant AJ, Kernell D. *Neuromuscular fatigue.* Amsterdam: 1993.

57. Sahlin K, Broberg S. Adenine nucleotide depletion in human muscle during exercise: causality and significance of AMP deamination. *International Journal of Sports Medicine* 1990; **11**: S62–7.

1.2 Nutrition

1.2.1 Diet and sports performance

Clyde Williams

Introduction

Interest in the influences of food on the capacity for physical activity is as old as mankind. From earliest times, certain foods were regarded as essential preparation for physical activity, whether this was for confrontation on the battlefields of history or competition in the Stadia of Ancient Greece;[1] the aim being to achieve greater strength, power, and stamina than the opposition. These aspirations are also those of the modern sportsperson, and so it is not surprising that the interest in the links between food and physical performance continue to be of as much interest to the Olympians of today as it was to those of antiquity.

A greater understanding of the physiology of exercise, in general, and fatigue, in particular, has allowed us to begin to take the mystery out of the links between food and fitness. Fatigue is a consequence of failing to match energy production with expenditure in working muscles. However, clearer insights into human energy balance have begun to show how and when nutritional strategies can help redress this mismatch between energy expenditure and energy production. These research findings are translated into dietary recommendations for sportspeople by an increasing number of well-qualified and experienced sports dietitians. Sports dietitians are now essential members of ever-expanding teams who support sportsmen and women in their pursuit of success in sport.

Although the aim of sports nutrition is to understand the influence of diet on sports performance, there are, unfortunately, only a few studies on the links between food intake and sports performance *per se*. There are so many factors which influence performance that nutritional scientists have shied away from undertaking studies based on the outcome of sports competitions. Therefore, most of our current knowledge is largely an extrapolation from the results of well-controlled laboratory studies. Even so, there is still a dearth of information on the influences of nutrition on specific sports skills *per se*. Nevertheless, the contribution of nutrition is to help delay fatigue for as long as possible and, in so doing, postpone the deterioration of skill during the latter stages of competition.

People who participate in sport, whether simply for pleasure, recreation, or as a profession, do not immediately think of themselves as athletes. This is because in Europe the term is reserved for those who participate in track and field athletics, or simply because they do not train hard enough to feel that they warrant the label of 'athlete'. Nevertheless, for the purpose of this chapter, 'athlete' will be used as the generic term for those people who undertake training in preparation for participation in sport, irrespective of the level of the competition.

Some general considerations

In seeking general principles to guide the nutritional preparation of athletes, it is helpful to classify sports according to the rate and amount of energy expenditure they require. Rate of energy expenditure is as an important characteristic of the simple classification process, as is overall energy expenditure, because it provides an insight into the reasons for fatigue in that sport. For this reason, the terms 'aerobic' and 'anaerobic' are often used by sports scientists to describe activities which are common to several sports. However, these labels should not be taken too literally because there are no activities which rely entirely on one or other of these two cellular routes to energy production. Endurance, power, and multiple-sprint sports are other ways of grouping sports with similar energy demands and, possibly, nutritional needs. Endurance sports include long-distance running, swimming, cycling, race walking, and cross-country skiing. Power sports typically include weightlifting, judo, shot and discus throwing, whereas the multiple-sprint sports include football, rugby, hockey, basketball, and tennis. The latter sports involve a mixture of brief periods of exercise of maximum intensity followed by recovery periods of rest or light activity.

The rapidly growing literature on sports nutrition is largely made up of laboratory studies describing the influences of nutritional intervention on exercise performance. Cycling and treadmill running are the two main forms of exercise used in laboratory-based nutritional studies. The performance criteria most commonly used are: (1) time to exhaustion while performing exercise at a predetermined, constant intensity; and (2) fastest time to complete an exercise task, such as completing a predetermined amount of work or running a predetermined distance. The former criterion is an assessment of endurance capacity, whereas the latter is a simulation of competition and so can be described as 'performance' rather than just 'capacity' for exercise.

The distinction between exercise capacity and performance is a functional one which helps us to understand more clearly the conditions under which nutritional strategies have improved performance. For example, nutritional interventions improve endurance capacity; however, the improvements in endurance performance during simulated competitions may not be of the same order of magnitude. Of course, endurance capacity is an essential ingredient of fitness for endurance competitions. Success in endurance competitions depends not only on a large endurance capacity but also on tactical experience, optimum environmental conditions, and robust

Table 1 Examples of daily intakes of energy, carbohydrate (CHO), fat, and protein, expressed as grams and as percentage (%) of energy intakes, of well-trained male athletes

Sport (n)		Energy (kcal)	CHO (g)	Fat (g)	Protein (g)	Reference
Distance runners	(10)	3034	396 49%	115 34%	128 17%	3
Marathon runners	(19)	3570	487 52%	128 32%	128 15%	6
Soccer players	(8)	4952	596 47%	217 39%	170 14%	62
Soccer players	(26)	2632	354 51%	93 32%	103 16%	140
Soccer players	(25)	3062	397 48%	118 35%	108 14%	140
Swimmers	(22)	5222	596 45%	248 43%	166 12%	141
Swimmers	(9)	3072	404 55%	102 30%	108 15%	142
Weight-lifters	(19)	3640	399 43%	155 39%	156 18%	6

psychology. However, the reasonable assumption is that if a nutritional intervention improves endurance capacity then it will also improve endurance performance, but not necessarily to the same extent.

Diet

Health professionals recommend a diet which provides us with at least 50 per cent of our daily energy intake in the form of carbohydrates, 35 per cent or less from fats, and the remainder from proteins. The widely held view is that we should move from high-fat, meat-based diets to those that contain more carbohydrates, fresh fruits, and vegetables.[2] The people who appear to comply most closely with these dietary recommendations are endurance athletes, whereas athletes in other sports tend to have diets which are not very different from those consumed by the population at large.[3-6] Sport has not evolved 'special diets' for its athletes. Where differences in athletes' diets exist, they are mainly differences in the amount, rather than the type, of food they consume. As an illustration of this point, Tables 1 and 2 give examples of the energy and macronutrient intakes of athletes from some widely different sports. Even athletes from the same sport have a different energy intake and often the percentage energy intake of a nutrient is a poor guide to the amount eaten.

Much effort and co-operation is required to accurately assess energy intakes and composition of habitual diets (see refs 3 and 4 for reviews). Athletes must weigh and record all they eat and drink for 1 or 2 weeks. Although this is the 'gold standard' method, it is not without its problems, not least of which is the full co-operation of the athletes. Furthermore, when this information has been gathered, it provides only a snapshot of the athletes' food intake over, at most, 1 or 2 weeks of the year. Therefore, for the purpose of assessing the general adequacy of an athlete's diet, sports dietitians use simple dietary recall methods or food diaries rather than the weighed food-intake method. When this broad-brush approach to dietary assessment uncovers a problem, then the effort and resources required to obtain more detailed information is usually justified. The most commonly encountered problems are those associated with the perceived need to lose weight as a means of improving performance (see Chapters 1.2.3 and 1.2.5).

In an attempt to provide sound advice for athletes about their nutritional needs, an International Consensus Conference[7] was convened to consider the available research on the links between food, nutrition, and sports performance. The conference concluded that the most significant influence on performance was the size of an athlete's pre-exercise carbohydrate stores. The reason for this conclusion is the strong link between glycogen depletion and fatigue during prolonged heavy exercise. Therefore, they recommended that the carbohydrate content of an athlete's diet should be between 60 and 70 per cent of their daily energy intake, 30 per cent or less from fat, and 10 to 15 per cent from proteins.[7] However, the recommended high consumption of carbohydrate-containing foods was not intended to be part of the habitual diet of athletes but to be part of the nutritional preparation for prolonged heavy exercise.

These dietary recommendations can be achieved effectively by using a food-exchange system. This concept is based on the allocation of food to six groups in which servings of different foods have the same energy value (Appendix: Tables 3, 4, 5, 6, 7, 8, and 9) Those wishing to decrease their fat intake and increase their carbohydrate intake, for example, are directed to decrease the meat intake by cutting out some meat exchanges and replacing them with the equivalent number of carbohydrate exchanges. For example, the daily energy and nutrient intake of a young, female distance runner whose diet has been altered to increase her carbohydrate intake is

Table 2 Examples of daily intakes of energy, carbohydrate (CHO), fat, and protein, expressed as grams and as percentage (%) of energy intakes, of well-trained female athletes

Sport (n)		Energy (kcal)	CHO (g)	Fat (g)	Protein (g)	Reference
Distance runners	(18)	2151	296 55%	62 29%	86 16%	5
Distance runners— amenorrhoeic	(12)	2151	344 60%	67 27%	74 13%	143
Distance runners— eumenorrhoeic	(33)	2489	352 53%	97 35%	81 12%	143
Swimmers	(21)	3573	428 48%	164 41%	107 12%	141
Swimmers	(11)	2130	292 56%	63 28%	79 16%	142

shown in Table 5 (Appendix). She was able to increase her carbohydrate intake without changing her daily energy intake, simply by choosing different yet familiar foods with similar energy values. Whenever possible, dietary manipulation of this kind should be undertaken with the guidance of a sports dietitian, particularly if athletes are trying to lose weight in preparation for competition. Failing this, then athletes should at least consult some of the available texts which will help translate these recommendations into meals.[8–10]

Types of carbohydrate

Bread, potatoes, pasta, rice, and vegetables are often called complex carbohydrates, whereas foods that have a low-fibre content and contain a significant proportion of simple sugars, such as glucose, sucrose, and fructose, are referred to as simple carbohydrates. The common assumption is that the simple carbohydrates rapidly increase blood glucose concentration after they are eaten, unlike the complex carbohydrates. However, this is not the case with all simple carbohydrates or, indeed, all complex carbohydrates.

A metabolically more informative way of describing carbohydrates is one which describes the degree to which they raise blood glucose concentrations. Carbohydrates which produce a large increase in blood glucose concentration are classified as having a high glycaemic index.[11] A glycaemic index is given to a carbohydrate by comparing the area under a glucose–time curve following the ingestion of 50 g of the nutrient. The reference value of 100 is assigned to the changes in blood glucose concentration following the ingestion of 50 g of glucose. Carbohydrates which have a high glycaemic index are glucose, white bread, rice, sweet corn, and potatoes, whereas low glycaemic-index carbohydrates are apples, dates, peaches, fructose, and milk ice-cream. Fructose is a simple sugar but has a glycaemic index of less than 60. The glycaemic index provides additional information about a carbohydrate, which is particularly useful when designing diets to deliver glucose to working muscles rapidly.[12]

The idea that eating large amounts of carbohydrate will lead to

increased body fat still persists in the minds of many people including athletes, coaches, and team physicians. Nevertheless, there is some basis for their views even in the face of some of the new information about carbohydrate nutrition. For example, a carbohydrate intake greater than about 800 g is necessary before the body begins to convert this carbohydrate into fat.[13] Even then, the conversion of carbohydrate into fat is only about 75 per cent efficient. In contrast, the fat we eat is efficiently stored as fat in the body's adipose tissue. However, if we eat more than we expend, then we will store the excess as fat and carbohydrate, and so gain in bodyweight. Even loyally following the recommendations of health professionals to eat a low-fat diet will lead to an increase in body fat if our energy intake exceeds our energy expenditure. In trying to maintain our energy balance, such that our energy intake does not exceed energy expenditure, we are helped by the fact that overeating is less likely when we eat a high-carbohydrate diet.

Consuming meals which contain high proportions of fat appear to lead to a greater degree of overeating than when we eat meals containing mainly carbohydrates.[14] Furthermore, when we eat a high-carbohydrate meal, we oxidize more carbohydrate during the hour following the meal whether or not this postprandial period includes exercise. The same holds true after eating meals containing large amounts of protein.[15] This appears not to be the case when we eat meals containing large amounts of fat which may provide part of the answer to the question of why in the United Kingdom and the United States of America people are becoming fatter while seemingly eating less. However, recent studies suggest that the fat in our meal may have more of an influence on the amount of fat subsequently oxidized than was formerly believed to be the case.[16] If this is so, then the increase in obesity is largely the result of a decrease in physical activity rather than in the composition and size of our meals.

We are encouraged to eat less fat and more carbohydrates, but we should not overlook the fact that fat plays several important roles in our diets. Fat is the body's most efficient fuel. It contributes 9 kcal (37 kJ) per gram to energy metabolism, whereas the equivalent value for carbohydrate is 4 kcal (17 kJ), and protein is also 4 kcal (17 kJ). Fat is also a carrier for the fat-soluble vitamins A, D, E, and K, and it provides the essential fatty acids linolenic acid and linoleic acid. These are essential because they form integral parts of cell membranes, particularly the membranes of nerve cells. Furthermore, we must not overlook the fact that fat, in relatively small quantities, contributes to the attractive taste of many foods.

Many athletes share the same beliefs as the first Olympians about the beneficial values of high-protein diets. There is a long-held, but misguided, belief that athletes who want to develop strength must consume large quantities of meat. The World Health Organization (WHO)[17] recommends a daily protein intake of 1 g/kg bodyweight (BW). However, the protein intakes of even female endurance athletes, who are not normally preoccupied with gaining strength, are about 1.5 g/kg BW/ day, and so they are well above the World Health Organization (WHO) recommendations. However, those recommendations may be too low for athletes involved in prolonged heavy training. These athletes should eat the equivalent of 1.2 to 1.7 g protein/kg BW/day.[18]

Dietary protein provides us with 20 amino acids from which all the cells in the body and their structural contents are created. They are the body's building blocks which contribute to the repair and reproduction of tissues; they also contribute to physiological regulation by the formation of hormones and enzymes. Of the 20 amino acids, 8 must be provided by our diet because they cannot be manufactured by our own metabolism. High-protein foods such as meat, eggs, and fish contain all the essential amino acids and are, therefore, regarded as being of high biological value. Cereals and vegetables contain only some of the essential amino acids and so are of low biological value. Combining several of the low biological foods to make a meal is a strategy for overcoming the limited number of essential amino acids present in vegetables and cereals. This mutual supplementation of dietary protein is an effective way of obtaining a full complement of essential amino acids without contributions from meat and meat products.

A well-balanced vegetarian diet does not impair endurance capacity, in particular, and physical fitness, in general. For example, the endurance capacity of non-vegetarians was no different after they had consumed a lacto-ovovegetarian diet for 6 weeks than before changing their diet.[19] Although there were no signs of iron deficiency after 6 weeks on a vegetarian diet, it is worth remembering that non-haem iron found in vegetables is less readily absorbed than animal haem iron. The large fibre intake which is characteristic of the diets of vegetarians may influence the absorption of some essential nutrients such as iron and calcium (i.e. negative effect on the absorption of these essential minerals).

Athletes who eat a wide variety of foods in sufficient quantity to cover their daily energy expenditures do not require vitamin and mineral supplements. There is no good evidence to suggest that vitamin and mineral[20,21] supplementation of a well-balanced diet improves performance. However, the diets of people who are trying to lose weight are, of necessity, low in energy. Low-energy diets, even if they contain the recommended proportions of carbohydrate, fat, and protein, can lead to vitamin and mineral deficiency. Therefore, those people who are physically active and on low-energy diets are most at risk and should seek the advice of a sports dietitian. Of particular concern are sportswomen who reduce their energy intake

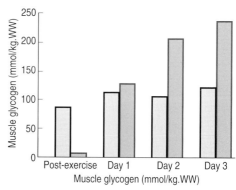

Fig. 1 Human muscle glycogen concentrations (mmol/kg WW) before and after prolonged heavy single leg exercise, for the active leg (dark shading) and the resting leg (light shading). (Modified after ref 24.)

and so run the risk of not consuming enough iron- and calcium-containing foods.

Carbohydrate-rich diets

A high-carbohydrate diet increases the stores of liver and muscle glycogen. Glycogen is a polymer of glucose which is described in terms of the amount of glucose released during hydrolysis, namely as millimoles of glucosyl units per kilogram of muscle. For example, human skeletal muscle has a glycogen concentration in the range 60 to 150 mmol glucosyl units/kg wet weight (WW) or 258 to 645 mmol glucosyl units/kg dry weight (DW).*

The size of the liver glycogen store depends on whether the person is fed or fasted. When fed, an adult man with a liver weighing about 1.8 kg has a liver glycogen concentration of approximately 550 mmol glucosyl units (WW), whereas after an overnight fast the concentration of glycogen falls to about 200 mmol WW. After a number of days on a high-carbohydrate diet, the liver glycogen concentration can increase to as much as 1000 mmol (WW).[22] Interestingly, however, an overnight fast does not appear to lower human muscle glycogen concentration as is the case with liver glycogen.[23]

Eating a high-carbohydrate diet in the days after exercise increases muscle glycogen stores to values which are greater than pre-exercise concentrations. This supercompensation of muscle glycogen is a local phenomenon because it only occurs in the previously active muscles (Fig. 1).[24] At least two dietary methods have been devised to exploit the fact that a carbohydrate-rich diet for 3 to 4 days after exercise to exhaustion results in larger muscle glycogen concentrations than pre-exercise values. In the original method, athletes were required to exercise to exhaustion a week before competition and then eat a very low-carbohydrate diet for the following 3 days; thereafter they would change to a high-carbohydrate diet for the 3 days before competition. This dietary and exercise manipulation produced high pre-exercise glycogen concentrations, especially in moderately to well-trained athletes.[25] However, 3 days on the low-carbohydrate diet is particularly unpleasant and athletes found that they could not train hard during these few days. This inability to continue to train reasonably hard in the week before competition tended to undermine the confidence of athletes. There-

---

* Many studies report glycogen concentrations, and those of the glycolytic intermediates, as dry weight values because they freeze-dry their muscle samples before analysis. Freeze-dried muscle samples are easier to handle and analyse than fresh muscle. On the basis that the water content of human skeletal muscle is approximately 77 per cent, wet-weight concentrations can be converted to dry-weight values by using a conversion factor of 4.3.

fore, other approaches to precompetition carbohydrate or glycogen loading were sought.

Sherman *et al.* recommended that athletes should taper their training in the week before competition, and during the 3 days before the event they should increase their carbohydrate intake.[26] The daily carbohydrate intake should be increased to about 550 g which for a 70 kg athlete translates to about 8 g/kg BW. This method produces the same high pre-exercise muscle glycogen concentrations as the traditional method of carbohydrate loading, and is far more tolerable and hence acceptable to athletes.

Pre-exercise diet and endurance capacity

Christensen and Hansen[27] were the first to provide detailed reports on the links between diet and exercise capacity. Their studies clearly showed the benefits of eating a high-carbohydrate diet before prolonged exercise. Almost 30 years later, Bergstrom *et al.*[28] examined the influence of different nutritional states on glycogen storage following prolonged heavy exercise. They found that a diet low in carbohydrate, and high in fat and protein for 3 days after prolonged submaximal exercise, produced a delayed muscle glycogen resynthesis, but when this was followed by a high-carbohydrate diet for the same period of time, glycogen supercompensation occurred (Fig. 2). This dietary manipulation not only increased the pre-exercise muscle glycogen concentration but also resulted in a significant improvement in endurance capacity of about 46 per cent (Fig. 3).

Ahlborg *et al.* also demonstrated the link between endurance capacity, during cycling, and pre-exercise muscle glycogen concentration.[29,30] They found a correlation of 0.87 between initial muscle glycogen concentrations and endurance times for their nine subjects. The importance of muscle glycogen during prolonged exercise was also confirmed in subsequent studies which showed that fatigue occurs when muscle glycogen concentrations are reduced to low values.[31–34]

The benefits of carbohydrate loading before prolonged submaximal exercise have been shown mainly during cycling. There are only a few studies on the influence of carbohydrate loading on running performance, and not all the available evidence supports the recommended dietary practice. Therefore, it is worth considering the results of a selection of the available studies on carbohydrate

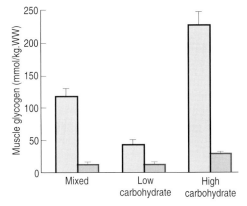

Fig. 2 Human muscle glycogen concentration (mmol/kg WW) before and immediately after prolonged submaximal cycling to exhaustion after a mixed diet, 3 days on a diet low in carbohydrate and high in protein and fat, and finally after 3 days on a high-carbohydrate diet (mean ± SD). (Modified after ref. 28.)

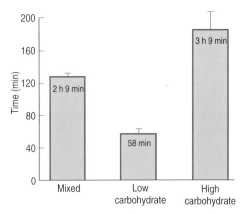

Fig. 3 Exercise time to exhaustion (min) after a mixed diet, 3 days on a diet low in carbohydrate and high in protein and fat, and finally after 3 days on a high-carbohydrate diet (mean ± SD). (Modified after ref. 28.)

loading in order to understand more clearly the conditions under which increasing the body's carbohydrate stores has a positive influence on performance.

Goforth *et al.*[35] reported that carbohydrate loading increased the endurance time of nine well-trained runners from 120 to 130 min at treadmill speeds equivalent to 80 per cent of $\dot{V}O_2$max. The carbohydrate-loading procedure was well controlled and the isocaloricity of each phase of the dietary manipulation was achieved using a combination of liquid and solid foods. The carbohydrate intake of the control diet was quite high and so this, together with the high relative exercise intensity (per cent of $\dot{V}O_2$max), may explain why there was only a 9 per cent increase in endurance capacity. This increase in performance was quite modest in comparison with the improvements of about 40 to 50 per cent reported in the cycle ergometer studies carried out during the late 1960s.[28,29]

A clear benefit from increasing the carbohydrate content of runners' diets is achieved when the exercise intensity is less intense. Brewer *et al.*[36] modified the normal diets of 30 runners during the 3 days following a treadmill run to exhaustion at 70 per cent of $\dot{V}O_2$max by providing either additional protein, complex carbohydrates, or simple carbohydrates to the runners' normal meals. The 'complex' carbohydrate group supplemented their normal mixed diet with bread, potatoes, rice, or pasta. The 'simple' carbohydrate group ate their normal mixed diet but increased their carbohydrate intake with chocolates, whereas the control group ate their normal diet to which was added extra protein and fat to ensure that the overall energy intake was the same for all three groups. After 3 days of recovery, the runners completed a second treadmill time trial to exhaustion. Running times increased after both types of high-carbohydrate diets. The complex carbohydrate group improved their running times by 26 per cent, and the simple carbohydrate group improved by 23 per cent. However, there was no improvement in the performance times of the control group, confirming that the carbohydrate content of the diet is the important nutrient and that the changes were not simply the consequence of a greater energy intake.

Not all studies on endurance capacity during submaximal running have shown benefits from dietary carbohydrate loading. Madsen *et al.*[37] reported that carbohydrate loading increased muscle glycogen concentrations in the gastrocnemius muscles of their subjects by 25 per cent. Their subjects ran to exhaustion on a level treadmill at speeds equivalent to 75 per cent to 80 per cent $\dot{V}O_2$max on two occasions. The time to exhaustion on the first trial, after the subjects consumed their normal mixed diet, was 70 min, whereas after carbohydrate loading they recorded 77 min. However, this 10 per cent improvement in endurance capacity was not statistically significant. The amount of muscle glycogen used by the gastrocnemius muscles was the same in both trials. Furthermore, the average glycogen concentrations at exhaustion, after the control and carbohydrate trials, were almost the same (553 and 434 mmol glucosyl units/kg DW, respectively). These values are what might be expected at the start of exercise rather than at exhaustion. Histochemical examination of samples from the gastrocnemius muscles of the runners did not show selective glycogen depletion in any of the type I or type II fibres. Therefore, selective glycogen depletion in one or other of the fibre populations in the gastrocnemius muscles was probably not the cause of fatigue. Hence, it is difficult to offer reasons why these runners did not continue, unless, of course, glycogen depletion occurred in the other muscle groups which also play a central role in running, such as the soleus and the quadriceps.

In a more recent study, very low glycogen concentrations were found in biopsy samples of the quadriceps muscles of young men after they had run to exhaustion.[38] The glycogen concentrations were as low as those normally found in the quadriceps of cyclists at exhaustion (< 25 mmol/glucosyl units/kg WW) and these occurred in the type I fibres. Contrary to the view that low glycogen concentration in the gastrocnemius, rather than the quadriceps muscles, is the limitation to running performance,[39] the study of Tsintzas *et al.* clearly shows that at the point of fatigue the quadriceps muscles of runners are glycogen-depleted.[38]

In the study of the influence of carbohydrate loading on submaximal endurance capacity, whether cycling or running, the assumption has been made that females will have a similar increase in muscle glycogen concentrations, as has been repeatedly shown for males. The assumption has only recently been put to the test. Tarnopolsky *et al.* compared the responses to carbohydrate loading of seven endurance-trained men with those of seven similarly trained women.[40] Dietary carbohydrate intake was increased to 75 per cent of daily energy intake for 4 days, after which both the men and the women cycled to exhaustion at 85 per cent $\dot{V}O_2$max. The muscle glycogen concentration in the quadriceps of the men increased by 41 per cent and their performance time improved by 45 per cent. In contrast, the women showed no increase in their muscle glycogen concentration nor in their endurance capacity. The study also confirmed earlier studies by these authors that during submaximal exercise, well-trained women use more fat as an energy substrate than well-trained men.[41] Therefore, there is clearly a need to undertake further studies in order to establish the efficacy of the carbohydrate-loading procedure for women.

Pre-exercise diet and endurance performance

Studies on submaximal constant-pace exercise to fatigue (endurance capacity) provide opportunities to examine the influences of dietary changes on fuel utilization, thermoregulation, and exercise tolerance without the complication of changes in exercise intensity. However, athletes do not always maintain a constant pace through-

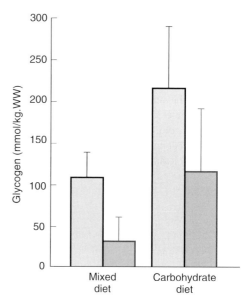

Fig. 4 Human muscle glycogen concentration (mmol/kg WW) before (light bars) and immediately after (dark bars) a 30-km cross-country race before which runners consumed either their normal mixed diets or undertook dietary carbohydrate loading in preparation for the race (mean ± SD). (Modified after ref. 34.)

out an endurance race. An athlete's pace is influenced by maximum oxygen uptake, his or her training status, the duration of the race, and the general feelings of fatigue. Several studies have tried to examine the influence of carbohydrate loading on performance under race conditions, and others have simulated race conditions in laboratories to provide a better understanding of the mechanism(s) responsible for improvements in performance.

One of the most informative field studies on the influence of dietary manipulation on endurance performance was undertaken by Karlsson and Saltin.[34] They addressed the question of whether or not an increased pre-exercise glycogen concentration improves running speed as well as endurance capacity during a 30-km cross-country race. Of the two groups of runners used: one group undertook carbohydrate loading according to the original form of this procedure,[25] prior to the race, while the other group remained on their normal mixed diet. In the second part of the study, the race conditions were re-created for the 10 runners, 3 weeks later, and the dietary preparation of the two groups was reversed. The time taken to complete the 30-km race was improved by 8 min (135.0 min compared with 143.0 min) when the subjects increased their pre-race muscle glycogen concentrations by carbohydrate loading. Their running speeds were not improved during the early part of the race as a consequence of carbohydrate loading, but they were able to sustain their optimum pace for longer. Interestingly, postexercise glycogen concentrations after carbohydrate loading were similar to the pre-exercise values of the runners when they were eating their normal mixed diets (Fig. 4). Therefore, the dietary preparation for the race provided glycogen stores which were more than adequate for muscle metabolism under these conditions. Thus, as a result of the pre-race carbohydrate loading, the performance of these athletes was not limited by the availability of muscle glycogen.

In a more recent study, the influence of carbohydrate loading on running performance during a simulated 30-km race was conducted using a laboratory treadmill.[42] One of the aims of this study was to determine at what point during the race runners began to show signs of fatigue, and how this was modified by dietary manipulation. The treadmill was instrumented so that the subjects controlled their own speeds using a lightweight, hand-held switch. Changes in speed, time, and distance elapsed were all displayed on a computer screen in full view of the subjects. The runners were divided into two groups after the first 30-km treadmill time trial. One group increased their carbohydrate intake during the 7-day recovery period, whereas the other group ate additional protein and fat in order to match the increased energy intakes of the carbohydrate group. Of the nine runners in the carbohydrate group, eight had faster times for 30 km than during their first attempt, and better times than the control group. Even though the carbohydrate group ran faster than the control group, after carbohydrate loading, they had lower adrenaline concentrations than during their first run. This unexpected result was attributed to their ability to maintain normal blood glucose concentrations throughout the race after carbohydrate loading. Plasma noradrenaline concentrations increased, as expected, during the simulated 30-km races following normal dietary conditions and after carbohydrate loading.

Long-distance cycling performance also benefits from an increased pre-exercise muscle glycogen concentration. Widrick *et al.*[43] reported that eight endurance-trained cyclists completed a 65-km laboratory time trial in 118.7 min when they had high pre-exercise muscle glycogen concentrations (170 mmol/kg WW), whereas they completed the distance in 123 min when they began exercise with lower glycogen concentrations (108 mmol/kg WW). Although the pre-exercise muscle glycogen concentrations were different before these time trials, it is worth noting that even the lower glycogen values were well within the normal range.

The improvement in endurance cycling performance after carbohydrate loading has been confirmed in a more recent study using a slightly different time trial. Rauch *et al.*[44] reported that increasing the daily carbohydrate intake of eight well-trained cyclists from 6.2 to 10.5 g/kg BW for 3 days increased their pre-exercise muscle glycogen concentrations by 47 per cent. The cyclists completed 2 h of cycling at an intensity equivalent to 75 per cent $\dot{V}O_2$max which included five, 1-min sprints, at 20-min intervals; thereafter they attempted to complete the greatest distance in the remaining 60 min of the test. Their average speed and distance covered during the 60-min performance test was greater after carbohydrate loading than after 3 days on a normal carbohydrate diet (38 compared with 33 km/h).

Carbohydrate loading does not appear to be of help under all conditions. Sherman *et al.*[26] studied the influence of high pre-exercise muscle glycogen concentrations on performance during an endurance race. Here, three different dietary procedures were used to prepare for the races: a low-carbohydrate diet followed by 3 to 4 days on a high-carbohydrate diet (low/high) (104 g compared with 542 g of carbohydrate); a normal mixed diet followed by the same period on a high-carbohydrate diet (mixed/high) (352 g compared with 542 g of carbohydrate); and a normal mixed diet for the whole of the preparatory period before the race (mixed/mixed) 353 g of carbohydrate). Both the carbohydrate-loading procedures (low/high and mixed/high) increased muscle glycogen concentrations in the gastrocnemius muscles of the runners prior to the races. The subjects who consumed their normal mixed diet throughout the week before the race also showed increased muscle glycogen

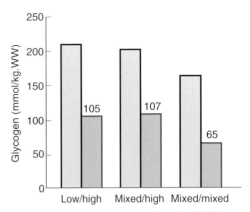

Fig. 5 Human muscle glycogen concentrations (mmol/kg WW) of a group of well-trained runners after three indoor 20.9-km races on a 200-m track following three dietary methods of increasing muscle glycogen concentrations. The numbers refer to the amount of glycogen used in each race (mmol/kg WW). (Modified after ref. 26.)

concentrations, but not to the same extent as in the carbohydrate-loading trials (Fig. 5). They found no differences in performance times for six well-trained endurance athletes who completed the three 20.9 km races on an indoor 200-m track. The running times for the three races were 83.5 min (low/mixed), 83.63 min (mixed/high), and 82.95 min (mixed/mixed), respectively. Therefore the muscle glycogen concentrations of the subjects were more than sufficient to meet the demands imposed upon them by the 20.9 km races. It is clear from this study, however, that well-trained runners need only taper their training in preparation for races of half-marathon distance. They do not need to undertake any dietary manipulation in preparation for races of this or shorter distances.

A similar conclusion was drawn by Pitsiladis *et al.*[45] from a study of the influences of carbohydrate loading on running performance during a 10-km treadmill time trial. The six well-trained runners achieved similar times irrespective of whether the pre-race diet was high (48.8 min) or low (48.6 min) in carbohydrate.

When the duration of exercise is no more than about an hour, carbohydrate loading and the subsequent increase in muscle glycogen stores do not appear to improve endurance performance. For example, Hawley *et al.*[46] increased the muscle glycogen concentrations of six well-trained cyclists by 23 per cent by carbohydrate loading. The cyclists then completed as great a distance as possible in 1 hour. Although pre-exercise muscle glycogen concentrations were higher after carbohydrate loading, there was no difference in the distance covered during the time trial (40.4 compared with 40.2 km).

Pre-exercise diets and high-intensity exercise

Although carbohydrate loading does not appear to influence performance during submaximal exercise lasting no more than an hour, there are some reports that it may improve performance during high-, but not maximal-, intensity exercise. Maughan and Poole[47] reported a 36 per cent improvement in cycling time to exhaustion (6.65 min compared with 4.87 min), at 105 per cent $\dot{V}O_2$max, after undergoing the traditional carbohydrate-loading procedure. A subsequent study concluded that the improvement in exercise tolerance

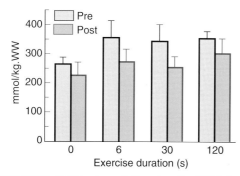

Fig. 6 Human muscle glycogen concentrations (mmol/kg DW) before and after maximal exercise of different durations: (from left to right) 6 s and 30 s of cycling, 30 s of sprinting on a non-motorized treadmill, and 120 s of running on a motorized treadmill (mean ± SEM).

may have been a consequence of an increased buffering capacity rather than the result of the additional glycogen stores.[48] In a similar study, Pizza *et al.* showed that running time to exhaustion at an intensity equivalent to 100 per cent $\dot{V}O_2$max improved from 4.7 to 5.06 min when their subjects tapered their training and increased their carbohydrate intake during 3 days before the test.[49]

It is difficult to offer a reason for these improvements in endurance capacity during exercise lasting only several minutes. Glycogen availability is clearly not a limitation during exercise of such short duration.[50] Some evidence for this conclusion is illustrated in Fig. 6, which is a summary of a series of studies on muscle glycogen changes during exercise of maximal intensity and different durations. It shows: the muscle glycogen concentrations before and immediately after 6 s and 30 s of maximal exercise during cycling, using a modified Wingate protocol;[51] glycogen concentrations before and after 30 s of sprint running on a non-motorized treadmill during which the loss of glycogen is more rapid in type II than in type I fibres;[52] and glycogen concentrations before and after 120 s of running on a motorized treadmill, at speeds equivalent to 110 per cent $\dot{V}O_2$max.[53,54] It is not surprising then that carbohydrate loading does not improve performance during two to three bouts of exercise of this intensity and duration.[55,56]

Repeated brief periods of maximal exercise make significant demands on muscle glycogen stores during the first several sprints, but, thereafter, muscle glycogen appears to be used more economically, probably because of a greater reliance on aerobic rather than anaerobic metabolism.[57] For example, in a series of 10 maximal sprints of 6-s duration and 30-s recovery on a cycle ergometer, glycogen degradation was reduced by half during the last sprint (Fig. 7). This glycogen sparing is probably the consequence of an increase in the aerobic metabolism of glycogen and free fatty acids. Nevertheless, had these sprints continued, then muscle glycogen concentrations would have been reduced to critically low levels thus limiting exercise performance. Therefore, it is reasonable to assume that well-stocked carbohydrate stores before prolonged intermittent high-intensity exercise would provide an advantage by postponing the early onset of fatigue.

Bangsbo *et al.*[59] showed that an increased carbohydrate intake, prior to a field test involving running patterns common to soccer, improves performance. Their subjects were seven professional soccer players who performed two tests, one after their normal mixed diet and the other after 2 days on a high-carbohydrate diet (65 per

cent carbohydrate, that is 602 g/day).[60] The field test consisted of two parts. During the first part, the subjects performed 46 min of walking and running, simulating the activity pattern common to soccer. The second part was a performance run on a laboratory treadmill. The subjects ran continuously at high (15 s) and low (10 s) speeds on a treadmill until exhaustion. After the high-carbohydrate diet, the subjects were able to run 0.9 km further (17.1 km) than when the test was performed after a normal mixed diet (16.2 km). The results of this study endorse the recommendations of Saltin[61] and Jacobs *et al.*[62] that soccer players should increase their carbohydrate intake as part of their match preparation.

A similar message comes from a study of ice-hockey players who raised their pre-exercise muscle glycogen concentrations by 12 per cent after precompetition carbohydrate loading.[63] The group of players who increased their muscle glycogen stores covered greater distances during the game, and at faster speeds, than the control group. The overall improvement in physical performance after carbohydrate loading was attributed to the differences in pre-exercise glycogen concentrations. It is reasonable to conclude that performance during sports which involve prolonged intermittent maximal exercise of brief duration will benefit from precompetition carbohydrate loading.

High-fat diets and exercise performance

High-fat diets may induce muscle to adapt to using a greater proportion of fat during prolonged exercise, and so spare the body's limited glycogen stores. Lambert *et al.*[64] reported that after 2 weeks on a high-fat diet (67 per cent fat, 7 per cent carbohydrate, and 26 per cent protein), their subjects had a greater endurance capacity, during submaximal exercise (about 60 per cent $\dot{V}O_2$max), than they exhibited after 2 weeks on a high-carbohydrate diet (74 per cent carbohydrate, 12 per cent fat, and 14 per cent protein). The endurance capacity of the subjects following the high-carbohydrate diet was 42 min, whereas the exercise time to exhaustion after the high-fat diet was 80 min. The exercise time for the carbohydrate trial was far too short for an exercise intensity of only 60 per cent $\dot{V}O_2$max. The explanation may be in the order of testing; the submaximal endurance test was performed after the high-intensity exercise test.

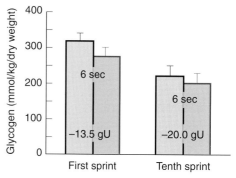

Fig. 7 Human muscle glycogen concentrations (mmol/kg DW) before and after the first and tenth 6-s period of maximal exercise (sprint) on a cycle ergometer. Each sprint was separated by a resting recovery of 30 s. Glycogen utilization in the first and tenth sprints are shown as glycosyl units per kg muscle mass (mmol/kg DW) (mean ± SD). (Modified after ref. 58.)

The cyclists on the high-carbohydrate diet performed the submaximal endurance test after completing more work during the previous high-intensity exercise test than when they were on the high-fat diet.[64] Therefore, they began the endurance test at a disadvantage, and so the study was not a true comparison of the endurance capacities of the cyclists on the two types of diets.

In a more recent study, Helge et al.[65] examined the influence of 7 weeks of endurance training on endurance capacity when their subjects ate diets which were either high in fat (62 per cent daily energy intake) or in carbohydrates (65 per cent daily energy intake). During the eighth week both groups ate a high-carbohydrate diet. However, the endurance capacity of the high-fat group was inferior to that of the high-carbohydrate group, not only after 7 weeks but also after a week on a high-carbohydrate diet. The authors suggest that a high-fat diet is less than optimal for full adaptation to endurance training.[65]

A high-fat diet during the day before prolonged exercise does not appear to improve performance when compared with a high-carbohydrate diet. Starling et al.[66] fed seven well-trained cyclists a high-fat (68 per cent of daily energy intake) and a high-carbohydrate (83 per cent of daily energy intake) diet during the 12 h following 2 h of cycling at 65 per cent $\dot{V}O_2$max. After an overnight fast they completed a 1600-kJ performance test on a cycle ergometer in as fast a time as possible. The previous day's high-fat diet resulted in a poorer time trial performance (139 min) than when the diet was high in carbohydrate (117 min).

Eating a high-fat, rather than a high-carbohydrate, meal 3 to 4 h before exercise is not recommended as a nutritional preparation for endurance competitions because these meals take longer to digest. Nevertheless, if high-fat meals do lead to glycogen sparing, then they would be expected to delay the onset of fatigue in a similar manner to consuming carbohydrate-rich meals before exercise.[67] A recent study attempted to answer this question by comparing the endurance performances of subjects following isocaloric high-fat or high-carbohydrate meals 4 h before submaximal exercise.[68] The pre-exercise meals contained approximately 280 g of carbohydrate in the high-carbohydrate meal and 84 g in the high-fat meal. The 10 endurance runners were required to exercise for 2 h on a cycle ergometer at 65 per cent $\dot{V}O_2$max, and thereafter the external workload was increased to the equivalent of 80 per cent $\dot{V}O_2$max for each subject. The time to exhaustion at 80 per cent $\dot{V}O_2$max was used to assess the endurance capacity of the subjects in the two trials. The times to exhaustion after the high-carbohydrate and high-fat pre-exercise meals were 128 min and 122 min, respectively. There was no statistically significant differences between these endurance times on the high- and low-carbohydrate meals.[68] Although gastrointestinal disturbances were not reported in this cycling study, this would probably not be the case when subjects were required to run after such a high-fat meal.

Precompetition meals

In most laboratory studies on the influence of diet and exercise capacity, subjects undergo an overnight fast before undertaking exercise tolerance tests. However, prolonged fasting before exercise is not usual practice for athletes because they normally have a meal a few hours before competition. The advice they are offered is to eat an easy to digest high-carbohydrate meal no later than 3 to 4 h before competition. There is some evidence to support this recommendation but only a few studies have used real meals rather than liquid preparations.

In one such study, subjects ate a breakfast consisting of bread, cereal, milk, and fruit juice (200 g carbohydrate) 4 h before cycling to exhaustion.[69] This meal increased pre-exercise muscle glycogen concentration by 15 per cent. The performance test required the subjects to cycle for 45 min at 80 per cent $\dot{V}O_2$max and then to cycle as fast as possible for 15 min. The total work accomplished during the last 15 min of the test was greater after the pre-exercise meal than it was following the non-meal trial.

The carbohydrate content of pre-exercise meals is also important. Sherman et al.[70] showed that although small amounts of carbohydrate (46 g and 156 g) consumed 4 h before intermittent cycling improved endurance capacity, a larger amount of carbohydrate (312 g) was even more effective. A meal containing 312 g of carbohydrate is larger than the amount normally consumed by athletes before exercise. Athletes' breakfasts usually contain about 100 to 120 g of carbohydrate.[71] Nevertheless, a compromise must be reached between eating sufficient carbohydrate to benefit performance but without causing gastrointestinal disturbances during subsequent exercise. Sherman et al.[70] avoided these potential gastrointestinal problems by liquidizing the pre-exercise meals given to their subjects. Furthermore, they used cycling rather than running, and so the potential for gastrointestinal disturbances was further reduced.

Although these studies confirm the principle that a large carbohydrate intake 3 to 4 h before exercise improves endurance capacity, compared with pre-exercise fasting, care has to be taken when translating this principle into practice. High-carbohydrate foods in large amounts may cause gastrointestinal disturbances, and so one way around this potential problem is to supplement precompetition meals with carbohydrate solutions. This nutritional strategy even allows athletes to take in carbohydrate to good effect as late as 1 h before exercise. Sherman et al.[72] showed that performance is improved during submaximal cycling lasting longer than 90 min, when a solution containing the equivalent of 1.1 to 2.2 g/kg BW of carbohydrate is consumed 1 h before exercise.

If eating a carbohydrate meal 3 to 4 h before exercise causes gastrointestinal discomfort during exercise, then an alternative is to drink a carbohydrate solution (5 g/kg BW) 3 h before exercise and every 20 min during exercise.[73] Wright et al. compared the cycling time to exhaustion when their subjects either ingested carbohydrate before exercise, ingested carbohydrate during exercise, undertook a combination of both, or exercised without carbohydrate.[73] Endurance capacity increased to a greater extent when their cyclists drank a carbohydrate solution before and during exercise than when they exercised without carbohydrate (18 per cent and 32 per cent, respectively). However, the greatest increase in endurance capacity (44 per cent) was achieved when the cyclists ingested carbohydrate solutions before and during exercise.

A similar result was reported by Chryssanthopoulos and Williams[74] for runners. They found that when runners combined a high-carbohydrate breakfast (2.5 g carbohydrate/kg BW) 3 h before exercise with drinking a carbohydrate–electrolyte solution (6.9 per cent) during a run to exhaustion, endurance capacity was greater than when they ran after a high-carbohydrate breakfast alone.

The pre-exercise meal contained the equivalent of 2.5 g/kg BW of carbohydrate. This high-carbohydrate meal, 3 h earlier, increased muscle glycogen concentration in the vastus lateralis muscle of runners by 11 per cent. The carbohydrate consumed could not all be accounted for by the increase in muscle glycogen concentration. Therefore, at the end of the 3-h postprandial period some of the carbohydrate was still undergoing digestion and absorption, and some would have been deposited in the liver as glycogen. The pre-exercise carbohydrate meal and the carbohydrate–electrolyte solution increased running time by 9 per cent (125 min) more than when only the meal was given (115 min), and 21 per cent more than when the runners had an overnight fast (103 min) before exercise.

Chryssanthopoulos et al. extended the observations of Wright et al.[73] by comparing the influences of a pre-exercise meal with no-meal on endurance running performance during a 30-km treadmill time trial.[75] The pre-exercise meal provided the runners with the equivalent of 2 g/kg BW of carbohydrate in the form of white bread, cereal, sugar, jam, and orange juice. During the time trial, 4 h later, the runners ingested only water. In the no-meal trial the runners ingested 10 ml/kg BW of a liquid placebo instead of breakfast, and immediately before the 30-km time trial they drank 8 ml/kg BW of a 6.9 per cent commercially available carbohydrate–electrolyte solution. They also drank 2 ml/kg BW of this same solution every 5 km during the simulated race. The performance times for the 30 km race were identical for the two trials (C, i.e. no meal, but carbohydrate; 121.7 min compared with M, i.e. meal plus water during exercise 121.8 min).

Composition of pre-exercise meals

The metabolic response to carbohydrate ingestion during exercise is different because of the glycaemic indices of the carbohydrates in the preceding meals,[76] and so the choice of carbohydrate in pre-competition meals could have an effect on subsequent performance.

In one study on the influence of high and low glycaemic-index carbohydrate foods on exercise capacity, the low glycaemic-index carbohydrate appeared to improve endurance capacity to a greater extent than the high glycaemic-index food. In this study, Thomas et al.[77] used lentils as the low glycaemic-index food, potatoes as the high glycaemic-index food, and compared the responses to those obtained after drinking a glucose solution or plain water. The meals and solutions were ingested 1 h before cycling to exhaustion at an exercise intensity of between 65 and 70 per cent $\dot{V}O_2$max. The carbohydrate content of the meals and glucose solution was equivalent to 1 g/kg BW and the volume was adjusted to 400 ml. The exercise times for the lentils, the potato, the glucose, and the water trials were 117 min, 97 min, 108 min and 99 min, respectively. There was a clear difference in exercise time for the lentils trial, but there were no differences in performance times between the potato, the glucose, or the water trials. What the authors did not address in this study was the different rates of digestion and absorption of the three carbohydrates within the hours before the start of exercise; nor the fact that they had only matched the amount of carbohydrate ingested in these trials, but did not account for the other nutrients in the lentils and potatoes, namely protein.

A more recent study addressed the question of whether or not there are performance benefits to eating low glycaemic-index carbo-

hydrate meals before exercise. Febbraio and Strewart[78] fed their subjects instant mash potatoes (made up in water) the high glycaemic-index carbohydrate, and lentils as the low glycaemic carbohydrate (1 g/kg BW), and as control meals the authors used jelly. The three conditions were assigned in random order and 'meals' were consumed 45 min before exercise. The exercise test required the six subjects to cycle at 70 per cent $\dot{V}O_2$peak for 2 h thereafter, they cycled as fast as possible to complete the greatest amount of work in 15 min. There were no differences in the muscle glycogen concentrations at the start of exercise nor any differences at the end of the performance test on the three occasions. The total amount of work accomplished during the last 15-min period was not different between the three conditions. Although these results are different to those reported by Thomas et al.,[77] a comparison cannot be made because different performance criteria were used in each study. Thomas et al. assessed endurance capacity, whereas Febbraio and Strewart[78] assessed total work done in a fixed time (endurance performance).

Paradoxical early onset of fatigue

Although recent studies support the practice of consuming carbohydrate-containing solutions during the hour before exercise, there is a popular, yet misguided, view that this practice will lead to an early onset of fatigue. This idea is based on the results of only two studies. In the first study, runners completed a 30-min run on a motorized treadmill on three occasions. In the first trial they drank a concentrated glucose solution (25 per cent) 45 min before submaximal treadmill running in order to depress plasma free fatty acid concentrations; in the second trial they drank water; and in the third their plasma free fatty acid concentrations were raised prior to exercise, by a high-fat meal, to examine the influence on glycogen utilization. The utilization of muscle glycogen was greater after the runners drank the concentrated glucose solution than after the other two conditions.[79]

When a glucose solution of the same concentration (25 per cent) was ingested 30 min before cycling to exhaustion, at an intensity equivalent to 80 per cent $\dot{V}O_2$max, exercise time was reduced by 19 per cent compared with the values obtained in a control trial in which the cyclists consumed only water.[80] This paradoxical early onset of fatigue was explained as the consequence of a reduction in fatty acid mobilization, induced by hyperinsulinaemia, which in turn led to an increased rate of glycogen degradation to cover the short-fall in ATP production from fat metabolism. However, more recent studies on the influence of glucose intake 30 to 60 min before exercise have not confirmed that this practice causes a decrease in endurance capacity either during cycling[81-83] or running.[84,85] Endurance running capacity is not impaired after drinking a 25 per cent glucose solution, 30 min before exercise, even though there is a marked rise and fall in blood glucose concentration early during prolonged exercise (Fig. 8). What is interesting is that runners who have a significant fall in blood glucose concentration following the pre-exercise ingestion of concentrated carbohydrate solutions are unaware that they are transiently hypoglycaemic (Williams et al., unpublished). Even consuming carbohydrate in the form of a chocolate bar 30 min, or indeed 5 min, before prolonged submaximal exercise has no detrimental effect on endurance capacity[86] and may even improve performance.[69] Therefore there is no basis for sug-

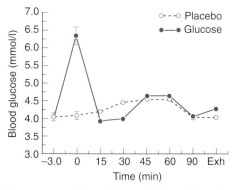

Fig. 8 Blood glucose concentrations during treadmill running to exhaustion (70 per cent $\dot{V}O_2$max) after drinking a concentrated glucose solution (25 per cent) and a placebo 30 min before exercise. (Modified after ref. 85.)

gesting that the pre-exercise ingestion of carbohydrate within the hour before exercise will decrease exercise capacity, other than the results of one study reported almost two decades ago.[80]

Carbohydrate intake during exercise

Endurance capacity

The importance in delaying the onset of severe dehydration during prolonged exercise is all too often overlooked by athletes, especially during training sessions. Dehydration is potentially far more of a risk to performance and health than is depletion of muscle glycogen (see Chapter 1.2.2). Drinking carbohydrate–electrolyte solutions during exercise is an effective way of trying to off-set severe dehydration and provide fuel for energy metabolism.

Consuming carbohydrate foods or fluids immediately, rather than within the hour, before prolonged submaximal exercise, does not cause hyperinsulinaemia or a reduction in endurance performance.[87] The increase in plasma noradrenaline levels at the start of exercise probably inhibits or blunts the release of insulin from the Islets of Langerhans.[88] Therefore, an increase in blood glucose concentration during exercise does not produce the same rise in plasma insulin concentration as when we are at rest.

Drinking carbohydrate-containing solutions immediately before and during exercise improves endurance capacity during cycling.[89–94] Even delaying the consumption of carbohydrate solutions until late in exercise, when muscle glycogen availability is reduced, delays fatigue and so improves endurance capacity.[93,95,96] Coggan and Coyle[93] showed that cyclists improved their exercise time by 36 min when they ingested a carbohydrate solution (3 g/kg BW) after 135 min of exercise. Endurance capacity is also improved during running when carbohydrate–electrolyte solutions are ingested immediately before and throughout exercise.[38,97,98]

The amounts which appear to be effective in improving endurance capacity vary widely between studies. For example, Bjorkman et al.[90] reported an improvement in endurance capacity of 18 per cent (137 min compared with 116 min) when their active but untrained subjects drank a 7 per cent glucose solution (250 ml) every 20 min, equivalent to 52.5 g/h during cycling to exhaustion at an intensity of 68 per cent $\dot{V}O_2$max. In a similar study, Coyle et al.[91]

showed that well-trained cyclists improved their exercise time to exhaustion by 33 per cent (3 h compared with 4 h) at a similar exercise intensity (70 per cent $\dot{V}O_2$max) when ingesting a carbohydrate solution every 20 min, at a rate which was twice as great (100 g/h) as that reported by Bjorkman et al.[90] In contrast, Maughan et al.[94] showed that cycling time to exhaustion improved by 29 per cent (90.8 min compared with 70.2 min) when their subjects drank a dilute carbohydrate–electrolyte solution (4 per cent); however, when they drank a concentrated glucose solution (36 per cent), their performance was no different from their endurance capacity during a water trial.

It is difficult to explain why such a range of concentrations and dosages of carbohydrate solutions are all so effective in improving endurance performance. There may be a threshold concentration, above which the additional carbohydrate is stored in the liver or indeed contributes to glycogen synthesis in non-active muscle fibres.[99] Of course, to be on the safe side, athletes may adopt the approach that if a recommended amount is effective, then twice that amount may be even more effective. However, during cycling or any sport where bodyweight is supported, gastrointestinal discomfort does not occur to the same extent after drinking large volumes of fluids as it does during running. Therefore, the question about the optimum volume and concentration of a carbohydrate solution is very real for sports involving running or walking, where gastrointestinal disturbances have a greater potential to impair performance than during cycling.

Endurance performance

Drinking a carbohydrate–electrolyte solution immediately before and throughout an endurance race improves performance. Tsintzas et al. showed that 30-km road racing times were improved when a group of runners (seven) drank a carbohydrate–electrolyte solution immediately before and throughout the race.[100] Their performance time, when they drank the 5 per cent carbohydrate–electrolyte solution, was 128 min, whereas when they drank a water placebo they completed the 30 km in 131 min (i.e. 128.3±19.9 min vs. 131.2±18.7 min; statistically significant, at $p<0.01$). In a longer endurance race, Millard-Stafford et al.[101] found that when their runners ingested a 7 per cent carbohydrate–electrolyte solution throughout a 40-km run, they completed the last 5 km faster than when they ingested a placebo solution in similar quantities. Running performance during the last half of a treadmill marathon was also improved when well-trained, ultradistance runners drank a 5.5 per cent carbohydrate–electrolyte solution throughout the simulated race.[102]

Although the consensus view is that carbohydrate loading does not improve performance when the duration of a race is about an hour or less, drinking carbohydrate–electrolyte solutions immediately before and during simulated races may improve performance. For example, Millard-Stafford et al.[103] found that the last 1.6 km of a 15-km treadmill time trial in the heat was completed in a faster time when their subjects drank a carbohydrate–electrolyte solution (cf. water placebo).

Similar improvements have been found in cycling performance when carbohydrate–electrolyte solutions are ingested before and during about an hour of exercise. For example, in a recent cycling study the authors assessed the influence of drinking a glucose-electrolyte solution (7.9 per cent) on the time to complete a fixed amount of work. The 19 endurance-trained cyclists took 58.7 min to complete the set task, whereas when they drank the same volume of a placebo the performance time was slower (60.15 min) (i.e. 58.74±0.52 min vs. 60.15±0.65 min; significantly different, $p < 0.001$).[104]

This study confirms an earlier finding of Below et al. who were also unable to offer an explanation for the improvement in the 1-h cycling performance test of their well-trained subjects.[105] Here, eight cyclists completed a performance test which required them to cycle for 50 min at 80 per cent $\dot{V}O_2$max before completing a predetermined amount of work as fast as possible. The authors examined four conditions, namely drinking a large volume of fluid during exercise, no fluid, carbohydrate, and no carbohydrate. The performance times were 6.5 per cent faster during the large volume compared with the small volume trials, and 6.3 faster for the carbohydrate compared with the no carbohydrate trials.[105]

The duration of exercise in these studies probably did not present a severe challenge to the subjects' muscle glycogen stores. One possible explanation for the improvements in performance during exercise of relatively short durations is that the ingested carbohydrate delayed what has been described as 'central fatigue'. An increase in one of the brain's neurotransmitters (serotonin, 5-HT) is believed to contribute to a decreased drive to continue exercise (see ref. 106). Drinking a carbohydrate solution decreases the concentration of plasma free fatty acids. Fatty acids are transported throughout the systemic circulation bound to plasma albumin which also binds the amino acid tryptophan. When tryptophan crosses the blood–brain barrier, it is a precursor for the formation of serotonin. However, when tryptophan is bound to albumin it is no longer free to cross the blood–brain barrier, and so the lower the plasma concentration of fatty acids the greater the number of available binding sites on albumin. Whether or not the carbohydrate supplied to the subjects had a positive influence on serotonin metabolism, and hence central fatigue,[106] has yet to be established. What is evident is that carbohydrate–electrolyte solutions of between 5 and 8 per cent ingested in amounts equivalent to between 30 and 60 g/h generally improve cycling and running performance.

Glycogen sparing

One explanation for the improvement observed in performance following the ingestion of carbohydrate–electrolyte solutions is that the exogenous carbohydrate helps to maintain a high rate of carbohydrate oxidation and prevents a fall in blood glucose concentrations during exercise. However, another possible mechanism is that the exogenous carbohydrate has a glycogen sparing effect on the endogenous glycogen stores. Bjorkman et al.[90] found that their subjects used less glycogen as a result of their carbohydrate intake during cycling exercise than when they drank only water. In another more recent cycling study, Yaspelkis and Ivy also reported evidence of muscle glycogen sparing which occurred when their subjects drank a carbohydrate solution during prolonged intermittent exercise.[107]

In contrast, Coyle et al.[91] showed quite clearly that the rate and amount of glycogen used in working skeletal muscles was the same during the carbohydrate and the water trials in which trained cyc-

lists exercised to exhaustion. Time to exhaustion increased by an hour when the cyclists drank a carbohydrate solution throughout the 4 h of exercise. However, during the carbohydrate trial the muscle glycogen concentration at exhaustion was the same after 4 h as it was after 3 h. This suggests that carbohydrate intake during the first 3 h of submaximal cycling did not lead to glycogen sparing, but the additional hour of exercise was at the expense of the exogenous carbohydrate supply. Coggan and Coyle[93] conclude from a review of the studies on carbohydrate ingestion, muscle glycogen, and endurance performance that the available evidence does not support the proposal that glycogen sparing is the reason for the improved exercise capacity. However, this conclusion was based on a review of cycling studies; the same conclusion may not be true of running.

Glycogen sparing occurs in the quadriceps of runners when they drink a carbohydrate–electrolyte solution throughout prolonged exercise. In a study by Tsintzas et al.[38] muscle biopsy samples were obtained from eight runners before and after they had run to exhaustion on a motorized treadmill at an exercise intensity equivalent to 70 per cent $\dot{V}O_2$max. During the first run they drank a placebo solution, whereas during the second run they drank a 5.5 per cent carbohydrate–electrolyte solution, before (8 ml/kg BW) and at 20-min intervals (2 ml/kg BW) throughout the run. During the second run, three biopsy samples were obtained from each of the subjects. An additional muscle sample was taken at the time the runners fatigued in the first run. As in previous studies using the same carbohydrate–electrolyte solution, all the subjects ran longer (132 min) than they did when they drank the placebo solution (104 min). Analyses of type 1 and type II muscle fibres showed that there was a 25 per cent reduction in glycogen utilization in the type I fibres during the carbohydrate trial compared with that in the placebo trial (Fig. 9).

Glycogen sparing occurs early in exercise and is not confined to the period late in exercise when muscle glycogen concentration is low. Tsintzas et al.[108] showed that drinking a carbohydrate–electrolyte solution (5.5 per cent) in the first hour of exercise results in a lower rate of glycogen utilization in type I fibres of the quadriceps muscles of active young men (Fig. 10). In a subsequent study designed to examine the performance advantages of glycogen sparing early in exercise, 11 trained men drank the same 5.5 per cent carbohydrate–electrolyte solution for the first hour of a run to exhaustion and then changed to drinking water for the remainder of the run.[97] Their endurance capacity was significantly better (124.5 min) when they drank the carbohydrate–electrolyte solution than when they drank only water (109.6 min) for the entire exercise period. This clear evidence of glycogen sparing, as a consequence of drinking a carbohydrate–electrolyte solution immediately before exercise, contributes to our understanding of the mechanisms responsible for the improvements in both endurance running capacity[98] and running performance[87,100,102,103]

Providing carbohydrate solutions for participants in multiple-sprint sports such as soccer also appears to improve performance. Kirkendall et al.[109] filmed a soccer game in which a group of players consumed a concentrated carbohydrate solution (approximately 15.5 per cent) before the game and at half-time. The players who drank the carbohydrate solution covered more ground during the second half of the game than those players who consumed a sweet placebo solution. Leatt and Jacobs[110] provided soccer players with a

7 per cent glucose polymer solution before a game and found that they used almost 40 per cent less muscle glycogen than the players who drank the same amount of a placebo solution.

In a 90-min field test designed to simulate the same activity pattern that occurs in a soccer match, Nicholas et al.[111] reported that soccer players were able to run longer when they drank a commercially available sports drink (6.9 per cent carbohydrate) than when they drank a water placebo. Furthermore, in a subsequent study Nicholas et al. found that glycogen utilization was greatest in type II fibres and that the overall use of glycogen was 21 per cent less during the carbohydrate trial (193 compared with 244 mmol glucosyl units/kg DW) (Nicholas, unpublished observations). This example of glycogen sparing during prolonged intermittent exercise involving sprinting, jogging, and walking supports an earlier report of muscle glycogen sparing in soccer players. Leatt and Jacobs reported that soccer players completed a game with 39 per cent more muscle glycogen than the control group. The five soccer players in the carbohydrate group drank 500 ml of a 7 per cent glucose polymer solution 10 min before the game and the same amount at half-time, whereas the five soccer players in the control group drank the same volume of a placebo solution at the same times.[110] Thus the available evidence suggests that there are performance benefits

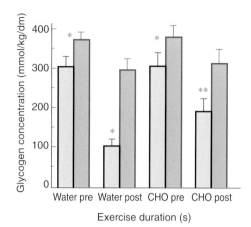

Fig. 10 Muscle glycogen concentrations (mmol/kg DW) in type I (open bars) and type II (filled bars) before and immediately after 60 min of treadmill running at 70 per cent $\dot{V}O_2$max during two trials. During one trial the runners drank water immediately before and at 20-min intervals throughout exercise (Water pre and Water post), and during the other trial they drank a 5.5 per cent carbohydrate–electrolyte solution immediately before and at 20-min intervals throughout exercise (CHO pre and CHO post). Asterisks denote significant differences between the pre-exercise glycogen concentrations in type I and type II muscle fibres (*) ($p < 0.05$) and the significantly greater ($p < 0.05$) amount of postexercise glycogen in the type I fibres after 60 min of running in the carbohydrate trial compared with the glycogen concentrations in the same population of fibres at the end of the water trial (CHO post compared with Water post).[108]

to be gained, during prolonged multiple-sprint sports, from drinking carbohydrate–electrolyte solutions before and during exercise.

Diet and recovery from exercise

Recovery from exercise is not a passive process. Tissues undergo repair and reproduction, fluid balance is restored, and substrate stores are replaced. Carbohydrate replacement is one of the most important events during recovery. Restocking muscle glycogen stores can take as long as 2 days,[112] although shorter recovery times are possible when initial glycogen stores are not high,[62,113] or where carbohydrate intake is increased immediately after exercise and for the duration of the recovery period.

Immediately after exercise, muscle membrane permeability to glucose is increased. Exercise changes the characteristics of the sarcolemma such that glucose permeability is improved and muscle has an increased insulin sensitivity. The two effects appear to be additive, and are linked with an increase in the protein mainly responsible for the transport of glucose through the sarcolemma, namely GLUT 4.[114] In addition, glycogen synthase, the enzyme complex responsible for glycogen synthesis, is also in its most active form immediately after exercise. There is an inverse relationship between muscle glycogen concentration and the concentration of glycogen synthase in the active form.[115,116] The specificity of this relationship has been highlighted in a study which examined, both biochemically and histochemically, the activity of this enzyme in samples of different populations of muscle fibres obtained from subjects who had exercised to exhaustion. The activity of glycogen synthase was greatest in the type I fibres, that is to say the slow-contracting oxidative fibres.[116] Type I fibres are more involved during submaximal exercise during cycling[117] and during running[38] than type II fibres.

Muscle biopsy samples taken from a group of professional football players immediately after a soccer match showed a range of

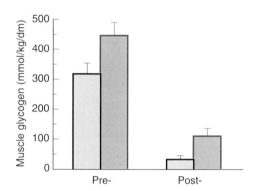

Water trial: constant pace running to exhaustion

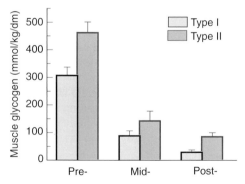

CHO trial: constant pace running to exhaustion

Fig. 9 The upper panel shows the muscle glycogen concentrations (mmol/kg DW) in type I (lightly shaded bars) and type II (darkly shaded bars) fibres of runners pre- and postrunning to exhaustion (70 per cent $\dot{V}O_2$max) during which they drank water throughout. The lower panel shows glycogen concentrations in type I and type II muscle fibres of the same runners pre- and postrunning to exhaustion (70 per cent $\dot{V}O_2$max), and also at the same time as they fatigued during the water trial (mid-) during which they drank a 5.5 per cent carbohydrate–electrolyte solution (mean ± SEM). (Modified after ref. 38.)

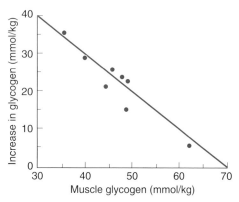

Fig. 11 Relationship between postmatch muscle glycogen concentrations (mmol/ kg WW) in professional soccer players and the increase after a 24-h recovery during which the players ate a high-carbohydrate diet.[62]

glycogen concentrations. Those players with very low, postexercise glycogen concentrations had the greatest increase in glycogen concentration a day later. Those players with a moderate level of muscle glycogen at the end of the game replaced only a relatively small amount of glycogen during the recovery period (Fig. 11).[62] Although the duration of exercise plays a significant part in activating glycogen synthase after exercise,[118] a low, postexercise muscle glycogen concentration may have the more influential role.[113] Of course, these two influences are not mutually exclusive because a low, postexercise glycogen concentration is a consequence of prolonged exercise.

Obviously, the rate at which glucose is transported across the muscle membrane will play a large part in dictating the rate of glycogen resynthesis. McCoy et al.[119] reported that a postexercise carbohydrate intake equivalent to 2.0 g/kg BW, and every 2 h for the first 6 h of recovery, was directly reflected in GLUT 4 and glycogen synthase I activities. However, the amount of GLUT 4 transporter proteins may ultimately make more of a contribution to glycogen resynthesis than glycogen synthase activation.[120]

The highest glycogen resynthesis rate occurs during the first few hours of recovery (see ref. 121 for a review). Blom et al.[122] found that the maximum rate of glycogen resynthesis occurred when their subjects consumed the equivalent of 0.7 g/kg BW of carbohydrate every 2 h during the first 6 h of recovery. This amounts to about 50 g of carbohydrate every 2 h for a person weighing 70 kg. Drinking a carbohydrate solution, which provided the equivalent to 2 g/kg BW, immediately after prolonged heavy exercise produced a muscle glycogen resynthesis rate of about 5 to 6 mmol/kg per h.[123] This rate of glycogen resynthesis (about 5 per cent an hour) is about 300 per cent greater than under conditions where no carbohydrate is ingested immediately after exercise. When carbohydrate intake was delayed for 2 h, the rate of glycogen resynthesis was 47 per cent slower than when carbohydrate was provided immediately after exercise. These and other studies are the basis for the recommendation that the optimum amount of carbohydrate needed for rapid postexercise glycogen resynthesis is about 1 g/kg BW, which should be consumed immediately after exercise and at 2 h intervals until the next mealtime. However, the timing of the postexercise ingestion of carbohydrate may not be as crucial as first reported by Ivy et al.[123] Parkin et al.[124] reported that there was no difference in the glycogen concentrations after 8 and 24 h when their subjects either

consumed carbohydrate immediately after exercise or delayed it for 2 h into recovery. Nevertheless, drinking a carbohydrate solution immediately after exercise provides not only carbohydrate for glycogen resynthesis but it also begins the rehydration process (see Chapter 1.2.2). Sports drinks are more effective as rehydration agents than either water or some of the most popular soft drinks.[125]

The type of carbohydrate in the recovery meals is also an important consideration for those who want to replace their muscle glycogen stores quickly. Kiens[19] compared the muscle glycogen resynthesis rates when her subjects were fed either high or low glycaemic foods. After their muscle glycogen stores were reduced by prolonged cycling, seven well-trained athletes were fed a diet for 2 days in which 70 per cent of their energy was obtained from either high or low glycaemic foods. The postexercise diet of high glycaemic foods produced a glycogen resynthesis rate which restored the carbohydrate store to 70 per cent of pre-exercise concentrations within 6 h, whereas the low glycaemic carbohydrate diet restored muscle glycogen stores to only 34 per cent of their pre-exercise values.

Similar results were obtained by Burke et al.[126] who fed their subjects a recovery diet which provided them with the equivalent of 10 g/kg BW of carbohydrate over a 24-h period. The recovery diet was divided into four equal meals, containing either high or low glycaemic-index carbohydrate foods. Muscle glycogen resynthesis was greater after the high glycaemic-index carbohydrate meals than after the low ones. These studies contribute to the evidence which supports the recommendation that glycogen resynthesis after exercise is most rapid when athletes consume high glycaemic-index carbohydrates.

Adding some protein to the carbohydrate solution increases the rate of postexercise glycogen synthesis to a greater extent than can be achieved with a carbohydrate solution alone.[127] The addition of protein increases the concentrations of plasma insulin to a greater extent than when only a carbohydrate solution is consumed after exercise. An increased insulin concentration will not only increase the transport of glucose into muscle cells, but will also help restore the potassium balance across muscle membranes. A ratio of 3:1 carbohydrate to protein supplement was used in these recovery studies, but the optimum mixture of these two macronutrients has yet to be determined.

There are conditions, other than low-carbohydrate diets, which can interfere with glycogen resynthesis. Hard training or prolonged competition causes residual fatigue which is often accompanied by muscle soreness and lethargy. The extreme stress of exercise and competition may lower the plasma concentrations of the body's natural anabolic hormones.[128] Testosterone has been shown to play a role in converting the inactive glycogen synthase into its active form[115] and so the depression of this hormone may delay the replenishment of the muscle's carbohydrate store.[128] Extreme muscle soreness is the result of damaged muscle fibres and the inflammatory response which is associated with the healing process. Glycogen resynthesis is delayed in skeletal muscle fibres that have experienced microtrauma as a result of too much eccentric activity.[129] But consuming carbohydrate (1 g/kg BW) immediately after exercise and 1 h later decreases the breakdown in myofibrillar protein which normally occurs following repeated knee extensor exercise.[130] This exercise is a common feature of strength training and so the obvious question is whether or not postexercise carbohydrate ingestion will lead to a more rapid adaptation to this type of training.

Diet, recovery, and performance

When several days separate periods of exercise or participation in sport, a normal mixed diet containing about 4 to 5 g/kg BW of carbohydrate is sufficient to replace liver and muscle glycogen stores. However, daily training or competition makes considerable demands on the body's carbohydrate stores. Even when the daily carbohydrate intake is 5 g/kg BW, cycling or running for an hour each day gradually delays the daily restoration of muscle glycogen stores.[131] Increasing the carbohydrate intake to 8 g/kg BW per day may not be enough to prevent a significant reduction in muscle glycogen concentrations after five successive days of hard training.[132] These studies underline the importance of prescribing adequate amounts of carbohydrate for athletes in training and justifies the need for more frequent recovery days between periods of intense training.

We now know more about what factors influence the rate of muscle glycogen resynthesis than we know about the impact of restoring our carbohydrate stores on our fitness during subsequent exercise. Keizer et al.[133] examined this question in a systematic way. They showed that muscle glycogen stores can be replenished in 22 h by administering either liquid or solid carbohydrates during the first 5 h of recovery. After the first 5 h, their subjects consumed foods which were consistent in composition and quantity with their normal diets. The amounts of carbohydrate ingested during the 22-h recovery period was 580 g for the group taking liquid carbohydrates and 602 g for the group taking the solid form. Before and after the recovery period, an incremental cycle ergometer test was used to assess the maximum physical work capacity of the subjects. Their maximum physical work capacity was 7 per cent lower after 24 h of recovery, even though their glycogen stores had returned to pre-exercise values. Therefore, it appears that replenishment of muscle glycogen concentration alone is not sufficient to restore maximal work capacity. One additional practical observation from this study was that when the subjects were allowed to eat ad libitum after exercise, their muscle glycogen concentrations were significantly lower than when their food was prescribed and prepared for them.

Nevill et al.[134] came to a similar conclusion to Keizer et al.[133] after studying the influence of a high-carbohydrate recovery diet on the multiple-sprint performance of a group of games players. Using a non-motorized treadmill, games players completed 30 maximal sprints of 6-s duration separated by a recovery period of 114 s. Between each sprint, the subjects walked and jogged on the treadmill. Mean power output decreased by 8.8 per cent over the 30 sprints. The recovery diet of the subjects was modified without changing their daily energy intakes. Their carbohydrate intakes were 322 g (4.6 g/kg BW), 80 g (1.1 g/kg BW), and 644 g (8.7 g/kg BW) for those consuming the normal mixed diet, the low-carbohydrate diet, and the high-carbohydrate diet, respectively. There were no overall differences in power output between each group after the 24 h, and all performances were poorer than on the day before. However, if only the first nine sprints on the second day are considered, then the high-carbohydrate group performed significantly better than the other two groups. It seems that performance during brief high-intensity exercise may not be restored along with carbohydrate stores.

In contrast, endurance running capacity is restored after a day's recovery, when the daily carbohydrate and energy intake is increased. For example, when runners ate a high-carbohydrate diet (9 g/kg BW) after completing 90 min of treadmill running at speeds equivalent to 70 per cent $\dot{V}O_2$max, they were able to repeat this training run the following day, whereas runners who ate their normal mixed diets, with additional energy in the form of extra fat and protein, could only complete 78 per cent of the 90-min run.[135] Using the same high-carbohydrate recovery diet, six games players were able to improve on their previous day's performance in a prolonged, intermittent high-intensity, shuttle-running test. However, when the identical test was repeated on a different occasion after they had eaten a recovery diet consisting of their normal foods plus additional energy, in the form of protein and fat, these players were unable to even match their previous day's performance.[136]

Even when the recovery period is as little as 4 h, drinking a carbohydrate solution, in the amount recommended to increase muscle glycogen resynthesis, helps, but does not entirely restore, endurance capacity. Runners who completed 90 min of treadmill running were able to run for a further 62 min after a 4-h rest, during which they drank the equivalent of 1 g/kg BW of carbohydrate from a sports drink immediately after exercise and again after 2 h of recovery. In contrast, a control group drank the same volume of a sweet placebo (using aspartame as artificial sweetener) during the recovery period after which they could only run for 40 min.[137] However, providing runners with the equivalent of 3 g/kg BW of carbohydrate during the same recovery period does not improve performance beyond that which was achieved with the lower amount of carbohydrate.[138]

There are clear benefits to be gained from drinking a carbohydrate solution immediately after exercise, even when the recovery period is very short. Coggan and Coyle[139] showed that when their subjects were given a glucose solution during exercise, 20 min after cycling to exhaustion at 70 per cent $\dot{V}O_2$max, they were able to continue for longer than when they consumed only water. During three recovery trials, their subjects (1) consumed a water placebo, or (2) consumed a glucose polymer solution (3 g/kg BW), or (3) received a glucose infusion throughout the subsequent exercise. The glucose infusion was included as an effective way of maintaining normal blood glucose concentrations during prolonged exercise. Endurance capacity was significantly greater after carbohydrate ingestion (26 min) and after glucose infusion (43 min) than after ingesting a water placebo (10 min). However, even though glucose infusion maintained the blood glucose concentrations of the cyclists, it did not restore their exercise capacity to its former value. Thus, the unanswered question is: why does fatigue occur even when the provision of exogenous carbohydrate is sufficient to maintain blood glucose concentrations and cover the rate of glucose metabolism in working muscles?

Summary

The clear message from over a half a century of research on the links between food, nutrition, and exercise capacity is that next to natural talent and appropriate training, a high-carbohydrate diet and adequate fluid intake, to avoid dehydration, are the two most important elements in the formula for successful participation in sport. Of course, there is an underlying assumption that athletes normally eat a well-balanced diet made up of a wide variety of foods and containing sufficient energy to cover their needs. Nutritional strategies to support training and help recovery from exercise will only be fully effective when they are used by athletes who regularly eat a well-balanced diet.

Appendix

Table 3 Carbohydrate (CHO) exchanges

The specific weights of all of these food items contain CHO exchange (high or medium) and are interchangeable

Amount (g)	Food description	Energy (kcal)	CHO (g)
High			
20 (3 tbs)	Cornflakes	74	17
20 (5 tbs)	Rice Krispies	75	18
25 (2)	Ryvita/crispbread	80	18
100 (2 egg sized)	Boiled potatoes	80	20
100 (1 small)	Jacket potatoes	85	20
60 (heaped tbs)	Boiled rice	74	18
65	Boiled spaghetti	76	17
130 (1/3 tin)	Spaghetti in tomato sauce	77	16
100 (3 tbs)	Sweetcorn	76	16
130	Jelly (made-up)	77	18
25 (1 slice)	Swiss roll	76	16
24 (2)	Jaffa cakes	88	16
Medium			
20 (3 tbs)	Fruit 'n Fibre	70	15
22 (1)	Shredded Wheat	72	15
20 (3 tbs)	Shreddies	66	15
30 (5 tbs)	Bran cereal	82	13
20 (heaped tbs)	Porridge oats (raw wt)	80	15
20 (heaped tbs)	Muesli	74	13
20 (3)	Cream crackers	88	14
20 (1)	Weetabix	68	14
20 (2/3 slice)	White bread	70	15
30 (1 slice)	Wholemeal bread	65	13
15 (1)	Sweet biscuits (e.g. digestives)		
70 (large scoop)	Mashed potatoes	83	13
50 (1 small)	Roast potatoes	79	14
30 (3)	Chips	76	11
100 (3 tbs)	Processed peas	80	14
125 (3 tbs)	Baked beans	80	13
80 (2 tbs)	Cooked pulses (e.g. lentils)	76	14
75 (1/2 pot)	Fruit yoghurt (low-fat)	72	14
80 (1/5 tin)	Canned rice pudding	73	12
35 (tbs)	Fruit crumble	73	13
20 (1/2 indiv)	Fruit pie (individual)	74	11
20 (1/4 slice)	Plain fruit cake	71	12
20 (1)	Jam tart (individual)	77	13
20 (3 heaped tsp)	Drinking choc/Horlicks	76	15
100 (3 tbs)	Frozen peas (boiled)	69	10

Table 4 Meat exchanges

The specific weights of all of these food items contain one meat exchange and are interchangeable

Amount (g)	Food description	Energy (kcal)	CHO (g)
50 (thick slice)	Lean beef (cooked wt)	78	0
35 (tbs)	Minced beef	80	0
35 (1 cube)	Stewed beef	78	0
30 (1 small)	Beefburgers	79	2
35 (thin slice)	Corned beef	76	0
60 (2 tbs)	Bolognese sauce	83	2
40 (thick slice)	Lean roast lamb	76	0
60 (cutlet)	Lean lamb chop	74	0
60 (sml chop)	Lean pork chop	80	0
25 (1 thin)	Grilled pork sausage	80	3
60 (2 thin slices)	Lean ham	72	0
30 (1 rasher)	Grilled bacon (lean)	88	0
25 (2 tsps)	Liver pâté/sausage	78	1
35 (sml slice)	Fried liver	81	1
25 (1/8 small tin)	Tuna fish in oil (drained)	73	0
67 (1/3 small tin)	Tuna fish in brine (drained)	80	0
80 (med fillet)	Grilled white fish	76	0
50 (2)	Sardines in tomato sauce	86	0
20 (sml chunk)	Cheddar cheese	81	0
75 (2 tbsp)	Cottage cheese	81	0
25 (sml chunk)	Edam/Gouda cheese	85	0
30 (1/2)	Fried egg	70	0
60 (1)	Boiled egg	88	0
35 (1/2)	Scrambled egg	86	0
40 (2/3 egg)	Omelette	76	0
50 (1)	Poached egg	78	0
55 (lge slice)	Roast chicken	83	0
55 (lge slice)	Roast turkey	77	0

Table 5 Fat exchanges

The specific weights of all the food items contain one fat exchange and are interchangeable

Amount (g)	Food description	Energy (kcal)	CHO (g)
10 (pat)	Margarine/butter	73	0
20 (2 pats)	Low-fat spread (e.g. Gold)	73	0
30 (3 pats)	Very low-fat spread	81	0
20 (sml chunk)	Cheddar cheese	81	0
20 (2 tsp)	Cream cheese	88	0
30 (lge triangle)	Cheese spread	85	0
17 (sml chunk)	Stilton cheese	79	0
35 (2 tbsp)	Single cream	74	1
12 (med)	French dressing	79	0
10 (heaped tsp)	Mayonnaise	72	0
15 (15)	Peanuts/other nuts	86	1
35 (1/4)	Avocado pear	78	1

Table 6 Milk exchanges

The specific weights of all the food items contain one milk exchange and are interchangeable

Amount (g)	Food description	Energy (kcal)	CHO (g)
150 (sml glass)	Whole milk	98	7
200 (1/3 pint)	Semi-skimmed milk	98	10
250 (lge glass)	Skimmed milk	83	13
75 (1/4 carton)	Custard	88	13
50 (sml scoop)	Icre cream	83	10
150 (sml bowl)	'Cream of . . .' soup	80	9
150 (pot)	Yoghurt (natural)	84	11

Table 7 Fruit exchanges

The specific weights of all the food items contain one fruit exchange and are interchangeable

Amount (g)	Food description	Energy (kcal)	CHO (g)
125 (med)	Apple (with core)	44	12
50 (1/2)	Banana (flesh only)	47	12
80 (16)	Grapes	48	12
140 (med)	Orange (no skin)	49	12
200 (sml)	Grapefruit (no skin)	44	11
200 (slice)	Honeydew melon	42	10
75 (2 tbsp)	Stewed fruit with sugar	50	13
150 (4 tbsp)	Stewed fruit, no sugar	48	12
50 (1/8 tin)	Tinned fruit in syrup	49	13
120 (wine glass)	Unsweetened orange juice	46	11
40 (med)	Orange squash	43	11
70 (1/5 can)	Lucozade	48	13
200 (med glass)	Lemonade	42	11
100 (1/3 can)	Coca cola	39	11
20 (1/3 measure)	Ribena (concentrate)	46	12
15 (heaped tsp)	Marmalade or jam	39	10
15 (heaped tsp)	Honey	43	12
10 (2 tsp)	Sugar	40	11
20 (2 tbsp)	Raisins	50	12

Table 8 Miscellaneous

These goods contain more than one exchange which must be included in your daily allowance

Amount (g)	Food description	Exchanges
70 (1 mini)	Cheese and tomato pizza	1 med CHO + 1 fat
25 (1/4 slice)	Cheesecake	1/2 med CHO + 1 fat
45 (1/2)	Doughnut	1 med CHO + 1 fat
100 (lge portion)	White sauce	1 med CHO + 1 fat
50 (1 sml)	Pancakes	1 med CHO + 1 fat
75 (sml slice)	Meat pie	1 med CHO + 1 meat + 1 fat
75 (1/2 small)	Cornish pastie	1 med CHO + 1 meat + 1 fat
25 (bag)	Potato crisps	1 med CHO + 1 fat
20 (1/3 bar)	Mars bar, Snickers, etc.	1 med CHO + 1 fat
32 (2/3 bar)	Chocolate bar	1 med CHO + 1 fat

Table 9 Dietary changes

	Normal diet	Recommended diet
Energy (kcal)	2130	2120
Protein (g)	96	94
Protein (%)	**18**	**18**
Fat (g)	95	56
Fat (%)	**40**	**24**
CHO (g)	241	331
CHO (%)	**42**	**58**
Alc (g)	0	0
Alc (%)	**0**	**0**
Exchanges		
High CHO	7	8
Med CHO	5	5
Meat	6	6
Fruit	2	9
Fat	5	0
Milk	3	3
Foods removed from diet		
20 g (2 pats) butter		3 fat exchanges
10 g (heaped tsp) mayonnaise		1 fat exchange
60 g (3 small chunks) Cheddar cheese		2 fat + 1 meat exchange
Foods added to diet		
30 g (2 heaped tsp) jam		2 fruit exchanges
24 g (2) jaffa cakes		1 high-CHO exchange
75 g (2 heaped tbsp) cottage cheese)		1 meat exchange
120 g (wine glass) orange juice		1 fruit exchange
200 g (av. glass) lemonade		1 fruit exchange
150 g (2 small) bananas		3 fruit exchanges

References

1. Schobel H. *The Ancient Olympic Games.* New York: Van Nor-strand, 1965: 325.
2. DHSS. Committee on Medical Aspects. *Diet and cardiovascular disease.* London: HMSO, 1984.
3. Grandjean A. Macronutrient intake of US athletes compared with the general population and recommendations made for athletes. *American Journal of Clinical Nutrition* 1989; **49**: 1070–6.
4. Hawley J, Dennis S, Lindsay F, Noakes T. Nutritional practices of athletes: are they sub-optimal? *Journal of Sports Science* 1995; **13**: S75–S81.
5. van Erp-Baart A, Saris W, Binhorst R, Vos J, Elvers J. Nationwide survey on nutritional habits in elite athletes: Part I. energy, carbo-hydrate, protein and fat intake. *International Journal of Sports Medicine* 1989; **10**: 3–10.
6. Burke L, Gollan R, Read R. Dietary intakes and food use of groups of elite Australian male athletes. *International Journal of Sport Nutrition* 1991; **1**: 378–94.
7. Devlin JT, Williams C. Foods, nutrition and sports performance; a final consensus statement. *Journal of Sports Science* 1991; **9** (Suppl. 9): iii.
8. Inge K, Brukner P. *Food for sport.* London: Kingswood Press, 1988: 242.
9. Clark N. *Nancy Clark's sports nutrition guidebook.* Champaign, IL: Leisure Press, 1990: 322.
10. Burke L. *The complete guide to food for sports performanced.* 2nd edn. Sydney: Allen and Unwin, 1995: 374.
11. Jenkins DJA, Thomas DM, Wolever MS, *et al.* Glycemic index of foods: a physiological basis for carbohydrate exchange. *American Journal of Clinical Nutrition* 1981; **34**: 362–6.

12. Coyle E.F. Timing and method of increased carbohydrate intake to cope with heavy training, competition and recovery. *Journal of Sports Science* 1991; **9** (Suppl.): 29–52.

13. Acheson K, Schutz Y, Bessard T, Anantharaman K, Flatt J-P, Jequier E. Glycogen storage capacity and *de novo* lipogenesis during massive carbohydrate overfeeding in man. *American Journal of Clinical Nutrition* 1988; **48**: 240–7.

14. Flatt J, Ravussin E, Acheson K, Jequier E. Effects of dietary fat on postprandial substrate oxidation and on carbohydrate and fat balance. *Journal of Clinical Investigation* 1985; **76**: 1019–24.

15. Abbott W, Howard B, Christin L, *et al.* Short term energy balance: relationship with protein, carbohydrate and fat balance. *American Journal of Physiology* 1988; **255**: E332–E337.

16. Whitley H, Humphreys S, Samra J, *et al.* Metabolic responses to isoenergetic meals containing different proportions of carbohydrate and fat. *British Journal of Nutrition* 1997; **78**: 15–26.

17. FAO/WHO/UNU. *Energy and protein requirements.* Geneva: World Health Organization, 1985

18. Lemon PWR. Protein and amino acid needs of the strength athlete. *International Journal of Sport Nutrition* 1991; **1**: 127–45.

19. Kiens B. Translating nutrition into diet: diet for training and competition. In: Macleod DAD, Maughan RJ, Williams C, Madeley CR, Sharp J, CM, Nutton RW, eds. *Intermittent high intensity exercise: preparation, stresses and damage limitation.* London: E. and F.N. Spon, 1993: 175–82.

20. van der Beek EJ. Vitamin supplementation and physical exercise performance. *Journal of Sports Science* 1991; **9** (Suppl.): 77–90.

21. Clarkson PM. Minerals: exercise performance and supplementation in athletes. *Journal of Sports Science* 1991; **9** (Suppl): 91–116.

22. Nilsson LH, Hultman, E. Liver glycogen in man—the effect of total starvation or a carbohydrate-poor diet followed by carbohydrate refeeding. *Scandinavian Journal of Clinical and Laboratory Investigation* 1973; **32**: 325–30.

23. Maughan RJ, Williams C. Differential effects of fasting on skeletal muscle glycogen content in man and on skeletal muscle in the rat. *Proceedings of the Nutrition Society* 1981; **40**: 45A.

24. Bergstrom J, Hultman E. Muscle glycogen synthesis after exercise: an enhancing factor localized to the muscle cell in man. *Nature* 1966; **20**: 309–10.

25. Astrand P-O. Diet and athletic performance. *Federation Proceedings* 1967; **26**: 1772–7.

26. Sherman W, Costill D, Fink W, Miller J. Effect of exercise–diet manipulation on muscle glycogen and its subsequent utilization during performance. *International Journal of Sports Medicine* 1981; **114**: 114–18.

27. Christensen EH, Hansen O. Arbeitsfahigkeit und Ehrnahrung. *Skandinavisches Archiv fur Physiologie* 1939; **81**: 160–75.

28. Bergstrom J, Hermansen L, Hultman E, Saltin B. Diet, muscle glycogen and physical performance. *Acta Physiologica Scandinavica* 1967; **71**: 140–50.

29. Ahlborg B, Bergstrom J, Brohult J, Ekelund L-G, Hultman E, Maschio G. Human muscle glycogen content and capacity for prolonged exercise after different diets. *Forsvarsmedicin* 1967; **3**: 85–99.

30. Ahlborg B, Bergstrom J, Ekelund L-G, Hultman E. Muscle glycogen and muscle electrolytes during prolonged physical exercise. *Acta Physiologica Scandinavica* 1967; **70**: 129–42.

31. Hermansen L, Hultman E, Saltin B. Muscle glycogen during prolonged severe exercise. *Acta Physiologica Scandinavica* 1967; **71**: 129–39.

32. Costill DL, Gollnick PD, Jansson ED, Saltin B, Stein EM. Glycogen depletion pattern in human muscle fibres during distance running. *Acta Physiologica Scandinavica* 1973; **89**: 374–83.

33. Gollnick PD, Armstrong RB, Saubert CW IV, Sembrowich WL, Shepherd RE, Saltin B. Glycogen depletion patterns in human skeletal muscle fibers during prolonged work. *Pflügers Archiv* 1973; **344**: 1–12.

34. Karlsson J, Saltin B. Diet, muscle glycogen and endurance performance. *Journal of Applied Physiology* 1971; **31**: 203–6.

35. Goforth HW, Hodgdon JA, Hilderbrand RL. A double blind study of the effects of carbohydrate loading upon endurance performance. *Medicine and Science in Sport and Exercise* 1980; **12**: 108A.

36. Brewer J, Williams C, Patton A. The influence of high carbohydrate diets on endurance running performance. *European Journal of Applied Physiology* 1988; **57**: 698–706.

37. Madsen K, Pedersen PK, Rose P, Richter EA. Carbohydrate supercompensation and muscle glycogen utilization during exhaustive running in highly trained athletes. *European Journal of Applied Physiology* 1990; **61**: 467–72.

38. Tsintzas K, Williams C, Boobis L, Greenhaff P. Carbohydrate ingestion and single muscle fiber glycogen metabolism during prolonged running in men. *Journal of Applied Physiology* 1996; **81**: 801–9.

39. Costill DL, Jansson E, Gollnick PD, Saltin B. Glycogen utilization in leg muscles of men during level and uphill running. *Acta Physiologica Scandinavica* 1974; **91**: 475–81.

40. Tarnopolsky M, Atkinson S, Phillips S, Macdougall J. Carbohydrate loading and metabolism during exercise in men. *Journal of Applied Physiology* 1995; **78**: 1360–8.

41. Tarnopolsky LJ, MacDougall JD, Atkinson SA, Tarnopolsky MA, Sutton JR. Gender differences in substrate for endurance exercise. *Journal of Applied Physiology* 1990; **68**: 302–7.

42. Williams C, Brewer J, Walker M. The effect of a high carbohydrate diet on running performance during a 30-km treadmill time trial. *European Journal of Applied Physiology* 1992; **65**: 18–24.

43. Widrick JJ, Costill DL, Fink WJ, Hickey MS, McConnell GK, Tanaka H. Carbohydrate feedings and exercise performance: effect of initial muscle glycogen concentration. *Journal of Applied Physiology* 1993; **74**: 2998–3005.

44. Rauch L, Roger I, Wilson G, *et al.* The effects of carbohydrate loading on muscle glycogen content and cycling performance. *International Journal of Sport Nutrition* 1995; **5**: 25–36.

45. Pitsiladis Y, Duignan C, Maughan R. Effect of alterations in dietary carbohydrate intake on running performance during a 10 km treadmill time trial. *British Journal of Sports Medicine* 1996; **30**: 226–31.

46. Hawley J, Palmer G, Noakes T. Glycogen content and utilization during 1-h cycling performance. *European Journal of Applied Physiology* 1997; **75**: 407–12.

47. Maughan RJ, Poole DC. The effects of a glycogen-loading regimen on the capacity to perform anaerobic exercise. *European Journal of Applied Physiology* 1981; **46**: 211–19.

48. Maughan RJ, Greenhaff PL. High intensity exercise performance and acid–base balance: the influence of diet and induced metabolic alkalosis. *Medicine and Science in Sport and Exercise* 1991; **32**: 147–65.

49. Pizza F, Flynn M, Duscha B, Holden J, Kubitz E. A carbohydrate loading regimen improves high intensity, short duration exercise performance. *International Journal of Sport Nutrition* 1995; **5**: 110–16.

50. Hargreaves M, Finn J, Withers RT, *et al.* Effect of muscle glycogen availability on maximal exercise performance. *European Journal of Applied Physiology* 1997; **75**: 188–92.

51. Lakomy HKA. The use of a non-motorized treadmill for analysing sprint performance. *Ergonomics* 1987; **30**: 627–37.

52. Greenhaff P, Nevill M, Soderlund KLB, Williams C, Hultman E. Energy metabolism in single muscle fibres during maximal sprint exercise in man. *Journal of Physiology* 1992; **446**: 15–16.

53. Boobis LH, Williams C, Wootton SA. Influence of sprint training on muscle metabolism during brief maximal exercise in man. *Journal of Physiology* 1983; **342**: 36–7.

54. Nevill M, Boobis L, Brooks S, Williams C. Effect of training on muscle metabolism during treadmill sprinting. *Journal of Applied Physiology* 1989; **67**: 2376–82.

55. Wootton SA, Williams C. Influence of carbohydrate-status on performance during maximal exercise. *International Journal of Sports Medicine* 1984; **5**: S126–S127.

56. Jenkins D, Palmer J, Spillman D. The influence of dietary carbohydrate on performance of supramaximal intermittent exercise. *European Journal of Applied Physiology* 1993; **67**: 309–14.

57. Essen B, Kaijser L. Regulation of glycolysis in intermittent exercise in man. *Journal of Physiology* 1978; **281**: 499–511.

58. Gaitanos GC, Williams C, Boobis LH, Brooks S. Human muscle metabolism during intermittent maximal exercise. *Journal of Applied Physiology* 1993; **75**: 712–19.

59. Bangsbo J, Norregaard L, Thorsoe F. The effect of carbohydrate diet on intermittent exercise performance. *International Journal of Sports Medicine* 1992; **13**: 152–7.

60. Costill D, Miller J. Nutrition for endurance sport: carbohydrate and fluid balance. *International Journal of Sports Medicine* 1980; **1**: 2–14.

61. Saltin B. Metabolic fundamentals of exercise. *Medicine and Science in Sport and Exercise* 1973; **15**: 366–9.

62. Jacobs I, Westlin N, Karlsson J, Rasmusson M, Houghton B. Muscle glycogen and diet in elite soccer players. *European Journal of Applied Physiology* 1982; **48**: 297–302.

63. Akermark C, Jacobs I, Rasmusson M, Karlsson J. Diet and muscle glycogen concentration in relation to physical performance in Swedish elite ice hockey players. *International Journal of Sport Nutrition* 1996; **6**: 272–84.

64. Lambert E, Speechly D, Dennis S, Noakes T. Enhanced endurance in trained cyclists during moderate intensity exercise following 2 weeks adaptation to a high fat diet. *European Journal of Applied Physiology* 1994; **69**: 287–93.

65. Helge J, Richter E, Kiens B. Interaction of training and diet on metabolism and endurance during exercise in man. *Journal of Physiology* 1996; **492**: 293–306.

66. Starling R, Trappe T, Parcell A, Kerr C, Fink W, Costill D. Effects of diet on muscle triglyceride and endurance performance. *Journal of Applied Physiology* 1997; **82**: 1185–9.

67. Rennie MJ, Winder WW, Holloszy JO. A sparing effect of increased plasma fatty acids on muscle and liver glycogen content in the exercising rat. *Biochemical Journal* 1976; **156**: 647–55.

68. Okano G, Sato Y, Takumi Y, Sugawara M. Effect of 4h pre-exercise high carbohydrate and high fat meal ingestion on endurance performance and metabolism. *International Journal of Sports Medicine* 1996; **17**: 530–4.

69. Neufer PD, Costill DL, Flynn MG, Kirwan J, Mitchell J, Houmard J. Improvements in exercise performance: effects of carbohydrate feedings and diet. *Journal of Applied Physiology* 1987; **62**: 983–8.

70. Sherman W, Brodowicz G, Wright D, WKA, Simonsen J, Dernbach A. Effects of 4h pre-exercise carbohydrate feedings on cycling performance. *Medicine and Science in Sport and Exercise* 1989; **21**: 598–604.

71. Piearce L. Dietary habits of football players. In: Macleod DAD, Maughan RJ, Williams C, Madeley CR, Sharp JC, Nutton RW, eds. Intermittent high intensity exercise. London: E. and F.N. Spon, 1993: 159–73.

72. Sherman W, Peden M, Wright D. Carbohydrate feedings 1 h before exercise improves cycling performance. *American Journal of Clinical Nutrition* 1991; **54**: 866–70.

73. Wright D, Sherman W, Dernbach AR. Carbohydrate feedings before, during, or in combination improve cycling endurance performance. *Journal of Applied Physiology* 1991; **71**: 1082–8.

74. Chryssanthopoulos C, Williams C. Pre-exercise carbohydrate meal and endurance running capacity when carbohydrates are ingested during exercise. *International Journal of Sports Medicine* 1997. (In press.)

75. Chryssanthopoulos C, Williams C, Wilson W, Asher L, Hearne L. Comparison beween carbohydrate feedings before and during exercise on running performance during a 30-km treadmill time trial. *International Journal of Sport Nutrition* 1994; **4**: 374–86.

76. Horowitz JF, Coyle EF. Metabolic responses to pre-exercise meals containing various carbohydrates and fat. *American Journal of Clinical Nutrition* 1993; **58**: 235–41.

77. Thomas D, Brotherhood J, Brand J. Carbohydrate feeding before exercise: effect of glycemic index. *International Journal of Sports Medicine* 1991; **12**: 180–6.

78. Febbraio M, Strewart K. CHO feeding before prolonged exercise: effect of glycemic index on muscle glycogenolysis and exercise performance. *Journal of Applied Physiology* 1996; **82**: 1115–20.

79. Costill D, Coyle E, Dalsky G, Evans W, Fink W, Hoopes D. Effects of elevated plasma FFA and insulin on muscle glycogen usage during exercise. *Journal of Applied Physiology* 1977; **43**: 695–9.

80. Foster C, Costill D, Fink W. Effects of pre-exercise feedings on endurance performance. *Medicine and Science in Sport and Exercise* 1979; **11**: 1–5.

81. Devlin JT, Calles-Escandon J, Horton ES. Effects of pre-exercise snack feeding on endurance cycle exercise. *Journal of Applied Physiology* 1986; **60**: 980–5.

82. Gleeson M, Maughan R, Greenhaff P. Comparison of the effects of pre-exercise feeding of glucose, glycerol and placebo on endurance and fuel homeostasis in man. *European Journal of Applied Physiology* 1986; **55**: 645–53.

83. Vanzant R, Lemon P. Pre-exercise sugar feeding does not alter prolonged exercise muscle glycogen or protein catabolism. *Canadian Journal of Applied Physiology* 1997; **22**: 267–79.

84. McMurray R, Wilson J, Kitchell B. The effects of fructose and glucose on high intensity endurance performance. *Research Quarterly on Exercise and Sport* 1983; **54**: 156–62.

85. Chryssanthopoulos C, Hennessy L, Williams C. The influence of pre-exercise glucose ingestion on endurance running capacity. *British Journal of Sports Medicine* 1994; **28**: 105–9.

86. Calles-Escandon J, Devlin JT, Whitcomb W, Horton ES. Pre-exercise feeding does not affect endurance cycle exercise but attenuates post-exercise starvation-like response. *Medicine and Science in Sport and Exercise* 1991; **23**: 818–24.

87. Williams C, Nute MG, Broadbank L, Vinall S. Influence of fluid intake on endurance running performance. *European Journal of Applied Physiology* 1990; **60**: 112–19.

88. Porte D, Williamson R. Inhibition of insulin release by norepinephrine in man. *Science* 1966; **152**: 1248–50.

89. Ivy JL, Miller W, Dover V, *et al.* Endurance improved by ingestion of a glucose polymer supplement. *Medicine and Science in Sports and Exercise* 1983; **15**: 466–71.

90. Bjorkman O, Sahlin K, Hagenfeldt L, Wahren J. Influence of glucose and fructose ingestion on the capacity for long-term exercise in well-trained men. *Clinical Physiology* 1984; **4**: 483–94.

91. Coyle EF, Coggan AR, Hemmert MK, Ivy JL. Muscle glycogen utilization during prolonged strenuous exercise when fed carbohydrate. *Journal of Applied Physiology* 1986; **61**: 165–72.

92. Okano G, Takeda H, Morita I, Katoh M, Mu Z, Miyake S. Effect of pre-exercise fructose ingestion on endurance performance in fed men. *Medicine and Science in Sport and Exercise* 1987; **20**: 105–9.

93. Coggan AR, Coyle EF. Metabolism and performance following carbohydrate ingestion late in exercise. *Medicine and Science in Sport and Exercise* 1989; **21**: 59–65.

94. Maughan RJ, Fenn CE, Leiper JB. Effects of fluid, electrolyte and substrate ingestion on endurance capacity. *European Journal of Applied Physiology* 1989; **58**: 481–6.

95. Wahren J. Substrate utilization by exercising muscle in man. *Progress in Cardiology* 1973; **2**: 255–80.

96. Bonen A, Malcolm SA, Kilgour RD, MacIntyre KP, Belcastro AN. Glucose ingestion before and during intense exercise. *Journal of Applied Physiology* 1981; **50**: 766–71.

97. Tsintzas K, Williams C, Wilson W, Burrin J. Influence of carbohydrate supplementation early in exercise on endurance running capacity. *Medicine and Science in Sport and Exercise* 1996; **28**: 1373–9.

98. Wilber R, Moffatt R. Influence of carbohydrate ingestion on blood glucose and performance in runners. *International Journal of Sport Nutrition* 1992; **2**: 317–27.

99. Kuipers H, Keizer HA, Brouns F, Saris WHM. Carbohydrate feeding and glycogen synthesis during exercise in man. *European Journal of Applied Physiology* 1987; **410**: 652–6.

100. Tsintzas K, Liu R, Williams C, Campbell I, Gaitanos G. The effect of carbohydrate ingestion on performance during a 30-km race. *International Journal of Sport Nutrition* 1993; **3**: 127–39.

101. Millard-Stafford LM, Sparling PB, Rosskope LB, Dicarlo L J. Carbohydrate–electrolyte replacement improves distance running performance in the heat. *Medicine and Science in Sport and Exercise* 1992; **24**: 934–40.

102. Tsintzas O, Williams C, Singh R, Wilson W, Burrin J. Influence of carbohydrate–electrolyte drinks on marathon running performance. *European Journal of Applied Physiology* 1995; **70**: 154–60.

103. Millard-Stafford M, Rosskopf L, Snow T, Hinson B. Water versus carbohydrate–electrolyte ingestion before and during a 15 km run in the heat. *International Journal of Sport Nutrition* 1997; **7**: 26–38.

104. Jeukendrup A, Brouns F, Wagenmakers A, Saris W. Carbohydrate–electrolyte feedings improve 1h time trial cycling performance. *International Journal of Sports Medicine* 1997; **18**: 125–9.

105. Below P, Mora-Rodriguez R, Gonzalez-Alonso J, Coyle E. Fluid and carbohydrate ingestion independently improve performance during 1h of intense exercise. *Medicine and Science in Sport and Exercise* 1995; **27**: 200–10.

106. Davis J. Central and peripheral factors in fatigue. *Journal of Sports Science* 1995; **13**: S49–S53.

107. Yaspelkis BB, Ivy JL. Effect of carbohydrate supplements and water on exercise metabolism in the heat. *Journal of Applied Physiology* 1991; **71**: 680–7.

108. Tsintzas O-K, Williams C, Boobis L, Greenhaff P. Carbohydrate ingestion and glycogen utilization in different muscle fibre types in man. *Journal of Physiology* 1995; **489**: 243–50.

109. Kirkendall D, Foster C, Dean J, Grogan J, Thompson N. Effect of glucose polymer supplementation on performance of soccer players. In: Reilly T, Lees A, David K, Murphy W, eds. *Science and football*. London: E. and F.N. Spon, 1988: 33–41.

110. Leatt PB, Jacobs I. Effect of glucose polymer ingestion on glycogen depletion during a soccer match. *Canadian Journal of Sports Science* 1989; **14**: 112–16.

111. Nicholas C, Williams C, Lakomy H, Phillips G, Nowitz A. Influence of ingesting a carbohydrate–electrolyte solution on endurance capacity during intermittent, high-intensity shuttle running. *Journal of Sports Science* 1995; **13**: 283–90.

112. Piehl K. Time course of refilling of glycogen stores in human muscle fibres following exercise-induced glycogen repletion. *Acta Physiologica Scandinavica* 1974; **90**: 297–302.

113. Zachwieja JJ, Costill DL, Pascoe DD, Robergs RA, Fink WJ. Influence of muscle glycogen depletion on the rate of resynthesis. *Medicine and Science in Sports and Exercise* 1991; **23**: 44–8.

114. Wallberg-Henriksson H, Constable SH, Young DA, Holloszy JO. Glucose transport into rat skeletal muscle: interaction between exercise and insulin. *Journal of Applied Physiology* 1988; **65**: 909–13.

115. Adolfsson S, Ahren K. Control mechanisms for the synthesis of glycogen in striated muscle. In: Pernow B, Saltin B, eds. *Muscle metabolism during exercise*. New York: Plenum Press, 1971: 257–72.

116. Piehl K, Adolfsson S, Nazar K. Glycogen storage and glycogen synthetase activity in trained and untrained muscle of man. *Acta Physiologica Scandinavica* 1974; **90**: 779–88.

117. Vollestad N, Vaage O, Hermansen L. Muscle glycogen depletion patterns in Type I and subgroups of Type II fibres during prolonged severe exercise in man. *Acta Physiologica Scandinavica* 1984; **122**: 433–41.

118. Yan Z, Spencer M, Katz A. Effect of low glycogen on glycogen synthase in human muscle during and after exercise. *Acta Physiologica Scandinavica* 1992; **145**: 345–52.

119. McCoy M, Proietto J, Hargreaves M. Skeletal muscle Glut 4 and post-exercise muscle glycogen storage in humans. *Journal of Applied Physiology* 1996; **80**: 411–15.

120. Nakatani A, Han D-H, Hansen P, *et al*. Effect of endurance exercise training on muscle glycogen supercompensation in rats. *Journal of Applied Physiology* 1997; **82**: 711–15.

121. Robergs R. Nutrition and exercise determinants of postexercise glycogen synthesis. *International Journal of Sport Nutrition* 1991; **1**: 307–37.

122. Blom P, Hostmark AT, Vaage O, Kardel KR, Maehlum S. Effect of different post-exercise sugar diets on the rate of muscle glycogen synthesis. *Medicine and Science in Sports and Exercise* 1987; **19**: 491–6.

123. Ivy JL. Muscle glycogen synthesis before and after exercise. *Sports Medicine* 1991; **11**: 6–19.

124. Parkin J, Carey M, Martin I, Stojanovska L, Febbraio M. Muscle glycogen storage following prolonged exercise: effect of timing of ingestion of high glycemic index food. *Medicine and Science in Sports and Exercise* 1997; **29**: 220–4.

125. Gonzalez-Alonso J, Heaps CL, Coyle EF. Rehydration after exercise with common beverages and water. *International Journal of Sports Medicine* 1992; **13**: 399–406.

126. Burke L, Collier G, Hargreaves M. Muscle glycogen storage after prolonged exercise: effect of the glycaemic index of carbohydrate feedings. *Journal of Applied Physiology* 1993; **75**: 1019–23.

127. Zawadzki K, Yaspelkis B III, Ivy J. Carbohydrate–protein complex increases the rate of muscle glycogen storage after exercise. *Journal of Applied Physiology* 1992; **72**: 1854–9.

128. Johansson C, Tsai L, Hultman E, Tegelman R, Pousette A. Restoration of anabolic deficit and muscle glycogen consumption in competitive orienteering. *International Journal of Sports Medicine* 1990; **11**: 204–7.

129. O'Reilly KP, Warhol MJ, Fielding RA, Frontera WA, Meredith CN, Evans WWJ. Eccentric exercise-induced muscle damage impairs muscle glycogen repletion. *Journal of Applied Physiology* 1987; **63**: 252–6.

130. Roy B, Tarnopolsky M, Macdougall J, Fowles J, Yarasheski K. Effect of glucose supplement timing on protein-metabolism after resistance training. *Journal of Applied Physiology* 1997; **82**: 1882–8.

131. Pascoe DD, Costill DL, Robergs RA, Davis JA, Fink WJ, Pearson DR. Effects of exercise mode on muscle glycogen restorage during repeated days of exercise. *Medicine and Science in Sports and Exercise* 1990; **22**: 593–8.

132. Kirwan JP, Costill DL, Mitchell JB, *et al*. Carbohydrate balance in competitive runners during successive days of intense training. *Journal of Applied Physiology* 1988; **65**: 2601–6.

133. Keizer H, Kuipers H, van Kranenburg G. Influence of liquid and solid meals on muscle glycogen resynthesis, plasma fuel hormone

response, and maximal physical working capacity. *International Journal of Sports Medicine* 1987; **8**: 99–104.

134. Nevill ME, Williams C, Roper D, Slater C, Nevill AM. Effect of diet on performance during recovery from intermittent sprint exercise. *Journal of Sports Science* 1993; **11**: 119–26.

135. Fallowfield J, Williams C. Carbohydrate intake and recovery from prolonged exercise. *International Journal of Sport Nutrition* 1993; **3**: 150–64.

136. Nicholas C, Hawkins R, Green P, Williams C. Carbohydrate intake and recovery of intermittent running capacity. *International Journal of Sport Nutrition* 1997. (In press.)

137. Fallowfield J, Williams C, Singh R. The influence of ingesting a carbohydrate–electrolyte solution during 4 h recovery from prolonged running on endurance capacity. *International Journal of Sport Nutrition* 1995; **5**: 285–99.

138. Fallowfield J, Williams C. The influence of a high carbohydrate intake during recovery from prolonged constant pace running. *International Journal of Sport Nutrition* 1997; **7**: 10–25.

139. Coggan A, Coyle E. Reversal of fatigue during prolonged exercise by carbohydrate infusion or ingestion. *Journal of Applied Physiology* 1987; **63**: 2388–95.

140. Maughan R. Energy and macronutrient intakes of professional (soccer) players. *British Journal of Sports Medicine* 1997; **31**: 45–7.

141. Berning J, Troup J, Van Handel P, Daniels J, Daniels N. The nutritional habits of young adolescent swimmers. *International Journal of Sport Nutrition* 1991; **1**: 240–8.

142. Hawley JA, Williams MM. Dietary intakes of age-groups swimmers. *British Journal of Sports Medicine* 1991; **25**: 154–8.

143. Deuster P, Kyle S, Moser P, Vigersky R, Singh A, Schoomaker E. Nutritional intakes and status of highly trained amenorrheic and eumenorrheic women runners. *Fertility and Sterility* 1986; **46**: 636–43.

1.2.2 Fluid and electrolyte loss and replacement in exercise

R. J. Maughan and Susan M. Shirreffs

Introduction

Recent decisions to hold a number of major sporting events (including the 1994 Soccer World Cup in Florida, the 1996 Olympic Games in Atlanta, and the 1998 Commonwealth Games in Kuala Lumpur) in venues where participants will be exposed to conditions of high heat and humidity have given a new impetus to the study of the physiology of exercise in the heat. With this has come a recognition that much of what we know about the limitations to exercise performance relates to exercise carried out in temperate or even cool conditions, and may not apply to the athlete competing in a hot, humid environment. Whatever the environmental conditions, fatigue is an inevitable accompaniment of exercise if the exercise is sufficiently intense or prolonged, but the nature of the fatigue process will be influenced by many factors. The most important of these is undoubtedly the intensity of the exercise in relation to the capacity of the individual, and the most effective way to delay the onset of fatigue and improve performance is by a systematic programme of training. In temperate conditions, the primary cause of fatigue in exercise lasting more than 1 hour but not more than 4 to 5 hours is usually the depletion of the body's carbohydrate reserves.[1]

This time-scale covers most ball games such as football, hockey, and tennis, and also individual events such as marathon running. Systematic training results in many adaptations to the cardiovascular system and to the muscles, allowing them to increase the extent to which they can use the relatively unlimited fat stores as a fuel and thus spare the rather small amounts of carbohydrate which are stored in the liver and in the muscles. Where the availability of carbohydrate fuel limits exercise, this will result in an improved performance.

Many other factors will, however, influence performance, and among these are the environmental conditions under which the exercise is performed. When the ambient temperature and humidity are high, the capacity to perform prolonged exercise is reduced: Galloway and Maughan have reported that subjects who were able to exercise for a mean time of 93 min at an ambient temperature of 11°C were exhausted after 82 min when the ambient temperature was 21°C, and after only 52 min when the temperature was increased to 30°C.[2] In this situation, dehydration and thermoregulatory problems rather than substrate depletion seem likely to be the cause of fatigue. At rest, the rate of heat production by the body is low, but at high work rates, metabolic heat production can exceed 80 kJ/min (20 kcal/min), and highly trained athletes can sustain these work rates for more than 2 h. The rate of sweating necessary to lose this heat load will result in a rapid loss of body water with an associated loss of electrolytes.

Fluid loss and temperature regulation

Fluid loss during exercise is linked to the need to maintain body temperature within narrow limits. The resting oxygen consumption of a normal adult is about 250 ml/min, corresponding to a rate of heat production of about 70 W. Thermoregulation is primarily achieved by behavioural mechanisms: the amount of clothing worn is adjusted or the ambient temperature is changed so that the rate of heat production is balanced by the rate of heat loss. During exercise, the rate of heat production can be increased to many times the resting level. Although this does not pose a problem in events of short duration, it represents a major threat to the endurance athlete. In an event such as running on the level, the rate of heat production is determined primarily by running speed and body mass, with individual variations in mechanical and metabolic efficiency being of secondary importance. Running a marathon in 2 h 30 min requires an oxygen consumption of about 4 l/min to be sustained throughout the race for the average runner with a body mass of 70 kg. When the ambient temperature is higher than skin temperature, heat will also be gained from the environment by physical transfer. In spite of this, marathon runners normally maintain body temperature within 2–3°C of the resting level, indicating that heat is being lost from the body almost as fast as it is being produced.

At high ambient temperatures, the only mechanism by which heat can be lost from the body is evaporation of sweat secreted on to the skin surface, and even at low ambient temperatures high sweat rates are sometimes necessary to prevent an excessive rise in body temperature.[3] Evaporation of 1 litre of water from the skin will remove 2.4 MJ (580 kcal) of heat from the body. To balance the rate of metabolic heat production by evaporative loss alone in a 2 h 30 min marathon runner with a body mass of 70 kg would therefore

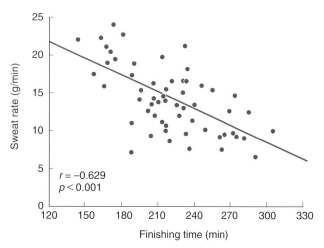

Fig. 1 Mean sweat rate in relation to finishing time in 59 male runners who completed a marathon (42.2 km) race on a cool (12°C) day. Sweat rate was calculated from the change in body weight after correction for fluid intake and respiratory water loss. Although there was a good relationship between sweat rate and running speed, there was a large variation between individuals, and there was no relationship between total sweat loss and finishing time for the race. (Reproduced from ref. 3, with permission.)

require sweat to be evaporated from the skin at a rate of about 1.6 l/h: at such high sweat rates, an appreciable fraction drips from the skin without evaporating, and a sweat secretion rate of about 2 l/h is likely to be necessary to achieve this rate of evaporative heat loss. This is possible, but would result in the loss of 5 litres of body water, corresponding to a loss of more than 7 per cent of body mass for a 70 kg runner. Even in cool conditions, sweat losses may be high when the exercise intensity is high or the duration long: in a marathon held on a cool (12°C) day, mean sweat losses measured on 59 male runners were estimated to be approximately 3.5 litres, with a large inter-individual variability, even when the running speed was the same (Fig. 1).

Some water will also be lost by evaporation from the respiratory tract, and this will also contribute to heat dissipation, though this mechanism is much less important in man than it is in animals such as the dog: this may reflect the limited evaporative capacity resulting from a thick coat of body hair. During hard exercise in a hot dry environment, respiratory water loss can be significant,[4] even though it is not generally considered to be a major heat loss mechanism in man. The rise of 2 to 3°C in body temperature which normally occurs during marathon running means that some of the heat produced is stored, but the effect on heat balance is minimal: for a 70 kg runner a rise in mean body temperature of 3°C—about the maximum tolerable increase—would reduce the total requirement for evaporation of sweat by less than 300 ml.

It is often reported that exercise performance is impaired when an individual is dehydrated by as little as 2 per cent of body mass, and that losses in excess of 5 per cent of body mass can decrease the capacity for work by about 30 per cent.[5] Prior dehydration will impair the capacity to perform high intensity exercise as well as endurance activities.[6,7] Nielsen et al. showed that prolonged exercise, which resulted in a loss of fluid corresponding to 2.5 per cent of body weight, resulted in a 45 per cent fall in the capacity to perform high-intensity exercise. It may be that even very small fluid

deficits impair performance but the methods used are not sufficiently sensitive to detect small changes.

Fluid losses are distributed in varying proportions among the plasma, extracellular water, and intracellular water. The decrease in plasma volume which accompanies dehydration may be of particular importance in influencing work capacity; blood flow to the muscles must be maintained at a high level to supply oxygen and substrates, but a high blood flow to the skin is also necessary to convect heat to the body surface where it can be dissipated.[8] When the ambient temperature is high and blood volume has been decreased by sweat loss during prolonged exercise, there may be difficulty in meeting the requirement for a high blood flow to both these tissues. In this situation, skin blood flow is likely to be compromised, allowing central venous pressure and muscle blood flow to be maintained but reducing heat loss and causing body temperature to rise.[9]

These factors have been investigated by Coyle and his colleagues: their results clearly demonstrate that increases in core temperature and heart rate during prolonged exercise are graded according to the level of hypohydration achieved.[10] They also showed, however, that the ingestion of fluid during exercise increases skin blood flow, and therefore thermoregulatory capacity, independent of increases in the circulating blood volume.[11] Plasma volume expansion using dextran/saline infusion was less effective in preventing a rise in core temperature than was the ingestion of sufficient volumes of a carbohydrate-electrolyte drink to maintain plasma volume at a similar level. More recently, Riebe et al. compared intravenous infusion with oral ingestion of the same volume of saline solution for recovery after dehydrating exercise which induced a loss of approximately 4 per cent of body mass.[12] There was no difference in the plasma-volume responses between the two fluid intake methods and there was no difference in core-temperature responses in a further 20 min period of walking.

Electrolyte loss in sweat and the effects on body fluids

The sweat which is secreted on to the skin contains a wide variety of organic and inorganic solutes, and significant losses of some of these components will occur where large volumes of sweat are produced. The electrolyte composition of sweat is variable, and the concentration of individual electrolytes as well as the total sweat volume will influence the extent of losses. The normal concentration ranges for the main ionic components of sweat are shown in Table 1, along with their plasma and intracellular concentrations for comparison. A number of factors contribute to the variability in the composition of sweat: methodological problems in the collection procedure, including evaporative loss, incomplete collection, and contamination with skin cells, account for at least part of the variability, but there is also a large biological variability.

The sweat composition undoubtedly varies between individuals, but can also vary within the same individual depending on the rate of secretion, the state of training and the state of heat acclimation.[16] In response to a standard heat stress, the sweat rate increases with training and acclimation and the electrolyte content decreases. These adaptations are generally considered to allow improved thermoregulation while conserving electrolytes. There are, however, some puzzling aspects: where the sweat rate is sufficient to keep the skin wet, further increases in the sweat rate will increase the amount

Table 1 Concentration (mmol/l) of the major electrolytes in sweat, plasma, and intracellular water. These values are taken from a variety of sources, but are based primarily on those reported by Pitts,[13] Lentner,[14] and Schmidt and Thews[15]

	Sweat (mmol/l)	Plasma (mmol/l)	Intracellular (mmol/l)
Sodium	20–80	130–155	10
Potassium	4–8	3.2–5.5	150
Calcium	0–1	2.1–2.9	0
Magnesium	< 0.2	0.7–1.5	15
Chloride	20–60	96–110	8
Bicarbonate	0–35	23–28	10
Phosphate	0.1–0.2	0.7–1.6	65
Sulphate	0.1–2.0	0.3–0.9	10

of water which drips from the skin without evaporation but will not further increase the rate of evaporative heat loss.

In spite of the variations which do occur, the major electrolytes in sweat, as in the extracellular fluid, are sodium and chloride (Table 1), although the sweat concentrations of these ions are invariably lower than those in plasma. Contrary to what might be expected, Costill reported an increased concentration of sodium and chloride in sweat content with increased flow: this was attributed to a reduced opportunity for reabsorption in the sweat duct.[17] Verde *et al.*, however, found that the sweat concentration of these ions was unrelated to the sweat flow rate.[18] Acclimation studies have shown that elevated sweating rates are accompanied by a decrease in the concentration of sodium and chloride in sweat in spite of the increased flow rate.[19,20] The potassium content of sweat appears to be relatively unaffected by the sweat rate, and the magnesium content is also unchanged or perhaps decreases slightly. These apparently conflicting results demonstrate some of the difficulties in interpreting the literature in this area. Differences between studies may be due to differences in the training status and degree of acclimation of the subjects used as well as differences in methodology: some studies have used whole-body washdown techniques to collect sweat, whereas others have examined local sweating responses using ventilated capsules or collection bags. There are differences in the composition of sweat from different regions of the body,[21,22] and the values obtained by regional collection also differ from those obtained by the whole body washdown technique.[23] The use of improved sweat collection techniques should now give the opportunity to resolve these issues.

Because sweat is hypotonic with respect to body fluids, the effect of prolonged sweating is to increase the plasma osmolality, which may have a significant effect on the ability to maintain body temperature. A direct relationship between plasma osmolality and body temperature has been demonstrated during exercise.[24,25] Hyperosmolality of plasma, induced prior to exercise, has been shown to result in a decreased thermoregulatory effector response; the threshold for sweating is elevated and the cutaneous vasodilator response is reduced.[26] In short-term (30 min) exercise, however, the cardiovascular and thermoregulatory response appears to be inde-

pendent of changes in osmolality induced during the exercise period.[27] The changes in the concentration of individual electrolytes are more variable, but an increase in the plasma sodium and chloride concentrations is generally observed in response to both running and cycling exercise. Exceptions to this are rare and occur only when excessively large volumes of drinks low in electrolytes are consumed over long time-periods; these situations are discussed further below.

The plasma potassium concentration has been reported to remain constant after marathon running,[28,29] although others have reported small increases, irrespective of whether drinks containing large amounts of potassium,[30] or no electrolytes,[31,32] were given. Much of the inconsistency in the literature relating to changes in the circulating potassium concentration can be explained by the variable time taken to obtain blood samples after exercise under field conditions; the plasma potassium concentration rapidly returns to normal in the post-exercise period.[33] Laboratory studies, where an indwelling catheter can be used to obtain blood samples during exercise, commonly show an increase in the circulating potassium concentration in the later stages of prolonged exercise. The potassium concentration of extracellular fluid (4–5 mmol/l) is small relative to the intracellular concentration (150–160 mmol/l), and release of potassium from liver, muscle, and red blood cells will tend to elevate plasma potassium levels during exercise in spite of the losses in sweat.

The plasma magnesium concentration is unchanged after 60 min of moderate intensity cycling exercise,[34] but Rose *et al.*[35] observed a 20 per cent fall in the serum magnesium concentration after a marathon race and attributed this to a loss in sweat; a fall of similar magnitude was reported by Cohen and Zimmerman[32]. A larger fall in the serum magnesium concentration has been observed during exercise in the heat than at neutral temperatures,[36] supporting the idea that losses in sweat are responsible. There are, however, reports that the fall in plasma magnesium concentration that occurs during prolonged exercise is a consequence of redistribution, with uptake of magnesium by red blood cells,[37] active muscle,[17] or adipose tissue[38]. Although the concentration of potassium and magnesium in sweat is high relative to that in the plasma, the plasma content of these ions represents only a small fraction of the whole-body stores; Costill and Miller[39] estimated that only about 1 per cent of the body stores of these electrolytes was lost when individuals were dehydrated by 5.8 per cent of body mass.

There have been some reports of differences in sweating function and in sweat composition between men and women (see Brouns *et al.*[40] for review), but it is not altogether clear to what extent this apparent gender difference can be accounted for by differences in training and acclimation status. There are some differences between children and adults in the sweating response to exercise and in sweat composition. The sweating capacity of children is low, when expressed per unit surface area, and the sweat electrolyte content is low relative to that of adults,[41] but the need for fluid and electrolyte replacement is no less important than in adults. Indeed, in view of the evidence that core temperature increases to a greater extent in children than in adults at a given level of dehydration, the need for fluid replacement may well be greater in children.[42]

An extensive review of the literature on sweat composition and sweat electrolyte losses has been completed by Brouns *et al.*:[40] these authors have suggested that, during exercise, the upper limit for replacement of electrolytes lost in sweat can be determined in relation to the losses. It does appear, however, that the variation between individuals and between conditions may be so large as to preclude any meaningful recommendations. It is also unclear whether there is any good evidence to show benefits resulting from replacement during exercise of any electrolyte other than perhaps sodium.

Control of water and electrolyte balance

The excretion of some of the waste products of metabolism and the regulation of the body's water and electrolyte balance are the primary functions of the kidneys. Excess water or solute is excreted, and where there is a deficiency of water or electrolytes, these are conserved until the balance is restored. Under normal conditions, the osmolality of the extracellular fluid is maintained within narrow limits; since this is strongly influenced by the sodium concentration, sodium and water balance are closely linked.

At rest, approximately 15 to 20 per cent of the renal plasma flow is continuously filtered out by the glomeruli, resulting in the production of about 170 litres of filtrate per day. Most (99 per cent or more) of this is reabsorbed in the tubular system, leaving about 1 to 1.5 litres to appear as urine. The volume of urine produced is determined primarily by the action of antidiuretic hormone (**ADH**) which regulates water reabsorption by increasing the permeability of the distal tubule of the nephron and the collecting duct to water. ADH is released from the posterior lobe of the pituitary in response to signals from the supraoptic nucleus of the hypothalamus: the main stimuli for the release of ADH, which is normally present only in low concentrations, are an increased signal from the osmoreceptors located within the hypothalamus, a decrease in blood volume, which is detected by low-pressure receptors in the atria, and by high-pressure baroreceptors in the aortic arch and carotid sinus. An increased plasma angiotensin concentration will also stimulate ADH output.

The sodium concentration of the plasma is regulated by the renal reabsorption of sodium from the glomerular filtrate. Most of the reabsorption occurs in the proximal tubule, but active absorption also occurs in the distal tubules and collecting ducts. A number of factors influence the extent to which reabsorption occurs, and among these is the action of aldosterone, which promotes sodium reabsorption in the distal tubules and enhances the excretion of potassium and hydrogen ions. Aldosterone is released from the kidney in response to a fall in the circulating sodium concentration or a rise in plasma potassium; aldosterone release is also stimulated by angiotensin which is produced by the renin–angiotensin system in response to a decrease in the plasma sodium concentration. Angiotensin thus has a twofold action, namely on the release of aldosterone as well as ADH. Atrial natriuretic factor (ANF) is a peptide synthesized in and released from the atria of the heart in response to atrial distension. It increases the glomerular filtration rate and decreases sodium and water reabsorption leading to an increased loss: this may be important in the regulation of extracellular volume, but it seems unlikely that ANF plays a significant role during exercise. Regulation of the body's sodium balance has profound implications for fluid balance, as sodium salts account for more than 90 per cent of the osmotic pressure of the extracellular fluid.

Loss of hypotonic fluid as sweat during prolonged exercise usually results in a fall in blood volume and an increased plasma osmolality: both these changes act as stimuli for the release of ADH.[43] The plasma ADH concentration during exercise has been reported to increase as a function of the exercise intensity.[44] Renal blood flow is also reduced in proportion to the exercise intensity and may be as low as 25 per cent of the resting level during strenuous exercise.[45] These factors combine to result in a decreased urine flow during, and usually for some time after, exercise.[45] It has been pointed out, however, that the volume of water conserved by this decreased urine flow during exercise is small, probably amounting to no more than 12 to 45 ml/h.[46]

The effect of exercise is normally to decrease the renal excretion of sodium and to increase the excretion of potassium, although the effect on potassium excretion is rather variable.[46] These effects appear to be largely due to an increased rate of aldosterone production during exercise.[45] Although the concentrations of sodium, and more especially of potassium, in the urine are generally high relative to the concentrations in extracellular fluid, the extent of total urinary losses in most exercise situations is small.

Fluid replacement during exercise

The ability to sustain a high rate of work output requires that an adequate supply of carbohydrate substrate be available to the working muscles. Thus fluid ingestion during exercise has the twin aims of providing a source of carbohydrate fuel to supplement the body's limited stores and of supplying water to replace the losses incurred by sweating. Increasing the carbohydrate content of drinks will increase the amount of fuel which can be supplied, but will tend to decrease the rate at which water can be made available;[47] where provision of water is the first priority, the carbohydrate content of drinks will be low, thus restricting the rate at which substrate is provided. The composition of drinks to be taken will therefore be influenced by the relative importance of the need to supply fuel and water; this in turn depends on the intensity and duration of the exercise task, on the ambient temperature and humidity, and on the physiological and biochemical characteristics of the individual athlete. Carbohydrate depletion will result in fatigue and a reduction in the exercise intensity which can be sustained, but is not normally a life threatening condition. Disturbances in fluid balance and temperature regulation have potentially more serious consequences, and it may be, therefore, that the emphasis for the majority of participants in endurance events should be on proper maintenance of fluid and electrolyte balance.

Availability of ingested fluids

The first barrier to the availability of ingested fluids is the rate of gastric emptying, which controls the rate at which fluids are delivered to the small intestine and the extent to which they are influenced by the gastric secretions. The rate of emptying is determined by the volume and composition of fluid consumed. The volume of the stomach contents is a major factor in regulating the rate of emptying, and the rate of emptying of any solution can be increased by increasing the volume present in the stomach; emptying follows an exponential time course, and falls rapidly as the volume remaining in the stomach decreases.[48-50] Where a high rate of emptying is desirable, this can be promoted by keeping the volume high by repeated drinking.[51] Dilute solutions of glucose will leave

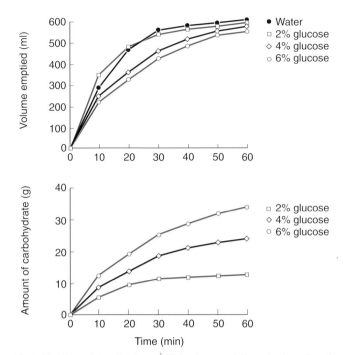

Fig. 2 Gastric emptying of water and dilute glucose solutions after ingestion of a fixed volume of 600 ml. The upper panel shows the volume of liquid emptied from the stomach, and the lower panel shows the amount of glucose emptied. Measurements were made at 10 min intervals by a double sampling gastric aspiration method. (Reproduced from ref. 52, with permission.)

the stomach almost, but not quite, as fast as plain water; the rate of emptying is slowed in proportion to the glucose content, and concentrated sugar solutions will remain in the stomach for long periods. There has been some debate as to the concentration of carbohydrate at which an inhibitory effect on gastric emptying is first observed: the conflicting results reported in the literature are caused, at least in part, by deficiencies in the methodology employed in some studies. It appears that glucose concentrations as low as 40 g/l will have some slowing effect on the rate of gastric emptying.[52]

It has been proposed that the rate of emptying of nutrient solutions is regulated so as to provide a constant rate of energy delivery to the intestine,[53] but it is clear from Fig. 2 that the rate of energy delivery from glucose solutions of different concentrations is not constant, but varies over time for any given solution and is proportional to the glucose concentration of the drinks. Even though the volume emptied is decreased as the glucose concentration increases, the amount of glucose emptied is increased with more concentrated solutions; this has implications for situations where the primary need is for water to replace sweat losses or where the aim is to supply large amounts of substrate without consideration of fluid replacement.

An increasing osmolality of the gastric contents will tend to delay emptying, and there is some evidence that substitution of glucose polymers for free glucose, which will result in a decreased osmolality for the same carbohydrate content, may be effective in increasing the volume of fluid and the amount of substrate delivered to the intestine. The differences, however, are generally small, with the exception of a report by Foster et al.,[54] who found that the rate of emptying of a 5 per cent glucose polymer solution was about one-third faster than that of a 5 per cent solution of free glucose; the results of this study may, however, be misleading as no account was taken of the volume of fluid secreted into the stomach, and this is now known to be greater for solutions of free glucose than for polymers (Sole and Noakes, 1989; Rehrer 1990).[51,55] Sole and Noakes found no significant difference in emptying rates between 5 per cent polymer and free glucose solutions, and Naveri et al.[56] made the same observation on 3 per cent solutions. With more concentrated solutions, Foster et al.[54] found no differences between polymer and free glucose solutions in the concentration range 10 to 40 per cent, but Sole and Noakes[55] found that 15 per cent polymer solutions emptied faster than the corresponding free glucose solution. The interpretation of many of these studies is complicated by the use of a variety of different carbohydrate sources and by the presence or absence of electrolytes. More recently, Vist and Maughan[47] have shown that there is an acceleration of emptying when glucose polymer solutions are substituted for free glucose solutions with the same energy density. At low (about 4 per cent) concentrations, this effect is small, but it becomes appreciable at higher (18 per cent) concentrations; where the osmolality is the same (as in the 4 per cent glucose solution and 18 per cent polymer solution), the energy density is shown to be of far greater significance in determining the rate of gastric emptying. It thus appears that the results are rather variable, but it is worth noting that there are no reports of polymer solutions being emptied more slowly than free glucose solutions with the same energy density; even when the difference is not significant, there is a tendency for faster emptying of polymer solutions.

The temperature of ingested drinks has been reported to have an influence on the rate of emptying, and in the past it has been recommended that drinks should be chilled to promote gastric emptying.[57] This recommendation is based on a study by Costill and Saltin,[58] who gave subjects 400 ml of a dilute glucose solution at temperatures ranging from 5 to 35°C: the volume emptied in the first 15 min after ingestion was approximately twice as great for the solution at 5°C as for the solution at 35°C. More recent reports, however, have cast some doubt on the importance of temperature in affecting emptying of liquids. Sun et al.[59] gave isosmotic orange juice at different temperatures, and found that the initial emptying rate for cold (4°C) drinks was slower than for drinks given at body temperature (37°C): the emptying rate for warm (50°C) drinks was not significantly different from that for the other two drinks. McArthur and Feldman[60] have also recently shown that the emptying rate for coffee drinks given at 4, 37, or 58°C was not different. Lambert and Maughan[61] used a tracer technique to show that fluids ingested at high temperature (50°C) appear in the circulation slightly faster than if they are chilled (4°C) before ingestion; this technique takes into account the effects of beverage temperature on both gastric emptying and intestinal absorption.[62] Other factors, such as pH, may have a minor role to play. Although there is some evidence that emptying is hastened if drinks are carbonated,[63] more recent results suggest that carbonation has no effect:[64] it is probable that light carbonation as used in most sports drinks does not influence the gastric emptying rate, but a greater degree of carbonation, as used in many soft drinks, may be effective by raising the intragastric pressure. Zachwieja et al.[65] have shown that carbonated and non-carbonated carbohydrate (10 per cent) solutions were equally effective in

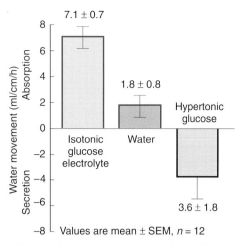

Fig. 3 Absorption rate of water in the upper part of the small intestine when per-fused with water, a dilute glucose electrolyte solution and with a concentrated glu-cose solution. The dilute glucose electrolyte solution results in a stimulation of water uptake, and the hypertonic glucose solution causes a net secretion of water into the intestine.

improving cycling performance relative to water administration: there was no effect of carbonation on the rate of gastric emptying or on the reported prevalence of gastrointestinal symptoms. Lambert et al.[66] did report a greater sensation of stomach fullness in exer-cising subjects drinking a carbonated 6 per cent carbohydrate solu-tion relative to the same drink without carbonation, but there was no apparent effect on physiological function.

Absorption of glucose occurs in the small intestine, and is an active, energy-consuming process linked to the transport of sodium. There is no active transport mechanism for water, which will cross the intestinal mucosa in either direction depending on the local osmotic gradients. The rate of glucose uptake is dependent on the luminal concentrations of glucose and sodium, and dilute gluco-se–electrolyte solutions with an osmolality which is slightly hypo-tonic with respect to plasma will maximize the rate of water uptake.[67] Solutions with a very high glucose concentration will not necessarily promote an increased glucose uptake relative to more dilute solutions, but, because of their high osmolality, will cause a net movement of fluid into the intestinal lumen (Fig. 3). This results in an effective loss of body water and will exacerbate any pre-existing dehydration. Other sugars, such as sucrose[68] or glucose polymers[69,70] can be substituted for glucose without impairing glu-cose or water uptake. In contrast, the absorption of fructose is not an active process in man: it is absorbed less rapidly than glucose, is not associated with sodium co-transport, and promotes less water uptake.[71]

Several studies have shown that exercise at intensities of less than about 70 per cent of $\dot{V}O_2$max has little or no effect on intestinal function, although both gastric emptying and intestinal absorption may be reduced when the exercise intensity exceeds this level.[58,72] These studies have been reviewed and summarized by Brouns et al.[73]

Some more recent results, using an isotopic tracer [^{2}H] tech-nique to follow ingested fluids, have suggested that there may be a decreased availability of ingested fluids even during low-intensity exercise: a decreased rate of appearance in the blood of a tracer for

water added to the ingested drinks indicated a decreased rate of appearance of the tracer at an exercise intensity of 40 per cent of $\dot{V}O_2$max.[74]

The factors regulating intestinal absorption of substrate, electro-lytes and water and the effects of exercise on these processes have recently been reviewed by Schedl et al.[75]

Metabolic effects of carbohydrate ingestion during exercise

Once emptied from the stomach and absorbed in the small intestine, carbohydrates ingested during exercise will enter the blood glucose pool, either directly or after metabolism in the liver. In the later stages of prolonged exercise, a fall in the circulating glucose concen-tration is commonly observed, and ingestion of glucose during exer-cise will maintain or raise the blood glucose concentration compared with the situation where no glucose is given.[76–78] Sugars other than glucose are commonly used in the formulation of sports drinks, and there is some justification for their inclusion, as similar effects are seen with short-chain length (3–10 glucosyl units) glu-cose polymers,[79–84] sucrose,[85] or mixtures of sugars.[86–88]

One of the aims of ingesting carbohydrate during exercise is to spare the limited muscle glycogen stores, as there is a good relation-ship between the availability of muscle glycogen and endurance cap-acity.[89] It is not clear how effectively this aim can be achieved, nor indeed whether sparing of muscle glycogen is necessary for ingested carbohydrate to be effective in increasing endurance capacity. It has been reported that glucose solutions providing 1 g glucose per kg body mass can reduce the rate of muscle glycogen utilization by about 30 per cent during 90 min of bicycle exercise at 65 to 70 per cent of $\dot{V}O_2$max.[78] In more prolonged (4 h) exercise consisting of low intensity cycle exercise interspersed with high intensity sprints, Hargreaves et al.[90] fed subjects hourly with either a flavoured pla-cebo or drinks containing 43 g of sucrose together with small amounts of fat and protein: the rate of muscle glycogen utilization was not different between the two trials in the first h, but over the following 3 h was about 37 per cent lower on the fed trial. Some other studies, which have employed a variety of exercise models and have fed different types and amount of carbohydrate during exer-cise, have shown no effect of carbohydrate feeding during exercise on the rate of muscle glycogen utilization.[81,84,91,92] The reason for these different results is not clear, and may be partly explained by differences in the type and amount of carbohydrate given, by the different exercise models used, and by differences in the training status of the subjects. Nutritional status may also be important, and Flynn et al.[93] found that carbohydrate feeding during exercise had no effect on the rate of muscle glycogen breakdown when this was elevated prior to exercise by a carbohydrate-loading procedure.

The ready availability of ingested carbohydrate as a fuel for the working muscles is demonstrated by the numerous studies which have followed the appearance in expired air of carbon isotopes added as tracers. Oxidation of ingested glucose can account for about half of the total carbohydrate oxidation after 1 to 2 h of walking at 50 per cent of $\dot{V}O_2$max;[94] after 3 to 4 h, ingested glucose can supply as much as 90 per cent of the total carbohydrate oxidation.[95] In this situation, there is clearly some sparing of endogenous carbohydrate, but it is not clear if the results can be applied to exercise at higher intensities, where it appears that total carbohydrate turnover is increased when exogenous carbohydrates are given.

Effects of fluid ingestion on performance

The effects of feeding different types and amounts of beverages during exercise have been extensively investigated using a wide variety of experimental models. Not all of these studies have shown a positive effect of fluid ingestion on performance, but, with the exception of a few investigations where the composition of the drinks administered was such as to result in gastrointestinal disturbances, there are no studies showing that fluid ingestion will have an adverse effect on performance.

Laboratory studies—cycling

Laboratory investigations into the ergogenic effects of the administration of carbohydrate–electrolyte drinks during exercise have usually relied upon changes in physiological function during submaximal exercise or on the exercise time to exhaustion at a fixed work rate as a measure of performance. While this is a perfectly valid approach in itself, it must be appreciated that there are difficulties in extrapolating results obtained in this way to a race situation in which the work load is likely to fluctuate as the pace, the weather conditions, and the topography vary, and where tactical considerations and motivational factors are involved. It is possible to demonstrate large differences in the time for which a fixed work load can be sustained in laboratory tests when carbohydrate solutions are given during exercise: in one study, for example, a 30 per cent increase (from 3 h to 4 h) was seen.[81] In a simulated race situation, where a fixed distance had to be covered as fast as possible, the advantage would translate to no more than a few per cent, and in a real competition it would probably be even less. Even a few per cent, however, is often the difference between a world-class performance and a mediocre one. To take account of some of these factors, some recent investigations have used exercise tests involving intermittent exercise, simulated races, or prolonged exercise followed by a sprint finish. Because different exercise tests and different solutions and rates of administration have been used in these various studies, comparisons between them are difficult. Some have included a trial where no fluids were given, whereas others have compared the effects of test solutions with trials where plain water or flavoured placebo drinks were given. These studies have been the subject of a number of extensive reviews which have concentrated on the effects of administration of carbohydrates, electrolytes, and water on exercise performance; however, the results of the individual studies will not be considered in detail here.[96–99] These studies have generally reported an improvement in performance with the ingestion of carbohydrate-containing drinks; although this does not always reach statistical significance, there are no reports of adverse effects on performance.

Ingestion of water alone or of carbohydrate-free electrolyte solutions can also improve performance. Walsh et al.[100] reported that ingestion of dilute (20 mmol/l) saline during 1 h of exercise was effective in improving performance in a subsequent ride to exhaustion at 90 per cent of $\dot{V}O_2$max compared with a trial where no fluid was given. Below et al.[101] have also shown water to be effective in

improving performance in a similar situation: they found that water and carbohydrate provision during exercise acted independently to improve performance, and the effects were found to be additive. In more prolonged exercise, water may be as effective as nutrient–electrolyte solutions in maintaining cardiovascular and thermoregulatory function:[102,103] it is clear, however, that the addition of carbohydrate can reduce the rate of decline of muscle glycogen concentration, which may be important.[104]

Laboratory studies—treadmill exercise

As with studies performed during cycling exercise many different exercise models have been used to investigate the effects of the administration of carbohydrate–electrolyte solutions during walking and running. Again, conflicting results have been obtained in that a significant effect of glucose ingestion has not always been observed. Sasaki et al.[85] found that running time at 80 per cent of $\dot{V}O_2$max was increased, compared with a placebo trial, by ingesting 90 g of sucrose in a volume of 500 ml. Macaraeg[105] reported an increased endurance time during running at 85 per cent of maximum heart rate when a 7 per cent carbohydrate–electrolyte solution was given, providing 84 g of carbohydrate in a volume of 1.2 litres, compared with either a no-drink or water-only trial. In contrast to these results, however, Fruth and Gisolfi[106] gave subjects a placebo or 150 g of glucose or fructose as a 10 per cent solution during treadmill running at 70 per cent of $\dot{V}O_2$max; running time on the fructose trial was less than on the other two runs, but there was no difference in running time between the glucose and placebo trials. Riley et al.[107] also found no difference in running time when a 7 per cent carbohydrate–electrolyte solution was given compared with a placebo trial; in this study subjects fasted for 21 h before exercise tests, and the first drink was given 20 min before exercise. In a study of very prolonged walking, Ivy et al.[108] reported an increased walking time (299 min) when 120 g of glucose polymer was given in a volume of 1.5 litres compared with a placebo trial (268 min).

Williams[109] and Williams et al.[110] have used an experimental model in which the subject is able to adjust the treadmill speed while running; the subject can then be encouraged either to cover the maximum distance possible in a fixed time or to complete a fixed distance in the fastest time possible. They showed that ingestion of 1 litre of a glucose polymer-sucrose (50 g/l) solution did not increase the total distance covered in a 2 h run, but that the running speed was greater over the last 30 min of exercise when carbohydrate was given compared with a placebo trial.[109] They observed a similar effect when a carbohydrate solution (50 g of glucose–glucose polymer, or 50 g of fructose–glucose polymer) or water was given in a 30 km treadmill time trial.[110] The running speed decreased over the last 10 km of the water trial, but was maintained in the other two runs; there was no significant difference between the three trials in the time taken to cover the total distance. As with cycling exercise, the conclusion must be that the ingestion of carbohydrate-containing drinks is generally effective in improving performance.

Field studies

There are many practical difficulties associated with the conduct of field trials to assess the efficacy of ergogenic aids, which accounts for the fact that few well-controlled studies of the effects of administration of glucose–electrolyte solutions have been carried out in this way. The main problem is with the design of an adequately controlled trial; where a cross-over design is used, this is likely to be confounded by changes in the environmental conditions between trials, and the use of parallel control and test groups raises the difficulty of matching the groups. Many of the early studies purporting to show beneficial effects of the ingestion of carbohydrate-containing solutions on performance in events such as cycling, canoeing, and soccer were so poorly designed that the results are of no value.

Cade et al.[111] gave subjects no fluids or approximately 1 litre of hypotonic saline or a glucose–electrolyte solution during a 7 mile course consisting of walking and running at an ambient temperature of 32 to 34°C. None of the subjects completed the course when no fluid was given, and the mean distance covered was 4.7 miles; when saline was given, they covered 5.5 miles and all subjects completed the 7 mile course when given the glucose–electrolyte solution.

Studies where matched groups of competitors consumed 1.4 litres of either water or a glucose–electrolyte solution during a marathon race[112] or 1.4 litres of different carbohydrate-containing drinks during marathon and ultramarathon races[92] have shown no differences between the groups in finishing time. In the study of Maughan and Whiting,[112] subjects were matched on the basis of their anticipated finishing times. Many of these individuals had not previously completed a marathon, so these times must be considered unreliable. None the less, the mean finishing time for the runners ($n=43$) drinking the carbohydrate–electrolyte solution was 220 ± 40 min compared with a predicted finishing time of 220 ± 35 min; for the group drinking water ($n=47$) actual finishing time was 217 ± 32 min and predicted time was 212 ± 32 min. In this race 24 runners (60 per cent) in the carbohydrate–electrolyte group ran faster than expected, compared with 19 (40 per cent) in those drinking water.

More recently, in a simulated road race, held over a distance of 30 km, Tsintzas et al.[113] gave runners, either a commercially formulated 5 per cent carbohydrate solution or plain water and found an improved (by a mean of 2.9 min) performance for the carbohydrate-solution group (difference in performance was statistically significant).

Other exercise models

Performance is more difficult to assess in complex tasks, such as those involved in most sports, but the assumption is that an improved exercise tolerance will lead to an improved playing performance in most games. Because of the difficulties in assessing performance, there is relatively little information on the effects of dehydration and rehydration on performance in complex tasks. Leatt[114] gave 1 litre of a 7 per cent glucose polymer solution or a flavoured placebo to football (soccer) players during a practice game. During the match, the group who had been given carbohydrate utilized 31 per cent less glycogen than the placebo group. No measure of performance of the two groups was made, but it was proposed that a beneficial effect would be experienced in the later stages of the game by the players taking the glucose polymer. Nicholas et al.[115] simulated the running pattern of ball games using an intermittent high-intensity shuttle-running test: ingestion of a carbohydrate–electrolyte drink was effective in improving performance compared with a trial where a non-carbohydrate placebo was given.

Practical issues in fluid replacement during exercise

Many factors affect the need for fluid replacement during exercise. The composition of the fluid, as well as the volume and frequency of drinks, that will confer the greatest benefit during exercise will depend very much on individual circumstances. As with most physiological variables, there is a large interindividual variability in the rates of fluid loss during exercise under standardized conditions and also in the rates of gastric emptying and intestinal absorption of any ingested beverage. Marathon runners competing under the same conditions and finishing in the same time may lose as little as 1 per cent or as much as 5 per cent of body mass, even though their fluid intake during the race is the same.[3] Under more controlled conditions, Greenhaff and Clough[116] found that sweat rate during 1 h of exercise at a work load of 70 per cent $\dot{V}O_2$max and an ambient temperature of 23°C ranged from 426 to 1665 g/h. It would seem logical that the need for fluid (water) replacement is greater in the individual who sweats profusely; thus any guidelines as to the rate of fluid ingestion and the composition of fluids to be taken must be viewed with caution when applied to the individual athlete. Sweat rate in activities such as running can be predicted from estimates of the energy cost of running, as used by Barr and Costill,[117] but these do not explain the variation which is observed between individuals. A more reliable method might be for the individual to measure body mass before and after training, or simulated competition and to estimate sweat loss from the change in body mass.

Many individuals and organizations have issued recommendations as to the most appropriate fluid replacement regimens.[57,118–120] Olsson and Saltin[118] recommended 100 to 300 ml of a 5 to 10 per cent sugar solution every 10 to 15 min during exercise; they also suggested that the temperature of ingested fluids should be 25°C. At the extreme ends of this range, this would give an intake each h of 400 to 1800 ml of liquid and 20 to 180 g of sugar. In 1975 the American College of Sports Medicine published a Position Statement on the prevention of heat injuries during distance running, in which an intake of 400 to 500 ml of fluid 10 to 15 min before exercise was recommended:[119] although no figures were given, it was also suggested that runners ingest fluids frequently during competition and that the sugar and electrolyte content of drinks should be low (2.5 per cent and 10 mmol/l sodium respectively) so as not to delay gastric emptying. A revised version of these guidelines continued to recommend hyperhydration prior to exercise by the ingestion of 400 to 600 ml of cold water 15 to 20 min before the event.[57] The recommendations as to intake during a race were more specific than previously: cool water was stated to be the optimum fluid, and an intake of 100 to 200 ml every 2 to 3 km was suggested, giving a total intake of 1400 to 4200 ml at the extremes. Again, taking these extreme values, it is unlikely that the élite runners could tolerate a rate of intake of about 2 l/h, and equally unlikely that an intake of 300 ml/h would be adequate for the slowest competitors except when the ambient temperature was low. A recent revision of the guidelines now recommends pre-exercise consumption of about 400 to 600 ml of water about 2 h before exercise, thus allowing time for the excretion of excess ingested water.[120] The recommendations for fluid intake during exercise are no longer given as absolute values, but rather it is stated that athletes should attempt to match their fluid losses during exercise, or, if this is not possible, they should consume the maximum amounts that can be tolerated. The fluids consumed should be cooler than ambient temperature and be flavoured to promote consumption. For events of less than 1 h duration, plain water should be sufficient, but for events of longer duration, carbohydrate ingestion at a rate of 30 to 60 g/h and sodium at a concentration of 22 to 30 mmol/l should be included.

Exercise intensity and duration

The rate of metabolic heat production during exercise is dependent on the exercise intensity and body mass; in activities such as running or cycling this is a direct function of speed. Although there do seem to be some differences between individuals in the energy cost of running at a fixed speed, the significance, if any, of these apparent differences in mechanical efficiency is not clear.[121] The rate of the rise in body temperature during the early stages of exercise and the steady-state level which is eventually reached are both proportional to the metabolic rate. The rate of sweat production is therefore also closely related to the absolute work load. In many sports, including most ball games, short bursts of high-intensity activity are separated by variable periods of rest or low-intensity exercise, and the sweating rate is likely to be a function of the mean power output.

The time for which high-intensity exercise can be sustained is necessarily rather short; the factors limiting exercise performance where the duration is in the range of about 10 to 60 min are not clear, but is does seem that substrate availability is not normally a limiting factor and that performance will not be improved by the ingestion of carbohydrate-containing beverages during exercise. Also, even though the sweat rate may be high, the total amount of water lost by sweating is likely to be rather small. Accordingly there is generally no need for fluid replacement during very high-intensity exercise, although it is difficult to define a precise cut-off point. In one study, however, the effects of an intravenous infusion of saline during cycle ergometer exercise to exhaustion at an exercise intensity equivalent to 84 per cent of $\dot{V}O_2$max were investigated.[122] In the control trial a negligible amount of saline was infused, whereas an infusion rate of about 70 ml/min was used in the other trial. The saline infusion was effective in reducing the decrease in plasma volume which occurred during the initial stages of exercise, although it did not completely abolish this response, and the core temperature and heart rate at the point of exhaustion were both lower in the infusion trial. There was no effect on endurance time which was the same in both trials. The endurance times were, however, short (20.8 and 22.0 min for the infusion and control trials, respectively), although the range was large (from about 9 to 43 min), and these results support the idea that fluid provision will not benefit exercise performance when the exercise duration is short.

There are also likely to be real problems associated with any attempt to replace fluids orally during very intense exercise. The rate of gastric emptying, which is probably the most important factor in determining the fate of ingested fluid, is impaired when the exercise intensity is high, as described above. Even at rest, the maximum rates of gastric emptying which have been reported are only about half the saline infusion rate (70 ml/min) used in the study of Deschamps et al.[122] and are commonly much less than this. To achieve a high rate of fluid delivery from the stomach, it is necessary to ingest large volumes, and any attempt to do so when the exercise intensity exceeds about 80 per cent of $\dot{V}O_2$max would almost certainly result in nausea and vomiting.

At lower exercise intensities, the duration of exercise is inversely related to the intensity. In an activity such as running, this holds true for populations as much as for individuals. As the distance of a race increases, so the pace that an individual can sustain decreases;[123] equally, in an event such as a marathon race where all runners complete the same distance, the slower runners are generally exercising at a lower relative (as a percentage of $\dot{V}O_2$max) and absolute work intensity.[124] Because the faster runners are exercising at a higher work load, in absolute as well as in relative terms, their sweat rate is higher, although this effect is offset to some extent by the fact that they generally have a lower body mass—because the faster runners are active for a shorter period of time; however, the total sweat loss during a marathon race is unrelated to finishing time.[3] The need for fluid replacement is therefore much the same, irrespective of running speed, in terms of the total volume required, but there is a need for a higher rate of replacement in the faster runners. Among the fastest marathon runners, sweat rates of about 30 to 35 ml/min can be sustained for a period of about 2 h 15 min by some runners. The highest sustained rates of gastric emptying reported in the literature are greater than this, at about 40 ml/min.[58,125] These gastric emptying measurements were made on resting subjects, and it is possible that there may be some inhibition of gastric emptying at the exercise intensity (about 75 per cent of $\dot{V}O_2$max) at which these elite athletes are running.[58] In the slower runners, the exercise intensity does not exceed 60 per cent of $\dot{V}O_2$max, and gastrointestinal function is unlikely to be impaired relative to rest.[49,87] In these runners, sweat rates will also be relatively low.[3]

Although in theory, therefore, it should be possible to meet the fluid loss by oral intake, gastric emptying rates of fluids are commonly much lower than the maximum figures quoted above, and it is inevitable that most individuals exercising hard, particularly in the heat, will incur a fluid deficit.

Composition of drinks

The American College of Sports Medicine's 1996 Position Stand on exercise and fluid replacement no longer recommends that plain water is the optimum fluid for ingestion during endurance exercise,[120] taking into account some of the evidence presented above indicating that there may be good reasons for taking drinks containing added substrate and electrolytes. In prolonged exercise, performance is improved by the addition of an energy source in the form of carbohydrate; the type of carbohydrate does not appear to be critical, and glucose, sucrose and oligosaccharides have all been shown to be effective in improving endurance capacity. Some studies have suggested that long chain glucose polymer solutions are more readily used by the muscles during exercise than are glucose or fructose solutions,[126] but others have found no difference in the oxidation rates of ingested glucose or glucose polymer.[51,127] Massicote et al.[127] also found that ingested fructose was less readily oxidized than glucose or glucose polymers. Fructose in high concentrations is best avoided because of the risk of gastrointestinal upset. The argument advanced in favour of the ingestion of fructose during exercise, namely that it provides a readily available energy source but does not stimulate insulin release and the consequent inhibition of fatty acid mobilization, is in any case not well founded: insulin secretion is suppressed during exercise.

The optimum concentration of sugar to be added to drinks will depend on individual circumstances. High carbohydrate concentrations will delay gastric emptying, thus reducing the amount of fluid available for absorption: very high concentrations will result in the secretion of water into the intestine and thus actually increase the danger of dehydration. High sugar concentrations (>10 per cent) may also result in gastrointestinal disturbances. Where there is a need to supply an energy source during exercise, however, increasing the sugar content of drinks will increase the delivery of carbohydrate to the site of absorption in the small intestine. As the carbohydrate concentration increases, the volume emptied from the stomach is reduced but the amount of carbohydrate emptied is increased.

The available evidence indicates that the only electrolyte that should be added to drinks consumed during exercise is sodium, which is usually added in the form of sodium chloride. Sodium will stimulate sugar and water uptake in the small intestine and will help to maintain extracellular fluid volume. Most soft drinks of the cola or lemonade variety contain virtually no sodium (1–2 mmol/l); sports drinks commonly contain 10 to 25 mmol/l; oral rehydration solutions intended for use in the treatment of diarrhoea-induced dehydration, which may be fatal, have higher sodium concentrations, in the range 30 to 90 mmol/l. A high sodium content, although it may stimulate jejunal absorption of glucose and water, tends to make drinks unpalatable, and it is important that drinks intended for ingestion during or after exercise should have a pleasant taste in order to stimulate consumption. Specialist sports drinks are generally formulated to strike a balance between the twin aims of efficacy and palatability, although it must be admitted that not all achieve either of these aims.

When the exercise duration is likely to exceed 3 to 4 h, there may be advantages in adding sodium to drinks to avoid the danger of hyponatraemia, which has been reported to occur when excessively large volumes of low sodium drinks are taken. It has often been reported that the fluid intakes of participants in endurance events are low, and it is recognized that this may lead to dehydration and heat illness in prolonged exercise when the ambient temperature is high. Accordingly, the advice frequently given to participants in endurance events is that they should ensure a high fluid intake to minimize the effects of dehydration. Most carbohydrate–electrolyte drinks intended for consumption during prolonged exercise also have a low electrolyte content, with sodium and chloride concentrations typically between 10 and 20 mmol/l. While this might represent a reasonable strategy for providing substrates and water (although it can be argued that a higher sodium concentration would enhance water uptake and that a higher carbohydrate content would increase substrate provision), these recommendations may not be appropriate in all circumstances.

Physicians dealing with individuals in distress at the end of long-distance races have become accustomed to dealing with hyperthermia associated with dehydration and hypernatraemia, but it has become clear that a small number of individuals at the end of very prolonged events may be suffering from hyponatraemia in conjunction with either hyperhydration[5,128–130] or dehydration.[131]

All the reported cases have been associated with ultramarathon or prolonged triathlon events; most of the cases have occurred in events lasting in excess of 8 h, and there are few reports of cases where the exercise duration is less than 4 h. Noakes et al.[128] reported four cases of exercise-induced hyponatraemia; race times were between 7 and 10 h, and post-race serum sodium concentrations were between 115 and 125 mmol/l. Estimated fluid intakes were between 6 and 12 litres, and consisted of water or drinks containing low levels of electrolytes; estimated total sodium chloride intake during the race was 20 to 40 mmol. Frizell et al.[130] reported even more astonishing fluid intakes of 20 to 24 litres of fluids (an intake of almost 2.5 l/h sustained for a period of many h, which is in excess of the maximum gastric emptying rate that has been reported) with a mean sodium content of only 5 to 10 mmol/l in two runners who collapsed after an ultramarathon run and who were found to be hyponatraemic (serum sodium concentration 118–123 mmol/l). Hyponatraemia as a consequence of ingestion of large volumes of fluids with a low sodium content has also been recognized in resting individuals. Flear et al.[132] reported the case of a man who drank 9 litres of beer, with a sodium content of 1.5 mmol/l, in the space of 20 min; plasma sodium fell from 143 mmol/l before to 127 mmol/l after drinking, but the man appeared unaffected. In these cases, there is clearly a replacement of water in excess of losses with inadequate electrolyte replacement. Noakes[133,134] has suggested that in situations such as this, a significant amount of sodium may move into the volume of unabsorbed fluid in the intestinal lumen, thus resulting in hyponatraemia. In competitors in the Hawaii Ironman Triathlon who have been found to be hyponatraemic, however, dehydration has also been reported to be present.[131] Fellmann et al.[135] reported a small but statistically significant fall in serum sodium concentration, from 141 to 137 mmol/l, in runners who completed a 24-h run, but food and fluid intakes were neither controlled nor measured.

These reports are interesting and indicate that some supplementation with sodium chloride may be required in extremely prolonged events where large sweat losses can be expected and where it is possible to consume large volumes of fluid. The recently revised recommendations of the American College of Sports Medicine,[120] do now encourage drinks to have a sodium concentration of 22 to 30 mmol/l for longer duration events. This should not, however, divert attention away from the fact that electrolyte replacement during exercise is not a priority for most participants in most sporting events, nor from the fact that most collapsed runners will be found to be hypernatraemic. Where immediate verification of a collapsed athlete's serum sodium concentration is not possible, it is probably safer to assume that this will be elevated and that intravenous fluid replacement may be warranted.

Sodium is also necessary for post-event rehydration, which may be particularly important when the exercise has to be repeated within a few hours: if drinks containing little or no sodium are taken, plasma osmolality will fall, urine production will be stimulated and most of the fluid will not be retained. When a longer time interval between exercise sessions is possible, replacement of sodium and other electrolytes will normally be achieved as a result of intake from the diet without additional supplementation. Post-exercise rehydration and restoration of electrolyte balance are discussed in more detail below.

It is often stated that there is an advantage to taking chilled (4°C) drinks as this accelerates gastric emptying and thus improves the availability of ingested fluids. The most recent evidence (which is quoted above) however, suggests that the gastric emptying rate of hot and cold beverages is not markedly different. In spite of this, there may be advantages in taking cold drinks, as the palatability of most carbohydrate–electrolyte drinks is improved at low temperatures.

Consumption of caffeine seems to exert some diuretic influence when consumed over a prolonged period of rest and it may be thought that caffeine would have negative effects on fluid balance status during exercise. However, this does not seem to be the case when caffeine-containing drinks are consumed during prolonged, moderate-intensity cycle exercise in a warm environment.[136] Also, the same authors reported that there was no effect of the caffeine-containing drinks on heart rate and sweat rate, rectal temperature or plasma volume changes during a period of exercise.[137]

Environmental conditions

The ambient temperature and wind speed will have a major influence on the physical exchange of heat between the body and the environment. When ambient temperature exceeds skin temperature, heat is gained from the environment by physical transfer, leaving evaporative loss as the only mechanism available to prevent or limit a rise in body temperature. The increased sweating rate in the heat will result in an increased requirement for fluid replacement. Other precautions such as limiting the extent of the warm-up prior to competition and reducing the amount of clothing worn will help to reduce the sweat loss and hence reduce the need for replacement. For endurance events at high ambient temperatures, there may also be a need to reduce the exercise intensity if the event is to be successfully completed.

When the humidity is high, and especially in the absence of wind, evaporative heat loss will also be severely limited. In this situation, exercise tolerance is likely to be limited by dehydration and hyperthermia rather than by the limited availability of metabolic fuel. Suzuki[138] reported that exercise time at a work load of 66 per cent $\dot{V}O_2$max was reduced from 91 min when the ambient temperature was 0°C to 19 min when the same exercise was performed in the heat (40°C). In an unpublished study in which 6 subjects exercised to exhaustion at 70 per cent $\dot{V}O_2$max on a cycle ergometer, we found that exercise time was reduced from 73 min at an ambient temperature of 2°C to 35 min at a temperature of 33°C. Exercise time in the cold was increased by ingesting a dilute glucose–electrolyte solution, but in the heat, the exercise duration was too short for fluid intake to have any effect on performance.

More recently, it has been shown that there is clearly an optimum temperature for the performance of prolonged exercise: Galloway and Maughan[2] measured time to exhaustion in subjects exercising on a cycle ergometer at a power output that required approximately 70 per cent $\dot{V}O_2$max, and found that the exercise time at an ambient temperature of 11°C was longer than was the case when the ambient temperature was either higher or lower (Fig. 4). Although fatigue at these work intensities is generally considered to result from depletion of the muscle glycogen stores, this is clearly not the case when the ambient temperature is high: the rate of carbohydrate oxidation was not different during exercise at different ambient temperatures.

From these studies, we can conclude that the supply of water should take precedence over the provision of substrate during exer-

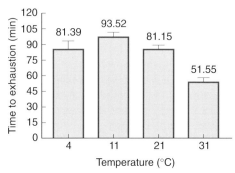

Fig. 4 Exercise time to exhaustion during cycle exercise at a power output requiring approximately 70 per cent of $\dot{V}O_2$max at different ambient temperatures. Exercise time at 11°C was significantly longer than at all other temperatures, and exercise time at 31°C was significantly shorter than at all other temperatures.

cise in the heat. There may therefore be some advantage in reducing the sugar content of drinks, to perhaps 2 to 5 per cent, and in increasing the sodium content, to something in the range 30 to 50 mmol/l. Conversely, when exercise is undertaken in the cold, fluid loss is less of a problem, and the energy content of drinks might usefully be increased.

State of training and acclimation

It is well recognized that both training and acclimation will confer some protection against the development of heat illness during exercise in the heat. Although this adaption is most marked in response to training carried out in the heat,[139] endurance training at moderate environmental conditions will also confer some benefit. Among the benefits of training is an expansion of the plasma volume.[140] Although this condition is recognized as a chronic state in the endurance trained individual, an acute expansion of plasma volume occurs in response to a single bout of strenuous exercise: this effect is apparent within a few h of completion of exercise and may persist for several days.[141,142] This post-exercise hypervolaemia should be regarded as an acute response rather than an adaptation, although it may appear to be one of the first responses to occur when an individual embarks on a training regimen. Circulating electrolyte and total protein concentrations are normal in the endurance-trained individual in spite of the enlarged vascular and extracellular spaces, indicating an increased total circulating content.[143]

The increased resting plasma volume in the trained state allows the endurance trained individual to maintain a higher total blood volume during exercise,[144] allowing for better maintenance of cardiac output, albeit at the cost of a lower circulating haemoglobin concentration. In addition, the increased plasma volume is associated with an increased sweating rate which limits the rise in body temperature.[145] These adaptive responses appear to occur within a few days of exposure to exercise in the heat, although, as pointed out above, this may not necessarily be a true adaptation. In a series of papers reporting the same study, Mitchell et al.,[145] Wyndham et al.,[146] and Senay et al.[147] followed the time course of changes in men exposed to exercise (40–50 per cent $\dot{V}O_2$max for 4 h) in the heat (45°C) for 10 days. Although there were marked differences between individuals in their responses, resting plasma volume increased progressively over the first 6 days, reaching a value about 23 per cent greater than the control, with little change thereafter. The main adaptation in terms of an increased sweating rate and an improved thermoregulatory response (with body temperature lower by 1°C and heart rate lower by 30 beats/min in the later stages of exercise) occurred slightly later than the cardiovascular adaptations, with little change during the first 4 days.

Although there is clear evidence that acclimation by exercise in the heat over a period of several days will improve the thermoregulatory response during exercise, this does not affect the need to replace fluids during the exercise period. Better maintenance of body temperature is achieved at the expense of an increased sweat loss. Although this allows for a greater evaporative heat loss, the proportion of the sweat which is not evaporated and which therefore drips wastefully from the skin is also increased.[145] A high sweat rate may be necessary to ensure adequate evaporative heat loss, but it does seem that many individuals have an inefficient sweating mechanism: even in the unacclimated state their rate of sweat secretion appears to greatly exceed the maximum evaporative capacity. The athlete who trains in a moderate climate for a competition to be held in the heat will, however, be at a disadvantage because of his inability to sustain a high sweat rate.

Post-exercise rehydration

Replacement of water and electrolyte losses during the post-exercise period may be of crucial importance when repeated bouts of exercise have to be performed; the ingestion of carbohydrate at this time is also important when the exercise has resulted in a significant reduction in the body's liver and muscle glycogen stores. The need for replacement will obviously depend on the extent of the losses incurred during exercise, but it will also be influenced by the time and nature of subsequent exercise bouts. Rapid rehydration may also be important in events such as wrestling, boxing, and weightlifting where competition is by weight category: competitors in these events frequently undergo acute thermal and exercise-induced dehydration to make the weight. The practice of acute dehydration to make weight should be discouraged, as it reduces exercise performance even when some restoration of the deficit is achieved[148] and increases the risk of heat illness,[149–151] but it will persist and hence there is a need to maximize rehydration in the time available.

In an early study where a dehydration of 4 per cent of body mass was induced in resting subjects by heat exposure, consumption over a 3 h period of a volume of fluid equal to that lost did not restore plasma volume or serum osmolality within 4 h.[152] Ingestion of a glucose–electrolyte solution, however, did result in greater restoration of plasma volume than did plain water: this was accompanied by a greater urine production in the water trial. Where the electrolyte content of drinks is the same it appears that the addition of carbohydrate (100 g/l) or carbonation has no effect on the restoration of plasma volume over a 4 h period after sweat loss corresponding to approximately 4 per cent of body mass.[64] Gonzalez-Alonso et al.[153] have shown that a dilute carbohydrate–electrolyte solution (60 g/l carbohydrate, 20 mmol/l Na+, 3 mmol K+) is more effective in promoting post-exercise rehydration than either plain water or a low–electrolyte diet cola—the difference between the drinks was primarily a result of differences in the volume of urine produced and there was a suggestion in this study that the caffeine content of the diet cola may have exerted a negative effect because of its potential diuretic properties.

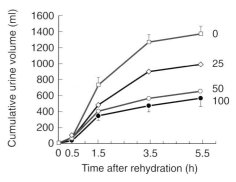

Fig. 5 Cumulative urine output after dehydration (equivalent to 2 per cent of body mass) induced by exercise in the heat followed by ingestion of a fixed volume (equal to 3 per cent of body mass) of fluid containing 0 to 100 mmol/l sodium. (Reproduced from ref. 156, with permission.)

Ingestion of plain water in the post-exercise period results in a rapid fall in the plasma sodium concentration and in plasma osmolality.[154] These changes have the effect of reducing the stimulus to drink (thirst) and of stimulating urine output, both of which will delay the rehydration process. In the study of Nose et al.,[154] subjects exercised at low intensity in the heat for 90 to 110 min, inducing a mean dehydration of 2.3 per cent of body mass, and then rested for 1 h before beginning to drink. Plasma volume was not restored until after 60 min when plain water was ingested together with placebo (sucrose) capsules. In contrast, when sodium chloride capsules were ingested with water (without sucrose) to give a saline solution with an effective concentration of 0.45 per cent (77 mmol/l), plasma volume was restored within 20 min. In the NaCl trial, voluntary fluid intake was higher and urine output was less; 71 per cent of the water loss with dehydration was retained within 3 h compared with 51 per cent in the plain water trial. The delayed rehydration in the water trial appeared to be a result of a loss of sodium, accompanied by water, in the urine caused by depressed plasma renin activity and aldosterone levels.[155]

More recently, a systematic evaluation of the effects of replacing a fixed volume of fluid with different sodium concentrations has been reported.[156] In this study, subjects were dehydrated by intermittent exercise in the heat until 2 per cent of body mass was lost; they then consumed a volume of fluid equivalent to 1.5 times the sweat loss: these drinks contained 0, 25, 50, or 100 mmol/l sodium. Urine output over the next few hours was inversely related to the sodium content of the ingested fluid (Fig. 5).

It is clear from the results of these studies that rehydration after exercise can only be achieved if the sodium lost in sweat is replaced as well as the water, and it might be suggested that rehydration drinks should have a sodium concentration similar to that of sweat. Since the sodium content of sweat varies widely, no single formulation will meet this requirement for all individuals in all situations. The upper end of the normal range for sodium concentration (80 mmol/l), however, is similar to the sodium concentration of many commercially produced oral rehydration solutions (**ORS**) intended for use in the treatment of diarrhoea-induced dehydration, and some of these are not unpalatable. The ORS recommended by the World Health Organization for rehydration in cases of severe diarrhoea has a sodium content of 90 mmol/l. By contrast, the sodium content of most sports drinks is in the range of 10 to

25 mmol/l and is even lower in some cases; most commonly consumed soft drinks contain virtually no sodium. In terms of maintaining the drive to drink it has recently been shown that drinks containing sodium at moderate concentrations (25 mmol/l) are more effective than either plain water, which removes the osmotic stimulus for thirst or a 50 mmol/l sodium drink which removes the volume-dependent dipsogenic stimuli.[137]

The requirement for sodium replacement stems from its role as the major ion in the extracellular fluid. It has been speculated that inclusion of potassium, the major cation in the intracellular space, would enhance the replacement of intracellular water after exercise and thus promote rehydration.[157] It appears that inclusion of potassium may be as effective as sodium in retaining water ingested after exercise-induced dehydration, in spite of the rather low levels of potassium lost in sweat. The addition of either ion will significantly increase the fraction of the ingested fluid which is retained, but, when the volume of fluid ingested is equal to that lost during the exercise period, there is no additive effect of including both ions as would be expected if they acted independently on different body fluid compartments.[158] This effect may, however, be a result of the rather small volume of fluid ingested, and the difficulty in further reducing the urine output; to achieve an effective rehydration not only should the composition of the fluid be considered, but rather the volume ingested should be more than the sweat volume lost if hydration status is to be restored.[159] The ingestion of the necessary electrolytes need not come from the beverage itself, however, and if solid food is consumed together with an adequate fluid volume (for instance, with water or a soft drink), effective rehydration can ensue.[160]

Some degree of temporary hyperhydration appears to result when drinks with high (100 mmol/l) sodium concentrations are ingested. An alternative strategy which has been attempted with the aim of inducing an expansion of the blood volume prior to exercise is to add glycerol to ingested fluids. Glycerol exerts an osmotic effect; its mechanism of action seems to be due to the increased plasma osmolality raising vasopressin levels with a concomitant reduction in urine flow rate and free water clearance, together with a direct effect of increasing the osmotic concentration gradient in the kidney medulla, therefore resulting in increased water reabsorption.[161] It seems that the glycerol is evenly distributed between the body's major fluid compartments: fluid ingested with the glycerol equilibrates between the intracellular and extracellular fluid compartments.[162] The elevated osmolality of the extracellular space may, however, result in some degree of intracellular dehydration, the implications of which are unknown.[163] It might be expected that the raised plasma osmolality may have negative consequences for thermoregulatory capacity,[164] although the available evidence at present seems to indicate that this is not the case.[165,166] Glycerol feeding before or during exercise has been shown not to improve the capacity to perform prolonged exercise.[163,167] In contrast to these earlier papers, however, there have been some recent suggestions of improved performance after the administration of glycerol and water prior to prolonged exercise.[165]

Conclusions

During exercise in warm or hot environments, body temperature will rise and losses of water and electrolytes, in the form of sweat, will be incurred. Both hyperthermia and dehydration are known to impair exercise performance, but their effects can be limited by appropriate fluid intake. Fluid ingestion is aimed at supplying a source of energy, usually in the form of carbohydrate, as well as helping to maintain hydration status. Drinks that have been shown to be most effective usually contain carbohydrate (at a concentration of 2–10 per cent) and sodium (typically at about 20–25 mmol/l), but the optimum formulation is likely to depend on the duration and intensity of the event, the environmental conditions, and the characteristics of the individual. As well as being effective in improving performance, drinks should be palatable to encourage consumption, as athletes generally fail to consume an adequate volume of fluid.

There is a need to ensure that exercise does not begin with the individual in a state of hypohydration: the kidneys, however, are generally effective in preventing an increase in the normal body water content. After exercise, replacement of the body's carbohydrate stores and restoration of fluid balance are essential parts of the recovery process. Failure to ensure this will impair performance in subsequent exercise bouts. Fluids should be ingested in a volume in excess of the sweat loss, and should contain sufficient sodium to replace that lost in sweat if recovery time before the next exercise session is limited and no solid food is to be consumed.

References

1. Hargreaves M. Carbohydrates and exercise. *Journal of Sports Sciences* 1991; **9** (Special Issue): 17–28.
2. Galloway SDR, Maughan RJ. Effects of ambient temperature on the capacity to perform prolonged cycle exercise in man. *Medicine and Science in Sports and Exercise* 1997; **29**: 1240–9.
3. Maughan RJ. Thermoregulation and fluid balance in marathon competition at low ambient temperature. *International Journal of Sports Medicine* 1985; **6**: 15–19.
4. Mitchell JW, Nadel ER, Stolwijk JAJ. Respiratory weight losses during exercise. *Journal of Applied Physiology* 1972; **34**: 474–6.
5. Saltin B, Costill DL. Fluid and electrolyte balance during prolonged exercise. In Horton ES, Terjung RL, eds. *Exercise, nutrition, and metabolism.* New York: Macmillan, 1988: 150–8.
6. Nielsen B, Kubica R, Bonnesen A, Rasmussen IB, Stoklosa J, Wilk B. Physical work capacity after dehydration and hyperthermia. *Scandinavian Journal of Sports Sciences* 1981; **3**: 2–10.
7. Armstrong LE, Costill DL, Fink WJ. Influence of diuretic-induced dehydration on competitive running performance. *Medicine and Science in Sports and Exercise* 1985; **17**: 456–61.
8. Nadel ER. Circulatory and thermal regulations during exercise. *Federation Proceedings* 1980; **39**: 1491–7.
9. Rowell LB. *Human circulation.* New York: Oxford University Press, 1986.
10. Montain SJ, Coyle EF. Influence of graded dehydration on hyperthermia and cardiovascular drift during exercise. *Journal of Applied Physiology* 1992; **73**: 1340–50.
11. Montain SJ, Coyle EF. Fluid ingestion during exercise increases skin blood flow independent of increases in blood volume. *Journal of Applied Physiology* 1992; **73**: 903–10.
12. Riebe D, Maresh CM, Armstrong LA, *et al.* Effects of oral and intravenous rehydration on ratings of perceived exertion and thirst. *Medicine and Science in Sports and Exercise* 1997; **29**: 117–24.
13. Pitts RF. *The physiological basis of diuretic therapy.* Springfield: CC Thomas, 1959.
14. Lentner C, ed. *Geigy Scientific Tables.* 8th edn. Basle: Ciba-Geigy Limited, 1981.

15. Schmidt RF, Thews G, eds. *Human physiology*. 2nd edn. Berlin: Springer-Verlag, 1989.

16. Leithead CS, Lind AR. *Heat stress and heat disorders*. London: Casell, 1964.

17. Costill DL. Sweating: its composition and effects on body fluids. *Annals of the New York Academy of Sciences* 1977; **301**: 160–74.

18. Verde T, RJ Shephard, P Corey, R Moore. Sweat composition in exercise and in heat. *Journal of Applied Physiology* 1982; **53**: 1540–5.

19. Allan JR, Wilson CG. Influence of acclimatization on sweat sodium secretion. *Journal of Applied Physiology* 1971; **30**: 708–712.

20. Kobayashi Y, Ando Y, Takeuchi S, Takemura K, Okuda N. Effects of heat acclimation of distance runners in a moderately hot environment. *European Journal of Applied Physiology*. 1980; **45**: 189–98.

21. Costa F, Calloway DH, Margen S. Regional and total body sweat composition of men fed controlled diets. *American Journal of Clinical Nutrition* 1969; **22**: 52–8.

22. Mickelsen O, Keys A. The composition of sweat, with special reference to the vitamins. *Journal of Biological Chemistry* 1943; **149**: 470–90.

23. van Heyningen R, Weiner JS. A comparison of arm-bag sweat and body sweat. *Journal of Physiology* 1952; **116**: 395–403.

24. Greenleaf JE, Castle BL, Card DH. Blood electrolytes and temperature regulation during exercise in man. *Acta Physiologica Polonica* 1974; **25**: 397–410.

25. Harrison MH, Edwards RJ, Fennessy PA. Intravascular volume and tonicity as factors in the regulation of body temperature. *Journal of Applied Physiology* 1978; **44**: 69–75.

26. Fortney SM, Wenger CB, Bove JR, Nadel ER. Effect of hyperosmolality on control of blood flow and sweating. *Journal of Applied Physiology* 1984; **57**: 1688–95.

27. Fortney SM, Vroman NB, Beckett WS, Permutt S, LaFrance ND. Effect of exercise hemoconcentration and hyperosmolality on exercise responses. *Journal of Applied Physiology* 1988; **65**: 519–24.

28. Meytes I, Shapiro Y, Magazanik A, Meytes D, Seligsohn U. Physiological and biochemical changes during a marathon race. *International Journal of Biometeorology* 1969; **13**: 317.

29. Whiting PH, Maughan RJ, Miller JDB. Dehydration and serum biochemical changes in runners. *European Journal of Applied Physiology* 1984; **52**: 183–7.

30. Kavanagh T, Shephard RJ. Maintenance of hydration in 'post-coronary' marathon runners. *British Journal of Sports Medicine* 1975; **9**: 130–5.

31. Costill DL, Branam G, Fink W, Nelson R. Exercise induced sodium conservation: changes in plasma renin and aldosterone. *Medicine and Science in Sports and Exercise* 1976; **8**: 209–13.

32. Cohen I, Zimmerman AL. Changes in serum electrolyte levels during marathon running. *South African Medical Journal* 1978; **53**: 449–53.

33. Stansbie D, Tomlinson K, Potman JM, Walters EG. Hypothermia, hypokalaemia and marathon running. *Lancet* 1982; **ii**: 1336.

34. Joborn H, Åkerström G, Ljunghall S. Effects of exogenous catecholamines and exercise on plasma magnesium concentrations. *Clinical Endocrinology* 1985; **23**: 219–26.

35. Rose LI, Carroll DR, Lowe SL, Peterson EW, Cooper KH. Serum electrolyte changes after marathon running. *Journal of Applied Physiology* 1970; **29**: 449–51.

36. Beller GA, Maher JT, Hartley LH, Bass DE, Wacker WEC. Serum Mg and K concentrations during exercise in thermoneutral and hot conditions. *The Physiologist* 1972; **15**: 94.

37. Refsum HE, Meen HD, Stromme SB. Whole blood, serum and erythrocyte magnesium concentrations after repeated heavy exercise of long duration. *Scandinavian Journal of Clinical and Laboratory Investigation* 1973; **32**: 123–7.

38. Lijnen P, Hespel P, Fagard R, Lysens R, Vanden Eynde E, Amery A. Erythrocyte, plasma and urinary magnesium in men before and after a marathon. *European Journal of Applied Physiology* 1988; **58**: 252–6.

39. Costill DL, Miller JM. Nutrition for endurance sport. *International Journal of Sports Medicine* 1980; **1**: 2–14.

40. Brouns F, Saris WHM, Schneider H. Rationale for upper limits of electrolyte replacement during exercise. *International Journal of Sport Nutrition* 1992; **2**: 229–38.

41. Meyer F, Bar-Or O, MacDougall D, Heigenhauser GJF. Sweat electrolyte loss during exercise in the heat: effects of gender and maturation. *Medicine and Science in Sports and Exercise* 1992; **24**: 776–81.

42. Bar-Or O. Temperature regulation during exercise in children and adolescents. In: Gisolfi CV, DR Lamb, eds. *Perspectives in exercise science and sports medicine*. Vol 2: Youth, exercise, and sport. Indianapolis: Benchmark Press, 1989: 335–62.

43. Castenfors J. Renal function during prolonged exercise. *Annals of the New York Academy of Sciences* 1977; **301**: 151–9.

44. Wade CE, Claybaugh JR. Plasma renin activity, vasopressin concentration and urinary excretory responses to exercise in men. *Journal of Applied Physiology* 1980; **49**: 930–6.

45. Poortmans J. Exercise and renal function. *Sports Medicine* 1984; **1**: 125–53.

46. Zambraski EJ. Renal regulation of fluid homeostasis during exercise. In: Gisolfi CV, Lamb DR, eds. *Perspectives in exercise science and sports medicine*. Volume 3: Fluid homeostasis during exercise. Carmel, IN: Benchmark Press, 1990: 247–80.

47. Vist GE, Maughan RJ. The effect of osmolality and carbohydrate content on the rate of gastric emptying of liquids in man. *Journal of Physiology* 1995; **486**: 523–31.

48. Leiper JB, Maughan RJ. Experimental models for the investigation of water and solute transport in man: implications for oral rehydration solutions. *Drugs* 1988; **36** Suppl 4: 65–79.

49. Rehrer NJ, Beckers E, Brouns F, Ten Hoor F, Saris WHM. Exercise and training effects on gastric emptying of carbohydrate beverages. *Medicine and Science in Sports and Exercise* 1989; **21**: 540–9.

50. Rehrer NJ, Janssen GME, Brouns F, Saris WHM. Fluid intake and gastrointestinal problems in runners competing in a 25-km race and a marathon. *International Journal of Sports Medicine* 1989; **10** Suppl 1: S22–S25.

51. Rehrer NJ. *Limits to fluid availability during exercise*. Haarlem: De Vrieseborsch, 1990.

52. Vist GE, Maughan RJ. The effect of increasing glucose concentration on the rate of gastric emptying in man. *Medicine and Science in Sports and Exercise* 1994; **26**: 1269–73.

53. Brener W, Hendrix TR, McHugh PR. Regulation of the gastric emptying of glucose. *Gastroenterology* 1983; **85**: 76–82.

54. Foster C, Costill DL, Fink WJ. Gastric emptying characteristics of glucose and glucose polymers. *Research Quarterly* 1980; **51**: 299–305.

55. Sole CC, Noakes TD. Faster gastric emptying for glucose-polymer and fructose solutions than for glucose in humans. *European Journal of Applied Physiology* 1989; **58**: 605–12.

56. Naveri H, Tikkanen H, Kairento A-L, Harkonen M. Gastric emptying and serum insulin levels after intake of glucose-polymer solutions. *European Journal of Applied Physiology* 1989; **58**: 661–5.

57. American College of Sports Medicine. Position stand on prevention of thermal injuries during distance running. *Medicine and Science in Sports and Exercise* 1984; **16**: ix–xiv.

58. Costill DL, Saltin B. Factors limiting gastric emptying during rest and exercise. *Journal of Applied Physiology* 1974; **37**: 679–83.

59. Sun WM, Houghton LA, Read NW, Grundy DG, Johnson AG. Effect of meal temperature on gastric emptying of liquids in man. *Gut* 1988; **29**: 302–5.

60. McArthur KE, Feldman M. Gastric acid secretion, gastrin release, and gastric temperature in humans as affected by liquid meal temperature. *American Journal of Clinical Nutrition* 1989; **49**: 51–4.

61. Lambert CP, Maughan RJ. Effect of temperature of ingested beverages on the rate of accumulation in the blood of an added tracer for water uptake. *Scandinavian Journal of Medicine and Science in Sports* 1992; **2**: 76–8.

62. Murray R, Bartoli WP, Eddy DE, Horn MK. Gastric emptying and plasma deuterium accumulation following ingestion of water and two carbohydrate-electrolyte beverages. *International Journal of Sports Nutrition* 1997; **7**: 144–53.

63. Lolli G, Greenberg LA, Lester D. The influence of carbonated water on gastric emptying. *New England Journal of Medicine* 1952; **246**: 490–2.

64. Lambert CP, Costill DL, McConnell GK, *et al*. Fluid replacement after dehydration: influence of beverage carbonation and carbohydrate content. *International Journal of Sports Medicine* 1992; **13**: 285–92.

65. Zachwieja JJ, Costill DL, Beard GC, Robergs RA, Pascoe DD, Anderson DE. The effects of a carbonated carbohydrate drink on gastric emptying, gastrointestinal distress, and exercise performance. *International Journal of Sport Nutrition* 1992; **2**: 239–50.

66. Lambert GP, Blieler TL, Chang RT, Johnson AK, Gisolfi CV. Effects of carbonated and noncarbonated beverages at specific intervals during treadmill running in the heat. *International Journal of Sport Nutrition* 1993; **2**: 177–93.

67. Wapnir RA, Lifshitz F. Osmolality and solute concentration—their relationship with oral rehydration solution effectiveness: an experimental assessment. *Pediatric Research* 1985; **19**: 894–8.

68. Spiller RC, Jones BJM, Brown BE, Silk DBA. Enhancement of carbohydrate absorption by the addition of sucrose to enteric diets. *Journal of Parenteral and Enteral Nutrition* 1982; **6**: 321.

69. Jones BJM, Brown BE, Loran JS, Edgerton D, Kennedy JF. Glucose absorption from starch hydrolysates in the human jejunum. *Gut* 1983; **24**: 1152–60.

70. Jones BJM, Higgins BE, Silk DBA. Glucose absorption from maltotriose and glucose oligomers in the human jejunum. *Clinical Science* 1987; **72**: 409–14.

71. Fordtran JS. Stimulation of active and passive sodium absorption by sugars in the human jejunum. *Journal of Clinical Investigation* 1975; **55**: 728–37.

72. Fordtran JS, Saltin B. Gastric emptying and intestinal absorption during prolonged severe exercise. *Journal of Applied Physiology* 1967; **23**: 331–5.

73. Brouns F, Saris WHM, Rehrer NJ Abdominal complaints and gastrointestinal function during long-lasting exercise. *International Journal of Sports Medicine* 1987; **8**: 175–89.

74. Maughan RJ, Leiper JB, McGaw BA. Effects of exercise intensity on absorption of ingested fluids in man. *Experimental Physiology* 1990; **75**: 419–21.

75. Schedl HP, Maughan RJ, Gisolfi CV. Intestinal absorption during rest and exercise: implications for formulating oral rehydration beverages. *Medicine and Science in Sports and Exercise* 1994; **26**: 267–80.

76. Costill DL, Bennett A, Branam G, Eddy D. Glucose ingestion at rest and during prolonged exercise. *Journal of Applied Physiology* 1973; **34**: 764–9.

77. Pirnay F, Crielaard JM, Pallikarakis N, *et al*. Fate of exogenous glucose during exercise of different intensities in humans. *Journal of Applied Physiology* 1982; **53**: 1620–4.

78. Erickson MA, Schwartzkopf RJ, McKenzie RD. Effects of caffeine, fructose, and glucose ingestion on muscle glycogen utilisa-

79. Ivy J, Costill DL, Fink WJ, Lower RW. Influence of caffeine and carbohydrate feedings on endurance performance. *Medicine and Science in Sports* 1979; **11**: 6–11.

80. Coyle EF, Hagberg JM, Hurley BF, Martin WH, Ehsani AH, Holloszy JO. Carbohydrate feeding during prolonged strenuous exercise can delay fatigue. *Journal of Applied Physiology* 1983; **55**: 230–5.

81. Coyle EF, Coggan AR, Hemmert MK, Ivy JL. Muscle glycogen utilisation during prolonged strenuous exercise when fed carbohydrate. *Journal of Applied Physiology* 1986; **61**: 165–72.

82. Maughan RJ, Fenn CE, Gleeson M, Leiper JB. Metabolic and circulatory responses to injestion of glucose polymer and glucose/electrolyte solutions during exercise in man. *Journal of Applied Physiology* 1987; **56**: 356–62.

83. Coggan AR, Coyle EF. Effect of carbohydrate feedings during high-intensity exercise. *Journal of Applied Physiology* 1988; **65**: 1703–9.

84. Hargreaves M, Briggs CA. Effect of carbohydrate ingestion on exercise metabolism. *Journal of Applied Physiology* 1988; **65**: 1553–5.

85. Sasaki H, Maeda J, Usui S, Ishiko T. Effect of sucrose and caffeine ingestion on performance of prolonged strenuous running. *International Journal of Sports Medicine* 1987; **8**: 261–5.

86. Murray R, Eddy DE, Murray TW, Seifert JG, Paul GL, Halaby GA. The effect of fluid and carbohydrate feedings during intermittent cycling exercise. *Medicine and Science in Sports and Exercise* 1987; **19**: 597–604.

87. Mitchell JB, Costill DL, Houmard JA, Flynn MG, Fink WJ, Beltz JD. Effects of carbohydrate ingestion on gastric emptying and exercise performance. *Medicine and Science in Sports and Exercise* 1988; **20**: 110–15.

88. Carter JE, Gisolfi CV. Fluid replacement during and after exercise in the heat. *Medicine and Science in Sports and Exercise* 1989; **21**: 532–9.

89. Ahlborg B, Bergstrom J, Brohult J, Ekelund L-G, Hultman E, Maschio E. Human muscle glycogen content and capacity for prolonged exercise after different diets. *Forsvarsmedicin* 1967; **3**: 85–99.

90. Hargreaves M, Costill DL, Coggan A, Fink WJ, Nishibata I. Effect of carbohydrate feedings on muscle glycogen utilisation and exercise performance. *Medicine and Science in Sports and Exercise* 1984; **16**: 219–22.

91. Fielding RA, Costill DL, Fink WJ, King DS, Hargreaves M, Kovaleski ME. Effect of carbohydrate feeding frequencies on muscle glycogen use during exercise. *Medicine and Science in Sports and Exercise* 1985; **17**: 472–6.

92. Noakes TD, Adams BA, Myburgh KH, Greeff C, Lotz T, Nathan M. The danger of an inadequate water intake during prolonged exercise. A novel concept re-visited. *European Journal of Applied Physiology* 1988; **57**: 210–19.

93. Flynn MG, Costill DL, Hawley JA, Fink WJ, Neufer PD, Fielding RA, Sleeper MD. Influence of selected carbohydrate drinks on cycling performance and glycogen use. *Medicine and Science in Sports and Exercise* 1987; **19**: 37–40.

94. Pirnay F, Lacroix M, Mosora F, Luyckx A, Lefebvre P. Glucose oxidation during prolonged exercise evaluated with naturally labeled [^{13}C]glucose. *Journal of Applied Physiology* 1977; **43**: 258–61.

95. Pallikarakis N, Jandrain B, Pirnay F, *et al*. Remarkable metabolic availability of oral glucose during long-duration exercise in humans. *Journal of Applied Physiology* 1988; **60**: 1035–42.

96. Coyle EF, Coggan AR. Effectiveness of carbohydrate feeding in delaying fatigue during prolonged exercise. *Sports Medicine* 1984; **1**: 446–58.

97. Lamb DR, Brodowicz GR. Optimal use of fluids of varying formulations to minimize exercise-induced disturbances in homeostasis. *Sports Medicine* 1986; **3**: 247–74.

98. Murray R. The effects of consuming carbohydrate-electrolyte beverages on gastric emptying and fluid absorption during and following exercise. *Sports Medicine* 1987; **4**: 322–51.

99. Maughan RJ. Effects of CHO-electrolyte solution on prolonged exercise. In: Lamb DR, MH Williams, eds. *Perspectives in exercise science and sports medicine.* Vol 4: Ergogenics: the enhancement of sport performance. Carmel, IN: Benchmark Press, 1991: 35–85.

100. Walsh RM, Noakes TD, Hawley JA, Dennis SC. Impaired high intensity cycling performance time at low levels of dehydration. *International Journal of Sports Medicine* 1994; **15**: 392–8.

101. Below PR, Mora-Rodriguez R, Gonzalez-Alonso J, Coyle EF. Fluid and carbohydrate ingestion independently improve performance during 1 h of intense exercise. *Medicine and Science in Sports and Exercise* 1995; 27: 200–10.

102. Levine L, Rose MS, Francesconi RP, Neufer PD, Sawka MN. Fluid replacement during sustained activity: nutrient solution vs. water. *Aviation Space and Environmental Medicine* 1991; **62**: 559–64.

103. Barr SI, Costill DL, Fink WJ. Fluid replacement during prolonged exercise: effects of water, saline or no fluid. *Medicine and Science in Sports and Exercise* 1991; **23**: 811–17.

104. Yaspelkis BB, Ivy JL. Effect of carbohydrate supplements and water on exercise metabolism in the heat. *Journal of Applied Physiology* 1991; **71**: 680–7.

105. Macaraeg PVJ. Influence of carbohydrate electrolyte ingestion on running endurance. In: Fox EL, ed. *Nutrient utilisation during exercise.* Columbus, OH: Ross Laboratories, 1983: 91–6.

106. Fruth JM, Gisolfi CV. Effects of carbohydrate consumption on endurance performance: fructose versus glucose. In: Fox EL, ed. *Nutrient utilisation during exercise.* Columbus, OH: Ross Laboratories, 1983; 68–75.

107. Riley ML, Israel RG, Holbert D, Tapscott EB, Dohm GL. Effect of carbohydrate ingestion on exercise endurance and metabolism after a 1-day fast. *International Journal of Sports Medicine* 1988; **9**: 320–4.

108. Ivy JL, Miller W, Dover V, *et al.* Endurance improved by ingestion of a glucose polymer supplement. *Medicine and Science in Sports and Exercise* 1983; **15**: 466–71.

109. Williams C. Diet and endurance fitness. *American Journal of Clinical Nutrition* 1989; **49**: 1077–83.

110. Williams C, Nute MG, Broadbank L, Vinall S. Influence of fluid intake on endurance running performance: a comparison between water, glucose and fructose solutions. *European Journal of Applied Physiology* 1990; **60**: 112–19.

111. Cade R, Spooner G, Schlein E, Pickering M, Dean R. Effect of fluid, electrolyte, and glucose replacement on performance, body temperature, rate of sweat loss and compositional changes of extracellular fluid. *Journal of Sports Medicine and Physical Fitness* 1972; **12**: 150–6.

112. Maughan RJ, Whiting PH. Factors influencing plasma glucose concentration during marathon running. In: Dotson CO, Humphrey JH, eds. *Exercise physiology.* Volume 1. New York: AMS Press, 1985: 87–98.

113. Tsintzas K, Liu R, Williams C, Campbell I, Gaitanos G. The effect of carbohydrate ingestion on performance during a 30-km race. *International Journal of Sport Nutrition* 1993; **3**: 127–39.

114. Leatt P. The effect of glucose polymer ingestion on skeletal muscle glycogen depletion during soccer match-play and its resynthesis following a match. M Sc Thesis, University of Toronto, 1986.

115. Nicholas CW, Williams C, Lakomy HKA, Phillips G, Nowitz A. Influence of ingesting a carbohydrate-electrolyte solution on endurance capacity during intermittent, high-intensity shuttle running. *Journal of Sports Sciences* 1995; **13**: 283–90.

116. Greenhaff PL, Clough PJ. Predictors of sweat loss in man during prolonged exercise. *European Journal of Applied Physiology* 1989; **58**: 348–52.

117. Barr SI, Costill DL. Water: can the endurance athlete get too much of a good thing. *Journal of the American Dietetic Association* 1989; **89**: 1629–32.

118. Olsson KE, Saltin B. Diet and fluids in training and competition. *Scandinavian Journal of Rehabilitation Medicine* 1971; **3**: 31–8.

119. American College of Sports Medicine. Position statement on prevention of heat injuries during distance running. *Medicine and Science in Sports* 1975; **7**: vii–ix.

120. American College of Sports Medicine. Position stand on exercise and fluid replacement. *Medicine and Science in Sports and Exercise* 1996; **28(1)**: i–vii.

121. Maughan RJ. Physiology and nutrition for middle distance and long distance running. In: Lamb DR, Knuttgen HG, Murray R, eds. *Perspectives in exercise science and sports medicine.* Vol 7: Physiology and nutrition for competitive sport. Carmel, IN: Cooper Publishing, 1994: 329–72.

122. Deschamps A, Levy RD, Cosio MG, Marliss EB, Magder S. Effect of saline infusion on body temperature and endurance during heavy exercise. *Journal of Applied Physiology* 1989; **66**: 2799–804.

123. Davies CTM, Thompson MW. Aerobic performance of female marathon and male ultramarathon athletes. *European Journal of Applied Physiology* 1979; **41**: 233–45.

124. Maughan RJ, Leiper JB. Aerobic capacity and fractional utilisation of aerobic capacity in élite and non-élite male and female marathon runners. *European Journal of Applied Physiology* 1983; **52**: 80–7.

125. Duchman SM, Blieler TL, Schedl HP, Summers RW, Gisolfi CV. Effects of gastric function on intestinal composition of oral rehydration solutions. *Medicine and Science in Sports and Exercise* 1990; **22** (Suppl): S89.

126. Noakes TD. The dehydration myth and carbohydrate replacement during prolonged exercise. *Cycling Science* 1990; **1**: 23–9.

127. Massicote D, Peronnet F, Brisson G, Bakkouch K, Hillaire-Marcel C. Oxidation of a glucose polymer during exercise: comparison with glucose and fructose. *Journal of Applied Physiology* 1989; **66**: 179–83.

128. Noakes TD, Goodwin N, Rayner BL, Branken T, Taylor RKN. Water intoxication: a possible complication during endurance exercise. *Medicine and Science in Sports and Exercise* 1985; **17**: 370–5.

129. Noakes TD, Norman RJ, Buck RH, Godlonton J, Stevenson K, Pittaway D. The incidence of hyponatremia during prolonged ultraendurance exercise. *Medicine and Science in Sports and Exercise* 1990; **22**: 165–70.

130. Frizell RT, Lang GH, Lowance DC, Lathan SR. Hyponatraemia and ultramarathon running. *Journal of the American Medical Association* 1986; **255**: 772–4.

131. Hiller WDB. Dehydration and hyponatraemia during triathlons. *Medicine and Science in Sports and Exercise* 1989; **21**: S219–S221.

132. Flear CTG, Gill CV, Burn J. Beer drinking and hyponatraemia. *Lancet* 1981; **ii**: 477.

133. Noakes TD. The hyponatremia of exercise. *International Journal of Sport Nutrition* 1992; **2**: 205–28.

134. Noakes TD. Hyponatraemia during distance running: a physiological and clinical interpretation. *Medicine and Science in Sports and Exercise* 1993; **24**: 403–5.

135. Fellmann N, Sagnol M, Bedu M, *et al.* Enzymatic and hormonal responses following a 24 h endurance run and a 10 h triathlon race. *European Journal of Applied Physiology* 1988; **57**: 545–53.

136. Wemple RD, Lamb DR, McKeever KH. Caffeine vs caffeine-free sports-drinks: effect on urine production at rest and during prolonged exercise. *International Journal of Sports Medicine* 1997; **18**: 40–6.

137. Wemple RD, Morocco TS, Mack GW. Influence of sodium replacement on fluid ingestion following exercise-induced dehydration. *International Journal of Sport Nutrition* 1997; **7**: 104–16.

138. Suzuki Y. Human physical performance and cardiocirculatory responses to hot environments during sub-maximal upright cycling. *Ergonomics* 1980; **23**: 527–42.

139. Senay LC. Effects of exercise in the heat on body fluid distribution. *Medicine and Science in Sports* 1979; **11**: 42–8.

140. Hallberg L, Magnusson B. The aetiology of sports anaemia. *Acta Medica Scandinavica* 1984; **216**: 145–8.

141. Davidson RJL, Robertson JD, Galea G, Maughan RJ. Haematological changes associated with marathon running. *International Journal of Sports Medicine* 1987; **8**: 19–25.

142. Robertson JD, Maughan RJ, Davidson RJL. Changes in red cell density and related parameters in response to long distance running. *European Journal of Applied Physiology* 1988; **57**: 264–9.

143. Convertino VA, Brock PJ, Keil LC, Bernauer EM, Greenleaf JE. Exercise training-induced hypervolemia: role of plasma albumin, renin and vasopressin. *Journal of Applied Physiology* 1980; **48**: 665–9.

144. Convertino VA, Keil LC, Greenleaf JE. Plasma volume, renin, and vasopressin responses to graded exercise after training. *Journal of Applied Physiology* 1983; **54**: 508–14.

145. Mitchell D, Senay LC, Wyndham CH, van Rensburg AJ, Rogers GG, Strydom NB. Acclimatization in a hot, humid environment: energy exchange, body temperature, and sweating. *Journal of Applied Physiology* 1976; **40**: 768–78.

146. Wyndham CH, Rogers GG, Senay LC, Mitchell D. Acclimatization in a hot, humid environment: cardiovascular adjustments. *Journal of Applied Physiology* 1976; **40**: 779–85.

147. Senay LC, Mitchell D, Wyndham CH. Acclimatization in a hot humid environment: body fluid adjustments. *Journal of Applied Physiology* 1976; **40**: 786–96.

148. Burge CM, Carey MF, Payne WR. Rowing performance, fluid balance, and metabolic function following dehydration and rehydration. *Medicine and Science in Sports and Exercise* 1993; **25**: 1358–64.

149. Claremont AD, Costill DL, Fink WJ, Vanhandel P. Heat tolerance following diuretic induced dehydration. *Medicine and Science in Sports and Exercise* 1976; **40**: 6–11.

150. Saltin B. Circulatory response to submaximal and maximal exercise after thermal dehydration. *Journal of Applied Physiology* 1964; **19**: 1125–32.

151. Sawka MN, Francesconi RP, Pandolf KB, Young AJ. Influence of hydration level and body fluids on exercise performance in the heat. *Journal of the American Medical Association* 1984; **252**: 1165–9.

152. Costill DL, Sparks KE. Rapid fluid replacement following thermal dehydration. *Journal of Applied Physiology* 1973; **34**: 299–303.

153. Gonzalez-Alonso J, Heaps CL, Coyle EF. Rehydration after exercise with common beverages and water. *International Journal of Sports Medicine* 1992; **13**: 399–406.

154. Nose H, Mack GW, Shi X, Nadel ER. Role of osmolality and plasma volume during rehydration in humans. *Journal of Applied Physiology* 1988; **65**: 325–31.

155. Nose H, Mack GW, Shi X, Nadel ER. Involvement of sodium retention hormones during rehydration in humans. *Journal of Applied Physiology* 1988; **65**: 332–6.

156. Maughan RJ, Leiper JB. Effects of sodium content of ingested fluids on post-exercise rehydration in man. *European Journal of Applied Physiology* 1995; **71**: 311–19.

157. Nadel ER, Mack GW, Nose H. Influence of fluid replacement beverages on body fluid homeostasis during exercise and recovery. In: Gisolfi CV, Lamb DR, eds. *Perspectives in exercise science and sports medicine*. Volume 3: Fluid homeostasis during exercise. Carmel, IN: Benchmark, 1990: 181–205.

158. Maughan RJ, Owen JH, Shirreffs SM, Leiper JB. Post-exercise rehydration in man: effects of electrolyte addition to ingested fluids. *European Journal of Applied Physiology* 1994; **69**: 209–15.

159. Shirreffs SM, Taylor AJ, Leiper JB, Maughan RJ. Post-exercise rehydration in man: effects of volume consumed and drink sodium content. *Medicine and Science in Sports and Exercise* 1996; **28**: 1260–71.

160. Maughan RJ, Leiper JB, Shirreffs SM. Restoration of fluid balance after exercise-induced dehydration: effects of food and fluid intake. *European Journal of Applied Physiology* 1996; **73**: 317–25.

161. Freund BJ, Montain SJ, Young AJ, *et al*. Glycerol hyperhydration: hormonal, renal, and vascular fluid responses. *Journal of Applied Physiology* 1995; **79**: 2069–77.

162. Riedesel ML, Allen DL, Peake GT, Al-Qattan K. Hyperhydration with glycerol solutions. *Journal of Applied Physiology* 1987; **63**: 2262–8.

163. Gleeson M, Maughan RJ, Greenhaff PL. Comparison of the effects of pre-exercise feeding of glucose, glycerol and placebo on endurance and fuel homeostasis in man. *European Journal of Applied Physiology* 1986; **55**: 645–53.

164. Thecomata A, Nagashima K, Nose H, Morimoto T. Osmoregulatory inhibition of thermally induced cutaneous vasodilation in passively heated humans. *American Journal of Physiology* 1997; **273**: R197–R204.

165. Montner P, Stark DM, Riedesel ML, *et al*. Pre-exercise glycerol hydration improves cycling endurance time. *International Journal of Sports Medicine* 1996; **17**: 27–33.

166. Latzka WA, Sawka MN, Matott RP, Staab JE, Montain SJ, Pandolf KB. Hyperhydration: Physiologic and thermoregulatory effects during compensable and uncompensable exercise-heat stress. *US Army Technical Report*. Alexandria, VA: Defense Technical Information Center, Cameron Station, 1996; T96–6.

167. Miller JM, Coyle EF, Sherman WM, *et al*. Effect of glycerol feeding on endurance and metabolism during prolonged exercise in man. *Medicine and Science in Sports and Exercise* 1983; **15**: 237–42.

1.2.3 Making weight for sports participation

Mikael Fogelholm and Wim H.M. Saris

Body weight, fatness, and athletic performance

Body size, structure, and composition are separate, yet interrelated, aspects of the wide diversity of physiological demands required in different sports. For instance, the height of élite male basketball players frequently exceeds 200 cm, sometimes even 210 cm, whereas female gymnasts are short, even less than 150 cm.

In addition to height, body mass and composition also affect physical performance. It is widely believed by athletes and coaches that there are 'ideal' body weights and compositions for specific sports. Again, the extremes are well known: Japanese sumo-wrestlers may weigh more than 200 kg, while the lightest Olympic wrestlers are less than 48 kg.

The term 'ideal' implies that there is a known optimal combination of body fat and fat-free mass for a specific sport. However, optimal body composition for an athlete is very difficult to define, because many other factors contribute to successful athletic performance.[1]

The association between weight and height for a large cohort of Finnish Olympic (141 males, 45 females) and subélite (190 males, 173 females) athletes is shown in Fig. 1 (Hiilloskorpi and Fogelholm, unpublished results). The male athletes' weight varied between 45 and 125 kg, while the range among female athletes was from 35 to 85 kg.

The difference between predicted (based on the association between weight and height) and actual body weight gives an indication if a certain type of sport favours light or heavy athletes. The Finnish athletes in the above cohort represented various types of sports, such as endurance events (running, cross-country skiing, orienteering, triathlon), weight-class sports (wrestling, judo, karate, weightlifting), sports requiring speed and power (sprints, throwing events, jumping for distance or height), aesthetic disciplines (gymnastics, figure-skating, ballet), and ball games (soccer, ice hockey, volleyball, basketball, badminton). Aesthetic athletes were, on average, 3 to 4 kg lighter than predicted from their height (Fig. 2). Male endurance athletes were also light. Athletes in weight-class sports and ballgames were, in general, heavier than predicted.

The subélite athletes' body-fat content (as per cent of body weight, **BF per cent**) was estimated by skinfold thickness (Fig. 3).

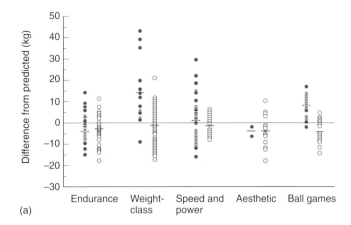

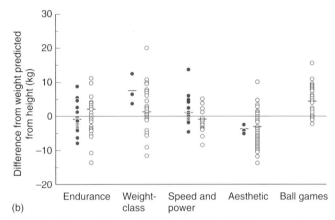

Fig. 2 The difference between actual and predicted weight (from regression equation between height and weight) in Finnish male (a) and female (b) athletes. Dark circles indicate élite, open circles subélite athletes (Hiilloskorpi and Fogelholm, unpublished data).

The ballgame athletes had the highest BF per cent in both sexes. In relation to other events among the same sex, the female aesthetic athletes were the leanest. However, the endurance, weight class, and speed and power groups also included very lean athletes (estimated at less than 7 BF per cent in males and less than 15 BF per cent in females). Comparable results were found in a nationwide study in élite athletes in the Netherlands.[2]

Reasons for weight reduction in athletes

Competitive athletes control their body weight for four main reasons:

1. Most athletes in weight-class events compete at weights far lighter than their natural weight. Reduction of body weight is necessary, because failure to 'make weight' results in disqualification from competition. Examples of weight-class sports are wrestling, judo, karate, weightlifting, boxing, and light-weight rowing.

2. Reduction of body weight and fat mass may be considered advantageous for aesthetical reasons (appearance). Typical examples of 'aesthetic' sports are gymnastics, diving, figure skating, and bodybuilding. The reasons for weight control in

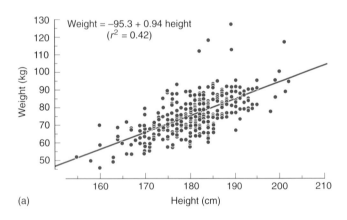

(a)

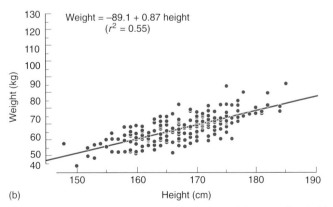

(b)

Fig. 1 Weight as a function of height in 331 Finnish male (a) and 218 female (b) athletes (Hiilloskorpi and Fogelholm, unpublished data).

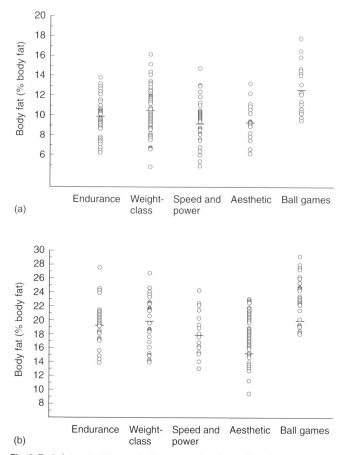

(a)

(b)

Fig. 3 Body-fat content (per cent of body weight), estimated by skinfold thickness, in 175 Finnish male (a) and 176 female (b) athletes (Hiilloskorpi and Fogelholm, unpublished data).

classical ballet are similar to those in gymnastics and figure skating.

3. Reduced body weight or relative fat mass is expected to bring about a physiological advantage, that is to improve physical performance. This is the most important reason for weight reduction in running, cross-country skiing, road cycling, and jumping for height or distance. Improved physical performance might be another reason behind weight reduction in weight-class and 'aesthetic' sports.

4. Increased body mass, preferably increased fat-free body weight, might be advantageous when a sports activity requires a high absolute-power output to resist, for instance the inertia of another body, or to overcome an external object. Examples are heavyweight wrestling, boxing, judo, and Rugby football. Ultra-long distance swimmers might benefit from a relatively high fat mass, because of the effects of fat on thermal insulation and buoyancy. However, the number of athletes who want to increase their body mass is lower compared with the number who want to reduce their weight.

Weight reduction is used throughout the whole of the athletic population, by males and females, by lean and muscular athletes, by endurance athletes, strength athletes, and sprinters, and by adolescent and adult athletes. Moreover, techniques for and the magnitude

of weight loss are highly variable. The only common factor seems to be that—from a clinical viewpoint—athletes trying to cut down their weight are not obese.

In fact, athletes with aesthetic performance elements, and some endurance and weight-class athletes, are already lighter and leaner, compared with untrained individuals and even with other athletes (Figs 2 and 3). Moreover, the preservation of an athlete's fat-free body compartment is very critical for peak performance. Finally, energy restriction might adversely affect recovery processes during intense training. Consequently, the physiological basis and critical elements of weight reduction in athletes are different from those found in obese people.[3]

Athletes lose weight either rapidly or gradually. In this chapter, striving for the target weight in less than one week is called 'rapid weight reduction'. Longer (7 days or more) reduction periods are called 'gradual'. The main difference is that gradual weight reduction is accomplished by a negative energy balance, whereas dehydration (negative water balance) is a necessary part of rapid weight loss.

This chapter will describe techniques for the two weight reductions mentioned above, their physiological effects, and effects on performance. In addition, potential health hazards of different weight-loss techniques are also considered. Finally, athletes in weight-class, aesthetic, and other sports are offered recommendations for weight control and reduction. Some aspects related to weight reduction in athletes are also partly covered in Chapters 1.2.2 and 1.5.

Rapid weight reduction and athletic performance

Rapid weight-reduction techniques

Rapid weight reduction is used mainly by athletes in weight-class events. It is a technique for achieving the target weight during a short period, sometimes even during a few hours. Fluid and food restriction and exercise wearing rubber or plastic suits are the most frequently practised methods among American college wrestlers (Fig. 4).[4] These techniques are also typical in experimental studies (Table 1).

About 90 per cent of the college wrestlers used food and fluid restriction on at least a weekly basis (Fig. 4). More than 60 per cent

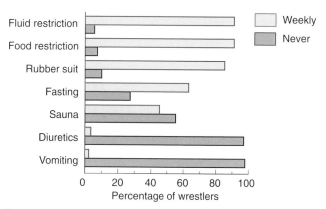

Fig. 4 The proportion (per cent) of college wrestlers using different rapid weight-reduction methods on a weekly basis, or never using these techniques. (Data from ref. 4.)

Table 1 Methods for rapid weight loss by active dehydration

Duration (h)	Loss (kg)	Loss (%)	Method of weight loss	Ref.
12	3.3	4.9	Exercise, energy intake 3.0 MJ/day	5
24	3.2	4.5	Dehydration (energy intake?)	6
48	3.4	4.7	Dehydration (energy intake?)	6
48	2.3	3.4	Exercise, low-energy diet	7
50	3.2	5.0	Exercise, low-energy diet	8
59	4.4	6.0	Exercise, energy intake 5.6 MJ/day	9
60	3.0	3.8	Fasting (0.6 MJ/day), diuretics	10
72	3.6	5.0	Dehydration (energy intake?)	6
72	4.0	4.6	Exercise, sauna, energy intake 9.1 MJ/day	11
96	4.3	6.3	Exercise, energy intake 8.6 MJ/day	12
96	6.0	8.0	Exercise, energy intake 3.4 MJ/day	13
96	4.3	5.8	Dehydration (energy intake?)	6

Columns: Duration of rapid weight loss (in hours); amount of weight loss (in kg and as percentage of body weight); method of weight loss (fluid restriction not mentioned separately); ref., reference.

of the wrestlers fasted every week to control their weight. To make a certain weight-class, the methods described above are probably intensified before major competitions. Competitive wrestlers in Finland typically reduce their weight by 5 to 10 per cent before competitions 15 to 20 times per year.

Restricting fluid intake is an essential part of rapid weight reduction. In contrast, the energy intake during rapid weight reduction appears to be highly variable, with reported values ranging from an almost total fast (0.6 MJ (140 kcal)/ day)[10] to a nearly unrestricted 9.1 MJ (2200 kcal)/day.[11] It is not clear to what extent energy intake affects rapid weight loss, but fluid restriction is presumably more important than reduced energy intake. Because sodium intake is associated with water retention, salt (sodium chloride) restriction will speed up the rate of rapid weight loss.

More than 80 per cent of the college wrestlers questioned used exercise in rubber suits to control their weight on a weekly basis (Fig. 4). Wrestlers usually jog, wrestle, and carry out calisthenics without replacing the fluid lost in sweating. Hence, the preparation for weight-class sports is totally different from the preparation of endurance athletes, who reduce training and fill up their carbohydrate and fluid stores before competition.

In two studies, male wrestlers reduced their body weight by 4 to 5 per cent within 12 to 24 h.[5,6] In other studies (see Table 1), a combination of increased exercise (usually in rubber suits) and diet and fluid restriction resulted in a 4 to 8 per cent loss of body weight in 48 to 96 h. Dehydration has also been achieved by exercising in a heated chamber (30 °C).[8]

Weight can be reduced by 2 to 4 per cent in less than 2.5 h by sauna.[10,14] Nevertheless, compared with exercise and dietary restriction, sauna is less popular among wrestlers both in the USA (Fig. 4) and in Europe. If used, intermittent sauna at 80 to 85 °C is recommended: for example, two sessions of three sauna periods of 15 min each with a 5 min break between periods and a 30 min break

between the sessions.[10] The reason for intermittent, rather than continuous, sauna is that during the breaks sweat is dried off the body, and the body is cooled by shaking a towel in front of the wrestler. Cooling and drying is needed to minimize an excessive rise of body temperature.

Another method of losing about 2 to 4 per cent of body weight is through the use of diuretics, for instance 0.5 to 1.7 frusemide/kg body weight.[7,10,15] However, diuretics are regarded as doping and their use is banned. Moreover, the results are not very impressive, compared to other rapid weight-reduction techniques. Consequently, the use of diuretics among young wrestlers is infrequent (Fig. 4).

Methods normally regarded as rapid (fasting, diet pills, self-induced vomiting, laxatives, diuretics) are occasionally used to speed up gradual weight reduction. In a study among 182 intercollegiate female athletes, 32 per cent practised at least one of the pathogenic 'weight control' methods mentioned above.[16] Female cross-country skiers[17] and gymnasts[18] also use pathogenic weight-control methods. These findings are not restricted to adult athletes, because a high proportion (15 per cent) of young (9- to 18-year-old) female swimmers have been found to control their weight with pathogenic methods.[19] Although the data on weight control in males, other than wrestlers is scarce, it seems that female athletes are more prone to using pathogenic weight-control methods.[19,20]

Usually the weigh-in takes place 2 to 20 h before a weight-class competition. The interval depends on the sport (for example, 2 h in judo, 15 to 20 h in international wrestling tournaments) and the age of the athletes (young wrestlers have a shorter interval than older ones). The magnitude of weight regain (as a percentage of the weight lost) varies between 21 per cent in 1 h[8] and 42 to 100 per cent in 3 to 5 h.[9,13,14] In an actual wrestling competition, the average weight gain between the weigh-in and the competition (20 h) was 3.7 kg or 5.3 per cent of the weigh-in weight.[21]

Table 2 Summary of the effects of rapid weight reduction on athletic performance. Results are grouped by the time for rehydration (time difference between the weigh-in and the competition)

	Rehydration 0–3 h	Rehydration 5–24 h
Maximal aerobic capacity	Maintained or reduced	?
Submaximal aerobic capacity	Reduced	?
Anaerobic capacity	Usually reduced	Maintained
Muscle endurance and strength	Maintained or reduced (depends on muscle group)	Maintained

Rapid weight reduction and sports performance

Aerobic endurance capacity (time to exhaustion on a submaximal working intensity or maximal workload reached during an incremental exercise test) deteriorates after dehydration with diet–exercise, sauna, or diuretic manipulation (Table 2).[5,7,15] Deterioration of aerobic capacity was 5 per cent after the use of diuretics and 10 per cent after dietary restriction.[5,15] In one study, the decline in performance was more marked after using diuretics than after weight reduction with diet–exercise or sauna.[7] Similarly, a 12 to 80 h fast has detrimental effects on submaximal endurance capacity.[22]

Both maintained[7,13,15] and lowered[5,7] maximal oxygen uptake capacities ($\dot{V}O_2$max, l/min) after rapid weight loss have been reported. A combined effect of the magnitude and rapidity of weight loss might be the most logical explanation behind these divergent results: negative effects were found after a 4.2 to 4.9 per cent weight loss in 12 to 24 h, whereas a smaller (1.6 to 3.4 per cent in 2 to 48 h) or slower (8.0 per cent in 96 h) weight loss did not change $\dot{V}O_2$max.

Maximal anaerobic power usually decreases following a rapid weight loss by dehydration. A 30 to 60 s maximal test on a cycle ergometer, the Wingate test, is often used for testing anaerobic power. Both maintained[23] and lowered[5] performances have been reported. A specific test to simulate wrestling was used in three studies. The 2-min 'CSU wrestling performance test' involved jumps, rolls, walking, running, etc.[8] The other test consisted of 6-min arm-cranking with alternating intensity.[11,12] Decreased performance was noted in all three studies after rapid weight reduction without subsequent rehydration, except after a high-carbohydrate diet.[12]

A short rehydration period (1.0 to 3.5 h) did not return anaerobic performance to normal levels in the 2-min wrestling test.[8] However, when exercise tests were carried out after 5 to 24 h rehydration, anaerobic performance was not significantly affected.[8,9]

Muscle-endurance and maximal-strength tests have involved both isometric and isotonic contractions. Decreased performance after dehydration was reported in several studies.[5,10,13,14] However, the effects vary with muscle group.[5,14]

A short rehydration time (1 to 3 h) after dehydration does not necessarily normalize muscle function.[13,14] In contrast, a 5 to 24 h recovery and rehydration period seems to be sufficient to recover muscle strength and vertical jumping height after rapid weight reduction.[9,10]

Physiological consequences of rapid weight reduction

A considerable fluid loss is evident in all rapid methods of weight reduction. The effect on plasma osmolality is dependent on the weight-reduction technique: sweating results in hyperosmotic hypovolaemia, while diuretics lead to iso-osmotic hypovolaemia. Hyperosmolality and reduced plasma volume affect thermoregulation and increase core temperature both during rest and exercise.[24] Responses to hypohydration seem to be more prominent during additional heat stress.

After fluid loss, cardiac output and stroke volume are decreased and the reduced plasma volume limits oxygen transportation to the working muscles.[25] Slow nutrient exchange, waste removal, and heat dissipation might also affect longer anaerobic work.[26] A very short anaerobic performance, on the other hand, is not likely to be affected by passive dehydration, such as sauna.[23]

Liver and muscle glycogen stores are almost emptied during the first days of marked energy restriction or starvation, because the energy needs cannot be totally covered by lipolysis. Therefore, in weight reduction accomplished by exercise-induced sweating and dietary restriction, not only body hydration, but also muscle glycogen stores may be affected.[13] Reduced availability of muscle glycogen impairs endurance performance (see Chapter 1.2.1) and may also affect anaerobic energy production and performance.[27] Glycogen stores may be preserved, at least partially, by a sufficient carbohydrate intake during weight loss. In one study,[12] rapid weight reduction decreased performance only in connection with a low-carbohydrate diet, a result that supports the above hypothesis.

Diuretics and sauna have negative effects on plasma volume and thermoregulation,[24] whereas dietary restriction and increased exercise also affect glycogen stores.[13] Despite reduced glycogen stores, however, both practical observations[4] and results[7] from laboratory studies suggest that active dehydration impairs anaerobic performance and strength less than passive methods. Consequently, wrestlers use active dehydration much more than passive techniques.[4]

Even short-term, low-carbohydrate diets, particularly in combination with unrestricted protein intake, may affect the blood's buffer systems by reducing the base-excess.[12,27,28] In one study, work capacity (3 to 6 min) during heavy exercise was reduced by 16 per cent after a 3-day, low-carbohydrate diet.[28] The decrement in work capacity was even greater (28 per cent) after a combination of glycogen depletion by exercise, and a low-carbohydrate, high-protein diet for 3 days.[27] The above results suggest that both reduced glycogen availability and buffer capacity affect performance during short-term heavy exercise after rapid weight reduction.

Glycogenolysis is an important, if not the predominant form of energy production during muscle endurance tests. Therefore the same mechanisms (reduced muscle glycogen content and blood base-excess) may affect both anaerobic performance and muscle endurance. In contrast, it is more difficult to explain decreased muscle strength. The muscle is fairly self-contained for short-term, maximal efforts, and is not dependent on effective nutrient exchange. Therefore a decrease in blood flow should not impair performance.[29] Moreover, muscle ATP and creatine phosphate concentrations are not affected by rapid weight reduction.[13] Hence, a reduced amount of high-energy phosphate compounds hardly explain reduced muscle strength.

Considerable amounts of electrolytes are lost through sweating (see Chapter 1.2.2) which could affect muscle function. The evidence is, however, scarce. A calculation of resting muscle-membrane potentials, at various levels of dehydration to a 6 per cent weight loss, showed no alterations in membrane excitability.[30,31] Moreover, nerve-impulse propagation was not impeded. Urinary electrolyte losses during rapid weight reduction are also unlikely to be large enough to affect muscle function.[6,15] Finally, unaltered serum electrolyte concentrations after a combined dehydration and rehydration protocol were found in Finnish wrestlers and judo athletes.[9]

Many young wrestlers feel mood alterations (increased fatigue, anger, anxiety) when 'making weight'.[4] Psychological factors may obviously affect performance. Perhaps athletes find weight reduction by active dehydration psychologically more acceptable than sauna-induced dehydration. This could be one explanation for the popularity of active dehydration,[4] despite its negative effects on muscle glycogen[13] and blood base-excess.[12]

Although rehydration reduces the magnitude of fluid deficit, weight regain does not predict whether performance will return to euhydrated levels or not. During a short (1 to 4 h) rehydration, weight gain was 21 to 100 per cent, but performance did not return to normal levels.[8,13,14] During 5 to 24 h rehydration (and recovery), most of the performance variables returned to the euhydrated level, despite that only 11 to 73 per cent of the weight loss was regained.[8-10] Consequently, total water loss, by itself, might not be the predominant factor causing a reduction in anaerobic, sprint and strength performance. For instance, fluid is first absorbed to the extracellular water space, and regain of the intracellular water and electrolyte balance might take longer. A longer recovery is also probably needed for muscle glycogen resynthesis and normalization of the blood's buffering capacity.

The above, predominantly negative, physiological effects of rapid weight reduction provide enough arguments to discourage the use of these types of techniques to try to improve performance. Nevertheless, it is very difficult to convince athletes of this. In some sports, such as wrestling, rapid weight reduction has been, and still is, an important part of the traditional preparation for a competition. Athletes might be 'bound' to these traditions, and breaking the traditional practice is very difficult, especially for young and inexperienced athletes.

Possible health hazards

Studies in developing countries show that under extremely adverse nutritional conditions, the bone growth of children may be inhibited and maturation delayed.[32] Excessive exercise could theoretically exaggerate the stress of malnutrition. Unfortunately, very little is known about growth in young athletes, who might have marginal nutrient intakes chronically or periodically.

Anthropometric growth patterns of 477 high-school wrestlers in the United States were recently investigated.[33] Very few differences in growth patterns between the wrestlers and a national representative sample of adolescents were found. The results suggest that, despite regular weight reductions, high-school wrestling does not affect normal growth. One explanation might be that the dietary restrictions are only brief and compensated for by a higher energy intake after competitions.

Lower resting energy expenditure (REE) in wrestlers with large weight fluctuations (weight-cycling) has been found in a cross-sectional study.[34] It was proposed that a persistent reduction of REE could increase the susceptibility for obesity. However, subsequent longitudinal studies did not confirm the suggestion that REE would be permanently decreased in weight-cyclers.[29]

Dehydration increases the specific gravity of urine, but this change is transient.[6] The same study[6] also showed an increased excretion of leucine aminopeptidase, an indicator of kidney damage. Moreover, dehydration increases the concentration of calcium and oxalate in the urine. This condition might lead to the formation of kidney stones in individuals with defects in calcium or oxalate excretion. Recently, a case of serious kidney-stone pathology in a young, female élite gymnast was recorded during the Dutch national team selection (Saris, personal observations). However, it is uncertain whether repeated dehydration procedures cause any damage to kidneys later in life.[26]

Abuse of thiazide or loop diuretics may cause hypokalaemia and metabolic acidosis, which increases the risk for severe cardiac disorders.[35] In addition to hypokalaemia, the frequent use of laxatives are associated with a wide variety of medical problems of the gastrointestinal tract, such as loss of colonic peristalsis and bleeding.[35] Consequently, the use of diuretics and laxatives should be strongly discouraged for both medical and sports ethical reasons.

Gradual weight reduction and athletic performance

Weight reduction and physical performance in obese people

Obesity, together with associated metabolic disturbances (high blood pressure, hypercholesterolaemia, glucose intolerance), are prevailing health problems of the modern Western society. The effects of a restricted energy intake (weight-reducing diet) or increased physical exercise on weight loss, composition of weight loss, and physical performance, in obese people, are briefly reviewed below. A thorough review of weight reduction in the obese is beyond the scope of this chapter, and readers are referred to excellent reviews on this topic.[3,36-38]

Table 3 Weight loss and energy intake in athletes during gradual weight reduction

Duration (week)	Rate of loss (kg/week)	Total loss (kg)	Loss as per cent of weight	FFM loss (%)	Energy intake (kJ/kg)	Ref.
1.0	3.6	3.6	4.6	39	75	43
1.0	4.0	4.0	4.9	67	75	43
1.0	2.4	2.4	3.1	33	88	44
3.0	1.2	3.7	5.0		98	9
3.0	1.6	5.0	8.1	16	87	45
3.0	1.6	5.0	8.8	10	94	45
3.7	2.4	8.9	10.0		93	46
3.7	0.8	3.0	4.4		127	46
3.7	1.9	7.1	8.0	32	100	47
3.9	0.7	2.7	4.7		117	48
7.0	0.6	4.3	7.8	51	134	49
8.0	0.8	6.0	6.3	58	215	50
9.0	0.6	5.4	9.0	26		17
12.0	0.3	3.4	5.2	47	108	51

Columns: Duration of weight reduction (weeks); rate of weight loss (kg/week); weight loss (as kg and percentage of body weight); loss of fat-free body mass (as per cent of total weight loss); daily energy intake; ref., reference.

Obesity (increased body-fat mass) is ultimately caused by a long-term, positive energy balance. Usually most (70 to 80 per cent) of the energy surplus is stored as fat, and the remaining as fat-free supporting tissue.[39] Conversely, weight loss, including both fat and fat-free body compartments, is achieved by a negative energy balance.

Weight reduction is usually achieved by a low-energy diet (5 to 7 MJ/day, 1200 to 1600 kcal/day) for a period of 2 to 12 months. An average weekly weight loss is 0.5 kg, out of which about 75 per cent is fat.[36] Very low energy diets (VLED), also referred to as very low calorie diets (VLCD), are specially designed for a more rapid weight loss. The daily energy intake of a very low energy diet is 1700 to 3300 kJ (400 to 800 kcal), providing at least 50 g protein and 40 g carbohydrate. Very low energy diets are eaten for 8 to 16 weeks,[40] and a typical weight loss is 10 to 25 kg (more than 1 kg/week). VLED and VLCD are commercially available, low-energy diets.

The fat to fat-free body mass ratio in weight reduction by commercially available VLED is 3:1, that is to say similar to the weight reduction achieved by low-energy diets.[41,42] During the first week or two of a severely energy-restricted diet, however, the proportional loss of fat-free mass is greater (about 50 per cent of the total weight loss), because of rapid losses of water and glycogen.[42]

The weight reductions achieved by aerobic exercise programmes in obese people, while on a weight-maintenance diet, are only modest (2 to 4 kg).[36,38] Practically all of this weight loss is fat mass. Resistance training leads to a fat loss of 1 to 2 kg, but to a similar increase in fat-free body mass.[36] Hence, body weight in obese people is hardly affected by resistance training.

Physical exercise is often used as a supplement to a low-energy diet or VLED in weight-reduction programmes. The additional effects of exercise on weight loss or the maintenance of fat-free body mass are positive, although moderate.[36,38] In a recent meta-analysis,[36] the average weight loss in obese, sedentary subjects, while on a low-energy diet, was 0.5 kg/week. The corresponding weight reductions in people undertaking additional aerobic or resistance exercise was 0.7 and 0.4 kg/wk, respectively. The mean weekly weight losses on VLEDs were 1.2 kg (sedentary), 1.5 kg (aerobic), and 1.4 kg (resistance). Fat-free mass loss in sedentary subjects was approximately 25 per cent of the total weight loss, while the corresponding proportion in exercising obese subjects was 15 to 20 per cent.

In obese people, energy restriction alone does not affect maximal oxygen uptake, whereas the effects on submaximal aerobic endurance are divergent.[3] Muscle strength in obese people is not usually affected by weight reduction. Adding aerobic exercise to a weight-reducing diet has positive effects on both maximal and submaximal aerobic capacity.[41] Resistance training, when used as a supplement to energy restriction, improves obese people's muscle strength, even in combination with energy restriction.[3]

Gradual weight reduction in athletes

Gradual weight reduction has been examined in a limited number of studies (Table 3), of which four were case reports.[45,47,49,50] Data on female athletes are scarce.[17,48] The duration of weight reduction varied between 1 and 12 weeks. The amount of weight lost (3 to 10 per cent of body weight, on average) was similar to rapid methods (see Table 1). Weekly weight loss was from a slow 0.3 kg to a considerable 3.8 kg. It seems that athletes are able to reduce their weight by dietary means at a similar rate as obese subjects.

Reduction of dietary energy intake was the primary technique used to achieve a gradual weight loss. The daily energy content of a weight-reducing diet was typically between 75 and 134 kJ/kg body weight (20 to 30 kcal/kg). For athletes with body weights of 55 and 80 kg, a weight-reducing diet would thus contain approximately 5500 kJ (1300 kcal) and 8000 kJ (1900 kcal) per day, respectively. In general, the fat content was low (12 to 33 per cent of the total energy intake, En per cent) and both protein and carbohydrate contents high.

Not surprising, the lower the energy intake, the faster the weekly weight loss (Table 3). Diets with less than 100 kJ/kg (less than 25 kcal/kg) body weight resulted in more than a 1 kg/week weight loss. A more moderate energy restriction (105 to 135 kJ/kg) led to a weight reduction of approximately 0.5 kg/wk. Information on daily exercise was inadequate, but most subjects in the above studies were involved in daily competitive wrestling or bodybuilding training.

A peculiar exception to studies with restricted energy intake during gradual weight reduction was one case report:[50] a male body-builder had a daily energy intake of 215 kJ/kg (29.4 MJ or 7000 kcal/day) and yet lost weight (0.75 kg/week). He was reported to train 5 h daily to accomplish the weight-reduction schedule.

There are two main reasons why increased activity is not the typical method for forced weight-reduction in athletes: first, in lean, untrained subjects,[52] and in athletes,[53] increased energy expenditure seems to be spontaneously counterbalanced by changes in energy intake, so that individuals remain in energy balance. Moreover, while endurance athletes show a considerable seasonal variation in energy expenditure,[53] large changes might be more difficult for weight-class athletes and gymnasts.

Gradual weight reduction and physical performance

The effects of gradual weight reduction on aerobic performance in athletes are seemingly dependent on the way that aerobic capacity is expressed. Maximal oxygen uptake capacity, as l/min, deteriorates[17,49] or remains unchanged.[45] In contrast, when expressed in relation to body weight (ml/kg per min), maximal oxygen uptake might even increase.[45,49] Nevertheless, in a Norwegian study,[17] a training-induced increase in weight-related maximal oxygen uptake was found in weight-stable controls, but not in élite skiers who reduced their body weight by 9 per cent in 9 weeks.

Changes in anaerobic performance are related to the weight-reducing diet's carbohydrate content. When reducing weight gradually with a 'normal-carbohydrate diet' (the proportion of carbohydrates was 50 En per cent and carbohydrate intake was 2.5 g/kg), anaerobic performance was impaired.[44] Similarly, reduced uphill running capacity was found in two wrestlers after gradual weight reduction.[45] In contrast, anaerobic performance was not affected after gradual weight loss with a higher (3.2 to 4.1 g/kg) daily intake of carbohydrate.[9,44]

The effects of gradual weight reduction on muscle endurance and strength are variable. Isometric muscle endurance was reduced,[43,45] whereas isotonic endurance was unaffected after gradual weight reduction.[43] An adequate dietary carbohydrate intake might be important for the preservation of muscle endurance in strength tests,[43] particularly when expressed against body weight. Vertical jumping performance seems to improve rather than worsen after gradual weight reduction.[9,45]

Physiological consequences of gradual weight reduction

Carbohydrate and protein balance

Carbohydrate balance plays a central role in maintaining an athlete's performance and training capacity during heavy training. For instance, in a study on swimmers during an extremely strenuous training period, an inability to sustain increased training load was associated with relatively normal (5.3 g/kg) dietary carbohydrate intake and reduced muscle glycogen stores.[54] Symptoms of over-training were not observed with a higher carbohydrate intake (8.2 g/kg). In extreme cases, such as professional cyclists, a carbohydrate intake approaching 12 g/kg body weight might be needed to ensure restorage of muscle glycogen stores in 24 h after strenuous exercise.[55]

During both rapid[12] and gradual[43,44] weight reduction, dietary carbohydrate intake seems to have an important role in preserving physical performance. Assuming a typical weight-reducing diet with 100 kJ (25 kcal)/kg body weight, a high carbohydrate proportion (70 En per cent) would provide 4.2 g/kg (1 g carbohydrate = 16.7 kJ). This amount is clearly low for endurance athletes,[54,55] but might barely be enough to keep weight-class athletes and gymnasts in carbohydrate balance during weight reduction. However, during both gradual and rapid weight reduction, the daily carbohydrate intake is typically only 2.5 to 3.5 g/kg.[43–45,47,51]

Negative protein balance and reduced muscle mass are both concerns during energy restriction. Decreased serum prealbumin and retinol-binding protein concentration, and a decreased ratio between essential amino acids and total amino acids, has been reported in wrestlers during the competition season.[51] It was suggested that liver protein synthesis might have been reduced due to a low protein intake.[51]

A higher protein intake (1.6 g/kg), instead of the standard recommendation (0.8 g/kg) might be needed to maintain the body nitrogen balance during weight reduction with a low-energy diet (6100 kJ/day).[43] Nitrogen balance studies are, however, difficult to carry out, and the results are variable. In another study, a protein intake of 1.0 g/kg was enough to maintain nitrogen balance in boxers during a 9-day weight reduction (6.7 MJ/day).[56]

In most of the gradual weight-reduction studies on athletes, the proportion of fat-free mass loss to total weight loss was 26 to 67 per cent (Table 3). Compared with obese people,[36] athletes seem to lose proportionally more fat-free mass during weight reduction, perhaps because of their initially lower fat mass.[42] Nevertheless, because of the lack of precision in assessing small body-composition changes accurately (see Chapter 1.5), this interpretation should be taken cautiously.

Vitamin and mineral balance

Vitamin and mineral intakes are strongly associated with total energy intake.[57,58] The close relation between energy and iron intake in 419 élite Dutch athletes is shown in Fig. 5. Consequently, it is logical that dietary vitamin and mineral intakes are low particularly during gradual weight reduction.[9,59] Because athletes are overly concerned with their micronutrient intake even during weight maintenance, additional worry about micronutrient balance during weight reduction is to be expected.

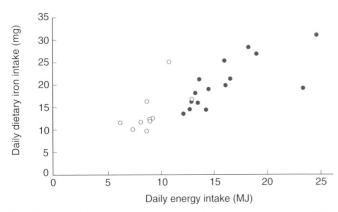

Fig. 5 The association between energy and iron intake in various groups of Dutch athletes. Dark circles, males; open circles, females. (Data from refs 2 and 57.)

Little is known about micronutrient status during gradual weight reduction in athletes (for aspects of electrolyte balance during rapid weight loss). In a study of Finnish male wrestlers and judo athletes, erythrocyte enzyme activities and serum concentrations were used as indicators of micronutrient status during weight loss.[9] Indicators for thiamin, riboflavin, potassium, iron, and zinc status did not change during a 3-week dieting period without micronutrient supplementation. Changes in indicators for vitamin B₆ and magnesium showed negative responses.

Vitamin B₆, a cofactor for glycogen phosphorylase, and magnesium, an activator for kinases, are needed for glycolysis. Therefore, an impaired status might have affected anaerobic performance. Nevertheless, no changes in two Wingate tests separated by 30 min were found.[9] Although these results did not exclude the possibility of altered vitamin B₆ and magnesium status, the negative changes seen did not affect performance.

Micronutrient balance is under strong homeostatic regulation. Adaptive mechanisms are likely to prevent functional disturbances unless a negative vitamin and mineral balance is exceptionally marked and persistent. Indirect evidence for the above has been obtained from anorexia nervosa patients, who typically eat very little and exercise vigorously: blood concentrations of vitamins and minerals in anorectics are relatively sustained, excluding rare findings of decreased serum zinc concentration.[35] Analogously, unaltered serum vitamin and mineral concentrations were found in élite female ballet dancers with a reported energy intake of 7000 MJ (1670 kcal)/day.[60]

Even after a 2- to 4-month weight-reduction period, plasma concentrations of haemoglobin, sodium, calcium, magnesium, copper, zinc, and chloride in 11 bodybuilders were found to be within the reference ranges.[59] Nevertheless, because almost all of the above subjects used micronutrient supplements, the question of dietary supplement needs during long (more than 1 month) weight reductions is still open. Consequently, a low-dose, multivitamin–mineral supplementation may be recommended for athletes during long weight reductions with restricted energy intake.

Androgen hormones

Serum testosterone concentration in male wrestlers has been found to decrease during the competitive season, perhaps as a consequence of undernourishment.[61] Certain hormones (for example, testosterone) are believed to amplify anabolic processes and recovery after exercise.[62] A decrease in free or total testosterone in serum, and an increase in serum cortisol concentration, has been used as indicators of overtraining, although their validity has been questioned.[62]

Hormonal strain (serum cortisol concentration) after exhaustive exercise seemed to be less prominent following a high-carbohydrate (7.3 g/kg) than after a low-carbohydrate (3.7 g/kg) diet.[63] Hence, the role of carbohydrates in maintaining physical performance during weight reduction might, at least partly, be associated with a more positive anabolic–androgen balance.

Possible health hazards

Endocrine disorders in female athletes

Heavy training and a weight-reducing diet might stress the female endocrine system and affect both sports performance and health. Hormonal changes, originating from a suppression in the hypothalamic–pituitary–gonadal axis, often lead to menstrual disorders, such as amenorrhoea (0 to 3 cycles per year) and oligomenorrhoea (4 to 9 cycles per year).[64] Typical findings in amenorrhoeic athletes are decreased serum oestradiol and progesterone levels, and altered luteinizing hormone and follicle-stimulating hormone secretory patterns.

Both weight loss and strenuous exercise affect reproductive hormone secretion in untrained females.[65] The effects correlate with age (more marked in younger subjects) and with the amount of weight loss.[65] In contrast to the common belief, a fixed, 'critical', amount or percentage of body fat, needed for regular menstruation, has not been established.[66]

Among athletes, the prevalence of amenorrhoea is greatest in disciplines such as running and gymnastics, in which a lean body is regarded as necessary for optimal performance.[64] The aetiology of amenorrhoea in competitive athletes is not entirely understood, but it is probably linked to weight loss, very intense training, and psychological strain.[66,67] Especially in young gymnasts and figure-skaters, an immature hypothalamic–pituitary–gonadal axis increases the susceptibility for menstrual dysfunction.[65,66]

An increased risk for stress fractures has been associated with menstrual irregularities in female athletes.[68] Endocrine disorders during adolescence might also have long-term consequences; in females, the peak bone mineral content is reached during late adolescence (between the ages of 15 and 20 years).[69] Endocrine dysfunction during this critical growth period might lead to lower peak bone mass and to an increased risk for postmenopausal osteoporosis.[68]

Weight control during puberty could theoretically affect biological maturation. Girl gymnasts are indeed smaller and they mature later than girls of a comparable age in sports without the pressure of being lean, for instance swimming.[70] It is, though, difficult to separate the effects of physical strain, energy restriction, and genetic predisposition to delayed puberty.[70] Especially so, because the relationship between dietary intake and growth is inadequately documented.

Although participation in sport does not seem to interfere with growth, it is recommended that the growth diagrams (height-for-age, weight-for-age, weight-for-height) of athletes at risk (for example, gymnasts and figure-skaters) are routinely monitored during puberty. Low height-for-age and weight-for-height parameters in girl gymnasts are to be expected at any chronological age.[71] However, if there is a sudden retardation in the normal growth pattern, determinants of energy and nutrient balance (training volume and intensity, dietary intake) should be examined carefully.

Dieting and weight reduction: risk for eating disorders?

Dieting and weight reduction in athletes have been linked to an increased risk of subclinical and clinical eating disorders (anorexia nervosa, bulimia nervosa).[72,73] The main arguments behind this hypothesis are the associations between dieting and eating disorders, in general,[74] and the results of an apparently increased prevalence for eating disorders in athletes participating in sports where there is great pressure for a lean body habitus.[75]

Eating disorders are seemingly most prevalent among female runners, gymnasts, and ballet dancers.[72,73,75] However, because almost all studies used self-administered questionnaires to assess behaviour and attitudes associated with eating problems, the real prevalence of clinical eating disorders is not known. Even less is known about eating disorders in male athletes, but rowers and wrestlers in low-weight classes might be considered a high-risk population.[76,77] The above results support the hypothesis that weight or appearance-dependent sports include factors that increase the risk for disordered eating and even for clinical eating disorders.

In a Norwegian study, 103 female athletes, previously classified as being at risk for eating disorders, were interviewed.[78] A group of 30 athletes, not identified as having a risk for eating disorders, were used as controls. Of the at-risk athletes 85 per cent were dieting, but only 10 per cent of them had received guidance for weight loss. All of the dieting athletes wanted to improve performance by weight loss, but 40 per cent also wanted to look better. Only 27 per cent of the controls were dieting, and 75 per cent of them had guidance. Appearance was a reason for weight reduction in only 25 per cent of the control athletes. Evidently, dieting without guidance, and with an intention to improve appearance, may be risk factors for the development of eating disorders in female athletes.

Appearance seems to be a typical motivation for weight control in female athletes, whereas males are solely interested in performance.[19,78] For instance, eating problems in wrestlers seem to be associated with making weight before competitions, because preoccupation with food almost disappears after the season.[4]

Practical recommendations for athletes and coaches

The concept of ideal body weight and composition

Body weight composition and competition success

Body composition is, to a certain extent, related to success in events where the body has to be moved against gravity (running, jumping), or where a lean appearance is required for aesthetic reasons. Concern about individual variability has led to recommended body-fat ranges rather than one 'optimal' value.[1] Even so, there appears to be

no evidence showing that an athlete's competitive success could be improved simply by reducing his or her weight to within the recommended range. Evidently, genetic endowment and strenuous training are the main reasons for both low body-fat content and competitive success.

An optimal body-fat range for physical performance and for appearance are not necessarily identical. A muscular, technical, and flexible female gymnast might be physically competent, but her competition success would be modest because she 'does not look good'. Only athletes achieving both physical requirements and aesthetic norms are successful at an international élite gymnastic level.

In wrestling, the association between body weight discrepancy (weight difference between the two opponents) and performance is unclear.[79] The argument for weight reduction is usually to increase strength, speed, and leverage in relation to other lighter competitors. However, the success in a wrestling tournament is not clearly related to weight increase after rehydration or to weight discrepancy between opponents.[79] Hence, the importance of reaching a lower weight-class, or to be heavier than the opponent, might be an overstatement.

Problems in estimating body-fat content

The uncertain associations between body composition and athletic performance is further complicated by problems of obtaining reliable values for body composition. Estimates of body composition are calculated by equations which contain components from measured body properties, such as body density, skinfold thicknesses, or impedance.[80] Some mathematical functions include assumptions of the physicochemical properties of the body, other equations are based on regression analyses (see Chapter 1.5).

The problems of estimating body composition are well illustrated in the admirable effort of finding valid anthropometric equations for estimating the minimum weight for high-school wrestlers (The Midwest wrestling study).[81,82] The starting point for this study was to prevent the health risks connected with dehydration and severe energy restriction, often characteristic of weight-class sports. The final aim was to use population-specific skinfold equations to predict 'minimal wrestling weight', corresponding to a body-fat content of 5 per cent.

In a large cross-validation study, 16 prediction equations were compared with underwater weighing.[81] All anthropometric and underwater weighing measurements were carefully standardized across the five collaborating laboratories. Therefore, this study showed the smallest possible error with these prediction equations.

A total of five equations appeared to be superior to all the others.[81] Of these five, two are presented in Table 4. Using these best prediction equations, the minimal standard error of fat-free mass estimate was approximately 1.7 kg for the lightweight wrestling group.[82] Hence, the estimated fat-free mass of 95 per cent for the lightweight group of wrestlers would be within ±3.4 kg (2×1.7 kg) of the result obtained by underwater weighing. Nevertheless, use of other equations, application of the wrestler equation in other athletes, and less standardized techniques will enlarge the random error and probably also introduce a systematic error. In general, individual errors in predicting an athlete's body component (fat or fat-free mass), even with the above equation, may be larger than 4 kg.

Table 4 Two recommended equations for predicting body composition in wrestlers[81]

(1) $BD = 1.0344 - (0.000554 \times [TC_{SF} + AS_{SF} + AB_{SF}]) + (0.0358 \times HT) + (0.000896 \times BT_{DM}) - (0.000949 \times BI_{DM}) + (0.000664 \times FA_{CF}) - (0.000648 \times CA_{CF})$

(2) $BD = 1.0973 - (0.000815 \times [TC_{SF} + SS_{SF} + AB_{SF}]) + (0.00000084 \times [\{TC_{SF} + SS_{SF} + AB_{SF}\}^2])$

$BF (\%) = (495/BD - 450)$

Abbreviations: BD, body density (g/cm³); $BF(\%)$, body fat proportion (% of body weight); HT, height (cm); AB_{SF}, abdomen skinfold (mm); AS_{SF}, anterior supriiliac skinfold (mm); SS_{SF}, subscapular skinfold (mm); TC_{SF}, triceps skinfold (mm); CA_{CF}, calf circumference (cm); FA_{CF}, flexed arm circumference (cm); BI_{DM}, bi-iliac diameter (cm); BT_{DM}, bitrochanteric diameter (cm).

Recommendations for weight-class sports

If the time between weigh-in and actual competition is less than 5 h, rapid weight loss should not exceed 4 per cent of body weight (Table 5). If the time for recovery and dehydration is longer than 5 h, a 4 to 8 per cent rapid weight reduction will probably not impair performance. There are no data on greater weight reductions. An extreme heat stress, caused by hot weather or a poorly air-

Table 5 Weight-control recommendations for sports

Weight-class sports

- Maximal limits for weight-loss are: 8% of body weight, if the time between weigh-in and the competition is 5–24 h; otherwise 4%.

- Combine rapid and gradual weight reduction.

- Follow a 4–7 MJ (1000–1600 kcal)/day diet with high-carbohydrate content (60–70 En% and > 4 g/kg per day) even during the rapid weight-loss phase.

- Consume carbohydrate-electrolyte drinks, together with carbohydrate-rich snacks, to restore your glycogen and water balance between the weigh-in and the competition.

- Avoid excessive postcompetition weight gain by well-balanced dietary habits.

Other sports

- Set reasonable, motivated weight goals.

- Follow a high-carbohydrate (60–65 En%), low-fat (20–25 En%), low-energy diet with a minimum daily energy intake of 100 kJ (24 kcal)/bodyweight.

- Fasting, crash diets with very low-energy content, or pathogenic weight-control methods (vomiting, laxatives, etc.) are *strictly* forbidden.

- Increase the daily amount of aerobic exercise, if possible.

- Recommended rate of weekly weight loss is 0.5–1.0 kg, maximal rate is 1.5 kg/week.

- Do not reduce weight during intensive endurance training.

- Prevent unnecessary weight gain by eating a well-balanced, high-carbohydrate diet.

En% = the proportion in the total energy intake

conditioned competition arena, is likely to amplify the negative effects of dehydration.[24]

Compared to gradual weight reduction, an advantage of a rapid technique might be a better predictability of the effort required for achieving the weight goal. A short period of diet and fluid restriction may also be mentally easier than many weeks of gradual weight loss. In contrast, a clear disadvantage is the repeated need for weight loss in tournaments of several days' duration.

For some reason, not fully apparent from scientific research, weight-class athletes prefer active rather than passive dehydration. A minimal duration for 4 to 8 per cent weight reduction might be 3 days, whereas a less than 4 per cent weight loss can be achieved in 2 days. Forced sweating and a simultaneous fluid restriction seems to be the most important factor in achieving fast weight losses. Because dietary carbohydrates might prevent some reduction in performance,[5,12] a daily energy intake of at least 100 to 120 kJ/kg or 4200 to 6700 kJ (1000 to 1600 kcal), and with a high-carbohydrate content (60 to 70 En per cent or 250 to 300 g/day), is recommended even during rapid weight reduction.

Rehydration after rapid weight loss is extremely important. There is little doubt that an optimal rehydration drink should contain glucose and electrolytes, particularly sodium (see Chapter 1.2.2). A high sodium concentration (50 to 60 mmol/l) seems to optimize fluid retention.[83] However, if an athlete finds the salty taste unpalatable, a larger volume of a normal glucose–electrolyte drink (sodium concentration 20 to 30 mmol/l) will also restore the fluid balance.[83]

A distinct advantage of gradual weight reduction is that during tournaments weight is maintained much better than after dehydration procedures. On the other hand, strenuous training in combination with a deficient diet might lead to training fatigue (overtraining) and to micronutrient, such as iron, deficiencies. Moreover, it is likely that the magnitude of weight loss by dieting is more difficult to predict. Lengthy dietary restrictions might also be mentally difficult.

To minimize the negative effects of gradual weight reduction on recovery, the diet should contain sufficient carbohydrates (at least 4 to 5 g/kg per day). Loss of some fat-free mass seems inevitable, despite a high-protein intake. Vitamin and mineral supplements are not needed, provided that the duration of energy restriction is less than 1 month. During energy restriction and weight reduction of longer duration, a low-dose (daily intakes close to the dietary recommendations), multivitamin–mineral supplementation may be considered.

A recommended option for weight-class athletes is to combine a gradual (not more than 5 per cent of body weight loss within 1 month) and rapid weight loss (2 to 5 per cent of body weight, as little as possible if the recovery between weigh-in and the competition is less than 5 h). Weight-class athletes should also be educated about how to prevent an excessive rise in body weight after competitions by consuming a well-balanced diet, and to reconsider the need for competing in a weight-class far below their natural weight.

Weight control and reduction in other sports

A reasonable way of establishing weight, body-fat percentage, or skinfold goals for athletes would be to use individual follow-up. It might then be possible to notice individual relationships between body weight or composition and performance. A significant (beyond the methodological error) increase in weight or body fat might warrant a gradual weight reduction towards the level earlier associated with maximal performance.

After establishing a reasonable weight goal, the recommended technique is a gradual weight reduction by negative energy balance (Table 5). A daily energy intake of 100 kJ/kg would lead to a weight loss of approximately 1 kg/week. There is no evidence that a slightly faster (1.5 kg/week) or slower (0.5 kg/week) weight loss would be more beneficial or harmful.

Pathogenic methods (fasting, vomiting, laxatives, diuretics, etc.) must not be used. To avoid the development of eating disorders, the weight loss should be professionally guided and not intensified by any psychological pressure, such as forbidding competitions before the weight goal has been reached.

Decreased energy intake should mainly be achieved by reduced fat intake. To ensure resynthesis of muscle glycogen after daily training, the dietary carbohydrate proportion should be maintained as high as possible, at least at 60 to 65 En per cent. On a long-term basis, a diet with a higher carbohydrate proportion (70 En per cent) might be difficult to follow. Because intense endurance exercise is particularly dependent on glycogen resynthesis (see Chapter 1.2.1) weight reduction during strenuous endurance-training periods is not recommended.

References

1. Wilmore JH. Eating and weight disorders in the female athlete. *International Journal of Sport Nutrition* 1991; 1: 104–17.
2. van Erp-Baart AMJ, Saris WHM, Binkhorst RA, Vos JA, Elvers JWH. Nationwide survey on nutritional habits in elite athletes. Part I. Energy, carbohydrate, protein and fat intake. *International Journal of Sports Medicine* 1989; 10: S3–10.
3. Walberg JL. Aerobic exercise and resistance weight-training during weight reduction. Implications for obese persons and athletes. *Sports Medicine* 1989; 7: 343–56.
4. Steen SN, Brownell KD. Patterns of weight loss and regain in wrestlers: has the tradition changed? *Medicine and Science in Sports and Exercise* 1990; 22: 762–8.
5. Webster S, Rutt R, Weltman A. Physiological effects of a weight loss regimen practised by college wrestlers. *Medicine and Science in Sports and Exercise* 1990; 22: 229–34.
6. Zambraski EJ, Foster DT, Gross PM, Foster DT, Gross PM, Tipton CM. Iowa wrestling study: weight loss and urinary profiles of collegiate wrestlers. *Medicine and Science in Sports* 1976; 8: 105–8.
7. Caldwell JE, Ahonen E, Nousiainen V. Differential effects of sauna-, diuretic- and exercise-induced hypohydration. *Journal of Applied Physiology: Respiratory, Environmental and Exercise Physiology* 1984; 57: 1018–23.
8. Klinzing JE, Karpowicz W. The effect of rapid weight loss and rehydration on a wrestling performance test. *Journal of Sports Medicine and Physical Fitness* 1986; 26: 149–56.
9. Fogelholm GM, Koskinen R, Laakso J, Rankinen T, Ruokonen I. Gradual and rapid weight loss: effects on nutrition and performance in male athletes. *Medicine and Science in Sports and Exercise* 1993; 25: 371–7.
10. Viitasalo JT, Kyröläinen H, Bosco C, Alen M. Effects of rapid weight reduction on force production and vertical jumping height. *International Journal of Sports Medicine* 1987; 8: 281–5.
11. Hickner RC, Horswill CA, Welker JM, Scott J, Roemmich JN, Costill DL. Test development for the study of physical perform-

12. Horswill CA, Hickner RC, Scott JR, Costill DL, Gould D. Weight loss, dietary carbohydrate modifications, and high intensity, physical performance. *Medicine and Science in Sports and Exercise* 1990; 22: 470–6.
13. Houston ME, Marrin DA, Green HJ, Thomson JA. The effect of rapid weight loss on physiological functions in wrestlers. *Physician and Sportsmedicine* 1981; 9: 73–8.
14. Torranin C, Smith DP, Byrd RJ. The effect of acute thermal dehydration and rapid rehydration on isometric and isotonic endurance. *Journal of Sports Medicine and Physical Fitness* 1979; 19: 1–7.
15. Armstrong LE, Costill DL, Fink WJ. Influence of diuretic-induced dehydration on competitive running performance. *Medicine and Science in Sports and Exercise* 1985; 17: 456–61.
16. Rosen LW, McKeag DB, Hough DO, Curley V. Pathogenic weight-control behavior in female athletes. *Physician and Sportsmedicine* 1986; 14: 79–86.
17. Inger F, Sundgot-Borgen J. Influence of body weight regulation on maximal oxygen uptake in female elite athletes. *Scandinavian Journal of Medicine and Science in Sports* 1991; 1: 141–6.
18. Rosen LW, Hough DO. Pathogenic weight-control behaviours of female college gymnasts. *Physician and Sportsmedicine* 1988; 16: 141–4.
19. Dummer GM, Rosen LW, Heusner WW, Roberts PJ, Counsilman JE. Pathogenic weight-control behaviours of young competitive swimmers. *Physician and Sportsmedicine* 1987; 15: 75–85.
20. Sykora L, Grilo CM, Wilfley DE, Brownell KD. Eating, weight, and diet disturbances in male and female lightweight and heavyweight rowers. *International Journal of Eating Disorders* 1993; 14: 203–11.
21. Scott JR, Horswill CA, Dick RW. Acute weight gain in collegiate wrestlers following a tournament weigh-in. *Medicine and Science in Sports and Exercise* 1994; 26: 1181–5.
22. Aragon-Vargas LF. Effects of fasting on endurance exercise. *Sports Medicine* 1993; 16: 255–65.
23. Jacobs I. The effects of thermal dehydration on performance of the Wingate anaerobic test. *International Journal of Sports Medicine* 1980; 1: 21–4.
24. Sawka MN, Francesconi RP, Young AJ, Pandolf KB. Influence of hydration level and body fluids on exercise performance in the heat. *Journal of the American Medical Association* 1984; 7: 1165–9.
25. Lamb DR, Brodowicz GR. Optimal use of fluids of varying formulations to minimise exercise-induced disturbances in homeostasis. *Sports Medicine* 1986; 3: 247–74.
26. Horswill CA. Applied physiology of amateur wrestling. *Sports Medicine* 1992; 14: 114–43.
27. Greenhaff PL, Gleeson M, Whiting PH, Maughan RJ. Dietary composition and acid-base status: limiting factors in the performance of maximal exercise in man? *European Journal of Applied Physiology* 1987; 56: 444–50.
28. Greenhaff PL, Gleeson M, Maughan RJ. The effects of dietary manipulation on blood acid-base status and performance of high intensity exercise. *European Journal of Applied Physiology* 1987; 56: 331–7.
29. Horswill CA. Weight loss and weight cycling in amateur wrestlers: implications for performance and resting metabolic rate. *International Journal of Sport Nutrition* 1993; 3: 245–60.
30. Costill DL, Cote R, Fink WJ, Van Handel P. Muscle water and electrolyte distribution during prolonged exercise. *International Journal of Sports Medicine* 1981; 2: 130–4.
31. Costill DL, Cote R, Fink W. Muscle water and electrolytes following varied levels of dehydration in man. *Journal of Applied Physiology* 1976; 40: 6–11.
32. Saris WHM. Nutritional concerns for the young athlete. In:

Rutenfranz J, Mocellin R, Klimt F, eds. *Children and exercise.* Champaign, IL: Human Kinetics, 1986: 11–19.

33. Housh TJ, Johnson GO, Stout J, Housh DJ. Anthropometric growth patterns of high school wrestlers. *Medicine and Science in Sports and Exercise* 1993; **25**: 1141–50.

34. Steen SN, Oppliger RA, Brownell KD. Metabolic effects of repeated weight loss and regain in adolescent wrestlers. *Journal of the American Medical Association* 1988; **260**: 47–50.

35. Pomeroy C, Mitchell JE. Medical issues in eating disorders. In: Brownell KD, Rodin J, Wilmore JH, eds. *Eating, body weight and performance in athletes.* Malvern: Lea and Febiger, 1992: 202–21.

36. Garrow JS, Summerbell CD. Meta-analysis: effects of exercise, with or without dieting, on the body composition of overweight subjects. *European Journal of Clinical Nutrition* 1995; **49**: 1–10.

37. Poehlman ET, Melby CL, Goran MI. The impact of exercise and diet restriction on daily energy expenditure. *Sports Medicine* 1991; **11**: 78–101.

38. Saris WHM. Exercise with and without dietary restriction and obesity treatment. *International Journal of Obesity* 1995; **19**: S113–16.

39. Saris WHM. Effects of energy restriction and exercise on the sympathetic nervous system. *International Journal of Obesity* 1995; **19**: S17–23.

40. American Dietetic Association. Position of the American Dietetic Association: very-low-calorie weight loss diets. *Journal of the American Dietetic Association* 1990; **90**: 722–6.

41. Saris WHM, van Dale D. Effects of exercise during VLCD diet on metabolic rate, body composition and aerobic power: pooled data of four studies. *International Journal of Obesity* 1989; **13**: 169–70.

42. Prentice AM, Goldberg GR, Jebb SA, Black AE, Murgatroyd PR, Diaz EO. Physiological responses to slimming. *Proceedings of the Nutrition Society* 1991; **50**: 441–58.

43. Walberg JL, Leidy MK, Sturgill DJ, Hinkle DE, Tichey SJ, Sebolt DR. Macronutrient content of a hypoenergy diet affects nitrogen retention and muscle function in weight lifters. *International Journal of Sports Medicine* 1988; **9**: 261–6.

44. McMurray RG, Proctor CR, Wilson WL. Effect of caloric deficit and dietary manipulation on aerobic and anaerobic exercise. *International Journal of Sports Medicine* 1991; **12**: 167–72.

45. Maffulli N. Making weight: a case study of two elite wrestlers. *British Journal of Sports Medicine* 1992; **26**: 107–10.

46. Hickson JF, Coleman AE, Frank PR, Gordon DE, Kish K. Four strategies for body weight control in athletics. *Nutrition Research* 1989; **9**: 1109–17.

47. Hickson JF, Johnson TE, Lee WL, Sidor RJ. Nutrition and the precontest preparations of a male bodybuilder. *Journal of the American Dietetic Association* 1990; **90**: 264–7.

48. Walberg-Rankin J, Edmonds CE, Gwazdkauskas FC. Diet and weight changes of female bodybuilders before and after competition. *International Journal of Sport Nutrition* 1993; **3**: 87–102.

49. Widerman PM, Hagan RD. Body weight loss in a wrestler preparing for competition: a case report. *Medicine and Science in Sports and Exercise* 1982; **14**: 413–18.

50. Manore MM, Thompson J, Russo M. Diet and exercise strategies of a world-class bodybuilder. *International Journal of Sport Nutrition* 1993; **3**: 76–86.

51. Horswill CA, Park SH, Roemmich JN. Changes in the protein nutritional status of adolescent wrestlers. *Medicine and Science in Sports and Exercise* 1990; **22**: 599–604.

52. Woo R, Pi-Sunyer FX. Effects of increased physical activity and voluntary intake in lean women. *Metabolism* 1985; **34**: 836–41.

53. Fogelholm M, Rehunen S, Gref C-G, *et al.* Dietary intake and thiamin, iron and zinc status in elite Nordic skiers during different training periods. *International Journal of Sports Nutrition* 1992; **2**: 351–65.

54. Costill DL, Flynn MG, Kirwan JP, *et al.* Effects of repeated days of intensified training on muscle glycogen and swimming performance. *Medicine and Science in Sports and Exercise* 1988; **20**: 249–54.

55. Saris WHM, van Erp-Baart MA, Brouns F, Westerterp KR, ten Hoor F. Study on food intake and energy expenditure during extreme sustained exercise: the Tour de France. *International Journal of Sports Medicine* 1989; **10**: S26–31.

56. Morita Y, Igawa S, Takahashi H, Tomida K, Hirota K. Effects of rapid weight reduction on protein metabolism and physical performance (in Japanese). *Annals of Physiological Anthropology* 1991; **10**: 25–33.

57. van Erp-Baart AMJ, Saris WHM, Binkhorst RA, Vos JA, Elvers JWH. Nationwide survey on nutritional habits in elite athletes. Part II. Mineral and vitamin intake. *International Journal of Sports Medicine* 1989; **10**: S3–10.

58. Fogelholm M. Vitamins, minerals and supplementation in soccer. *Journal of Sports Sciences* 1994; **12**: S23–7.

59. Kleiner SM, Bazzarre TL, Litchford MD. Metabolic profiles, diet, and health practices of championship male and female bodybuilders. *Journal of the American Dietetic Association* 1990; **90**: 962–7.

60. Cohen JL, Potosnak L, Frank O, Baker H. A nutritional and hematologic assessment of elite ballet dancers. *Physician and Sportsmedicine* 1985; **13**: 43–54.

61. Strauss RH, Lanese RR, Malarkey WB. Weight loss in amateur wrestlers and its effects on serum testosterone levels. *Journal of the American Medical Association* 1985; **254**: 3337–8.

62. Kuipers H, Keizer H. Overtraining in elite athletes. Review and directions for the future. *Sports Medicine* 1988; **6**: 79–92.

63. Anderson RA, Bryden NA, Polansky MM, Thorp JW. Effects of carbohydrate loading and underwater exercise on circulating cortisol, insulin and urinary losses of chromium and zinc. *European Journal of Applied Physiology* 1991; **63**: 146–50.

64. De Souza MJ, Metzger DA. Reproductive dysfunction in amenorrheic athletes and anorexic patients: a review. *Medicine and Science in Sports and Exercise* 1991; **23**: 995–1007.

65. Schweiger U, Laessle R, Pfister H, *et al.* Diet-induced menstrual irregularities: effects of age and weight loss. *Fertility and Sterility* 1987; **48**: 746–51.

66. Loucks AB. Athletics and menstrual dysfunction in young women. In: Gisolfi CV, Lamb DR, eds. *Perspectives in exercise science and sports medicine. Volume 2: Youth, exercise and sport.* Indianapolis: Benchmark Press, Inc., 1989: 513–38.

67. Highet R. Athletic amenorrhea. An update on aetiology, complications and management. *Sports Medicine* 1989; **7**: 82–108.

68. Constantini NW. Clinical consequences of athletic amenorrhea. *Sports Medicine* 1994; **17**: 213–23.

69. Haapasalo H, Kannus P, Stevänen H, *et al.* Development of mass, density, and estimated mechanical characteristics of bones in Caucasian females. *Journal of Bone and Mineral Research* 1996; **11**: 1751–60.

70. Mansfield MJ, Emans SJ. Growth in female gymnasts: should training decrease during puberty? *Journal of Pediatrics* 1993; **122**: 237–40.

71. Peltenburg AL, Erich ML, Zonderland ML, Bernink MJE, van den Brande JL, Huisveld IA. A retrospective growth study of female gymnasts and girl swimmers. *International Journal of Sports Medicine* 1984; **5**: 262–7.

72. Leon GR. Eating disorders in female athletes. *Sports Medicine* 1991; **12**: 219–27.

73. Wilmore JH. Body weight standards and athletic performance. In: Brownell KD, Rodin J, Wilmore JH, eds. *Eating, body weight and performance in athletes.* Malvern: Lea and Febiger, 1992: 315–29.

74. Hsu LKG. *Eating disorders.* New York: The Guilford Press, 1990.

75. Sundgot-Borgen J. Prevalence of eating disorders in elite female athletes. *International Journal of Sport Nutrition* 1993; **3**: 29–40.

76. Enns MP, Drewnowski A, Grinker JA. Body composition, body size estimation, and attitudes towards eating in male college athletes. *Psychosomatic Medicine* 1987; **49**: 56–64.

77. Thiel A, Gottfried H, Hesse FW. Subclinical eating disorders in male athletes. A study of the low weight category in rowers and wrestlers. *Acta Psychiatrica Scandinavica* 1993; **88**: 259–65.

78. Sundgot-Borgen J. Risk and trigger factors for the development of eating disorders in female elite athletes. *Medicine and Science in Sports and Exercise* 1994; **26**: 414–19.

79. Horswill CA, Scott JR, Dick RW, Hayes J. Influence of rapid weight gain after the weigh-in on success in collegiate wrestlers. *Medicine and Science in Sports and Exercise* 1994; **26**: 1290–4.

80. Wang Z-M, Heshka S, Pierson RN, Heymsfield SB. Systematic organization of body-composition methodology: an overview with emphasis on component-based methods. *American Journal of Clinical Nutrition* 1995; **61**: 457–65.

81. Thorland WG, Tipton CM, Lohman TG, *et al*. Midwest wrestling study: prediction of minimal weight for high school wrestlers. *Medicine and Science in Sports and Exercise* 1991; **23**: 1102–10.

82. Lohman TG. *Advances in body composition assessment*. Champaign, IL: Human Kinetics, 1992.

83. Maughan RJ, Leiper JB. Sodium intake and post-exercise rehydration in man. *European Journal of Applied Physiology* 1995; **71**: 311–19.

1.2.4 Nutritional ergogenic aids/ supplements and exercise performance

Melvin H. Williams

Introduction

The popularity of sport is a worldwide phenomenon, and athletes who are triumphant may receive substantial personal and financial rewards. Athletes at all levels of competition, from the élite international performer to the local 10 km-road race, age–group award contender, are attempting to attain their personal best in order to be successful. Currently there are literally scores of different organized competitive sports, and each sport demands sport-specific task characteristics that are important for success, such as strength, power, endurance, and agility, among others. Often such task characteristics are referred to as exercise performance or physical performance tasks, and these terms will be used interchangeably with sport performance in this review.

Genetic endowment with sport-specific task characteristics is an important criterion for success in any given sport. Specific sport training is another. An athlete may inherit the necessary sport-specific task characteristics, but performance will not be optimized if the athlete has not received appropriate sport-specific training. At the United States Olympic Training Center, and at other national sport training facilities, the training programme of the élite athlete usually involves three major elements: (1) training for physical power; (2) training for mental strength; and (3) training for a mechanical edge.

These three factors all relate to human energy: the capacity we have to move our bodies, including the diverse movement patterns in sport. Physical power relates to energy production; mental strength refers to energy control; and mechanical edge represents energy efficiency. Physical power, or energy production, is the crux of the three, because mental strength simply helps control energy production and a mechanical edge provides the most efficient application of energy to the desired movement. In essence, physical power for human movement is provided by three distinct energy systems. The adenosine triphosphate–phosphocreatine (**ATP–PCr**) energy system is designed to replace ATP very rapidly. It is the predominant energy system in very short-duration, high-power events, ranging from 1 to 20 seconds or so, such as the shot put, the 100 m race in running, and the 50 m sprint in swimming. The lactic acid energy system involves a series of reactions for the rapid breakdown of muscle glycogen (glycolysis) when the oxygen supply is limited (anaerobic conditions); lactic acid is produced, but in the process ATP is generated rapidly. The lactic acid system (anaerobic glycolysis) is the predominant energy system in short-duration, high-intensity events lasting from 30 to 120 s, such as the 400 and 800 m races in running, and the 100 and 200 m races in swimming. The oxygen energy system involves the complete combustion of either carbohydrate or fat via the Krebs cycle and an electron transport system. Although both carbohydrate (aerobic glycolysis) and fat (aerobic lipolysis) may be used as fuel sources for the oxygen system, carbohydrate is the more efficient, that is to say it produces more ATP per unit of oxygen than does fat. The oxygen system predominates in prolonged endurance events lasting from 5 min to several hours, such as a 5-km road race, a 1500-m swim, or very prolonged endurance events such as the 26.2-mile (42.2 km) marathon run.

Although the sport coach (trainer) is primarily responsible for optimizing the athlete's physical power for competition, sport scientists may also contribute significantly to the athlete's total preparation. Sport physiologists may monitor various metabolic and physiological responses during training to enhance the development of physical power. Sport psychologists may teach the athlete appropriate psychological strategies to increase mental strength. Sport biomechanists may improve the athlete's technique or equipment to provide a mechanical edge. Sport physicians, sport nutritionists and, in some cases, sport pharmacologists, may complement the scientific approach to training the athlete. The total training programme for the élite athlete is designed to maximize the opportunities for success.

Athletes may also resort to other means in attempts to enhance sport success beyond that attainable through genetics and training. These means are often referred to as ergogenic aids, or ergogenics, and may include a variety of approaches to modify favourably physical power, mental strength, and mechanical efficiency. Ergogenics can be grouped into five categories:[1]

(1) pharmacological aids, or drugs, such as anabolic steroids;

(2) physiological aids, or normal body constituents, such as sodium bicarbonate;

(3) psychological aids, or mental techniques, such as hypnosis;

(4) mechanical or biomechanical aids, such as aerodynamically designed bicycles; and

(5) nutritional aids, such as special dietary supplements.

The legality of specific ergogenic aids is determined by specific athletic-governing bodies, such as the International Olympic Committee (**IOC**) and its specific sport federations. In general, most pharmacological agents that may enhance performance, known as doping, are prohibited. Some physiological aids such as erythrocyte infusion (blood doping) are prohibited, while others are not, for example ingestion of sodium bicarbonate. Mechanical or biomechanical aids (if accepted by the sport federation) and psychological aids are generally legal. No nutrient or dietary supplement is currently prohibited unless the supplement contains a prohibited pharmacological agent, such as ephedrine which can be found in some commercial dietary supplements.

Pharmacological, physiological, and nutritional aids are designed to be taken into the athlete's body, mostly orally, to exert their purported ergogenic effect. Because the use of illegal pharmacological and physiological ergogenics may be grounds for suspension from sport competition, there has been considerable research in attempts to find effective, legal nutritional ergogenic aids that may enhance physical power, increase mental strength, or provide a mechanical edge.

The six major classes of nutrients in the foods we eat (carbohydrates, fats, proteins, vitamins, minerals, and water) subserve three general physiological functions in the body: they provide energy, promote growth and development, and regulate metabolic processes. Although each class of nutrients may serve many functions in the body, in general, carbohydrate and fat provide energy, protein is important for growth and development, while vitamins, minerals, and water help regulate metabolic processes. Within each major class of nutrients there are a number of essential and nonessential nutrients, each with specific functions in the body; for example, the human organism needs 13 specific vitamins and about 20 minerals.

In the past, a balanced diet of wholesome, natural foods was the main means by which athletes obtained essential nutrients. However, vitamins and minerals became available commercially as individual nutrients were identified, isolated, and mass-produced. Because many vitamins and minerals are important to those physiological processes relevant to sport performance, they were among the first dietary supplements to be marketed to athletes. In more recent years, increased research and knowledge relative to the interaction of nutrition and sport performance, coupled with rapid advances in nutritional biotechnology, have led to the development of a variety of dietary supplements targeted to physically active individuals. Specific nutrients which may possess pharmaceutical properties when consumed in adequate amounts, for instance vitamin E supplementation to prevent unwanted lipid peroxidation during exercise, have been termed nutraceuticals. Plant extracts which may elicit physiological effects favourable to exercise performance, for example ginseng and resistance to the stress of exercise, are known as phytochemicals. Other dietary supplements may be designed to augment the store of endogenous physiological substances which are involved in those metabolic reactions important to exercise, for example ubiquinone 50 (CoQ10) and oxidative processes, because

they are either found in small amounts in the diet or formed in the body in small amounts. Often, dietary supplements for athletes contain multiple ingredients.

Table 1 lists various nutrients, plant compounds, commercial supplements, and associated nutritional products which have been studied for their potential ergogenic properties. As discussed in other chapters in this textbook, some have been found to be effective, such as carbohydrate and fluid replenishment in prolonged aerobic endurance events. Most nutritional ergogenics in Table 1 are thought to enhance physical power via one of the three basic functions of nutrients, namely: directly supplying a source of energy; promoting the development of power-generating tissues; or regulating the energy metabolism pathways. For example, creatine supplementation may help to increase endogenous levels of creatine phosphate, an important source of energy in short-term, high-intensity exercise. It has been suggested that amino-acid supplementation, such as arginine and ornithine, enhances the development of muscle mass in attempts to increase muscle power. Carnitine supplementation theoretically will enhance fatty acid utilization during exercise, sparing muscle glycogen for later use during endurance events. Some nutrients may also be used to increase mental energy or provide a mechanical edge. Branched-chain amino-acid supplementation is thought to prevent central nervous system (mental) fatigue during prolonged aerobic exercise, while chromium supplementation is postulated to reduce excess body fat, which would improve mechanical efficiency in sports where the bodyweight must be moved efficiently, such as running.

In the past, and even today, the use of purported nutritional ergogenics was based primarily on folklore, individual testimony, unsupported theoretical considerations, and poorly controlled experimental research. Most likely, an athlete would not use an ergogenic if it was ineffective. But how does the athlete know whether or not a specific ergogenic will enhance his or her sport performance? Several lines of evidence may be used, but the most compelling would be consistent findings in properly designed laboratory and field research investigations.

A legitimate rationale must exist for the use of the purported nutritional ergogenic; that is to say, the ergogenic, theoretically, should be able to influence favourably physiological, psychological, or biomechanical factors associated with enhanced performance in specific sport characteristics. Given such a justification, Sherman and Lamb[2] enumerated a number of experimental design considerations for use when investigating the efficacy of nutritional ergogenics, including an appropriate subject population, valid and reliable tests for dependent variables, random or matched assignment of subjects to treatments, double-blind protocol, placebo-control, crossover design (if possible), control of extraneous factors during the experimental period, and appropriate statistical techniques.

In all scientific disciplines, the most reputable data appear in peer-reviewed scientific journals—the three most common sources of data being individual studies, reviews by experts, and meta-analyses by statisticians—and sports science does not differ in this respect. Although individual studies provide the principal data points, a single study does not provide conclusive evidence that an ergogenic is either effective or ineffective for its stated purpose. Reviews of previously published individual studies provide a stronger foundation, but the conclusion may be influenced by the

Table 1 Some nutrients, plant compounds, commercial substances, and associated products investigated for potential ergogenic properties

Alcohol	Coenzyme Q₁₀ (ubiquinone 50)	Multivitamins/ multiminerals
Amino acid	Creatine	
Arginine		Octacosanol
Aspartates	Dihydroxyacetone	
Branched-chain	and pyruvate (DHAP)	Protein
Leucine		
Isoleucine	Dimethylglycine	Smilax
Valine		
Glutamine	Fats	Soldium bicarbonate
Glycine	Medium chain triglycerides	
Lysine		Spirulina
Ornithine	Fatty acids	
Tryptophan	Omega-3	Vitamins
		Beta-carotene
Antioxidants	Gamma oryzanol	Folic acid
		Niacin
Bee pollen	Ginseng	Pantothenate
		Pyridoxine
Caffeine	Glycerol	Riboflavin
		Thiamin
Calcium pangamate	Guarana	Vitamin B₁₂
		Vitamin B₁₅
Carbohydrates	Honey	Vitamin C
Fructose		Vitamin E
Glucose	Insosine	
Glucose polymers		Water
Soluble starches	Lecithin	
Sucrose		Wheatgerm oil
	Minerals	
Carnitine	Boron	Yohimbine
	Chromium	
Choline	Iron	
	Magnesium	
	Phosphates	
	Potassium	
	Sodium	
	Vanadium	
	Zinc	

reviewer's orientation. Meta-analyses of an adequate number of previously published individual studies provide the strongest evidence, for a meta-analysis provides a summary statistic which is derived from the statistical analyses of all the included studies. Unfortu-

nately, there are few meta-analyses available relative to the ergogenic efficacy of purported nutritional ergogenics. A number of well-documented reviews are available for some nutritional ergogenics, but for others there may be too few published reports on which to base a review.

Space does not permit coverage of all the putative ergogenics listed in Table 1, nor does it permit a detailed analysis of specific studies which have investigated each nutrient. Thus, this review will provide a broad overview of the efficacy of purported nutritional ergogenics. For some nutrients and dietary supplements, for example sodium bicarbonate and iron, there is a substantial research database involving well-controlled studies and detailed reviews. However, the database for others contains numerous studies which possess experimental design flaws (for example, ginseng), or where reports are somewhat limited (for example, chromium and ubiquinone 50 known as coenzyme Q₁₀ in the United States). This review will highlight some of the principal nutritional ergogenics in five major classes of nutrients (carbohydrates, fats, proteins, vitamins, and minerals) and other dietary supplements marketed to physically active individuals.

Carbohydrate

Carbohydrate is the preferred fuel for exercise during high-intensity, anaerobic endurance exercise, such as running a 400-m race, because it is the only fuel source for the lactic acid energy system. Carbohydrate is also the preferred fuel for exercise during high-intensity, aerobic endurance exercise, such as performing at 70 to 80 per cent of the maximal aerobic capacity, near the anaerobic threshold in trained endurance athletes, because for each litre of oxygen consumed, carbohydrate will provide more energy compared to the oxidation of fat or protein. The role of carbohydrate in exercise is detailed elsewhere in this volume, but it should be noted that numerous reviews[3-7] have documented a beneficial effect of carbohydrate supplementation prior to and during prolonged aerobic endurance exercise. Carbohydrate may also help to prevent a drop in blood levels of branched-chain amino acids (**BCAA**) and to maintain a low, free tryptophan:BCAA ratio. An increase in this ratio may facilitate the entry of tryptophan into the brain where it may increase the formation of serotonin, a neurotransmitter believed to be associated with the development of fatigue.

Carbohydrate metabolic byproducts

In glycolysis, glucose is converted into pyruvate via a series of enzymatic reactions. One theory of fatigue suggests that enzyme inactivation occurs at one of the stages in glycolysis, thus blocking the formation of pyruvate for entrance into the Krebs cycle (see Chapter 1.1.4). Thus, the ingestion or infusion of glucose metabolic byproducts beyond the blocked enzyme may bypass this limiting enzyme and provide substrate to deter the onset of fatigue. However, only a few studies have investigated the potential ergogenic effect of carbohydrate metabolites. Myers et al.[8] found that the infusion of fructose 1,6-diphosphate did not influence the metabolic responses to exercise at 70 per cent $\dot{V}O_2$max. However, in two separate studies, Stanko et al.[9,10] reported significant ergogenic effects following the ingestion of dihydroxyacetone and pyruvate (**DHAP**), a combination of two 3-carbon metabolic byproducts of glycolysis. In untrained males, the ingestion of 100 g DHAP daily for 7 days, compared with a placebo of 100 g of Polycose (a glucose polymer), increased time to exhaustion in an arm ergometer endurance task at 60 per cent $\dot{V}O_2$peak and in a leg cycle ergometer task at 70 per cent $\dot{V}O_2$peak. Even though the subjects consumed 55 to 70 per cent of their diet as carbohydrates, the DHAP supplement may have increased performance by providing more glucose to the muscle, either by increasing extraction of glucose from the blood or by increasing muscle glycogen concentrations. Although these were well-designed studies, more research is needed with trained individuals or athletes.

Fats

Fats belong to a class of compounds known as lipids. The major lipids in human nutrition are triglycerides, phospholipids, and cholesterol. Although phospholipids and cholesterol are very important substances involved in the regulation of human metabolism, the triglycerides are of primary interest for exercise because they may be used as a source of energy. They may be stored as energy reserves in various body tissues, most notably the adipose and muscle tissues.

Triglycerides are a major energy reserve in the human body, and chronic aerobic-exercise training leads to an increased utilization of triglycerides as fuel during exercise, one of the factors that may contribute to improved aerobic-exercise endurance. Free fatty acids (FFA) provide energy only via oxidative processes, and they may be derived from muscle triglycerides or mobilized from adipose tissue triglycerides for delivery by the circulation to the muscle. Because the rate at which FFA are oxidized in the muscle may be partly dependent on their concentration in the blood plasma, several techniques have been used to increase plasma FFA levels , including the infusion of triglyceride emulsions and the ingestion of medium-chain triglycerides (MCTs). Although these practices may increase plasma FFA, in a recent review Sherman[11] noted that there were insufficient data to support an ergogenic effect. Sherman further noted that it would actually be more prudent to advise endurance athletes to consume a diet that is largely carbohydrate to optimize training and competitive performance, as well as health.

Some dietary supplements derived from fats or lipids, such as wheatgerm oil, omega-3 fatty acids, glycerol, and choline, as well as other substances that may influence FFA metabolism, such as caffeine and carnitine, have been studied for their ergogenic potential and are discussed later in this chapter.

Protein and amino acids

Protein

Protein is one of the most important nutrients in human nutrition for it not only serves as the structural foundation for the body, but also governs most of its functions. Some possible roles of protein relative to sport performance include the formation of muscle protein (structural tissue), the formation of haemoglobin to transport oxygen, (transport function), the formation of enzymes involved in energy metabolism (enzyme activity), the formation of neurotransmitters (neural function), and catabolism (energy source).

Protein supplements have been recommended to athletes to enhance nitrogen retention and increase muscle mass, to prevent protein catabolism during prolonged exercise, to prevent sports anaemia, to support an increased synthesis of haemoglobin, myoglobin, oxidative enzymes, and mitochondria during aerobic train-

ing, and to restore protein which may be lost in the sweat and urine during exercise. In general, research into protein supplementation has shown no beneficial effects on strength, power, hypertrophy of muscle, or physiological work capacity; although several studies have reported greater gains in bodyweight.[12] Recent reviews by leading investigators recommend augmented protein intake in weightlifters, maturing young athletes attempting to gain muscle mass, and endurance athletes. Although this issue is still being studied, current research reviews[13,14] suggest that athletes may need slightly more protein than the RDA. Values for strength-type athletes suggest approximately 1.4 to 1.8 g per kg bodyweight, whereas recommended amounts for endurance athletes are approximately 1.2 to 1.4 g per kg bodyweight. Such values may be easily obtained in the typical athlete's diet, particularly if the athlete selects nutrient-dense foods as the source of daily energy intake.

Amino acids

Although adequate dietary protein will provide us with the recommended daily intake of all 20 amino acids, a number of specific individual amino acids have been used for ergogenic purposes because they may modify physiological processes when taken in large amounts.

Arginine, ornithine, and lysine

Supplementation with arginine, ornithine, and lysine has been used in attempts to increase human growth hormone (hGH) and insulin secretion, the theory being to increase lean-muscle mass and strength. However, current data, including results from several well-controlled studies in experienced weightlifters, do not support an ergogenic effect of these amino acids on human growth hormone levels, body composition, or various measures of muscular strength or power.[15-17]

Tryptophan

Segura and Ventura.[18] suggested that tryptophan supplementation may increase serotonin secretion and tolerance to pain. In this study, when 12 athletes ingested 1200 mg of tryptophan 24 h prior to testing on a treadmill run, it was found that not only was the time to exhaustion increased by 49 per cent at 80 per cent of $\dot{V}O_2$max, but that this was also accompanied by significant reductions in the ratings of perceived exertion (RPE). However, there was no effect on $\dot{V}O_2$ peak and the performance times were highly variable. Stensrud et al.[19] replicated this study using 49 well-trained male runners, although their subjects ran to exhaustion at 100 per cent $\dot{V}O_2$max. They reported no significant effects of tryptophan supplementation on performance. Additionally, van Hall et al.[20] reported that tryptophan supplements (approximately 3.9 g) provided during performance had no effect on cycle time to exhaustion at 70 to 75 per cent maximal power output in endurance-trained male athletes.

Branched-chain amino acids (BCAA)

BCAA supplementation has been postulated to enhance exercise performance by decreasing the free tryptophan (f-TRP):BCAA ratio in plasma. In contrast to the Segura–Ventura[18] hypothesis, Newshome[21] suggests that high levels of brain serotonin may actually induce fatigue, and that a high f-TRP:BCAA ratio will increase the formation of brain serotonin. Since BCAA compete with tryptophan for entry into the brain, elevated levels of BCAA may prevent fatigue. In a recent review, Davis[22] noted there is convincing evidence that exercise-induced increases in the f-TRP:BCAA ratio are associated with increased brain serotonin and the onset of fatigue during prolonged exercise, but that the effects of BCAA supplementation on exercise performance are mixed, with the few published studies often suffering from methodological flaws. However, several well-controlled studies have shown that BCAA supplementation does not appear to improve endurance performance. Similar to the tryptophan study cited previously, van Hall et al.[20] found that neither low (about 7.8 g) nor high (about 23.4 g) doses of BCAA provided during performance had any effect on time to exhaustion at 70 to 75 per cent maximal power output in endurance-trained male athletes. Varnier et al.[23] also reported that, in a progressive test to exhaustion, the infusion of BCAA to moderately trained, glycogen-depleted subjects did not improve endurance performance. Furthermore, Madsen et al.[24] found that BCAA supplements (18 g), when added to a glucose solution and provided before and during exercise, exerted no significant effect on 100-km cycling performance in well-trained cyclists.

Aspartates

Potassium and magnesium aspartates are salts of aspartic acid, an amino acid. Aspartate supplements have been studied for a possible ergogenic potential because they are believed to increase fatty acid metabolism and spare muscle glycogen, mitigate the accumulation of ammonia (associated with fatigue), or improve psychological motivation. Williams[12] reviewed the available literature and noted that the effect of aspartate supplementation on physical performance is equivocal. However, about 50 per cent of the available studies have indicated that these salts can enhance performance. For example, Wesson et al.[25] reported that 10 g of aspartates consumed over a 24-hour period increased endurance capacity by over 15 per cent in trained athletes, noting also increased blood levels of free fatty acids and decreased levels of blood ammonia. Additional research is needed to study the potential ergogenicity and underlying mechanisms of aspartate supplements.

Vitamins

Vitamins are complex organic compounds that influence a wide variety of metabolic functions important to exercise. Several are of particular interest.

1. Vitamins of the B complex (notably thiamin, riboflavin, and niacin) serve as coenzymes in the energy metabolic pathways of carbohydrate and fat in muscle.

2. Vitamin B_6 (pyridoxine) is involved in protein metabolism.

3. Vitamin B_{12} and folic acid are critical for the formation of red blood cells.

4. Beta-carotene, vitamin C, and vitamin E are antioxidants, which may help prevent lipid peroxidation during exercise.

A vitamin deficiency may adversely affect physical performance, and studies have shown that if vitamin supplementation corrects such a deficiency then exercise performance will improve. However, several recent major reviews of the literature[26-28] support the view that vitamin supplements are unnecessary for athletes or other physically active individuals who have a well-balanced diet with an adequate energy intake.

On the other hand, some studies have shown that specific vitamin supplements can have beneficial effects in certain conditions. In a well-controlled study, Bonke[29] reported that thiamin, pyridoxine, and cobalamin supplementation (60 to 200 times the RDA) enhanced performance in pistol shooting. They postulated that the vitamins induced brain serotonin secretion and a resultant relaxing, anxiolytic effect, thus decreasing hand tremor.

Numerous studies have been conducted to investigate a possible protective effect of antioxidant supplements (beta-carotene, vitamin C, vitamin E), either separately or in combination, against muscle tissue damage (presumably lipid peroxidation induced by reactive oxygen species) associated with strenuous exercise. While the results of these studies appear promising, several recent reviews[30-32] note that although physically trained individuals may have a greater need for antioxidants, further research is needed to determine whether antioxidant supplements prevent exercise-induced lipid peroxidation and muscle tissue damage. It is has been suggested that antioxidants, particularly vitamin E, enhance aerobic endurance performance, possibly by preventing the peroxidation of the red blood-cell membrane during exercise and optimizing oxygen delivery to the muscles. Although most studies investigating the influence of vitamin E supplementation on oxygen dynamics and exercise performance at sea level have reported no ergogenic effects, several studies have shown that vitamin E supplementation may enhance oxygen utilization during exercise at altitude.[12] These studies should be regarded as preliminary and additional research is needed for confirmation.

Minerals

Several minerals are involved in critical metabolic or physiological processes associated with exercise, and it has been postulated that they may have significant effects on various aspects of sports performance. For example, minerals may help to transport oxygen to the tissues, may function as metalloenzymes essential for energy production, or may serve as electrolytes involved in the regulation of numerous physiological processes, such as muscle contraction. Although all minerals may play a role in a variety of metabolic and physiological processes, only those minerals that have received research attention or consideration relative to possible ergogenic effects are reviewed.

Phosphorus (phosphates)

In the body, dietary phosphates are incorporated into many compounds that are involved in energy metabolism, such as ATP as an energy substrate, thiamin pyrophosphate as a vitamin cofactor, sodium phosphate as a buffer, and 2,3-diphosphoglycerate for RBC function. All these roles could provide ergogenic potential, but the most researched theory involves the effect of phosphate salt supplementation on 2,3-diphosphoglycerate levels (**2,3-DPG**). Increased levels of 2,3-DPG could facilitate the release of oxygen from haemoglobin and possibly enhance aerobic endurance exercise performance. About 12 studies have been conducted to look at the effects of phosphate salt supplementation on physical performance, and the results are clearly equivocal. Nevertheless, four well-controlled studies[33-36] have reported that phosphate supplementation may enhance exercise performance, although the underlying mechanism has not been clarified. For example, 2,3-DPG did not increase in all studies. Increased maximal oxygen uptake and improved performance on bicycle ergometer exercise tests are the most consistent findings, and although these results are impressive, several reviewers recommend additional research before any solid recommendations can be made to athletes.[37,38]

Magnesium

Magnesium is a component of over 300 enzymes, some involved in the regulation of muscle contraction, oxygen delivery, and protein synthesis. Several studies have investigated the effect of magnesium supplementation on performance and have been the focus of some brief reviews.[12,39,40,] While some studies suggest that magnesium may enhance muscular strength, possibly by increased protein synthesis, and improve running economy, other studies report no beneficial effects on similar performance parameters. Reviewers note possible confounders such as the magnesium status (possible deficiency state) of the subjects before supplementation and the form of magnesium supplementation; for example, the aspartate component may be the effective ergogenic in magnesium aspartate and not the magnesium. All reviewers indicate that more research is needed to evaluate the effects of magnesium supplementation on physical performance.

Iron

Iron is one of the most critical minerals with implications for sports performance. Iron is a component of haemoglobin, myoglobin, cytochromes, and various enzymes in the muscle cells, all of which are involved in oxygen metabolism during aerobic-exercise energy production. Some female athletes, particularly those involved in weight-control sports, do not consume adequate amounts of iron in their daily diet and may experience either iron-deficiency anaemia or iron-deficiency without anaemia. Iron-deficiency anaemia afflicts a small percentage of female athletes; correcting an iron-deficiency anaemia with an iron supplement will improve performance.[39] Iron-deficiency without anaemia is a condition of normal haemoglobin levels, but reduced levels of serum ferritin. Iron supplementation will usually restore serum ferritin to normal, and although a few studies have reported improvement in running performance, the majority of the studies find no effects on $\dot{V}O_2max$ or various performance measures.[12,39] Iron supplementation to individuals with a normal haemoglobin and iron status does not enhance performance.[12]

Chromium

Chromium is considered to be an integral component of the glucose tolerance factor; it may affect carbohydrate, lipid, and protein metabolism since it is believed to enhance the activity of insulin. Theoretically, chromium could possibly improve the regulation of blood glucose during exercise, enhance the storage of muscle glycogen prior to exercise, and increase muscle uptake of amino acids. Although chromium supplementation might improve insulin sensitivity and help regulate carbohydrate metabolism more effectively during exercise, no research has been uncovered which has studied this effect. Most of the research has focused on the role of chro-

mium in modifying body composition, possibly enhancing the anabolic effect of insulin by incorporating more amino acids into muscle and modifying fat metabolism to lose excess body fat. Early research findings with college students and college football players suggested that chromium supplementation could help reduce body fat and increase body mass.[41] However, these studies have been criticized for improper methodology: mainly the use of skinfolds to determine body composition and no control of diet or other physical activity.[39,42] In a later study, Evans and Pouchnik[43] studied the effect of chromium tripicolinate or chromium dinicotinate on the body composition of males and females involved in an aerobics class for 12 weeks, noting a more beneficial effect of the chromium tripicolinate on lean body mass; however, there was no control group in this study. More contemporary research, using improved experimental protocols including hydrostatic weighing, basically replicated these studies but have not supported their findings.[44,45] Nevertheless, exercise may increase chromium excretion from the body; carbohydrate metabolism may increase the use of chromium; and diets containing substantial amounts of highly processed foods may be low in chromium. These factors may predispose an athlete to a chromium deficiency. If chromium supplements cure a chromium deficiency, performance may be improved. More research is needed, particularly in aerobic endurance-type events.

Boron

Boron has been marketed to bodybuilders as a potent anabolic agent, suggesting boron supplementation may increase serum testosterone levels; an exaggerated claim based on a study in postmenopausal women in whom a boron deficiency was created.[46] However, Nielsen[46] noted that boron supplements did not increase serum testosterone in healthy males. Furthermore, a recent study of bodybuilders reported no significant effects of boron supplementation on serum testosterone, lean body mass, or strength.[47]

Selenium

Selenium is a component of several enzymes, particularly glutathione peroxidase (**Gpx**) which is an important cellular antioxidant enzyme. Theoretically, selenium supplementation could prevent peroxidation of the RBC membrane and muscle cell substructures involved in oxygen metabolism, possibly enhancing aerobic-exercise performance. As noted previously, antioxidant supplements have not been shown to prevent lipid peroxidation universally. However, some studies with selenium supplementation have shown an enhancement of glutathione peroxidase status and/or reduced lipid peroxidation in athletes involved in prolonged aerobic exercise;[48-50] although, only one study evaluated the effects on performance, and there was no effect on a prolonged exercise task.[50]

Zinc, copper, and vanadium

Zinc is a component of over 100 enzymes, some of which are involved in functions important to physical performance, for example muscle energy production and protein synthesis. Copper is a component of many enzymes deemed important to exercise processes, including the proper use of iron in the formation of haemoglobin, cytochrome activity, and antioxidant activity.

Vanadium may play a role in enzymatic activity, possibly exerting insulin-like effects on glucose metabolism, enhancing glycogen synthesis and inhibiting protein degradation. Vanadium has been advertised for its potential anabolic effect.

The effect of zinc and copper supplementation on physical performance has been reviewed recently,[40,48] but only two studies with zinc and none with copper were uncovered, a rather limited database. In one study, the effects of zinc supplementation on muscular strength and endurance in sedentary women were equivocal, with some measures improving and others not being affected. In another study, zinc supplementation with approximately 33 mg/day for 30 days had no effect on $\dot{V}O_2$max.

The effect of vanadium supplementation on physical performance in humans has not been studied extensively. In a well-designed, placebo-controlled study, Fawcett *et al.*[51] reported no significant increases in anthropometrical or body composition measures in weight-training athletes during 12 weeks' oral vanadyl sulphate supplementation (0.5 (mg/kg)/day). Although both the placebo and vanadyl sulphate groups improved in four strength tests (bench press and leg extension; 1 repetition maximum (maximal amount of weight an individual can lift one time or **RM**) and 10 RM each), the vanadyl sulphate group increased strength at a faster rate for the first 4 weeks in the 1 RM extension test. There were no differences in the other strength tests. The investigators noted that this may be an anomaly, but additional research is needed to confirm this modest improvement in strength.

Multivitamin/mineral supplements

As with individual vitamin and mineral supplements, supplementation with a combination of both will not improve physical performance in athletes or other physically active individuals who have a well-balanced diet with an adequate energy intake.

Williams,[52] citing four recent well-controlled studies, found no significant ergogenic effect of prolonged multivitamin/mineral supplementation to physically active individuals. In particular, Telford *et al.*[53] found that a multivitamin/mineral supplement, containing 100 to 5000 per cent of the RDA for assorted vitamins and minerals, had no effect on either laboratory- or field sport-specific and common tests of exercise performance in highly trained athletes at the Australian Institute of Sport.

Food drugs, commercial dietary supplements, and other purported nutritional ergogenics

Several food drugs, such as caffeine and sodium bicarbonate, may be classified as nutritional ergogenics, as may numerous dietary supplements marketed to athletes. In the United States of America, the Dietary Supplement Health and Education Act of 1994,[54] defines a dietary supplement as a product added to the total diet that contains at least one of the following ingredients: a vitamin, mineral, herb or botanical derivative, amino acid, metabolite, and/or a constituent, extract, or combination of any ingredient described above. The products can be ingested in any form (tablet, capsule, powder, softgel, gelcap, or liquid), must be labelled as a dietary supplement, and cannot be represented for use as a conventional food or sole item of a meal or diet. Some may contain caffeine and sodium bicarbonate.

Caffeine

Caffeine is a stimulant drug, but because it is a natural constituent of several beverages that are consumed daily, it may be construed as a nutritional ergogenic. A therapeutic dose is between 100 and 300 mg and a 150 ml cup of coffee contains 100 to 150 mg.

Several recent reviews[55-57] have detailed theoretical mechanisms underlying the ergogenic potential of caffeine, but two of the more important appear to be its ability to stimulate the central nervous system and increase adrenaline secretion. Caffeine may also enter the muscle cell and exert favourable effects on calcium and enzyme activity. Resultant effects could include psychological arousal, increased cardiac output, increased mobilization and utilization of free fatty acids as an energy source during exercise, as well as enhanced muscle contractility.

There are literally hundreds of studies which have investigated the ergogenic potential of caffeine. Based on several recent reviews,[12,55-57] caffeine is recognized as an effective ergogenic aid for various types of physical performance. Caffeine may reduce reaction time, particularly if fatigued. Although an earlier review[58] indicated that caffeine has little effect on strength, power, speed, or local muscle endurance, a more contemporary review[55] cites several recent studies providing evidence of an ergogenic effect on such performance variables. More research is needed to confirm these findings. Caffeine may enhance performance in aerobic-exercise endurance tasks. In more prolonged events, this effect may be due to increased adrenaline levels, which may spare muscle glycogen by mobilizing free fatty acids. Although research findings are not in total agreement, caffeine may possibly increase plasma FFA levels during exercise, and this may lead to an enhanced FFA oxidation from both plasma FFA and FFA released from muscle triglycerides. Caffeine may also enhance performance in aerobic-exercise events of shorter duration, such as a 1500 m run, which would not be dependent on muscle glycogen sparing. In such cases, psychological stimulation may be the underlying mechanism. Indeed, recent research revealed that caffeine ingestion may increase work output at a standardized psychological rating of perceived exertion.[59]

It should be noted that in competitive sports, caffeine is regarded as a controlled substance; certain amounts are permitted because of its presence in commonly ingested beverages, but excess amounts constitute grounds for disqualification. However, the amounts used in studies providing evidence of an ergogenic effect are lower than the amount considered by the IOC to be doping.

Sodium bicarbonate

Sodium bicarbonate is a physiological/biochemical buffer found naturally in the body. It is considered a medicine for the treatment of gastric acidity. However, it may be regarded as a nutritional ergogenic because, as baking soda, it may be added to various recipes. Additionally, it is marketed in various forms and combinations as a dietary supplement to athletes. The popular literature has referred to sodium bicarbonate supplementation by various terms, including soda loading, soda doping, and buffer boosting. In high-intensity, anaerobic-exercise tasks, such as a 400-m race, the accumulation of lactic acid is associated with the onset of fatigue. Theoretically, sodium bicarbonate supplementation could increase natural levels in the body and more effectively buffer lactic acid, thus delaying the onset of fatigue in high-intensity, anaerobic exercise dependent on the lactic-acid energy system.

The effect of sodium bicarbonate supplementation on physical performance has been studied for over 50 years. Both laboratory and field studies have investigated its ergogenic potential. The typical protocol is to provide a dose of about 0.3 g sodium bicarbonate per kg bodyweight about 1 h prior to the exercise task, which is usually designed to elicit fatigue in 1 to 3 min.

Many studies have been conducted over the years, and about half have revealed positive effects. Several recent detailed reviews[60-64] have concluded that sodium bicarbonate is an effective ergogenic. Additionally, a recent meta-analysis[65] reported a significant effect size in high-intensity, anaerobic-exercise tasks favouring sodium bicarbonate when compared with placebo. In general, sodium bicarbonate supplementation may increase plasma pH, reduce acidosis in the muscle cell, and improve performance in high-intensity exercise tasks lasting from 1 to 7 min, particularly in repetitive tasks with short recovery intervals; in the meta-analysis,[65] there was a mean improvement of 27 per cent in studies that measured exercise time to exhaustion.

The exact mechanism by which sodium bicarbonate may elicit an ergogenic effect has not been determined. Other substances containing sodium (for example, sodium citrate, trisodium phosphate, and even sodium itself) have also been shown to improve performance.[52]

L-*Carnitine*

L-Carnitine is a water soluble, vitamin-like compound that may affect various physiological functions important in exercise; most of the effects are ergogenic in nature, but some are possibly ergolytic.[52,66] A primary function of L-carnitine is to facilitate the transfer of free fatty acids into the mitochondria to help promote FFA oxidation and thus provide energy. Theoretically, L-carnitine supplementation could enhance free fatty acid oxidation and help to spare the use of muscle glycogen, which, it is suggested, might improve prolonged aerobic-endurance capacity. In addition, the role of L-carnitine supplementation may be to facilitate the oxidation of pyruvate, which could reduce lactic acid accumulation and improve anaerobic-endurance exercise performance.[52] On the other hand, the increased oxidation of glucose could lead to an earlier depletion of muscle glycogen stores thereby impairing performance, an ergolytic effect.[66]

Although L-carnitine supplementation will increase plasma levels of carnitine, it has not been shown to consistently increase muscle carnitine levels.[52,66] The data are equivocal relative to the effects of L-carnitine supplementation on free fatty acids during exercise and $\dot{V}O_2max$, with some studies providing evidence of enhanced free fatty acid utilization and increased $\dot{V}O_2max$ and other studies showing no effect on energy metabolism.[32,52] On the other hand, research data clearly indicate that L-carnitine supplementation does not affect lactic acid accumulation in an ergogenic fashion. .[32,52] In general, where studies included physical performance measures, L-carnitine supplementation was not shown to enhance either aerobic- or anaerobic-exercise performance.[32,52] However, further research is needed to investigate the potential ergogenic effects of L-carnitine on prolonged, aerobic-endurance exercise tasks, such as marathon running, and to test for the possibility of muscle glycogen sparing and subsequent improved performance.

Ubiquinone 50 (coenzyme Q10)

Although it is a lipid, ubiquinone 50 (coenzyme Q10 or CoQ10) has characteristics in common with a vitamin. It is located primarily in the mitochondria of, for example, heart and muscle cells, and is involved in the processing of oxygen for the production of cellular energy. Ubiquinone 50 (CoQ10) is also an antioxidant. Bucci[67] cites six studies showing the beneficial effects of ubiquinone 50 (CoQ10) supplementation in various subject populations, but these studies appeared in the proceedings of a conference and do not appear to have been published in peer-reviewed journals. Moreover, each study suffered one or more experimental design flaws, for instance no control group.[12] A recent review of six well-controlled scientific studies involving ubiquinone 50 (CoQ10) supplementation, either administered alone or in combination with other putative ergogenic nutrients, indicated that although blood levels of ubiquinone 50 (CoQ10) may be increased, there was no effect on serum lactate levels, oxygen uptake, cardiac function, or anaerobic threshold during submaximal exercise; in addition, serum lactate levels and oxygen uptake during maximal exercise were unaffected. Moreover, there was no effect on time to exhaustion on a bicycle ergometer.[12]

Creatine

Creatine is a nitrogen-based organic compound which can be obtained in the diet, primarily in meat products, or formed in the body from several amino acids. In the muscle cell, creatine combines with phosphate to form creatine phosphate, a high energy compound and a main component of the ATP–PCr energy system. Creatine supplementation is postulated to increase muscle stores of phosphocreatine, an energy substrate for very short-term intense exercise, which may better maintain ATP turnover during exercise.[68]

The effect of creatine supplementation on physical performance has only been studied extensively in recent years. Both laboratory and field studies have investigated its ergogenic potential. The typical protocol is to supplement the diet with 20 to 25 g creatine monohydrate per day for about 5 to 6 days. A variety of exercise protocols have been employed, primarily very short-term, intense, repetitive exercise tasks using the ATP–PCr energy system, but effects of supplementation have also been studied relative to more prolonged exercise tasks utilizing the lactic acid and oxygen energy systems.

Two recent reviews suggest that creatine supplementation may be an effective ergogenic.[68,69] Although not all studies have shown beneficial effects, some well-controlled studies do indicate that creatine supplementation may increase muscle creatine and phosphocreatine content, and this may significantly improve performance in very short-term, intense, repetitive exercise tasks that would be dependent primarily on the ATP-PCr energy system. However, since these studies were mostly laboratory-based, involving repeated exercise bouts with limited recovery time between repetitions, additional research is needed to investigate the ergogenic potential in actual field-performance tests. The limited research available does not support an ergogenic effect of creatine supplementation on single bouts of maximal sport performance, such as a 60 m dash or 25 to 50 m swim sprints.[70]

Additionally, some research suggests creatine supplementation may enhance performance in exercise tasks dependent on the lactic acid energy system, but, again, more research is needed.[70] On the other hand, increased body mass is often noted following creatine supplementation, which may be linked to a possible impairment in endurance-running performance.[69]

In general, although current data tend to support the ergogenicity of creatine supplementation, few well-controlled studies have been performed to date and further research, particularly in the field, is still needed.

Inosine

Inosine is a nucleoside, and, based on some *in vitro* research, it has been suggested that inosine supplementation increases the amount of 2,3-diphosphoglycerate (**2,3-DPG**) in red blood cells. Increased levels of 2,3-diphosphoglycerate may facilitate the release of oxygen from the red blood cells to the muscle and enhance aerobic endurance exercise. Advertisements in bodybuilding magazines have also suggested inosine supplementation may increase muscle concentrations of ATP. Only two well-controlled studies have evaluated the purported ergogenic effect of inosine supplementation. Williams *et al.* found that 2 days of inosine supplementation (6000 mg/day) exerted no significant effect on heart rate, ventilation, oxygen consumption, or lactic acid production in highly trained runners during both submaximal and maximal exercise, nor was there any effect on performance in a 3-mile treadmill run for time.[71] Recently, Starling and colleagues reported that 5 days of inosine supplementation (5000 mg/day) did not influence peak power, end power, a fatigue index, total work, or post-test lactate levels in competitive male cyclists undertaking several cycle ergometer exercise tasks.[72] In both studies, inosine supplementation actually impaired performance in some of the tests, including run time to exhaustion in a peak oxygen uptake test[71] and time to fatigue in a supramaximal cycling sprint.[72]

Choline

Choline is a naturally occurring amine which may exist in a free state in body cells, or be a constituent of lecithin and other phospholipids. Choline is involved in fat metabolism and as a methyl donor may enhance creatine synthesis, but it has been studied for its ergogenic potential primarily because of its role as a precursor for acetylcholine, an important neurotransmitter.

Serum choline levels decreased nearly 40 per cent in runners completing a 42.2 km marathon,[73] the investigators suggesting that such reductions could elicit a reduction in acetylcholine release and impaired performance. Other investigators noted that lecithin supplementation helped prevent a decrease in serum choline levels in triathletes and adolescent runners following long-term, hard physical stress, but they did not evaluate the effects on performance.[74] No studies of choline supplementation and physical performance were presented in a recent review.[32] Subsequent to this review, a double-blind, placebo-controlled, crossover study in trained male cyclists, using a single dose of 2.43 g choline bitartrate, reported that although there was a significant increase in serum choline

levels, compared to the placebo there were no significant ergogenic effects on time to exhaustion in either a high-intensity (150 per cent $\dot{V}O_2$max) or a prolonged (70 per cent $\dot{V}O_2$max) cycle exercise test.[75] At the present time, there are no data to support choline supplementation as an effective ergogenic, but, again, further research is still needed.

Glycerol

Glycerol is an alcohol derived from triglycerides. Glycerol–water supplementation may be a more effective hyperhydration technique than water-hyperhydration alone, and by increasing body water stores, it may enhance exercise performance under heat-stress environmental conditions. Several well-controlled studies have compared water-hyperhydration with glycerol–water hyperhydration and have reported greater body retention of fluids, reduction in the thermal stress of exercise, lower heart rate, lower rectal temperature, and improved performance in cycling endurance task with the latter.[70] Contrarily, other recent studies have not reported any beneficial effects of glycerol-hyperhydration on cycle ergometer endurance performance.[70] Research data with glycerol supplementation are preliminary in nature and although some initial data are impressive, more research is needed.

Omega-3 fatty acids (Omega-3 FA)

Omega-3 fatty acids, particularly eicosapentanoic (**EPA**) and docosahexaenoic (**DHA**) fatty acids from fish oils, are polyunsaturated fats that have been postulated to be ergogenic because of several possible physiological effects in the body. One theory suggests omega-3 fatty acids may be incorporated into the RBC membrane, making it less viscous and less resistant to flow, while another theory proposes that one of the byproducts of omega-3 FA metabolism, prostaglandin E_1, may elicit a vasodilatory effect. Both of these effects could facilitate the delivery of oxygen to muscle cells and enhance aerobic endurance capacity. However, only one study has been uncovered which has studied this issue, and no significant effects were shown.[76] Additionally, prostaglandin E_1 has also been suggested to increase human growth hormone secretion, which could have anabolic effects. However, there are no peer-reviewed scientific data to support an anabolic effect of omega-3 fatty acid supplementation on body composition or on measures of strength and power.[12]

Plant extracts

Numerous plant and herb extracts possess pharmacological properties which may possess ergogenic properties. For example, caffeine can be extracted from plants, and as noted previously, may be an effective ergogenic for a variety of athletic endeavours. Although a number of plant extracts have been marketed to athletes for their purported ergogenic potential, one of the most popular is ginseng.

Ginseng

Ginseng is a generic term encompassing a wide variety of compounds derived from the plant family Araliaceae. The ergogenic effect of ginseng is attributed to specific glycosides, also referred to as ginseng saponins or ginsenosides. The specific physiological effects of ginseng extracts depend on the plant species, including: Chinese or Korean ginseng (*Panax ginseng*), American ginseng (*Panax quinquefolium*), Japanese ginseng (*Panax japonicum*), and

Russian/Siberian ginseng (*Eleutherococcus senticosus*). Although the mechanism underlying the alleged ergogenicity of ginseng on physical performance has not been delineated, theories include stimulation of the hypothalamic–pituitary–adrenal cortex axis and increased resistance to the stress of exercise, enhanced myocardial metabolism, increased haemoglobin levels, vasodilation, increased oxygen extraction by muscles, and improved mitochondrial metabolism in the muscle, all of which, theoretically, could enhance aerobic exercise performance.[77]

However, there are very few well-controlled studies supporting an ergogenic effect of ginseng supplementation. Bahrke and Morgan,[78] in their major recent review, indicated that because of methodological and statistical shortcomings, there is no compelling evidence to indicate that ginseng supplementation consistently enhances human physical performance and so there remains a need for well-designed research to address this issue. One recent well-designed study did find an ergogenic effect of Geriatric Pharmaton (a preparation including ginseng G115 and other elements, including dimethylaminoethanol) on various physiological variables, including $\dot{V}O_2$max, and performance during the Bruce treadmill protocol.[79]

However, the investigators noted that the ergogenic effect is attributed to the total preparation used, namely Geriatric Pharmaton, and not to the standardized ginseng G115; some research has supported a beneficial effect of dimethyaminoethanol bitartrate, possibly by favourably affecting the choline–acetylcholine complex. Moreover, several recent, appropriately designed, (double-blind, placebo control, matched group) studies have reported no benefits in endurance performance. For example, no significant ergogenic effects were associated with 6-weeks *Eleutherococcus senticosus* Maxim L (**ESML**) supplementation on any metabolic, psychological, or performance parameters measured in both a submaximal and maximal aerobic exercise task, including heart rate, $\dot{V}O_2$, $\dot{V}_E$, $\dot{V}_E/\dot{V}O_2$, and respiratory exchange ratio (**RER**) during both exercise and recovery, ratings of perceived exertion during exercise, serum lactate levels following exercise, and run time to exhaustion in a maximal test.[77] Nevertheless, as yet, few well-controlled studies have investigated the effect of ginseng supplementation on exercise performance and further research is still needed.

Wheatgerm oil (octacosanol)

Wheatgerm oil is extracted from the embryo of wheat and is a good source of octacosanol, an alcohol isolate alleged to possess ergogenic properties. Although the mechanism underlying the purported ergogenic effect of wheatgerm oil (or octacosanol) has not been determined, Cureton,[80] its principal advocate, has suggested it could enhance glycogen metabolism and oxygen uptake, and would therefore be most useful in endurance exercise tasks. Most of the support for the reported beneficial effects of wheatgerm oil is presented in *The physiological effects of wheat germ oil on humans in exercise*,[80] a compilation of unpublished master's theses and other published articles emanating from the same research facility. Although this text does present a case in support of wheatgerm oil supplementation, the design and interpretation of these studies has been questioned and studies conducted in other research facilities have shown no positive benefits from wheatgerm oil supplementation.[81] Unfortunately, no research relative to this issue has been conducted for over 20 years.

Bee pollen

Bee pollen is a mixture of vitamins, minerals, amino acids, and other organic substances. Its putative ergogenic effect is based on anecdotal reports, suggesting supplementation may facilitate recovery during repeated training bouts.

Theoretically, improved training would enhance competitive performance. However, six well-controlled studies have shown that bee pollen supplementation will not improve physiological responses to exercise, including maximal oxygen uptake and endurance capacity.[12] In particular, one study evaluated the rate of recovery from repeated bouts of strenuous exercise in highly trained runners and reported no significant effect of varying doses of bee pollen, evidence not in support of bee pollen's theoretical value to athletes.[82]

Gamma oryzanol, yohimbine, smilax, guarana, kola nuts, and ephedra

Several plant extracts have been used in attempts to increase serum levels of testosterone or human growth hormone, possibly enhancing the anabolic effect of resistance exercise training. Three compounds marketed to athletes include: gamma oryzanol, a ferulic acid ester derived from rice bran oil; yohimbine (yohimbe), a nitrogen-containing alkaloid from the bark of the yohimbe tree; and smilax, an extract of phytosterols from the dried roots of *Smilax officinalis*, or various forms of sarsaparilla. No peer-reviewed studies have been discovered that have investigated the effect of these plant extracts on body composition or measures of strength or power. In a review, Wheeler and Garleb[83] reported that no scientific evidence has been published indicating that phytosterols or gamma oryzanol possess anabolic–androgenic activity. Based on animal research, they speculated that gamma oryzanol might actually decrease serum testosterone levels.

Other plant extracts are used for their stimulatory effects. Guarana and kola nuts contain caffeine, and although no research has been uncovered which has investigated supplementation effects on physical performance, the effects may be comparable to those elicited by caffeine, as discussed previously. Ephedra, also known as *ma huang*, is a stimulant comparable to ephedrine, whose use is prohibited by the IOC. Most supplements marketed as *ma huang* or ephedra are actually the synthetic form of ephedrine,[84] which may be grounds for disqualification.

Summary

Proper nutrition, including an adequate intake of energy and all essential nutrients, is an important factor to help optimize physical performance. A balanced diet consisting of wholesome, natural foods is the key to proper nutrition, and is the main recommendation of most sport nutritionists to help prevent a nutrient deficiency and an impairment in performance. However, athletes and other physically active individuals may consume nutrient and dietary supplements for a variety of reasons, for instance to provide 'nutritional insurance' or for other purported health benefits. In some cases, such as those athletes involved in weight-control sports associated with low-energy intakes, supplements may help to deter specific nutrient deficiencies.

But athletes also take supplements in the hope of increasing sport or physical performance. Nutritional ergogenics have been used since time immemorial, and will continue to be used as long as athletes believe they may gain a competitive advantage. However, before using such supplements for their purported ergogenic effects, one should address the following questions.

1.   Is it effective? If the supplement has not been shown to be effective, either by appropriately designed research or repeated personal experiences, there is no reason to buy it.

2.   Is it safe? Most nutrient and dietary supplements are presumed to be safe if consumed in recommended dosages. However, athletes often believe that if one is good, 10 are better, and may take amounts in excess of normal needs and recommendations.[85] Excess amounts of common nutrients, such as vitamin A, iron, zinc, and selenium, etc. may be toxic. Some plant or herb extracts may pose health risks to some individuals; for example, there are several case reports of anaphylactic shock reactions in susceptible individuals following ingestion of bee pollen. Other agents, when used inappropriately, may actually impair performance, such as a diarrhoea in response to sodium bicarbonate.

3.   Is it legal? Most nutritional ergogenics are considered legal because they are regulated as food or dietary supplements, not drugs. However, the caffeine in some dietary supplements, such as guarana, may be grounds for disqualification if consumed in excess. Synthetic forms of ephedrine in *ma huang* preparations are also prohibited.

4.   Is it ethical? One of the stipulations of the IOC doping legislation is that any physiological substance taken in abnormal quantity with the intention of artificially and unfairly increasing performance should be construed as doping. Some dietary supplements, such as creatine, may fall under this stipulation. Caffeine, in currently legal doses, has been shown to enhance performance. Although legal, are these, and possibly others, to be construed as doping agents? Might their use raise ethical concerns for athletes who desire to excel on their own merits?

Athletes should be allowed to utilize any effective, safe, and legal nutritional supplement in attempts to enhance physical power, mental strength, and athletic performance, just as they should be able to use the most effective and legal equipment specific to their sport which may provide a mechanical edge. To avoid an ethical dilemma, athletic governing bodies should make specific regulations regarding the use of nutrients or dietary supplements as they relate to the antidoping legislation currently in place.

References

1.   Williams MH. *Beyond training. How athletes enhance performance legally and illegally.* Champaign, IL: Leisure Press, 1989.
2.   Sherman W, Lamb D. Introduction to the Gatorade Sports Science Institute Conference on Nutritional Ergogenic Aids Supplement. *International Journal of Sport Nutrition* 1995; **5**: Siii–iv.
3.   Coggan A, Swanson S. Nutritional manipulations before and during endurance exercise: Effects on performance. *Medicine and Science in Sports and Exercise* 1992; **24**: S331–5.
4.   Costill D, Hargreaves M. Carbohydrate nutrition and fatigue. *Sports Medicine* 1992; **13**: 86–92.
5.   Coyle E. Carbohydrate feeding during exercise. *International Journal of Sports Medicine* 1992; **13**: (Suppl. 1) S126–8.
6.   Sherman W. Carbohydrate meals before and after exercise. In: Lamb D, Williams M, eds. *Ergogenics: The enhancement of sport performance.* Dubuque, IA: Brown and Benchmark, 1991, 1–34.
7.   Williams C. Macronutrients and performance. *Journal of Sports Sciences* 1995; **13**: S1–10.
8.   Myers JJ, Atwood S, Forbes M, *et al.* Effect of fructose 1,6-diphosphate infusion on the hormonal response to exercise. *Medicine and Science in Sports and Exercise* 1990; **22**: 102–5.
9.   Stanko R, Robertson R, Galbreath R, Reilly J, Greenwalt K, Goss F. Enhanced leg exercise endurance with a high-carbohydrate diet and dihydroxyacetone and pyruvate. *Journal of Applied Physiology* 1990; **69**: 1651–66.
10. Stanko R, Robertson R, Spina R, Reilly J, Greenwalt K, Goss F. Enhancement of arm exercise endurance capacity with dihydroxyacetone and pyruvate. *Journal of Applied Physiology* 1990; **68**: 119–23.
11. Sherman W. Fat loading: The next magic bullet? *International Journal of Sport Nutrition* 1995; **5**: S1–12.
12. Williams M. *Nutrition for fitness and sport* (4th edn). Dubuque IA: Brown and Benchmark, 1995.
13. Lemon P. Do athletes need more dietary protein and amino acids? *International Journal of Sport Nutrition* 1995; **5**: S39–61.
14. Tarnopolsky M. Protein, caffeine and sports. Guidelines for active people. *Physician and Sportsmedicine* 1993; **21**: 137–49.
15. Fogelholm M, Naveri H, Kiilavuori K, Harkonen M. Low-dose amino acid supplementation: No effects on serum human growth hormone and insulin in male weightlifters. *International Journal of Sport Nutrition* 1993; **3**: 290–7.
16. Lambert M, Hefer J, Millar R, MacFarlane P. Failure of commercial oral amino acid supplements to increase serum growth hormone concentrations in male bodybuilders. *International Journal of Sport Nutrition* 1993; **3**: 298–305.
17. Mitchell M, Dimeff R, Burns B. Effects of supplementation with arginine and lysine on body composition, strength and growth hormone levels in weightlifters. *Medicine and Science in Sports and Exercise* 1993; **25**: S25 (Abstract).
18. Segura R, Ventura J. Effect of L-tryptophan supplementation on exercise performance. *International Journal of Sports Medicine* 1988; **9**: 301–5.
19. Stensrud T, Ingjer F, Holm H, Stromme S. L-tryptophan supplementation does not improve running performance. *International Journal of Sports Medicine* 1992; **13**: 481–5.
20. van Hall G, Raaymakers J, Saris W, Wagenmakers A. Ingestion of branched-amino acids and tryptophan during sustained exercise in man: failure to affect performance. *Journal of Physiology* 1995; **486**: 789–94.
21. Newsholme E. Physical and mental fatigue: Metabolic mechanisms and importance of plasma amino acids. *British Medical Bulletin* 1992; **48**: 477–95.
22. Davis JM. Carbohydrates branched-chain amino acids and endurance: The central fatigue hypothesis. *International Journal of Sport Nutrition* 1995; **5**: S29–38.
23. Varnier M, Sarto P, Martines D, *et al.* Effect of infusing branched-chain amino acid during incremental exercise with reduced muscle glycogen content. *European Journal of Applied Physiology* 1994; **69**: 26–31.
24. Madsen K, MacLean D, Kiens B, Christensen D. Effects of glucose, glucose plus branched-chain amino acids, or placebo on bike performance over 100 km. *Journal of Applied Physiology* 1996; **81**: 2644–50.
25. Wesson M, McNaughton L, Davies P, Tristram S. Effects of oral administration of aspartic acid salts on the endurance capacity of trained athletes. *Research Quarterly for Exercise and Sport* 1988; **59**: 234–9.
26. Keith R. Vitamins and physical activity. In: Wolinsky I, Hickson J,

eds. *Nutrition in exercise and sport*. Boca Raton, FL: CRC Press, 1994, 159–83.

27. van der Beek E. Vitamin supplementation and physical exercise performance. *Journal of Sports Sciences* 1991; **92**: 77–9.

28. Williams M. Vitamin supplementation and athletic performance. *International Journal for Vitamin and Nutrition Research* 1989 (Suppl.); **30**: 161–91.

29. Bonke D. Influence of vitamins B_1, B_6, and B_{12} on the control of fine motoric movements. *Bibliotheca Nutritio et Dieta* 1986; **38**: 104–9.

30. Goldfarb A. Antioxidants: Role of supplementation to prevent exercise-induced oxidative stress. *Medicine and Science in Sports and Exercise* 1993; **25**: 232–6.

31. Kanter M. Free radicals, exercise, and antioxidant supplementation. *International Journal of Sport Nutrition* 1994; **4**: 205–20.

32. Kanter M, Williams M. Antioxidants, carnitine and choline as putative ergogenic aids. *International Journal of Sport Nutrition* 1995; **5**: S120–31.

33. Cade R, Conte M, Zauner C, *et al*. Effects of phosphate loading on 2,3-diphosphoglycerate and maximal oxygen uptake. *Medicine and Science in Sports and Exercise* 1984; **16**: 263–8.

34. Kreider R, Miller G, Williams M, Somma C, Nassar T. Effects of phosphate loading on oxygen uptake, ventilatory anaerobic threshold, and run performance. *Medicine and Science in Sports and Exercise* 1990; **22**: 250–6.

35. Kreider R, Miller G, Schenck D. *et al*. Effects of phosphate loading on metabolic and myocardial responses to maximal and endurance exercise. *International Journal of Sport Nutrition* 1992; **2**: 20–47.

36. Stewart I, McNaughton L, Davies P, Tristram S. Phosphate loading and the effects on $\dot{V}O_2$max in trained cyclists. *Research Quarterly for Exercise and Sport* 1990; **61**: 80–4.

37. Kreider R. Phosphate loading and exercise performance. *Journal of Applied Nutrition* 1992; **44**: 29–49.

38. Tremblay M, Galloway S, Sexsmith J. Ergogenic effects of phosphate loading: Physiological fact or methodological fiction? *Canadian Journal of Applied Physiology* 1994; **19**: 1–11.

39. Clarkson P. Minerals: Exercise performance and supplementation in athletes. *Journal of Sports Sciences* 1991; **9**: 91–116.

40. Lukaski H. Micronutrients (magnesium, zinc and copper): Are mineral supplements needed for athletes? *International Journal of Sport Nutrition* 1995; **5**: S74–83.

41. Evans G. The effect of chromium picolinate on insulin controlled parameters in humans. *International Journal of Biosocial and Medical Research* 1989; **11**: 163–80.

42. Lefavi R, Anderson R, Keith R, Wilson G, McMillan J, Stone M. Efficacy of chromium supplementation in athletes: Emphasis on anabolism. *International Journal of Sport Nutrition* 1992; **2**: 111–22.

43. Evans G, Pouchnik D. Composition and biological activity of chromium–pyridine carboxylate complexes. *Journal of Inorganic Biochemistry* 1993; **49**: 177–87.

44. Clancy S, Clarkson P, DeCheke M, *et al*. Effects of chromium picolinate supplementation on body composition strength and urinary chromium loss in football players. *International Journal of Sport Nutrition* 1994; **4**: 142–53.

45. Hallmark M, Reynolds T, DeSouza C, Dotson C, Anderson R, Rogers M. Effects of chromium supplementation and resistive training on muscle strength and lean body mass in untrained men. *Medicine and Science in Sports and Exercise* 1996; **28**: 139–144.

46. Nielsen F. Facts and fallacies about boron. *Nutrition Today* 1992; **27**: 6–12.

47. Ferrando A, Green N. The effect of boron supplementation on lean body mass, plasma testosterone levels, and strength in male bodybuilders. *International Journal of Sport Nutrition* 1993; **3**: 140–9.

48. Clarkson P, Haymes E. Trace mineral requirements for athletes. *International Journal of Sport Nutrition* 1994; **4**: 104–19.

49. Tessier F, Hida V, Favier A, Marconnet P. Muscle GSH-Px activity after prolonged exercise training and selenium supplementation. *Biological Trace Element Research* 1995; **47**: 279–85.

50. Tessier F, Margaritis I, Richard M, Moynot C, Marconnet P. Selenium and training effects on the glutathione system and aerobic performance. *Medicine and Science in Sports and Exercise* 1995; **27**: 390–6.

51. Fawcett J, Farquhar S, Walker R, Thou T, Lowe G, Goulding A. The effect of oral vanadyl sulfate on body composition and performance in weight-training athletes. International Journal of Sport Nutrition 1996; **6**: 382–90.

52. Williams M. Nutritional ergogenics in athletics. *Journal of Sports Sciences* 1995; **13**: S63–74.

53. Telford R, Catchpole E, Deakin V, Hahn A, Plank A. The effect of 7 to 8 months vitamin/mineral supplementation on athletic performance. *International Journal of Sport Nutrition* 1992; **2**: 135–53.

54. Rosenberg IH, ed. Dietary supplements: Recent chronology and legislation. *Nutrition Reviews* 1995; **53**: 31–6.

55. Graham T, Rush J, van Soeren M. Caffeine and exercise: Metabolism and performance. *Canadian Journal of Applied Physiology* 1994; **19**: 111–38.

56. Nehlig A, Debry G. Caffeine and sports activity: A review. *International Journal of Sportsmedicine* 1994; **15**: 215–23.

57. Spriet L. Caffeine and performance. *International Journal of Sport Nutrition* 1995; **5**: S84–99.

58. Williams J. Caffeine, neuromuscular function and high-intensity exercise performance. *Journal of Sports Medicine and Physical Fitness* 1991; **31**: 481–9.

59. Cole K, Costill D, Starling R, Goodpaster B, Trappe S, Fink W. Effect of caffeine ingestion on perception of effort and subsequent work production. *International Journal of Sport Nutrition* 1996; **6**: 14–23.

60. Heigenhauser G, Jones N. Bicarbonate loading. In: Lamb D, Williams M, eds. *Ergogenics: Enhancement of performance in exercise and sport*. Dubuque IA: Brown and Benchmark, 1991, 183–212.

61. Horswill C. Effects of bicarbonate, citrate, and phosphate loading on performance. *International Journal of Sport Nutrition* 1995; **5**: S111–19.

62. Linderman J, Gosselink K. The effects of sodium bicarbonate ingestion on exercise performance. *Sports Medicine* 1994; **18**: 75–80.

63. Maughan R, Greenhaff P. High intensity exercise performance and acid–base balance: The influence of diet and induced metabolic alkalosis. *Medicine and Sport Science* 1991; **32**: 147–65.

64. Williams M. Bicarbonate loading. *Sports Science Exchange* 1992; **4**: 1–4.

65. Matson L, Tran SV. Effects of sodium bicarbonate ingestion on anaerobic performance: A meta-analytic review. *International Journal of Sport Nutrition* 1993; **3**: 2–28.

66. Wagenmakers A. L-carnitine supplementaion and performance in man. *Medicine and Sport Science* 1991; **32**: 110–27.

67. Bucci L. *Nutrients as ergogenic aids for sports and exercise*. Boca Raton, FL: CRC Press, 1993.

68. Greenhaff P. Creatine and its application as an ergogenic aid. *International Journal of Sport Nutrition* 1995; **5**: S100–10.

69. Balsom P, Soderlund K, Ekblom B. Creatine in human with special reference to creatine supplementation. *Sports Medicine* 1994; **18**: 268–80.

70. Williams M. *The ergogenics edge: Pushing the limits of sport performance*. Champaign, IL: Human Kinetics, 1998.

71. Williams M, Kreider R, Hunter D, *et al*. Effect of inosine supplementation on 3-mile treadmill performance and $\dot{V}O_2$peak. *Medicine and Science in Sports and Exercise* 1990; **22**: 517–22.

72. Starling R, Trappe T, Short K, *et al.* The effect of inosine supplementation on aerobic and anaerobic cycling performance. *Medicine and Science in Sports and Exercise* 1996; **28**: 1193–8.

73. Conlay L, Sabounjian L, Wurtman R. Exercise and neuromodulators: Choline and acetylcholine in marathon runners. *International Journal of Sports Medicine* 1992; **13**: S141–2.

74. von Allworden H, Horn S, Kahl J, Feldheim W. The influence of lecithin on plasma choline concentrations in triathletes and adolescent runners during exercise. *European Journal of Applied Physiology* 1993; **67**: 87–91.

75. Spector S, Jackman M, Sabounjian L, Sakkas C, Landers D, Willis W. Effect of choline supplementation on fatigue in trained cyclists. *Medicine and Science in Sport and Exercise* 1995; **27**: 668–73.

76. Brilla L, Landerholm T. Effect of fish oil supplementation and exercise on serum lipids and aerobic fitness. *Journal of Sports Medicine and Physical Fitness* 1990; **30**: 173–80.

77. Dowling E, Redondo D, Branch J, Jones S, McNabb G, Williams M. Effect of *Eleutherococcus senticosus* on submaximal and maximal exercise performance. *Medicine and Science in Sports and Exercise* 1996; **28**: 482–9.

78. Bahrke MS, Morgan WP. Evaluation of the ergogenic properties of ginseng. *Sports Medicine* 1994; **18**: 229–48.

79. Pieralisi G, Ripari P, Vecchiet L. Effects of a standardized ginseng extract combined with dimethylaminoethanol bitartrate, vitamins, minerals, and trace elements on physical performance during exercise. *Clinical Therapeutics* 1991; **13**: 373–82.

80. Cureton T. *The physiological effects of wheat germ oil on humans in exercise.* Springfield, IL: CC Thomas, 1972.

81. Williams M. *Nutritional aspects of human physical and athletic performance.* Springfield, IL: CC Thomas, 1985.

82. Woodhouse M, Williams M, Jackson C. The effects of varying doses of orally ingested bee pollen extract upon selected performance variables. *Athletic Training* 1987; **22**: 26–8.

83. Wheeler K, Garleb K. Gamma oryzanol–plant sterol supplementation: metabolic endocrine and physiologic effects. *International Journal of Sport Nutrition* 1991; **1**: 170–7.

84. Ostgarden J. Rocket fuel. *Bicycling* 1995; **36** (7): 92–3.

85. Burke L, Read R. Dietary supplements in sport. *Sports Medicine* 1993; **15**: 43–65.

1.2.5 Eating disorders in athletes

Jorunn Sundgot-Borgen and Roald Bahr

Introduction

Eating disorders can have long-lasting physiological and psychological effects and may even be fatal. Symptoms of eating disorders are more prevalent among athletes than non-athletes, at least among women. Data on males are limited. Athletes competing in sports where leanness or a specific weight are considered important for performance are at increased risk of developing eating disorders. However, studies show that some female athletes competing in sports where weight is considered less important also suffer from weight or eating disorders. Psychological, biological, and social factors interrelate to produce the clinical picture of eating disorders. Recent studies indicate that specific risk factors for the development of eating disorders occur in some sport settings.

This chapter reviews the definitions, diagnostic criteria, prevalence, and risk factors for the development of eating disorders in sport. Practical implications for the identification and treatment of eating disorders in athletes are also discussed.

Definitions and diagnostic criteria

According to the revised third edition (**DSM-III-R**) of the *Diagnostic and statistical manual of mental disorders* by the American Psychiatric Association,[1] eating disorders are characterized by gross disturbances in eating behaviour. They include anorexia nervosa, bulimia nervosa, and eating disorder not otherwise specified.

Athletes constitute a unique population and special diagnostic considerations should be made when working with this group.[2–4] An attempt has been made to identify the group of athletes who show significant symptoms of eating disorders, but who do not meet the DSM-III-R criteria for anorexia nervosa, bulimia nervosa, or eating disorder not otherwise specified.[2] These athletes have been classified as having a subclinical eating disorder termed anorexia athletica. Health care professionals should be aware of the normal needs, expectations, and performance demands of athletes as this awareness and experience may be helpful in both diagnosis and treatment.[4] It is assumed that many cases of anorexia nervosa and bulimia nervosa begin as subclinical variants of these disorders. Early identification and treatment may prevent development of the full disorder.[5] Finally, subclinical cases are more prevalent than those meeting the formal diagnostic criteria for anorexia nervosa, bulimia nervosa or binge eating disorder.

Anorexia nervosa

Anorexia nervosa is characterized by a refusal to maintain body weight over a minimal level considered normal for age and height, a distorted body image, an intense fear of fatness or weight gain, while being underweight and having amenorrhoea (Table 1). Individuals with anorexia nervosa 'feel fat', while in reality they are underweight.[1]

Bulimia nervosa

Bulimia nervosa is characterized by binge eating (rapid consumption of a large amount of food in a discrete period of time) and purging. This typically involves consumption of high-energy foods, usually eaten inconspicuously or secretly. By relieving abdominal discomfort through vomiting, the individual can continue the binge.[1] The DSM-IV diagnostic criteria for bulimia nervosa include: recurrent episodes of binge eating, inappropriate behaviour to prevent weight gain, the occurrence of binge eating and inappropriate compensatory behaviours at least twice a week for at least 3 months, and self-evaluation based on body shape and weight (Table 2).[6]

Eating disorder not otherwise specified

The category of eating disorder not otherwise specified is for disorders of eating that do not meet the criteria for any specific eating disorder. Examples of eating disorders not otherwise specified are listed in Table 3, and this category acknowledges the existence and importance of a variety of eating disturbances.[4]

Anorexia athletica

The term anorexia athletica was first introduced by Pugliese *et al.*[7] The main feature of anorexia athletica is an intense fear of gaining weight or becoming fat, even though an individual is already lean (at least 5 per cent less than expected normal weight for age and height for the general female population). Weight loss is accomplished by a reduction in energy intake, often combined with extensive or compulsive exercise. The restrictive energy intake is below that required to maintain the energy requirements of the high training volume.[8] In addition to normal training to enhance performance in sport, athletes with anorexia athletica exercise excessively or compulsively to purge their bodies of the effect of eating. These athletes frequently report binge eating and the use of vomiting, laxatives, or diuretics. The binge eating is usually planned, and included in a strict training and study schedule. The definition of a binge used by an athlete with anorexia athletica is usually within the daily energy requirements for unaffected athletes. Since it is often difficult for elite athletes to have time for more than two meals, some athletes do not meet their energy requirements.[8] The criteria for anorexia athletica listed in Table 4 include a modification of the original criteria introduced by Pugliese et al.[7]

Some athletes with anorexia athletica also meet the criteria of eating disorder not otherwise specified. Most athletes have a higher percentage of lean body mass than age-matched non-athletes. A body weight of more than 5 per cent lower than expected could indicate that an athlete is too lean. Athletes with anorexia athletica usually indicate that they need to lose weight because of the requirements of their sport, often motivated by directions from their coach.

Prevalence of eating disorders in athletes

Data on the prevalence of eating disorders in athletic populations is limited and equivocal. Most studies have looked at preoccupation with food, obsessive preoccupation with weight, disturbed body image, or the use of pathogenic weight control methods. Almost all investigators who have attempted to study this issue have used surveys or inventories to estimate the prevalence of eating disorders, and few have obtained response rates that permit firm conclusions to be drawn.

There are gender differences in the prevalence of eating disorders in the general population.[9] Anorexia nervosa is approximately one-tenth as common in males as it is in females.[10] Studies of the prevalence of bulimic behaviour in college students indicate a prevalence of 0 to 5 per cent in males compared with 5 to 10 per cent in females.[10] However, Andersen[10] argues that more males are afflicted than previously assumed. It is not clear whether the gender differences observed in the general population also exist among athletes, since most studies deal with female athletes only. This could reflect a higher prevalence among females, or the bias of researchers.

There is insufficient data on male athletes to establish the prevalence of specific problems across sports or across levels of ability within sports. The studies necessary to define causal relationships between athletic participation, personality variables, and eating disturbances in males have not been done. Studies are needed in which prevalence is defined in males and females in the same sports at equivalent levels of training and competition.[11] A summary of the studies conducted to date have been presented previously.[11]

Female athletes

Estimates of the prevalence of the symptoms of eating disorders and the existence of eating disorders among female athletes range from less than 1 per cent to as high as 62 per cent.[12-15] Estimates vary greatly depending on whether they are based on self-reports or clinical interviews, and on the athletic population investigated. Only one study have used clinical evaluation and the American Psychiatric Association criteria applied across athletes and controls.[15] Data from that study showed that the prevalence of DSM–III–R diagnosed anorexia nervosa is 1.3 per cent, which is somewhat higher than the prevalence reported for non-athletes. Diagnosed bulimia nervosa was 8.2 per cent among Norwegian female élite athlete, which was within the prevalence reported among non-athletes. The prevalence within each sport category, however, was significantly different.[15] The prevalence of anorexia nervosa seems to be within the same range as that reported previously,[10] whereas bulimia nervosa and subclinical eating disorders seem to be more prevalent among athletes (17 per cent in athletes and 5 per cent among non-athletes).[15]

Existing studies vary in whether they measure behaviour, attitudes, body image, or factors thought to be associated with eating disorders. Studies examining pathological behaviour and attitudes are fairly consistent in showing a higher prevalence than that of

---

Table 1 Diagnostic criteria for anorexia nervosa[6]

A. Refusal to maintain body weight at or above a minimally normal weight for age and height (e.g. weight loss leading to maintenance of body weight less than 85 per cent of that expected; or failure to make expected weight gain during period of growth, leading to body weight less than 85 per cent of that expected)

B. Intense fear of gaining weight or becoming fat, even though underweight

C. Disturbance in the way in which one's body weight or shape is experienced, undue influence of body weight or shape on self-evaluation, or denial of the seriousness of the current low body weight

D. In postmenarcheal females, amenorrhoea, i.e. the absence of at least three consecutive menstrual cycles. (A woman is considered to have amenorrhoea if her periods occur only following hormone administration, such as oestrogen)

Specify type:
Restricting type: During the episode of anorexia nervosa, the person has not regularly engaged in binge eating or purging behaviour (i.e. self-induced vomiting or the misuse of laxatives, diuretics, or enemas)
Binge eating/purging type: During the current episode of anorexia nervosa, the person has regularly engaged, in binge eating or purging behaviour (i.e. self-induced vomiting or the misuse of laxatives, diuretics, or enemas)

Table 2 Diagnostic criteria for bulimia nervosa[6]

A. Recurrent episodes of binge eating. An episode of binge eating is characterized by both of the following: (i) eating, in a discrete period of time (e.g. within any 2-h period), an amount of food that is definitely larger than most people would eat during a similar period of time in similar circumstances; and, (ii) a sense of lack of control over eating during the episode (e.g. a feeling that one cannot stop eating or control what or how much one is eating)

B. Recurrent, inappropriate compensatory behaviour in order to prevent weight gain, such as: self-induced vomiting; misuse of laxatives, diuretics, or other medications; fasting; or excessive exercise

C. The binge eating and inappropriate compensatory behaviours both occur, on average, at least twice a week for 3 months

D. Self-evaluation is unduly influenced by body shape and weight

E. The disturbance does not occur exclusively during episodes of anorexia nervosa

Specify type:
Restricting type: The person regularly engages in self-induced vomiting or the misuse of laxatives, diuretics, or enemas.
Non-purging type: The person uses other inappropriate compensatory behaviours, such as fasting or excessive exercise, but does not regularly engage in self-induced vomiting or the misuse of laxatives, diuretics, or enemas.

Table 3 The category of eating disorder not otherwise specified[6]

1. All of the criteria for anorexia nervosa are met except the individual has regular menses
2. All of the criteria for anorexia nervosa are met except, despite significant weight loss, the individual's current weight is in the normal range
3. All of the criteria for bulimia nervosa are met except binges occur at a frequency of less than twice a week or a duration of less than 3 months
4. An individual of normal body weight regularly engages in inappropriate compensatory behaviour after eating small amounts of food (e.g. self-induced vomiting after the consumption of two cookies)
5. An individual who repeatedly chews and spits out, but does not swallow, large amounts of food
6. Binge-eating disorder: recurrent episodes of binge eating in the absence of inappropriate compensatory behaviours characteristic of bulimia nervosa

DSM-III diagnosed eating disorders.[15] The frequency of eating disorder problems reported by Rucinski[16] and Rosen and Hough[17] (48 per cent and 32 per cent, respectively) is much higher than the frequency reported when athletes have been clinically evaluated.[15] Despite the methodological weaknesses, existing studies are consistent in showing that symptoms of eating disorders and pathogenic weight control methods are: (i) more prevalent in female athletes than non-athletes and (ii) more prevalent in sports in which leanness or a specific weight are considered important than among athletes competing in sports where these factors are considered less important.[2,17-24]

Male athletes

Results from existing studies on male athletes indicate that the frequency of eating disturbances and pathological dieting practices varies from none to 57 per cent, depending on the definition used and the population studied.[14,16,18,25,26]

No studies on male athletes and eating disorders have used the American Psychiatric Association criteria to diagnose male athletes with different degrees of eating disturbances. Therefore, the true prevalence of clinically diagnosed eating disorders is not known.

A number of years ago concerns were raised about the rapid, frequent, and severe weight loss and regain cycles in male wrestlers.[27] Both the American College of Sports Medicine[28] and the American Medical Association[29] have issued position stands warning against the dangers of these practices in wrestlers. Thus, most of the studies on male athletes that have attempted to determine the use of pathological weight control methods and eating disorders have been performed on athletes competing in weight dependent or weight-class sports, such as wrestling, rowing, martial arts, and body building.[9,11] Only a limited number of studies have examined the frequency of pathological weight control or eating disorders

Table 4 Diagnostic criteria for anorexia athletica[15]

1.	Weight loss greater than 5 per cent of expected body weight	+
2.	Delayed puberty (no menstrual bleeding at age 16, i.e. primary amenorrhoea)	(+)
3.	Menstrual dysfunction (primary amenorrhoea, secondary amenorrhoea, and oligomenorrhoea)	(+)
4.	Gastrointestinal complaints	(+)
5.	Absence of medical illness or affective disorder explaining the weight reduction	+
6.	Distorted body image	(+)
7.	Excessive fear of becoming obese	+
8.	Restriction of food (less than 1200 kcal/day)	+
9.	Use of purging methods (self-induced vomiting, laxatives, and diuretics)	(+)
10.	Binge eating	(+)
11.	Compulsive exercise	(+)

+, Absolute criteria; (+), relative criteria.

among male athletes representing some of the endurance-type sports or ball games.

In a study by Blouin and Goldfield,[30] body builders reported significantly greater body dissatisfaction, a high drive for bulk, a high drive for thinness, and increased bulimic tendencies when compared with runners and athletes in the martial arts. They also reported frequent use of anabolic steroids and the most liberal attitudes towards using steroids were among bodybuilders with symptoms of eating disorders.

Sykora et al.[25] compared eating, weight, and dieting disturbances in male and female lightweight and heavyweight rowers. Females displayed more disturbed eating and weight control methods than did males. Male rowers were more affected by weight restriction than were female rowers, probably because they gained more weight during the off-season. Lightweight males showed greater weight fluctuation during the season and gained more weight during the off-season than did lightweight females and heavyweight males and females.

. There are many similarities between male athletes and males with eating disorders, including the preoccupation with body size and shape.[9] However, data suggest that male athletes with eating disorders are special cases, even when compared with other male athletes.[9] Although both groups place a high value on changing body weight and shape as a means of achieving athletic goals, and both groups demonstrate compulsive and perfectionistic personality traits, only the males with eating disorders demonstrate distinctive and diagnosable psychopathology. Also, males with eating disorders tend to continue in a self-sustaining way in their abnormal thinking and behaviour, even when the environment changes. A number of male athletes tend to have temporary, situation-related symptoms that improve during off-season. For example, those competing in weight-class sports have frequent and large cycles of weight loss that can have enduring medical consequences. However, most tend to normalize these behaviours when not in season.[10]

Methodological problems

Measurements

Most of the studies published on prevalence have used individually developed questionnaires or standardized instruments such as the Eating Disorder Inventory[31] and The Eating Attitude Test[32] to assess eating problems in athletes. Both the Eating Disorder Inventory and the Eating Attitude Test have been tested for reliability and validity.[31,32] However, the validity of the Eating Attitude Test has not been tested in athletes. In one study, 89 per cent of the athletes who were classified as at risk by the Eating Disorder Inventory also met the criteria of anorexia nervosa, anorexia athletica, or bulimia nervosa when interviewed.[2]

The weight questionnaire was developed to assess eating, dieting, and weight control practices in athletes competing in weight controlled sports such as wrestling and rowing. This is the only instrument developed specifically for athletes, and it has been shown to meet strict criteria for validity and reliability.[26] This instrument could be used in most sports with minor adjustments.

Self-reports versus clinical interviews

When data from self-reports and clinical interviews were compared by Sundgot-Borgen,[2] the results showed that elite athletes under-report the use of purging methods such as laxatives, diuretics, and vomiting, and overreport the use of binge eating in the questionnaire. Furthermore, athletes underreport the prevalence of eating disorders in the questionnaire. Most of those athletes who report having an eating disorder claim that they suffer from anorexia nervosa, while generally most meet the criteria for bulimia nervosa or subclinical eating disorders.

The erroneous reporting may be explained by a number of factors. First, many athletes and non-athletes are probably not familiar with the definitions of the different eating disorders, which most individuals only associate with anorexia. People with bulimia, whose weight is within accepted limits, may therefore not realize they have an eating disorder, and do not report it. The underreporting by the athletes may also be due to their fear of being discovered by their coach or other people important to them or their athletic career. For an athlete, the diagnosis of eating disorders may, in addition to the problems associated with such a disorder, result in their losing a place on a team. Also, athletes tend to report fasting and strict dieting, pathogenic weight control methods that indicate they have a certain control, while practising vomiting, which indicates a loss of control. Another reason may be that some attitudes and behaviours characteristic of eating disorders are accepted by many athletes and coaches in particular sports. Thus, there is a need to validate self-report measures in athletic populations, and identify the conditions under which self-reports of eating disturbances are most likely to be accurate.[11]

To determine whether an athlete actually suffers from any of the eating disorders described above, an interview with a clinician is necessary to assess an athlete's physical and emotional condition, and whether this interferes with everyday functioning.

Groups investigated

Few of the existing studies on prevalence of eating disorders in athletes have clearly defined the population investigated, making it difficult to compare them. Investigators have grouped athletes according to sports that emphasize leanness and those that do not. It has been concluded that the prevalence of eating disorder symptoms is higher among those competing in sports considered to emphasize leanness.[23,34] Studies indicate that this grouping of athletes representing different sports could affect the validity of the data. For example, Sundgot-Borgen[2] studied athletes representing 35 different sports which were divided into six groups: technical, endurance, aesthetic, weight-dependent, ball games, and power sports. Each group comprised sports or events that have similar demands. The prevalence of eating disorders was significantly higher among athletes competing in aesthetic and weight-dependent sports than among other sport groups where leanness is considered less important (Fig. 1). A significant difference in the prevalence of eating disorders between the sports in the endurance group was also found (Fig. 2).[2]

However, using this method of comparing sports is not entirely consistent because of divergent methods. Dummer et al.[18] targeted swimmers because of their strong concerns with weight and shape, whereas Sundgot-Borgen and Corbin[23] used swimmers as controls because they are in a sport that emphasizes leanness. However, research on elite athletes is generally limited by small sample sizes, and grouping of elite athletes from sports with similar demands

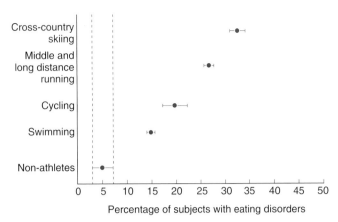

Fig. 1 Prevalence of eating disorders in female élite athletes representing technical sports (n = 98), endurance sports (n = 119), aesthetic sports (n = 64), weight-dependent sports (n = 41), ball games (n = 183), and power sports (n = 17), and non-athletes (n = 522). The data are shown as means and 95 per cent confidence intervals.

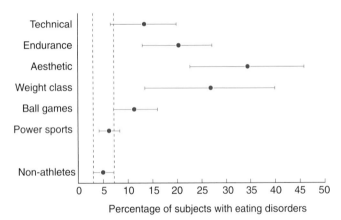

Fig. 2 Prevalence of athletes meeting the criteria for anorexia nervosa, anorexia athletica, or bulimia nervosa in cross-country skiing (n = 22), middle- and long-distance running (n = 15), cycling (n = 10), swimming (n = 20), and orienteering (n = 13). These athletes are among those comprising the endurance group in Fig. 1. The data are shown as means and 95 per cent confidence intervals.

would be helpful. Therefore, there is a need for large scale, epidemiological studies using consistent measures to define the prevalence of eating disorders in various sports or sport groups, and to develop a standardized way to group sports to obtain more representative data. Grouping considerations should include how the performance in each sport is evaluated (subjectively or objectively), whether it is weight classed, whether it is a team or individual sport, the age group in question, and the particular season of the year.[15]

Élite versus non-élite athletes

It is not established whether élite athletes are at greater risk for eating disorders than non-élite athletes. Few studies have specified the competitive level of the athletes investigated. It is assumed that some risk factors (such as intense pressure to be lean, increased training volume, and perfectionism) are more pronounced in élite athletes. However, it may be assumed that élite athletes would have difficulty performing with an eating disorder, since performance

would suffer. It is therefore possible that the prevalence of eating disorders and related problems is even higher among athletes who fail to stay at a high performance level. Hamilton et al.[20] found that less-skilled dancers in the United States reported significantly more eating problems than the more-skilled dancers. However, firm conclusions cannot be drawn without longitudinal studies with a careful classification and description of the competitive level of the athletes investigated.

Risk factors for the development of eating disorders

Psychological, biological, and social factors are implicated in the development of eating disorders.[34,35] Personality, hunger intensity, and activity level contribute to the psychological predisposition. Difficulties in a child's early relationship with the caregiver may create an additional psychological predisposition.[36] Social factors, especially the cultural phenomenon of equating thinness with success in women, may also contribute.[31] When an individual with a substantial predisposition begins a strict diet, it can become a self-perpetuating, self-reinforcing process.[36] It has been claimed that female athletes appear to be more vulnerable to eating disorders than the general female population, because of additional stresses associated with the athletic environment.[24] General and sport-specific risk factors are given in Fig. 3.

The attraction to sport hypothesis

It has been suggested that sport or specific sports attract individuals who are anorexic before commencing their participation in sports, at least in attitude if not in behaviour or weight.[4] These individuals seem to use or abuse exercise to expend extra energy or to justify their abnormal eating and dieting behaviour. Others have suggested that many anorexic individuals are attracted to sports in which they can hide their illness.[37] The attraction to certain sports, such as running and cross-country skiing, may be related to the emphasis on and acceptance of thinness and high training volumes in those sports. The stereotyped standards of body shape of some sports, such as gymnastics or long-distance running, make it difficult for observers to notice when a particular athlete has lost too much weight. These common and accepted weight standards help athletes to hide their problem and delay the intervention.[4] The 'attraction to sport' hypothesis appears to have merit in that it covers individuals who already have an eating disorder or are at high risk for developing an eating disorder. However, élite gymnasts, for example, are picked to begin intensive, high-level training at the age of 6 years, 10 years before developing an eating disorder. Therefore, it would not appear that these individuals were attracted to gymnastics because of a desire for thinness.[4]

Exercise and the inducement of eating disorders

A biobehavioural model of activity-based anorexia nervosa was proposed in a series of studies by Epling and Pierce[38] and Epling et al.[39] They suggest that dieting and exercising initiate the anorexic cycle, and that as many as 75 per cent of the cases of anorexia nervosa are exercise induced. Specifically, they contend that strenuous exercise tends to suppress appetite, which serves to decrease the value of

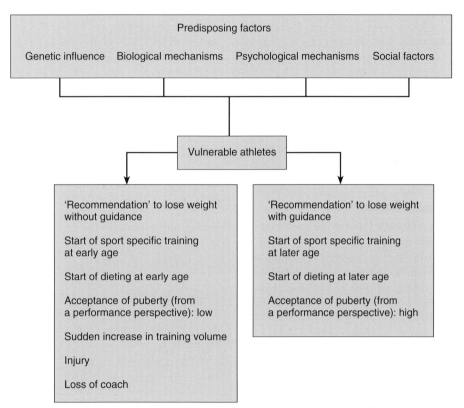

Fig. 3 General and sport-specific factors that can contribute to the development of eating disorders in athletes.

food reinforcement. As a result, food intake decreases, while the motivation for more exercise increases.

A recent study reported that élite endurance athletes with eating disorders could not give any specific reason why they developed an eating disorder.[15] However, many reported that with a sudden increase in training volume, a significant amount of weight was lost, and anorexia nervosa or anorexia athletica developed.[15] Costill[40] found that some athletes who increased their training volume experienced energy deprivation. Furthermore, it has been claimed that appetite may be truly diminished, in part as a result of changes in endorphin levels.[41] Thus, it has been speculated that the increased training load may induce an energy deprivation in endurance athletes, which in turn may elicit biological and social reinforcements leading to the development of eating disorders.[15] Data from a study by Brownell et al.[11] indicated that the training intensity plays a significant role in the development of eating disorders for male runners. However, not all individuals with anorexia nervosa exercise, and the hypothesis of exercise-induced anorexia nervosa does not explain bulimia nervosa. Thus, longitudinal studies with close monitoring of the training volume, and type and intensity of the training in athletes representing different sports are needed before the question regarding the role played by different sports in the development of eating disorders can be answered.

Early start of sport-specific training

It is claimed that an individual's natural body type inherently steers the athlete to an appropriate sport;[42] but it is also suggested that the greater the extent to which an athlete's body deviates from the ideal for a particular sport, the greater the risk that the athlete will

develop an eating disorder.[11] Also, starting sport-specific training at a prepubertal age may prevent athletes from choosing the sport most suitable for their adult body type. Athletes with eating disorders have been shown to start sport-specific training at an earlier age than athletes who do not meet the criteria for eating disorders.[15]

Hamilton et al.[20] suggested that dancers who have passed a stringent process of early selection (girls who are enrolled in late childhood and where rigid standards for weight, body shape, and technique must be constantly met) may be more naturally suited to the thin body image demanded by ballet directors, and therefore are less at risk. Furthermore, a personal history or family history of overweight may be a risk factor for disordered eating, because it poses an obstacle to achieving the thinness demanded by some activities, such as modern rhythmic gymnastics, gymnastics, and long-distance running. The family history should be taken into account when girls choose to compete in a sport at a high level.

Dieting and body weight cycling

Athletes reduce body weight for several reasons: to compete in a lower weight class, to improve aesthetic appearance, or to increase physical performance.[15] Most athletes in weight-class events compete in a class below their natural body weight. Reduction of body weight is necessary because failure to 'make weight' results in disqualification from competition. Examples of weight-class sports are boxing, judo, karate, lightweight rowing, weight lifting, and wrestling. Also, a reduction of body weight and fat mass is considered advantageous in the aesthetic sports. Examples of aesthetic sports are body building, dancing, diving, figure skating, and gymnastics.

Extra weight is thought to impair performance and detract from appearance in the eyes of judges. This provides an incentive for extreme dieting. Finally, a reduced body weight and relative fat mass is expected to increase physical performance capacity. This is the predominant reason for body weight reduction in endurance sports such as running, cross-country skiing, road cycling, and jumping events for height or distance. Improved physical ability might also be an additional argument behind body weight reduction in weight-class and aesthetic sports. Dieting and the use of pathogenic weight control methods are more prevalent among athletes competing in sports in which leanness or extreme leanness are considered important for optimal performance.[15,23,43]

Weight reduction and extreme methods are used by males and females; lean and muscular athletes; endurance athletes, strength athletes, and sprinters; adolescent and adult athletes. The techniques used and the magnitude of weight loss may vary widely. The only common factor seems to be that athletes trying to reduce body weight are not obese. Consequently, the effects of weight reduction on the physiology and performance of athletes are likely to differ from those found in obese individuals.[43,44]

Weight cycling usually occurs in athletes who wish to keep weight at a certain level, but have difficulty accomplishing this. An example may be a gymnast who wishes to have a low weight to get the best score from the judges. During the off-season their weight increases, and restricted eating or additional exercise may be necessary to restore the desired weight. Such athletes frequently engage in cycles where they keep their body weight low for periods, but then gain weight due to their restraint weakness or when physiological processes result in a restoration of a higher body weight.[11] In addition to the pressure to reduce weight, athletes are often pressed for time, and they have to lose weight rapidly to make or stay on the team. As a result they often experience frequent periods of restrictive dieting or weight cycling.[15]

Such periods have been suggested as important risk or trigger factors for the development of eating disorder in athletes.[15,42] Relatively little information is available on the physiological adaptation of athletes who have restricted their diet or have experienced weight cycling over a period of time.

Steen et al.[45] reported that wrestlers who gain and lose weight repeatedly during training and competition have significantly lower resting metabolic rate than non-wrestlers of similar weight, height, and body fat content. It is not known whether the repeated weight gain and losses result in a lower resting metabolic rate, or if there is a subgroup of wrestlers with a low resting metabolic rate prior to their history of weight cycling.[45]

Personality factors

The characteristics of a sport (such as emphasis on leanness or individual competition) may interact with the personality traits of the athlete to start and perpetuate an eating disorder.[36] Some of the personality traits exhibited by athletes in general are similar to traits manifested by many patients with eating disorders. For example, both groups tend to be characterized by high self-expectation, perfectionism, persistence, and independence.[46] It may be that these qualities, which enable these individuals to succeed in sports, also place athletes more at risk of developing eating disorders.[49] Williamson et al.[47] examined a psychosocial model of risk factors for developing eating disorder symptoms in female college athletes. This model suggests that social pressure for thinness from coaches and peers, combined with anxiety about athletic performance and negative self-appraisal of athletic achievement, is associated with increased concern about body size and shape. Excessive concern about body size mediates these antecedent risk factors and eating disorder symptoms.

Williamson et al.[47] concluded that eating disorders in collegiate athletes are multidetermined, and are not simply a function of the emphasis on thinness in some women's sports, or the personality characteristics of some young women. More likely, several risk factors must occur during the same time period to cause overconcern with body size and shape, which in turn leads to pathological eating, dieting, and purgative habits.

Traumatic events

Some athletes with eating disorders who experience a significant weight loss without intending to lose weight report that they had lost their coach or changed coach prior to the weight loss period.[15] These athletes describe their coaches as being vital to their future athletic career.

Other athletes have reported that they developed eating disorders as a result of an injury or illness that left them temporarily unable to continue their normal level of exercise, as previously described by Katz.[41] An injury can hamper treatment and aftercare in the athlete with an existing disorder and tends to curtail the athlete's exercise and training. As a result, the athlete may gain weight due to less energy expenditure; or, even if weight gain does not occur, the athlete may develop an irrational fear of weight gain. In either case, the athlete may begin to diet as a means of compensating.[4]

Injured athletes are also likely to become depressed. If they are predisposed to have an eating disorder, this depression can play a role in the development of the disorder in at least two ways. First, depression often changes a person's eating patterns by increasing or decreasing appetite and energy intake. Second, the athlete could use the eating disorder in an attempt to manage their depression.[4]

Thus, the loss of a coach or unexpected illness or injury can probably be regarded as traumatic events similar to those described as trigger mechanisms for eating disorders in non-athletes.[5] Sexual abuse by male coaches has also been reported as a possible explanation for the development of eating disorders among some female elite athletes.[15]

The impact of coaches and trainers

Pressure to reduce weight has been the general explanation for the increased prevalence of eating disorders among athletes. When an athlete is not performing as well as a coach believes he or she should, the coach will look for an explanation and a solution. Unfortunately, many coaches decide to have an athlete lose weight based on how the athlete looks. It is possible for an individual to look heavy, be heavy, and still have relatively low body fat. Unfortunately, too many coaches focus on what the scale reads when the athlete is weighed. In this case, the athlete may lose weight, but not increase performance.[4,8] A number of investigations report that athletes started dieting after coaches had advised a reduction in weight.[22] Many of these

Table 5 The different reasons for the development of eating disorders reported by athletes with eating disorders[15]

Reason given	Athletes with eating disorders (%)
Prolonged periods of dieting	37
New coach	30
Injury/illness	23
Casual comments	19
Leaving home/failure at school or work	10
Problem in relationship	10
Family problems	7
Illness/injury to family members	7
Death of significant others	4
Sexual abuse (by coach)	4

Multiple answers were allowed; 15 per cent did not give any specific reason.

athletes are young and extremely impressionable. For them such a recommendation could be seen as a necessary step to achieve success in their sport. Rosen and Hough[17] reported that 75 per cent of young athletes who were told by their coaches that they were too heavy started using pathological weight loss methods. However, they did not report how many of these young athletes actually developed eating disorders. In a study comparing athletes with eating disorders with those not suffering from eating disorders, results showed that among those who had been told to lose weight, but had not developed eating disorders, 75 per cent had received guidance during the weight loss, compared with 10 per cent of those who had developed eating disorders.[15] Therefore, it is not necessarily dieting *per se*, but whether the athlete receives guidance or not, that is important. The different reasons for the development of eating disorders reported by high-level athletes with eating disorders are presented in Table 5.

A few studies have examined the educational level among athletes, coaches, and athletic trainers.[8,48,49] Findings indicate that too few of the coaches have a formal education in sport.[8,51,52] In Norway, only half of the coaches in charge of the female élite athletes have a formal education in physical education and sports. Of those who reportedly supervised athletes during weight loss periods, only coaches with a formal education in sport or physical education followed recommended routines. Furthermore, the coaches in high-prevalence sports (such as aesthetic and weight-dependent sports) had less formal education.[15]

The higher prevalence of eating disorders in those groups can probably not be explained by the low percentage of educated coaches alone, but there may be a connection. For example, the use of pathological weight control methods, such as vomiting, laxatives, and diuretics, were recommended more frequently by coaches without formal physical education. Finally, this study showed that coaches with a formal physical education have a significantly better knowledge of eating disorders. This enables them to recognize the

signs and symptoms of athletes who may have or may develop eating disorders.[15]

Nevertheless, most researchers agree that coaches do not cause eating disorders in athletes, although through inappropriate coaching, the problem may be triggered or exacerbated in vulnerable individuals.[24] Therefore, in most cases the role of coaches in the development of eating disorders in athletes should be seen as a part of a complex interplay of factors.

Rules

Health care personnel and representatives of those sports governing bodies where eating disorders are known to be a problem, should examine the rules and regulations of their sport. Eligibility criteria, rules, judging procedures, and coaching standards should be evaluated to determine if changes could diminish the pressure on athletes to strive for unrealistic and dangerously low body weights. An example of a serious approach to solving problems of this type is the action taken recently by the Women's Tennis Association in increasing the age for full participation on the professional circuit to 18 years. In the aesthetic sports, changes in the judging criteria should be considered. Teaching coaches and athletes about the dangers of eating disorders and the importance of good nutrition, without addressing the need to alter the rigorous weight standards imposed on them, is almost worthless. Eating disorders will always be a problem in young athletes involved in sports where weight and leanness are considered important for performance, unless age and body fat limits for participation are introduced.

Medical issues

Eating disorders can result in serious medical problems, and can even be fatal. Often, signs and symptoms of eating disorders are ignored or trivialized until serious medical damage has occurred.[4] Bulimia nervosa differs from anorexia nervosa in that medical complications result from different sources. Whereas most complications of anorexia nervosa occur as a direct or indirect result of starvation, complications of bulimia nervosa occur as a result of binge eating and purging.[4] Hsu,[50] Johnson and Connor,[51] and Mitchell[52] provide information on the medical problems encountered in patients with eating disorders.

Studies have reported mortality rates from less than 1 per cent to as high as 18 per cent in patients with anorexia nervosa in the general population.[4] Regardless of how mortality is measured, death is usually attributable to fluid and electrolyte abnormalities, or suicide.[11] Mortality in bulimia nervosa is less well studied, but deaths do occur, usually secondary to the complications of the binge–purging cycle or suicide. Mortality rates of eating disorders among athletes are not known. However, a number of cases of top level athletes representing gymnastics, running, cross-country, alpine skiing, and cycling have been reported in the media. Five (5.4 per cent) of those diagnosed in the Sundgot-Borgen[15] study reported that they had tried to commit suicide.

For years, athletes have used and abused drugs to control weight.[4] Some athletes use dieting, bingeing, vomiting, sweating, and fluid restriction for weight control. It is clear that many of these behaviours exist on a continuum, and may present health hazards for the athlete. Laxatives are probably the type of drug most commonly abused by athletes with weight and eating disorders. From 4

Table 6 Physical symptoms of athletes with anorexia nervosa or anorexia athletica

1. Significant weight loss beyond that necessary for adequate sport performance
2. Amenorrhoea or menstrual dysfunction
3. Dehydration
4. Fatigue beyond that normally expected in training or competition
5. Gastrointestional problems (i.e. constipation, diarrhoea, bloating, postprandial distress)
6. Hyperactivity
7. Hypothermia
8. Bradycardia
9. Lanugo
10. Muscle weakness
11. Overuse injuries
12. Reduced bone mineral density
13. Stress fractures

Modified after Thompson and Trattner-Sherman.[4]

to 75 per cent of athletes[15] reportedly abuse laxatives. Abuse of laxatives is an ineffective method of weight loss, because the weight loss that occurs is due to temporary fluid loss rather than prevention of nutrient absorption.[11] Long-term high-dose abuse of various diet pills is uncommon in eating disorder patients in general, and infrequently reported among athletes. Ipecac is used by some patients with eating disorders to induce vomiting. The normal fluctuation in weight during the menstrual cycle or a pressure to reduce weight fast can lead to initiation of diuretic use. Eight per cent of the Norwegian élite athletes suffering from eating disorders reported use of diuretics.[15] It should be noted that diet pills often contain drugs in the stimulant class, and that both these and diuretics are banned by the International Olympic Committee as doping agents.

Identifying athletes with anorexia nervosa and anorexia athletica

Most individuals with anorexia nervosa or anorexia athletica do not realize that they have a problem, and therefore do not seek treatment on their own. These athletes might consider seeking help only if their performance is levelling off.

Usually a coach or parent will call and ask how to approach the problem. Physical and psychological characteristics listed in Tables 6 and 7 may indicate the presence of anorexia nervosa or anorexia athletica. The presence of some of these characteristics does not mean that an athlete is anorexic, but the likelihood of the disorder being present increases with the number of characteristics that a particular athlete displays.[4]

Identifying athletes with bulimia nervosa

Most athletes suffering from bulimia nervosa are at or near normal weight. Bulimic athletes usually try to hide their disorder until they feel that they are out of control, or when they realize that the disorder negatively affects sport performance. Therefore, the team support staff must be able to recognize the physical symptoms and psychological characteristics listed in Tables 8 and 9. The presence of some of these characteristics does not necessarily indicate the presence of the disorder. However, the likelihood of the disorder being present increases as the number of characteristics increases.[4]

The effect of eating disorders on athletic performance

The nature and the magnitude of the effect of eating disorders on athletic performance are influenced by the severity and chronicity of the eating disorder and the physical demands of the sport. For example, anorexia nervosa will probably have different effects on an endurance athlete such as a distance runner, than on an athlete in a less aerobic sport such as gymnastics.

A number of studies have shown that both athletic controls and athletes suffering from eating disorders, who need to keep lean to improve performance, consume surprisingly low amounts of energy.[52-54] Athletes with eating disorders, except for some of the athletes with bulimia nervosa, consume diets low in energy and key nutrients.[8] However, the effects of the low energy intake on protein balance have not been studied in detail.

Athletes know that the quickest way to lose weight is by losing body water. Water is essential for the regulation of body temperature, and a dehydrated athlete becomes overheated and fatigued more easily. It has been shown that loss of endurance and co-ordination due to dehydration impairs exercise performance.[55]

Reduced plasma volume, impaired thermoregulation and nutrient exchange, decreased glycogen availability and decreased buffer capacity in the blood are plausible explanations for reduced performance in aerobic, anaerobic, and muscle endurance work, especially after rapid weight reduction. It is more difficult to explain decreased muscle strength found in some studies.[43,56]

Absolute maximal oxygen uptake (measured as litres/min) is

Table 7 Psychological and behavioural characteristics of athletes with anorexia nervosa and anorexia athletica[4,15]

1. Anxiety, both related and unrelated to sport performance
2. Avoidance of eating and eating situations
3. Claims of 'feeling fat' despite being thin
4. Resistance to weight gain or maintenance recommended by sport support staff
5. Unusual weighing behaviour (i.e. excessive weighing, refusal to weigh, negative reaction to being weighed)
6. Compulsiveness and rigidity, especially regarding eating and exercise
7. Excessive or obligatory exercise beyond that required for a particular sport
8. Exercising while injured despite prohibitions by medical and training staff
9. Restlessness—relaxing is difficult or impossible
10. Social withdrawal from team-mates and sport support staff, as well as from people outside sports
11. Depression
12. Insomnia

Table 8 Physical symptoms of athletes with bulimia nervosa[4]
1. Callus or abrasion on back of hand from inducing vomiting
2. Dehydration, especially in the absence of training or competition
3. Dental and gum problems
4. Oedema, complaints of bloating, or both
5. Electrolyte abnormalities
6. Frequent and often extreme weight fluctuations (i.e. mood worsens as weight goes up)
7. Gastrointestinal problems
8. Low weight despite eating large volumes
9. Menstrual irregularity
10. Muscle cramps, weakness, or both
11. Swollen parotid glands

unchanged or decreased after rapid body weight loss, but maximal oxygen uptake expressed in relation to body weight (ml/kg per min) may increase after gradual body weight reduction.[43,57] Anaerobic performance and muscle strength are typically decreased after rapid weight reduction with or without 1 to 3 h of rehydration. When tested after 5 to 24 h of rehydration, performance is maintained at euhydrated levels.[58,59]

Psychological factors may also affect performance. Many young wrestlers feel mood alterations (increased fatigue, anger, or anxiety) when attempting to lose body weight rapidly.[60]

The long-term effects of body weight reduction and eating disorders in athletes are not clear. Biological maturation and growth has been studied in girl gymnasts before and during puberty: there

Table 9 Psychological and behavioural characteristics of athletes with bulimia nervosa[4]
1. Binge eating
2. Agitation when bingeing is interrupted
3. Depression
4. Dieting that is unnecessary for appearance, health, or sport performance
5. Evidence of vomiting unrelated to illness
6. Excessive exercise beyond that required for the athlete's sport
7. Excessive use of the restroom
8. Going to the rest room or 'disappearing' after eating
9. Self-critical, especially concerning body, weight, and sport performance
10. Secretive eating
11. Substance abuse—whether legal, illegal, prescribed, or over-the-counter drugs, medications, or other substances
12. Use of laxatives or diuretics (or both) that is unsanctioned by medical or training staffs

are sufficient data to conclude that young female gymnasts are smaller and mature later than similar females from sports which do not require extreme leanness, such as swimming.[61,62] It is, however, difficult to separate the effects of physical strain, energy restriction, and genetic predisposition to delayed puberty. Nevertheless, a prospective study on athletes representing 'at risk' sports that provides information on dietary intake, training, and growth in young gymnasts and wrestlers would clarify the issue.

Besides increasing the likelihood of stress fractures, early bone loss may prevent normal peak bone mass to be achieved. Thus, after the typical postmenopausal period, former athletes with frequent or longer periods of amenorrhoea may again be at high risk of sustaining fractures. Studies on bone density in former female gymnasts, ballet dancers, and runners would provide more information on this potential health hazard.[59]

The psychological and medical features and consequences of eating disorders among athletes and non-athletes have been described and discussed in detail elsewhere.[4,11,41] Laboratory abnormalities and characteristic endocrine abnormalities of eating disorders are discussed by Katz.[43]

A drawback in studies on body weight reduction in athletes is that the relationship between performance test results and actual competitive performance are not clear.[43] Most investigators have used athletes in weight-class events as study participants. More longitudinal data on gradual body weight reduction in endurance athletes and participants in aesthetic sports is clearly needed.

Case histories

Female athlete with anorexia nervosa

Anne was a 22-year-old cross-country skier who competed at international level (168 cm in height, 47 kg in weight, and with 8 per cent body fat). She initially presented for treatment with menstrual dysfunction (amenorrhoea for the previous 2 years). She met all the DSM-IV[6] criteria for anorexia nervosa. When asked in the initial session about her eating, she denied any difficulty, but she was thin and claimed that the weight loss was related to an increase in training volume during the last year. When asked to do a 7-day-weight registration, she admitted that she was following a restricted regimen of vegetables and grains, about 800 kcal daily. She ate only at specific times, usually the same three or four foods each day. During this period, she trained for 4 h each day, skiing, running, and weight-training. She and her coach both believed that she could perform better at her present weight. She had started dieting 3 years earlier, and in the first season Anne enhanced her performance level despite the restricted eating, and used her sport to rationalize her training and eating regimens the following years. She developed a stress fracture 1 month prior to consultation (possibly due to 3 years of menstrual dysfunction), and had difficulty following the alternate training plan designed by the team's physical therapist. The coach explained that his athlete was actually suffering from an eating disorder, and therefore not allowed to compete. In the case of Anne, the reason for the development of an eating disorder was due to the intense wish of enhancing performance. Since no deep psychological trauma could explain her eating disorder, a psychologist was not included in the treatment team from the beginning. The nutritionist, her coach, and Anne carefully planned her eating and training schedule. To resume menses and reduce the risk of further loss of bone mass, oral contraceptives were prescribed by the gynae-cologist. Anne reduced her training from 12 h a week to 6 h, using non-weight bearing activities. After 2 months her energy intake was above 1300 kcal, and she gradually increased weight. Six months after the initial consultation, she was still improving, but struggling with the reduced training load and her fear of losing control of her eating behaviour.

Male athlete with bulimia nervosa

Erik was an 18-year-old ski jumper (172 cm in height, 60 kg in weight). He sought treatment, reporting that he had been bingeing and purging 3 to 16 times a week for the last 2 years. He met all the DSM-IV[6] criteria for bulimia nervosa. He had no doubt that the demand to 'make ideal weight' for ski jumping was the precipitating factor in his disorder. Before his involvement in ski jumping, he had no concerns about his weight and had never dieted. To make weight, Erik usually restricted his diet to about 800 kcal, induced vomiting, and used extreme amounts of laxatives. The reason for seeking treatment was that he had experienced fatigue cramps during the last season, and his coach claimed that he was not as focused as usual. Since his eating behaviour was extremely chaotic, he was referred to a cognitive treatment therapist who worked closely with the sports nutritionist. Erik had to relearn what, how much, and when to eat. The nutritionist followed the treatment plan suggested by Clark.[63] At the time of writing, Erik is still in treatment. He has learned how to be more at peace with himself and with food. He still fights the urge to binge, but he is improving.

Treatment of eating disorders

Unfortunately, few have discussed the specific issue of athletes and treatment of eating disorders. Therefore, this section mainly relies on the experiences described by Thompson et al.,[4] Clark,[63] and our own experiences from treatment of élite athletes suffering from eating disorders. Since most patients suffering from eating disorders are female, the patient will be referred to as she.

Once coaches, team-mates, or health care staff suspect that an athlete has an eating problem, questions about referral and arrange-ment for treatment, implementation of the therapeutic regimen, monitoring of specific therapeutic strategies, and arranging for follow-up should arise.[4] The formal treatment of athletes with eating disorders should be undertaken only by qualified health care professionals. Ideally, these individuals should also be familiar with, and have an appreciation for, the sport environment.[4,63]

It has been our experience that, in some ways, admitting to having an eating disorder is more threatening for the athlete with bulimia nervosa or bulimic symptoms than for those suffering from anorexia nervosa or anorexia athletica. Many athletes with bulimic symptoms have binged and purged for years, and regard their disorder as a disgusting habit.

Athletes are more likely to accept the idea of going for a consultation than committing to ongoing treatment.[4] Athletes with eating disorders usually resist treatment until they reach a point of despair, at which time they are more willing to accept help.[63] An appointment for an evaluation should be made as soon as possible because the athlete's fear and ambivalence about treatment may make her change her mind if given the opportunity.[4] Getting the athlete to accept a referral for an evaluation is sometimes a significant accom-

plishment in itself, but then getting her to participate in formal treatment may be quite another challenge. However, if the presence of an eating disorder is confirmed in the evaluation, then the eating disorder specialist providing the evaluation can play a major role in convincing the athlete of the need for treatment and can begin to motivate the individual for treatment.[4]

The success of the treatment plan must be based on establishing a trusting relationship between the athlete and the care providers. This includes respecting the athlete's desire to be lean for athletic performance, and expressing a willingness to work together to help the athlete be lean and healthy. The treatment team needs to listen to the athlete's fears and irrational thoughts about food and weight, then present a rational approach for achieving self-management of healthy diet and weight.[63]

Refusal of medical examination

If the athlete does not accept the initial referral or does not even admit that a problem exists, it is probably best not to push too hard at this point unless you believe the athlete is at risk medically. Schedule a medical examination at this point to determine her risk in this regard. If the athlete continues to refuse this examination, prohibit training and competition until she undergoes such an examination.[4] Give her information concerning a healthier weight. Ask her if she is having difficulty sleeping, or is feeling depressed, weak, tired, or irritable, and if she has lost her menstrual cycle. If she admits to these problems, suggest that they may all be related to her eating or weight control behaviour.

According to Thompson et al.,[4] the athlete should not be allowed to practise or compete until she agrees to the evaluation, but as a part of the team or the programme she must still attend practices and competitions. Suspension is not a good solution for several reasons. First, if the athlete is suspended, she may train on her own, which in some cases may be more dangerous because no one will be monitoring her exercise. Second, preventing the athlete from participating in her sport may further reduce her self-esteem. Third, control is a key issue for the individual with an eating disorder. She may view the suspension as an attempt by others to control.[4]

The athlete's family may be involved in the process of getting the athlete into treatment. One factor affecting this involvement is the athlete's age—the younger the athlete, the more the family's involvement is recommended. Certainly, one would anticipate more involvement with younger athletes.[4]

Treatment for the athlete who agrees to participate can involve a variety of types and modes and may vary as to goals, duration, and intensity.

Inpatient versus outpatient

Treatment for an eating disorder can involve either inpatient or out-patient treatment, or both. The decision regarding the appropriate treatment mode for the athlete is usually made by the professional health care providers involved in her care. Generally, most individuals with anorexia nervosa require at least some inpatient treatment, although the health care provider may try outpatient treatment if the individual's weight is stable and not extremely low and she is not purging.[50] Conversely, most individuals with bulimia nervosa can and should be treated on an outpatient basis.[52]

Types of treatment

Whether the athlete is in inpatient or outpatient treatment, he or she is likely to be involved in several modes of treatment. Typically, these include individual, group, and family therapy. Nutritional counselling and pharmacotherapy may also be included as adjuncts to the treatment regimen.

Individual psychotherapy

The therapist works only with the person with the eating disorder. The issues they deal with may vary somewhat depending on the therapist's particular theoretical orientation. Typically, the therapist tries to determine the exact nature of the individual's eating difficulties and how they might be most effectively changed. The therapist then tries to implement a change process. One issue that athletes need to deal with in therapy is how their sport or sport participation may be contributing to the maintenance of the eating disorder.[4]

Group therapy

The athlete will be part of a group made up of other individuals with eating disorders. Group treatment can benefit the athlete in many ways. It allows the athlete an opportunity to discover that she is not alone—that others have a similar problem. It gives the individual a support group that understands her feelings and eating problem. Group therapy provides a safe environment for the athlete to practise the new skills and attitudes she has learned.[4]

Family therapy

This includes the patient and part or all of her immediate family. The family rather than the individual is the focus of treatment. A primary goal in family therapy is to modify maladaptive family interactions, attitudes, and dynamics to decrease the need for, or the function of, the eating disorder in the family.[4]

Family issues and how they relate to the athlete's eating disorder are sometimes related to the patient's status as an athlete. For example, an athlete may believe that the only way she can gain her parent's acceptance is through exceptional sport performance. As a result, the athlete may be willing to resort to the methods of anorexia or bulimia to achieve and maintain a suboptimal or even unhealthy body weight. The modification of such a dysfunctional relationship between family needs, the eating disorder, and sport should be a focus in family therapy.[4]

Nutritional counselling

This is often part of a multimodal treatment approach. Most of the athletes with eating disorders have practised abnormal eating behaviours, and their attitudes about eating are often based on myths and misconceptions. Individuals with eating disorders do not remember what constitutes a balanced meal or 'normal' eating. The dietitian's primary roles involve providing nutritional information and assisting in meal planning.

Pharmacotherapy

This is sometimes useful in the treatment of eating disorders, especially bulimia nervosa. Using pharmacological agents to treat patients with eating disorders is a matter of clinical judgement by the treating doctor or psychiatrist.[4]

Treatment goals and expectations

The primary focuses of treatment are normalizing weight and eating behaviours, modifying unhealthy thought processes that maintain the disorder, and dealing with the emotional issues in the individual's life that in some cases create a need for the disorder. Athletes have the same general concerns as non-athletes about increasing their weight, but they also have concerns from a sport standpoint. What they think is an ideal competitive weight, one that they believe helps them be successful in their sport, may be significantly lower than their treatment goal weight. As a result, athletes may have concerns about their ability to perform in their sport following treatment.

The severity and chronicity of the disorder, regardless of type, affect the length of treatment, as do complicating personality factors. It may take months or years to recover from an eating disorder. Generally, anorexia nervosa requires a longer treatment time than bulimia nervosa. For athletes to complete treatment successfully, they must be able to trust the individuals involved in managing and treating their difficulties. A violation of confidentiality can destroy that trust. Some athletes may not want anyone associated with their sport to be involved in or receive information about their treatment. These athletes may need to have a special relationship with their therapist in which only the therapist is privy to certain information.[4]

In our experience, we have found that most athletes are willing to allow a coach or other support staff at least minimal contact with the therapist. Some others very much want the coach involved and view this as evidence of caring and concern on the part of the coach.

Team-mates of an athlete with an eating disorder are often aware of the problem and may also know that the athlete is in treatment. Information about the athlete with an eating disorder should be handled as the affected athlete desires. Some athletes may not want their parents to know about their disorder. Therapists cannot release information even to parents without the individual's consent, except under special circumstances and in the case of minors.

Training and competition

Once an athlete has been evaluated and the health care professionals have determined that she needs treatment, several issues that relate to training and competition arise. The most important question is whether the athlete should be allowed to continue to train and compete while recovering from the disorder.

Thompson et al.,[4] recommend suspension for athletes who refuse to be evaluated for an eating disorder. They based this recommendation on the premise that the athlete's health takes precedence over sport performance, and without an evaluation it is difficult or impossible to determine accurately the athlete's health risk.

The athlete in treatment

Athletes with an eating disorder should not compete until the health care professionals working with her decide it is safe. This decision can come at any point during the treatment process. Thompson et al.[4] state a number of reasons why the athlete should not compete until cleared to do so. First, depending on the nature and severity of the disorder, competing while suffering from an eating disorder may place the athlete at greater risk medically or psychologically. Second, sport may play a significant role in the disorder such that the athlete's participation in sport may help to maintain or perpetuate it. In addition, allowing an athlete to compete while affected by an eating disorder may give her the message that sport performance is more important than her health.

Generally, athletes are not recommended to compete during treatment. However, in some cases it may be permissible for the athlete to continue competing before successfully completing treatment. However, several important issues must be considered, the most important of which include diagnosis, the severity of the disorder, the type of sport, and the competitive level.

The medical risk of competing for an anorexic athlete is considerable. This is usually also true for athletes suffering from bulimia nervosa. In certain circumstances it may be acceptable for some athletes with milder symptoms, such as anorexia athletica or eating disorder not otherwise specified, to compete before they have completed treatment.

The athlete who is being considered for continuing competition while in treatment must undergo extensive medical and psychological evaluations. These evaluations must indicate that the athlete is not at risk medically and that competition will not increase her risk either medically or psychologically.[4]

Health maintenance standards

If the athlete meets the criteria just mentioned, the bottom-line standards regarding health maintenance must be imposed to protect the athlete. The treatment staff determine these and individually tailor them according to the athlete's particular condition. These standard may vary between individual athletes or by sport.

At a minimum, athletes should maintain a weight of no less than 90 per cent of 'ideal' weight, not sport related, but health related. The athlete should eat at least three balanced meals a day, consisting of enough energy to sustain the pre-established weight standard the dietician has proposed. Athletes who have been amenorrhoeal for 6 months or more should undergo a medical examination to consider hormone replacement therapy.[41] In addition, bone mineral density should be assessed and results should be within normal range.

To continue competition and training the following list represents what Thompson et al.[4] believe are the minimal criteria in this regard: (i) the athlete must agree to comply with all treatment strategies as best as she can; (ii) the athlete must genuinely want to compete; (iii) the athlete must be closely monitored on an ongoing basis by the medical and psychological health care professionals handling her treatment and by the sport-related personnel who are working with her in her sport; (iv) treatment must always take precedence over sport; and (v) if any question arises at any time regarding whether the athlete is meeting or is able to meet the preceding criteria, competition is not to be considered a viable option while the athlete is in treatment.[4]

Limited training while in treatment

If the criteria mentioned above for competing cannot be met, or if competition rather than physical exertion is a problem, some athletes who are not competing may still be allowed to engage in limited training. The same criteria used to assess the safety of competition apply (i.e. diagnosis, problem severity, type of sport, competitive level, and health maintenance).

We believe that continuing in training and competition could have some advantages for some athletes. Some athletes will be motivated in treatment by the opportunity to continue training.

If the athlete is ready to get over her disorder, allowing her to continue with her sport with minimal risk when she really wants to continue can enhance the motivation for and the effect of treatment. For some athletes, allowing them to train or compete is a source of well being or self-esteem.[4]

Decision to compete

Some athletes should be allowed to compete while in aftercare if not medically or psychologically contraindicated. It is extremely important to examine whether the athlete really wants to go back to competitive sport. If so, she should be allowed to compete as soon as she feels ready for it when finishing treatment and if she is in good health.[4]

Prevention of eating disorders in athletes

Since the exact causes of eating disorders are unknown, it is difficult to draw up preventive strategies. Coaches should realize that they can strongly influence their athletes. Coaches or others involved with young athletes should not comment on an individual's body size, or require weight loss in young and growing athletes. Without offering further guidance, dieting may result in unhealthy eating behaviour or eating disorders in highly motivated and uninformed athletes.[64] Early intervention is also important, since eating disorders are more difficult to treat the longer they progress. However, most important of all is the prevention of circumstances or factors which could lead to an eating disorder. Therefore, professionals working with athletes should be informed about the possible risk factors for their development; early signs and symptoms of eating disorders; the medical, psychological, and social consequences of these disorders; how to approach the problem if it occurs; and what treatment options are available. This improves awareness and facilitates early detection and intervention. While coaches, parents, and athletes can learn to identify symptoms that indicate risk, diagnosis and treatment should only be made by a physician or psychologist.

Weight loss recommendation

Most athletes do not have an ideal body composition for their sport. A change in body composition and weight loss can be achieved safely if the weight goal is realistic and based on body composition rather than weight-for-height standards. Use of the skinfold appraisal techniques is recommended, because of the large time and equipment demands required when using hydrostatic weighing. The following recommendations for safe weight loss in athletes have been modified from Eisenman et al.[64]

Identify realistic weight goals

Athletes must consume sufficient energy to avoid the loss of muscle tissue, and should start a weight loss programme well before the season begins. Changes in body composition should be monitored on a regular basis.

Monitor weight

The coach or others educated in weight control methods should set realistic goals that address methods of dieting, rate of weight change, and a reasonable target range of weight and body fat. After the athlete has reached the target weight and percentage of body fat, the coach should continue to monitor weight and body composition to detect any continued or unwarranted losses or weight fluctuations. Weigh-ins and other measurements of body composition should be done in private to reduce the stress, anxiety, and embarrassment of public assessment.

Provide nutritional guidance

The coach should not tell athletes to lose weight without providing them with proper nutritional guidance. Rather, the coach should provide a total nutritional programme that includes general nutrition counselling, as well as help in appropriate methods of weight loss and weight gain. If the coach has no education in nutrition, a registered dietician should be involved to plan individual diets that are nutritionally adequate. Throughout this process, the role of overall good nutrition practices in optimizing performance should be emphasized.

Be aware of symptoms

If athletes exhibit symptoms of an eating disorder, they should be confronted with the possible problem.

Seek professional help

Coaches should not try to diagnose or treat eating disorders, but they should be specific about their suspicions and talk with the athlete about the fears or anxieties they may be having about food and performance. Medical evaluation should be encouraged and the athlete supported and reassured that a team position will not be affected if not medically initiated (i.e. if the medical exam and laboratory tests indicate that exercise is not harmful for her).

Be a team member

The coach should assist and support the athlete during treatment.

Conclusions

The prevalence of eating disorders is higher among athletes than non-athletes, but the relationship to performance or training level is unknown. Additionally, athletes competing in sports where leanness or a specific weight are considered important are more prone to eating disorders than athletes competing in sports where these factors are considered less important. Therefore, it is necessary to examine anorexia nervosa, bulimia nervosa, and subclinical eating disorders, and the range of behaviours and attitudes associated with eating disturbances in athletes to learn how these clinical and subclinical disorders are related.

Interesting suggestions about possible sport-specific risk factors for the development of eating disorders in athletes exist, but large-scale longitudinal studies are needed to learn more about risk factors and the aetiology of eating disorders in athletes at different competitive levels and within different sports.

The formal treatment of athletes with eating disorders should be undertaken only by qualified health care professionals. Ideally, these individuals should also be familiar with, and have an appreciation for, the sport environment.

More knowledge about the short- and long-term effects of eating disorders upon the health and performance of athletes is needed.

References

1. American Psychiatric Association. *Diagnostic and statistical manual of mental disorders*, 3rd edn rev. Washington DC: American Psychiatric Association, 1987: 65–9.
2. Sundgot-Borgen J. Prevalence of eating disorders in female elite athletes. *International Journal of Sport Nutrition* 1993; **3**: 29–40.
3. Szmuckler GI, Eisler I, Gillies C, Hayward ME. The implications of anorexia nervosa in a ballet school. *Journal of Psychiatric Research* 1985; **19**: 177–81.
4. Thompson RA, Trattner-Sherman R. *Helping athletes with eating disorders*. Champaign, IL: Human Kinetic, 1993.
5. Bassoe HH. Anorexia/bulimia nervosa: the development of anorexia nervosa and of mental symptoms. Treatment and the outcome of the disease. *Acta Psychiatrica Scandinavica* 1990; **82**: 7–13.
6. American Psychiatric Association. *Diagnostic and statistical manual of mental disorders*, 4th edn. (DSM-IV). Washington DC: American Psychiatric Association, 1994: 1–2.
7. Pugliese MT Lifshitz F, Grad G, Fort P, Marks-Katz M. Fear of obesity. A cause of short stature and delayed puberty. *New England Journal of Medicine* 1983; **309**: 513–18.
8. Sundgot-Borgen J, Larsen S. Nutrient intake and eating behavior of female elite athletes suffering from anorexia nervosa, anorexia athletica and bulimia nervosa. *International Journal of Sport Nutrition* 1993; **3**: 431–42.
9. Andersen AE. Eating disorders in males: a special case. In: Brownell KD, Rodin J, Wilmore JH, eds. *Eating, body weight and performance in athletes. Disorders of modern society*. Philadelphia: Lea and Febiger, 1992: 172–88.
10. Andersen AE. Diagnosis and treatment of males with eating disorders. In: Andersen AE, ed. *Males with eating disorders*. New York: Brunner/Mazel, 1990: 133–62.
11. Brownell KD, Rodin J, Wilmore JH. Prevalence of eating disorders in athletes. In: Brownell KD, Rodin J, Wilmore JH, eds. *Eating, body weight and performance in athletes. Disorders of modern society*. Philadelphia: Lea and Febiger, 1992: 128–43.
12. Gadpalle WJ, Sandborn CF, Wagner WW. Athletic amenorrhea, major affective disorders and eating disorders. *American Journal of Psychiatry* 1987; **144**: 939–43.
13. Warren BJ, Stanton AL, Blessing DL. Disordered eating patterns in competitive female athletes. *International Journal of Eating Disorders* 1990; **5**: 565–9.
14. Burckes-Miller ME, Black DR. Male and female college athletes. Prevalence of anorexia nervosa and bulimia nervosa. *Athletic Training* 1988; **2**: 137–40.
15. Sundgot-Borgen J. Risk and trigger factors for the development of eating disorders in female elite athletes. *Medicine and Science in Sports and Exercise* 1994; **4**: 414–19.
16. Rucinski A. Relationship of body image and dietary intake of competitive ice skaters. *Journal of the American Dietetic Association* 1989; **89**: 98–100.
17. Rosen LW, Hough DO. Pathogenic weight-control behaviors of female college gymnasts. *Physician and Sports Medicine* 1988; **9**: 141–4.
18. Dummer GM *et al.* Pathogenic weight-control behaviors of young competitive swimmers. *Physician and Sports Medicine* 1987; **5**: 75–6.
19. Hamilton LH, Brocks-Gunn J, Warren MP. Sociocultural influences on eating disorders in professional female ballet dancers. *International Journal of Eating Disorders* 1985; **4**: 465–77.
20. Hamilton LH, Brocks-Gunn J, Warren MP, Hamilton WG. The role of selectivity in the pathogenesis of eating problems in ballet

dancers. *Medicine and Science in Sports and Exercise* 1988; **20**: 560–5.

21. Rosen LW, McKeag DB, Hough DO. Pathogenic weight-control behaviors in female athletes. *Physician and Sports Medicine* 1986; **14**: 79–86.

22. Smith NJ. Excessive weight loss and food aversion in athletes simulating anorexia nervosa. *Pediatrics* 1980; **1**: 139–42.

23. Sundgot-Borgen J, Corbin CB. Eating disorders among female athletes. *Physician and Sports Medicine* 1987; **15**: 89–95.

24. Wilmore JH. Eating and weight disorders in female athletes. *International Journal of Sport Nutrition* 1991; **1**: 104–17.

25. Sykora C, Grilo CM, Wilfly DE, Brownell KD. Eating, weight, and dieting disturbances in male and female lightweight and heavyweight rowers. *International Journal of Eating Disorders* 1993; **2**: 203–11.

26. Steen SN, Brownell KD. Current patterns of weight loss and regain in wrestlers: has the tradition changed? *Medicine and Science in Sports and Exercise* 1990; **22**: 762–8.

27. Tipton CM, Theng TK, Paul WD. Evaluation of the Hall methods for determining minimal wrestling weights. *Journal of the Iowa Medical Society* 1969; **59**: 571–4.

28. American College of Sport Medicine. Position stand on weight loss in wrestlers. *Medicine and Science in Sports and Exercise* 1976; **8**: XI–XIII.

29. American Medical Association, Committee on the Medical Aspects of Sports. Wrestling and weight control. *Journal of the American Medical Association* 1967; **201**: 541–3.

30. Blouin AG, Goldfield GS. Body image and steroid use in male bodybuilders. *International Journal of Eating Disorders* 1995; **2**: 159–65.

31. Garner DM, Olmsted MP, Polivy J. *Manual of eating disorder inventory.* Odessa: Psychological Assessment Resources, 1984.

32. Garner DM, Garfinkel PE. An index of symptoms of anorexia nervosa. *Psychological Medicine* 1979; **9**: 273–9.

33. Mallick MJ, Whipple TW, Huerta E. Behavioral and psychological traits of weight-conscious teenagers: a comparison of eating disordered patients and high- and low-risk groups. *Adolescence* 1987; **22**: 157–67.

34. Garfinkel PE, Garner DM, Goldbloom, DS. Eating disorders implications for the 1990's. *Canadian Journal of Psychiatry* 1987; **32**: 624–31.

35. Katz JL. Some reflections on the nature of the eating disorders. *International Journal of Eating Disorders* 1985; **4**: 617–26.

36. Wilson T, Eldredge KL. Pathology and development of eating disorders: implications for athletes. In: Brownell KD, Rodin J, Wilmore JH, eds. *Eating, body weight and performance in athletes. Disorders of modern society*, Philadelphia: Lea and Febiger, 1992: 115–27.

37. Sacks MH. Psychiatry and sports. *Annals of Sports Medicine* 1990; **5**: 47–52.

38. Epling WF, Pierce WD. Activity based anorexia nervosa. *International Journal of Eating Disorders* 1988; **7**: 475–85.

39. Epling WF, Pierce WD, Stefan L. A theory of activity based anorexia. *International Journal of Eating Disorders* 1983; **3**: 27–46.

40. Costill DL. Carbohydrate for exercise: dietary demands for optimal performance. *International Journal of Sports Medicine* 1988; **9**: 1–18.

41. Katz JL. Eating disorders in women and exercise. In Shangold M and Mirken G, eds. *Physiology and sports medicine.* Philadelphia: Davis Company, 1988: 248–63.

42. Brownell KD, Steen SN, Wilmore JH. Weight regulation practices in athletes: analysis of metabolic and health effects. *Medicine and Science in Sports and Exercise* 1987; **6**: 546–56.

43. Fogelholm M. Effects of bodyweight reduction on sports performance. *Sports Medicine* 1994; **4**: 249–67.

44. Walberg JL. Aerobic exercise and resistance weight-training during weight reduction. Implications for obese persons and athletes. *Sports Medicine* 1989; **7**: 343–56.

45. Steen SN, Oppliger RA, Brownell KD. Metabolic effects of repeated weight loss and regain in adolescent wrestlers. *Journal of the American Medical Association* 1988; **260**: 47–50.

46. Yates A. *Compulsive exercise and eating disorders.* New York: Brunner/Mazel, 1991.

47. Williamson DA, Netemeyer RG, Jackman LP, Andersen DA, Funsch CL, Rabalis JY. Structural equation modeling of risks for the development of eating disorder symptoms in female athletes. *International Journal of Eating Disorders* 1995; **4**: 387–93.

48. Wolf EMB, Wirth JC, Lohman TG. Nutritional practices of coaches in the Big Ten. *Physician and Sports Medicine* 1975; **2**: 112–24.

49. Parr RB, Porter MA, Hodgson SC. Nutrient knowledge and practice of coaches, trainers, and athletes. *Physician and Sports Medicine* 1984; **3**: 127–38.

50. Hsu, L.K.G. *Eating disorders.* New York: Guilford Press, 1990.

51. Johnson C, Connor SM. *The etiology and treatment of bulimia nervosa.* New York: Basic Books, 1987.

52. Mitchell, J.E. *Bulimia nervosa.* Minneapolis: University of Minnesota Press, 1990.

53. Erp-Bart AMJ *et al.* Energy intake and energy expenditure in top female gymnasts. In: Brinkhorst *et al.*, eds. *Children and exercise XI.* Champaign, IL: University Park Press, 1985: 218–23.

54. Welch PK, Zager KA, Endres J. Nutrition education, body composition and dietary intake of female college athletes. *Physician and Sports Medicine* 1987; **15**: 63–74.

55. Webster S, Rutt R, Weltman A. Physiological effects of weight loss regimen practiced by college wrestlers. *Medicine and Science in Sports and Exercise* 1990; **22**: 229–33.

56. Housten ME, Marrin DA, Green HJ. The effect of the rapid weight loss on physiological functions in wrestlers. *Physician and Sports Medicine* 1981; **9**: 73–8

57. Ingjer F, Sundgot-Borgen J. Influence of body weight reduction on maximal oxygen uptake in female elite athletes. *Scandinavian Journal of Medicine and Science in Sports* 1991; **1**: 141–6.

58. Klinzing JE, Karpowicz W. The effect of rapid weight loss and rehydration on a wrestling performance test. *Journal of Sports Medicine and Physical Exercise* 1986; **26**: 149–56.

59. Fogelholm GM, Koskinen R. Laakso J. Gradual and rapid weight loss: effects on nutrition and performance in male athletes. *Medicine and Science in Sport Exercise* 1993; **25**: 371–7.

60. Armstrong LE, Costill DL, Fink WJ. Influence of diuretics induced dehydration on competitive running performance. *Medicine and Science Sports and Exercise* 1985; **17**: 456–61.

61. Mansfield MJ, Emans SJ. Growth in female gymnasts: should training decrease during puberty? *Pediatrics* 1993; **122**: 237–40.

62. Theintz MJ, Howald H, Weiss U. Evidence of a reduction of growth potential in adolescent female gymnasts. *Journal of Pediatrics* 1993; **122**: 306–13.

63. Clark N. How to help the athlete with bulimia: practical tips and case study. *International Journal of Sport Nutrition* 1993; **3**: 450–60.

64. Eisenman PA, Johnson SC, Benson JE. *Coaches guide to nutrition and weight control*, 2nd edn. Champaign, IL: Leisure Press, 1990.

1.3 Kinesiology

1.3.1 Biomechanics as applied to sports

Benno M. Nigg

Introduction

Biomechanics is the science that studies external and internal forces acting on a biological system and the effects produced by these forces.

The discipline of biomechanics can be subdivided into particular directions including:

(1) anatomical biomechanics, studying movements of joints and muscular contribution to these movements;

(2) neurophysiological biomechanics, studying muscular control as well as reflex and feedback mechanisms; and

(3) mechanical biomechanics, studying the mechanical aspect of human movement by analysing motion and by assessing internal and/or external forces.

This chapter concentrates on mechanical biomechanics, which is concerned with forces, moments, accelerations, velocities, energy, momentum, and other mechanical expressions associated with Newton's three laws of motion. The aim is to help the reader learn to analyse and assess human movement from a biomechanical perspective, and to look at human movement from a biomechanical viewpoint.

Biomechanical questions can be subdivided into two groups: those dealing with performance, and those dealing with load, overload, and associated injuries. Both types of question may require basic or applied research to answer them.

Selected examples of biomechanical topics and questions related to performance are as follows.

1. How is it possible for an athlete to jump over 8 m? Or, in a more general sense, what are the factors that determine the performance of a long jumper? Can these factors be modified through training to improve performance?

2. Gymnasts, divers, and trampolinists perform somersaults with twists. Often they make specific movements with their arms when starting the twisting movement in the air. How can an athlete initiate a twisting movement during a somersault, and can movement during the flight phase be modified to improve performance? (It should be noted that there are athletes with no arms who perform twisting somersaults.)

3. Sport shoes vary in their construction depending on the sport activity. What are the factors determining performance in a particular sport activity, and can performance be enhanced by sport shoe design? Is it possible to construct shoes which return energy during running?

4. Amputees walking with a prosthesis may desire a walking style which is similar to that of non-amputees. What are the possibilities for differentiating between normal and abnormal human gait? What are the main factors characterizing normal gait, and can they be learned by the amputee?

5. Performance in sports often depends on forces produced by the muscles. What are the rules governing muscular force production? How can muscular forces be transferred into power output to enhance performance?

Examples of biomechanical topics and questions related to load and overload on the human locomotor system are as follows.

1. Forces acting on the anatomical structures of a skier are assumed to be quite high. How high are such forces in specific structures of the human body? How do forces acting on articular cartilage in the knee joint, for instance, compare with the critical limits of articular cartilage? Can strategies be developed to reduce these forces?

2. Tennis is played on clay, concrete, asphalt, artificial turf, sand-filled artificial turf, natural grass, and other surfaces. How does the surface influence the forces acting on specific anatomical structures of a tennis player? Are certain surfaces less likely to produce particular injuries than others?

3. Shin splints (pain at the anterior aspect of the tibia) are common in runners. Long-distance runners, sprinters, and even basketball and volleyball players are often affected by this injury. There are different theories about the aetiology of this condition. Is the type of movement related to the occurrence of shin splints? Are anthropometric factors associated with the development of shin splints?

4. In many sport activities, bones are broken, ligaments are torn, and cartilages are destroyed. Injuries occur in acute situations and as a result of chronic overloading. Arthritis as a result of repeated microdamage to cartilage, for instance, is assumed to be such a chronic 'injury'. What mechanisms are responsible for these injuries? What are the critical limits for human tissue, such as bone, cartilage, ligament, tendon, etc., for acute and chronic injuries? Does age affect these limits?

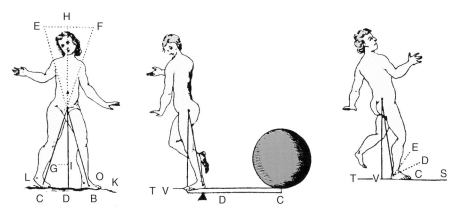

Fig. 1 Forces acting on the human body, an illustration from Borelli's book *De motu animalium*. (Reproduced from ref. 1, with permission.)

In the following sections we attempt to provide insight into the possibilities for answering such questions. The purpose of this chapter is to illustrate how biomechanics can be used to study human movement or, in more popular terms, to outline how one can look at human movement through biomechanical spectacles.

Selected historical highlights

Aristotle (384 BC–322 BC), a Greek philosopher and 'natural scientist', introduced the term 'mechanics' and is considered to be the initiator of mechanics as we understand it at present. He can be considered the first biomechanist since he wrote about the movement of living beings. It is obvious that his view of the science of nature and mechanical principles is different from the current understanding. However, in his time his ideas aimed at understanding nature, and particularly human movement, were unique and are considered an important step in the development of the understanding of human movement and of the factors influencing it.

Ambroise Paré (1510–90) developed prostheses for legs, hands, and arms. They were often used for soldiers who had lost parts of their upper or lower extremities. Paré was among the first to apply biomechanics to improve the life of the handicapped. He can be considered as one of the first biomechanists or bioengineers.

Alphonso Borelli (1608–79), an Italian scientist, is considered the 'father of biomechanics'. He was a student of Galileo Galilei and had degrees in medicine and mathematics. This enabled him to understand the human body anatomically and to develop the necessary mathematical models to describe human movement mechanically. His research in biomechanics was published in the book *De motu animalium*.[1] He was probably the first to perform gait analysis and to determine the centre of mass of the human body. An illustration from *De motu animalium* is shown in Fig. 1. Borelli discussed many different aspects of human movement as related to the externally visible motion of animals or humans. He described the function of muscles, formulated mechanical lemmas to explain the movements produced by muscles, explained the function of muscles for the motion of the knee joint, and discussed the influence of the direction of the muscle fibres on force production by this muscle. Furthermore, he discussed standing, walking, jumping, flying, and swimming. He formulated his findings or hypotheses in the form of propositions.

Isaac Newton (1642–1727) formulated the mechanical principles which are still used for classical mechanics. Newtonian mechanics is the foundation of biomechanics related to human movement. Newton was not a full-time physicist or a natural scientist. His main interest was in philosophy, and it is said that he considered his involvement in physics more as a burden than as an interesting task.

Étienne-Jules Marey (1830–1904) developed various techniques such as film analysis and pressure-measuring devices which could be applied to biomechanical research. His contribution to the field of biomechanics was not to propose solutions to basic questions as his predecessors had done. Rather it consisted of the development of methodologies and techniques to quantify human movement. His pressure-measuring device (Fig. 2) was the first attempt to quantify

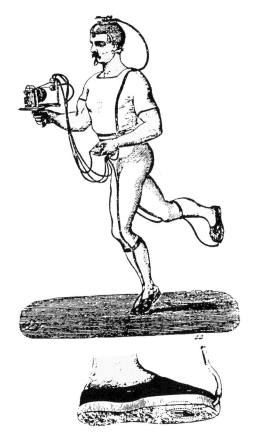

Fig. 2 Test subject with a pneumatic device to quantify pressure underneath the foot as developed by Marey. (Reproduced from ref. 3, with permission.)

forces acting on the foot of a subject during movement. He also developed chronophotography.

Elftmann developed a method of quantifying the centre of pressure under the foot during gait (published in 1938, see ref. 23).

In 1965, Paul estimated internal forces in the human hip joint.[2] One of the difficulties in the estimation of internal forces is that the human locomotor system has more force-carrying structures crossing a joint than are needed to perform a specific movement, which results in a mathematical system with more unknowns than equations. Paul solved this problem by reducing the actual number of muscles crossing a joint to equal the number required to perform the movement in question (reduction method).

Hatze[4] expanded the mainly mechanical approach to modelling the human body during movement by developing a model which included a comprehensive mechanical, physiological, and neurological approach.

Currently, several thousand researchers are active in the field of biomechanics, covering fields such as cardiac biomechanics, fluid biomechanics, injury biomechanics, muscle biomechanics, orthopaedic biomechanics, rehabilitation biomechanics, sport biomechanics, and tissue biomechanics.

Mechanics

Classical mechanics is based on Newton's three laws: the law of inertia (first law); the law of action (second law); and the law of reaction (third law).

Mechanics can be subdivided into statics and dynamics. Dynamics is usually subdivided into kinematics and kinetics. Kinematics describes position, displacement, velocity, and acceleration without an indication of the cause of the movement. Kinetics relates the forces acting on a body to its mass and motion. Conventionally, kinetic analysis predicts the motion of a mass for known forces (direct dynamics) or determines the forces required to produce a given motion (inverse dynamics). The study of statics goes back to the Greek philosophers. The first significant contribution to the study of dynamics was made by Galileo Galilei (1564–1642). His experimental findings on the topic of uniformly accelerated bodies formed the basis for Newton's fundamental laws of motion.

Statics

Force

Most of our ideas about force are associated with exertion of muscular forces on objects. The meaning of force seems clear because force is experienced every day, whether it be sitting in a chair, pushing against a resistance, jumping, or walking. Force is considered as a 'push' or 'pull' exerted by one body on another. Effects produced by forces can be listed and are descriptions (not definitions). In a static sense, force can be described as follows.

If 'something' is able to keep a spring stretched, this 'something' is called a force.

In biomechanics the expressions external and internal forces are used. To distinguish between external and internal forces the system of interest must first be defined.

Forces acting upon the system of interest are called external forces.

Forces acting within the system of interest are called internal forces.

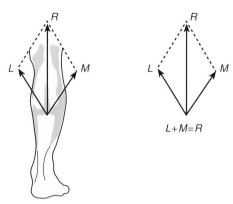

Fig. 3 Illustration of a resultant vector *R* resolved into its components *L* and *M*. (Adapted from ref. 5, with permission).

If, for instance, the human body is the system of interest, all the forces acting upon the human body are external forces (for example, gravity, ground reaction force, air resistance), while all the forces acting within the body are internal forces (for example, joint forces, muscle forces, tendon and ligament forces). If, however, the forearm and hand comprise the system of interest, the joint forces in the elbow joint would be external forces.

If the human body is considered to be the system of interest, typical external forces would be gravitational forces, frictional forces, ground reaction forces, and contact forces. Typical internal forces would include bone-to-bone forces in joints, tendon insertion forces, muscular forces, and ligament forces.

Forces acting upon or within the human body while at rest can be called 'static forces'. When a person is standing on both legs the force bodyweight is acting. Bodyweight and body mass are not the same. Bodyweight is analytically determined from body mass by using Newton's second law. To a first approximation the acceleration is 10 m/s². This value will be used in all the following examples. Thus the bodyweight for a human with the mass of 50 kg is 500 N, and the bodyweight for a human with the mass of 80 kg is 800 N (where N is the symbol for 1 newton).

Often the forces are expressed in units of bodyweight (**BW**). Examples of static forces expressed in bodyweight are as follows:

- force in hip joint (standing on both legs) = 0.5 BW
- force in hip joint (standing on one leg) = 3–5 BW
- force in the Achilles tendon (one leg/toe) = 3–6 BW.

Forces (like all vectors) are often resolved into components in the direction of the axes of the chosen coordinate system. Sometimes these axes are related to body posture. Typical conventions used in this text are listed above. Forces may also be resolved into components relative to surfaces. In joints, one often distinguishes between forces perpendicular to the joint surface (normal forces) and forces tangential to the surface. Forces in muscles may be resolved with respect to the line of action of muscle fibres (Fig. 3).

Moment of force

If the system of interest is not a particle but a rigid body with length, width, and height (dimensions), forces can produce two types of movements: translation and/or rotation. In order to describe the effects of forces which can produce a rotation, the quantity 'moment of force' or 'moment' is introduced. The symbol for moment is M, where M is a vector:

$$M = \text{moment of force} = \text{moment} = \text{torque}.$$

The magnitude of the moment of F about an axis O is:

$$M_O = d_O F;$$

where:
M_O is the magnitude of the moment with respect to point O, d_O is the perpendicular distance from 0 to the line of action of F, and F is the magnitude of force acting on the body. The units of F are newtons (N), the units of d_O are metres (m), and the units of M_O are newton metres (N.m).

Examples of moments

The following numbers are given for an average body mass of 80 kg. The moment produced by the Achilles tendon with respect to the ankle joint while standing on one leg on the toes is about 7 to 14 N.m. The moment produced by the (idealized) bodyweight about the sagittal hip joint axis while standing on one leg is about 5 to 10 N.m. The moment of the (idealized) biceps and brachialis tendon for an assumed mass of 1 kg and an assumed forearm mass of 2 kg is about 0.56 N.m.

Equilibrium of rigid bodies

If a body is at rest and remains at rest it is said to be in equilibrium. In this case the vector sum of all the forces and moments acting on the body is equal to zero:

$$F_1 + F_2 + \ldots + Fn = \Sigma \, Fi = O \;\; i = 1, \ldots, n,$$

$$M_1 + M_2 + \ldots + Mn = \Sigma \, Mi = O \;\; i = 1, \ldots, n.$$

These equations will be used in the following to estimate internal forces in static situations. The examples will be restricted to two-dimensional questions.

Example of internal forces

To illustrate how the concept of equilibrium can be applied to biomechanical problems the equilibrium equations will be used to calculate muscle and joint forces for a two-dimensional example. A subject is standing on the forefoot of one leg illustrated in Fig. 4. We wish to determine the bone-to-bone force in the ankle joint and the force in the Achilles tendon.

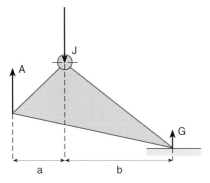

Fig. 4 Free-body diagram of a human foot while standing on the forefoot.

Assumptions

1. The problem can be solved two-dimensionally.

2. There is one joint to the neighbouring segment—the ankle joint which is idealized as a hinge joint. The human foot is considered as one rigid body.

3. The forces acting are as follows (in scalar form): ground reaction force $g = 800$ N; force in the Achilles tendon $a =$ unknown; force in the ankle joint $J =$ unknown.

4. All forces act in vertical direction.

5. The distance of the forces from the ankle joint are $a = 0.04$ m and $b = 0.12$ m.

6. Friction in the ankle joint and on the ground can be neglected.

7. The weight of the foot can be neglected.

Solution

The following equilibrium equation can be formulated for the moments with respect to an axis through the ankle joint (note that the force J does not produce a moment about the ankle joint since its line of action is through the axis of the ankle joint):

$$-aA + bG = 0.$$

The only unknown is a; therefore:

$$A = (b/a)g$$

$$A = 2400 \text{ N.}$$

The following equilibrium equation can be formulated for the forces:

$$A + G - J = 0.$$

The only unknown is J; therefore:

$$J = A + G$$

$$J = 3200 \text{ N.}$$

It should be noted that in this example the joint and muscle forces are larger than the ground reaction force. This result is typical of the relationship between internal and external forces.

Dynamics

Kinematics

Movement, in general, is subdivided into translational and rotational movement. A motion is said to be a translation if any straight line within a body keeps the same orientation for any time ti throughout the motion. The mechanical quantities which are used to describe translational movement are position, displacement, velocity, and acceleration.

The acceleration which is frequently used is the earth acceleration or the acceleration due to gravity. The value for the acceleration due to gravity is 9.81 m/s² and is referred to as $1/g$. In many practical applications, and for simplicity, the acceleration due to gravity g is often approximated as 10 m/s². This approximation is used consistently throughout this chapter.

Table 1 Speeds for various movements

Body part	Velocity (m/s)	Movement
CM	30	Take-off in ski-jumping
CM	10	Average speed in sprinting
CM	4.5	Free fall from $H = 1$ m
CM	7.7	Free fall from $H = 3$ m
Heel	2–3	Landing speed in running
Toe	1–2	Landing speed in running
Hand	30	Javelin (maximal speed)
Foot	20	Football kick

CM, centre of body mass.

Examples of speeds and accelerations for various movements are summarized in Tables 1 and 2.

Translational movement

Translational considerations can be appropriate for the analysis of running. The average speed in running can be written as:

$$v_a = \text{distance}/\text{time} = (\text{stride length}) \times (\text{stride frequency}).$$

For each step the average speed depends on the stride length and the stride frequency. Therefore an increase in stride length and/or stride frequency can be used to increase average running speed. This has been supported experimentally[6] for changes in running speed between 3 and 4 m/s (Fig. 5). However, stride lengths and stride frequencies cannot be increased indefinitely. The increase in stride length may be limited by the fact that the centre of mass is increasingly lowered with an increase in the stride length. Thus additional work must be done for the increased vertical movement of the centre of mass. The increase in frequency is limited by the muscular strength and/or the inertia of the masses involved. While the masses involved usually only change slightly for a given athlete, the muscular strength may increase substantially.

Table 2 Accelerations for various movements

Body part	Acceleration (g)	Movement
Hand	5–10	Boxing (active movement)
Hand	30–60	Boxing (passive impact)
Tibia	10–30	Landing on room surface from 0.5 m
Tibia	30–50	Skiing (30 km/h, squatting)
Hip	2–3	Skiing (30 km/h, squattting)
Head	1–2	Skiing (30 km/h, squatting)
Tibia	5–10	Skiing (30 km/h, standing)
Tibia	200	Skiing (100 km/h, squatting)
CM	0.4	Sprint start

CM, centre of body mass.

The following set of equations can be used to calculate displacements, speeds, accelerations, and time intervals for movements with constant acceleration:

$$x = x_0 + v_0 + \tfrac{1}{2} at^2;$$

$$v = v_0 + at.$$

The following three equations can be derived from equations 1 and 2:

$$x - x_0 = \tfrac{1}{2} t (v + v_0);$$

$$x - x_0 = (\tfrac{1}{2} a) (v^2 - v_0^2);$$

$$a = \tfrac{1}{2}(v^2 - v_0^2)/(x - x_0);$$

where x_0 is the initial displacement, x is the final displacement, v_0 is the initial speed, v is the final speed, a is the constant acceleration, and t is the time interval between initial and final time.

Examples for movement with (assumed) constant acceleration

1. Determine the average acceleration of a javelin in a world-class throw if the approach speed of the athlete's hand is 5 m/s, the release speed of the javelin from the hand is 30 m/s, and the distance over which the javelin is accelerated is 2 m.

Known:	v_0	=	5 m/s
	v	=	30 m/s
	x_0	=	0 m
	x	=	2 m
Unknown:	a	=	?

Solution

Use equation 5:

$$a = \tfrac{1}{2}(900 - 25)/(2 - 0)\text{m/s}^2 = 218.77 \text{ m/s}^2.$$

The average acceleration of the javelin is about 220 m/s² or about 22 G. The actual maximum acceleration in javelin throwing is higher than the average acceleration estimated in this example. A realistic estimate for the maximum acceleration is about twice the calculated average acceleration. This can be illustrated by assuming a triangle distribution of the acceleration–time curve.

2. Determine the take-off speed of a world-class high jumper assuming that the jumper's centre of mass at take-off is at 1.05 m, that it clears the bar by 10 cm, and that the cleared bar is at 2.45 m.

Known:	x_0	=	1.05 m
	x	=	2.55 m
	v	=	0 m/s
	a	=	-10 m/s²
Unknown	v_0	=	?

Solution

Use equation 5 and solve it for v_0:

$$2a(x - x_0) = v^2 - v_0^2.$$

Now

$$v = 0.$$

Therefore:

$$
\begin{aligned}
v_0 &= [-2a(x - x_0)]^{1/2} \\
&= (20 \times 1.5)^{1/2} \text{ m/s} \\
&= 5.5 \text{ m/s}.
\end{aligned}
$$

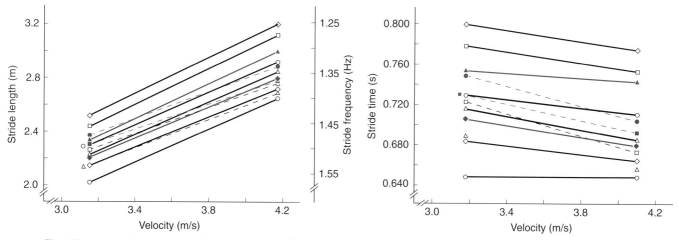

Fig. 5 Measures of stride lengths and stride frequencies for athletes running at different speeds on a treadmill. (Adapted from ref. 6, with permission.)

The take-off speed of the centre of mass for a world-class high jump is about 5.5 m/s.

3. Determine the average acceleration for a sprinter, assuming that he/she accelerates from no movement to a speed of 10 m/s in the first 20 m.

Known:
v_0 = 0 m/s
v = 10 m/s
x_0 = 20 m

Unknown: a = ?

Solution
Use equation 5:

$$a = 100/40 \text{ m/s}^2 = 2.5 \text{ m/s}^2.$$

If $x = 0$, then:

$$a = 1/2(v^2 - v_0^2)/(x - x_0) = 1/2(100 - 0)/(0 - 20) = 1/2(100/20) = 1/2(5) = 2.5$$

The average acceleration of a world-class sprinter for the first 20 m is about 2.5 m/s^2 or about 0.25 g. The maximum acceleration for a sprint start is about twice the average acceleration which corresponds to about 5 m/s^2 or 0.5 G.

Rotational movement

A motion is said to be a rotation if any straight line within a rigid body changed its direction during the motion. A normal movement is usually a combination of translation and rotation. In what follows rotations are studied independent of translations. The magnitudes of the mechanical quantities used to describe rotational movements are angular position, angular displacement, angular velocity, and angular acceleration. Rotational movements of the foot or parts of the foot as measured during running are used to illustrate the application of rotational analysis to human movement.

The foot is a complex anatomical structure consisting of 26 bones. It possesses unique qualities. It can be rigid or flexible depending on the task performed. The talus plays a critical role in the mechanics of the link between the lower leg and the foot. On the proximal side it connects to the lower leg. On the distal side it connects to the foot. The joint between the tibia and the talus is called the ankle joint, talocrural joint, or talotibial joint. To a first approximation, it is considered to be a hinge joint and to lie approximately

in the frontal plane. Measurements[7] have shown that the ankle joint is slightly oblique. The ankle joint axis is rotated laterally in the transverse plane, and inclined downwards and laterally since the fibular malleolus (on the outside) lies more posteriorly (towards the back side) and extends more distally (towards the extremities) than the tibial malleolus. Consequently, rotation around the ankle joint produces dominantly plantar-flexion/dorsiflexion, but additionally some minor components or inversion/eversion and adduction/abduction.

The joint between the talus and the calcaneus is known as the subtalar joint. (It should be noted that the talus has additional joints with the navicular bone (the talonavicular joint) and with the cuboid bone (the talocuboid joint). (These joints are not discussed in the following.) It appears to be well established that the motion between the talus and the calcaneus is a rotation about a single oblique axis, the subtalar joint axis.[7] The 'average' subtalar joint axis is inclined upwards anteriorly by approximately 42 degrees and inclined medially approximately by 16 degrees (Fig. 6). A rotation about the subtalar joint axis includes components for inversion/eversion, adduction/abduction, and dorsiflexion/plantar-flexion. The rotation about the subtalar joint axis is known as pronation or supination. It is difficult to distinguish *in vivo* between rotations about the ankle and about the subtalar joint.

It has been speculated that many running injuries are related to excessive eversion (or pronation). For this reason a methodology has been developed to quantify angles and changes in angles in the lower extremities (Fig. 7). The method uses projections of markers which are fixed on the human leg and the shoe into the frontal and the sagittal plane. The projected angle which proved to be most frequently implicated in running injuries was the Achilles tendon angle, the angle between the lower leg and the calcaneus.[8] The following examples for running concentrate on this angle.

The two variables used most frequently are the initial pronation and the maximal pronation. The initial pronation is defined as the change in the Achilles tendon angle during the first tenth of ground contact. The maximal pronation is defined as the total change in the Achilles tendon angle between first contact and maximum pronation. It should be noted that the measured variable does not quantify pronation and/or eversion accurately because of the two-dimensional limitation.

It has been shown in a prospective study[9] that more than 50 per cent of all running injuries are associated with excessive values in maximal pronation. Furthermore, it has been shown[8] that the pronatory movement of the foot can be influenced significantly by the shoe (Fig. 8). The maximal pronation for subject A was 21 degrees in his personal shoe. However, when using a special (laboratory) shoe which was built to reduce pronation, maximal pronation could be reduced to only 12 degrees in this subject. The effect is even more pronounced for subject B who shows an excessive maximal pronation of 31 degrees in his personal shoe.

One method of influencing the pronatory movement is to change the construction of the shape of the heel on the lateral side of the running shoe. A second approach is to use different material densities in the construction of the heel of the shoe. The effect of these two strategies on pronation has been studied using nine shoes which were identical except in their heel shape and their material composition in the heel.[10] The shapes (on the lateral side) used were flared, neutral, and rounded. The material compositions used were a combination of 'soft' on the outside and 'medium hardness' on the inside (shore A 25/35, dual-density EVA), a 'medium hardness' shoe sole (shore A 35, single-density EVA), and a 'hard' shoe sole (shore A 70/45, dual-density polyurethane).

The results of the study show that the 'initial pronation' can be reduced by changing (a) the geometry of the lateral side of the heel (reduce the lever) or (b) the material hardness of the heel of the shoe (soft on the outside and hard on the inside).

Initial biomechanical research dealing with sport shoe development concentrated primarily on the ankle and subtalar joint. Limited additional research has been performed for the metatarsalphalangeal joints. However, studies of the foot have revealed that there is an additional possibility of rotation about the longitudinal axis of the foot. If the heel is fixed, the forefoot can be rotated through about 35 degrees into inversion and about 15 degrees into eversion (Fig. 9). This movement is possible because the first three rays and the talus form one 'connected structure' and the fourth

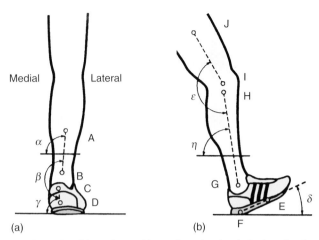

Fig. 7 Illustration of the angles used in two-dimensional analysis of running shoes: (a) posterior view; (b) lateral view.

and fifth ray together form a second connected structure (Fig. 10). The relative movement of these connected structures allows torsion of the forefoot with respect to the rearfoot.

This aspect is important since each joint of the lower extremities (hip, knee, ankle, subtalar, etc.) provides an additional possibility for the absorption of forces during locomotion. However, the conventional shoe constructions are rather stiff in the midfoot area and do not allow for torsional movement of the foot. Consequently, rotation of the forefoot with respect to the rearfoot is restricted, and the

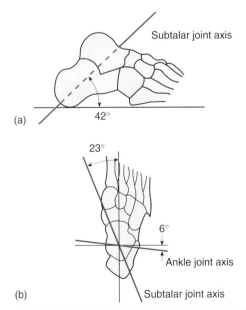

Fig. 6 Illustration of the ankle and subtalar joint axes. (a) Lateral view; (b) superior view. (Adapted from ref. 7, with permission.)

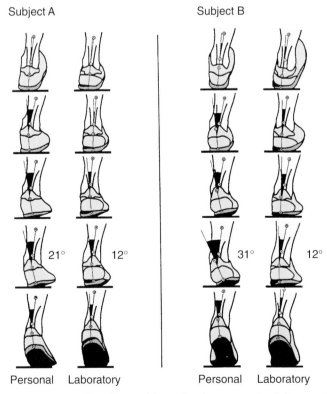

Fig. 8 Illustration of the influence of the running shoe on pronation during ground contact in running at a speed of 4 m/s (heel–toe running). The picture sequences should be read from the top to the bottom.

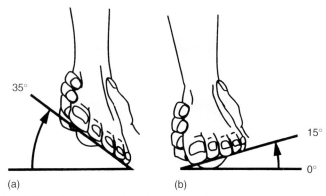

Fig. 9 Illustration of inversion (a) and eversion (b) of the forefoot for a fixed position of the rearfoot. (Adapted from ref. 11, with permission.)

ankle and subtalar joint complex must primarily compensate to provide the necessary additional rotation. This may result in excessive loading situations. If an athlete lands in an everted position on his/her forefoot (for example, landing on the foot of a team-mate in volleyball or landing on uneven ground in cross-country running), the rearfoot must follow the forefoot eversion and excessive strain may occur on the medial side of the ankle joint complex. This would not occur in the barefoot situation since the forefoot would rotate torsionally with respect to the rearfoot.

The barefoot movement of the foot in the example above is assumed to be less stressful than the same movement in a shoe. Consequently, a solution for the sport shoe has been proposed[12,13] by cutting the shoe sole in the midfoot area (torsion groove), allowing torsional movement of the forefoot with respect to the rearfoot to occur. Additionally, a stiff element has been added (torsion bar) to prevent the shoe from flexing in the midfoot area since the midfoot does not allow for this movement. Research showed that this torsional concept provides a shoe which allows the foot to move more in the way that it would move in a barefoot situation, which is assumed to reduce the overall load in the foot complex.

Kinetics

As outlined earlier, the quantity 'force' cannot be defined but only described. In a dynamic sense force can be described as follows:

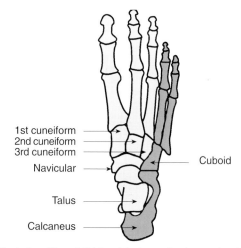

Fig. 10 Illustration of the subdivision of the human foot into two functional units.

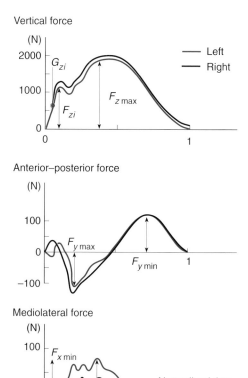

Fig. 11 Example for the components of the ground reaction force during running at a speed of 4 m/s for one subject and one trial (left and right foot).

If 'something' is able to accelerate (or decelerate) a mass, this 'something' is called a force in a dynamic sense.

A force acting on a mass can produce translational and/or rotational motion. The mass which is moved has a resistance against changes in its state of motion. For translation this resistance is proportional to the mass. For rotation this resistance is proportional to the moment of inertia.

Ground reaction forces

Force platforms are commonly used in biomechanics. They are measuring devices which quantify the forces exerted by subjects onto them. Often, they are installed in the ground and the forces measured with them are called ground reaction forces. The force vector is resolved into three components: a vertical component Fz, an anteroposterior component Fy, and a mediolateral component Fx.. Figure 11 illustrates the three components of the ground reaction force during one ground contact for heel–toe running at a speed of 3.5 m/s. The time axis is normalized. The initial value 0 is the time of first ground contact and the final value 1 is the time of last ground contact. Different aspects of ground reaction forces may be of interest and are discussed in the following.

The force components are associated with the acceleration of the centre of mass in the corresponding directions. The vertical force component describes the acceleration of the centre of mass in the vertical direction. Analogous statements are appropriate for the two horizontal components.

The vertical force component for heel–toe running usually has two force peaks. The first vertical peak occurs about 5 to 30 ms after first ground contact. It is called the vertical impact force peak and is referred to here as Fz_i. Similar peaks may occur in the two horizontal force–time curves. Impact forces can be defined as follows:

Impact forces are forces due to a collision of two objects with a maximum earlier than 50 ms after first contact of the two objects.

In running, impact forces are connected to the landing of the heel of the foot on the ground. The time to occurrence and the magnitude of the impact force peak depends on various factors such as the running speed, the style of running, the geometrical shoe construction, and the material properties of the shoe sole. For running barefoot on steel the impact peak occurs about 5 to 10 ms after first contact, and for running with a soft-soled running shoe on asphalt the impact peak occurs about 20 to 30 ms after first contact. Running on a soft sandy beach would show no impact peak at all.

The second peak in the vertical force–time curve for heel–toe running is called the vertical active force peak and is referred to in this text as Fz_a. Similar peaks may occur in the two horizontal force– time curves. Active forces can be defined as follows:

Active forces are forces due to movement which is entirely controlled by muscular activity.

In running at a speed of 4 m/s vertical active force peaks occur at about two to three times bodyweight. Fz_a occurs in the middle of the stance phase which is about 100 to 200 ms after first ground contact.

The force in the anteroposterior direction has two parts. In the first half of ground contact the foot pushes in the anterior direction. Consequently, the reaction force from the force platform is directed in the posterior direction (backwards). In the second half of the ground contact the foot pushes in the posterior direction. Consequently, the reaction force from the force platform is directed in the anterior direction.

The force in the mediolateral direction has two parts. It can be directed towards the medial side (inwards), which corresponds to a positive force, or towards the lateral side (outwards), which corresponds to a negative force (Fig. 11). The typical pattern of the mediolateral force in heel–toe running initially shows, for a short time, a reaction force in the lateral direction followed by a force of longer duration in the medial direction.

Forces in the vertical and anteroposterior direction show a small variability, while force components in the mediolateral direction show a large variability. Additionally, ground reaction forces for left and right are often different, which suggests that the movement may not be symmetrical. It has been shown that world-class runners show significant differences in their ground reaction forces for left and right feet.

Values of externally measured impact forces have been reported in the literature over the last 15 years. A summary of the reported values is shown in Fig. 12. The external impact forces were assessed using force platforms. The internal impact forces were estimated using mathematical models of the human body together with kinematic and kinetic data from experiments. As shown, external vertical impact force peaks can exceed 10 BW. Internal impact peaks have been estimated to be as high as 6 BW in running and 10 BW for landings in gymnastics. It is speculated that such forces may be close to or exceed limits beyond which damage to anatomical structures may occur.

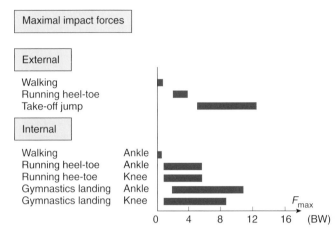

Fig. 12 Summary of the magnitude of the measured external and estimated internal impact force peaks.

Values of active forces which have been reported by various authors are shown in Fig. 13. Maximal active force peaks acting on the feet of athletes during various sports activities have been measured with force platforms and do not appear to exceed 4 BW. Internal active forces, estimated from mathematical models, were reported to be larger than the external forces. Maximal forces in the ankle joint during running and sprinting have been estimated to be 10 to 13 BW.[14,15]

A two-dimensional model of the human body in sprinting may explain the difference in magnitude of the internal and external active force peaks. The external force during push-off in sprinting acts with a moment arm (lever) of about 20 cm with respect to the ankle joint axis. The main reaction to this moment on the posterior side of the leg is provided by the Achilles tendon. The moment arm (lever) of the Achilles tendon to the ankle joint axis is about 5 cm. Consequently, the force in the Achilles tendon must be about four times the ground reaction force.

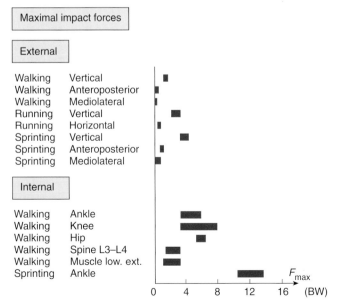

Fig. 13 Summary of the magnitudes of the measured external and estimated internal active force peaks as reported in the literature by various authors.

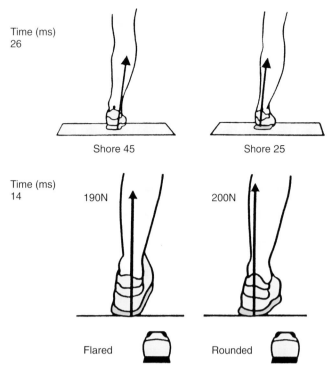

Fig. 14 Illustration of the effects of changes in midsole material and heel geometry on the location of the line of action of the resultant ground reaction force.

Impact force peaks are affected by the geometric construction and the material properties of the heel of the shoe. Results of the running shoe project which were discussed earlier with respect to angular kinematics are discussed below for kinetics. Results of this experiment show that geometry, as well as material, influences the magnitude of the external vertical impact force peaks. The effect of the material is more pronounced for flared heels but is minimal for rounded heels. The maximal differences in external vertical impact force peaks are between 20 and 25 per cent.

Kinetics and kinematics

Kinetics and kinematics must be combined to allow estimations of the effects of external forces. Internal forces acting on structures of the human locomotor system are associated with external forces. If a force acts with a small moment arm, the moments produced about that joint axis are small. If a force acts with a large moment arm, the forces acting in structures of the human body may be a multiple of the external forces. An example of the combination of kinematics and kinetics for heel–toe running is illustrated in Fig. 14.

The (idealized) joint axes are indicated by points in the figure, which is an oversimplification of the actual situation. However, the example illustrates that the ground reaction force produces positive and negative (left- and right-turning) moments about the ankle and the knee joint. Furthermore, the sign of the moment about one joint changes several times, throughout foot contact, thus producing changing loads for specific structures of the athlete's leg. Consequently, one can expect changes of compression and tension in the tibia, for example, and changes between high and low forces in the gastrocnemius, soleus, and tibialis anterior muscles and the corresponding tendons during one ground contact.

A graphical representation of the posterior view (Fig. 14) illus-

trates the influence of the midsole hardness on the relative position of the external ground reaction force with respect to the foot. The general finding as derived from this figure can be summarized as follows. The differences are significant during the first half of ground contact but not during the last half. The ground reaction force is close to the longitudinal foot axis for a soft shoe-sole material (shore 25) while a harder material (shore 45) has a ground reaction force towards the lateral side of the shoe. Consequently, one expects larger internal forces in the tendon–muscle structures and in the ligaments around the subtalar joint for the harder shoe compared with the softer shoe.

It has been speculated that the loading of the lower extremities with respect to possible acute and/or chronic injuries is reduced when the external force acts with a small moment arm compared with an external force acting with a large moment arm. On the basis of the results mentioned above, there are at least two possible methods of influencing the external forces during landing in running when wearing the shoe. Both possibilities influence the relative position of the line of action of the force with respect to the foot. One approach uses a soft material for the sole of the heel on the lateral side or for the whole heel (Fig. 14(a)). Another possibility uses a rounded or neutral geometrical shape on the lateral heel of the running shoe (Fig. 14(b)). The two solutions have advantages and disadvantages. The soft heel material may be compressed totally under the applied load (bottoming out), which would result in excessive impact forces. Possible increases in impact force peaks may be as high as 30 to 50 per cent. The rounded heel increases the impact peaks by about 10 to 20 per cent. Both changes in shoe construction seem to have the effect of increasing the external ground reaction forces. The increases are in a range from zero to about 60 per cent. In order to understand the effect of such changes in shoe construction, models can be developed which are able to estimate the internal forces in the anatomical structures of interest. On the basis of literature data it seems that increases in the moment arm of the acting force with respect to the subtalar joint axis may increase the internal forces by several hundred per cent. Consequently, it seems to be appropriate to work with the rounded (or neutral) heel geometry to reduce the initial pronatory effects of ground reaction forces.

Linear momentum

Consider a particle of mass m acted upon by a force F. Replacing the acceleration by the time derivative of the velocity, one can write Newton's second law as:

$$\Sigma F = m\frac{dv}{dt};$$

or, if we assume that the mass is constant,

$$\Sigma F = m\frac{d(mv)}{dt};$$

and:

$$mv = L;$$

where L is the linear momentum of the system and has units of kilogram metres per second (kg/(m/s)).

The force acting on a particle with the mass m is equal to the rate of change of its linear momentum:

$$\int_{t_2}^{t_1} F(t)\, dt \text{ (impulse)} = mv_2 - mv_1 = \text{(change in (linear) momentum)};$$

where F is the force acting on the particle, m is the mass of the particle, v_2 is the velocity of the particle at time t_2, and v_1 is the velocity of the particle at time t_1.

Linear momentum is of mechanical importance as it can be written in the form of the principle of conservation of linear momentum, which can be recognized as another form of Newton's first law.

If the resultant force acting on a particle is zero, the linear momentum of the particle remains constant, in both magnitude and direction, and the change in momentum is zero.

Example

A subject is standing on a frictionless cart which stands on a horizontal plane. The subject throws a brick (mass m_1) in the horizontal direction from the cart. What happens to the person (mass m_2) and the cart (mass m_3)?

Assumptions

1. The cart can move without friction along the line determined by the throw of the brick.

2. The subject and cart have no relative movement and can be considered as one mass m_4.

3. The masses m_4 and m_1 can be considered as particles and the problem can be dealt with as a two-dimensional problem.

4. No external forces act on the system cart–subject–brick. Air resistance can be neglected.

5. The following values are assumed for the numerical calculations: $m_4 = 100$ kg; $m_1 = 10$ kg; $v_1 = 10$ m/s (in the positive y axis direction).

6. The brick is thrown in the positive y direction. The problem can be solved one-dimensionally.

Solution

Let the times just before and just after the brick has been thrown be t_1 and t_2, respectively. Then:

$$\int_{t_2}^{t_1} F_y(t)\, dt = 0 = (m_4 v_4 + m_1 v_1)_2 - (m_4 v_4 + m_1 v_1)_1$$

momentum of the system after the throw	momentum of the system before the throw $= 0$

$$m_4 v_4 + m_1 v_1 = 0$$

$$v_4 = -(m_1/m_4) v_1$$

$$v_4 = -1 \text{ m/s}.$$

The cart and the subject will move with a velocity of 1 m/s in the direction opposite to the brick (negative y axis).

Work and energy

Work

Work done on a body by the action of an external force producing a motion is an important concept that has been developed in physics.

The term 'work' as used in physics is a mechanical term. It is defined as follows:

The work done by a force that acts on a body is equal to the product of the magnitude of the force and the distance that the body moves in the direction of the acting force, while the force is being applied to the body.

This is expressed as:

$$W = \int_{d_2}^{d_1} F\, ds.$$

Work for a constant force in rectilinear motion is:

$$W = F\, dF;$$

where W is the work, F is the force, and dF is the distance travelled in the direction of the force while the force is being applied.

Work in a mechanical sense, work in a physiological sense, and work in daily life may have different meanings. A person standing in an airport and holding two suitcases in his/her hands does no mechanical work. However, physiologically he/she does work as can be measured by his/her oxygen consumption. A person sitting in a chair in an office developing new marketing strategies 'works' in the sense of the daily use of the term (at least he/she is paid for it). His/her muscles are active at a low level. Consequently, the physiological work is not zero. However, the mechanical work is zero as long as he/she does not move.

Different forms of mechanical work are distinguished:

work against gravity	$W_{\text{gr}} = -mg\Delta H$
work to deform a spring	$W_{\text{sp}} = \frac{1}{2}kx^2$
work to accelerate a mass	$W_{\text{acc}} = \frac{1}{2}mv^2.$

The unit of work is kg m^2/s^2 = joule (J).

The term 'calorie' or 'kilocalorie' is often used in discussions of losing weight or the mechanical work done during competition. The connection between joules and kilocalories (kcal) is:

$$1 \text{ J} = 2.4 \times 10^{-4} \text{ kcal} = 0.00024 \text{ kcal}.$$

Energy

Energy is the capacity (ability) to perform work.

A body has energy if it has the ability to alter the state or the condition of another body. For example, a flying football has energy because it is able to move or deform another object. A diver standing on the diving board at a height above the ground has energy because of his/her position. When diving, the body will accelerate and attain a certain speed when hitting the water. The body is able to move with water and consequently it has energy.

Different forms of mechanical energy are distinguished:

kinetic translation	$E_{\text{kint}} = \frac{1}{2} mv^2$
kinetic rotation	$E_{\text{kinro}} = \frac{1}{2}I\omega^2$
potential gravity	$E_{\text{potgr}} = mgH$
potential spring	$E_{\text{potsp}} = \frac{1}{2}kx^2$

where m is the mass, v is the speed, I is the moment of inertia, g is the earth acceleration, H is the height, k is the spring constant, and x is the deformation of spring. The unit of energy is the same as the unit for work. There are other forms of energy such as chemical, electrical, thermal, nuclear, etc.

One of the main laws of physics is the conservation of energy. In general, a group of bodies is selected arbitrarily and called a 'system'. The law of conservation of energy applies to such an arbitrarily selected system.

The sum of all the energies in a 'system' remains constant.

An example of a mechanical system is a trampolinist. The system is the athlete and the trampoline. An athlete jumping down into a trampoline will rebound. At the start, the athlete has a potential energy due to the position. Next, this potential energy will decrease and the kinetic energy will increase. When contacting the trampoline the potential and the kinetic energy will decrease to zero and the energy is used to deform/stretch the trampoline (spring). This potential energy is then given back and the athlete is accelerated upwards. However, the final height will be less than the initial height since part of the energy is lost in heat due to friction in the trampoline.

In a scientific sense the law of conservation of energy holds for all forms of energy. This is obvious in the subsequent example of a marathon runner. Without energy from outside (food and beverages), an athlete is able to do work of about 1500 kcal (about 6 250 000 J). Consequently, a marathon runner must eat and drink since the total energy needed for a marathon is about 2500 kcal (about 10 400 000 J).

Example

The work done by a runner during a marathon is of the order of about 2000 to 2500 kcal. One may be interested in the additional work an athlete must perform due to the weight of his/her running shoes. The example in this section estimates the additional work for an additional shoe mass of 200 g per shoe.

Assumptions

1. The two forms of additional work of interest are the work against gravity and the work in order to accelerate the shoe.

2. Each foot is lifted 0.2 m in each step.

3. The maximal speed of the swinging leg is 7 m/s.

4. The step length (left toe to right toe) is 2 m which corresponds in a marathon to about 21 000 steps.

Solution For additional work against gravity:

$$W = nmgH;$$

where $n = 21\,000$, $m = 0.2$ kg, and $H = 0.2$ m. Therefore:

$$W = 21\,000 \times 0.2 \text{ kg} \times 10 \text{ m2/s}^2 \times 0.2 \text{ m}$$

$$= 8400 \text{ J or about 2 kcal.}$$

For additional work for acceleration of the foot:

$$W = n\left(\tfrac{1}{2}\,mv^2\right)$$

$$= 21\,000 \times 0.5 \times 0.2 \text{ kg} \times 49 \text{ m}^2/\text{s}^2$$

$$= 102\,900\text{J or about 25 kcal.}$$

The mechanical work needed to accelerate the foot is about 10 times greater than the work against gravity. This suggests that, in running, the movement of the extremities during running is critical with respect to the mechanical work done. The additional work to accelerate an additional mass of 0.2 kg on each foot is about 100 000 J or about 25 kcal. This corresponds to about 1 per cent of

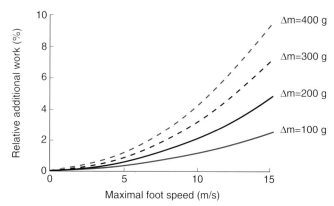

Fig. 15 Relative additional work due to acceleration of additional shoe mass as a function of the maximal speed of the foot.

the total physiological work done during a marathon. If work and time are related linearly this could correspond to an additional 1 to 1.5 min in the total marathon time.

The relative additional work due to the acceleration of the additional shoe mass depends on the actual running speed and on the actual added mass (Fig. 15). An increase in mass corresponds to a linear increase in work required. An increase in speed for a given mass corresponds to a quadratic increase of the required work. Mass considerations for shoes for high-performance athletes become increasingly important for sports with high speeds. However, considerations of the effect of shoe mass on performance is less important for recreational marathon runners.

The mechanical estimation of the additional work due to the acceleration of the additional mass of the shoe assumes that everything is kept constant when changing speed and/or mass. This is obviously a simplification since kinematics, kinetics, and internal muscular activities probably change. Also, the acceleration phase is followed by a deceleration phase, which in itself needs additional work which may well be of the same order of magnitude as the acceleration work. Therefore the estimated additional work is inaccurate. However, the estimate seems to be on the conservative side.

Biomaterials (bone and cartilage)

General comments

The human body is constructed of different materials such as bone, cartilage, ligament, tendon, muscle, and other soft tissues. Based on their function, the different anatomical components of the human body can be divided into two groups: the first group comprises the passive structures (bone, cartilage, ligament, tendon) and the second group comprises the only active elements, the muscles. The passive structures do not produce force, while the active structures do.

The importance of the musculoskeletal system is documented by its various functions. This system is one important tool which can be used to influence the environment. The effects of actions due to the musculoskeletal system can be mechanical (for example, walking, jumping) and also psychological (for example, expression of joy or pain by facial expression).

In this section we provide some insight into mechanical aspects of construction and function of some of these anatomical structures.

Table 3 Historical highlights in understanding the construction and functioning of bone

1855	Breithaupt	Described stress fractures in military recruits of a Prussian military unit
1856	Fick	Bone is a passive structure; the surrounding muscles determine the form bone
	Virchow	Bone plays an active role in developing its form and structure
1862 1863	Volkmann Hüter	Pressure inhibits bone growth and release of pressure promotes it
1867	van Meyer	Relationship between architecture and function of bone
1867	Culman	Similarity of the trabecular arrangement in bone to that of a crane; in both cases the principle of highest efficiency and economy is used
1870	Wolff	Interdependence between form and function of bone; physical laws have strict control over bone growth
1883	Roux	Orientation of the trabecular system corresponds to the direction of tension and compression stresses and is developed using the principle of maximum economy of use of material (as Wolff); architecture of bone follows good engineering principles
1897	Stechow	First radiographic verification of stress fractures

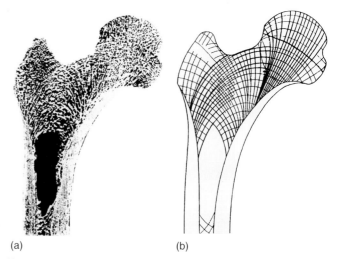

Fig. 16 (a) Picture of the cross-section of a femur illustrating the architecture of the upper end of a femur of a 31-year-old male and (b) schematic representation of the same picture. (Reproduced from ref. 17, with permission.)

Space considerations limit the section to the description of bone and cartilage.

Bone

Selected historical highlights
The understanding of the construction and functioning of bone and bone growth made significant progress in the second half of the nineteenth century. Selected important contributions are listed in Table 3.

Various illustrations of bone have been published, showing the similarity of theoretical constructions of three-dimensional trajectorial systems and the actual arrangement of the trabeculae in the human bone (Fig. 16).

General comments
The entire human skeleton of an adult consists of 206 distinct bones (Table 4). The structural functions of bone are as follows:

(1) to provide support for the body against gravity;

(2) to act as a lever system to transfer muscular forces;

(3) to act as protection for vital internal organs.

In addition to the structural functions, bone has metabolic functions (for example, as a repository for calcium).

Bone cells produce two types of tissue, poorly organized woven

bone and highly organized lamellar bone. Woven bone has a lower mineral content than lamellar bone and forms rapidly during periods of intensive growth such as adolescence, fracture healing, or periods of rapid bone remodelling. Lamellar bone forms more slowly than woven bone and characteristically comprises thin layers of bone with collagen arranged in a perpendicular matrix. Cortical or compact bone is hard and predominates in the long bones. Trabecular, cancellous, or spongy bone is softer than cortical bone and predominates in bones of the axial skeleton (for instance, vertebrae, ribs).

The bones are divisible into four classes: long, short, flat, and irregular. The long bones consist of a hollow cylindrical shaft and two extremities. Examples are the humerus, tibia, fibula, and femur. Long bones are found in the extremities and form a system of levers to transfer forces. The short bones are roughly cubical and are spongy except on their surfaces, where they are compact. Examples of short bones are the carpal and tarsal bones. It is assumed that their function is mainly to provide strength. The flat bones are, as the term indicates, bones where the osseous structure is expanded into broad flat plates. These bones are composed of two thin layers of compact bone with spongy bone enclosed between them.

Table 4 Bones in the human skeleton

Part	Number of bones
Vertebral column, sacrum, and coccyx	26
Cranium	8
Face	14
Auditory ossicles	6
Hyoid bone, sternum, and ribs	26
Upper extremities	64
Lower extremities	62
Total	206

Examples of flat bones include the sternum, ribs, skull bones, ilium, and scapula. The main function of flat bone is to provide protection or a large area for the attachment of tendons or ligaments. The irregular bones are of irregular shape. They consist of a compact outer layer and a spongy inner layer of bone. Their shape seems to be adapted to a special function. Examples of irregular bones include the ischium, pubis, maxilla, and vertebrae.

Wolff's law of functional adaptation

In his classic publication in 1892, Wolff wrote:[16]

The shape of bone is determined only by the static stressing . . . Only static usefluity and necessity or static superfluity determine the existence and location of every bony element and, consequently of the overall shape of the bone.

Two comments are appropriate in the context of these statements.

1. Stress may have different effects on bone. It can effect growth as seen in the healing process of a fracture or it can have an inhibitory effect causing absorption of bone. Such atrophy can occur when stress is absent, constant, excessive or when periods of pressure exceed periods of release.

2. Growth of bone is influenced by heredity, among other factors. If a person has an inherited bone deformity, stress will not change the inherited form.

Considerations of this kind suggest that Wolff's law of the functional adaptation of bone should be restated in a more general way. Stress is not the only factor which determines bone growth, but it plays a major role. Thus Wolff's law can be modified as follows:

Physical laws are a major factor influencing bone growth.

Physical properties of bone

The terms used in this section are defined as follows.[17] The density of a material is its mass per unit volume. The mineral content is the ratio of the unit weight of the mineral phase of bone to the unit weight of dry bone. The water content is the ratio of extracted water divided by the volume of the specimen (bone). The elastic modulus E is the ratio of stress divided by strain:

$$\sigma = E\,\varepsilon;$$

where the units of E are N/m² or pascals (Pa). The tensile strength or ultimate tensile strength is the maximal force in tension that a material can sustain before failure. The compressive strength or ultimate compressive strength is the maximal force in compression a material can sustain before failure.

Selected physical properties of bone (and other selected materials for comparison) are summarized in Table 5.

The elastic modulus E represents the stress needed to double the length of an object. The elastic modulus is a constant which describes the material characteristic. It does not suggest that the particular material can in fact be stretched to its double length. However, this constant can be used to determine the ultimate strength of a material. For bone the typical values for E are as follows: trabecular (spongy) bone, 10^9 Pa = 1 GPa; cortical (compact) bone, 2×10^{10} Pa = 20 GPa; metals, 10^{11} Pa = 100 GPa.

For bone, the elongation to fracture requires only a small fraction of this doubling length. As a guide one can write:

$$F_{\text{fracture}} = (1/200)\,F_{\text{double}}.$$

Table 5 Physical properties of bone

Variable	Comment	Magnitude	Unit
Density	Cortical bone	1700–2000	kg/m³
	Cortical bone	1.7–2.0	g/cm³
	Lumbar vertebra	600–1000	kg/m³
	Water	1000	kg/m³
Mineral content	Bone	60–70	%
Water content	Bone	150–200	kg/m³
Elastic modulus E	Femur	11–28	GPa
Cortical bone, tensile strength	Femur	80–150	MPa
	Tibia	95–140	MPa
	Fibula	93	MPa
Cortical bone, compressive strength	Femur	131–224	MPa
	Tibia	106–200	MPa
Compressive strength	Wood (oak)	40–80	MPa
	Limestone	80–180	MPa
	Granite	160–300	MPa
	Steel	370	MPa

Example

Using the information given above one can estimate the ultimate tensile force required to break a trabecular bone. Calculate the ultimate tensile force for trabecular bone in general and for the femur in particular.

Assumptions

E	=	10^9 Pa
A	=	1 mm² = 10^{-6} m² for general calculation
$\Delta L/L_O$	=	1/200
A_{tib}	=	800 mm² = 8×10^{-4} m².

Solution What force is needed to break a bone sample with a diameter of 1 mm²?

ε	=	$(1/E)\sigma = (1/E)(F/A)$
	=	$\Delta L/L_O$
F	=	$(1/L_O)\Delta L E\,A$
F	=	$(1/200) \times 10^9 \times 10^{-6}$
F	=	5 N.

A force of 5 N is needed to break a bone of 1 mm² cross-section in tension. For a bone of 800 mm² cross-section (femur in the part where it is not hollow) a force of about 4000 N is needed to break it in tension.

The ultimate forces for tension and compression are different. The ultimate force for compression $F_u(\text{compr})$ is about 30 per cent higher than the ultimate force for tension $F_u(\text{tension})$:

$$F_u(\text{compr}) = 1.3 F_u(\text{tension}).$$

Table 6 Estimation of maximal stress

Cross-section	Maximal stress for tension or compression σ_{be} (MPa)	Maximal stress for torsion σ_{tor} (MPa)
Solid circle	$32M_{be}/\pi D^3$	$16M_{tor}/\pi D^3$
Hollow circle	$32M_{be}D/\pi(D^4 - d^4)$	$16M_{tor}D/\pi(D^4 - d^4)$

M_{be}, bending moment responsible for compression and tension.
M_{tor}, moment responsible for torsion.
$D = 2R$, outer diameter of bone.
$d = 2r$, inner diameter of the hollow bone.

There is only a small region of elongation where bone follows a linear law between force and elongation (Hooke's law). Beyond this limit, deformation and force are no longer arithmetically proportional, and when force is removed bone does not return to its original form but some deformity remains. This is demonstrated in conditions such as osteomalacia or rickets.

Estimation of stress

Maximal stress for compression, tension, or torsion can be estimated for bone of circular cross-section by using the formulae in Table 6.

Example

An idealized bone has the shape illustrated on the left of Fig. 17. The cross-section is assumed to be circular. The radius of the bone column is $R = 1$ cm and a constant force of 100 N is acting as illustrated at a distance $2R$ from the axis of the bone. Estimate the maximal tensile and compressive stress at the cross-section S.

If the force F acts as illustrated in Fig. 17, the bone will be bent to the right. Consequently, the right bone surface will show compression and the left will show tension.

Assumptions

1. The weight of the bone can be neglected.

2. Bone is isotropic (same material properties over the whole bone).

3. The problem can be treated two-dimensionally.

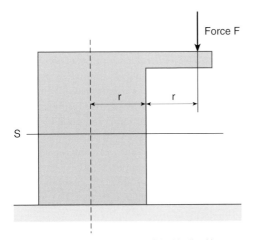

Fig. 17 Schematic illustration of the idealized bone.

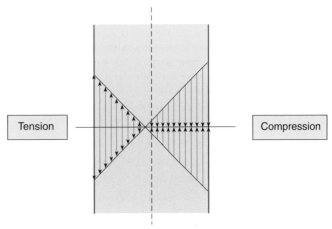

Fig. 18 Stress distribution due to a bending force F at the cross-section S.

4. Bending moments are defined to be positive.

$$\sigma_{comp} = \sigma_{ax} + \sigma_{be}$$
$$\sigma_{tens} = \sigma_{ax} - \sigma_{be}$$
$$\sigma_{ax} = F/\pi R^2$$
$$\sigma_{be} = 32M_{be}/\pi D^3 = (32F \times 2R)/(\pi \times 8R^3) = 8F/\pi R^2.$$

Consequently:

$$\sigma_{comp} = 9F/\pi R^2$$
$$\sigma_{tens} = -7F/\pi R^2.$$

Hence:

$$\sigma_{comp} = 2.87 \text{ MPa} = 2.87 \text{ N/mm}^2$$
$$\sigma_{tens} = 2.23 \text{ MPa} = 2.23 \text{ N/mm}^2.$$

The stress distribution in a cross-section of the bone structure discussed is illustrated in Fig. 18.

The actual maximal compression stress is greater than the actual maximal tension stress. The result is in the same direction as the previously mentioned result, which indicates that the ultimate compression stress is about 30 per cent higher than the ultimate tension stress. It is possible that the higher ultimate stress for compression is a result of an adaptation.

The stresses estimated due to bending in the above example are about an order of magnitude larger than the axial stresses. This illustrates that the geometry of the acting forces is extremely important. If the resultant force is not acting along the axis of a bone, the total stress on the surface of the bone increases and can easily reach multiples of the stresses produced by the axial forces.

This has at least four practical implications.

1. Joint forces which do not act along a bone axis are often compensated for by muscular forces reducing the maximal stresses on the surface of the bone.

2. Misalignment of the skeleton may require an increased muscular compensation to reduce the maximal stresses on the

bone surfaces. In cases of muscular atrophy as a consequence of injury or ageing, this balance may be disturbed and excessive stresses on the bone surfaces may develop which may lead to fractures.

3. Movements where external forces do not act along the bone axes on the human body (e.g. forces on the foot in different shoes) may produce high internal stresses on the bone surfaces.

4. Commonly, bone is loaded in different modes (tension, compression, torsion, and shear).

Bone and load

Bone can be loaded in different modes—compression, tension, shear, and torsion. Usually, a combination of all these forms of loads are present in bone during human locomotion. The different forms of loading of one finite bone element may change continuously during one ground contact.

Fracture of bone may occur for a variety of reasons:

(1) excessive forces;

(2) weak material;

(3) small bone diameter;

(4) excessive frequency of repetition of load application;

(5) reduced time of recovery between load application.

Bone needs a stimulus. However, the stimuli in the form of forces acting on bone must be in an optimal range.

Integrity of bone

As a living tissue, bone responds to physical, environmental, and biological events. Bone modelling occurring during childhood and adolescence determines the shape and length of bones. In the adult, bone remodelling predominates and provides a continual turnover of bone matrix and bone mineral. Some of the most important factors affecting bone integrity include hormonal, physical, nutritional, ageing, and pathological factors.

Hormonal factors

The hormones primarily responsible for calcium metabolism and thus skeletal metabolism are collectively referred to as the calciotropic hormones. These hormones respond to changes in serum calcium balance and will sacrifice calcium from the skeleton in order to restore calcium homeostasis. A second group of hormones, the reproductive hormones, include the female sex hormone oestrogen (E2), the male sex hormone testosterone, and progesterone. They act as critical hormones for the balance of the skeletal metabolism. Finally, bone integrity is influenced by a number of other hormones (for example, thyroid hormones).

Physical factors

Bone integrity is influenced by mechanical loading which affects local stress. Studies with animals and humans have demonstrated that bone responds to low and high mechanical stress and associated strain. The response of bone to stress and strain (modelling, remodelling) depends on the age of the organism and the magnitude, duration, and repetition of the imposed mechanical stress and strain.

Nutritional factors

Bone integrity is influenced by nutritional quality and quantity. Calcium is one of the most widely reported nutritional requirements for optimal bone growth, development, and maintenance. In addition, bones require protein, vitamin C, magnesium, boron, zinc, and, in fact, most of the nutritional components of food.

Age-related factors

The ageing process indirectly influences skeletal integrity through its impact on hormonal balance, digestion of dietary products, and the degree of physical activity a person engages in. Reproductive function, most obviously in women but also in men, decreases with age. Additionally, calcitonin levels and the production of vitamin D metabolites decrease with increasing age, and thus may affect the adequate absorption of ingested calcium.

Pathological factors

Bone integrity is influenced directly or indirectly by many pathological conditions. Chronic asthma, for instance, results in severe reduction of bone mass in children who are treated with glucocorticosteroids. Diseases such as osteomalacia and osteoporosis have a direct impact on bone remodelling and thus skeletal integrity.

Cartilage

Selected historical highlights

Many outstanding contributions to the understanding of the construction and the functioning of cartilage were made in the latter part of the nineteenth century and the first half of the twentieth century. Selected examples are given in Table 7.

General comments

Cartilage consists of cells (chondrocytes) which are embedded in an extracellular matrix. As described in *Gray's Anatomy*, cartilage is a non-vascular structure which is found in various parts of the human body. The articulating surfaces of bones are covered with articular cartilage (the main focus of this section). Additionally, cartilage is found in various tubes (nostrils, ears) which are to be kept permanently open. Cartilage is classified according to its structure as white fibrocartilage, yellow fibrocartilage, and hyaline cartilage.

White fibrocartilage consists of white fibrous tissue and cartilaginous tissue. The fibrous tissue is mainly responsible for flexibility and toughness, the cartilaginous tissue for elasticity. White fibrocartilage is found in intervertebral discs and articular discs.

Yellow fibrocartilage consists of cartilage cells and a matrix which is pervaded in every direction. It can be found in the external ear, the Eustachian tubes, and other areas.

Hyalin cartilage is the main focus of this section. The word hyalin derives from the Greek word *hyalos*, which means glass.

Hyalin cartilage consists of a gristly mass of firm consistency, bluish colour, and considerable elasticity. Hyalin cartilage is externally covered by a fibrous membrane, the perichondrium. It contains no nerves. Hyalin articular cartilage is specialized connective tissue and consists of three elements: cells, intercellular matrix (hyalin substance), and a fibre system.

The schematic representation (Fig. 19) shows the main course of the collagenous fibrils in articular cartilage. The lines of the collagenous fibrils are perpendicular to the underlying bony surface of the deep layers. They bend sharply in the transitional zone and run parallel to the cartilage surface in the superficial zone where they act

Table 7 Historical highlights in understanding the construction and function of cartilage

1851	Weber	Thickness of articular cartilage is proportional to the pressure it must sustain
1860	Virchow	Intercellular matter in hyaline cartilage is perfectly homogeneous and as clear as water
1876	Rauber	Modulus of elasticity of cartilage is 0.9 kg/mm² = 0.9 MPa
1887	Morner	Discovered a substance with a high sulphur content which he called condroit
1898	Hultzkranz	Joint cartilage is under less tension in the transverse than in the longitudinal direction
1907	Fischer	Cartilage can be compressed: results from specimens are from 5 to 2.5 mm and from 2.5 to 1 mm
		Cartilage deformation increases the contact area in a joint and increases the possible range of motion
		Within the limits of its normal function, cartilage can fully regain its normal shape after release of pressure
1911	Fick	Greater elasticity always develops in the direction of joint motion; where the joint pressure is concentrated, the tension lines always run radially from the point of greatest pressure
1948	Fairbank	Menisectomy results in overloading the articular surface locally with increasing compression of the cartilage and an increase of friction of about 20%

Table 8 Physical properties of cartilage

Variable	Magnitude	Unit
Density	1300	kg/m³
	1.3	g/cm³
Water content (wet)	75	%
Organic content (wet)	20	%
Organic content (dry)	90	%
Coefficient of friction (dry)	0.0025	
Ultimate stress	5	MPa
	500	N/cm²

pressure and dilates. Fluid flows out when the tissue is under compression. The mechanical properties of articular cartilage alter with changes in its fluid content. The movement of the fluid in and out of the cartilage seems to be the principal way that cartilage obtains its nutrients.

Physical properties of cartilage

Articular cartilage exhibits a viscoelastic response to loads. Creep and stress relaxation are typical mechanical reactions of cartilage to loads. The viscoelastic response depends on the intrinsic viscoelastic properties of the fibre matrix and the frictional drag arising from the interstitial fluid. Articular cartilage has mechanical material properties which change as a function of load. Selected physical properties of cartilage are summarized in Table 8.

The friction coefficient of articular cartilage is the lowest friction coefficient measured for any solid material. No technology has yet been developed which would permit the construction of materials with a lower friction coefficient.

The numbers for ultimate stress indicate an order of magnitude. They are based on data from Yamada[20] and indicate the stress beyond which irreversible structural damage will occur to the cartilage tissue.

Cartilage deforms under load. Figure 20 shows a typical deformation–time curve based on an experiment performed by Hirsch.[21] A constant force of 10 N is applied to patellar cartilage for about 5 min. Fluid is initially squeezed out of the cartilage and a deformation close to the maximal deformation in these 5 min is reached

as a protecting net. The thickness of articular cartilage increases with increasing local stress and is inversely proportional to the congruency of the joint surfaces. The patellar cartilage, for instance, is thickest at the sagittal crest (up to 6 mm).

Articular cartilage is a viscoelastic material. It is rather porous and the interstitium (space between the collagenous fibres) is filled with fluid (about 60 to 80 per cent of the wet weight) which moves in and out under stress. Fluid flows in when the tissue is not under

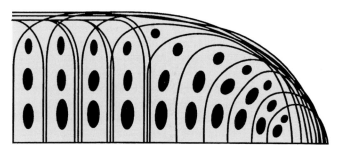

Fig. 19 Schematic representation[18] showing the main course of the collagenous fibrils in articular cartilage and arcual arrangement of fibrils with the chondrium drawn as dark ovals.[19]

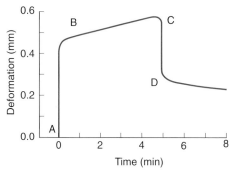

Fig. 20 Deformation–time curve for healthy patellar cartilage. (Adapted from ref. 19, with permission.)

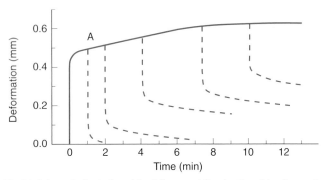

Fig. 21 Schematic illustration of the influence of the duration of loading on the deformation of cartilage. The applied force was 5 N and the area of contact was 10.6 mm². (Adapted from ref. 19 with permission.)

quickly. After unloading at about 5 min, the cartilage does not return immediately to its original thickness but needs time to recover. A second experiment under similar conditions (Fig. 21) underlines the importance of the duration of loading. Loading with a constant force for about 1 min allows cartilage to recover its original form in about another minute. However, when the cartilage was loaded with the same force for 2 min it had not recovered after 6 min. In general, the longer the loading of cartilage, the slower is the recovery. An example of this compression effect is the change of body height as a function of the time of the day. Humans are 1 to 2 cm taller in the morning than in the evening.

Several mechanical functions are often suggested for articular cartilage, including mobility in the joints, stress distribution in the joints, and shock absorption of impact forces. The appropriateness of such suggestions is discussed below.

The suggested function of mobility in the joints seems to be well supported by the fact that articular cartilage has the lowest friction coefficient measured for two solid materials, and the observation that joint range of motion is increased when cartilage is compressed.

The suggested function of stress distribution in the joints seems to be well supported by the fact that the contact area increases substantially due to the compression of articular cartilage. Consequently, the local stress is reduced.

The suggested function of shock absorption of impact forces seems to have less support. The human body during locomotion has a soft-tissue pad of about 1.5 cm thickness at the heel which can be compressed up to about 1 cm. The thickness of articular cartilage is only a few millimetres. Additionally, articular cartilage can only be compressed by about 1 to 2 mm. Furthermore, articular cartilage in the load-bearing joints of the lower extremities is compressed after a few minutes of standing, walking, or running, and the possible compression due to impact loading is reduced. Consequently, it is suggested that the suggested function of shock absorption is not appropriate and that the following holds.

The two main functions of articular cartilage are: (1) providing mobility in the joints; and (2) distributing stress in the joints and thus minimizing peak stresses on subchondral bone.

The average stress in the hip joint has been estimated for two groups of subjects, subjects who needed a hip replacement because of arthritis and normal subjects of the same age and gender.[21] The estimation found an average stress during walking of 5 MPa for the subjects with arthritis and 1 MPa for the normal subjects with no

sign of arthritis. This finding suggests that excessive load may be associated with arthritis and that daily stress situations in joints may be close to the ultimate stresses for cartilage. The following example illustrates this point.

Example
Calculate the maximal average stress in the tibiofemoral joint for running.

Assumptions

1. Maximal bone-to-bone force for running F_{knee} = 4000 N.

2. Contact area of the tibiofemoral joint A = 10 cm²

3. Ultimate compression stress for cartilage σ_u = 5 MPa.

4. The stress is equally distributed over the total contact area.

Solution The actual maximal average stress in the tibiofemoral joint is:

σ = F_{knee}/A

σ = 4000 N/10 cm² = 400 N/cm² = 4 MPa.

Comment The result supports the previous statement that loading of articular cartilage may often be close to the ultimate stress limits during sport activities.

Articular cartilage is an example of functional efficiency. The lubrication efficiency is of a superior magnitude to the best lubrication mechanisms known in modern engineering. Additionally, the functional efficiency is maintained throughout life in most humans. This is remarkable considering that cartilage is only a few millimetres thick and has limited repair capabilities. If one compares the functional efficiency of articular cartilage with many modern mechanical devices, one rarely finds something which is at the same efficiency level as cartilage.

Integrity of articular cartilage

The integrity of any living organism depends largely on the nutrients it obtains. In normal adult articular cartilage, the nutrients required by the chondrocytes are derived from the synovial fluid. The nutrients must travel a significant distance to reach the cells. The transport occurs by diffusion and/or convection. Cartilage deformation in response to joint loading plays an important role in this process.

The integrity of articular cartilage is significantly influenced by joint motion. It has been shown that the biochemical composition, the tensile properties, and the swelling properties of articular cartilage depend strongly on whether or not the tissue is normally subjected to load. Ingelmark and Ekholm[22] showed an increase of 12 to 13 per cent in the thickness of knee cartilage in animals after running for 10 min compared with the thickness after 60 min of immobilization. However, stress on articular cartilage can be excessive. It is speculated that 'fatigue wear' due to an accumulation of microscopic damage within the cartilage material may occur. A further mechanism responsible for creating excessive stress is speculated to be associated with joint impact loading.[24] One theory suggests that the time between impact forces (for example, in running) is too short for cartilage to recover and that the mechanical properties of cartilage are reduced and make it prone to injuries. Another theory suggests that impact loading may be particularly dangerous when cartilage is not loaded (for example, in the morning) and cannot adjust properly by increasing the contact area and consequently reducing the local stresses. The exact mechanisms are not well understood. Nevertheless, impact forces are assumed to be a major factor in the aetiology of damage to articular cartilage.

A number of studies have shown a gradual decrease in material characteristics with age. This change is assumed to be associated with changes in the relative content of collagen and proteoglycan. In the case of osteoarthritis the change is not only in the relative content but is also associated with chaotic changes in the collagen ultrastructure and the proteoglycan organization.

Articular cartilage can rarely be repaired. Research is underway to study possibilities of repairing and/or regrowing articular cartilage. However, current knowledge does not make it possible to repair cartilage in most applications.

References

1. Borelli GA. *On the movement of animals* (*De motu animalium*). Macquet P, transl. Berlin: Springer Verlag, 1989.
2. Paul JP. Bioengineering studies of the forces transmitted by joints. In: Kennedy RM, *Engineering analysis, biomechanics and related bioengineering topics*. Oxford: Pergamon, 1965: 369–80.
3. Marey EJ. *La photographie du movement*. Paris: Centre Georges Pompidou, Musée National d'Art Moderne, 1977.
4. Hatze H. *Myocybernetic control models of skeletal muscle*. Pretoria: University of South Africa, 1981.
5. Williams M, Lissner HR. *Biomechanics of human movement*. Philadelphia: WB Saunders, 1977: 23
6. Cavanagh P, Kram R. Stride length in distance running: velocity, body dimensions, and added mass effects. *Medicine and Science in Sports and Exercise* 1989; **21**: 467–79.
7. Inman VT. *The joints of the ankle*. Baltimore: Williams and Wilkins, 1976: 37
8. Nigg BM. *Biomechanics of running shoes*. Champaign, IL: Human Kinetics, 1986.
9. Bahlsen, AH. The etiology of running injuries: a longitudinal, prospective study. PhD Thesis, University of Calgary, 1988.
10. Nigg BM, Bahlsen AH. Influence of heel flare and midsole construction on pronation, supination and impact forces for heel–toe running. *International Journal of Sport Biomechanics* 1988; **4**: 205–19.
11. Debrunner HU. *Orthopaedisches Diagnostikum*. Stuttgart: Thieme, 1978.
12. Segesser B, Stuessi E, Stacoff A, Kaelin X, Ackermann R. Torsion—ein neues Konzept intramuscular Sportschuhbau. *Sportverletzung–Sportschaden* 1989; **3**: 167–82.
13. Stacoff A, Denoth J, Kaelin X, Segesser B. The torsion of the foot in running. *International Journal of Sport Biomechanics* 1989; **5**: 375–89.
14. Baumann W, Stucke H. Sportspezifische Belastungen aus der Sicht der Biomechanik. In: Cotta H, Krahl H, Steinbrück K, eds. *Die Belastungstoleranz des Bewegungsapparates*. Stuttgart: Thieme, 1980: 55–64.
15. Scott SH, Winter DA. Internal forces at chronic running injury sites. *Medical Science in Sports and Exercise* 1990; **22**: 357–69.
16. Wolff J. *The law of bone remodelling*. Maquet P, Furlong R, transl. Berlin: Springer-Verlag, 1986.
17. Cowin SC, ed. *Bone mechanics*. Boca Raton: CRC Press, 1989.
18. Benninghoff, A. *Lehrbuch der Anatomie des Menschen*. München: Lehmann, 1939.
19. Hirsch C. A contribution to the pathogenesis of chondromalacia of the patella. *Acta Chirurgia Scandinavica*. (From Steindler A. *Kinesiology of the human body*. Springfield IL: Charles C. Thomas, 1977.)
20. Yamada H. *Strength of biological materials*. Baltimore: Williams and Wilkins, 1970.
21. Legal H, Reinecke M, Ruder H. Zur biostatischen Analyse des Hüftgelenkes. *Zeitschrift für Orthopaedie and Ihre Grenzgebiete* 1980; **118**: 804–15.
22. Ingelmark BE, Ekholm R. A study on variations in the thickness of articular cartilage in association with rest and periodical load. *Uppsala Läkareförenings Förhandlingar* 1948; **53**: 61. (From Astrand P, Rodahl K. *Physiological bases of exercise. Textbook of work physiology*. New York: McGraw-Hill, 1977.)
23. Elftman H. The force exerted by the ground in walking. *Arbeitsphysiologie* 1938; **125**: 357–66.
24. Mow WC, Rosenwasser M. Articular cartilage: Biomechanics. In: Woo SL-Y, Buckwalter JA, eds. *Injury and repair of the musculoskeletal soft tissues*. Park Ridge, IL: American Academy of Orthopedic Surgeons, 1988.

1.3.2 Strength and power

Henryk K.A. Lakomy

Introduction

This chapter will focus on those factors which determine the maximum strength that a muscle can generate and will go on to consider how muscle develops power. The chapter will conclude by examining how power output is measured during maximum-intensity exercise of short duration.

Strength

Strength is defined as the maximum force or torque that a muscle, or a group of muscles, can exert on the associated skeletal structure. However, as the muscles may perform maximal effort during isometric, concentric, or eccentric actions (explained later) and as the latter two actions can be performed across a wide spectrum of speeds, the type and speed of movement must be specified when measuring strength. This chapter will examine the structure of skeletal muscle and a number of factors which affect the maximum ability of muscle to generate force.

Traditionally the term 'contraction' has been used to describe the action of a muscle generating force. This term is confusing as the muscle does not always shorten whilst stimulated. In this chapter, therefore, the term muscle 'action' will be used to describe muscle in its active state.[1]

Architecture of skeletal muscle

Skeletal, or voluntary, muscle is composed of individual cells called muscle fibres. Groups or fibres are bundled together to form fascicles. Each muscle fibre is cylindrical with a diameter of 10 to 100 μm. The average fibre length is 30 mm, ranging from less than 1 mm up to as long as 300 mm. The fibre is enclosed within a thin plasma membrane called the sarcolemma. Each muscle cell contains up to several thousand rod-shaped structures called myofibrils. The myofibrils are 1 to 2 μm in diameter. They are arranged in parallel

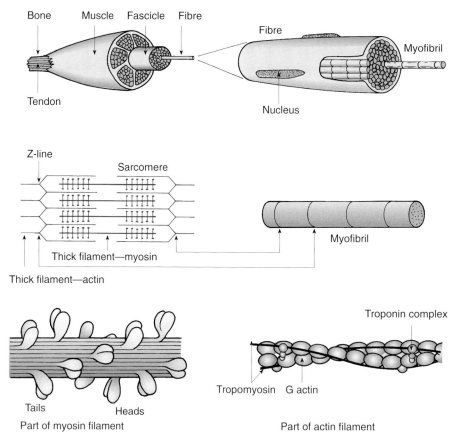

Fig. 1 The structure of skeletal muscle.

with each other and are usually as long as the muscle fibre. In turn, the myofibrils are made up of a series of repeating units called sarcomeres laid end to end.[2] It is the sarcomere that is the basic contractile unit of the cell (Figs 1 and 2).[3]

Within each sarcomere there are two main types of protein filaments. Thin filaments are made up of two chains of G actin which are polymerized into strands of F actin. The two chains are twisted to form a helix. Two rod-like protein structures, called tropomyosin, are twisted around these helical chains and are bound to the chains at intervals by a complex called troponin. In the absence of calcium ions the troponin complex holds the tropomyosin in a position which covers the active sites on the actin filaments. At the extremes of each sarcomere one end of the actin filaments are attached to form the Z line, which are spaced about 2.5 μm apart. The other ends of the filaments are unattached and extend into the heart of the sarcomere forming a symmetrical pattern. The length of the actin filaments is controlled by the protein nebulin which lies alongside it.

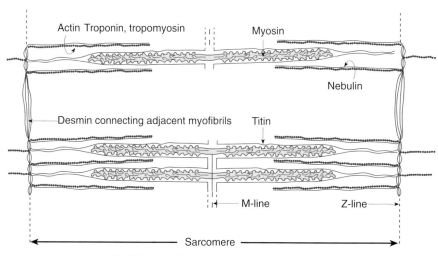

Fig. 2 Proteins of the sarcomere. (Adapted from ref. 24.)

The thick filaments are made up of approximately 200 to 250 myosin molecules. Each molecule of myosin is made up of a 'tail' or shaft with two heads at one end. The molecules are arranged in bundles so that all the tails point to the centre of the fibre and all the heads protrude from the filament towards its end. The centre of the filament where there are no heads present is called the bare zone. The arrangement of the filament allows the heads of each myosin filament to interact with the binding sites of six actin filaments. The myosin filaments are held in place in the middle of the sarcomere by a large, highly elastic protein called titin.

Calcium is stored in an elaborate structure called the sarcoplasmic reticulum. The sarcoplasmic reticulum envelopes the myofibrils. At the location of each Z line the surface of the fibre is invaginated creating a tube-like structure called the T tubule. This tubule is in 'contact' with the sarcoplasmic reticulum, and an action potential passing down it will cause the sarcoplasmic reticulum to release the calcium ions stored within it. The concentration of calcium ions in the sarcoplasmic reticulum is about 10^5 times higher than in the remainder of the cell. When released these ions will diffuse throughout the sarcomere, with some attaching to the binding sites on the troponin complex. If no further impulse arrives the calcium ions are pumped rapidly back to the sarcoplasmic reticulum. Resting concentrations of calcium are restored within approximately 30 ms.

Excitation−contraction coupling

The sliding-filament theory, which has become accepted as the mechanism of muscle action, was described by Huxley in 1957.[4] A stimulus of sufficient magnitude passing down the motor neurone results in a transmitter substance called acetylcholine to be released at the end of its axon. The acetylcholine diffuses across the synaptic cleft between the axon and the surface of the fibre and binds on to the receptor sites on the muscle fibre. This causes an action potential to be created which rapidly spreads across the entire surface of the muscle fibre. This electrical signal passes down the T tubules and on to the sarcoplasmic reticulum, possibly through protein complexes called 'junctional feet'. Once stimulated, the sarcoplasmic reticulum releases its stored calcium. The free calcium ions diffuse into the myofibril and some bind on to the receptor sites on the troponin complex causing it to move which results in translocation of the tropomyosin, thus exposing the previously covered binding sites on the actin filaments. Heads of the adjacent myosin filaments, which are in a high-energy state, bind on to these exposed sites creating crossbridges. Immediately upon attachment the myosin heads 'swivel' through an arc, known as the conformational change or power stroke, which results in the actin filaments being moved by a sliding motion past the myosin filaments. It is this conformational change which creates the tension in the muscle. The myosin heads, which as a result of the power stroke are now in a low-energy stage, detach from the binding sites on the actin filament in the presence of ATP. Activated by the myosin ATPase located in the myosin head the ATP hydrolyses to provide energy to return the myosin heads to their high-energy state. If calcium is still present the binding sites remain exposed and the crossbridge cycle can continue. If, however, reuptake of the calcium into the sarcoplasmic reticulum has occurred then the binding sites become covered preventing further crossbridge formation. During a dynamic action a sufficient rate of

stimulation occurs which allows each head to cycle several hundred times per second enabling the filaments to slide past each other at speeds up to 12 to 18 µm/s. In an active muscle, tension is produced by the concerted action of more than 10^9 myosin heads interacting with actin asynchronously. During excitation up to 50 per cent of possible crossbridges are attached at any time, with the actual number decreasing with increasing speed of muscle shortening (Fig. 3).

When the muscle is stretched whilst active it performs an eccentric muscle action. During this type of action the rate of hydrolysis of ATP is substantially decreased, by up to 75 per cent, compared with concentric actions. As approximately 70 per cent of the ATP utilized in the muscle cell can be attributed to myosin ATPase it appears that virtually no crossbridge cycling is taking place at all during eccentric actions. During these actions the myosin heads are being torn from the actin filaments without the power stroke or conformational change taking place. Maximum eccentric actions are therefore performed with substantially lower energy demands than either isometric or concentric actions.[5]

To allow the force created by the crossbridges formed within a single sarcomere to be transmitted to the tendons and skeletal system, a similar number of crossbridges must be created in each sarcomere in series with it. If this were not the case the shortening occurring in one sarcomere would simply result in lengthening of another in which insufficient crossbridges had been created. Therefore, the force transmitted to the tendon is that generated by the weakest sarcomere in the myofibril chain. Although it is known that sarcomeres display differential rates of activity it can be assumed, for most practical purposes, that a neural stimulus activates the whole myofibril equally and therefore the tension created by each myofibril can be regarded as being equal to that produced by a single constituent sarcomere. The overall tension developed by the muscle is the sum of all the myofibrils activated in parallel with each other. The more myofibrils activated the greater will be the number of crossbridges being created and the higher will be the overall tension developed by the muscle.

Maximum speed of muscle shortening is influenced by myofibril length. The greater the length the greater the number of sarcomeres linked together. The sarcomeres connected in series with each other have an additive effect and therefore the greater the number the higher will be the maximum rate of muscle shortening.

The maximum tension that a muscle can generate depends on a number of factors which are discussed below.

Level and type of muscle activation

A muscle is subdivided into motor units.[6] Each motor unit is made up of a number of fibres innervated by a single motor neurone. The number of fibres comprising a motor unit can range from less than 10 to more than 1000. The excitation of a single motor neurone will result in the action of all the muscle fibres innervated by this neurone. The tension of the whole muscle reflects the number of motor units being recruited at any time within it. With increasing recruitment of motor units the number of active fibres increases, resulting in the excitation of more crossbridges thereby increasing muscle tension. Each active fibre will make a different contribution to the overall muscle tension depending on its size and type. In general, the larger the cross-sectional area of the fibre the greater will be the

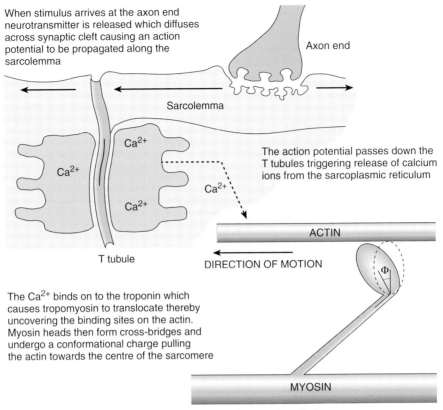

When stimulus arrives at the axon end neurotransmitter is released which diffuses across synaptic cleft causing an action potential to be propagated along the sarcolemma

Axon end

Sarcolemma

The action potential passes down the T tubules triggering release of calcium ions from the sarcoplasmic reticulum

T tubule

DIRECTION OF MOTION

ACTIN

MYOSIN

The Ca²⁺ binds on to the troponin which causes tropomyosin to translocate thereby uncovering the binding sites on the actin. Myosin heads then form cross-bridges and undergo a conformational charge pulling the actin towards the centre of the sarcomere

Fig. 3 Excitation–contraction coupling—a schematic diagram.

number of parallel myofibrils. When stimulated, the larger fibre will therefore be able to develop more tension than one with a smaller cross-sectional area. Fibres can also be classified according to the way in which they respond to a stimulus. Some develop high levels of tension quickly following activation but they fatigue relatively easily. These types of fibres are termed fast-twitch fibres (type II) and have properties making them most suited to short bursts of activity in which high-power outputs or speeds of movement are required. In contrast, slow-twitch fibres (type I) develop tension more slowly and have a longer decay time. These fibres are specialized for activity of extended duration as they are more fatigue resistant. When a standard number of sarcomeres of each fibre type are compared (cat muscle) an approximate 2.5-fold difference in the maximum rate of shortening is found.[7] As the different fibre types show clear differences in maximum speed of shortening, their ability to produce tension is affected by the speed of limb movement. However, in a maximal static muscle action the force developed is independent of the fibre type and is only dependent on the cross-sectional area.[8,9]

The range of average values for the tension produced by muscle is 15 to 42 N/cm² with 22.5 N/cm² most often used as the mean value for homogenous muscle.[10,11]

The manner in which a muscle is stimulated affects the magnitude of the tension it develops. A one-off stimulation of the motor units results in a muscle twitch (Fig. 4), resulting in a low force production lasting only a fraction of a second. If, however, the stimulus is repeated sufficiently quickly (20 to 30 Hz), twitches overlap resulting in optimum tension development called tetanus. Tetanic muscle actions are those which are most frequently required

during sporting activity and it is this type of action which will be considered in this chapter.

The level to which a muscle has been activated can be examined by monitoring the electrical activity within the muscle. This can be achieved by placing electrodes on prepared sites on the skin and measuring the potential difference between these electrodes. The potential difference reflects the electrical activity of the muscles directly beneath the electrodes (**EMG**). Figure 5 shows the relationship between the muscle tension and level of activation (expressed as integrated EMG). The illustration shows that as activation increases so does the tension developed by the muscle. This relationship remains consistent for all types of muscle action being performed.[12]

Angle of pennation

The fibres of many muscles in the body lie parallel to the long axis of the muscle. These are called longitudinal or fusiform muscles, and

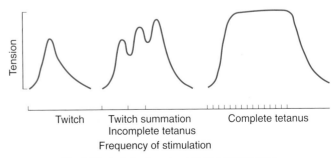

Twitch   Twitch summation
          Incomplete tetanus

Complete tetanus

Frequency of stimulation

Fig. 4 Effect of stimulus rate on tension development.

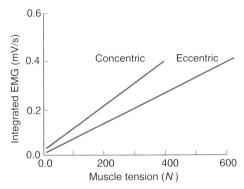

Fig. 5 The relationship between muscle tension and integrated EMG.

the line of pull of the fibres is the same as that of the whole muscle. In other muscles the fibres within it are arranged to be at an angle relative to the line of pull of the muscle. These are called pennated muscles, and the angle between the line of pull of the whole muscle and that of the muscle fibres is called the angle of pennation.

Figure 6 shows a very simple model of how an increase in the angle of pennation results in more fibres per unit volume of muscle. The active muscle will therefore be able to create a greater number of crossbridges for a given volume resulting in an increased force production. The force produced, however, is in the direction of the muscle fibres and, consequently, only a proportion of the force produced is transmitted along the line of pull of the muscle. If F is the force produced by the muscle fibres then the tension developed in the muscle tendon is $F\cos\theta$ where θ is the angle of pennation. The efficiency of the pull of the fibres in the desired direction decreases with increasing angle of pennation. Figure 5 shows the way in which the proportion of the force F being transmitted to the tendon (relative tension) is affected by an increasing angle of pennation. The

Angle of pennation	0	30	60
No. of fibres (=n)	12	16	27
Relative no. of fibres	100	133	225
Efficiency of angle of pull (=e) (%)	100	87	50
Relative tension ($n \times e$) (%)	100	116	113
Relative average length of fibres (=l) (%)	100	75	44
Effective length of fibres ($l \times e$) (%)	100	65	22

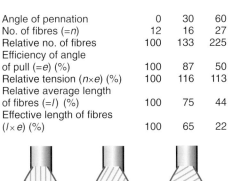

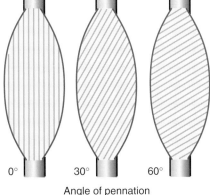

Angle of pennation

Fig. 6 The effect of pennation on the ability of muscle to generate tension.

result of the increasing number of active fibres combined with a decreasing efficiency of pull due to increased pennation is that the tension transmitted to the tendons is maximized at angles of pennation between 30 and 45 degrees.

There is however a 'trade-off' for having the fibres pennated. Although the maximum tension improves with pennation, the range that a muscle can shorten decreases due to the average length of the muscle fibres becoming shorter. This decrease is further magnified when the direction of the fibres which are angled to the desired line of shortening is considered. The maximum rate of muscle shortening decreases with increasing pennation angle. Those muscles which require a large range of movement without the need for high-force outputs, such as the Sartorius muscle, have evolved with fibres which are not pennated. If, however, force, not range, is important then muscles have evolved that have significantly pennated fibres. Examples of pennated muscles are those of the quadriceps femoris group and the deltoids. It should be noted that the actual relationship between the angle of pennation and the development of force is more complex than the simple model described above.[13]

Force–length relationship

The length of the muscle, or more particularly the length of the sarcomere, at the time of its action is a factor which not only affects the number of crossbridges that can be created but also the contribution that the elastic structures of the muscle can make to the overall tension development. The number of crossbridges that can be formed is dependent on the extent of the overlap between the actin and myosin filaments. At the natural resting length of the muscle (l), a sarcomere length of approximately 2.85 μm, the overlap of the filaments is near optimal for crossbridge formation. If the muscle is stretched then the overlap decreases until at approximately 4.2 μm, (150 per cent of l) there can be no crossbridges formed at all.[14] If, in contrast, the muscle is permitted to shorten, then the actin filaments start to overlap one other. This happens at a sarcomere length of less than 2.6 μm. This actin-filament overlap reduces the number of sites available to the heads of the myosin filaments, thereby reducing the overall magnitude of possible tension development.

Muscle tension, however, is not governed exclusively by the active crossbridges. As the muscle is physically stretched beyond its resting length several muscle tissues are themselves being stretched, resulting in tension being created in these elastic structures. This is regarded as the passive component of muscular force production, and the contribution it makes to the overall tension is related to the magnitude of the stretch. The resultant muscle tension is the sum of the active and passive components, as shown in Fig. 7. It should be noted that *in vivo* the range of muscle sarcomere lengths (functional range) is approximately 80 to 120 per cent of l.

Type and speed of muscle action

There are three possible results of recruiting a muscle.

1. *Concentric action.* In this type of action the distance between the origin and insertion of the muscle becomes shorter. The tension developed by the muscle produces a torque exceeding that resisting movement.

2. *Isometric action.* Although the muscle is active the distance between the origin and insertion of the muscle does not

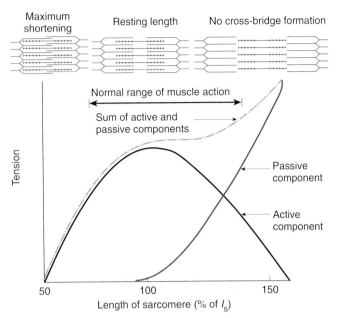

Fig. 7 The relationship between sarcomere length and active, passive, and total tension generation.

change. The muscle torque matches the resistance applied to the limb, resulting in no movement. It should be noted that although there is no overall length change of the entire muscle there will be some shortening of the sarcomeres and some stretching of the elastic structures in series with those sarcomeres, for example tendons, connective tissue.

3. *Eccentric action.* In this type of action the tension developed by the active muscle produces less torque than that caused by the resistance. The result is that the muscle is forced to lengthen, increasing the distance between the origin and insertion of the muscle.

This section of the chapter will examine the effects of both type and velocity of muscle action on the maximum tension that the muscle can generate.

It has been well established that during concentric actions, as the velocity of muscle shortening increases, the maximum tension that can be produced decreases. The relationship between maximum tension and velocity of shortening was first described by Fenn and Marsh.[15] This relationship was further explained by Hill[16] and is shown in Fig. 8. Although muscle actions *in vivo* do not appear to follow the curves predicted by Hill's equation exactly, the characteristic inverse relationship between force and velocity is found to occur.[17] The maximum speed of shortening (V_{max}) occurs when the load is zero. Greater maximum force is produced (P_o) for isometric actions, when no muscle shortening takes place, than for concentric actions. If the external torque applied to the limb increases further, the limb is forced to move in the direction opposite to that during the concentric action. The maximum tension developed in the muscle is found to increase above that generated during the isometric or concentric actions. Further increase in external torque will result in an increased velocity of muscle lengthening and an increase in muscle tension until a plateau is reached. Any further increase in load will increase the velocity of lengthening without an

increase in maximum tension. If the speed of lengthening becomes too great then 'failure' to maintain tension occurs. Hill's equation does not describe eccentric muscle actions.

It was originally suggested that some of the changes in maximum muscle tension with differing velocities of shortening and lengthening could be accounted for by the effects of internal resistance or viscosity of the muscle. This has, however, been shown not to be a significant factor. Variation in the duration of crossbridge attachment may combine with the magnitude of the forces produced (called impulse) to account for the changes seen. When the muscle is shortening the time taken for the conformational change in the myosin head during the power stroke diminishes with increasing velocity of shortening. The effect of increasing the speed of shortening will be to decrease both the peak force produced and the time of attachment, thereby reducing the impulse created by each crossbridge. The number of crossbridges created at any instant also decreases with an increasing speed of shortening. As the overall muscle tension is the sum of the contributions of each active crossbridge then peak tension will decrease with increased muscle shortening speed. During eccentric muscle actions the myosin heads are also attempting to undergo conformational changes; however, during these actions the myosin heads are being forced to move in the opposite direction. Detachment of the crossbridges is caused by the myosin head being 'ripped from' the binding site on the actin filament resulting in high forces being created. These large forces, coupled with a long duration of attachment, result in the very high muscle tensions generated during eccentric actions. The forcing of the myosin head in the wrong direction will cause significant deformation of the filaments which may well account for some of the muscle damage associated with this type of muscle action.

Angle of insertion

The strength of a muscle group is often determined by measuring the external torque or moment being produced. This torque is a function of the tension (T) created by the muscle which is transmitted to the skeleton by the muscle tendon, the angle of insertion of the tendon on the bone ($\emptyset$), and the distance of the point of inser-

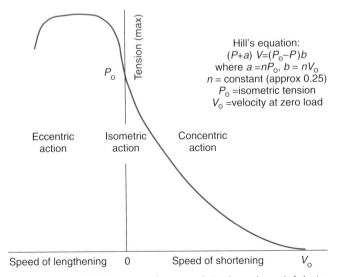

Fig. 8 The relationship between maximum muscle tension and speed of shortening/lengthening during concentric, isometric, and eccentric muscle actions.

tion from the axis of rotation of the associated joint (*d*). It is calculated from the equation:

Torque = *Td* sinO.

The angle of insertion of the muscle tendon on the bone changes as the limb moves through its range of movement. As a consequence, a muscle generating a constant tension will produce an external torque that varies as the limb moves, as shown in the strength curve in Fig. 9. The optimum position for torque production is when the angle of insertion is 90 degrees.[18] The situation is, however, complicated by the force–length relationship described earlier, as the length of the muscle will change with limb movement which, in turn, will affect the tension being developed within the muscle.

The net external effect is therefore a combination of the maximum tension that the muscle can generate, the angle of insertion on the bone, and any change in the distance from the joint axis from the point of muscle insertion. Movement at a joint is rarely caused by the action of a single muscle, Usually a group of muscles act together to produce the movement. As the torque produced by each muscle varies with joint angle, then the resultant (sum) of all the torques of the active muscles also varies with the angle of the joint.

Stretch–shortening cycle

In dynamic activities muscles seldom perform a single isolated muscle action. More often there is a combination of actions resulting from the large interaction with the applied external forces. By combining actions it is possible to create a sequence of movements resulting in increased force production. Cavagna *et al.* clearly describe how greater tension can be produced in a concentric muscle action if it is preceded by active stretching.[19] This sequence of events is called the stretch–shortening cycle.[20]

The enhanced force production produced when the stretch-shortening cycle is performed is due to several factors:

1. At the start of the main action the muscle tension is greater

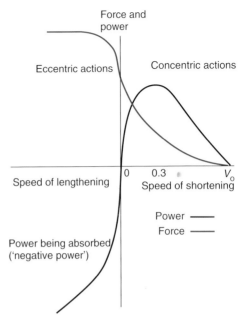

Fig. 10 The power–velocity relationship of muscle.

than would be possible if the preceding muscle stretch (eccentric action) was not performed.

2. Energy stored during stretching of the elastic components of the muscle can be subsequently recovered during the concentric phase of the action.[21]

3. The time course of tension build-up is optimized.

4. Uninhibited activation of the muscle occurs due to the invocation of the myotactic stretch reflex.

In order to achieve maximum muscle tension during the main phase of the activity, the pattern of prior muscle action must be performed in the correct sequence. The limbs must first perform a counter movement in the direction opposite to the main action. Muscle activity occurs to overcome the momentum of the counter movement, resulting in an eccentric action whilst the muscle is being forcibly stretched. This eccentric action must be immediately followed, without pause, by a forceful concentric action of the same muscles. Without the active prestretch preceding the main action, shortening will rely almost exclusively on the contractile structures of the muscle with no contribution from its elastic properties, thereby greatly attenuating the maximum tension that could be produced.[22]

Power

The strength of a muscle has been clearly shown to be influenced by the speed of action of the muscle. In contrast, power, which is the rate at which work is performed, incorporates the speed of movement and relies on it. Power is defined as the product of the applied force and the velocity of movement. As the maximum force produced by a muscle has been shown to be a function of both the type of muscle action being performed and the speed of muscle shortening/lengthening (Fig. 8), it is therefore not surprising that maximum power output is also governed by these factors. Figure 10

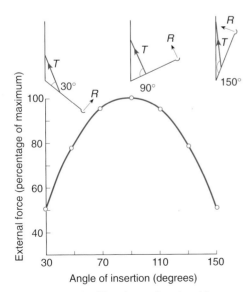

Fig. 9 The effect of the angle of insertion on the external torque produced by a muscle generating constant maximum tension. (After ref. 23.)

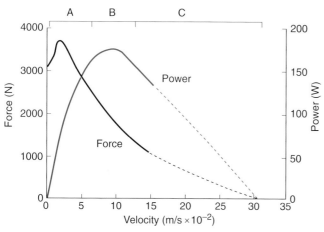

Fig. 11 The force–velocity and power–velocity relationships of the knee extensors performing concentric contractions.

shows the profile of maximum power output with muscle action speed.

Speed/type of muscle action

It can be seen in Fig. 11, where the muscle is acting concentrically, that the speed of shortening markedly influences the maximum power that can be produced. In this figure, speed of action is represented by pedalling speed. Peak power occurs at approximately $0.3 \dot{V}_0$, where $\dot{V}_0$ is the maximum speed of muscle action. Exercise with muscle action velocities falling in the bands marked A and C in Fig. 3 will result in a power output below optimum. Greatest power output will occur when the speed of contraction falls within band B; for example, during cycling this speed represents a pedalling speed of approximately 110 rev./min.[25]

For isometric actions no external power output can be produced as the contraction velocity is zero. In contrast, the greatest levels of power values are measured during eccentric actions. However, it should be noted that the muscle is absorbing power rather than producing it.

Exercise duration

Figure 12 shows that the average power output declines with increasing duration of activity. The decline in power output during maximal, short-term (sprint) exercise has been associated with several metabolic changes in the exercising muscle, such as a decrease in muscle phosphocreatine (**PCr**)[26], a corresponding increase in inorganic phosphate (P_i) and its diprotonated form $H_2PO_4^-$, and a marked fall in muscle pH.[27] Although the accumulation of H^+, P_i, and $H_2PO_4^-$ in the muscle cell may directly impair the activation of the contractile mechanism, experiments have suggested that the decline in power output may be related to the inability to regenerate ATP at the required rates.[28] Maximum rates of ATP regeneration are required during sprint exercise. The average rate of ATP regeneration from anaerobic sources during a 6 s sprint on a cycle ergometer is as high as 14.9 mmol/kg dm/s (dm = dry muscle)[29] and a mean value of 7.5 mmol/kg dm/s during a sprint lasting 30 s.[30,31] This high rate of required ATP regeneration results in a 60 to 80 per cent fall in phosphocreatine, a decline of approximately 30 per cent

in ATP concentration, and a severalfold increase in lactate during a 30 s sprint.

Since PCr can regenerate ATP at very high rates, and its concentration in the muscle is limited, fatigue during short-term, high-intensity exercise may be related to PCr availability. However, there is a simultaneous decline in pH due to the rise in muscle H^+ concentration which will contribute to fatigue. The decline in power output is linked, in part, to these two mechanisms.

Experiments on multiple sprint activities, in which short bouts of maximal exercise are interspersed by periods of recovery, have shown that PCr resynthesis is important for the recovery of power output and that this recovery has taken place despite a continued reduced muscle pH. This would suggest that the muscle PCr content is possibly more important to the production of power output in activities lasting only a few seconds than the H^+ concentration.[32] The muscle pH, however, plays an important role in reducing the rate of recovery of PCr during the rest interval, thereby influencing subsequent performance.

Measurement of power output

Many sports are characterized by their need for short bursts of maximal power output. A high proportion of the required energy is provided by anaerobic metabolism. It is important to realize that 'it is impossible to measure the rates at which muscles produce and transfer energy internally. Only the external manifestations of the energy are capable of being measured.'[33] In this chapter, only tests which measure either the external power output of the body or the rate of energy transfer to external devices are discussed.

The two components of anaerobic performance of most interest are peak and mean external power output. Peak power output is the maximum rate at which energy is transferred to the external system. The mean power output is the total work done during the performance test divided by the time taken. The total work done in tests lasting for a minimum of 30 s is sometimes termed the 'anaerobic capacity'.[34,35] The term 'capacity' implies that there is a finite exhaustible store of energy that can be used for anaerobic energy metabolism and that tests can determine the size of these stores.[36] This author believes that neither of these statements can be sup-

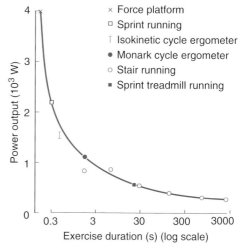

Fig. 12 Relationship between maximum power output and exercise duration for various activities.

ported and therefore, other than when referring to published texts, values of mean power output and total work done will be discussed rather than anaerobic capacity.

Tests of increasing duration

Margaria *et al.*[37] reported that supramaximal exercise of 10 to 15-s duration could be performed without a significant elevation in blood lactate. This suggested that maximal exercise lasting up to 10 s would use energy derived solely from alactic anaerobic sources and therefore that tests of up to this duration could measure these alactic energy sources. Boobis *et al.*[38] and Jacobs *et al.*[39] showed, using muscle-biopsy techniques, that maximum exercise of 6- and 10-s duration, respectively, resulted in significantly elevated concentrations of muscle lactate, suggesting that glycolysis did in fact occur within these time frames. Therefore, it is evident that it is not possible to test the 'alactic' and 'lactic' acid components of energy production independently as both systems appear to be active throughout such tests. No attempt will be made to apportion energy provision from these sources.

Vertical jump test
Tests lasting only a fraction of a second have been shown to result in the highest values of power output. The most common test is the vertical jump test in which the maximum height that the centre of mass of the body is raised during a maximal, standing vertical jump (with counter-movement) is used as an indicator of the power generated in the knee and hip extensors.[40] The instantaneous values of force and velocity required to calculate the power generated are determined using force platforms. It is assumed that the force accelerating the centre of mass is equal to the reaction force applied to the force plate minus the bodyweight. By integrating the resultant acceleration with respect to time, we can obtain the instantaneous value of the velocity of the centre of mass. Instantaneous power output is calculated from the product of the accelerating force and velocity of the centre of mass.[41-43] Davies and Young,[44] using this technique, showed a high correlation ($r = 0.92$) between the height achieved in the jump and the peak power output generated.

However, the vertical jump test has been strongly criticized as not being a valid method for measuring power output.[45] The main criticism is that jumping is an impulsive activity, with the height jumped being a function of the product of force and time and not the product of force and velocity.

Single dynamic movement of a limb
Isokinetic dynamometers are able to give instantaneous information on torque and limb position (angle) at predetermined angular velocities of the limb. Power is calculated from the product of torque T and the preset angular velocity ω. This can be shown to be the same as the product of force F and velocity $\dot{V}$:

$$F = T/r;$$

and

$$\dot{V} = \omega r;$$

where r is the length of the lever arm. Therefore:

$$F\dot{V} = T/r \, \omega r = T\omega$$

Perrine[33] showed that the maximum peak power of the knee extensors occurs at angular velocities around 240 deg/s (range 192 to 288 deg/s) This is approximately 34 per cent of the projected

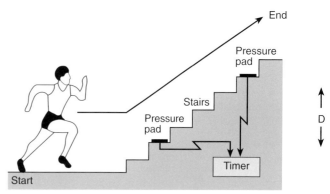

Fig. 13 Margaria step test.

maximum unloaded velocity of the limbs of 832 deg/s. This value of 34 per cent is close to that which would be predicted from the power–velocity relationship of muscle discussed earlier. Perrine[33] also reported unpublished observations of volleyball players showing a correlation coefficient of 0.87 between the peak total leg power per unit bodyweight and the vertical jump height. A high correlation was also found between peak leg power and 100-yard sprint time for women sprinters.

Margaria step test
Margaria *et al.*[46] proposed a test in which anaerobic power is measured over an activity lasting approximately 3 s. The test requires the subjects to sprint up a flight of ordinary stairs, two steps at a time, as quickly as possible after a run-up of 2 m (Fig. 13). It is assumed that the subject attains maximum speed prior to reaching the first step and that the running speed remains constant throughout the stair climb. The time taken to run up an even number of stairs is accurately measured, usually using pressure mats resting on the steps. The subjects are instructed to maintain their normal sprinting posture throughout the test. It is assumed that all the external work is done in raising the centre of mass of the body and that this rise is the same as the level difference D between the steps. The power output of the subject is calculated from the formula:

$$\text{power} = F\dot{V} = m_b g D/t;$$

where m_b is the mass of the subject (kg), g is the acceleration due to gravity (9.81 m/s²), D is the level difference, and t is the time taken. The test–retest coefficient has been found to be high ($r = 0.85$ to 0.9) with a variability over a 5-week period of less than 2 per cent.[46-48]

It has been shown that the power output during this type of test can be increased by having the subjects run with weight packs on their backs. This increase in power output has been shown to range from 10 per cent with a loading of 33 per cent of bodyweight[49] to 16 per cent with a loading of 40 per cent of bodyweight.[50]

Modifications to the original protocol have been proposed. For example, Kalamen[51] had the subjects take three steps at a time after a run-up of 6 m. In this test, however, the number of 'measured steps' is the same as in the Margaria protocol.

Bosco jump test
This test, which examines the power generated whilst jumping, was suggested by Bosco *et al.*[52] The test duration (T_s) is from 15 to 60 s and requires the exact determination of the time spent in the air during a series of repeated maximum jumps. The performer

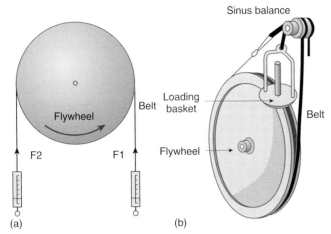

Fig. 14 (a) The frictional forces applied to a strap brake. (b) The modern system adopted by Monark-Crescent AB, which uses the sinus balance to apply a known frictional loading to the flywheel.

attempts to jump as high and as many times as possible during the test period. An instrument pad is required to determine the number (*n*) of jumps performed and the total 'flight' or non-contact time F_t. The average power *W* generated during the test is calculated from:

$$W = F_t \ T_s^2 / 4n(T_s - F_t).$$

It is important that the amount of hip and knee flexion is standardized and that the jumps are performed without interruption. Bosco *et al.*[52] showed high correlations between the power output for a 15-s jump test and the results of a 60-m sprint ($r = 0.84$) and a 15-s cycle ergometer test ($r = 0.87$). A power index can be obtained by dividing the average power obtained by the mass of the performer (kg).

Cycle ergometry

In 1954 von Dobeln[53] described a cheap, but accurate, cycle ergometer which used the principle of the sinus balance to 'weigh' the resistive torques being applied to the flywheel of the ergometer. A steel band was attached to the back wheel of a stationary cycle to give a cylindrical surface to which a strap brake was fitted, the pull of which could be adjusted. The frictional force acting on the strap brake to retard the flywheel is the difference between the forces at the two ends of the belt (Fig. 14).

The work done by a mechanical system is given by the product of the applied force and the distance travelled by the point of application of the force. Once the sinus balance has been calibrated using known forces, the work done can be calculated from the formula:

$$W \text{ (J)} = BR(N) \times \text{flywheel circumference (m)} \times NR;$$

where *BR(N)* is the balance reading and *NR* is the number of flywheel revolutions. The power output is then calculated by dividing the work done by the time taken to do the work. Monark-Crescent AB have developed a range of friction-loaded cycle ergometers based on the von Dobeln ergometer in which the sinus balance is replaced by a suspended weight. When the sinus wheel is free to rotate and the applied load is *L* (N), the von Dobeln equation becomes:

$$W \text{ (J)} = L \text{ (N)} \times \text{flywheel circumference (m)} \times NR.$$

This formula enables us to calculate power output:

$$\text{power output } (W) = Lt;$$

The duration of the exercise must be considered when deciding on the test protocol to be used. Gollnick and Hermansen[54] showed that an exercise duration of 10 s was too short to tax the anaerobic processes fully. Although increasing the duration of the exercise will place greater demands on the anaerobic processes, it will also proportionally increase contributions to energy provision from anaerobic metabolism. Gollnick and Hermansen calculated the relative contributions of anaerobic metabolism to the total energy output during maximal exercise. They found that for the first 10 s of exercise the anaerobic contribution was approximately 83 per cent. This value dropped to approximately 60 per cent, 40 per cent, and 20 per cent for exercise durations of 1 min, 2 min, and 5 min, respectively. Katch[55] reported that 90 per cent of $\dot{V}O_2$max was reached in approximately 60 s during supramaximal exercise. As the aerobic system clearly does not achieve steady state in activities lasting only a few seconds, the contribution made to the total energy production by aerobic metabolism in this type of exercise is difficult to measure precisely, requiring the determination of the oxygen debt which occurred during the test. Although there is general agreement that the tests of 'anaerobic capacity' must be of maximal intensity throughout, there has been no standardization of the duration of the exercise, with test durations lasting from 20 to 240 s having been proposed. The work by Margaria *et al.*[37,46] has greatly influenced the decisions that researchers have made regarding the duration of such tests. They estimated that the maximum lactic acid production was reached after 40 to 60 s of maximal exercise. Katch *et al.*[56] examined test durations of 40 and 120 s on the Monark cycle ergometer and found that the total cumulative work at 40 s had a high correlation ($r = 0.95$) with the total cumulative work in 120 s. They also stated that 'it can be calculated that by 40 s the work rate drops to a level that is within the 'aerobic range' of oxygen requirements'.

Using the findings described above, coupled with the developmental work by Cumming[57] and Ayalon *et al.*,[47] Bar-Or[34] described a test protocol which has become known as the 'Wingate test' or the anaerobic work test. This test requires the subject to cycle at maximum speed against a predetermined resistance for 30 s. The resistance is set at 75 N per 1000 N bodyweight. During the test the number of flywheel revolutions for each 5-s period is monitored. Using the von Dobeln equation described earlier the power output for each 5-s period of the test could be calculated, as could the total work done during the test.

In the protocol described by Bar-Or[34] the subjects start to pedal as fast as possible against a very low resistance which is increased to the required level during the first 2 to 3 s of the test. Many researchers have subsequently replaced this 'flying start' with either a stationary start or a 'rolling start' at a predetermined submaximal speed, with maximum effort commencing once the required load has been introduced. Irrespective of the method used to start the test, the subject works as hard as possible throughout the test with no attempt made at 'pacing' or energy conservation. Toe clips are used to hold the feet on the pedals. The subjects must remain seated throughout the test.

Three indices of anaerobic performance are calculated from the test.

1. Maximal anaerobic power: the highest 5-s power output. This index reflects the peak power generated by the active muscles.

2. Anaerobic capacity: the total work done in the 30-s test.

3. Fatigue index: the difference between the highest and lowest 5-s power outputs divided by the elapsed time.

The test–retest reliability of the protocol was checked for various age, sex, and fitness groups both on the same day and over a period of up to 2 weeks. For tests repeated on the same day correlation coefficients of 0.95 to 0.98 were obtained. Over the 2-week period correlation coefficients of 0.90 to 0.93 were calculated even when environmental conditions were modified. It was concluded that the test was highly reliable.

The method of calculation of power output in the 'Wingate test' has been criticized.[58] This method does not include the work being done in transferring kinetic energy to and from the flywheel of the ergometer. In order to calculate the total power output being generated correctly, the work done against the frictional load, as described by von Dobeln, must be added to the work done in accelerating the flywheel:

$$\text{total power output} = PO_{\text{TOT}} = PO_{\text{FL}} + PO_{\text{AF}};$$

where PO_{FL} is the power output against the frictional load, PO_{AF} is the power output required to accelerate the flywheel, and:

$$PO_{\text{TOT}} = \omega\,(Lr + I\,d\omega/dt);$$

where I is the moment of inertia of the flywheel which is obtained by performing a mechanical run-down test. L is the applied load and r is the radius of the flywheel.

It is clear from the equation for total power output that the angular acceleration $d\omega/dt$ of the flywheel must be known. To achieve this, the speed of the flywheel must be constantly monitored by a computer and the instantaneous values of flywheel acceleration calculated. A simple, but effective, computerized system for monitoring flywheel speed is described by Lakomy.[58] It comprises a small d.c. generator which is driven by the flywheel. The voltage output from the generator, which is proportional to the speed of revolution ($r^2 = 0.998$), is logged by the computer. The computer is able to monitor the flywheel speed and acceleration and therefore to calculate the correct power output.

When the corrected method of calculation is applied to the standard Wingate test, that is to say where the subject is pedalling at maximum speed before the load is applied, the power output at any time during the test is found to be less by a small (up to 6.2 per cent), but significant, amount than that calculated by the conventional method[59] because of the recovery of kinetic energy from the flywheel as it decelerates throughout the test. When a stationary or low-speed rolling start is used, large discrepancies in power output between the two methods of calculations are found. Using a loading recommended by Bar-Or[34] of 75 N per 1000 N bodyweight and a rolling start of 60 pedal rev./min, it was found that not only were the corrected 1-s averaged peak power values approximately 32 per cent higher than the uncorrected values but that peak power output occurred on average 2.1 s earlier.[60] Examination of the Wingate indices revealed that, when using the low-speed start, the uncorrected values of the maximal anaerobic power and fatigue index were greatly underestimated when compared with the correct val-

ues. However, the total work done in the 30 s, defined as anaerobic capacity, was found to be independent of the method of calculation ($p < 0.005$).

Many researchers have attempted to optimize the power output generated during cycle ergometer tests by varying the frictional loads being applied to the flywheel whilst using the uncorrected method of calculation.[56,61-63] All found that peak power output was sensitive to changes in applied load and that it increased with increasing loads up to approximately 100 N per 1000 N bodyweight. In contrast with these findings, Lakomy[64] has shown that when the corrected method of calculation is used the peak power output is independent of the load used. Irrespective of the method of calculation, however, it appears that a loading of approximately 105 N per 1000 N of bodyweight will result in the greatest amount of work being done during the test.

In addition to the single continuous exercise tests on the cycle ergometer, multiple sprint tests have been developed. In many sports, such as rugby, soccer, hockey, basketball, and volleyball, the performer is required to exercise at maximum or near-maximum intensities for a few seconds with these bouts of activity being interspersed with periods of recovery. The ergometer-based multiple sprint tests are designed to investigate the response of the body to such activities. These tests attempt to mimic the sporting situation. The duration of the sprints and the recovery time can be linked to a temporal analysis of sport. An example of a test protocol was that adopted by Wootton and Williams[65] to examine the influence of recovery duration on repeated 6-s sprints. In this test, five 6-s maximal sprints were performed with rest intervals of either 30 or 60 s against loading of 75 N per 1000 N bodyweight. They found that the capacity to perform repeated bouts of maximal exercise was markedly influenced by the preceding number of sprint bouts and the duration of recovery. In such tests the decline in peak and mean power output per sprint is used to describe the fatigue taking place.

An alternative multiple sprint protocol requires the subject to perform a fixed amount of work whilst performing maximally (Loughborough sprint test).[60] The time taken for each sprint is recorded, with the fatigue taking place being described by the increase in this time. Figure 15 shows a typical example of the time taken to perform set amounts of work, with 100 per cent being the total amount of work that could be performed in a single 6-s sprint.

Dynamic power has been investigated using isokinetic cycle ergometry.[66] On such ergometers the pedalling speed is controlled and the forces exerted on the pedal cranks are detected by foil strain gauges and transmitted to a computer. Torque, work, and power are calculated for each leg in every pedal stroke to obtain data on maximal power and decline in power over the test period, expressed as a fatigue index. All the tests described for the friction-loaded cycle ergometer can also be performed with isokinetic ergometers.

Critical power

A contrasting system for measuring anaerobic work capacity and critical power has been developed by Moritani et al.[67] based on the test proposed by Monod and Scherre.[68] The test involves a series of exhaustive exercises on the cycle ergometer at a range of intensities during which the total amount of work and the time to exhaustion are measured. The test's exercise intensities ranged from 170 to

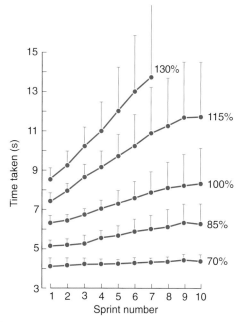

Fig. 15 The time taken to perform a series of fixed work sprints with 30 s of recovery between sprints ($n = 8$; mean ± SD).

360 W 'depending on bodyweight and level of fitness' so that the durations of the exercise (to exhaustion) lasted approximately 1 to 10 min. The pedalling rate was set at 70 rev./min. The test was terminated immediately when the subject was unable to maintain cadence (that is to say when the pedalling speed dropped to 65 rev./min). A regression equation was generated such that the x and y values were the duration of the exercise and the product of exercise tensity W and exercise duration, respectively. The slope of the relationship obtained was termed the critical power and the intercept was termed the anaerobic work capacity. The authors suggested that critical power is the exercise intensity which can just be maintained without exhaustion, while anaerobic work capacity is the total amount of work that can be performed utilizing only stored energy sources within the muscle. They further claim that critical power is significantly correlated ($p < 0.01$) with the ventilatory threshold ($r = 0.927$) and with the physical work capacity at the fatigue threshold ($r = 0.869$), which has been defined as the highest constant-power output that requires no increase in electromyographical activity of the major muscles involved for its maintenance.[67] Although four exercise intensities over a period of 2 days were used to determine the regression equation, Moritani et al.[67] concluded that critical power and anaerobic work capacity could be estimated with reasonable accuracy using only two exercise bouts. They qualified this statement by stipulating that the two bouts should be chosen with care, so that they produce exhaustion between 1 and 10 min and differ by at least 5 min. They feel that 'the adoption of this protocol would reduce demands on the subject and investigator thereby improving the practicality of the critical power test in the laboratory and field settings'.

Nebelsick-Gullett et al.[69] examined the relationship between anaerobic work capacity and anaerobic capacity (**AC**) from the critical power and Wingate tests, respectively. Anaerobic work capacity and AC were found to be significantly ($p < 0.05$) related ($r = 0.74$). There was no significant difference ($p < 0.05$) between test–retest

means for critical power or anaerobic work capacity. Test–retest correlations for critical power ($r = 0.94$) and anaerobic work capacity ($r = 0.87$) led Nebelsick-Gullett et al.[69] to conclude that the critical power test was a reliable technique for measuring anaerobic capacity as well as the maximum rate of fatigueless work.

Sprint running

Sprint running, in contrast with sprint cycling, is a weight-bearing activity. Therefore the cycle ergometer may be of limited value to those interested in the evaluation of sprint running. Thomson and Garvie[70] described a laboratory test in which subjects sprinted for 15, 30, 45, and 60 s on a motor-driven treadmill up a 5 per cent gradient at a speed which would produce exhaustion at around 60 to 70 s. The energy expenditure was determined by indirect calorimetry combining the measurement of oxygen uptake with those of peak lactate concentrations.[71] In the sprinters the mean total energy expended in the sprint to exhaustion was 63.9 kcal, of which 72.3 per cent was calculated to be derived from anaerobic metabolism. In contrast, the corresponding values for the marathon runners were 52.8 kcal and 62.9 per cent. The anaerobic work done was then subdivided into alactic (mean 48 per cent) and lactacid (mean 52 per cent) components. These total energy expenditure results were highly correlated with the subject's sprinting performance over 329 m ($r = 0.82$, $p < 0.01$, $n = 14$). The conclusion drawn was that the protocol provided a direct quantitative measurement of anaerobic capacity and partitioned the alactic and lactacid components. It was also sensitive enough to distinguish between groups of subjects (trained vs. untrained, sprinters vs. endurance) and between subjects within a specific group.

In contrast with the indirect calorimetry test of Thomson and Garvie,[70] an ergometer for the direct measurement of power output during sprint running has been described.[64,72] The ergometer was based on a non-motorized treadmill which: (1) allowed the subjects to sprint at speeds similar to those achieved in sprint running; (2) allowed the same variability in instantaneous work rate during sprinting that cycle ergometers permit during cycling; and (3) enabled instantaneous values of power output to be determined throughout the sprint.

The external forces generated by a sprinter can be resolved into vertical and horizontal components. The vertical component raises the centre of gravity during each stride so that leg recovery can take place. Fukunaga et al.[73] found that for a given runner the vertical component of the work being done was independent of the running speed. The horizontal or 'propulsive' component moves the runner along the ground; the greater this propulsive component the faster the sprinter will cover the ground. Therefore the sprinter attempts to maximize his work rate in this direction. Ideally, the total work done by the sprinter, namely the sum of the vertical and horizontal components, should be monitored when evaluating the physiological demands of sprinting. It is extremely difficult to measure the vertical component of the work done during sprinting, and so the instrumented ergometer measured only the horizontal component of the work rate, that is to say the component that actually maintains treadmill motion.

A commercially available non-motorized treadmill (Woodway model AB), which normally slopes backwards, was levelled by placing its rear feet on supports (Fig. 16). All four feet were anchored securely to a baseboard to prevent excessive lateral movement dur-

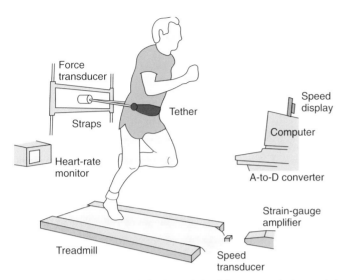

Fig. 16 Non-motorized treadmill for the analysis of the power output generated during sprint running.

ing use. Measurement of the propulsive force was achieved by applying Newton's third law of motion which states that for every action there is an equal and opposite reaction. If the sprinter does not move relative to the ground, then the force that the sprinter applies to the treadmill belt must be equal to the horizontal component of the restraining force in the harness. The horizontal restraining tether was connected to a force transducer. The output from the force-transducer amplifier and the treadmill belt speed was continuously monitored by a computer. The rate at which work was being done to move the treadmill, namely the horizontal power output, was calculated from the product of the restraining force and the belt speed. This calculation assumes that the error resulting from the points of force application and measurement not being the same is small, and that little of the subject's weight is detected as a horizontal force due to forward lean.

At the conclusion of a test the following information was calculated and displayed:

(1) the mean propulsive power for each second of the sprint;

(2) the mean propulsive power for the sprint duration;

(3) the total propulsive work done;

(4) a fatigue index defined as the difference between the peak and the lowest propulsive power output values expressed as a percentage of the peak value.

The same test indices that were described for the cycle ergometer could also be measured on the sprint ergometer.

Peak propulsive power outputs were found to occur during the acceleration phase of the sprint. Mean 1-s values in excess of 1 kW were commonly obtained, with within-stride instantaneous values (0.025 s average) often in excess of 3 kW. Fukunaga *et al.*[73] have shown that this propulsive power represents approximately 80 per cent of the total power output, with the remaining 20 per cent required for the work against gravity.

According to Cheetham *et al.*[74] 'This laboratory-based method for studying sprint running offers an additional way of investigating human response to brief periods of high-intensity exercise.'

References

1. Cavanagh PR. On 'muscle action' vs. 'muscle contraction'. *Journal of Biomechanics* 1988; **22**: 69.

2. Partridge LD, Benton LA. Muscle, the motor. In: Brookhart JM, Mountcastle VB, Brooks VB, Geiger SR, eds. *Handbook of Physiology*: Section 1. The Nervous System. Bethesda, MD: American Physiological Society, 1981: 43–106.

3. Barany M. ATPase activity of myosin correlated with speed of muscle shortening. *Journal of General Physiology* 1967; **50**: 197–216.

4. Huxley AF. Muscle structure and theories of contraction. *Progress in Biophysics and Biophysical Chemistry* 1957; **7**: 255–318.

5. Curtin NA, Davies RE. Very high tension with very little ATP breakdown by active skeletal muscle. *Journal of Mechanochemical Cell Motility* 1975; **3**: 147–54.

6. Burke RE. Motor units: anatomy, physiology and functional organisation. In: Brooks VB, ed. *Handbook of Physiology*. Section I, The nervous system II. Washington, DC: American Physiological Society, 1981: 345–422.

7. Spector SA, Gardiner PF, Zernicke RF, Roy RR, Edgerton VR. Muscle architecture and force–velocity characteristics of the cat soleus and medial gastrocnemius: Implications for motor control. *Journal of Neurophysiology* 1980; **44**: 951–60.

8. Close RI. Dynamic properties of mammalian skeletal muscle. *Physiological Reviews* 1972; **52**: 128–97.

9. Saltin B, Gollnick PD. Skeletal muscle adaptability: significance of metabolism and performance. In: Peachet L, ed. *Handbook of Physiology*. Bethesda: American Physiological Society, 1983: 555–631.

10. Edgerton VR, Roy RR, Apor P. Specific tension of human elbow flexor muscles. In: Saltin B, ed. *Biochemistry of exercise*. Champaign, IL: Human Kinetics, 1986: 487–500.

11. Wickiewicz TL, Roy RR, Powell PL, Perrine JJ, Edgerton VR. Muscle architecture and force–velocity relationships in humans. *Journal of Applied Physiology* 1984; **56**: 435–43.

12. Bigland B, Lippold OCJ. The relation between force, velocity and integrated electrical activity in human muscles. *Journal of Physiology* 1954; **123**: 214–24.

13. Otten E. Concepts and models of functional architecture in skeletal muscle. *Exercise and Sports Sciences Review* 1988; **16**: 89–137.

14. Gordon AM, Huxley AF, Julian FJ. The variation in isometric tension with sarcomere length in vertebrate muscle fibres. *Journal of Physiology* 1966; **184**: 170–92.

15. Fenn WO, Marsh BS. Muscular force at different speed of shortening. *Journal of Physiology* 1935; **85**: 277–97.

16. Hill AV. The heat of shortening and the dynamic constants of muscle. *Proceedings of the Royal Society B* 1938; **126**: 136–95.

17. Wilkie DR. The relationship between force and velocity in human muscle. *Journal of Physiology* 1950; **110**: 248–80.

18. Singh M, Korpovich PV. Strength of forearm flexors and extensors. *Journal of Applied Physiology* 1968; **25**: 177–80.

19. Cavagna GA, Saibene FP, Margaria R. Effect of negative work on the amount of positive work performed by an isolated muscle. *Journal of Applied Physiology* 1965; **20**: 157.

20. Norman RW, Komi PV. Electromechanical delay in skeletal muscle under normal movement conditions. *Acta Physiologica Scandinavica* 1970; **106**: 241–8.

21. Shorten MR. Muscle elasticity and human performance. In: van Gheluwe B, Atha J, eds. *Current research in sports sciences. Medicine and sports science*. Basel: Karger, 1987; **25**: 1–18.

22. Cavanagh GA, Dusman B, Margaria R. Positive work done by the previously stretched muscle. *Journal of Applied Physiology* 1968; **20**: 157–8.

23. Komi PV. Relationship between muscle tension, EMG and velocity of contraction under concentric and eccentric work. In: Desmedt JE, ed. *New developments in electromyography and clinical neurophysiology.* Basel: Karger, 1973; **1**: 596–600.

24. Billeter R, Hoppeler H. Muscular basis of strength. In: Komi PV, ed. *Strength and power in sport.* Oxford: Blackwell Scientific, 1992: 39–63.

25. Katz A, Sahlin K, Henriksson. Muscle ATP turnover rate during isometric contractions in humans. *Journal of Physiology* 1985; **60**: 1839–42.

26. Baker AJ, Carson PJ, Green AT, Miller RG, Weiner MW. Influence of human muscle length on energy transaction studied by 31P-NMR. *Journal of Applied Physiology* 1992; **73**: 160–5

27. Sahlin K, Ren JM. Relationship of contracting capacity to metabolic changes during recovery from a fatiguing contraction. *Journal of Applied Physiology* 1989; **67**: 648–54

28. Gaitanos GC, Williams C, Boobis LH, Brooks S. Human muscle metabolism during sprint running. *Journal of Applied Physiology* 1993; **75**: 712–19

29. Bogdanis GC, Nevill ME, Lakomy HKA, Boobis LH. Muscle metabolism during repeated sprint exercise in man. *Journal of Physiology* 1994; **475**: 25P

30. Nevill ME, Boobis LH, Brooks SA, Williams C. Effect of training on muscle metabolism during treadmill sprinting. *Journal of Applied Physiology* 1989; **67**: 2376–82.

31. Bogdanis GC, Nevill ME, Boobis LH, Lakomy HKA, Nevill AM. Recovery of power output and muscle metabolites following 30 s of maximal sprint cycling in man. *Journal of Physiology* 1995; **482.2**: 467–80.

32. McCartney N, Heigenhauser GJ, Jones NL. Power output and fatigue of human muscle in maximal cycling exercise. *Journal of Applied Physiology* 1983; **55**: 218–24.

33. Perrine JJ. The biophysics of maximal muscle power outputs: Methods and problems and measurement. In: Jones NL, McCartney N, McComas AJ, eds. *Human muscle power.* Champaign, IL: Human Kinetics, 1986: 15–25.

34. Bar-Or O. A new anaerobic capacity test—characteristics and applications. *Proceedings of the 21st World Congress of Sports Medicine*, Brasilia, 1978: 1–27.

35. Katch VL, Weltman A. Interrelation between anaerobic power output, anaerobic capacity and anaerobic power. *Ergonomics* 1979; **22**: 325–32.

36. Simoneau J, Lortie G, Boulay M, Bouchard C. Test of anaerobic alactacid and lactacid capacities: description and reliability. *Canadian Journal of Applied Sport Sciences* 1983; **8**: 266–70.

37. Margaria R, Cerretelli RP, Mangili F. Balance and kinetics of anaerobic energy release during strenuous exercise in man. *Journal of Applied Physiology* 1964; **21**: 1662–4.

38. Boobis L, Williams C, Wootton S. Human muscle metabolism during brief maximal exercise. *Journal of Physiology (London)* 1982; **338**: 21–2P.

39. Jacobs I, Tesch Per, Bar-Or O, Karlsson J, Dotan R. Lactate in human skeletal muscle after 10 and 30 s of supramaximal exercise. *Journal of Applied Physiology* 1983; **55**: 365–7.

40. Cavagna GA. Force platforms as ergometers. *Journal of Applied Physiology* 1975; **39**: 174–9.

41. Davies CTM, Rennie R. Human power output. *Nature (London)* 1968; **217**: 770–1.

42. Offenbacher EL. Physics and the vertical jump. *American Journal of Physics* 1970; **38**: 7.

43. Davies CTM. The aerobic and anaerobic components of work during submaximal exercise on a bicycle ergometer. *Ergonomics* 1971; **14**: 257–63.

44. Davies CTM, Young K. Effects of external loading on short term power output in children and young male adults. *European Journal of Applied Physiology* 1984; **52**: 351–4.

45. Adamson GT, Whitney RJ. Critical appraisal of jumping as a measure of human power. In: Vredenbregt J, Wartenweiler J, ed. *Medicine and sport*, Vol. 6: *Biomechanics* II. Basel, Karger, 1971: 208–11.

46. Margaria R, Aghemo, P, Rovelli E. Measurement of muscular power (anaerobic) in man. *Journal of Applied Physiology* 1966; **21**: 1662–4.

47. Ayalon A, Inbar O, Bar-Or O. Relationships among measurements of explosive strength and anaerobic power. In: Nelson RC, Morehouse CA, ed. *International series on sports sciences*, Vol. 1. *Biomechanics* IV: *Proceedings of the fourth international seminar on biomechanics.* Baltimore, MD: University Park Press, 1974: 572–7.

48. Sawka MN, Tahamount MV, Fitzgerald PI, Miles DS, Knowlton RG. Alactic capacity and power: reliability and interpretation. *European Journal of Applied Physiology* 1980; **41**: 93–9.

49. Kitiwaga K, Suzuki M, Miyashita M. Anaerobic power output of young obese men: comparison with non obese men and the role of excess fat. *European Journal of Applied Physiology* 1980; **43**: 229–34.

50. Caiozzo VJ, Kyle CR. The effect of external loading upon power output in stair climbing. *European Journal of Applied Physiology* 1980; **44**: 217–22.

51. Kalamen J. Measurement of maximum muscular power in man. PhD Thesis, Ohio State University, 1968.

52. Bosco C, Luhtanen P, Komi P. A simple method for measurement of mechanical power in jumping. *European Journal of Applied Physiology* 1983; **50**: 273–82.

53. von Dobeln W. A simple bicycle ergometer. *Journal of Applied Physiology* 1954; **7**: 222–4.

54. Gollnick PD, Hermansen L. Biochemical adaptations to exercise: anaerobic metabolism. In: Wilmore JH, ed. *Exercise and sports science reviews.* New York: Academic Press, 1973: 1–43.

55. Katch VL. Kinetics of oxen uptake and recovery for supra maximal work of short duration. *Zeitschrift für Angewandte Physiologie* (international edition) 1973; **31**: 197–201.

56. Katch VL, Weltman A, Martin R, Gray L. Optimal test characteristics for maximal anaerobic work on the cycle ergometer. *Research Quarterley* 1977; **48**: 319–27.

57. Cumming GR. Correlation of athletic performance and aerobic power in 12–17 year old children with bone age, calf muscle, total body potassium, heart volume and two indices of anaerobic power. In: Bar-OR O, ed. *Pediatric work physiology.* Natanya: Wingate Institute, 1974: 109–37.

58. Lakomy HK. An ergometer for measuring the power generated during sprinting. *Journal of Physiology* 1984; **354**: 33P.

59. Bassett DR Jr. Correcting the Wingate test for changes in kinetic energy of the ergometer flywheel. *International Journal of Sports Medicine* 1989; **10**: 446–9.

60. Lakomy HK. Measurement of external power output during high intensity exercise. PhD Thesis, Loughborough University, 1988.

61. Evans J, Quinney H. Determinations of resistance settings for anaerobic power testing. *Canadian Journal of Applied Sports Sciences* 1981; **6**: 43–56.

62. Nadeau M, Brassard A, Cuerrier JP. The bicycle ergometer for muscle power testing. *Canadian Journal of Applied Physiology* 1983; **8**: 41–6

63. Nakamura Y, Yoshiteru M, Miyashita M. Determination of the peak power output during maximal brief pedalling bouts. *Journal of Sports Science* 1986; **3**: 181–7.

64. Lakomy HK. Effect of load on corrected peak power output generated on friction loaded cycle ergometers. *Journal of Sports Sciences* 1985; **3**: 240.

65. Wootton SA, Williams C. The influence of recovery duration on repeated maximal sprints. In: Knuttgen HG, Vogel JA, Poortmans JR, ed. *Biochemistry of exercise. International series on Sports Sciences.* Champaign, IL: Human Kinetics, 1983: 269–73.

66. McCartney N, Heigenhauser GJ, Sargeant A, Jones NL. A constant velocity ergometer for the study of dynamic muscle function. *Journal of Applied Physiology* 1983; **55**: 212–17.

67. Moritani T, Nagata A, De Vries H, Muro M. Critical power as a measure of physical work capacity and anaerobic threshold. *Ergonomics* 1981; **24**: 338–50.

68. Monod H, Scherre J. The work capacity of a synergic muscular group. *Ergonomics* 1965; **8**: 329–38.

69. Nebelsick-Gullett L, Housh T, Johnson G, Bauge S. A comparison between methods of measuring anaerobic work capacity. *Ergonomics* 1988; **31**: 1413–19.

70. Thomson JM, Garvie KJ. A laboratory method for the determination of anaerobic energy expenditure during sprinting. *Canadian Journal of Applied Sport Sciences* 1981; **6**: 21–6.

71. Margaria R, Cerretelli P, di Prampero PE, Massari C, Torelli G. Kinetics and mechanisms of oxygen debt contraction in man. *Journal of Applied Physiology* 1963; **18**: 371–7.

72. Lakomy HK. The use of a non-motorised treadmill for analysing sprint performance. *Ergonomics* 1987; **30**: 627–37.

73. Fukunaga T, Matsuo A, Yuas K, Fujimatsu H, Asahina K. Mechanical power output in running. In: Asmussen E, Jorgensen K, eds. *Biomechanics VI-B. International Series on Biomechanics.* Baltimore, MD: University Park Press, 1978: 17–22.

74. Cheetham ME, Williams, Lakomy HK. A laboratory running test: metabolic responses of sprint and endurance trainined athletes. *British Journal of Sports Medicine* 1985; **19**: 81–4.

1.4 Sport psychology

Lew Hardy and Graham Jones

Introduction

The beginnings of sport psychology in the western world can be traced back at least as far as 1897 to Triplett's studies on the effects of the presence of other people on performance.[1] However, despite the prodigious work of Coleman Griffith in the 1920s (see, for example, ref. 2), sport psychology did not really become established as a scientific discipline until the mid-1960s, when the International Society of Sport Psychology (1965), the North American Society for the Psychology of Sport and Physical Activity (1967), and the European Federation of Sport Psychology (1968) were formed. Early work in sport psychology had a strong research emphasis. However, during the last 15 years sport psychologists have also become heavily involved in applied work with athletes on the maximization of performance. In most countries, this has led to inevitable territorial disputes over who is qualified to do what. Essentially, sport psychologists, who generally have first degrees in sports science and higher degrees in (sport) psychology, claim that psychologists, who generally have first (and sometimes higher) degrees in psychology but no background in sports science, do not have the necessary knowledge of sports science. Conversely, of course, psychologists claim that sport psychologists do not have the necessary breadth of knowledge in psychology (see below).

A rather more constructive development has been the shift in research emphasis away from behavioural approaches towards more process-oriented cognitive approaches. This shift in emphasis follows the lead of mainstream psychology, and has been accompanied by the adaptation and adoption of many cognitive behavioural methods from mainstream psychology.[3-6] Other positive developments include the establishment of the subdiscipline of exercise psychology, and sustained improvements in the quality of both research output and applied work with performers.

Current areas of interest in sport psychology are diverse, but include the identification of factors which influence participation and performance; the development of psychological strategies to enhance performance; the influence of involvement in sport and exercise upon psychological well being; the psychology of children involved in sport; and the development of ecologically valid methodologies to answer applied questions in the field. However, in view of the space constraints that operate upon a review chapter such as this, it is perhaps inevitable that some aspects of sport psychology have been omitted. Indeed, the present authors would readily admit that they have somewhat arbitrarily divided the chapter into six general sections, which must, at least, partially reflect their own areas of interest. These six sections focus upon motivation, stress and performance, individual differences, interpersonal relationships, exercise psychology, and mental training. Each section provides a review of the current state of knowledge in that area, and then attempts to identify some of the important issues that are likely to be addressed by sport psychologists over the next few years.

Motivation

In behavioural terms, motivation is concerned with the strength or intensity dimension of behaviour. Furthermore, according to motivation theories, this energy is determined by the biological and social needs of the organism.[7] It is often suggested that motivation theories are concerned with the reasons why people behave in certain ways, and to some extent this is true. However, there are many explanations of people's behaviour that do not depend upon needs for their explanatory power; for example, the Social Learning Theory explains how acts of violence can be brought about by a process similar to mimicry, simply by repeated observation of such acts.[8] Strictly speaking, these are not motivation theories, although the precise distinction between such (social) cognitive theories and motivation theories is not always a very clear one.

Motives for participation

Early research on motivation in sport examined reasons for participation, and indicated that the majority of young (North American) performers had multiple reasons for their involvement. The most commonly identified reasons were needs for affiliation, to develop skill, for excitement, to succeed, and for fitness/health.[9] More contemporary researchers[10] have reduced these needs to three more-fundamental reasons: the activities have intrinsic value (enjoyment); they are claimed to have positive health benefits; and/or they provide opportunities for participants to gain feelings of competence. It is perhaps worth noting that this latter explanation is as much cognitive in nature as it is motivational.

Other research examining the reasons why young people 'drop out' from sport has identified four motives for achievement in sport: namely, to demonstrate competence; to master the task; to gain social approval; and to experience enjoyment and excitement.[11,12] This research suggests that young children are motivated by task mastery and social approval rather than a need to feel competent; but as they grow older so they acquire a greater need to demonstrate competence.[7] Furthermore, Roberts[11] has argued that the existing evidence suggests that children are likely to 'drop out' of sport if their prime motive for participation is to demonstrate their competence by beating others. The extent to which this finding can be generalized to other cultures is as yet unclear.[12] However, recent research[13] suggests that these findings probably do not generalize to all performers from all cultures, and in particular do not generalize to élite performers.

An interesting question in the area of motives for participation is why people pursue dangerous sports such as climbing, caving, skin diving, parachuting, and motor racing. One possible explanation is that such performers are high sensation seekers[14] who indulge in dangerous activities for 'arousal jags'.[15] An alternative explanation has been put forward by Solomon.[16] He proposed that although performers habituate to the fear that precedes the performance of dangerous activities, their secondary reaction of elation and satisfaction upon completion of the activity is increased with successive presentations of the feared stimulus (namely the dangerous activity). This secondary effect then becomes the motive for continued involvement. Whilst Bakker *et al.*[10] have suggested that this theory has considerable potential for explaining participation in dangerous sports, from a cognitive viewpoint it could be argued that it simply replaces one 'black box' with another. More precisely, it does not explain why the secondary response to negative stimuli does not habituate with repeated presentations of the stimulus; nor does it really explain why people choose to take part in sports where the negative stimulus is physical danger, rather than in competitive sports where the negative stimulus is ego-threat.

A rather different sort of explanation can be deduced from the work of Piet (cited by Bakker *et al.*[10]) and that of Lester.[17] Following a qualitative study of élite Himalayan mountaineers, Lester concluded that such people often find the normal interpersonal situations of everyday life stressful. Coupled with Piet's finding that one of the major reasons given for mountaineering was the great feeling of competence generated by controlling stress responses, this suggests that such mountaineers may have a very strong need to demonstrate their competence at dealing with stressful situations precisely *because* they find many situations in everyday life stressful. Having said all this, direct empirical tests of both this and Solomon's[16] theory have yet to be performed.

Intrinsic and extrinsic motivation

As indicated above, behaviour can be initiated and maintained for a variety of reasons. Similarly, the rewards that people receive as a result of participating in sport can also be very varied; for example, praise, prizes, financial rewards, satisfaction, enjoyment, and a sense of achievement. Some of these rewards are external to the task, whilst others are apparently inherent in performing the task itself.[9] Behaviour which is maintained by rewards that are intrinsic to the task is said to be intrinsically motivated, whilst behaviour that is maintained by rewards extrinsic to the task is said to be extrinsically motivated. However, the situation is much more complex than this, since external rewards can sometimes enhance subsequent intrinsic motivation and sometimes reduce it. This paradox has been superbly illustrated by Casady:

[An]old man lived alone on a street where boys played noisily every afternoon. One day the din became too much, and he called the boys into his house. He told them he liked to listen to them play, but his hearing was failing and he could no longer hear their games. He asked them to come around each day and play noisily in front of his house. If they did he would give them each a quarter. The youngsters raced back next day and made a tremendous racket in front of the house. The old man paid them, and asked them to return the next day. Again they made noise, and again the old man paid them for it. But this time he gave each boy only 20 cents, explaining that he was running out of money. On the following day, they got only 15 cents each. Furthermore, the old man told them, he would reduce the fee to five cents each on the 4th day. The boys became angry and told the old man that they would not be back. It was not worth the effort, they said, to make noise for only five cents a day. (ref. 18, p. 52)

De Charms[19] and Deci[20] attempted to explain this phenomenon by arguing that humans have an innate need to feel competent and self-determining (namely that they determine which behaviours they will, or will not, engage in). Based upon this assumption, Deci and Ryan's Cognitive Evaluation Theory[7] proposes that external rewards will enhance intrinsic motivation for a particular activity whenever the information that is contained in them infers an increase in self-competence *and* self-determination. Conversely, extrinsic rewards which convey information indicating a decrease in self-competence, or which attempt to control the performer and thereby decrease self-determination, will lead to a reduction in intrinsic motivation. These basic predictions of Cognitive Evaluation Theory have now received considerable empirical support in the literature.[7,21]

Cognitive Evaluation Theory has attracted considerable attention in the context of sport because the success and failure that are implicit in competitive activities can be regarded as rewards that are essentially external to the task of performing.[7,22] Unfortunately, a detailed review of this research is beyond the scope of this chapter. However, the implications of Cognitive Evaluation Theory for sport include:

(1) performers should be actively involved in the decision-making processes that determine their training and competition programme;

(2) performers should be encouraged to set goals that are not easily influenced by others. These goals should be difficult, but must be realistic, so that performers have the maximum chance of achieving objectives that they perceive to be worthwhile (see later section on Mental training);

(3) rewards should be used to provide information about performers' competence, not to control their behaviour. In particular, simply rewarding success and punishing mistakes may well lead to a decrease in the intrinsic motivation of performers.

Attributions

Attributions are the reasons which people perceive to be the causes of events such as success or failure in sport. Weiner's attribution theory[23] proposed that attributions for success and failure could be classified along two dimensions: stability and locus of causality. The stability dimension is relatively straightforward and refers to the extent to which the attributed quality is stable across time. The locus of causality dimension is also relatively straightforward to define in the context of attributions; however, rather confusingly, this definition differs from that used by Cognitive Evaluation Theorists.[7] In the attribution literature, locus of causality refers simply to whether the cause was internal or external to the individual concerned. For example, the attribution of a given success to innate ability would be classified as internal and stable, because innate ability is clearly internal to the performer and should not change a great deal across time. Other stereotypical attributions for success and failure include: effort (internal and unstable); task difficulty (external and stable); and luck (external and unstable). Essentially, Weiner's theory predicted that the locus of causality of attributions influences the intensity of the affective response to the outcome, whilst the stability of attributions determines the performer's expectations for future success or failure. Subsequent theorizing[24,25] led to the identification of two further attributional dimensions. The first of these, controllability, was non-orthogonal to Weiner's earlier dimensions and was hypothesized to be concerned with the moral judgements that people make in relation to success and failure. The second dimension, globality, referred to the extent of generalizability of the cause to other areas of behaviour. Considerable research has now been conducted in sport settings using the two basic attributional dimensions, although rather less has been performed on controllability and globality.[26,27] In summary, this research suggests that attributions may be important determinants of affective responses to success and failure,[26,28,29] expectations regarding future performance,[30,31] and intrinsic motivation.[7]

Other research has shown that people's needs and expectancies influence the attributions that they make. In particular, the need to preserve self-esteem may lead performers to employ a self-serving bias when making attributions for success and failure such that they generally give more internal attributions for success, but more external attributions for failure.[32] Similarly, team cohesion may lead to a team-serving bias in attributions for success and failure.[33] Finally, social factors may also influence attributions, since publicly declared attributions have been found to show less self-serving bias than private attributions.[27]

In 1983, Rejeski and Brawley commented that attribution research in sport had to that date been quite narrow in focus.[27] In particular, they criticized its preoccupation with applying Weiner's 1972 theory[23] to the study of self-attributions for achievement outcomes. In 1997, this criticism still largely stands, the only real difference being that the literature now applies Weiner's 1979 theory[24] to the study of self-attributions for achievement outcomes. This is unfortunate, because attributions seem to form an important part of most cognitive and motivational theories of emotion and behaviour, both personal and interpersonal. Furthermore, at an applied level, attributions appear to be closely related to performers' motivational states and also to influence their subsequent behaviours. Finally, personal construct theorists[34] would probably argue that current trends towards subjects mapping their own attributions on to attributional dimensions provided by the experimenter[27,35] should be extended to subjects defining their own attributional dimensions (personal construct system). Sport psychologists appear to be largely unaware of the potential of personal construct theory to both researchers and practitioners alike (for exceptions, see refs 36,37).

Withdrawal

Apart from research which was discussed earlier into the reasons why young people 'drop out' from sport, this is a much under-researched area. Examination of the effects of enforced withdrawal from sports participation in the health-related exercise domain has led some researchers to propose that performers can become 'addicted' to exercise or sport.[38] Various reasons for this dependency have been proposed, including the release of beta-endorphins during and after exercise[39] (see also later section on Exercise psychology). However, the magnitude of the problem is frequently sensationalized, and several researchers have emphasized the need to distinguish between commitment and addiction.[40,41]

It seems to be generally accepted that psychological factors play an important part in recovery from injury,[42] and the psychological response to injury has been likened to a grief response. However, whilst theories and models abound,[43–45] relatively little high-quality empirical evidence is yet available. That which is available[46–48] suggests that high levels of skill in goal-setting, self-talk, and imagery might help performers to adhere better to the rehabilitation process and recover faster from injury.

Research has also been conducted on the psychological symptoms of staleness in performers following 'overtraining'.[49] This research has largely relied on measuring disturbances from the so-called 'iceberg' mood profile that élite performers may possess. The underlying idea behind this research was that, once identified, training loads could be adjusted according to psychological moods to minimize the risk of placing too great a training load on athletes. However, the 'iceberg' profile is not without its critics,[50] whilst sports scientists and physicians working in the field generally acknowledge that staleness results from the total sum of stressors that the athlete has to deal with, not just the training load. More recent research on overtraining[51] has adopted a more complete approach to monitoring which includes mood state as just one of a number of psychological variables.

There are some clear similarities between staleness, or over-stressing, in athletes and psychological burnout in coaches and other service professions. However, whilst there is an established literature on burnout in the service professions, and even some literature on burnout in coaches,[52,53] there is, as yet, only a small empirical literature on burnout in sports performers.[54–56] This literature suggests that performers are most vulnerable to burnout when they have perfectionist tendencies, are personally disorganized, have poor cognitive restructuring strategies, and their sport is organized in such a way as to disempower them by giving them few choices and little self-determination.

Current situation

Despite the fact that motivation was one of the earliest areas to be investigated in sport psychology, many interesting and far-reaching questions still await an acceptable answer. In the area of motives for participation, there is a need to perform prospective studies to explore further the generalizability of Roberts'[11] finding that children who compete in sport to beat other people are more likely to 'drop out' than other children. Another interesting question, which has not yet been satisfactorily answered, relates to the reasons why people pursue dangerous sports.

Although the area of intrinsic motivation is one of the few aspects of motivation to receive serious attention from researchers, there is still an urgent need for longitudinal studies that explore the cyclical nature of the relationships that exist between goal orientations, rewards, attributions, self-competence, and intrinsic motivation (cf. ref. 57). Furthermore, such studies may throw some light on the different roles that may be assumed by extrinsic rewards at different stages during the development of intrinsic motivation. Other research on attributions in sport might focus upon actor–observer differences in attributions, attributions for interpersonal as well as achievement outcomes, and the mapping of attributions on to subjects' own personal construct systems.

The whole area of withdrawal from sport is in need of development. In particular, there is an urgent need for research into the role that active regeneration, and other preventive and curative strategies, might have in helping athletes to avoid and recover from overstressing.[58] Related to this is a need for further empirical research addressing the question of how athletes might best cope with the stressors of injury[42,43,46] and retirement. Finally, there is also a need to explore further the differences between, and commonalities of, commitment and addiction.[41]

Stress and performance

The recent publication of texts on the specialized topic of stress[59] and anxiety[60,61] reflects the considerable amount of research attention devoted to this area in recent years. This endeavour to gain a greater understanding of stress and sports performance represents an extension of the early interest in social facilitation.

Social facilitation

Social facilitation is one of the oldest and most studied topics in social psychology. However, whilst the study of audience effects upon motor performance was a popular area of research for many years, it was also plagued by a general inability to explain the inconsistent findings which were produced. It was not until 1965 that Zajonc[62] made significant progress towards resolving the situation by explaining the previously inconsistent findings in terms of the emission of dominant responses (a construct of drive theory) as a function of the increased drive or generalized arousal elicited by the mere presence of an audience; that is, the increased arousal caused by the presence of an audience enhanced performance on well-learned tasks but impaired performance on poorly-learned tasks. Zajonc's classic paper rekindled interest in this area, and the subsequent upsurge in social facilitation research led to Cottrell *et al.*'s[63] re-statement of Zajonc's proposals. These authors argued that the mere presence of others was not necessarily arousing, and that the audience had to be perceived by the performer to have the potential to evaluate performance in order for arousal to be increased and the hypothesized effects to occur. These developments, in the latter half of the 1960s, encouraged sport psychologists to gain a greater knowledge of the interaction between performers' social environments, their skill levels, and performance. By the 1970s, three different aspects of social facilitation had been identified and studied using different paradigms: audience effects; coaction effects; and competition effects (see ref. 64 for a review). Much of this research was laboratory-based and involved non-interactive audiences. However, researchers experienced considerable difficulty in achieving experimental control over the many variables operating; for example, personality, nature and difficulty of the task, perception of the 'threat' or the 'challenge' of the situation, etc. Other research examined interactive audience effects in more ecologically valid field settings, and studied factors such as home advantage[65], audience size[66] and spectator mood.[67] However, due largely to methodological problems, social facilitation research has become unfashionable and more recent work has turned towards examining some of the specific variables which are thought to underlie social facilitation effects.

Competitive state anxiety and performance

Research into competitive state anxiety may be divided into three general areas: the nature and temporal patterning of the competitive state anxiety response; the antecedents or precursors of anxiety; and the relationship between anxiety and performance.

Nature and temporal patterning of the state anxiety response

The competitive state anxiety concept itself has formed the focus of much recent research effort, and opinion has generally fallen into line with the clinical and test anxiety literature in which the anxiety response has been separated into cognitive and somatic components.[68,69] The current multidimensional conceptualization of competitive state anxiety stems largely from the work of Martens *et al.*[70] and their development of the Competitive State Anxiety Inventory-2 (CSAI-2), a competition-specific questionnaire which measures cognitive and somatic anxiety components, together with self-confidence. The inclusion of anxiety and self-confidence as independent scales is interesting since they were largely viewed as representing opposite ends of the same continuum in earlier literature. Borkovec,[71] for example, described self-confidence as simply an epi-phenomenon resulting from a lack of anxiety. Conversely, Bandura[72] proposed that anxiety was an epi-phenomenon resulting from a lack of self-confidence, or self-efficacy. However, factor analysis of Martens *et al.*'s CSAI-2 revealed orthogonal anxiety and self-confidence factors which suggests that they should be regarded as being independent rather than bipolar in nature.

The CSAI-2 has been employed to examine the precompetition temporal patterning of its three components during the time leading up to competition. The findings have been fairly consistent in showing that cognitive anxiety remains relatively stable prior to competition; somatic anxiety, on the other hand, tends to increase rapidly close to the start of the event. Self-confidence is generally less consistent during the precompetition period, but the theoretical predictions are that neither cognitive anxiety nor self-confidence are likely to change unless expectations of success change during this period. Recent research findings have shown, however, that the patterning of the multidimensional competitive state anxiety components may differ as a function of individual difference variables, including skill level,[70] type of sport,[70,73] and sex.[74]

Whilst the CSAI-2 has facilitated the development of knowledge about the competitive state anxiety response, it is, like many other state anxiety measures, based on a somewhat limited conceptualization of the anxiety response in that it measures only the intensity of the symptoms and not what has been referred to as 'direction', in terms of how the symptoms are interpreted along a 'facilitative–debilitative to performance' continuum.[75,76] Anxiety has been largely viewed as negative and detrimental to performance, particularly in the North American sport psychology literature. However, as Mahoney and Avener's findings from gymnastics indicated,[77] anxiety can also be seen as a stimulant to enhanced performance. More recent findings have supported this notion.[78-80] The ways in which sports performers perceive their competitive state anxiety responses is clearly an area that warrants further research.

Antecedents of competitive state anxiety

It has been proposed that identification of the precursors of competitive state anxiety may provide a valuable means of determining effective methods for achieving optimal performance states.[81] Whilst some research has examined the predictors of unidimensional anxiety (see ref. 82), relatively little research has been carried out in the context of multidimensional anxiety. The antecedents of cognitive anxiety and self-confidence are hypothesized to be those factors in the environment which are related to the athlete's expectations of success, including perception of one's own and opponent's ability. Cues which elicit elevated somatic anxiety, on the other hand, are thought to be non-evaluative, of shorter duration, and consist mainly of conditioned responses to stimuli, such as changing-room preparation and precompetition warm-up routines.[70,81] Findings reported by Jones et al., from a sample of good distance runners,[83] suggested that cognitive anxiety and self-confidence do share some common antecedents which contribute to performance expectations, but that there are also factors which may be unique to each. Furthermore, findings reported by Jones et al. suggest that the antecedents of cognitive anxiety and self-confidence may differ between male and female sports performers.[84]

Anxiety–performance relationship

The general lack of precise definitions of and, consequently, distinctions between key concepts such as arousal and anxiety has meant that precise identification of the relationship between anxiety and performance has proved elusive. Many researchers have debated the merits of Drive Theory and the Inverted-U Hypothesis, but both of these approaches have been based on the assumption that the anxiety–performance relationship can be explained as a function of changes in a very general arousal system. Despite equivocal research findings and problems associated with using stress, arousal, and anxiety almost interchangably in this context, the Inverted-U Hypothesis continues to form the focal point of discussions on anxiety and performance in many sport psychology textbooks. However, recent papers by Neiss[85] and Jones and Hardy[86] have raised numerous objections to the validity of the assumptions underlying the Inverted-U Hypothesis, particularly when viewed in the context of sports performance.

The adoption of a multidimensional approach to anxiety has been an encouraging and important step forward in the empirical examination of the anxiety–performance relationship in sport psychology (see refs 70 and 87 for reviews) as it has also meant the adoption of much more precise definitions and terminology. This has, in turn, led to an increasing number of studies which have attempted to examine the relationship between the specific components of the competitive state anxiety response and sports performance.[81,88,89] Burton,[88] for example, carried out a study on swimmers and found the following results: cognitive anxiety was related to performance in the form of a negative linear trend, with performance deteriorating as cognitive anxiety increased; somatic anxiety was related to performance by a quadratic trend, thus supporting Gould et al.'s earlier finding,[89] and suggesting the existence of an inverted U-shaped curve although not in terms of a general, undifferentiated arousal system; self-confidence was related to performance by a positive linear trend.

Some more recent work has moved away from examining global sports performance and has adopted Hockey and Hamilton's[90] 'broad band' approach to examine the effects of anxiety on different subcomponents of performance, such as working memory and anaerobic output.[91] What is becoming increasingly clear from this line of research is that competitive state anxiety does not necessarily impair performance and can, in some circumstances, enhance it.

The application to sport of models developed within the 'mainstream' psychological literature, such as Apter's Reversal Theory[92] (see also ref. 93), Sanders' model of stress and performance,[94] and Humphreys and Revelle's model of personality, motivation, and performance[95] (see also ref. 96), has also proved encouraging for advancing our knowledge of the competitive anxiety–performance relationship. Furthermore, Hardy and Fazey's Catastrophe Model[97] of the relationship between competitive state anxiety and sports performance represents a behavioural application of Zeeman's mathematically based Catastrophe Theory[98] (see ref. 99 for a review). Hardy and Fazey's proposals stem from a dissatisfaction with the multidimensional anxiety theory's attempt to explain the anxiety–performance relationship by means of two main effects (namely separate effects of cognitive and somatic anxiety). They argue, instead, that performance effects are determined by a complex interaction between cognitive anxiety and physiological arousal. Their model has gained some empirical support.[100,101]

Finally, Gould and Krane[102] have commented on the almost over-reliance on quantitative information in the pursuit of an understanding of the anxiety–performance relationship. They advocated the use of in-depth interviews with athletes in conjunction with questionnaires to gain a broader perspective of their experiences. Recent studies which have employed this type of methodology have unearthed some interesting findings.[103,104] Certainly, this approach has been lacking and is worthy of greater research attention.

Current situation

Recent research into stress and performance within the realms of sport psychology has resulted in some encouraging conceptual and methodological advances. Current issues include: measuring both the 'intensity' and the 'direction' of competitive state anxiety symptoms, and examining their relationships with performance; identifying the antecedents of anxiety as a function of individual difference variables such as sex and sport; investigating the complex interaction between cognitive anxiety and somatic anxiety, and in particular testing the predictions of Hardy and Fazey's Catastrophe Model;[97] adopting both quantitative and qualitative research methodologies in order to gain a clearer picture of the relationship between stress and performance in sport. Finally, Jones[105] has argued that researchers in this area have been too preoccupied with examining the influence of anxiety in sport and that relatively little is known about how other emotions are related to performance.

Individual differences

The study of individual differences has been popular in sport psychology research. This section considers four individual difference variables which have formed the focus of much of this research attention; these are, personality, sex and gender, cognitive style, and skill level.

Personality

The area of personality in sport has been the subject of considerable interest since the late 1960s when it represented the first area of sport psychology to receive systematic research attention.[106] Personality research has centred largely around the person/situation debate, focusing on whether traits or environmental factors are the primary determinants of behaviour. Much of the early work adopted the trait approach (see, for example, ref. 107), in which traits were viewed as being stable across both time and situations. Mischel,[108] however, later argued that environmental factors were better predictors of behaviour. Current thinking favours an approach in which person and situation factors interact (see, for example, ref. 109). The person–situation debate has continued to be very evident in the sport psychology literature (see, for example, ref. 110), although as early as 1975, Martens[111] had concluded that the interactional approach was the one that should be favoured in future research.

Unfortunately, research in this area has been plagued by a number of problems, leading Bakker et al.[10] to observe that: '… in spite of the fact that no other topic in the field of sport psychology has received quite so much attention as the relationship between sport and personality, the findings are not particularly impressive' (p. 54). The reasons for this have been discussed at length by Martens[111] and Morgan,[112] and include: a generally atheoretical approach; poor sampling procedures; inappropriate instrumentation; and interpretive errors. Martens[111] reported that only 10 per cent of the empirical studies which he had reviewed involved any experimental manipulation, whilst 89 per cent were correlational in nature and lacking any inferences of causality.

However, in an examination of trends and issues that have emerged since 1975, Vealey[106] has portrayed a somewhat brighter picture of the situation: '… sport personality research in the last 14 years has become more theoretical and more balanced methodologically' (p. 226). In particular, the proportion of studies using correlational methods had decreased to 68 per cent, whilst the proportion using experimental methods had increased to 28 per cent of the studies examined. In addition, Vealey emphasized that significant advances had been made in the form of establishing theoretical bases in several areas, including anxiety, self-confidence, and motivation.

In the case of anxiety, for example, advances in the conceptualization of competitive trait anxiety and, in particular, the development of the Sport Competition Anxiety Test[113] have formed the basis of a considerable amount of research. Furthermore, Smith et al.[114] have recently developed a multidimensional measure of competitive trait anxiety, the Sport Anxiety Scale, thus keeping abreast with current developments in competitive state anxiety research (see section on Stress and performance). Other measures of personality which have recently been developed as a result of similar theoretical advances include measures of self-confidence (for example, the Trait Sport-Confidence Inventory[115]) and motivation (for example, the Sport Orientation Questionnaire[116]).

Sex and gender

Following the convention used by Deaux,[117] this section distinguishes between sex, based upon the biological distinction, and gender, which refers to the psychological characteristics associated with males and females. This appears to be an important distinction within the context of both mainstream and sport psychology.

The influential work of Maccoby and Jacklin[118] on sex differences showed males to be more aggressive and to have greater mathematical and spatial ability than females, whereas females have greater verbal ability. However, a meta-analysis by Hyde[119] showed that sex differences accounted for less than 5 per cent of the variance in mathematical and spatial ability. In a similar vein, Gill[120] has argued that sex differences are unlikely to be a powerful predictor of behaviour in sport, and that social psychological aspects of gender in sport are more valid predictors.

Gender differences in sport have generally been found in the areas of achievement orientations, achievement cognitions, and competitive anxiety. Gill[121] concluded that females seem to focus more on personal goals and standards which reflect a non-competitive achievement orientation, whereas males focus more on interpersonal comparisons and winning. Research findings have also demonstrated that females tend to score higher on competitive trait anxiety[113,121] and multidimensional competitive state anxiety than males.[84] Finally, Gill et al.[122] have proposed that competitive sport situations exaggerate gender differences in achievement cognitions, with females generally reporting less confidence and lower expectations of success than males. This is in line with Lenney's[123] assertions that these differences vary according to the task and situation, with gender differences being particularly evident in tasks perceived as masculine; sport has been generally considered a male domain,[124] a gendered cultural form that has been dominated by males and masculinity.[125]

The reference to 'masculinity' introduces an extension to gender research which has been relatively popular in recent years, namely gender role orientation. Gender role concerns the psychological traits of masculinity and femininity, which are not dependent at all on sex; males and females can possess both masculine and feminine traits. The plethora of gender role research which emerged in the 1970s was in part due to the development of the Bem Sex Role Inventory[126] and the Personality Attributes Questionnaire.[127] Although these measures have been used widely in sport psychology research, several criticisms have been levelled at them, limiting the usefulness of the research that they have generated (see ref. 120).

Cognitive style

Individual differences in sports performers' cognitive styles have attracted a notable amount of research interest. One of the most prominent cognitive style typologies was developed by Nideffer[128] in the context of attentional style. He proposed that attentional style exists along two dimensions: width (that is to say broad versus narrow) and direction (namely internal versus external), based upon which attentional focus was classified into four types: broad–external; broad–internal; narrow–external; narrow–internal. Nideffer's Test of Attentional and Interpersonal Style (TAIS)[128] was developed to measure individual differences in ability to use the various attentional styles and has proved popular in sport psychology research. However, Nideffer's typology makes no distinction between relevant and irrelevant information so that the validity of the TAIS is questionable. Furthermore, Van Schoyk and Grasha's[129], and Albrecht and Feltz's[130], findings showed that sport-specific measures of attentional style were more valid and reliable than the TAIS. Both of these studies also raised questions about the factor structure of Nideffer's model.

Landers[131] was very critical in his assessment of the worth of the TAIS in sport psychology research, advocating less reliance on questionnaire measures and greater emphasis on physiological and behavioural measures of attention in sport. Several studies have been carried out to examine physiological concomitants of attention in sport (for example ref. 132; see ref. 133 for a review). Behavioural measures of perception have also been used (for example ref. 134) and have proved equally encouraging.

Associative versus dissociative attentional strategies were identified as a cognitive style dimension which distinguished élite from non-élite marathon runners.[135] Specifically, élite runners were generally found to use associative strategies whereby their direction of attention was internalized towards the body's feedback signals, whilst non-élite runners tended to use dissociative strategies in which attention was externalized. It is likely, however, that runners, whether élite or non-élite, do not use solely one or the other but a combination of the two. In any case, subsequent research has shown that associative strategies are not necessarily superior.[136]

Skill level

In an area of study where skill level is clearly a crucial factor, it is not surprising that it has been the focus of considerable research interest. This research has mainly concentrated on differences between élite and non-élite sports performers which are evident across a broad range of areas. In the case of anxiety, for example, differences have been found in both the patterning and perceptions of anxiety. Élite performers have generally been found to experience their highest levels of anxiety prior to the event, whilst non-élite performers experience their highest levels during performance.[77,137] In addition to this apparent ability of élite performers to control anxiety during the crucial moments of competition, Mahoney and Avener[77] have also reported that élite gymnasts used their anxiety as a stimulant to better performance, whereas the less successful gymnasts aroused themselves into near panic states.

Other areas in which skill level differences are evident include imagery, attention, and perceptuomotor factors. Orlick and Partington[138] have reported that successful Olympians make greater use of imagery than their less successful counterparts. Mahoney and associates have also suggested that élite performers may make greater use of internal and kinaesthetic imagery as opposed to external imagery than non-élite performers. Élite performers have also been found to be superior on the following perceptuomotor factors: the ability to 'chunk' and recall elements of structured ball games (for example ref. 140); the use of advanced visual cues (for example ref. 141); and decision time and accuracy (for example ref. 140).

Current situation

Due to the large number of individual difference variables operating in sport, it has not been possible to consider all of them in this section. Research in those areas selected demonstrates that the situation is very complex and that there is still much to be learned. One of the major problems with the research which has been carried out is that the vast majority is descriptive. There is a clear need for the use of causal analyses in future research in this area.

Interpersonal relationships in sport

At least four different types of relationship can be identified which are of interest to sport psychologists. These are between coaches and their performers, between different performers in the same team, between performers and their parents, and between coaches and the parents of performers. Unfortunately, despite the obvious importance of the latter two relationships, very little empirical research has, as yet, been published in these areas.[142] Consequently, this review will focus strongly on the other two areas.

The coach as a leader

Following 'The Great Man' theory of leaders, early research attempted to identify personality differences between successful and less successful coaches. This research suffered from many of the same deficiencies as early trait personality research on sports performers,[111] not the least of which was that it ignored the potential influence of situational factors, and the performers who were being 'led', upon the leadership process.[143] More recent research has been based on a person-by-situation model of behaviour, and has been dominated by the work of Chelladurai. Chelladurai[144] presented a multidimensional model of leadership in sport that emphasized three factors: the personal characteristics of the leader; the group members' needs and desires; and the demands of the situation. The major prediction of the model was that performance and satisfaction are a positive function of the degree of congruence between three different aspects of leadership: the leader's actual behaviour, the leader behaviour preferred by the group, and the leader behaviour required by the situation. Furthermore, according to the model, these different leader behaviours are influenced by the antecedents of leader characteristics, the group members' characteristics, and situational characteristics.

In order to measure coaches' leadership behaviours, Chelladurai and Saleh[145] developed the Leadership Scale for Sports (LSS). This consists of five subscales which assess training and instruction behaviours, democratic behaviours, autocratic behaviours, social support behaviours, and rewarding behaviours (positive feedback). It is worth noting that three of these behaviours focus upon an end-product (training and instruction, social support, and reward), whilst the other two focus upon a process (the means by which decisions will be made). The LSS has now been used to examine the influence of several antecedents on preferred leader behaviour and satisfaction with actual leader behaviour. These have included gender differences,[146] experience,[147] task characteristics,[148,149] organizational variables,[143] and cultural differences.[150] The findings of these studies have been generally supportive of Chelladurai's multidimensional conceptualization of leadership behaviour in sport,[151] and have also shown that performers generally prefer coaching that emphasizes training and instruction, together with positive feedback. This latter finding replicates earlier results obtained with different paradigms.[152,153] Furthermore, some studies[146,147] have also shown that experienced performers prefer more social support than inexperienced performers, and that males prefer more social support than females. However, it is, as yet, unclear whether this latter finding is a true reflection of gender differences, or due to the fact that female athletes often train with a male coach.

The coach as a decision maker

Humanistic orientations towards participation in decision making[20] led to claims that coaches are generally autocratic and insensitive.[154] However, researchers in organizational psychology[155] have argued that participation is not always the most appropriate decision-making strategy for a leader or manager to use. In line with these arguments, Chelladurai and Haggerty[156] proposed a model of decision making that matched seven situational attributes of problems to one of three decision-making processes. The seven situational attributes were time pressure, quality requirements, the coach's knowledge, problem complexity, acceptance requirement, coach's power, and group integration; whilst the three decision-making processes were autocratic, participative, and delegative. Subsequent tests of this model indicated that the delegative style of decision making was not acceptable to performers of either gender.[157] However, a revised version of the original model which replaced the delegative style of decision making with varying degrees of autocratic and democratic decision making did receive support.[158] Other results which are of relevance to this model include findings that: autocratic decision-making processes are both preferred and more effective under conditions of external stress;[159] male athletes show a greater preference for autocratic decision making than female athletes;[136] and older, more experienced, athletes show a greater preference for autocratic decision making than younger, less experienced athletes.[147]

Group dynamics

Like much of the more recent competitive stress and performance literature, interest in group cohesion in sport developed out of research into social facilitation,[64] group motivation,[160] and the Ringelmann effect (later known as 'social loafing').[161] The term 'social loafing' refers to the reductions in effort that have been observed when a group of individuals work together on a task. These effects have been demonstrated across a wide range of tasks in both males and females, but appear to be alleviated by identifiability, the uniqueness of the individual's contribution to the group, group cohesion, and the personal meaning of the task. Nevertheless, social loafing has been shown to be a reliable phenomenon that exists even when tasks are personally meaningful.[162] The converse of social loafing has also been demonstrated,[160] with subjects demonstrating enhanced rather than diminished effort when working in groups.

These findings clearly require some sort of conceptual model in order to be understood. Carron[163] provided such a model which related personal, environmental, and leadership factors to team factors, group cohesion, and personal and group outcomes. Carron's model enables some of the rather equivocal findings regarding team effects upon performance to be tentatively explained.[120] Much of the early literature on team cohesion had utilized the Team Cohesiveness Questionnaire[164] which contains items that directly rate the individual's attraction to the group, and items that tap interpersonal attraction between individuals. Most of the studies that have demonstrated negative effects for team cohesion on performance have used an interpersonal measure of cohesion, whilst those producing positive effects have used a direct measure of attraction to group.[120]

Other important factors in Carron's model[163] include the interactive nature of the task, the compatibility of the group members, group norms regarding performance, team goals, and the crudeness and conceptual distance of the criterion measure of performance from the independent variables of interest.[120,165] Another area of interest is the circularity of the cohesion–performance relationship. Although the literature is replete with all the design problems that are implied by Carron's model, the findings generally suggest a stronger influence for performance upon cohesion than for cohesion upon performance.[165]

More recent research on team cohesion has viewed it as a multidimensional construct. Yukelson and associates developed the Multidimensional Sport Cohesion Instrument[166] for measuring cohesion in basketball teams. Factor analysis of the instrument yielded four factors: attraction to the group; valued roles; quality of teamwork; and unity of purpose. Similarly, Carron and associates developed the Group Environment Questionnaire[167] which evaluates attraction to group and integrated group activity along both task and social dimensions. The interested reader will be able to identify links between these two factor structures.

Several researchers have now used the Group Environment Questionnaire to demonstrate a relationship between team cohesion and adherence to physical activity,[168] group resistance to disruption,[169] collective efficacy,[170] and competitive state anxiety[171] in performers of different ability levels. Widmeyer et al.[172] have also examined the effects of group size (both in terms of action-unit size and total number of players on the team) upon group cohesion, enjoyment, and performance. Their results indicated that cohesion, enjoyment, and performance were all decreased in large groups, and suggested the possibility that these effects may be mediated by a lack of influence/responsibility felt by members of large teams, together with poor coordination of the team effort.

Aggression

Aggression has not proved to be an easy construct to define. The present authors will follow Silva's lead[173] and define it narrowly as overt behaviours which are intended to psychologically or physically injure another person or oneself. In using this definition, it is important to distinguish between hostile aggression where the primary goal of the action is to injure, and instrumental aggression where the behaviour is directed at the target for some means other than the injury itself. Instrumental aggression is often allowed by the rules of sport, whereas hostile aggression is generally prohibited. Finally, it is necessary to distinguish between aggression and assertiveness. Assertive behaviours are purposeful, goal-directed behaviours where there is no intention to harm.

At least three different types of aggression theory can be distinguished in the literature[120]: instinct theories; drive theories; and social learning theories. Instinct theories are usually based on territorial defence, and propose that aggressive energy builds up as a result of the 'territorial invasions' that naturally occur during social interactions. Drive theories argue that aggressive drives arise from the frustration that occurs as a result of any blocking of goal-directed behaviour. Social learning theories argue that aggression is a learned response that is acquired through direct reinforcement or observational learning. Instinct and drive theories are currently very unfashionable, largely because they predict that sport should have a cathartic effect upon aggression by providing a constructive outlet for naturally occurring aggressive energy or drive. Empirical research that has addressed this question has been distinctly equivocal.[120,174,175] However, it should be noted that Berkowitz, one of the most prominent researchers in the area, has proposed that learned and innate sources of aggression coexist.[176] Evidence in favour of the social learning theory position is much stronger both in terms of direct reinforcement and observational learning of aggression.[120] Bandura[8] has also argued that disinhibition and de-individuation of the target for aggression could be an important feature of the development of aggression. Eventually, the target of the aggression becomes so stripped of all favourable characteristics that any form of aggression appears to be perfectly justifiable.

Research on the antecedents of aggression also favours the influence of situational factors in the triggering of aggressive behaviours. Such factors include the norms and values of the sport, the coach's goal orientation, the period of the game, the stage of the season, and the state of the game.[10,177] Other factors that are thought to influence aggression include physical appearance,[178] experience,[179,180] and gender;[181] although the influence of gender has been disputed.[182] Unfortunately, research on the effects of aggression upon performance is somewhat confounded by the use of either non-experimental field study designs,[183] or provocation to manipulate aggression.[184] A considerable quantity of research has been performed by van der Brug's group on the situational factors that elicit aggression in spectators.[10] However, this research tends towards being sociological rather than psychological in nature, and will not be reviewed here.

Finally, Gill has presented a reasoned argument that sport is neither a 'good' nor a 'bad' influence upon moral development. It simply provides opportunities for moral judgement ('good' or 'bad') to be developed.[120] This hypothesis has been empirically explored by Bredemeier and associates who have shown that appropriately structured sport experience can indeed aid moral development.[185]

Current situation

It should be clear from the research that has just been reviewed that both Chelladurai's model of leadership behaviour in sport,[144] and Chelladurai and Haggerty's[156] model of decision-making styles in sport offer considerable promise for future research. Research on the latter model[158] has shown that situational factors account for approximately three times more of the variance in performers' preferred decision-making styles than individual differences in preferred styles. It has also suggested that performers may prefer democratic styles of decision making in less than 20 per cent of the situations which are commonly encountered in sport. As to whether these preferences result from social evolutionary processes or from considerations of performance effectiveness remains unclear. In the light of these findings, it is disappointing that several of the studies reviewed have examined rather global preferences and trends in coaches' leader behaviours, without really exploring the details of the situation-by-group member interaction across different situations that occur in sport. Future research should also explore the situational discrepancy hypothesis in terms of both group performance and performer satisfaction, as well as the necessity and sufficiency of Chelladurai and Haggerty's seven situational attributes.

The processes underlying group dynamics are necessarily complex; nevertheless, progress in this area was held up for a long time by the lack of a theoretical framework. The work which has been reviewed on Carron's conceptual model[163] therefore represents a fairly significant step forward. However, much remains to be learned about the group dynamics of sports teams, and Carron's is not the only conceptual model that has been proposed.[186] Having said all this, it can be at least tentatively concluded that groups which are not too large and have clearly defined team goals, but which recognize and value the individual contributions made by their members, are most likely to maximize their potential.

Psychological research into aggression proved difficult to review because, although there is a considerable body of research on the topic, much of it seems to sit on the sociology side of the social psychology 'fence'. From psychological research by Berkowitz[176] and Bandura[8] it is known that aggressive behaviours can be acquired by observation and direct reinforcement, but little is known about the psychological processes that trigger these behaviours. It is also known that watching sport does not have a cathartic effect by releasing aggressive urges in spectators. However, despite claims to the contrary,[120] the available literature does not indicate that participation in sport has no cathartic effect upon performers. It merely indicates that a cathartic effect has not been reliably demonstrated. Considering that interventions generally exert their greatest effects upon 'extreme' populations, together with the ethical problems that would have to be overcome to design an experiment to test the catharsis hypothesis in, for example, men who regularly abuse their wives, this inability of the empirical literature to demonstrate a cathartic effect is perhaps unsurprising. Finally, on a rather positive note, the recent work of Bredemeier et al.[185] exploring the potential of appropriately structured sport environments for moral development appears most promising.

Exercise psychology

The role that exercise plays in the prevention of physical health problems has long been recognized by both health professionals and scientists. A significant development in this area during the last decade has been the recognition that exercise also has a potentially very important role to play in both the prevention and treatment of mental health problems. This development, which has largely been associated with the recent growth in health psychology and broadening of research interests in the sport and exercise sciences, has led to the emergence of 'exercise psychology'.[187] The increasing prominence of exercise psychology during the 1980s is reflected in the publication of texts on such specialized topics as exercise and mental health[188] and exercise adherence.[189] A significant move in sport psychology was that in 1988 the flagship journal of sport psychology in North America, *The Journal of Sport Psychology*, was re-named *The Journal of Sport and Exercise Psychology*. The two major areas of research which have emerged in exercise psychology are exercise and mental health, and exercise motivation.

Exercise and mental health

Despite general assertions in the literature that exercise and mental health are positively related in both clinical and non-clinical populations, there is a significant lack of evidence to suggest that this relationship is anything more than associative. The dearth of evidence to imply causality is largely due to problems in research methodology, and the lack of longitudinal studies in particular.[190,191]

None the less, Biddle and Fox[187] have identified three areas in which the link between exercise and mental health appears to be relatively robust: a reduction in anxiety[192,193] and depression;[194] an enhancement of self-esteem,[195] particularly in the subdomain of physical self-esteem;[187] and improved reactivity to stress (see ref. 196 for a meta-analytical review). All of the benefits discussed are related predominantly to aerobic exercise, the most popular exercise activities being running (see, for example, ref. 197) and swimming (see, for example, ref. 198).

In an attempt to draw together research findings and to unravel specific details of the relationship between exercise and mental health, the American National Institute of Mental Health produced a series of consensus statements of the state of current knowledge and future research needs (see ref. 188). These were summarized by Biddle and Fox[187] as follows.

Current knowledge

1. Exercise is associated with reduced state anxiety.

2. Exercise has been associated with a decreased level of mild to moderate depression.

3. Long-term exercise is usually associated with reductions in traits such as neuroticism and anxiety.

4. Exercise may be an adjunct to the professional treatment of severe depression.

5. Exercise results in the reduction of various stress indices.

6. Exercise has beneficial emotional effects across all ages and in both sexes.

Research questions

1. What is the role of exercise in primary prevention?

2. What is the effect of exercise on the rehabilitation of people with physical and mental disorders?

3. What are the mechanisms that mediate the effects of exercise on stress?

4. What are the effects of exercise on the stress reactivity of different groups, such as those differing by age, sex, socioeconomic status, and personality?

5. What are the optimal exercise doses required to produce effective responses to mental stress?

6. What is the effect of exercise compared with other interventions?

7. What are the effects of exercise on the mental health of children?

8. What are the mechanisms underlying exercise effects?

The identification of the mechanisms underlying the relationship between exercise and mental health is clearly crucial to understanding the specific details of the relationship. Recent proposals in this context include muscle relaxation, thermogenesis effects and brainwave pattern change,[199,200] release of endogenous opiates,[201] and enhancement of self-esteem[202] and mastery (see ref. 187).

A question of primary concern, of course, relates to the comparison of the effect of exercise with other interventions. In particular, there is a need to know whether exercise provides anything more than a 'time-out'.[203] Whilst several researchers (see, for example, refs 204, 205) have compared exercise with other types of intervention, the findings are somewhat equivocal, leading Biddle[206] to state:

'... despite impressive survey data (Stephens, 1988)[207], and theoretically sound speculation on the mechanisms of mental health effects from exercise (Dishman, 1985[208], 1986[209]; Morgan and O'Connor, 1988[190]), there remains some doubt about the uniqueness of exercise effects and whether other interventions might not be equally effective. The challenge is there ....' (p. 6).

Finally, it should be emphasized that exercise may not always be associated with mental health benefits and can sometimes have negative psychological effects.[191] Steinberg et al.[210] cited evidence which they interpreted as suggesting that regular physical exercise which becomes compulsive can be viewed as a form of dependence or addiction similar to addiction to opiates and other drugs.[211] For example, Morris et al.[212] found that male runners deprived of running for 2 weeks produced withdrawal syndrome, although in a form milder than one would expect from opiate withdrawal. This is clearly a cause for concern amongst exercise psychologists and requires extensive systematic investigation. However, as has already been stated in the section on Motivation, it is important that future research clearly defines addiction in such a way as to distinguish between commitment and addiction;[213] for example, mothers who are separated from their children frequently demonstrate considerable distress, but does this mean that they are addicted to them?

Exercise motivation

Despite the now wide acceptance of the mental health benefits of exercise, surveys have suggested that a very disappointing proportion of the population (probably no more than 50 per cent) are involved in any significant amount of exercise (see, for example, ref. 214). Biddle and Fox[187] further noted that a still smaller proportion are likely to undertake an exercise programme or schedule which will significantly enhance health (it should be noted here that the intensity, frequency, and duration of exercise required to produce health benefits remains an area for debate). This situation is exacerbated still further by the fact that relatively few of those who do begin an exercise programme will persist for very long. In fact, the rapidly expanding amount of research examining adherence to exercise seems to have firmly established that 50 per cent of those who enrol in a supervised exercise programme can be expected to drop out in the first 3 to 6 months.[215,216] Interestingly, those people who would benefit most from exercise (such as the obese) tend to be the very people who drop out.[217]

Early research which attempted to identify factors important in decisions to initiate and adhere to exercise suffered from the lack of a theoretical underpinning. More recently, however, researchers have become increasingly 'theoretically-driven', examining models based upon beliefs, attitudes, and self-perceptions.[187] The Health Belief Model[218] together with Fishbein and Ajzen's theory of reasoned action[219] have formed the basis of research into beliefs and attitudes, whilst self-esteem, attribution theory, locus of control, and self-efficacy theory have been amongst the self-perception theories that have been examined.[220] Bandura's social cognitive theory[221] is also becoming increasingly prominent, with the most studied mechanism within the theory being self-efficacy. In fact, studies by Dzewaltowski[222] and Dzewaltowski et al.[223] showed social cognitive theory (self-perception based) to be a better predictor of exercise behaviour than the theory of reasoned action (beliefs and attitudes based).

The different approaches to exercise motivation reflect the general lack of consensus among researchers over the definition of motivation.[224] Recently, emphasis has been placed on defining the concept of motivation itself, with Duda[225] proposing a broad-based definition involving three components: direction; intensity; and persistence. Clearly, exercise motivation will continue to provide a fertile area for research in the foreseeable future. However, one issue which will have to be addressed is the definition of adherers and drop-outs as this has also been a source of inconsistency in studies to date.

Current situation

Exercise psychology is clearly an area of massive growth and development. It is beyond the scope of this chapter to discuss the many applications of exercise psychology, other than to note that it has proved to be of great interest and benefit in rehabilitation (see, for example, ref. 226), corporate (for example ref. 227), therapeutic (for example ref. 194), and educational (for example ref. 228) settings. However, many issues remain to be addressed, including: the examination of causal relationships between exercise and mental health; the examination of factors affecting exercise adherence; antecedent factors influencing exercise commitment and dependence; the efficacy of exercise versus other forms of therapeutic intervention; and the intensity, frequency, and duration of exercise required for mental health benefits. Clearly, well-designed longitudinal studies are required to address such issues. Finally, while the vast majority of the literature and research findings in this area have emanated from North America, the generalization of this work to other populations and cultures has yet to be determined.

Mental training

The last 10 years has seen an increasing acceptance of mental training as an integral part of the preparation for peak performance, so that sport psychologists working alongside national squads and teams have now become the norm rather than the exception. Research on peak performance and ideal performance states is still in its infancy; however, retrospective studies of peak performance[229] suggest that a number of factors may contribute to such performances. These include intentionality on the part of the performer, clear focus upon the task, total absorption in the task, effortless concentration, feelings of the body performing on its own without fatigue, loss of fear, and certainty of success. Similarly, research into the differences between élite and non-élite performers[77,138,139] has identified that élite performers have clear daily goals, less anxiety, greater confidence, higher levels of motivation, and superior attention control strategies than their less successful colleagues.

Following Vealey,[230] the present authors will make a distinction between advanced psychological skills, such as anxiety control, and basic psychological skills such as goal-setting, imagery, physical relaxation, and self-talk. However, unlike Vealey,[230] we do not view basic psychological skills as simply methods. Rather, we will view them as psychological skills in their own right. The first part of the section will discuss basic psychological skills, and then the rest of the section will focus upon their use and application in the development of anxiety control, activation control, self-confidence, motivation, and attention control.

Basic psychological skills

Goal-setting

Much of the empirical literature on goal-setting has been provided by organizational psychology. It has also been claimed that many of these findings should generalize to sport settings.[231] However, Beggs[232] has quite rightly pointed out that there are a number of important differences between occupational organizations and sport which may well impede generalizations. Nevertheless, following an extensive review of the relevant literature, Beggs concluded that goal-setting was potentially a valuable tool for athletes and coaches. The available literature suggests that a number of factors need to be controlled if goal-setting is to exert such a beneficial influence upon performance.[231-234] Essentially, these are that goals must identify specific targets that lie largely within the performer's own control, that the performer is committed to, and that the performer perceives to be realistic and worthwhile. Furthermore, long-term goals should be broken down into short-term goals, and positive feedback must be available to the performer for the goal-setting process to work.

At least three different types of goal can be identified in the literature.[233,235] Outcome goals focus upon the outcomes of particular events and usually (but not always) involve social comparisons of some sort; for example, finishing a race in seventh place. Performance goals specify an end-product of performance that will be achieved by the performer relatively independently of other performers; for example, running a 5-minute mile. Finally, process-oriented goals specify the processes in which the performer will engage in order to perform at an optimal level; for example, maintaining perceived exertion at a rating of 14 for 1 mile. Whilst outcome goals may possess great motivational value for performers in the short term, Roberts[11] and others have argued that, ultimately, such goals are likely to lead performers to 'drop out' from sport. Burton[233] has also shown that outcome goals are associated with higher levels of competitive state anxiety than performance goals. Consequently, sport performers are usually encouraged to set performance, rather than outcome, goals for their performances. Little research has so far been performed on process-oriented goals, but the available data[236,237] suggest that they may have benefits over and above performance goals in terms of limiting competitive state anxiety and maximizing performance in sport.

Imagery

Imagery can be defined as a symbolic sensory experience that may occur in any sensory mode. However, the visual, kinaesthetic, and auditory modes seem likely to be the most relevant to sport. The majority of research that has examined the use of imagery in sports settings has utilized a learning paradigm. The consensus of this research is that mental practice of a motor task is certainly better than no practice at all.[238] A smaller number of studies have investigated the immediate effects of (multimodal) imagery upon performance, either in conjunction with relaxation,[239] or without it.[240] Again, the consensus of these studies is that imagery can exert a beneficial effect upon performance. It has also been suggested that imagery can be used to initiate relaxation,[68] and enhance self-confidence.[72,241] However, to date, direct empirical support for these suggestions is limited.[242,243]

Traditionally, several theories have been called upon to explain the effects of mental rehearsal upon motor performance, including symbolic learning theory, psychoneuromuscular theory, and the activation set hypothesis.[226] However, all these theories have been extensively criticized on both conceptual and empirical grounds.[10,238,240,244,245] Furthermore, following an excellent critique of imagery research in sport psychology, Murphy[244] concluded that earlier theorizing on imagery effects had been greatly hampered by its preoccupation with the effects of mental rehearsal upon motor performance. He argued that theories were required which acknowledged the importance of psychophysiology in the imagery process and the meaning of the image for the individual.[246,247]

Physical relaxation

Physical relaxation has long been used as a means of anxiety control, often in the form of progressive muscular relaxation[248] or one of its derivatives.[249,250] Furthermore, physical relaxation is also included as a part of most stress-management programmes,[251-253] and has been readily adapted to mental training in sports settings.[235,254] Whilst there is relatively little literature that shows a direct effect for relaxation upon sports performance, there is a considerable literature that demonstrates the anxiety-reducing properties of relaxation and the efficacy of cognitive-behavioural strategies involving relaxation, imagery, and positive self-talk (for reviews, see refs 4,68,255).

A number of researchers have examined the relationship between relaxation and imagery.[239,256-258] Although the results of these investigations are equivocal, it is widely accepted that relaxation enhances imagery and imagery can be used to relax. However, Weinberg et al.[258] interpreted their data as suggesting that the ideal activation state for mentally rehearsing a task depends upon the nature of the task. Whatever the case, relaxation can be regarded as one of the basic psychological skills that are involved in more complex skills such as anxiety and attention control.

Self-talk

Several researchers have shown that thought content and self-statements are important predictors of sports success (for a review, see ref. 13). The precise reasons for this relationship are not known, although it seems likely that self-confidence[72] and anxiety control[252,259] are at least partially involved. Furthermore, despite the strong emphasis that mental training programmes often place upon the development of 'appropriate' self-talk,[260] relatively few controlled studies have been performed that would enable any sort of empirically based operationalization of the word 'appropriate' to be attempted. However, it is known that positive self-talk has a beneficial effect upon performance;[261] that thought-stopping techniques can be used to modify negative self-statements;[262] that self-statements can be used to trigger desired actions more effectively;[263] and that self-statements can be used to provide self-reward.[7] It is also thought that self-statements can be used to increase effort,[260] mod-

ify mood,[235] and control attention[264] (see also the earlier discussion of process-oriented goals).

Use and application of basic psychological skills

Anxiety control

As indicated earlier, the state anxiety response is currently conceptualized to have at least two components: cognitive anxiety (worry); and somatic anxiety (perceptions of physiological arousal). Traditionally, these different modes of anxiety were thought to be optimally controlled by matching relaxation strategies to the response system in which the anxiety response principally occurred.[68] For example, meditation and imagery-based strategies might be used to control cognitive anxiety, whilst progressive muscular relaxation might be used to control somatic anxiety.[265] However, more recent research has suggested that, in practice, the different types of anxiety rarely occur in total isolation,[61] and that some sort of multimodal stress-management strategy is likely to be necessary.[3]

Most multimodal stress-management programmes currently employed in sports settings are derivatives of Meichenbaum's stress inoculation training,[252] or Smith's[253] stress-management training. Programmes are usually characterized by helping performers learn how to use positive self-statements and physical relaxation when they are confronting a problem, imagery to rehearse their coping strategy, and process-oriented goals to enable them to reward themselves for successfully engaging in the coping process regardless of the outcome of their coping efforts.[4] The available empirical literature[3] suggests that such multimodal stress-management strategies are generally effective in controlling anxiety, but are perhaps not quite so effective at enhancing performance under stressful conditions. There are a number of theoretical reasons why this might be, most of which revolve around the question of whether or not high states of physiological arousal are beneficial to performance.[3,93,100]

Activation control

This aspect of psychological preparation is not generally well understood. In order to consider more fully the issue of optimal physiological arousal, it is necessary to distinguish between activation and physiological arousal. The work of Pribram and McGuinness[266] suggests that physiological arousal is best viewed as a temporary response to any input to the organism. Its primary purpose is to energize the perceptual processes. Conversely, activation is best viewed as a preparatory readiness to respond, which includes the preparation of a motor response. Pribram and McGuinness[266] also present evidence that the arousal and activation functions are the responsibilities of different neural networks of the brain. The implications of this line of research for mental training are important, since it suggests that increases in general physiological arousal are likely to be beneficial to performance only to the extent that such increases assist the performer to obtain the desired activation pattern. For some tasks, therefore, 'psyching up' strategies will be effective, whilst for others they will be ineffective.[258,267] Furthermore, the likelihood of such activation strategies being successful will almost certainly depend upon their precise content, a fact that does not always seem to have been appreciated by sport psychologists or performers. Individual differences in cognitive style may also be an important variable to consider in determining an appropriate activation strategy. Consequently, mental training programmes usually include strategies based on self-talk and imagery which performers can adapt to meet their own personal needs.[3]

Self-confidence

Self-confidence has been thought to be an important influence on performance for a number of years,[72,268] and more recent research has confirmed this importance.[88,139] Research suggests that this relationship is cyclical. Confident performers set more difficult goals which they persist at until they have achieved them, thereby gaining feelings of competence and increased self-confidence.[269] Bandura's theory of self-efficacy[72] (situationally specific self-confidence) has received considerable support in sport and other settings.[13,115,221] Essentially, the theory predicts that the strongest influence upon self-efficacy is previous experience of success, followed by vicarious experience, verbal persuasion, and physiological arousal in that order. Consequently, most mental training which is focused on enhancing self-confidence teaches performers to:

(1) break down long-term goals into short-term goals which are within their control so as to maximize their experience of success;

(2) regularly mentally rehearse succeeding at their goals so as to maximize the vicarious experience of success;

(3) use positive self-talk to encourage themselves and reinforce their feelings of self-confidence.

Motivation

Most serious athletes seem to be naturally highly motivated towards their sport. However, extremely high levels of motivation may be necessary to produce the consistently high-quality training sessions that are essential for success in some sports.[13,138,139] Furthermore, maintaining motivation throughout the duration of a long season, during periods of injury, or following setbacks to the training programme may severely tax the motivational skills of even the most élite performers. One of the major reasons for this is probably best explained by Deci and Ryan's cognitive evaluation theory.[7]

According to cognitive evaluation theory, human beings have an innate need to feel competent and self-determining. In accordance with these needs athletes commit themselves to difficult and demanding goals, the achievement of which will lead to enhanced feelings of competence and greater intrinsic motivation towards their sport. Consequently, any disruption to the achievement of these goals is highly likely to lead to reductions in motivation by a reversal of this cycle. It is also worth noting the involvement of self-confidence in this motivational cycle. Greater self-confidence means that athletes are likely to set and achieve more difficult goals,[221,269] which then increase feelings of self-competence and intrinsic motivation. In view of these findings, mental training for motivation often focuses upon encouraging performers to set goals that are within their control in order to increase the likelihood of success, and upon attributional retraining to encourage performers to attribute their failures and setbacks to external factors or to unstable internal factors.[13,24,31,270] Positive self-talk and self-reward are clearly also important techniques to develop.

Finally, a cautionary word is in order regarding the role of goals in the motivational process. As Beggs[232] has pointed out, goals are something of a 'double edged sword' in sport, since they can themselves become a source of additional stress and anxiety if performers do not adjust them when circumstances change. Anecdotal evidence suggests that this can present a serious problem for committed athletes. One implication of this seems to be that athletes should be taught how to set process-oriented goals that focus on emotional control as well as performance goals that focus upon the end-product of successful performance. They should also be taught how to regularly evaluate their goals and be flexible enough to adjust them when appropriate without losing their commitment to their goals.[235,271] Having said all this, very little empirical research[236] has directly addressed these questions.

Attention control

The need for totally focused concentration is frequently cited by athletes as one of the primary requirements of high-level performance.[13,59] However, the means by which such control of attention might be achieved are far from well understood. Attention has been conceptualized by empirical researchers in a number of different ways: in terms of single versus multiple resources;[272] in terms of scanning, focus, and selectivity;[273] and in terms of breadth and direction.[128] However, the research that has been generated by these conceptualizations is no more than suggestive as regards the control of attention.[13] In practice, desensitization to the competition environment, via simulation training and heavy overlearning, is thought to be a fundamental requirement.[59] Both association and dissociation strategies have been shown to be of potential benefit to performance,[274,275] and some sort of dissociation from stressful stimuli is a common part of many stress-management training programmes.[254] Élite athletes report using process-oriented goals and detailed, well-rehearsed, competition plans as part of their attention control strategies.[13,59,133,138] However, there is also counter-evidence[13] which suggests that process-oriented goals could lead to a breakdown in performance because they encourage performers to try and consciously control actions that would be much better performed automatically.

Current situation

Mental training has become established as an important aspect of sport psychology. Furthermore, there is evidence that mental training can be an effective means of enhancing competitive performance.[13] However, empirical research into the optimal content of mental training programmes is still in its infancy. In particular, there is an urgent need for research on: the means by which attention can be controlled and concentration enhanced; the precise role of physiological arousal and activation in the performance of different sports tasks; the means by which activation states can be modified in a controlled fashion if this is appropriate; the use of goal-setting with complex tasks in sports settings; and the role of process-oriented goals in stress management and attention control. Furthermore, in recent years a number of distance-learning, mental training packages have been published which purport to enhance athletes' mental skills. Most of these packages consist of either a book, or a book plus audio cassette tapes. There is a need to evaluate the effectiveness of these packages, when used both with and without tutorial support, and also a need to identify those factors that influence adherence to mental training programmes generally.[276]

Conclusions

This chapter has reviewed our current state of knowledge in six areas of sport psychology: motivation; stress and performance; individual differences; interpersonal relationships; exercise psychology; and mental training. As indicated in the introduction to the chapter, it is perhaps inevitable that some important topics have been omitted or only very briefly considered; for example, some would no doubt argue that the psychology of children in sport and the female athlete should have received more prominent positions in the review. Nevertheless, the authors feel that this remains a fairly broad, if not an all-embracing, review of current activity in sport psychology.

At the end of each section, a number of important issues and research questions have been identified. Many of these issues and questions are quite fundamental, and the consequences of their investigation are likely to be far-reaching. It should be clear from all this that the current rate of development in sport psychology, at both a professional and an academic level, is very rapid indeed. Furthermore, this progress looks set to continue until at least the end of this century.

References

1. Triplett N. Dynamogenic factors in pacemaking and competition. *American Journal of Psychology* 1897; **9**: 507–33.
2. Griffith CR. *Psychology of athletics.* New York: Scribners, 1928.
3. Burton D. Multimodal stress management in sport: current status and future directions. In: Jones JG, Hardy L, eds. *Stress and performance in sport.* Chichester: John Wiley, 1990: 171–201.
4. Mace R. Cognitive behavioural interventions in sport. In: Jones JG, Hardy L, eds. *Stress and performance in sport.* Chichester: John Wiley, 1990: 203–30.
5. Straub WF, Williams JM. Cognitive sport psychology: historical, contemporary and future issues. In: Straub WF, Williams JM, eds. *Cognitive sport psychology.* Lansing, New York: Sport Science Associates, 1984: 3–10.
6. Straub WF, Williams JM (eds). *Cognitive sport psychology.* Lansing, New York: Sport Science Associates, 1984.
7. Deci EL, Ryan RM. *Intrinsic motivation and self-determination in human behavior.* New York: Plenum Press, 1985.
8. Bandura A. *Aggression, a social learning analysis.* Englewood Cliffs, NJ: Prentice-Hall, 1973.
9. Carron AV. *Motivation: implications for coaching and teaching.* London, Ontario: Sport Dynamics, 1984.
10. Bakker FC, Whiting HTA, van der Brug H. *Sport psychology: concepts and applications.* Chichester: John Wiley, 1990.
11. Roberts GC. The growing child and the perceptions of competitive stress in sport. In: Gleeson G, ed. *The growing child in competitive sport.* London: Hodder and Stoughton, 1986: 130–44.
12. Whitehead J. Achievement goals and drop-out in youth sports. In Gleeson G, ed. *The Growing Child in competitive Sport.* London: Hodder and Stoughton, 1986: 240–247.
13. Hardy L, Jones G, Gould D. Understanding *Psychological preparation for sport: theory and practice of elite performers.* Chichester: John Wiley, 1996.
14. Robinson DW. Stress seeking: Selected behavioral characteristics of elite rock climbers. *Journal of Sport Psychology* 1985; 7: 400–4.
15. Carruthers M. *The western way of death.* London: Davis-Poynter, 1974.
16. Solomon RL. The opponent-process theory of acquired motivation. *American Psychologist* 1980; **35**: 691–712.
17. Lester JT. Wrestling with the self on Mount Everest. *Journal of Humanistic Psychology* 1983; **23**: 31–41.
18. Casady M. The tricky business of giving rewards. *Psychology Today* 1974; 8: 52.
19. De Charms R. *Personal causation: the internal affective determinants of behavior.* New York: Academic Press, 1968.
20. Deci EL. *Intrinsic motivation.* New York: Plenum Press, 1975.
21. Deci EL, Ryan RM. A motivational approach to self: Integration in personality. In Dienstbier R, ed. *Nebraska symposium on motivation: Vol. 38, Perspectives of motivation.* Lincoln, NA: University of Nebraska Press, 1991: 237–88.
22. McAuley E, Duncan T, Tammen VV. Psychometric properties of the Intrinsic Motivation Inventory in a competitive sport setting: A confirmatory factor analysis. *Research Quarterly for Exercise and Sport* 1989; **60**: 48–58.
23. Weiner B. *Theories of motivation: from mechanism to cognition.* Chicago: Rand-McNally, 1972.
24. Weiner B. A theory of motivation for some classroom experiences. *Journal of Educational Psychology* 1979; **71**: 3–25.
25. Abramson LY, Seligman MEP, Teasdale JD. Learned helplessness in humans: Critique and reformulation. *Journal of Abnormal Psychology* 1978; **87**: 49–74.
26. Biddle SJH. Attributions. In: Singer RN, Murphey M, Tennant LK, eds. *Handbook on research in sport psychology.* New York: Macmillan, 1993: 437–64.
27. Rejeski WJ, Brawley LR. Attribution theory in sport: Current status and new perspectives. *Journal of Sport Psychology* 1983; **5**: 77–99.
28. McAuley E, Duncan TE. Causal attributions and affective reactions to disconfirming outcomes in motor performance. *Journal of Sport and Exercise Psychology* 1989; **11**: 187–200.
29. McAuley E, Duncan TE. Cognitive appraisal and affective reactions following physical achievement outcomes. *Journal of Sport and Exercise Psychology* 1990; **12**: 415–26.
30. Carver CS, Scheier MF. Outcome expectancy, locus of attribution for expectancy, and self-directed attention as determinants of evaluations and performance. *Journal of Experimental Social Psychology* 1982; **18**: 184–200.
31. Dweck CS. Achievement. In: Lamb LE, ed. *Social and personality development.* New York: Holt, Rinehart and Winston, 1978: 114–30.
32. Scanlan TK, Passer MW. Self-serving biases in the competitive sport setting: An attributional dilemma. *Journal of Sport Psychology* 1980; **2**: 124–36.
33. Brawley LR. Attributions as social cognitions: Contemporary perspectives in sport. In: Straub WF, Williams JF, eds. *cognitive sport psychology.* Lansing, New York: Sport Science Associates, 1984: 212–30.
34. Bannister D, Fransella F. *Inquiring man: the theory of personal constructs.* London: Croom Helm, 1986.
35. Benson MJ. Attributional measurement techniques: Classification and comparison of approaches for measuring causal dimensions. *The Journal of Social Psychology* 1989; **129**: 307–23.
36. Butler RJ. Psychological preparation of Olympic boxers. In Kremer J, Crawford W, eds. *The psychology of sport: theory and practice.* Occasional Paper. Leicester: The British Psychological Society, 1989: 74–84.
37. Butler RJ, Hardy L. The performance profile: theory and application. *The Sport Psychologist* 1992; **6**: 253–64.
38. Veale MW. Exercise dependence. *British Journal of Addiction* 1987; **82**: 735–40.
39. Dishman RK, ed. *Exercise adherence: its impact on public health.* Champaign, IL: Human Kinetics, 1988.
40. Morgan WP, O'Connor PJ. Exercise and mental health. In: Dishman RK, ed. *Exercise adherence: its impact on public health.* Champaign, IL: Human Kinetics, 1988: 91–121.

41. Summers JJ, Hinton ER. Development of scales to measure participation in running. In: Unestahl LE, ed. *Contemporary sport psychology.* Orebro, Sweden: VEJE, 1986.

42. Heil, J. *Psychology of sport injury.* Champaign, IL: Human Kinetics, 1993.

43. Evans L, Hardy L. Sport injury and grief responses: A review. *Journal of Sport and Exercise Psychology* 1995; **17**: 227–45

44. Anderson CA, Williams JM. A model of stress and athletic injury: prediction and prevention. *Journal of Sport and Exercise Psychology* 1988; **10**: 721–86.

45. Wiese-Bjornstal DM, Smith AM. Counselling strategies for enhanced recovery of injured athletes within a team approach. In: Pargman D, ed. *Psychosocial bases of sport injuries.* Morgantown, WV: Fitness Information Technology, 1993: 149–82.

46. Ievleva L, Orlick T. Mental links to enhanced healing. *The Sport Psychologist* 1991; **5**: 25–40.

47. Wiese DM, Weiss MR, Yukelson DP. Sport psychology in the training room: A survey of athletic trainers. *The Sport Psychologist* 1991; **5**: 15–24.

48. Taylor A, May S. Threat and coping appraisal as determinants of compliance to sports injury rehabilitation: an application of protection motivation theory. *Journal of Sports Sciences* in press.

49. Morgan WP, Costill DL, Flynn MG, Raglin JS, O'Connor PJ. Mood disturbance following increased training in swimmers. *Medicine and Science in Sports and Exercise* 1988; **20**: 408–14.

50. Cockerill IM, Nevill AM, Lyons N. Modelling mood states in athletic performance. *Journal of Sports Sciences* 1991; **9**: 205–12.

51. Murphy SM, Fleck SJ, Dudley G, Callister R. Psychological and performance concomitants of increased volume training in elite athletes. *Journal of Applied Sport Psychology* 1990; **2**: 34–50.

52. Taylor AH, Daniel JV, Leith L, Burke RJ. Perceived stress, psychological burnout and paths to turnover intentions among sport officials, *Journal of Applied Sport Psychology* 1990; **2**: 84–97.

53. Kelley BC. A model of stress and burnout in collegiate coaches: Effects of gender and time of season. *Research Quarterly for Sport and Exercise* 1994; **65**: 48–58.

54. Coakley J. Burnout among adolescent athletes: A personal failure or a social problem? *Sociology of Sport Journal* 1992; **9**: 271–85.

55. Gould D, Tuffey S, Udry E, Loehr J. Burnout in junior elite tennis players: Qualitative content analysis and case studies. *The Sport Psychologist*, in press.

56. Gould D, Udry E, Tuffey S, Loehr J. Burnout in junior elite tennis players: A quantitative psychological assessment. *The Sport Psychologist*, in press.

57. Kelly HH, Michela JL. Attribution theory and research. *Annual Review of Psychology* 1980; **31**: 459–501.

58. Paikov VB. Means of restoration in the training of speed skaters. *Soviet Sports Review* 1985; **20**: 9–12.

59. Jones JG, Hardy L, eds. *Stress and performance in sport.* Chichester: John Wiley, 1990.

60. Hackfort D, Spielberger CD. *Anxiety in sports: an international perspective.* Washington: Hemisphere, 1989.

61. Martens R, Vealey RS, Burton D, eds. *Competitive anxiety in sport.* Champaign, IL: Human Kinetics, 1990.

62. Zajonc RB. Social facilitation. *Science* 1965; **149**: 269–74.

63. Cottrell NB, Wack NB, Sekerak GJ, Rittle RH. Social facilitation of dominant responses by the presence of an audience and the mere presence of others. *Journal of Personality and Social Psychology* 1968; **9**: 245–50.

64. Landers DM, McCullagh PD. Social facilitation of motor performacne. *Exercise and Sport Sciences Reviews* 1976; **4**: 125–62.

65. Baumeister RF. Choking under pressure: self-consciousness and paradoxical effects of incentives on skilful performance. *Journal of Personality and Social Psychology* 1984; **46**: 610–20.

66. Schwartz B, Barsky SF. The home advantage. *Social Forces* 1977; **55**: 641–61.

67. Thirer J, Rampey MS. Effects of abusive spectators' behavior on performance of home and visiting inter-collegiate basketball teams. *Perceptual and Motor Skills* 1979; **48**: 1047–54.

68. Davidson RJ, Schwartz GE. The psychobiology of relaxation and related states: a multiprocess theory. In: Mostofsky D, ed. *Behavioural control and modification of physiological activity.* Englewood Cliffs, NJ: Prentice-Hall, 1976: 399–442.

69. Liebert RM, Morris LW. Cognitive and emotional components of test anxiety: a distinction and some initial data. *Psychological Reports* 1967; **20**: 975–8.

70. Martens R, Burton D, Vealey RS, Bump LA, Smith DE. Development and validation of the Competitive State Anxiety Inventory-2. In: Martens R, Vealey RS, Burton D, eds. *Competitive anxiety in sport.* Champaign, IL: Human Kinetics, 1990: 117–90.

71. Borkovec TD. Physiological and cognitive processes in the regulation of anxiety. In: Schwartz G, Shapiro D, eds. *Consciousness and self-regulation: advances in research (Vol 1).* New York: Phelem, 1978: 261–312.

72. Bandura A. Self-efficacy: toward a unifying theory of behavioural change. *Psychological Review* 1977; **84**: 1475–82.

73. Krane V, Williams JM. Performance and somatic anxiety, cognitive anxiety and confidence changes prior to competition. *Journal of Sport Behavior* 1987; **10**: 47–56.

74. Jones JG, Swain A, Cale A. Gender differences in precompetition temporal patterning and antecedents of anxiety and self-confidence. *Journal of Sport and Exercise Psychology* 1991; **13**: 1–15.

75. Jones JG. Recent developments and current issues in competitive state anxiety research. *The Psychologist* 1991; **4**, 152–5.

76. Jones JG. More than just a game: research developments and issues in competitive anxiety in sport. *British Journal of Psychology* 1995; **86**, 449–78.

77. Mahoney MJ, Avener M. Psychology of the elite athlete: an exploratory study. *Cognitive Therapy and Research* 1977; **1**: 135–41.

78. Jones JG, Hanton S, Swain, ABJ. Intensity and interpretation of anxiety symptoms in elite and non-elite sports performers. *Personality and Individual Differences* 1994; **17**, 657–63.

79. Jones JG, Swain ABJ. Predispositions to experience facilitative and debilitative anxiety in elite and non-elite performers. *The Sport Psychologist* 1995; **9**, 202–12.

80. Jones JG, Hanton S. Interpretation of competitive anxiety symptoms and goal attainment expectancies. *Journal of Sport and Exercise Psychology* 1996; **18**, 144–57.

81. Gould D, Petlichkoff L, Weinberg RS. Antecedents of, temporal changes in, and relationships between CSAI-2 subcomponents. *Journal of Sport Psychology* 1984; **6**: 289–304.

82. Scanlan TK. Competitive stress and the child athlete. In: Silva, JM, Weinberg, RS, eds. *Psychological foundations of sport.* Champaign, IL: Human Kinetics, 1984.

83. Jones JG, Swain A, Cale A. Antecedents of multidimensional competitive state anxiety and self-confidence in elite intercollegiate middle-distance runners. *The Sport Psychologist* 1990; **4**: 107–18.

84. Jones JG, Swain A, Cale A. Gender differences in precompetition temporal patterning and antecedents of anxiety and self-confidence. *Journal of Sport and Exercise Psychology* 1991; **13**: 1–15.

85. Neiss R. Reconceptualizing arousal: psychobiological states in motor performance. *Psychological Bulletin* 1988; **103**: 345–66.

86. Jones JG, Hardy L. Stress and cognitive functioning in sport. *Journal of Sports Sciences* 1989; **7**: 41–63.

87. Parfitt CG, Jones JG, Hardy L. Multidimensional anxiety and performance. In: Jones JG, Hardy L, eds. *Stress and performance in sport.* Chichester: John Wiley, 1990: 43–80.

88. Burton D. Do anxious swimmers swim slower? Reexamining the elusive anxiety-performance relationship. *Journal of Sport and Exercise Psychology* 1988; **10**: 45–61.

89. Gould D, Petlichkoff L, Simons J, Vevera M. Relationship between Competitive State Anxiety Inventory-2 subscale scores and pistol shooting performance. *Journal of Sport Psychology* 1987; **9**: 33–42.

90. Hockey GRJ, Hamilton P. The cognitive patterning of stress states. In: Hockey GRJ, ed. *Stress and fatigue in human performance.* Chichester: John Wiley, 1983: 331–62.

91. Parfitt CG, Hardy L. Further evidence for the differential effects of competitive anxiety upon a number of cognitive and motor subsystems. *Journal of Sports Sciences* 1987; **5**: 62–3 (abstract).

92. Apter MJ. *The experience of motivation: the theory of psychological reversals.* London: Academic Press, 1982.

93. Kerr JH. Stress in sport: reversal theory. In: Jones JG, Hardy L, eds. *Stress and performance in sport.* Chichester: John Wiley, 1990: 107–31.

94. Sanders AF. Towards a model of stress and human performance. *Acta Psychologica* 1983; **53**: 64–97.

95. Humphreys MS, Revelle W. Personality, motivation, and performance: a theory of the relationship between individual differences and information processing. *Psychological Review* 1984; **91**: 153–84.

96. Jones JG. A cognitive perspective on the processes underlying the relationship between stress and performance in sport. In: Jones JG, Hardy L, eds. *Stress and performance in sport.* Chichester: John Wiley, 1990: 17–42.

97. Hardy L, Fazey JA. *The inverted-U hypothesis—a catastrophe for sport psychology and a statement of a new hypothesis.* Paper presented at the Annual Conference of the North American Society for the Psychology of Sport and Physical Activity, Vancouver, Canada, 1987.

98. Zeeman EC. Catastrophe theory. *Scientific American* 1976; **234**: 65–83.

99. Hardy L. Testing the predictions of the cusp catastrophe model of anxiety and performance. *The Sport Psychologist* 1996; **10**, 140–56.

100. Hardy L, Parfitt CG. A catastrophe model of anxiety and performance. *British Journal of Psychology* 1991; **82**: 163–78.

101. Hardy L, Parfitt CG, Pates J. Performance catastrophes in sport: A test of the hysteresis hypothesis. *Journal of Sports Sciences* 1994; **12**, 327–34.

102. Gould D, Krane V. The arousal–athletic performance relationship: current status and future directions. In: Horn T, ed. *Advances in sport psychology.* Champaign, IL: Human Kinetics, 1992: 119–42.

103. Gould D, Jackson SA, Finch L. Sources of stress in national figure skaters. *Journal of Sport and Exercise Psychology* 1993; **15**, 134–59.

104. Gould D, Jackson SA, Finch L. Life at the top: The experiences of US national champion figure skaters. *The Sport Psychologist* 1993; **7**, 354–74.

105. Jones JG. More than just a game: Research developments and issues in competitive anxiety in sport. *British Journal of Psychology* 1995; **86**, 449–78.

106. Vealey RS. Sport personology: a paradigmatic and methodological analysis. *Journal of Sport and Exercise Psychology* 1989; **11**: 216–35.

107. Cattell RB. *Description and measurement of personality.* Yonkers-on-Hudson, New York: World, 1946.

108. Mischel W. *Personality and assessment.* New York: John Wiley, 1968.

109. Magnusson D, Endler NS. Interactional psychology: present status and future prospects. In: Magnusson D, Endler NS, eds. *Personality at the cross-roads: current issues in interactional psychology.* Hillsdale, NJ: Erlbaum, 1977: 3–31.

110. Fisher AC. New directions in sport personality research. In: Silva, JM, Weinberg, RS, eds. *Psychological foundations of sport.* Champaign, IL: Human Kinetics, 1984: 70–80.

111. Martens R. The paradigmatic crisis in American sport personology. *Sportwissenschaft* 1975; **1**: 9–24.

112. Morgan WP. The trait psychology controversy. *Research Quarterly for Exercise and Sport* 1980; **51**: 50–76.

113. Martens R. *Sport Competition Anxiety Test.* Champaign, IL: Human Kinetics, 1977.

114. Smith RE, Smoll FL, Schutz RW. Measurement and correlates of sport-specific cognitive and somatic trait anxiety: the Sport Anxiety Scale. *Anxiety Research* 1990; **2**: 225–36.

115. Vealey RS. Sport-confidence and competitive orientations: preliminary investigation and instrument development. *Journal of Sport Psychology* 1986; **8**: 221–46.

116. Gill DL, Deeter TE. Development of the Sport Orientation Questionnaire. *Research Quarterly for Exercise and Sport* 1988; **59**: 191–202.

117. Deaux K. Sex and gender. *Annual Review of Psychology* 1985; **36**: 49–81.

118. Maccoby E, Jacklin C. *The psychology of sex differences.* Dubuque, IA: William C. Brown, 1974.

119. Hyde JS. How large are cognitive gender differences? A meta-analysis using w^2 and d. *American Psychologist* 1981; **36**: 892–901.

120. Gill DL. *Psychological dynamics of sport.* Champaign, IL: Human Kinetics, 1986.

121. Gill DL. Gender differences in competitive orientation and sport participation. *International Journal of Sport Psychology* 1988; **19**: 145–59.

122. Gill DL, Gross JB, Huddleston S, Shifflett B. Sex differences in achievement cognitions and performance in competition. *Research Quarterly for Exercise and Sport* 1984; **55**: 340–6.

123. Lenney E. Women's self-confidence in achievement settings. *Psychological Bulletin* 1977; **84**: 1–13.

124. Harris DV. Femininity and athleticism: conflict or consonance. In Sabo, Runfola, Jock, eds. *Sports and male identity.* Englewood Cliffs, NJ: Prentice-Hall 1980; 222–39.

125. Theberge N. Sport and women's empowerment. *Women's Studies International Forum*, 1987; **10**: 387–93.

126. Bem SL. The measurement of psychological androgyny. *Journal of Consulting and Clinical Psychology* 1974; **42**: 155–62.

127. Spence JT, Helmreich RL, Stapp J. The Personality Attributes Questionnaire: a measure of sex role stereotypes and masculinity-feminity. *JSAJ Catalogue of Selected Documents in Psychology* 1974; **4**: 127.

128. Nideffer RM. Test of attentional and interpersonal style. *Journal of Personality and Social Psychology* 1976; 34: 394–404.

129. Van Schoyk SR, Grasha AF. Attentional style variations and athletic ability: the advantages of a sports-specific test. *Journal of Sport Psychology* 1981; **3**: 149–65.

130. Albrecht RR, Feltz DL. Generality and specificity of attention related to competitive anxiety and sport performance. *Journal of Sport Psychology* 1987; **9**: 231–48.

131. Landers DM. Beyond the TAIS: alternative behavioral and psychophysiological measures for determining an internal vs external focus of attention. Paper presented at the NASPSPA Conference, Gulfpark, MS, 1975.

132. Boutcher SH, Zinsser NW. Cardiac deceleration of elite and beginning golfers during putting. *Journal of Sport and Exercise Psychology* 1990; **12**: 37–47.

133. Boutcher SH. The role of performance routines in sport. In: Jones JG, Hardy L, eds. *Stress and performance in sport.* Chichester: John Wiley, 1990: 231–45.

134. Allard F, Graham S, Paarsalu MT. Perception in sport: basketball. *Journal of Sport Psychology* 1980; **2**: 14–21.

135. Morgan WP, Pollock ML. Psychologic characterization of the elite distance runner. *Annals of the New York Academy of Sciences* 1977; **301**: 382–403.

136. Gill DL, Strom EH. The effect of attentional focus on perform-

ance of an endurance task. *International Journal of Sport Psychology* 1985; **16**: 217–23.

137. Fenz W. Coping mechanisms and performance stress. In: Landers DM, ed. *psychology of sport and motor behavior II*. University Park, PA: Pennsylvania State University, 1975: 3–24.

138. Orlick T, Partington J. Mental links to excellence. *The Sport Psychologist* 1988; **2**: 105–30.

139. Mahoney MJ, Gabriel TJ, Perkins TS. Psychological skills and exceptional athletic performance. *The Sport Psychologist* 1987; **1**: 181–99.

140. Starkes JL. Skill in field hockey: the nature of the cognitive advantage. *Journal of Sport Psychology* 1987; **9**: 146–60.

141. Abernethy B, Russell DG. Expert–novice differences in an applied selective attention task. *Journal of Sport Psychology* 1987; **9**: 326–45.

142. Smoll FL, Magill RA, Ash MJ, eds. *Children in sport*. 3rd edn. Champaign, IL: Human Kinetics, 1988.

143. Weiss MR, Friedrichs WD. The influence of leader behaviours, coach attributes, and institutional variables on performance and satisfaction of collegiate basketball teams. *Journal of Sport Psychology* 1986; **8**: 332–46.

144. Chelladurai P. Leadership in sports. In: Silva JM, Weinberg RS, eds. *Psychological foundations of sport*. Champaign, IL: Human Kinetics, 1984: 329–39.

145. Chelladurai P, Saleh SD. Dimensions of leader behavior in sports: Development of a leadership scale. *Journal of Sport Psychology* 1980; **2**: 34–45.

146. Chelladurai P, Saleh SD. Preferred leadership in sports. *Canadian Journal of Applied Sport Science* 1978; **3**: 85–92.

147. Chelladurai P, Carron AV. Ahtletic maturity and preferred leadership. *Journal of Sport Psychology* 1983; **5**: 371–80.

148. Chelladurai P. Discrepancy between preferences and perceptions of leadership behavior and satisfaction of athletes in varying sports. *Journal of Sport Psychology* 1984; **6**: 27–41.

149. Reimer, HA, Chelladurai, P. Leadership and satisfaction in athletics. *Journal of Sport and Exercise Science* 1995; **17**: 276–93.

150. Chelladurai P, Imamura H, Yamaguchi Y, Oinuma Y, Miyauchi T. Sport leadership in a cross-national setting: The case of Japanese and Canadian university athletes. *Journal of Sport and Exercise Psychology* 1988; **10**: 374–89.

151. Chelladurai, P. Leadership. In Singer RN, Murphey M, Tennant LK, eds. *Handbook on research in sport psychology*. New York: Macmillan, 1993: 647–71.

152. Tharp RG, Gallimore R. What a coach can teach a teacher. *Psychology Today* 1976; **9**: 74–8.

153. Smoll FL, Smith RE. Leadership research in youth sports. In: Silva JM, Weinberg RS, eds. *Psychological foundations of sport*. Champaign, IL: Human Kinetics, 1984: 371–86.

154. Hendry LB. Human factors in sport systems: Suggested models for analysing athlete–coach interaction. *Human Factors* 1974; **16**: 528–44.

155. Vroom VH, Yetton RN. *Leadership and decision-making*. Pittsburgh: University of Pittsburgh Press, 1973.

156. Chelladurai P, Haggerty TR. A normative model of decision styles in coaching. *Athleic Administrator* 1978; **13**: 6–9.

157. Chelladurai P, Arnott M. Decision styles in coaching: Preferences of basketball players. *Research Quarterly for Exercise and Sport* 1985; **56**: 15–24.

158. Chelladurai P, Haggerty TR, Baxter PR. Decision style choices of university basketball coaches and players. *Journal of Sport and Exercise Psychology* 1989; **11**: 201–15.

159. Rosenbaum LL, Rosenbaum WB. Morale and productivity consequences of group leadership style, stress, and type of task. *Journal of Applied Psychology* 1971; **55**: 343–88.

160. Zander A. *Motives and goals in groups*. New York: Academic Press, 1971.

161. Latane B, Williams KD, Harkins SG. Many hands make light work: The causes and consequences of social loafing. *Journal of Personality and Social Psychology* 1979; **37**: 823–32.

162. Hardy CJ, Latane B. Social loafing in cheerleaders: Effects of team membership and competition. *Journal of Sport and Exercise Psychology* 1988; **10**: 109–14.

163. Carron AV. Cohesiveness in sport groups: Interpretations and considerations. *Journal of Sport Psychology* 1982; **4**: 123–38.

164. Martens R, Landers DM, Loy JW. *Sport cohesiveness questionnaire*. Unpublished report, University of Illinois at Urbana-Champaign.

165. Widmeyer WN, Carron AV, Brawley LR. Group cohesion in sport and exercise. In: Singer RN, Murphey M, Tennant LK, eds. *Handbook on research in sport psychology*. New York: Macmillan, 1993: 672–92.

166. Yukelson D, Weinberg R, Jackson A. A multidimensional sport cohesion instrument for intercollegiate basketball players. *Journal of Sport Psychology* 1984; **6**: 103–17.

167. Carron, AV, Widmeyer, WN, Brawley, LR. The development of an instrument to assess cohesion insport teams: The Group Environment Questionnaire. *Journal of Sport Psychology* 1985; **9**: 275–94.

168. Carron AV, Widmeyer WN, Brawley LR. Group cohesion and individual adherence to physical activity. *Journal of Sport and Exercise Psychology* 1988; **10**: 127–38.

169. Brawley LR, Carron AV, Widmeyer WN. Exploring the relationship between cohesion and group resistance to disruption. *Journal of Sport and Exercise Psychology* 1988; **10**: 199–213.

170. Spink KS. Group cohesion and collective efficacy of volleyball teams. *Journal of Sport and Exercise Psychology* 1990: **12**: 301–11.

171. Prapavessis H, Carron, AV. The effect of group cohesion on competitive state anxiety. *Journal of Sport and Exercise Psychology* 1996; **18**: 64–74.

172. Widmeyer WN, Brawley LR, Carron AV. The effects of group size in sport. *Journal of Sport and Exercise Psychology* 1990; **12**: 177–90.

173. Silva JM. Understanding aggressive behavior and its effects upon athletic performance. In: Straub WF, ed. *Sport psychology: an analysis of athlete behavior*. Ithaca, NY: Mouvement, 1980: 177–86.

174. Leith LM. The effect of various physical activities, outcome, and emotional arousal on subject aggression scores. *International Journal of Sport Psychology* 1989; **20**: 57–66.

175. Nosanchuk TA. The way of the warrior: the effects of traditional martial arts training on aggressiveness. *Human Relations* 1981; **34**: 435–44.

176. Berkowitz L. Some determinants of impulsive aggression; role of mediated association with reinforcements for aggression. *Psychological Review* 1974; **81**: 165–76.

177. Stephens DE, Bredemeier BJL. Moral atmosphere and judgements about aggression in girls' soccer: Relationships among moral and motivational variables. *Journal of Sport and Exercise Psychology* 1996; **18**: 158–73.

178. Frank MG, Gilovich T. The dark side of self- and social perception: black uniforms and aggression in professional sports. *Journal of Personality and Social Psychology* 1988; **54**: 74–85.

179. Bredemeier BJ. Moral reasoning and the perceived legitimacy of intentionally injurious acts. *Journal of Sport Psychology* 1985; **7**: 110–24.

180. Ryan MK, Williams JM, Wimer B. Athletic aggression: perceived legitimacy and behavioral intentions in girls' high school basketball. *Journal of Sport And Exercise Psychology* 1990; **12**: 48–55.

181. Silva JM. The perceived legitimacy of rule violating behavior in sport. *Journal of Sport Psychology* 1983; **5**: 438–48.

182. Frodi A, Macauley J, Thome PR. Are women always less aggressive than men? A review of the experimental literature. *Psychological Bulletin* 1977; **84**: 638–60.

183. McCarthy JF, Kelly BR. Aggression, performance variables, and anger self-report in ice-hockey players. *Journal of Psychology* 1978; **99**: 97–101.

184. Silva JM. Behavioral and situational factors affecting concentration and skill performance. *Journal of Sport Psychology* 1979; **1**: 221–7.

185. Bredemeier BJ, Weiss MR, Shields DL, Shewchuk RM. Promoting moral growth in a summer sport camp: the implications of theoretically grounded instructional strategies. *Journal of Moral Education* 1986; **15**: 212–20.

186. McGrath JE. *Groups: interaction and perfomance.* Englewood Cliffs, NJ: Prentice-Hall, 1984.

187. Biddle SJH, Fox KR. Exercise and health psychology: emerging relationships. *British Journal of Medical Psychology* 1989; **62**: 205–16.

188. Morgan WP, Goldston SE, eds. *Exercise and mental health.* Washington, DC: Hemisphere, 1987.

189. Dishman RK. *Exercise adherence: its impact on public health.* Champaign, IL: Human Kinetics, 1988.

190. Morgan WP, O'Connor PJ. Exercise and mental health. In: Dishman RK, ed. *Exercise adherence: its impact on public health.* Champaign, IL: Human Kinetics, 1988: 91–122.

191. Taylor CB, Sallis JF, Needle R. The relation of physical activity and exercise to mental health. *Public Health Reports* 1985; **100**: 195–202.

192. Berger B, Owen D. Stress reduction and mood enhancement in four exercise modes: swimming, body conditioning, hatha yoga, and fencing. *Research Quarterly for Exercise and Sport* 1988; **59**: 148–59.

193. Raglin JS, Morgan WP. Influence of exercise and quiet rest on state anxiety and blood pressure. *Medicine and Science in Sports and Exercise* 1987; **19**: 456–63.

194. Greist JH. Exercise intervention with depressed patients. In: Morgan WP, Goldston SE, eds. *Exercise and mental health.* Washington, DC: Hemisphere, 1987: 117–21.

195. Gruber JJ. Physical activity and self-esteem development in children: a meta-analysis. In: Stull G, Eckert H, eds. *Effects of physical activity on children.* Champaign, IL: Human Kinetics, 1986.

196. Crews DJ, Landers DM. A meta-analytic review of aerobic fitness and reactivity to psychosocial stressors. *Medicine and Science in Sports and Exercise* 1987; **19** (Suppl.): S114–S120.

197. Harris DV. Comparative effectiveness of running therapy and psychotherapy. In: Morgan WP, Goldston SE, eds. *Exercise and mental health.* Washington, DC: Hemisphere, 1987: 123–30.

198. Berger B. Stress levels in swimmers. In: Morgan WP, Goldston SE, eds. *Exercise and mental health.* Washington, DC: Hemisphere, 1987: 139–43.

199. de Vries HA. Tension reduction with exercise. In: Morgan WP, Goldston SE, eds. *Exercise and mental health.* Washington, DC: Hemisphere, 1987: 99–104.

200. Hatfield BD, Landers DM. Psychophysiology in exercise and sport research: an overview. *Exercise and Sport Sciences Reviews* 1987; **15**: 351–87.

201. Harber VJ, Sutton JR. Endorphins and exercise. *Sports Medicine* 1984; **1**: 154–71.

202. Sonstroem RJ. Exercise and self-esteem. *Exercise and Sport Sciences Reviews* 1984; **12**: 123–55.

203. Bahrke MS, Morgan WP. Anxiety reduction following exercise and meditation. *Cognitive Therapy and Research* 1978; **2**: 323–33.

204. Berger B, Friedman E, Eaton M. Comparison of jogging, the relaxation response, and group interaction for stress reduction. *Journal of Sport and Exercise Psychology* 1988; **10**: 431–47.

205. Long BC, Haney CJ. Long-term follow-up of stressed working men: a comparison of aerobic exercise and progressive relaxation. *Journal of Sport and Exercise Psychology* 1988; **4**: 461–70.

206. Biddle SJH. Introduction. In: *Sport, health, psychology and exercise symposium.* London: Sports Council/ Health Education Authority, 1990: 5–7.

207. Stephens T. Physical activity and mental health in the United States and Canada: evidence from four population surveys. *Preventive Medicine* 1988; **17**: 35–47.

208. Dishman RK. Medical psychology in exercise and sport. *Medical Clinics of North America* 1985; **69**: 123–43.

209. Dishman RK. Mental health. In: Seefeldt V, ed. *Physical activity and well-being.* Reston: AAHPERD, 1986.

210. Steinberg H, Sykes EA, Morris M. Exercise addiction: the opiate connection. In: *Sport, health, psychology and exercise symposium.* London: Sports Council/ Health Education Authority, 1990: 161–66.

211. Veale MW. Exercise dependence. *British Journal of Addiction* 1987; **82**: 735–40.

212. Morris M, Steinberg H, Sykes EA, Salmon P. Temporary deprivation from running produces 'withdrawal' syndrome. In: *Sport, health, psychology and exercise symposium.* London: Sports Council/ Health Education Authority, 1990: 161–71.

213. Sheehan G. The best therapy. *Physician and Sportsmedicine* 1983; **11**: 43.

214. Sports Council. *Sport in the community: the next ten years.* London: The Sports Council, 1982.

215. Dishman RK. Compliance/adherence in health-related exercise. *Health Psychology* 1982; **1**: 237–67.

216. Morgan WP. Involvement in vigorous physical activity with special reference to adherence. *Proceedings of the NCPEAM/ NAPECW National Conference* 1977: 235–46.

217. Dishman RK, Gettman LR. Psychobiologic influences on exercise adherence. *Journal of Sport Psychology* 1980; **2**: 295–310.

218. Janz NK, Becker MH. The Health Belief Model: a decade later. *Health Education Quarterly* 1984; **11**: 1–47.

219. Fishbein M, Ajzen I. *Belief, attitude, intention and behavior: an introduction to theory and research.* Reading, MA: Addison-Wesley, 1975.

220. Sonstroem RJ. Psychological models. In: Dishman RK, ed. *Exercise adherence: its impact on public health.* Champaign, IL: Human Kinetics, 1988: 125–53.

221. Bandura A. *Social foundations of thought and action.* Englewoood Cliffs, NJ: Prentice-Hall, 1986.

222. Dzewaltowski DA. Toward a model of exercise motivation. *Journal of Sport and Exercise Psychology* 1989; **11**: 251–69.

223. Dzewaltowski DA, Noble JM, Shaw JM. Physical activity participation: social cognitive theory versus the theories of reasoned action and planned behaviour. *Journal of Sport and Exercise Psychology* 1990; **12**: 388–405.

224. Kleinginna PR, Kleinginna AM. A categorized list of motivation definitions with a suggestion for a consensual definition. *Motivation and Emotion* 1981; **5**: 263–91.

225. Duda JL. Goal perspectives and behavior in sport and exercise settings. In: Ames C, Maehr M, eds. *Advances in motivation and achievement (Vol. 6).* Greenwich, CT: JAI Press, in press.

226. Oldridge NB. Compliance with exercise in cardiac rehabilitation. In: Dishman RK, ed. *Exercise adherence: its impact on public health.* Champaign, IL: Human Kinetics, 1988: 283–304.

227. Shephard RJ. Exercise adherence in corporate settings: personal traits and program barriers. In: Dishman RK, ed. *Exercise adherence: its impact on public health.* Champaign, IL: Human Kinetics, 1988: 305–19.

228. Corbin CB. Youth fitness, exercise and health: there is much to be done. *Research Quarterly for Exercise and Sport* 1987; **58**: 308–14.

229. Ravizza K. Peak experience in sport. *Journal of Humanistic Psychology* 1977; **17**: 35–40.

230. Vealey RS. Future directions in psychological skills training. *The Sport Psychologist* 1988; **2**: 318–36.

231. Locke EA, Latham GP. The application of goal setting to sports. *Journal of Sport Psychology* 1985; **7**: 205–22.

232. Beggs WDA. Goal setting in sport. In: Jones JG, Hardy L, eds. *Stress and performance in sport*. Chichester: John Wiley, 1990: 135–70.

233. Burton D. The Jeckyl/Hyde nature of goals: Reconceptualising goal setting in sport. In Horn T, ed. *Advances in sport psychology*. Champaign, IL: Human Kinetics, 1992: 267–97.

234. Hardy L, Nelson D. Self-regulation training in sport and work. *Ergonomics* 1988; **31**: 1673–83.

235. Hardy L, Fazey JA. *Mental training*. Leeds: The National Coaching Foundation, 1990.

236. Kingston KM, Hardy L. When are some goals more beneficial than others, *Journal of Sport Sciences* 1994, **12**: 198–9.

237. Kingston KM, Hardy L. Factors affecting the salience of outcome performance and process goals in golf. In: Cochran AJ, Farally MR, eds. *Science and Golf II*, London: Chapman and Hall, 1994: 144–9.

238. Feltz DL, Landers DM. The effects of mental practice on motor skill learning and performance: a meta-analysis. *Journal of Sport Psychology* 1983; **5**: 25–57.

239. Suinn RM. Imagery and sports. In: Straub WF, Williams JM, eds. *Cognitive sport psychology*. Lansing, New York: Sports Science Associates, 1984: 253–72.

240. Ainscoe M, Hardy L. Cognitive warm-up in a cyclical gymnastics skill. *International Journal of Sport Psychology* 1987; **18**: 269–75.

241. Weinberg RS, Gould D, Jackson A. Expectations and performance: an empirical test of Bandura's self-efficacy theory. *Journal of Sport Psychology* 1979; **1**: 320–31.

242. Moritz SE, Hall CR, Martin K. What are confident athletes imaging?: An examination of image content. *The Sport Psychologist*, in press.

243. Vadocz EA, Hall CR. The cognitive and motivational functions of images in the anxiety-performance relationship. *Journal of Applied Sport Psychology*, in press.

244. Murphy SM. Models of imagery in sport psychology: A review. *Journal of Mental Imagery* 1990; **14**: 153–72.

245. Pylyshyn Z. The imagery debate: analog media versus tacit knowledge. In: Block N, ed. *Imagery*. Cambridge, MA: MIT press, 1981: 151–205.

246. Lang PJ. A bio-informational theory of emotional imagery. *Psychophysiology* 1979; **17**: 179–92.

247. Ahsen A. ISM: The triple code model for imagery and psychophysiology. *Journal of Mental Imagery* 1984; **8**: 15–42.

248. Jacobson E. *Progressive relaxation*. Chicago: University of Chicago Press, 1930.

249. Bernstein DA, Borkovec TD. *Progressive relaxation: a manual for the helping professions*. Champaign, IL: Research Press, 1973.

250. Ost LG. Applied relaxation: description of an effective coping technique. *Scandinavian Journal of Behaviour Therapy* 1988; **17**: 83–96.

251. Wolpe J. *Psychotherapy by reciprocal inhibition*. Stanford, CA: Stanford University Press, 1958.

252. Meichenbaum DH. *Cognitive-behaviour modification*. New York: Plenum Press, 1977.

253. Smith RE. A cognitive-affective approach to stress management training for athletes. In: Nadeau CH, Halliwell WR, Newell KM, Roberts GC, eds. *Psychology of motor behavior and sport—1979*. Champaign, IL: Human Kinetics, 1980: 54–72.

254. Unestahl LE. *Inner mental training*. Orebro, Sweden: Veje Publications, 1983.

255. Cooke LE, Alderson GJK. *Stress and anxiety in sport*. Sheffield: Pavic Publications, 1986.

256. Hamberger K, Lohr J. Relationship of relaxation training to the controllability of imagery. *Perceptual and Motor Skills* 1980; **51**: 103–10.

257. Singer JL. *Imagery and daydream methods in psychotherapy and behavior modification*. New York: Academic Press, 1974.

258. Weinberg R, Seabourne T, Jackson A. Arousal and relaxation instructions prior to the use of imagery. *International Journal of Sport Psychology* 1987; **18**: 205–14.

259. Ellis A. Self-direction in sport and life. *Rational living* 1982; **17**: 27–33.

260. Rushall BS. The content of competition thinking. In: Straub WF, Williams JM, eds. *Cognitive sport psychology*. Lansing, NY: Sports Science Associates, 1984: 51–62.

261. Van Raalte JL, Brewer BW, Rivera PM, Petitpas AJ. The relationship between observable self-talk and competitive junior tennis players' match performances. *Journal of Sport and Exercise Psychology* 1994; **16**: 400–15.

262. Meyers AW, Schleser RA. A cognitive behavioral intervention for improving basketball performance. *Journal of Sport Psychology* 1980; **2**: 69–73.

263. Silva JM. Performance enhancement in sport environments through cognitive intervention. *Behaviour Modification* 1982; **6**: 433–63.

264. Schmid A, Peper E. Techniques for training concentration. In: Williams JM, ed. *Applied sport psychology: personal growth to peak performance*. Palo Alto, CA: Mayfield, 1986: 271–84.

265. Schwarz EE, Davidson RJ, Goleman DJ. Patterning of cognitive and somatic processes in the self-regulation of anxiety: effects of medication versus exercise. *Psychosomatic Medicine* 1978; **40**: 321–8.

266. Pribram KH, McGuinness D. Arousal, activation and effort in the control of attention. *Psychological Review* 1975; **82**: 116–49.

267. Shelton TO, Mahoney MJ. The content and effect of 'psyching-up' strategies in weight lifters. *Cognitive Therapy and Research* 1978; **2**: 275–84.

268. Mahoney MJ. Cognitive skills and athletic performance. In: Kendall PC, Hollon SD, eds. *Cognitive behavioral interventions*. New York: Academic Press, 1979: 423–43.

269. Locke EA, Frederick E, Bobko P, Lee C. Effect of self-efficacy, goals, and strategies on task performance. *Journal of Applied Psychology* 1984; **69**: 241–51.

270. Forsterling F. Attributional retraining: a review. *Psychological Bulletin* 1985; **98**: 495–512.

271. Harris DV, Harris BL. *The athlete's guide to sports psychology: mental skills for physical people*. New York: Leisure Press, 1984.

272. Eysenck MW. *Attention and arousal: cognition and performance*. Berlin: Springer-Verlag, 1982.

273. Wachtel PL. Conceptions of broad and narrow attention. *Psychological Bulletin* 1967; **68**: 417–29.

274. Morgan WP, Horstman DH, Cymerman A, Stokes J. Facilitation of physical performance by a cognitive strategy. *Cognitive Therapy and Research* 1983; **7**: 251–64.

275. Schomer HH. Mental strategy training programme for marathon runners. *International Journal of Sport Psychology* 1987; **18**: 133–51.

276. Bull SJ. Personal and situational influences on adherence to mental skills training. *Journal of Sport and Exercise Psychology* 1991; **13**: 121–32.

1.5 Anthropometry and the assessment of body composition

Peter R. M. Jones and N. G. Norgan

Introduction

Anthropometric and body composition techniques allow the body's size and shape and the masses and proportions of its constituents to be described. This information is helpful in acquiring a greater understanding of those attributes which contribute to performance in sport. Physical performance, for example speed, strength, and endurance, depends strongly on the amount of force-producing tissue, the application of forces through the levers of the limbs, and the adaptations to training.

The significance of information about the size, shape, and body composition of athletes is that it correlates with performance and may also indicate 'condition' and 'potential'. In athletics in particular, achievement and success require a particular body configuration; elite sprinters, middle-distance runners, and long-distance runners tend to have characteristic sizes and shapes, although inevitably there are exceptions. Anthropometric and body composition information can therefore contribute to decisions concerning the sport or event in which an individual is most likely to succeed and help in the development of appropriate training schedules and in the management and rehabilitation of those with sports-related injuries. Variation in the intensity of training and the periodic attainment of peaks may be accompanied by changes in size and/or composition which reflect relatively subtle changes in energy balance not readily apparent from measuring body mass alone. Indices of body fatness can contribute to the assessment of the state of training of a sportsman or sportswoman.

Anthropometry and body composition have long been indispensable measurements in exercise and sports science, as they have in human biology, and the proximity and interrelations of the two disciplines have been mutually beneficial. The study of body composition has benefited from investigations of sports participants. An early stimulus to the development of reproducible measurements of body fatness was the now familiar observation that American professional footballers could be classified as overweight and unfit for military service not because of excess fatness but because of muscularity and skeletal frame size. This led Behnke and colleagues to introduce a method for the measurement of body specific gravity which provided estimates of fat content of the body.[1]

Numerically, the majority of sports participants are not the elite or competitive sports people but modern-day urban dwellers with regular working hours who want an enjoyable activity that brings a sense of well being and may help in regaining or maintaining fitness and appropriate body weight. Anthropometric and body composition techniques must therefore be applicable to the general population and relevant to the monitoring of health status in general. However, the extreme physiques of elite sportspeople test the methodology, leading to improvements which benefit both sport and science. For example, body composition studies in athletes have emphasized the needs and the benefits of multicomponent models of body composition (see later in this chapter).

This chapter considers the techniques available to describe body size, shape, and composition in sports medicine and recommends the use of a minimum of six basic anthropometric parameters. In addition, the validity of the underlying assumptions when dealing with sportsmen and sportswomen is considered.

Rationale for taking size, shape, and body composition measurements

Physicians have been prominent in the history of constitutional investigation, especially in studies of the relationships between morphology and susceptibility to disease. Damon[2] reviewed the history of human classification and defined constitution as the sum total of the morphological, physiological, and psychological characters of an individual, in large part determined by heredity but influenced in varying degrees by environmental factors.

The characteristics of body physique associated with success in sports and other types of physical activity have always greatly interested scientists, artists, sports writers, and others. There have been numerous studies which have used measurements describing the morphology of sportsmen to focus on the descriptions and comparisons within and between sporting groups and athletic events. A review by Tittel and Wutscherk[3] cited over a hundred studies and to date we must add at least another hundred.

We would expect to find that the most successful sportsmen and sportswomen have physical characteristics best suited to their particular sport, and that differences in morphology and physique will highlight the importance of measuring aspects of physique such as a somatotype. This general hypothesis has been stated by Tanner,[4] who reported that an appropriate body build and composition was important to success in athletic competition.

Early anatomists noted four different body types: (i) the fat abdominal type, (ii) the strong muscular type, (iii) the tall slender-chested thoracic form, and (iv) the more rounded and larger headed cephalic type. Later writers contrasted the well-rounded and compact form of the pyknic contestant with the muscular athletic build and the long, thin asthenic leptosome. In the 1940s Sheldon, a pioneer in this area, moved away from the strict typology by introducing the concept of three discrete and continuous variables—endomorphy, mesomorphy, and ectomorphy—to describe the varieties of human physique.[5] Unfortunately, this promising somatotype method came to be virtually abandoned because of the inflexibility in the technique and Sheldon's rigid adherence to his concept of the unchanging, genetically determined somatotype. However, important and sound concepts underlie his original method, and modifications to it by Heath and Carter have produced an extremely useful and widely used research technique for the study of variation in human physique.

The Heath–Carter method uses the somatotype as a phenotypic rating. This allows not only for changes over time, but also recognizes that each of the rating scales for the three components are open ended and apply to physiques of both sexes. The selected anthropometric measurements bring objectivity to the rating scores. Technical issues of this hybrid methodology have been published. The photoscopic and the anthropometric somatotype methods have been described by Carter and Heath.[6]

Measurements of body composition are important in many of the disciplines which contribute to sports medicine. They can, for example, provide sensitive indices of body fatness and therefore a means of describing relatively subtle changes in energy balance which are not readily apparent from measuring body mass alone but which have the potential to influence performance or, in the longer term, health. During an intensive training programme the body density can increase, which is indicative of a reduction in body fat content that, at the same time, would be supported by a reduction in the skinfold thicknesses observed.

The amount of fat in the body is often expressed as a percentage of fat, or the proportion of the mass of fat to the total body mass. Fat distribution may vary considerably even between people with exactly the same percentage of body mass as fat, and some may have a larger proportion of fat subcutaneously whilst others may have a larger proportion internally. Similarly, some people may have a larger proportion of subcutaneous fat on the limbs as opposed to the thorax and abdomen.

Customization

Anthropometry—its contribution to sports medicine management

A considerable number of physiotherapists in sports medicine clinics use anthropometry in the everyday treatment and rehabilitation of the injured athlete. It is important to understand what kind of anthropometric and body composition techniques are available and useful as well as how they can be applied to aid the clinical practitioner and answer some of the injured athlete's problems.

Muscle has an important protective role in the function and sta-

bilization of joints. If muscle strength and function are reduced because of pain following injury, new damage can occur more easily. Changes in muscle circumference with strength-related exercises pre- and postoperatively, as well as during and after rehabilitation, can be monitored by measuring circumferences of the quadriceps femoris and hamstring muscle groups at levels of 50, 100, and 150 mm proximal to the superior patella border with the leg straight and the muscles relaxed. These types of muscle bulk measurements would also be invaluable in the assessment of postoperative treatment following menisectomy by arthroscopy for anterior cruciate, medial, and lateral ligament injuries. It is usual to compare the measurements of the injured limb with those of the contralateral limb.

Where knee pain occurs in tibialis anterior disease, chondromalacia patellae, which has several synonyms including runner's knee, jogger's knee, and cyclist's knee to name but a few, it is usual to see a small difference in the total leg length. This in turn often reflects abnormalities associated with discrepant leg lengths leading to pelvic tilting and hence spinal deformities such as scoliosis or compensatory spinal curvature. It also gives rise to unequal stride length causing pelvic rotation. To identify this condition the subjects are measured in the standing position using a long levelling device placed on skin marks over the anterior superior iliac spines (Fig. 1). Two measurements are then made on each leg from the anterior superior iliac spines to the medial malleolus or datum using a flexible steel tape. Packing boards, 5 or 10 mm in thickness, can be placed under the feet in order to achieve a horizontal pelvic level and hence a correct leg length. These measurements can also be obtained from radiological techniques, provided that the subject's posture is carefully standardized during the examination. However, this method of measurement is undesirable owing to additional radiation hazards, especially where the gonads are unprotected during the procedure.

For severe injuries to the shoulder requiring surgical replacement, it is helpful to measure total arm length. This is measured, using marked points, from the inferior border of the acromial process (acromiale) to the distal point of the ulna bone (Fig. 1).

Most joint angles (shoulder, spine, elbow, wrists, hips, knees, and ankles) can be measured using a goniometer. This is particularly useful in cases of suspected hypermobility very often seen in gymnasts. In runners, excessive pronation of the ankle joint is associated with high injury risk.

Anthropometry for biomechanics

The segmental lengths of the body's limbs are known to have a significant effect on the performance of sportsmen. For example, élite endurance runners differ from non-runners not only in factors such as muscle fibre types but also in the mechanics of the limb levers, in particular the ratios of the sitting height to subischial length (leg length) and its divisions (upper and lower leg). Body mechanics are of prime importance in throwing, and the optimal body physique of throwers can be readily interpreted from the study of the mechanics of athletic activities.[7] For example, the length of the humerus, radius, and ulna contribute to the ultimate mechanical advantage which is gained by these skeletal levers and their muscles, thereby affecting the force and speed of movement and the speed of objects delivered by these lever systems.

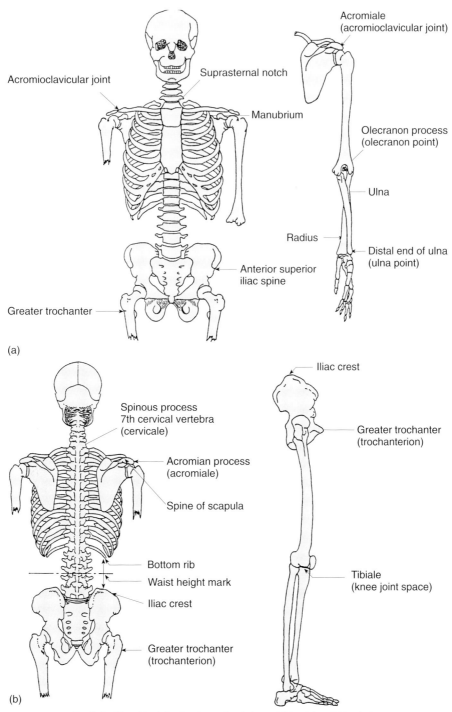

Fig. 1 Position of body landmarks on the skeleton: (a) front view, (b) back view.

Many muscles and joints in the body act as third-class levers, that is levers in which the fulcrum is farther away from the object to be raised than from the point where the force is being applied. For example, the biceps brachii muscle is inserted into the bicipital aponeurosis and radial tuberosity in a very mechanically disadvantageous way close to the elbow joint. Therefore it follows that a sportsman with a biceps brachii inserted 2 or 3 cm distal to the elbow joint would have considerable mechanical advantages, by permitting heavier loads to be raised, over other throwers. However, it must be remembered that for throwing a balance must be found between strength and speed and the mass of the projectile. This analogy also applies to the lower appendicular system and has implications for running.

The role of anthropometry in measuring the length of these lever systems seems to be important. What is perhaps more important is the role of new technology such as ultrasound which could be applied to demonstrate the actual points where tendons insert into the bones in relation to the joint space. This may reveal individual differences that exist in leverage arrangement and therefore help us to understand more clearly the differences in performance.

Anthropometry, body composition, and performance

There is no doubt that certain shapes, configurations, and compositions are more appropriate and conducive to success in particular sports, events, or team positions. However, determinism should be avoided. The exceptions are almost as well known as the generalizations. The practice of selection for teams or squads based on certain anthropometric or compositional criteria may reflect more a coach's intuition of the degree of application in diet control or training effort than the importance or advantage of characteristics as an indicator of training or for a team role.

In theory, the strength, speed, and possibly endurance are expected to be related to the amount of skeletal muscle. However, a simple linear single-stage model is far too simplistic to account for much of the variation in élite performance. Other biological, anatomical, and psychological factors are also involved, requiring a multicomponent, multistage, non-linear model. Therefore many variables intervene between anthropometry, body compositions, and performances, for example the level of training and the degree of motivation. It should come as no surprise that the relationships are less strong than might be expected on first sight. There are other reasons for the unexpectedly weak relationships between size and performance. First, the common index of size and composition is the fat-free mass. This is a heterogeneous entity, largely consisting of water. Indices such as skeletal muscle mass or lean leg volume are more appropriate. Second, individuals of different sizes are compared as per kilogram body weight or per kilogram fat-free mass, but this is inappropriate as the relationship is not directly proportional. There is a significant intercept term. This means that, for example, the VO_2 max of small lean individuals would be higher (per kilogram fat-free mass) than those of larger individuals without any necessary difference in other performance variables.

Measurements and calculations

The measurements on anthropometry and body composition that may be used in sports medicine are discussed in this section.

Weight and height

Weight and height are the two cardinal measurements of size. They are also widely used as indices of overweight and obesity. Although weight alone or weight and height in combination cannot distinguish between overweight due to excess fat and the muscular athlete or between the underweight of the ill or undernourished and the lean thin endurance runner, they remain the primary descriptive characteristics and should be recorded in all investigations or treatments.

Body mass is widely used as an index of body size and composition, but without other anthropometric measurements its application in the assessment of fatness is limited because it may be fat or lean. It is impossible to discriminate between fatness or leanness on the basis of height and body mass alone. Changes in body mass over a period of time in an adult are more useful as the height and frame size will be constant. However, without further measurements it is still impossible to tell whether the change in body mass is due to a change in fat or muscle. This is particularly true in an exercise or training programme where there is likely to be a change in muscle mass. During inactivity or habitual training the body mass may remain relatively constant, although inactivity often produces a gradual body mass gain. Daily changes in body mass, which could be plus or minus 1 kg, are most likely to be due to variations in the amount of body water or gastrointestinal contents. Tables of excess body mass developed by insurance companies have been used for many years as a simple index of obesity.[8]

In terms of assessing overweight and obesity, the current popular reference values are those of the Metropolitan Life Insurance Company. They are derived from the data on mortality and longevity from more than 25 North American insurance companies for over 4 million men and women insured between 1954 and 1972. Ninety per cent of the weights were obtained by actual weighing and those with major diseases were excluded. A range of weights is given for three frame sizes at each height for the two sexes. The frame sizes are determined by measurement of elbow breadth. The data for the references were not derived from insurance company data but were collected separately in the National Health and Nutrition Examination Surveys. The interquartile range, the range of the 50 per cent of the population in the middle of the range, is used for the medium frame category and the lower and upper quartiles are used for small and large frames. The weight ranges reflect the lowest mortality at each height.

Although the objective assessment of an index of frame size is an improvement, it should be remembered that it was not measured in the insured persons. The wide ranges for each frame size and height should highlight the fact that this is an imprecise approach. Many factors affect weight. The data on the insured population may not be representative of the general or sports populations. Interestingly, the difference between weights for height associated with the lowest mortality and average weights decreased markedly between 1959 and 1979. Weights for height were some 6 to 7 kg higher but remained below average weights. These weight increases were 10 per cent for short men and women, 5 per cent for medium men and women, and 1 per cent for tall men and women. Furthermore, the weight for a given height associated with the lowest mortality increases with age by some 4 to 5 kg per decade for individuals of average height. There is no systematic sex difference in the weight ranges. Thus weight standards ought to be adjusted for age.

Frame size

The rationale for categories of frame size is that the greater the frame size, the greater the lean body mass will be for a given height and therefore the greater the total weight can be without increasing the risk from adiposity.

The elbow breadth (biepicondylar humerus) is most commonly used. It is easily accessible, it is unaffected by adiposity, and normative data are available. The measurement technique is described below and standard values are given by the Metropolitan Life Insurance Company, New York.

Indices of fatness and leanness

Relative weight

Relative weight (ratio of body weight to midpoint of the weight range for the appropriate sex, height, and frame size) has been used to categorize overweight and obesity in different individuals. Obesity has been defined as more than 120 per cent of standard weight. However, the move is away from reference-based comparators with all their problems to independent indices such as weight-to-height ratios. However, the cut-offs for these usually require recourse to the insurance company data.

Weight-to-height ratios

The simplicity of measurement and availability of normative data have contributed to the widespread use of these indices in population studies and in the clinics. The body mass index (W/H^2, kg/m^2), or Quetelet's index, is widely used as a simple assessment of fatness and leanness in Western populations. It correlates with fatness more highly ($r = 0.7$) than indices such as W/H or W/H^3 and is poorly correlated with height. This index is useful because it is relatively independent of height, although the requirement for height independence has recently been challenged. The addition of age to the body mass index improves the estimations of the percentage of the body mass as fat.

Weight is more fat-free mass than fat mass, and, not surprisingly, the body mass index is also well correlated with fat-free mass. Also, it does not discriminate between fat-free mass and fat mass so that it cannot separate the muscular from the overweight or obese. For an individual gaining or losing weight, or for setting targets, body mass index may offer no real advantage over weight as height remains constant and changing body mass index is determined by changing weight. Some endurance athletes have very low body mass indices within the range that nutritionists would interpret as chronic energy deficiency, which may well be the case. This raises the question of form versus function and the importance of long-term outcomes (see below).

Waist-to-hip circumference ratio

The site of deposition of fat is an independent risk factor for health, as important as the amount of fat. The ratio of the waist circumference to the hip circumference is a measure of intra-abdominal fatness. The waist-to-hip circumference ratio is a risk factor in cardiovascular disease.

Skinfold thickness

This measurement is the thickness of a so-called double fold of skin and underlying subcutaneous adipose tissue under a calliper jaw pressure of 10 g/mm^2. Skinfold thickness, when measured properly, correlates well ($r = 0.8$–0.9) with hydrostatic weighing, with a low standard error of estimate, that is 3 to 4 per cent of the body weight as fat. Their value in estimating percentage body weight as fat in young adults is well documented. Measurements of limb, trunk, and other skinfolds can be used to detect changes in fat distribution.

Proportionality

Size, shape, and composition cannot be described by single variables. Each has several components. The portrayal of multidimensional data is usually diagrammatic, for example somatograms, '0'-scales deviation.[9] The reference data may be obtained from national studies, data collected in single laboratories, or data for single groups of sportspeople. These methods have considerable merit theoretically, but have not proved to be popular with users as opposed to researchers.

Body density

One of the most accurate estimations of body composition is obtained from body density determined by hydrostatic weighing. Here, body density is calculated from body mass divided by body volume. An inexpensive system to measure body volume by underwater weighing has been described by Jones and Norgan.[10] The apparatus is transportable and does not require dedicated space as it is easily stored. It consists of a 3.5 m^3 cylindrical tank containing water heated to 35 to 36°C. A lightweight plastic chair is suspended from a calibrated force transducer mechanically protected against excess weights. The filtered output allows underwater weight to be measured to 0.02 kg in habituated subjects and to 0.05 kg in others.

Subjects are equipped with a snorkel and trained to submerge themselves gently to avoid water movement and undue weight oscillation. They learn to expire maximally underwater and carry out the rebreathing sequence needed to measure residual volume after the underwater weight has been taken. Residual volume is measured by the three-breath nitrogen dilution method at the same time as the weight is taken. After the necessary procedures have been learned by the subject, the measurements are made in duplicate or until two results agree to within 1 per cent fat. In our experience in a large series of middle-aged men and women, satisfactory results were obtained in two trials in 40 per cent of subjects and in three trials in 55 per cent of subjects. If more than three trials are required, the reasons for the variations should be established (e.g. fluctuating weight, poor rebreathing) before accepting duplicates. The learning and measurement of body density together with the associated anthropometry take about an hour. Subjects who are unfamiliar with immersion in water, such as non-swimmers, may require a greater degree of habituation in order to give consistent readings. In two separate studies on women aged 20 to 70 years and 35 to 55 years only 4 out of the total of 100 were unable to participate in underwater weighing.

The body density D (kg/m^3) is given by

$$D = \frac{\text{mass in air}}{[(\text{mass in air } - \text{mass in water})/\text{density of water}] - RV} \times 10^3$$

The residual volume RV (litres) at body pressure, ambient temperature, saturated with water vapour (BTPS) is given by

$$RV = 3.000 \times \frac{N - 0.5}{80 - N} \times \frac{Bp}{Bp - 47} \times \frac{310}{273 + t} - DS$$

when using 3 litres of dry 99.5 per cent oxygen (0.5 per cent nitrogen) at room temperature t (°C); Bp is the barometric pressure, and the saturated water vapour pressure at 37°C has a value of 47. *DS* is the dead space of the snorkel and tap, and the nitrogen content of alveolar air is assumed to be 80 per cent. N is the nitrogen content obtained by subtraction after measuring the oxygen and carbon dioxide in the expired and rebreathed air. Siri's equation, the most widely accepted equation for converting body density to body composition, is based on the assumption that fat has a known density of 900 kg/m^3 and that the fat-free mass density is, on average, 1100 kg/m^3.

The proportion (*ffm*) of the body weight that is fat free is given by Siri's equation:[11]

$$ffm = 1 - \left(\frac{4950}{D}\right) - 4.5$$

and the fat-free mass is given by

$$FFM = ffm \times body\ weight$$

Estimation procedures

Estimation of body density

The technique of hydrostatic weighing imposes severe restrictions of both practicality and convenience, so that the alternative procedure of estimating density from skinfold thicknesses is used for most purposes.

A skinfold measurement includes the double thickness of the dermis and the underlying subcutaneous adipose tissue. The sum of four skinfold thicknesses, invariably biceps, triceps, subscapular, and suprailiac, can be used to estimate body density and hence total body fat or fat-free mass. Many equations are available. For the general population, we recommend the equations of Durnin and Womersley[12] and of Jackson et al.[13] These equations are given in Appendix 1. The authors provide similar equations for individual skinfolds and all combinations of the four used in the Appendix, where the standard errors of estimation (SEEs) were 7.3 to 12.5 kg/m^3. Jackson and Pollock's equation for men aged 18 to 60 years is

$$D = 1109.4 - 0.827x + 0.0016x^2 - 0.257\ (age)$$

where x is the sum of chest, abdomen, and thigh skinfolds.[14] The SEE is 7.7 kg/m^3. The authors provide validated equations for the sum of seven skinfolds (the three above plus axilla, triceps, thigh, and suprailiac) transformed to natural logarithms and waist and forearm circumference.

Their equation for women aged 18 to 55 years is

$$D = 1099.5 - 0.993x + 0.0023x^2 - 0.139\ (age)$$

where x is the sum of triceps, thigh, and suprailiac skinfolds.[13] The SEE is 8.6 kg/m^3. The authors provide validated equations for the sum of four skinfolds (those listed above plus abdomen), seven skinfolds (the preceding plus chest, axilla, and subscapular), the natural logarithm of the sum of skinfolds, and the gluteal circumference.

All these equations have been cross-validated and have proved to be widely applicable. The suprailiac site of Durnin and Womersley differs from the usual site by being just above the iliac crest in the midline. The abdominal site described by Jackson and Pollock is adjacent to the umbilicus as opposed to the usual site of 50 mm to the left.[14] For the best estimate, it may be necessary to follow the site description given by the original authors. Whichever technique is used, this should be recorded in the reports of the study.

However, there may be inherent dangers in the use of equations which are derived from populations whose physical characteristics differ markedly from those of athletes. Evidence about the applicability of the commonly used equations to this special group is available from cross-validation surveys. Thorland et al.[15] compared 17 equations for estimating body density from skinfolds, circumferences, and diameters in adolescent male athletes and 15 equations for adolescent female athletes. Linear and quadratic forms gave acceptable accuracy for males whilst only quadratic equations did so for females. The male adolescent athletes seemed more similar in terms of body density to non-athletic populations than did the

females. This could explain why the estimations from equations were more applicable to males than females.

Sinning and coworkers[16,17] conducted similar studies using 265 male athletes and 79 female athletes. Of a total of 21 equations, only those of Jackson and Pollock gave estimates of percentage body fat which did not differ significantly from values obtained by hydrostatic weighing.[14] Overall, the equations tended to overestimate the percentage of body mass as fat in men. For women, the equation of Jackson et al.[13] which relied on four skinfolds gave a mean percentage of fat identical to that derived from hydrostatic weighing. No other equation was sufficiently accurate and, as in the men, there was a tendency towards overestimation.

The available evidence therefore suggests that, in athletes, the quadratic equations are more generalizable than the logarithmic or linear equations. If subjects with a greater range of age and density had been studied, this advantage might have been even more pronounced. Nevertheless, estimations derived from some linear equations were sound, for example Sloan's equation in men, whilst some based on quadratic equations were poor.

Estimation of limb cross-sectional areas

Estimates of limb muscle plus bone areas correlate well with strength and can be calculated from

$$A = (C - \pi S/10)^2/4\pi$$

where A is muscle plus bone area (cm^2), C is limb circumference (cm), and S is the appropriate limb skinfold or mean skinfold (mm). This formula can be applied to the mid-upper arm, the thigh, and the calf at the levels described in the next section. For the upper arm, the upper arm circumference and the biceps and triceps skinfolds are required. For the mid-thigh, the thigh circumference and the anterior thigh and posterior thigh skinfolds are measured. For the calf, the calf circumference and the medial and lateral calf skinfolds are required. It is recommended that two skinfolds should be taken at each level.

Subcutaneous adipose tissue (SCAT) areas can be calculated by subtracting A from the total limb area:

$$SCAT = C^2/4\pi - A\ cm^2$$

Anthropometric techniques and instrumentation

The techniques and methods of measuring anthropometry and body composition variables that are useful in sports medicine or related studies are described in this section. The descriptions include the anatomical landmarks, sites, and conventions adopted. Precision and accuracy of measurement are crucial in anthropometry to evaluate measurements, particularly if serial measurements are made to categorize changes. More commonly, measurements are compared with norms or reference values of some type. The deviation from the reference can be calculated or a series of deviations for a series of measurements can be determined, leading to a scale or profile.

Basic anthropometric techniques

The basic anthropometric techniques are as follows:

- body mass (weight)
- stature (height)
- biepicondylar humerus
- upper arm circumference
- triceps skinfold
- subscapular skinfold

By convention, measurements are taken on the left side of the body where appropriate. Some measurements require landmarks to be identified and marked. These are given at the beginning of the measurement. In many cases an observer can greatly assist the measurer and check the technique.

Body mass (kg)

The apparatus required is a weighing machine. The subject should be lightly clothed. The weight of the clothes or representative garments should be recorded and subtracted from the body mass.

Stature (height) (mm)

The apparatus required is a stadiometer (wall-mounted stadiometer or portable anthropometer). The landmark is the Frankfort plane—the position of the head when the imaginary line from the lower border of the left orbit to the upper meatus is horizontal.

The subject should stand on a horizontal platform with the heels together, stretching upwards to the full extent. Gentle upward pressure is exerted on the mastoid processes by the measurer who encourages the subject to 'stand tall, take a deep breath, and relax'. The subject's back should be as straight as possible, which can be achieved by rounding or relaxing the shoulders and manipulating the posture. The head is held in the Frankfort plane. Either the horizontal arm of the anthropometer or a counterweighted board is brought down on the subject's head. If an anthropometer is used, one measurer should hold the instrument vertical with the horizontal arm in contact with the subject's head, while another applies gentle upward pressure. The subject's heels must be watched to ensure that they do not leave the ground.

Biepicondylar humerus (cm)

The apparatus required is an anthropometer or sliding calliper. The subject's arm is bent at a right angle and the width across the outermost parts of the lower end of the humerus is taken. The measurement is usually oblique since the medial epicondyle of the humerus is lower than the lateral.

Upper arm circumference (cm)

The apparatus required is a tape. The landmark is a horizontal mark on the left upper arm, measured halfway between the inferior border of the acromial process and the tip of the olecranon process, with the arm flexed at a right angle.

The measurement is performed with the arm relaxed and hanging beside the body, and the hand supinated. When measuring a circumference the tape should be at right angles to the long axis and contact with the skin should be continuous along the tape, but the skin should not be compressed.

Skinfold thicknesses (mm)

The skinfold is picked up vertically between thumb and forefinger and the calliper jaws are applied at exactly the level marked. The measurement is read 2 s after full pressure of the calliper jaws is applied to the skinfold; if a longer interval is allowed, the reading may 'creep'. Skinfold callipers are used for the measurements.

The landmark for the triceps skinfold measurement is the same as that for the upper arm thickness. The skinfold is picked up at the back of the arm about 1 cm above the level described for the upper arm thickness, directly in line with the olecranon process.

For measurement of the subscapular skinfold, the subject stands with shoulders relaxed and arms by his or her sides. The inferior angle of the scapula is located and the skinfold is lifted, slightly inclined downwards and laterally in the natural cleavage lines.

Additional anthropometric techniques

The choice of additional measurements will depend on how comprehensive a description of size and an estimation of composition are required. This is likely to be influenced by the time, resources, and personnel available, and whether the measurements are made in the laboratory or the field. The following additional anthropometric measurements could be useful where the aims of the study have been carefully considered in relation to either the size or shape of sports competitors.

Chest circumference (cm)

The apparatus required is a tape. The circumference is measured horizontally at the junction of the third and fourth sternebrae. The arms are raised to allow the tape to be passed round the trunk and lowered once it is in position. The measurement is taken during normal light breathing in mid-inspiration.

Waist circumference (cm)

The apparatus required is a tape. The landmark is in the mid-axillary line at the midpoint between the costal margin and iliac crest. This is often the natural waist. The tape is lowered from the position in which the chest circumference is measured to the level of the waist marking.

Hip circumference (cm)

The apparatus required is a tape. The subject stands with feet together and at an angle of approximately 15°. The tape is lowered to the level of the trochanters, which is used as a guide for location of the maximum hip circumference. The observer ensures that the tape remains horizontal, while the tape is raised and lowered until the maximum circumference is found.

Mid-thigh circumference (cm)

The apparatus required is a tape. The landmark is the mid-thigh. With the subject sitting, the mark is at the point between the centre of the inguinal crease and the proximal border of the patella.

The subject stands with the weight on the right leg and the left leg relaxed and slightly bent. The measurement is made round the thigh level with the landmark.

Calf circumference (cm)

The apparatus required is a tape. The subject sits with his lower limbs relaxed. The maximal horizontal circumference is measured, using the belly of the gastrocnemius as a guide.

Sitting height (m)

The apparatus required is an anthropometer or sitting height table. The measurement is made with the subject's back stretched up straight, sitting on a table top with the feet hanging down unsupported over the edge; the backs of the knees should be directly above the edge of the table. Extension of the spine should be encouraged in the same way as for stature. Gentle upward pressure is applied under the chin; the muscles of the thighs and buttocks should be relaxed. The head is held as in the measurement of stature and the anthropometer is stood vertically in contact with the back at the sacral and interscapular regions. If a sitting height table is used, the movable backboard is brought into contact with the subject's back and the headboard is lowered to rest firmly against the head.

Biacromial diameter (cm)

The apparatus required is an anthropometer. The landmark is the inferior edge of the most lateral border of the acromial process.

To give maximum shoulder width the subject stands with shoulders relaxed by pulling the shoulders slightly downwards and forwards. Standing behind the subject, the measurer feels for the outside edge of the acromial process of the shoulder blade which can be detected as a ridge just above the shoulder joint. The measurer then places the edge of one arm of the anthropometer along the lateral border of one acromial process and brings the other arm of the anthropometer inwards until its edge rests on the lateral border of the opposite acromial process.

Bi-iliac diameter (cm)

The apparatus required is an anthropometer. The subjects stands with heels together and the anthropometer arms are brought into contact with the iliac crests at the place which gives the maximum diameter. The measurement should always be taken with the measurer standing behind the subject. As in measurements of the biepicondylar humerus and the biacromial diameter, sufficient pressure should be applied so that the calliper blades compress the soft tissues.

Biceps skinfold (mm)

The apparatus required is a skinfold calliper. The landmark is as for the measurement of the upper arm circumference.

The skinfold is measured with the subject's arm relaxed by the side with the palm facing forward. It is measured on the anterior of the arm, over the belly of the biceps muscle, at the level of the mid-upper arm marking described for the upper arm circumference measurement.

Suprailiac skinfold (mm)

The apparatus required is a skinfold calliper. The landmark is the iliac crest. The most prominent superior border of the iliac crest is in the mid-axillary line. The skinfold is picked up vertically approximately 1 cm above the landmark.

Mid-anterior thigh skinfold (mm)

The apparatus required is a skinfold calliper. The landmark is the mid-thigh. With the subject sitting, a mark is made midway between the inguinal crease and the proximal border of the patella as for the measurement of the mid-thigh circumference.

The subject stands with the weight on the right leg so that the left leg is relaxed. The skinfold is taken vertically, in the midline, on the anterior aspect of the thigh at the level of the mid-thigh marking.

Some of these measurement descriptions are based on the guide to field methods prepared for the Human Adaptability Section of the International Biological Programme and subsequently updated.[18] These sources contain descriptions of other anthropometric measurements used mainly in growth and physical anthropology and detailed descriptions of instruments. A further source of measurement descriptions is the recent manual edited by Lohman et al.[19] A feature of this well-illustrated publication is that the technique, purpose, literature, reliability, and sources of reference data are given for each measurement, and the recommendations are likely to be adopted widely, at least in North America.

Instruments

A list of instruments, together with the names and addresses of the supplier, that are suitable for undertaking anthropometric measurements such as stature (height), lengths, breadths, girths, and skinfold thicknesses, either in the laboratory or for field studies, can be found in Appendix 2.

Other body composition techniques

Other body composition techniques, including two relatively new pieces of equipment that can be used either in the field or laboratory, are described in this section. They are useful as quick and socially acceptable body composition measurements where a change in value is of more interest than an answer in absolute terms.

Bioelectrical impedance analysis

The measurement of human body composition by bioelectrical impedance analysis treats the body as consisting of two compartments: the fat-free mass and the fat mass. The fat-free mass contains virtually all the electrolytes and body fluids which are involved in conduction, so that the impedance of the body can be used as an estimate of fat-free mass. The impedance of a conductor is related to its length and cross-sectional area:

$$Z = r \, L/A$$

where Z is the impedance in ohms (Ω), r is the volume resistivity (Ω cm), L is the length of the conductor (cm), and A is its area (cm^2). Multiplying by L/L gives

$$Z = r \, L^2/AL$$

where AL will be equal to the volume V:

$$Z = r \, L^2/V \text{ or } V = r \, L^2/Z$$

The key assumptions are that the body geometry is a simple cylinder, that body temperature is constant and that electrolytes and water are uniformly distributed.

Bioelectrical impedance was not used in the evaluation of human body composition until 1981 when Nyboer developed a tetrapolar electrode method.[20] Four electrodes, placed on the dorsal surfaces of the hands and feet, are used to minimize the contact impedance. A current of 800 mA at 50 kHz is applied at the distal electrodes, and the voltage drop at the proximal electrodes is measured. Operators should be aware that displacement of the electrodes by 1 cm at the wrist and the ankle will produce a combined change in impedance of 4.1 per cent, equivalent to a 3 per cent change in body mass as fat. As the technique is dependent upon the water content of the body, factors which may alter body water content, such as alcohol consumption and exercise before measurement, are avoided. Regression equations have been developed relating total body water (measured by D²O dilution) to impedance measurements (usually as Ht^2/Z). These also include anthropometric variables to reflect body geometry. Here, and with near-infrared interactance described below, there is debate as to the relative contributions of anthropometry and the body's electrical propoerties. As the total body water forms a relatively constant proportion of the fat-free mass, the latter can be calculated from total body water and fat mass calculated from the difference between body mass and fat-free mass.

The technique has been frequently and critically reviewed.[21,22] A number of instruments to measure impedance are available, and a number of equations have been developed to estimate body composition from impedance values. When compared with densitometry, the SEE of percentage body fat calculated using various instruments and equations has been reported to vary widely, between 2.7 and 6.1 per cent. Some workers have found bioelectrical impedance analysis to be a better predictor of hydrostatically determined body fat than anthropometry (SEE 3.5 per cent) and a better predictor of changes in body water and fat-free mass than anthropometry. Bioelectrical impedance, like most body composition estimation techniques, performs less well at the ends of the range of body composition. As this is where most sportspeople lie, there is a case for population-specific estimations equations.

The latest development is of multifrequency bioelectrical impedance.[23] The frequency of the current determines whether it crosses the cell membrane and indexes extracellular water and total body water. What these studies show is that intracellular fluid has a higher specific resistivity than extracellular fluid, thus highlighting that the simple impedance approach is always dependent on the distribution of water between the two main compartments.

The cost-effectiveness of bioelectrical impedance analysis equipment, relative to its accuracy, must be seriously questioned. It is unlikely that improvements in a 'high tech' design will overcome the limitations caused by the shape of the human body.

Bioelectrical impedance is popular because it is inexpensive, simple to use, and its precision is good. Its limitations are often overlooked in the enthusiasm of adopting and using a technique with such advantages.

Near-infrared interactance

Near-infrared interactance involves irradiating a sample in the near-infrared spectrum and determining the proportion of energy transmitted which returns to the detector. The interactance theoretically depends on the distance through which the radiation travels, as well as the physical properties of the substance irradiated, according to the Beer–Lambert law:

$$\text{interactance} = I/I^0 = 10^{-kcL} \text{ or } \log^{10}(I/I^0) = kcL$$

where I is the intensity of radiation emerging, I^0 is the intensity transmitted, k is the molar absorption coefficient, c is the molar concentration, and L is the path length through which the radiation travels.

Each substance has its own absorption spectrum with characteristic peaks. For example, there is a peak for fat and a trough for water at 930 nm, and a peak for water and a trough for fat at 970 nm. These absorption spectral differences can be exploited for measurement of human body composition because adipose tissue is high in fat and muscle is high in water content. The relative absorptions at two wavelengths, at one of which there is a greater absorption for fat

and at the other a greater absorption for muscle, can be used to obtain information about relative proportions of fat and muscle. The radiation used is non-ionizing and of low intensity, and so the measurement is harmless.

A commercial instrument, the Futrex 5000 (Futrex Inc.), is available. It consists of a light wand with four infrared-emitting diodes, two emitting radiation at a wavelength of 940 nm and two at 950 nm. These illuminate a circular diffusing ring which allows radiation to be emitted evenly. In the centre is a silicon detector which measures the intensity of re-emitted light. The light wand is attached to a Hitachi microprocessor from which the optical density readings ($\log 1/I$) can be read. The manufacturers have calibrated each machine against their own hydrostatic weighing measurements to allow estimation of percentage body fat from optical density readings at the biceps for, body weight, height, sex, and activity level. This method had an SEE of 3 per cent body fat in a cross-validation group of 17 men and women when a sophisticated computerized spectrophotometer was used. The criterion method was based on isotope dilution assessment of total body water. Modelling of the performance of a low cost, portable apparatus suggests an SEE of 3 to 4 per cent body fat. Comparisons of estimates of percentage fat measurements by Futrex 5000 with hydrostatic weighing in 39 males and females gave an SEE of 3.1 per cent fat for males and 4.3 per cent for females.

A number of studies have found the accuracy of near-infrared interactance to be similar to, or poorer than, that of skinfolds, with overestimation in leaner and underestimation in fatter subjects.[24-27] Several factors may contribute to this poor accuracy. Measurement is made at the biceps site only—using multiple sites has not been found to improve body composition estimates. Addition of interactance data does not greatly improve prediction of body fat above other variables in the prediction equations: gender, weight, height, and activity level.[26,27] Interactance at the two wavelengths measured is very highly correlated, and including a second wavelength does not improve prediction of body fat.[26] Moreover, work at our laboratory has found that although interactance is correlated with subcutaneous adipose tissue thickness, skinfold thickness has a better correlation with the latter.[28]

Despite some of these limitations, body composition assessments using near-infrared technology are in widespread use by health care professionals, fitness trainers, and medical assessors, whose advice athletes and non-athletes seek to gain information about body fatness and the changes required to maintain the levels recommended for everyday life and for participation in sport.

A more advanced body composition analyser, the Futrex 6000, has been under development for the past 3 years and is currently being evaluated by two laboratories in the United States. It contains a light wand with six infrared-emitting diodes measuring a broader range of wavelengths at 866, 871, 878, 938, 945, and 952 nm, in an attempt to better discriminate fat and water.

Isotope dilution

Measurement of body water alone by single-labelled (deuterium-labelled) water has provided information on body composition. The analytical standard error is about 1 litre of water, equivalent to 1.4 kg of fat-free mass. Factor analysis of data in patients suggests that values for fat-free mass obtained from body water have more random errors than those from skinfolds.[29] Equilibration periods of 3 to 5 h may be a consideration for some investigators.

Naturally occurring and induced radiation

These techniques require apparatus beyond the scope of most laboratories. Detection of the naturally occurring γ-radiation from potassium allows a measurement of body potassium content with a standard error of 4 per cent, equivalent to more than 2 kg of fat-free mass. The calculation of fat-free mass from potassium content has evoked more controversy than other body composition technique.

In vivo neutron activation analysis provides a means of estimating the body content of up to seven elements (potassium, carbon, calcium, nitrogen, phosphorus, sodium, and chlorine) with one whole-body irradiation. The precision (standard deviation of repeated measures) of fat-free mass and fat mass measurements of 0.7 kg is similar to that for body density, but more confidence may be justified in these more direct measurements of multiconstituents. The use of ionizing radiation and the expense are obstacles to widespread adoption, and its main value may be in the validation of other methods.

Total body electrical conductivity

This is another method with bulky, expensive apparatus. Values for SEE of 1.4 kg fat-free mass have been reported. Direct carcass analysis of pigs suggest an SEE value of 2.8 kg fat-free mass. Recent cross-validation trials have shown this technique to underestimate percentage body fat by 3.6 per cent in 117 males aged 20 to 90 years and 0.8 per cent in 178 females aged 19 to 89, when compared with underwater weighing.[30]

Computed tomography and magnetic resonance imaging

Computed tomography (**CT**) and magnetic resonance imaging (**MRI**) are newer methods of imaging with great potential but limited applicability. As with other approaches, the high cost restricts the availability of these methods and CT also uses ionizing radiation. These methods provide cross-sectional views of the body and a series of scans can be used to provide estimates of fat mass and fat-free mass and to establish regional fat distribution. MRI accurately quantifies adipose tissue *in vivo* in 75-kg pigs.[31] It is safe to use with children and may eventually supersede CT scanning in the field of body composition, although its long scan time is a disadvantage. The immediate value of these methods to the field has been in validating existing and new simpler techniques, as in the case of CT and limb cross-sectional areas. van der Kooy and Seidell[32] have produced a good practical guide to the imaging techniques for the study of body composition. New advances have been made in the field of CT, importantly the current scan range can now be displayed on the monitor in real time and the topogram can be ended as soon as the desired volume has been attained. This novelty thus prevents unnecessary patient exposure to radiation.

Soft tissue radiography

This provides an accurate assessment of regional, particularly appendicular, body composition provided that care is taken with tissue magnification, subject positioning, and subject protection from X-radiation. The method should not be used with children and has become less popular because of the radiation exposure, the limited number of sites that can be measured, and the development of other non-hazardous techniques.

Ultrasound

Ultrasound methods directly measure the depth of adipose and muscle tissue thickness by passing high- frequency sound waves through the skin–fat layer and then reflecting them back off the fat-–muscle and/or muscle–bone interface. Calibration of the ultrasound system is important and is achieved by measuring the time taken for the echo to return to the transducer and converting this to a distance measurement that assumes the velocity of ultrasound in soft tissue is 1450 m/s in adipose tissue and 1580 m/s in muscle. A-scan (amplitude-modulated) ultrasound is not a new technique but several portable machines are now available. Ideally, ultrasound should provide measurements of single, uncompressed, subcutaneous, adipose tissue thickness avoiding the interference of varying tissue compressibility from skinfold callipers. To achieve this, uniform and constant transducer pressure at the skin surface is essential. The identification of the tissue interfaces can be difficult at some sites and in some individuals, but improved instrumentation, particularly displays, help overcome this problem. For the estimation of body density, the SEE using subcutaneous adipose tissue from ultrasound is only 0.5 kg/m³ lower than that from skinfolds. Apart from measurements on obese people, when the expense, measurement time, and absence of extensive validation trials and reference data are taken into account, ultrasound does not prove to be superior to callipers. Ramirez has reviewed the area.[33]

Photon absorptiometry, broadband ultrasonic attenuation, and contact ultrasonic broadband attenuation

Measurement of bone mineral by the absorption of monoenergetic photon energy from radionuclides is useful for investigating the composition of its fat-free mass. Single-photon absorptiometry of limb bones such as the radius can be made with portable apparatus in the field. Correct positioning of the limb is crucial for high precision and accuracy. As an estimate of skeletal mass, it has an error of 10 per cent. Dual-photon absorptiometry has a high precision (2 to 3 per cent) in humans and accuracy of 1 per cent for skeletons. The error of estimate compared with *in vivo* neutron activation analysis is 113 g of total body mineral, that is about 2 per cent. However, the apparatus is expensive and difficult to transport.

Bone density measurements by ultrasound are usually made at the calcaneus or patella since they have a high percentage of cancellous bone and the medial and lateral sides are approximately parallel. The new approaches of broadband ultrasonic attenuation use non-ionizing radiation and portable equipment. Coefficients of variation ranging from 2 to 5 per cent have been reported. Broadband ultrasonic attenuation is stated to reflect both bone mineral content and structural parameters.[34]

Dual energy X-ray absorptiometry (DEXA)

This technique was introduced in 1989 and has become a valuable research tool for assessing axial and appendicular bone mineral density and or fat/muscle content of the whole body or body segments *in vivo*. It was a natural development of dual-photon absorptiometry and uses two photon energies to allow for different absorber thickness and inhomogeneities overlying the sites of measurement in the lumbar spine, neck of the femur, and distal radius. The X-ray source permits greater photon flux and so measurements are quicker and more precise (about 1 per cent) than with dual-photon absorptiometry, although the results are very highly correlated.

DEXA is still being developed as a reliable method for soft tissues. It has been described as a boon, but most workers regard any elevation to the gold standard of body composition methods as premature.[35] It is not free from assumptions about hydration or of the proportions of protein to water and its accuracy for soft tissue is questionable.[36] There is variability between instruments of different manufacturers in methods of calibration, data acquisition and analysis, and in the results obtained when the same subjects are measured in the three main types of analysers. In the case of bone mineral density, the difference due to the different calibration procedures is as much as 12 to 15 per cent. Frequent software upgrades make comparability of machines, studies, and methods difficult. The advantages of DEXA are that it is quick and that the radiation dose is low. Difficulties may be experienced accommodating large individuals in scanners. The data obtained include cross-sectional areas of lean and fat and volumes of tissues that can be calculated from serial scans.

Applications
Applicability of methods

Anthropometry involves simple objective measurement without inherent assumptions, although there are exceptions to this in the calculations of areas and volumes where perfect circles, cones, or pyramids are assumed to represent parts of the body. However, the estimation of body composition *in vivo* requires assumptions about the relationships of the proportions of constituents of the body. These relationships differ in the sexes, change with age, differ between and within performers, and during training, etc. The significance of these variations to the accuracy of the estimates of body composition needs to be considered. Fortunately, in sports, the individual and changes in the individual, rather than the group, are usually the units of interest to coaches, doctors, or selectors.

The transformation of physical values of density, resistivity, interactance, and ultrasound attenuation, and the chemical values of water, potassium, or calcium content, to whole or regional body composition estimates requires the relationships between them to be established. Many have been defined for young adult men and women, but not for elite athletes or the other stages of the life-span.

The water and mineral contents of fat-free mass are lower in children than in adults. In athletes with high proportions of muscle, fat-free mass density is lower. In both of these cases fatness will be overestimated. Body densities of more than 1100 kg/m³ have been described, that is negative body fat contents. These examples indicate the inapplicability of the methods to every situation.

To overcome problems such as these, multicomponent models and methods of body composition measurement have been introduced. Commonly, two or more measurements of body density, water content, and mineral content will be taken and fatness and leanness calculated. This improves the accuracy of the estimate. The fundamental equations expressing the relationships between body composition and constituents are reformulated and applied to new groups. This is exemplified by the new equations available for calculating the body composition of children.[37] Suggested revisions to Siri's equation for age, level of nutrition, and activity have appeared over many years, but the evidence for modifications was weak as the topic is characterized by widespread circularity of reasoning. Methods that require constancy of proportions of constituents in order to be valid are used to show that the proportions change or differ.

Effects on body composition

Of the variable fat-free mass components, for example total body water, protein, and osseous minerals, the one most likely to have the greatest effect on body composition determinations is the skeleton. The substantial body of evidence that bone mineral density is markedly higher in sportsmen and sportswomen than in their less active contemporaries calls into question the validity and applicability of Siri's equation to estimate the percentage of body mass as fat.

Other factors, such as ethnic group, age, and sex, influence the density of the fat-free mass. For example, a decrease in the degree of osseous mineralization of about 1 per cent per year occurs after the age of 50. Durnin and Womersley[12] have calculated that a 15 per cent decrease in the body mineral content results in a fall in the density of the fat-free mass of about 6 kg/m³, approximately a 15 per cent error on percentage body fat. The potential extent of the distortion of the estimates of fat-free mass in athletes is of a similar order if one assumed, quite reasonably, that athletes possessed 18 per cent higher bone mineral density than the population from which Siri's equation was based. Such changes play an important role in influencing the validity of body fat estimations from body density measurements. This has been clearly shown when spuriously low values for the percentage of body mass as fat have been reported for athletes by using conventional methods of estimation.

Thus it follows that if sports participants have denser bones and muscles, this will result in an underestimation of their body fat. Conversely, if osteoporosis is present in the skeleton, this reduces the bone density and leads to overestimation of the body fat.

Applicability to changing states
Acute
Many sports competitions are based on weight classes. Individuals attempt to perform at the top end of a weight category as weight is usually an advantage and determinant of performance. Frequently, participants will have to 'make the weight'—lose a kilogram or more to meet the requirement.

The composition of weight loss depends on the deviation and degree of water and energy balance. The initial weight loss and high weight loss in a short time will predominantly consist of water or lean tissue. Neither of these are consistent with optimum functioning. Proper and improper weight loss programmes have been the topic of a position statement of the American College of Sports Medicine.[38]

In this context, these weight loss procedures, although accurately reflected by weight changes, compromise the body composition measurements. The composition of the fat-free mass is altered and affects the interpretations of density and body water measurements, and probably also alters measurements of skinfolds, bioelectrical impedance analysis, and near-infrared interactance. Thus, in acute weight loss, weight changes do not reflect losses of lean or fat and the accuracy of body composition measurements is also affected. The way forward would be to regard these losses as water, often associated with losses of lean tissue or diminution of the glycogen stores. The arithmetic of the energy balance equation should be checked before any claims for sizeable fat losses are claimed.

Chronic

Longer-term efforts by sports participants to modify body composition involve reducing the fat content by strict control of food intake and, to a greater or lesser degree depending on the sport, to increase leanness or muscularity by conditioning, particularly weight training. Both methods are widespread in recreational participants and elite athletes.

There is more information in the literature on weight loss than on any other aspect of human energetics. Unfortunately, it concentrates on attempts by persons who are overweight or obese to move towards the midpoint of the range. Sports participants are attempting to move beyond this to the end of the range. Whereas the arithmetic and efficiency of energy utilization remain unchanged, the composition of tissue lost, and hence the extent to which weight loss compromises estimates of body composition and changes in composition, depends on the initial body composition. In underfeeding studies of at least 4-week duration, the proportion of lean in weight loss was negatively and exponentially related to initial fatness. Dieting alone is an inappropriate weight loss strategy for most athletes. Some exercise to maintain or increase leaness is required. The common experience of weight loss and resistance training regimes is of modest changes that reverse easily. The dedicated participant is more successful, as evinced by the well-known changes in body form and muscle development and definition unaided by artificial means. However, the exact role of agents such as anabolic steroids in modifying body composition remains controversial.

Changes in body composition need to be greater than 1 kg to be detected by current methods. Gains of lean tissue of more than 3 to 5 kg occur slowly and might best be reflected by serial weight measurements. Measurements of total body water would be less affected by changing compositions and could be used to determine whether the changes could be ascribed to lean tissue.

Contemporary issues

Hazards of thinness

Much is known of the dangers of raised morbidity and mortality in persons who are overweight or obese but, in contrast, little is known about the dangers of thinness, natural or induced. The relationships between mortality and body mass index are J-shaped. The body mass index associated with the lowest mortality increases with age. It is commonly assumed that the raised mortality at low body mass index arises from individuals with existing but unrecognized disease or from smokers with their lower body weights. There is a higher than expected mortality from pneumonia and influenza, malignant neoplasms, suicides, and hypertensive heart disease. However, observations such as the increase in life expectancy of populations over the last 200 years coinciding with an increase in body weight, and the rise in the body mass index with lowest mortality in the 1959 and 1979 insurance company data suggest that thinness may have other ill-defined risks. Although induced extreme leanness is regarded by coaches and athletes as increasing performance in, for example, middle-distance running, a fitness–health dichotomy follows the hazards of thinness. The groups at risk may be jockeys, runners, and ballet dancers, who participate for many years, and gymnasts.

The association of disturbance of menstruation and other aspects of reproductive function in women athletes is well known and has been reviewed repeatedly.[39] Concerns about the effects of prolonged hard training and dieting on bone mineral content have also arisen.

Body composition and menstrual status in athletes: the hazards of estimations

Many women athletes with high training loads develop menstrual irregularities such as secondary oligomenorrhoea or amenorrhoea. The condition is also common (up to 50 per cent) in ballet dancers, but less so in swimmers and cyclists. Frisch and McArthur[40] proposed that a minimum level of fat is required to initiate menarche (17 per cent) and to maintain regular menstrual function (22 per cent). It is suggested that adequate energy stores as fat are required for successful pregnancy and lactation and this trigger has evolved. The mechanism may be a degree of conversion of androgens to oestrogens in the adipocyte affecting steroid feedback to the hypothalamus or pituitary gland. The evidence advanced for the hypothesis included the observations that girls who mature early usually weigh more than their peers, that body weight at menarche is independent of menarcheal age, that both ballet dancers and females with anorexia have a high incidence of amenorrhoea, and that very obese men have raised serum oestradiol, decreased serum testosterone, and an increased conversion of androstanedione to oestrone.

The hypothesis of Frisch and colleagues that body fat is a determinant of mature sexual function in women was anchored on the lower variability in fatness than in body weight at menarche, yet this is also true at other ages during growth. Other evidence against the hypothesis is the considerable ranges in weight and fatness at menarche and in groups of eumenorrhoeal and amenorrhoeal athletes. Also, changing training status without alteration of body weight or fatness and the development of changing menstrual function indicates an absence of a link between body composition and menstrual function. Thus, increasing the training distance of runners or introducing training to the untrained resulted in the majority developing abnormal menses. Conversely, ballet dancers report resuming menstruation on vacation or during injury. Thus the stress of the exercise appears a more likely determinant of menstrual function than critical levels of weight or fatness. The mechanism may be neural rather than hormonal, although other hormone responses such as prolactin may be involved. A predisposition to abnormalities may remain. A greater proportion of amenorrhoeal athletes report a prior history of irregular menses than is the case in eumenorrhoeal athletes.

Frisch and coworkers estimated body fatness from measurements of height and weight using a regression equation to estimate body water and from that percentage fat. This equation was based on data from 27 girls and 18 young women that had not been cross-validated and, like all estimation equations, it performs less well at the ends of the range. In particular, it is not accurate for women with less than 22 per cent fat. The work of Frisch and her colleagues has been criticised on statistical grounds of improper data analysis and interpretation of results. When measurements are made with body composition estimates that are more reliable, controlling for age, size, training load, and fitness, percentage fat values in amenorrhoeal and eumenorrhoeal runners are identical.

This is not the end of the question, however, as athletes may differ from non-athletes in the composition of fat-free mass, affecting estimates of body composition by the traditional techniques usually regarded as reliable. This is not a problem if amenorrhoeal and eumenorrhoeal athletes are equally affected, but low bone mass (osteopenia) is more common in amenorrhoeal athletes than in those with normal functions. Percentage fat will be overestimated if the bone mineral content is less than that assumed.

Osteoporosis

Osteoporosis is a disease characterized by low bone mass and microarchitectural deterioration of bone tissue, leading to enhanced bone fragility and a consequent increase in fracture risk. It is a complex multicausal chronic disease with major, worldwide, health care implications in Europe and North America, recognized by the World Health Organization.[41] The condition is most common in postmenopausal women, with serious consequences for at least one-third of older (>50 years) women and 15 to 20 per cent of older (>50 years) men. The incidence of osteoporotic fracture is increasing faster than can be explained by the increase in age of the population.[42]

Physical inactivity is associated with increased risk of osteoporotic fracture,[43] so it has been suggested that physical activities and sports may be effective in optimizing bone mass, thus reducing the incidence of osteoporosis. Evidence of the association of long-term habitual exercise with bone mineral content and density largely comes from studies in athletes. Cross-sectional studies show that athletes, particularly those who are strength trained, have greater bone mineral density than non-athletes. In addition, strength, muscle mass, and maximal oxygen uptake correlate with bone density.[44] Cross-sectional studies, however, are liable to selection bias: Dalen and Olsson[45] showed that mineral content of the calcaneus, humerus, radius, and ulna in a group of cross-country runners was higher by 20 per cent than that in non-runners matched for age and body size. Whilst these differences may be due in part to mechanical stresses imposed by exercise, the fact that some of these sites were not stressed during running confirms the importance of constitutional differences between athletes and others. However, a higher mineral content of cortical bone has been found in the dominant arm compared to the non-dominant arm in unilateral exercises such as tennis.[46] Longitudinal studies indicate that lack of weight bearing, imposed by long-term bed rest, results in marked bone loss,[47] whereas strength training and high-impact endurance training increase bone density.[48] However, amenorrhoea associated with intensive endurance training may lead to decreased trabecular bone density in premenopausal female athletes.

In conclusion, the increased bone mass observed in athletes may be partly due to selection bias. Longitudinal studies confirm that taking up a programme of exercise or sport does provoke modest increases in bone mass, although the beneficial effects of increased mechanical loading may be counteracted by oestrogen deficiency in athletic amenorrhoea.

Concluding comments

Anthropometric and body composition techniques are becoming commonplace in the sports medicine clinic and the human performance laboratory. The size, shape, and composition of athletes and recreational sports participants correlate with performance and indicate condition and potential. To yield precise, reliable, and, most importantly, useful information, standardized measurement procedures are essential. The validity of the information is strongly dependent on the applicability of these techniques to the sports population and particularly the elite athlete. This has been considered but is an area that will change rapidly as more information becomes available. Future trends are likely to be towards multidimensional scaling systems and multicomponent descriptions of body composition based on population-specific approaches. The coexistence of anthropometry and body composition measurements with exercise and sports science has been mutually beneficial and synergistic, and this is also likely to be the case in the future.

Appendix 1
Recommended equations for the estimation of the body density of men and women

$D = a + b(x)$ where $x = \log^{10}$ sum (biceps, triceps, subscapular, and suprailiac skinfolds) and D is the density; a and b are given in the table below.

Age (years)	Men		Women	
	a	b	a	b
17–19	1162.0	63.0	1154.9	67.8
20–29	1163.1	63.2	1159.9	71.7
30–39	1142.2	54.4	1142.3	63.2
40–49	1162.0	70.0	1133.3	61.2
50 +	1171.5	77.9	1133.9	64.5
17–70	1176.5	74.4	1156.7	71.7

Reproduced from ref. 12 with permission from Cambridge University Press.

The authors provide similar equations for individual skinfolds and all combinations of the four used here. The SEE values were 7.3 to 12.5 kg/m³. SEE values for other groups will be higher (see text).

For men aged 18 to 60 years:

$$D = 1109.4 - 0.827x + 0.0016x^2 - 0.257 \text{ (age)}$$

where x is the sum of chest, abdomen, and thigh skinfolds and SEE = 7.7 kg/m³.[14] The authors provide validated equations for the sum of seven skinfolds (those above plus axilla, triceps, thigh, and suprailiac) transformed to natural logarithms and waist and forearm circumference.

For women aged 18 to 55 years:

$$D = 1099.5 - 0.993x + 0.0023x^2 - 0.139 \text{ (age)}$$

where x is the sum of triceps, thigh, and suprailiac skinfold and SEE = 8.6 kg/m³.[13] These authors provide validated equations for the sum of four skinfolds (those above plus abdomen), seven skinfolds (the preceding plus chest, axilla, subscapular), natural logarithm of the sum of skinfolds, and gluteal circumference.

Appendix 2
Instruments

List of instruments, together with the names and addresses of the supplier:

Harpenden stadiometer	Holtain Ltd, Crosswell,
Harpenden anthropometer	Crymmych, Dyfed SA41 3UF,
Harpenden sitting height table	Wales
Harpenden bicondylar callipers	
Flexible 2-m measuring tapes	
Holtain skinfold callipers	
GPM (Martin type)	Pfister Import–Export Inc.,
Anthropometer	450 Barell Avenue, Carlstadt,
	NJ 07072, USA
	Owl Industries Ltd,
	177 Idema Road,
	Markham, Ontario L3R 1A9,
	Canada
Harpenden skinfold callipers	British Indicators Ltd, Quality
	House, 46–56 Dumfries Street,
	Luton, Beds LU1 5BP, UK
	H. E. Morse Co., 455 Douglas
	Avenue, Holland, MI 49423,
	USA
Harpenden electronic read-out	HUMAG Research Group,
incorporating computer system	Department of Human
(HEROICS) skinfold callipers	Sciences, Loughborough
	University, Loughborough,
	Leics LE11 3TU, UK
CMS weighing scales	CMS Weighing Equipment
	Ltd, 18 Camden High Street,
	London NW1 0JH, UK
Salter weighing scales	Salter International,
	Measurement Ltd, George
	Street, West Bromwich, Staffs,
	UK
Toledo electronic scales	Toledo Scale, 431 Ohio Pike,
	Suite 302, Way Cross Office
	Park, Toledo, OH, USA
Linen measuring tape	Pfister Import–Export Inc.,
	450 Barell Avenue, Carlstadt,
	NJ 07072, USA
Anthropometric tape measure	County Technology Inc., PO
	Box 87, Gays Mill, WI 54631,
	USA

References

1. Behnke AR, Feen BG, Welham WC. The specific gravity of healthy men: body weight/volume as an index of obesity. *Journal of the American Medical Association* 1942; **118**: 495–501.
2. Damon A. Constitutional medicine. In: Von Meering O, Kasdan L, eds. *Anthropology and the behavioural and health sciences*. Pittsburgh: University of Pittsburgh Press, 1970: 179–95.
3. Tittel K, Wutscherk H. *Sportanthropometrie*. Leipzig: Barth, 1972.
4. Tanner JM. *The physique of the Olympic athlete*. London: Allen & Unwin, 1964.
5. Sheldon WH (with the collaboration of SS Stevens and WB Tucker). *The varieties of human physique*. New York: Harper and Brothers, 1940.
6. Carter JL, Heath BH. *Somatotyping—development and applications*. Cambridge University Press, 1990.
7. Dyson GHG. *The mechanics of athletics*, 2nd edn. University of London Press, 1963.
8. Metropolitan Life Insurance Company. 1983 Metropolitan height and weight tables. *Statistical Bulletin of the Metropolitan Life Insurance Company* 1983; **64**: 1–9.
9. Ross WD, Ward R. Proportionality of Olympic athletes. In: Carter JEL, ed. *Physical structure of Olympic athletes*. Part II. *Kinanthropometry of Olympic athletes*. Basel: Karger, 1984: 110–43.
10. Jones PRM, Norgan NG. A simple system for the determination of human body density by underwater weighing. *Journal of Physiology* 1974; **239**: 71–3P.
11. Siri WE. The gross composition of the body. *Advances in Biological and Medical Physics* 1956; **4**: 239–80.
12. Durnin JVGA, Womersley J. Body fat assessed from total body density and its estimation from skinfold thickness: measurements on 481 men and women aged from 16 to 72 years. *British Journal of Nutrition* 1974; **32**: 77–97.
13. Jackson AS, Pollock ML, Ward A. Generalized equations for predicting body density of women. *Medicine and Science in Sports and Exercise* 1980; **12**: 175–82.
14. Jackson AS, Pollock ML. Generalized equations for predicting body density of men. *British Journal of Nutrition* 1978; **40**: 497–504.
15. Thorland WG, Johnson GO, Tharp GD, Housh TJ, Cisar CJ. Estimation of body density in adolescent athletes. *Human Biology* 1984; **56**: 339–48.
16. Sinning WE *et al*. Validity of generalized equations for body composition analysis in male athletes. *Medicine and Science in Sports and Exercise* 1985; **17**: 124–30.
17. Sinning WE, Wilson JR. Validity of generalized equations for body composition in women athletes. *Research Quarterly* 1984; **55**: 153–60.
18. Weiner JS, Lourie JA. *Practical human biology*. London: Academic Press, 1981.
19. Lohman TG, Roche AF, Martorell R, eds. *Anthropometric standardisation reference manual*. Champaign, Illinois: Human Kinetics.
20. Nyboer J. Percent body fat measured by four terminal bioelectrical impedance and body density methods in college freshmen. *Proceedings of the 5th International Conference in Bioelectrical Impedance, Tokyo, Japan, August 1981*.
21. Baumgartner RN, Chumlea WC, Roche AF. Bioelectric impedance for body composition. *Exercise and Sports Sciences Review* 1990; **18**: 193–224.
22. Heitmann BL. Impedance: a valid method in assessment opf body composition. *European Journal of Clinical Nutrition* 1994; **48**: 228–40.
23. Deurenberg P, Tagliabue A, Schouten FJM. Multifrequency impedance for the prediction of extracellular water and total body water. *British Journal of Nutrition* 1995; **73**: 349–58.

24. Elia M, Parkinson SA, Diaz E. Evaluation of near infra-red interactance as a method for predicting body composition. *European Journal of Clinical Nutrition* 1990; **44**, 113–21.

25. Fuller NJ, Jebb SA, Laskey MA, Coward WA, Elia M. Four-component model for the assessment of body composition in humans: comparison with alternative methods, and evaluation of the density and hydration of fat-free mass. *Clinical Science* 1992; **82**: 87–693.

26. Hortobágyi T, Israel RG, Houmard JA, McCammon MR, O'Brien KF. Comparison of body composition assessment by hydrodensitometry, skinfolds, and multiple site near-infrared spectrophotometry. *European Journal of Clinical Nutrition* 1992; **46**: 205–11.

27. Wilmore KM, McBride PJ, Wilmore JH. Comparison of bioelectrical impedance and near-infrared interactance for body composition assessment in a population of self-perceived overweight adults. *International Journal of Obesity* 1994; **18**: 375–81.

28. Brooke-Wavell K, Jones PRM, Norgan NG, Hardman AE. Evaluation of near intra-red interactance for assessment of subcutaneous and total body fat. *European Journal of Clinical Nutrition* 1995; **49**: 57–65.

29. Burkinshaw L. Measurement of body composition *in vivo*. In: Orton CG, ed. *Progress in medical radiation physics*, Vol. 2. New York: Plenum Press, 1985: 113–37.

30. Pierson RN *et al*. Measuring body fat: calibrating the rulers. Intermethod comparisons in 389 normal Caucasian subjects. *American Journal of Physiology* 1991; **261**: E103–8.

31. Fowler PA, Fuller MF, Glasbet CA, Cameron GG, Foster MA. Validation of the *in vivo* measurment of adipose tissue by magnetic resonance imaging of lean and obese pigs. *American Journal of Clinical Nutrition* 1992; **56**: 7–13.

32. van der Kooy K, Seidell JC. Techniques for the measurement of visceral fat: a practical guide. *International Journal of Obesity* 1993; **17**: 187–96.

33. Ramirez ME. Measurement of subcutaneous adipose tissue using ultrasound images. *American Journal of Physical Anthropology* 1992; **89**: 347–57.

34. Langton CM. The role of ultrasound in the assessment of osteoporosis. *Clinical Rheumatology* 1994; **13**: 13–17.

35. Roubenoff R, Kehysias JJ, Dawson-Hughes B, Heymsfield SB. Use of dual-energy X-ray absorptiometry in body composition studies: not yet a 'gold standard'. *American Journal of Clinical Nutrition* 1993; **58**: 589–91.

36. Kohrt WM. Body composition by DXA: tried and true? *Medicine and Science in Sports and Exercise* 1995; **27**: 1349–353.

37. Lohmann TG. Applicability of body composition techniques and constants for children and youths. *Exercise and Sports Sciences Review* 1986; **2**: 29–57.

38. American College of Sports Medicine. Position statement on proper and improper weight loss programs. *Medicine and Science in Sports and Exercise* 1983; **15**: ix–xiii.

39. Loucks AB, Horvath SM. Athletic amenorrhea: a review. *Medicine and Science in Sports and Exercise* 1985; **17**: 56–72.

40. Frisch RE, McArthur JW. Menstrual cycles: fatness as a determinant of minimum weight for height necessary for their maintenance of onset. *Science* 1974; **185**: 949–51.

41. WHO study group. Assessment of fracture risk and its application to screening for postmenopausal osteoporosis. *WHO technical report series* 843, 1994, Geneva.

42. Martin AD, Silverthorn KG, Houston CS, Bernhardson S, Wajda A, Roos LL. Trends in fracture of the proximal femur in two million Canadians: 1972–1984. *Clinical Orthopaedics and Related Research* 1991; **266**: 111–18.

43. Cummings SR *et al*. Risk factors for hip fracture in white women. *New England Journal of Medicine* 1995; **332**: 767–73.

44. Suominen H. Bone mineral density and long term exercise. An overview of cross-sectional athlete studies. *Sports Medicine* 1993; **16**: 316–30.

45. Dalen N, Olsson KE. Bone mineral content and physical activity. *Acta Orthopaedica Scandinavica* 1974; **45**: 170–4.

46. Kannus P, Haapasalo H, Sievanen H, Oja P, Vuori I. The site-specific effects of long-term unilateral activity on bone mineral density and content. *Bone* 1994; **15**: 279–84.

47. Leblanc AD, Schneider VS, Evans HJ, Engelbretson DA, Krebs JM. Bone mineral loss and recovery after 17 weeks of bed rest. *Journal of Bone Mineral Research* 1990; **5**: 843–50.

48. Chilibeck PD, Sale DG, Webber CE. Exercise and bone mineral density. *Sports Medicine* 1995; **19**: 103–22.

2

Sport and the environment

2.1 The underwater environment

David Elliott

Introduction

There are about 50 000 sports divers in the United Kingdom and, according to the American 'Diver Alert Network', about 3 million in the United States. There are more than 100 diving fatalities each year in the United States alone, and no reliable estimate is available on the prevalence of diving illnesses.

The problems and challenges imposed by the underwater environment are many and complex. The sport of diving is universal, and an understanding of the effects of this environment is essential, for example, when deciding upon the fitness of apparently healthy individuals to participate in underwater sports.

The sport of diving

There are two quite distinct underwater activities to be considered. Each shares the challenge of raised environmental pressure, but the physiological responses and sequelae can be very different. The two activities are separated by the simple distinction of whether the individual is relying upon his breath-hold duration for his excursion underwater or whether, when submerged, he is able to breath from some form of breathing apparatus.

Breath-hold diving includes snorkel diving in which the use of a J-shaped tube enables a person to breathe while face down on the surface of the water. This equipment together with a mask and fins is cheap and readily available to the young, the casual, and the untrained. Snorkelling is associated with many hazards but, though it is not safe, the risks are fewer than those of SCUBA diving.

The well-trained and experienced breath-hold diver can achieve remarkable underwater excursions and it is in this area in particular that the competitive element has arisen. Depth alone is a challenge, and the achievement of more than 105 m (350 feet) on a single breath is associated with a risk of death by drowning that only the foolish would accept. Speed through the water is important in competitive spear-fishing, a breath-hold activity which is still practised in parts of the Mediterranean, whereas competitive underwater photography demands breath-hold control.

The use of self-contained underwater breathing apparatus (SCUBA) requires more than a bottle of compressed air. The air cylinder is pressurized to around 150 bar (15 MPa) and passes through a first-stage regulator on the cylinder and a pressure hose to the second-stage regulator on the mouthpiece. This regulator provides compressed air to the diver on inspiratory demand at an adequate flow and at the same pressure as the surrounding water. The SCUBA diver will also have a snorkel, for swimming on the surface, a mask, fins, and a weight belt with extra weight to compensate for the buoyancy of a thermally protective wet-suit or dry-suit. A knife, a watch, and a depth gauge are carried, and a buoyancy vest is worn. This does not simply act as a life-jacket at the surface but also, by adjusting the volume of compressed air within it, serves as a buoyancy compensator while at depth.

There is a minority of sports divers who use breathing gases other than compressed air. Closed- circuit breathing apparatus using pure oxygen provides a lesser bulk which can facilitate the negotiation of narrow passages when diving in caves. This type of apparatus, which is also favoured by video and film cameramen because of its lack of bubbles, is notoriously dangerous. It exposes the subject to a number of additional hazards not encountered with SCUBA. The increased partial pressure of oxygen can cause oxygen intolerance in the form of oxygen neurotoxicity resulting in shallow-water black-out. These are described later. The nature of the apparatus itself can lead to the accidental inhalation of a caustic mixture of soda lime and sea water. The soda lime normally removes all the carbon dioxide and thus also removes carbon dioxide accumulation which would normally act as a warning of gas supply failure. When this occurs the oxygen content of the recirculating gas can fall unnoticed by the diver who passes quietly through hypoxia to an anoxic death. This type of apparatus is rightly banned by many diving organizations.

Oxygen can also be used to enrich the air of self-contained equipment in order to prolong bottom-time or shorten decompression time. The use of enriched air 'nitrox' (EAN) requires special gas-mixing techniques and specific decompression procedures, and thus is not for the untrained. Oxygen can also be used during decompression stops to hasten the elimination of dissolved nitrogen. Increasingly, recreational divers are adopting advanced techniques previously used only by naval and commercial divers. These include the use of more than one gas mixture during a single deep dive and the use of semiclosed-circuit breathing apparatus.

The relative expense of SCUBA-diving equipment limits its availability, but it can be hired. Training is essential, but a 1-day 'dive-resort course' is too often provided without a proper pre-dive health check and, though better than no introductory supervision at all, this is regarded by many as inadequate.

Those who pursue SCUBA diving as a recreational sport not only need knowledge of the equipment in use, its failures, and its

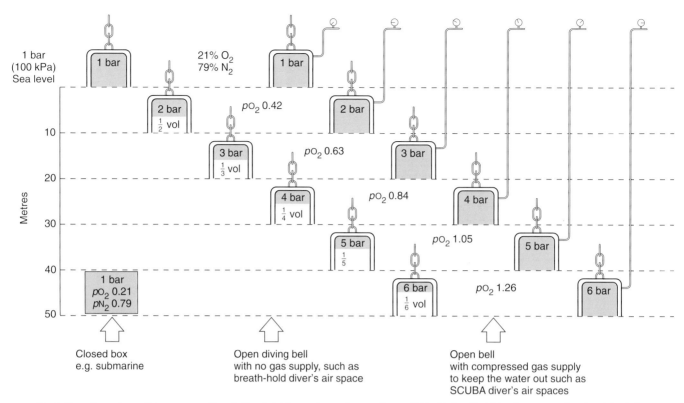

Fig. 1 The volume of gas within an open and inverted jar diminishes on descent in accordance with Boyle's law. If additional compressed gas is admitted, the volume within the jar can be kept constant. The particular pressure of the contained gases increases in proportion to the absolute pressure. If a closed pressure-proof box is submersed, the pressure and volume are maintained at the atmospheric level (1 bar = 100 kPa).

maintenance, but also need to understand the environmental hazards which they might encounter. They should pass a recognized training course of several days' duration and, after that, remain under a degree of direct supervision while progressing towards more advanced training courses. For all this they need to be mentally, physically, and medically fit. The professional sports diver is primarily concerned with instruction and requires to be in virtually perfect health.

Underwater sports are widely distributed; divers certainly do not confine their activities to coastal waters. For instance, in the United Kingdom nearly every major town has a branch of a sports diving club which holds weekly training sessions in a local swimming pool. These are usually well conducted and contribute to the safety performance of the sport. The geographical distribution of recreational diving is increased by diving training in lakes and reservoirs, wherever these are available. Practitioners may also encounter problems which arise when divers return by air from a vacation overseas. Altitude itself is also hazardous, and thus a diving sports injury can be susceptible to aggravation by bubble growth at a cabin altitude which is normally around 2440 m (8000 feet). Though a popular image of sports diving may be associated with tropical seas, the practice of diving medicine is in fact universal.

The environment

Water has a specific heat some 1000 times greater and a thermal conductivity 32 times greater than air, and so the exposed skin of the diver can be considered to be at the same temperature as the surrounding water. Thus those diving without any thermal protection

will become cold with time, even in the relatively warm waters of the Caribbean (30°C). The subjective threshold for feeling cold depends on many intrinsic factors, and each diver must determine the most suitable protection for the particular diving conditions. One effect of cold water on the face and body is to cause a bradycardia, a feature of the so-called 'diving reflexes'. These phenomena, although they are a topic of intense physiological research, they have no clinical significance and will not be described further.

Water isolates the individual. Though sound travels well through the water, verbal communication between divers is not normally possible and hand signals are needed. In water there is some magnifying distortion at the air–water interface of the diver's mask, but the water is not always clear and indeed when diving in certain locations, visibility can be zero. Water also contains unexpected currents and dangers, such as nylon fishing lines, wrecks, and caves. The surge of waves overhead will affect safe movement and constant vigilance is essential.

However, the feature of the underwater environment that provides most of the problems is that the weight of a 10-m column of water exerts an additional pressure equivalent to the earth's atmosphere above it. As a result of the pressure exerted at depth by the column of water above the diver, his body experiences effects which are in accordance with some fundamental physical laws (Fig. 1). Boyle's law states that the volume of a given mass of gas is inversely proportional to the pressure. Thus 1 litre of gas at sea level decreases to 0.25 litre at a depth of 30 m, where the pressure is four times atmospheric. Of importance to the diver are the effects of this upon his gas-containing spaces: barotrauma of decent and ascent, when those spaces are unable to compensate for the changes of pressure and volume, and changes of buoyancy as a result of gas volume changes. The application of Dalton's law, that the partial pressure of a gas in a mixture is equal to the product of its fractional concentration and the absolute pressure, shows that the partial pressures of oxygen and nitrogen in compressed air are doubled at a depth of 10 m, and these partial pressures increase proportionately at deeper depths.

Also, the weight of water is sufficient to create a pressure gradient of physiological significance to the diver, particularly when in a vertical orientation. Yet this pressure is not noticed subjectively. Whether salty or fresh, the density of water is approximately equivalent to that of the body, such that the diver feels neutrally buoyant. The redistribution of venous blood consequent upon this pressure gradient is one of the factors causing a physiological diuresis which, through dehydration, may contribute to subsequent decompression sickness.

For the SCUBA diver at any environmental pressure, buoyancy can be finely controlled by the volume of gas held in the chest. However, the support given to the body by being in the water almost eliminates proprioception; for example, if an episode of dizziness or vertigo occurs while underwater, there may be no proprioceptive clues and also no visual clues to orientation. To what might be a transient episode on land, the undersea environment contributes additional factors which may lead to a serious outcome.

Physical laws need to be fully understood by both the diver and his physician: Pascal's law which describes the transmission of pressure throughout a fluid, Dalton's law which describes the partial pressures of gases, and Henry's law which accounts for the uptake and distribution of gases, particularly nitrogen, from the lungs of a diver. Equally fundamental is Boyle's law which affects the air-containing spaces of the body. These are outlined where relevant in the following text.

The effects of submersion

Cellular effects

The body behaves as if it were a fluid and is regarded as incompressible. Within the shallow depths encountered by sports divers this can be considered true for practical purposes. Nevertheless the direct effects of pressure upon the cell and its constituents give rise to the serious 'high pressure nervous syndrome'[1] in professional divers at depths greater than some 200 m. At this depth and beyond there are also changes, for instance, in red-cell membranes and blood platelet aggregation[2] which show that, after a period at raised environmental pressure, humans are not the same physiologically as they were previously at the surface. While these deep diving phenomena may have little direct bearing on the clinical aspects of sports diving medicine, they do illustrate that mere exposure to the environmental pressure of sports diving is not without a possible physiological impact on a subsequent safe return to the surface.

Air-containing spaces

The effect of submersion upon the gas-containing spaces of the body is more obvious. The gas within them must follow Boyle's law and thus either reduce in volume with increased depth or, to maintain volume, be able to admit additional compressed gas. The adverse consequences of pressure–volume inequality are termed 'barotrauma' and can occur in both the compression and decompression phases of the dive.

The increased density of the gas also has an effect upon respiration: indeed, physical effort underwater tends to be ventilation limited. This limitation affects both expiration and inspiration. Maximum expiratory flow rate is diminished and at any depth is limited due to increased gas density. Thus the limitation is effort independent. Inspiratory flow is also diminished but this is dependent on effort. A diminished ventilation is associated with a raised arterial carbon dioxide tension. Another consequence of breathing gas at increased density is an increased respiratory heat loss. This loss is not so great that the inspiratory gas requires to be heated, as it is in deep oxyhelium diving, but is a significant drain on the body's thermal reserve during an air dive.

Buoyancy

The self-contained diver has equipment which, when properly used, can overcome changes in his buoyancy. A set of weights, which can easily be ditched in an emergency, counterbalance the natural buoyancy of the diver and his suit. A buoyancy compensator (BC) vest can be used for trimming buoyancy as the tank of compressed gas becomes lighter as the gas is used. Misuse of the air inflation of a dry suit, inadequate control of the buoyancy compensator, or unintentional release of the weights can lead to an unexpected, rapid, and hazardous return to the surface.

The breath-hold diver may carry a few weights, especially if he is wearing a wet-suit, but equipped normally with only mask, fins, and snorkel he is not capable of making buoyancy adjustments. His buoyancy is controlled by lung volume which, in order to prolong breath-hold duration, will be close to vital capacity when leaving the surface. On plunging down from the surface he quickly reaches a depth where Boyle's law has compressed the full chest and he has become negatively buoyant. It is not sufficiently widely known that, to return to the surface, the breath-hold diver may have to push off from the bottom or even swim his way back up. The importance of such instruction to novices seems obvious.

Latent hypoxia

Another cause of fatalities among breath-hold divers is considered to be excessive hyperventilation before descent. The advantages for breath-hold duration of eliminating carbon dioxide as far as possible seem obvious, but the unique circumstance of breath-hold diving make it hazardous. This is because hyperventilation cannot provide a significant increase in oxygen at the same time.

During the breath-hold dive, which is likely to be continued until the diver nears his carbon dioxide breakpoint, oxygen is being consumed. However, the depth of the dive means that the diminished oxygen level is at an increased partial pressure. Compression of the chest in accordance with Boyle's law further diminishes the desire for the next breath. In some instances, perhaps when the diver has overridden his carbon dioxide drive while chasing a fish, the oxygen is consumed further so that on ascent, with the concurrent fall in partial pressure of oxygen, hypoxia and unconsciousness supervene. To prevent this type of accident, no more than two or three deep respirations should precede any breath-hold dive.

Oxygen intolerance

The increased partial pressure of the respiratory oxygen content can lead to a risk of oxygen toxicity which can be manifest beyond 150 kPa in a neurological form as an epileptiform fit or, for longer duration beyond 50 kPa, as a pulmonary form with dyspnoea leading to pulmonary oedema. However, if divers use only compressed air, the threshold for either type of oxygen toxicity should not be reached. In 1990, one diver on air achieved a depth of 137 m (452 feet),[3] where the partial pressure of oxygen (309 kPa) is equivalent to '309 per cent' oxygen at the surface. This demonstrates the foolhardiness of sports record seekers who take unnecessary risks and encourage others to do so.

Only the use of pure oxygen, or of nitrox (oxygen-enriched air) can pose such threats at depths shallower than 50 m. Associated with the use of pure oxygen for diving is the phenomenon of 'shallow-water black-out', an otherwise unexplained loss of consciousness underwater thought to be due to a lowering of the syncope threshold and perhaps related to the vasoconstrictive effect of oxygen on cerebral blood flow.

Carbon dioxide effects

Carbon dioxide from extrinsic sources should never cause a problem for those using an open-circuit breathing apparatus, but nevertheless a number of experienced divers have been demonstrated to have become 'carbon dioxide retainers'. Such persons do not respond to an increased carbon dioxide tension, whether this arises intrinsically or extrinsically, and, while the increased carbon dioxide threshold might be thought of as an adaptive response, it can act synergistically with other factors to be one cause of apparently unexplained loss of consciousness underwater.

Nitrogen narcosis

Nitrogen is not an inert gas, and at increased partial pressure it behaves like an anaesthetic agent. Decreased performance and behaviour can be quantified at depths as shallow as 30 m, the limit recommended by some for inexperienced amateurs, and is the reason why even a professional diver should not use compressed air at depths greater than 50 m. Beyond such depths euphoria can make the individual irresponsible and less likely to be able to recover from a sudden emergency, thus converting a simple incident in the water into a potential fatality. Even when utterly foolish behaviour has been recorded on video, the diver may be quite unable to recall this after surfacing. However, nitrogen narcosis is directly related to its partial pressure and diminishes equally quickly on ascent. Though undoubtedly another contributory factor for underwater accidents, nitrogen narcosis is self-limiting and does not require any specific treatment.

Gas uptake and elimination

The other great problem in sports diving is the safe elimination of the respiratory gases dissolved from the alveoli into the body during the time spent at depth. The amount of gas which dissolves in a liquid is, in accordance with Henry's law, proportional to the partial pressure of that gas. The solubility of gases in the watery and fatty tissues is different and uptake depends on the dynamics of local circulation. Because of bubble formation, the dynamics of gas elimination are more complex than those of uptake. There are many mathematical models relating to the uptake and distribution of dissolved gas in the body but, whether presented to the diver as a printed table or as an on-line computer display, the theoretically safe decompression derived from such predictions cannot be guaranteed. The causative factors and consequences of an inadequate decompression have a clinical importance and will be discussed later.

The phases of submersion

The physiological and pathological effects of pressure, presented only in outline here, are reviewed elsewhere.[4] The clinical consequences of these effects can be considered separately in relation to the compression phase of a dive, the submerged phase, and the decompression phase which extends into a postdive phase for some hours. The subsequent descriptions will follow this sequence. Only a few of these clinical conditions affect the breath-hold diver, particularly those of compression barotrauma to the air-containing spaces of the body.

Compression illnesses

The air-containing spaces of the head (Fig. 2) are vulnerable to the effects of Boyle's law if the appropriate pressure and volume of the gas within them cannot be maintained during compression. Lack of patency of an orifice into an otherwise closed space denies access to it for additional compressed gas as required. The consequent reduction of relative pressure within that space leads to either a compensating ingress of transudate or rupture of one of its walls.

Middle ear barotrauma

Equalizing the pressure within the middle ear during descent is a procedure known to divers as 'clearing the ears'. Difficulty in doing this is very common. Boyle's law demands that sufficient gas enters the middle ear via the eustachian tube to prevent a relative underpressure there and the consequences of middle ear barotrauma or 'ear squeeze'.[5]

The unsupported medial third of the eustachian tube can become flattened during descent by relative overpressure before any symptoms of pain arise, and blockage of the normal tube cannot be reversed at a depth as shallow as 1 m. Experienced divers know this well and use an equalization manoeuvre immediately on leaving the surface in order to 'keep ahead of the pressure'. If this is unsuccessful and discomfort is felt, it is necessary to ascend to a shallow depth where the ears can be felt subjectively to clear. Another attempt to descend can then be made. It follows that any inflammation of the nasopharynx, whether due to infection or allergy, can reduce the patency of the tube and thereby inhibit pressure equalization.

Equilibration is commonly achieved using the Toynbee manoeuvre—blowing against closed lips and nose with an open glottis in order to raise the pressure sufficiently within the nasopharynx to encourage air to pass through the eustachian tube. The use of oral decongestants before diving is common and may also help, but the rebound phenomenon from nasal sprays can aggravate the problem. Experienced divers learn the Frenzel manoeuvre which is performed by a swallowing movement with a closed glottis, again with the lips and nose closed.

Failure to equilibrate middle ear pressure leads to damage ranging from a simple mild injection to rupture of the tympanic membrane (Fig. 3). A serosanguinous transudate may have occurred to compensate for the potential reduction in middle ear volume and may be seen through the drum as a fluid level, possibly full of bubbles. If this is the case, the person should not dive until the condition has resolved and a prophylactic antibiotic against secondary infection should be administered. Rupture of the ear-drum is more serious, and when it occurs underwater it carries the risk of immediate and debilitating vertigo if relatively cold water enters the middle ear. The individual should be given a prophylactic antibiotic and

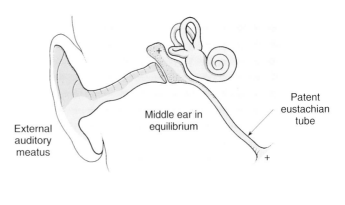

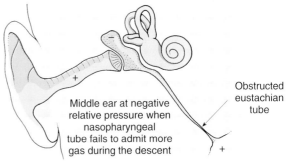

Fig. 3 The effect of an obstruction of the nasopharyngeal tube upon the pressure of the middle ear during descent.

should not dive for some 6 weeks until the drum is well healed and its mobility easily demonstrated subjectively or by observation.

Inner ear barotrauma

Persistent attempts to clear the ears on descent may cause a greater problem: round or oval window rupture. The pressure from a forced Toynbee or Valsava manoeuvre passes through the cerebrospinal fluid to the perilymph. Rupture of the window results in vertigo and possible total deafness. Its possible association with the forceful Toynbee or Valsava manoeuvres may help to distinguish it from the other causes of vertigo such as acute decompression illness. First aid is by bedrest with the head elevated. Some ear, nose, and throat surgeons may wish to operate immediately; others may wish to postpone the repair for a few days to allow for the possibility of spontaneous improvement. Persistent vertigo postdive or the onset, perhaps delayed by 12 h, of total sensineural hearing loss requires immediate surgery to close the fistula.[6]

Alternobaric vertigo

A more benign phenomenon is a sudden transient disorientation during the dive caused by an inequality of pressure between the right and left ears consequent upon the relative difficulty of air passing through one of the eustachian tubes. There may be a history of some difficulty in clearing the ears during the descent. However, in contrast with the possible association of round or oval window rupture with a forced Valsava or Toynbee manoeuvre, this form of barotrauma commonly manifests itself as transient vertigo after a relatively trouble-free period at depth, just at the start of the ascent. No treatment is required.

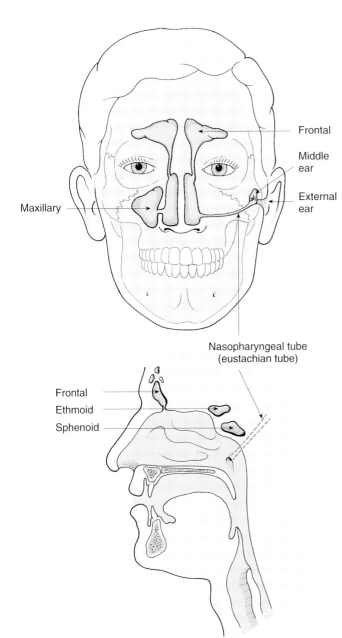

Fig. 2 The air-containing spaces of the head which are vulnerable to the effects of Boyle's law.

'Reversed' ear

The external auditory meatus may occasionally suffer from compression injury. This occurs if the meatus is closed by wax, an earplug, or some foreign body, or if it is covered by the impermeable hood of a dry suit. The consequent pressure change may rupture the tympanic membrane outwards.

Sinus and dental compression barotrauma

The free access of compressed air to the paranasal sinuses may be compromised by inflammatory conditions such as infection, allergy, or polyps. Pain may be referred from a sinus and can be intense. The affected sinus may fill with serosanguinous transudate, for which prophylactic antibiotics may be given, but usually there are no other effects.

Dental pains may be associated with compression of gas entrapped behind a filling or within an unhealthy tooth.

Thoracic compression

Even with the lungs filled to vital capacity before a breath-hold dive, it is obvious from Boyle's law that the lung volume must have diminished to residual volume long before the maximum recorded depth of 90 m was reached. However, it has been shown that, to compensate for the reduction of breath-hold pulmonary gas volume, the pulmonary blood volume can increase by as much as 1 litre at depths of 30 m.[7]

Coincidental illness and injury

There is always the small chance of acute illness developing during a dive, although this is much reduced if the diver has been previously screened for fitness to dive and also if he has been taught not to dive if feeling less than '100 per cent'. Conditions such as diabetes, which are absolute or relative contraindications for diving, are reviewed later. Many such conditions would, in their acute phase, be more hazardous if the patient were underwater at the time. Others, such as epilepsy and diabetes, would also be difficult to diagnose differentially from specific diving illnesses.

In practice, myocardial infarction among male sports divers over 50 years old is the most common coincidental condition and represents about 10 per cent of all recreational diving fatalities (Diver Alert Network, personal communication). Among professional divers there have been a number of cerebrovascular accidents at pressure, but there is no evidence that these occur other than by coincidence.

The final endpoint of many non-fatal diving accidents is near-drowning, perhaps complicated by hypothermia. These conditions are described in other chapters and all that needs to be emphasized here is that, if such a condition arises in a patient who has been diving, there may be an urgent need also to combat the effects of omitted decompression or of the embolic consequences of pulmonary barotrauma. Concurrent recompression of the ill diver is compatible with the management of most medical and surgical conditions. This is possible only if a recompression chamber is available and, if so, the appropriate procedures should be well known to the chamber staff and their medical adviser.

Physical injury underwater is uncommon in sports diving and needs to be managed in accordance with basic principles. Even if injured tissues bubble more than uninjured tissues on decompression, there are no special precautions required other than to complete any decompression profile to which the individual is obligated by the nature of the preceding dive.

Marine animal injury

Another hazard of sports diving, particularly in some locations, is from animals which injure divers by envenomation or direct physical attack. The majority of these animals are not aggressive and attack only in self-defence. Thus the prevention of injury can be achieved by good predive instruction.

Coelenterates

Coelenterates are very diverse in their variety, ranging from static corals to the mobile jellyfish. The common feature of many thousands of species is the nematocyst. This is a stinging cell which shoots out a coiled thread with a poisoned tip in order to immobilize its prey. The structure, action, and consequences to man of nematocysts varies from species to species.

The hazard to sports divers is largely defined by the geographical location of the diving, and the risk within these regions can be affected by the individual's own vigilance and behaviour.

Fire coral and stinging hydroids

These animals are static and thus sting only if touched by the diver. Recognition of their particular plant-like form and the avoidance of contact is thus an effective preventive measure. An immediate slight itch which is persistent for several days is the mildest manifestation. An extensive contact can result in a severe stinging with visible local inflammatory response. Any rubbing of the part can cause the discharge of more of the attached nematocysts and aggravate the condition. Fanning sea water with the hand over the affected part is the only recommended action to be taken to remove the nematocysts while the diver is still underwater. On return to the surface a liberal dowsing with vinegar should denature the toxic proteins and relieve symptoms. The application of alcohol on the part has been recommended, but the consensus view is that alcohol can aggravate the condition.

Coral is sharp and lacerations are common. These wounds may be painful and persistent because of the initial effects of the nematocysts and the likelihood of infection with marine pathogens. The wound can progress over several days to chronic ulceration. A culture of any organisms present should be made prior to the use of a topical antibiotic such as neomycin.

Portuguese man-of-war

Below its floating air sac, sometimes purple in colour, trail tentacles as long as 10 m. A sharp stinging sensation on contact is soon followed by intense pain which tracks centrally and may be associated with swelling of the axillary or inguinal lymph modes. The red weal of the original line of contact with the tentacle may be complicated by the bead-like string of very small blisters. Systemic manifestations are unusual, but hypotension, nausea and vomiting, abdominal cramps, irritability, confusion, and respiratory depression have been reported.[8]

Vinegar and the local application of lidocaine (lignocaine) ointment (5 per cent) are recommended as first-aid measures. Systemic support may be required as described below for the sea wasp.

Sea wasp or box jellyfish

The sea wasp, which is confined to the Indo-Pacific, is a venomous animal. Contact with as little as 7 cm of tentacle has led to death. Some 15 tentacles, up to 3 m long, trail below its box-shaped body which has sides up to 20 cm long. The pain is immediate and so intense that a number of victims have drowned at this early stage. Confusion may proceed to coma and death within 10 min. The prospect of survival increases after the first hour.

The clinical picture is well described elsewhere,[8] and, besides the severe pain, can include hypotension and shock with transient episodes of hypertension and rapid respiration. Respiratory distress, cyanosis, and pulmonary congestion also occur. The skin lesions and general irritability may persist for weeks.

First-aid measures include vinegar and the removal of tentacles, using gloves to do so. Local anaesthetic ointment and systemic analgesics should be provided and hydrocortisone given (100 mg, 2 hourly). Cardiopulmonary resuscitation may be needed, using oxygen and intermittent positive pressure respiration with intubation and general anaesthesia. Sea wasp antivenom is available in Australia, and it is obvious that the treatment of this condition, which is unknown in northern latitudes, is best left in experienced hands.

Prevention is vital. Consultation with knowledgeable local residents should help with the assessment of the risk which varies according to season and weather. In the same way as for the prevention of other milder stings, significant protection against unforeseen contact can be provided by wearing a wet-suit or other coverall at all times in hazardous waters.

Echinoderms

The sea-urchin is characterized by its many long spines which are brittle and break off on puncturing the diver's skin. Some of the spines are venomous, with systemic effects such as nausea and vomiting, and all can cause an uncomfortable wound. The calcareous material left under the skin may be absorbed in days or may persist for months. Since the spines are very difficult to remove intact it has been suggested that instead they are treated by the application of blunt trauma so that they are broken up and more readily absorbed.[8] It is also said that, for this particular inflammation, the conventional use of rest or immobilization is not as effective as activity.

Stingrays

Because of their habit of settling down and concealing themselves in the sand, stingrays provide an unexpected hazard to the inattentive diver. Though not aggressive to man, the stingray will defend itself by a sudden up-and-over flick of its tail which has a spine that is both sharp and venomous. The spine may penetrate the lung, the abdomen, or a major artery, with possibly fatal consequences. The venom from the spine enters the wound and can cause bradycardia, hypotension, a degree of cardiac ischaemia, and some respiratory depression. This too can be fatal but more usually regresses within 24 h.

The pain of the wound can be intense, but the venom is heat labile and much of the pain, and possibly some of the systemic consequences, can be relieved if the affected part is immersed in hot water (up to 50°C) for an hour or so. Debridement, with radiography to check for bone injury if this seems a possibility, and antibiotics are indicated.

Later systemic deterioration should be managed symptomatically.

Other stinging fish

The stonefish, which can be some 30 cm long, is well camouflaged and does not move away when approached. Its venomous spines are visible only when erect. The venom is vasoconstrictive, and thus remains fairly localized, but nevertheless can lead to muscular paralysis, respiratory depression, and cardiac arrest. The pain can be sufficiently excruciating to lead to death by drowning.

First-aid measures include immersion of the wound into hot water, because the toxin is heat labile, and cardiopulmonary support as necessary. An antivenom for stonefish is available in Australia but is not necessary for the milder venom of the related European weever fish. A local anaesthetic should be used without adrenaline.

The scorpion fish and other species differ from the stonefish in that they are not camouflaged but warn potential predators of their venomous capability by the use of bright colours. The manifestations are, in general terms, similar and the intensity depends upon the species and degree of envenomation. Even those fish with little or no venom, such as the surgeon fish, can inflict a wound which, contaminated by marine pathogens, can become necrotic and take months to heal.

Cone shell

The geographical distribution of venomous molluscs such as the cone shell is such that in Europe there is no such hazard and in warmer waters there is a hazard of which the consequences are known to locally resident medical practitioners. It is therefore advisable for the diver visiting a strange area to make himself aware of the risks and of any necessary first-aid measures.

The cone shell, which is visually attractive, up to 10 cm long, and found in shallow water, has a proboscis which can reach fingers on any part of its outer shell, and if the animal is in a pocket, can penetrate clothing. The mortality rate is some 25 per cent and children are particularly vulnerable. Neurological manifestations, particularly of vision, precede total paralysis of skeletal muscle, including respiration, which can occur within 30 min. Symptomatic support may lead to recovery in some 24 h.

Blue-ringed octopus

This octopus, which is confined to parts of the Indo-Pacific, has a tentacle spread of not more than about 20 cm, and usually less. Its blue striations may be noticed when the animal is excited, but its bite is said to be painless. Death by total paralysis can occur within minutes. Symptomatic cardiopulmonary support may be needed for many hours.

Electric fish

Electric eels and electric rays can discharge as much as 200 V, enough to disable a diver. Other than support, no particular treatment is required. Again, the diver should rely upon local knowledge to assess the risk and take preventive action.

Moray eels

These fish bite. They have a powerful body which they can use to anchor themselves in a hole in a rock and their teeth are angled inwards. They are usually docile and often fed by divers, but they can attack when provoked. Removal of a bitten hand from the mouth of an eel may be difficult and the injuries can be extensive.

Sharks

The vast majority of sharks are harmless. The same is true of the much maligned barracuda. However, a hazard can be present and this depends not only on species but also the particular location within the wider distribution of that species—some may be harmless in one area, such as the Caribbean, but dangerous elsewhere, for example California.

There is no substitute for local knowledge in assessing the potential risk to divers. If a shark attack occurs, the wound can be lethal. If the victim is recovered from the water and survives, first aid should be applied to the wound and, if the equipment is available, to the restoration of blood volume.

Other marine animals

The venomous sea-snake is another hazard of diving, but only in the Indo–Pacific. If envenomation occurs by a bite from some species, death by general ascending paralysis may occur within minutes in some cases, but the onset may be 24 h later in others. Immobilization and pressure bandages may defer the onset of symptoms. An antivenom is available and knowledgeable medical support is essential. Fortunately, the mouths of some snakes are too small to bite through clothing and a number of those bitten never develop signs of envenomation.

Crocodiles and related reptiles have a much wider geographical distribution. Divers have been killed by them and all should be regarded as dangerous, both on land and under water.

This overview of marine animals which are dangerous to divers is far from complete but does indicate to the specialist in sports medicine the breadth of knowledge that may be needed by a physician who provides medical support to any sports diving expedition.

Impaired consciousness under water

A number of factors which may lead to loss of consciousness in the water have been mentioned already, for instance latent hypoxia in breath-hold divers. There are many other possible causes of impairment or loss of consciousness under water.

It is rare for the content of the breathing gas to be a contributory factor for those using open-circuit compressed-air breathing apparatus. However, some carbon monoxide occasionally enters the air inlet of the compressor from the exhaust of its engine and, more rarely, it may be generated within an oil-lubricated compressor. Because the partial pressure of oxygen at depth is elevated at the time that the symptoms of carbon monoxide poisoning would otherwise become manifest, the onset of mental impairment may not commence until some time during the ascent to the surface.

Divers should also be aware that if moist compressed air is retained for some months within a steel tank, much of the oxygen may be used up in the formation of rust.

If open-circuit apparatus is being supplied with a premixed gas such as oxygen-enriched air, the mixture itself may be incorrect and cases of hyperoxia and anoxia have occurred.

Semiclosed-circuit or closed-circuit 'rebreather' breathing apparatus can lead to similar consequences. The presence of a carbon dioxide scrubber eliminates any drive to respiration due to carbon dioxide build-up. Thus failure of the oxygen supply can lead to an insidious loss of consciousness.

'Deep-water black-out' is a phenomenon among divers who go below about 70 m on air. The cause is unknown, but is probably due to a combination of the many factors present as such depths. These include increased oxygen partial pressure (more than 160 kPa at 70 m), nitrogen narcosis, and a build-up of carbon dioxide associated with the increased density of respiratory gases. Some of these divers are found to have an inadequate ventilatory response to carbon dioxide, and one common feature of these incidents is that the sudden loss of consciousness may occur during a period of hard physical work. If the victim retains his air supply he may recover quickly and there will be no serious consequences. However, underwater loss of consciousness is a hazardous event. There is also a small number of amateur divers who use air–helium mixtures (trimix) for descending beyond 50 m and sometimes to more than 200 m, particularly in caves. The physiological effects of deep dives bring additional neurological and respiratory hazards which may contribute to the fatalities which do occur at such depths.

Decompression barotrauma of paranasal and other spaces

The expansion of gas occurs within the air-containing spaces of the body during decompression in accordance with Boyle's law. If the gas cannot be naturally vented, its expansion may cause tissue damage or barotrauma. Expansion of the gases of the intestines does not usually cause any problem in sports divers but is sufficient to justify a recommendation that an unreduced inguinal hernia is a contraindication to diving.

The expansion of gas from the sinuses (Fig. 2) may occasionally be restricted by a polyp or by swelling. The result is facial pain and the expanded gas may escape into the subcutaneous tissue of the face or into the venous system. Though painful, there are usually no serious sequelae. The expansion of gas from the middle ear is not restricted by the flutter valve of the eustachian tube as it was during compression and, other than alternobaric vertigo which has been described already, no serious sequelae result. Gas retained within a tooth cavity has been know to blow out a dental filling explosively, which may be disconcerting but is not necessarily dangerous.

Pulmonary decompression barotrauma

Pulmonary barotrauma is a very serious event. Damage to the lungs by the expansion of the gases retained within them may cause severe local damage and may also cause arterial gas embolism because of disruption of the pulmonary vasculature (Fig. 4). These two principal consequences of lung overpressure are rarely seen together in

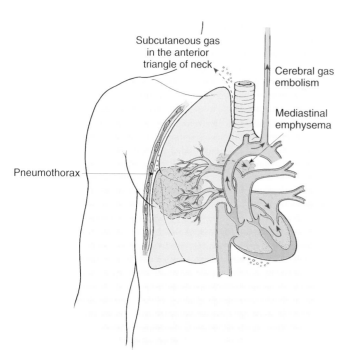

Fig. 4 The effects of localized pulmonary overpressure during ascent (pulmonary barotrauma): mediastinal emphysema and other extrapulmonary gas and arterial gas embolism.

one individual and, because the clinical features of gas embolism may be similar to the neurological features of a different decompression illness, known traditionally as 'decompression sickness', the neurological sequelae of both will be described together, later.

Pathogenesis of pulmonary barotrauma

Pulmonary barotrauma can occur in any type of diving but the subsequent course of events may be complicated by the additional presence of gas which became dissolved in the tissues during the diver's stay at raised environmental pressure. In contrast, cases arising from submarine escape training, a rapid procedure in which no significant gas load is acquired by the tissues, provide the classic clinical presentations of pulmonary barotrauma alone. In 200 000 buoyant ascents from submarine escape training in the Royal Navy there were 88 incidents, including five fatalities.[9]

The obvious cause of pulmonary barotrauma is failure to exhale respiratory gases during ascent. At a steady rate of ascent, the rate of volume expansion increases exponentially and it follows that, from whatever depth the diver ascends, the greatest hazard is close to the surface. Not much overpressure is required and cases of the associated complication of arterial gas embolism have been reported from an exposure as shallow as 1.5 m. Only a single breath of compressed gas is needed to place the lungs in hazard. Another reason for gas retention in the lungs is pulmonary pathology. The most obvious cause, such as asthma and chronic bronchitis, can be eliminated by a full and careful medical history and examination. A recent upper respiratory tract infection is a good temporary reason not to dive. Nevertheless, despite good training, correct procedures, and apparently good pulmonary fitness, cases are still all too frequent.

Another mechanism for localized pulmonary overpressure has been termed 'dynamic airway collapse'. When a rapid flow of gas is

driven through the airways by a relatively large pressure differential, the unsupported smaller airways may collapse. The air retained distally will continue to expand and may press upon nearby airways, compounding the condition.

Clinical manifestation

The expanded gas may escape (Fig. 4) by rupturing the pleura, possibly leading to bilateral tension pneumothoraces, or it may pass along the perivascular sheaths to the hilum of the lung. Such gas accounts for the finding of pneumomediastinum or pneumopericardium, each of which may be symptom free. Further tracking of the air can lead to its detection in the retroperitoneum by radiography or in the subcutaneous tissue of the anterior triangle of the neck by palpation. These findings, though not often present, are diagnostic.

The passage of expanded alveolar gas into the pulmonary circulation leads to arterial gas embolism, a condition which will be described with other neurological decompression illnesses.

A history of sudden respiratory embarassment on arrival at the surface is usually sufficient to make the diagnosis. Less severe cases may escape notice and, particularly if an associated neurological condition is treated by recompression to depth in a compression chamber, some may reveal themselves only later during the subsequent reduction of environmental pressure. Pulmonary manifestations may be relieved by recompression but the underlying condition will recur when decompression is resumed and experience shows that the onset will be at a deeper depth. Clinical examination of the chest within a compression chamber is made more difficult because raised environmental pressure distorts sound and because the performance of the medical examiner may be impaired by the effect of raised environmental pressure. Diagnostic aids such as radiography and ultrasound, suitably modified, are not always available for use in a compression chamber.

In 64 cases of barotrauma reviewed by the Royal Australian Navy,[10] 42 had clinical evidence of pulmonary damage, 21 had arterial gas embolism, and only 1 had both concurrently. Nevertheless, the urgency of treatment for neurological complications takes precedence and demands immediate recompression. Mediastinal emphysema has been observed radiologically in 1 per cent of asymptomatic healthy individuals following submarine escape ascents.

Treatment of pulmonary barotrauma

The management of pulmonary barotrauma is entirely symptomatic. The most urgent matter may be the relief of respiratory distress due to tension pneumothorax by use of a trochar and cannula with a Heimlich valve. This can, if necessary, be done while the patient is in a recompression chamber, but recompression is not required for the treatment of extra-alveolar gas alone. However, failure to recognize and relieve a unilateral pneumothorax in a compression chamber has led to at least one death. The treatment of the associated neurological manifestations will be described later.

Prevention

In addition to medical fitness screening of all divers and proper instruction, the recent introduction by some sports agencies of an arbitrary 'stop' for SCUBA divers at a depth of around 5 m is intended to reduce the risk of pulmonary barotrauma and arterial gas embolism due to ascent made too rapidly, often compounded by loss of buoyancy control. The need for a diver to stop in midwater at this depth encourages proper buoyancy control throughout the ascent.

The decompression illnesses

Nomenclature

There are at least two quite distinct causes of the acute illnesses that arise as a result of the reduction of environmental pressure which is experienced by the diver on returning to the surface. It has been customary to describe these illnesses as distinct entities, but the two conditions merely represent the extremes of what appears to be a continuous spectrum of manifestations which are end results of many pathogenetic pathways.

In order to present a logical description of these decompression illnesses it is necessary first to review the principal terms which have been in use for clinical cases and are still valid in describing pathology.

'Pulmonary barotrauma' is the damage to the lung, already described, which is due to the expansion of retained alveolar gas on ascent. The term can also be correctly applied to compression barotrauma—'squeeze' of the lungs associated with an uncorrected descent through the water of an old-fashioned helmet diver. Pulmonary compression barotrauma is not seen in sports SCUBA diving. The term 'pulmonary barotrauma' implies decompression and is also used to refer to the underlying lung pathology causing arterial gas embolism even when there is no clinical evidence of pulmonary damage in that individual.

'Arterial gas embolism' is usually used to refer to the carotid or vertebrobasilar embolism associated with pulmonary barotrauma. However, this use is not exclusive and arterial gas embolism can arise from other sources.

'Decompression sickness' is a term which was first used by [11]Matthews has since become identified with the clinical conditions associated with the release of gas as bubbles from the tissues in which it became dissolved during the dive.

'Decompression illness' has been adopted as a clinical term to include both of the major decompression disorders, together with other manifestations, such as those associated with a foramen ovale which is patent to otherwise innocuous venous gas emboli.

'Arterial gas embolism'

From accidents arising in the course of submarine escape training it is possible to define some characteristics of the neurological illness of decompression which occurs when there is no significant gas uptake in the tissues due to exposure to pressure. Features of this 'pure' form of gas embolism may be found in sports divers but there are differences, as noted by Kidd and Elliott.[12]

The causative exposure in all these naval cases was an excursion of around 2 min to a depth of not more than 30 m. Ascent rate through the water was at approximately 2 m/s, a rate at which the venting of the expanding alveolar gas also eliminates carbon dioxide build-up. The accidents occurred on arrival at the surface where the casualty's eyes may be seen to roll upwards. Onset might be delayed by a few minutes, sufficient for the individual to emerge from the water. The occurrence of one exceptional case after a surface interval of over 2 h can be explained by the speculation that a trapped volume of the lung expanded on ascent but, though under tension, did not burst until later.

The presenting manifestation in 65 cases was immediate unconsciousness in 30 and disorientation, giddiness, or observed unsteadiness in 20. Fifteen presented with a paresis: six of one arm, four of one leg, and five with a hemiparesis. Paraplegia, which is characteristic of what may be called 'spinal decompression sickness', was not seen in any of these neurological cases which had had no significant exposure to depth. Blindness developed later in a few victims. Thus the clinical picture may be similar to stroke, suggesting carotid embolism, but vertebrobasilar embolism is also invoked to explain some of the physical signs.[9]

It is important to appreciate that in this and similar series there were no cases of limb pain, no cutaneous manifestations, and no cases characteristic of multiple small venous emboli to the lungs (known as the 'chokes'), all of which conditions are considered to be components exclusively of 'decompression sickness' due to bubbles arising from dissolved gas. These will be described later. Similarly, non-specific constitutional disturbances are not reported in this rapidly progressive illness, but possibly because there is no time for them to be noticed during the rapid onset of neurological deficits.

A similar condition occurs in divers and retention of alveolar gas is a common cause of death from gas embolism in sports diving. While the associated features may include inexperience, inadequate training, equipment failure, and running out of air, the fundamental association seems to be with an ascent which is more rapid than usual. As will be discussed, the clinical picture and subsequent time-course may be more complex if the diver has acquired a significant gas load, but there are often sufficient similarities for the condition to have been called arterial gas embolism due to pulmonary overpressure in the past even though there may be a component in the final clinical picture due to dissolved gas.

After its rapid onset, the normal progression of gas embolism, as it occurs when there is no significant gas load, is either death or spontaneous resolution. Every case must be regarded as a medical emergency. The specific treatment will be described later.

'Decompression sickness'

In its classic form, many of the features of this condition are quite characteristic but there is a wide variety of clinical presentations.[13] On some occasions, there is also the possible contribution of alveolar gas emboli to the pathogenesis of what primarily is due to the evolution of dissolved gas from the tissues as bubbles. Another factor which may also modify the pathogenesis of decompression sickness is the presence of a small right-to-left shunt, such as a patent foramen ovale through which venous bubbles can pass to the arterial distribution with a potential for growth in size when they arrive in the peripheral tissues.

Some of the features of decompression illness, such as cutaneous manifestations, limb pain, and so-called 'chokes', are not found in submarine escape trainees, who have no significant gas load, but only in individuals who have had the opportunity to acquire a dissolved gas load.

Cutaneous decompression illness

A number of skin conditions may be associated with decompression illness. None is serious, but they can be uncomfortable and should be a warning of the possible onset of a more serious condition.

A simple itching of the skin has been linked to direct absorption of gas into the skin when it is exposed to compressed air during the time at pressure. This can occur in pressure-chamber dives and in those who wear a dry-suit during wet dives. This cutaneous condition does not arise in those areas of the skin that were wet throughout the dive. It is totally benign.

Cutis marmorata is the term given to a superficial red and/or purple blotchy rash, usually of the upper trunk. Itching may also be present. The 'marbling' appearance is thought to be due to vaso-dilation and then stasis. The rash whitens under local pressure. An urticarial response has also been described, but is not common.

Peau d'orange and possibly gross oedema occur and are considered to be due to the obstruction of the lymphatics and lymph glands by bubbles. This has been sufficiently gross to have been misdiagnosed as mumps, but usually is peripheral in distribution.

Constitutional symptoms

A general malaise may be indicated by a diver losing his appetite for his postdive meal, a warning of possibly more serious manifestations to come. In many persons it is not until they have been successfully treated by recompression that they realize how 'off colour' they have been feeling just previously. Fatigue that is disproportionate for the preceding physical exercise is said to be another warning of further manifestations.

Musculoskeletal decompression illness

Pain in the region of one or more large joints—'bends'—is the best known manifestation of decompression illness but is not always present. Indeed, though reported as the presenting symptom in up to 70 per cent of cases,[12] more recent analysis of sports diving at some treatment centres suggest limb pain in less than 25 per cent.[14]

Although the shoulders and the knees are the most commonly affected joints, pain can occur in the region of any synovial joint. In some the pain is mild and transient, while in others it may be intense. The pain may seem to flit from joint to joint and several joints may be affected in one individual. Pain is not easy to classify, but it has been considered that there may be two basic varieties—a superficial pain, fairly precisely located and close to the joint, and a deeper and more diffuse throbbing pain in the region of a joint. A 'niggle' may be defined arbitrarily as a pain which is already beginning to disappear within 10 min of onset. The course of established limb pain, if not treated, is that it slowly resolves over a period of several days, though in some cases it may persist for weeks.

The presence of some limitation of movement or of associated paraesthesiae must raise the possibility that there is also a neurological involvement, whereas the presence of redness or oedema in the vicinity of the joint suggests that the pathology is local.

Cardiopulmonary decompression illness

This condition, though not common, may become serious. It is believed to be due to the pulmonary embolism of many intravascular bubbles, and the onset usually occurs very soon after surfacing and may rapidly progress towards total cardiovascular collapse. The classic presentation is a sudden sharp retrosternal pain that limits deep inspiration and progressive dyspnoea. However, as in other conditions, the classic presentation is exceptional and early diagnosis can be difficult.

Neurological decompression illness

Almost any neurological manifestation can follow decompression and, classically, hemiplegia is associated with gas embolism due to pulmonary barotrauma, whereas paraplegia is associated with decompression sickness of the spinal cord. However, many cases are not so clearly distinguished and each of these classic presentations could be due to the other pathogenic mechanism.

A precise aetiological diagnosis is not possible. Since the emergency treatment for both conditions is essentially the same, all the neurological manifestations must be considered together.

Cerebral manifestations

The anatomical distribution of bubble-induced lesions is widespread and almost any presentation is possible. Psychotic disturbances, disorders of speech and of affect, generalized 'spaciness', and headaches are each presentations that, if they resolve rapidly on therapeutic recompression to raised environmental pressure, can be considered to be due to presence of bubbles. Such a response is diagnostic, but the failure of treatment does not eliminate the decompression bubble as the primary cause since the bubbles can quickly induce many secondary haematological and localized deficits.

Lesions of the individual cranial nerves, particularly V and VII, are uncommon but have been reported. Visual blurring is likely to be centrally located, and total blindness has been reported by several submarine escape trainees. As mentioned previously, the most common presentation in this particular category is sudden loss of consciousness on surfacing.

The vestibular presentation is characteristic of acute decompression illness. Often associated with ipsilateral deafness or tinnitus, and possibly with vomiting, the causative lesions are considered to occur most commonly in the cochlear and vestibular end-organs, though in some cases they may be more centrally located.

The most common peripheral presentation of neurological decompression illness is that usually ascribed to lesions of the spinal cord. While this might not be the site of the lesion in all such cases, there is a large amount of evidence to show that there are multilevel and multifocal discrete lesions which combine to produce paraplegia. This may be identified as being at a specific cord level but, more commonly, may be due to a more diffuse collection of deficits. The presence of a monoparesis or hemiparesis may be a consequence of cerebral gas embolism and, though less common than unconsciousness or disorientation, is a characteristic presentation in those who have just completed a rapid ascent through the water. In those who have also acquired a dissolved gas load during their dive, the clinical picture can be more complex. It is also known that a rapid ascent, perhaps because it initiates a number of intra-arterial bubbles of alveolar gas, may be followed by 'classic spinal cord' manifestations, even after a dive that did not infringe accepted no-stop decompression durations. There is also evidence that venous bubbles may bypass the pulmonary filter, where their gases are normally excreted, and enter the arterial circulation through a shunt.

The insidious onset of 'pins and needles' in the feet, a sensation of 'woolliness', or some slight weakness is a characteristic mode of onset for what will develop in minutes or hours into a serious paraplegia, possibly ascending to quadriplegia with respiratory difficulties. Retention of urine is common in such cases, and impotence and rectal incontinence may follow.

A sudden 'girdle' pain on one or both sides of the trunk is an uncommon but well-documented onset of acute neurological decompression illness, and is usually followed rapidly by complete loss of function below that level.

It must be concluded that any type of neurological lesion can occur after any dive profile. One single breath of compressed gas at depth is sufficient to expose the individuals to the hazard of 'burst lung' on ascent, but there is no report in the literature of a neurological deficit occurring from depths shallower than 1.5 m of sea water.

Hypovolaemia

Although haemoconcentration due to bubble-induced increased capillary permeability is a feature of serious decompression sickness, postural hypotension is not considered to be a presenting manifestation but develops later, as a complicating feature.

Latency and duration

While the onset of decompression illness may be immediate upon surfacing, or in some even while still making the ascent, a delay of some 36 h may occur before the first onset of symptoms. A failure to recognize or report the condition may account for latencies apparently longer than this. In one review, 85 per cent of neurological presentations occurred within 1 h.[15]

The time course of the illness is unpredictable. After the onset of the presenting manifestation, there may be a spontaneous recovery or the development of further symptoms or signs. Deterioration may be very rapid or take several hours. Recovery can be very slow and some neurological lesions may become permanent even when treated vigorously and expertly.

Treatment of the decompression illnesses

Early suspicion of the possible diagnosis and a contingency plan for urgent recompression are the essentials of good case management. The unpredictable progression of the illness and the diminution of its responsiveness to treatment if there is delay make the condition a medical emergency.[16]

The generally accepted view is that anything untoward which occurs after a dive should be considered as decompression illness unless it can be shown otherwise. There is a natural tendency for persons to look for some explanation for their symptoms other than 'bends'—a recent injury, for example, or possibly seasickness.

A recompression chamber is not always immediately available but, if it is, a return of the diver to raised environmental pressure can provide apparent complete relief almost instantaneously. Delay, even for further history and examination, is not justifiable in these circumstances. The history can be taken in detail later and the examination can be made at pressure to check for any residua before the necessary decompression commences. In some, the placement of

an intravenous line and urinary catheter may be performed, usually by the doctor associated with the recompression unit.

The remarkable reversal of unconsciousness or paraplegia is one reason why the bubble is still regarded as the primary pathological event; no other explanation of such a response seems feasible. However, the response may be incomplete or the patient may subsequently deteriorate, which are two reasons why there should be access to the patient at raised environmental pressure. Though used in places where nothing else is readily available, a one-compartment chamber has no facility to allow a doctor to 'lock in' with his patient. Thus the management of a tension pneumothorax during the subsequent return to the surface would become very difficult. One-man chambers which are transportable and which can then be locked on to a large pressure chamber elsewhere are available in some parts of the world.

A temptation for the patient's colleagues may be to return the stricken diver to the water, perhaps 'for extra stops'. This, for a number of reasons, may make the patient worse. Back in the water the ill diver may require physical support, there may be a limited duration of gas supply, and all concerned are likely to become very cold and treatment is likely to be too shallow and too brief to be of value. In-water recompression has been successful, but only when a pre-dive decision has been made to provide additional equipment for use in the event of this emergency. This includes dry suits for thermal protection, a large volume of oxygen, and full facemasks.[17] Even so, the recompression is limited in depth and duration and there is no access for ancillary treatment.

A two-compartment recompression chamber capable of taking the patient to an equivalent pressure of 50 m (165 feet) of sea water and providing oxygen-enriched mixtures or pure oxygen by means of a built-in breathing system is preferred and, indeed, required by regulations in some commercial circumstances.

Many decompression accidents occur at sea, miles from any recompression chamber. In these circumstances administration of 100 per cent oxygen by close-fitting mask is essential. Some advocate quickly tipping the subject head down 'to dislodge cerebral bubbles' but, if maintained, this procedure may lead to cerebral oedema. Plenty of fluids, preferably by mouth but intravenously if the subject is neurologically ill, are equally important. These should be continued until the urine is copious and colourless. A fluid balance sheet should also be kept. Catheterization and pleurocentesis may be required.

The use of drugs such as the corticosteroids to reduce cerebral oedema is less clear cut. There is as yet no consensus view on the appropriate dosage, and the efficacy of steroids is relatively unproven and depends upon reports of their use in analogous conditions.

There are, however, a number of contraindications and warnings. These include the use of analgesic nitrous oxide–oxygen mixtures because the nitrous oxide is known to diffuse rapidly into bubbles, thus enlarging them. The use of drugs such as acetylsalicyclic acid (aspirin) and heparin might enhance a haemorrhage within the inner ear. Valium might provide such good symptomatic relief that it would be tempting to omit subsequent recompression which is necessary for the underlying pathology.

A spontaneous recovery may be only transient. The evacuation of a 'recovered' casualty to a treatment centre is important because of the real possibility that a relapse and further deterioration will occur.

Evacuation must take into account the need to avoid exposing the patient to the compounding effects of diminished environmental pressure caused by either driving over a mountain pass or transport by aircraft. Whenever possible the patient should remain at an altitude below 150 m (500 feet).

As for all emergencies, preparedness is the key. When the emergency occurs, it is too late to begin planning. Not only should the correct first-aid equipment be available at the dive site and the potential methods of emergency transport arranged, but the recompression treatment centre must also be checked in advance in case it may be unavailable for casualties for some period of time. Once the subject is in a recompression chamber and being treated by a competent chamber crew, the details of the recompression should be left to the chamber's own doctor who should be well trained and experienced in such treatment. In cases of difficulty, whether at the contingency planning phase or in an emergency, there are a number of on-call physicians in several countries who can be reached for advice by telephone. These sources are known to those in the diver training organizations and, in most countries, to the coastguard and the navy also.

The emergency procedures must be planned in advance and each case treated as an emergency with aggressive optimism.

Fitness assessment

In order to minimize life-threatening underwater incidents, a number of predisposing medical conditions need to be recognized and some individuals advised to avoid this sport. For professional divers, particularly the sports diving instructor upon whom the life of a student in an underwater emergency may depend, the highest standards of physical, medical, and mental fitness are to be expected.[18] Indeed, the criteria on entry must be very strict since cardiopulmonary and other important functions are likely to deteriorate with age. For the amateur, who can choose when, where, and how to dive, there is a lesser demand for such perfection. Nevertheless, it is not only for the potential diver's own sake that some candidates should be medically disbarred from diving, but also for the sake of a diving partner ('buddy') upon whom the responsibility for a rescue would fall.

Those disorders which compromise the equalization of pressure or volume of the air-containing spaces during descent or ascent through the water provide the most obvious examples of medical conditions incompatible with this sport. Also, because of the need for continuous alertness in this unforgiving environment, any disorder that may lead to altered levels of consciousness or to erratic or irresponsible behaviour are likewise incompatible.

More difficult to evaluate are those disorders which have less obvious effects in diving. There are no clearly defined boundaries and, for conditions such as asthma or diabetes, there are both liberal and conservative interpretations. These relative contraindications to diving should be interpreted by a physician familiar with the environmental hazards and the nature of the diving to be undertaken. With recognition of the need for greater supervision and support while in the water, diving can be a suitable recreation for blind, paraplegic, and other handicapped sportspersons.

Thus the following examples (Table 1), which are more fully dis-

Table 1 Some conditions often assessed as contraindications to sports SCUBA diving

Ophthalmological

Inadequate visual acuity (unless diving in a category for the blind)

Ocular surgery within previous 12 months

Ear, nose, and throat

Inability to autoinflate the middle ear

Tympanic membrane perforation or aeration tubes

Obstruction to external ear equilibration

Menière's disease or other vertiginous conditions

Middle ear prostheses and stapedectomy

Inner ear surgery

Chronic mastoiditis

Deformity interfering with retention of mouthpiece

Laryngectomy or laryngocele; tracheostomy

Chronic sinusitis

Respiratory

History of spontaneous pneumothorax

Exercise or cold-induced asthma

Chronic obstructive pulmonary disease

Radiological blebs, bullae, or cysts

Sarcoidosis

Cardiovascular

History of myocardial infarction, angina, or other evidence of coronary artery disease

History of cerebrovascular accident

Unrepaired gross cardiac septal defects

Aortic or mitral stenosis; aortic coarctation

Complete heart block; fixed second-degree heart block

Exercise-induced tachyarrhythmias

Wolf–Parkinson–White syndrome with syncope or paroxysmal atrial tachycardia

Fixed-rate pacemakers; any drugs which inhibit cardiovascular response to exercise

Hypertension requiring drug treatment or with related retinal, cardiac, renal, or vascular findings

Inadequate exercise tolerance to cope with any physical emergency in water

Peripheral circulation

Any vascular disease that limits exercise tolerance

Gastrointestinal

Paraoesophageal or incarcerated sliding hiatal hernia

Any abdominal wall hernia with potential for gas trapping until surgically repaired

Hepatitis

Bleeding   *continued overleaf*

Table 1 continued..

Genitourinary

Pregnancy (or currently intended pregnancy)

Renal failure or transplant

Endocrine

Insulin-dependent diabetes mellitus

History of hypoglycaemic episodes even if not requiring insulin

Haematological

Sickle-cell disease

Haemophilia

Polycythaemia

Leukaemia

Unexplained anaemia

Central nervous system and psychiatric

Demyelinating diseases

History of head injury with more than 30 min unconsciousness or
 with post-traumatic amnesia for more than 1 h

Neurological deficits due to illness or injury unless fully investigated

History of epilepsy including childhood fits unless fully investigated

Neurological migraine

Myasthenia gravis

Transient ischaemic attacks

Psychosis, significant anxiety states, manic states

Severe depression, suicidal ideation

Alcoholism and use of mood-altering drugs

Musculoskeletal

Impediments of mobility or dexterity

cussed elsewhere,[18,19] apply to recreational divers. These examples, presented below by organ system, require very careful assessment.

Neurological system

The absence of any neurological illness or deficit is the obvious ideal for a diver candidate but, in sports diving in particular, there are conditions in which some allowances can be made without compromising safety. The safety of the individual is the prime consideration. Any possibility of a seizure under water, whether epileptic in origin or as a consequence of previous head injury, is a good example because it is likely to be associated with a loss of the mouthpiece and drowning. There is a secondary consideration, given that the condition is not a threat to immediate safety, which is the possible risk to subsequent health. For example, in multiple sclerosis the risk of associated decompression sickness from diving must be seen as potentially reducing still further the diminished function of the central nervous system, and there is also the potential problem that the sudden onset of neurological symptoms could provide dif-

ficulties in planning the diagnosis and management of decompression illness. Wise counselling should be used to persuade such persons to seek another sport.

Gastrointestinal system

An unreduced hernia may contain bowel and has the potential for barotrauma during ascent. No diving should be performed until it is fully repaired. Diverticulitis is similarly disqualifying. Ileostomies and colostomies carry no such risk and are compatible with diving.

Musculoskeletal system

Persons with paraplegia resulting from trauma can dive under close supervision provided that they have sufficient control over pulmonary function.

Bone necrosis, though an occupational hazard of professional diving, is a rare complication of sports diving. The lesions may be in the shaft of the long bones or juxta-articular, and the latter can lead to osteoarthritis of the shoulder or hip. Radiological evidence of asymptomatic dysbaric osteonecrosis is not, *per se*, a contraindication to further diving since the necrosis does not affect in-water safety. However, the presence of juxta-articular necrosis is of sufficient long-term concern to advise the individual to discontinue this activity in case further diving leads to deterioration of the condition.

Endocrine system

Insulin-dependent diabetes is not compatible with unrestricted diving even when there is no end-organ disease. Some gentle diving by dietary-controlled diabetics is safer, but the onset of unconsciousness during a dive or after surfacing is likely to make immediate diagnosis and management in the field rather difficult.

Pulmonary system

A history of spontaneous pneumothorax is disqualifying. Repetition is likely to result in a potentially fatal expanding pneumothorax during the return to the surface. Traumatic pneumothorax, especially with lung injury, is also a contraindication even when all pulmonary function tests are normal. Any respiratory disease is disqualifying; the possibility of gas retention behind a mucous plug or constricted airway is ever present. Normal pulmonary function during (and, in persons with asthma, after) hard exercise is essential for safe diving.

Vision

Those with good eyesight will find this important for tasks associated with diving such as reading gauges and finding the boat again after returning to the surface. Corrective lenses, contact lenses, and, when healed, lens implants are compatible with diving. Radical keratotomy may be susceptible to barotrauma within the facemask and is a relative contraindication.

Ear, nose, and throat

The ability to equalize middle ear pressures during descent is essential in diving. Middle ear disease, history of stapes surgery, or radical mastoidectomy are disqualifying. Provided that middle ear equalization is easy, a healed repair of the tympanic membrane is acceptable. Chronic sinusitis may well prevent pressure excursions.

Menière's disease is a contraindication; an attack during the dive could totally disorientate the diver in midwater, and if it occurred after the dive, management of the case would need to focus on the possibility of acute decompression sickness.

Dental health is advantageous because of the need to grip the mouthpiece of the underwater breathing apparatus even though this can also be done adequately after removal of partial dentures. Air pockets in carious teeth and behind fillings can cause local pain.

Cardiovascular system

Persons with controlled hypertension can dive, but those taking drugs like β-blockers that limit exercise should demonstrate their ability to reach 13 mets (metabolic equivalents) of exercise (around 45 ml of oxygen consumption per kg body weight per min), a level necessary in order to surmount most in-water difficulties.

A history of coronary insufficiency contraindicates recreational diving in which a maximal effort may be required unexpectedly.

Aortic and mitral stenosis are disqualifying. Mitral regurgitation and aortic insufficiency, as long as there is no left-ventricular dysfunction, are acceptable. Mitral valve prolapse with symptoms is also acceptable. Septal defects are not necessarily considered to be disqualifying even though there is a possibility of venous bubbles crossing to the left side. This is justified because the one-third of sports divers who have septal defects of some kind far exceeds those few (less than 0.1 per cent) who will ever suffer neurological decompression illness.

Arrhythmias are a particular cause of concern but the ultimate criterion is again the ability to sustain hard exercise.

References

1. Bennett PB, Rostain JC. The high pressure nervous syndrome. In: Bennett PB, Elliott DH, eds. *The physiology and medicine of diving*, 4th edn. London: WB Saunders, 1993: 194–237.
2. Hallenbeck J, Andersen JC. Pathogenesis of the decompression disorders. In: Bennett PB, Elliott DH, eds. *The physiology and medicine of diving*, 3rd edn. London: Baillière Tindall, 1982: 435–60.
3. Anonymous. Editorial. *Aquacorps* 1991; **2**: 1–3.
4. Bennett PB, Elliott DH, eds. *The physiology and medicine of diving*, 4th edn. London: WB Saunders, 1993.
5. Farmer JC. Otologic and paranasal sinus problems in diving. In: Bennett PB, Elliott DH, eds. *The physiology and medicine of diving*, 4th edn. London: WB Saunders, 1993: 267–300.
6. Pullen WF. Round window membrane rupture: a cause of sudden deafness. *Transactions of the American Academy of Ophthalmology and Otology* 1972; **76**: 1444–50.
7. Schaefer KE *et al.* Pulmonary and circulatory adjustment determining the limits of depths in breath-hold diving. *Science* 1968; **162**: 1020–3.
8. Edmonds C. Marine animal injuries. In: Bove AA, Davis JC, eds. *Diving medicine*. Philadelphia: WB Saunders, 1990: 115–37.
9. Elliott DH, Harrison JAB, Barnard EEP. Clinical and radiological features of 88 cases of decompression barotrauma. In: Shilling CW, Beckett MW, eds. *Underwater physiology VI, Proceedings of the 6th International Symposium on Underwater Physiology*. Bethesda: FASEB, 1978.
10. Gorman DF. Arterial gas embolism as a consequence of pulmonary barotrauma. In: Desola J, ed. *Diving and hyperbaric medicine. Proceedings of the 9th Congress of the EUBS*. Barcelona: CRIS, 1984: 347–68.
11. Matthews BHC. *Interim report on research on oxygen problems.* London: Air Ministry, 1939.
12. Kidd DJ, Elliott DH. Clinical manifestations and treatment of decompression sickness in divers. In: Bennett PB, Elliott DH, eds. *The physiology and medicine of diving and compressed air work*, 1st edn. London: Baillière, Tindall, and Cassell, 1969: 464–90.
13. Elliott DH, Moon RE. Manifestations of the decompression disorders. In: Bennett PB, Elliott DH, eds. *The physiology and medicine of diving*, 4th edn. London: WB Saunders, 1993: 481–505.
14. Bennett PB, Dovenbarger J, Corson K. Etiology and treatment of air diving accidents. In: Bennett PB, Moon RE, eds. *Diving accident management*. Bethesda: Undersea and Hyperbaric Medical Society, 1990: 12–22.
15. Francis TJR, Pearson RR, Robertson AG, Hodgson M, Dutka AJ, Flynn ET. Central nervous system decompression sickness: latency of 1070 human cases. *Undersea Biomedical Research* 1988; **15**: 403–17.
16. Davis JC, Elliott DH. Treatment of the decompression disorders. In: Bennett PB, Elliott DH, eds. *The physiology and medicine of diving*, 3rd edn. London: Baillière Tindall, 1983: 473–87.
17. Edmonds C, Lowry C, Pennefather J. Underwater oxygen treatment of decompression sickness. In: *Diving and subaquatic medicine*, 2nd edn. Mosman, NSW: Diving Medical Centre, 1981: 171–80.
18. Elliott DH, ed. *Medical assessment of fitness to dive.* London: Biomedical Seminars, 1995.
19. Bove AA, ed. *Bove and Davis' Diving medicine*, 3rd edn. Philadelphia: WB Saunders, 1997.

2.2 Immersion in cold water: effects on performance and safety

M.J. Tipton and F. St C. Golden

Introduction

Up to 10 million people participate in water-based leisure activities on a regular basis in the United Kingdom alone. For individuals involved in sporting activities which require deliberate immersion in cold water, such as swimming, wind surfing, triathlons, or diving, a knowledge of how such an immersion can influence performance, and how performance can be maintained in this environment is clearly advantageous. For others for whom immersion is not planned, such as sailors, canoeists, and fishermen, a knowledge of the hazards associated with immersion in cold water may be life-saving.

It is estimated that 140 000 people drown each year throughout the world;[1] in the United Kingdom the figure is approximately 700.[2,3] An understanding of the responses associated with cold-water immersion may be critical and should include knowledge of the methods of protecting against them. It is also important that anyone who may have to treat an immersion casualty appreciates the problems that may be encountered during rescue and subsequent management.

This chapter includes information on the responses associated with immersion and how they may influence performance or threaten life. Methods of protecting against the responses and treating those who become immersion casualties are also considered.

Thermoregulation: air versus water

Humans possess an intricate and integrated thermoregulatory system (Fig. 1) which, by varying heat production and heat loss, attempts to regulate the deep body temperature at a relatively constant temperature of about 36.9 °C (98.4 °C).

As humans are constantly producing heat as a by-product of metabolism, this must be lost to the environment for the total heat content of the body to remain constant. For someone to be in heat balance the following must apply:

$$M +/- R +/- C +/- K - E +/- W +/- S = 0;$$

where: M is metabolic rate, R is radiation, C is convection, K is conduction, E is evaporation, W is work, and S is body heat storage. Detailed descriptions of both the routes of heat exchange and the thermoregulatory system are outside the scope of the present chapter, but interested readers are referred to several excellent references which deal with these areas.[4–9]

Heat loss from the surface of the naked body follows the same basic principles in air and water: heat passes to the microenvironment adjacent to the skin by conduction and is carried away by convection. In still air, radiation and evaporation are the major pathways for heat loss; the contribution of convective heat loss is increased with air movement ('forced' convection). In water, evaporation of sweat cannot be used and heat loss due to radiation is negligible. Therefore the route of heat transfer in water is principally convective and partly conductive.

Although only two primary pathways for heat loss are available in water, humans cool two to five times more quickly in cold water compared to air at the same temperature.[10] Water temperature can be 11 °C higher than that of air and produces an equivalent physiological response.[11] Furthermore, thermoneutral temperature in water averages about 35 °C with a very narrow range,[12,13] this compares with about 26 °C and a broader range for still air.[13] (A thermoneutral temperature is one in which the deep body temperature remains stable and thermoregulation is achieved by variations in vasomotor tone alone.) Therefore a naked resting man will be unable to maintain his deep body temperature when immersed in water at a temperature regarded as thermoneutral in air.

The reason for these differences lies in the physical properties of air and water; the thermal conductivity of water is 25 times that of air, and water has a specific heat per unit volume that is approximately 4000 times that of air. Thus water, unlike air, provides practically no insulation at the skin-water interface. Therefore cooling is extremely effective in water and results in rapid dissipation of the heat which is delivered to the skin from the deeper tissues. As a consequence, skin temperature quickly approximates water temperature following cold-water immersion. In contrast, the lower cooling capacity of air often allows skin temperature to be adjusted independently of air temperature; therefore it can assist in the maintenance of heat balance.

The cooling capacity of water is reflected in the values which have been reported for the combined heat transfer coefficient for convection and conduction. In still water the value is between 44 and 230 W/m²/°C,[14–16] rising to 460 at rest in moving water and 580 during swimming at any speed.[16] These figures are difficult to obtain and vary greatly between studies largely because of methodological differences. However, they are at least two orders of magnitude greater than those reported for air.

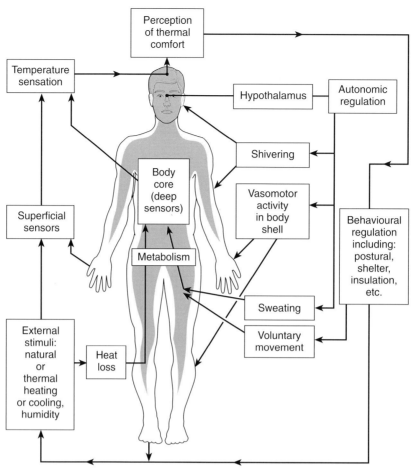

Fig. 1 Schematic diagram of temperature regulation in humans. The body 'shell' (the vasomotor labile region) is represented by the non-shaded area.

As a result of the capacity of water for removing heat from the surface of a naked body, heat loss must be largely limited by internal insulation between the deep and superficial tissues. Heat produced in the deep tissues of the body is transported to the skin surface by mass flow in blood and conduction through intervening body tissues to the skin. Therefore heat flux is determined by tissue conduction and the temperature gradient between the deep tissues and the skin.

Bullard and Rapp[17] have produced a theoretical model of heat conductance to the skin in which the flow of heat from the deep tissues to the skin is affected by two parallel resistors. One of these is 'variable' and is represented by the peripheral circulation, and the other is 'fixed' and is determined by the subcutaneous layer of fat.

As peripheral blood flow represents a 'variable' resistance, when this is at its lowest tissue conductance will also be at its lowest. In water at 13 °C forearm blood flow can be as low as 0.5 ml/(min/ 100 ml tissue).[18,19] This compares with values of around 17.6 ml/ (min/100 ml tissue) in water at 45 °C.[18]

There is general agreement that in lean individuals peripheral blood flow—and as a consequence tissue conductance—is lowest, and maximum insulation is achieved in water below 33 to 30 °C.[20-22] The comparative air temperature is 10 °C.[23] There is further evidence[21,24,25] to suggest that fatter individuals do not achieve maximum tissue insulation until they are immersed in much lower water temperatures, as low as 12 °C in some cases.[21]

As the 'variable' resistance is dependent on vasomotor activity, it can be influenced by factors such as exercise or shivering, both of which can increase peripheral blood flow and thereby increase tissue conductance. There is indirect evidence[19,26,27] to suggest that 70 to 90 per cent of the total body insulation of individuals at rest in cold water is provided by poorly perfused skeletal muscle. This is derived from the finding that maximum body insulation of a resting individual is approximately four times higher than would be predicted from fat insulation alone.

This has practical implications because skeletal muscle blood flow will increase significantly with exercise, including shivering. This increase will effectively remove the insulation provided by the muscle when poorly perfused. Thus the 'variable' resistance to heat flow depends on both muscular and cutaneous blood flow, with the former altering conductance and the latter the amount of heat delivered to the skin by mass flow.

The effectiveness of peripheral vasoconstriction in heat conservation is further improved by a reduction in the temperature of the arterial blood reaching the extremities, through countercurrent heat exchange between venae committes and arterial blood in the proximal portion of the limbs.[28] In water at 22 °C, heat loss from the hands and feet is negligible;[21] heat loss from the torso is transferred by conduction down the high thermal gradient over the short tissue pathway from the visceral organs to the body surface. Therefore most of the heat loss in relatively cold water takes place from the trunk rather than the limbs.

It has been suggested[29] that even fat individuals are at risk during immersion in very cold water (below 12 °C) as a result of a sudden increase in peripheral heat loss brought on by cold-induced vasodilatation. Lewis[30] first described cyclical fluctuations in skin temperatures of fingers immersed in cold water (10 to 12 °C). This response is caused by cold paralysis of vascular smooth muscle.[31] The resulting increase in perfusion by warm blood raises the vasoconstrictor muscle temperature, restoring its contractility and thus vasoconstrictor tone until it becomes subject to cold paralysis once more.

The classic, lobster-pink coloration of the skin seen following prolonged immersion in water below 12 °C is generally attributed to such cold-induced vasodilatation. However, the time delay evidenced in capillary filling of a blanched area of skin following digital pressure suggests that haemodynamic stasis and temperature impairment of oxygen dissociation, rather than high blood flow, are responsible for this red skin coloration. Presumably, proximal larger vessels are still vasoconstricted, thereby minimizing blood flow and thus the delivery of heat to the more superficial dilated vascular bed.

The evidence for increased heat loss due to cold-induced vasodilatation has generally been obtained from individuals who are warm but whose hands are immersed in cold water,[32] namely from those in whom proximal vasoconstriction is likely to be less intense. Such circumstances rarely apply during whole-body, cold-water immersion, and these authors do not consider cold-induced vasodilatation to be a significant route of heat loss during such immersions.

With regard to the 'fixed' resistance to heat flow, it is well known that individuals with thicker layers of subcutaneous fat cool more slowly in cold water than those with less fat.[33–35] The insulation provided by fat remains fairly constant with exercise because blood flow to fat is relatively low in all conditions.[36]

Peripheral vasoconstriction will slow the rate of heat loss in cold water but will not prevent an overall reduction in body heat stores and deep body temperature. In response to falling skin and deeper body temperatures, involuntary metabolic heat production through shivering is evoked in an attempt to maintain normal deep body temperature.[4] Both the magnitude and rate of change of skin and deep body temperature combine to stimulate shivering, the severity of which is reflected in oxygen consumption.[17,37] When skin temperature is low, oxygen consumption from shivering increases linearly as deep body temperature falls; the metabolic rate may increase and stabilize at a maximum value of approximately 1.5 l/min, that is to say approximately five times the resting level.[13,33,38]

Although shivering increases heat production, by increasing peripheral blood flow and the combined heat transfer coefficient at the skin-water interface, it may result in an overall reduction in the heat stores of a naked individual immersed in still water.

Responses to immersion in thermoneutral water

Head-out, seated immersion in thermoneutral water can produce profound changes in cardiovascular, renal, and endocrine functions. These effects are a direct result of the high density of the water and the differential hydrostatic pressure over the immersed body. A negative transthoracic pressure of about 14.7 mmHg is established[39] which will result in negative-pressure breathing. There is a ceph-

alad redistribution of blood which, within six heart beats of immersion, can increase central blood volume by up to 700 ml.[40–42] This is associated with enhanced diastolic filling, a raised right atrial pressure, and a 32 to 66 per cent increase in cardiac output due entirely to an increase in stroke volume, which itself is due to enhanced filling of the heart rather than alterations in afterload and contractility.[41,42] Heart rate has been reported to remain either unchanged or to decrease slightly following immersion.[41,43–45]

The increase in intrathoracic blood volume engorges the pulmonary capillaries and competes with air for space in the lung. The engorgement of the pulmonary capillaries results in a 30 to 50 per cent reduction in static and dynamic lung compliance, while pulmonary gas flow resistance is increased by 30 to 58 per cent and impedance by 90 per cent.[46,47] In conjunction with the increase in hydrostatic pressure on the chest, these alterations result in a 65 per cent increase in the work of breathing.[40]

Vital capacity is reduced by an average of 6 per cent, maximum voluntary ventilation by 15 per cent,[48] and expiratory reserve volume is reduced by an average of 66 per cent which results in a reduction of functional residual capacity.[46,49] The decrease in functional residual capacity and the increase in intrathoracic pooling of blood produces a small increase in pulmonary shunting and a small, but consistent, fall in the arterial partial pressure of oxygen.[50]

Opposing some of these reductions in lung function are an improved ventilation-perfusion ratio and improved diffusion capacity.[41,44] From the practical viewpoint there is little evidence that these changes in lung function threaten respiration in fit individuals.[51]

Most of the renal responses seen following immersion in thermoneutral water are due to the shift in blood volume which the body senses as hypervolaemia. These responses include: diuresis; natriuresis; and kaliuresis.[52,53,54] Diuresis is usually manifest by the first or second hour of immersion, and the natriuresis peaks by the fourth or fifth hour of immersion.[55]

In fully hydrated, sodium-replete individuals, head-out upright immersion can result in 200 to 300 per cent increases in sodium excretion and free-water clearance, with urine output reaching 350 ml/h leading to dehydration.[55]

It is concluded that immersion in water at thermoneutral temperature can result in profound alterations in the physiological function of the body. However, many of these responses are of long duration and vary with factors such as posture, activity, and level of hydration before and during immersion. It is this variability which makes it impossible to draw any firm conclusions about the effect that immersion *per se* may have on in-water performance, much of which is of relatively short duration.

Responses to immersion in cold water

Most of the alterations resulting from immersion in water at thermoneutral temperatures also occur in cold water. The changes in lung function remain and may be potentiated because of the effect of cooling on respiratory muscle function.[56]

Cardiac output increases by a similar amount (30 to 40 per cent) during prolonged immersion in cold compared to thermoneutral temperatures; on the basis of this it has been suggested that no further translocation of blood occurs with the vasoconstriction and venoconstriction seen during cold-water immersion.[57,58] However, cold and water pressure are thought to act additively to raise urinary output during cold-water immersion. Cold-induced diuresis accounts for one-third of the total response and is a result of cold-induced vasoconstriction.[59]

Despite a paucity of information, prolonged exposure to cold is thought to be a powerful stimulus for sympathetic nervous system activity and hormonal secretion in man.[60-62] Long-distance swimming in cold water may produce higher plasma concentrations of catecholamines, cortisol, and thyroxine and lower glucose, insulin, and growth hormone concentrations than those observed during comparable activities in thermoneutral environments.[61,63]

The response to short-term immersions is less clear. Little evidence of the release of catecholamines was found in early work. However, in more recent work employing modern analytical techniques significant increases have been found in plasma levels of noradrenaline and adrenaline after immersion in cold water for 1 to 2 min.[60,64,65,66,67] The release of noradrenaline from the sympathetic nervous system is closely correlated with metabolic rate during immersion; it can be quickly activated or suppressed on immersion or removal from cold water and is therefore thought to be evoked by changes in skin rather than deep body temperature.[60]

Hazardous responses

Short term

Sudden immersion in cold water evokes a group of cardiorespiratory responses which are collectively known as the 'cold shock' response. These responses, which have been reviewed,[68] are summarized in Fig. 2. They are initiated by rapid falls in skin temperature and are potentially extremely hazardous; they are probably responsible for the majority of deaths resulting from immersion in cold, open water.

Respiratory drive is enhanced on immersion in water cooler than 25 °C.[69] It is inversely related to water temperature, reaching a maximum level in water at a temperature of about 10 °C.[70] The respiratory responses include: an inspiratory 'gasp' response of between 2 and 3 litres,[70,71] and uncontrollable hyperventilation, which can result in a 10-fold increase of minute ventilation,[72] and significantly reduce the arterial tension of carbon dioxide.[65]

The respiratory drive evoked by cold-water immersion can reduce the maximum breath-hold times of normally clothed individuals to less than 10 s,[73] and significantly increases the chance of aspirating water and drowning during the first few minutes of immersion in choppy water. The hypocapnia caused by hyperventilation probably accounts for the tetany, disorientation, and clouding

of consciousness observed in individuals, including swimmers and canoeists, on cold-water immersion.[74-76]

There is an inspiratory shift in end-expiratory lung volume following cold-water immersion which can result in the occurrence of tidal breathing within 1 litre of total lung capacity.[69,70] This response makes breathing very difficult and probably contributes to the sensation of dyspnoea experienced on initial immersion.[69]

The initial cardiovascular responses to immersion include intense vasoconstriction, a 42 to 49 per cent increase in heart rate, and a 59 to 100 per cent increase in cardiac output.[64,77] As a result of these responses arterial and venous pressures are increased.

The early cardiovascular responses to immersion in cold water place a significant and sudden strain on the system and are a particular threat to people with coronary heart disease, in whom myocardial ischaemia is more likely to develop with sudden increases in cardiac workload. Hypertensive or aneurysmal individuals are also at risk from the sudden elevations in blood pressure caused by cold water immersion. The work of the heart, particularly the left ventricle, is increased on immersion in cold water; this can result in greater ventricular irritability and cardiac irregularities, and, on rare occasions, precipitate ventricular fibrillation.[78] Both ventricular and atrial ectopic beats have been reported on immersion in cold water.[78] They have also been reported in young healthy individuals on initial immersion in thermoneutral water,[41,51] when they are probably due to distension and acute straining of the right heart. This response, together with the increase in catecholamine secretion, probably contribute to the arrythmias seen on cold-water immersion. Recent evidence from the laboratory[79] also suggests that although the cold-shock response overrides the diving response in most people,[80,81] even when clothed,[81] the coexistence of these two responses can result in large numbers of supraventricular arrhythmias immediately following breath-holding during submersion in cold water; a similar situation occurs during snorkelling.

The diving response includes bradycardia, apnoea, and selective vasoconstriction and is evoked by immersion of the face in cold water and the consequent stimulation of the ophthalamic division of the trigeminal nerve.[82] Thus, the stimulae for both the cold-shock and diving responses are present during whole-body submersion, and it has been suggested that it is competition between the positive (sympathetic) chronotropic input to the heart of the cold-shock response and negative (parasympathetic) input of the diving response which is responsible for the arrhythmias.[79] From a practical point of view the clinical implications of these arrhythmias is unclear, given that they have been reported to be of short duration, that they are largely supraventricular in origin, and that they are asymptomatic. However, their occurrence may be significant in susceptible individuals, such as those with underlying conduction defects; it is clearly impossible to test this in the laboratory, but they may explain some of the hitherto inexplicable sudden immersion deaths.

Long term

Prolonged immersion in water at temperatures below thermoneutrality will inevitably result in hypothermia, that is to say a deep body temperature below 35 °C. Hypothermia is unlikely to be a problem within 30 min of immersion in water even as low as 5 °C, and times to the onset of hypothermia will vary between individuals for the reasons given in a later section. As a general rule, however,

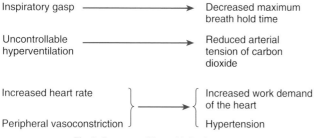

Fig. 2 Summary of the cold-shock response

the deep body temperature of those wearing ordinary clothing will have fallen to 35 °C after 1 h in water at 5 °C, after about 2 h in water at 10 °C and after 3 to 6 h in water at 15 °C.[83]

Before general hypothermia becomes established, locomotor impairment will produce a deterioration in swimming performance through delays in muscle cell-membrane repolarization as a consequence suboptimal temperatures for intracellular enzyme activity. The tone of both protagonist and antagonist muscle groups gradually increases to such a level that swimming becomes virtually impossible; shivering becomes intense and eventually the body tends to assume a semirigid, fetal attitude. Unless flotation aids are available, the individual will be unable to maintain his airway clear of the water and drowning will result before deep body temperature falls to a level where cardiac arrest from hypothermia would normally be expected to occur, namely a myocardial temperature below 28 °C, but more usually 24 to 26 °C.[84]

At cardiac temperatures below 28 °C the conduction velocity of the Purkinje tissue is slowed to approximate that of myocardial fibres. This predisposes the heart to ventricular fibrillation. If a flotation aid such as a life-jacket is available, then the airway should remain protected even when unconsciousness occurs due to hypothermia (at a deep body temperature of about 30 °C).

Normally an individual supported by a life-jacket will keep his back to the waves by paddling. However, once cold-induced locomotor incapacitation becomes established, there is a tendency for the relaxed body supported by a life-jacket to be turned to face the oncoming waves. Depending on the frequency and the steepness of the front of the waves, they may break or splash over the face and compromise the airway. Aspiration could result in coughing and hence uncontrollable inspiration, leading to drowning.

An exception to the general sequence of events outlined above can be found in long-distance outdoor swimmers who are habituated to cold water. Pugh and Edholm attributed the ability of these swimmers to withstand prolonged immersion in cold water, without apparent ill effect, to their unique combination of physical fitness and substantial thickness of subcutaneous fat.[33] This enabled them to maintain a steady work rate for several hours and to retain much of the heat produced within the body. However, many contemporary outdoor distance swimmers are not as fat as those described above.[33] Before the Windermere International Race in 1974, Golden[85] measured the skinfold thickness of eight swimmers. They were not excessively fat, yet all completed the 16.5 mile swim in water at 15 °C.

The winner of the race, a 16-year-old male (15.9 per cent fat, height 195 cm, weight 78 kg), completed the distance in 6 h 42 min; the remainder staggered in over the next 6 h (mean swim time, 9 h). None of the swimmers showed subjective signs of hypothermia—a remarkable feat for near-naked people, given that the estimated 50 per cent survival time for a fully clothed 70 kg man in water at 15 °C is approximately 6 h.[83]

In a subsequent experiment on three long-distance swimmers the value of cold habituation was clearly demonstrated.[86] Conversely, the apparent absence of cold habituation in other published accounts[63,87,88] may explain why some swimmers failed to complete the required distance because of hypothermia, despite relatively high water temperatures (18 to 19 °C) and short swim times (less than 3 h).[63,87]

Successful outdoor long-distance swimmers would thus appear to be those who are physically fit with a good swimming technique, moderately fat, and habituated to the water temperature at which they are to compete. Lean fast swimmers will be successful in warmer water, but in colder water fatter swimmers are likely to have an advantage.

A negative aspect of the habituation of distance swimmers may be that the incipient onset of hypothermia may go unnoticed in the absence of subjective discomfort and other signs such as shivering.[86] More research is required to identify the deep body temperature at which such individuals become distressed. The potential is there for them to become hypothermic before swimming is seriously impaired.[88] Then, with the cessation of swimming and therefore heat production, heat reserves from the deep body store will continue to be lost to the substantial heat sink in their subcutaneous fat, thereby reducing the interval of useful consciousness from the initial prodromal symptoms to collapse.

Hardwick[88] describes a semiconscious long-distance swimmer reluctantly being removed from the sea after almost 12 h and collapsing pulseless into unconsciousness on entry into the boat. Three years later the same swimmer attempted the identical swim in water around 13 °C; again, she had to be removed from the sea after 7 h:33 min. Throughout the swim her normal stroke rate of 60 strokes/min progressively declined to 45 strokes/min.

Post-immersion

In the absence of flotation assistance, loss of consciousness through hypothermia, uncomplicated by near-drowning, or pure hypothermic cardiac arrest is unlikely in immersion victims. Live hypothermic casualties, or near-drowned cold casualties, may suffer collapse and cardiac arrest during or shortly after the rescue process. This phenomenon, which has been termed 'circum-rescue collapse' although not yet fully understood has been reviewed by Golden et al.[89] Excluding those who may die shortly after rescue from hypoxia caused by drowning, there is evidence to suggest that circulatory collapse and cardiac arrest may occur during rescue as a result of a number of factors, of which the most important are:

- loss of hydrostatic assistance to venous return and the reimposition of the full effects of gravity;

- hypovolaemia caused by diuresis and intercompartmental fluid shifts;

- increased blood viscosity as a result of cooling;

- diminished work capacity of the hypothermic heart and reduced time for coronary filling;

- dulled baroreceptor reflexes;

- unattainable demands to perfuse skeletal muscle;

- psychological stress and pre-existing coronary disease.

It follows from the mechanisms suggested above that, during rescue, the greatest problems are likely to be encountered by those who are lifted vertically after prolonged immersion in a vertical position. Any problems are likely to be potentiated by a requirement for unnecessary activity by the casualty during rescue.

Lifting casualties in a horizontal position is likely to be less traumatic and, with the inevitable proviso, 'circumstances permitting', immersion victims should be handled with the utmost gentleness and as the potentially critically ill patients that they are.

Individual differences

One of the difficulties in describing the responses associated with immersion in cold water is the wide variation encountered between individuals. This is due, in part, to methodological differences between investigations which are reflected in both the way and the degree to which subjects have been cooled. In addition, differences in body morphology, sex, age, fitness, nutritional state, and previous exposure to cold are also major sources of variation. As might be expected, many of these factors are interrelated.

As mentioned previously, the fall in deep body temperature during cold-water immersion is inversely related to subcutaneous fat thickness. It has been estimated[38] that each additional per cent of body fat equates approximately with a 0.1 °C rise in deep body temperature. Additionally, as poorly perfused muscle makes a significant contribution to insulation at rest, differences in body mass are another potential source of variation between individuals during resting immersions.

As would be expected from a response evoked by skin receptors, there is no significant difference between the cold-shock responses of fat and lean individuals; however, increased fat thickness is associated with a smaller metabolic and cardiovascular response to prolonged cold-water immersion.[21,38] In fatter individuals the metabolic response to cold is primarily stimulated by receptors in the skin, whereas in leaner individuals there is usually also an input from deep body receptors as they cool.[21]

The ratio A_d/wt of surface area to weight may also be a cause of variation between the responses of individuals during cold-water immersion. A small ratio has been reported to reduce heat losses in both young[90] and adult groups.[91] In contrast, Toner *et al.*[92] conclude that, within a given population and sex, differences in A_d/wt have no effect on the responses observed during exercising or resting immersions.

The greater A_d/wt and lower thermoregulatory sensitivity of women may explain why, during cold-water immersion, the deep body temperatures of resting females fall by a greater amount than in males with similar subcutaneous fat thicknesses. The lower thermoregulatory thermosensitivity of women is evidenced by the smaller increase in their metabolism, compared to that of men, in response to reductions in deep body temperature by more than 1 °C.[38] Thus, although women have greater amounts of subcutaneous fat than men, as a consequence of their greater A_d/wt and lower thermoregulatory sensitivity, it has been calculated that lean women require twice the amount of fat of lean men to show similar changes in deep body temperatures in cold water.[38]

Despite these differences, women with similar fat thicknesses to men demonstrate roughly equivalent responses when exercising in cold water.[93,94] This is probably because the exercise enables women to produce similar levels of heat to men but, because of their greater thickness of fat over the active musculature[95] and a greater peripheral vasoconstriction,[96] they are better able to retain this heat. These morphological and physiological differences may be of limited benefit at rest, but are an advantage when exercise increases peripheral blood flow. During exercise immersions they compensate for the higher A_d/wt of women; during resting immersions they are counteracted by the less-sensitive metabolic response.

The initial respiratory response of females to cold-water immersion may be smaller than that of males,[97] although this is not generally agreed.[77,80]

Largely because of differences in the methodologies employed, a rather confused picture has emerged regarding the effect of age on the responses of individuals to cold. In general, it appears that ageing is accompanied by a diminished responsiveness to cold. This includes progressive weakening of the vasoconstrictor response,[98,99] possibly because of morphological changes in blood vessels[100] and a reduced shivering response.[101] Older men appear to have lower deep body temperatures on exposure to thermoneutral conditions[98,102] and are more susceptible to cold than younger people; on exposure to cold they do not prevent further falls in their initially low deep body temperatures.[102]

Although fitness does not appear to be related to the hormonal changes induced by cold-water immersion,[103] individuals with high levels of aerobic fitness do have attenuated initial respiratory and cardiac responses to such immersion.[104]

A cross-adaptation between fitness and the long-term thermoregulatory responses to immersion has been reported by several authors.[23,105] The major differences between very fit and less fit individuals appear to be that fitter individuals have a slightly reduced normal body temperature, they experience cold sensation and thermal discomfort at lower mean body temperatures, and they demonstrate a downward shift in their shivering thresholds as a consequence of a lowering of their thermoregulatory set point.[105,106]

Despite the downward shift in the shivering thresholds of fitter individuals, there is evidence[107] to suggest that the maximum intensity of shivering achievable by individuals is related to their maximum oxygen consumption $\dot{V}O_2$max. Furthermore, on exposure to cold air, rather than water, individuals may show a direct relationship between fitness, metabolic heat production, and skin temperature.[23,108] This may be due to the differences in the physical properties of air and water, or the type of training programme used to increase levels of fitness.

As suggested by the above discussion, many of the responses exhibited by fitter individuals on exposure to cold are similar to those occurring as a result of cold habituation. In the wide range of studies and methodologies which typify the field of human acclimatization to cold, a 'hypothermic' adaptation to cold is the most frequently reported response. This adaptation is characterized by a smaller metabolic response to cold, a greater fall in deep body temperature on exposure to cold, and, despite these alterations, a greater level of thermal comfort during exposure.[109,110] However, this response may not occur if individuals perform exercise which helps maintain deep body temperature during exposure to cold.[111]

Both the initial respiratory and cardiac responses to cold-water immersion can be significantly reduced by as few as six repeated immersions in cold water.[78,111]

Exercise in cold water

Effect of exercise on responses to cold water

The performance of gentle exercise during the first minutes of cold-water immersion does not prevent the cold-shock induced falls in the end-tidal partial pressure of carbon dioxide. At moderate and maximal levels of exercise, however, the fall can be reduced or reversed and therefore hyperpnoea rather than hyperventilation occurs.[75]

At an exercise intensity of 150 W or more the 70 to 90 per cent of total body insulation provided by poorly perfused muscle is almost completely eliminated by exercise hyperaemia.[112,113] This leaves the physical barriers of subcutaneous fat and skin as the principal sources of insulation. On the basis of this, body mass should give the best indication of the insulation available to an individual resting in cold water, and skinfold thickness should give the best indication of the insulation available when exercising.

Although exercise will increase heat loss, several factors will determine whether an individual will cool more or less quickly when exercising compared with resting during cold-water immersion. These factors include: water temperature; water agitation; exercise intensity; type of exercise performed; subcutaneous fat thickness; fitness; and clothing worn.

In general, at water temperatures above 25 °C, exercise requiring an oxygen consumption of about 1 litre/min will slow the rate of fall of deep body temperature of an average individual compared with resting immersions. Below 25 °C this intensity of exercise will accelerate the fall in deep body temperature.[34,114,115] In fat individuals, however, physical exertion has a smaller effect on falls in deep body temperature in water at temperatures as low as 5 °C,[114] although when either fat or thin men rest in water at a temperature at which they are just unable to stabilize deep body temperature, exercise increases their rates of fall of deep body temperature.[21]

Maximal or high-intensity exercise in cold water may result in slower rates of fall of deep body temperature than those seen with either lower intensity exercise[114] or during resting immersions.[13,38] Costill et al.[12] observed that when their well-conditioned, non-obese subjects performed high-intensity exercise (oxygen consumption of 3 l/min) in water at 17 °C, they showed a slight increase in deep body temperature after 20 min.

It might be expected that high-intensity exercise should be beneficial in cold water; convective heat losses are maximal when swimming at any speed and the insulation provided by poorly perfused muscle is lost at quite low levels of exercise. Thereafter, any further increases in heat production should be associated with relatively small increases in heat loss and result in a net heat gain.

Whole-body exercise has been employed in most of the studies where the effect of physical exertion on deep body temperature during cold-water immersion has been investigated. In the studies in which either leg-only or arm-only exercise has been examined,[104,116] the results suggest that leg-only exercise results in slower rates of fall in deep body temperature than resting immersions, and that the arms are a greater source of heat loss than the legs during high-intensity exercise. This might be expected as the arms have a surface area to mass ratio of approximately twice that of the legs[117] and a shorter conductive pathway from the centre to the surface of the limb. Furthermore, when they are not being exercised, the arms can be placed against the torso, thereby providing some insulation as well as reducing the overall surface area for convective heat loss.[104]

The number of factors determining the influence of exercise on deep body temperature during cold-water immersion, and their possible interactions, make it extremely difficult to give general advice concerning whether or not individuals should exercise following accidental immersion. It is fair to say that in most cases, and

in particular those involving lean people wearing few clothes in relatively still water, body movements should be avoided.

Effect of cold immersion on exercise performance

On immersion, exercise performance may be significantly impaired at first, as a result of the initial responses to cold. The respiratory responses can cause swimming failure within the first few minutes of immersion. High respiratory frequencies can make the synchronization of breathing and swim stroke impossible thus resulting in the inhalation of water.[118-120]

With the adaptation of the initial responses, after about 3 min of immersion, the next influence on performance is likely to be peripheral cooling. The hands are particularly susceptible to cooling largely because of their high ratio of surface area to mass and, to a lesser extent, their low level of local heat production and variable blood supply. Grip strength can be reduced very quickly following cold-water immersion,[121] and both tactile sensitivity and manual dexterity are also quickly affected.[122,123]

The effects of peripheral cooling are primarily due to alterations in muscle and nerve function. Low muscle temperature can affect several chemical and physical processes at the cellular level including metabolic rate, enzyme activity, calcium and acetylcholine release, diffusion rate, and series elastic components.[121] Muscle-fibre repolarization becomes adversely affected, resulting in an increased muscle tone of both protagonist and antagonist muscle groups.

The rate of conduction of nervous impulses is slowed, and the amplitude of action potentials is reduced with cooling.[124,125] This occurs at nerve temperatures below about 20 °C; in the ulnar nerve a reduction in conduction velocity of 15 m/s per 10 °C fall in local temperature can occur. Nerve block may present at different temperatures with different types of fibres;[126] in general, a local temperature of between 5 and 15 °C is required for 1 to 15 min. Such cooling of peripheral motor and sensory nerves leads to a dysfunction equivalent to peripheral paralysis.[125,127]

The result of these alterations is that maximal performance is reduced; maximum power output is reduced by 3 per cent per degree fall in muscle temperature[128,129] and mechanical efficiency is also reduced.[112]

In contrast with the reduction in maximum performance, muscle temperatures down to 27 °C increase the duration for which sustained contractions can be maintained. This may be due to a slower production and accumulation of the metabolites causing fatigue.[125] At muscle temperatures below 25 °C muscle fatigue occurs earlier as cooling begins to impair neuromuscular function in peripheral muscle fibres, leaving a smaller number of fibres to produce the same amount of force.[121]

The changes in neuromuscular function resulting from cooling explain, in part, the reduction in work capacity in cold water. Other reasons for this decline are the alterations in the central circulation and the reductions which occur in deep body temperature.

The shivering evoked by cold-water immersion raises oxygen consumption. This increases as more and more muscle groups are recruited as skin and deep body temperatures continue to fall. There is progressive involvement of the muscles of the neck, torso, and finally the extremities. It is possible for shivering to occur during exercise,[13,130] but it is progressively centrally inhibited with increasing exercise intensity.[130] Shivering has been reported to be 80 per cent suppressed by exercise at an intensity of 50 per cent $\dot{V}O_2$max[130] and totally suppressed at workloads requiring oxygen consumptions of between 1.2 and 1.4 l/min.[131,132] In contrast, higher oxygen consumptions have been noted in cold compared with neutral environments during exercise requiring oxygen consumptions of up to 2.0 l/min,[133,134] but not at 3.0 l/min in cold compared to thermoneutral water.[12]

Swimming and ergometry in cool and cold water result in an increased metabolic rate at a given work intensity and a decreased heart rate at a given oxygen consumption.[16,135,136] In water at 25 °C and 18 °C average oxygen consumption during arm and leg ergometry is increased by 9 per cent and 25.3 per cent, respectively, when compared to that seen in water at 33 °C. The increase in oxygen consumption is greater in leaner individuals.[58]

The twofold increase in the viscosity of water at 0 °C compared with 25 °C may contribute to the greater energy expenditure seen during swimming in cold water. However, this effect is compensated to some extent by the increased pulling power per stroke which results from the increase in water viscosity. Although the efficiency of each stroke may improve, the shivering and increased muscle tone during exercise in cold water may further reduce mechanical efficiency by increasing the activity of antagonist muscles.[130]

It can be concluded that during cold-water immersion shivering can coexist with exercise up to moderate intensities of exercise. This results in an increase in the energy cost of submaximal exercise in water cooler than 26 to 28 °C.[12,16] As shivering involves both protagonist and antagonist muscles simultaneously, it will itself impair performance.

Shivering may not only impair skilled performance, but the metabolic cost it adds to exercise can result in an more rapid depletion of carbohydrate and lipid energy sources and, as a consequence, an earlier onset of fatigue.[137-139]

$\dot{V}O_2$max, during ergometry or swimming, and maximum performance are both reduced during cold-water immersion.[16,58,136,140] The reduction in $\dot{V}O_2$max can occur in water with a temperature as high as 25 °C[112] and is approximately linearly related to deep body temperature,[136] with a 10 to 30 per cent reduction following a 0.5 to 2.0 °C fall in deep body temperature.[141] Maximal swimming performance can be reduced in water with a temperature as high as 26 °C.[16] In water at 18 °C the subjective sensations associated with exhaustive swimming are related to muscle function rather than cardiorespiratory distress.[16]

Associated with the decrease in $\dot{V}O_2$max in cold water, lactic acid appears in the blood at lower workloads and accumulates at a more rapid rate than in thermoneutral conditions.[136,140] With more profound cooling, however, this is also reduced due to muscle cooling and direct impairment of the processes responsible for the anaerobic production of energy.[134] These changes will all contribute to the degradation of performance in the cold.

A decrease in deep body temperature of 0.5 to 1.5 °C results in a reduction of 10 to 40 per cent in the capacity to supply oxygen to meet the increased requirements of activity.[141] The mechanisms proposed for this reduction and that observed in $\dot{V}O_2$max in cold water include temperature-dependent reductions in enzyme activity within the muscle, reduced oxygen transport due to decreased respiratory and/or cardiac function, and reduced muscle blood flow.[141]

As with immersion in thermoneutral water, there is little evidence to suggest that the alterations associated with cold-water immersion impair respiratory function to an extent that it interferes with oxygen uptake during exercise.[136,142]

With regard to cardiac function, once the cold-shock response has subsided, cold-water immersion reduces resting, submaximal, and maximal heart rates when compared with those seen in warm water.[136,140,143] Despite the reduction in heart rate, cardiac output appears to be maintained during submaximal exercise in cold water by an elevated stroke volume.[58,136,140] Both $\dot{V}O_2$max and maximum cardiac output[112] are reduced by 10 to 30 per cent in cold water, but the relationship between them remains linear and similar to that seen in warm water. There is little evidence to suggest that cardiac output limits $\dot{V}O_2$max in cold water.[141] With profound cooling however, β-receptor activity may be reduced by the direct effect of cold on cardiac muscle, and the reduction in $\dot{V}O_2$max may then be related to decreased heart rate, decreased cardiac output, and decreased oxygen delivery due to the reduced capacity of the heart to develop force.[134,141]

The early appearance of lactic acid in the blood and elevation in diastolic blood pressure seen during exercise in the cold suggests that oxygen delivery to the working muscle may be reduced in cold water. Marked reductions in skeletal muscle blood flow have been measured in subjects in cold water.[141] Therefore it is probable that the exercise hyperaemia seen in normal conditions is attenuated in cooled individuals by a sympathetically mediated vasoconstriction of muscle resistance vessels.[112,136,141] This will not only reduce oxygen delivery, but may also reduce the rate of removal of the end-products of metabolism; these, in turn, may then contribute to the impairment of performance.

It was noted above that immersion in thermoneutral water resulted in a reduction in plasma volume. In cold water this reduction may be as great as 24 per cent.[139] Such changes may further affect muscle perfusion and, as a result of dehydration, reduce work times and compromise thermoregulation.[12]

Therefore a major limitation on performance in the cold is thought to be a progressively lower muscle blood flow with cooling. If the oxygen requirements of the muscle remain the same, then local hypoxia will develop and impair work capacity.[144] This situation may be accentuated by a shift to the left in the oxygen dissociation curve as a result of cooling.[145]

It can be concluded that the performance of both short- and long-term exercise may be seriously impaired in cold water. In some cases this impairment may reach the point where survival is threatened.

Protection, augmentation of performance, and treatment

Protection

The use of specialist protective clothing, which either keeps the body dry and/or insulates it, will help to maintain both skin and deep body temperatures during cold-water immersion and thereby help to maintain performance and extend the time of useful consciousness and survival time (Fig. 3).[73,146-148] With such garments a

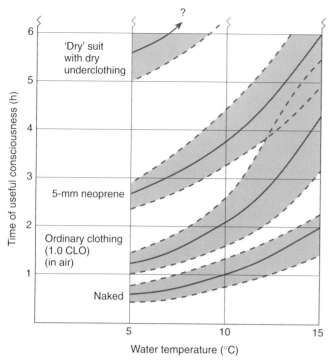

Fig. 3 Times of useful consciousness (deep body temperature 35 °C of individuals immersed in cold water in different clothing assemblies under laboratory conditions. (1 CLO = 0.155 °C/m².W; or the insulation provided by a business suit and standard undergarments.)

good fit is essential to prevent leakage or 'flushing' of water between the skin and garment; both these will significantly increase heat loss. Protection of the head is particularly important as the poor vasoconstrictor response in this region makes it a major area of heat loss.[149] Finally, shivering is more likely to make a positive rather than a negative contribution to the maintenance of body heat stores in individuals who are wearing specialist protective clothing designed to keep the surface of the skin dry and therefore reduce the heat-transfer coefficient at the skin.

If no 'external' insulation is available, the most important source of 'internal' insulation for a swimming man is subcutaneous fat. Pugh *et al.*[150] estimate that an extra 1 mm of subcutaneous fat may be equivalent to increasing water temperature by 1.5 °C. A thick layer of subcutaneous fat is especially useful if, as in many long-distance outdoor swimmers, it is coupled with a high level of aerobic fitness.[33,150] Such a combination allows heat production to be maintained at a high level and to be retained due to low tissue conductance. Pugh *et al.*[150] argue that a person who is not fat should not take up swimming because he or she will be unable to endure the cold; however, there is evidence to the contrary in a more recent study of long-distance outdoor swimmers.[86]

The advantage of an insulating layer of fat forms the rationale for covering the outdoor cold-water swimmer in grease. When swimming in cold water, where heat flows are high, it has been calculated that a 1-mm thick layer of lanolin or Vaseline, which has approximately the same thermal conductivity as fat, has the same effect as raising water temperature by about 1.5 °C.[17,150]

With the exception of increasing buoyancy, subcutaneous fat, as noted earlier, provides no protection against the initial cold-shock response because the receptors which initiate this response are located in the superficial subepidermal tissues, exterior to the subcutaneous fat. Apart from specialist protective clothing, the best protection against the cold-shock response to immersion is to habituate the response by repeated immersions in cold water.[111] Recent, as yet unpublished, evidence from the authors' laboratory confirms earlier work[111] which found that the initial ventilatory responses to immersion can be reduced by up to 60 per cent following just six 3-min immersions in cold water. The habituation produced is due to central nervous rather than peripheral alterations, and, within as yet undefined limits, is not specific to either the body region immersed or water temperature. This latter conclusion is based on the finding that repeated immersions in water at 15 °C reduce the responses evoked on immersion in water at 10 °C.

Cold habituation may be disadvantageous with regard to long-term immersions if a 'hypothermic' adaptation is developed; although skilled performance may improve due to increased thermal comfort and the attenuation of shivering, the consequent reduction in heat production could result in deep body temperature falling at a faster rate.[111,151] Because of the increased comfort associated with the 'hypothermic' type of adaptation there is a danger of the development of incipient hypothermia. Furthermore, it is unclear whether normal thermoregulatory responses are eventually actuated (decreased thermoregulatory threshold) with such an adaptation or whether they remain attenuated (decrease in 'gain' of thermoregulatory responses). Cold adaptation could be of use during long-term immersion if an 'insulative' adaptation were developed; this results in an increase in insulation on immersion[86,152,153] and a reduction in the rate of fall of deep body temperature. Unfortunately, the factors determining which type of adaptation is developed are not clear.

As mentioned previously, increasing fitness levels may be advantageous with regard to protecting against the long- and short-term responses to cold-water immersion. If all else fails, the initial responses can be attenuated by slowing the rate of entry into cold water, while swimming performance is significantly improved if the initial ventilatory responses are allowed to subside before swimming is commenced.[154] A fitter individual will also have a greater capacity to cope with the increased work requirements associated with exercise in cold water. With less fit individuals, the combination of the reduction in $\dot{V}O_2$max and increased oxygen requirements for submaximal work in the cold may seriously impair physical performance.

Maintenance of normal levels of muscle glycogen in large muscle groups may be an important factor in protection against the cold; it has been reported that low, skeletal muscle glycogen levels are associated with more rapid body cooling during cold-water immersion in humans.[155] However, the availability and compensatory use of other metabolic substrates may be an explanation for the failure of others to confirm this finding.[156,157] It would certainly appear that muscle glycogen levels that are higher than normal do not increase tolerance to cold.[155] It has been suggested that because of its relatively low intensity (approximately 25 per cent of $\dot{V}O_2$max), the carbohydrate utilized during shivering is primarily supplied by blood glucose.[158,159] Hypoglycaemia has, for many years, been associated with the inhibition of shivering and, as a consequence, more rapid reductions in deep body temperature and shorter survival times.[160-164] The evidence suggests that hypoglycaemia inhibits shivering via a central mechanism,[165] possibly involving a direct inhibitory effect of low glucose levels on the activity of multisensory neurones in the preoptic/anterior hypothalamic area of the brain.[166] The practical message is clear, during cold exposure, particularly over prolonged periods, adequate sugar intake is essential for the maintenance of normal thermoregulation.

Augmentation of performance

Special diets and pharmacological agents have both been suggested as means of improving cold tolerance in humans.[167-169] It is believed that fat-rich diets are superior to carbohydrate- or protein-rich diets with regard to the maintenance of body temperature in the cold.[167]

Drinking a moderate amount of alcohol (28 ml) before cold-water immersion reduces the rise in respiratory frequency, heart rate, and the number of extrasystoles seen on initial cold-water immersion;[170,171] it also improves morale. In addition, because the powerful cold-induced stimulus to vasoconstriction overcomes the vasodilatory effect of the alcohol, a moderate alcohol intake does not result in a faster rate of fall of deep body temperature during cold-water immersion.[171] Despite these potential 'advantages', the use of alcohol prior to cold-water immersion is not recommended because, when combined with exercise in a cold environment, alcohol induces hypoglycaemia which, in turn, leads to failure of the metabolic processes and, as a result, an accelerated onset of hypothermia and earlier impairment of performance.[162]

Finally, with regard to thermal comfort, heat flux, and maximal swimming performance, the optimal pool temperature for teaching and competitive short-distance swimming is 28 to 30 °C.[16,172] For longer distances, water temperature should be lowered to about 25 °C; this will enable thermal balance to be maintained. Outdoor, long-distance swimmers are advised to train in water at temperatures they expect to encounter in competitive events.

Treatment

Following rescue, the casualty should be quickly placed in a horizontal position while a general assessment of his condition is carried out and essential first aid or appropriate resuscitation given. The possibility of other injuries should always be considered, particularly in those cases not showing the expected response to early treatment. It is not uncommon to sustain a traumatic injury when falling into the water or during a capsize. The signs and symptoms of head or spinal injury, or ruptured viscera, may be concealed by confusion or unconsciousness from a subsequent near-drowning.

Management of the hypoxia, hypercapnia, and acidosis associated with near-drowning casualties is outside the scope of this chapter, but has been well reviewed elsewhere.[173] Controversy still surrounds the rewarming of hypothermic casualties; the authors' views, giving some simple guidelines, follow.

1. On rescue prevent further heat loss by providing adequate insulation both from the ground and from the ambient conditions.

2. If evacuation is not immediately possible and facilities are available, a casualty who is conscious, shivering, and uninjured, may be immersed to the neck in a bath of hot water. The temperature of the bath should approximate, but not exceed, 40 °C (comfortable to your elbow and to the casualty) and should be maintained at this temperature by constant stirring and adding hot water as necessary. This treatment will require a good reservoir of hot water.

3. Cessation of shivering will occur on, or shortly after, immersion, but this should not be interpreted as an indication that rewarming is complete. When subjectively warm, and just before warm flushing or sweating occurs, the casualty should be helped from the bath, dried, and placed in a warmed bed. When fully rested and recovered the casualty may be discharged.

4. An unconscious or semiconscious cold casualty should be regarded as being in a critical condition. The major objective of management is the prevention of further heat loss to facilitate passive metabolic rewarming, without stressing the cardiovascular system which may precipitate ventricular fibrillation. Therefore all movement of the casualty should be conducted slowly and carefully.

5. Normal cardiopulmonary resuscitation should be commenced on the way to hospital if indicated. Subsequent hospital management should be similar to that given to normothermic patients with the following provisos: death should not be diagnosed until the casualty is 'warm and dead'; cardioversion is unlikely to be successful until the myocardial temperature exceeds 28 °C; in fact, repeated attempts at defibrillation below this temperature are likely to damage the heart. Attempts at surface warming are contraindicated as they may result in 'rewarming collapse',[174] namely a fall in systemic blood pressure caused by peripheral local heat inducing vasodilatation before central reflex cardiovascular responses, dulled by hypothermia, are restored.

6. In patients in cardiac arrest, metabolic rewarming will be virtually non-existent, while surface rewarming will be too slow and largely ineffective. In such patients extracorporeal circulation, when available, has proved successful, as has the less sophisticated peritoneal dialysis. The dialysate should be warmed to 37 °C and external cardiac compression should be continued until the deep body temperature has risen above 28 to 30 °C when defibrillation can be attempted.

Summary

Immersion in cold water represents a profound change in the environment surrounding the body. The responses which are evoked by this change can significantly influence performance and, when extreme, can threaten survival. An understanding of these responses should help reduce the risk to, as well as maintain the performance of, those who participate in water-related activities.

References

1. Pleuckhahn VD. The aetiology of 134 deaths due to 'drowning' in Geelong during the years 1957–1971. *Medical Journal of Australia* 1972; **2**: 1183–7.
2. Home Office. *Report of the working party on water safety.* London: Her Majesty's Stationary Office, 1977.
3. Royal Society for the Prevention of Accidents. *Drownings in the UK 1987.* Birmingham: Royal Society for the Prevention of Accidents, 1988.
4. Burton AC, Edholm OG. *Man in a cold environment.* London: Edward Arnold, 1955.

5. Stlowijk JAJ, Hardy JD.Temperature regulation in man. *Pflugers Archiv* 1966; **291**: 129–62.

6. Bligh J. *Neuronal models of temperature regulation*. In: Bligh J, Moore RE, eds. *Temperature regulation*. Amsterdam, London: North Holland, 1972: 105–20.

7. Carlson LD, Hsieh CL. Temperature and humidity. In: Slonim NB, ed. *Environmental physiology*. Saint Louis: CV Mosby Co., 1974: 61–83.

8. Fox RH. Temperature regulation with special reference to man. In: Linden RJ, ed. *Recent advances in physiology*. London: Churchill Livingstone, 1974: 340–405.

9. Hensel H. Thermoreception and temperature regulation. *Monographs of the Physiological Society* No.38. London: Academic Press, 1981.

10. Hong SK. Thermal considerations. In: Shilling CW, Carlston CB, Mathias RA, eds. *The physician's guide to diving medicine*. New York, London: Plenum Press, 1984: 153–78.

11. Gagge AP. Standard operative temperature. A generalized temperature scale. Applicable to direct and partitional calorimetry. *American Journal of Physiology* 1940; **131**: 93–103.

12. Costill DL, Cahill PJ, Eddy D. Metabolic responses to submaximal exercise in three water temperatures. *Journal of Applied Physiology* 1967; **22**: 628–32.

13. Craig AB, Dvorak M. Thermal regulation during water immersion. *Journal of Applied Physiology* 1966; **21**: 1577–85.

14. Colin J, Timbal J, Guieu JD, Boutelier C, Houdas Y. Combined effects of radiation and convection. In: Hardy JD, Gagge AP, Stolwijk JAJ, eds. *Physiological and behavioural temperature regulation*. Springfield, Ill: CC Thomas, 1970: 81–96.

15. Witherspoon JM, Goldman RF, Breckenridge JR. Heat transfer coefficients of humans in cold water. *Journal of Physiology (Paris)* 1971; **63**: 459–62.

16. Nadel ER, Holmer I, Begh U, Astrand PO, Stolwijk JA. Energy exchanges of swimming man. *Journal of Applied Physiology* 1974; **36**: 465–71.

17. Bullard RW, Rapp GM. Problems of heat loss in water immersion. *Aeropace Medicine* 1970; **41**: 1269–77.

18. Barcroft H, Edholm OG. The effect of temperature on blood flow and deep temperature in human forearm. *Journal of Physiology* 1943; **102**: 5–12.

19. Rennie DW. Thermal insulation of Korean diving women and non-divers in water. In: Rahn H, Yokoyoma T, eds. *Physiology of breath-hold diving and the Ama of Japan*. Washington, DC: Publication 1341 NAS-NRC, 1965: 315–24.

20. Burton AC, Bazett HC. A study of the average temperature of the tissues, of the exchange of heat and vasomotor responses in man by means of a bath calorimeter. *American Journal of Physiology* 1936; **117**: 36–54.

21. Cannon P, Keatinge WR. The metabolic rate and heat loss of fat and thin men in heat balance in cold and warm water. *Journal of Physiology* 1960; **154**: 329–44.

22. Rennie DW, Covino BG, Howell GJ, Hong SH, Kang BS, Hong SK. Physical insulation of Korean diving women. *Journal of Applied Physiology* 1962; **17**: 961–6.

23. Bittel JHM, Nonotte-Varly C, Livecchi-Gonnot GH, Savourey GLMJ, Hanniquet AM. Physical fitness and thermoregulatory reactions in a cold environment in men. *Journal of Applied Physiology* 1988; **65**: 1984–9.

24. Smith RM, Hanna JM. Skinfolds and resting heat loss in cold air and water: temperature equivalence. *Journal of Applied Physiology* 1975; **39**: 93–102.

25. Toner MM, Holden WL, Foley ME, Bogart JE, Pandolf KB. Influence of clothing and body-fat insulation on thermal adjustments to cold water stress. *Aviation, Space and Environmental Medicine* 1989; **60**: 957–63.

26. Veicsteinas A, Ferretti GT, Rennie DW. Superficial shell insula-

tion in resting and exercising man in cold water. *Journal of Applied Physiology* 1982; **52**: 1557–64.

27. Park VS, Pendergast DR, Rennie DW. Decreases in body insulation with exercise in cold water. *Undersea Biomedical Research* 1984; **11**: 159–68.

28. Bazett HL, Love L, Newton M, Eisenberg L, Day R, Forster R. Temperature changes in blood flowing in arteries and veins in man. *Journal of Applied Physiology* 1948; **1**: 3–19.

29. Keatinge WR. *Survival in cold water*. Oxford: Blackwell Scientific, 1969.

30. Lewis T. Observations upon the reactions of the vessels of the human skin to cold. *Heart* 1930; **15**: 177–208.

31. Keatinge WR. Mechanism of adrenergic stimulation of mammalian arteries and its failure at low temperatures. *Journal of Physiology* 1964; **174**: 184–205.

32. Nelms JD, Soper JG. Cold vasodilatation and cold acclimatisation in the hands of British fish filleters. *Journal of Applied Physiology* 1962; **17**: 444–8.

33. Pugh LGC, Edholm OG. The physiology of Channel swimmers. *Lancet* 1955; **2**: 761–8.

34. Carlson LD, Hsieh ACL, Fullington F, Elsner RW. Immersion in cold water and total body insulation. *Journal of Aviation Medicine* 1958; **29**: 145–52.

35. Keatinge WR. The effect of subcutaneous fat and of previous exposure to cold on the body temperature, peripheral blood flow and metabolic rate of men in cold water. *Journal of Physiology* 1960; **153**: 166–78.

36. Rowell LB. *Human circulation. Regulation during physical stress*. New York: Oxford University Press, 1986.

37. Nielsen B. Metabolic reactions to changes in core and skin temperature in man. *Acta Physiologica Scandinavica* 1976; **97**: 125–38.

38. McArdle VTD, Magel JR, Gergley TJ, Spina RJ, Toner MM. Thermal adjustment to cold water exposure in resting men and women. *Journal of Applied Physiology* 1984; **56**: 1565–71.

39. Lin YC, Hong SK. Physiology of water immersion. *Undersea Biomedical Research* 1984; **11**: 109–11.

40. Hong SK, Cerretelli P, Cruz JC, Rahn H. Mechanics of respiration during submersion in water. *Journal of Applied Physiology* 1969; **27**: 535–8.

41. Arborelius M Jr, Balldin UI, Lilja B, Lundgren CEG. Hemodynamic changes in man during immersion with the head above the water. *Aerospace Medicine* 1972; **43**: 592–8.

42. Risch WD, Koubenec HJ, Beckmann U, Lange S, Gauer OH. The effect of graded immersion on heart volume, central venous pressure, pulmonary blood distribution, and heart rate in man. *Pflugers Archiv* 1978; **374**: 115–18.

43. Gauer OH, Henry JP. Neurohumeral control of plasma volume. In: Guyton AC, Crowley AW, eds. *Cardiovascular physiology II*. Baltimore, MD: University Park Press, 1976: 145–90.

44. Begin R, Epstein M, Sackner MA, Levinson R, Dougherty R, Duncan D. Effects of water immersion to the neck on pulmonary circulation and tissue volume in man. *Journal of Applied Physiology* 1976; **40**: 293–9.

45. Lin YC. Circulatory functions during immersion and breath-hold dives in humans. *Undersea Biomedical Research* 1984; **11**: 123–38.

46. Dahlback GO, Jonsson E, Liner MH. Influence of hydrostatic compression of the chest and intrathoracic blood pooling on static lung mechanics during head-out immersion. *Undersea Biomedical Research* 1978; **5**: 71–85.

47. Reid MB, Banzett RB, Feldman HA, Mead J. Reflex compensation of spontaneous breathing when immersion changes diaphragm length. *Journal of Applied Physiology* 1985; **58**: 1135–42.

48. Flynn ET, Camporesi EM, Nonnely SA. Cardiopulmonary responses to pressure breathing during immersion in water. In:

Lanphier EH, Rahn H, eds. *Man, water, pressure.* Buffalo: University of New York Press, 1975: 79–94.

49. Jarrett AS. Effect of immersion on intrapulmonary pressure. *Journal of Applied Physiology* 1965; **20**: 1261–6.

50. Craig AB, Dvorak M. Expiratory reserve volume and vital capacity of the lungs during immersion in water. *Journal of Applied Physiology* 1975; **38**: 5–9.

51. Epstein M, Johnson G, De Nunzio AG. Effects of water immersion on plasma catecholamines in normal humans. *Journal of Applied Physiology* 1983; **54**: 244–8.

52. Behn C, Gauer OH, Kirsch K, Eckert P. Effects of sustained intrathoracic vascular distension on body fluid distribution and renal excretion in man. *Pflugers Archiv* 1969; **313**: 123–35.

53. Gauer OH, Henry JP, Behn C. The regulation of extracellular fluid volume. *Annual Review of Physiology* 1970; **32**: 547–95.

54. Epstein M, Duncan DC, Fishman LM. Characterization of the natriuresis caused in normal man by immersion in water. *Clinical Science* 1972; **43**: 275–87.

55. Epstein M. Renal effects of head-out water immersion in man: Implications for an understanding of volume homeostasis. *Physiological Reviews* 1978; **58**: 529–81.

56. Choukroun M-L, Kays C, Varene P. Effects of water temperature on pulmonary volumes in immersed human subjects. *Respiration Physiology* 1989; **75**: 255–66.

57. Rennie DW, DiPrampero P, Cerretelli PC. Effects of water immersion on cardiac output, heart rate and stroke volume of man at rest and during exercise. *Medicina Dello Sport* 1971; **24**: 223–8.

58. McArdle WD, Magel JR, Lesmes GR, Pechar GS. Metabolic and cardiovascular adjustments to work in air and water at 18, 25 and 33°C. *Journal of Applied Physiology* 1976; **40**: 85–90.

59. Knight DR, Horvath SM. Urinary responses to cold temperature during water immersion. *American Journal of Physiology* 1985; **248**: R560–6.

60. Johnson DG, Hayward JS, Jacobs TP, Collis ML, Eckeson JD, Williams RH. Plasma norepinephrine responses of man in cold water. *Journal of Applied Physiology* 1977; **43**: 216–20.

61. Galbo H, Houston ME, Christensen NJ, Holst JJ, Neilsen B, Nygaard E, Suzuk J. The effect of water temperature on the hormonal response to prolonged swimming. *Acta Physiologica Scandinavica* 1979; **105**: 326–37.

62. Arnett EL, Watts DT. Catecholamine excretion in men exposed to cold. *Journal of Applied Physiology* 1960; **15**: 449–500.

63. Dulac S, Quimon A, DeCarutel D, Le Blanc J, Jobin M, Cote J, Brisson GR, Lavoie JM, Diamond P. Metabolic and hormonal responses to long-distance swimming in cold water. *International Journal of Sports Medicine* 1987; **8**: 352–6.

64. Manager WM, Wakim KG, Bollman JL. *Chemical quantitation of epinephrine and norepinephrine in plasma.* Springfield, IL: CC Thomas, 1959.

65. Keatinge WR, McIlroy MB, Goldfien A. Cardiovascular responses to ice-cold showers. *Journal of Applied Physiology* 1964; **19**: 1145–50.

66. Le Blanc J, Cote J, Jobin M, Labrie A. Plasma catecholamines and cardiovascular responses to cold and mental activity. *Journal of Applied Physiology* 1979; **47**: 1207–11.

67. Bohring M, Spies HF. *Pathogenesis of sudden death following water immersion (immersion syndrome).* Washington, DC: Technical Memorandum, National Aeronautic and Space Administration, 1981.

68. Tipton MJ. The initial responses to cold water immersion in man. *Clinical Science* 1989; **77**: 581–8.

69. Keatinge WR, Nadel JA. Immediate respiratory response to sudden cooling of the skin. *Journal of Applied Physiology* 1965; **20**: 65–9.

70. Tipton MJ, Stubbs DA, Elliott DS. Human initial responses to immersion in cold water at 3 temperatures and following hyperventilation. *Journal of Applied Physiology* 1991; **70**: 317–22.

71. Goode RC, Duffin J, Miller R, Romet TT, Chant W, Ackles A. Sudden cold water immersion. *Respiration Physiology* 1975; **23**: 301–10.

72. Tipton MJ, Golden, FStC. The influence of regional insulation on the initial responses to cold immersion. *Aviation Space and Environmental Physiology* 1987; **58**: 1192–6.

73. Tipton MJ, Vincent MJ. Protection provided against the initial responses to cold immersion by a partial coverage wet suit. *Aviation, Space and Environmental Physiology* 1989; **60**: 769–73.

74. Golden FStC, Hervey GR. A class experiment on immersion hypothermia. *Journal of Physiology* 1972; **227**: 35–6P.

75. Cooper KE, Martin S, Riben P. Respiratory and other responses in subjects immersed in cold water. *Journal of Applied Physiology* 1976; **40**: 903–10.

76. Baker S, Atha J. Canoeist's disorientation following cold immersion. *British Journal of Sports Medicine* 1981; **15**: 111–15.

77. Hayward JS, Eckerson JD. Physiological responses and survival time predictions for humans in ice-water. *Aviation, Space and Environmental Physiology* 1984; **55**: 206–12.

78. Keatinge WR, Evans M. The respiratory and cardiovascular response to immersion in cold and warm water. *Quarterly Journal of Experimental Physiology* 1961; **46**: 83–94.

79. Tipton MJ, Kelleher PC, Golden FStC. Supraventricular arrhythmias following breath-hold submersions in cold water. *Undersea and Hyperbaric Medicine* 1994; **21**: 305–13.

80. Hayward JS, Hay C, Matthews BR, Oveeweel CH, Radford DD. Temperature effect on the human dive response in relation to cold water near-drowning. *Journal of Applied Physiology* 1984; **56**: 202–6.

81. Tipton MJ. The effect of clothing on 'diving bradycardia' in man during submersion in cold water. *European Journal of Applied Physiology* 1989; **59**: 360–4.

82. Andersen HT. Physiological adaptations in diving vertebrates. *Physiological Reviews* 1966; **46**: 212–43.

83. Molnar GW. Survival of hypothermia by men immersed in the ocean. *Journal of the American Medical Association* 1946; **131**: 1046–50.

84. Alexander L. *The treatment of shock from prolonged exposure to cold, especially water.* Combined Intelligence Objectives Sub-Committee APO 413 C105, Item No. 24. London: Her Majesty's Stationary Office, 1945.

85. Golden FStC. Physiological changes in immersion hypothermia, with special reference to factors which may be responsible for death in the early rewarming phase. PhD Thesis, University of Leeds, 1979.

86. Golden FStC, Hampton IFG, Smith DJ. Lean long distance swimmers. *Journal of the Royal Naval Medical Service* 1980; **66**: 26–30.

87. Bergh U, Ekblom B, Holmer I, Gullstrand L. Body temperature response to a long distance swimming race. *International Series on Sport Sciences*, Volume 6. *Swimming Medicine IV.* Baltimore, MD: University Park Press, 1978: 342–4.

88. Hardwick RG. Two cases of accidental hypothermia. *British Medical Journal* 1962; **1**: 147–9.

89. Golden FStC, Hervey GR, Tipton MJ. Circum-rescue collapse: collapse, sometimes fatal, associated with rescue of immersion victims. *Journal of the Royal Naval Medical Service* 1991; **77**: 139–49.

90. Sloan REG, Keatinge WR. Cooling rates of young people swimming in cold water. *Journal of Applied Physiology* 1973; **35**: 371–5.

91. Buskirk ER, Kollias J. Total body metabolism in the cold. *New Jersey Academy of Science Special Symposium Issue* 1969: 17–25.

92. Toner MM, Sawka MN, Foley ME, Pandolf KB. Effects of body mass and morphology on thermal responses in water. *Journal of Applied Physiology* 1986; **60**: 521–5.

93. Hayward JS, Eckerson JD, Collins ML. Thermal balance and survival time prediction of man in cold water. *Canadian Journal of Physiology and Pharmacology* 1975; **53**: 21–32.

94. McArdle WD, Magel JR, Spina RJ, Gergley TJ, Toner MM. Thermal adjustments to cold-water exposure in exercising men and women. *Journal of Applied Physiology* 1984; **56**: 1572–7.

95. Edwards DAW. Differences in the distribution of subcutaneous fat with sex and maturity. *Clinical Science* 1951; **10**: 305–15.

96. Bollinger A, Schlumpf M. Finger blood flow in healthy patients of different age and sex and in patients with primary Raynauld's disease. *Acta Chirurgica Scandinavica (Suppl.)* 1976; **465**: 53–7.

97. Malkinson TJ, Martin S, Simper P, Cooper KE. Expired air volumes of males and females during cold water immersion. *Canadian Journal of Physiology and Pharmacology* 1981; **59**: 843–6.

98. Wagner JA, Robinson S, Marino RP. Age and temperature regulation of humans in neutral and cold environments. *Journal of Applied Physiology* 1974; **37**: 562–5.

99. Budd GM, Brotherhood JR, Hendrie AL, Jeffery SE. Effects of fitness, fatness, and age on men's responses to whole body cooling in air. *Journal of Applied Physiology* 1991; **71**: 2387–93.

100. Wagner JA, Matsushita K, Horvath SM. Effects of carbon dioxide inhalation on physiological responses to cold. *Aviation, Space and Environmental Medicine* 1983; **54**: 1074–9.

101. Horvath SM, Radcliffe CE, Hutt BK, Spurr GB. Metabolic responses of old people to a cold environment. *Journal of Applied Physiology* 1958; **8**: 145–8.

102. Wagner JA, Horvath SM. Cardiovascular reactions to cold exposures differ with age and gender. *Journal of Applied Physiology* 1985; **58**: 187–92.

103. Jacobs I, Romet T, Frim J, Hynes A. Effects of endurance fitness on responses to cold water immersion. *Aviation, Space and Environmental Medicine* 1984; **55**: 715–20.

104. Golden FStC, Tipton MJ. Human thermal responses during leg-only exercise in cold water. *Journal of Physiology* 1987; **391**: 399–405.

105. Baum E, Bruck K, Schwennicke HP. Adaptive modifications in the thermoregulatory system of long-distance runners. *Journal of Applied Physiology* 1976; **40**: 404–10.

106. Dressendorfer RM, Smith RM, Baker DG, Hong SK. Cold tolerance of long-distance runners and swimmers in Hawaii. *International Journal of Biometeorology* 1977; **21**: 51–8.

107. Golden FStC, Hampton IFG, Hervey GR, Knibbs AV. Shivering intensity in humans during immersion in cold water. *Journal of Physiology* 1979; **290**: 48P.

108. Adams T, Herberting EJ. Human physiological responses to a standard cold stress as modified by physical fitness. *Journal of Applied Physiology* 1958; **132**: 226–30.

109. Stanton-Hicks C, O'Connor WR. Skin temperatures of Australian Aborigines under varying atmospheric conditions. *Australian Journal of Experimental Biology and Medical Science* 1938; **16**: 1–18.

110. LeBlanc J. Evidence and meaning of acclimatization to cold in man. *Journal of Applied Physiology* 1956; **9**: 395–8.

111. Golden FStC, Tipton MJ. Human adaptation to repeated cold immersions. *Journal of Physiology* 1988; **396**: 349–63.

112. Rennie DW, Park Y, Veicsteinas A, Pendergast D. Metabolic and circulatory adaptation to cold water stress. In: Cerretelli P, Whipp B, eds. *Exercise bioenergetics and gas exchange*. Amsterdam: Elsevier/N. Holland, 1980: 315–21.

113. Strong LH, Gee GK, Goldman RF. Metabolic and vasomotor insulative responses occurring on immersion in cold water. *Journal of Applied Physiology* 1985; **58**: 964–77.

114. Keatinge WR. The effect of work and clothing on the maintenance

115. Beckman EL. Thermal protection during immersion in cold water. In: Lambertson LJ, Greenbaum LG, Jr, eds. *Proceedings of the second symposium on underwater physiology*. Washington, DC: Publication 1181 NAS-NRC, 1963.

116. Toner MM, Sawka NM, Pandolf KB. Thermal responses during arm and leg and combined arm–leg exercise in water. *Journal of Applied Physiology* 1984; **56**: 1355–60.

117. Burton AC. Human calorimetry II. The average temperature of the tissues of the body. *Journal of Nutrition* 1935; **9**: 261–80.

118. Glaser EM, Hervey GR. Swimming in very cold water. *Journal of Physiology* 1951; **115**: 14P.

119. Keatinge WR, Prys-Roberts C, Cooper KE, Honour AJ, Haight J. Sudden failure of swimming in cold water. *British Medical Journal* 1969; **1**: 480–3.

120. Golden FStC, Hardcastle PT. Swimming failure in cold water. *Journal of Physiology* 1982; **330**: 60–1P.

121. Vincent MJ, Tipton MJ. The effects of cold immersion and hand protection on grip strength. *Aviation, Space and Environmental Medicine* 1988; **59**: 738–41.

122. Bowen HM. Diver performance and the effects of cold. *Human Factors* 1968; **10**: 445–63.

123. Stang PR, Weiner EL. Diver performance in cold water. *Human Factors* 1970; **12**: 391–9.

124. Douglas WW, Malcolm JL. The effect of localized cooling on conduction in cat nerves. *Journal of Physiology* 1955; **130**: 53–71.

125. Clarke SJ, Hellon RF, Lind AR. The duration of sustained contractions of the human forearm at different muscle temperatures. *Journal of Physiology* 1958; **143**: 454–73.

126. Basbaum CB. Induced hypothermia in peripheral nerve: electron microscopic and electrophysiological observations. *Journal of Neurocytology* 1973; **2**: 171–87.

127. Vanggaard L. Physiological reactions to wet-cold. *Aviation, Space and Environmental Medicine* 1975; **46**: 33–6.

128. Bergh U, Ekblom B. Influence of muscle temperature on maximal muscle strength and power output in human skeletal muscles. *Acta Physiologica Scandinavica* 1979; **107**: 33–7.

129. Sergeant AJ. Effect of muscle temperature on leg extension force and short-term power output in humans. *European Journal of Applied Physiology* 1987; **56**: 693–8.

130. Hong SK, Nadel ER. Thermogenic control during exercise in a cold environment. *Journal of Applied Physiology* 1979; **47**: 1084–9.

131. Stromme S, Andersen KL, Elner RW. Metabolic and thermal responses to muscular exertion in the cold. *Journal of Applied Physiology* 1963; **18**: 756–63.

132. Andersen KL, Hart LS, Hammel HT, Sabean HB. Metabolic and thermal response of Eskimos during muscular exertion in the cold. *Journal of Applied Physiology* 1963; **18**: 613–18.

133. Hanna JN, Hill PMcN, Sinclair JD. Human cardiorespiratory responses to acute cold exposure. *Clinical and Experimental Pharmacology and Physiology* 1975; **2**: 229–38.

134. Bergh U. Human power at subnormal body temperatures. *Acta Physiologica Scandinavica* 1980; **478**: 1–39.

135. Nielsen B. Metabolic reactions to cold during swimming at different speeds. *Archives des Sciences Physiologiques* 1973; **27**: A207–11.

136. Holmer I, Bergh U. Metabolic and thermal response to swimming in water at varying temperatures. *Journal of Applied Physiology* 1974; **37**: 702–5.

137. Jacobs I, Romet TT, Kerrigan-Brown D. Muscle glycogen depletion during exercise at 9°C and 21°C. *European Journal of Applied Physiology* 1985; **54**: 35–9.

138. Shephard RJ. Adaptation to exercise in the cold. *Sports Medicine* 1985; **2**: 59–71.

139. Martineau L, Jacobs I. Muscle glycogen utilization during shivering thermogenesis in humans. *Journal of Applied Physiology* 1988; **65**: 2046–50.

140. Dressendorfer RH, Morlock JF, Baker DG, Hong SK. Effect of head-out water immersion on cardiorespiratory responses to maximal cycling exercise. *Undersea Biomedical Research* 1976; **3**: 177–87.

141. Pendergast DR. The effect of body cooling on oxygen transport during exercise. *Medicine and Science in Sports and Exercise* 1988; **20**: S171–6.

142. McMurray R, Horvath S. Thermal regulation in swimmers and runners. *Journal of Applied Physiology* 1979; **46**: 1086–92.

143. Denison DM, Wagner PD, Kingaby GL, West JB. Cardio-respiratory responses to exercise in air and under water. *Journal of Applied Physiology* 1972; **33**: 426–30.

144. Davies M, Ekblom B, Bergh U, Kanstrup-Jensen I-L. The effects of hypothermia on submaximal and maximal work performance. *Acta Physiologica Scandinavica* 1975; **95**: 201–2.

145. Gutierrec G, Warley AR, Dantzker DR. Oxygen delivery and utilization in hypothermic dogs. *Journal of Vascular Research* 1986; **60**: 751–7.

146. Goldman RF, Breckenridge BS, Reeves E, Beckman EL. 'Wet' versus 'dry' suit approaches to water immersion protective clothing. *Aerospace Medicine* 1966; **47**: 485–7.

147. Hayward JS. Thermal protection performance of survival suits in icewater. *Aviation, Space and Environmental Medicine* 1984; **55**: 212–15.

148. Tipton MJ, Stubbs DA, Elliott DS. The effect of clothing on the initial responses to cold water immersion in man. *Journal of the Royal Naval Medical Service* 1990; **76**: 89–95.

149. Froese G, Burton AC. Heat losses from the human head. *Journal of Applied Physiology* 1957; **10**: 235–41.

150. Pugh LGCE, Edholm OG, Fox FH, Wolff HS, Hervey GR, Hammond WH, Tanner JM. A physiological study of channel swimming. *Clinical Science* 1960; **19**: 257–73.

151. Muza SR, Young AJ, Sawka MN, Bogart JE, Pandolf KB. Respiratory and cardiovascular responses to cold stress following repeated cold water immersion. *Undersea Biomedical Research* 1988; **15**: 165–78.

152. Skreslet S, Aarefjord F. Acclimatization to cold in man induced by frequent scuba diving in cold water. *Journal of Applied Physiology* 1968; **24**: 177–81.

153. Park YS, *et al.* Time course of deacclimatization to cold water immersion in Korean women divers. *Journal of Applied Physiology* 1983; **54**: 1708–16.

154. Golden FStC, Hardcastle PT, Pollard CE, Tipton MJ. Hyperventilation and swim failure in man in cold water. *Journal of Physiology* 1986; **378**: 94P.

155. Martineau L, Jacobs I. Muscle glycogen availability and temperature regulation in humans. *Journal of Applied Physiology* 1989; **66**: 72–8.

156. Young AJ, Sawka MN, Neufer PD, Muza SR, Askew EW, Pandolf KB. Thermoregulation during cold water immersion is unim-

157. Martineau L, Jacobs I. Effects of muscle glycogen and plasma FFA availability on human metabolic responses in cold water. *Journal of Applied Physiology* 1991; **71**: 1331–9.

158. Romijn JA, Coyle EF, Sidossis LS, Gastaldelli A, Horowitz JF, Endert E, Wolte RR. Regulation of endogenous fat and carbohydrate metabolism in relation to exercise intensity and duration. *American Journal of Physiology* 1993; **265**: E391–92.

159. Vallerand AL, Zamecnik J, Jacobs I. Plasma glucose turnover during cold stress in humans. *Journal of Applied Physiology* 1995; **78**: 1296–302.

160. Cassidy GJ, Dworkin S, Finney WH. The action of insulin on the domestic fowl. *American Journal of Physiology* 1925; **75**: 609–15.

161. Premitt RL, Anderson GL, Musacchia XJ. Evidence for a metabolic limitation of survival in hypothermic hamsters. *American Journal of Physiology* 1972; **24**: 1279–83.

162. Haight JSJ, Keatinge WR. Failure of thermoregulation in the cold during hypoglycaemia induced by exercise and ethanol. *Journal of Physiology* 1973; **229**: 87–97.

163. Bennett T, Gale EAM, Green JH, MacDonald IA, Walford S. Insulin-induced hypoglycaemia inhibits shivering. *Journal of Physiology* 1980; **305**: 56P.

164. Passias TC, Meneilly GS, Mekjavic IB. Effect of hypoglycemia on thermoregulatory response. *Journal of Applied Physiology* 1996; **80**: 1021–32.

165. Gale EAM, Bennett T, Green HJ, MacDonald IA. Hypoglycaemia, hypothermia and shivering in man. *Clinical Science* 1981; **61**: 463–9.

166. Boulant JA, Silva NL. Multisensory hypothalamic neurons may explain interaction among regulatory systems. *News in Physiological Sciences* 1989; **4**: 245–8.

167. Kreider MB. Effect of diet on body temperature during sleep in the cold. *Journal of Applied Physiology* 1961; **16**: 239–42.

168. Wang LCH, Man SFP, Belcastro AN. Metabolic and hormonal responses in theophylline-increased cold resistance in males. *Journal of Applied Physiology* 1987; **63**: 589–96.

169. Vallerand AL, Jacobs I, Kavanagh MF. Mechanism of enhanced cold tolerance by an ephedrine–caffeine mixture in humans. *Journal of Applied Physiology* 1989; **67**: 438–44.

170. Franks CM, Golden FStC, Hampton IFG, Tipton MJ. The effect of blood alcohol on the initial responses to cold water immersion in humans. *European Journal of Applied Physiology* 1997; **75**: 279–81.

171. Keatinge WR, Evans M. Effect of food, alcohol, and hyoscine on body-temperature and reflex responses of men immersed in cold water. *Lancet* 1960; **2**: 176–8.

172. Robinson S, Somers A. Temperature regulation in swimming. *Journal of Physiology (Paris)* 1971; **63**: 406–9.

173. Modell JH. *Pathophysiology and treatment of drowning and near-drowning.* Springfield, IL: CC Thomas, 1971.

174. Golden FStC. Rewarming. In: Pozos RS, Wittmers LE, eds. *The nature and treatment of hypothermia.* Minneapolis: University of Minnesota Press, 1983: 194–208.

paired by low muscle glycogen levels. *Journal of Applied Physiology* 1989; **66**: 1809–16.

2.3 Altitude

James S. Milledge

Introduction

The study of high-altitude physiology and medicine is of interest to the student of sports medicine for a number of reasons.

First, as part of a general interest in human physiology, the response of the body to a reduction in oxygen availability is a fascinating example of adaptation. Since oxygen is such a vital substrate for animal life its lack affects every system of the body, although some systems are more sensitive than others. The central nervous system may be the most sensitive in terms of irreversible damage, but the musculocardiorespiratory system suffers in terms of function even under the mild hypoxia experienced at modest altitude, for example Mexico City (2300 m).

Second, altitude training for athletics is of great topical interest to all involved in coaching, and the questions of its efficacy, timing, duration, and optimum altitude are all of importance.

Also, with more and more people travelling to high altitude on trekking and climbing holidays the problems of mountain sickness are of interest to all those involved, including doctors asked to advise on such activities.

Of course, the high-altitude environment may include elements other than hypoxia which are deleterious to health. At extreme altitude cold is almost always a problem, whilst in many mountain regions at lower altitudes gastrointestinal problems, common to travellers world-wide, may well be greater than those of hypoxia. These aspects of the mountain environment are dealt with in other chapters. Therefore, this chapter is only concerned with the effects of hypoxia, and mainly with chronic hypoxia of some days', or longer, duration rather than hypoxia lasting only some minutes, which is the realm of aviation medicine.

The atmosphere

The composition of the air is the same all over the world (apart from local pollutants) and at all altitudes, namely about 21 per cent of oxygen and 79 per cent of nitrogen with small quantities of argon, carbon dioxide, and other trace gases. The problem humans face at altitude is not strictly the shortage of oxygen but its low partial pressure, which decreases exactly in line with the decreasing barometric pressure.

We live at the bottom of a sea of air and the barometric pressure is due to the weight of air above us. As we go up in altitude there is less air above and the pressure falls. If air were incompressible like water the fall in pressure would be linear with the rise in altitude, but because it is compressible the relationship is curvilinear. The relationship of pressure to altitude is further complicated by the fall in temperature with altitude. Finally, there are local variations of pressure and temperature which complicate matters even more.

Figure 1 shows the relationship of pressure to altitude according to the International Civil Aviation Organization (**ICAO**) Standard Atmosphere. This is a simplified model atmosphere in which certain assumptions are made regarding temperature, humidity, and pressure and their changes with altitude in order to arrive at a standard for calibrating aircraft altimeters. Altimeters are merely barometers calibrated in height. Aviation authorities are more interested in having all aircraft using the same calibration than in the actual pressure at any given height. There are other formulas for describing this relationship, for instance that of Zuntz *et al.*[1] which happens to fit the data from measurements of barometric pressure made in the Himalayas and Andes rather better than the ICAO model. Up to about 5500 m there is little difference, but at heights

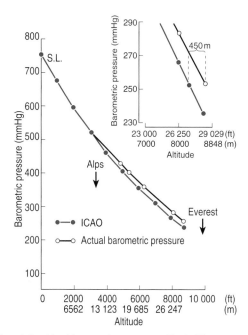

Fig. 1 The relationship of barometric pressure to altitude. The upper curve is calculated from the Zuntz1 formula, assuming a mean air column of 15 °C. The lower curve is from the IOAC Standard Atmosphere. The plotted points are from observations made on the ground in the Himalayas and Andes. (After Pugh.[2])

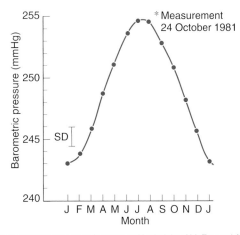

Fig. 2 Mean monthly pressures for 8848 m (the height of Mt Everest) from weather balloons released from New Delhi. The pressure measured on the summit of Everest (*) is also shown. (Reproduced from ref. 67 with permission.)

above this the difference becomes greater, until at the height of the summit of Everest it becomes very important. The ICAO line would predict a pressure of only 236 mmHg. When using the Zuntz formula one must guess the temperature. Pugh[2] calculated a pressure of 250 mmHg, assuming various temperatures at various heights, based on measurements made in the mountains. When it was actually measured on a day of good weather in October 1981 the pressure on the summit of Everest was found to be 253 mmHg.[3]

This difference of about 17 mmHg may not seem much, but at that altitude it is equivalent to about 470 m. Climbers not using supplementary oxygen reach the summit with a rate of climb of less than 50 m (vertical) per hour, so it is unlikely that Everest would ever have been climbed without oxygen had the pressure been only 236 mmHg. The difference between the Standard Atmosphere and the pressures measured in the mountains is greatest near the equator and least near the poles. For a full discussion of this phenomenon see ref. 3.

Pressure is highest in summer and lowest in winter. Figure 2 shows this seasonal variation based on measurements made above Delhi with weather balloons. The January figure of 243 mmHg means that Everest is, physiologically speaking, about 330 m higher in the winter than in the summer which, together with the cold and wind, makes Sherpa Ang Rita's winter oxygenless ascent in December 1987 even more remarkable.

The physiological response to hypoxia

The response of the body to hypoxia depends upon the rate and degree of the hypoxic stress. For instance, the effect on the pilot of a sudden loss of cabin pressure at 28 000 ft (8534 m) is quite different from the effect of a similar altitude on the climber who has spent some weeks at altitude. The pilot would lose consciousness in a few minutes (Fig. 3), whereas the climber not only remains conscious but is able to work out the route and climb upward, if rather slowly. Perhaps the surprising thing about hypoxia is how little it is felt at rest. Indeed, this is why it is so dangerous for an aviator. If the oxygen line becomes disconnected at high altitude the symptoms are so subtle that without training the pilot is likely to lose consciousness

before realizing the danger. The time to unconsciousness decreases with increasing altitude as shown in Fig. 3. At a height of the summit of Everest this is only about 2 min.

By contrast, the effect of hypoxia on an acclimatized person is much less. The main symptom is of breathlessness on exertion. The work rate used by climbers walking uphill at their preferred speed (at sea level) is about half maximum work rate. A ventilation of about 50 litres/min is required at sea level, whereas at 6300 m the rate is 160 litres/min, close to the maximum voluntary ventilation. Below this altitude the climber adopts a discontinuous pattern of climbing with pauses for breath. The difference between the pilot and the climber is due to a series of adaptive changes in the body known as acclimatization.

These changes occur in various systems and with varying time courses.

Figure 4 illustrates the futility of the question, 'How long is required for acclimatization?'. However, the most important changes are in the blood and cardiorespiratory systems, with a time course of days or weeks. These processes are described, as far as they are understood, in the next few sections.

Respiratory acclimatization

One of the most important mechanisms of acclimatization is the increase in ventilation which results in an increase in PaO_2 and a decrease in $PaCO_2$. Thus the decrease in inspired PO_2 due to lower barometric pressure is partially countered. This unconscious increase in breathing is brought about by changes in the chemical control of ventilation.

Hypoxia

Breathing is stimulated by both carbon dioxide and hypoxia. Normally at sea level the hypoxic stimulus to breathing is small. If the carotid bodies are removed ventilation falls by about 15 per cent so that the $PACO_2$ rises from the normal of 40 to 46 mmHg, only just outside the normal range. However, if acute hypoxia is imposed by breathing a hypoxic mixture there is normally an increase in ventilation, especially if CO_2 is added to the inspired mixture to prevent the $PACO_2$ from falling. This is called the hypoxic ventilatory response (**HVR**) and is linear with respect to arterial oxygen saturation (SaO_2) and hyperbolic with respect to PaO_2.

People born and bred at high altitude are found to have a blunted

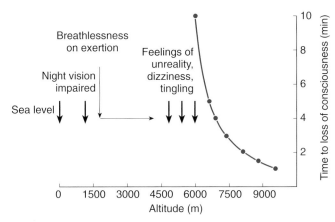

Fig. 3 Effect of sudden exposure to various altitudes on an unacclimatized subject.

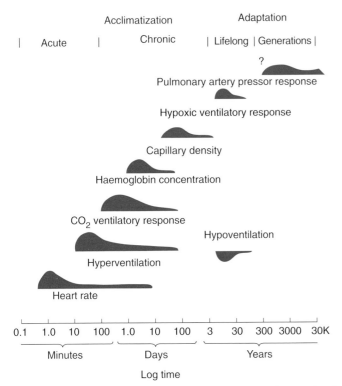

Fig. 4 Time courses of a number of acclimatization and adaptive changes plotted on a log time-scale, the curve for each response denoting the rate of change, fast at first then tailing off.

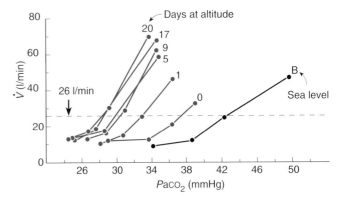

Fig. 5 Effects of acclimatization at 4340 m on the CO_2 ventilatory response. The numbers against each curve indicate the days at altitude. (After Kellogg.[68])

HVR compared to lowlanders. Their performance at altitude does not seem to be in any way impaired by this; on the contrary, they seem less prone to acute mountain sickness and to function very well at extreme altitude. Presumably having developed more fundamental changes, perhaps at the tissue level, they do not need the emergency response of hyperventilation that is useful to the lowlander. It is this late HVR adaptation which is shown in Fig. 4.

There is now good evidence that HVR increases over a period of about 3 weeks at altitude,[4] which may account for the continued increase in ventilation and decrease in $PACO_2$ observed during this period.

Carbon dioxide

If a subject is given a small percentage of CO_2 in the inspired gas, both alveolar and arterial PCO_2 increase, the central chemoreceptors in the brainstem are stimulated and the minute ventilation increases. Further increases in the inspired PCO_2 cause further rises in ventilation. This CO_2-stimulated increase in ventilation is called the CO_2 ventilatory response. The response is linear after an initial lag phase.

Figure 5 shows the results of such an experiment conducted at sea level and repeated at altitude. When going to altitude the slope shifts to the left. About half the eventual shift takes place within the first day at altitude, but it takes 2 to 3 weeks to complete the adaptive response. For a discussion of the mechanisms underlying these changes in the control of breathing see ref. 5.

The net result of these changes is that breathing is set at a higher level both at rest and during exercise. This reduces the difference between the inspired and alveolar PO_2 and thus mitigates the effects of reduced barometric pressure.

Lung diffusion

After inspired air has reached the alveolus, the next step in the oxygen-transport system is the diffusion of oxygen into the blood. The diffusing capacity of the lung does not increase as part of the acclimatization process, apart from a small increase due to the increased haematocrit.[6] This is unfortunate because the diffusion capacity is probably an important limiting factor to exercise at altitude. Highlanders born and reared at altitude do seem to have higher lung diffusing capacities.[7]

The cardiovascular response

Heart rate

On exposure to hypobaric oxygen the heart rate is increased both at rest and during exercise. With acclimatization the resting heart rate falls. At altitudes below about 4500 m it falls to within the sea-level range, above this altitude resting heart rates remain modestly elevated. A similar pattern is seen at submaximal work rates.

Figure 6 shows the heart rate at a fixed work rate in an individual at sea level and at intervals after arrival at altitude. In the fully acclimatized subject at altitudes up to 4300 m the heart rate for the same absolute work rate is the same as at sea level (or lower as in Fig. 6 if the study induces a training effect).

At higher altitudes, heart rates are higher than at sea level for low work rates, but equal to, or even lower, for high work rates.

Figure 7 shows this effect. It should also be noted that since maximum work rate is reduced and since heart rate is related to absolute work rate, the maximum exercise heart rate is progressively

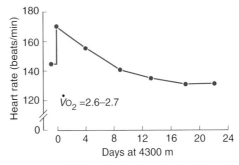

Fig. 6 The heart rate at a fixed work rate at sea level and at various days after arrival at altitude in one subject. (After Astrand and Astrand.[69])

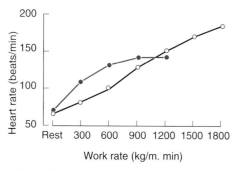

Fig. 7 Effect of increasing exercise on heart rate at sea level (○) and at an altitude of 5800 m (●) in one subject. (Redrawn from Pugh *et al.*[70])

reduced with increasing altitude. The maximum heart rate at an altitude equivalent to the summit of Everest was found to be only 118 beats/min compared with 180 to 200 beats/min at sea level[8]. This limitation of maximum heart rate is surprising since an increase in rate (and cardiac output) would increase oxygen supply to the working muscles. Presumably, it protects the myocardium from possible hypoxic damage.

Cardiac output, stroke volume, and contractility

When a person is exposed to hypobaric oxygen the early changes in cardiac output mirror the changes in heart rate, presumably reflecting sympathetic activity. In absolute terms, after acclimatization the cardiac output is the same as it is at sea level for any given work rate.[9,10] It follows that after acclimatization at moderate altitudes the stroke volume is unchanged from that at sea level, but is reduced at altitudes where the heart rates are elevated.

Indices of contractility, left and right filling pressures, and left ventricular ejection fraction were found to be well maintained even on exercise up to an equivalent altitude of 8000 m during Operation Everest II.[8]

Systemic blood pressure

In contrast to some animals, altitude hypoxia results in no increase in systemic blood pressure. Indeed, some studies report a reduction in blood pressure whilst others have found no change.[10] The rise in blood pressure with exercise is more pronounced than at sea level (Fig. 8), but the change is much less than for the pulmonary circulation.

Pulmonary hypertension

One of the most striking cardiovascular changes found at high altitude is pulmonary hypertension. This hypoxic pulmonary pressor response has been much studied since it was first reported in man by Motley *et al.*[11] Since it can be demonstrated in isolated lung preparations it is thought to be due to the release of mediators in the lung rather than any neurological mechanism. Despite so much research the actual mediator of this response is still unknown. Probably the main role of the response is in the fetus. Here the hypoxia is similar to a man on the summit of Mount Everest, and the response constricts the pulmonary circulation diverting blood via the ductus to the systemic circulation. After birth the response may also be important in diverting blood away from small areas of lung consolidation or collapse, thus maintaining better matching of blood flow and ventilation.

At altitude, with global hypoxia, the pressor response results in a

raised pulmonary artery pressure with very little benefit to the individual. Indeed, it merely puts strain on the right ventricle and may well be important in the genesis of acute pulmonary oedema of high altitude. It is of interest that the yak, an animal well adapted to high altitude, has little or no hypoxic pressor response unlike lowland cattle who have brisk responses.[12]

Most studies have looked at animals or man at rest, but probably the importance of this response is that the pressure goes up very significantly on exercise. Figure 8 shows the rise in resistance with increasing cardiac output during progressive exercise. At sea level there is very little rise in resistance, whereas at 8000 m there is a far greater rise with a smaller increase in cardiac output.

Pulmonary hypertension reverses in acute hypoxia as soon as the hypoxia is relieved; but after hypoxia of only a few weeks, oxygen breathing does not relieve the hypertension. Presumably, structural changes in the pulmonary artery have already taken place by this time. People native to high altitude also have raised pulmonary artery pressures, and they show muscularization of the pulmonary arterial tree and hypertrophy of the right side of the heart.[13]

The electrocardiogram (ECG) at altitude

The main changes in the ECG are due to the increased load on the right ventricle from pulmonary hypertension. There is a shift to the right and to the posterior in the QRS vector.[14] The standard leads show this right axis deviation and the T wave becomes inverted progressively across the chest leads. In general, these changes become more pronounced the higher the altitude and are seen in both low-

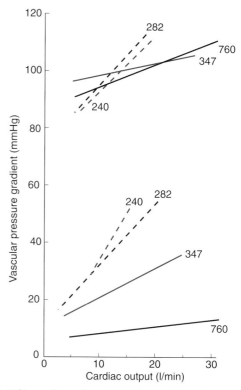

Fig. 8 Effect of increasing cardiac output during exercise on the mean pulmonary artery minus wedge pressure (lower) and on systemic artery minus right atrial pressure (upper) at sea level (760 mmHg) and at two higher equivalent altitudes. Hypoxia has a marked effect on the pulmonary but not on the systemic circulation. (Reproduced from ref.71 with permission.)

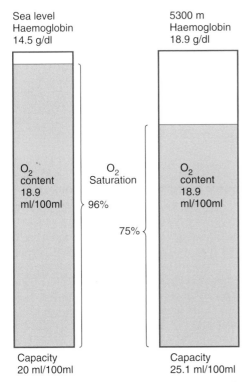

Fig. 9 The oxygen content of arterial blood in an acclimatized subject at 5300 m and at sea level. Despite the oxygen saturation falling to 75 per cent the oxygen content is the same as at sea level because of the increase in haemoglobin and therefore oxygen capacity.

and highlanders. They do not indicate cardiac dysfunction, nor do the inverted T waves have the sinister implication of ischaemia that they might have at sea level.

Haemoglobin and haematocrit

Probably the best-known effect of altitude is the increase in haemoglobin concentration in the blood of people and animals at high altitude. This is illustrated in Fig. 9 where it can be seen that, despite a reduced oxygen saturation, the oxygen content of the blood is maintained by the increased haemoglobin capacity. The mechanism for this increase is the rise in the concentration of erythropoietin due to hypoxia which stimulates the bone marrow to produce more red blood cells.

Figure 10 shows the time course of erythropoietin levels in a group of climbers going quite rapidly to altitude, together with their assent profile and the haematocrit. However, it is clear that the initial rise in haematocrit is mainly due to a reduction in plasma volume and that the erythropoietin-stimulated increase in red blood cells takes much longer.

Figure 11 shows the time course of the change in plasma volume, red cell mass, and blood volume. The rise in haemoglobin concentration levels out after about 6 weeks. At altitude the red cell mass was found to be still increasing after about 36 weeks and was 67 per cent higher than sea-level values. By this time the blood volume was 23 per cent above sea level values when corrected for the reduction in body weight.[15] Similar or greater red cell masses are found in people resident at high altitude.

There is some debate as to the importance of this mechanism in acclimatization. It has been argued that the evolutionary importance

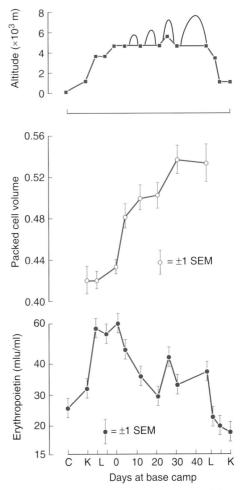

Fig. 10 The effect of ascent to altitude on the serum erythropoietin concentration (lower panel). Upper panel shows the altitude/time profile of ascent, the curved lines indicating ascents above base camp between sampling. The sample at 30 days was taken at 5500 m. Centre panel shows the packed cell volume (PCV). (C) control, sea level; (K) Kashgar, 1200 m; (L) Karakol lakes, 3500 m. (Reproduced from ref. 72 with permission.)

of this system is to deal with the problem of blood loss. The fact that altitude hypoxia activates the mechanism is fortuitous but adds little

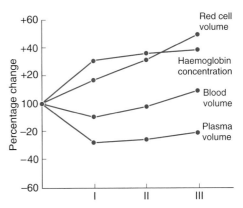

Fig. 11 Changes in haemoglobin concentration, red cell volume, and plasma volume in four subjects: I after 18 weeks at between 4000 and 5800 m; II after a further 3 to 6 weeks at 5800 m; III after a further 9 to 14 weeks at or above 5800 m. (After Pugh.[15])

benefit for the individual. It is pointed out that an increase in haemoglobin concentration increases the viscosity of blood and may reduce cardiac output. Further, it is argued that some altitude populations have very little increase in haemoglobin concentration, yet seem to perform well, and that within any group of climbers on an expedition there is no correlation between climbing performance and haemoglobin concentration. These considerations led Winslow and Monge to state that: 'Excessive polycythaemia serves no useful purpose. Indeed, it is doubtful whether there is any physiological value in "normal" polycythaemia at altitude.'[16]

However, it is becoming clear that an increase in haemoglobin concentration is an advantage in some athletic events even at sea level, so there can be little doubt that some increase is beneficial at altitude.

The endocrine response

The renin–aldosterone system

Aldosterone is probably the most important hormone in the regulation of sodium. It acts on the kidney causing retention of sodium. Exercise is a stimulus to renin and aldosterone release. If exercise of some hours' duration is taken, significant quantities of sodium are retained, especially if continued for some days.[17]

Altitude hypoxia has a variable effect on renin levels, but in all studies on resting subjects aldosterone levels have been found to be reduced. The response of aldosterone to the rise in renin is blunted with exercise. Subjects who develop acute mountain sickness have higher aldosterone levels on arrival at altitude (and more sodium retention) than subjects who are resistant to acute mountain sickness.

Atrial natriuretic peptide

Atrial natriuretic peptide (ANP) is secreted by the atria of the heart in response to stretching. Its effect on the kidneys is to promote a sodium diuresis. It is thought to play an important part in maintaining the constancy of the plasma volume in the face of a salt or water load. Hypoxia results in an increase in plasma levels of ANP, probably by both a direct effect on the heart and secondarily by causing an increase in pulmonary artery pressure and hence right atrial pressure. Exercise also causes an increase in ANP levels, therefore it would be expected that subjects climbing to altitude would have greatly increased levels. However, studies measuring ANP in subjects walking to altitude report only a modest rise.[18,19] The relationship with acute mountain sickness is an open one, with some studies showing a positive and some an inverse correlation. It probably does not play an important role in AMS.

Antidiuretic hormone

Altitude hypoxia in itself does not seem to cause any change in the level of the antidiurietic hormone in those free of acute mountain sickness. In those who do become sick levels are occasionally found to be elevated, especially if subjects actually vomit or have developed pulmonary oedema.[20] In this case, the rise is thought to be the effect of sickness rather than the cause. After acclimatization at 6300 m the antidiuretic hormone level was found to be low in the face of high osmolality, suggesting a reduced response of this system.[21]

Corticosteroids

On ascent to altitude there is stimulation of the adrenal cortex by ACTH with secretion of cortisol as part of a generalized stress reac-

tion. This response wanes over 5 to 7 days. After some weeks at altitude, up to 6300 m, cortisol levels and the response to ACTH is unchanged from the response at sea level.

Insulin and glucose control

Acute hypoxia causes a rise in glucose of about 1.7 mmol/l, followed by a fall towards control levels over about a week. In acclimatized subjects, fasting glucose levels tend to be lower than at sea level and insulin sensitivity is increased (as it is by athletic training).

The central nervous system and hypoxia

Psychomotor performance at altitude

Acclimatized subjects seem to perform well even at altitudes up to 6300 m. On the 1953 Everest expedition, Bourdillon completed *The Times* crossword puzzle in the Western Cwm (6300 m). But climbers find that any task, mental or physical, requires a much greater effort of will to start and complete. Sensitive tests of psychomotor function will detect diminution in function. At an altitude as low as 1524 m a test that depends on learning a novel task was found to show lower scores in subjects breathing air compared with subjects breathing oxygen,[22] although a more recent study showed no effect at this altitude.[23] A test of hand–eye co-ordination, moving a stylus along a groove as fast and accurately as possible, showed deterioration at 4000 m even after 10 months although there was some improvement after 25 months.[24] At higher altitudes, although simple well-learnt tasks can be carried out quite well, tests will bring out deficiencies in concentration, speed, and dexterity.

Psychomotor function after altitude exposure

Of equal interest as performance at altitude is the question of residual impairment after return to sea level. Anecdotally, it has been pointed out that many of those pioneer climbers of pre-war Everest expeditions who climbed above 8000 m without oxygen went on to have distinguished careers and lived to a ripe old age with mental faculties better than average, Professor Odel and Dr T. H. Somervell being outstanding examples. However, studies which have addressed this question rigorously have found some evidence of a decrease in some aspects of psychomotor performance after returning to sea level. Even 1 year after return from altitude, Townes *et al.*[25] found that a finger-tapping test and one out of four tests of memory were significantly reduced compared with scores before the expedition (two other aspects of memory were impaired immediately on return to low altitude but recovered within a year). These findings were confirmed in Operation Everest II, a chamber experiment, thus excluding the possibility that results could have been due to cold or dehydration, etc.[26]

Weight loss and anorexia

Anorexia and weight loss are features of life at high altitude. In the first few days at altitude anorexia, nausea, and vomiting are likely to be part of the syndrome of AMS. After a few days AMS passes, and below about 4500 m appetites are regained. But above about 5500 m most people complain of anorexia which, if anything, gets worse the longer they spend at these altitudes. Above 6500 m anorexia is almost universal and weight loss common. No doubt reduced calorific intake plays a part in the cause of this weight loss. Energy expenditure over the whole 24 h might be expected to be reduced at these altitudes since $\dot{V}O_2$max is reduced, climbing rates are slowed,

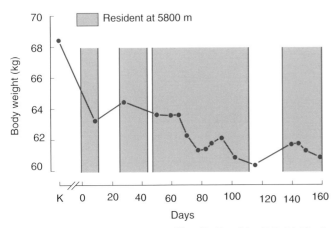

Fig. 12 Weight chart of one subject on the Silver Hut Expedition 1960–61. After the march out from Kathmandu (K) and the initial period of preparation he was in residence at 5800 m or at base camp, 4500 m. Note the loss of weight at 5800 m but weight gain during two breaks at 4500 m.

and even simple tasks of daily living are carried out slowly. However, recent studies using the double-labelled water technique (in which a dose of water is taken with both the H and O atoms labelled; urine is collected and the total CO_2 production over some days can be calculated) have indicated energy expenditure on Mount Everest (5300–8872 m) to be 3510 kcal, similar to that in the Alps (2500–4800 m).[27] When climbers have kept diaries of food eaten, intakes of 2200–3000 kcal have been estimated which should have resulted in only minimal loss of body weight, yet weight was lost at about 500 g/week. The weight chart of one well-acclimatized subject is shown in Fig. 12.

Most of the time was spent at 5800 m where weight was lost at just under 400 g/week. Descent to 4500 m on two occasions for only a few days resulted in weight gain. Arterial oxygen saturation would have been below 70 per cent at the higher altitude and above 70 per cent at the lower. This seems to be the crucial degree of hypoxaemia needed to produce this continued weight loss.

There are probably a number of causes for weight loss above about 5500 m. There is evidence that this degree of hypoxia causes some small bowel malabsorption. Climbers report that their stools tend to be greasy at very high altitude; patients with this degree of arterial desaturation due to congenital heart disease or severe lung disease had reduced xylose absorption which was improved when their hypoxia was corrected by surgery or oxygen breathing[28]. Boyer and Blume[29] found that in climbers at 6300 m xylose absorption was less than at sea level and faecal fat was increased. There is also some evidence of a reduction in muscle protein synthesis at altitude.[30]

Diet at altitude

Views on diet (not only at altitude) are strongly held, often the strength of opinion being inversely related to the strength of scientific evidence. Climbers at altitude often develop a preference for high-carbohydrate/low-fat diets. There is a good physiological reason for this since such a diet results in an increase in the respiratory quotient (**RQ**). This, in turn, means that for a given PCO_2 (or ventilation) the PO_2 will be higher. There is also the possibility that fat is less well absorbed than carbohydrate at altitude. In a study at 4300 m it was found that subjects on a high-carbohydrate diet had greater exercise endurance than subjects on a normal diet.[31]

There is no evidence that extra vitamins or minerals are beneficial if subjects are on a good mixed diet, with the possible exception of iron supplements for women. One study showed that in a group of subjects at 6542 m two women failed to show the expected increase in haematocrit. They had low serum iron.[32]

The major dietary problem at high altitude is anorexia. The sense of taste seems to be dulled and a craving for strong flavours, spicy foods, and more sugar develops. Fresh food, after a period eating preserved food, is also much desired. Every effort should be made to provide for these wishes on expeditions in order to maintain calorie intake and lessen weight loss.

Peripheral tissues
Capillary density

It would clearly be advantageous to increase the number of capillaries per unit of tissue volume since then the intercapillary distance would be decreased and the pathway for oxygen shortened. Increased vascularization has been reported in the brain, muscles, and liver of animals at high altitude. But, at least in the case of the muscles, the increased capillary density is probably due to a reduction in muscle fibre diameter. This, in turn, may be due to a combination of disuse, negative calorie balance, and reduced protein synthesis. The result is a loss of muscle bulk but with the same number of capillaries and therefore more capillaries per unit area.[33]

Muscles

Although there is reduction of muscle fibre size at altitude which must reduce muscle power, myoglobin concentration is increased in the muscle cell in the same way that haemoglobin concentration is increased in the blood. Men native to high altitude had 16 per cent higher myoglobin concentration than lowlanders.[34] Mitochondria have been reported to be increased in some animals but not in others nor in man.[35] These changes, together with an increase in capillary density, will all help to mitigate the effect of arterial hypoxaemia on oxygen transport in muscles.

Intracellular enzymes

A number of the enzymes essential to energy production from glucose and oxygen have been studied in muscle biopsies in men at high altitude. It seems that at intermediate altitudes (up to about 4500 m) levels of enzymes in the citric acid (Krebs') cycle are increased, but at more extreme altitudes (above 6000 m) they are reduced.[36] The changes at intermediate altitude are similar to those resulting from endurance training, and this lends support to the idea that in training the changes are caused by hypoxia in the exercising muscles.

Athletic performance at altitude

The effect of altitude on athletic performance depends upon the type of sport. The reduction in oxygen partial pressure with altitude increases fatigue and reduces the $\dot{V}O_2$max. This will reduce performance in sports that depend upon aerobic capacity. Thus times for middle- and long-distance running events will be increased. But sports that use mainly anaerobic capacity, such as weight lifting, will be unaffected below extreme altitudes.[37] Sports such as sprinting and throwing events will show increased performance because of the decrease in air density, which parallels the reduction in barometric pressure. These expected effects were borne out by the results in the

Table 1 Olympic Games—Mexico City 1968

Event	Winner	Time/distance	Comment
Long jump	Beamon	8 m 90 cm	World record
Pole vault	Seagren	5 m 40 cm	World record
100 m	Hines	9.95 s	World record
200 m	Smith	19.83 s	World record
400 m	Evans	43.86 s	World record
800 m	Doubell	1 min 44.3 s	World record
1500 m	Keino	3 min 39.9 s	Olympic record
3000-m steeplechase	Biwott	8 min 51 s	4% slower than world record
10 000 m	Temu	29 min 27 s	7% slower than world record
Marathon	Wolde	2 h 20 min 26 s	8.5% slower than world record

1968 Olympics held in Mexico City (2300 m) shown in Table 1 and Fig. 13.

Altitude and $\dot{V}O_2max$

Figure 14 shows the reduction of $\dot{V}O_2max$ with altitude. At 2300 m (the height of Mexico City) $\dot{V}O_2max$ is down to 84 per cent of the sea-level value. Thereafter $\dot{V}O_2max$ decreases with increasing altitude so that at the summit of Everest it is 25 per cent of sea level. With acclimatization there is an increase again in $\dot{V}O_2max$, which in one study was shown to be about 10 per cent from days 1 to 14 at 4300 m.[38]

Altitude and fatigue

There is a strong impression that in exercise involving work at rates below maximum, endurance is reduced at altitude. Endurance of this sort is much more difficult to study than $\dot{V}O_2max$ since it is so dependant upon motivation. For work at the same percentage of $\dot{V}O_2max$ there was a 10 per cent reduction in endurance time on the first day after arrival at 4300 m. but this was not statistically significant.[39] With acclimatization there was significant improvement over the first day. In practice, exercise is often attempted at roughly the same rate in absolute terms, that is to say at progressively higher percentages of the prevailing $\dot{V}O_2max$ as altitude increases. Of course, the endurance time under these conditions is much reduced. Thus an athlete attempting his normal training programme will find he becomes fatigued much more easily at altitude.

Altitude training

The idea that training at high altitude, for competitions to be held at low altitude, might be beneficial stems from two sources. First, the observation that a number of very successful middle- and long-distance runners (for example Keino and Wolde) came from areas of East Africa situated at altitudes of 1500 to 2000 m and that their life and training there might be part of the reason for their success. Second, the presumed benefit of developing an increased haemo-

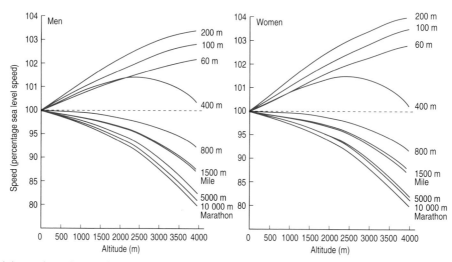

Fig. 13 Theoretical changes in running speeds over various distances with changes in altitude. Note that the scales are different above and below 100 per cent sea-level speed. (Reproduced from ref. 73 with permission.)

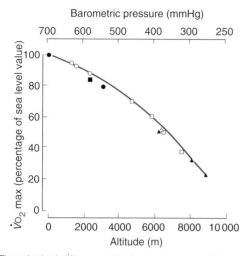

Fig. 14 The reduction in $\dot{V}O_2$max at altitude as a percentage of the sea-level value. The first three points are from a chamber study (unacclimatized subjects);[73] other points are from acclimatized lowland subjects. The 2300 m point is the mean (and SD) of five studies;[47,75-78] 3100 m point;[71] open triangles;[70] closed triangles.[67]

globin concentration or haematocrit (Hct) as a result of altitude hypoxia. The advantage of this increase achieved by blood transfusion (blood doping) or erythropoietin administration has been well reviewed by Williams,[40] but this practice is illegal.

There may well be some advantage in being born and bred at altitude in respect of these aerobic events, although it is not clear exactly which physiological parameters are important. It has been suggested that such people have a greater density of capillaries in their muscles. On the one hand, this is also achieved by any training. But on the other hand, altitude hypoxia, in lowlanders at least, causes a loss in muscle mass and the increase in density is merely due to a reduction in muscle fibre diameter. In any case, lowland athletes considering altitude training cannot achieve the effect of a lifetime of altitude exposure in just a few weeks or months. Highlanders also probably have higher pulmonary diffusing capacities and possibly greater ventilatory capacity.

The second reason to increase haematocrit is probably uppermost in the minds of those advocating altitude training.

The possible benefits of altitude training of a few weeks' duration are shown in Table 2 which also shows the disadvantages of training at altitude.

Haematocrit increase at altitude

Hypoxia stimulates the release of erythropoietin which, in turn, stimulates the bone marrow to produce more red blood cells. However, this process takes place over a number of months rather than days. The initial rise in haematocrit is almost entirely due to a reduction in plasma volume, namely haemoconcentration. This is an advantage to the acclimatizing subject in that it achieves a rapid increase in the oxygen-carrying capacity of the blood. However, the consequent reduction in blood volume may be part of the reason for the reduction in maximum cardiac output found at this stage of altitude exposure. More important, for the athlete contemplating altitude training for low altitude competition, is the point that as the plasma volume can be reduced rapidly on going to altitude so it can be increased as rapidly on coming down and the advantage in terms of haematocrit is lost in a few days.

In a person resident at altitude for months or years the red cell mass is increased by as much as 50 per cent of its normal sea-level value (Fig. 11). When such a person comes down to low altitude he retains this increased red cell mass for some weeks, therefore this could be of advantage in middle- and long-distance running events.

Other advantages of altitude training

The other possible advantages of altitude training listed in Table 2 are rather speculative. The fact that exercise requires much greater ventilation at altitude will mean that the muscles of respiration will be more stressed and therefore possibly the respiratory capacity might be increased, but there is no evidence for this. Training under hypoxic conditions might increase the local effects of training in the working muscles, namely their capillary density or metabolism in some way.

This possibility was explored by Davis and Sargeant[39] by having their subjects train one leg under normal oxygen and the other under hypobaric oxygen. There was no difference in the effect of training under these two conditions. A recent study of well-trained athletes who trained further at altitude for 2 weeks also found no increase in $\dot{V}O_2$max, but it did find some improvement in short-term running time.[41] Unfortunately, this study had no control group so the significance of the last finding is uncertain.

Disadvantages of altitude training.

The risk of acute mountain sickness is a possibility (see below). At best this will mean an interruption in training and at worst may mean a life-threatening illness and the need for evacuation to low altitude.

The reduction in maximum work capacity ($\dot{V}O_2$max) and the earlier onset of fatigue at altitude mean that training has to be less intensive than is possible at sea level.

Is altitude training worth it?

The short answer to this question is that at present it is not known. There have been few really good controlled trials, which is not surprising in view of the difficulty of conducting such trials and the large number of variables of altitude, time, and training schedules.

The trials which have been carried out have given conflicting results. Earlier studies, which mostly claimed to show that training at altitude was advantageous, were not controlled.[42,43] The improved performance could have been simply due to training at any altitude. Roskamm et al.[44] did use controls, they found that subjects trained at 2250 m improved their $\dot{V}O_2$max by 17.5 per cent compared with 6.4 per cent in subjects trained at sea level, for subjects at 3450 m the improvement was 10 per cent. The advantage for the altitude group was significant. Hanson et al.[45] also included sea-level controls, starting with unfit subjects ($\dot{V}O_2$max less than 40 ml/kg per min) they found no advantage in training at an altitude of 4300 m.

In well-trained subjects the picture is also unclear. Dill and Adams[46] found an increase in $\dot{V}O_2$max in high-school champion runners after 17 days at 3090 m, but there was no control sea-level group. A well-controlled, crossover study by Adams et al.[47] in experienced trained athletes ($\dot{V}O_2$max, 73 ml/kg per min average) showed no significant difference in performance (tested at sea level) between altitude (2300 m) and sea-level training. Each leg of the study was of 3 weeks' duration of intensive training.

Table 2 The possible advantages and disadvantages of training at altitude for events held at low altitude	
Advantages	**Disadvantages**
Increased haemoglobin concentration (Hct)	Risk of acute mountain sickness
Increased red cell mass	But only after months at altitude
Increased ventilatory capacity	Reduced $\dot{V}O_2$max
Increased capillary density	Reduced training intensity
	Reduced plasma volume

Recently, Levine and Stray-Gundersen[48] have conducted a well-controlled trial to test the idea of living at moderate altitude (2500 m) and going down each day to train at low altitude (1250 m) where training intensity could be maintained. This study comprised 39 well-trained competitive runners who, after a 2-week lead-in phase and 4 weeks supervised training in a camp at sea level, were randomized to one of three groups; living high and training low; living and training high; and living and training low (150 m). The outcome measures included a 5 km time trial, $\dot{V}O_2$max, and red cell mass. The results showed that both altitude groups increased their red cell mass by 9 per cent and $\dot{V}O_2$max by 5 per cent, the low altitude group showed no change. The 5 km time trial improved in all groups during sea-level training, but was only further improved by the additional training in the test group (living high, training low). In this group their time improved by a mean of 22.7 s, whereas it was 3.3 s slower in the living high, training high group. The improvement in time was proportional to the increase in red cell mass in the test group.

Conclusion from trials

Generally, the better controlled trials show no effect of altitude in enhancing the effect of training. If there is an effect it is probably best to train at modest altitudes, namely 2300 m, rather than any higher. On the strength of the one trial reported above it would seem that, for distance events at least, to live at about 2500 m and train at lower altitude below 1500 m is best.

Other aspects of altitude training

The optimum duration of stay at altitude is also unclear and there are no trials to guide us. At least 4 weeks at altitude would be necessary in order to increase red cell mass, but the reduction in training intensity for this period would almost certainly be disadvantageous.

How long before an important event should the athlete come down to low altitude? Again, there is no clear answer to this question. Most subjects following a prolonged period at high altitude feel rather 'slack' for a few days after coming down. Advocates of altitude training seem to agree on a minimum of 2 to 3 days, but some suggest 14 to 21.[49]

Acute mountain sickness

Acute mountain sickness (**AMS**) can be defined as a condition affecting previously healthy individuals who ascend rapidly to high altitude. There is a delay of a few hours to 2 days before symptoms develop. It is characterized by headache (usually frontal), nausea,

vomiting, irritability, malaise, insomnia, and poor climbing performance. In the simple or benign form the condition is self-limiting, lasting 3 to 5 days. After this time it does not recur at that given altitude, although it may do so if the subject goes higher. In a small proportion of individuals there may be progression to the malignant forms of AMS, namely high-altitude pulmonary (o)edema (HAPE) or high-altitude cerebral (o)edema (HACE), or a mixed form of both. If not treated, these conditions are frequently fatal in a matter of hours. They are considered below.

Incidence of AMS

The incidence of AMS depends upon altitude and the rate of ascent. With the increased accessibility of high-altitude resorts and the possibility of getting into high mountains in a very few days, the incidence of AMS is probably greater than in the leisured days of old. A recent survey in alpine huts showed an incidence of 9 per cent at 2850 m, 13 per cent at 3050 m, 34 per cent at 3650 m, and 53 per cent at 4559 m.[50] Amongst trekkers on the way to Everest base camp an incidence of 43 per cent was found at 4300 m,[51] and was higher in those who had flown into an airstrip at 2800 m than in those who had walked all the way (49 per cent vs 31 per cent).

Risk factors for AMS

Clearly hypoxia of more than a few hours' duration is required for the development of AMS and speed of ascent is important, but there is great variation in susceptibility. Amongst a group of people going together to high altitude there will be some unaffected, some mildly, and some severely affected. At present, there is no way to predict who is susceptible, except that past performance at altitude is a guide.[52] As Ravenhill observed in his classic paper published in 1913:[53]

'There is in my experience no type of man of whom one can say he will or will not suffer from puna [the South American term for AMS]. Most cases I have instanced were young men to all appearances perfectly sound. Young, strong and healthy men may be completely overcome. Stout, plethoric individuals...may not even have a headache'.

People of all ages, men and women seem to be equally affected. Fitness is no protection, indeed in that the fit are likely to ascend faster, they may be at greater risk. Any respiratory infection is probably a risk factor, and this may account for the person who has previously acclimatized well having trouble on another occasion. A brisk hypoxic ventilatory response would be expected to be protective; but while some studies seem to support this, others do not.[54] Certainly, high-altitude residents who have a blunted hypoxic ventilatory response are less prone to AMS than lowlanders. A brisk pulmonary artery pressor response to hypoxia may well be a risk factor for HAPE.

Mechanisms of AMS

Although hypoxia is obviously the starting point in the genesis of AMS it is not the immediate cause of the symptoms since these are delayed by several hours after arrival, whereas hypoxia is most severe in the first few minutes. It seems that hypoxia sets in train a mechanism which, in turn, after a few hours, produces symptoms. The symptoms are the same as those associated with raised intra-cranial pressure seen on neurosurgical wards, and, at least in cases of high-altitude cerebral oedema, there is good evidence of increased intracranial pressure. The most popular view is that even in simple AMS there is a degree of cerebral oedema (and often subclinical pulmonary oedema) which causes the symptoms of AMS. There is frequently dependent or periorbital oedema as well. All this points to some disturbance of fluid balance or capillary permeability throughout the body.

Other factors which should be accommodated in an overall scheme include ventilation on arrival at altitude. Earlier studies suggested that those with the highest PCO_2 on arrival at altitude (who have failed to lower their PCO_2 by hyperventilation) were likely to go on to develop AMS. Exercise is thought to be a risk factor, although this is yet to be rigorously tested. The effect of prolonged exercise of the type taken by mountaineers is to cause retention of sodium and water through activation of the renin–aldosterone system.[55] This may place subjects at risk of AMS.

Prevention of AMS

A slow rate of ascent is the best way to prevent AMS. A suggested rule is that above 3000 m, ascent should be not more than 300 m a day with a 'rest' day, when no height gain is made, every 3 days. But even this rate will be too fast for some and unnecessarily slow for others. An added rule must be: 'If symptoms of AMS develop, go no higher. If they become severe, go down.'

Acetazolamide and dexamethasone

In real life it is often not possible or practicable to plan for this rate of ascent. There may be no camp site between the valley floor and a pass 500 m higher. Some who know themselves to be slow acclima-tizers do not wish to delay their companions. In these situations it is justified to recommend the use of acetazolamide (Diamox). This drug, which is a carbonic acid anhydrase inhibitor, probably acts as a respiratory stimulant. It has been shown to increase PaO_2 and decrease $PaCO_2$, thus giving a sort of artificial respiratory acclima-tization. There have been a number of good, double-blind con-trolled trials which have shown that AMS is reduced in those taking the drug.[56] Of course, AMS, and even HAPE or HACE, is still pos-sible whilst taking the drug and common sense is still needed. The dose used in trials has usually been 250 mg every 8 h, but nowadays 250 mg or even 125 mg twice daily is usually recommended. The drug should be started not less than 24 h before a major gain in altitude. The side-effects of the drug include a mild diuresis which tends to diminish if the drug is continued; paraesthesia of the fin-gers and toes is almost universal. Some subjects find this distress-ing. Flushing, thirst, headache, rash, and blood dyscrasias are mentioned but are rare; finally, beer and all fizzy drinks taste flat!

The drug has been very widely used in the treatment of glaucoma for prolonged periods often at higher doses than are recommended for AMS prophylaxis, so its relative safety is assured.

Dexamethasone has been shown to be an effective prophylactic drug, but most would consider it unjustified to use it for this pur-pose.

Treatment

Simple or benign AMS is self-limiting and usually lasts about 3 days, so treatment is not essential; aspirin or paracetamol can be used to relieve headache, but these are not very effective. Recently, a placebo-controlled trial has shown ibuprofen to be effective.[57] Of course, if the condition progresses to HAPE or HACE then treat-ment is urgent, as indicated below.

High-altitude pulmonary oedema

In the great majority of cases AMS is a minor affliction which resolves in a few days. However, in a small proportion of people going to high altitude, the potentially lethal condition of HAPE or HACE, or a mixture of both, can develop. The incidence will depend on the rate of ascent and the population involved. Figures of 0.5 to 2.0 per cent of people going to altitude have been quoted. Individuals with a previous history of HAPE are at greater risk of developing subsequent problems.

Both lowlanders and people resident at high altitude are suscep-tible on return to altitude. Men and women of all ages can fall vic-tim, although there is an impression that the young male is more at risk than other groups. Athletic fitness affords no protection.

Clinical picture

Typically, the patient is a previously fit young man who has climbed rapidly to altitude and been very energetic on arrival. He suffers at least a moderate degree of AMS. He becomes more breathless than his companions. A cough develops, dry at first then productive of frothy white sputum later becoming tinged with blood. He may complain of chest discomfort. Crackles will be heard at the lung bases and there will be an increase in heart and respiratory rates. There may be peripheral oedema and raised jugular venous pres-sure. A right ventricular heave and accentuated pulmonary second heart sound may be detected. Over a few hours the condition deteri-orates; heart and respiration rates rise, breathing becomes 'bubbly', and cyanosis develops. Coma leads to death if no action is taken.

Investigations

The chest radiograph (Fig. 15) typically shows asymmetric blotchy opacities. These clear in a few days if the patient recovers. There is usually a mild pyrexia. The blood count usually shows a neutrophil leucocytosis. Blood gases show a reduced PO_2 and arterial oxygen saturation compared with fit individuals at the same altitude. The PCO_2 is variable but not significantly different from controls. The ECG shows tachycardia, peaked P waves, right axis deviation, and, in some cases, elevation of the S–T segment, all changes suggestive of pulmonary hypertension. Cardiac catheter findings confirm the high pulmonary artery pressure (81/49 mmHg in one study[58]), but normal wedge pressure. The cardiac output is normal. The oedema fluid is found to have a high protein content with concentrations approaching that of plasma.[59,60]

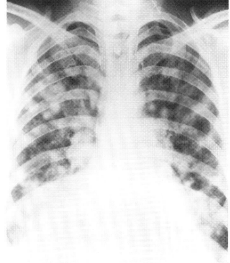

(a)

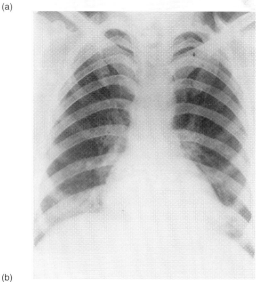

(b)

Fig. 15 Chest radiograph in a case of acute high-altitude pulmonary oedema showing typical blotchy asymmetric opacities. (By courtesy of Dr T. Norbu of Leh, Jammu, and Kashmir, India.)

Postmortem findings show the lungs to be oedematous, but the oedema is very patchy with areas of normal lung adjacent to areas of simple oedema and other areas of haemorrhagic oedema, the pattern corresponding with the radiographic appearance. There are many thrombi and fibrin clots in the small arteries and veins. The alveoli contain fluid, red cells, polymorphs, and macrophages and there may be hyaline membrane formation.

Mechanism of high-altitude pulmonary oedema

The mechanism of this condition is not clear. It is not that of acute left ventricular failure despite the clinical similarity. Catheter studies all agree in their finding of a normal wedge pressure. The most popular hypothesis, originally proposed by Hultgren et al.[61], is that the vasoconstriction is uneven in susceptible subjects who have been shown to have brisk hypoxic pulmonary artery pressor responses.[62] Those areas with greater vasoconstriction have reduced blood flow

and are protected. Those areas with less constriction therefore have a greatly increased blood flow. This torrential blood flow causes capillary damage—perhaps by sheer stress on the walls, perhaps by increased capillary pressure. Oedema then results. This accounts for the finding of pulmonary hypertension and the patchy nature of the oedema.

Various kinins are found in the oedema fluid[59]. The release of these potent chemicals are likely to increase permeability further as well as recruiting more leucocytes by chemotaxis.

Treatment

The most important measure in a case of HAPE is to evacuate the patient to lower altitude. A reduction in altitude of as little as 300 m may make all the difference. If this is impossible, or while awaiting evacuation, oxygen, if available, will help. A portable, lightweight, rubberized canvas hyperbaric chamber (the Gamow bag) is now available; the patient can be placed in this bag and the pressure increased by 2 p.s.i. (1406 kg/m²) using a foot pump. This has the effect, if the patient is at a typical base camp altitude (4000–4500 m), of reducing his equivalent altitude by almost 2000 m. There have been a number of case reports on the use of this bag in the treatment of HAPE and HACE with sometimes dramatic improvement. Bartsch et al.[63] have carried out a randomized controlled trial in 64 cases of AMS treated with 1 h of pressurization of either 193 mbar or 20 mbar (control). The genuine pressure treatment gave greater relief immediately, but over the 12 h follow-up period at 4600 m altitude there was no difference in the use of analgesics and at the end of the period no difference in symptom scores. It is also true that it requires considerable effort to keep pumping if there is limited manpower available. The bag may be valuable in improving a patient sufficiently to be able to walk down unaided. It is no substitute to descent.

Since pulmonary vasoconstriction is thought to be important in the genesis of the condition vasodilators have been tried, specifically the calcium channel blocker nifedipine has been shown to be beneficial.[64] A dose of 10 mg of nifedipine sublingually plus 20 mg of a slow-release oral preparation was used; however, since the sublingual drug can cause systemic hypotension it is probably best to stick to the oral form unless the situation is critical.

Diuretics have been advocated but seem to be losing favour amongst those who see many cases. Similarly, morphine and digoxin have been suggested, but again there is no evidence from controlled trials to support their use.

Outcome

In fully established cases of altitude sickness where evacuation is impossible or not carried out, the result is usually death within a few hours. In cases evacuated promptly signs and symptoms are usually relieved within minutes or hours, although the radiograph may take a few days to clear. Patients should be warned to be cautious in re-ascent to altitude, but many have been able to go back to altitude with no recurrence.

Summary

HAPE is a serious life-threatening condition. It may be avoided by following the rules for avoiding AMS, that is to say a slow ascent, going no higher if symptoms occur, and descending if symptoms persist or worsen. If diagnosed, descent as soon as possible is the first priority. The use of oxygen and nifedipine are likely to be beneficial, and a pressure bag (Gamow bag) may be useful as a temporary measure.

High-altitude cerebral oedema

The other malignant form of AMS is HACE. In the early stages this is indistinguishable from simple AMS with headache, nausea, and vomiting being the prominent symptoms. When ataxia (unsteadiness on walking) is added to this symptom cluster the line between benign and malignant AMS has probably been crossed. Truncal ataxia (unsteadiness even when sitting), hallucinations, clouding of consciousness, with various neurological signs including extensor plantar reflexes and papilloedema may follow. There are often signs of pulmonary oedema as well. Finally, the patient becomes unconscious and dies if not treated.

The incidence is rather lower than acute pulmonary oedema, Hacket and Rennie[51] give an incidence of 1.8 per cent (2.5 per cent for HAPE) in 278 trekkers passing through Pheriche (4243 m) on their way to Everest base camp.

The mechanism is presumably the same as simple AMS, but it is unclear why a few individuals progress to this lethal complication whereas the majority suffer only a self-limiting reversible condition. As with HAPE, lowlanders and highlanders, men and women of any age can become victims.

In the few cases where a postmortem has been carried out this has revealed evidence of antemortem cerebral oedema, raised intracranial pressure, and petechial haemorrhages. Venous thrombi have also been found.[65]

Treatment

This is similar to that in acute pulmonary oedema. The most important measure is to get the patient down from altitude. While awaiting evacuation, oxygen breathing or increasing the ambient pressure in a pressure bag helps, but often not very quickly in more severe cases. Dexamethasone 4 mg intramuscularly in severe cases and orally in less severe cases will help reduce the cerebral oedema.

Outcome

As in acute pulmonary oedema, descent often leads to rapid improvement. However, in some cases recovery is delayed for a number of days and there may even be permanent or at least long-lasting neurological defects.[66]

Chronic mountain sickness

There is also a condition known as chronic mountain sickness which is quite different. It affects residents of high altitude and consists of extreme polycythaemia, with haemoglobin concentrations up to 23 g/dl. The victims become slow mentally and physically and complain of headaches, dizziness, somnolence, fatigue, difficulty in concentration, etc. On going down to sea level, symptoms clear and the polycythaemia disappears, only to recur on return to their high-altitude homes. Venesection (at altitude) helps to reduce symptoms.

References

1. Zuntz N, Loewy A, Muller F, Caspari W. Atmospheric pressure at high altitudes. In: *Hokenklima und Bergwanderungen in ihrer Wirkung auf den Menschen.* Berlin: Bong and Co., 1906; 37–9. (Translation in West JB, ed. *High altitude physiology.* Stroudsburg, PA: Hutchinson Ross, 1981; 78–80.

2. Pugh LGCE. Resting ventilation and alveolar air on Mount Everest: with remarks on the relation of barometric pressure to altitude in mountains. *Journal of Physiology* 1957; **135**: 590–610.

3. West JB, Lahiri S, Maret KH, Peters RM Jr, Pizzo CJ. Barometric pressures at extreme altitudes on Mt. Everest: Physiological significance. *Journal of Applied Physiology* 1983; **54**: 1188–94.

4. Sato M, Severinghaus JW, Bickler P. Time course of augmentation and depression of hypoxic ventilatory response at altitude. *Journal of Applied Physiology* 1994; **77**: 313–16.

5. Ward MP, Milledge JS, West JB. *High altitude medicine and physiology.* 2nd edn. London: Chapman and Hall Medical, 1995; 69–97.

6. West JB. Diffusing capacity of the lung for carbon monoxide at high altitude. *Journal of Applied Physiology* 1962; **17**: 421–6.

7. Dempsey JA, Reddon WG, Birnbaum ML, *et al.* Effects of acute through life-long hypoxic exposure on exercise pulmonary gas exchange. *Respiratory Physiology* 1971; **13**: 62–89.

8. Reeves JT, Groves BM, Cymerman A, *et al.* Operation Everest II: Preservation of cardiac function at extreme altitude. *Journal of Applied Physiology* 1987; **63**: 531–9.

9. Pugh LGCE, Cardiac output in muscular exercise at 5800 m (19 000 ft). *Journal of Applied Physiology* 1964; **19**: 441–7.

10. Ward MP, Milledge JS, West JB. *High altitude medicine and physiology.* 2nd edn. London: Chapman and Hall Medical, 1995; 138.

11. Motley HL, Cournand A, Werko L, Himmelstein A, Dresdale D. Influence of short periods of induced acute anoxia upon pulmonary artery pressure in man. *American Journal Physiology* 1947; **150**: 315–20.

12. Harris P. Evolution, hypoxia and high altitude. In: Heath D. ed. *Aspects of hypoxia.* Liverpool: Liverpool University Press, 1986; 207–16.

13. Heath D and Williams DR. *High altitude medicine and pathology.* London: Butterworth, 1989; 102–14.

14. Milledge JS. Electrocardiographic changes at high altitude. *British Heart Journal* 1963; **25**: 291–8.

15. Pugh LGCE. Blood volume and haemoglobin concentration at altitudes above 18 000 ft (5800 m). *Journal of Physiology* 1964; **170**: 344–54.

16. Winslow RM, Monge C. *Hypoxia, polycythemia and chronic mountain sickness.* Baltimore: Johns Hopkins University Press, 1987; 203.

17. Williams ES, Ward MP, Milledge JS, Withey WR, Older MWJ, Forsling ML. Effect of exercise of seven consecutive days hill-walking on fluid homeostasis. *Clinical Science* 1979; **56**: 305–16.

18. Milledge JS, Beeley JM, McArthur S, Morice AH. Atrial natriuretic peptide, altitude and acute mountain sickness. *Clinical Science* 1989; **77**: 509–14.

19. Bartsch P, Shaw S, Franciolli M, Gnadinger MP, Weidmann P. Atrial natriuretic peptide in acute mountain sickness. *Journal of Applied Physiology* 1988; **65**: 1929–37.

20. Ward MP, Milledge JS, West JB. *High altitude medicine and physiology.* 2nd edn. London: Chapman and Hall Medical, 1995; 303–8.

21. Blume FD, Boyer SJ, Braverman LE, Cohen A, Dirkse J, Mordes JP. Impaired osmoregulation at high altitude: studies on Mt. Everest. *Journal of the American Medical Association* 1984; **252**: 524–6.

22. Denison DM, Ledwith F, Poulton EC. Complex reaction times at simulated cabin altitudes of 5000 feet and 8000 feet. *Aerospace Medicine* 1966; **57**: 1010–13.

23. Paul MA, Fraser WD. Performance during mild acute hypoxia. *Aviation, Space, and Environmental Medicine* 1994; **65**: 891–9.

24. Sharma VM, Malhotra MS, Baskaran AS. Variations in psycho-motor efficiency during prolonged stay at high altitude. *Ergonomics* 1975; **18**: 511–16.

25. Townes BD, Hornbein TF, Schoene RB, Sarnquist FH, Grant I. Human cerebral function at extreme altitude. In: West JB, Lahri S. eds. *High altitude and man.* Bethesda, MD: American Physiological Society, 1984; 31–6.

26. Hornbein TF, Townes BD, Schoene RB, Sutton JR, Houston CS. The cost to the central nervous system of climbing to extremely high altitude. *New England Journal of Medicine* 1989; **321**: 1714–19.

27. Westerterp KR, Kayser B, Brouns F, Herry J-P, Saris WHM. Energy expenditure climbing Mt. Everest. *Journal of Applied Physiology* 1992; **73**: 1815–19.

28. Milledge JS. Arterial oxygen desaturation and intestinal absorption of xylose. *British Medical Journal* 1972; **704**: 557–8.

29. Boyer SJ, Blume FD. Weight loss and changes in body composition at high altitude. *Journal of Applied Physiology* 1984; **57**: 1580–5.

30. Rennie MJ, Babji P, Sutton JR, *et al.* Effects of acute hypoxia on forearm leucine metabolism. In: Sutton JR, Houston CS, Jones NL, eds. *Hypoxia exercise and altitude.* New York: Alan Liss, 1983; 317–23.

31. Consolazio CF, Matoush LO, Johnson HL, Krzywicki HJ, Daws TA, Isaac GJ. Effects of high-carbohydrate diets on performance and clinical symptomatology after rapid ascent to high altitude. *American Journal of Clinical Nutrition* 1972; **25**: 23–9.

32. Richalet J-P, Soubervielle J-C, Antezana A-M, *et al.* Control of erythropoiesis in humans during prolonged exposure to the altitude of 6,542 m. *American Journal of Physiology* 1994; **266**: R756–64.

33. Ward MP, Milledge JS, West JB. *High altitude medicine and physiology.* 2nd edn. London: Chapman and Hall Medical, 1995; 203–7.

34. Reynafarje B. Myoglobin content and enzymatic activity of muscle and altitude adaptation. *Journal of Applied Physiology* 1962; **17**: 301–5

35. Ward MP, Milledge JS, West JB. *High altitude medicine and physiology.* 2nd edn. London: Chapman and Hall Medical, 1995; 208–9.

36. Ward MP, Milledge JS, West JB. *High altitude medicine and physiology.* 2nd edn. London: Chapman and Hall Medical, 1995; 210–13.

37. Narici MV, Kayser B. Hypertrophic response of human skeletal muscle to strength training in hypoxia and normoxia. *European Journal of Applied Physiology* 1995; **70**: 213–19.

38. Horstman D, Weiskopf R, Jackson RE. Work capacity during a 3-wk sojourn at 4,300 m: effects of relative polycythemia. *Journal of Applied Physiology* 1980; **49**: 311–18.

39. Davis CTM, Sargeant AJ. Effects of hypoxic training of normoxic maximal aerobic power output. *European Journal of Applied Physiology* 1974; **33**: 227–36.

40. Williams C. Haemoglobin—is more better? *Nephrology Dialysis Transplantation* 1995; **10** (Suppl. 2): 48–55.

41. Mizuno M, Juel C, Bro-Rasmussen T, *et al.* Limb skeletal muscle adaptation in athletes after training at altitude. *Journal of Applied Physiology* 1990; **68**: 496–502.

42. Balke B, Nagle J, Daniels J. Altitude and maximum performance in work and sports activity. *Journal of the American Medical Association* 1965; **194**: 646–9.

43. Faulkner JA, Kollias J, Favour CB, Buskirk ER, Balke B. Maximum aerobic capacity and running performance at altitude. *Journal of Applied Physiology* 1968; **5**: 685–91.

44. Roskamm F, Londry F, Samek L, Schlager M, Weidermann H, Reindell H. Effects of a standardised ergometer training program at three different altitudes. *Journal of Applied Physiology* 1969; **27**: 840–7.

45. Hanson JE, Vogel JA, Stelter GP, Consoazio F. Oxygen uptake in man during exhaustive work at sea level and high altitude. *Journal of Applied Physiology* 1967; **23**: 511–22.

46. Dill DB, Adams WC. Maximal oxygen uptake at sea level and at 3,090 metres altitude in high school champion runners. *Journal of Applied Physiology* 1971; **6**: 854–9.

47. Adams WC, Bernauer EM, Dill DB, Bowman JB. Effects of equivalent sea level and altitude training on VO2max and running performance. *Journal of Applied Physiology* 1975; **39**: 262–6.

48. Levine BD, Stray-Gundersen J. 'Living high—training low' The effect of high altitude acclimatisation with low altitude training on sea level performance in trained athletes. *Journal of Applied Physiology* 1997; **83**: 102–112.

49. Dick F. Relevance of altitude training. *Athletics Coach* 1979; **4**: 11–14.

50. Maggiorini M, Buhler B, Walter M, Oelz O. Prevalence of acute mountain sickness in the Swiss Alps. *British Medical Journal* 1990; **301**: 853–5.

51. Hacket PH, Rennie D. The incidence, importance and prophylaxis of acute mountain sickness. *Lancet* 1979; **ii**: 1449–54.

52. Forster P. Reproducibility of individual response to exposure to high altitude. *British Medical Journal* 1984; **289**: 1269.

53. Ravenhill TH. Some experiences of mountain sickness in the Andes. *Journal of Tropical Medicine and Hygiene* 1913; **20**: 313–22.

54. Milledge JS, Thomas PS, Beeley JM, English JSC. Hypoxic ventilatory response and acute mountain sickness *European Respiratory Journal* 1988; **1**: 948–51.

55. Milledge JS, Bryson EI, Catley DM, *et al.* Sodium balance, fluid homeostasis and the renin–aldosterone system during the prolonged exercise of hill walking. *Clinical Science* 1982; **62**: 595–604.

56. Ward MP, Milledge JS, West JB. *High altitude medicine and physiology.* 2nd edn. London: Chapman and Hall Medical, 1995; 377.

57. Broom JR, Stoneham MD, Beeley JM, Milledge JS, Hughes AS. High altitude headache: treatment with ibuprofen. *Aviation, Space, and Environmental Medicine* 1994; **65**: 19–20.

58. Antezanan G, Leguia G, Guzman AM, Coudert J, Spielvogel H. Haemodynamic study of high altitude pulmonary oedema (12 200 ft). In: Brendel W, Zink RA, eds. *High altitude physiology and medicine.* New York: Springer-Verlag, 1982; 232–41.

59. Hacket PH, Bertman J, Rodriguex G. Pulmonary oedema fluid protein in high-altitude pulmonary oedema. *Journal of the American Medical Association* 1986; **256**: 36.

60. Schoene RB, Swenson ER, Pizzo CJ, *et al.* The lung at high altitude: bronchoalveolar lavage in acute mountain sickness and pulmonary oedema. *Journal of Applied Physiology* 1988; **64**: 2605–13.

61. Hultgren HN, Robison MC, Wuerflein RD. Over perfusion pulmonary oedema. *Circulation* 1966; **34**: 132–3.

62. Yagi H, Yamada H, Kobayashi T, Sekiguchi M. Doppler assessment of pulmonary hypertension induced by hypoxic breathing in subjects susceptible to high altitude pulmonary oedema. *American Review of Respiratory Disease* 1990; **142**: 796–801.

63. Bartsch P, Merki B, Hofstetter D, Maggiorini M, Kayser B, Oelz O. Treatment of acute mountain sickness by simulated descent: a randomised trial. *British Medical Journal* 1993; **306**: 1098–101.

64. Oelz O, Maggiorini M, Ritter M, *et al.* Nifedipine for high altitude pulmonary oedema. *Lancet* 1989; **ii**: 1241–4.

65. Dickinson J, Heath D, Gosney J, Williams D. Altitude related deaths in seven trekkers in the Himalayas. *Thorax* 1983; **38**: 646–56.

66. Houston CS, Dickenson J. Cerebral form of high-altitude illness. *Lancet* 1975; **ii**: 758–61.

67. West JB, Boyer SJ, Graber DJ, *et al*. Maximal exercise at extreme altitudes on Mt. Everest: Physiological significance. *Journal of Applied Physiology* 1983; **55**: 688–98.

68. Kellogg RH. The Role of CO_2 in altitude acclimatisation. In: Cunningham DJC, Lloyd BB, eds. *The regulation of human respiration.* Oxford: Blackwell, 1963; 379–96.

69. Astrand P-O, Astrand I. Heart rate during muscular work in man exposed to prolonged hypoxia. *Journal of Applied Physiology* 1958; **13**: 75–80.

70. Pugh LGCE, Gill MB, Milledge JS, Ward MP, West JB. Muscular exercise at great altitudes. *Journal of Applied Physiology* 1964; **19**: 431–40.

71. Groves BM, Reeves JT, Sutton JR, *et al*. Operation Everest II: elevated high-altitude pulmonary resistance unresponsive to oxygen. *Journal of Applied Physiology* 1987; **63**: 521–30.

72. Milledge JS, Coates PM. Serum erythropoietin in humans at high altitude and its relation to plasma renin. *Journal of Applied Physiology* 1985; **59**: 360–4.

73. Peronnet F, Thibault G, Cousineau D-L. A theoretical analysis of the effect of altitude on running performance. *Journal of Applied Physiology* 1991; **70**: 399–404.

74. Squires RW, Buskirk ER. Aerobic capacity during acute exposure to simulated altitude, 914 to 2286 meters. *Medicine and Science in Sports and Exercise* 1982; **14**: 36–40.

75. Saltine B. Aerobic and anaerobic work capacity at an altitude of 2,250 metres. In: Goddard RF, ed. *International symposium on the effects of altitude on physical performance.* Chicago: The Athletic Institute, 1967; 97–102.

76. Pugh LGCE. Athletes at altitude. *Journal of Physiology* 1967; **192**: 619–46.

77. Faulkner JA, Daniels J, Balke B. Effects of training at moderate altitude on physical performance capacity. *Journal of Applied Physiology* 1967; **23**: 85–9.

78. Daniels J, Oldridge N. The effects of alternate exposure to altitude and sea level on world-class middle-distance runners. *Medicine and Science in Sport* 1970; **3**: 107–112.

2.4 Physiological and clinical consequences of exercise in heat and humidity

John R. Sutton and Martin W. Thompson*

Thermal effects and thermal regulation

The maintenance of internal temperature is a unique feature of birds and mammals which has only been acquired during the last 70 million years of evolution, but it is an adaption which makes these species largely independent of the external environment. The price we pay for this independence is a high metabolic rate that enables us to maintain our body temperature within a fairly narrow range, although the range for survival is much greater. What is interesting is that at 37 °C we are fairly close to the ceiling of thermal viability compared with the lower end of the temperature scale. Therefore it is not surprising that more elaborate temperature–regulating mechanisms are available to prevent overheating than to prevent over-cooling.

Figure 1 illustrates the normal responses of resting humans over a wide environmental range. The zone of minimum metabolism

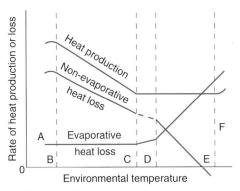

Fig. 1 Relationship between heat production, evaporative and non-evaporative heat loss, and deep body temperature in a homeothermic, as opposed to poikilo-thermic animal. A, zone of hypothermia; B, temperature of summit metabolism and incipient hypothermia; C, critical temperature; D, temperature of marked increase in evaporative loss; E, temperature of incipient hyperthermal rise; F, zone of hyper-thermia; CD, zone of minimum metabolism; and BE, either above or below this range thermoregulatory control is lost (hyper/hypothermia). These zones were defined by Mount.[1]

* It is with regret that we report the death of John R. Sutton prior to the preparation of this edition of the textbook. Much of his contribution to the first edition has been retained.

(CD), in the centre of the figure, is the range that requires the least thermoregulatory effort. As the environmental temperatures rise, heat production remains constant in the resting state and there is a major increase in evaporative heat loss by sweating. As the environmental temperature is lowered, evaporative heat loss virtually stops and there is a major increase in heat production, particularly induced by shivering. Exercise changes this balance dramatically by increasing the heat load, sometimes by as much as twentyfold.

There are three bidirectional avenues of thermal exchange between the body and the environment—conduction, convection, and radiation—and one unidirectional change, evaporation. This relationship is expressed by Winslow *et al.*'s heat–storage equation:[2]

$$S = M ñ R ñ C_V ñ C_D - E;$$

where S is heat storage, M is metabolic heat production, R is heat gained or lost through radiation, C_V is heat gained or lost by convection, C_D is heat gained or lost by conduction, and E is heat lost by evaporation. These are important physiological mechanisms, but it should be stated at the outset that behavioural factors in humans far outweigh their physical capabilities of withstanding environmental extremes, that is to say putting on or removing clothing, seeking shelter for environmental extremes.

Body core-temperature response to exercise

In 1938 Nielsen[3] put forward the idea that the magnitude of the body core-temperature rise in steady-state exercise was environmentally independent. He came to this conclusion after studying three subjects performing exercise at a variety of intensities under environmental conditions ranging from 5 °C to 36 °C and low humidity. These findings were extended and substantially supported by the work of Robinson *et al.*[4] and Lind.[5] In essence, the findings revealed the following:

1. With continuous work, the rectal temperature increased to a new equilibrium within 60 min.

2. The body temperature depended on the work rate and was higher the higher the work rate.

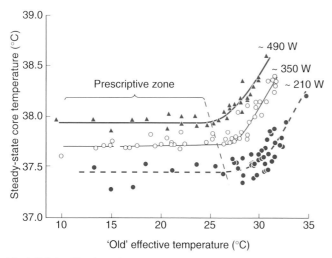

Fig. 2 Relationship of steady-state, core-temperature responses during exercise at three metabolic rates to the environmental conditions. (Reproduced from ref. 5, with permission.)

3. The time taken to reach an equilibrium temperature was longer the higher the exercise intensity.

4. Over a wide range of environmental temperatures the body core temperature was primarily related to work rate but independent of the environment.

Most of these studies concerned work at low intensities for prolonged periods and were often designed to examine the work environment rather than sport. However, it was appreciated that under extreme climatic conditions body temperature could continue to rise and that subjects might collapse. A further extension of this work was carried out by Lind,[5] who tried to examine the relationship between environmental conditions and work rate so that safe limits for work environments and work rates (as opposed to recreation) might be constructed. In many work environments, particularly mining, there would be additional problems related to clothing. Again, examining a wide range of ambient conditions and work rates, Lind[5] proposed the so-called prescriptive zone (Fig. 2). This prescriptive zone was determined statistically, and naturally there were marked individual variations. What might account for these individual differences? Astrand[6] was the first to report the importance of relative exercise intensity rather than absolute metabolic rate on the rise in body core temperature during exercise, and in 1966 these findings were extended by Saltin and Hermansen[7] (Fig. 3).

Further clarification of the relationship between exercise intensity and ambient conditions was provided by the studies of Davies[8] and Davies and Thompson.[9] Over a wide range of environmental conditions, with dry-bulb temperatures from 5 to 25 °C and relatively low humidity, they examined subjects exercising at between 20 and 90 per cent of $\dot{V}O_2$max and demonstrated a curvilinear relationship between steady-state body core temperature and relative intensity. Even at exercise intensities up to 65 per cent $\dot{V}O_2$max, the core temperature was largely independent of the dry-bulb temperature within the range 5 to 20 °C. These observations were consistent with those of Lind,[5] but at intensities of 85 per cent $\dot{V}O_2$max the prescriptive zone becomes smaller.

Most of these studies were performed using leg cycle ergomen-

try, but work by arm cranking suggests that the body core-temperature response may be more closely related to maximal oxygen uptake than relative work rate. As early as 1947, Asmussen and Nielsen[10] showed that for the same absolute work intensity performed by arm versus leg cycle ergometry, a lower rectal temperature was recorded in the former and that the difference became exaggerated as the metabolic rate increased. These observations brought out two points:

1. Different modes of exercise have an effect on the rate of body core-temperature increase.

2. More important is body core temperature, and could a rectal temperature be safely assumed to be a good reflection of the body core under all working conditions?

Nowadays, oesophageal temperature is probably considered to be a more reliable indicator of body core temperature. Oesophageal temperature is a more rapidly responding measurement for the onset of heat storage, however, a rectal temperature probe is better tolerated by subjects. In fact, when Nielsen[11] repeated these experiments using oesophageal temperature, the steady-state exercise temperatures seemed comparable under two exercise regimes.

So far the emphasis has been on the rates of increase in body core temperature under different ambient conditions. Clearly, while the importance of metabolic rate has dominated our considerations, as ambient conditions become more extreme, particularly as humidity increases, our major route of heat loss—and therefore our ability to thermoregulate in the heat—becomes ineffective. Evaporation accounts for the majority of our heat-losing abilities, but as the relative humidity approaches 100 per cent, this avenue of heat loss becomes increasingly reduced eventually falling to zero. A high sweat rate in the presence of a high, ambient vapour pressure will result in sweat drippage rather than evaporation limiting exercise performance under such conditions. There is a lack of research concerning the limits of the 'so-called' prescriptive zone imposed by increases in humidity. Data reported by Robinson[4] on several élite athletes competing in 5 to 10 km events, where the humidity and solar radiation were high and the ambient temperature was between 30 °C and 31 °C, showed that rectal temperature rose to 41 °C after about 15 to 30 minutes of running. These observations clearly show that a steep rise in core temperature occurs with the combination of humidity, heat, and intense exercise.

A particularly elegant study by MacDougall et al. contrasted the effects of different body core temperatures on fatigue.[12] In this study, six subjects exercised on a treadmill at 70 per cent of their $\dot{V}O_2$max. The thermal environment (normal, cool, and hot) was controlled using the lightweight water-perfused suit described by Rowell et al.[13] Each subject ran to exhaustion. All groups showed similar elevations in rectal temperature that failed to reach a plateau. However, the exercise time to exhaustion was different under the three conditions, with a mean of 75 min under normal conditions and 90.75 min when it was cool, but only 48.25 min under the hot conditions. An additional point of interest in this study was the increase in blood lactate levels, which was maximal under the hot conditions. Furthermore, immediately prior to exhaustion there was a fall in cardiac output predominantly due to a decrease in stroke volume.

The problem of circulatory regulation during exercise has

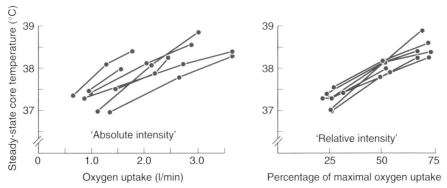

Fig. 3 Relationship of steady-state, core-temperature responses during exercise to the absolute (left) and relative (right) metabolic rates. (Reproduced from ref. 7, with permission.)

received much attention in recent years. The circulation has two increased demands imposed upon it when exercise is performed in a warm environment. In addition to delivering appropriate nutrients and oxygen to working muscle, there is also a need to perfuse the skin for thermoregulation. The conductance of heat from the exercising muscles to the skin requires a large blood flow to the skin, but without compromising muscle blood flow. To meet this demand a redistribution of the central vascular volume to peripheral regions occurs through a reduction in splanchnic and renal blood flow along with a gradual change in compliance of the capacitance vessels.[14,15] Problems of clinical significance may arise through ischaemia and hyperthermia as a result of extended visceral vasoconstriction during prolonged severe exercise.[16] Furthermore, the increase in cutaneous venous volume has been implicated as a potential limiting factor for prolonged exercise, especially when this circulatory adjustment is heightened by the addition of an environmental heat stress.[17]

During prolonged exercise a 'cardiovascular drift' occurs which is characterized by a continuous rise in heart rate, a continuous fall in stroke volume, and a progressive decline in arterial and central venous pressure.[18] It has been suggested that the high metabolic rates and elevated body temperatures encountered by competitive distance runners accentuates the 'cardiovascular drift' and may eventually result in either decreased cutaneous blood flow or a reduced cardiac output.[19] Rowell *et al.*[18] concluded that there is a hierarchy of homeostatic mechanisms which favour the maintenance of arterial blood pressure and circulation to the vital organs at the expense of skin vasodilation and thermoregulation. This certainly seems to be the case, and in a recent publication, Hales *et al.*[20] demonstrated a marked reduction in skin blood flow in collapsed runners when compared with their control counterparts. They postulated that the skin blood flow was reduced when the right-heart filling pressure fell and that this was the fundamental regulatory mechanism.

Females sweat at a lower rate than males[21-23] when their greater surface area to weight ratio is taken into account. Per unit volume of sweat produced, women reach a lower body core temperature than men, and thus have been considered to be the more efficient temperature regulators.[24] In a recent acute heat-stress study of males and females with identical cardiorespiratory fitness, surface area, and equal surface area to mass ratios, Avellini *et al.*[25] found that females during the follicular phase of the menstrual cycle had a lower sweat rate, a lower rectal temperature, and a lower heart rate than men. However, following 10 days of acclimatization the differences between the sexes were eliminated.

Heat acclimatization

Exercise-heat tolerance is invariably improved following heat acclimatization, which usually involves daily bouts of exercising in heat sufficient to raise the core temperature and stimulate profuse sweating. The critical stimulus appears to be the extent to which core temperature is elevated during each exercise bout which is a consequence of the total thermal load. The thermal load is related to the exercise intensity, environmental temperature, and the rate at which sweat can evaporate. Heat acclimatization is thus specific to the thermal load, and so the metabolic heat load incurred through regular bouts of exercise training in a cool environment provides only a partial contribution to exercise-heat tolerance. Further improvements are achieved through the combination of an environmental and metabolic heat load.

Repeated bouts of exercise-heat exposure on a daily basis provide a stimulus for changes in the cardiovascular and thermoregulatory systems. The changes that improve cardiovascular function in the heat do not appear to be directly related to the thermoregulatory changes. Nevertheless, the exercise-heat acclimatized subject experiences less circulatory strain and is better able to maintain thermoregulatory control during subsequent exercise-heat exposure. The classical physiological adjustments during exercise-heat acclimatization include:

- an expansion of plasma volume;

- earlier onset and increased rate of sweating;

- decreased core and skin temperature;

- enhanced skin blood flow with a lower vasodilation threshold;

- decreased heat storage;

- reduced heart rate.

Most of these adaptive responses occur in the first week of exercise-heat acclimatization and it has been reported that the state of training will effect the rate of adaptation.[26] Whether more extended periods of acclimatization (natural heat exposure) are warranted for the athlete preparing for competition in a hot environment is a moot point. Exercise–heat acclimatization can be a stressful stimulus for those normally residing in a cool environment if attention is not given to hydration, a high carbohydrate diet and rest/recovery. It is therefore advisable to increase the intensity, duration, and frequency of exercise–heat exposure progressively with the goal of completing 7 to 10 consecutive days of vigorous exercise in the heat of approximately 40 to 60 minutes duration to optimize the effects of acclimatization. The magnitude of these effects depends on the relative degree of heat acclimatization at the outset and the thermal load provided by the acclimatization programme. It is of interest to note that intermittent cold exposure does not hasten the loss of heat acclimation (artificial heat exposure).[27] In this regard, it is also of interest to note that acclimation to both heat and cold can be achieved simultaneously over the same period with bouts of exposure to heat and cold each day.[28]

People living in tropical climates show greater tolerance to hot, humid environmental conditions compared with inhabitants of more temperate climates.[4,29,30] However, it has been reported that naturally acclimatized people need to undergo intense exercise-heat stress to achieve similar adaptive responses to artificially acclimated subjects from temperate climates.[31-33] There are some indications that acclimatization brought about by living in a hot, humid environment for several years may result in a reduced rate of sweating and possible reduced circulatory strain.[29,30,34] There is difficulty in determining the relative benefits of acclimatization versus acclimation from the available published research, this centres on problems related to matching subjects in terms of their $\dot{V}O_2max$, body surface area, lean body mass, per cent $\dot{V}O_2max$ at exercise, and the varying heat tolerance/performance tests and environmental conditions used. These problems also relate, in a broader sense, to the vast number of exercise-heat acclimatization permutations reported in the extensive literature on this subject. Armstrong and Maresh[26] report that there have been more than 350 scientific studies on human heat acclimatization since 1930.

However, few studies have investigated the minimal exercise-heat exposure required to maintain the adaptive responses following an acclimation programme. Acclimation studies which have excluded the weekend (Saturday and Sunday) have reported a small decline in the adaptive response following the weekend, while a single exercise-heat exposure each week has been shown to be insufficient in provoking heat acclimation.[35,36] Reports vary from 18 to 28 days for almost complete loss of heat acclimatization following withdrawal of the heat stimulus.[37-39]

Clinical consequences of hyperthermia

Although an increase in body core temperature is a normal concomitant of exercise, the dividing line between normality and abnormality in absolute levels of body core temperature varies enormously. One of the most important issues is the site at which body core temperature is recorded. Rectal, oesophageal, and tympanic membrane temperatures can all differ considerably, although each of these is a more accurate reflection of the internal body tempera-

ture than the axillary or oral temperature. The last two can be particularly misleading. In the past, the use of oral or axillary temperatures has often been so erroneous as to lead clinicians to a diagnosis of hypothermia when, in fact, patients were hyperthermic (Fig. 4). In one patient, the oral temperature was 35.5 °C (96 °F) but the rectal temperature was 42 °C (108 °F).

The terms 'heat exhaustion' and 'heatstroke' are both used by the Medical Research Council of Great Britain and the World Health Organization, although differentiation between the two is often tenuous since they are part of a spectrum. Serious central nervous system dysfunction and multiple organ failure are probably the most important distinctive features of heatstroke.

In relation to exercise it is important to realize that the clinical picture differs greatly from the classic original description of heatstroke which included anhydrosis and a rectal temperature in excess of 41 °C. In hyperthermic states associated with 'fun runs' and any exercise of short duration, dehydration is not usually an issue; more than 85 per cent of all participants who collapse in fun runs are found to have cold and sweaty skin.

Heat cramps

Heat cramps are classically intermittent, of short duration, and often excruciating. Most commonly, they have been associated with prolonged exercise, sometimes over several hours or days; the cramps are thought to be related to an absolute or relative sodium deficiency when there has often been excessive water replacement in the absence of salt following a period of dehydration. This was observed in the steel mills in Ohio and also during the building of the Hoover dam.[40]

Heat syncope

Heat syncope is a common problem, and classically relates to the peripheral pooling of blood that occurs when a vasodilated person stops exercising after a run and the muscle pump action is eliminated. Venous return is therefore reduced and cardiac output—and hence cerebral blood flow—falls, resulting in syncope.

Heat exhaustion and heat stroke

Under extreme environmental conditions potential heat stroke is an ever present threat to many in the population, particularly to the aged, infirm, and infants, even when they are at rest.

One of the most graphic descriptions of heat stroke was reported when a British frigate docked at Liverpool in 1841. The weather gradually became warmer, the decks were constantly wetted, and every precaution taken to prevent heat exposure. However, in one day 30 men were lost, and it was stated that the decks resembled a slaughterhouse so numerous were the bleeding patients. This was probably one of the first descriptions of disseminated intravascular coagulation associated with heat stroke.

Nowadays, exercise-related heat stroke is more common in fun runs and short-duration events than in marathons and ultramarathons, and in its classic form is rapid in onset, has multiple organ pathology, and if not treated has a high morbidity and mortality. An

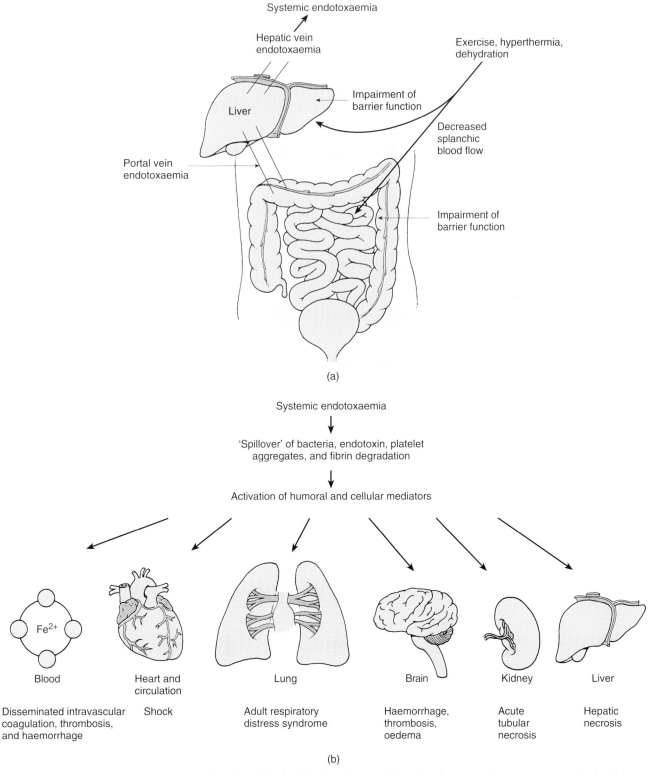

Fig. 4 (a) Mechanisms whereby exercise hyperthermia and dehydration lead to a decreased splanchnic blood flow with impairment of barrier function of the gut and liver—with development of systemic endotoxaemia. (b) The saga of biochemical events following systemic endotoxaemia and resulting cytokine cascade with production of multiorgan failure. (Based on an article by A. Ryan, 'Heat stroke and endotoxins sensitization in tolerance to endotoxins'. In: Gisolfi CV, Lamb DL, eds. *Perspectives in exercise science and sports medicine*. Indiana: Benchmark Press, 1993.)

additional crucial point to remember is that heat stroke can occur when environmental conditions are not extreme. Experience from the Sydney City to Surf race[41] shows that it is the young, fit amateur runner who seems to be at most risk. This is because the relative rate of exertion, not the environmental conditions, is a crucial factor in producing heat stroke in these individuals. When a person runs at more than 90 per cent of their own $\dot{V}O_2$max, their ability to thermo-regulate is impaired.

Pathophysiology of heat stroke

Similarities to septic shock

In a recent series of cases of heat stroke occurring in fun runs and football games, the clinical picture and the degree of organ damage was variable. In general, when the rectal temperature is comparable, tissue damage to various organs is greater in cases of exertional heat stroke than in those of classic heat stroke.[42] Although absolute core temperature is important, the length of time it is raised and the rate of change may be even more so. The integrity of the circulation also may well determine organ damage. As with hypotension, the additional ischaemic injury appears to potentiate the problem of heat stroke. Previously held ideas that heat stroke was due to the cellular toxicity of the heat *per se* and/or other reflex cardiovascular changes that might be derived from a poor cardiac-filling pressure in dehydrated subjects must now be modified. Recent evidence implicates endotoxin as an initial trigger in the sequence of events leading to clinical heatstroke.[43] Endotoxins are lipopolysaccharide–protein complexes (**LPS**) derived from the cell walls of Gram-negative bacteria (occasionally Gram-positive) and are extremely potent stimuli to the release of tumour necrosis factor (**TNF**) and interleukin-1 (**IL-la**).[44] These are endogenous pyrogens and are responsible for the shock and tissue injury associated with endotoxaemia.[45] During exercise, mild elevations of some of these trigger mediators occur, while in collapsed athletes endotoxin concentrations above 1 ng/ml have been reported.[46] There is inevitably evidence of liver and gastrointestinal damage in most heat stroke patients associated with the increase in endotoxin concentrations. In two fatal cases of heat stroke endotoxin concentration was reported to be 500 ng/ml.[47,48]

In patients with classic (not exertional) heat stroke, LPS, TNF, and IL-la were found to be markedly increased.[49] Although no control measurements were made, an interesting relationship was observed in these victims between increasing temperature and the plasma concentration of these mediators. Rectal temperature ranged from 40.6 to 43.3°C while the mean plasma concentration of endotoxin was 8.60 ± 1.19 ng/ml (±SE). Furthermore, the plasma concentration fell dramatically upon cooling. Although these were not exercising patients, the lessons almost certainly apply, perhaps even more so, to exertional heat stroke.

Current thinking suggests that the following sequence of events takes place. During exercise, especially if it is associated with hyperthermia, the relatively ischaemic bowel mucosa loses its barrier function which allows bacterial translocation in the gut to occur, resulting in portal vein endotoxaemia. If the liver also loses its barrier function then systemic endotoxaemia will occur, resulting in increased plasma concentrations of LPS which stimulate the release of interleukin-1a and tumour necrosis factor. These important mediators then stimulate a cytokine cascade; for example, complement pathways, intrinsic and extrinsic coagulation pathways, colony-stimulating factor, and interferon as well as numerous other cytokines. However, most evidence to date suggests that tumour necrosis factor and interleukin-1 are the primary mediators of endotoxic shock. Nevertheless, the situation may be ameliorated when an additional family of proteins (the so-called heat-shock proteins) are released; these may help to protect the organism from the destruc-tion mediators. Heat stroke proteins are acidic proteins of pI 5.0 to 6.5 and are classified according to molecular weight. This so-called heat-shock family of proteins include HSP28 and HSP70, which appear to provide protection against TNF cytotoxicity and may possibly inhibit the induction of IL-1 and TNF synthesis in LPS-stimulated cells. The synthesis of HSP70 in particular seems to be important in the acquired tolerance of mammalian cells to hyperthermia.

Of all the pathological features of heat stroke, it is the development of disseminated intravascular coagulation, together with rhabdomyolysis, which is probably responsible for the multiorgan pathology resulting in significant morbidity and mortality. In virtually all fatal cases of heat stroke, disseminated intravascular coagulation is concomitant. The following mechanisms are suggested.

1. The release of tissue thromboplastins as a result of extensive tissue injury stimulates the coagulation cascade by the extrinsic pathway and results in intravascular fibrin deposition.

2. A second possible mechanism is the induction of endothelial damage which then activates platelets and the coagulation cascade via the intrinsic pathway.[50,51]

3. Endotoxins released from the bowel stimulate the intrinsic and extrinsic coagulation pathways and also fibrinolysis.[49,52,53]

In a recent autopsy study of 10 patients who died following heat stroke, disseminated intravascular coagulation was thought to be causally related.[53] Rhabdomyolysis itself may produce a disseminated intravascular coagulation, and certainly with the release of myoglobin and uric acid it was thought to have been causally important in the development of progressive renal impairment and acute tubular necrosis.

Few organs escape involvement in heat stroke, but the effects on the brain usually determine the outcome; prolonged unconsciousness in a person with disseminated intravascular coagulation has a particularly bad prognosis.

The central nervous system

Effects on the central nervous system are common, and without some central nervous sytem impairment the diagnosis of heat stroke cannot be made. Most commonly there is a transient loss of consciousness, but this may be preceded by impaired judgement, irritability, and hallucinations. Other associated features include status epilepticus, oculogyric crisis, and cerebellar symptoms and hemiplegia. There may even be decerebrate posturing. The duration of unconsciousness is some indication of the prognosis, although even after 10 days to 3 weeks patients have regained consciousness and gone on to make a full neurological recovery. The pathological changes found in the central nervous system consist of oedema, congestion, and haemorrhages usually associated with disseminated intravascular coagulation.

The kidney

Oliguria, anuria, and acute renal failure with acute tubular necrosis are particularly common.[55,56] The role of rhabdomyolysis in acute renal failure has already been mentioned, but disseminated intravascular coagulation may also play a causative role and certainly renal impairment is well documented in patients in whom rhabdomyolysis is not particularly severe.[57] Some patients go on to develop a chronic interstitial nephritis.

The liver

Liver failure often occurs more than 24 h after the original impairment is evident. The patients will present with jaundice and biochemical or hepatocellular damage with increases in the liver enzymes aspartate aminotransferase (**AST**), alanine aminotransferase (**ALT**), and γ-glutamyl transferase (**GGT**) as well as elevations of alkaline phosphatase, indicative of liver excretory impairment. Pathological findings include perisinusoidal oedema and centrilobular necrosis; there can also be desquamation of the sinusoidal and lining cells and a ballooning and flattening of the microvilli.[58]

The lungs

Tachypnoea and alveolar hyperventilation are common in heat stroke; patients who develop fulminant pulmonary features usually have pulmonary oedema similar to that associated with the adult respiratory distress syndrome. Classically, the left-atrial, pulmonary-artery wedge pressure is low thus distinguishing it from cardiogenic pulmonary oedema. Such patients have a low $PaCO_2$ and are hypoxaemic with a widened $P(A-a)O_2$. Mechanical ventilation may be difficult as the lungs are stiff. As cardiovascular problems may also be present, occasionally cardiogenic pulmonary oedema can be associated with heatstroke.

Cardiovascular system

Most patients will have a sinus tachycardia and perhaps transient hypertension. Although in the early phase after admission to hospital, the circulatory state is unstable as the patients may have marked dehydration and fluid-compartment shifts. Therefore careful monitoring of central blood volume and cardiac filling pressures with the Swan–Ganz catheter is particularly valuable. Non-specific electrocardiographic changes have been reported including T-wave changes and prolonged or borderline QT interval. Pathologically, subendocardial, subpericardial, and myocardial haemorrhages are usually associated with disseminated intravascular coagulation; there can also be fragmentation and rupture of the muscle fibres in the presence of interstitial oedema.[53,54]

The blood

Disseminated intravascular coagulation, a consumption coagulopathy, is very common. Also known as defibrination syndrome, this is a haemorrhagic disorder where there is diffuse intravascular clotting resulting in a haemostatic defect due to excessive utilization of the coagulation factors and the platelets—hence the name consumption coagulopathy.[59] As mentioned earlier, Chao et al.[53] found disseminated intravascular coagulation associated in 10 consecutive fatal cases.

The two main clinical features are bleeding and organ damage due to ischaemia. The kidney failure previously reported may well be due to the occlusion of small vessels with fibrin deposits. A haemolytic anaemia can, in addition, be associated with the defibrination. Very rarely, there can also be early thrombosis of large veins and arteries.

Prevention and management of exertional heatstroke

I am of the opinion that in healthy subjects the only serious potential risk to life from violent exercise is heat-stroke. (Sir Adolphe Abrahams, *British Encyclopaedia of Medical Practice*, 1950.)

Forty years later this comment is just as relevant. Both participants and organizers of athletic events must bear in mind the possibility that a competitor's bizarre behaviour could be the result of heat stroke. The failure to appreciate that heatstroke could be the cause of erratic behaviour in athletes or the reason for changing consciousness in someone who has collapsed will delay the diagnosis and therefore the treatment. It cannot be emphasized too strongly that the speed with which the core temperature is returned to normal and the various other abnormalities are corrected will determine the outcome.

In most cases, the measurement of rectal temperature together with a full clinical assessment of the cardiovascular, respiratory, and neurological state is vital. Treatment must begin on site. All too often one hears race organizers alert a neighbourhood hospital to the fact that patients will be transported there in the event of some disaster. This results in great delay and often emergency-room physicians may be unaware of the likelihood of heatstroke, thus further delaying the institution of life-saving treatment.

Following the first City to Surf Race in Sydney in 1971 the following suggestions were made regarding race organization, medical support, and competitor education.[41]

Race organization

Organized races and sporting events should avoid the hottest summer months and the hottest part of the day. In the northern hemisphere early spring can be particularly hazardous as frequently there are unseasonably hot days. These comments apply to any athletic event.

Athlete education

The following points should be noted.

1. Training and fitness will improve thermoregulation during exercise.

2. Heat acclimatization—athletes are advised to train at the time of day when the competitions will be held. All too often training sessions will take place in the morning or evening although the competition will be held in the middle of the day. A minimum of 7 to 10 days of heat acclimatization is advisable.

3. Begin the competition hydrated—often football players and athletes will already be 1 and 2 litres down at the start of competition.

4. Only compete when well—hazards include any febrile or dehydrating illness such as upper respiratory tract infections and especially gastroenteritis.

5. During the race or fun run be aware of headache, nausea, dizziness, and lack of coordination. These are often the first

symptoms of heat injury, and the time taken from their onset to the loss of consciousness can be very brief.

6. Run within one's capabilities—in fun runs the victims tend to be younger, overenthusiastic amateur runners striving for a personal best time.

Medical organization and medical facilities

Ideally, medical facilities should be available on-site at competitions; the medical personnel should be capable of full-scale resuscitation and, in particular, should be able to cool and rehydrate the patient with intravenous therapy as described in detail elsewhere.[41]

Summary

Heat stroke is a serious and potentially fatal event. Organizers of various athletic competitions must be aware of the possibility that heat stroke could occur in the events—even on apparently cool days. Medical facilities must be available on-site and staff must have the ability to make the diagnosis and begin definitive treatment. The full-blown picture of heat stroke with multiorgan damage may be caused by endotoxaemia and be pathogenically akin to septic shock. Such an aetiology opens up new horizons in the mechanisms of thermal tolerance and intolerance and possible new approaches to the treatment of heat stroke.

The principal concern in the management of runners who collapse following a race is the establishment of an accurate diagnosis. Anyone who collapses to the ground has a temporary impairment of consciousness and is a potential candidate for heatstroke. Experience has taught us that an accurate measurement of core temperature is mandatory; however, axillary or oral readings can be very misleading and therefore taking oesophageal, tympanic, or, most practically, a rectal temperature is essential. Our practice has been to measure rectal temperature, and a wide range of values has been obtained for those who have collapsed. Clearly, not everyone who collapses suffers from heat exhaustion, but unless the rectal temperature is taken it is impossible to establish a logical course of action. As with any seriously ill patient, begin with the ABC (airway, breathing, and circulation). In most instances, airway, breathing, and circulation are functioning, but in the 1990 City to Surf Race in Sydney three individuals collapsed, were asystolic, and could not be resuscitated.[60]

Having established the diagnosis, the specific treatment is rapid rehydration and cooling. The administration of 1 to 2 litres of intravenous dextrose–saline in the first hour will restore the circulation and thus can be the most important step in the cooling process. A greater volume (3 to 4 litres) may be administered to these patients who have succumbed to heat stroke in the course of prolonged exercise. In addition, there is some advantage in placing cool packs over the large vessels of the neck, groin, and axilla.

The most effective means of rapid cooling is that established by Weiner and Khogali,[61] known as the Mecca Cooling Unit in which an atomized spray of warm water is directed on to the individual who is then fanned with warm air. This retains the vasodilation of the skin and allows rapid cooling to occur. In contrast, applying cold sheets or direct cold usually results in vasoconstriction with impairment of heat loss, thus ensuring further temperature elevation. Some sources advocate immersion in an ice-cold bath. This will certainly lower the body core temperature, but it is usually logistically difficult to treat large numbers of people in this way. Obviously, this would also expose patients and health-care workers to the risk of electrocution if defibrillators were used.

When the above approach is used most people who collapse in fun runs can be observed for an hour or more and then safely discharged. If their recovery is in question they should be transferred to a medical facility for further monitoring. Nevertheless, it should be emphasized that the emergency care of collapsed athletes must be performed on-site as any delay in establishing the diagnosis and start of treatment may increase morbidity and even mortality.

Where there is evidence of multiorgan damage and the developing saga of fulminant heat stroke, I would recommend bowel sterilization and an intravenous antibiotic regime appropriate for the treatment of Gram-negative sepsis.

References

1. Mount LE. Thermal neutrality. In: Monteith JL, Mount LE, eds, *Heat loss from animals and man*. London: Butterworths, 1974.
2. Winslow GEA, Herrington LP, Gagge AP. A new method of partitional calorimetry. *American Journal of Physiology* 1936; **116**: 641–7.
3. Nielsen M. Die regulation der korpetemperataur bei muskelarbeit. *Skandinavisches Archiv für Physiologie* 1938; **79**: 193–230.
4. Robinson S, Dill DB, Wilson JW, Nielsen M. Adaptations of white men and Negroes to prolonged work in humid heat. *American Journal of Tropical Medicine* 1941; **21**: 261–87.
5. Lind AR. A physiological criterion for setting thermal environmental limits for everyday work. *Journal of Applied Physiology* 1963; **18**: 51–6.
6. Astrand I. Aerobic work capacity in men and women. *Acta Physiologica Scandinavica* 1960; **49** (Suppl. 169): 64–73.
7. Saltin B, Hermansen L. Esophageal, rectal and muscle temperature during exercise. *Journal of Applied Physiology* 1966; **21**: 1757–62.
8. Davies CTM. Thermoregulation during exercise in relation to sex and age. *European Journal of Applied Physiology* 1979: **42**: 71–9.
9. Davies CTM, Thompson MW. Aerobic performance of female marathon and male ultramarathon athletes. *Journal of Applied Physiology* 1979; **41**: 233–48.
10. Asmussen E, Nielsen M. The regulation of the body-temperature during work performed with the arms and with the legs. *Acta Physiologica Scandinavica* 1947; **14**: 373–82.
11. Nielsen B. Thermoregulation during work in carbon monoxide poisoning. *Acta Physiologica Scandinavica* 1971; **82**: 98–106.
12. MacDougall JD, Reddan WG, Layton CR, Dempsey JA. Effects of metabolic hyperthermia on performance during heavy prolonged exercise. *Journal of Applied Physiology* 1974; **36**: 538–44.
13. Rowell LB, Brengelmann GL, Murray JA, Kraning KK, Kusumi F. Human metabolic responses to hyperthermia during mild to maximal exercise. *Journal of Applied Physiology* 1969; **26**: 395–402.
14. Johnson JM, Rowell LB. Forearm skin and muscle vascular responses to prolonged leg exercise in man. *Journal of Applied Physiology* 1975; **39**: 920.
15. Johnson JM. Regulation of skin circulation during prolonged exercise. The marathon: physiological, medical, epidemiological and psychological studies. *Annals of the New York Academy of Sciences* 1977; **301**: 195–212.
16. Dancaster CP, Whereat SJ. Fluid and electrolyte balance during the Comrades Marathon. *South African Medical Journal* 1971; **45**: 547–51.
17. Nadel ER, Wenger CB, Roberts MF, Stolwijk JAJ, Cafarelli E. Physiological defenses against hyperthermia of exercise. The marathon: physiological, medical, epidemiological and psycho-

logical studies. *Annals of the New York Academy of Sciences* 1977; 301: 98–109.

18. Rowell LB, Marx J, Bruce RA, Conn RD, Kusumi, F. Reductions in cardiac output, central blood volume and stroke volume with thermal stress in normal men during exercise. *Journal of Clinical Investigation* 1966; **45**: 1801–16.

19. Sawka MN, Knowlton RG, Critz JB. Thermal and circulatory responses to repeated bouts of prolonged running. *Medicine and Science in Sports* 1979; **11**: 177.

20. Hales JRS, Stephens FRN, Fawcett AA, *et al.* Lowered skin blood flow and erythrocyte sphering in collapsed fun-runners. *Lancet* 1986; **i**: 1494–5.

21. Fox RH, Lofstedt BE, Woodward PM, Erikkson E, Werkstrom B. Comparison of thermoregulatory function in men and women. *Journal of Applied Physiology* 1969; **26**: 444–53.

22. Hertig BA and Sargent F. Acclimatization of women during work in hot environments. *Federation Proceedings* 1963; **22**: 810–13.

23. Wyndham CH, Morrison JF, Williams CG. Heat reactions of male and female caucasians. *Journal of Applied Physiology* 1965; **20**: 357–64.

24. Drinkwater BL, Denton JE, Kupprat IC, Talag TS, Horvath SM. Aerobic power as a factor in women's response to work in hot environments. *Journal of Applied Physiology* 1976; **41**: 815–21.

25. Avellini BA, Kamon E, Krajewski JT. Physiological responses of physically fit men and women to acclimatization to humid heat. *Journal of Applied Physiology* 1980; **49**: 254–61.

26. Armstrong LE, Maresh CM. The induction and decay of heat acclimatization in trained athletes. *Sports Medicine* 1991; **12**: 302–12.

27. Stein HJ, Eliot JW, Boder RA. Physiological reactions to cold and their effects on the retention of acclimatization to heat. *Journal of Applied Physiology* 1949; **1**: 575–85.

28. Glaser EM, Shephard RJ. Simultaneous experimental acclimatization to heat and cold in man. *Journal of Physiology (London)* 1963; **36**: 419–25.

29. Eijkman C. Some questions concerning the influence of tropical climate on man. *Lancet,* 1924; **i**: 887–93.

30. Kuno Y. The acclimatization of the human sweat apparatus to heat. In: Kuno Y, ed. *Human perspiration.* Springfield, IL: CC Thomas, 1956; 318–35.

31. Ladell WSS. Acquired heat tolerance of temperate climate men living in the tropics. Abstracts of the *XVIII International Physiology Congress,* Copenhagen 1950; 320–2.

32. McPherson RK. Acclimatization status of temperate zone man. *Nature* 1958; **182**: 1240–1.

33. Ladell WSS. Inherent acclimatization of indigenous West Africans. *Journal of Physiology (London)* 1951; **112**: 15–16. (Abstr.)

34. Wyndham CH, Benade AJA, Williams CG, Strydom NB, Goldin A, Heyns AJA. Changes in central circulation and body fluid spaces during acclimatization to heat. *Journal of Applied Physiology* 1968; **25**: 586–93.

35. Leithead CS, Lind AR. *Heat stress and heat disorders.* London: Cassell and Co., 1964; 25.

36. Barnett MA, Maughan RJ. Response of unacclimatized males to repeated weekly bouts of exercise in the heat. *British Journal of Sports Medicine* 1993; **27**: 39–55.

37. Williams CG, Wyndham CH, Morrison JF. Rate of loss of acclimatization in summer and winter. *Journal of Applied Physiology* 1967; **22**: 21–6.

38. Pandolf KB, Burse RL, Goldman RF. Role of physical fitness in heat acclimatization decay and reinduction. *Ergonomics* 1977; **20**: 399–408.

39. Adams WC, Fox RH, Grimby G, Kidd DJ, Wolff HS. Acclimatization to heat and its rate of decay in man. *Journal of Applied Physiology* 1960; **152**: 26P–27P.

40. Talbot JH. Heat cramps. *Medicine, Baltimore* 1935; 323–76.

41. Richards D, Richards R, Schofield PJ, Ross V, Sutton JR. Management of heat exhaustion in Sydney's The Sun City-to-Surf fun runner. *Medical Journal of Australia* 1979; **2**: 457–61.

42. Knochel JP, Reed G. Disorders of heat regulation. In: Kleeman CR, Maxwell MH, Narin RG, eds. *Clinical disorders, fluid and electrolyte metabolism.* New York: McGraw-Hill, 1987; 1197–232.

43. Gathiram P, Wells MT, Raidoo D, Brock-Utne JD, Gaffin SL. Portal and systemic plasma lipopolysaccharide concentrations in heat-stressed primates. *Circulatory Shock* 1988; **25**: 223–30.

44. Old LJ. Tumor necrosis factor. Another chapter in the long history of endotoxin. *Nature (London)* 1987; **330**: 602–3.

45. Tracey KJ, Beutler B, Lowry SF, Merryweather J, Wolpe S, Milsarak IW, Hariri RJ, Fahey TJ, Zentella A, Albert JD, Shires GT, Cerami A. Shock and tissue injury induced by recombinant human cachetin. *Science* 1986; **234**: 470–4.

46. Brock-Utne JG, Gaffin SL, Wells MT, Gathiram P, Sohar E, James MF, Morrell DF, Norman RJ. Endotoxemia in exhausted runners after a long distance race. *South African Medical Journal* 1988; **73**: 533–6.

47. Graber DC, Reinhold RB, Breman JG, Harley RA, Hennigar GR. Fatal heat stroke. Circulating endotoxin and gram-negative sepsis as complications. *Journal of the American Medical Association* 1971; **216**: 1195–6.

48. Cardis DT, Reinhold RB, Woodruff PW, Fine J. Endotoxemia in man. *Lancet* 1972; **i**: 1381–6.

49. Bouchama A, Parhar RS, El-Yazigi A, Sheth K, Al-Sedairy S. Endotoxemia and release of tumour necrosis factor and interleukin 1 in acute heatstroke. *Journal of Applied Physiology* 1991; **70**: 2640–4.

50. Mustafa KY, Omer O, Khogali M, *et al.* Blood coagulation and fibrinolysis in heat stroke. *British Journal of Haematology* 1985; **61**: 517–23.

51. Sohal RS, Sun SC, Colcolough HL, *et al.* Heat stroke: an electron microscopic study of endothelial cell damage and disseminated intravascular coagulation. *Archives of Internal Medicine* 1968; **122**: 43–7.

52. Bosenberg AT, Brock-Utne JG, Gaffin SC, Wells MT, Blake GT. Strenuous exercise causes systemic endotoxemia. *Journal of Applied Physiology* 1988; **65**: 106–8.

53. Chao TC, Sinniah R, Pakiam JE. Acute heat stroke deaths. *Pathology* 1981; **13**: 145–56.

54. Clowes GHA, O'Donnell TF. Heat stroke. *New England Journal of Medicine* 1974; **291**: 564–7.

55. Hart LE, Egier BP, Shimizu AG, Tandan PJ, Sutton JR. Exertional heat stroke: The runner's nemesis. *Canadian Medical Association Journal* 1980; **122**: 1144.

56. Savdie E, Prevedoros H, Irish A, *et al.* Heatstroke following rugby league football. *Medical Journal of Australia* 1991; **155**: 636–9.

57. Kew MC, Abrahams C, Seftel HC. Chronic interstitial nephritis as a consequence of heatstroke. *Quarterly Journal of Medicine* 1970; **39**: 189–99.

58. Malamud N, Haymaker W, Custer RP. Heatstroke: a clinico-pathologic study of 125 fatal cases. *Military Surgery* 1946; **99**: 397–449.

59. Sutton JR, Coleman MK, Millar AP, Lazarus L, Russo P. The medical problems of mass participation in athletic competition: The 'City-to-Surf' race. *Medical Journal of Australia* 1972; **2**: 127.

60. Richards R, Richards D, Sutton JR. Exertion-induced heat exhaustion: an often overlooked diagnosis. *Australian Family Physician* 1992 (Jan.); **21**: 18–24.

61. Weiner JS, Khogali M. A physiological body cooling unit for treatment of heat stroke. *Lancet* 1980; **i**: 507–9.

2.5 Circadian rhythms

Thomas Reilly

Introduction

Physiological determinants of exercise performance are affected by circadian rhythms. Performance rhythms conform closely in phase with body temperature and also with the level of arousal. These rhythms have implications for élite athletes, for people performing exercise for health purposes, and for the optimal timing of training. They also have repercussions for team managers with responsibilities for the travel plans of athletes competing abroad. There are consequences for sports medicine personnel who must consider, for example, the effects of time of day on joint stiffness and pain perception. Additionally, some drug doses that are safe in the evening may have exaggerated effects if administered early in the morning. Circadian rhythms may be influenced by environmental factors such as ambient temperature, light and darkness, and so on. Endogenous rhythms persist during sleep deprivation, when they are superimposed on an underlying trend towards fatigue. Separate rhythms are desynchronized in time-zone transitions and during nocturnal shiftwork, and exercise capability is then temporarily impaired. Coping with desynchronization is helped by adopting different behavioural, dietary, or pharmacological strategies. Attempts to identify individuals with poor tolerance to sleep loss, shift work, or jet lag have largely been unsuccessful.

Biological rhythms should not be confused with 'biorhythms', a theory which has no scientific foundation. According to this theory there are three independent cycles which start for each individual at birth. A physical cycle determines vigour and has a cycle length of 23 days. A cycle of emotion has a period of 28 days, and there is supposedly also a cycle of intellectual ability with a period of 33 days. Halfway through each cycle there is a swing across the baseline from positive to negative. The theory predicts that sports performance will be benefited when cycles are positive and adversely affected when they are negative, but interpreting a mixture of the three rhythms is less straightforward. Advocates of the theory may point to outstanding sports successes (such as the Olympic Games victories of Mark Spitz and the first world record runs of Sebastian Coe) to justify their case, but the theory is easily discredited by retrospective analysis of athletic records. There is no basis for justifying its application to strenuous exercise and the scientific preparation of athletes. In contrast, the scientific study of biological rhythms, which is known as chronobiology, is now a respected field in its own right.

Chronobiology

Biological rhythms

Rhythms are an essential feature of nature and many aspects of human behaviour. Cyclical changes that recur regularly over a given length of time and are related to underlying physiological processes are referred to as biological rhythms. In humans the length of the cycles, known as the period, can range from small fractions of a second, such as in neural firing rates, to slower changes in close harmony with the lunar cycle (circamensal) or with the changes of the season (circannual). Rhythms associated with the solar day are called circadian. Rhythms with periods longer than a day are known as infradian and those recurring repeatedly within a day are known as ultradian.

In addition to the period or length, a rhythm is also characterized by its amplitude, which is equal to half of the variation from peak to trough, and its acrophase, which refers to the time that the peak occurs. The oscillation is deemed to occur around a midpoint which is called the mesor. Where observations are made at unequal intervals throughout 24 h, the mean value may differ from the mesor.

Circadian rhythms

Circadian rhythms influence biological function. They can have a profound impact on the performance of physical activity and athletic skills. The major determinant of the rhythms is the spin of the Earth about its vertical axis. Humans have adapted to this over the ages by timing the alternation of sleep and wakefulness to coincide with the periods of darkness and light, respectively. In turn, this pattern of rest and activity affects many physiological functions which slow down at night and accelerate with daylight. Human circadian rhythms have been established at levels ranging from cellular and tissue operations to whole-body functions. The myriad of rhythms in the body interact with each other and with the environment. The concept of homeostasis, accepted from the mid-nineteenth century and implying that the internal environment within the body is relatively constant, now acknowledges that the internal environment is constantly changing with a regular oscillatory behaviour. Indeed, the capacity for rhythmic change is accepted as an inherent characteristic of living organisms. Thus when the physiological responses to exercise assume a so-called steady state, this level may depend upon the time of day.

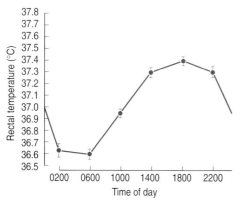

Fig. 1 The circadian rhythm in rectal temperature. Values shown are mean ± SD. (Reproduced from ref. 1, with permission.)

Rhythms in motor performance are closely linked to the circadian curve in body temperature (Fig. 1). Circadian rhythms may interact with habitual daily activities, and the persistence of rhythms in responses to submaximal and maximal exercise should be of interest to sports practitioners. Similarly, circadian variations in joint stiffness and flexibility are relevant to physical therapists. Factors limiting exercise performance, such as thermoregulation, motivation, and pain, may operate differentially according to the time of day. It is important to consider individual preferences for morning or evening effort and the extent to which some performances are vulnerable to ultradian influences. Of course, the existence of circadian rhythms is most easily acknowledged when they are disrupted through transmeridian flight, nocturnal shiftwork, or sleep loss.

Physiology of circadian rhythms

Body temperature and sleep–wake cycles

Those human circadian rhythms that result from changes in the environment are referred to as exogenous. The most prominent environmental changes are alternating day and night. The solar day dictates habits of sleep, rest, and activity, as well as work and leisure-time social activity. Ambient temperature varies with the time of day, potentially accentuating rhythms in physiological processes that are temperature dependent. Light is also an important factor in defining rhythm characteristics and it can be manipulated to alter certain circadian rhythms. These external factors serve to fine-tune rhythms into a 24-h period and are referred to as *Zeitgebers* or time-givers.

Certain rhythms persist when environmental conditions are kept constant or in circumstances devoid of time cues. The main ones are body temperature and the sleep–wake cycle. They are recognized as being self-sustaining in character and are referred to as endogenous rhythms. Their identification implicates a biological mechanism which times the duration and sequences of the processes involved, thereby operating as a clock. The characteristics of endogenous rhythms are not easily altered by changes in the environment; for example, the rhythm in body temperature persists under conditions of sleep deprivation.

When time cues are removed, which is possible within the Arctic Circle in summer, in isolation chambers, or in underground caves, endogenous rhythms drift to a period between 25 and 27 h. There

appear to be two master clocks, one controlling the body temperature cycle and the other the sleep–wake cycle. In conditions of continual isolation the temperature rhythm maintains its period of 25 to 26 h but the sleep–wake cycle drifts to a period of 33 h. This dissociation occurs after only 15 days of isolation.[2]

Many human circadian rhythms result from the combined influences of endogenous and exogenous factors. They are not present at birth but develop in the first year of life. The rhythms are entrained to an exact 24-h period by the *Zeitgebers*. There is probably a hierarchy of clocks, with those governing the body temperature and sleep–wake cycles being the major ones influencing many other rhythmic functions. The major clocks may synchronize the activities of other circadian functions in the manner of non-linear oscillators.[3] Many human performance measures tend to follow closely the circadian rhythm in body temperature,[4] but are also affected by the sleep–wake cycle and local physiological conditions within the active tissues.

Neural and hormonal influences (effects of light and dark)

The suprachiasmatic nucleus cells of the hypothalamus have been cited as the probable source of the master clock. In some animals there is a direct link between the suprachiasmatic nucleus and the retina.[3] There is also evidence of a centre in the lateral hypothalamic area with functions related to circadian rhythm in core temperature and crosslinked to the suprachiasmatic region.[5] The pineal gland is sensitive to changes in light intensity during the day, and important timekeeping functions are attributed to it. In this gland, which in simple organisms is thought to function as a third eye, light exerts time-giving properties via a special visual pathway that synapses with the suprachiasmatic nucleus.[6] The hormone melatonin is synthesized from serotonin in the pineal gland, although there is a secondary source of melatonin within the retina. Human melatonin levels are increased at night with plasma concentrations rising from about 2 pg/ml diurnally to a nocturnal peak approaching 60 pg/ml.[7] The activity of *N*-acetyltransferase, an enzyme associated with the synthesis of melatonin from serotonin, also shows a pronounced rhythmic fluctuation, with nocturnal activity exceeding daytime levels by a factor of over 1000.

Although environmental and body-temperature changes affect the circadian rhythm in arousal, the level of arousal is influenced mainly by the sleep–wake cycle and by neural traffic through the reticular activation formation in the brain. Circadian phase systems are not completely isolated from other time structures with different periodicities. Nevertheless, it is via environmental signals that rhythms are adjusted to an exact 24-h period.

In northern latitudes near and above the Arctic Circle the incidence of a malaise known as seasonal affective disorder increases when daylight hours are short. The condition is accompanied by decrements in psychomotor performance.[8] Exposure to bright or ultraviolet light may ameliorate the condition. Élite Scandinavian athletes tend to spend some time during their winter training in southern climates which are warmer and have longer hours of daylight. The shortened hours of daylight in winter affect the training of some athletes; for example, professional soccer players in England tend to train in the morning, whereas their matches are timed for the afternoon or at night under floodlights. Increasing the duration and intensity of exposure to daylight does seem to affect the phase of the circadian rhythm: in the northern hemisphere the peak occurs 55 min later in June than in December.[9] Changes in ambient temperature do not appear to alter the rhythm.

Rhythms in performance

Sports performance

Most athletic records are set in the late afternoon or evening. For example, world record performances by British athletes in 800 to 5000 m track races from 1979 to the end of the next decade took place between 19:00 and 23:00 h. This partly reflects the fact that record attempts are usually scheduled for evening meetings when the environmental temperature is more favourable for performance than at midday or in the early afternoon. Nevertheless, athletes tend to prefer evening contests and consistently achieve their top performances at this time of day.

This preference has also been manifested in the work rate of soccer players during indoor five-a-side games sustained for four days.[10] Observations on players showed that the pace of play reached a peak at about 18:00 h and a trough at 05:00 to 06:00 h. Feelings of fatigue were correlated negatively with levels of activity. The self-paced level of activity conformed closely to the curves in heart rate (Fig. 2) and in body temperature; this relationship persisted throughout successive days. The fact that the freely chosen level of exercise is highest at about the time the body-temperature rhythm reaches a peak has important implications for training as well as for certain competitive sports.

Soccer players are accustomed to playing in the evening and tend to feel at their best at this time. Competitive matches last at least 90 min, and the window of daytime during which professional players can function at their best probably stretches over a 4- to 6-h period from midafternoon to evening. The usual routine of professionals is to train in the morning. Soccer coaches might seriously consider altering this convention by timing the training so that players are taxed maximally in the afternoon or evening.

The same advice may not necessarily always apply to short-term

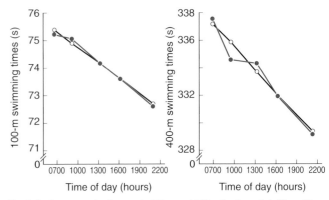

Fig. 3 Performance of swimmers in 100-m and 400-m front crawl at different times of day. The broken lines represent values fitted by a linear trend. (Reproduced from ref. 16, with permission.)

activity, particularly the 'explosive' events. Over the last 50 years the only two track and field world records to have been set in morning meetings were in the men's shot put and the women's javelin. French international sabre fencers had their best scores, as far as they related to speed and skill, around noon.[11] Explosive actions with substantial neuromotor components may be linked more closely to the arousal rhythm than to that of body temperature and perhaps reach a peak earlier in the day.

Sports contests are not amenable to the types of manipulation demanded by experimental designs. Consequently, research workers have tended to concentrate on the effects of time of day on performance in time trials or simulated contests. In the first systematic investigation of diurnal variation in performance, six runners, three weight-throwers, and three oarsmen performed better in the evening than in the morning.[12] Swimmers have produced faster times over 100 m at 17:00 h compared with 07:00 h in three out of four strokes studied.[13] The speed of running in a 5-min test varied in close correspondence to the circadian curve in body temperature.[14]

The better performances of swimmers in the evening also applies to multiple efforts. Performances in front crawl were found to be 3.6 per cent and 1.9 per cent faster for 400-m and repeated 50-m swim trials, respectively at 17:30 h than at 06:30 h.[15] This time-of-day effect was apparent throughout 3 days of partial sleep deprivation. Even after disrupted sleep swimmers can produce maximal efforts, at least if they are required to do so in the evening.

The diurnal variation in swimming performance is not entirely coincident with the circadian rhythm in core temperature. When front crawl times over 100 m and 400 m were examined at five different times of day from 06:00 h onwards, it was noted that performances improved steadily throughout the day.[16] There was no turning point evident before the final measurement at 22:00 h, even though body temperature had peaked some hours earlier (Fig. 3). This reinforces the observations that evening is best for sprint swimmers, particularly if time-trial results are attributed importance, such as in achieving championship qualifying standards.

There is a time window close to the acrophase of body temperature in which optimal performance in sports involving gross motor tasks can be attained. This can extend for 4 to 6 h provided that meals and rests are suitably fitted in during the daily routine. Sports requiring fast explosive efforts tend to peak earlier and may be

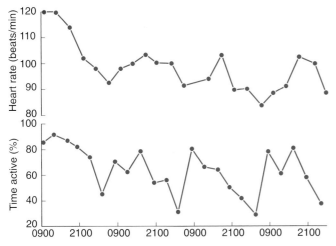

Fig. 2 Mean heart rate and percentage time active in four outfield indoor soccer players every 4 h. Monitoring of heart rate lagged the activity measurement by 1 h. Progression on the horizontal axis indicates successive days of play. (Reproduced from ref. 10, with permission.)

related to the sleep–wake clock rather than to body temperature. Consequently, practices where skills have to be acquired should be conducted early in the day or around midday, but more severe training drills and 'pressure training' practices are best timed for later in the day. It is acknowledged that sports performance is determined by many variables and there may be multiple performance rhythms. This can be further examined by looking at the existence of rhythms in components of sports performance.

Components of sports performance

Rhythms in motor performance tasks closely approximate the body-temperature curve. Performance rhythms are also related to the state of arousal: a low level of arousal predisposes towards errors and injury risk, whereas heightened arousal promotes readiness for intense physical efforts. Thus, mistakes in motor coordination that lead to accidents and injuries are more likely early in the day. Such occurrences later in the day could be due to fatigue resulting from time spent on the task, as in sailing or rally driving, for example.

Isometric muscle force, dynamic muscle activity, neuromotor performance, and gross motor performance are all subject to circadian rhythms.[14] The timing of the peaks tends to follow the phase of the body-temperature curve, although this does not imply that they are caused by the changes in temperature. Rhythms in grip strength and back strength have been replicated in dynamic muscular activity such as the vertical jump[14,17] and the standing broad jump. The variation in such tests attributable to the time of day ranges from about 3 per cent of the mean value for jumping to 6 to 10 per cent for isometric strength and to about 15 per cent for power output on a swim-bench. The amplitude of the rhythm increases with increasing complexity of the task. Although seemingly small in magnitude, an improvement in the order of 3 per cent can have a profound effect on competitive performance. As tests of this type are easy to administer, they can be employed as markers of circadian rhythm in monitoring the effects of desynchronization on performance.

The rhythm in muscular strength is robust and persists under conditions where subjects are deprived of sleep for four consecutive nights. The circadian variation in grip strength is greater than the effects of sleep loss on this function.[15,18] Although the normal rhythm in muscular strength is in phase with that of body temperature, the extent to which alterations in muscle temperature or in the motivation of subjects contribute to the rhythm is not clear. Muscle performance is optimal at a muscle temperature of around 39 °C and a core temperature of 38.3 °C.[19] Competitive athletes may elevate muscle temperature to this level as a result of warming up and so might override an inherent rhythm in muscle performance. Consequently, attention is directed towards a proper warm-up regimen in cases where competitors have to perform in the morning or at night (delayed start) when muscle temperature would otherwise be suboptimal. There is a strong motivational component to muscular strength, and experimental work comparing muscle performance under conditions of maximal voluntary contraction and in response to electrical stimulation is needed in order to establish whether the rhythm in strength is due to central or peripheral factors.

Muscle strength is usually measured by cable tensiometry, strain-gauge assemblies, or isokinetic machines. Although a circadian rhythm in strength is evident in human performance tests, the

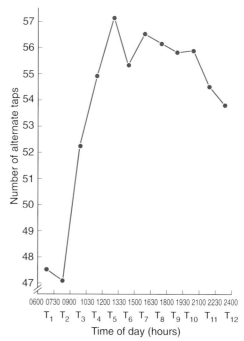

Fig. 4 Speed of tapping performance during the day showing a post-lunch dip in speed. (Reproduced from ref. 23, with permission.)

magnitude of the circadian variation in muscle performance may be beyond the sensitivity of contemporary computer-linked dynamometers. Isokinetic dynamometry has not always shown evidence of a significant rhythm in peak torque for fast and slow actions during maximum concentric and eccentric efforts of the knee extensors.[20] For circadian rhythms to be identified in such actions the measurement error must be small. Similarly, a vigorous warm-up can partly overcome the night-time troughs in performance. In leg exercise the anaerobic capacity (as measured by the Wingate test) is reduced by 8 per cent at 06:00 h compared with 14:00 h, whereas the peak power value is maintained well;[21] a decline in performance during the 30-s test suggests a motivational component in the circadian variation in anaerobic capacity. When all-out arm exercise for 30 s is preceded by a vigorous warm-up, there is no distinguishable rhythm in mean power or peak power.[22] Since such tests call for total subject compliance in producing maximal efforts, it is difficult to distinguish the motivational basis from a true biological rhythm as an explanation of the time-of-day effect.

Some psychomotor and muscular strength fluctuations show a bimodal pattern in their circadian rhythms. For example, tapping speed, indicated by moving a stylus as rapidly as possible between two plates, shows a slight dip in performance in the early afternoon (Fig. 4). This is referred to in occupational contexts as the 'post-lunch' dip, although it persists in some tasks even when no lunch is taken.[24] In the study of tapping performance, measurements were performed repeatedly throughout the working day over a 3-month span.

A similar fall has been noted in the isometric strength of the knee extensors.[25] In this study measurements were repeated at 2-h intervals throughout the normal period of wakefulness. It is only when performance tests are repeated frequently throughout the day that this afternoon decline, analogous to the post-lunch dip in ergo-nomic tasks, is observed. This transient decrement in performance might be due to an underlying 90-min cycle that prevails during sleep, and during the day comes closest to the surface of detection in the early afternoon.[26] It may also be linked with the turning point of circulating adrenaline and noradrenaline levels whose peak is attained at about this time.[27] Sports specialists who spread their training over, say, three or more separate sessions with long training times overall are the most likely to benefit from an afternoon nap.

Rhythms have been identified in sensory motor (reaction time), psychomotor (hand–eye coordination), sensory perceptual, cognitive, and psychological functions.[14,28-30] It is incorrect to generalize to a single performance rhythm since different types of task can show different circadian rhythms, depending largely on whether they are influenced by the body temperature or the sleep–wake clock.

To determine the links between performance rhythms and physiological processes it is necessary to examine: (1) the scale of circadian rhythms in resting conditions; and (2) the persistence of these rhythms during exercise.

Circadian rhythms in physiological functions

Physiological rhythms at rest

Many physiological parameters are known to show circadian rhythmicity. They include metabolic, cardiovascular, and endocrine functions. The metabolic functions showing cyclical changes include oxygen consumption ($\dot{V}O_2$), carbon dioxide production ($\dot{V}CO_2$), and minute ventilation ($\dot{V}_E$). The rhythms in $\dot{V}O_2$ and $\dot{V}CO_2$ have an amplitude of about 7 per cent of their mean resting value (Fig. 5), whereas that in $\dot{V}_E$ is about 11 per cent. Only about one-third of the variations in metabolism can be explained by the circadian rhythm in body temperature, despite the fact that the peaks occur close together in time.[13,14]

Cardiovascular functions also display a rhythm similar in shape to the body-temperature curve.[32] The peak in heart rate occurs earlier in the day than that of body temperature, but is close to the phase of the rhythm in circulating catecholamines. The peak-to-trough variation at rest is about 8 beats/min; this should be taken into account by athletes and their mentors when resting pulse rate is used as an index of either training state or overtraining. The catecholamine rhythms are probably closely related to changes in arousal; they have been shown to influence rifle-shooting performance and are negatively related to fatigue during the day.[33]

Output from endocrine glands, particularly the trophic hormones of the anterior pituitary, exhibit circadian rhythms. Some endocrine secretions, for example growth hormone, prolactin, and testosterone, peak during the night. There is no overall pattern to the rhythms that would help to explain the circadian curves in exercise performance. The rhythms in adrenaline and nonadrenaline are the most closely related to the performance curve.[33] The excretion of electrolytes is also closely related in phase to the body-temperature and performance rhythms. The diurnal changes in renal function have only marginal impact during exercise because of the relative shutdown of blood flow to the kidneys and the inactive muscles. Angiotensin and aldosterone are hormones linked not only with renal function but also with the circadian rhythm in blood

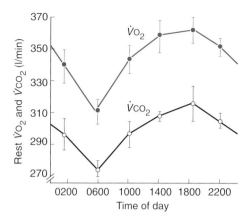

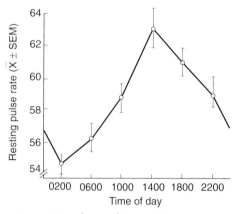

Fig. 5 Mean values (± SE) for $\dot{V}O_2$ and $\dot{V}CO_2$ at rest (top) and pulse rate pre-exercise (bottom) at six different times of the day. (Reproduced from ref. 31, with permission.)

pressure, although this function merits most consideration in contexts of exercise for health rather than élite sport.

Physiological responses to exercise

Submaximal exercise

Physiological rhythms detected at rest may be obliterated or attenuated, or maintained or amplified, under exercise conditions. Research reports can be marshalled to support all these possibilities. The conflict is partly due to a failure to control the environment adequately and to masking factors such as diet and previous activity of the subjects. When these variables are carefully considered, a consistent picture begins to emerge. For example, the heart-rate rhythm that is noted at rest is still evident during light and moderate exercise (Table 1). The consistency of its phase and amplitude applies to both leg[31,34] and arm[35] exercise.

The heart-rate rhythm is not paralleled by $\dot{V}O_2$ and $\dot{V}_E$ throughout the range of submaximal exercise intensities. This applies to arm exercise as well as leg exercise. In a longitudinal study of one subject, the rhythm in $\dot{V}O_2$ gradually faded away as the exercise intensity increased.[31] The rhythm at a moderate exercise level was accounted for by variations in bodyweight. No circadian rhythm was found for $\dot{V}CO_2$ or the respiratory exchange ratio during moderate exercise. This indicates that the choice of substrate as a fuel for exercising muscle is not determined by the time of day, once the

Table 1 Cosinor parameters for heart rate including rest, exercise, and recovery values ($n = 15$)

| | Heart rate (beats/min) | | | |
	Mean	Amplitude	p zero amplitude	Acrophase (95% confidence limits)
Rest	70	4	$p < 0.001$	13:50 (12:05–15:35)
Light exercise	105	4	$p < 0.001$	13:10 (11:15–15:05)
Medium exercise	134	4	$p < 0.001$	13:48 (11:44–15:52)
Maximum	181 ·	2	$p < 0.005$	14:10 (12:02–16:18)
3rd minimum	126	5	$p < 0.001$	14:04 (12:14–16:54)

Statistically significant rhythm was demonstrated in all cases ($p < 0.005$). Reproduced from ref. 34, with permission.

diet, environmental temperature, and activity are controlled. The rhythms in $\dot{V}O_2$ and $\dot{V}CO_2$ may no longer be detectable once the exercise intensity reaches about 50 per cent of $\dot{V}O_2$max.[34]

The most robust rhythm seems to be that of $\dot{V}_E$ which is amplified at light and moderate exercise intensities.[31] Even when $\dot{V}_E$ is expressed as the ventilation equivalent of oxygen (Fig. 6), the rhythm is clearly evident.[36] This may partly explain the mild dyspnoea sometimes associated with exercising in the early morning. At vigorous exercise intensities, the point at which $\dot{V}_E$ begins to increase disproportionately to $\dot{V}O_2$, does not vary with the time of day.[31]

The temperature in soft tissues around the joints can affect their resistance to motion and this could alter the energy cost of exercise. The muscular efficiency, which represents the mechanical work done as a percentage of its energy cost, can be computed as gross or net efficiency. Where more than one steady rate of exercise is performed, the delta efficiency (which considers the increment in work done in relation to the increment in energy expended) can be calculated. For a given exercise mode the muscular efficiency is influenced more by the work rate and the mode of computation than by the time of day.[31] The greater joint viscosity at night does not sig-

nificantly affect the time required to attain 'steady state' metabolic conditions during submaximal exercise.[36]

Responses of catecholamines, aldosterone, cortisol, and plasma renin activity have been examined during 25 min of exercise at 60 per cent of $\dot{V}O_2$max.[37] Time of day generally did not affect the hormonal or haemodynamic responses to exercise, with the exception that plasma renin activity was markedly higher during exercise at 16:00 h compared with 04:00 h. This was thought to reflect a greater vasoconstrictor activity in the cutaneous blood vessels.

Maximal physiological responses

When maximal values are being attributed to measurements, the question arises as to whether the ceiling of physiological function was reached during the exercise test. Consequently, recognized criteria are applied when assessing $\dot{V}O_2$max. Otherwise, data collected during graded exercise to volitional exhaustion may merely reflect the reluctance of subjects to work at $\dot{V}O_2$max at night. For a well-trained individual with a body mass of 70 kg the normal amplitude of the $\dot{V}O_2$ rhythm at rest would be less than 0.5 per cent of the mean maximal value. It is difficult to detect this against the background of biological variation and measurement error associated with assessing $\dot{V}O_2$max. Therefore, it should not be surprising that the most carefully conducted studies fail to show circadian variation in $\dot{V}O_2$max. This applied when 12 different times of day and duplicate measurements at each time point were used.[38] It also applied to a longitudinal design used to eliminate variability between subjects and to results of a cross-sectional approach:[31,34] the coefficient of variation of $\dot{V}O_2$max was found to be 2.9 per cent. In these studies it was concluded that $\dot{V}O_2$max is a stable function, independent of time of day. This is in sharp contrast to the value predicted from submaximal heart rate (Fig. 7), which shows an error in estimating $\dot{V}O_2$max that is not acknowledged when the maximal function is predicted from a submaximal test.

The circadian rhythm in $\dot{V}_E$, which is apparent during light and moderate exercise, similarly disappears under maximal aerobic conditions, at least for leg exercise. In arm exercise the highest metabolic measurements generally do not demonstrate a plateau and are lower than observed at $\dot{V}O_2$max because of the decreased muscle mass involved. Consequently, the highest measurements during arm exercise are referred to as peak rather than maximal values. During the performance of arm ergometry the $\dot{V}O_2$ peak and high-

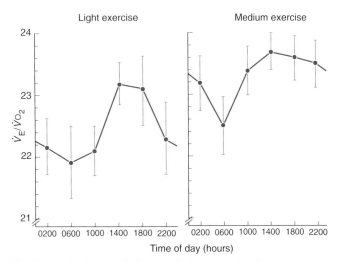

Fig. 6 The rhythm in the ventilation equivalent of oxygen at light and medium exercise intensities. (Reproduced from ref. 36, with permission.)

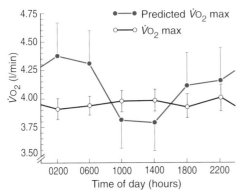

Fig. 7 The contrast between results measured for $\dot{V}O_2$max throughout the day and values predicted from heart-rate response to submaximal exercise. (Reproduced from ref. 28, with permission.)

est heart rate demonstrate a circadian rhythm, the highest values being observed close to the crest time of rectal temperature.[35] The results reflect a rhythm in the total work performed.

Studies of the maximal heart rate during exercise have consistently shown an influence of the time of day.[32] The circadian rhythm is similar in phase to that noted at rest and submaximal exercise, but its amplitude is reduced. A circadian rhythm in recovery heart rate is evident soon after maximal exercise ceases.[32,34] Therefore fitness indices, such as the Harvard test score, could contain an error as large as 5 per cent due to the time of day that the test is performed. This also means that self-monitoring of post-exercise pulse rates by athletes and coaches is subject to at least this degree of error.

In view of the stability of $\dot{V}O_2$max throughout the solar day, a rhythm in maximal aerobic power cannot explain time-of-day effects in all-out performance such as 400-m swim trials and 5-min shuttle runs. The effects might be accounted for by an ability to sustain a fixed exercise intensity for longer in the evening. Exercise to voluntary exhaustion at an intensity close to $\dot{V}O_2$max does exhibit circadian variation.[39] Subjects tested on a cycle ergometer exercised for longer in the evening (22:00 h) than in the morning (06:30 h), with the mean values being 436 and 260 s, respectively. The subjects also tolerated higher blood lactate levels in the evening as a result of the increase in total work performed at that time.

It is possible that rhythms in vigorous exercise performance may be due to a combination of motivation and psychological drive that is reflected in anaerobic power output. There is a circadian rhythm in power output in a stair-run test, although its amplitude is only 2.5 per cent.[21] This is compatible with the circadian variation in body temperature, as maximal anaerobic exercise is impaired by about 5 per cent for each 1 °C fall in core temperature.[40] Some studies of anaerobic efforts using the Wingate test have failed to show a significant rhythm in anaerobic power and capacity for leg[21] and arm[22] exercise, although a fall in anaerobic capacity (mean power output over 30 s) at night without a corresponding decline in peak power output (highest power output in the first 5 s) was noted in the study of leg exercise. A comprehensive warm-up procedure employed prior to experimental tests can swamp underlying rhythms. The sensitivity of such tests may be insufficient to detect performance rhythms that are small in magnitude. As there is no objective physiological criterion that maximal anaerobic capacity is being employed in tests such as the Wingate model, results may be

due mainly to motivation. This would account for the large diurnal variation in performance in those studies reporting positive findings. Power outputs 5 to 8 per cent higher in the day compared with the night have been reported. Even when this difference in performance between 06:00 and 14:00 h is observed, data throughout the whole day may not conform to a significant rhythm.[22] Power output over 30 s on a swim-bench does exhibit a circadian rhythm. The acrophase for peak power and mean power (anaerobic power and anaerobic capacity) was found to occur at 16:20 h with amplitudes of the rhythms being 14 per cent and 11 per cent, respectively.[41] These rhythms were linked to both the body-temperature and subjective-alertness curves, and so the relative effects of these two influences could not be determined. They supplement the observations of circadian variation in short-term efforts such as those required in isometric muscle strength and dynamic jump tests.[14,17]

Thermoregulation

Core temperature (reflected in oral, oesophageal, tympanic, or rectal temperature) possesses an endogenous rhythm and so is used in chronobiological studies as a physiological marker of rhythmicity. This rhythm persists during exercise. A 5 per cent impairment in maximal anaerobic power would be predicted at night due solely to the fall in core temperature. The optimal time of day would be in the evening when muscle and core temperatures are at their peaks.

This rationale may not apply to sustained high-intensity exercise, such as marathon running, in hot conditions. In such instances thermoregulatory requirements may limit endurance performance. This supports the practice of starting marathon races in the morning rather than in the afternoon in hot climates, although the argument has been based solely on the lower environmental heat stress in the morning. The ideal ambient temperature for marathon running is around 13 °C. In cold and wet conditions, a morning start would place the slower performers at increased risk of hypothermia. The advantage of starting sustained exercise at a core temperature which would normally be suboptimal is that the onset of heat stress is delayed and the overall strain on thermoregulatory mechanisms is reduced. Experimental support for this view is available.[42] Precooling oesophageal temperature by 0.4 °C and mean skin temperature by 4.5 °C before 60 min of submaximal exercise causes a 6.8 per cent overall increase in work rate compared with control conditions.

There is a significant interaction between work rate during exercise of 60–90 min duration and the time of day.[43,44] In the evening when body temperature is highest, subjects choose greater work rates at the beginning of the exercise period at this time of day compared to in the morning. However, as the body temperature rises above optimal levels during the evening exercise, the work rate begins to drop. In the morning, the work rate gradually increases as body temperature rises towards optimal levels until, at the end of the exercise, the work rates chosen in the morning are higher than the corresponding evening values. In cold and wet conditions however, individuals operating at very light exercise intensities (for instance, charity runners in marathon runs) may be at an increased risk of hypothermia in the morning. Their low work rates may be inadequate for the maintenance of heat balance due to the high loss of heat to the cold environment.[45] In such conditions, appropriate

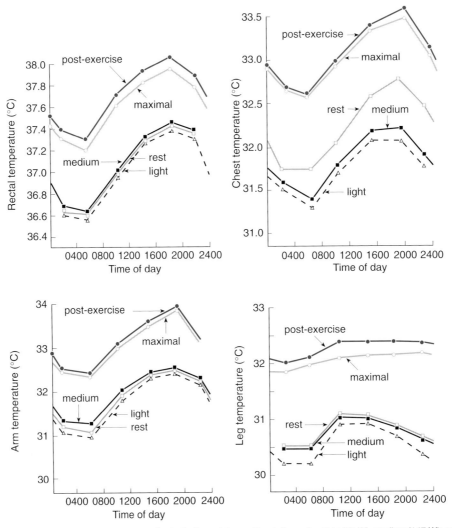

Fig. 8 Mean values for rectal and skin temperatures according to the time of day and level of exercise: light (82 W); medium (147 W); and maximal. Rest and post-exercise values are included. (Reproduced from ref. 47, with permission.)

clothing is needed to safeguard against a dangerous drop in the body's temperature.

The circadian rhythm in core temperature during exercise represents a fixed thermal load superimposed on the resting baseline temperature.[41] This occurs despite a circadian variation in the mean skin temperature for the onset of sweating and in blood flow to the skin.[46] The rhythm in rectal temperature apparent at rest persists in phase and amplitude at different levels of exercise. There are closely related cyclical changes in rectal and skin temperatures.[47] The time course of changes in skin temperature varies with the body surface location, and the rhythm in the exercising limb tends to disappear during exercise because of the convective airflow created by the leg movements (Fig. 8).

Physical factors in circadian rhythms and exercise

Spinal shrinkage

There are physical as well as physiological factors that vary with the time of day and these have implications for exercise. On the one

hand, the day–night cycle of activity and rest provides an alternation of weight bearing associated with the upright posture and, on the other, recovery while sleeping. Weight bearing imposes compressive loading on the spine and leads to a loss of disc height primarily because of extrusion of water through the disc wall.[48] This loss of height is known as shrinkage and is reflected in measurements of changes in stature using appropriate apparatus. Spinal shrinkage during the day is about 1 per cent of stature.[49] The circadian rhythm in shrinkage is of the same order of magnitude in females,[50] but is more erratic in subjects with back-pain syndrome.[51]

The data in Fig. 9 conform to a cosine curve but a power function best fits the shrinkage during the day, with the rate of loss declining as the discs stiffen.[50] Shrinkage is reversed at night whilst recumbent, with the rate of regain in height being greater in the first part of the night's sleep. An endogenous rhythm in stature could be reinforced or masked by the changes in posture and spinal loading between day and night. The rate of reversal of shrinkage suggests that circadian variation in stature is largely attributable to spinal loading and unloading rather than to an endogenous rhythm.[49]

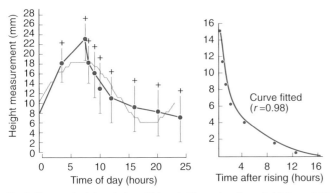

Fig. 9 Changes in stature during a 24-h period from a baseline set at 7.5 mm (left). The solid line indicates mean observations with 95 per cent confidence limits. The power function relating time since rising from sleep to the same data for loss of height is shown on the right. This curve overlaps the observed changes in height almost perfectly. (Reproduced from ref. 50, with permission.)

The loss of disc height could render the spine more vulnerable as its stiffness increases,[52] thus making weightlifting and similar activities more hazardous as stature recedes throughout the day. Loss in height alters the dynamic response characteristics of the disc and so there is a time-of-day effect on the shrinkage resulting from a fixed exercise regimen. Losses of height as a result of a 20-min, circuit weight-training regimen are greater at 07:30 h than at 23:00 h. The disc was found to be a more effective shock absorber in the morning when shrinkage was 5.4 mm compared with a mean value of 4.3 mm in the evening.[50] This greater stiffness in the evening is partly compensated for by greater back muscle strength. A high negative correlation was found between back strength and height lost: the greater the muscle strength, the less height was lost.

The habitual activity level and the postures engaged in can influence the amount of shrinkage during the day. Intervention procedures for unloading the spine prior to heavy physical training in the evening have been advocated. An example is the Fowler position at rest with the trunk supine and the legs raised to rest on a bench. Gravity-inversion systems have also proved effective,[53,54] although the spinal distension that is induced before exercise is quickly lost once a strenuous exercise regimen is undertaken.[55]

Joint stiffness and flexibility

Other physical factors that are known to vary with the time of day to affect muscular function are joint stiffness and flexibility. The former refers to resistance to motion, whilst the latter indicates range of movement about a joint. There is circadian variation in stiffness of the knee joint, with increased stiffness observed late in the evening and early in the morning.[56] Stiffness increases as body temperature decreases, and so the curve may be related to the fall in body temperature towards the end of the day. It may also be affected by activity patterns during the course of the day.

There is a circadian variation in trunk flexibility[16] and hip flexibility.[28] Trunk flexibility measurements were made five times during the day between 07:00 h and 22:00 h. Trough values were observed first thing in the morning and peak values in the middle of the day (13:00 h).[16] Circadian variation has also been found in lumbar flexion and extension, passive straight-leg raising, glenohumeral lateral rotation, and the distance from fingertip to floor in forward flexion.

The mean acrophase was 18:10 h, although individual peaks ranged from midday to near midnight.[57]

Diseased joints may exert an influence on the circadian rhythm in musculoarticular function. The peak and trough times of the rhythm in the grip strength of patients with rheumatoid arthritis have been found to be similar to those in healthy subjects.[58] Despite this normality in phase, the peak-to-trough variation may be affected: the peak-to-trough difference in rheumatoid arthritic patients is approximately three times the normal range.[59] The magnitude of this variation is reduced with corticosteroid administration, but the timing of the rises and falls in muscular strength is unaffected.[60] The rhythms in muscular strength help to explain the variations in propensity towards physical activity in these patients during the day.

Subjective strain

Perceived exertion

A circadian variation in the subjective reaction to exercise might explain why performance is generally better in the evening than in the morning. The perception of effort does not seem to vary at light ergometric loads up to 150 W, although the slope of the relationship between heart rate and perceived exertion changes with the time of day.[32] Ratings of exertion have been studied at treadmill running speeds eliciting heart rates of 130, 150, 170 beats/min.[38] As the heart-rate response to a fixed submaximal exercise intensity is lowest at night, it follows that more exercise can be performed at a given heart rate at that time. The higher subjective ratings reported at night may be due to the work rate and not to an inherent variation in effort perception.

The circadian variation in the rating of exertion is evident once a high steady rate of exercise is reached. In one investigation of circadian variation in perceived exertion a significant result was found only at one submaximal load (245 W), although several lower exercise levels were rated.[61] This is supported by findings of others whose subjects first cycled at 40 per cent of $\dot{V}O_2$max for 5 min before cycling to exhaustion at 95 per cent of $\dot{V}O_2$max at two different times of day, 06:30 h and 22:00 h.[39] No difference in perceived exertion with time of day was noted at either work rate, although the higher work rate was sustained for longer in the evening to the point where the same endpoint (exhaustion) was reached. The findings offered support for the concept of a motivational component in the circadian variation in exercise performance.

The predisposition of athletes towards exercise can be examined in another way, namely by allowing them to choose an exercise intensity that they are prepared to tolerate for a predetermined period. This self-selected work rate exhibits a circadian rhythm that is in phase with the body-temperature rhythm.[62] In fact it may be more strongly influenced by the arousal cycle. It reinforces the recommendation that strenuous training regimens are best carried out in the late afternoon or evening to obtain optimal compliance from athletes.

Submaximal exercise is perceived to be harder in the morning than in the evening under conditions of partial sleep loss. The time-of-day effect is greater in magnitude than the effect of sleep loss.[15,18] The results suggest that changes in the subjective reactions to exercise with time of day may be tied more closely to the rhythm of arousal than to that of body temperature.

A standard circuit of weight training was rated as harder when conducted at 07:30 h compared with 22:00 h. In this instance, the perceived exertion was negatively correlated to back strength ($r = -0.59$), which was higher in the evening than in the morning.[50]

An alternative paradigm which employs light work bouts every 4 h for 24 h may include a cumulative fatigue effect. With this experimental protocol, exercise was rated harder at night and perceived exertion was marginally elevated in the afternoon.[14,26] This may represent a subharmonic in the circadian rhythm of biological arousal, which is sometimes reflected in a postlunch dip in performance[24,26] and in a siesta particularly in Hispanic cultures.

The fact that a set exercise regimen is perceived as harder in the morning than in the evening[50,61] has implications for timing of training. It would be logical to suggest that greater training loads would be tolerated in the evening compared with earlier in the day. However, caution should be expressed before arriving at any generalizations, since the effects of warm-up, occupational activity during the day, individual characteristics, and the nature of the training stimulus need to be considered. One longitudinal study[63] attempted to establish whether the training effect due to a fixed exercise bout differed with time of day. Although there was some evidence of the specificity of adaptation due to the time of day, no substantial circadian variations in the training effect accrued.

Pain perception

There is also a circadian variation in pain perception that might be relevant in the context of sport injury. Self-ratings of pain intensity in patients with painful conditions show definite patterns throughout the waking day. Minimum levels of pain are noted in the morning, with a more or less steady increase during the day to a peak during the evening.[64] Laboratory investigations have shown similar findings, with subjects becoming more sensitive and the pain perception threshold falling as the day proceeds. The highest threshold for epicritic pain is noted at about 03:00 to 06:00 h, and that for more diffuse pain at 11:00 h.[65] These observations have implications for the prescription of analgesics for a variety of sports injuries and other painful conditions.

Time estimation

Estimation of how quickly time passes is also influenced by the time of day.[66] The usual method of time estimation is to ask subjects to count to themselves at a 1-s rate for 60 s. The rhythm in subjective time perception is related to a chemical-clock hypothesis: the higher the body temperature, the quicker the chemical reaction, and the faster the internal clock, the faster the speed of counting. The chemical-clock theory is supported by observations that lowering body temperature in divers leads to overestimation of time lapsed.[67] Whether the circadian variation in time estimation affects coordination tasks entailing fine timing of actions or prolonged efforts where motivation may decline has not been investigated.

Individual differences

There is some evidence that the phasing of circadian rhythms is affected by personality. Introverts tend to be better performers in the morning, whereas extroverts are more sluggish at this time. The latter make up for this by reaching a peak level of performance later

in the day and staying alert for longer in the evening. The body-temperature curves of these different personalities show a similar form, but that of the introvert peaks earlier in concordance with the performance curves. However, the difference in acrophase between these extremes of personality is only about 1 h.[68]

Age and state of fitness influence human circadian rhythm characteristics. Older athletes tend to have an earlier acrophase in their performance than younger athletes and are less affected by an early morning start to races.[43,69,70] Highly trained individuals tend to have higher amplitudes in their rhythms compared to inactive subjects, the main difference being that the athletes have lower trough values.[43,71] This may be due to sleep characteristics of athletes which differ from sedentary individuals in electroencephalograph patterns.[43]

Individual variability has also been described according to how people phase their habitual activities throughout the day. Circadian phase types have been referred to as 'larks' (morning types) and 'owls' (evening types), indicating a preference for morning or evening work.[72] This preference is likely to be a more influential factor than personality in minor variations in rhythms between subjects, since the majority of people do not exhibit extreme personalities. Being a morning type is more important than extroversion in determining individual differences in the phase of circadian rhythms.[73] The existence of morning and evening types among athletes has not been systematically examined. Most responses to exercise on a cycle ergometer do not differ between the two circadian phase types.[74] This finding also applies to swimmers whose circadian rhythms in power output on a swim-bench are unrelated to circadian phase types.[37] Apparently healthy subjects may commonly display internal desynchronization of a set of circadian rhythms. Competitive athletes with internally synchronized rhythms generally have a better chance of being victorious than individuals with internal desynchronization. This was confirmed in a study of French fencers participating in the 1984 Olympic Games.[11] External desynchronization of rhythms is affected by nocturnal shift work and travelling across time zones. These, together with disruptions due to sleep loss, are discussed next.

Desynchronization

Jet lag

Desynchronization refers to the disruption of circadian rhythms which become out of phase with each other. Rhythms are externally desynchronized if the individual switches to a nocturnal work schedule or rapidly crosses a series of time zones. The physiological rhythms affected include body temperature, the sleep–wake cycle, pulse rate, ventilation, arterial pressure, diuresis, and excretion of electrolytes.[75] The disorientation that results is known as jet lag, and symptoms include fatigue and general tiredness, inability to sleep at night, loss of appetite, loss of concentration, decreased drive, headache, and general malaise. Jet lag can impair the performances of athletes on busy competitive schedules until the major rhythms have all adjusted to the new time zone.[76,77]

Westward travel, when time is extended, tends to be easier to adjust to than travelling in an easterly direction. This reflects the fact that in conditions where the major environmental signals are absent, the period is lengthened to 25 to 27 h.[3] Performance of psychomotor and athletic skills tends to suffer more after eastward than

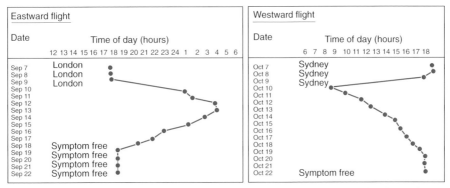

Fig. 10 Time of day at which oral temperature attained a peak plotted according to local time on outward (eastward) and return (westward) journeys between England and Australia. A stopover of one night in Singapore occurred on both journeys. The points were determined using cosinor analysis of data collected throughout each day on one subject. (Reproduced from ref. 77, with permission.)

after westward flights. The difference may be negligible if the time-zone shift is 9 to 12 h or near maximal (Fig. 10).

Data on rugby players after travelling to Australia showed a diminution in muscular strength until jet-lag symptoms abated.[78] Recommendations were that training should best be performed about midday until the body's rhythms were resynchronized. In crossing fewer time zones (phase shifts of 3 to 5 h) it is advisable to train within the window of time when rhythms in the home and in the local country are above the mesor. For these medium-range phase shifts this time would be midday after a westward flight and in the evening after an eastward flight.

Coping with jet lag

A variety of strategies has been suggested for offsetting the effects of jet lag. The first is to tune-in mentally to the new local time as soon as possible. This can be done during the flight by altering one's watch, missing meals if inappropriately timed, and avoiding alcoholic and other diuretic drinks such as strong coffee. It is also advisable to drink plenty of fruit juices to avoid the dehydrating effects of inspiring dry cabin air.[75]

Altering bedtime for a few days before departure in the direction of intended travel and for a few days after arrival is sometimes suggested as a means of lessening the disruptive effects of travelling across time zones. Bedtime is delayed for a few nights prior to travelling westwards, with the opposite applying before flying east. Since only the behaviour and sleep-wake cycles, and not environmental variables, are adjusted, the alterations in phase of the new biological rhythms occur at a slower rate than in time-zone transition. The entrainment rate for alertness is faster than for core temperature, but even after 8 days on a 3- to 5-h shift of the sleep-wake cycle the adjustment of the alertness rhythm is incomplete. Entrainment of physiological, performance, and psychological variables in response to phase advance and phase delay of the sleep-wake cycle is easier with phase delay of the cycle, simulating preparation for westward travel, than with phase advance. The following conclusions can be drawn: shifting the sleep-wake cycle alters rhythms in accord with the direction of the shift; however, the adjustment is incomplete and motor performance is compromised during the course of such adaptive changes, with both mean and amplitude being depressed.

Sleep is a stronger synchronizer of circadian rhythms than are mealtimes or social activities. Consequently, prolonged napping at

the new location should be avoided as this operates against adaptation by anchoring the rhythm in its previous phase.[79] This tactic of anchoring or maintaining circadian rhythms at the time phase of the country of departure is used by non-sports personnel who regularly cross time zones for short spells abroad. Its use by sports practitioners would be feasible on flying in for single contests, but might be counteracted by the effects of 'travel fatigue'.

Minor tranquillizers (the benzodiazepines) are effective in inducing sleep but not necessarily good at keeping the individual asleep. Also, hangover effects cannot be discounted.[76] Melatonin capsules taken in the evening, by local time in the new time zone, may reduce the symptoms of jet lag.[43] Their use should require the careful timing of ingestion according to whether the body clock should be delayed or advanced. Besides, the consequences of athletes using melatonin have not been studied.

It is important to use natural signals such as light to help resynchronize rhythms. These include both natural daylight and bright artificial light. These work to link the arousal and sleep-wake cycles to the new environment. Exercise stimulates catecholamine production and increases alertness, and is an effective resynchronizer. Moderate exercise is recommended, even on the day of arrival, unless it is very late in the evening local time. It switches the traveller quickly into local time cues, and is also a good antidote to travel fatigue.

The best plan is to ensure that the athletes arrive in the country of destination in good time for physiological and performance rhythms to resynchronize. Empirical data on runners crossing the Atlantic support the wisdom of allowing one day for each time-zone shift to enable adaptation to occur. The coping strategies already outlined should help to shorten this time. Rhythms in potassium excretion may take longer than this to readjust,[4] as might rhythms in complex skills such as pistol shooting.[80] Where possible, friendly matches should be arranged in the early stages of team tours and the important competitions scheduled later when complete resynchronization should have occurred.

Shift work

About 20 per cent of workers in technologically advanced countries are on some form of shift-work system. Inevitably, this number includes sports participants. Although some British and Irish distance runners have gained Olympic representation whilst employed on nocturnal shift-work systems, these have tended to be fast-rotating shifts rather than predominantly nightwork.

Training programmes and the performances of athletes will be disturbed by the desynchronization of rhythms that shift work causes. The extent of the disturbances depends on the type of shift system employed and whether the individual is allowed to sleep during the shift when 'on call' but not actively engaged. Performances adversely affected include muscular strength, simple motor tasks, and memory-loaded tasks.[81]

Difficulty in ensuring good quality sleep during time off work is a major problem. Apart from sleep disturbances, gastrointestinal problems linked with unusual mealtimes constitute a major source of discomfort. Long-term issues may be more related to health than to the fitness of nocturnal shift workers.

About one-third of workers are intolerant to shift work, and this intolerance is linked to the degree to which rhythms are internally synchronized. Individuals with large amplitudes in their rhythms, and who therefore adjust slowly to altered schedules, are at an advantage in fast-rotating shifts.[81] Physical activity contributes to strengthen the internal synchronization,[71] and athletes are more tolerant of nocturnal shift work than are non-athletes.

The rate at which circadian rhythms revert to their normal cycles seems to be much faster than their adaptation to nocturnal shift work.[82] Even so, it would be advisable to leave a substantial period of time between the termination of nightwork and participation in a major sporting event. Individuals with serious sporting aspirations will experience difficulty in realizing their ambitions if their occupations demand working at night. The fast-rotating form of shift-work systems leaves them with some opportunities to organize training and competition schedules. Further, a consistently high level of performance requires a change to daytime work or to full-time engagement in sport. These moves allow the individual to establish the kind of daily routine into which training and competitive programmes, social activity, and leisure can be slotted to harmonize with the body's endogenous rhythms.

The sleep–wake cycle

Sleep and exercise

Sleep incorporates a cycle of stages that recurs about every 90 min (the order in which the various stages appear is not necessarily consistent from cycle to cycle). The use of electroencephalography (**EEG**) and electro-oculography (**EOG**) has provided insights into underlying events. The two major types of sleep are rapid eye movement (**REM**) sleep, which comprises roughly 20 per cent of total sleep and is discernible by EOG, and non-REM sleep which is subdivided into four stages. Stage 1 characterizes the EEG after sleep onset, following which sleep increases progressively in depth. Stage 2 is longer than any other stage and usually precedes or follows REM, the phase when dreaming occurs. Stages 3 and 4 together are known as slow-wave sleep (**SWS**) because of their low-frequency, high-amplitude EEG waves. Early in sleep SWS predominates; REM sleep dominates later.

Although the mean length of human sleep is about 8 h, there is a large variation between individuals in the amount taken, with the coefficient of variation being about 30 per cent. Athletes assume that sound sleep on a regular and habitual basis is an essential part of preparing for top performances. Professional soccer players spend a lot of time resting, meriting the title '*Homo recumbans*'.[83] Duration is not the only characteristic of a good night's sleep, since restfulness (indicated by relative movements) and latency (indicated by the time between lights out and the onset of Stage 2) are important aspects. Aerobically fit athletes display shorter sleep latencies and longer sleep periods than normal, as well as a tendency towards greater levels of SWS.[84] To what extent these features reflect the contemporary lifestyles of élite athletes and other characteristics rather than aerobic fitness is undetermined.

Sleep patterns of athletes were monitored at times when they were aerobically fit and when they were deemed to be unfit: profiles were compared with sedentary controls.[85] Elevated Stage 3 SWS in fit athletes was compensated for by opposite changes in Stage 4. The biological significance of this shift is unknown. The athletes tended to have a longer sleep duration and more non-REM sleep, although the time spent in bed was similar to the inactive controls. The athletes had a longer REM latency which was associated with a higher level of SWS in the first cycle of sleep. As the differences between the athletes and non-athletes could not be ascribed to aerobic fitness, it appears that the sleep profiles reflected a trait in athletes rather than an effect of training.

Residual fatigue from daytime exercise is believed to alleviate many problems in sleeping. Subjective reactions after exercise indicate a greater degree of tiredness and sleepiness and, if the exercise is not too vigorous, subjects feel that they sleep better. The intensity and duration of exercise may affect subsequent sleep, as does the interval for recovery before retiring to bed. If vigorous exercise is conducted late in the evening, particularly by unfit individuals, the effect may be a delay in sleep onset rather than an induction of sleep. Physiological recovery processes begin once exercise is ended, and the elevations in metabolism and body temperature induced by exercise may delay the onset of sleep. Also, soreness after running on hard surfaces or as a result of physical-contact activities may cause discomfort to a level that prevents restful sleep.

Sleep is an enigma, in the sense that there is no consensus among sleep researchers about its essential function. One school of thought relates sleep to the restitution of the body's tissues.[86] Tissue restitution theories have been linked with heightened mitosis during sleep and elevated growth-hormone secretion during SWS stages. An alternative view is that the need for sleep is specific to nerve cells.[87] The argument for the latter is based on the observations that tissue restitution proceeds during wakefulness, even after exhausting exercise, and convincing evidence such as increased protein turnover in sleep is lacking. Nevertheless, it is obvious that sleep is essential, and this need is apparent when we consider how human operations deteriorate with severe loss of sleep.

Sleep deprivation

There is an interaction between sleep loss and circadian rhythms in that impairments in human performance during sleep deprivation are most pronounced at night. In self-paced activity, consisting of four-a-side indoor soccer sustained for 3 to 4 days, the activity level peaked at about 18:00 h, coinciding with the daily high point of body temperature. Other variables that followed this curve include grip strength[11] and choice reaction time.[88] The circadian rhythm persists for as many days as the individual can be kept awake. Over 3 to 5 days of total sleep deprivation, there is a trend towards deterior-

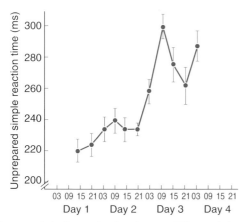

Fig. 11 Unprepared simple reaction time (mean ± SD) recorded on 10 sleep-deprived subjects every 6 h for 4 days of indoor soccer play.

ating performance (Fig. 11) upon which the circadian rhythm is superimposed.[77] For the purposes of statistical analysis this trend has to be removed prior to establishing circadian rhythms by, for example, cosinor or Fourier analysis.[89] The trend is not evident in all functions: gross muscular performances, such as isometric strength, are highly resistant to effects of sleep loss, despite the decrease in muscle enzyme activity noted after the first night.[90] In contrast, cognitive functions are easily affected. Complex and challenging tasks are less affected than monotonous repetitive ones, and strong motivation may overcome the effects of sleep loss, at least for short periods. Nevertheless, after 4 days of sustained activity in which only 2 h sleep were allowed, military subjects were deemed to be ineffective as soldiers.[91] This conclusion was based on their performance on a 1-km assault course, in shooting tests, and a 3-km run; provision of a high-energy diet was unsuccessful in offsetting these impairments. The decline is likely to have been a fatigue effect rather than attributable to sleep loss; soldiers who are deprived of sleep for 2 to 3 nights but are not physically fatigued can perform highly demanding tasks at the same work rate as fresh troops.[92]

In one study subjects were kept awake for 64 h under conditions of isolation from external time cues. Activity was classed as sedentary and was kept as constant as possible, as was the intake of food and liquids.[93] Adrenaline secretion showed a pronounced circadian rhythm, with the rhythm in noradrenaline levels being relatively weaker (based on amplitude as a percentage of the mean value). The circadian rhythms in cardiovascular variables (blood pressure, heart rate, contractility, T-wave amplitude, and QRS, PQ, and QT intervals) observed under normal conditions were effectively obliterated, suggesting that alternating between sleeping and waking is their main determinant. The experimental design could not rule out the existence of self-sustained rhythms in cardiovascular variables since the continuous wakefulness may have concealed low-amplitude endogenous rhythms. Other studies have shown an apparent haemodilution with sleep deprivation, which may be associated with a slight decline in $\dot{V}O_2$max.[94]

There is also an interaction between sleep loss and environmental stressors, although this effect is not linear. For example, the effects of sleep deprivation are compounded by heat, whereas noise can offset them.[95] In humans, the urinary excretion of melatonin follows a circadian pattern during sleep deprivation when subjects are exposed to light, but excretion levels increase with increased sleep loss.[91]

Subjects deprived of sleep for 1 to 3 nights begin to exhibit psychotic-like symptoms and bizarre behaviour. They also experience temporary visual illusions. In such circumstances meaningful physical activity becomes difficult to sustain without error. Sailors will be unreliable on watch duty when suffering from such severe sleep loss. It has been suggested that naturally occurring brain amines may play a role in the cycles of behaviour and mood associated with prolonged sleep deprivation. A circadian rhythm was found in phenylethylamine levels in the urine of sleep-deprived footballers playing indoors: by the third successive night without sleep, the concentrations of this substance being excreted were found to approach the values typically observed in psychiatric patients.[96] Fortunately, such prolonged periods of sleeplessness are experienced only rarely. They may be met by sports medical personnel on hospital duty. In military recruits, where such regimens are imposed during training, similar trends superimposed on a circadian rhythm in catecholamine excretion have been noted.[27] The curve in catecholamine levels coincided with the rises and falls in the accuracy of shooting performance.

Partial sleep loss

Partial sleep loss or disrupted sleep is a more common problem than complete sleep deprivation. It can affect athletes who are restless through anxiety, sailors and yachtsmen during prolonged competitions, and athletes with children who themselves have unsettled sleeping patterns. In view of the variability between individuals in the usual amount of sleep taken, tolerance of sleep loss, sensitivity of laboratory measures of performance to the effects of sleep deprivation, and so on, inferences from experimental investigations must be made with caution. Effects of partial sleep loss also depend on motivation, task complexity, stage of sleep most affected, and other factors.[97]

Faculties associated with SWS may be unimpaired unless the duration of sleep is 3 h or less.[98] Consequently, the effects of a nightly ration of 2.5 h of sleep were examined on a battery of psychomotor, work capacity, and mental-state tests over 3 nights of sleep loss and after one night of subsequent recovery.[88] A 3-day control period was used in a counterbalanced design to eliminate an order effect. Functions that required fast reactions were found to deteriorate significantly. This applied to anaerobic power output in a stair run and choice reaction time at rest and during exercise on a cycle ergometer. Physical exercise attenuated the effects of sleep loss on reaction time, suggesting the benefits of manipulating arousal level by means of a warm-up. This beneficial effect is likely to be short lived and exercise is less effective in offsetting sleep loss when the disruptions continue over days. Limb speed, as measured by a reciprocal tapping task, also becomes steadily worse over successive days of partial sleep loss.[88]

Gross motor tasks such as grip strength, lung function, and treadmill run time were unaffected by sleep restriction. As the restricted sleep regimen was found to affect the more complex motor coordination tasks whilst leaving gross motor functions relatively intact, the data support the 'nerve restitution' theory of sleep.[95]

These effects of partial sleep loss found in males are replicated in female subjects.[21] These subjects were also limited to 2.5 h of sleep for three successive nights in a counterbalanced experimental design: performances were measured each morning (07:00 to 09:00 h) and each evening (19:00 to 21:00 h). A circadian rhythm was noted in the majority of measures; for gross motor function this effect was greater than that of sleep loss. The perceived exertion during cycling at 60 per cent of $\dot{V}O_2$max showed both a diurnal variation and an underlying trend towards increased subjective strain. This coincided with the observations on the sleepiness of subjects, self-rated before exercise. The reduced subjective ratings on the final experimental morning may be explained by anticipation of the end of the experiment.

That sleep is needed more for 'brain restitution' rather than for 'tissue restitution' is further supported by observations on the effects of partial sleep deprivation on swimmers.[18] The sleep ration was restricted to 2.5 h a night for three consecutive nights. Performance over 400 m and over four successive 50-m swims was maintained throughout the experimental period. Swimming times were faster in the evening (17:30 h) compared with the morning (06:30 h), replicating the findings that the time-of-day effect on gross motor functions exceeds that of sleep loss.[18] The most pronounced effects of the restricted sleep regimen were deteriorations in mood over the period of the investigation.

Despite the fact that muscular strength may be retained during consecutive days of partial sleep loss, the quality of training may be adversely affected. This applies to training sessions with repeated or multiple maximal efforts, as occurs in weight-training programmes. Thus maximal performances can be reproduced in weight-training exercises executed in the early parts of the session, but the quality of performance declines towards the end.[98] The reasons for this are attributed to deteriorations in mood with successive nights of deprived sleep.

A paradoxical result of partial sleep loss is that some tasks show an improvement.[99] Hand steadiness, for example, is generally better after loss of sleep. This is attributable to a decrease in spontaneous contraction of the involved muscles as a result of reduced muscle tone. Similarly, tasks with high loadings on short-term memory appear to improve with sleep deprivation owing to a tendency to code information acoustically for mental storage and recall in laboratory tests.[88] Thus care is needed in designing and interpreting sleep-deprivation studies and in making assumptions about the effects of disrupted sleep on athletic performance. Individuals forced to reduce their normal sleep ration may adapt to their shortened sleep length without any consequences for exercise performance, provided that the reduction does not exceed about 2 h. Otherwise they may need to reorganize their daily routine to accommodate an afternoon nap. How practical this is depends on personal and occupational circumstances.

Napping

Ultradian cycles with 90-min periods are identifiable during sleep and may be latent during wakefulness. This may explain subharmonics within the circadian phase system, as evidenced in the 'post-lunch dip' in performance.[4,26] To what extent this drop can be offset by napping or reorganization of the work–rest schedule of activity has not been adequately investigated. Individuals on short sleep durations for some time derive considerable refreshment from short naps.[14,100]

It is known that prolonged napping at an inappropriate time can delay resynchronization of rhythms after abrupt phase shifts.[73] A study of nocturnal shift workers showed that a 1-h nap at 02:00 h was less effective than caffeine in maintaining performance in a range of tasks overnight.[101]

Often, we hear people claim that they were unable to sleep during the night. Such accounts need independent corroboration. Short periods of sleep snatched unwittingly during the night do serve a restorative function. Individuals deprived of sleep for some time derive considerable benefit from such naps, and those deprived of sleep for 2 to 4 days usually recover from their ordeal after uninterrupted sleep for a complete night. A nap could counteract the fall in arousal underlying any subharmonic in the performance curve linked to ultradian rhythms. There has been no substantive research on the refreshing effects of napping on subsequent exercise performance. A nap taken early in the day should be better than a late afternoon nap (provided that the individual can fall asleep), unless performance is late in the evening. A late afternoon nap would contain more SWS and less REM sleep, and would take longer to rouse from than a nap taken earlier. In preparing mentally for competition, athletes would generate the drive to overcome this de-arousal. Advocation of a nap depends on factors such as timing of the contest, precompetition feeding, and individual preferences.

Sleeplessness

Although true insomnia is rare, a large number of people—perhaps 10 to 15 per cent of the population—do have difficulty in sleeping. Causes may include anxiety, depression, bereavement, stress, overwork, or environmental noise such as motor vehicle traffic. Some of these problems are transient and self-limiting; others may persist and become chronic.

It is generally thought that exercise promotes sleep and so it is recommended as therapy for individuals having difficulty in sleeping. The effect of exercise is likely to be indirect, promoting sleep by alleviating the anxieties that prevented it. Athletes do exhibit different sleep patterns from those of sedentary individuals according to observations of their EEG. However, EEG characteristics are only marginally altered with a regimen of physical training. Strenuous exercise shortly before retiring to sleep is likely to raise arousal rather than induce drowsiness because of the increased levels of circulating catecholamines. Thus exercise as therapy for sleeping problems should not be strenuous and should be performed earlier rather than later in the evening.

The usual prescription for insomnia is a sleeping pill. People taking sedatives or hypnotics for a prolonged period develop a dependence on them and the drugs lose their effectiveness. Minor tranquillizers (the benzodiazepines) are probably now being over-prescribed in Europe and North America. Habitual users become dependent on benzodiazepines and suffer severe symptoms if treatment is suddenly stopped. Normal doses also impair reaction time and mental concentration the morning after they have been taken.[102,103] They also affect muscular performance, notably in movements at high velocities. Consequently, their prescription for athletes should be considered only in cases of dire necessity.

Non-pharmacological methods of treating sleeplessness include hypnotherapy. Biofeedback of skin resistance and EEG may also be employed to train the individual to overcome the emotional tension that prevents sleep. Psychological techniques such as visualization of tranquil scenes, concentration on relaxing muscle activity, and deep breathing provide alternative treatments. Stimulus control therapy refers to a mental strategy whereby bed and sleeplessness are dissociated: the individual goes to bed only when sleepy, avoids eating, reading, or watching television in the bedroom, and does not 'sleep in' in the morning. Sensible eating and drinking habits (such as avoiding large meals, heavy alcoholic beverages, or caffeine late at night) should also promote sleep and so help 'knit up the ravell'd sleeve of care'.

References

1. Reilly T. Circadian rhythms in muscular activity. In: Marconnet P, Komi PV, Saltin B, Sejersted OM, eds. *Muscle fatigue mechanisms in exercise and training.* Basel: Karger, 1992; 218–22.

2. Wever R. Zur Zeitgeber-Stärke eines Licht-Dunkel-Wechsels fur dier circadiase periodic des Menschen. *Pflügers Archiv* 1970; **321**: 133–42.

3. Minors DS, Waterhouse JM. *Circadian rhythms and the human.* Bristol: John Wright, 1981.

4. Colquhoun WP. *Biological rhythms and human performance.* New York: Academic Press, 1971.

5. Folkard S, Minors DS, Waterhouse JM. Is there more than one internal clock in man? *Journal of Physiology,* 1983; **341**: 50P.

6. Moore-Ede MC. Jet lag, shift work and maladaptation. *News in Physiological Sciences* 1986; **1**: 156–60.

7. Arendt J, Minors DS, Waterhouse JM. *Biological rhythms in clinical practice.* London: John Wright, 1989.

8. Sherer MA, Weingartner H, James SP, Rosenthal NE. Effects of melatonin on performance testing in patients with seasonal affective disorder. *Neuroscience Letters* 1985; **58**: 277–82.

9. Horne JA, Coyne I. Seasonal changes in the circadian variation of oral temperature during wakefulness. *Experientia* 1975; **31**: 1296–8.

10. Reilly T, Walsh TJ. Physiological, psychological and performance measures during an endurance record for 5-a-side soccer play. *British Journal of Sports Medicine* 1981; **15**: 122–8.

11. Reinberg A, Proux S, Bartal JP, Levi F, Bicakova-Rocher A. Circadian rhythms in competitive sabre fencers: internal desynchronisation and performance. *Chronobiology International* 1985; **2**: 195–201.

12. Conroy RTWL, O'Brien M. Diurnal variation in athletic performance. *Journal of Physiology* 1974; **236**: 51P.

13. Rodahl A, O'Brien M, Firth PGR. Diurnal variation in performance of competitive swimmers. *Journal of Sports Medicine and Physical Fitness* 1976; **16**: 72–6.

14. Reilly T. Human circadian rhythms and exercise. *Critical Reviews in Biomedical Engineering* 1990; **18**: 165–80.

15. Sinnerton S, Reilly T. Effects of sleep loss and time of day in swimming. In: MacLaren D, Reilly T, Lees A, eds. *Biomechanics and medicine in swimming: swimming science VI.* London: Spon, 1992; 399–405.

16. Baxter C, Reilly T. Influence of time of day on all-out swimming. *British Journal of Sports Medicine* 1983; **17**: 122–7.

17. Reilly T, Down A. Circadian variation in the standing broad jump. *Perceptual and Motor Skills* 1986; **62**: 830.

18. Reilly T, Hales AJ. Effects of partial sleep deprivation on performance measures in females. In: Megaw ED, ed. *Contemporary ergonomics.* London: Taylor and Francis, 1988; 509–14.

19. Astrand PO, Rodahl K. *Textbook of work physiology.* New York: McGraw-Hill, 1986.

20. Cabri J, Clarys JP, De Witte B, Reilly T, Strass D. Circadian variation in blood pressure responses to muscular exercise. *Ergonomics* 1988; **31**: 159–66.

21. Reilly T, Down A. Investigation of circadian rhythms in anaerobic power and capacity of the legs. *Journal of Sports Medicine and Physical Fitness* 1992; **32**: 342–7.

22. Reilly T, Down A. Time of day and performance on all-out arm ergometry. In: Reilly T, Watkins J, Borms J, eds. *Kinanthropometry III.* London: Spon, 1986; 296–300.

23. Stockton ID, Reilly T, Sanderson FH, Walsh TJ. Investigation of circadian rhythms in selected components of sports performance. *Bulletin of the Society of Sports Sciences* 1980; **1**: 14–15.

24. Rutenfranz J, Colquhoun WF. Circadian rhythms in human performance. *Scandinavian Journal of Work and Environmental Health* 1979; **5**: 167–77.

25. Wit A. *Zayanienia regulacji w procesie rozwoju siły miesnionej na przykladzie zawodnikow uprawiajacych podnoszenie ciezarow.* Warsaw: Institute of Sport, 1979.

26. Horne JA, Gibbons H. Effect on vigilance and sleepiness of alcohol given in the early afternoon ('post lunch') vs early morning. *Ergonomics* 1991; **34**: 67–77.

27. Akerstedt, T. Altered sleep/wake patterns and circadian rhythms. *Acta Physiologica Scandinavica* 1979; Suppl. 469.

28. Reilly T. Circadian rhythms and exercise. In: Macleod D, Maughan RJ, Nimmo M, Reilly T, Williams C, eds. *Exercise benefits, limits and adaptations.* London: Spon, 1987; 346–66.

29. Shephard RJ. Sleep, biorhythms and human performance. *Sports Medicine* 1984; **1**: 11–37.

30. Winget CM, De Roshia CW, Holley DC. Circadian rhythms and athletic performance. *Medicine and Science in Sports and Exercise* 1985; **17**: 498–516.

31. Reilly T, Brooks GA. Investigation of circadian rhythms in metabolic responses to exercise. *Ergonomics* 1982; **25**: 1093–197.

32. Reilly T, Robinson G, Minors DS. Some circulatory responses to exercise at different times of day. *Medicine and Science in Sports and Exercise* 1984; **16**: 477–82.

33. Froberg J, Karlsson CG, Levi L. Circadian variation in performance, psychological ratings, catecholamine excretion and diuresis during prolonged sleep deprivation. *International Journal of Psychobiology,* 1972; **2**: 23–36.

34. Reilly T, Brooks GA. Selective persistence of circadian rhythms in physiological responses to exercise. *Chronobiology International* 1990; **7**: 59–67.

35. Cable T, Reilly T. Influence of circadian rhythms on arm exercise. *Journal of Human Movement Studies* 1987; **13**: 13–27.

36. Reilly T. Circadian variation in ventilatory and metabolic adaptations to submaximal exercise. *British Journal of Sports Medicine* 1982; **16**: 115–16.

37. Stephenson LA, Kolka MA, Francesconi R, Gonzalez RR. Circadian variations in plasma renin activity, catecholamines and aldosterone during exercise in women. *European Journal of Applied Physiology* 1989; **58**: 756–64.

38. Faria IE, Drummond BJ. Circadian changes in resting heart rate and body temperature, maximal oxygen consumption and perceived exertion. *Ergonomics* 1982; **25**: 381–6.

39. Reilly T, Baxter C. Influence of time of day on reactions to cycling at a fixed high intensity. *British Journal of Sports Medicine* 1983; **17**: 128–30.

40. Bergh U, Ekblom B. Influence of muscle temperature on maximal muscle strength and power in human skeletal muscles. *Acta Physiologica Scandinavica* 1979; **107**: 33–7.

41. Reilly T, Marshall S. Circadian rhythms in power output of swimmers. *Journal of Swimming Research* 1991; **7**: 11–13.

42. Hessemer V, Langusch D, Bruck K, Bodeker RK, Breidenbach T. Effects of slightly lowered body temperature on endurance performance in humans. *Journal of Applied Physiology—Respiratory, Environmental and Exercise Physiology* 1984; **57**: 1731–7.

43. Atkinson G, Reilly T. Effect of age and time of day on preferred work-rates during prolonged exercise. *Chronobiology International* 1995; **12**: 121–9

44. Reilly T, Garrett R. Effects of time of day on self-paced performances of prolonged exercise. *Journal of Sports Medicine and Physical Fitness* 1995; **35**: 99–102.

45. Reilly T, Atkinson G, Waterhouse J. *Biological rhythms and exercise.* Oxford: Oxford University Press, 1997.

46. Stephenson LA, Winger CB, O'Donovan BH, Nadel ER. Circadian rhythm in sweating and cutaneous blood flow. *American Journal of Physiology* 1984; **246**: R321–4.

47. Reilly T, Brooks GA. Exercise and the circadian variation in body temperature measures. *International Journal of Sports Medicine* 1986; **7**: 358–62.

48. Tyrrell AR, Reilly T, Troup JDG. Circadian variation in stature and the effects of circuit weight-training. *Spine* 1985; **10**: 161–4.

49. Reilly T, Tyrrell A, Troup JDG. Circadian variation in human stature. *Chronobiology International* 1984; **1**: 121–6.

50. Wilby J, Linge K, Reilly T, Troup JDG. Spinal shrinkage in females: Circadian variation and the effects of circuit weight-training. *Ergonomics* 1987; **30**: 47–54.

51. Garbutt G, Boocock MG, Reilly T, Troup JDG. Application of spinal shrinkage to subjects with low back pain. In: Duquet W, Day JAP, eds. *Kinanthropometry* IV. London: Spon, 1993; 114–18.

52. Adams MA, Dolan P, Hutton WP, Porter RW. Diurnal changes in spinal mechanics and their clinical significance. *Journal of Bone and Joint Surgery* 1990; **72B**: 266–70.

53. Troup JDG, Reilly T, Eklund JAE, Leatt P. Changes in stature with spinal loading and their relation to the perception of exertion or discomfort. *Stress Medicine* 1985; **1**: 303–7.

54. Leatt P, Reilly T, Troup JDG. Unloading the spine. In: Oborne D, ed. *Contemporary ergonomics.* London: Taylor and Francis, 1985; 227–32.

55. Boocock MG, Garbutt G, Reilly T, Linge K, Troup JDG. Effect of gravity inversion on exercise induced spinal loading. *Ergonomics* 1988; **31**: 1631–8.

56. Wright V, Dawson D, Longfield MD. Joint stiffness—its characterisation and significance. *Biology and Medicine in Engineering* 1969; **4**: 8–14.

57. Gifford LS. Circadian variation in human flexibility and grip strength. *Australian Journal of Physiotherapy* 1987; **33**: 3–9.

58. Harkness JA, Richter MB, Panagi GS, Van de Pette K, Unger A, Pownall R, Geddani M. Circadian variation in disease activity in rheumatoid arthritis. *British Medical Journal* 1982; **284**: 551–4.

59. Job-Deslondre C, Reinberg A, Delbarre F. Chrono-effectiveness of indomethacin in four patients suffering from an evolutive osteo-arthritis of hip or knee. *Chronobiologia* 1983; **10**: 245–54.

60. Reinberg A, Briere L, Fraboulet G., *et al.* Clinical chronopharmacology, of ACTH 1–17.111. Effects of fatigue, oral temperature, heart rate, grip strength and bronchial potency. *Chronobiologia* 1981; **8**: 101–15.

61. Ilmarinen J, Ilmarinen R, Korhonen O, Nurminen M. Circadian variation of physiological functions related to physical work capacity. *Scandinavian Journal of Work and Environmental Health* 1980; **6**: 112–22.

62. Coldwells A, Atkinson G, Reilly T, Waterhouse J. Self-chosen work-rate determines day–night differences in work capacity. *Ergonomics* 1993; **36**: 313.

63. Hill DW, Cureton KJ, Collins MA. Circadian specificity in exercise training. *Ergonomics* 1989; **32**: 79–82.

64. Procacci P, Corte MD, Zoppi M, Marascu M. Rhythmic changes of the cutaneous pain threshold in man. A general view. *Chronobiologia* 1974; **1**: 77–96.

65. Strempel H. Circadian cycles of epicritic and protopathic pain threshold. *Journal of Interdisciplinary Cycle Research* 1977; **8**: 276–80.

66. Ptaff D. Effects of temperature and time of day on time judgements. *Journal of Experimental Psychology* 1968; **76**: 419–22.

67. Baddeley AD. Time estimation at reduced body temperature. *American Journal of Physiology* 1966; **79**: 475–9.

68. Blake MJF. Relations between circadian variation of body temperature and introversion–extroversion. *Nature (London)* 1967; **215**: 896–7.

69. Atkinson G, Coldwells A, Reilly T, Waterhouse J. An age-comparison of circadian rhythms in physical performance and mood states. *Journal of Interdisciplinary Cycle Research* 1992; **23**: 186–8.

70. Atkinson G, Coldwells A, Reilly T, Waterhouse J. The influence of age on diurnal variations in competitive cycling performance. *Journal of Sports Sciences* 1994; **12**: 127.

71. Atkinson G, Coldwells A, Reilly T, Waterhouse J. A comparison of circadian rhythms in work performance between physically active and inactive subjects. *Ergonomics* 1993; **36**: 273–81.

72. Horne JA, Ostberg O. Individual differences in human circadian rhythms. *Biological Psychology* 1977; **5**: 179–90.

73. Vidacek S, Kaliterna L, Tadosevic-Vidacek B, Folkard S. Personality differences in the phase of circadian rhythms: a comparison of morningness and extroversion. *Ergonomics* 1988; **31**: 873–8.

74. Hill DW, Cureton KJ, Collins MA, Grisham SC. Diurnal variations in responses to exercise of 'morning types' and 'evening types'. *Journal of Sports Medicine and Physical Fitness* 1988; **28**: 213–19.

75. Winget CM, De Roshia CW, Markley CL, Holley DC. A review of human physiological performance changes associated with desynchronosis of biological rhythms. *Aviation, Space and Environmental Medicine* 1984; **54**: 132–7.

76. De Looy A, Minors D, Waterhouse J, Reilly T, Tunstall Pedoe D. *The coach's guide to competing abroad.* Leeds: National Coaching Foundation, 1988.

77. Reilly T. Time zone shift and sleep deprivation problems. In: Torg JS, Welsh RP, Shephard RJ, eds. *Current theory in sports medicine,* Vol. 2. Toronto: BC Decker 1990, 135–9.

78. Reilly T, Mellor S. Jet lag in student Rugby League players following a near-maximal time-zone shift. In: Reilly T, Lees A, Davids K, Murphy WJ, eds. *Science and football.* London: Spon, 1988; 249–56.

79. Minors DS, Waterhouse JN. Anchor sleep as a synchroniser of abnormal routines. *International Journal of Chronobiology* 1981; **7**: 165–88.

80. Antal LC. The effects of the changes of the circadian body rhythm on the sports shooter. *British Journal of Sports Medicine* 1975; **9**: 9–12.

81. Reinberg A, Vieux N, Andlauer P. *Night and shift work: biological and social aspects.* Oxford: Pergamon, 1980.

82. Van Loon JH. Diurnal body temperature curves in shift workers. *Ergonomics* 1963; **6**: 267–73.

83. Reilly T, Thomas V. Estimated daily energy expenditures of professional association footballers. *Ergonomics* 1979; **22**: 541–8.

84. Griffin SJ, Trinder J. Physical fitness, exercise and human sleep. *Psychophysiology* 1978; **15**: 447–50.

85. Paxton SJ, Turner J, Montgomery I. Does aerobic fitness affect sleep. *Psychophysiology* 1983; **20**: 320–24.

86. Oswald I. Sleep as a restorative process: human clues. *Progress in Brain Research* 1980; **53**: 279–88.

87. Horne JA. *Why we sleep: the function of sleep in humans and other mammals.* Oxford: Oxford University Press, 1988.

88. Reilly T, Deykin T. Effects of partial sleep loss on subjective states, psychomotor and physical performance tests. *Journal of Human Movement Studies* 1983; **9**: 157–70.

89. Thomas V, Reilly T. Circulatory, psychological and performance variables during 100 h of paced continuous exercise under conditions of controlled energy intake and work output. *Journal of Human Movement Studies* 1975; **1**: 149–55.

90. Vondra K, Brodan V, Bass A, Kuhn E, Tersinger J, Andel M, Veselkova A. Effects of sleep deprivation on the activity of selected metabolic enzymes in skeletal muscle. *European Journal of Applied Physiology* 1981; **47**: 41–6.

91. Rognum TO, Varedal F, Rodahl K, Opstad PK, Knudsen-Baas O, Kindt E, Withey WR. Physical and mental performance of soldiers during prolonged heavy exercise combined with sleep deprivation. *Ergonomics* 1986; **29**: 859–67.

92. Myles WS, Romet TT. Self-paced work in sleep deprived subjects. *Ergonomics* 1987; **30**: 1175–84.

93. Ahnve S, Theorell T, Akerstedt T, Fröberg JE, Halberg F. Circadian variations in cardiovascular parameters during sleep deprivation. *European Journal of Applied Physiology* 1981; **46**: 9–19.

94. Akerstedt T, Fröberg JE, Friberg Y, Wetterberg L. Melatonin excretion, body temperature and subjective arousal during 64 h of sleep deprivation. *Psychoendocrinology* 1979; **4**: 219–25.

95. Wilkinson RT. Some factors influencing the effect of environmental stressors upon performance. *Biological Bulletin* 1969; **72**: 260–72.

96. Reilly T, George A. Urinary phenylethylamine levels during three days of indoor soccer play. *Journal of Sports Sciences* 1983; **1**: 70.

97. Reilly T. Exercise and sleep: an overview. In: Watkins J, Reilly T, Burwitz L, eds. *Sports science.* London: Spon, 1986; 414–19.

98. Reilly T, Piercy M. The effect of partial sleep deprivation on weight-lifting performance. *Ergonomics* 1994; **37**: 107–15.

99. Plyley MJ, Shephard RJ, Davis GM, Goode RC. Sleep deprivation and cardiorespiratory function. *European Journal of Applied Physiology and Occupational Physiology*, 1987; **56**: 338–44.

100. Dinges DF, Orne MT, Whitehouse WG, Orne EC. Temporal placement of a nap for alertness. Contributions of circadian phase and prior wakefulness. *Sleep* 1987; **10**: 313–29.

101. Rogers AS, Spencer MB, Stone BM, Nicholson AN. The influence of a 1 h nap on performance overnight. *Ergonomics* 1989; **32**; 1193–205.

102. Reilly T. Alcohol, anti-anxiety drugs and exercise. In: Mottram DR, ed. *Drugs in sport.* London: Spon, 1988; 127–56.

103. Reilly T. Alcohol: its influence in sport and exercise. In: Reilly T, Orme M, eds. *The clinical pharmacology of sport and exercise.* Amsterdam: Elsevier, 1997: 281–92.

3

Medical aspects of exercise and sport

3.1 Cardiac adaptations to exercise training

Antonio Pelliccia and Barry J. Maron

Introduction

Sporting activities and athletic training have become an integral part of everyday life for a substantial segment of the Western population. As a result, there has been a growing scientific interest in the effects of training on the different organ systems. A large body of research has been focused on the consequences of systematic athletic training and competition on the cardiovascular system. We describe this complex remodelling process, including the intrinsic adaptive changes of cardiac cells, the gross morphological ventricular changes and the altered functional properties, as well as the adaptation of coronary vascular supply.

Intrinsic myocardial adaptations induced by exercise training

In normal hearts, the law of Laplace establishes the reciprocal relations between left ventricular volume, pressure, and myocardial wall tension, as follows:

$$\text{Wall tension} = \text{Pressure} \times \text{Radius}.$$

Wall stress expresses the wall tension for unit area of ventricle, and can be derived from the above law as follows:

$$\text{Wall stress} = \text{Pressure} \times \text{Radius} / \text{Wall thickness}.$$

Alteration of myocardial wall stress, as occurs in exercise, is the trigger to events leading to adaptive left ventricular remodelling. The exercise-induced stretching of the ventricular wall increases the stress on myocytes which initiates a cascade of events leading to adaptive growth of contractile proteins.[1] When isolated cardiac muscle cells are stretched, transcriptional activity and protein synthesis is increased, and particular genes are expressed that may ultimately alter the cardiac phenotype.[2] How altered haemodynamic load may influence changes in gene and protein expression is still an area of intensive investigation; however, it appears that events leading to myocyte growth include cytoplasmic signal transduction ('second messengers'), which in turn activates nuclear proteins ('third messengers'). Altered expression of actin and myosin is thought to depend, in part, on these transcription factors. Also responsible for cardiac hypertrophy is the up-regulation of growth factors, including basic fibroblastic growth factor and transforming growth factor-β_1.[3]

The degree and duration of altered wall stress is responsible for the different adaptive responses of myocytes.[4] In animal and human studies it has been shown that the magnitude of myocyte growth, and eventually the extent of ventricular hypertrophy, depends primarily on the degree of haemodynamic overload.[4,5] The capacity of mitochondria to increase in size and activity may also regulate the response of contractile proteins; indeed, the extent to which mitochondria increase the production and delivery of oxygen may determine the type of myosin isozymes that are synthesized. When the haemodynamic overload is particularly prolonged and intense, excessive growth results with massive synthesis of contractile elements, relatively low density of mitochondria and capillaries, and increased content of connective tissue.[6] This is also the case when haemodynamic overload is applied abruptly, such as in experimentally induced aortic stenosis.[4,6]

It should be emphasized, however, that these features of myocardial adaptation are derived from models exposed to pathological conditions of pressure or volume overload, which are considerably different from those associated with exercise conditioning.[7-9] The haemodynamic load associated with chronic exercise, instead, presents certain characteristics that make it unique: (i) it usually consists of combined volume and pressure load, although the contribution of each can differ greatly in dynamic (aerobic) and static (anaerobic) exercise; (ii) it is of low intensity and short duration in untrained individuals, and increases progressively during training as the athlete's fitness improves; (iii) the duration is limited, and usually does not exceed 6 to 7 h daily, even in elite athletes who are exposed to the most prolonged and intensive training; and (iv) it affects the heart globally, inducing adaptive changes in the right and left ventricle, as well as in the atria.

Further support for the physiological nature of cardiac remodelling in conditioned individuals derives from animal studies that have documented the intrinsic functional changes in trained hearts. The major findings of these studies are that myosin ATPase activity and the rate of sarcoplasmic turnover of calcium ions are enhanced in conditioned hearts.[7,9-11]

A direct relationship exists between the rate of myosin ATPase activity and the maximum shortening velocity of contractile elements. It is of particular note that in cardiac hypertrophy induced by exercise training, a consistent and significant increase of myosin ATPase activity has been described,[7,9–15] while in pathological hypertrophy myosin ATPase activity is usually depressed.[15] In the hypertrophied hearts of trained animals, most of the myosin isozymes comprise the V1 isoform (characterized by an increased rate of ATP hydrolysis), which is eventually responsible for improved contractility.[4,15] This myosin ATPase activity has been found to increase in proportion to the intensity and duration of training.[16] Differences in ATPase activity in trained compared with untrained hearts become evident after 6 weeks and reach their peak after 8 weeks of intensive endurance training.[16] However, the observed changes are reversible after approximately 2 weeks of complete detraining.[16]

The largest cellular concentration of calcium ions is contained in the sarcoplasmic reticulum, where it is structurally bound with high-affinity proteins. The amount of calcium ions determines the number of cross-bridges established among contractile filaments and the tension developed during systole. Sarcoplasmic reticulum of conditioned hearts may transport calcium ions more rapidly and to a greater extent than in sedentary hearts, allowing for a greater availability of calcium ions to contractile elements during systole.[10,12,14–17] During diastolic relaxation, the rate of calcium reuptake controls the decrease of ventricular wall tension, and this process is faster in conditioned hearts.[10–12,15–17] Therefore, intrinsic adaptations occur in conditioned hearts that provide for an increased velocity of fibre shortening and maximum tension developed during systole, as well as for increased velocity of fibre relaxation during diastole.

Changes in left ventricular morphology associated with exercise training

Left ventricular gross morphological changes associated with exercise training have been extensively evaluated in the last two decades by echocardiography, a technique particularly suitable for non-invasive, prospective studies in athletes. These studies have described left ventricular morphology in a variety of athletes and have provided information on mechanisms, features, and the limits of physiological adaptation to athletic conditioning.[18–33]

Different cardiac dimensions in athletes engaged in varied sporting disciplines have been attributed primarily to the stimulus provided from different conditioning programmes. These differences, however, may also be related to other determinants, such as body size (and lean body mass), gender and age,[34,35] as well as genetic factors.[36] The majority of published studies have been based on a limited number of athletes, usually restricted to men and confined to a small number of athletic disciplines. Therefore the specific impact of the type of sport and these constitutional determinants on cardiac morphological changes in athletes have not been completely assessed previously.

The impact of type of sport

The hypothesis that different forms of left ventricular remodelling may occur in athletes dependent upon the nature of their athletic conditioning was first proposed by Morganroth et al.[18] The increased size of the left ventricular cavity in endurance athletes

(e.g. long-distance runners and swimmers) was considered to be the result of chronic volume overload, while increased thickness of the left ventricular wall in resistance athletes (e.g. shot-putters and wrestlers) was thought to be the result of chronic pressure overload. This model of cardiac adaptation to exercise training, which resembles the left ventricular remodelling seen in patients with chronic volume or pressure overload, achieved wide recognition. However, several subsequent echocardiographic studies, encompassing a variety of athletic populations of different sporting disciplines and level of achievement, have shown a more varied spectrum of cardiac morphological adaptation to training. These observations include increased thickness of the left ventricular wall associated with an enlarged cavity in certain elite endurance athletes[26,29,31,32] and, in contrast, absence of a substantial thickening of the left ventricular wall in elite resistance athletes.[23,33,37,38]

In this regard, we utilized a multivariate statistical analysis to assess the impact of type of sporting activity (separately from that of constitutional determinants) in a large population of 947 elite Italian athletes, women and men, training and competing in 29 different sporting disciplines.[33] Our findings were: (i) the type of sport was an independent determinant of cardiac dimensions, and (ii) different sporting disciplines showed a widely varying impact on left ventricular cavity size and wall thickness (Table 1; Fig. 1). Specifically, endurance disciplines (e.g. cycling, cross-country skiing, rowing, canoeing, and swimming) proved to have the strongest impact on left ventricular cavity size and wall thickness. Cycling, in particular, had the greatest effect on left ventricular cavity enlargement, and rowing had the greatest effect on left ventricular wall thickening. Power disciplines (e.g. weightlifting) showed a disproportionately larger impact on left ventricular wall thickness than on cavity size. Mixed (aerobic and anaerobic) disciplines, such as soccer, field-hockey, and tennis showed a moderate and relatively equal impact on left ventricular cavity dimension and wall thickness. Finally, primarily technical disciplines with low metabolic expenditure (such as equestrian sports or yachting) showed no or only a marginal effect on left ventricular morphology.

Mechanisms by which exercise training modifies left ventricular dimensions

Left ventricular remodelling varies in different sporting disciplines largely as a result of the different intensities and durations of the haemodynamic load associated with exercise training.[24,25,39,40] In athletes engaged in predominantly endurance disciplines (such as cycling, cross-country skiing, rowing, and canoeing) cardiac output greatly increases during peak exercise up to 30 litre/min or more, and is maintained at such a level for substantial periods of time during conditioning.[39,41] This is made possible by the large increase in stroke volume due to reduced afterload and greatly increased preload. Also, a marked increase in systolic blood pressure, to 200 mmHg or more, has been recorded in rowers during strenuous exercise.[42] Left ventricular remodelling in endurance trained athletes is characterized by substantial cavity enlargement and moderate wall thickening. Absolute values of cavity size are above upper normal limits and not uncommonly fall in a range compatible with primary pathological conditions, such as dilated cardiomyopathy.[43] Absolute values of wall thickness are usually greater than in seden-

Table 1 Normal values for left ventricular cavity size, wall thickness, and mass index in 947 elite athletes, according to their sport activity[a]

Sport	Male	Female	Total	Percentage of overall group	Age (year)	Body surface area (m²)	Left ventricular measures[b]		
							LVED	Maximal wall thickness (mm)	Mass index (g/m²)
Rowing	92[c]	3	95	10.0	21 ± 4	2.04 ± 0.1	56.0 ± 3	11.3 ± 1.3	121 ± 22
Track[d]	66	23	89	9.4	26 ± 4	1.79 ± 0.1	51.4 ± 4	9.8 ± 1.2	101 ± 24
Cycling[e]	49	15	64	6.7	20 ± 3	1.86 ± 0.1	54.8 ± 5	10.4 ± 1.1	115 ± 23
Soccer	62	0	62	6.5	24 ± 4	1.95 ± 0.1	54.9 ± 4	9.9 ± 0.7	105 ± 17
Canoeing	52	8	60	6.3	20 ± 3	1.92 ± 0.1	54.5 ± 3	10.5 ± 1.5	110 ± 21
Roller skating	32	26	58	6.1	19 ± 2	1.73 ± 0.1	49.0 ± 4	9.0 ± 1.0	85 ± 17
Swimming	26	28	54	5.7	19 ± 3	1.81 ± 0.1	53.0 ± 4	9.3 ± 1.2	98 ± 23
Volleyball	36	15	51	5.4	20 ± 4	2.08 ± 0.1	53.7 ± 3	9.4 ± 1.0	88 ± 14
Pentathlon	36	14	50	5.3	19 ± 4	1.77 ± 0.1	52.4 ± 4	9.2 ± 0.9	98 ± 18
Tennis	32	15	47	5.0	17 ± 2	1.76 ± 0.1	50.0 ± 3	9.1 ± 1.0	88 ± 16
Fencing	31	11	42	4.4	22 ± 3	1.85 ± 0.1	51.7 ± 5	9.2 ± 1.3	92 ± 23
Alpine skiing	24	8	32	3.4	21 ± 2	1.89 ± 0.1	52.0 ± 3	8.9 ± 0.9	87 ± 15
Cross-country skiing	24	7	31	3.3	24 ± 4	1.77 ± 0.1	54.5 ± 4	9.6 ± 0.8	107 ± 19
Equestrian events	23	5	28	3.0	28 ± 6	1.78 ± 0.1	50.4 ± 3	9.0 ± 0.8	87 ± 14
Team handball	9	17	26	2.7	22 ± 2	1.86 ± 0.1	51.8 ± 4	8.5 ± 0.9	80 ± 13
Yachting	20	4	24	2.5	27 ± 4	1.88 ± 0.1	51.2 ± 4	9.0 ± 0.8	85 ± 15
Roller hockey	23	0	23	2.4	22 ± 2	1.92 ± 0.1	53.4 ± 3	9.7 ± 0.9	99 ± 17
Water polo	21	0	21	2.2	24 ± 2	2.03 ± 0.1	54.7 ± 3	10.7 ± 0.6	110 ± 15
Tae kwon do	14	3	17	1.8	21 ± 2	1.76 ± 0.1	50.6 ± 4	8.7 ± 1.2	85 ± 17
Wrestling and judo	14	2	16	1.7	24 ± 3	1.93 ± 0.2	52.6 ± 5	10.2 ± 0.9	100 ± 14
Bobsledding	16	0	16	1.7	26 ± 3	2.08 ± 0.1	55.1 ± 2	9.6 ± 0.5	96 ± 7
Boxing	14	0	14	1.5	22 ± 4	1.85 ± 0.2	52.5 ± 3	9.8 ± 1.0	101 ± 16
Diving	7	4	11	1.2	23 ± 3	1.71 ± 0.1	49.6 ± 3	8.7 ± 1.1	83 ± 15
Field weight events[f]	8	1	9	0.9	24 ± 3	2.26 ± 0.1	55.5 ± 4	10.0 ± 0.5	91 ± 8
Weightlifting	7	0	7	0.7	24 ± 2	1.96 ± 0.1	53.2 ± 3	10.4 ± 0.7	100 ± 9

[a] Plus minus values are means ± SD.

[b] LVED denotes transverse left ventricular end-diastolic dimension. Generally accepted normal limits of echocardiographic left ventricular dimensions for a population of young persons without evidence of cardiovascular disease are as follows: end-diastolic dimension, 40 to 54 mm; maximal wall thickness, 8 to 12 mm; and mass index, ≤ 134 g/m².

[c] Includes 32 lightweight and 60 heavyweight rowers.

[d] Includes 40 sprinters (≤ 200 m), 16 middle-distance runners (400 to 1500 m), 12 long-distance runners (3000 m to marathon), 8 walkers, and 13 participants in the high jump, long jump, triple jump, and pole vault.

[e] Includes 42 pursuit and 22 road cyclists.

[f] Includes three who competed in the shot put, three in discus, two in javelin, and one in hammer throw.

(Reprinted by permission of *The New England Journal of Medicine*, Pelliccia *et al*: The upper limit of physiologic cardiac hypertrophy in highly trained elite athletes. *New England Journal of Medicine* 1991; **324**: 295–301. Copyright 1991. Massachussets Medical Society. All rights reserved.)

tary subjects, but only rarely exceed upper normal limits and fall in a range compatible with the diagnosis of hypertrophic cardiomyopathy.[31]

In athletes engaged in primarily resistance (power) disciplines, such as weightlifting, powerlifting, or throwing events, skeletal muscle tension is markedly increased during exercise, causing sig-

nificant reduction of peripheral blood flow when it exceeds 70 per cent of maximal voluntary contraction.[44] As a consequence, enhanced sympathetic neural activity increases systolic arterial pressure in the attempt to restore blood flow.[45] The magnitude of the blood pressure response is related to the intensity of exercise, to the size of the recruited muscle,[46] and to the increased intrathoracic and

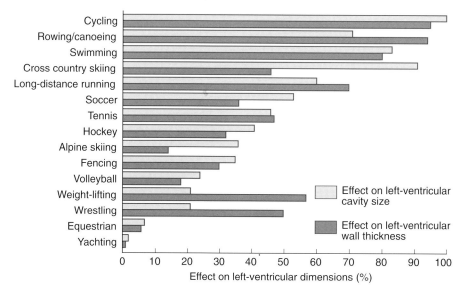

Fig. 1 Effect of different types of sport on left ventricular cavity dimension and wall thickness, as a percentage of maximum (from results of multivariate analysis of cardiac dimensions in 947 elite athletes[33]). Abbreviations: Hockey, field-hockey.

intra-abdominal pressure associated with the Valsalva manoeuvre.[47] Intra-arterial measurements have recorded peak values of 320 and 240 mmHg for systolic and diastolic blood pressure, respectively, during repetitive weightlifting exercise.[48] Left ventricular remodelling in resistance trained athletes is characterized by mild thickening of the left ventricular wall (in which absolute values do not usually exceed the upper normal limits) and no significant change of cavity size.[23,37,38,49]

There is some concern that a more substantial thickening of the left ventricular wall may develop in power athletes when resistance training is associated with the abuse of androgenic anabolic steroids. Such drugs are known to promote protein synthesis and induce cardiac hypertrophy in animal models, which is reversible upon the discontinuation of drugs.[50,51] However, only a few longitudinal echocardiographic studies support the hypothesis that regular self-administration of these hormones for long periods, at a dosage of several times the therapeutic range, is associated with a mild, but significant increase of left ventricular wall thickness and mass.[52-54] Other reports, however, do not show any substantial thickening of the left ventricular wall in power athletes taking androgenic anabolic steroids.[37,49,55-57]

In athletes engaged in mixed (aerobic and anaerobic) disciplines, such as soccer, field hockey, and rugby, exercise training usually alternates short periods of intensive muscular work (during which a moderate volume and pressure overload occurs) and periods of recovery. Morphological adaptation of the left ventricle in these athletes is usually characterized by a moderate enlargement of absolute cavity size, and a mild increase in absolute wall thickness, which usually does not exceed normal limits.[31]

Finally, in athletes engaged in technical disciplines, such as yachting, table tennis, and equestrian events, significant increases of heart rate and systolic blood pressure (due to neurosympathetic activation) may occur at crucial phases of competition. For example, in yachtsmen during regattas, or in horse riders during cross-country competition, heart rates may reach 200 beats/min.[58,59] However, no prolonged or sustained pressure and/or volume overload usually occurs and no significant morphological changes in the left ventricle have been observed in such athletes.[31]

The impact of constitutional factors

Body size

Substantial evidence exists that cardiac dimensions are closely related to body dimensions. In several species of mammals, from rats to horses, heart weight is related proportionally to body weight.[34] Indeed, cardiac dimensional growth observed in humans from adolescence to adulthood shows a close relationship to increasing body size.[35,60] Finally, regression equations that allow calculation of the 95 per cent prediction interval for cardiac dimensions as a function of body weight as well as age have been established.[61] In our series of 947 highly trained athletes, body size (expressed as body surface area) proved to be the strongest constitutional determinant of left ventricular cavity dimension and wall thickness, accounting for more than 50 per cent of the variability in these dimensions.[33]

Age

Ageing represents an independent determinant of cardiac dimensions in athletes, regardless of type of sport and body size.[33] Among subjects of different ages engaged in the same sporting discipline, senior athletes (who had begun exercise training programmes at a young age) had larger cardiac dimensions than did their junior team-mates.[22,62] This difference was probably due to a variety of factors, including the cumulative effect of several years of intensive athletic conditioning, as well as the cardiac adaptation to body growth associated with the passage from adolescence to adulthood.

Structural and functional cardiovascular changes that normally occur with advanced age, such as increased systolic blood pressure, absolute and relative thickening of the left ventricular wall, and decreased Doppler ratio of early:late diastolic filling pattern, have been attributed to the increasing vascular and myocardial stiffness and resistance to left ventricular ejection.[63] Exercise training may partially limit this morphological and functional remodelling associated with ageing; elderly endurance athletes usually have an

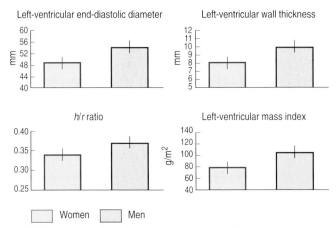

Fig. 2 Left ventricular dimensions assessed by echocardiography in 600 female elite athletes (light bars) and 738 male elite athletes (dark bars) (from results of studies[69] and[31]). Abbreviations: h/r ratio, relative wall thickness; calculated as the average of left ventricular septal and posterior free wall thicknesses divided by the internal cavity radius.

enlarged left ventricular cavity and a normal Doppler diastolic transmitral filling pattern, similar to that found in young athletes.[64]

Gender

The majority of previous studies describing cardiac dimensions in athletes have rarely included a sizeable group of women, and the data on gender-related differences in cardiac adaptation to training are relatively scarce.[28] Previous echocardiographic studies showed increases in left ventricular cavity (average 7 per cent) and wall thickness (average 20 per cent) in female athletes engaged mostly in running, swimming, or ball games compared with sedentary controls.[65-68] Recently, we had the opportunity to evaluate 600 highly trained female athletes participating in 27 different sporting disciplines.[69] In comparison to matched, untrained controls, the athletes had a larger left ventricular cavity (average plus 6 per cent) and maximal wall thickness (average plus 14 per cent). The absolute size of the left ventricular cavity exceeded normal limits (i.e. greater than 54 mm) in 8 per cent of elite female athletes and, rarely (1 per cent), was markedly enlarged (60 mm or more). In contrast, the absolute thickness of the left ventricular wall remained within normal limits (i.e. 12 mm or less) in all subjects. The most marked dimensional changes were found in female athletes engaged in cycling, cross-country skiing, rowing, and canoeing, as also observed in male athletes.[31]

The absolute values of left ventricular cavity size and wall thickness were lower (by 10 per cent and 23 per cent, respectively) in female athletes in comparison with male athletes of the same age, ethnic origin, sporting discipline, and training load (Fig. 2). This difference appears to be of clinical relevance with regard to left ventricular wall thickening: in fact, none of the female athletes,[69] but 2 per cent of the male athletes[31] had a wall thickness of 13 mm or greater. Gender-related differences of absolute cardiac dimensions in athletes are probably related to several factors: (i) lower absolute body size (and lean body mass) in women; differences in left ventricular mass between the sexes are reduced when body surface area is taken into account and eventually abolished when lean body mass is considered;[70] (ii) different haemodynamic responses to exercise in

women and men; women show lower absolute cardiac output at peak exercise due to lower stroke volume;[34,71-73] the systolic blood pressure response to exercise is also lower in women during both dynamic and isometric exercise;[74,75] and (iii) different endocrine milieu in women and men; specific receptors for oestrogens and androgens are present on cardiac muscle cells, and those hormones have an opposing effect on the promotion of cardiac protein synthesis.[76] It is reasonable to assume that the greater abundance of androgenic anabolic hormones in men may enhance cardiac protein synthesis in the presence of haemodynamic load, such as during exercise training. In fact, experimental studies have shown that male animals generate greater left ventricular mass than females when subjected to exercise training, and this difference can be abolished by orchidectomy and restored with testosterone replacement.[77] Furthermore, among hypertensive human subjects, women usually show less increase in left ventricular mass than men, given the same age, race, and level of hypertension.[78]

Finally, the influence of genetic endowment on athletic performance is suggested by the finding that aerobic power (maximum oxygen uptake) is determined in part by genetic factors.[34,79,80] In view of the close relationship of oxygen uptake and cardiac output, the possibility also exists that cardiac dimensions and performance in athletes may be an expression of inheritance. In an attempt to evaluate the influence of genetic and environmental determinants on cardiac morphology, Fagard *et al.* studied aerobic power and left ventricular dimensions in monozygotic and dizygotic male twins.[80] Their study showed that genetic control was significant for maximum oxygen uptake and skinfold thickness, as well as heart rate and systolic blood pressure. Inheritance, however, had little effect on left ventricular cavity size and wall thickness.[80] Therefore, it seems that environmental determinants (primarily exercise training) have a much stronger impact than genetic factors on the cardiac remodelling observed in athletes.

Changes in left ventricular function associated with exercise training

Systolic performance

There is evidence that left ventricular systolic performance may be improved in exercise trained hearts, by a greater stroke volume at rest and during exercise, and enhanced contractility during maximal exercise. In animal models, isolated papillary muscles are often used when evaluating myocardial mechanics. However, these studies have yielded contradictory results, with either increased, decreased, or unchanged indices of performance observed in trained hearts.[7,11] Other studies have evaluated ventricular performance in open-chest animals, and have demonstrated improvement with training in some indices of systolic function, such as peak isometric tension.[7,11] In the model developed by Scheuer *et al.*[81,82] consisting of an isolated and intact heart exposed to increased preload, the stroke volume and cardiac output were significantly larger in trained animals. Other indices of systolic performance, such as peak velocity of fibre shortening and maximum rate of ventricular pressure change in a time unit (dp/dt), as well as ejection fraction, were also greater in conditioned hearts. Similarly, other studies have shown that indices of left ventricular systolic performance, although not significantly different under basal conditions, are improved in trained hearts in conditions of acute volume or pressure overload or hypoxia.[7,11,83,84]

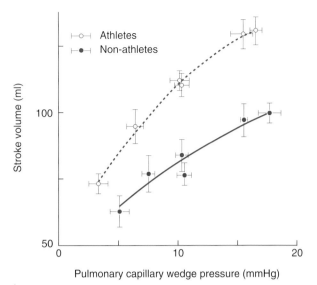

Fig. 3 Variations in left ventricular stroke volume in response to change in pulmonary capillary wedge pressure (index of the left ventricular end-diastolic pressure), assessed comparatively in endurance athletes (open circles) and untrained controls (filled circles). Athletes show a significantly greater stroke volume for any level of pulmonary capillary wedge pressure. (Reproduced with permission from Levine *et al.* Left ventricular pressure–volume and Frank–Starling relations in endurance athletes. Implications for orthostatic tolerance and exercise performance. *Circulation* 1991; **84**: 1016–23. Copyright 1991 American Heart Association.)

This functional improvement was also found in the absence of left ventricular remodelling, suggesting that it is independent of the Starling mechanism and more likely the consequence of intrinsic myocardial adaptations, such as the increased myosin ATPase activity and rate of sarcoplasmic calcium turnover.[7,11,81,82]

It is more difficult to evaluate changes in left ventricular function in trained athletes because assessments of systolic performance by non-invasive techniques lack precision. Indeed, widely used indices of systolic function, such as ejection fraction and fractional shortening, appear to be similar at rest in athletes and in untrained matched controls.[32] The relation of rate-corrected velocity of left ventricular shortening to end-systolic wall stress (an echocardiographically derived index of systolic performance that is independent of loading conditions) has been found consistently to be within normal limits in the individual athlete and similar in trained runners, swimmers, powerlifters, and control subjects.[52]

While indices of left ventricular systolic function remain unchanged under basal conditions, these values are increased in trained athletes under conditions of haemodynamic overload. Levine *et al.*[85] assessed the relation of left ventricular systolic performance to filling pressure in endurance athletes and sedentary controls. Left ventricular filling was artificially altered using either low, body negative pressure (decreased preload) or rapid saline infusion (increased preload); their results show that athletes were able to increase stroke volume disproportionately for any given change in central blood volume and ventricular filling pressure (Fig. 3). In other words, athletes showed an increased systolic reserve when compared with untrained controls.

Dynamic (aerobic) exercise
Differences between trained athletes and sedentary controls may become evident when left ventricular function is examined during exercise. The haemodynamic response to dynamic exercise (as evaluated by radionuclide ventriculography and two-dimensional echocardiography) shows that changes in stroke volume and cardiac output differ when trained athletes are compared with controls,[86–90] as exemplified in Fig. 4. In athletes, stroke volume increases during submaximal exercise more than in untrained controls due to a greater increase in end-diastolic volume and to more efficient utilization of the Frank–Starling mechanism. At peak exercise, when any further increase in cardiac output depends on enhanced contractility,[90] athletes still showed greater ventricular efficiency, probably by virtue of the intrinsic myocardial adaptations.[7,11]

Static (anaerobic) exercise
The haemodynamic response to static exercise has been evaluated in trained weightlifters and untrained matched individuals, in whom heart rate, stroke volume, and cardiac output showed similar changes.[91] In another study, trained body-builders showed a lower heart rate and blood pressure response to the same relative intensity of isometric exercise than less intensively trained body-builders and individuals who were not resistance trained.[92] Possible explanations for a lower blood pressure response to static exercise include resetting of the thresholds of peripheral baroreceptors, or decreased sympathetic drive in well-trained body-builders,[92] and differences from other strength-trained athletes may also be related to differing training programmes of body-builders. Thus, most of the improvement of performance in static (anaerobic) exercise after strength training appears to be independent of cardiovascular response and primarily the consequence of skeletal muscle adaptations.

Diastolic performance
Myocardial diastolic performance has been examined in athletes using non-invasive techniques, i.e. digitized M-mode echocardio-

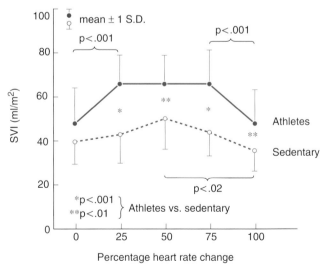

Fig. 4 Changes in stroke volume index (stroke volume in relation to body surface area) during dynamic exercise in athletes (filled circles) and sedentary controls (open circles). In athletes, the stroke volume index shows an early increase during submaximal exercise and a significantly higher value compared with sedentary controls. At maximal exercise, the stroke volume index decreases in athletes and in controls, but is still significantly greater in athletes. (Reproduced with permission of the American College of Cardiology, from Ginzton *et al.* Effect of long-term high intensity aerobic training on left ventricular volume during maximal upright exercise. *Journal of the American College of Cardiology* 1989; **14**: 364–71)

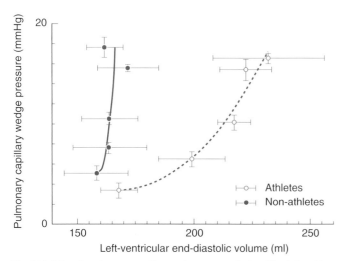

Fig. 5 Variations in pulmonary capillary wedge pressure (index of the left ventricular enddiastolic pressure) in relation to changes of left ventricular end-diastolic volume, assessed comparatively in endurance athletes (open circles) and untrained controls (filled circles). The athletes show a significantly larger left ventricular end-diastolic volume for any level of end-diastolic pressure. (Reproduced with permission from Levine *et al*. Left ventricular pressure–volume and Frank–Starling relations in endurance athletes. Implications for orthostatic tolerance and exercise performance. *Circulation* 1991; **84**: 1016–23. Copyright 1991 American Heart Association.)

graphy, Doppler echocardiography, and radionuclide angiocardiography. Normal values for echocardiographically derived indices (such as peak rate of ventricular chamber enlargement and wall thinning) have been reported in highly trained athletes engaged in a variety of sporting disciplines.[37,67,93-98] Doppler-derived indices of left ventricular filling have been found consistently to be within normal limits, even in the presence of substantial left ventricular structural remodelling related to conditioning, and not significantly different in athletes and untrained subjects.[95,96,98] In a few studies, an increased ratio of early to late diastolic peak flow velocity has been described in well-trained athletes, probably as a response to reduced heart rate.[99]

Some evidence exists, however, that left ventricular diastolic properties are improved in trained individuals. In the study of Levine *et al*.[85] the relation of left ventricular end-diastolic pressure and volume was assessed in endurance athletes and untrained controls in various conditions of loading. Their results indicate that athletes had lower end-diastolic pressure for any given volume compared with controls (Fig. 5). As a consequence, athletes showed a greater diastolic reserve by virtue of the capacity to increase left ventricular diastolic volume more than untrained subjects for the same filling pressure. Similarly, in animal models the left ventricular relaxation time and rate of fall in end-diastolic pressure have been found to be shorter in trained hearts.[81,82] In these animals, improvement in indices of diastolic function appears to have been largely due to the increased rate of sarcoplasmic calcium transport.[7,11,81,82]

In man, some studies suggest that indices related to diastolic function may be improved in endurance trained athletes during dynamic exercise.[100-104] Digitized echocardiograms obtained during aerobic exercise showed a faster relaxation of the left ventricular wall in trained runners compared with untrained controls.[100,102] Doppler-derived indices of diastolic function, such as early diastolic

peak of filling rate and normalized peak lengthening rate, have also been found greater in endurance athletes at peak dynamic exercise.[101,103,104] Therefore, these reports suggest that diastolic left ventricular filling is improved in athletes during exercise, and this functional achievement contributes substantially to increased stroke volume.[104]

Upper limits of physiological left ventricular adaptation to exercise training and relevance to diagnosis of primary cardiac diseases

Previous echocardiographic studies have shown that absolute values for left ventricular dimensions are increased in athletes in comparison with matched untrained controls, by an average of 10 per cent for cavity size and 15 per cent for wall thickness.[28] These differences are relatively small and absolute left ventricular dimensions usually remain within the accepted normal limits for adults without heart disease,[61] and generally differ from dimensions found in patients with structural cardiac diseases, such as cardiomyopathy or valvular heart disease.

In elite athletes, however, left ventricular cavity dimensions and, in some instances, wall thicknesses may be increased above the upper normal limits predicted by age and body size.[61] A left ventricular wall thickness of 13 mm or more, morphologically compatible with primary pathological hypertrophy such as hypertrophic cardiomyopathy,[105] occurs in about 2 per cent of elite athletes,[31] and left ventricular cavity dilatation (end-diastolic dimension of 60 mm or more) in a range morphologically compatible with primary dilated cardiomyopathy[106-108] occurs as frequently as 14 per cent of elite athletes.[43] In such circumstances, the morphological features of the athlete's heart unavoidably raise the differential diagnosis between physiological adaptation to athletic conditioning and cardiac pathological conditions.[109] These observations are of particular relevance because an incorrect diagnosis of cardiac disease may lead to unnecessary withdrawal of an athlete from competition. On the other hand, the correct diagnosis of certain cardiovascular diseases may be the basis for disqualification of an athlete from competition, in a effort to minimize the risk of sudden cardiac death related to sports activity.[110]

Differential diagnosis of athlete's heart and hypertrophic cardiomyopathy

Hypertrophic cardiomyopathy is a primary cardiac disease of which the most characteristic morphological feature is a hypertrophied non-dilated left ventricle in the absence of cardiac or systemic disease capable of producing left ventricular hypertrophy.[105] Its prevalence is estimated to be 0.1 to 0.2 per cent.[111] The differential diagnosis of athlete's heart and hypertrophic cardiomyopathy is of crucial importance because sudden death may be the initial clinical event in young people with hypertrophic cardiomyopathy, often in relation to physical activity.[112] At present, there is no single approach that will clearly distinguish between the two in all instances, although several criteria appear useful in this regard, as summarized in Fig. 6.

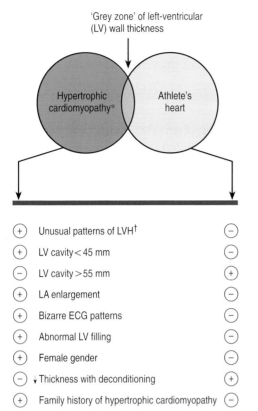

'Grey zone' of left-ventricular (LV) wall thickness

	Hypertrophic cardiomyopathy* / Athlete's heart	
(+)	Unusual patterns of LVH†	(−)
(+)	LV cavity < 45 mm	(−)
(−)	LV cavity > 55 mm	(+)
(+)	LA enlargement	(−)
(+)	Bizarre ECG patterns	(−)
(+)	Abnormal LV filling	(−)
(+)	Female gender	(−)
(−)	↓ Thickness with deconditioning	(+)
(+)	Family history of hypertrophic cardiomyopathy	(−)

Fig. 6 Flow chart showing criteria used to distingush hypertrophic cardiomyopathy (HCM) from athlete's heart when the left ventricular (LV) wall thickness is within the shaded zone of overlap consistent with both diagnoses. * Assumed to be the non-obstructive form of HCM in this discussion since the presence of substantial mitral valve systolic motion would confirm *per se* the diagnosis of HCM. + May involve a variety of abnormalities, including heterogeneous distribution of left ventricular hypetrophy (LVH) in which the asymmetry is prominent, and adjacent regions may be of greatly different thicknesses, with sharp transitions evident between segments; also, patterns in which the anterior ventricular septum is spared from the hypertrophic process and the region of predominant thickening may be in the posterior portion of the septum or anterolateral or posterior free wall. LA, left atrial. (Reproduced with permission from Maron *et al.* Cardiac disease in young trained athletes. Insights into methods for distingushing athlete's heart from structural heart disease, with particular emphasis on hypertrophic cardiomyopathy. *Circulation* 1995; **91**: 1596–601. Copyright 1995 American Heart Association.)

Left ventricular morphology (Fig. 7)

Extent of hypertrophy

The question of differential diagnosis usually arises when an athlete shows left ventricular wall thickness within the grey zone of 13 to 15 mm.[28] The maximum wall thickness found in elite, highly trained athletes is 15 to16 mm, and probably represents the upper limit of physiological left ventricular wall thickening.[31] By contrast, in patients with hypertrophic cardiomyopathy, including those who are asymptomatic and involved in athletic activities, measures of thickness cover a broad range of values from 15 to 60 mm and average 22 mm.[105,113–115] However, a minority of patients with hypertrophic cardiomyopathy show relatively little hypertrophy (wall thickness 13 to 15 mm[28,116]) and, therefore, the single morphological criterion of maximum wall thickness may not differentiate physiological from pathological hypertrophy in all instances.

Patients with hypertrophic cardiomyopathy demonstrate a marked increase in left ventricular wall thickness during adoles-

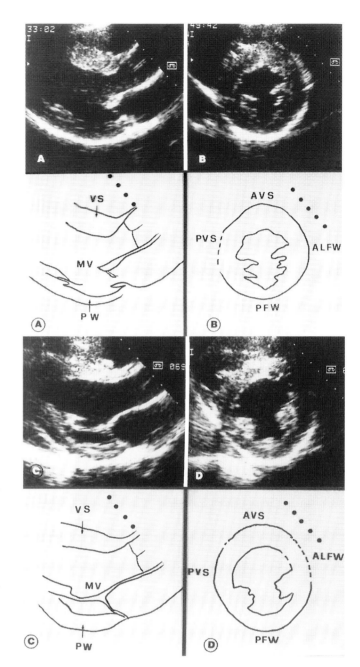

Fig. 7 Comparative echocardiographic images of left ventricular hypertrophy characteristics of hypertrophic cardiomyopathy (A, B) and athlete's heart (C, D). Parasternal long axis (A) and short axis (B) views and respective schematic drawings of the left ventricle, at the same calibration, from an 18-year-old asymptomatic patient with hypertrophic cardiomyoapthy who plays volleyball. In comparison, the same views and schematic drawings (C, D) from a 25-year-old élite rower with physiological left ventricular hypertrophy. In the subject with hypertrophic cardiomyopathy, the maximum thickness is 18 mm in the anterior ventricular septum, but the posterior free wall is 8 mm, resulting in a markedly asymmetric distribution of hypertrophy. In the rower, the maximum ventricular septal thickness is 15 mm and there is a more symmetric distribution of hypertrophy. The left ventricular cavity is within normal limits (48 mm) in the patient, but is enlarged (58 mm) in the rower. Abbreviations: ALFW, anterolateral free wall; AVS, anterior ventricular septum; MV, mitral valve; PFW / PW, posterior free wall; PVS, posterior ventricular septum; VS, ventricular septum. (Reprinted with permission of *Cardiology Clinics, The athlete's heart* 1992; Vol. 10: 267–79.)

cence, but this may not reach a maximum until full physical maturation and development is achieved.[117] Therefore, serial echocardiographic studies may be needed to show the evolution of left ventricular wall thickening in young athletes with suspected hypertrophic cardiomyopathy.

Distribution of hypertrophy
The distribution of the hypertrophy seen in the athlete's heart is symmetrical and regular. Although the different segments of the left ventricular wall may not be thickened to an identical degree (maximum wall thickness is usually in the anterior ventricular septum), differences between contiguous segments of the left ventricle are generally very small (less than 2 mm) and the overall pattern of myocardial hypertrophy appears homogeneous.[31] In contrast, in patients with hypertrophic cardiomyopathy, the distribution of hypertrophy is characteristically asymmetric and heterogeneous.[105,113,115] Also, while the anterior portion of the ventricular septum is usually the most thickened segment, not uncommonly, other regions of the left ventricle may show the greatest degree of thickening. Furthermore, contiguous portions of the left ventricular wall often show striking differences in thickness, and abrupt transitions between adjacent segments of the wall frequently occur.[105,113,115]

Left ventricular cavity size
In athletes with physiological wall thickening, the size of the left ventricular cavity is consistently enlarged (end-diastolic cavity diameter of 55 mm or more).[31] The shape of the left ventricular cavity appears normal, with the mitral valve positioned typically within the cavity and no evidence of left ventricular outflow tract obstruction. However, in patients with hypertrophic cardiomyopathy, including those who are asymptomatic, the size of the left ventricular cavity is small or within normal limits (end-diastolic cavity diameter of less than 45 mm[105,113-115]). The left ventricular cavity is enlarged (to 55 mm or more) only in those adult patients with evidence of progressive systolic dysfunction and wall thinning (end-stage phase).[118] Therefore, in some cases, it may be possible to distinguish physiological from pathological hypertrophy if the size of the left ventricular cavity is either less than 45 mm or more than 55 mm. However, when absolute cavity size falls between these two extremes, this size criterion does not reliably discriminate between physiological and pathological hypertrophy.

Dynamic changes in left ventricular hypertrophy
Serial echocardiographic studies may show dynamic changes in left ventricular wall thickness associated with variations in the intensity of training.[119-121] Of note, in elite and highly trained rowers examined both at the peak of their conditioning (when maximum wall thickness averaged 13 to 15 mm) and subsequently after 3 months of deconditioning, a significant reduction in wall thickness (by 2 to 5 mm; mean 3) was documented.[121] By contrast, in pathological conditions such as hypertrophic cardiomyopathy, no substantial changes in wall thickness should occur in response to changes in the level of physical activity. Consequently, a brief period of forced deconditioning combined with serial echocardiographic studies may be useful in distinguishing physiological from primary pathological hypertrophy. This approach requires high-quality echocardiographic images and the inconvenience of temporary interruption in training which many athletes are not prepared to accept.[109]

Left ventricular filling
Indices of left ventricular filling may be useful in distinguishing athlete's heart from hypertrophic cardiomyopathy. Trained athletes with left ventricular hypertrophy consistently show a normal left ventricular filling pattern.[95,96,98] In contrast, abnormalities in relaxation and filling time have been described as characteristic features of hypertrophic cardiomyopathy, present in up to 80 per cent of patients.[122,123] Typically, the normal rapid-filling phase of early diastole is significantly prolonged in cardiomyopathy and is associated with a decrease in chamber volume. There is also an apparent compensatory increase in the contribution of the atrial systole to overall left ventricular filling. Consequently, the Doppler transmitral diastolic waveform shows a slowed deceleration of early diastolic flow velocity associated with an increased late (atrial) peak flow velocity, and a reversed early to late diastolic peak flow velocity ratio. In hypertrophic cardiomyopathy, diastolic dysfunction is usually unrelated to the severity or distribution of left ventricular hypertrophy,[122] and may be present in those with only mild hypertrophy and with no symptoms.[124]

Therefore, in an athlete with borderline left ventricular hypertrophy, the presence of an abnormal Doppler diastolic waveform helps to support the diagnosis of hypertrophic cardiomyopathy, whereas a normal Doppler filling pattern does not distinguish between hypertrophic cardiomyopathy and athlete's heart.

Integrated backscatter signal
Evaluation of the acoustic properties of the myocardium has been proposed to distinguish the myocardial hypertrophy of athlete's heart from hypertrophic cardiomyopathy.[125,126] Endurance athletes with increased left ventricular mass show a normal myocardial tissue reflectivity,[126] while most asymptomatic patients with hypertrophic cardiomyopathy, including those with mild and localized hypertrophy, show increased intensity of the ultrasound signal from the left ventricular wall.[125] At present, it is uncertain whether these differences reliably distinguish the athlete's heart from cardiac disease in the individual subject and, although promising, this technique is presently confined to research settings and has not achieved wide clinical use.

Type of sport
Knowledge of the type of athletic training may be helpful in distinguishing physiological from pathological hypertrophy. Marked left ventricular wall thickening is virtually limited to elite, highly-trained athletes engaged in endurance disciplines (primarily rowing, canoeing, and cycling).[31] Consequently, absolute increase of left ventricular wall thickness (13 mm or more) in an athlete training in most other sporting disciplines is unlikely to represent the effect of conditioning alone and would suggest pathological hypertrophy.

Gender
Gender itself may be a useful criterion for discriminating physiological from pathological hypertrophy. Physiological left ventricular wall thickening (13 mm or more) is virtually confined to male athletes.[31] In a large population of 600 élite women athletes, engaged in

a variety of sporting disciplines, none showed wall thickening greater than 12 mm, in a range compatible with the diagnosis of hypertrophic cardiomyopathy.[69] On the other hand, men and women with hypertrophic cardiomyopathy do not differ with regard to the morphological expression of the disease, either in terms of maximum wall thickness (mean: 22 mm in both sexes), distribution of left ventricular hypertrophy, or number of hypertrophied segments.[115] This feature probably largely reflects the fact that hypertrophic cardiomyopathy is a primary, genetically determined, myocardial disease. Therefore, the finding of borderline wall thickness (i.e. 13 to 15 mm) in a female athlete is unlikely to be the consequence of athletic conditioning itself and is more likely the expression of pathological hypertrophy.

Electrocardiogram

In a large proportion of athletes with physiological left ventricular hypertrophy a variety of electrocardiographic abnormalities can be found, not uncommonly mimicking those of hypertrophic cardiomyopathy, such as markedly increased QRS voltage, T-wave inversion, and abnormal Q waves.[127,128] In patients with hypertrophic cardiomyopathy, the 12-lead electrocardiogram is abnormal in the vast majority of patients (95 per cent or more of cases),[129] showing a wide variety of patterns which are often bizarre.[129-131] However, no particular electrocardiographic pattern is specific for hypertrophic cardiomyopathy and in the individual subject the 12-lead electrocardiogram may not discriminate between athlete's heart and pathological hypertrophy.

Familial transmission and genetic screening

The most definitive evidence for the presence of hypertrophic cardiomyopathy in an athlete with increase in wall thickness probably comes from the demonstration of this disease in a relative.[132] Therefore, echocardiographic screening for affected family members represents a potential method for resolving this diagnostic uncertainty. However, absence of echocardiographic evidence for hypertrophic cardiomyopathy in family members does not exclude occurrence of the sporadic form.[132]

In recent years, a variety of genetic defects have been found in association with familial hypertrophic cardiomyopathy and have raised the possibility of DNA-diagnosis in athletes with borderline hypertrophy. At present, disease-causing mutations have been identified in genes located on chromosomes 1, 11, 14, and 15; these genes encode the sarcomere proteins cardiac troponin-T, myosin binding protein-C, β-myosin heavy chain, and α-tropomyosin, respectively.[133-137] Recently, mutations in the troponin-I gene have been reported. Furthermore, a large number of mutations for each of these abnormal genes have been described.[137] In most cases, different families have been shown to have different mutations and some of these have been associated with an unfavourable natural history and clinical course.[135] In consideration of the substantial genetic heterogeneity of hypertrophic cardiomyopathy and the relatively complex, time consuming, and expensive techniques necessary for genetic screening, identification of the disease-causing mutations is, at present, quite laborious and not routinely available for clinical practice.

Differential diagnosis of athlete's heart and idiopathic dilated cardiomyopathy

Idiopathic dilated cardiomyopathy is a primary myocardial disease characterized by marked left ventricular dilatation and systolic dysfunction. The prevalence of this cardiac disorder has been estimated to be 0.4 per cent of the general population.[138] Left ventricular cavity dimensions show a broad range of absolute values and in a few instances the degree of dilatation may be minimal.[106,107,139] The magnitude of impairment in left ventricular systolic function is also variable, and in the early stages of the disease may be minimal under resting conditions.[106,108,140,141]

On the other hand, left ventricular cavity size may be markedly increased (end-diastolic transverse diameter of 60 mm or more) in a proportion of highly trained, elite athletes (about 15 per cent).[43] In these individuals, the question of differential diagnosis between idiopathic dilated cardiomyopathy and physiological left ventricular enlargement of the athlete's heart may arise.[109]

Left ventricular morphology (Fig. 8)

Physiological left ventricular cavity enlargement in athletes is associated with similar enlargement of the right ventricular cavity and also of the atrial chambers, as an expression of global cardiac remodelling induced by the haemodynamic load of exercise training. The maximum left ventricular end-diastolic cavity dimension seldom exceeds 70 mm, and this probably represents the upper limit of physiological left ventricular enlargement.[43] On the other hand, in patients with dilated cardiomyopathy, left ventricular enlargement usually predominates and may be substantial, as an expression of primary myocardial disease.[139-141] In addition, the enlarged left ventricular cavity in athletes maintains the normal ellipsoid shape, while the left ventricular cavity in patients with dilated cardiomyopathy usually becomes more spherical and is associated with impaired muscle contractility.[142,143] In dilated cardiomyopathy, mitral regurgitation is also common due to annular dilatation and distortion of the mitral ring.

Left ventricular function

In athletes with physiological left ventricular dilatation, global systolic function is normal, and regional wall motion abnormalities are absent.[43] Therefore, in an athlete with left ventricular cavity dilatation, evidence of systolic dysfunction is the most reliable criterion for differentiating athlete's heart from a primary pathological condition, such as idiopathic dilated cardiomyopathy.[139-43]

Type of sport

In assessing whether an enlarged left ventricular cavity in an athlete represents a physiological or pathological condition, knowledge of the athlete's training profile may also be useful. Long-term and intensive training in largely aerobic disciplines (primarily cycling, cross-country skiing, canoeing, rowing, and soccer) has been shown to represent a strong and independent determinant for physiological enlargement of the left ventricular cavity.[43]

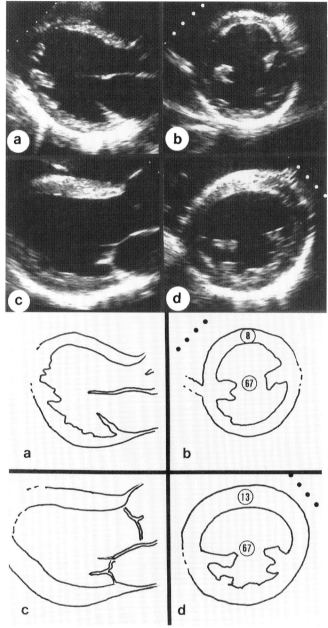

Fig. 8 Comparative echocardiographic images of left ventricular dilatation in idiopathic dilated cardiomyopathy (a, b) and an extreme expression of athlete's heart (c, d). Parasternal long axis (a), short axis (b) and respective schematic drawings of the left ventricle from a 20-year-old asymptomatic patient with idiopatic dilated cardiomyoapthy. In comparison, the same views (c and d, respectively) at the same calibration from a 26-year-old élite rower, who was a participant at the Olympic Games. In both the patient and the elite athlete, the left ventricular cavity is dilated to the same extent (67 mm); however, the ventricular septum and free wall are relatively thin (8 mm) in the patient, but are increased (up to 13 mm) in the rower. In the patient, the mitral valve and papillary muscles are superiorly located due to dilatation of the inferior left ventricular cavity; in the athlete, the mitral valve is normally located within the left ventricular cavity.

Electrocardiogram

A wide range of electrocardiographic alterations have been described in association with both physiological left ventricular dilatation[128] and idiopathic dilated cardiomyopathy.[144,145] However, no particular pattern is specific for idiopathic dilated cardiomyopathy and, in the individual athlete, the analysis of a 12-lead electrocardio-

gram may not reliably discriminate between athlete's heart and this pathological condition.

Right ventricular morphological changes associated with exercise training

The complex geometry of the right ventricular chamber makes the precise definition of its anatomical adaptive changes to athletic training challenging. In addition, its retrosternal position makes the assessment with echocardiography difficult, and other expensive techniques, such as magnetic resonance imaging, may be more suitable for right ventricular imaging.

A few echocardiographic studies have described a significant enlargement of the right ventricular and atrial chambers in endurance athletes, compared with untrained matched controls.[19,20,146,147] The planimetric area of the right ventricle (assessed in the apical four-chamber view) was increased by 26 per cent, and the left ventricular area was 20 per cent greater (with no difference in the ratio of right to left ventricular area in athletes and untrained subjects).[146] Right ventricular free wall thickness was also greater (by 22 per cent), as was the area of the right atrium (by 44 per cent), in athletes compared with untrained controls.[146] Other echocardiographic studies have shown that the right ventricular shape in athletes is normal and the overall increase in the right ventricular cavity is symmetrical.[147]

We have assessed the impact of different sporting disciplines on right ventricular dimensional changes in elite athletes engaged in 12 different athletic activities (A. Pelliccia and A. Spataro, unpublished data). Our results showed that right ventricular (as well as atrial) dimensions were greater in endurance athletes compared with resistance athletes or untrained controls (Table 2). The magnitude of right ventricular enlargement in these athletes differed as a consequence of the different haemodynamic load associated with athletic conditioning; the greatest enlargement was found in cyclists, rowers, and cross-country skiers (Fig. 9). Indeed, a positive linear correlation was evident in these athletes between the dimensional increase of the right and left ventricle.

Right ventricular function in athletes

The right ventricular response to exercise was assessed in normal subjects by combining the carbon dioxide rebreathing method with first-pass radionuclide angiocardiography.[148] At rest, the right ventricle showed larger end-diastolic and end-systolic volumes, but lower ejection fraction than the left ventricle (49 ± 3 per cent compared with 72 ± 3 per cent). Right ventricular ejection fraction increased during exercise by an average of 20 per cent, but at peak exercise was still lower than in the left ventricle.[148]

Studies evaluating right ventricular function in athletes are scarce and little information is available regarding the possible differences from untrained subjects. Endurance athletes, examined upon completion of the Hawaiian Ironman Triathlon,[149] showed increased right ventricular end-diastolic (+ 13 per cent) and end-

Table 2 Right ventricular dimensions in male, elite, endurance and resistance athletes compared with untrained controls*

	Endurance athletes (n = 80)	Resistance athletes (n = 57)	Untrained controls (n = 12)	p < 0.05
RV end-diastolic transverse dimension (cm)	4.1 ± 0.3	3.8 ± 0.4	3.9 ± 0.2	a, b
RV end-diastolic longitudinal dimension (cm)	7.9 ± 0.3	7.9 ± 0.6	7.5 ± 0.5	b, c
RV end-diastolic area (cm²)	26.2 ± 3.6	25.0 ± 3.8	23.5 ± 3.4	a, b
RA end-systolic area (cm²)	21.4 ± 3.3	18.7 ± 3.3	16.7 ± 2.0	a, b, c

* As assessed by two-dimensional echocardiography in the four-chamber apical view.
Abbreviations: RV, right ventricle; RA, right atrium.
Endurance athletes included: 25 cyclists, 24 rowers, 9 canoeists, 8 cross-country skiers, 5 middle- and long-distance runners, 5 walkers, and 4 marathon runners. Resistance athletes included: 17 alpine skiers, 14 volleyball players, 11 sprinters, 8 weightlifters, 4 jumpers, and 3 throwers.
Statistical significance of the differences (p < 0.05) is shows as: a = endurance athletes compared with untrained controls, b = endurance athletes compared with resistance athletes, c = resistance athletes compared with untrained controls.

systolic (+ 15 per cent) dimensions compared with baseline measurements, while right atrial size was slightly decreased (− 6 per cent) and Doppler-derived right ventricular inflow velocities were increased. However, even after such extreme exercise, global right ventricular systolic function was within normal limits and without evidence of wall motion abnormalities in each athlete.[149]

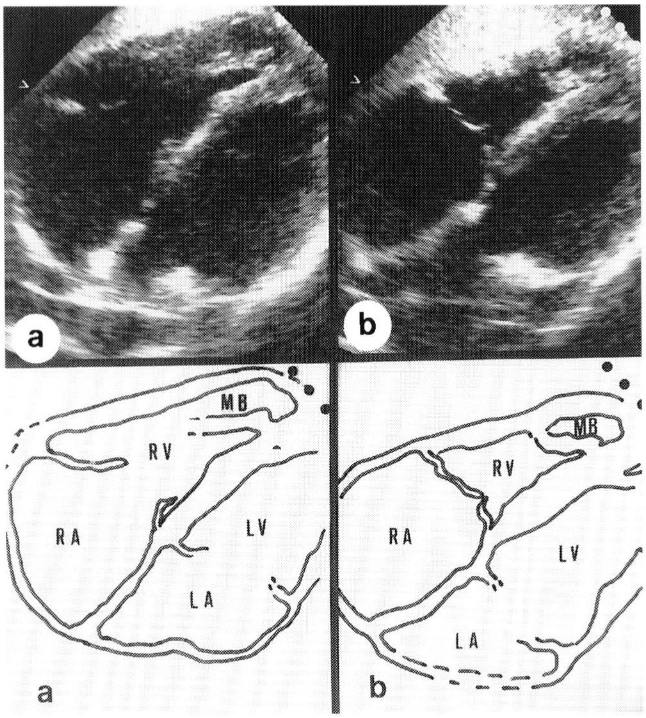

Fig. 9 Subcostal, two-dimensional, echocardiographic stop-frame images of the right ventricle (and respective schematic drawings) at end-diastole (a) and end-systole (b), from a 28-year-old élite cyclist. The end-diastolic right ventricular cavity (a) appears substantially and globally enlarged (transverse diameter is 50 mm); the end-systolic stop-frame image (b) shows a normally reduced cavity dimension (transverse diameter is 32 mm) and absence of regional wall motion abnormalities. Abbreviations: LA, left atrium; LV, left ventricle; MB, moderator band; RA, right atrium; RV, right ventricle.

In summary, the remodelling of the right heart observed in athletes includes enlargement of ventricular and atrial chambers, associated with mild increase in wall thickness, and normal systolic function at rest and during exercise. This physiological adaptation to exercise training differs from changes occurring in primary right ventricular disease, such as arrhythmogenic right ventricular dysplasia and may be utilized to differentiate these two entities.

Differential diagnosis of athlete's heart and arrhythmogenic right ventricular dysplasia (ARVD)

Arrhythmogenic right ventricular dysplasia (or cardiomyopathy) is a primary myocardial disease that is characterized pathologically by fatty or fibro-fatty replacement of right ventricular myocardium, and clinically by ventricular tachyarrhythmias and sudden death.[150] The prevalence of this disorder appears to be very low (estimated 1 in 10 000).[151] The disease is often (in about 30 per cent of cases) familial, and in these pedigrees transmission is autosomal dominant, with incomplete penetrance and variable phenotypic expression.[152] Recently, three different loci responsible for the disease have been identified on chromosomes 14, 1, and 2.[151,153] Sporadic forms, however, account for up to 70 per cent of the cases described.

The most characteristic pathological features of ARVD are the prominent degenerative changes affecting the right ventricle. The histological hallmark of the disease is myocyte death with fibro-fatty replacement in the right ventricular wall, which may be massive or only segmental.[154,155] In young patients myocytes are replaced predominantly by fibrous tissue, while in adults fatty replacement is more substantial.[156] Recently, cell death of the apoptosis type has been reported in the right ventricular wall of patients dying from ARVD.[157] Focal areas of inflammatory cells may also be present. The sites of right ventricular involvement are usually at the apex, in the infundibular region, and in the posterobasal wall, described as the 'triangle of dysplasia'.[150]

The arrhythmogenicity of ARVD is probably based on these histological abnormalities. The widespread and irregular disruption

Table 3 Criteria for diagnosis of right ventricular dysplasia

I *Global and/or regional dysfunction and structural alterations*[a]	IV *Depolarization/conduction abnormalities*
Major	Major
Severe dilatation and reduction of right ventricular ejection fraction with no (or only mild) LV impairment	Epsilon waves or localized prolongation (> 110 ms) of the QRS complex in right precordial leads (V1–V3)
Localized right ventricular aneurysms (akinetic or dyskinetic areas with diastolic bulging)	Minor
Severe segmental dilatation of the right ventricle	Late potentials (signal averaged ECG)
Minor	V *Arrhythmias*
Mild global right ventricular dilatation and/or ejection fraction reduction with normal left ventricle	Minor
Mild segmental dilatation of the right ventricle	Left bundle branch block type ventricular tachycardia (sustained and non-sustained) (ECG, Holter, exercise testing)
Regional right ventricular hypokinesia	Frequent ventricular extrasystoles (more than 1000/24 h) (Holter)
II *Tissue characterization of walls*	VI *Family history*
Major	Major
Fibrofatty replacement of myocardium on endomyocardial biopsy	Familial disease confirmed at autopsy or surgery
III *Repolarization abnormalities*	Minor
Minor	Familial history of premature sudden death (< 35 years) due to suspected right ventricular dysplasia.
Inverted T waves in right precordial leads (V2 and V3) (people aged more than 12 years; in absence of right bundle branch block)	Familial history (clinical diagnosis based on present criteria)

[a] Detected by echocardiography, angiography, magnetic resonance imaging, or radionuclide scintigraphy. ECG, electrocardiogram; LV, left ventricle.

(From: McKenna WJ, *et al.* Diagnosis of arrhythmogenic right ventricular dysplasia/cardiomyopathy. *British Heart Journal* 1994; **71**: 215–218. Reproduced with permission of BMJ Publishing Group.)

of the electrical wavefront through the fibro–fatty areas likely represents the basis of potentially malignant re-entrant ventricular tachyarrhythmias. Exercise could trigger these arrhythmias, through the mechanical stretching of right ventricular walls by increased preload, and by increasing sympathetic drive.[151] Sudden and unexpected death, not uncommonly related to physical exercise, may be the initial clinical presentation of this disease.[154]

While the clinical recognition of ARVD is of crucial importance for the prevention of sudden death in athletes, early diagnosis may be particularly difficult, especially in the absence of symptoms or impaired cardiac performance. Recently, standardized diagnostic criteria have been proposed,[158] based on the presence of major and minor criteria, encompassing clinical, morphological, electrocardiographic, and genetic factors (Table 3). According to these recommendations, the diagnosis of ARVD requires the presence of two major, or one major plus two minor, or four minor criteria.

Echocardiographic features of ARVD may include: (i) global dilatation of the right ventricular chamber, associated with depressed systolic function (in absence of left ventricular dilatation and/or systolic dysfunction) or, more frequently, (ii) segmental morphological alterations, such as localized thinning of wall and right ventricular akinetic or dyskinetic areas (usually in the subtricuspid inferobasal wall), dilatation of the right ventricular outflow tract, enlargement of the apex, and abnormal pattern and reflectivity of trabeculae and moderator band.[159,160]

In athlete's heart, right ventricular enlargement may be substantial (particularly in highly trained, endurance athletes) and in the same range of absolute dimensions as ARVD. However, right ventricular cavity enlargement in athletes is associated with similar dimensional increase of the left ventricle. Physiological remodelling of the right ventricle induced by exercise training symmetrically affects the outflow and inflow tracts, and segmental alterations, such as wall thinning, aneurysms, or wall motion abnormalities (as occur in ARVD), are not present. Finally, right ventricular function in athletes is normal at rest and during exercise.

Magnetic resonance imaging (**MRI**) is uniquely suited for the detection and localization of the high-intensity signal from adipose tissue within the right ventricular wall, which represents the pathological hallmark of ARVD. Moreover, MRI can provide better definition of the right ventricular anatomy than echocardiography and, in patients with ARVD, potentially permits quantitative assessment of the wall thinning and cavity enlargement. Therefore, MRI appears to be the most reliable non-invasive diagnostic technique for ARVD;[161,162] however, limitations of this technique emanate from the high cost and its restricted availability to selected medical centres.

The 12-lead electrocardiogram in patients with ARVD usually shows prolonged QRS duration (more than 110 ms), most prominent in lead V1,[155] often associated with a pattern of incomplete right bundle branch block; this pattern, however, has low specificity for differentiating ARVD from athlete's heart. In up to 75 per cent of selected patients with ARVD presenting with ventricular tachyarrhythmias,[155,163] and in most of those dying suddenly,[151] the pattern of inverted T waves in the anterior precordial leads V1 to V3 is present. This finding has been considered by some investigators as a marker of the disease,[151,154,155] with the extent of precordial T-wave inversion related to the degree of right ventricular enlargement. The occurrence of T-wave inversion in the anterior precordial leads is uncommon in normal adults, but it may be found occasionally (about 2 per cent) in a population of elite athletes without evidence of ARVD.[128] Consequently, in the individual athlete there is no single electrocardiographic pattern that will definitively differentiate ARVD from athlete's heart.

Adaptations of coronary circulation associated with exercise training

The determinants of coronary blood flow under physiological conditions are the pressure gradient between the aorta and right atrium and the coronary vascular resistance. The pressure gradient in normal individuals depends primarily on the level of aortic pressure (which, in fact, is not substantially altered by exercise conditioning). Three types of coronary resistances are known: (i) basal resistance, i.e. the impedance to flow offered by the coronary vascular bed during diastole, that depends primarily on the luminal diameter of the epicardial coronary arteries; (ii) autoregulatory resistance, that results from tonic control of muscular media layer of the extramural and intramural coronary arteries; and (iii) compressive resistance, due to the squeezing of intramyocardial vessels during systole, that regulates specifically the blood flow directed to the subendocardium.

There is substantial evidence that exercise training is associated with a series of adaptations that eventually result in improved blood flow capacity, dependent on: (i) morphological changes of the coronary vessels (increasing the luminal dimensions of extramural coronary arteries and the number of capillaries);[11,164,165] (ii) neurohumoral control of the coronary vascular resistance (altering the vascular responsiveness to vasoconstrictor and vasodilator agents);[166,167] and (iii) prolonging diastolic period, due to training-induced bradycardia.

Morphological adaptation of the extramural coronary arteries

A large number of studies examining several species of animals have consistently shown with different techniques that exercise training increases the luminal cross-sectional area of epicardial coronary arteries, reducing the basal resistance and impedance to coronary blood flow. Tepperman and Pearlman[168] and Stevenson et al.,[169] using vinyl acetate casts of the coronary tree, demonstrated a dimensional increase and higher ratio of coronary cast-weight to heart-weight in animals undergoing endurance training. Subsequently, Ho et al.[170] showed that the largest increase of coronary cast-weight (+ 21 per cent) and ratio of heart-weight to body weight (+ 23 per cent) was present in endurance trained animals, while resistance trained animals showed only mildly increased coronary cast-weight (+ 6 per cent) and ratio of heart-weight to body-weight (+ 6 per cent) in comparison with untrained controls.

Luminal cross-sectional area of epicardial coronary arteries was measured by coronary angiography or at autopsy in several animal models. Leon and Bloor[171] showed that the area of proximal left and right coronary arteries increased by 27 per cent in rats undergoing a 10-week, daily swimming programme. A subsequent 4-week period of total deconditioning caused the epicardial coronary cross-sectional area to return to basal value.[171] Similar changes were observed by Haslam et al.[172] Wyatt and Mitchell [173] prospectively evaluated the changes of circumflex coronary artery cross-sectional area in dogs during a 12-week conditioning and a 6-week deconditioning period. Luminal cross-sectional area was significantly increased at peak training (by about 10 per cent), and decreased to a similar extent after detraining. Kramsh et al.[174] compared monkeys trained for a long period (42 months) and fed with an atherogenic diet with untrained animals on either normal or atherogenic diets. The proximal left main and right coronary arteries were significantly larger (and with substantially less atherosclerotic lesions) in trained monkeys than in both groups of untrained animals.

In humans, there are only anecdotal reports on the morphological adaptations of coronary arteries in trained subjects. Frequently cited is the report based on the autopsy of Clarence DeMar (Mr Marathon), who engaged in marathon running for half a century of his life, in which the epicardial coronary arteries were found to be 'two or three times the normal size'.[175] Also, Mann et al. [176]showed that highly physically active Masai tribesmen have as much coronary atherosclerosis as Western white men, but maintained a patent coronary lumen because of larger overall size of the epicardial coronary arteries. More recently, non-invasive visualization of the ostia and proximal portions of the main coronary arteries has been possible with echocardiography;[177,178] endurance trained runners have been shown to have larger epicardial coronary arteries than untrained controls.[179] In a systematic echocardiographic study of 125 elite athletes,[180] we demonstrated a positive correlation between the outer dimensions of the proximal left and right coronary arteries and the left ventricular wall thicknesses ($r = 0.68$; $p < 0.001$) and mass ($r = 0.50$; $p < 0.001$). Athletes engaged in endurance sporting disciplines, such as canoeing, rowing, and cycling showed the greatest absolute dimensions of epicardial coronary arteries (Fig. 10).

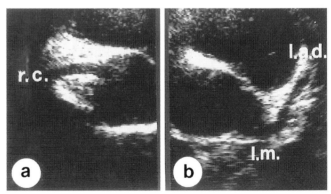

Fig. 10 Transthoracic two-dimensional echocardiographic images of the ostium and proximal course of the epicardial right (a) and left (b) coronary arteries, from a 30-year-old, highly trained cyclist. In panel a is shown the ostium of the right coronary artery (r.c.), located at 10 o'clock of the aortic ring and extending transversely in the proximal course. In panel b is shown the ostium and course of the left main (l.m.) coronary artery, originating at 5 o'clock from the aortic ring and, after the bifurcation, proceeding superiorly as the left anterior descending (l.a.d.) coronary artery.

Morphological adaptation of the microcirculatory bed

There is substantial evidence that, in response to exercise training, capillary growth also occurs (i.e. angiogenesis) when the coronary arteries enlarge and left ventricular mass increases. Changes in the capillary vascular bed associated with chronic exercise have been reported in a number of studies with several species of animals. Poupa and Rakusan [181] showed that animals of similar species, but with a largely different physical habit (such as hares and rabbits), have significantly different heart weight and capillary density. Leon and Bloor [171] reported that endurance trained rats had a larger capillary density, as well as increased capillary to fibre ratio, compared with untrained controls. The capillary growth was larger in animals undergoing daily (rather than semi-weekly) exercise training, as was the increase of heart weight and coronary artery cross-sectional area. [171] A similar increase in capillary density was described in dogs after a 12-week conditioning period, and was reversed after 6 weeks of deconditioning. [173] However, the most convincing evidence that exercise training is responsible for angiogenesis derives from studies with [³H]thymidine as a radioactive marker. [182,183] Ljungqvist and Unge[182] studied three groups of rats exposed to different haemodynamic loads, experimentally produced by: (i) swimming training, (ii) renal hypertension, and (iii) aortic valve stenosis. Swimming was the strongest stimulus for new capillary proliferative activity in both the ventricles; increased labelling of [³H]thymidine was evident in capillary cells after 2 weeks of regular conditioning and reached the highest level after 4 weeks. However, a 2-month deconditioning period reduced the nuclear incorporation of capillary cells to baseline value. In rats exposed to pathological pressure loads, only a mild increase of [³H]thymidine incorporation was found in capillary cells, but incorporation of the radioactive tracer was significantly increased also in cells from the interstitium, suggesting an increased production of connective tissue elements. [182]

Age is a limiting factor for proliferation of the microvascular bed; older animals show a reduced, but not absent, capability of microcirculation growth in response to exercise training. [184,185] Tomanek[184] examined groups of young, mature, and senescent rats undergoing a 12-week training programme. The capillary density decreased in all animals with ageing, but was higher in the trained animals of all ages (+ 11 per cent in young, + 7 per cent in mature and + 9 per cent in senescent animals).

Intensity of exercise training is also a determinant for growth of the capillary bed. The vast majority of studies that report increased capillary network have been based on exercise training of moderate intensity, and it has been suggested that strenuous training (or overtraining) may compromise the mechanisms that stimulate capillary proliferation. [186]

It is worth emphasizing that cellular mechanisms leading to capillary proliferation are quite complex. Although growth factors may be involved, endothelial stretching induced by increased myocardial blood flow is probably the most potent stimulus for angiogenesis. [165] Mechanical stretching of endothelial cells triggers a cascade of biochemical events leading to capillary proliferation. Training-induced bradycardia may also be a determinant of angiogenesis, because it prolongs the time that capillaries spend in a dilated state and prolongs the stretching stimulus on endothelial cells.

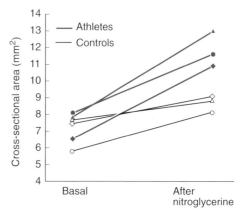

Fig. 11 Comparative changes of cross-sectional coronary area after pharmacologically induced vasodilation in ultra-endurance runners (filled boxes) and untrained controls (open boxes). At baseline, the cross-sectional area of coronary arteries is not significantly different in athletes and controls, but after administration of nitroglycerine the cross-sectional area of epicardial coronary arteries is substantially greater in athletes than in controls. Symbols: circles, right coronary artery; triangles, left anterior descending coronary artery; squares, circumflex coronary artery (Modified from results of the study.[85])

Neurohumoral control of coronary vascular resistance

In the last decade evidence has been growing that exercise training is associated also with alterations in the neurohumoral control of coronary vascular resistance, characterized by an enhanced vasodilatory response to different stimuli. This functional resetting occurs in large epicardial coronary arteries and small resistance arterioles.

Epicardial coronary arteries

Differences in the vasomotor control of epicardial coronary arteries in trained animals were initially described in 1985 by Bove and Dewey. [187] Vasoconstriction as a response to intracoronary infusion of phenylephrine was reduced, and the percentage reduction of coronary luminal size was significantly less in trained animals. [187] Similar results were achieved, more recently, by Parker *et al.*[166] utilizing preparations of epicardial coronary arteries exposed to increasing concentrations of noradrenaline. In contrast, the vasodilator response was significantly enhanced in trained animals by either α-adrenergic blockade or infusion of adenosine. [166,188]

Recently, Haskell *et al.*[189] reported that the vasodilatory response was enhanced in trained athletes. The authors assessed the epicardial coronary cross-sectional area at rest and after pharmacologically induced vasodilation in ultraendurance runners compared with sedentary controls. The coronary cross-sectional area was similar at rest, but increased significantly more after pharmacologically induced vasodilation in the athletes (58 compared with 32 per cent) (Fig. 11).

Resistance arterioles

In small resistance arterioles, the most evident effect induced by exercise training is endothelium-dependent vasorelaxation[190] in response to adrenergic agents, as well as adenosine and bradykinin. [166,191] Most evidence indicates that flow-induced vasodilation in resistance arterioles is dependent on the integrity of endothelium, and training is likely to enhance the release of endothelium-derived relaxing factors, such as bradykinin. On the other hand, the contractile response of smooth muscle cells induced by acetylcholine is less evident in endurance trained animals.[166]

Morphological and functional adaptations of the coronary circulation described here represent the basis for increased coronary reserve in exercise trained hearts. Coronary reserve has been assessed directly in a few animal studies by measuring blood flow with microspheres, at rest and after pharmacologically induced vasodilation.[192,193] Trained hearts show a significantly larger increase of coronary blood flow for any degree of perfusion pressure.[193] In trained hearts, the increased coronary reserve allows a more uniform distribution of blood flow across the myocardium, also when myocardial oxygen consumption is substantially increased, such as during peak exercise.[194]

References

1. Komuro I *et al.* Streching cardiac myocytes stimulates protooncogene expression. *Journal of Biological Chemistry* 1990; **265**: 3595–8.

2. Buttrick PM. Role of hemodynamic load in the genesis of cardiac hypertrophy. In: Fletcher GF, ed. *Cardiovascular response to exercise.* Mount Kisco, New York: Futura Publ. Co. Inc., 1994: 101–10.

3. Brand T, Schneider MD. Peptide growth factors as determinants of myocardial development and hypertrophy. In: Fletcher GF, ed. *Cardiovascular response to exercise.* Mount Kisco, New York: Futura Publ. Co. Inc., 1994: 59–99.

4. Wikman-Coffelt J, Parmley WW, Mason DT. The cardiac hypertrophy process. Analyses of factors determining pathological vs. physiological development. *Circulation Research* 1979; **45**: 697–707.

5. Laks MM, Morady F, Swan HJC. Temporal changes in canine right ventricular volume, mass, cell size and sarcomere lengths after banding of pulmonary artery. *Cardiovascular Research* 1974; **8**: 106–11.

6. Bartosova D *et al.*. The growth of the muscular and collagenous parts of the rat heart in various forms of cardiomegaly. *Journal of Physiology (London)* 1969; **200**: 285–95.

7. Scheuer J, Tipton CM. Cardiovascular adaptations to physical training. *Annual Review of Physiology* 1977; **39**: 221–51.

8. Anversa P, Ricci R, Olivetti G. Quantitative structural analysis of the myocardium during physiologic growth and induced cardiac hypertrophy: a review. *Journal of the American College of Cardiology* 1986; **7**: 1140–9.

9. Scheuer J, Buttrick PM. The cardiac hypertrophic responses to pathologic and physiologic loads. *Circulation* 1987; **75**: I63–68.

10. Penpargkul S, Malhotra A, Schaible T, Scheuer J. Cardiac contractile proteins and sarcoplasmic reticulum in hearts of rats trained by running. *Journal of Applied Physiology* 1980; **48**: 409–13.

11. Schaible TF, Scheuer J. Cardiac adaptations to chronic exercise. *Progress in Cardiovascular Diseases* 1985; **27**: 297–324.

12. Bahn A, Scheuer J. Effects of physical training on cardiac actomyosin adenosine triphosphate activity. *American Journal of Physiology* 1972; **223**: 1486–90.

13. Bahn A, Malhotra A, Scheuer J. Biochemical adaptations in cardiac muscle: effects of physical training on sulfhydryl groups of myosin. *Journal of Molecular and Cellular Cardiology* 1975; **7**: 435–42.

14. Baldwin KM, Winder WW, Holloszy JO. Adaptation of actomyosin ATPase in different types of muscle to endurance exercise. *American Journal of Physiology* 1975; **229**: 422–6.

15. Scheuer J, Bhan AK. Cardiac contractile proteins. Adenosine triphosphatase activity and physiological function. *Circulation Research* 1979; **45**: 1–12.

16. Scheuer J, Bhan AK, Penpargkul S, Malhotra A. Effects of physical training and detraining on intrinsic cardiac control mechanisms. *Advances in Cardiology* 1976; **18**: 15–26.

17. Tibbits G, Koziol BJ, Roberts NK, Baldwin KM, Barnard RJ. Adaptation of the rat myocardium to endurance training. *Journal of Applied Physiology* 1978; **44**: 85–9.

18. Morganroth J, Maron BJ, Henry WL, Epstein SE. Comparative left ventricular dimensions in trained athletes. *Annals of Internal Medicine* 1975; **82**: 521–4.

19. Roeske WR, O'Rourke RA, Klein A, Leopold G, Karliner JS. Noninvasive evaluation of ventricular hypertrophy in professional athletes. *Circulation* 1976; **53**: 286–92.

20. Gilbert CA, Nutter DO, Felner JM, Perkins JV, Heymsfield SB, Schlant RC. Echocardiographic study of cardiac dimensions and function in the endurance trained athlete. *American Journal of Cardiology* 1977; **40**: 528–33.

21. Ikaheimo MJ, Palatsi IJ, Takkunen JT. Noninvasive evaluation of the athletic heart: sprinters versus endurance runners. *American Journal of Cardiology* 1979; **44**: 24–30.

22. Nishimura T, Yamada Y, Kawai C. Echocardiographic evaluation of long-term effects of exercise on left ventricular hypertrophy and function in professional bicyclists. *Circulation* 1980; **61**: 832–40.

23. Longhurst JC, Kelly AR, Gonyea WJ, Mitchell JH. Echocardiographic left ventricular masses in distance runners and weight lifters. *Journal of Applied Physiology* 1980; **48**: 154–62.

24. Longhurst JC, Kelly AR, Gonyea WJ, Mitchell JH. Chronic training with static and dynamic exercise: cardiovascular adaptation and response to exercise. *Circulation Research* 1981; **48** (Suppl. I): I171–8.

25. Keul J, Dickuth HH, Simon G, Lehmann M. Effect of static and dynamic exercise on heart volume, contractility, and left ventricular dimensions. *Circulation Research* 1981; **48** (Suppl. I): I162–70.

26. Fagard R, Aubert A, Lysens R, Staessen J, Vanhees L, Amery A. Noninvasive assessment of seasonal variations in cardiac structure and function in cyclists. *Circulation* 1983; **67**: 896–901.

27. Fagard R, Aubert A, Staessen J, Van den Eynde E, Vanhees L, Amery A. Cardiac structure and function in cyclists and runners. Comparative echocardiographic study. *British Heart Journal* 1984; **52**: 124–9.

28. Maron BJ. Structural features of the athlete heart as defined by echocardiography. *Journal of the American College of Cardiology* 1986; **7**: 190–203.

29. Douglas PS, O'Toole ML, Hiller WD, Reicheck N. Left ventricular structure and function by echocardiography in ultraendurance athletes. *American Journal of Cardiology* 1986; **58**: 805–9.

30. Fisher AG, Adame TD, Yahowitz FG, Ridges JD, Orsmond G, Nelson AG. Noninvasive evaluation of world class athletes engaged in different modes of training. *American Journal of Cardiology* 1989; **63**: 337–41.

31. Pelliccia A, Maron BJ, Spataro A, Proschan MA, Spirito P. The upper limit of physiologic cardiac hypertrophy in highly trained elite athletes. *New England Journal of Medicine* 1991; **324**: 295–301.

32. Fagard RH. Impact of different sports and training on cardiac structure and function. In: Maron BJ, ed. *The athlete's heart. Cardiology Clinics* 1992: 241–56.

33. Spirito P *et al.* Morphology of the 'athlete's heart' assessed by echocardiography in 947 elite athletes representing 27 sports. *American Journal of Cardiology* 1994; **74**: 802–6.

34. Astrand PO, Rodahl K. *Textbook of work physiology.* New York: McGraw Hill, 1986: 391–411.

35. Gardin JM, Savage DD, Ware JH, Henry WL. Effect of age, sex, body surface area on echocardiographic left ventricular wall mass in normal subjects. *Hypertension* 1987; **9** (Suppl. II): II36–9.

36. Adams TD *et al.* Heritability of cardiac size: an echocardiographic and electrocardiographic study of monozygotic and dizygotic twins. *Circulation* 1985; **71**: 39–44.

37. Pearson AC *et al.* Left ventricular diastolic function in weight-lifters. *American Journal of Cardiology* 1986; **58**: 1254–9.

38. Pelliccia A, Spataro A, Caselli G, Maron BJ. Absence of left ventricular wall thickening in athletes engaged in intense power training. *American Journal of Cardiology* 1993; **72**: 1048–54.

39. Ekblom P, Hermannsen L. Cardiac output in athletes. *Journal of Applied Physiology* 1968; **25**: 1968–73.

40. Cooper G IV, Kent RL, Uboh CE, Thompson EW, Marino TA. Haemodynamic versus adrenergic control of cat right ventricular hypertrophy. *Journal of Clinical Investigation* 1985; **75**: 1403–14.

41. Rosiello RA, Mahler DA, Ward JL. Cardiovascular responses to rowing. *Medicine and Science in Sports and Exercise* 1987; **19**: 239–45.

42. Clifford PS, Hanel B, Secher NH. Arterial blood pressure response to rowing. *Medicine and Science in Sports and Exercise* 1994; **26**: 715–19.

43. Pelliccia A, Maron BJ, Culasso F, Spataro A, Caselli G. Upper limits of physiologically induced left ventricular cavity enlargement due to athletic training. *Circulation* 1994; **90** (abstract): I165.

44. Humphreys PW, Lind AR. The blood flow through active and inactive muscles of the forearm during sustained handgrip contractions. *Journal of Physiology* (*London*) 1963; **166**: 120–31.

45. Mitchell JH. Neural control of the circulation during exercise. *Medicine and Science in Sports and Exercise* 1990; **22**: 141–54.

46. Mitchell JH, Schibye B, Payne FCIII, Saltin B. Response of arterial blood pressure to static exercise in relation to muscle mass, force development, and electromyographic activity. *Circulation Research* 1981; **48**: 170–5.

47. MacDougall JD, McKelvie RS, Moroz DE, Sale DG, McCartney N, Buick F. Factors affecting blood pressure during heavy weight lifting and static contractions. *Journal of Applied Physiology* 1992; **73**: 1590–7.

48. MacDougall JD, Tuxen D, Sale DG, Moroz JR, Sutton JR. Arterial blood pressure response to heavy resistance exercise. *Journal of Applied Physiology* 1985; **58**: 785–90.

49. Longhurst JC, Stebbins CL. The isometric athlete. In: Maron BJ, ed. *The athlete's heart. Cardiology Clinics* 1992: 281–94.

50. Melchert RB, Welder AA. Cardiovascular effects of androgenic-anabolic steroids. *Medicine and Science in Sports and Exercise* 1995; **27**: 1252–62.

51. Pesola MK. Reversibility of the hemodynamic effects of anabolic steroids in rats. *European Journal of Applied Physiology* 1988; **58**: 125–31.

52. Colan SD, Sanders SP, Borow KM. Physiologic hypertrophy: effects on left ventricular systolic mechanics in athletes. *Journal of the American College of Cardiology* 1987; **9**: 776–83.

53. Urhausen A, Holpes R, Kindermann W. One and two-dimensional echocardiography in body builders using anabolic steroids. *European Journal of Applied Physiology* 1989; **58**: 633–40.

54. Sachtleben TR, Berg KE, Elias BA, Cheatham JP, Felix GL, Hofschire PJ. The effects of anabolic steroids on myocardial structure and cardiovascular fitness. *Medicine and Science in Sports and Exercise* 1993; **25**: 1240–5.

55. Salke RC, Rowland TW, Burke EJ. Left ventricular size and function in bodybuilders using anabolic steroids. *Medicine and Science in Sports and Exercise* 1985; **17**: 701–4.

56. Zuliani U, Bernardini B, Catapano A, Campana M, Cerioli G, Spattini M. Effects of anabolic steroids, testosterone and HGH on blood lipids and echocardiographic parameters in body builders. *International Journal of Sports Medicine* 1989; **10**: 62–6.

57. Thompson PD *et al.* Left ventricular function is not impaired in weight-lifters who use anabolic steroids. *Journal of the American College of Cardiology* 1992; **19**: 278–82.

58. Bernardi M, Felici F, Marchetti M, Marchettoni P. Cardiovascular load in off-shore sailing competition. *Journal of Sports Medicine and Physical Fitness* 1990; **30**: 127–31.

59. Granata M, Danese M, Ziantoni P. Heart rate recording in the riders and horses during training and three-day events official competition. In: *Sports, medicine and health. Proceedings of XXIV World Congress of Sports Medicine. Excerpta Medica* 1990: 1010–14.

60. Epstein M, Goldberg SJ, Allen HD, Konecke L, Wood J. Great vessels, cardiac chamber and wall growth patterns in normal children. *Circulation* 1975; **67**: 1124–9.

61. Henry WL, Gardin JM, Ware JH. Echocardiographic measurements in normal subjects from infancy to old age. *Circulation* 1980; **62**: 1054–61.

62. Wieling W, Borghols EAM, Hollander AP, Danner SA, Dunning AJ. Echocardiographic dimensions and maximal oxygen uptake in oarsmen during training. *British Heart Journal* 1981; **46**: 190–5.

63. Lakatta EG, Mitchell JH, Pomerance A, Rowe GG. Human aging: changes in structure and function. *Journal of the American College of Cardiology* 1987; **10** (Suppl.): 42A–47A.

64. Douglas P, O'Toole M. Aging and physical activity determine cardiac structure and function in the older athlete. *Journal of Applied Physiology* 1992; **72**: 1969–73.

65. Zeldis SM, Morganroth J, Rubler S. Cardiac hypertrophy in response to dynamic conditioning in female athletes. *Journal of Applied Physiology* 1978; **44**: 849–52.

66. Pollak SJ *et al.* Echocardiographic analysis of elite women distance runners. *International Journal of Sports Medicine* 1987; **8**: 81–3.

67. Fagard R, Van Den Broeke C, Vanhees L, Staessen J, Amery A. Noninvasive assessment of systolic and diastolic left ventricular function in female runners. *European Heart Journal* 1987; **8**: 1305–11.

68. Riley-Hagan M, Peshock RM, Stray-Gundersen J, Katz J, Ryschon TW, Mitchell JH. Left ventricular dimensions and mass using magnetic resonance imaging in female endurance athletes. *American Journal of Cardiology* 1992; **69**: 1067–74.

69. Pelliccia A, Maron BJ, Culasso F, Spataro A, Caselli G. The athlete's heart in women. Echocardiographic characterization of highly trained elite female athletes. *Journal of the American Medical Association* 1996; **276**: 211–15.

70. Devereux RB *et al.* Standardization of M-mode echocardiographic left ventricular anatomic measurements. *Journal of the American College of Cardiology* 1984; **4**: 1222–30.

71. Zwiren LD, Cureton KJ, Hutchinson P. Comparison of circulatory responses to submaximal exercise in equally trained men and women. *International Journal of Sports Medicine* 1983; **4**: 255–9.

72. Higginbotham MB, Morris KG, Coleman E, Cobb R. Sex-related differences in the normal cardiac response to upright exercise. *Circulation* 1984; **70**: 357–66.

73. Mitchell JH, Tate C, Raven P. Acute responses and chronic adaptation to exercise in women. *Medicine and Science in Sports and Exercise* 1992; **24** (Suppl.): S258–65.

74. Gleim GW, Stachenfeld NS, Coplan NL, Nicholas JA. Gender differences in the systolic blood pressure response to exercise. *American Heart Journal* 1991; **121**: 524–30.

75. Petrofsky JS, Burse RL, Lind AR. Comparison of physiological responses of women and men to isometric exercise. *Journal of Applied Physiology* 1975; **38**: 863–8.

76. McGill HC, Anselmo VC, Buchnan JM, Sheridan PJ. The heart is a target for androgen. *Science* 1980; **207**: 775–7.

77. Koenig H, Goldstone A, Lu CY. Testosterone-mediated sexual dimorphism of the rodent heart. Ventricular lysosomes, mitochondria, and cell growth are modulated by androgens. *Circulation Research* 1982; **50**: 782–7.

78. Garavaglia GE, Messerli FH, Schmieder RE, Nunez BD, Oren S. Sex differences in cardiac adaptation to essential hypertension. *European Heart Journal* 1989; **10**: 1110–14.

79. Bouchard C *et al.* Aerobic performance in brothers, dizygotic and monozygotic twins. *Medicine and Science in Sports and Exercise* 1986, **18**: 639–46.

80. Fagard R, Van Den Broeke C, Bielen E, Amery A. Maximum oxygen uptake and cardiac size and function in twins. *American Journal of Cardiology* 1987; **60**: 1362–7.

81. Bersohn MM, Scheuer J. Effects of physical training on end-diastolic volume and myocardial performance of isolated rat hearts. *Circulation Research* 1977; **40**: 510–16.

82. Schaible TF, Scheuer J. Effects of physical training by runnning or swimming on ventricular performance of rat hearts. *Journal of Applied Physiology* 1979; **46**: 854–60.

83. Codini MA, Yipintsoi T, Scheuer J. Cardiac responses to moderate training in rats. *Journal of Applied Physiology* 1977; **42**: 262–6.

84. Dowell RT, Cutilleta AF, Rudnik MA, Sodt PC. Heart functional responses to pressure overload in exercised and sedentary rats. *American Journal of Physiology* 1976; **230**: 199–204.

85. Levine BD, Lane LD, Buckey JC, Friedman DB, Blomqvist CG. Left ventricular pressure–volume and Frank–Starling relations in endurance athletes. *Circulation* 1991; **84**: 1016–23.

86. Rubal BJ, Moody JM, Damore S, Bunker SR, Diaz NM. Left ventricular performance of the athletic heart during upright exercise: a heart rate-controlled study. *Medicine and Science in Sports and Exercise* 1986; **18**: 134–40.

87. Crawford MH; Petru MA, Rabinowitz C. Effect of isotonic exercise training on left ventricular volume during upright exercise. *Circulation* 1986; **72**: 1237–43.

88. Ginzton LE, Conant R, Brizendine M, Laks MM. Effect of long-term high intensity aerobic training on left ventricular volume during maximal upright exercise. *Journal of the American College of Cardiology* 1989; **14**: 364–71.

89. Percy RF, Conetta DA, Miller AB. Echocardiographic assessment of the left ventricle of endurance athletes just before and after exercise. *American Journal of Cardiology* 1990; **65**: 1140–4.

90. Mitchell JH., Raven PB. Cardiovascular adaptation to physical activity. In: Bouchard C, Shepard R, Stephens T, eds. *Physical activity, fitness and health: International Proceedings and Consensus Statement.* Champaign, Illinois: Human Kinetics Publ., 1994: 286–99.

91. Longhurst JC, Kelly AR, Gonyea WJ, Mitchell JH. Cardiovascular responses to static exercise in distance runners and weight lifters. *Journal of Applied Physiology* 1980; **49**: 676–83.

92. Fleck SJ. Cardiovascular adaptations to resistance training. *Medicine and Science in Sports and Exercise* 1988; **20** (Suppl): S146–51.

93. Granger CB, Karimeddini MK, Smith VE, Shapiro HR, Katz AM, Riba AL. Rapid ventricular filling in left ventricular hypertrophy. I. Physiologic hypertrophy. *Journal of the American College of Cardiology* 1985; **5**: 862–8.

94. Colan SD, Sanders SP, MacPherson D, Borow KM. Left ventricular diastolic function in elite athletes with physiologic cardiac hypertrophy. *Journal of the American College of Cardiology* 1985; **6**: 545–9.

95. Fagard R, Van den Broeke C, Bielen E, Vanhees L, Amery A. Assessment of stiffness of the hypertrophied left ventricle of bicyclists using left ventricular inflow Doppler velocimetry. *Journal of the American College of Cardiology* 1987; **9**: 1250–4.

96. Lewis JF, Spirito P, Pelliccia A, Maron BJ. Usefulness of Doppler echocardiographic assessment of diastolic filling in distinguishing 'athlete's heart' from hypertrophic cardiomyopathy. *British Heart Journal* 1992; **68**: 296–300.

97. Finkelhor RS, Hanak LJ, Bahler RC. Left ventricular filling in endurance-trained athletes. *Journal of the American College of Cardiology* 1986; **8**: 289–94

98. Missault L *et al.*. Cardiac anatomy and diastolic filling in professional road cyclists. *European Journal of Applied Physiology* 1993; **66**: 405–8.

99. Harrison MR, Clifton GD, Pennel AT, DeMaria AN, Cater A. Effect of heart rate on left ventricular diastolic transmitral flow velocity patterns assessed by Doppler echocardiography in normal subjects. *American Journal of Cardiology* 1991; **67**: 622–7.

100. Fagard R, Van den Broeke C, Amery A. Left ventricular dynamics during exercise in elite marathon runners. *Journal of the American College of Cardiology* 1989; **14**: 112–18.

101. Nixon JV, Alasdair RW, Porter TR, Roy V, Arrowood JA. Effects of exercise on left ventricular diastolic performance in trained athletes. *American Journal of Cardiology* 1991; **68**: 945–9.

102. Matsuda M, Sugishita Y, Koseki S, Ito I, Akatsuka T, Takamatsu K. Effect of exercise on left ventricular diastolic filling in athletes and nonathletes. *Journal of Applied Physiology* 1983; **55**: 323–8.

103. Brandao MUP, Wajngarten M, Rondon E, Giorgi CP, Hironaka F, Negrao CE. Left ventricular function during dynamic exercise in untrained and moderately trained subjects. *Journal of Applied Physiology* 1993; **75**: 1989–95.

104. Gledhill N, Cox D, Jamnik R. Endurance athlete's stroke volume does not plateau: major advantage is diastolic function. *Medicine and Science in Sports and Exercise* 1994; **26**: 1116–21.

105. Maron BJ, Bonow RO, Cannon RO, Leon MB, Epstein SE. Hypertrophic cardiomyopathy. Interrelations of clinical manifestations, pathophysiology and therapy. *New England Journal of Medicine* 1987; **316**: 780–9, 844–52.

106. Michels VV *et al.*. The frequency of familial dilated cardiomyopathy in a series of patients with idiopathic dilated cardiomyopathy. *New England Journal of Medicine* 1992; **326**: 77–82.

107. Gavazzi A *et al.* The spectrum of left ventricular size in dilated cardiomyopathy: clinical correlates and prognostic implications. *American Heart Journal* 1993; **125**: 410–22.

108. Redfield MM, Gersh BJ, Bailey KR, Rodeheffer RJ. Natural history of incidentally discovered, asymptomatic idiopathic dilated cardiomyopathy. *American Journal of Cardiology* 1994; **74**: 737–9.

109. Maron BJ, Pelliccia A, Spirito P. Cardiac disease in young trained athletes: insights into methods for distinguishing athlete's heart from structural heart disease, with particular emphasis on hypertrophic cardiomyopathy. *Circulation* 1995; **91**; 1596–601.

110. Maron BJ, Mitchell JH. Revised eligibility recommendations for competitive athletes with cardiovascular abnormalities: the introduction to Bethesda Conference 26. *Journal of the American College of Cardiology* 1994; **24**: 846–8.

111. Maron BJ, Gardin JM, Flack JM, Gidding SS, Kurosaki TT, Bild DE. Prevalence of hypertrophic cardiomyopathy in a general population of young adults. Echocardiographic analysis of 4111 subjects in the CARDIA study. *Circulation* 1995; **92**: 785–9.

112. Maron BJ, Roberts WC, McAllister HA, Rosing DR, Epstein SE. Sudden death in young athletes. *Circulation* 1980; **62**: 218–29.

113. Maron BJ, Gottdiener JS, Epstein SE. Patterns and significance of the distribution of left ventricular hypertrophy in hypertrophic cardiomyopathy: a wide angle, two-dimensional echocardiographic study of 125 patients. *American Journal of Cardiology* 1981; **48**: 418–28.

114. Maron BJ, Klues H. Surviving competitive athletics with hypertrophic cardiomyopathy *American Journal of Cardiology* 1994; **73**: 1098–104.

115. Klues HG, Schiffers A, Maron BJ. Phenotypic spectrum and patterns of left ventricular hypertrophy in hypertrophic cardiomyopathy: morphologic observations and significance as assessed by two-dimensional echocardiography in 600 patients. *Journal of the American College of Cardiology* 1995; **26**: 1699–708.

116. Maron BJ, Kragel AH, Roberts WC. Sudden death due to hypertrophic cardiomyopathy in the absence of increased left ventricular mass. *British Heart Journal* 1990; **63**: 308–10.

117. Maron BJ, Spirito P, Wesley Y, Arce J. Development and progression of left ventricular hypertrophy in children with hypertrophic cardiomyopathy. *New England Journal of Medicine* 1986; **315**: 610–14.

118. Spirito P, Maron BJ, Bonow RO, Epstein SE. Occurrence and significance of progressive left ventricular wall thinning and relative cavity dilatation in patients with hypertrophic cardiomyopathy. *American Journal of Cardiology* 1987; **60**: 123–9.

119. Ehsani AA, Hagberg JM, Hickson RC. Rapid changes in left ventricular dimensions and mass in response to physical conditioning and deconditioning. *American Journal of Cardiology* 1978; **42**: 52–6.

120. Martin WH III, Coyle EF, Bloomfield SA, Enshani AA. Effects of physical deconditioning after intense endurance training on left ventricular dimensions and stroke volume. *Journal of the American College of Cardiology* 1986; **7**: 982–9.

121. Maron BJ, Pelliccia A, Spataro A, Granata M. Reduction in left ventricular wall thickness after deconditioning in highly trained Olympic athletes. *British Heart Journal* 1993; **69**: 125–8.

122. Spirito P *et al*. Diastolic abnormalities in hypertrophic cardiomyopathy: relation to magnitude of left ventricular hypertrophy. *Circulation* 1985; **72**: 310–16.

123. Maron BJ, Spirito P, Green KJ, Wesley YE, Bonow RO, Arce J. Noninvasive assessment of left ventricular diastolic function by pulsed Doppler echocardiography in patients with hypertrophic cardiomyopathy. *Journal of the American College of Cardiology* 1987; **10**: 733–42.

124. Nihoyannopoulos P *et al*. Diastolic function in hypertrophic cardiomyopathy: relation to exercise capacity. *Journal of the American College of Cardiology* 1992; **19**: 536–40.

125. Lattanzi F *et al*. Quantitative assessment of ultrasonic myocardial reflectivity in hypertrophic cardiomyopathy. *Journal of the American College of Cardiology* 1991; **17**: 1085–90.

126. Lattanzi F *et al*. Normal ultrasonic myocardial reflectivity in athletes with increased left ventricular mass. *Circulation* 1992; **85**: 1828–34.

127. Zehender M, Meinertz T, Keul J, Just H. ECG variants and cardiac arrhythmias in athletes: clinical relevance and prognostic importance. *American Heart Journal* 1990; **119**: 1378–91.

128. Pelliccia A *et al*. Clinical significance of abnormal electrocardiographic patterns in elite athletes: the impact of gender and cardiac morphologic adaptations to training. *Circulation* 1996; Suppl. I (abstract): I 326

129. Maron BJ, Wolfson JK, CirÒ E, Spirito P. Relation of electrocardiographic abnormalities and patterns of left ventricular hypertrophy identified by two-dimensional echocardiography in patients with hypertrophic cardiomyopathy. *American Journal of Cardiology* 1983; **51**: 189–94.

130. Lemery R, Kleinebenne A, Nihoyannopoulos P, Aber V, Alfonso F, McKenna WJ. Q waves in hypertrophic cardiomyopathy in relation to the distribution and severity of right and left ventricular hypertrophy. *Journal of the American College of Cardiology* 1990; **16**: 368–74.

131. Alfonso F, Nihoyannopoulos P, Stewart J, Dickie S, Lemery R, McKenna WJ. Clinical significance of giant negative T waves in hypertrophic cardiomyopathy. *Journal of the American College of Cardiology* 1990; **15**: 965–71.

132. Maron BJ, Nichols PF III, Pickle LW, Wesley YE. Patterns of inheritance in hypertrophic cardiomyopathy: assessment by M-mode and two-dimensional echocardiography. *American Journal of Cardiology* 1984; **53**: 1087–94.

133. Geisterfer-Lowrance AAT *et al*. A molecular basis for familial hypertrophic cardiomyopathy: a β-cardiac myosin heavy chain gene missense mutation. *Cell* 1990; **62**: 999–1006.

134. Rosenzweig A *et al*. Preclinical diagnosis of familial hypertrophic cardiomyopathy by genetic analysis of blood lymphocites. *New England Journal of Medicine* 1991; **325**: 1753–60.

135. Watkins H *et al*. Characteristics and prognostic implications of myosin missense mutations in familial hypertrophic cardiomyopathy. *New England Journal of Medicine* 1992; **326**: 1108–14.

136. Thierfelder L *et al*. α-Tropomyosin and cardiac troponin T mutations cause familial hypertrophic cardiomyopathy: a disease of the sarcomere. *Cell* 1994; **77**: 701–12.

137. Watkins H *et al*. Mutations in the cardiac myosin binding protein-C gene on chromosome 11 cause familial hypertrophic cardiomyoapthy. *Nature Genetics* 1995; **11**: 434–7.

138. Codd MD, Sugrue DD, Gersh BJ, Melton LJ III. Epidemiology of idiopathic dilated and hypertrophic cardiomyopathy: a population based study in Olmsted County, Minnesota, 1975–1984. *Circulation* 1989; **80**: 564–72.

139. Keren A *et al*. Mildly dilated congestive cardiomyopathy. Use of prospective diagnostic criteria and description of the clinical course without heart transplantation. *Circulation* 1990; **81**: 506–17.

140. Sugrue DD, Rodeheffer RJ, Codd MB, Ballard DUJ, Fuster V, Gersh BJ. The clinical course of idiopathic dilated cardiomyopathy: a population-based study. *Annals of Internal Medicine* 1992; **117**: 117–23.

141. Lauer MS, Evans CE, Levy D. Prognostic implications of subclinical left ventricular dilatation and systolic disfunction in men free of overt cardiovascular disease (the Framingham heart study). *American Journal of Cardiology* 1992; **70**: 1180–4.

142. O'Cruz IA, Daly DP, Hand RC. Left ventricular shape in idiopathic dilated cardiomyopathy and cardiomyopathy with or without only mild ventricular dilatation. *American Journal of Cardiology* 1992; **69**: 1499–501.

143. Douglas PS, Morrow R, Ioli A, Reichek N. Left ventricular shape, afterload and survival in idiopathic dilated cardiomyoapathy. *Journal of the American College of Cardiology* 1989; **13**: 311–15.

144. Roberts WC, Siegel RJ, McManus BM. Idiopathic dilated cardiomyopathy: analysis of 152 necropsy patients. *American Journal of Cardiology* 1987; **60**: 1340–55.

145. Wilensky RL *et al*. Serial electrocardiographic changes in idiopathic dilated cardiomyopathy confirmed at necropsy. *American Journal of Cardiology* 1988; **62**: 276–83.

146. Hauser AM, Dressendorfer RH, Vos M, Hashimoto Y, Gordon S, Timmis G. Symmetric enlargement in highly trained endurance athletes: a two-dimensional echocardiographic study. *American Heart Journal* 1985; **109**: 1038–44.

147. Zeppilli P *et al*. Right heart in athletes. In: Dagianti A, Feigembaum H, eds. *Echocardiography 1988*. Amsterdam: Elsevier Science, 1988: 173–7.

148. Mahler DA, Matthay RA, Snyder PE, Pytlik L, Zaret BL, Loke J. Volumetric responses of right and left ventricles during upright exercise in normal subjects. *Journal of Applied Physiology* 1985; **58**: 1818–22.

149. Douglas PS, O'Toole M, Hiller Douglas W, Reichek N. Different effects of prolonged exercise on the right and left ventricles. *Journal of the American College of Cardiology* 1990; **15**: 64–9.

150. Marcus FI *et al*. Right ventricular dysplasia: a report of 24 adult cases. *Circulation* 1982; **65**: 384–7.

151. Nava A, Corrado D, Oselladore L. Cardiomyopathies, myocarditis and sport. In: Pelliccia A, Caselli G, Bellotti P, eds. *Advances in sports cardiology*. Milan: Springer-Verlag Italia, 1997: 90–7.

152. Nava A *et al*. Familial occurrence of right ventricular dysplasia. A study involving nine families. *Journal of the American College of Cardiology* 1988; **12**: 1222–8.

153. Rampazzo A *et al*. The gene for arrhythmogenic right ventricular cardiomyopathy maps on chromosome 14q23-q24. *Human Molecular Genetics* 1994; **3**: 959–62.

154. Thiene G, Nava A, Corrado D, Rossi L, Pennelli N. Right ventricular cardiomyopathy and sudden death in young people. *New England Journal of Medicine* 1988; **318**: 129–33.

155. Marcus FI, Fontaine G. Arrhythmogenic right ventricular dysplasia/cardiomyopathy: a review. *Pacing and Clinical Electrophysiology* 1995; **18**: 1298–1314.

156. Daliento L *et al*. Arrhythmogenic right ventricular cardiomyopathy in young versus adult patients: similarities and differences. *Journal of the American College of Cardiology* 1995; **25**: 655–64.

157. Basso C, Thiene G, Corrado D, Angelini A, Nava A, Valente ML. Arrhythmogenic right ventricular cardiomyoapthy. Dysplasia, dystrophy, or myocarditis? *Circulation* 1996; **94**: 983–91.

158. McKenna WJ *et al*. Diagnosis of arrhythmogenic right ventricular dysplasia/cardiomyopathy. *British Heart Journal* 1994; **71**: 215–18.

159. Kisslo J. Two-dimensional echocardiography in arrhythmogenic right ventricular dysplasia. *European Heart Journal* 1989; **10** (Suppl. D): 22–6.

160. Scognamiglio R *et al*. Relevance of subtle echocardiographic findings in the early diagnosis of the concealed form of right ventricular dysplasia. *European Heart Journal* 1989; **10** (Suppl. D): 27–8.

161. Ricci C *et al*. Magnetic resonance imaging in right ventricular dysplasia. *American Journal of Cardiology* 1992; **70**: 1589–95.

162. Blake LM, Scheinman MM, Higgins CB. MR features of arrhythmogenic right ventricular dysplasia. *American Journal of Radiology* 1994; **162**: 809–12.

163. Metzger JT, de Chillou C, Cheriex E, Rodriguez L-M, Smeets JLRM, Wellens HJJ. Value of the 12-lead electrocardiogram in arrhythmogenic right ventricular dysplasia, and absence of correlation with echocardiographic findings. *American Journal of Cardiology* 1993; **72**: 964–7.

164. Scheuer J. Effects of physical training on myocardial vascularity and perfusion. *Circulation* 1982; **66**: 491–5.

165. Tomanek RJ. Exercise-induced coronary angiogenesis: a review. *Medicine and Science in Sports and Exercise* 1994; **26**: 1245–51.

166. Parker JL, Oltman CL, Muller JM, Myers PR, Adams HR, Laughlin MH. Effects of exercise training on regulation of tone in coronary arteries and arterioles. *Medicine and Science in Sports and Exercise* 1994; **26**: 1252–61.

167. Laughlin MH, McAllister RM, Jasperse JL, Crader SE, Williams DA, Huxley VH. Endothelium-mediated control of the coronary circulation. *Sports Medicine* 1996; **22**: 228–50.

168. Tepperman J, Pearlman D. Effects of exercise and anemia on coronary arteries of small animals as revealed by the corrosion-cast technique. *Circulation Research* 1961; **9**: 576–84.

169. Stevenson JA, Feleki V, Rechnitzer P, Beaton JR. Effect of exercise on coronary tree size in the rat. *Circulation Research* 1964; **15**: 265–9.

170. Ho KW, Roy RR, Taylor JF, Heusner WW, Van Huss WD. Differential effects of running and weight-lifting on the coronary arterial tree. *Medicine and Science in Sports and Exercise* 1983; **15**: 472–7.

171. Leon AS, Bloor CM. Effects of exercise and its cessation on the heart and its blood supply. *Journal of Applied Physiology* 1968; **24**: 485–90.

172. Haslam RW, Cobb RB. Frequency of intensive, prolonged exercise as a determinant of relative coronary circumflex index. *International Journal of Sports Medicine* 1982; **3**: 118–21.

173. Wyatt Hl, Mitchell J. Influences of physical conditioning and deconditioning on coronary vasculature of dogs. *Journal of Applied Physiology* 1978; **45**: 619–25.

174. Kramsch DM, Aspen AJ, Abramawitz BM, Kreimendahl T, Hood WB. Reduction of coronary atherosclerosis by moderate conditioning exercise in monkeys on an atherogenic diet. *New England Journal of Medicine* 1981; **305**: 1483–9.

175. Currens JH, White PD. Half a century of running. Clinical, physiologic and autopsy findings in the case of Clarence DeMar. *New England Journal of Medicine* 1961; **256**: 988–93.

176. Mann GV, Shaffer RD, Rich A. Physical fitness and immunity to heart disease in Masai. *Lancet* 1965; **ii**: 1308–10.

177. Weyman AE, Feigenbaum H, Dillon JC, Johnston KW, Eggleton RC. Noninvasive visualization of the left main coronary artery by cross-sectional echocardiography. *Circulation* 1976; **54**: 169–74.

178. Vered Z *et al*.. Two-dimensional echocardiographic analysis of proximal left main coronary artery in humans. *American Heart Journal* 1986; **112**: 972–6.

179. Zeppilli P, Rubino P, Manno V, Cameli S, Palmieri V, Gorra A. Visualizzazione ecocardiografica delle arterie coronarie in atleti di resistenza. *Giornale Italiano di Cardiologia* 1987; **17**: 957–65.

180. Pelliccia A, Spataro A, Granata M, Biffi A, Caselli G, Alabiso A. Coronary arteries in physiological hypertrophy: echocardiographic evidence of increased proximal size in elite athletes. *International Journal of Sports Medicine* 1990; **11**: 120–6.

181. Poupa O, Rakusan K. The terminal microcirculatory bed in the heart of athletic and non-athletic animals. In: Evang K, Andersen KL, eds. *Physical activity in health and disease*. Baltimore: Williams & Wilkins, 1966: 18–29.

182. Ljungqvist A, Unge G. The proliferative activity of the myocardial tissue in various forms of experimental cardiac hypertrophy. *Acta Pathologica et Microbiologica Scandinavica (A)* 1973; **81**: 233–40.

183. Ljungqvist A, Unge G. Capillary proliferative activity in myocardium and skeletal muscle of exercised rats. *Journal of Applied Physiology* 1977; **43**: 306–7.

184. Tomanek RJ. Effects of age and exercise on the extent of the myocardial capillary bed. *Anatomical Record* 1969; **167**: 55–62.

185. Bloor CM, Leon AS. Interaction of age and exercise on the heart and its blood supply. *Laboratory Investigation* 1970; **22**: 160–5.

186. Anversa P, Beghi C, Levicky V, McDonald L, Kikkawa Y, Olivetti G. Effects of strenuous exercise on the quantitative morphology of left ventricular myocardium in the rat. *Journal of Molecular and Cellular Cardiology* 1985; **17**: 587–95.

187. Bove AA, Dewey JD. Proximal coronary vasomotor reactivity after exercise-training in dogs. *Circulation* 1985; **71**: 620–5.

188. Laughlin MH, Overholser KA, Bhatte M. Exercise training increases coronary transport reserve in miniature swine. *Journal of Applied Physiology* 1989; **67**: 1140–9.

189. Haskell WL, Sims C, Myll J, Bortz W, St. Goar FG, Alderman EL. Coronary artery size and dilating capacity in ultradistance runners. *Circulation* 1993; **87**: 1076–82.

190. DiCarlo SE, Blair WR, Bishop VS, Stone HL. Daily exercise enhances coronary resistence vessel sensitivity to pharmacological activation. *Journal of Applied Physiology* 1989; **66**: 421–8.

191. Muller JM, Myers PR, Tanner A, Laughlin MH. The effect of exercise training on sensitivity of porcine coronary resistance arterioles to bradykinin. *FASEB Journal* 1991; **5**: A658.

192. Lauhlin MH, Diana JN, Tipton CM. Effects of exercise training on coronary reactive hyperemia and blood flow in the dog. *Journal of Applied Physiology* 1978; **45**: 604–10.

193. Laughlin MH. Effects of exercise training on coronary transport capacity. *Journal of Applied Physiology* 1985; **58**: 468–76.

194. Overholser KA, Laughlin MH, Bhatte MJ. Exercise training-induced increase in coronary transport capacity. *Medicine and Science in Sports and Exercise* 1994; **26**: 1239–44.

3.2 The lung in sport

Mark Harries

Acid/base balance and the lung

The energy for muscular activity derives from a cycle of chemical reactions in which ingested carbon-based fuels (glucose and fatty acids) are oxidized liberating carbon dioxide and forming carbonic acid in the tissues. Carbonic acid is in dynamic equilibrium with its dissociation products and with CO_2, a reaction catalysed by the enzyme carbonic anhydrase. The high solubility of CO_2 compared with oxygen (more than 20 times), coupled with the wide distribution of carbonic anhydrase ensures that it can always be mopped up in the tissues regardless of its rate of production. What is more, the capacity of the lung to dispose of CO_2 can always overwhelm the metabolic acidosis resulting from the oxidative processes that produce it.

Higher energy demands can be met, although only over very short periods, by metabolizing glucose anaerobically with the hydrolysis of pyruvate to lactate. The reaction is reversible, so that when oxygen becomes available lactate can be converted back to pyruvate which can then enter the citric acid (Krebs') cycle. Lactate that is not metabolized diffuses from muscle and begins to accumulate in plasma at levels beyond 4 mmol/l, a point referred to as the lactate inflection point, beyond which plasma levels begin to rise steeply with further physical activity. The resulting metabolic acidosis (reflected in a fall in plasma bicarbonate levels) stimulates the carotid body chemoreceptors to increase respiratory rate. As ventilation increases, arterial CO_2 is driven down towards ambient levels returning arterial pH towards normal. In summary, during light to moderate exercise arterial pH should never fall and arterial CO_2 should never rise. However, heavier exertion is restricted by the metabolic acidosis resulting from an accumulation of lactate which cannot be oxidized immediately (Fig. 1).

Pulmonary gas exchange

The lung may be regarded as a membrane two cells thick, the alveolar and capillary endothelium with blood on one side and alveolar air on the other. The membrane covers a surface area roughly that of a tennis court, and offers no barrier to diffusion, therefore oxygen and CO_2 can pass across freely down a concentration gradient. At rest, alveolar ventilation (Va) is perfectly matched with perfusion (Q), and air and blood are always on opposite sides of the membrane at the same time (Fig. 2). Oxygen is only sparingly soluble in plasma, but this situation is transformed by the presence of haemoglobin, each gram of which takes up around 1.306 ml of oxygen with every pass through the lungs (see below). Oxygenation of erythro-

cytes takes only a fraction of a second, with full saturation achieved during first pass. The pulse oximeter may record falls down to 95 per cent saturation, although only at the limits of physical capability in élite athletes. Desaturation is thought to represent a limitation to gas diffusion introduced by the alveolar–capillary membrane during exercise at these very high levels.[1] Larger falls in haemoglobin percentage saturation indicate a mismatch of ventilation with perfusion (Va/Q defect) indicating in a physiological right to left shunt (Fig. 3).

Alveolar and arterial gas tensions

Transcutaneous measurement of arterial blood-gas tensions and haemoglobin percentage saturation is now possible, bringing it well within the reach of most laboratories. The concept of gas-pressure measurements in blood and alveolar air is easier to understand if a metric scale is used instead of a mercury column. Thus the pressure exerted by one atmosphere, that is 760 mm of mercury (mmHg), is close to 100 kilopascals (kPa). The partial pressures of oxygen (PaO_2), carbon dioxide ($PaCO_2$), and of nitrogen (PaN_2) in alveolar air expressed in kilopascals (kPa) can then be translated to their percentage representations in the gas mixture. For example, ambient air contains 21 per cent oxygen, so the partial pressure of oxygen in air at sea level is 21 kPa. There is a small amount of water vapour, depending on the relative humidity, and virtually no CO_2, the rest is made up with nitrogen, so the PaN_2 will be around 79 kPa (100 minus 21). Alveolar air contains around 5 per cent CO_2, derived from the oxidation of muscle fuels which diffuses in from venous blood, and is also fully saturated with water vapour. Hence, the partial pressure of oxygen in alveolar air falls to around 12 kPa because of the displacement by CO_2 (5.0 kPa) and the volume occupied by water vapour (6 kPa). Since the alveolar–capillary membrane offers no barrier to diffusion, arterial gas tensions match the partial pressures of the gases found in alveolar air.

Arterial carbon dioxide tensions

Underventilation of the alveoli results in an accumulation of CO_2 in arterial blood with a rise in the $PaCO_2$ above 5.0 kPa. Conversely, by hyperventilating while at rest, CO_2 can be expired faster than it is produced, driving the $PaCO_2$ down towards (though never reaching) ambient levels. Any rise in arterial CO_2 is a powerful stimulus to the respiratory centre and the respiratory rate rises to return the $PaCO_2$ towards normal. Arterial CO_2 therefore reflects the level of

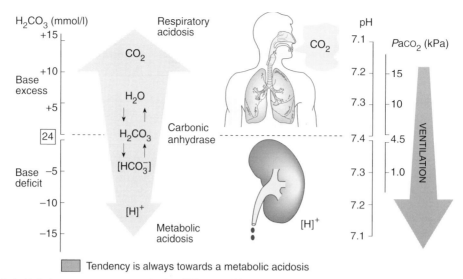

Tendency is always towards a metabolic acidosis

Fig. 1 All metabolic (oxidative) processes generate carbonic acid from the CO_2 evolved when glucose and fats are burned. Despite this, during light to moderate exercise the normal lung can void all the CO_2 that is generated, ensuring that arterial pH remains neutral and that arterial CO_2 never rises much above 5.0 kPa. Plasma bicarbonate (known as base) is maintained at around 24 mmol/l, showing neither a deficit nor an excess of base. (1) Metabolic acidosis (downward displacement of the dashed line). Heavier exercise demands can be met over short periods by metabolizing glucose anaerobically, with lactate the product. This results in a rapid addition of protons (hydrogen ions), but wild swings in pH are resisted by the capacitance of various buffering agents, of which bicarbonate is but one. The extent to which the bicarbonate buffer is indented is known as the base deficit and provides a clearer indication of the number of protons added to the system than does any fall in pH. Arterial pH is maintained at the cost of a base deficit. For example, a lactic acidosis sufficient to cause a fall in plasma bicarbonate from 24 to 14 mmol/l, (a base deficit of 10: namely, 24 minus 14) might result in a pH fall to only 7.25. Any larger fall in arterial pH is thus contained, at the same time stimulating an increase in ventilation which voids more CO_2 and returns pH towards normal (a compensated metabolic acidosis). The kidneys are the major organs of proton (acid) excretion. Failure of the kidneys to excrete protons (renal failure) can lead to a metabolic acidosis that can no longer be buffered (an uncompensated metabolic acidosis). (2) Respiratory acidosis (upward displacement of the dashed line). Contrasting with a metabolic acidosis, which forms the major limitation to continued heavy exertion, respiratory acidosis is never seen in normal individuals during exercise. It is caused by a failure to excrete CO_2 due to underventilation of the alveoli (respiratory failure), and leads to a rise in arterial CO_2 levels above 5 kPa and a rise in plasma bicarbonate (a base excess). Chronic respiratory acidosis (that is, chronic respiratory failure) is a common finding in chronic bronchitis, but, unlike severe metabolic acidosis, this can always be compensated for by the buffers.

alveolar ventilation and should never rise, even at the limits of physical exertion. CO_2 retention is highly abnormal and is seen only in respiratory failure or in those with irreversible obstructive disease of the airways, for instance in chronic bronchitis.

Arterial oxygen tensions

Arterial oxygen tension can be raised a little by hyperventilating (simply the result of lowering the CO_2 content), but it cannot reach

much above 15 kPa because of the constant partial pressure of the water vapour in the alveoli (6 kPa). Indeed, arterial oxygen can only be raised appreciably in one of two ways. First, by increasing the inspired oxygen fraction (F_iO_2, which measures 0.21 in air) or secondly, by increasing the ambient pressure. The reverse is also true; for example, atmospheric pressure at the altitude of Mexico City is around 80 kPa, which means an inspired oxygen partial pressure of only 17 kPa (21 per cent of 80), although, of course, the F_iO_2 remains a constant 0.21. This fall in arterial oxygen tension was suf-

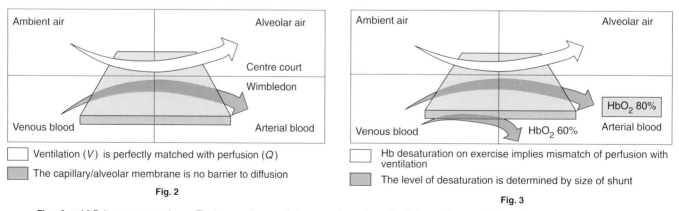

Fig. 2

Fig. 3

Figs. 2 and 3 Pulmonary gas exchange. The lung may be regarded as a membrane two cells thick, covering roughly the surface area of a tennis court with air on one side (ventilation; Ve) and blood (perfusion; Q) on the other. If the following assumptions are made of the normal lung—ventilation and perfusion are perfectly matched, the alveolar-capillary membrane offers no barrier to gas diffusion, and haemoglobin becomes fully saturated with oxygen (100 per cent saturation) during each pass—it follows that any mismatching of ventilation with perfusion (Ve/Q mismatch) represents a physiological right to left shunt, gas tensions in the alveoli match those in found arterial blood, and a fall in haemoglobin saturation during exercise represents a diffusion limitation.

ficient to reduce the times of nearly all the endurance events at the Mexico Olympics, while athletes in the short-distance track, throwing, and jumping competitions prospered in the thinner atmosphere due to the reduced air resistance. A fall in arterial oxygen tension should not occur during exercise if the lung is normal, even though haemoglobin per cent saturation may fall a little at the limits of physical endurance.

The importance of haemoglobin to tissue oxygen delivery

Tissue oxygen delivery is the product of cardiac output, haemoglobin concentration, per cent haemoglobin saturation (assumed to be 100 per cent), and the oxygen-combining capacity of haemoglobin. On this, Nunn[2] states:

Until 1963 the value (oxygen combining power of haemoglobin) was taken to be 1.34 ml/g. Following the precise determination of the molecular weight of haemoglobin, the theoretical value of 1.39 ml/g was derived and passed into general use. However, it gradually became clear that this value was not obtained when direct measurements of haemoglobin concentration and oxygen capacity were compared. After an exhaustive study of the subject, Gregory[3] proposed the value of 1.306 ml/g for human adult blood.

These differences, although small, are physiologically significant. Assuming a haemoglobin of 15 g/dl, with cardiac output around 40 l/min, and the erythrocytes fully saturated, a calculation based upon the higher figure would mean that tissue oxygen delivery could theoretically reach 8.34 l/min instead of a true 7.8 l/min. Haemoglobin concentration is linearly related to oxygen delivery,[4] and this has a critical impact on performance. For example, a shift of haemoglobin within the normal range, say from 11 to 18 g/dl, increases tissue oxygen delivery by a factor of 1.6. Raising the haemoglobin concentration gives an advantage in the endurance sports, particularly when these take place at altitude.[5]

Increasing the haemoglobin concentration is one of the strategies behind altitude training, but this gives rise only to modest increases (around 1 to 2 g/dl). For a bigger advantage, illicit means must be sought. Erythropoietin is a hormone produced by the kidney that has powerful stimulant effects on the bone marrow. There is little doubt that it has been used to raise haemoglobin prior to competition, but it is very difficult to detect in urine. Homologous red blood cell transfusion cannot be detected at all. During the 1984 Olympic Games in Los Angeles, the American cycling team came from nowhere, and, contrary to expectations and form, swept the board. Some months later it was revealed that seven of the successful team members had received a blood transfusion the night prior to competition.[6]

Paradoxically, highly trained athletes may have a haemoglobin concentration at or below the lower limit of normal. This reflects an increase in plasma volume due to heavy training. Blood samples were drawn for the first time at an Olympic Games in Albertville. If the results are to be believed, the haemoglobin levels found to measure around 19 and 20 g/dl must surely raise concerns.

Breathing capacity

Ventilatory capacity is expressed as the product of breath frequency and breath volume measured over 1 min (MV l/min; MV, minute volume). It is linearly related to oxygen consumption (VO_2 l/min);

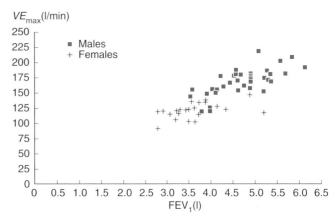

Fig. 4 Relationship between minute variation and oxygen consumption. Expired ventilation per minute (VE l/min) was measured at the point when oxygen consumption was maximal (VO_2max l/min) in 99 Olympic class athletes. These group data show that, for individuals with normal lung function, a high VO_2 can only be achieved if the minute volume is also large ($R = 0.94$). Any impairment in ventilation such as occurs in asthma will cause a fall in the minute volume. This may also result in a fall in maximal oxygen consumption. (Data from the British Olympic Medical centre.) VO_2max = (VEmax × 0.0263) + 0.4384 ($R = 0.94$)

high aerobic power demands a high ventilatory capacity (Fig. 4). Over short periods, say 10 s, ventilation can always be raised above that which is sustainable (maximum sustainable ventilatory capacity; **MSVC**) to reach maximum voluntary ventilation (**MVV**). For sedentary individuals, MSVC is around 50 to 80 per cent of MVV.[7,8] But élite athletes can maintain a ventilatory capacity much closer to their maximum voluntary ventilation than this; for example, 90 per cent of MVV in the case of élite oarsmen.

For oarsmen, breath frequency is linked to stroke rate reaching around 66 ± 7 breaths per minute during sustained maximal exercise. Female rowers breathe at a slightly lower rate—62 ± 6 breaths per min, roughly one breath per second. The average breath volume for rowers is around 50 per cent of the volume that can be forcibly expired in one second (**FEV₁**). Hence, maximum sustainable ventilatory capacity can be estimated simply by knowing FEV_1 (0.5 FEV_1 × 60 l/min). Track athletes breathe at a slightly higher rate and also access a greater proportion of their FEV_1 each breath. For them, a closer approximation can be reached by adding a factor of 23; (0.5 FEV_1 × 60 + 23 l/min). The greatest absolute minute volumes are breathed by the biggest athletes. The highest recorded by any athlete at the British Olympic Medical Centre was 284 l/min, clocked up by an oarsman (FEV_1 around 7.5 l).

Maximum effort flow–volume curve

The capacity to increase ventilation is limited ultimately by resistance to airflow imparted by the convolutions of the bronchial tree rather than by any intrinsic weakness of the diaphragm or chest-wall musculature. The increase in ventilation that can be achieved when reducing gas density by replacing nitrogen with helium is evidence for this.[9] Conversely, ventilatory capacity is reduced when bronchial constriction results in an increase in airway resistance to inhaled gases; for example, during an asthma attack.

The upper limit to gas-flow rates in the airways varies at different points in the respiratory cycle, describing a loop on the volume axis known as the 'static maximum effort flow–volume curve'.[10] This is generated during a forced expiratory manoeuvre from full

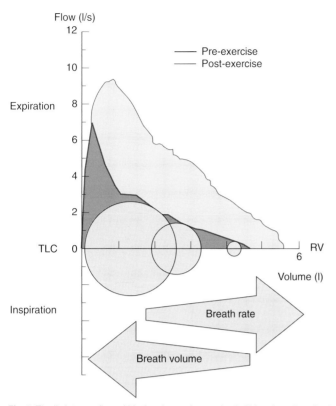

Fig. 5 The limit to gas flow within the airways is contained within a loop described on the volume axis. The loop is generated by breathing out forcibly from full inspiration (i.e. total lung capacity, **TLC**) to full expiration (residual volume, **RV**) followed immediately by a full forced inspiration. On inspiration the bronchioles lengthen and widen, returning to their dimensions by elastic recoil during expiration. Thus the principal factor limiting ventilation is always resistance to airflow in expiration. The limit to expiratory airflow is reached taking large volume breaths slowly, or by breathing faster but taking smaller breaths. In this example, flow loops are recorded in the same subject before and 5 min after a 3-min run. The postexercise loop is typical of exercise-induced asthma with collapse of the small airways due to a rise in intrathoracic pressure. Minute ventilation must fall because of an obligatory reduction in breath volume.

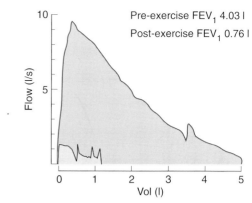

Fig. 6 Flow loops were recorded before and 5 min after a vigorous 3-min run in a world-class runner complaining of poor performance due to breathing difficulties. Postexercise expiratory flow (the inspiratory loop is not recorded) is so restricted that the athlete was scarcely able to hold a conversation. Spikes in the flow pattern are due to coughing. These were even seen pre-exercise, providing a strong indication that this was an asthmatic subject.

inspiration (total lung capacity) out to full expiration (residual volume) followed at once by a forced inspiratory effort returning to total lung capacity. Airflow rate measured at the mouth (l/min) peaks at total lung capacity (peak expiratory flow, **PEF**) close to the beginning of expiration, falling to zero at the end (residual volume, **RV**). The average is best defined as the flow rate recorded at mid-expiration (**MEF** 50 per cent); that is to say, when 50 per cent of vital capacity still remains in the lung. On inspiration the bronchioles lengthen and widen, returning to their original dimensions by elastic recoil in expiration (Fig. 5). Thus airway resistance is always lower during inspiration than expiration. In summary, it is expiratory effort that marks the limit to breathing capacity, not inspiratory, exposing the folly of wearing nasal strips in the belief that opening the nose improves ventilation by reducing inspiratory resistance.

During light to moderate exertion, inspiration and expiration are equal in length, but as the level of exercise increases, expiration occupies a greater proportion of the respiratory cycle (because this is where the greater resistance to airflow is encountered) and it also becomes a more active process. Any obstruction of the airways not only further prolongs the expiratory phase, but also demands a greater expiratory effort, with the result that pressure rises within the thorax. Respiratory bronchioles that are unsupported by cartil-

age then tend to collapse (pressure-dependent airway collapse) causing a fall in mid-expiratory flow (MEF 50 per cent) and producing a highly characteristic peaking and scalloping in the expiratory portion of the flow loop. Any shrinkage in the size of the maximum effort, flow–volume curve is important because it means that the envelope within which ventilation can take place is smaller and, hence, minute volume must fall, thereby reducing muscle oxygen delivery.

Clearly, the limits of flow can be reached either by increasing respiratory rate or breath volume, but not both. The respiratory frequency/breath volume ratio at maximal sustainable ventilatory capacity is remarkably consistent in any one subject, but varies widely between individuals, ranging from 16 to 25 in male rowers and 19 to 36 in females. Those with a low breath frequency/volume ratio breathe more slowly but with larger breath volumes; since this is a ratio, subject size should be unimportant. Maximum voluntary ventilation is invariably reached by increasing the frequency/breath volume ratio; in other words, by breathing faster but taking smaller breaths. Strategies which alter the timing of breathing pattern with physical activity (namely, that change respiratory–locomotor coupling) could have important implications for training and competition.[11] Specifically, aerobic efficiency might be improved by doubling the respiratory rate (and reducing breath volume), while increasing the strike rate but shortening lever or stride length.

Asthma and exercise testing

The most important features of asthma in sport are that airway narrowing always worsens as a result of exertion, and that all asthmatics wheeze on exercise.[12] Asthma has an impact both on performance and on training by shrinking the size of the flow/volume loop. Minute ventilation then falls with a fall in oxygen delivery which, on occasions, may be incapacitating (Fig. 6). Between 15 and 20 per cent of athletes attending the British Olympic Medical Centre complaining of underachievement blame their poor performance on problems with breathing.

An exercise test should form an essential part of the work-up of any athlete whose performance is below par. Running in the open air is a more potent stimulus to bronchial constriction than exercising on a cycle or treadmill ergometer. The reasons for this are complex

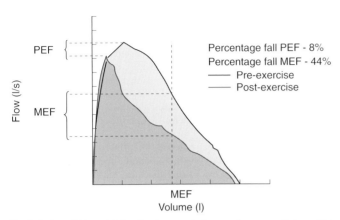

Fig. 7 As bronchial constriction develops, expiration requires more effort resulting in a rise in pressure within the chest. Bronchioles unsupported by cartilage tend to collapse, causing a greater fall in flow at mid-expiration (MEF 50 per cent) post-exercise and may provide the earliest indication of an asthmatic tendency. In the example shown, the fall recorded in peak flow was only 8 per cent, a negative exercise test. But this is clearly an asthmatic subject because the fall in midflow is over 40 per cent.

and related, in part, to climatic conditions. Cold dry air causes more bronchial constriction than warm moist conditions. Air pollutants also play a part, particularly ozone and the oxides of nitrogen and sulphur that form as a result of the action of sunlight on exhaust gases.

The exercise test must be rigorous enough to raise the heart rate to around 80 per cent of the maximum that can be achieved (approximately 220 minus the subject's age in years). The duration of the test is also important. It should last at least 3 min but not much longer than 5 min. Normal subjects may show a short-lived bronchial dilatation on stopping, but a fall in FEV_1 or peak flow of more than 15 per cent occurring 5 to 10 min after exercise confirms exercise-induced asthma. Earlier diagnostic clues are revealed in the shape of the flow–volume curve, which shows peaking and scalloping of the expiratory loop postexercise (due to pressure-dependent airway collapse), and occasionally oscillations due to coughing.[13] A fall in midexpiratory flow (MEF 50 per cent) is invariably greater than any fall seen either in FEV_1 or PEF, thus providing a sensitive indicator of the asthmatic tendency (Fig. 7).

The role of allergy in asthma and rhinitis

Allergy is a state of altered reactivity in the host that results from interactions between an antigen and antibody. An antigen is an agent that stimulates the production of antibody, which it does by first penetrating the mucous epithelium either of the respiratory or gastrointestinal tracts. To do this, an antigen must be soluble in water. The antibody classically associated with allergy is immunoglobulin E (**IgE**), a product of the B lymphocytes that is controlled for by a gene locus on Chromosome 11q.[14,15] A greater proportion of IgE antibody is bound to specific Fc receptors concentrated on the surface of the circulating basophils and also to mast cells located in the stroma immediately beneath the epithelial surface.

Measuring total IgE is not a useful test, it tends to be high in those with multiple allergies, especially in the presence of eczema, but provides little additional information. Specific IgE, which is

present in extremely small quantities in the unbound state in peripheral blood, can be detected using the laboratory-based radioallergosorbant test (**RAST**). However, in clinical practice, skin-prick tests are the more pragmatic. They can be performed in the consulting room and the result available within 10 min. In this case, a soluble extract of antigen is inoculated through the skin to reach the mast cells beneath. If the antigen is recognized by the IgE molecules on the mast-cell surface, calcium channels in the mast-cell membrane are opened providing the signal to release histamine, **sRS-A** leukotrienes (slow-reacting substance of anaphylaxis), kinins, and chemoattractant factors for neutrophils and eosinophils. The release of histamine provides the earliest evidence of mast-cell activation in the skin, with dilatation of the surrounding capillaries causing a flare, followed by a leak of plasma causing intradermal oedema resulting in a wheal. The inflammatory response signalled by the arrival of neutrophils takes a further 4 h to develop. In the lung these events account for the timing of both the immediate and the late asthmatic responses. Continued exposure to antigen (such as ragweed or grass pollens) ensures that symptoms are perpetuated.[16]

The use of skin-prick tests is of some value if the offending agent can be avoided. Examples include danders shed by household pets, but pollens and, to an extent, house-mite antigens cannot be avoided during normal day-to-day living. Individuals born with a tendency to raise IgE antibody against common environmental antigens are termed atopic. Excessive antibody production is associated with eczema and with an increased sensitivity to a wider variety of antigens. Allergic reactions of the airways begin in the nose because this is where allergens such as pollens or house dust first alight and are filtered out. The inflammatory reaction caused by mast-cell discharge blocks the nose resulting in a switch to mouth breathing. This gives allergens direct access to the lower respiratory tract where the same inflammatory response gives rise to asthma instead. A blocked nose is a nuisance, but it does not limit aerobic performance since, when breathing with the mouth open, the greatest resistance to airflow is in the bronchioles and not in the upper airways.

Medicines that improve asthma and those to avoid

Steroids

Asthma (of which exercise-induced asthma is just a symptom) is an inflammatory condition of the airways.[17] Inhaled corticosteroids form the mainstay of anti-inflammatory treatment in the airways.[18] Breath-actuated, drug-delivery systems are preferred by many because they rely less on technique than metered dose inhalers and therefore give a better drug delivery.[19] These include, beclomethasone diproprionate (Diskhaler) and budesonide propionate (Turbohaler). Medication is effective when given morning and evening and the daily dose should not exceed 1600 μg. In the current climate, it is wise to supply the athlete with a letter stating the condition that is being treated, the drug, the dosage, and the delivery system. Severe asthma may require a course of systemic treatment, but oral medication is banned. Any medical officer wishing to use oral steroid medication should appeal to the IOC Medical Commission with a letter explaining the exceptional circumstances under which treatment has been given. If an appeal has not been both lodged and approved, it is likely that an athlete found to have been taking systemic steroids will be disqualified and suspended.

Beta agonists

Drugs with selective beta-adrenergic stimulant properties (beta agonists) form an adjunct to steroid therapy and are effective when taken about 10 min before exercise. These include salbutamol and terbutaline, but must be inhaled only. In common with steroid treatment, beta agonists may not be taken in tablet form. All drugs with alpha-adrenergic stimulant actions given by whatever route are banned by the IOC Medical Commission. These include adrenaline, noradrenaline, isoprenaline, fenoterol, and phenylpropanolamine. Cromoglycate taken by inhalation inhibits exercise-induced asthma and may be useful, especially in children.

References

1. Rasmussen J, Hanel B, Diamant B, Secher NH. Muscle mass effect on arterial desaturation after maximal exercise. *Medicine and Science in Sports and Exercise* 1991; **23**: 1349–52.
2. Nunn JF. *Applied respiratory physiology*. 3rd edn. Cambridge: Butterworth, 1987.
3. Gregory IC. The oxygen and carbon monoxide capacities of fetal and adult blood. *Journal of Physiology* 1974; **236**: 625.
4. Spiet LL, Gledhill N, Froese AB, Wilkes DL. Effect of graded erythrocythaemia on cardiovascular and metabolic responses to exercise. *Journal of Applied Physiology* 1986; **60**: 1942–8.
5. Sawka MN, Joyner MJ, Miles DS, Robertson RJ, Spriet LL, Young AI. The use of blood doping as an ergogenic aid. American College of Sports Medicine: Position stand. *Medicine and Science in Sports and Exercise* 1996; **28**: 1–8.
6. Klein GH. Blood transfusion and athletics: games people play. *New England Journal of Medicine* 1985; **312**: 854–6.
7. Freedman S. Sustained maximum voluntary ventilation. *Respiration Physiology* 1970; **8**: 230–44.
8. Shephard RJ. The maximum sustained voluntary ventilation in exercise. *Clinical Science* 1967; **32**: 167–76.
9. Ward SA, Whipp JB, Poon CS. Density-dependant air flow and ventilatory control in exercise. *Respiration Physiology* 1982; **49**: 267–77.
10. Jensen JE, Lyager S, Pendersen OF. The relationship between maximum ventilation, breathing patterns and mechanical limitation of ventilation. *Journal of Physiology* 1980; **309**: 521–32.
11. Caretti DM, Szlyk PC, Sils VI. Effects of exercise modality on patterns of ventilation and respiratory timing. *Respiration Physiology* 1992; **90**: 201–11.
12. McFadden ER, Hejal R. Asthma. *Lancet* 1995; **345**: 1215–20.
13. Harries MG. Pulmonary limitations to performance in sport. *British Medical Journal* 1994; **309**: 113–15.
14. Cookson WOCM, Sharp PA, Faux JA, Hopkin JM. Linkage between immunoglobulin E responses underlying asthma and chromosome 11q. *Lancet* 1989; **i**: 1292–4.
15. Wilkinson J, Holgate ST. Candidate gene loci in asthmatic and allergic inflammation. *Thorax* 1996; **51**: 3–8.
16. Boushey HA, Holtzman MJ, Sheller JR, Nadel JA. Bronchial hyperreactivity. *American Review of Respiratory Disease* 1980; **121**: 389–93.
17. Barnes PJ. A new approach to the treatment of asthma. *New England Journal of Medicine* 1989; **321**: 1517–27.
18. Woodhead M (ed.). Guidelines on the management of asthma. *Thorax* 1993; **48**: s1–24.
19. Derom E, Pauwels R. Bioequivalence of inhaled drugs. *European Respiratory Journal* 1995; **8**: 1634–6.

3.3 Infections in sports medicine

Geoffrey Pasvol

Competitive sport requires peak performance, and even minor physical or psychological injury can blunt achievement. Although physical injury remains one of the most important hazards to good athletic performance, infections of many varieties can lead to deterioration in competitive ability for a number of reasons. Whilst some infections may be of a major acute nature, it is often minor or chronic low-grade infections that are implicated in the unexplained failures of top athletes. Unfortunately, it is the latter that on a numerical basis are of relatively greater importance, and yet our knowledge of them is sadly deficient.

Whilst infections are commonly associated with early childhood and old age, a number of factors predispose the predominantly young-adult sportsperson to infection. These include reduced immunity as a result of stress and overtraining (see below), close contact with other sportspeople facilitating person-to-person spread, trauma especially of the skin, foreign travel, and sexual activity. Most of the infections encountered in the physically young and fit are of a minor nature, but their effect on performance may be considerable.[1] One particularly fascinating area of recent interest has been the effects of both exercise and psychological stress on the immune system and, in turn, their effect on resistance or susceptibility to infection.[2,3]

Exercise, stress, and immunity

Moderate exercise

It is believed by many that moderate exercise protects against infection, apart from its many other beneficial effects such as those on the cardiovascular system and the psychological well being of the individual. Certainly studies of the effect of moderate exercise in mice would indicate enhanced humoral immunity when compared with controls. However, most studies when undertaken in man vary in the selection and the level of fitness of the subjects under scrutiny, making direct comparison difficult.[4] Moderate exercise increases the granulocyte count which could result from haemoconcentration, mobilization of the marginal granulocyte pool, or release of these cells from the bone marrow. These effects may, in turn, be the result of increased catecholamine and cortisol levels observed during exercise. However, whether increased granulocyte counts result in functional improvement is not clear, and in one study the granulocytes obtained from well-trained athletes were functionally indistinguishable from those of sedentary individuals. Exercise also appears to increase the numbers of circulating lymphocytes, especially T-cells. As with granulocyte function however, there is no conclusive evidence that these exercise-induced raised counts alter host defence to any important extent. Moreover, it has been shown that exercise-induced leukocytosis is short-lived. Plasma levels of α-interferon, interleukin-1, endorphin, and met-enkephalin all increase during exercise. Moderate exercise has no major effect on immunoglobulin or complement levels. Thus, although a number of changes within the immunological system have been noted in moderate exercise, the basic question of whether these changes contribute to resistance to infection remains unanswered.

Overtraining (see also Chapter 3.6)

Whilst moderate exercise stimulates the immune system without any clear beneficial or harmful effect, overtraining appears to have a deleterious effect on the host immune response and may ultimately be a limiting factor in athletic performance.[5] Overtraining is often blamed by top athletes for frequent persistent colds, sore throats, and influenza-like illnesses which can lead to states resembling the postviral fatigue syndrome. An athlete might miss an entire sports season or give up sport altogether because of such infections.

A number of changes in the immune system have been documented in intense exercise. The salivary immunoglobulins IgA and IgM appear to be suppressed for up to 24 h, which could, perhaps, account for the anecdotal statements by athletes that severe exercise increases their susceptibility to upper respiratory tract infections. Similar changes can also occur in students during an examination period. Low resting levels of IgG have also been found in élite ultra-distance runners at the end of the season. Natural killer cell activity appears to be decreased for up to 24 h after severe exercise, largely due to a decrease in the percentage of these cells, although on a per cell basis, natural killer activity is increased. Whilst T lymphocytes are increased by exercise, there is some evidence that the ratio of CD4 to CD8 cells may be reduced, and that in fact these T cells may be incapable of responding normally to mitogens. Low lymphocyte counts (< 1500 per microlitre) have been found in marathon runners at rest. Maximal physical exercise was found to reduce bactericidal and adherence capacity of neutrophils and monocytes when compared to controls.[6] Overtrained Olympic athletes were found to have significantly lower plasma glutamine levels when compared to controls, and glutamine is regarded as an important substrate for lymphocyte metabolism.[7] Whilst all these observations could account for a temporary susceptibility to infection during overtraining, they provide no information on functional outcome.

There are limited data which would support the argument that strenuous exercise leads to increased susceptibility to infection. In mice infected with coxsackievirus B, for example, enforced exercise increased mortality from 5 per cent in the non-exercised to 50 per cent in the exercised group. Monkeys exercised during incubation of the poliomyelitis virus had a higher incidence of paralysis than controls. In an outbreak of poliomyelitis in the United States, all nine boys who became ill were participating in strenuous sports. In a study of 150 ultramarathon runners, symptoms of respiratory tract infections were most common in those who had achieved the fastest times and who as a group had the highest weekly training mileages.

Psychological stress

A complicating factor in immunity to infection in sport is psychological stress, particularly when competitive sport is involved, since this type of stress is thought to result in immunosuppression.[8] Anecdotes abound of individuals who become ill following stressful situations. Many studies over the last 20 years have indicated that psychological stress and psychiatric illness can compromise immunological function, and it appears that the final common pathway is via stimulation of adrenocortical secretion by adrenocorticotrophin (**ACTH**) and the sympathetic nervous system with the subsequent release of catecholamines. The field of psychoneuroimmunology is a relatively recent one.[2] Overall, the complex relationship between moderate or excessive exercise, psychological stress, and disease makes it extremely difficult to predict the final outcome of these interacting factors.

Specific infections

The young sportsperson is most susceptible to those infections which are spread mainly by droplets (for example, upper respiratory tract infections), via the orofaecal route (for example, hepatitis A and E), or occasionally by sexual activity (for example, hepatitis B or HIV). Whilst common acute bacterial infections generally have few sequelae, viral infections, although initially milder, may produce longer lasting effects which often compromise athletic performance.

Upper respiratory tract infections

Upper respiratory tract infections can be extremely worrisome to the athlete, especially when they become recurrent. They are mostly commonly due to viruses such as enteroviruses (for example, echovirus and coxsackieviruses A and B), adenoviruses, and influenza viruses, and therefore frequent consumption of antibiotics for these infections is often unnecessary. Upper respiratory infection due to the newly identified *Chlamydia pneumoniae* has gained recent notoriety in involving Swedish orienteers and leading to a myocarditis. Unfortunately, there are very few cost-effective and rapid methods available to distinguish the different upper respiratory tract infections from one another, other than by throat swab culture for β-haemolytic streptococci (Plate 1) or a heterophile antibody (Paul–Bunnell) test for infectious mononucleosis. Viral culture and serology in the diagnosis of other causes of an acute upper respiratory tract infection are seldom helpful. In any event, infectious mononucleosis and bacterial pharyngitis can coexist.

Management

Symptomatic relief using analgesics, antihistamines, or decongestants may help in some cases. A throat swab should be taken for culture in all athletes with an upper respiratory tract infection and a positive result can usually be obtained within 24 h. Group A β-haemolytic streptococcal sore throats are amenable to treatment with penicillin, or erythromycin in the case of penicillin allergy. Recently, cephalosporins have been shown to be even better at streptococcal clearance. Treatment should continue for at least 10 days to avoid recurrence.

The major issue which arises with regard to sport is whether an individual with an upper respiratory tract infection should refrain from exercise. The conventional guidance is that in the presence of fever, tachycardia at rest, or severe myalgia or lethargy, athletes should not participate in sport. There is still controversy as to whether premature resumption of exercise leads to delayed recovery or a postviral fatigue condition. The occurrence of complications, such as that of a sudden arrhythmia following exercise during a viral illness, has been overemphasized, and sudden cardiac death in the presence of a viral myocarditis is a rare event.[9] Sudden cardiac deaths during exercise are more commonly due to hypertrophic cardiomyopathy or undetected coronary artery disease.

Tetanus

Although rare, tetanus can be fatal and it is essential that all sportspeople who are vulnerable to 'dirty' wounds should ensure that their immunization status is up to date. Infection is caused by the organism *Clostridium tetani*. All wounds should demand careful consideration of whether a booster vaccination, human tetanus immunoglobulin, and/or an antibiotic is indicated. Attention to appropriate prophylaxis after injury is certainly required where the last immunization was more than 10 years ago, the injured person did not receive a full course of vaccination, or the wound involves an appreciable amount of devitalized tissue, is a penetrating wound, where contact with soil or manure is evident, or in the presence of sepsis.

The glandular fevers

The glandular fevers include a number of conditions grouped together because of similarities in clinical presentation, including sustained fever and glandular enlargement. Amongst the more important are infectious mononucleosis (due to the Epstein–Barr virus), toxoplasmosis, and cytomegalovirus infection. To this should be added the primary seroconversion illness of HIV infection, which may be similar in presentation but is more often accompanied by a rash (Plate 2).

The glandular fevers are important in sportspeople for a number of reasons. First, the condition is common in this age group in developed countries. Second, the glandular fevers may predispose to certain complications which are of particular relevance to sportspeople, for example splenic rupture or myocarditis. Finally, the glandular fevers have achieved some notoriety as being one group of infections which may lead on to a post 'viral' fatigue syndrome.

Infectious mononucleosis

Infectious mononucleosis due to the Epstein–Barr virus is an important and common infection in athletes, affecting mainly adolescents and young adults in developed countries, and young children, often asymptomatically, in developing countries. Spread of the infection is mainly via intimate close contact, and for this reason isolation of proven or suspected cases is unnecessary when it occurs in the context of a large sports gathering.

The most common clinical presentation is a sore throat (Plates 3 and 4) with fever and generalized lymphadenopathy with or without an enlarged spleen. In a minority of cases a diffuse maculopapular rash may be present (Plate 5). Patients may present with jaundice, a haematological disorder (for instance, thrombocytopenia or haemolytic anaemia), or any neurological disorder ranging from an encephalitis to a peripheral neuropathy.

Complications

There are two complications of this disease which are of particular relevance to athletes.

Splenic rupture Up to 40 per cent of cases of traumatic splenic rupture have occurred in athletes who have or have subsequently been found to have infectious mononucleosis. Whilst rupture occurs mostly in patients with an enlarged spleen, it may occur in the absence of splenomegaly. Moreover, there appears to be no correlation between the severity of infectious mononucleosis and the risk of rupture.

Persistent fatigue Whilst the majority of episodes of infectious mononucleosis are of relatively short duration (about 2 to 6 weeks), there appear to be a few cases in whom symptoms, predominantly those of fatigue and lethargy, persist for an indefinite period. These cases may comprise a proportion of individuals with the chronic fatigue syndrome (see below).

Diagnosis

The diagnosis of infectious mononucleosis is made on the basis of:

(1) the clinical findings;

(2) the presence of a significant percentage (at least 15 per cent) of atypical lymphocytes on a peripheral blood film; and

(3) a positive heterophile antibody test for infectious mononucleosis.

The heterophile antibody test identifies the ability of the patient's serum to agglutinate horse red cells, and to reduce the number of false positivities the serum is first preabsorbed with guinea-pig kidney cells. It must be remembered that the test may be negative during the first week or two of illness, and that in a proportion of cases (10 to 15 per cent) the tests for such heterophile antibodies might remain negative.

The patient's serum may also be tested for antibodies against the viral capsid antigen. A positive viral capsid antigen IgM would indicate a current infection and this remains positive for about 2 months. A positive IgG test (whatever the titre) only indicates past infection unless a fourfold rise or fall can be demonstrated which would indicate a more recent infection.

Some patients may have a coexistent group A streptococcal throat infection, and for this reason throat swabs for bacterial culture should be taken. Most cases of infectious mononucleosis will have abnormal liver function tests, especially the transaminases and lactate dehydrogenase. The serology of chronic fatigue due to Epstein–Barr virus has not been consistent, but has included increased antibodies to both Epstein–Barr virus early antigen, and Epstein–Barr virus capsid antigen IgM.

Management

In the main, infectious mononucleosis lasts for 2 to 6 weeks and is self-limiting. Treatment is mainly symptomatic. If the throat swab turns out to be positive for group A streptococci, this should be treated with penicillin or an oral cephalosporin. If the patient is penicillin hypersensitive then erythromycin should be used. Treatment should continue for at least 10 days to avoid recurrence. Ampicillin or amoxycillin should be avoided as in over 90 per cent of cases with infectious mononucleosis patients develop a florid, often troublesome rash.

Good evidence for the usefulness of corticosteroids in infectious mononucleosis has only been established in the case of obstructive pharyngitis where the patient has difficulty in speaking, swallowing, or breathing. The usefulness of corticosteroids in cases with hepatitis, neurological, or haematological involvement is unproven. In particular, steroids have not been shown to reduce the risk of splenic rupture or to shorten the course of those with fatigue thought to be due to the Epstein–Barr virus.

Return to sporting activity after infectious mononucleosis should always be graded and limited to the exercise tolerance of the patient.[10] Total bedrest is unnecessary and may even delay recovery, as was demonstrated in a controlled trial amongst university students.[11] Since the risk of splenic rupture is greatest in the first months following infectious mononucleosis, strenuous exercise and alcohol consumption should be avoided during this period. A more cautious return to activity is advisable in contact sports such as rugby and wrestling, and these sports should not be resumed before resolution of splenic enlargement.

Toxoplasmosis

Toxoplasma gondii is another organism which may produce a glandular fever syndrome with fever, hepatosplenomegaly, and generalized or localized lymphadenopathy. This intracellular protozoan infection is most commonly acquired from animals, especially cats (via ingestion of the cysts in their faeces), and undercooked or raw meat. Most infections in man are asymptomatic. Up to 60 per cent of healthy adults in certain countries (for example, France) may be antibody-positive without any past history of illness. Clinical presentation as a glandular syndrome is the most common observation in young adults and is generally self-limiting. However, it has recently gained notoriety in being implicated in the prolonged fatigue and poor performance of certain outstanding athletes and as an opportunistic infection in patients infected with the HIV virus.

Diagnosis

The clinical diagnosis of toxoplasmosis can be confirmed by serology, and a fourfold rise or fall in the toxoplasma latex test or a positive toxoplasma IgM regardless of titre is indicative of recent infection, although a few cases of 'chronic' toxoplasmosis where the toxoplasma IgM titre remains elevated have been documented. A positive latex or IgG titre may occasionally be very high, but without a fourfold rise or fall a current or recent infection cannot be confirmed.

Table 1 Commoner causes of hepatitis in humans

Organism	Transmission route
Hepatitis A virus	Orofaecal
Hepatitis B virus	Blood or sexual contact
Hepatitis C virus	Blood; sexual contact not common
Hepatitis D virus	Only in the presence of hepatitis B virus
Hepatitis E virus	Orofaecal
Non-A, non-B hepatitis (NANB)	Presumed orofaecal
Less common	
Epstein–Barr virus	
Cytomegalovirus (CMV)	
Toxoplasma gondii	
Leptospira spp.	

Management

Most infections with *Toxoplasma* are self-limiting and do not require specific treatment. However, when systemic signs are severe and prolonged the patient may be treated with a combination of pyrimethamine (25 mg daily by mouth) and sulphadiazine (0.5 to 1 g four times a day by mouth), given for up to 4 weeks. However, there is no good evidence that such treatment is beneficial in the immunocompetent host or when the disease is believed to be chronic. A full blood count, looking out for a leukopenia and thrombocytopenia, should be carried out weekly during treatment.

Cytomegalovirus

Glandular fever syndrome due to cytomegalovirus is even less frequent in the immunocompetent individual than toxoplasma infection, but it may present with a syndrome that is indistinguishable from that caused by the Epstein–Barr virus or toxoplasma. The illness is usually self-limiting and the treatment in such cases is symptomatic only. Occasionally, the presentation is that of jaundice.

Hepatitis

Acute hepatitis may be due to a number of causes (Table 1) and is not an uncommon infection in the young-adult sportsperson.

Hepatitis A

Hepatitis A virus is a relatively common cause of hepatitis in the young adult, and a subclinical infection may occur in many cases. Spread is via the orofaecal route. Nausea, loss of appetite, vomiting, and abdominal pain often precede the appearance of jaundice by a number of days and it is during this period that the individual is most infectious. The urine becomes dark due to the presence of bilirubin and the stools light due to intrahepatic cholestasis. Jaundice may then appear and remain for a few days or weeks followed by a variable period to complete recovery. Hepatitis A is contagious and spreads rapidly. However, by the time jaundice appears the need to isolate the patient in order to prevent spread is usually unneces-sary as viral excretion is decreasing and may no longer be detectable.

Diagnosis

The diagnosis of hepatitis A is made clinically with confirmation in the laboratory of a positive hepatitis A virus IgM antibody test. The illness can be monitored by the measurement of liver-function tests such as the transaminases and lactate dehydrogenase, but these do not necessarily correlate with the severity of disease or outcome. A positive hepatitis A virus IgG on its own indicates past infection only.

Management

The treatment of hepatitis A virus infection is symptomatic. Close contacts of those who have not had the infection may be given passive protection with gammaglobulin. The usual dose is 250 mg given intramuscularly. Gammaglobulin has been shown to reduce the severity and duration of illness in those exposed, especially when given early. Hepatitis A vaccine can be used in seronegative subjects at increased risk, which in the case of sportspeople amounts to travel to countries of medium to high endemicity or those who stay for more than 3 months (see below).

Patients with hepatitis A virus infection should rest and only participate in limited activities until the symptoms have subsided, but they need not wait until their liver function tests have returned to normal. Moderate activity even with abnormal tests has been shown to have no deleterious effect on the rate of recovery or relapse in hepatitis A virus infection. Whilst alcohol has been traditionally prohibited during most acute forms of hepatitis and into convalescence, there are no data to suggest that moderate alcohol intake leads to a worsening of acute hepatitis or predisposes to chronic hepatitis.

Hepatitis B

Hepatitis B virus (**HBV**) is a relatively rare infection amongst athletes and the major risk occurs via sexual contact. There is also the minimal risk of spread via contact sports. The prodromal symptoms are similar to hepatitis A virus infection, but occasionally there may be a preceding skin rash and/or arthralgia. In the context of hepatitis B and sport, the precautions taken by first-aid workers and accompanying sports staff should be similar to those outlined for HIV infection as laid out below. If exposed to the blood of a known infected individual then the use of hepatitis B vaccine (usually 500 International Units for adults) to confer active immunity as well as specific hepatitis B immunoglobulin (**HBIG**) should be used. These should be given at different sites. Immunization with HBIG does not suppress an active immune response to the vaccine.

Treatment of acute cases is symptomatic and the majority recover spontaneously. Return to sporting activity must be graded and full activity should not be resumed until the symptoms have subsided. Careful follow-up of patients with hepatitis B virus infection is important to ensure that they eliminate the virus, and do not develop any of the important sequelae of infection such as chronic carriage (occurring in 5 to 10 per cent of cases), chronic active hepatitis, cirrhosis, and hepatoma. Patients with any of these sequelae require further specialist follow-up since, at the present time, treatment with interferon may be indicated according to infection status and can eradicate infection in up to 40 per cent of those treated. There is, as yet, no indication that chronic carriers of hepatitis B virus should be prevented from participating in sport, except in close contact sports such as boxing, wrestling, and rugby.

Hepatitis C

The hepatitis C virus has recently gained much publicity. It is transmitted primarily by blood and blood products and many haemophiliacs and intravenous drug abusers are infected, but sexual contact does not appear to be a major route of spread. Clinically, there is little to distinguish it from the other causes of viral hepatitis. The diagnosis is made serologically, which may take up to 6 months after infection to become positive. Hepatitis C virus is an important cause of hepatitis as infection can lead to prolonged liver dysfunction and cirrhosis. However, it is uncommon amongst sportspeople. Treatment with interferon is beneficial in patients selected on a number of laboratory and histopathological criteria.

Hepatitis E

Hepatitis E virus is now known to be responsible for some cases of enterically transmitted non-A, non-B hepatitis. The virus has now been identified and cloned. Serological tests, albeit insensitive, are now available. Hepatitis E appears to be particularly common in the Indian subcontinent but probably occurs worldwide.

Chronic fatigue syndrome

The chronic fatigue syndrome has now become a major area of controversy, especially because of the debate as to whether it is of organic or functional origin. Whatever its cause it is of major importance to sportspeople.[12] Undoubtedly some, if not most, individuals suffer from a variable period of fatigue, malaise, and depression after viral illnesses such as influenza, infectious mononucleosis, and hepatitis. However, the extent to which more prolonged symptoms may be attributed to a viral infection remains open to debate. In 1991 an operational definition for the chronic fatigue syndrome was published, this emphasizes a primary complaint of fatigue of at least 6 months' duration in the absence of neurological signs with myalgia, psychiatric symptoms, and previous viral infection as commonly associated features, although none are exclusions or necessary for the diagnosis.[13]

Attributing a cause to chronic fatigue syndrome has been difficult and it is almost certain that it is a heterogeneous group of conditions. However, evidence in favour of an organic cause include a number of objective laboratory parameters, some of which are highly specialized and have only been used in the context of research. These include the finding of abnormal muscle biopsies in some of these patients, together with the finding of virus particles in muscle. Abnormal intracellular acidosis in the muscles of the forearm has been detected using magnetic resonance imaging. Antibodies to the coxsackievirus and a component viral antigen (**VP1**) have been found in increased frequency in patients with chronic fatigue syndrome. Markers of persistent Epstein–Barr virus infection such as an IgM response to the viral capsid antigen, absence of a response to the Epstein–Barr nuclear antigen (**EBNA** antibody negativity), and increased response to the early antigen (EA antibody) have been presented as evidence for prolonged fatigue following infectious mononucleosis. Toxoplasmosis has also achieved publicity with regards to its potential for producing prolonged symptoms, and a few individuals may continue to maintain levels of IgM in their serum which might indicate continued replication of the organism. Brucellosis is a good example where a persistent infection is commonly thought to produce prolonged symptoms.

Equally, there are abundant data which argue against an organic cause for chronic fatigue syndrome. In one study of 100 adults with chronic fatigue nearly 70 per cent were found to have a psychiatric disorder that was thought to be the cause of their fatigue; 5 per cent had medical conditions (for example, a seizure disorder, sleep apnoea, polmyalgia, and asthma), while in 30 per cent the cause of chronic fatigue was unexplained.[14] Many other published studies have shown a clear association between chronic fatigue syndrome and self-reported depression and anxiety.

In many cases patients are able to date their illness back to an upper respiratory tract infection or a diarrhoeal illness. This is followed by a variable period of symptoms such as fatigue, muscle weakness and pain, poor concentration, sleep abnormalities, irritability, joint pain, headaches, forgetfulness, painful lymph glands, photophobia, sore throat, etc. These can often be severe enough to produce gross impairment of athletic performance.

Management

None of the interventions used in controlled studies such as aciclovir or steroids for Epstein–Barr virus infection, definitive treatment outside the acute phase for toxoplasmosis, or more generalized treatment such as gammaglobulins have been shown to be of benefit in chronic fatigue syndrome. Treatment with magnesium has been used, as have interventions to eradicate yeast infection by diet, the use of antifungals or bacteria, such as *Lactobacilli* spp. However, these treatments have not as yet been supported by adequate studies. Treatment should be directed towards the relief of symptoms. In all cases a positive and optimistic attitude towards outcome, coupled with continued support and reassurance, is of far greater importance in the gradual return to full activity. Sportspeople should exercise within their effort-tolerance limits and increase their exercise in a graded fashion. There is no evidence to support the concept of total bedrest.

Infections of the skin

The skin is one of the main barriers to infection. However, in sport because of increased exposure to infection due to travel, close contact with others, friction and another forms of trauma, and increased sweating, the skin becomes particularly susceptible to infection. Whilst seemingly trivial in the first instance, such infections can become a major limiting factor in athletic performance.

Viral infections

Molluscum contagiosum

Molluscum contagiosum is due to a pox virus, and the lesions can be very easily recognized by their characteristic umbilicated appearance (Plate 6).

A number of strategies are available for the treatment of this infection.

1. Liquid nitrogen can be used locally on the lesions to good effect.

2. An orangestick may be used to release the cheesy material from the lesion.

3. Podophylline, 25 per cent, can be applied to the lesions once or twice weekly.

Herpes simplex infections

In sports where there is close contact, for example in rugby and wrestling, it is possible for an individual who is herpetic to transmit the virus to a team-mate or to the opposition leading to the well-known lesions of herpes gladiatorum or 'scrumpox' (Plate 7). Those dealing with athletes such as masseurs and physiotherapists might also contract the infection by contact with clients. When lesions occur on the fingers (herpetic whitlow) they may be especially painful. In the primary herpes infection systemic features may be severe (Plate 8) with a high fever, malaise, and prostration. In secondary recurrences the lesions generally produce only a local problem with characteristic clustered vesicles on an erythematous base. Herpes simplex infections may occasionally trigger more generalized erythema multiforme-type lesions and sometimes full-blown Stevens–Johnson syndrome with mucous membrane involvement.

Management

The acute management of primary infection may require an oral antiviral drug such as valiciclovir or famciclovir. In secondary infections the antiviral drug may be given orally for several days (usually about 5 to 7 days). In severe cases, especially in cases of primary infection, antivirals may need to be given parenterally, which at the current time limits one to the use of aciclovir. A topical antiviral preparation is not as effective.

Prophylaxis

Many athletes who suffer from cold sores may wish to avoid attacks during important sporting events and therefore the use of prophylactic antiviral agents could be considered. Many regimens have been devised although, particularly for the newer antivirals, these need to be tailored. Aciclovir, 400 mg twice a day, is a useful starting dose for prophylaxis, particularly during periods of competition and stress.

Warts (verrucas)

Warts may be a particular nuisance if they occur at sites which interfere with a specific sport. Warts are due to infection by the group of viruses known as the papovaviruses. Many warts will disappear of their own accord, but obviously further treatment might be indicated in athletes especially if they occur at sites on the body which may interfere with performance.

1. Wart paints—a number of these exist and many of them contain salicylic acid.

2. Liquid nitrogen cryotherapy can be used for warts.

3. Where warts are particularly problematical they may be curetted or surgically removed.

Bacterial infections

Streptococcal and staphylococcal infections

Streptococcal and staphylococcal infections of the skin are especially common and most often due to *Streptococcus pyogenes* or *Staphylococcus aureus*. Whilst, as a general rule, streptococcal infections tend to produce erythema and widely spreading lesions often with blistering (for example, in cellulitis and erysipelas) (Plate 9), staphylococcal infections are often more focal and produce pus (for example, in the case of boils and furuncles) (Plate 10). The clinical description is often that of a cellulitis, which may be due to either organism. It is often difficult to distinguish between the two without culturing wound swabs. Impetiginous lesions with widespread scabs could be due to either. When the lower limb is involved, the portal of entry in sportspeople is often due to athlete's foot.

Diagnosis

The diagnosis of a streptococcal or staphylococcal skin lesion is most often a clinical one, although culturing wound swabs may occasionally be of help particularly if pus is present. If the infection becomes systemic, a blood culture may be positive.

Management

Streptococcal or staphylococcal infections may often spread rapidly, particularly in the case of impetigo, and need to be urgently treated. The patient needs to be isolated because of easy person-to-person spread. For localized lesions, treatment with oral penicillin and flucloxacillin in combination is usually adequate, although parenteral antibiotics may be required especially if there are signs of systemic involvement. Systemic involvement is indicated by the clinical state of the patient, for instance a raised temperature and raised white-cell count, ESR, C-reactive protein, etc. For patients who are penicillin hypersensitive, a macrolide antibiotic such as erythromycin or clarithromycin may be used. Meticulous care should be paid to handwashing to avoid local spread of the infection.

Recurrent skin and ear infections

Some sportspeople become carriers of staphylococci which often lead to recurrent infection, especially if they gain access to small cuts and abrasions. Such individuals should pay meticulous care to bathing, and in some cases may need to use an antiseptic skin cleanser daily, such as povidone iodine (Betadine®), together with an antibiotic nasal cream, for example chlorhexidine and neomycin (Naseptin®), applied three times a day to the nostril for 10 days in order to eradicate the carriage of staphylococci.

Otitis externa can be a particular problem in swimmers and is easily diagnosed in the patient who has a painful ear with discharge and characteristic erythematous findings on examination of external auditory meatus. The infecting organisms may be a mixture of Gram-positive and -negative organisms and may require topical treatment with an antibiotic which is not used systemically (such as neomycin or clioquinol). Application of a local cream or ear drops containing an antibiotic and a steroid may be given for 7 to 10 days. If the infection does not clear within this period, specialist advice should be sought.

Fungal infections

Fungal infections are particularly problematical in sites where sweat and moisture accumulate.

Athlete's foot (tinea pedis) and ringworm (tinea corporis)

Athlete's foot characteristically presents as peeling of the skin with fissuring and sometimes secondary infection, especially between the 4th and 5th toes (Plate 11). It is often associated with blisters on the feet, so-called podopomphylix. The most common infections are due to *Tricophyton rubrum* and *Epidermophyton floccosum*, although infection due to other fungi also occur. The fissuring may be painful, but the most important complication of athlete's foot is secondary bacterial infection, and it is not uncommon that the seedling for ascending lymphangitis or cellulitis is athlete's foot.

Fungal infection of the skin on the trunk and limbs (tinea corporis) produces a characteristic round plaque with a raised edge, scaling and central clearing (Plate 12).

Management

Treatment involves meticulous washing of the feet together with careful drying thereafter. A hair-dryer can be useful. Application of an antifungal cream (such as cotrimazole, itraconazole, or econazole) is effective. More recently, the use of oral terbinafine has been advocated in these infections especially if the lesions are in a difficult site, are severe, or are extensive. A 2- to 6-week course of terbinafine is necessary.

Tinea unguium

Nail infection (tinea unguium; Plate 13) is far more difficult to treat. First, it needs accurate diagnosis with skin and nail-plate scrapings or clippings which can then be examined microscopically with potassium hydroxide. Whilst griseofulvin used to be the treatment of choice, terbinafine has now been shown to produce better results and requires shorter treatment times (between 6 weeks and 3 months)

Tinea versicolor

Tinea versicolor is caused by the fungal form of *Malassezia furfur*. The lesions are typical, producing areas of discoloured patches which are often scaly at the edges (Plate 14). Diagnosis is clinical and can be confirmed by means of skin scrapings. The treatment consists of the application of selenium sulphide (Selsun®) shampoo. However the antifungal imidazole creams are also effective. Terbinafine has also been effective in eradicating this infection.

Sexually transmitted diseases and HIV infection

Sexually transmitted diseases and HIV are common in many parts of the world and therefore sportspersons should be educated about the risks of infection. The risk may be reduced, but not abolished, by avoiding unprotected sexual intercourse, using good-quality condoms, practising 'safer sex' techniques, and being wary of alcohol-related loss of inhibitions.

Infection by HIV and the disease it causes (**AIDS**) is now a global health problem. Sportspeople generally have the same risk of infection as the general population, but travel abroad and increased sexual activity may increase this risk. The risks are proportional to the prevalence of HIV-positive individuals in a given population which, in turn, differs from place to place. In certain countries AIDS will become the major killer of individuals between 15 and 45 years of age. The number of AIDS cases and HIV-positive individuals is growing rapidly and is often inadequately documented so that published figures are often misleading. Whilst initially the at-risk groups included homosexual and bisexual men, intravenous drug abusers, haemophiliacs, transfusion recipients, prostitutes, and sexual partners of all these, infection has now spread into the heterosexual population so it is no longer possible to predict reliably who may be at risk.

Having said this, however, the risks of contracting HIV infection in sport-related activities must be exceedingly small and, to date, no cases have been reported. The risk to sportspeople must lie mainly in sexual intercourse, and in this respect the regular use of condoms and the restriction in the number of sexual partners must be advocated. The sharing of razors and toothbrushes has the theoretical possibility of transmitting the virus and should be discouraged. At the same time, it should be emphasized that normal social contact, the sharing of changing facilities, and swimming pools constitute no risk of infection.

There are no documented cases of the spread of HIV infection by contact sports. However, cases have been recorded where seroconversion occurred following contact of infected blood with open skin lesions. Thus this route could theoretically pose a risk.

In injuries resulting from bleeding of wounds, participants should be aware of the risk and in all cases such wounds should be covered or the player excluded from further participation. All participants, first-aid workers, and accompanying sports staff should realize that, outside sexual contact and other high-risk practices, the risks of acquiring HIV infection are very small, but general recommendations for treating injuries on the sportsfield are listed in Table 2.

Travel abroad

Wherever and whenever travel is undertaken for sport, business, or leisure, there is an increased risk of mortality and morbidity. Not surprisingly, excess mortality abroad is mainly due to traffic accidents and drowning rather than the scourges of exotic infectious diseases. In one study of 2500 deaths of American travellers of all ages whilst abroad, 50 per cent were due to cardiovascular events, 25 per cent due to injury of one kind or another, and only 1 per cent due to infection, although it should be noted that these data referred to travellers whilst abroad and not to illnesses which manifested after return. However, this does emphasize the need for anyone travelling abroad to have adequate medical insurance.

Table 2 General recommendations for handling injuries on the sportsfield involving sportspersons who may be HIV-positive[19]

1. Assume that all casualties are HIV-positive.
2. Wear gloves for all procedures involving contact with blood or other body secretions.
3. Cover all cuts and abrasions where possible.
4. Wear protective glasses where blood may be splashed into the face.
5. Wash skin immediately after contamination with blood or secretions.
6. Dispose of sharps safely: never attempt to re-sheathe needles.
7. Dispose of waste materials by burning.
8. Contaminated clothes should be presoaked in hot (> 70 °C) soapy water for 30 min and then washed in a hot-cycle washing machine; alternatively, they may be soaked in household bleach (1 in 10 dilution) or Milton® solution for 30 min.
9. All contaminated equipment or surfaces may be treated with bleach as above.
10. Communal items in the first-aid kit no longer have a place in the care of injured sportspeople (e.g. bucket and sponge).
11. No cases of HIV infection transmitted by mouth-to-mouth resuscitation have been recorded; however, simple devices which prevent direct contact between the operator and patient are now available to assist in ventilation.

Table 3 Morbidity and mortality of certain infections in 1 000 000 non-immune travellers visiting developing countries for 1 month[20]

Infection	Incidence	Mortality
Malaria (without chemoprophylaxis)		
West Africa	24 000	480
East Africa	15 000	300
Hepatitis A	3 000	3
Hepatitis B	800	16
Typhoid		
Overall	30	0.3
India	300	3
Poliomyelitis	1	0.2
Cholera	3	0.06

Travellers to developing countries suffer a high morbidity which is mainly due to diarrhoeal disease. The relative risk of some other infections is shown in Table 3. Malaria outstrips the others by far. The most frequent occurring disease preventable by immunization is hepatitis A followed by hepatitis B. The risk of acquiring cholera abroad is exceedingly small. Moreover, some of the illnesses may only be minor (for example, a short episode of traveller's diarrhoea), some will only manifest themselves a good time after return from abroad (for example, hepatitis), while others can be extremely severe and even life-threatening (for example, cerebral malaria).

Many of the measures (immunization or prophylaxis) taken against these diseases are not without side-effects; and although these are often minor, they are sufficient to interfere with sports performance. Thus if these agents are to be administered they should be given as early as possible before the time of competition. In the final analysis, when instituting preventive measures, it is judicious to consider the benefits and to weigh these against the side-effects, costs, and inconvenience caused. Not all the measures implemented are completely effective. No antimalarial can provide absolute protection; gammaglobulin is said to prevent only 70 to 90 per cent of clinical attacks and cholera vaccine is only 60 to 70 per cent effective. It is also often difficult to decide whether or not to give a preventive measure, largely because of insufficient information available on the risks. Thus it is often the case that where the risks and costs are thought to be small, the particular preventive measure is administered. Certainly pretravel advice with regard to food hygiene, exposure to insect bites, etc. is as important as measures that are ultimately instituted such as vaccination or drug prophylaxis.

Travellers' diarrhoea

Travellers' diarrhoea is by far the most common illness afflicting travellers and varies with destination: below 8 per cent in the United States, Canada, Northern and Central Europe, Australia, and New Zealand; 8 to 20 per cent in the Caribbean, Southern Europe, Israel, Japan, and South Africa; 20 to 55 per cent in developing countries.

Enterotoxigenic *Escherichia coli* are most commonly responsible. A wide range of other bacteria, viruses, and protozoa make up the remainder (Table 4).

Symptoms most frequently start on the third day abroad—20 per cent will have a second bout during the second week. The symptoms, apart from watery diarrhoea of varying degree, include cramps, nausea, vomiting, fever in a few cases, and sometimes frank dysentery. Passage of blood and/or mucus implies bowel inflammation or ulceration and raises the likelihood of an invasive organism such as *Shigella* species or *Entamoeba histolytica*, although *Salmonella* and *Campylobacter* spp. can produce such a picture. Giardiasis has a longer and often more variable incubation period (frequently measured in weeks rather than days), and often produces persistent diarrhoea, flatulence, abdominal distension, and lactose intolerance. Cyclospora as a cause of travellers diarrhoea is a recent finding, especially in travellers to Nepal.

Management
Prevention
Dietary precautions such as care in selecting well-cooked food and consumption of only fresh fruit and vegetables which require peeling are particularly important. Salads and uncooked shellfish are considered high risk. Only sterilized water should be consumed, including tooth-brushing and ice in drinks. Because of their low pH, bottled carbonated drinks are safe. However, studies have shown that travellers very soon relinquish these restrictions and eat salads, use ice cubes in drinks, and even consume raw or under-cooked foods.

Prophylaxis
Many drugs have been proposed for the prophylaxis of travellers' diarrhoea, but only antimicrobials such as cotrimoxazole, trimethoprim, and ciprofloxacin have been shown to have proven efficacy. However, the medical profession has been reluctant to advocate

Table 4 Principal causes of traveller's diarrhoea

Bacteria

Enterotoxigenic *Escherichia coli* (ETEC)

Shigella spp.

Salmonella spp.

Campylobacter jejuni

Vibrio cholerae

Non-cholera vibrios, e.g. *V. parahaemolyticus*

Viruses

Rotavirus

Small round viruses, e.g. Norwalk agent

Protozoa

Giardia lamblia

Entamoeba histolytica

Cyrptosporidium parvum

Cyclospora cayetanensis

their widespread use, mainly because of fears of the development of resistant organisms. Prophylactic antimicrobials may be indicated in athletes who are staying abroad for less than 2 weeks and in whom it is vital that peak performance is assured.

Treatment

In most cases the management of travellers diarrhoea is symptomatic. The patient should rest and drink plenty of clear fluids especially water with sugar and electrolytes (for example, Dioralyte®). A simple alternative can be made by adding a pinch of salt and a teaspoon of sugar to 250 ml of bottled water. Potassium can be provided by fruit juice. Milk should be avoided when symptoms are severe. Painful spasms may be treated with co-phenotrope (Lomotil®) (four tablets at once then two every 4 h until the diarrhoea has stopped) or loperamide (Imodium®) (two capsules at once and then one with each diarrhoeal motion). These drugs should be used with caution and only for short periods, since nausea, vomiting, and sedation are associated with increasing doses, especially in the presence of renal impairment. The use of codeine and morphine has been banned by the International Olympic Committee. If used, the dose is codeine phosphate (two 30 mg tablets every 4 h until the diarrhoea has stopped). All these antidiarrhoeal agents may prolong the course of shigella and salmonella infections, and should not be used where invasive disease is suspected (for example, when blood or mucus are present in the stool).

If antimicrobials are required the drug of choice would be ciprofloxacin (500 mg twice daily for 3 days) since it would cover the majority of gut pathogens, including *Campylobacter* spp. Both cotrimoxazole (960 mg twice daily) and trimethoprim (200 mg twice daily) taken for 5 days have been shown to be effective in the treatment of travellers' diarrhoea.

Giardias is best treated with a single dose of tinidazole (Fasigyn®) (2 g and the same dose repeated after a week).

Malarial chemoprophylaxis

The spread of drug-resistant *Plasmodium falciparum* malaria has complicated malarial chemoprophylaxis, as well as the awareness that some of the more effective combination drugs such as Fansidar®, Maloprim®, and amodiaquine (Camoquin®), may have severe, and sometimes fatal, side-effects. There has also been some concern with regard to the occurrence of moderate neuropsychiatric side-effects due to mefloquine (Lariam®) which may modify one's use of this drug.[15] Thus the risk of contracting malaria in any given country or situation needs to be constantly weighed against the risk of developing a serious reaction to the drug. In the absence of adequate data this becomes difficult.[16] However, it appears that compliance is of extreme importance—whilst those who comply poorly may have a similar rate of attack to unprotected individuals, poor compliers have an increased relative risk of death.

It is most important to emphasize to travellers that antimosquito measures are probably as important as antimalarial chemoprophylaxis. Thus in endemic areas travellers should take the following precautions:

(1) sleep in properly screened rooms;

(2) use mosquito nets without holes which are tucked in under the mattress well before nightfall;

(3) wear long-sleeved clothing and long trousers when out of doors after sunset;

(4) consider using other adjuncts such as insect spray (usually containing permethrin), mosquito coils, or repellents such as diethyltoluamide (**DEET**).

A brief guide to antimalarial chemoprophylaxis is shown in Table 5. If there is any doubt, specialist advice should be sought. Chemoprophylaxis should start at least a week before departure (to ensure adequate blood levels and to evaluate any potential side-effects), whilst away, and for 4 weeks after return. The simplest and safest regimen to use at present (1997) for most malarial endemic parts of the world is chloroquine (Nivaquine® or Avloclor®, two tablets (150 mg base each) once a week, together with proguanil (Paludrine®, two tablets (200 mg) daily. These drugs have only minor side-effects, the commonest being gastrointestinal and difficulty in visual accommodation in the case of chloroquine, and mouth ulcers with the use of proguanil. Mefloquine may be used when travelling in Papua New Guinea and The Solomon Islands. Travellers to sub-Saharan Africa may use mefloquine, 250 mg (1 tablet) weekly. However, this should only be used for trips lasting longer than 2 weeks and where the risks of disease outweigh the risks of associated adverse neuropsychiatric side-effects of intermediate severity—these are believed to be more frequent with mefloquine than say chloroquine and proguanil.[15]

More detailed and specialist advice should be sought in other circumstances of malarial chemoprophylaxis, as follows:

(1) long-term visitors;

(2) children under 12 years of age;

(3) individuals with drug allergies;

(4) pregnancy;

(5) underlying medical conditions and medication.

The possibility of malaria should be considered in any person with a fever who is or has been in a malarious area whether or not they have been taking antimalarial chemoprophylaxis. At present, no antimalarial agent can guarantee absolute protection.

Vaccination of travellers

Vaccination of travellers has become routine and is often undertaken without any consideration of the risks or benefits involved.[17,18] Such an analysis is often impossible for a given individual, even when the destination is known. Furthermore, there is often no time before departure to complete a vaccination schedule (for example, hepatitis B). In this circumstance it should be regarded that, where indicated, some vaccination is better than none. A brief outline of the use of vaccination for travellers is given in Table 6.

Poliomyelitis and tetanus

Vaccination against poliomyelitis and tetanus should be kept up to date since these illnesses occur worldwide. It is recommended that polio be updated every 10 years where travel to developing countries is involved and tetanus every 10 years up to a maximum of five vaccinations. Booster doses at less than 10-year intervals are not recommended since they have not been shown to be necessary and they

Table 5 Brief guidelines for malarial chemoprophylaxis[16]

Chemoprophylaxis	Area to be visited	Dose/comments
None	North Africa (Morocco, Algeria, Tunisia, Libya, tourist areas of Egypt) Tourist areas of South-East Asia (Thailand, Philippines, Hong Kong, Singapore, Bali, China)	
Chloroquine or	Middle East (including summer months in rural Egypt and Turkey) Central America, rural Mauritius	300 mg base (2 tablets once per week)
proguanil (Paludrine[R])		200 mg once per day
Chloroquine and proguanil	Sub-Saharan Africa, Indian subcontinent, Afghanistan and Iran, South America	Doses as above
Mefloquine (Lariam[R])	Papua New Guinea, Solomon Islands and Vanuatu, sub-Saharan Africa	250 mg (one tablet) once a week. An alternative to chloroquine and proguanil in areas of high risk. Possible increased risk of neuropsychiatric side-effects
Doxycycline	Mefloquine-resistant areas of South-East Asia (e.g. Thai–Cambodian, Thai–Myanmar borders)	100 mg per day

can lead to unpleasant local reactions which could certainly interfere with sporting performance. Even when given, vaccination should be administered well ahead of a sporting event.

Typhoid

Typhoid vaccine is no longer as unpleasant as it was previously. It is now a monovalent vaccine against *Salmonella typhi* only (that is to say, not against Paratyphi A and B as before). An intradermal injection of 0.1 ml to 0.2 ml has been shown to be as effective as 0.5 ml given intramuscularly. This regimen also appears to reduce the side-effects of redness and swelling at the site of injection and the more generalized symptoms of an influenza-like illness. The risk of contracting the disease is variable depending on the destination, nutritional characteristics, duration of stay, and gastric acidity (assumed to be normal in healthy athletes). The vaccine is only regarded as 70 to 80 per cent effective and needs to be given on two occasions a month apart. A booster is recommended every 3 years, but this will depend on circumstances. Areas of 'high risk' appear to be the Middle East, Africa, and Asia, especially the Indian subcontinent. Amongst American citizens, for example, travel to Mexico accounted for the majority of cases. Only 7 per cent of those American citizens contracting typhoid had been vaccinated.

Recently, two further vaccines for typhoid have become available.

The first, an oral vaccine, has the advantage of being more acceptable and the second, a subunit vaccine, is said to have fewer side-effects and needs to be given only once rather than twice for the primary course. However, both are expensive.

The oral vaccine is a live, attenuated strain of *S. typhi* (strain Ty21A) and can be used for the active immunization of adults and children who are more than 6 years old. A capsule is swallowed before a meal with a cold or lukewarm drink on alternate days for three doses, and the manufacturers advise that the capsules should not be chewed but swallowed immediately. The reported side-effects are few but mild nausea, vomiting, abdominal cramps, diarrhoea, and urticaria may occur. The same contraindications as for other live vaccines apply. As with other typhoid vaccines, this vaccine is not 100 per cent effective and travellers should still take precautions against contact or ingestion of potentially contaminated food or water. A limiting factor in its use remains the cost.

The second typhoid vaccine is the subunit vaccine prepared from the Vi capsular polysaccharide of *S. typhi* and has the advantage of a single-dose schedule which protects for 3 years. It is also said to have a lower incidence of local and systemic reactions compared with the standard whole-cell inactivated typhoid vaccine. However, the vaccine is not licensed for children under 18 months of age and is more expensive than the standard vaccine.

Table 6 Some more commonly used vaccines for travel abroad

Vaccine	Dose	Comments
Polio*	3 drops	Primary course: 3 doses 1 month apart.
		Boost every 10 years
Tetanus (adsorbed tetanus toxin)	0.5 ml subcutaneously	Primary course: 3 doses 1 month apart. Boost every 10 years up to maximum 5 vaccinations unless at special risk.
Typhoid		
(a) Monovalent typhoid vaccine	0.5 ml intramuscularly for first dose, than 0.2 ml intradermally	Primary course: 2 doses preferably a month and not less than 10 days apart.
		Boost every 5 years unless at special risk.
(b) Live oral typhoid* vaccine strain Ty21A	3 enteric-coated capsules on alternate days	Boost every 3 years unless at special risk
(c) Vi capsular polysaccharide typhoid vaccine	0.5 ml subcutaneously or intramuscularly once only	Single boost every 3 years
Cholera	0.5 ml intramuscularly (first dose), then 0.1 ml intradermally	Primary course: 2 doses preferably a month and not less than 10 days apart
		Booster every 6 months
Yellow fever*	0.5 ml subcutaneously	Single injection from a recognized yellow fever centre with certificate (valid 10 days after vaccination for 10 years)
Hepatitis A (human diploid cell)	1 ml intramuscularly	Primary course: a single dose (> 1440 ELISA units for hepatitis A protein). For immunity up to 10 years, booster at 6–12 months
Hepatitis B	1 ml intramuscularly	Primary course: 0, 1, and 6 months
		One booster at 3–5 years
Rabies (human diploid cell vaccine)	1 ml intramuscularly or 0.1 ml intradermally**	Primary course: 3 doses 1 month apart.
		Booster every 2–3 years

* Indicates live vaccine

** Not standard recommendation but probably as effective, cheaper and less likely to cause side-effects.

Cholera

The use of cholera vaccine remains controversial. Cholera vaccines are only about 60 to 70 per cent effective and last for only 3 to 6 months. The risk for travellers contracting cholera is extremely low (Table 2). Certain countries sporadically demand a certificate of vaccination against cholera and it has been argued that possession of a certificate is more relevant than the vaccine itself. Sportsmen are unlikely to work or live in highly endemic areas which may from time to time demand vaccination. In 1973 the WHO waived the requirement for a cholera vaccination certificate. Vaccination, if given, should be by deep subcutaneous or intramuscular injection using two doses administered a month apart. The first dose is given by intramuscular injection (0.5 ml), whereas all subsequent doses are given intradermally. Intradermal vaccination results in fewer side-effects but may result in less protection. On balance, cholera vaccine is not necessary for ordinary tourists or sportspeople visiting most countries.

Hepatitis

Other than malaria, hepatitis A emerges as the disease in which intervention can be most effective in travellers. Since the incubation period may be prolonged (up to 2 months), symptoms may only begin well after return from abroad, but the effects on high-level sporting performance may be marked. Active vaccination against hepatitis A is now available and should ultimately replace the use of gammaglobulin. The hepatitis A vaccine consists of a formaldehyde-inactivated hepatitis A virus (HM 175 strain) grown on human diploid cells and absorbed on aluminium hydroxide as adjuvant. The immunization regimen consists of two doses of 1 ml of vaccine given intramuscularly spaced 2 to 4 weeks apart, and provides anti-HAV antibodies for at least 1 year. To obtain more persistent immunity for up to 10 years, a 1 ml booster is recommended 6 to 12 months after the initial dose. The reported side-effects so far have been mild and amount to mainly local symptoms. Because of the expense, travellers should first be screened for HAV antibodies before receiving the vaccine. Those who possess HAV IgG do not need the vaccine.

Administration of pooled gammaglobulin, as a cheaper alternative to hepatitis vaccine, is usually given in a dose of 250 mg intramuscularly to those travelling abroad for 2 months or less, and 500 mg to those who will be abroad for longer than 2 months. Gammaglobulin is given as late as possible before departure to maintain antibody levels as high as possible whilst at risk of infection. It is important to emphasize that from the point of view of the risk of HIV infection, injection of gammaglobulin is entirely safe and that no cases of transmission of HIV have ever been reported using these preparations.

Vaccination against hepatitis B in sportspeople is not, as yet, considered routine. However, with increasing knowledge of the safety of the vaccine, falling costs, and an indication of the definite risk in the travelling population (Table 2), it may become more routinely administered. Vaccination (1 ml intramuscularly) should be given at time zero, 6 weeks, and 6 months; an adequate antibody response is confirmed by taking serum at 2 to 4 weeks after the last dose and checking for adequate antibody levels.

Yellow fever

This is the only vaccine regarded by the World Health Organization as requiring an International Certificate of Immunization for travellers to sub-Saharan Africa and certain parts of South America. A single dose of 0.5 ml is given subcutaneously. It is a safe and effective vaccine and is valid for 10 years beginning 10 days after vaccination.

Other vaccines

From time to time, indications to give other vaccines might arise. These will include diphtheria, influenza, Japanese B encephalitis, measles, meningococcal vaccine, plague, typhus, tick-borne encephalitis, and rabies. All of these would require further specialist advice according to the circumstance.

References

1. Roberts J, Wilson J, Clements G. Virus infections and sports performance—a prospective study. *British Journal of Sports Medicine* 1988; **22**: 161–2.
2. Ader R, Cohen N, Felten D. Psychoneuroimmunology: interactions between the nervous system and the immune system. *Lancet* 1995; **345**: 99–103.
3. Simon H. The immunology of exercise. A brief review. *Journal of the American Medical Association* 1984; **252**: 2735–8.
4. Keast D. Exercise and the immune response. *Sports Medicine* 1988; **5**: 248–67.
5. Budgett R. The overtraining syndrome. *British Medical Journal* 1994; **309**: 465–8.
6. Lewicki R, Tchorzewski H, Majewska E, Nowak Z, Baj Z. Effect of maximal physical exercise on T-lymphocyte subpopulations and on interleukin (IL1) and interleukin 2 (IL2) production *in vitro*. *International Journal of Sports Medicine* 1988; **9**: 114–17.
7. Parry-Billings M, Blomstrand E, McAndrew N, Newsholme E. A communicational link between skeletal muscle, brain, and cells of the immune system. *International Journal of Sports Medicine* 1990; **11**: S122–8.
8. Khansari D, Murgo A, Faith R. Effects of stress on the immune system. *Immunology Today* 1990; **11**: 170–4.
9. Liberthson R. Sudden death from cardiac causes in children and young adults. *New England Journal of Medicine* 1996; **334**: 1039–44.
10. Haines J. When to resume sports after infectious mononucleosis. How soon is safe? *Postgraduate Medicine* 1987; **81**: 331–3.
11. Dalrymple W. Infectious mononucleosis—II. Relationship of bedrest and activity to prognosis. *Postgraduate Medical Journal* 1964; **35**: 345–9.
12. Budgett R. The post-viral fatigue syndrome in athletes. In: Jenkins R, Mowbray J, eds. *Post-viral fatigue syndrome*. London: Wiley, 1991: 345–62.
13. Sharpe M, Archard L, Banatvala J. Chronic fatigue syndrome: guidelines for research. *Journal of the Royal Society of Medicine* 1991; **84**: 118–22.
14. Manu P, Lane T, Matthews D. The frequency of chronic fatigue syndrome in patients with chronic fatigue. *Annals of Internal Medicine* 1988; **109**: 554–6.
15. Barrett P, Emmins P, Clarke P, Bradley D. Comparison of adverse events associated with the use of mefloquine and combinations of chloroquine and proguanil as antimalarial prophylaxis: postal and telephone survey of travellers. *British Medical Journal* 1996; **313**: 525–8.
16. Bradley D, Warhurst D. Malaria prophylaxis: guidelines for travellers from Britain. *British Medical Journal* 1995; **310**: 709–14.
17. Department of Health. *Health information for overseas travel*. London: HMSO, 1995.
18. WHO. *International travel and health*. Vaccination requirements and health advice. Geneva: World Health Organization, 1997.
19. Payne S, ed. *Medicine, sport and the law*. Oxford: Blackwell Scientific Publications, 1990.
20. Steffen R. Travel medicine—Prevention based on epidemiological data. *Transactions of the Royal Society of Tropical Medicine and Hygiene* 1991; **85**: 156–62.

3.4 Drug abuse

David A. Cowan

Introduction

There are so many powerful medications available today that we have almost come to expect that there is a 'pill for every ill'. People often think that many of these substances can act as ergogenic aids to put one into a supranormal position, the position required by sportsmen and women if they are to succeed.

It may sometimes be difficult to distinguish ethically why the use of some medicines, for instance vitamins, amino acids, and minerals, are considered by sport as permissible whereas the use of others, for instance amphetamine, are not. The improvement in performance that an athlete may require to win an event is often extremely small and less than the level of significance which may be demonstrated by normal methods of measurement. For example, the 4 min mile was broken by Sir Roger Bannister in 1954 with a time of 3 min 59.4 s (before electronic time-keeping). In 1981 Sebastian Coe reduced the record to 3 min 47.33 s and in 1985 Steve Cram beat this with a time of 3 min 46.32 s. Thus Cram's performance was 5.5 per cent better than Bannister's and 0.4 per cent better than Coe's, averaging less than 0.2 per cent per year. In 1993 Noureddine Morceli knocked nearly 2 s off Cram's record with a time of 3 min 44.39 s. Even so, this is less than 1 per cent improvement achieved in 8 years. Therefore, it is hardly surprising that, when a scientific test fails to show a difference between a placebo or a comparator drug in an athletic performance, the sports community fails to consider this as relevant. Less this comparison be misconstrued, it should not be taken to imply that any of these record-breakers have ever misused any drug. Coyle[1] has pointed out that a good training programme is the most effective means of improving physical performance and estimates that, in previously sedentary individuals, improvements of 50 per cent in muscle strength or speed are achievable in long-distance running events.

International Olympic Committee rules

To determine what is and what is not acceptable in sport one must look at the doping regulations; the word 'doping' is the accepted term for drug abuse in sport. The International Olympic Committee (**IOC**) provides a set of doping regulations which have been adopted by all Olympic sports and by most international federations.

The current IOC list of prohibited classes of substances and prohibited methods is given in the Appendix to this chapter. It is divided into three groups:

I. *Prohibited classes of substances*, which comprise the main groups of substances whose administration is banned by most international federations.

II. *Prohibited methods*, which include blood doping and pharmacological, chemical, and physical manipulation.

III. *Classes of drugs subject to certain restrictions*, which cover additional classes controlled by certain sports, for example alcohol in shooting, or whose use may be permitted only under specially controlled conditions, for example corticosteroids.

Acceptability of drug control programmes

Drug control programmes implemented by most sports governing bodies include the collection and analysis of urine samples from their competitors. Although the great majority of athletes accept the need for controls and indeed wish drug control to succeed, those who are taking banned substances do not wish this use to be detected. In addition, too many people are prepared to sell these substances on the black market and to provide information about their use. The *Underground steroid handbook* circulated in California is just one such example. Korkia and Stimson[2] have explored the extent of anabolic steroid use in Great Britain. They report that the most important sources of information about anabolic steroids were friends, followed by underground handbooks and dealers.

At present, urine is collected in drug controls to determine whether a substance from any of the IOC banned classes may have been taken, but there is much discussion about collecting blood from athletes. Although in order to ensure that a valid sample has been collected most protocols require that the athlete be observed providing the urine sample, the collection is otherwise non-invasive and may be collected by sampling officers who have no medical training.

Effectiveness of analytical methods

Some indication of what may be detected is apparent by inspecting the findings of IOC accredited laboratories (Table 1). These figures do not necessarily represent the scale of misuse. Most of the samples

Table 1 IOC accredited laboratories:
(a) Summary of samples analysed 1986 to 1995

Year	Number of samples	Number of negative samples	Number of analytically positive A-samples	Percentage	No. of laboratories
1986	32 982	32 359	623	1.89	18
1987	37 882	37 028	854	2.25	21
1988	47 069	45 916	1153	2.45	20
1989	52 371	51 165	1206	2.30	20
1990	71 341	70 409	932	1.31	21
1991	84 088	83 283	805	0.96	21
1992	87 808	86 815	993	1.13	23
1993	89 166	87 944	1222	1.37	23
1994	93 680	92 402	1278	1.36	24
1995	93 938	92 422	1516	1.61	24

(b) Summary of identified substances 1986 to 1995

Year	Stimulants		Narcotics		Anabolic steroids		β-Blockers		Diuretics		Masking agents		Peptide hormones		Others	
		%		%		%		%		%		%		%		%
1986	177	26.3	23	3.4	439	65.3	31	4.6	2	0.3	—	—				
1987	300	31.9	55	5.8	521	55.4	32	3.4	9	1.0	24	2.6				
1988	420	31.0	58	4.3	791	58.5	8	0.6	57	4.2	19	1.4				
1989	508	40.4	76	6.1	611	48.6	6	0.5	45	3.6	10	0.8				
1990	340	32.0	62	5.8	579	54.4	8	0.8	37	3.5	6	0.6	1	0.1	31	2.9
1991	221	23.9	72	7.8	552	59.7	10	1.1	47	5.1	1	0.1	1	0.1	21	2.3
1992	277	22.1	102	8.2	717	57.3	12	1.0	70	5.6	22	1.8	4	0.3	47	3.8
1993	331	22.8	46	3.2	940	64.7	11	0.9	65	4.5	7	0.4	4	0.3	48	3.3
1994	347	24.0	42	2.9	891	61.6	15	1.0	63	4.4	8	0.6	3	0.2	77	5.3
1995	310	18.9	34	2.1	986	60.2	14	0.9	59	3.6	3	0.2	9	0.5	224	13.7

NB Some samples contain more than one substance from banned classes.

have been collected at competitions and may be biased by the sampling protocol, for example, by sampling athletes coming in first, second, and third for one event. The detectability of the substance depends not only on the analytical technique employed and the limit of detection of the substance but also on its elimination profile, which may be represented by the plasma half-life, and on its formulation. For example, cocaine has a plasma half-life of about 1 h, caffeine has a plasma half-life of about 3.5 h, whereas an oily injection of a nandrolone ester has a half-life of about 22 days.

The Medical Commission of the International Olympic Committee (IOC) has stated that it wishes to control those drugs which may be harmful when misused and to do this with the minimum interference to their normal therapeutic use. Far more drugs are permitted than are banned; this is very different from the sport of horse racing where nearly everything that is not a normal nutrient is banned.

The number of samples collected worldwide has increased over the last few years but seems to have reached a plateau of less than 94 000, representing only a very small proportion of athletes in top-level sport. Approximately 1 to 2.5 per cent of the samples analysed have been found to contain one or more substances from the banned classes. The commonest group of banned substances detected has been the anabolic steroids, with testosterone being the commonest substance in that group and nandrolone the second most common over the last 5 years. The ephedrines are the most frequently found

substances in the stimulant category. It should be noted that β-blockers are controlled only in certain sports and hence the figures relating to their finding depends on whether participants in those sports have been tested. Cannabis is the most commonly found substance in the 'others' category and is controlled only in certain sports.

Performance-enhancing effects of the substances controlled in sports

For convenience, the performance-enhancing effects and the side-effects of the substances controlled in sport will be discussed grouped under the various IOC categories. In addition, a brief description of the methods of detection currently used by IOC accredited laboratories will be given. Although the categories are intended to represent pharmacological classifications, they are very broad descriptions.

Analytical methods

The analytical methods used to detect and to confirm the presence of substances banned in sport rely very much on chromatography to separate the various components extracted from the urine sample. Immunoassays are sometimes used for certain substances, such as benzoylecgonine (the metabolite of cocaine) and cannabinoids, and at present are the only suitable methods for the detection of the protein hormones. With the exception of human chorionic gonadotrophin, the IOC requires the use of mass spectrometry to confirm the presence of the substance before issuing a formal analytical report. Unless the IOC accepts other confirmatory methods, or advances in mass spectrometry make it possible to use the technique for protein hormones, the presence of most substances from this class cannot be confirmed.

Prohibited classes of substances

Stimulants

The first of the IOC categories of the prohibited classes of substances is called 'stimulants'. Examples of substances which are included in this category are cocaine, amphetamine, the ephedrines, and caffeine.

Cocaine

Despite cocaine being a widely used recreational drug, there appears to be no reported studies of its effects on athletic performance. The drug acts on catecholaminergic neurones in preventing reuptake of both noradrenaline and dopamine.[3] The physiological effects are similar to those of amphetamine, but the mood effects are more profound.

Immunoassays for benzoylecgonine, the main metabolite found in urine, are the most convenient methods to screen for cocaine since they can be applied directly to a small volume of urine (0.1 ml). Any sample which fails this screen are submitted for confirmatory analysis using gas chromatography coupled to mass spectrometry (**GC–MS**). For this confirmation, a somewhat complex extraction and chemical derivatization procedure has to be followed to make the sample suitable for GC–MS analysis.

Amphetamine

The term amphetamine is often used to describe amphetamine itself and the homologous substances methylamphetamine, dimethylamphetamine, benzylamphetamine, and other substances known as 'masked amphetamines' which are metabolized to amphetamine in the body. The term is sometimes used incorrectly to describe ephedrine and its homologues (which are discussed in a separate paragraph below) probably because some immunoassays for amphetamine crossreact with the ephedrines, thus giving rise to possible misinterpretation of the results.

Amphetamines have been shown to enhance certain sporting performances. For example, amphetamines administered 2 to 3 h before a swimming competition produced an increase in time to exhaustion and a small but consistent increase in speed.[4] Other studies have shown that sprinting speed and muscular strength are unaffected by amphetamines.[5,6] Large doses in rats[7] (10 to 20 mg/kg) have been effective in increasing time to exhaustion in swimming, whereas doses of 1.25 to 5 mg/kg have produced no significant effect. Treadmill endurance tests have given similar results.[8]

Amphetamine can be detected readily by extracting the urine with diethyl ether at pH 13 and by gas chromatography of the extract using a nitrogen-selective detector.

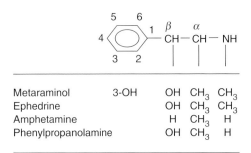

Metaraminol	3-OH	OH	CH₃	CH₃
Ephedrine		OH	CH₃	CH₃
Amphetamine		H	CH₃	H
Phenylpropanolamine		OH	CH₃	H

Fig. 1 Structure–activity relationship of ephedrine.

Ephedrines

Although most people accept the need to control drugs such as amphetamine and cocaine, the necessity for restricting the use of the 'ephedrines', namely ephedrine, pseudoephedrine, and phenylpropanolamine, is frequently questioned. These substances are readily available in most countries in over-the-counter 'cold remedies' because the national regulatory authorities consider their use by the public to be relatively safe.

Consideration of the structure–activity relationship of the ephedrines aids the understanding of their effects as sympathomimetics relative to the endogenous neurotransmitter noradrenaline.[9] Substitution at the amino terminal group (Fig. 1) increases β-receptor activity, and the smaller the substituent the greater is the selectivity for α-receptor activity. However, N-methylation increases the potency compared with the corresponding primary amine. The presence of hydroxyl groups in the 3 and 4 positions of the aromatic ring results in maximal α- and β-receptor activity. The absence of the polar phenolic hydroxyl groups permit the compound to cross the blood–brain barrier more readily, producing greater central activity. Thus, amphetamine, ephedrine, and phenylpropanolamine exhibit considerable central nervous system activity.

Substitution on the α-carbon atom blocks metabolism by monoamine oxidase, allowing these sympathomimetics to persist in nerve terminals and hence prolonging the stimulation of the release of noradrenaline from storage sites. A hydroxyl group on the β-carbon atom tends to decrease central nervous system activity because of reduced lipid solubility. Thus phenylpropanolamine, which is probably the weakest sympathomimetic of the ephedrines, has more marked α-activity than β-activity because it is a primary amine and because of the hydroxyl group on the β-carbon atom. It has considerable, but often underestimated, central nervous system activity because of the absence of aromatic substituents. However, this activity is less than that of amphetamine because of the β-substituent which reduces the lipid solubility. Phenylpropanolamine induces hypertension characterized by an increase in cardiac output, peripheral vascular resistance, stroke volume, ejection fraction, and a decrease in heart rate.[10] Even in normal individuals a typical dose of 75 mg can have a significant effect, severe hypertension is common after excessive dose and may result in hypertensive encephalopathy, intracerebral haemorrhage, and death.

The ephedrines can be readily detected, like amphetamine, by extracting the urine with diethyl ether at pH 13 and by gas chromatography of the extract using a nitrogen-selective detector. IOC accredited laboratories are advised to ignore small concentrations of ephedrines provided that the pH and specific gravity of the urine is within normal limits.

Caffeine

There is a lack of good dose–response data for caffeine, and the evidence for its stimulant effect on the central nervous system is conflicting. However, caffeine has been shown to have direct effects on muscle contraction during exercise *in vivo*. At low stimulation frequencies, increased muscle tension was observed 1 h after 50 mg caffeine was administered orally, but there was no apparent change in endurance time.[11] Most studies have used a single dose of caffeine ranging from less than 1 mg/kg to more than 14 mg/kg. Caffeine tolerance may be an explanation of the conflicting results. However, considering the published data, doses greater than 400 mg are probably capable of increasing endurance and physical performance.

The mechanism for its action is also not certain. Caffeine has been shown to increase calcium permeability which is essential for muscle contraction.[12] Its action on the central nervous system may mask fatigue and increase the capacity for sustained intellectual effort.[13] Although it may decrease reaction time, fine motor co-ordination and the ability to judge distance may be impaired. It stimulates the medullary respiratory centres but may produce emesis via the central nervous system.

Caffeine significantly increases the availability of free fatty acids from fat by lipolysis.[14,15] When available, fatty acids are the primary substrate for aerobic metabolism, thus sparing glycogen. Unlike fatty acids, glucose (produced from glycogen) can be metabolized either aerobically or anaerobically, and thus the glycogen spared by the alternative metabolism of fatty acids can be made available at a time when the oxygen supply to the tissues is insufficient for aerobic metabolism.[16]

Caffeine has been shown *in vitro* to produce a translocation of intracellular calcium to inhibit phosphodiesterase, thus producing an accumulation of cyclic nucleotides, and also to block the actions of adenosine at adenosine receptors. Among other actions, adenosine strongly inhibits hormone-induced lipolysis, reduces the release of noradrenaline from nerve endings, and may inhibit the release of excitatory neurotransmitters in the central nervous system. The concentrations of caffeine required for the translocation of intracellular calcium and the inhibition of phosphodiesterase are greater than are thought to be achieved from a therapeutic dose.[17] Thus this leaves the blocking of the adenosine receptor as at least one of the most likely routes for caffeine's actions.

The IOC makes it an offence to have a urinary caffeine concentration greater than 12 mg/l (60 μmol/l) and this may be exceeded with a 400 mg dose. Only about 1 per cent of administered caffeine appears in the urine unchanged; most is metabolized in the liver. A significant proportion of caffeine is *N*-demethylated to form dimethylxanthines, and the concurrent administration of a dimethylxanthine, such as theophylline or theobromine (found in chocolate), may reduce the metabolism of caffeine.[18] The concentration of caffeine in urine is readily measured by high-pressure liquid chromatography (**HPLC**) with ultraviolet (**UV**) detection at 280 nm.

β₂-Agonists

The IOC Medical Commission recognizes that the choice of medication in the treatment of asthma and respiratory ailments has posed many problems. Some years ago, ephedrine and related substances were administered quite frequently. However, these substances are prohibited because they are classed in the category of 'sympathomimetic amines' and therefore considered as stimulants. However, the IOC permits the use of certain specified β₂-agonists in aerosol form, namely salbutamol, salmeterol, and terbutaline. These are substances which act relatively selectively at the β₂-adrenergic receptor sites in human bronchial muscle and have relatively little activity at cardiac β₁-adrenoreceptor sites.

Narcotic analgesics

The second category of the prohibited classes of substances is the narcotic analgesics. Narcotic analgesics are not perceived by most people as ergogenic drugs. The chronic use of narcotics might seem to lead to an impairment of athletic skills. However, the available evidence does not support this assumption. No significant difference has been demonstrated between age-matched controls and addicts in tests of motor strength, rapid alternating movements, eye–hand co-ordination, visual perception, and cognitive skills.[19] Encephalins and endorphins are endogenous peptides with potent analgesic activity which bind to the sites in the brain to which morphine and other potent analgesics bind avidly. A correlation between exercise and endorphin activity has been demonstrated.[20] Much of the euphoria experienced by athletes, sometimes known as a 'runner's high', can be explained by a release of some of these endogenous opiates. Individuals who participate in running may even have a type of addiction to these endogenous opiates.[21] On stopping exercising many athletes experience symptoms including anxiety, restlessness, irritability, nervousness, muscle twitching, and sleep disturbances which may be an 'abstinence syndrome'.

According to the IOC Medical Commission there is evidence indicating that narcotic analgesics have been and are being abused in sports and hence should banned. The IOC also justifies their ban on the use of these substances because of the international restrictions affecting the movement of these compounds, and comments that their action is in line with the regulations and recommendations of the World Health Organization (**WHO**) regarding narcotics.

Many of the narcotic analgesics appear in the urine as glucuronic acid conjugates and some (for example, morphine) are amphoteric aminophenols which require hydrolysis of the conjugate before extraction with a moderately polar solvent such as ether plus propan-2-ol (9:1 v/v) at pH 9.2 to 9.5 which is close to the isoelectric point of the aminophenols. Production of chemical derivatives is usually necessary to facilitate good chromatography, and the derivatized extract may be screened by gas chromatography with a nitrogen-selective detector or by GC–MS with selected ion monitoring (**SIM**).

Anabolic agents

Anabolic androgenic steroids

Although the misuse of anabolic steroids was originally thought to be a problem unique to competitive heavy sports, there is increasing evidence that they are being misused in endurance events and increasingly by body builders. A survey in the United States[22] revealed that more than 6 per cent of high-school males had taken anabolic steroids to make them appear more masculine to their girl friends.

Testosterone is the principal biologically active androgen circulating in the blood of both men and women, although women pro-

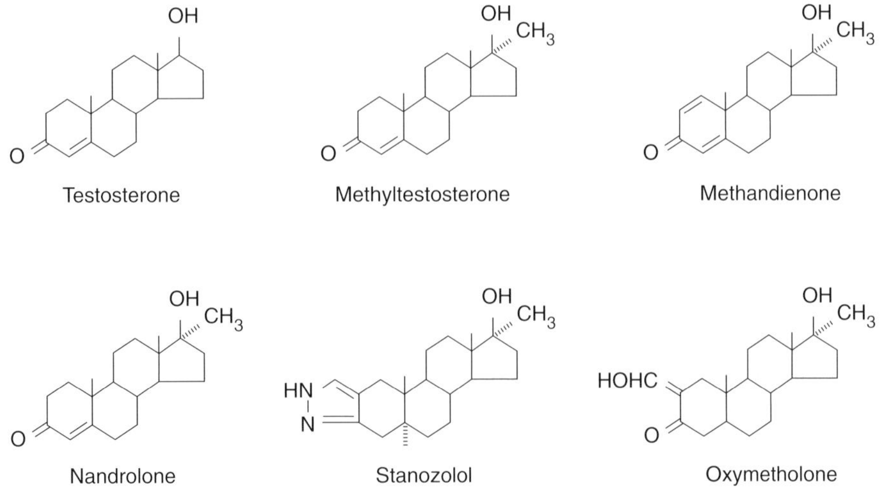

Fig. 2 Structure of testosterone and some synthetic anabolic steroids.

duce about one-twentieth of the amount produced by men. The 5α-reduced form of testosterone is a more potent androgen than testosterone. The reduction predominates in androgen-dependent tissues, for example the prostate, seminal vesicles, and epididymus. Gonadotrophin–releasing hormone (**GnRH**) stimulates the release of luteinizing hormone (**LH**) which, in turn, stimulates the production of testosterone. Circulating androgens exert a negative feedback on the adenohypophysis and hypothalamus, suppressing LH and GnRH release and thus controlling the production of the androgens.

Many chemical modifications of testosterone (Fig. 2) have been attempted to alter the anabolic to androgenic ratio (or more muscle per whisker) in order to reduce the virilizing androgenic effects or to make the substance orally active. Alkylation at the C17 position reduces hepatic oxidative metabolism and makes the compound orally active, for example 17α-methyltestosterone and methandienone. Removal of the methyl group at C10 produces nandrolone (19-nortestosterone) which exhibits more anabolic than androgenic activity. Other modifications to increase the anabolic-to-androgenic ratio are the inclusion of a second double bond in the A ring (for example methandienone), attachment of a pyrazole ring to the A ring (stanozolol), or a hydroxymethylene group at C2 (oxymetholone). Despite these modifications, it has not proved possible to remove the androgenic (virilizing) effects from these synthetic steroids which is why this group is called the anabolic androgenic steroids.

Many studies attempting to demonstrate a positive effect of anabolic steroids on sports performance have been conducted over the last 40 years and the reader should consult one of the number of reviews on the subject for more details.[23-25] Perhaps the firmest conclusion that can be drawn from these studies is that if anabolic steroids do have any effect, then their effect is small. Although fluid retention, and hence increase in bodyweight, may be one of the first effects observed with anabolic steroid use, some studies have shown a significant increase in body size and weight which is not due to fluid retention. These studies have observed experienced weight-lifters who continued training while taking anabolic steroids and whose strength was also shown to increase more than when they were not taking anabolic steroids. A recent study by Bhasin *et al.*[26]

in which the independent effects of testosterone and exercise were controlled, reached the conclusion that supraphysiological doses of testosterone, especially when combined with strength training, increase fat-free mass and muscle size in normal men. Generally, the actions of anabolic steroids that would benefit the athlete are due to anabolic, anticatabolic, and motivational or behavioural effects. Athletes can develop a negative nitrogen balance during excessive training, and anabolic steroids may block the effects of the glucocorticoids released from the adrenal cortex in response to the stress of training. Anabolic steroids stimulate erythropoiesis, but it is questionable whether the effect is sufficiently significant to enhance performance. However, now that erythropoietin produced by recombinant DNA technology is readily available, despite being more expensive, this is more likely to be misused to increase haemoglobin production.

Adverse effects of anabolic steroids include testicular atrophy, sterility, virilization, and gynaecomastia, and in adolescents premature closure of the epiphyses resulting in permanent short stature. Dermatological disorders include oily skin and acne, hirsutism, and alopecia.[27] Behavioural effects,[28] including major depression or psychosis,[29] may occur quite frequently. Choi *et al.*[30] have reviewed the subject. In addition, common adverse effects in females include amenorrhoea, hirsutism, enlargement of the larynx with consequent deepening of the voice, clitoral hypertrophy, and breast atrophy.[31] Anabolic steroids decrease serum high-density lipoprotein cholesterol (**HDL-C**) and either do not change or increase low-density lipoprotein cholesterol (**LDL-C**). Thus, the LDL-C to HDL-C ratio will usually increase, and this is a cardiovascular risk factor.[32] Cases of stroke and infarction may reflect an altered thrombogenesis caused by the use of anabolic steroids.[33] These and other adverse effects of anabolic steroids are discussed in the review by Hickson *et al.*[34]

Testosterone

At present, only an untimed urine sample is available from an athlete to determine whether doping with a prohibited substance has occurred. All that is required for detecting the use of synthetic anabolic steroids is the unequivocal identification of the parent compound or its diagnostic metabolite in the urine. In the case of natural hormones, where they or their metabolites are normally present in urine, detection depends on the effect of administration upon the system controlling their endogenous secretion and the consequent alterations in the pattern of steroid excretion. The administration of supraphysiological doses of testosterone to men results in the inhibition of LH release and, as a consequence, inhibition of the secretion of testosterone and other testicular steroids. The resulting decrease in the urinary excretion rates of LH and its 17-epimer epitestosterone (17α-hydroxyandrost-4-en-3-one), together with the increase in that of testosterone (from the injection), is reflected by elevated ratios of testosterone to epitestosterone[35] and testosterone to LH[36] in urine. A testosterone to epitestosterone ratio greater than 6 is not allowed under the regulations of the IOC (see Appendix) and may result in disqualification of the athlete and disciplinary action. It is possible to evade detection by the administration of combined testosterone–epitestosterone preparations. In normal men, 30 times more testosterone compared with epitestosterone is produced endogenously, but only 1 per cent of testosterone is excreted unchanged compared with 30 per cent of epitestosterone, resulting in a urinary testosterone to epitestosterone ratio of unity. It follows that athletes could take supraphysiological doses of testosterone with epitestosterone in a ratio of about 30:1 and still maintain a normal urinary ratio. Franke and Berendonk[37] report that VEB Jenapharm have produced preparations of epitestosterone propionate since 1983. Since there is no apparent pharmaceutical use for epitestosterone, one is left with the conclusion that this former East German state-owned pharmaceutical company was producing the formulation solely to help beat doping-control tests. In comparison with the testosterone to epitestosterone ratios, the testosterone to LH ratios would be expected to be abnormally high, and in the United Kingdom the ratio of testosterone to LH is measured in addition to that of testosterone to epitestosterone. LH measurement may also be important in the detection of the administration of dihydrotestosterone, which is a particularly active metabolite of testosterone.[38]

Some male athletes who have denied using testosterone have produced testosterone to epitestosterone ratios between 6 and 9.[39] The possibility that these individuals excrete smaller quantities of epitestosterone, perhaps due to an enzymatic deficiency in their biosynthesis of epitestosterone, must not be excluded. These athletes would be expected to have normal urinary testosterone to LH ratios because the homeostatic mechanism tends to keep the concentration of testosterone in the blood constant. A dynamic endocrine test[40,41] has been developed to help to distinguish whether an individual with an abnormally large testosterone to epitestosterone ratio may be a biological outlier or has administered testosterone. The IOC now requires a review of previous tests, subsequent tests, and any results of endocrine investigations, before a sample is declared positive. The IOC states that if previous tests are not available, the athlete should be tested unannounced at least once each month for 3 months.

Dihydrotestosterone

Administration of dihydrotestosterone, an active metabolite of testosterone, also inhibits LH secretion,[42] but, because of the reduced excretion of testosterone as well as of LH and epitestosterone, it is unlikely to alter these ratios significantly. Thus dihydrotestosterone is a likely candidate for use by athletes. Furthermore, dihydrotestosterone can be regarded as more potent than testosterone since it is

known to bind more strongly than testosterone to the androgen receptor.[43]

Under normal circumstances the concentration of circulating testosterone in men is as much as 10 times that of dihydrotestosterone, so that in skeletal muscle testosterone is the predominant ligand bound to the androgen receptor. In contrast with muscle, sexual tissue contains much greater 5α-reductase activity which converts testosterone to dihydrotestosterone. In these tissues dihydrotestosterone is bound by the receptor, thus amplifying the effect of circulating testosterone. Therefore large plasma concentrations of dihydrotestosterone (for example following dihydrotestosterone administration) would have a greater effect in muscle compared with sexual tissue, thereby giving dihydrotestosterone a greater myotrophic to androgenic ratio than testosterone.

The IOC has not, as yet, named a specific test as evidence of dihydrotestosterone administration. However, several workers have proposed methods based on the relative concentrations of dihydrotestosterone, 5α-androstane-3α,17β-diol (3α-diol), and 5α-androstane-3β,17β-diol (3β-diol), compared with that of testosterone, 5β-androstane-3α,17β-diol (5β-diol), epitestosterone, and LH.[44,45]

β₂-Agonists

The IOC states that, when administered systemically, β₂-agonists may have powerful anabolic effects. Clenbuterol is a β-selective adrenergic agonist which is probably the most potent of this group. It has been shown to stimulate the deposition of body protein and inhibit that of body fat in animals.[46] It has a very small therapeutic dose in man (10 to 40 μg/day) and a relatively long half-life of about 30 h. Its anabolic and antilipogenic actions are mechanistically distinct, and there is growing concern that it is being misused in sport for its anabolic properties. One study[47] on young men administered salbutamol in a slow-release formulation showed a significant increase in strength of certain skeletal muscles.

Diuretics

The most obvious reason why athletes may misuse diuretics is to lose body fluid and hence bodyweight rapidly in order to be able to compete in a lower weight category in those sports where weight is controlled, for instance judo, boxing, and rowing. The second and somewhat more obscure reason for misusing diuretics is to reduce the urinary concentration of drugs through rapid diuresis to decrease the likelihood of detection of those drugs in a urine test. Diuretics listed as examples by the IOC include the potent loop-diuretics frusemide and bumetanide as well as thiazide diuretics such as hydrochlorothiazide and benzthiazide. These substances cause a pronounced diuresis resulting in a rapid loss of body water. The carbonic anhydrase inhibitor diuretic acetazolamide also increases urinary pH and will thereby reduce the excretion rate of basic drugs. For example, the peak excretion rate of the stimulant drug phentermine is delayed from the normal 2 to 4 h after administration to 30 to 36 h.[48,49] There appears to be no study which indicates any enhancement in performance as a result of diuretic use.

Despite their effect on reducing the concentration of other substances in urine, the diuretics producing this effect are readily detectable. The urine can be extracted with an organic solvent at acid and also at alkaline pH, and the extracts combined and analysed by HPLC, or the extract can be chemically derivatized and analysed by GC–MS. Alternatively, a solid-phase extraction of the urine can be used followed by derivatization or by direct extractive alkylation and GC–MS analysis.[50]

Peptide and glycoprotein hormones and analogues

In 1989 the IOC Medical Commission introduced the new prohibited class of 'peptide hormones and analogues' which include human chorionic gonadotrophin (hCG) and related compounds, adrenocorticotrophic hormone (ACTH), human growth hormone (hGH), all the releasing factors of these listed hormones, and erythropoietin. Most of these hormones are produced endogenously, and several are now produced synthetically using recombinant DNA technology. In each case, the administered substance is identical with that produced naturally. Currently there are no IOC approved definitive tests for these hormones, but highly specific immunoassays combined with suitable purification techniques may be sufficient to warrant IOC approval. Indeed, the IOC in their Medical Code[51] state that a validated immunoassay may be used to detect and to quantify hCG and that a second different immunoassay is required for confirmation. Kicman and Cowan have reviewed the misuse and detection of peptide hormones in sport.[52]

Human chorionic gonadotrophin

Human chorionic gonadotrophin is a glycopolypeptide secreted in large amounts by the developing placenta (chorion) and by certain types of tumour. Although hCG and LH are immunologically distinct, these two gonadotrophins have essentially the same biological action at the cellular level. The approximate molecular weight of hCG is 37 000 Da and that of LH is 28 000 Da with very similar α-subunits in primary structure. The hCG α-subunit consists of 92 amino acids and has two carbohydrate moieties which are branch-chained to asparagine residues, giving an average total molecular weight of 14 500 Da. The β-subunit of hCG consists of 145 amino-acid residues with 30 additional residues at the C-terminal region compared with the β-subunit of LH. It is within this region that a specific antigenic determinant is located which allows for immunological distinction as opposed to biological distinction between hCG and LH.

Attached to the β-hCG subunit are six carbohydrate moieties, giving an average total molecular weight of 22 000 Da. Two branch-chain moieties are linked to asparagines and four are linked to serines within the unique C-terminal peptide region.

The complete molecule has eight carbohydrate moieties in total, making it approximately 30 per cent by weight in carbohydrate content. Each moiety contains two attached N-acetylneuraminic acid groups, which is a sialic acid, giving rise to 16 sialic acids per hCG molecule. However, there is microheterogeneity in the carbohydrate content of the gonadotrophins which have not yet been fully characterized, hence the total number of sialic acid groups per hCG molecule will only represent an average amount and this number will vary between reported studies. The greater number of sialic acid groups on hCG leads to a greater ionization constant and hence a smaller pI value when compared with the other gonadotrophins. The pI of hCG is about 3.5 and that of LH about 5.5.

Small concentrations of hCG or hCG-like material have been measured in pituitary and urine extracts, and have also been found in the serum of normal men (less than 60 years of age, < 1.3 IU/l; more than 60 years < 2.3 IU/l) and non-pregnant women (premenopausal, < 1.0 IU/l; postmenopausal, < 4.8 IU/l).[53] The biochemical and endocrinological features of hCG, together with its detection and misuse in sport, have been reviewed by Kicman et al.[54]

In the male, LH and hCG interact with specific target receptors on the surface of Leydig cells in the testes. The hormone-bound receptors activate cyclic AMP and calcium-ion secondary messenger systems which, in turn, activate various protein kinases, finally stimulating steroidogenesis and protein synthesis. Phospholipid metabolites, in particular the leukotrienes, may also act as secondary messengers in LH/hCG-induced steroidogenesis. hCG stimulation of testicular steroidogenesis in healthy adult men is very rapid. A 50 per cent increase in plasma testosterone concentration has been measured 2 h after an intramuscular injection of 6000 IU of hCG.[55] However, there is no direct correlation between plasma concentrations of hCG and testosterone; the rise in plasma testosterone is biphasic. Pharmaceutical preparations of hCG may be used by some male athletes to stimulate testosterone production and also to prevent testicular atrophy during and after prolonged courses of androgen administration. The use of pharmaceutical preparations of LH are not as suitable for these purposes because of the much shorter plasma half-life of LH and the small amount supplied per ampoule (for instance 75 IU) compared with hCG (for instance 5000 IU) (1 IU of hCG has approximately the same biological activity as 1 IU of LH). The administration of hCG has been banned by the IOC since December 1987.

Various immunometric assays are available to measure the presence of hCG in urine. The use of an ultrafiltration method may be suitable as part of a confirmatory procedure.[56] However, at present, it is not possible to determine by assaying hCG in urine whether a concentration greater than normal has arisen from hCG administration or from pregnancy or an hCG-secreting tumour.

Growth hormone

Human growth hormone is secreted episodically by the somatotrope cells of the anterior pituitary. The major physiological form is a single-chain peptide with a molecular weight of 22 000 (22 kDa) consisting of 191 amino-acid residues and two intrachain disulphide bridges. Several variants of hGH also exist, possibly due to artefacts generated by proteolytic digestion in the pituitary, enzymatic processing, and the formation of dimers and oligomers. Also a 20 kDa form exists which may result from variation in the processing of the mRNA precursor.

No studies to date have shown an increase in strength or endurance in association with growth hormone (GH) administration.[57,58] Prior to puberty, excessive GH gives rise to gigantism. The sufferer tends to die in early adult life from infection, debility, or hypopituitarism. After puberty and closure of the long bones, excessive GH can cause acromegaly with characteristic features such as spade-like hands, lengthened and thickened jaw, coarse and leathery skin, increase in coarse body hair, and enlargement of the heart.[59]

GH release is stimulated by a variety of substances including GH-releasing hormone, noradrenaline, adrenaline (and hence stress), levodopa, arginine, and insulin (hypoglycaemia), and by sleep. Blood concentrations are reduced by somatostatin and by insulin-like growth factor-1 (**IGF**-1).

The mechanism of action of GH is far from fully understood. The GH receptor is widely distributed throughout the body and has been identified on the cell-surface membranes of hepatocytes, adipocytes, fibroblasts, lymphocytes, and chondrocytes.[60] GH has been shown, using rat hepatocytes, to cause phosphorylation of certain proteins. This has been demonstrated to be important for the proliferation, differentiation, and growth processes, and can alter enzymatic activity and cytoskeletal mobility and may modulate events in the nucleus such as gene expression.

GH has a short half-life of 20 to 30 min. The production of growth hormone currently utilizes recombinant DNA technology and although initially it was not an exact duplication, with the end amino acid being methionine, it now has an identical sequence. Thus it would be extremely difficult to devise a test based on the detection of GH itself to prove that it had been administered in contravention of the rules of sport. Following acute GH administration, serum insulin-like growth factor (IGF) binding protein 2 (**IGFBP**-2) has been shown[61] to decrease and the ratios of serum IGF-1/IGFBP-2 and IGFBP-3/IGFBP-2 to increase. These ratios may form the basis of a test to detect GH administration in sport. However, many factors affect endogenous GH production. A large multicentre study, known as GH-2000, funded by the European Union and by the IOC led by Professor Peter Sonksen at St Thomas' Hospital in London, aims to develop a test in time for the Olympic Games in 2000 to be held in Sydney, Australia.

Erythropoietin

Erythropoietin is an acidic glycoprotein hormone mainly secreted by the kidney consisting of a 166 amino-acid chain. It has an estimated molecular weight of 34 000 Da and exists in two distinguishable forms, α and β. The α and β forms have a carbohydrate content of approximately 31 per cent and 24 per cent by weight, respectively. These two forms of erythropoietin have similar biological and antigenic properties.

Erythropoietin exerts a specific-receptor-mediated effect on committed erythroid stem cells, inducing these target cells (colony-forming unit or erythroid) to proliferate approximately 30 times into mature erythrocytes. The mechanism by which erythropoietin causes its target cells to undergo division and maturation is not fully understood, although high- and low-affinity receptors have been identified and signal transduction may involve Ca^{2+} and arachidonic acid. Erythropoietin production is regulated by the relative amount of oxygen in arterial blood; serum erythropoietin concentration increases in hypoxia and decreases in hyperoxia. Nevertheless, erythropoiesis is also stimulated by blood loss despite normal arterial oxygen pressure, which has led to the hypothesis that it is tissue oxygen tension, as determined by the supply of and demand for oxygen by cells, which regulates erythrocyte production rather than arterial oxygen *per se*.

The mean serum erythropoietin concentration in normal individuals is 35 IU/l, whereas individuals with aplastic anaemia may have erythropoietin concentrations up to approximately 3000 IU/l and individuals with anaemia caused by renal disease have erythropoietin concentrations which are abnormally small. However, individuals with polycythaemia vera may have normal or small serum erythropoietin concentrations. Hypopituitarism and hypothyroidism reduce metabolic rate and erythropoiesis.

With the recent success in producing recombinant human erythropoietin, sufficient quantities are now available for patient treatment (for example anaemia due to renal failure) and is obtainable as a licensed product from pharmaceutical manufacturers. Recombinant human erythropoietin is of therapeutic value when endogenous erythropoietin production is less than expected for the degree of haemoglobin and/or the volume of erythrocytes in relation to whole blood (haematocrit), and provided that erythroid progenitors are available. The average dose necessary to maintain the haematocrit between 30 and 36 per cent in anaemic dialysis patients is 50 IU/kg bodyweight administered three times weekly. Recombinant human erythropoietin may also be administered to patients wanting to deposit blood for transfusion during elective surgery.

Erythrocyte production increases dramatically in response to the administration of supraphysiological doses of recombinant human erythropoietin. Maximal oxygen uptake has been shown to increase in healthy individuals who have undergone erythrocyte infusion to induce a state of erythrocythaemia. Therefore athletes may choose to use recombinant human erythropoietin or erythrocyte infusion (blood doping) to increase their oxygen uptake in the hope of improving their endurance capacity and recovery during training and competition. In contrast with patients who constantly require recombinant human erythropoietin replacement therapy, an athlete would only need a short course of recombinant human erythropoietin to gain a possible advantage against fellow competitors. Thus, relative to the expense of recombinant human erythropoietin replacement therapy, the cost of recombinant human erythropoietin abuse to gain a short-term sporting advantage would be small.

Erythropoietin has minimal toxicity and has been used in clinical trials up to doses of 500 IU/kg/day. Recombinant human erythropoietin appears not to be immunogenic. Some patients report a sensation of cold and ache in the long bones 1 to 2 h after recombinant human erythropoietin administration. In patients receiving recombinant human erythropoietin there may be an increase in peripheral vascular resistance which may lead to hypertension. In athletes who induce erythrocythaemia by recombinant human erythropoietin administration or blood doping, there is a danger of thrombosis and haemorrhage.

Although erythropoietin administration is included in an IOC banned doping class and blood doping in a doping method, currently there is no IOC approved confirmatory procedure to detect these practices. To detect erythropoietin doping simply by determining abnormally high serum erythropoietin concentrations using specific immunoassay techniques may not be effective due to the short half-life of recombinant human erythropoietin of approximately 4 to 6 h when administered intravenously. Only about 10 per cent of erythropoietin is excreted into the urine. However, as erythropoietin administration or blood doping would be expected to raise erythrocyte count, haemoglobin concentration, and haematocrit, the measurement of these parameters could be used as criteria for the detection of both types of practice. Additionally, a serum erythropoietin concentration below or above the normal range could be used as an additional criterion in the detection of erythropoietin administration or blood doping. Nevertheless, this profile may be indistinguishable from that of athletes who have undergone high-altitude training. In any case, the informed athlete would know that the effect of erythropoietin administration would result in a sustained increase in the erythrocyte population long after administration had ceased, since the average life of erythrocytes is about 110 days. The detection of erythropoietin administration by determining abnormal erythropoietin concentrations, whether in blood or urine, may therefore be difficult because the athlete could take steps to avoid giving a sample while abnormal concentrations are present in his or her body, for example by going on 'holiday'. An approach which shows great promise has been described by Gareau et al.[62] Their proposed method is based on the determination of the ratio of soluble transferrin receptor to ferritin in blood. This appears to remain significantly greater than basal for 2 weeks post-erythropoietin administration and thus overcomes the difficulty of detection caused by the very short half-life of this glycoprotein.

Adrenocorticotrophic hormone

Adrenocorticotrophic hormone (**ACTH**) is a polypeptide released from the corticotrope cells of the anterior pituitary, resulting in stimulation of the secretion of adrenal androgens as well as the glucocorticoids. It is composed of 39 amino acids and has a molecular weight of 4500 Da. However, only the first 24 N-terminal amino acids are necessary for full biological activity, and it is this synthesized form, called tetracosactrin (for example Synacthen®), which is used for diagnostic purposes. Pituitary-derived ACTH (for example Acthar®) is now only supplied in the United Kingdom as an unlicensed product.

The non-therapeutic administration of corticosteroids prompted the IOC Medical Commission to ban their use except for topical treatment, inhalation therapy, and local or intra-articular injections. Therapeutic use of corticosteroids may be particularly beneficial in the treatment of local inflammation and pain associated with sports injuries, but such treatment may cause some entry of these drugs into the bloodstream. However, any systemic effects are likely to be insignificant except with topical applications where treatment can occasionally result in suppression of the hypothalamic–pituitary–adrenal axis and Cushing's syndrome.[63] As ACTH stimulates the secretion of cortisol and other glucocorticoids into the systemic circulation, the administration of ACTH is considered to be equivalent to an oral, intramuscular, or intravenous application of a corticosteroid and hence is banned.

The predominant therapeutic use of tetracosactrin is for the differential diagnosis of adrenocortical failure. However, ACTH replacement therapy is not suitable in the treatment of secondary adrenocortical insufficiency, not least because tetracosactrin is not orally active, and in such cases treatment is with cortisol or a synthetic analogue (for example prednisolone). Tetracosactrin is also used for short-term therapy to induce an excessive secretion of glucocorticoids rapidly, for example in severe asthma attacks. The depot form of tetracosactrin is used in cases where the results of short-term stimulation with tetracosactrin for the diagnosis of adrenocortical insufficiency has been inconclusive or in patients who are unable to tolerate glucocorticoid therapy.

Currently, there is no IOC approved method to detect ACTH administration; detection of ACTH is a complex problem as it is particularly liable to rapid degradation by endopeptidases present in the blood, resulting in the excretion of inactive oligopeptides. Hence the development of a confirmatory test using urine samples is unlikely. However, with the future possibility of blood as well as urine samples being collected from athletes, detection could be based on chromatographic methods followed by immunoassays to distinguish between serum ACTH and tetracosactrin. Clinically, special steps are taken for analytes such as ACTH and tetracosactrin, which are susceptible to enzyme degradation in serum or plasma. Plasma is immediately separated in a refrigerated centrifuge and then stored at –20 °C, or lower, throughout storage and transport and only thawed prior to analysis. Clearly, this approach is not practical for collecting samples at competitions and training venues, and alternative procedures for maintaining stability need to be investigated. A more feasible approach could include the presence of enzyme inhibitors in the sample collection tube together with reducing agents such as dithiothreitol, since ACTH is also particularly susceptible to oxidation at methionine residues.[64]

Releasing factors

These are neuropeptide hormones secreted episodically by the hypothalamus, which in turn regulate the secretion of LH, hGH, and ACTH by the anterior pituitary. A single administration of any of these releasing hormones or their analogues stimulates a prompt dose-related response in the secretion of the corresponding pituitary hormone. The response is of short duration and, to maintain the effect, the dose and timing of repeated administration is critical as sustained high concentrations of GnRH or corticotrophin-releasing factor (**CRF**) suppress the release of the associated pituitary hormones due to the down-regulation of receptors. Thus the chronic use of GnRH and CRF are disadvantageous to the athlete as the pituitary requires the pulsatile release of these hormones to respond normally. None the less, long-term pulsatile administration of GnRH or one of its analogues could be used by male athletes in an attempt to stimulate and maintain testicular function during and after prolonged courses of androgen administration. In contrast with GnRH and CRF, continued exposure to GH-releasing hormone causes only partial down-regulation of the corresponding receptors, probably because of the continuing pulsatile secretion of somatostatin. With the future availability of GH-releasing hormone for therapeutic use, athletes may administer supraphysiological doses of this releasing hormone or its more potent analogues to increase their secretion of GH.

Doping methods

Blood doping

Following the revelations after the Olympic Games in Los Angeles in 1984 that the United States cycling team had received blood transfusions, the practice of blood doping in sport was banned by the IOC. Although older studies failed to show clear improvements in performance, this may be because refrigerated citrated blood deteriorates whereas modern procedures enable the freezing of red blood cells to preserve them indefinitely with minimum deterioration. Following infusion of 900 ml of autologous red blood cells collected some 7 weeks previously, highly trained élite athletes experienced increases in run time to exhaustion (35 per cent), $\dot{V}O_2$max (5 per cent), and haemoglobin (7 per cent).[65]

Any form of induced erythrocythaemia increases the risk (like the clinical condition of polycythaemia), of hypertension, congestive heart failure, and stroke.

The detection of heterologous blood doping requires a blood sample and proof that the detected phenotypes differ from those of the individual sampled. In this case, all that may be required is proof of the presence of heterologous erythrocytes. This is the principle employed in the Finnish approach.[66] The detection of autologous blood doping is far more complex. At present, the most likely approach to detect blood doping, and also erythropoietin administration, would seem to be to determine a haematocrit threshold value which may not be exceeded. This would need to be set at different values for males and females, and further differentials would probably be necessary since haemoglobin is known to vary widely between athletes.[67] Of course, this approach would control high-altitude training, but it would be difficult to deal with individuals, such as Mexicans, who live at high altitudes.

Pharmaceutical, chemical, and physical manipulation

The IOC ban pharmaceutical (pharmacological), chemical, and physical methods which alter the integrity and validity of the urine sample collected in a doping control. Specifically, as a pharmacological method, they ban probenecid and related compounds. They also ban substances which alter testosterone and epitestosterone measurements and cite epitestosterone application or bromantan administration as examples. A conjugated hydroxylated metabolite of bromantan coelutes with epitestosterone in the commonly used GC–MS screening procedures. As a foreign substance banned by the IOC which is readily detected, it is relatively easy to control. However, since epitestosterone is produced endogenously, the mere presence cannot constitute an offence. Very little guidance is available as how to distinguish 'application' from endogenous production, although the use of combustion isotope ratio mass spectrometry is probably the most incontrovertible method.

Probenecid

Probenecid inhibits the transport of organic acids across epithelial barriers, and this is of greatest importance in the renal tubule where the tubular secretion of many drugs and their metabolites is inhibited. However, the excretion of uric acid is increased since its reabsorption in the renal tubule is inhibited by probenecid. Many anabolic steroids are excreted as glucuronic acid conjugates and probenecid can reduce their renal clearance and hence urinary concentration. To be effective, about 2 g of probenecid needs to be taken and it is not difficult for the laboratory to detect its presence in a urine sample.

Classes of drugs subject to certain restrictions

Alcohol

The IOC does not prohibit the use of alcohol. However, because the governing body of some sports such as pistol shooting and motor racing limit alcohol use, the IOC will determine breath or blood alcohol levels at the request of an International Federation.

Marijuana

Although the IOC does not ban marijuana, tests were carried out at the Olympic Games held in Seoul in 1988 for the presence of its metabolites in urine, and this will be continued at subsequent Games if so requested by an International Federation.

Local anaesthetics

The IOC permits the use of certain injectable local anaesthetics such as procaine, xylocaine, and carbocaine, but not cocaine, by local or intra-articular injections when medically justified. The IOC Medical Commission requires the details including diagnosis, dose, and route of administration to be submitted immediately in writing to them. There is no ban on the topical use of local anaesthetics.

Corticosteroids

One of the important effects of glucocorticoids is on the central nervous system processes which underlie behaviour.[68] In both patients with Addison's disease and Cushing's syndrome psychiatric disturbances are often manifested. In Cushing's syndrome depression is more commonly manifested than mania, but curiously the converse is often the case in patients treated with corticosteroid therapy.[69] Corticosteroid treatment can result in mood-elevating, energizing effects, and upon treatment withdrawal the symptoms of tiredness, malaise, and depression.[70] These effects have some analogies with those observed with amphetamine administration and withdrawal. Consequently, corticosteroids may be misused in sport for their immediate psychoendocrine effects in overcoming tiredness and lethargy and to give a 'pepped-up' feeling during training and competition. Short-term use of tetracosactrin, by stimulating excessive corticosteroid secretion, would be expected to give similar effects. Of course, long-term administration of either tetracosactrin or corticosteroids would diminish performance because of the inducement of protein catabolism resulting in skeletal muscle wasting and weakness.

The IOC permits the use of corticosteroids by inhalational therapy to treat asthma and allergic rhinitis, and also allows the use of aural, opthalmological, and dermatological preparations and intra-articular injections. However, written notification must be given to the IOC Medical Commission to justify such use medically.

By analogy with synthetic androgens, the approach to detecting the presence of synthetic glucocorticoids, such as dexamethasone or prednisolone, in athletes' urine is straightforward. Likewise, athletes may switch from using synthetic glucocorticoids to administering tetracosactrin and cortisol to evade detection. As with testosterone, detection of tetracosactrin and cortisol administration must be based on more than elevated concentrations of these hormones alone. The problem is further compounded in that the secretion of ACTH and cortisol increase in response to stress during strenuous exercise.[71,72]

A detection method for cortisol administration using the urinary ratios of the isomer 11β-hydroxyaetiocholanolone (3α,11β-dihydroxy-5β-androstan-17-one) to the isomer 11β-hydroxyandrosterone (3α,11β-dihydroxy-5α-androstan-17-one), defined as the 5β:5α ratio, has been investigated.[73] Cortisol and the androgen 11β-hydroxyandrostenedione (11β-hydroxyandrost-4-en-3,17-one) are exclusively secreted by the adrenals, but cortisol is metabolized in greater amounts to 11β-hydroxyaetiocholanolone (5β) compared with 11β-hydroxyandrosterone (5α), whereas the reverse is the case for 11β-hydroxyandrostenedione. The study showed that the 5β:5α ratio was a useful criterion of cortisol administration and that

Table 2	IOC Medical Commission: sports to be tested for β-blockers	
Winter Games	**Summer Games**
Biathlon	Archery
Bobsled	Diving and synchronous swimming
Luge	Modern pentathlon—shooting only
Ski jumping	Sailing—match race, helms only
	Shooting

tetracosactrin stimulation, to mimic the physiological response to stress, only caused a small increase in this ratio. The minor effect of tetracosactrin administration on the 5β:5α ratio was encouraging, but it meant that athletes could evade detection by switching from cortisol to tetracosactrin administration.

β-Blockers

In normal individuals β-blockers adversely affect both anaerobic endurance and aerobic power as measured by VO_2max, endurance, and time for a 2 km run.[74] Athletes in events such as archery and shooting may gain an advantage from the anxiolytic, bradycardic, and antitremor effects of the β-blockers.

The IOC Medical Commission has reviewed the therapeutic indications for the use of β-blocking drugs and considers that there is a wide range of effective alternative preparations available to control hypertension, cardiac arrhythmias, angina pectoris, and migraine. Because of the continued misuse of β-blockers in some sports where physical activity is of no or little importance, it reserves the right to test those sports which it deems appropriate and states that these are unlikely to include endurance events. As examples, the IOC lists the lipid-soluble β-blockers such as propranolol, which may act via the central nervous system and have anxiolytic activity, as well as those which are water soluble, such as atenolol, nadolol, and sotalol, and hence are not centrally active. Some β-blockers such as atenolol and metoprolol have less effect on the $β_2$ (bronchial) receptors and are relatively cardioselective but not cardiospecific. These agents are not exempted from control, and hence presumably the IOC wish to control β-blockers because of their effect of slowing the heart rate. Table 2 indicates those sports which, in September 1987, the IOC Medical Commission decided would be tested for β-blockers at the Olympic Games.

Most β-blockers are excreted as glucuronic acid conjugates of the parent substance and its metabolites. Urine samples can be screened for β-blockers following enzyme hydrolysis of the conjugates and then by solvent extraction at alkaline pH and analysis by HPLC, or the extract may be chemically derivatized and analysed by GC–MS. Alternatively, a solid-phase extraction of the urine can be used followed by GC–MS of the derivatized extract.

Miscellaneous substances

Bicarbonate

People have used bicarbonate with the aim of increasing the buffering capacity of blood; hence to counteract the build-up of lactic acid resulting from anaerobic glycolysis which would inhibit glycolysis and cause fatigue. Provided that the exercise is not primarily aerobic and the dose is adequate, bicarbonate has been shown to enhance exercise time to exhaustion.[75] Large amounts are required (more than 300 mg/kg) which will cause diarrhoea in most subjects. Chronic administration can cause hypercalcaemia and alkalosis which can cause changes in electrolyte balance and respiration, potentially with serious consequences.

Bicarbonate has previously been used to alkalinize the urine in order to increase the reabsorption of basic drugs in the renal tubules and hence to reduce the urinary excretion and therefore concentration of these substances. However, modern analytical methods are sufficiently sensitive to make this technique ineffective in evading detection. At the present time the use of bicarbonate is not normally controlled in sport, although urinary pH is sometimes checked at the time of sample collection.

Concluding remarks

This chapter serves to illustrate the variety of substances which have been used in sport in an attempt to enhance performance. The athlete does not appear to be deterred by any lack of scientific evidence that the substance is efficacious nor by the documented risk of potentially hazardous side-effects. The whole area is dynamic, advancing as science advances. There is a definite need to improve our understanding of whether and how these substances work and, although many are detectable by current analytical methods, new techniques are needed to meet and to anticipate the new challenges. Ultimately, however, what is accepted use and what represents misuse is a moral question to be answered not by science but by all of us in society and especially by those in sport.

Appendix

International Olympic Committee Medical Code

Prohibited classes of substances and prohibited methods 31 January 1997

Doping contravenes the ethics of both sport and medical science. Doping consists of:

(1) the administration of substances belonging to prohibited classes of pharmacological agents; and/or

(2) the use of various prohibited methods.

I. *Prohibited classes of substances*

    A. Stimulants

    B. Narcotics

    C. Anabolic agents

    D. Diuretics

    E. Peptide and glycoprotein hormones and analogues

II. *Prohibited methods*

    A. Blood doping

    B. Pharmacological, chemical, and physical manipulation

III. *Classes of drugs subject to certain restrictions*

    A. Alcohol

B.   Marijuana

C.   Local anaesthetics

D.   Corticosteroids

E.   Beta-blockers

I: Prohibited classes of substances

A. Stimulants Prohibited substances in class A include the following examples:

amineptine, amiphenazole, amphetamines, bromantan, caffeine*, cocaine, ephedrines, fencamfamin, mesocarb, pentetrazol, pipradrol, salbutamol**, salmeterol**, terbutaline**, . . . and related substances

* For caffeine the definition of a positive result depends on the concentration of caffeine in the urine. The concentration in urine may not exceed 12 micrograms per millilitre.
** Permitted by inhaler only and must be declared in writing, prior to the competition, to the relevant medical authority.
NOTE: All imidazole preparations are acceptable for topical use, e.g. oxymetazoline. Vasoconstrictors (e.g. adrenaline) may be administered with local anaesthetic agents. Topical preparations (e.g. nasal, ophthalmological) of phenylephrine are permitted.

B. Narcotics Prohibited substances in class B include the following examples:

dextromoramide, diamorphine (heroin), methadone, morphine, pentazocine, pethidine, ... and related substances
NOTE: Codeine, dextromethorphan, dextropropoxyphene, dihydrocodeine, diphenoxylate, ethylmorphine, pholcodine, and propoxyphene are permitted.

C. Anabolic agents The anabolic class includes: (1) anabolic androgenic steroids (**AAS**) and (2) β_2-agonists.
Prohibited substances in class C include the following examples:

1. Anabolic androgenic steroids clostebol, dehydroepiandrosterone (**DHEA**), fluoxymesterone, metandienone, metenolone, nandrolone, oxandrolone, stanozolol, testosterone*, . . . and related substances
* The presence of a testosterone (T) to epitestosterone (E) ratio greater than six (6) to one (1) in the urine of a competitor constitutes an offence unless there is evidence that this ratio is due to a physiological or pathological condition, e.g. low epitestosterone excretion, androgen-producing tumour, enzyme deficiencies.

In the case of T/E higher than 6, it is mandatory that the relevant medical authority conduct an investigation before the sample is declared positive. A full report will be written and will include a review of previous tests, subsequent tests, and any results of endocrine investigations. In the event that previous tests are not available, the athlete should be tested unannounced at least once per month for three months. The results of these investigations should be included in the report. Failure to co-operate in the investigations will result in declaring the sample positive.

2. β_2-Agonists When administered systemically, β_2-agonists may have powerful anabolic effects:
clenbuterol, fenoterol, salbutamol, salmeterol, terbutaline, ... and related substances

D. Diuretics Prohibited substances in class D include the following examples:
acetazolamide, bumetanide, chlortalidone, etacrynic acid, frusemide, hydrochlorothiazide, mannitol*, mersalyl, spironolactone, triamterene, . . . and related substances
* Prohibited by intravenous injection.

E. Peptide and glycoprotein hormones and analogues Prohibited substances in class E include the following examples:

(1) chorionic gonadotrophin (hCG—human chorionic gonadotrophin);

(2) corticotrophin (ACTH);

(3) growth hormone (hGH, somatotrophin).

(All the respective releasing factors of the above-mentioned substances are also prohibited.)

(4) erythropoietin (**EPO**)

II: Prohibited methods
The following procedures are prohibited:

Blood doping Blood doping is the administration of blood, red blood cells, and related blood products to an athlete. This procedure may be preceded by withdrawal of blood from the athlete who continues to train in this blood-depleted state.

Pharmacological, chemical, and physical manipulation Pharmacological, chemical, and physical manipulation is the use of substances and of methods which alter, attempt to alter, or may reasonably be expected to alter the integrity and validity of urine samples used in doping controls, including, without limitation, catheterization, urine substitution and/or tampering, inhibition of renal excretion such as by probenecid and related compounds, and alterations of testosterone and epitestosterone measurements such as epitestosterone application or bromantan administration.

The success or failure of the use of a prohibited substance or method is not material. It is sufficient that the said substance or procedure was used or attempted for the infraction to be considered as consummated.

III: Classes of drugs subject to certain restrictions

A. Alcohol In agreement with the International Sports Federations and the responsible authorities, tests may be conducted for ethanol. The results may lead to sanctions.

B. Marijuana In agreement with the International Sports Federations and the responsible authorities, tests may be conducted for cannabinoids (e.g. marijuana, hashish). The results may lead to sanctions.

C. Local anaesthetics Injectable local anaesthetics are permitted under the following conditions:

(1) Bupivacaine, lidocaine, mepivacaine, procaine, etc. are used but not cocaine. Vasoconstrictor agents (e.g. adrenaline) may be used in conjunction with local anaesthetics.

(2) Only local or intra-articular injections may be administered.

(3) Only when medically justified. The details, including diagnosis, dose, and route of administration, must be submitted prior to the competition or, if administered during the competition, immediately after injection, in writing to the relevant medical authority.

D. Corticosteroids The use of corticosteroids is banned except:

(1) for topical use (aural, dermatological, and ophthalmological) but not rectal;

(2) by inhalation;

(3) by intra-articular or local injection.

The IOC Medical Commission has introduced mandatory reporting of athletes requiring corticosteroids by inhalation during competitions. Any team doctor wishing to administer corticosteroids by local or intra-articular injection, or by inhalation, to a competitor must give written notification prior to the competition to the relevant medical authority.

E. β-Blockers Some examples of β-blockers are:
acebutolol, alprenolol, atenolol, labetalol, metoprolol, nadolol, oxprenolol, propranolol, sotalol, ... and related substances
In agreement with the rules of the International Sports Federations, tests will be conducted in some sports at the discretion of the responsible authorities.

List of examples of prohibited substances
The International Non-Proprietary Name (**INN**), Proposed INN, or Recommended INN is listed and, where different, the British Approved Name is given in parentheses.
CAUTION: This is not an exhaustive list of prohibited substances. Many substances that do not appear on this list are considered banned under the term 'and related substances'.

Stimulants
amfepramone (diethylpropion), amineptine, amiphenazole, amphetamine, bromantan, caffeine, cathine, cocaine, cropropamide, crotetamide (crotethamide), ephedrine, etamivan (ethamivan), etilamphetamine, etilefrine, fencamfamin, fenetylline (fenethylline), fenfluramine, heptaminol, mefenorex, mephentermine, mesocarb, methamphetamine (methylamphetamine), methoxyphenamine, methylenedioxyamphetamine, methylephedrine, methylphenidate, nikethamide, norfenfluramine, parahydroxyamphetamine, pemoline, pentetrazol, phendimetrazine, phentermine, phenylpropanolamine, pholedrine, pipradrol, prolintane, propylhexedrine, pseudoephedrine, salbutamol, salmeterol, strychnine, terbutaline.

Narcotics
dextromoramide, diamorphine (heroin), hydrocodone, methadone, morphine, pentazocine, pethidine.

Anabolic agents
boldenone, clenbuterol, clostebol, danazol, dehydrochlormethyltestosterone, dehydroepiandrosterone (DHEA), dihydrotestosterone, drostanolone, fenoterol, fluoxymesterone, formebolone, mesterolone, metandienone (methandienone), metenolone (methenolone), methandriol, methyltestosterone, mibolerone, nandrolone, nore-thandrolone, oxandrolone, oxymesterone, oxymetholone, salbutamol, salmeterol, stanozolol, terbutaline, testosterone, trenbolone.

Diuretics
acetazolamide, bendroflumethiazide (bendrofluazide), bumetanide, canrenone, chlortalidone (chlorthalidone), etacrynic acid (ethacrynic acid), frusemide (furosemide), hydrochlorothiazide, indapamide, mersalyl, spironolactone, triamterene.

Masking agents
bromantan, epitestosterone, probenecid.

Peptide hormones
ACTH, erythropoietin (**EPO**), hCG, hGH.

β-Blockers
acebutolol, alprenolol, atenolol, betaxolol, bisoprolol, bunolol, labetalol, metoprolol, nadolol, oxprenolol, propranolol, sotalol.

References

1. Coyle EF. Ergogenic aids. *Clinical Sports Medicine* 1984; **3**: 731–42.
2. Korkia P, Stimson GV. Anabolic steroid use in Great Britain: an exploratory investigation. London: HMSO, 1993: ISBN 1 874676 05 4
3. Kuchenski R. Biochemical actions of amphetamine and other stimulants. In Creese I, ed. *Stimulants: neurochemical, behavioral, and clinical perspectives*. New York: Raven Press, 1983: 31–61.
4. Smith GM, Beecher HK. Amphetamine sulfate and athletic performance. I. Objective effects. *Journal of the American Medical Association* 1959; **170**: 542–57.
5. Williams MH. *Drugs and athletic performance*. Springfield, IL: Charles C Thomas, 1974.
6. Chandler JV, Blair SN. The effects of amphetamines on selected physiological components related to athletic success. *Medicine and Science in Sports and Exercise* 1980; **12**: 65–9.
7. Bhagat B, Wheeler N. Effect of amphetamine on the swimming endurance of rats. *Neuropharmacology* 1973; **12**: 711–13.
8. Gerald MC. Effects of (+)-amphetamine on the treadmill endurance performance of rats. *Neuropharmacology* 1978; **17**: 703–4.
9. Bravo EL. Phenylpropanolamine and other over-the-counter vasoactive compounds. *Hypertension* 1988; **11** (Suppl. II): 7–10.
10. Pentel PR, Asinger RW, Benowitz NL. Propranolol antagonism of phenylpropanolamine-induced hypertension. *Clinical Pharmacology and Therapeutics* 1985; **37**: 488–94.
11. Lopes JM, Aubier M, Jardim J, Aranda JV, Macklem PT. Effect of caffeine on skeletal muscle function before and after fatigue. *Journal of Applied Physiology: Respiratory, Environmental and Exercise Physiology* 1983; **54**: 1303–5.
12. Wood DS. Human skeletal muscle: analysis of Ca^{2+} regulation in skinned fibers using caffeine. *Experimental Neurology* 1978; **58**: 218–30.
13. Goldstein A, Warren R, Kaizer S. Psychotropic effects of caffeine in man. I. Individual differences in sensitivity to caffeine-induced wakefulness. *Journal of Pharmacology and Experimental Therapeutics* 1965; **149**: 156–9.
14. Costill DK, Dalsky GP, Fink WJ. Effects of caffeine ingestion on metabolism and exercise performance. *Medicine and Science in Sports* 1978; **10**: 155–8.
15. Ivy JL, Costill DL, Fink WJ, *et al*. Influence of caffeine and carbohydrate feedings on endurance performance. *Medicine and Science in Sports* 1979; **11**: 6–11.
16. O'Neill FT, Hynak-Hankinson MT, Gorman T. Research and application of current topics in sports nutrition. *Journal of the American Dietetic Association* 1986; **86**: 1007–15.

17. Rall TW. Evolution of the mechanism of action of methylxanthines: from calcium mobilizers to antagonists of adenosine receptors. *Pharmacologist* 1982; **24**: 277–87.

18. Trang JM, Blanchard J, Conrad KA, Harrison GG. Relationship between total body clearance of caffeine and urine flow rate in elderly men. *Biopharmaceutics and Drug Disposition* 1985; **6**: 51–6.

19. Brown R, Partington J. A psychometric comparison of narcotic addicts with hospital attendants. *Journal of General Psychology* 1942; **27**: 71.

20. Appenzeller O, Standefer J, Appenzeller J, *et al.* Neurology of endurance training. V. Endorphins. *Neurology (NY)* 1980; **30**: 418–19.

21. Glasser W. *Positive addiction.* New York: Harper and Row, 1976.

22. Terney R, McLain LG. The use of anabolic steroids in high school students. *American Journal of Diseases in Children* 1990; **144**: 99–103.

23. Haupt HA, Rovere GD. Anabolic steroids: a review of the literature. *American Journal of Sports Medicine* 1984; **12**: 469–84.

24. Wilson JD. Androgen abuse by athletes. *Endocrine Reviews* 1988; **9**: 181–99.

25. Ryan AJ. Athletics. In: Kochakian CD, ed. *Anabolic–androgenic steroids. Handbook of experimental pharmacology.* New York: Springer-Verlag, 1976: **43**, 525–34 and 723–5.

26. Bhasin S, Storer TW, Berman N, *et al.* The effects of supraphysiologic doses of testosterone on muscle size and strength in normal men. *New England Journal of Medicine* 1996; **335**: 1–7.

27. Scott MJ Jr, Scott MJ III. Dermatologists and anabolic–androgenic drug abuse. *Cutis* 1989; **44**: 30–5.

28. Choi PYL, Parrott AC, Cowan D. High-dose anabolic steroids in strength athletes: effects upon hostility and aggression. *Human Psychopharmacology* 1990; **5**: 349–56.

29. Pope, HG Jr, Katz, DL. Bodybuilder's psychosis. *Lancet* 1987; **i**: 863.

30. Choi P, Parrott AC, Cowan DA. Adverse behavioural effects of anabolic steroids in athletes: a brief review. *International Journal of Sports Medicine* 1989; **1**: 183–7.

31. Strauss RH, Liggett MT, Lanese RR. Anabolic steroid use and perceived effects in ten weight-trained women athletes. *Journal of the American Medical Association* 1985; **253**: 2871–5.

32. Hurley BF, Seals DR, Hagberg JM, *et al.* High-density-lipoprotein cholesterol in bodybuilders v powerlifters. Negative effects of androgen use. *Journal of the American Medical Association* 1984; **252**: 507–13.

33. Ferenchick GS. Are anabolic steroids thrombogenic? *New England Journal of Medicine* 1990; **322**: 476.

34. Hickson RC, Ball KL, Falduto MT. Adverse effects of anabolic steroids. *Medical and Toxicological Adverse Drug Experience* 1989; **4**: 254–71.

35. Donike M, Bärwald KR, Klosterman K, Schänzer W, Zimmermann J. The detection of exogenous testosterone. In: Heck H, Hollmann W, Liesen H, eds. *Sport: Leistung und Gesundheit.* Köln: Deutcher Artze-Verlag, 1983: 293–300.

36. Kicman AT, Brooks, RV, Collyer, SC, *et al.* Criteria to indicate testosterone administration. *British Journal of Sports Medicine* 1990; **24**: 253–64.

37. Franke WW, Berendonk, B. Hormonal doping and androgenization of athletes: a secret proram of the German Democratic Republic government. *Clinical Chemistry* 1997; **43**: 1262–79.

38. Southan GJ, Brooks RV, Cowan DA, Kicman AT, Unnadkat N, Walker CJ. Possible indices for the detection of the administration of dihydrotestosterone to athletes. *Journal of Steroid Biochemistry and Molecular Biology* 1992; **42**: 87–94.

39. Catlin DH, Hatton CK. Use and abuse of anabolic and other drugs for athletic enhancement. *Advances in Internal Medicine* 1991; **36**: 399–424.

40. Kicman AT, Oftebro H, Walker C, Norman N, Cowan DA. Potential use of ketoconazole in a dynamic endocrine test to differentiate between biological outliers and testosterone use by athletes. *Clinical Chemistry* 1993; **39**: 1798–803.

41. Oftebro H, Jensen J, Mowinckel, Norli HR. Establishing a ketoconazole suppression test for verifying testosterone administration in the doping control of athletes. *Journal of Clinical Endocrinology and Metabolism* 1994; **78**: 973–7.

42. Stewart-Bentley M, Odell W, Horton R. The feedback control of luteinizing hormone in normal adult men. *Journal of Clinical Endocrinology and Metabolism* 1974; **38**: 545–53.

43. Toth M, Zakar T. Relative binding affinities of testosterone, 19-nortestosterone and their 5α-reduced derivatives to the androgen receptor and to other binding proteins: a suggested role of 5α reductive steroid metabolism in the dissociation of 'myotrophic' and 'androgenic' activities of 19-nortestosterone. *Journal of Steroid Biochemistry* 1982; **17**: 653–60.

44. Kicman AT, Coutts SB, Walker CJ, Cowan DA. Proposed confirmatory procedure for detecting 5α-dihydrotestosterone doping in male athletes. *Clinical Chemistry* 1995; **41**: 1617–27.

45. Donike M, Ueki M, Kuroda Y, *et al.* Detection of dihydrotestosterone (DHT) doping: alterations in the steroid profile and reference ranges for DHT and its 5α-metabolites. *Journal of Sports Medicine and Physical Fitness* 1995; **35**: 235–50.

46. Reeds PJ, Hay SM, Dorward PM, *et al.* The effect of β-agonists and antagonists on muscle growth and body composition of young rats (Rattus sp.). *Comparative Biochemistry and Physiology* 1988; **89C**: 337–41.

47. Martineau L, Horan MA, Rothwell NJ, Little RA. Salbutamol, a β2-adrenoceptor agonist, increases skeletal muscle strength in young men. *Clinical Science* 1992; **83**: 615–21.

48. Delbeke FT, Debackere M. The influence of diuretics on the excretion and metabolism of doping agents. II. Phentermine. *Arzneimittel-forschung Drug Research* 1986; **36**: 134–7.

49. Delbeke FT, Debackere M. The influence of diuretics on the excretion and metabolism of doping agents. III. Etilamfetamine. *Arzneimittel-forschung Drug Research* 1986; **36**: 1413–16.

50. Lisi AM, Trout GJ, Kazlauskas R. Screening for diuretics in human urine by gas chromatography–mass spectrometry with derivatisation by direct extractive alkylation. *Journal of Chromatography* 1991; **563**: 257–70.

51. IOC Medical Code. Lausanne: International Olympic Committee, 1995, ISBN 92 9149 003 2.

52. Kicman AT, Cowan DA. Peptide hormones and sport: misuse and detection. *British Medical Bulletin* 1992; **48**: 496–517.

53. Stenman U, Alfthan A, Ranta T, Vartianen E, Jalkanen J, Seppala M. Serum levels of human chorionic gonadotropin in nonpregnant women and men are modulated by gonadotropin-releasing hormone and sex steroids. *Journal of Clinical Endocrinology and Metabolism* 1987; **64**: 730–6.

54. Kicman AT, Brooks RV, Cowan DA. Human chorionic gonadotrophin and sport. *British Journal of Sports Medicine* 1991; **25**: 73–80.

55. Saez JM, Forest MG. Kinetics of human chorionic gonadotropin-induced steroidogenic response of the human testis. I. Plasma testosterone: implications for HCG stimulation test. *Journal of Clinical Endocrinology and Metabolism* 1979; **49**: 278–83.

56. Cowan DA, Kicman AT, Walker CJ, Wheeler MJ. Effect of administration of human chorionic gonadotrophin on criteria used to assess testosterone administration in athletes. *Journal of Endocrinology* 1991; **131**: 147–54.

57. Vanhelder WP, Radomski MW, Goode RC. Growth hormone responses during intermittent weight lifting exercise in men. *European Journal of Applied Physiology* 1984; **53**: 31–4.

58. Vanhelder WP, Casey K, Goode RC, *et al.* Growth hormone regulation in two types of aerobic exercise of equal oxygen uptake. *European Journal of Applied Physiology* 1986; **55**: 236–9.

59. Daughaday WH. The anterior pituitary. In: Wilson JD, Foster DW, eds. *Williams textbook of endocrinology*, 7th edn. Philadelphia: WB Saunders, 1985: 568–613.

60. Hughes JP, Friesen HG. The nature and regulation of the receptors for pituitary growth hormone. *Annual Review of Physiology* 1985; **47**: 483–99.

61. Kicman AT, Miell JP, Teale JD, *et al*. Serum insulin-like growth factor (IFG-1) and IGF binding proteins 2 and 3 as potential markers of doping with human growth hormone. *Clinical Endocrinology* 1997; **47**: 43–50.

62. Gareau R, Audran M, Baynes RD, *et al*. Erythropoietin abuse in athletes. *Nature* 1996; **380**: 113.

63. Haynes RC. Adrenocorticotropic hormone; adrenocortical steroids and their synthetic analogs; inhibitors of the synthesis and actions of adrenocortical hormones. In: *Goodman and Gilman's pharmacological basis of therapeutics*. 8th edn. New York: Pergamon Press, 1990: 1431–62.

64. Chard T. Requirements for binding assays—extraction of ligand from biological fluids, and collection and storage of samples. In: Burdon RH, van Knippenberg PH, eds. *An introduction to radioimmunoassay and related techniques*. Amsterdam: Elsevier, 1987: 137–52.

65. Buick FJ, Gledhill N, Froese AB, *et al*. Effect of induced erythrocythaemia on aerobic work capacity. *Journal of Applied Physiology* 1980; **48**: 636–42.

66. Videman T, Sistonen P, Stray-Gundersen J, Lereim I. Experiences in blood dope testing at the 1989 world cross-country ski championships in Lahti, Finland. In: Bellotti P, Benzi G, Ljungqvist A, eds. *Official Proceedings of IInd International Athletic Foundation World Symposium on Doping in Sport—1989*. London: International Athletic Foundation, 1990: 5–12.

67. Clement DB, Asmundson RG, Medhurst CW. Hemoglobin values: comparative survey of the 1976 Canadian Olympic team. *Canadian Medical Association Journal* 1977; **117**: 614–16.

68. McEwen BS. Influences of adrenocortical hormones on pituitary and brain function. In: Baxter JD, Rousseau GG, eds. *Glucocorticoid hormone action*. Berlin: Springer-Verlag, 1979: 467–92.

69. Rose RM. Psychoendocrinology. In: Wilson JD, Foster DW, eds. *Williams textbook of endocrinology*. Philadelphia: WB Saunders, 1985: 653–81.

70. Myles AB, Daly JR. Corticosteroid withdrawal. In: *Corticosteroid and ACTH treatment*. London: Edward Arnold, 1974: 89–97.

71. Few JD. Effect of exercise on the secretion and metabolism of cortisol in man. *Journal of Endocrinology* 1974; **62**: 341–53.

72. Kuoppasalmi K, Näveri H, Härkönen M, Adlercreutz H. Plasma cortisol, androstenedione, testosterone and luteinizing hormone in running exercise of different intensities. *Scandinavian Journal of Clinical and Laboratory Investigation* 1980; **40**: 403–9.

73. Southan GJ, Brooks RV. The detection of synthetic and natural corticosteroids. In: Shipe JR, Savory J, eds. *Drugs in competitive athletes*. Oxford: Blackwell Scientific, 1991: 33–7.

74. Kaiser P. Physical performance and muscle metabolism during β-adrenergic blockade in man. *Acta Physiologica Scandinavica* 1984; **536** (Suppl): 1.

75. Wilkes D, Gledhill N, Smyth R. Effect of acute induced metabolic alkalosis on 800m racing time. *Medicine and Science in Sports and Exercise* 1983; **15**: 277–80.

3.5 Gender verification and the place of XY females in sport

Malcolm A. Ferguson-Smith

Introduction

In the Olympic Games of ancient Greece which date from the eighth century BC, the athletes had to abide by strict rules. They had to be free men, not slaves, without criminal conviction, and had to have trained for 10 months. Strict penalties for bribery, cheating, and for transgressing the rules were exacted and all athletes affirmed by solemn oath at the start of the Games that they were eligible to compete. Only male athletes took part and the custom was that they, and later also their trainers, entered the stadium naked. Women could not take part or even watch the Games on penalty of death. However, women could enter teams into the equestrian events. Women also took part in their own Games, the Heraia, in honour of the goddess Hera. The Heraia were short foot races for which only virgins were eligible, and the event was held separately from the Olympic Games. It was a great honour to take part in the Olympic Games and to win the crown of wild olive branches. This was the only prize, although all champions were glorified throughout Greece.

When the modern Olympic Games were revived in 1896, Baron Pierre de Coubertin followed the ancient tradition and only male athletes competed. Perhaps he foresaw problems with eligibility for women. None the less, in 1912 women swimmers were accepted at the Stockholm Olympics and by 1928 in Amsterdam women were competing separately in most athletic events. It has been accepted, and is well documented that there are substantial differences in performance between men and women.[1,2] These differences tend to be less in highly trained athletes but they are sufficient to justify the continued segregation of men and women in all but a few sports. Equestrian events, yachting, and shooting remain the only exceptions.

Success in sport is not only the result of dedication and intense training. Athletes of both sexes tend to have inherent physical advantages over the average person in terms of stature, body build, and neurological and motor attributes. These inherent factors are genetically determined and often direct the athlete to a particular sport. Tall athletes have obvious advantages in netball and long jump whereas short and squat athletes tend to excel in weightlifting and in some field events. Some of these attributes, especially height, are influenced by the sex chromosomes, but the main differences in performance between male and female athletes can be attributed to the increased muscle mass in males due to the action of androgenic steroids (especially testosterone) secreted by the testes. This hormonal difference is the main justification for separating the sexes in sport. In a few sports such as boxing and weightlifting, weight is used to classify athletes so that they can compete with one another on a fair basis. A similar argument might be advanced for classifying high and long jumpers by height. However, there would appear to be a limit to the quest for absolute fairness in sport, and genetically determined height is not at present regarded as a reasonable criterion.

Notwithstanding the high moral standards of the Olympic athlete, it is natural for a competitor to wish to maximize the chances of success by whatever permissible means are available. Intensive training and improved diet are obviously acceptable, but measures which involve taking steroids to increase the muscle mass or erythropoietin to increase the red blood cell count amount to cheating, may be damaging to health, and are rightly proscribed. However, pressures on individual athletes are great. It is not only a matter of individual prestige as in ancient Greece, but there are also other factors including national and political pressure, the prospect of financial gain, self-aggrandizement, and other personal motives, which sometimes lead the athlete to cheat even in the most recent times when sophisticated methods for screening athletes for anabolic steroid use, for example, are routinely employed at international events.

The introduction of gender verification

The anecdotal evidence that on several international occasions individuals competed as females who later changed their sexual identity to live as men, and even father children, has undoubtedly led to rumour and innuendo about those successful female athletes considered to have increased muscle mass, a male habitus, and hirsutism. It was frequently suggested that some form of verification was necessary to ensure that males were not masquerading as females. As early as 1948, the British Women's Amateur Athletic Association required a doctor's letter verifying the sex of women competitors. This was later dropped as being too ineffective against a determined imposter.

There are at least six well-documented examples of individuals who were said to have testes and competed successfully in international women's events.[3]

1. The earliest recorded case was the winner of the women's 100-m sprint in the 1932 Olympic Games in Los Angeles. Forty-eight years later she was killed in a shooting incident and at autopsy was found to have testes.[4] It is not recorded whether she was virilized and it is probable that she had the androgen insensitivity syndrome.

2. The winner of the women's 800-m race and world record holder in 1934 was found to be a male pseudohermaphrodite who had a sex change operation at the age of 30 years. From the account of the operation it is clear that there was considerable virilization of the external genitalia, and thus the diagnosis may not have been androgen insensitivity.[5]

3. A high jumper who came fourth in the Berlin Olympics in 1936 was barred from competition by the German Athletic Federation after the 1938 European Championships in Vienna, when she was found to have both male and female organs. It is reported that the Nazi youth movement had forced the athlete to pose as a women for 3 years.[6] He returned to male gender thereafter.

4. Two members of the women's relay team that came second in the European Championships in 1946 subsequently had sex change operations and lived afterwards as men.[6] One fathered several children.

5. In 1964 another runner broke world track records in races for women at 400- and 800-m distances which were never ratified. He was later recognized by his father as the son he had lost in the war.[7] This may have been an example of a male simply masquerading as a female.

6. The winner of the women's world downhill ski title in 1966 was identified as being male as a result of a medical examination in 1967.[7] This revealed undescended testes and, after surgical correction, the skier married and became a father.

In several of these cases there is documentation of ambiguity of the external genitalia and testicular maldescent. The diagnosis of male intersex seems likely and their androgen levels may have contributed to their success. They were regarded as having an unfair physical advantage over normal women athletes and there was considerable pressure on the various international organizations of sport to ensure that this apparent cheating did not occur in the future. The anecdotes also alerted competitors to the possibility of males masquerading as females and, as indicated above, anybody with an apparently masculine body habitus tended to be regarded with suspicion.

Rumours of this sort were rife at the Rome Olympics in 1960 and this prompted the International Olympic Committee (**IOC**) to consider establishing rules of eligibility for women athletes in order to ensure that the athletes were competing on an equal basis, considering their physical status.[8] At the same time there was growing concern about the use of hormones and stimulant drugs by athletes, and this led to the introduction of measures designed to stop all forms of cheating.

The drug problem and gender verification of women athletes were both considered by the IOC at the 1964 Olympic Games in Tokyo. A decision was taken to form a Medical Commission to take charge of medical aspects, including the taking of drugs. Competitors were required in future to sign statements accepting the arrangements for drug and 'femininity' controls before they were admitted to the Games. This was to protect the athletes' health, to ensure fair play and equal conditions for all and, in the case of gender verification, to eliminate cases in which a genetic alteration leading to masculinization in a competitor registered as a female gave the competitor an unfair advantage. It was specifically intended that persons with intersexuality or hermaphroditism should be barred from competition. The signed statement also served to absolve the organizers from responsibility should an athlete be debarred in error.

The early attempts at gender verification were clumsy and insensitive. The first was made at the European Athletics Championships in Budapest in 1966. Women athletes were required to undergo a parade in the nude in front of three gynaecologists.[9] All 234 competitors passed the test but it was noted that five world record holders failed to appear at the Championships. Their absence was unexpected, and it was widely assumed that this was because they believed that they might have failed the test. However, with hindsight it seems more likely that they had been using anabolic steroids. They included a double Olympic champion in the shot put and discus, a double Olympic champion in the 80-m hurdles and pentathlon, a European long jump champion, a European 400-m champion, and an Olympic high jump champion.

In the Commonwealth Games in Kingston in 1966, the femininity control took the form of a manual examination of the external genitalia by a gynaecologist.[10] This treatment created great indignation among the athletes. Further resentment was expressed at the Pan American Games in Winnipeg in 1967, when another 'on sight' inspection was carried out by three doctors sitting at a desk in front of which each athlete was asked to pull up her shirt and push down her pants.[9] It is not known if any of these athletes were barred. These degrading forms of examination have made a lasting impression on the athletic community and have led to resistance to any form of clinical examination in the context of eligibility control.

The sex chromatin test

The experience with these forms of physical examination prompted the IOC to follow the advice of Bunge and adopt the buccal smear test as an alternative method of femininity control.[11] The test involves scraping a sample of epithelial cells from inside the cheek with a wooden spatula, and transferring the cells to a microscope slide which is then fixed and stained to reveal the presence or absence of the Barr body in the epithelial cell nuclei. The Barr body (or X chromatin) is a small dense mass of chromatin which can be observed under the oil immersion lens of a light microscope in approximately 30 per cent of nuclei in female somatic cells (Fig. 1). It represents one of the two X chromosomes which is genetically inactive and becomes condensed within the nucleus. Male cells do not show the Barr body as they have only one active X chromosome. The test therefore indicates the number of X chromosomes in the cell nucleus and thus the sex chromosome constitution of the individual, normally XX in females and XY in males. As the short arm

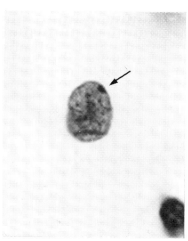

Fig. 1 The nucleus of a buccal smear cell showing the X chromatin or Barr body (arrowed) which represents the condensed, inactivated X chromosome characteristic of cells with two X chromosomes. Approximately 30 per cent of cells in a buccal smear from a normal female will show such an X-chromatin body; male cells do not have X chromatin.

of the Y chromosome carries the primary genetic determinants for the development of testes, normally only individuals with a Y chromosome develop as males. Male differentiation occurs because the testes secrete the male hormones necessary for the development of male internal ducts including prostate and seminal vesicles, and male external genitalia consisting of penis and scrotum. In the absence of a Y chromosome and testes, the individual develops along female lines. The sex chromatin test might therefore be considered a satisfactory means of distinguishing XY males from XX females and thus of detecting males who are attempting to masquerade as females. Unfortunately, there are two problems. First, it is possible to make a technical mistake, particularly if the sample has not been properly collected and fixed. XX females may be wrongly classified as male, and XY males may be missed. Both errors have occurred during the course of femininity control, the former with disastrous results for the unfortunate athlete. Second, there are several genetic disorders which interfere with the normal process of sexual development and lead to individuals of normal appearance but with paradoxical sex chromatin (and sex chromosome) findings. These cases illustrate the principle that a person's anatomical sex (and thus social and legal sex) is the most important factor in establishing gender, which need not necessarily conform to the chromosomal sex as determined by the sex chromatin test.

The most important genetic conditions that cause problems in femininity control occur in individuals who have an apparently normal male chromosomal constitution but who develop to adulthood as perfectly normal-looking girls. These individuals are sometimes referred to in the medical literature as XY females. They are quite easily recognized after puberty because they fail to menstruate and remain infertile; in some the breasts fail to form and the vulva and vagina do not mature. Many, however, grow into normal women with well-developed breasts and, as they are healthy (apart from being amenorrhoeal) and sometimes taller than average, they tend to do well in sport. In fact, tests for feminity control suggest that at least 1 in 500 women athletes have one or other of these conditions and are, unknowingly, XY females.[3] The two most common types of

XY female are those with gonadal dysgenesis, in which only vestiges of the gonads remain and no male hormones are produced, and those with the androgen insensitivity syndrome (or testicular feminization syndrome) in which the uterus is not formed and the tissues fail to be masculinized by the normal amounts of male hormone produced by intra-abdominal testes.

Gonadal dysgenesis

The individual with XY gonadal dysgenesis has normal female internal and external genitalia but fails to mature at the time of puberty as the ovaries are only represented by thin streaks of ovarian tissue, which cannot secrete sufficient oestrogenic steroids. Estimation of serum hormones therefore reveals low levels of oestrogens and high levels of gonadotrophins. There is usually little or no breast development and no menstruation. As the streak gonads are liable to malignant change (gonadoblastoma, dysgerminoma) arising from nests of abnormal XY germ cells, it is usual to remove the streak gonads in late adolescence or early adulthood. Secondary sexual characteristics can be induced by regular replacement therapy with oestrogens to the point of inducing withdrawal bleeding from the uterus; as induced menstruation serves no useful purpose it is often avoided. Oocyte donation and *in vitro* fertilization have allowed a number of affected women to have children. Because of the genetic determinants for stature carried by the Y chromosome,[12] women with XY gonadal dysgenesis are taller than the average and may do well in sport. The author knows of a successful hockey player with the condition, but it is not known how often femininity controls have debarred individuals with gonadal dysgenesis from international sport. It should be emphasized that the streak gonads do not secrete male hormone and that those affected show no evidence of masculinization. They have no advantage in sport over other women of the same height.

There are several genetic causes of XY gonadal dysgenesis. Some cases lack male determinants because of mutations within the testis-determining region of the Y chromosome.[13] Others are due to X-linked and autosomal mutations. Similar conditions in animals are known to be due to mutations of the autosomes.

Androgen insensitivity syndrome

Those with the androgen insensitivity syndrome are also XY females who tend to be taller than average women. The condition may be recognized occasionally in childhood because of the presence of testes in the labia or because the child develops an inguinal hernia. Most cases, however, are not recognized until adolescence when the presenting feature is failure to menstruate despite the development of breasts and other secondary sex characteristics. Gynaecological examination reveals that the uterus is absent and that the vagina is only one-third its normal length, ending blindly in the absence of the cervix uteri. Male internal genital (Wolffian) ducts remain undeveloped. Normal-sized testes are usually found in the pelvis or at the internal inguinal ring. As these cryptorchid testes are liable to malignancy (usually dysgerminoma), they should be removed once secondary sex characteristics are fully developed. Scanty pubic and axillary hair is a characteristic sign which should alert the clinician to the correct diagnosis in the adult. It is estimated that the frequency of the condition is approximately 1 in 62 000 males.

The androgen insensitivity syndrome is due to mutations of the androgen receptor gene carried by the X chromosome. Normal androgen receptors are not present in the tissue cells which therefore cannot respond to the normal amounts of testosterone produced by the testes. Consequently, the external genitalia, secondary sex characteristics, and musculature are female.

As the development of sex hair is also dependent on the presence of normal androgen receptors, pubic and axillary hair is sparse. The tissues are unresponsive to treatment with androgenic steroids, and this is one condition in which anabolic steroids have no effect in building up muscle mass. Serum hormone estimations will reveal levels of testosterone within the normal male range.

The above description applies to the complete androgen insensitivity syndrome, but it has been apparent for many years that there are variants due to different mutations at the same X-linked locus. These appear to be 'leaky' mutations in that the abnormal androgen receptors formed are capable of handling small amounts of male hormone, sufficient to cause virilization of the external genitalia and a normal distribution of pubic and axillary hair. These variants are referred to as the incomplete androgen insensitivity syndrome. There is no evidence that the amount of masculinization produced has a significant effect on athletic performance.

As androgen insensitivity is inherited as an X-linked recessive trait, it is usually transmitted through normally fertile women (who may have a patchy distribution of sex hair) to half their XY offspring. Enquiry should therefore be made for the condition in sisters and maternal aunts of affected individuals.

The androgen insensitivity syndrome is the most common abnormality detected by sex chromatin tests for gender verification in sport. Although those detected are aware of their amenorrhoea, they have had no doubts about their femininity and the pronouncement that they are genetic males comes as a complete shock. The response is invariably to withdraw from competition in great distress and to reject any further testing or examination. The Medical Commission of the IOC recommend that those affected with the complete syndrome are eligible to compete, but that before doing so they must submit to chromosome analysis, gynaecological examination, and hormone tests to ensure that there is no masculinization which might indicate that they have an unfair advantage over normal women. Despite the worthy intentions of the IOC Medical Commission, it is clear that athletes who have failed the sex chromatin test are often too distressed to follow their advice and as a result have been disqualified unjustly. The IOC Medical Commission must accept responsibility for this as they have failed, until recently, to provide any clear guidelines to medical committees at international events as to the eligibility of athletes with androgen insensitivity or one of its variants.

While almost all such athletes retire permanently from their sport, one recent case has aroused special interest in that the athlete concerned has fought successfully against the decision and has been granted an eligibility certificate. This has not been without considerable personal distress and humiliation. The case concerns an athlete in the 60-m hurdles who 'passed' the sex chromatin test at the 1983 World Championships in Helsinki. However, another test was taken at the World Student Games in Kobe (Japan) in 1985 and the athlete was found to have androgen insensitivity and debarred.[14] This led to the withdrawal of her university scholarship and unwelcome publicity in the press. After 4 months waiting for the results of endocrine tests, the athlete was confirmed to be a woman, although infertile. Her case was argued before the Medical Committee of the International Amateur Athletic Federation (**IAAF**) in 1988 and she was pronounced eligible to compete in future. The case illustrates the fallibility of the sex chromatin test, the level of ignorance among sports physicians about the eligibility rules, and the trauma experienced by individual athletes caught by an unjust and ineffective system.

Sex chromosomal abnormalities

The sex chromatin test may give a paradoxical result in individuals who have gross numerical or structural abnormalities of the sex chromosomes. One of the best known of these conditions is Turner's syndrome in which those affected have primary amenorrhoea, short stature, and may have developmental malformations including webbing of the neck. Gonadal dysgenesis is invariably present and is the cause of the sexual infantilism. Chromosome analysis reveals a 45,X karyotype without a Y chromosome. As there is only one X chromosome, the Barr body is absent from somatic cell nuclei and, therefore, affected individuals fail the sex chromatin test. The short stature and developmental disabilities are such as to preclude success in most sports and there is no record of anyone with Turner's syndrome being debarred. However, variants of Turner's syndrome are not uncommon where chromosome analysis reveals a more complex sex chromosome constitution and those affected may be normal in height and have few disabilities. Some are chromosomal mosaics, that is their somatic cells are made up of two or more cell lines with different karyotypes. The most common are 45,X/46,XX and 45,X/46,XY mosaics. The latter may have rudimentary testes and ambiguous genitalia associated with significant levels of androgens. Other cases have structural rearrangements of the X or Y chromosomes including deletions, isochromosomes, and duplications; these are often accompanied by 45,X mosaicism. It is clear that those with only X rearrangements would have no advantage over normal women in sports, but those whose Y chromosome rearrangements lead to testis differentiation and masculinization may well have increased muscle mass and might be considered to be at an advantage, although this is doubtful.

Of more relevance to the present discussion are a group of individuals with Klinefelter's syndrome. These are infertile males with small testes (and commonly gynaecomastia) due to a 47,XXY karyotype. Most of those affected are rather taller than average males and tend to show clinical evidence of androgen deficiency such as diminished body hair and reduced frequency of shaving. However, many cases are fully masculinized and the muscle mass would be regarded as normal for an average male. As in Turner's syndrome, sex chromosome mosaicism is not uncommon, usually either 46,XY/47,XXY or 46,XX/47,XXY. In the latter case, the presence of a normal female cell line may lead to ambiguity of the internal and external genitalia and a few cases have been described of true hermaphrodites with both ovarian and testicular tissue.

One of the first women to be excluded from international events because she failed the current femininity test would appear to have had 46,XX/47,XXY mosaicism. This athlete won gold and bronze medals at the Tokyo Olympics in 1964 and held the world record for the women's 100 m. In 1966 she passed the inspection at the European Games at Budapest, but in the following year in Kiev was ruled ineligible for the European Cup women's track and field competition. On this occasion the test involved a close inspection of the external genitalia. A six-man medical commission investigated her case and karyotype analysis revealed cells with a 47,XXY sex chromosome complement.[9] It is understood that gonads had been removed at an earlier stage and that she was being treated with oestrogens. She was disqualified from competing in women's athletics and in 1970 the IAAF removed her name from the record books. It is of interest to consider what would have happened during the time the sex chromatin test was used for gender verification. She would have passed the test and would not have been required to submit to a gynaecological examination or chromosome analysis. It follows that she would have been eligible to compete and her name would be honoured still in world athletics. Instead she has suffered public humiliation and lived for much of her life as a recluse.

Another group of infertile patients, known as XX males, have a rather similar condition to Klinefelter's syndrome. Chromosome analysis reveals an apparently normal female karyotype but molecular studies show that the testis-determining part of the Y chromosome has been transferred to one of the two X chromosomes. The Barr body test is positive, but the individual usually develops as a normal-appearing male. Height is within the normal female range, gynaecomastia is frequent and, in a few cases, the genitalia are ambiguous.[15] It is possible that in those cases with ambiguity of the genitalia, the abnormality at birth is sufficient to raise enough doubt about the gender and the sex for the individual to be reared as female. In the closely related condition of XX true hermaphroditism, individuals in about half of the cases are raised as females. Once again it is doubtful if the degree of masculinization due to the testicular development can confer an advantage in terms of muscle mass over normal women, although the ambiguous phenotype may be a cause for genuine concern among competitors. Of course, all individuals in this group would pass the sex chromatin test and would therefore not be detected unless the more recent, polymerase chain reaction test for the sex-determining region (**SRY**) of the Y chromosome is used (see below).

Male intersex

The term male intersex (or male pseudohermaphrodite) is used to describe individuals with testes who have ambiguity of the external genitalia and who are assigned female gender at birth usually because of inadequate development of the penis. Although they are reared as girls, problems frequently arise because of masculinization at puberty. In some cases orchidectomy is performed and others undergo sex change operations in adolescence. The IOC believe that there have been cases where such individuals have been selected for training as women athletes and have been deprived of proper treatment. There appears to be no documentation of this in the medical literature. However, it is likely that in some of the early reports of males competing in women's events, the individuals concerned have had a variety of untreated male intersexuality.

Male intersexes have varying degrees of testicular development and usually respond at least partially to androgens secreted by the testes. In addition to the cases of incomplete androgen insensitivity and the cases of sex chromosome mosaicism mentioned above, there are several rare conditions which must be considered in the differential diagnosis. In 5α-reductase deficiency there is defective virilization of the external genitalia at birth because the testes are unable to convert testosterone to dihydrotestosterone. This leads to perineal hypospadias and a blind-ending perineal opening resembling a small vagina. In most families the ambiguity of the external genitalia is sufficient to lead to assignment of female gender at birth. However, at puberty, masculinization of the external genitalia occurs due to the action of testosterone and there is no breast development. The testes enlarge and semen can be produced, although beard growth may be less than normal. Many patients undergo reassignment of sex and live as males; others undergo orchidectomy and continue in the female gender. The condition is inherited as an autosomal recessive disorder limited to males, that is male sibs have a one in four risk of being affected.

The testicular regression syndrome is also likely to be a sex-limited autosomal recessive disorder. The condition occurs in XY individuals and is due to regression of the embryonic testes. If this occurs, early sex differentiation is female with hypoplasia of the müllerian ducts and normal female external genitalia. If testicular regression occurs later, there may be absence of the uterus and tubes and mild masculinization of the external genitalia. Occasionally, the phenotype is entirely male with absence of testes (anorchia).

Congenital adrenal hyperplasia

There are a number of metabolic defects which lead to virilization in women in the form of hirsutism and increased muscle mass. The best-known example is 21-hydroxylase deficiency, an autosomal recessive disorder found in at least 1 in 20 000 births. The most severe form results in virilization of the female fetus before birth and precocious puberty in boys. The metabolic defect is due to a failure to convert 17-hydroxyprogesterone to 11-deoxycortisol in the adrenal cortex. Lack of cortisol production induces the anterior pituitary to secrete ACTH which in turn leads to hyperplasia of the adrenal cortex and overproduction of adrenal androgens. The affected newborn female has normal ovaries and internal genital ducts but may appear as a male with well-developed penis (and penile urethra) but empty scrotum. Affected males are normal at birth but develop penile enlargement and pubic hair in early childhood; rapid growth is followed by early closure of the epiphyses and short stature. These changes can be prevented by cortisone therapy which suppresses ACTH production. Milder forms of 21-hydroxylase deficiency appear to be quite common in infertile, but otherwise healthy, adult women.[16] They tend to be muscular, have a male body habitus, and are often hirsute. The diagnosis is made by the estimation of urinary hormone levels following ACTH stimulation.

Female athletes who are well built, muscular, and masculine in bodily habitus are often suspected of having a mild form of congenital adrenal hyperplasia. Those affected with 21-hydroxylase deficiency are, of course, genetic females and, as they would pass the femininity control, are unlikely to be recognized. There is certainly no record of an affected individual excelling in any sport and thus it is not known whether the suspicions are unfounded. Affected males might also benefit in sport from the additional adrenal androgens, but information on this is also not available.

Male transsexuals

Males who have severe problems of gender identity may seek a sex change operation with removal of testes and genitalia and often with the construction of an artificial vagina. Replacement therapy with oestrogens may allow such male transsexuals to appear and to live as women. At least two male transsexuals have taken part in women's national events and both have aroused considerable interest in the sporting media. In 1976, a player who had previously undergone a sex change operation was allowed to enter the United States Open Tennis Tournaments after a Supreme Court Justice ruled that she was now a female.[17] That this was a controversial decision was evident from the subsequent action of the United States Tennis Association which required those entering their tournaments to pass the sex chromatin test. (This requirement has since been abandoned.) The United States Golf Association discussed the same issue in 1988 when a male transsexual was accepted for entry to the qualifying rounds of the Mid-Amateur Championship and United States Women's Open Golf Tournament. The question at issue was whether or not a person who had bilateral orchidectomy and 7 years of treatment with oestrogens could be regarded as having any advantage over normal women competitors in a golf tournament. The outcome of these discussions is not known.

While many people would regard the male transsexual as being eligible on the grounds that she was now registered and living as a female without the advantage of male androgens, the case of a male transvestite would appear to be quite different. No physical sex reassignment has been made and it would not be realistic to allow anyone who chooses to cross-dress to masquerade as a female athlete.

In India there is a large sect of individuals (numbering half a million) known as the Hegira or eunuchs who live together in small communities throughout the continent and practise their own special religious rites. Their origin can be traced back several centuries to the custom of abandoning newborn infants with sexual ambiguity to the care of this sect who come to collect their 'new member' whenever they hear about such a birth. In more recent times the membership has been augmented by stealing and forcibly castrating male children and by admitting transvestites. The Hegira earn their living by telling fortunes, giving advice on curing infertility, by entertaining at family weddings and births, and by prostitution. It is not impossible that the more athletic of the castrated eunuchs could be recruited into sport, or that castration and reassignment of sex might be used to obtain the financial benefits associated with success in sport. However unrealistic this might seem to be, it would seem important to exclude even the remotest possibility that a young male athlete might be persuaded to undergo a sex change operation for such a purpose.

The introduction and use of sex chromatin tests

The buccal smear test was first tried out in a small proportion of athletes chosen at random at the Winter Olympic Games in Grenoble in 1968. The apparent success of the procedure led to its use among almost 1000 female competitors in the Olympic Games in Mexico City the same year. There is no official information about the results of testing on either of these occasions as the IOC Medical Commission has taken a decision to maintain strict secrecy about sex chromatin findings in order to avoid innuendo and rumour. However, it is understood that while one athlete failed the test in Grenoble there were no ineligible athletes in Mexico City. Technical

and organizational problems at the Mexico City Games may have led to incomplete testing[18] and thus the failure to prevent 'ineligible' persons from competing. The situation was reviewed by the IOC before the Olympic Games in Munich in 1972 and stricter guidelines were introduced. In addition to the Barr body test, the buccal smears were also tested for fluorescent Y chromatin revealed by quinacrine staining. The Y body represents the heterochromatic and fluorescent distal segment of the long arm of the Y chromosome which is visible in about 80 per cent of male nuclei. As it varies in size between individuals, it is sometimes difficult to detect and can be missed altogether. In addition, other non-sex chromosomes may occasionally carry large variant fluorescent segments which stain with quinacrine and can be confused with the Y chromatin. Thus false-positive and false-negative results are common, and it is recorded that a swimmer at the World Student Games in 1985 failed the femininity control because of such a false-positive result on the Y-chromatin test.[19] She was told that she might not be able to have children and suffered considerable anxiety and distress before detailed chromosome analysis at home some months later revealed that the fluorescent spot was due to a variant autosome which had no clinical significance.

It is known that 3 of the 1280 female athletes at the Munich Games failed the X- and Y-chromatin tests, but no details are available.[18] The tests apparently did not prevent all attempts at fraud for it is alleged that one of the Asian women's volleyball teams included a man.[9] Eighteen hundred tests were performed at the 1976 Olympics in Montreal; while some reports suggest that all results were normal, another more reliable source indicates that four athletes were found to be ineligible. No information is available about the numbers tested at the Moscow Olympics in 1980, although two athletes are thought to have failed the femininity control. In 1984, 6 athletes out of approximately 2500 failed the test at Los Angeles and several others failed at the Winter Olympics in Calgary. There is no information available on the results of testing at the 1988 Olympic Games in Seoul.

The above information on the results of sex chromatin testing at the Olympic Games has been gleaned largely from unofficial sources and may therefore be unreliable. The best estimate suggested that at least 1 in 500 athletes fail the sex chromatin test.[3] As indicated earlier in this chapter, the available information suggests that the diagnosis in the majority of cases is the androgen insensitivity syndrome in XY females. Although athletes with this condition are eligible to compete, they cannot do so without submitting themselves to further investigation and, almost without exception, it seems that they have chosen not to submit to additional testing and examination (see above). Consequently, these athletes have been debarred unjustly from competition and have suffered needless distress and anxiety. On the other hand, there is no evidence that the tests have either identified males masquerading as females, or intersex individuals who have a substantial advantage over normal females due to male hormones.

The author believes that athletes who have to submit to gender verification by sex chromatin tests have a right to the complete information about results of such testing in the past, so that they may understand the limitations of the test and the problems that may occur. Correct information should be made available about the number of athletes who have failed the sex chromatin test, the number who have returned for further investigation after failing the test, the diagnoses obtained on complete investigation, the number of athletes who have retired from competition without returning for further investigation, and the number of tests which gave incorrect results. This information can be supplied without relating it to individual competitions and thus there need be no concern about breaching confidentiality or initiating rumours about individual athletes. The IOC Medical Commission are believed to have the necessary records to provide this data, but until 1993 have not responded positively to requests to make summaries available (see below).

Recent developments

The buccal smear test was introduced as a scientific and practical means of femininity control which avoided the need for the demeaning types of genital inspection which were so resented by athletes in 1966 to 1967. However, the use of sex chromatin was criticized as early as 1968 by Dr K.L. Moore, one of the pioneers of nuclear sex determination,[20] as being an inappropriate measure of the gender of an individual. In a letter to the British Olympic Committee declining an invitation to undertake sex chromatin tests for the Commonwealth Games in Edinburgh in 1970, the author of this chapter pointed out that there was a greater possibility of detecting an unsuspecting female with androgen insensitivity than a normal male masquerading as a female. It was further suggested that if the athletes found a physical inspection by a physician unacceptable, it would be wiser to drop the establishment of sex as a criterion than to use a wholly inappropriate test. The same view has been taken by a number of medical geneticists and others,[21,22] and experience over the past 25 years has fully substantiated all the fears that were expressed. The current position of the IOC Medical Commission is that femininity control has been successful in that it has stopped the rumour and innuendo that was rife among sportswomen in the 1960s and that it has deterred individuals with an unfair advantage from competing in women's events. Athletes have in general been satisfied with the system as they believe that individuals have been deterred from cheating by a test which does not invade their privacy. However, owing to the secrecy imposed about those unjustly debarred from competition, most athletes are unaware of the serious deficiencies of the present system.

In the face of the determination of the IOC to continue with the sex chromatin test, the author and others have subsequently agreed to undertake gender verification by sex chromatin testing on the grounds that they can help ensure that those who fail the test can be advised promptly and correctly. In this way a number of athletes with androgen insensitivity have been granted eligibility certificates in good time to compete without anyone other than the athlete and the scientists involved in the testing being aware of the diagnosis. Not all those involved in testing are adequately informed about these matters (particularly at the national level) and so it cannot be guaranteed that mistakes and tragedies can always be avoided. Indeed, competitors continued to be debarred unjustly despite such efforts. Clearly, a more rational approach to gender verification was needed.

In November 1990 the International Athletic Foundation (**IAF**) convened an international group of individuals concerned with gender verification in sport at a Workshop in Monte Carlo. The membership included sports physicians, former world-class female athletes, a medical geneticist, paediatrician, obstetrician, pathologist, psychiatrist, and several representatives of international governing bodies of sport including a representative of the IOC Medical Commission. The Workshop was chaired by Professor Arne Ljungqvist, Chairman of the IAAF Medical Committee, and its aim was to review the system of gender verification, discuss the need for it in sport and, if necessary, propose more suitable alternative methods. The group made a number of important recommendations for submission to the IAAF and IOC.[23] These are summarized below.

1. That the general information concerning the results of sex chromatin testing since 1968 be made available in a form which protected the confidentiality of individual athletes. It was felt that lack of such data prevented the athletic community from a proper consideration of the need for gender verification and the problems associated with it.

2. That the purpose of gender verification was to prevent normal men from masquerading as women in women's competition. XY females who were raised as girls and live with female gender should not be excluded. Individuals undergoing male–to–female sex reassignment before puberty should not be excluded. Decisions about male transsexuals who have been reassigned to female gender after puberty should be made by the relevant medical body within the sports organization concerned.

3. In view of the unfair exclusion of women athletes in the past due to erroneous sex chromatin testing and medical ignorance, gender verification by this means should be abandoned. So long as concerns exist about males masquerading as females, a revised and medically sound form of eligibility certification is required.

4. All men and women selected to participate in international competition should have a medical examination, performed under the auspices of the respective national organization and according to international guidelines, to ensure that there is no form of ill health or physical reason why it would not be in their interest to compete. The examination would include a simple inspection of the external genitalia and the certificate issued after the examination should be entitled the 'Health and Gender Certificate'.

5. Quality control must be conducted at international competition to combat possible abuse. This should be done randomly and by repeating the examination conducted at national level. The number of examinations should be strictly limited and, once undertaken, should not be required of the same athlete again.

The important conclusion of the Workshop was that female competitors are eligible irrespective of their genetic, chromosomal, gonadal, or hormonal sex. Those who have some form of masculinization due to any cause other than taking drugs are not to be barred from women's events. This includes for example 21-hydroxylase deficiency, 5α-reductase deficiency, androgen insensitivity, and all forms of sex chromosomal mosaicism provided that the individual has been reared as a female. Only those individuals (of whatever

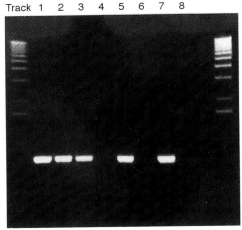

Track 1 2 3 4 5 6 7 8

Fig. 2 Gel electrophoresis showing the presence of amplified DNA from the SRY gene in five of eight tracks. Tracks 4, 6 and 8 contain no SRY fragment and are from XX individuals; the remaining tracks are from XY individuals. Tracks on either side contain size markers.

genetic sex) who have been reared as male are ineligible. The opinion of the Workshop was that any form of genetic testing, whether by sex chromatin or the more modern, polymerase chain reaction technique using Y-specific DNA probes, was inappropriate.

The IAF Council considered and approved the recommendations of the Monte Carlo Workshop in January 1991 and implemented the new procedures at the IAAF World Championships in Athletics in Tokyo in August 1991. Thus, 16 of the 20 teams who had at least 20 participants (male and female) had conducted a full health check on all athletes before they went to Tokyo. Women athletes who had not been subjected to a health check at home and who did not already carry an eligibility certificate took part in the health check. Although male participants were not examined in Tokyo, at least 556 of the 925 male athletes had had a health check at home. Most of the major countries participating in Tokyo had understood the new procedures very well. However, some athletes saw the health check as an unwelcome return to the unacceptable genital examinations used for gender verification over 25 years ago, and there was uncertainty among team physicians about what constituted a health check.

The IOC Medical Commission considered the Monte Carlo report in February 1991 and decided to recommend to the IOC Executive Board that they accept the proposal to allow National Olympic Committees to issue health certificates. The Medical Commission could not agree to accept the proposals in full and recommended that a sex test should continue to be carried out on all female athletes at the Olympic Games. A decision was taken to use the polymerase chain reaction test at the 1992 Winter Olympics in Albertville and so check the validity of the health and gender certificates issued by the National Olympic Committees.

At the Albertville Games 557 women athletes were tested by polymerase chain reaction amplification of the SRY (sex-determining region of the Y chromosome) gene (Fig. 2) using an appropriate control.[24] Two samples from the inside of the left and right cheeks were taken from each athlete by women assistants and the laboratory tests were run under rigorous conditions. It was stated that the test was 99 per cent reliable and polymerase chain reaction amplification

is known to have failed in only a comparatively small number of cases. This implies that in five or six cases an erroneous result was obtained and that an unstated number of tests had to be repeated. None the less, in 98 per cent of cases the results were available within 24 h. The Medical Commission of the IOC required those involved to undertake not to disclose the results; the number of those who failed the eligibility test and were disqualified is therefore unknown.

More complete details are known about the arrangements for gender verification at the 1992 Summer Olympics in Barcelona thanks to the kind co-operation of Dr A. Garciá Herreros, who was in charge of the testing, and to the IOC Medical Commission who permitted the author to have access to the unattributed results; neither the names of the athletes nor the events in which they competed were divulged so that full confidentiality was preserved.[25] Two samples of buccal mucosal cells were taken from both sides of the mouth of each female competitor. One sample was tested using the polymerase chain reaction for a repetitive DNA sequence (DYZ1) carried by the Y chromosome as well as a control sequence for mitochondrial DNA (Mit). It was expected that the DYZ1 sequence would be present exclusively in XY individuals and that the Mit sequence would give a positive reaction in all individuals irrespective of their sex chromosome constitution. However, 12 of the samples from the 2406 female athletes gave a positive result with the DYZ1 sequence. When these 12 samples were retested on duplicate samples for the DYZ1 sequence, the positive results were confirmed in all except one (false-positive) case. When the 11 true-positive samples were tested for the testis-determining SRY-specific sequence, only 5 gave a positive result. The five athletes from whom these samples were taken were asked to attend for physical examination. Four athletes had clinical findings consistent with the diagnosis of an XY female. All were allowed to compete and so it is presumed that the likely diagnosis was the androgen insensitivity syndrome. One athlete refused clinical examination and withdrew from the competition. A press report refers to this athlete who is reputed to be the mother of three children born after normal pregnancies, but this is not confirmed. An additional athlete, who was known to be SRY positive before the Barcelona Games, was diagnosed as having androgen insensitivity and allowed to compete without retesting.

These results indicate that 1 in 401 (6 of 2407) of the female athletes had a test result positive for the SRY sex-determining gene. This is a higher frequency that the 1 in 504 tentatively estimated from anecdotal information obtained from previous international events.[3] The six athletes in whom the buccal cell samples were positive for the DYZ1 sequence carried by the Y chromosome but negative for the SRY sequence raise interesting questions. It is possible that their genotypes contain fragments of the Y chromosome, present either as a chromosomal rearrangement or as an additional abnormal Y chromosome, carrying Y-linked genes influencing height.

It is reported that 711 samples failed to give results using the polymerase chain reaction test for either the Y-specific sequence or the Mit control sequence. Retesting using purified DNA from the samples gave good results except in three cases which had to be resampled. A recall rate of 1 in 800 would seem reasonably satisfactory in such circumstances.

In May 1992, the IAAF convened a second Working Group in

London to consider the views of team physicians and others on the working of the health check proposal. Health checks had proved difficult to document and the use of Health and Gender Certificates seemed unpopular and impracticable. All agreed that in view of the arrangements in place for doping control, which required athletes to void a urine sample in the presence of an observer, there was no longer any need for an additional inspection for gender verification to exclude males masquerading as females. The Group recommended unanimously to the IAAF Council that femininity certification was no longer required. This recommendation was formally accepted at the annual meeting of the IAAF Council in Toronto on the 29 to 31 May 1992. Members of the IAAF were advised to monitor the health of their athletes before participation in international events, but this was not compulsory and certificates were no longer to be issued. In June 1993, the organizers of the 1993 World University Games announced that, following representations from the IAAF and others, they had decided to abandon any form of gender verification at the Games in Buffalo. By September 1995 only 4 of 37 Olympic Sports Federations consulted about the matter were known to be conducting sex testing at their own World Championships or similar competitions; however nine Federations failed to respond (Professor Arne Ljungqvist, personal communication). The four Federations that had not abandoned mandatory testing are the International Skiing Federation, the International Basketball Federation, the International Volleyball Federation and the International Weightlifting Federation. Sex testing has also been abandoned at the Commonwealth Games and by the European Handball Association. The Women's Tennis and Ladies Professional Golf Associations no longer require routine gender verification but reserve its use in the event of a challenge concerning the eligibility of a particular athlete.

Despite the widespread agreement to abandon mandatory genetic sex testing, some athletes believe that this may lead to the return of cheating by males masquerading as females or by individuals with disorders of sex determination who may have unfair advantage in competition due to high testosterone levels. A group of 16 Olympic and international-class athletes (mostly long distance runners) petitioned the IAAF in 1994 to reintroduce gender verification at 'high-stakes events' such as marathon races with large prize money, World Championships, and Olympic Games.[26] They proposed that all competitors should sign a statement agreeing to testing following the event should they be among the medalists or money winners. Testing would include a genetic test on buccal smear cells and a gynaecological examination, followed by further blood tests if the results were in doubt. Prize money could not be dispensed without gender verification. They regarded the buccal smear alone as an unfair test of gender and argued that observation of athletes voiding urine for doping control was ineffective for gender verification as experience showed that in many cases no one was watching closely enough. They claimed that cursory medical examinations by national team physicians often do not extend below the waist. It is understood that the athletes were not only concerned about males masquerading as females but also had concerns that some transsexuals with intact testes may try to compete. They believed that anyone found to have 5-α reductase deficiency should also be excluded. With regard to the alternative method of challenging athletes of questionable gender, the consensus was that this places an

unfair burden on both the accused and the accuser. Routine high-stakes testing would make the challenge method unnecessary.

It is clear that these petitioners of the IAAF were unconvinced by the medical arguments that XY females had no unfair advantage over other athletes of similar height and build, and that doping control as practised was insufficient to detect a determined male imposter. Endocrinologists view with alarm their suggestion that blood tests might be introduced to measure hormone levels. Apart from the additional costs and the ethical problem of blood sampling, there are considerable difficulties in interpreting the variable blood levels which will be found; and these are likely to lead to more problems than the tests are designed to resolve.

These concerns, and the anxiety that innuendo about gender problems might return should gender verification be abandoned, have led the IOC to maintain its resolve to continue genetic testing at the Olympic Games. Although the medical and scientific community in Norway declined to co-operate with testing at the 1994 Winter Games in Lillehammer, the commercial unit responsible for testing at the 1992 Winter Games in Albertville were charged to conduct the testing again. No information is available about the results on this occasion.

A significant change in the arrangements for testing was introduced at the 1996 Olympic Games in Atlanta. Responsibility for both the laboratory and subsequent clinical investigations was given by the Atlanta Committee for the Olympic Games to the Division of Medical Genetics at the Emory University School of Medicine situated in Atlanta. Dr L.G. Elsas, a certified medical geneticist, was appointed Medical Director for Gender Verification and his priorities were to prevent masquerading males from competing and to ensure that no harm was done to females with anticipated problems of intersex. A full account of the arrangements and results have been published in the *Journal of the Medical Association of Georgia*.[27] Fifty volunteers were recruited for sample collection and laboratory processing; all were females to avoid possible accidental contamination of samples by males. All buccal mucosal cell samples were collected within a few days of the opening ceremony in the Polyclinic at the Olympic Village, except for 242 that were collected at outreach stations in Columbus, Savanna, and Ocoee. Of the 3387 athletes who were issued with gender verification cards, 296 did not require testing as they had certificates from previous Olympic games. All samples were analysed and reported within 48 h, with an average turn-round time of 22 h. Once again the presence of the SRY gene was used as a marker of male genetic sex, and an autosomal gene (galactose-1-phosphate uridyltransferase) was used as the control to confirm adequate DNA amplification in all samples. Eight out of 3387 female athletes (1 in 423) tested positive and agreed to further clinical evaluation. Seven of the eight had the androgen insensitivity syndrome; four had the incomplete and three the complete syndrome. With the exception of one with incomplete and one with the complete syndrome, who were unaware of their problem, all had had bilateral gonadectomy at least 3 months prior to the Olympic Games in Atlanta. Care was taken to avoid anxiety and letters were written to team physicians explaining the results and, where necessary, recommending further medical evaluation after the games. One of the eight athletes was found to have 5-α reductase deficiency; she had had gonadectomy previously and so there was no question about her being eligible to compete. Thus, all eight who

Olympic Games	Number of athletes tested	Number with positive test (%)	Frequency
Munich, 1972	1280	3 (0.23)	1 in 426
Montreal, 1976	1800	4 (0.22)	1 in 450
Los Angeles, 1984	2500	6 (0.24)	1 in 416
Barcelona, 1992	2406	6 (0.25)	1 in 401
Atlanta, 1996	3387	8 (0.24)	1 in 423
Total	11,373	27 (0.24)	1 in 421

Table 1 Results of genetic testing for gender verification at various Olympic Games

NB The figures for other Olympic Games are not available to the author.

tested positive for SRY were given gender verification certificates and went on to compete.

At the time of testing, all female athletes at the Atlanta Games were handed a questionnaire written in both English and French asking whether in their view testing of females should be continued in future Olympics and whether or not they were made anxious by the testing procedure. Of the 928 athletes who responded, 82 per cent felt that testing should be continued and 94 per cent indicated that they were not made anxious by the procedure; however, 46 athletes stated that they were made anxious. The main aims of the verification process were therefore satisfactorily achieved; no males were found to masquerade as females, and all females who were found to be SRY positive were able to compete. While a similar proportion of females failed the test as in previous Olympics (Table 1), it is noteworthy that on this occasion no mistakes were made and no athlete was unjustly barred from competition.

The organizers of the genetic testing at Atlanta noted that US$150 000 was needed to provide the laboratory testing alone, and that this cost did not include the time given voluntarily by 50 professionals who donated from 18 to 90 days to accomplish the programme. They concluded from their results and from their experience of the cost and complexity of the procedure, that genetic screening of all female athletes should be abandoned in future and replaced by random, standardized medical examinations by a consultative organization of physicians preapproved by the IOC and the Olympic Programme Sports Federations and well ahead of competition. Athletes, sports governors, and sports physicians should be educated about sex differentiation disorders and their appropriate medical care. Such a practice would allow evaluation of intersex problems and the institution of gonadectomy and oestrogen replacement therapy (which is the recommended and established treatment for these disorders) in ample time before any major event.

While the author of this chapter is sympathetic to the conclusions of the gender testing team at Atlanta, he remains unconvinced that gender verification by special medical examination is necessary in future. It is agreed that athletes and sports physicians should be fully advised about disorders of sex differentiation as described in these pages, if only to ensure that athletes with these conditions receive appropriate medical advice. This view was endorsed by the Women's Sports Foundation who passed a resolution in April 1997 that chromosomal screening for gender verification should be abandoned. Since then, the Norwegian parliament has taken the decision

that genetic testing for the purpose of gender verification in sport is illegal in Norway (Professor Arne Ljungqvist, personal communication). Meanwhile, the IOC have referred the matter for a legal opinion; it is understood that the recommendation was that there is to be no change at present, although the matter will be kept under continuous review. Perhaps it is not too much to hope that the matter may be resolved by the IOC before the new millennium, and in time for the Olympic Games in Sydney.

Why are XY females over-represented among athletes?

It is appropriate to consider in more detail the basis for the increased frequency of XY females among athletes in comparison with the general population. Higher testosterone levels can be excluded as an explanation in almost all cases, as gonadectomy is part of the treatment in incomplete androgen insensitivity and other forms of male intersex. Individuals with complete androgen insensitivity are unresponsive to testosterone, while those with gonadal dysgenesis produce no testosterone. Another explanation might be that XY females are invariably amenorrhoeal, but the possibility that this might confer an advantage seems remote. In any case, many athletes become amenorrhoeal during intensive training.

The author believes that a more likely explanation is that XY females are selected on the basis of their stature. Although this will be largely a matter of conjecture until anthropometric data are available on XY female athletes for comparison with other athletes, there is good circumstantial evidence in favour of this view. It is known from clinical research that XY female patients with either androgen insensitivity or pure gonadal dysgenesis have a mean adult height on average 10 cm more than normal female controls (and patients with XX gonadal dysgenesis) and only 2 cm less than normal male controls.[28] The effect is largely, if not entirely, due to determinants for stature carried by the differential region of the Y chromosome. There is a large standard deviation from the mean and the range in XY females is known to extend to at least 183 cm. One might expect XY female athletes to be at the upper end of the range observed in XY female patients. The importance of Y-linked genes on adult height is further supported by the observation that XX males are on average 9 cm shorter than normal Y-bearing males.[15]

Athletes who are XY females are therefore likely to be taller than average women but not necessarily taller than other athletes, as all must be equally selected on the basis of their physical attributes. The only information available on this point comes from the height records of female athletes at Atlanta (Dr L.J. Elsas, personal communication). The mean height of the 8 SRY+ve athletes was 175 cm (range 167 to 184 cm) which, although uncontrolled, is consistent with the hypothesis that stature is the important variable. It would clearly be of interest to compare the athletic abilities of XY female athletes with XX female athletes matched for height to determine if other factors also played a part. However, the opportunities for such studies would seem to be remote.

Selection in favour of tall athletes undoubtedly occurs in many types of sport and it would not be surprising that XY females are among those chosen. Genes important for stature are not only present on the Y chromosome, but also occur on the X chromosome and on several autosomes. Variation in stature due to Y-linked genes cannot be distinguished from variation due to genes on other chromosomes. These factors are part of the inherent characteristics of every athlete and no one would suggest that they be used to determine who should or should not compete in any particular event.

Conclusion

In view of the above, one must conclude that the most likely explanation for the observation that XY females are found more frequently among athletes than in the general population is due to their increased stature. As athletes do not compete on the basis of their stature, there would seem to be no reason to exclude athletes that are tall due to Y-linked genes. The only other reason for gender verification is to exclude males from masquerading as females, but, as far as is known, genetic testing has never detected an instance of this within at least the last 30 years. Despite the fear of some athletes, the opportunity for such deception, given doping control and the type of sports clothing now in use, seems remote. At the very most, the only change that might be required to ensure that cheating does not occur is a more rigorous enforcement of the requirements for doping control; those charged with observing urine collection need to be given the responsibility for notifying cases of questionable gender. The sooner athletes realize that genetic tests are irrelevant, are highly discriminating, and have subjected a substantial number of women unnecessarily to emotional and social injury, the sooner it will be possible to achieve international competition among women according to the best principles of the Olympic tradition.

References

1. Wilmore JH. The application of science to sport: physiological profiles of male and female athletes. *Canadian Journal of Applied Physiology* 1979; **27**: 25–31.
2. Dyer KF. The trend of the male–female performance differential in athletics, swimming and cycling, 1948–1976. *Journal of Biosocial Science,* 1977; **9**: 325–8.
3. Ferguson-Smith MA, Ferris EA. Gender verification in sport: the need for change? *British Journal of Sports Medicine* 1991; **25**: 17–21.
4. Anonymous. Athlete's sex secret. *The Guardian* 1981; **Jan 26**.
5. Tachezy R. Pseudohermaphroditism and physical efficiency. *Journal of Sports Medicine and Physical Fitness* 1969; **9**: 119–22.
6. Donohoe T, Johnson N. Drugs and the female athlete In: *Foul Play.* Oxford: Basil Blackwell, 1986; 66–79.
7. Ryan AJ. Sex and the singles player. *Physician and Sports Medicine* 1976; **4**: 39–41.
8. Hay E. Sex determination in putative female athletes. *Journal of the American Medical Association* 1972; **221**: 998–9.
9. Larned D. The femininity test: a woman's first Olympic hurdle. *Womensports* 1976; **3**: 8–11, 41.
10. Turnbull A. Woman enough for the Games? *New Scientist* 1988; **Sep 15**: 61–4.
11. Bunge RG. Sex and the Olympic Games. *Journal of the American Medical Association* 1960; **173**: 196.
12. Ferguson-Smith MA. Genotype–phenotype correlations in individuals with disorders of sex determination and development including Turner's syndrome. In: Goodfellow PN, Lovell-Badge R, eds. *Sex determination and the mammalian Y chromosome. Seminars in Development Biology* 1991; **2**: 265–76.
13. Berta P *et al.* Genetic evidence equating SRY and the testis determining factor. *Nature* 1990; **348**: 448–50.
14. Sakamoto H, Nakanoin K, Komatsu H, Michimoto T, Takashima E, Furuyama J. Femininity control of the XXth Universiade in Kobe, Japan. *International Journal of Sports Medicine* 1988; **9**: 193–5.
15. Ferguson-Smith MA, Cooke A, Affara NA, Boyd E, Tolmie JL. Genotype–phenotype correlations in XX males and their bearing on current theories of sex determination. *Human Genetics* 1990; **84**: 198–202.
16. New M, Levine LS. Recent advances in 21-hydroxylase deficiency. *Annual Review of Medicine* 1984; **35**: 649–53.
17. Caldwell F. Victorious in court, she's defeated on court. *Physician and Sports Medicine* 1977; **5**: 26–8.
18. Schwinger E. Problems of sex differentiation in athletics. *Atleticastudi* 1981; **5**: 72–80.
19. Carlson A. Chromosome count. *Ms* (New York) 1988; **Oct**: 40–4.
20. Moore KL. The sexual identity of athletes. *Journal of the American Medical Association* 1968; **205**: 787–8.
21. de la Chapelle A. The use and misuse of sex chromatin screening for 'gender identification' of female athletes. *Journal of the American Medical Association* 1986; **256**: 1920–3.
22. Simpson JL. Gender testing in the Olympics. *Journal of the American Medical Association* 1986; **256**: 1938.
23. Ljungqvist A, Simpson JL. Medical examination for health of all athletes replacing the need for gender verification in international sports. *Journal of the American Medical Association* 1992; **267**: 850–2.
24. Dingeon B, Hamon P, Robert M, Schamasch P, Pugeat M. Sex testing at the Olympics. *Nature* 1992; **358**: 447.
25. Serrat A, Garcia de Herreros A. Determination of genetic sex by PCR amplification of Y-chromosome specific sequences. *Lancet* 1993; **341**: 1593.
26. Heinonen J. A decent proposal. Keeping Track. *International Track and Field Newsletter* 1994; **24 (March)**.
27. Elsas LJ, Hayes RP, Muralidharan K. Gender verification at the Centennial Olympic Games. *Journal of the Medical Association of Georgia* 1997; **86**: 50–4.
28. Ogata T, Matsuo N. Comparison of adult height between patients with XX and XY gonadal dysgenesis: support for a Y specific growth gene(s). *Journal of Medical Genetics* 1992; **29**: 539–41.

3.6 The overtraining syndrome

Richard Budgett, Linda Castell, and E.A. Newsholme

Background to the problem

Any prolonged deterioration in performance is of major concern to athletes and will often lead them to seek help from a sports medicine doctor. Athletes are used to feeling fatigued due to the physical and mental stresses of training and competition, but they do expect to recover within a few days. If they fail to recover, respond negatively to training, and especially if they suffer from a cluster of other symptoms, they may be diagnosed as suffering from the so-called 'overtraining syndrome'.[1] This is also described as burn-out, staleness, and chronic fatigue in athletes, but it should really be viewed as an under-recovery syndrome since some sufferers are training no more than their fit colleagues.[2–5]

The intensity and volume of training is very important,[6] as high-intensity exercise with little rest (intensive interval work) is the most likely to precipitate an overtraining syndrome. It is extremely rare in sprinters because their training involves frequent, long rest periods.[7,8]

The primary complaint is that of reduced performance. As many as 10 to 20 per cent of élite swimmers are described as suffering from symptoms of this syndrome each year.[9] Other causes, such as the fatigue associated with infectious mononucleosis, myocarditis should be included.[10]

Definition of overtraining

Over-reaching is a term that describes the effects of hard training which, when followed by adequate rest, leads to recovery with supercompensation and an improvement in performance. It is a normal part of most training programmes.[1] By contrast, overtraining that leads to the overtraining syndrome can only be diagnosed in retrospect since an athlete may recover from very hard training—in which case it was over-reaching. The overtraining syndrome can be defined as a state of prolonged fatigue and underperformance caused by a failure to recover from hard training and competition.[10] Underperformance should be measured objectively using an appropriate ergometer or by checking the athlete's training and competition history. Symptoms must have lasted at least 2 weeks despite adequate rest, with no other identifiable medical cause.[11] This contrasts with the diagnosis of chronic fatigue syndrome in which similar symptoms typically can last for more than 6 months.[12]

Clinical presentation and the overtraining syndrome

Many sportsmen and women train very hard to compete even at club level, so fatigue due to the stress of training is not confined to Olympic athletes.[13] The overtraining syndrome is most common in endurance athletes such as middle- and long-distance runners, cyclists, swimmers, triathletes, rowers, and cross-country skiers. It is seen less frequently in repetitive sprint sports/games such as football, rugby, tennis, and badminton, and is only in sprinters or power athletes.[14,15]

Symptoms

Athletes often describe being able to keep-up at the beginning of a race but are unable to lift the pace or sprint for the line. They also complain of fatigue, heavy muscles, and depression. Sleep disturbance is known to be important in chronic fatigue syndrome. Direct questioning reveals poor sleep in over 90 per cent of cases, with reports of difficulty getting to sleep, waking in the night, nightmares, and waking unrefreshed.[16] Other common symptoms include: increased anxiety, irritability, and emotional lability; loss of appetite with weight loss; loss of competitive drive, energy, purpose, and libido; raised resting pulse rate and excessive sweating. Upper respiratory tract infections (**URTI**), frequently recur each time the athlete returns to training after a period of inadequate rest.[1] Some distinguish overtraining syndrome between sympathetic and parasympathetic forms, for example, by anxious and excited athletes or by depressed or phlegmatic athletes, respectively.[14] Although any combination is possible.

Signs

Signs are often linked with an associated illness, for example, cervical lymphadenopathy. There may be an increased postural drop in blood pressure and postural rise in heart rate.[17] Underperformance can be confirmed by demonstrating a reaction in maximal power output (VO_2max), and an increase in submaximal oxygen consumption and pulse rate with a slow recovery to normal after exercise.[16] Precipitating factors in overtraining include:

- intensive interval training;
- sudden increases in training;
- heavy monotonous training;
- physical and psychological stress.

Training patterns

There is often a recent history of an increase or change in training.[18] As the competitive summer season approaches many athletes switch from low-intensity winter training to high-intensity summer training with intensive interval work. This involves 1 to 6 min of hard exercise repeated several times interspersed with short periods of rest.[19] The stress of competition and selection pressures may also be contributory factors.[1] Sudden increases in training can also be contributory, especially if there is inadequate time for recovery.[20] Heavy, monotonous training without cyclical variation (called periodization) can also lead to burn-out.[2] Most athletes should be able to recover within 2 weeks of exhaustive training (as in a typical training camp) as long as they started in a non-fatigued state.[21] In addition, psychological stresses and physical stresses may also reduce the ability to recover from, or respond to, heavy training.[15]

Clinical investigations

The aim of clinical investigations is to exclude other causes of chronic fatigue and often to reassure the athlete, since there is no diagnostic test available. Any battery of tests depends on a sensible approach to clinical possibilities guided by the history and examination. A routine haematological screen may be all that is necessary, but occasionally more extensive investigations are needed in order to exclude serious disease such as viral myocarditis. A history of recurrent URTIs, allergic rhinitis, or exercise-induced wheeze, provide an indication for lung function testing.[10] Haemoglobin and haematocrit levels fall as a normal response to heavy training due to haemodilution, and do not affect performance.

Plasma creatine kinase activity is an unreliable measure of overtraining since there is a 50-fold individual variation in the response to hard exercise.[17] Viral titres must be shown to rise to make a diagnosis of postviral illness. A positive Paul–Bunnell test for infectious mononucleosis is highly suggestive of Epstein–Barr viral infection.

Changes in red blood cells magnesium concentration or concentrations of other trace elements have also been linked to the overtraining syndrome. However, the widespread use of supplements by athletes has not been observed to date to offer any protection from chronic fatigue.[5]

Over-reaching

Much of the literature on overtraining describes investigations of athletes who are, in fact, over-reaching. Athletes are followed through periods of very heavy short-duration training sessions and recovery. With a normal physiological response to over-reaching, performance is maintained and normally improves after a brief rest. Raised plasma cortisol and creatine kinase levels (from damaged muscle) and decreased testosterone levels, therefore leading to a lower testosterone:cortisol ratio are also seen. Muscle glycogen stores are depleted and the resting heart rate rises.[21] The profile of mood state (**POMS**) questionnaire indicates reduced vigour and increased tension, depression, anger, fatigue, and confusion.[23] These changes are proportional to training load and do not necessarily reflect an abnormal response.

Hormonal changes

The role of hormones in the overtraining syndrome is unclear. However, the levels of several hormones are known to vary directly with exercise and also to affect immune function. Adrenaline has been shown to mediate many of the same effects on immune cells *in vitro* as seen postexercise *in vivo*. In addition, cortisol levels rise more in overtrained athletes than in controls (those who were not overtrained). Salivary cortisol levels (reflecting free-cortisol) in a group of swimmers were shown to rise as training was increased over a 6-month period, and were significantly higher in stale, underperforming athletes. This correlated with depressed mood state.[24]

It has been suggested that athletes fail to recover from hard training because of a change in the balance of anabolism to catabolism. A low testosterone:cortisol ratio has been suggested as a marker for the overtraining syndrome, but since this falls as a normal response to hard training only a very low ratio is diagnostically useful. There may be no change during heavy training, despite reduced performance and depressed mood state.[24] In one report, the (prohibited) use of anabolic steroids has been used to treat the overtraining syndrome.[25] A reduced hormonal response to insulin-induced hypoglycaemia has also been reported.[26]

Lehmann *et al.* followed eight middle-distance runners who became overtrained. These athletes showed changes in a number of parameters including reduced plasma free fatty acid and raised plasma creatine kinase levels.[27] They showed a rise in noradrenaline levels for the same workload and a 30 per cent fall in basal nocturnal plasma dopamine, noradrenaline, and adrenaline levels which correlated with symptoms, suggesting a way of monitoring overtraining. In addition, the 24-h cortisol level was reduced by 30 per cent. A later study showed a 50 per cent fall in basal nocturnal dopamine, noradrenaline, and adrenaline levels, suggesting an impairment in the response of the sympathetic nervous system to stress.[28]

Hooper *et al.* studied overtrained swimmers and found that noradrenaline levels were higher in this group than in controls (those who were not overtrained), particularly during tapering. There was no change in the cortisol level.[9] A later study showed that plasma catecholamine levels and stress ratings (by questionnaire) predicted staleness, and a 'well being rating' questionnaire during tapering predicted performance.[11]

Training and psychology

Morton used a complex mathematical model to optimize the periodization of athletic training. He concluded that training intensity and spacing of training were the most important factors. For maximum performance, and for minimizing the risk of overtraining, intensive training on alternate days over a 150-day season, with a build-up over the first half and taper over the second half, was found to be the optimum. This was more effective than moderate training throughout the whole year.[29]

Fry *et al.* advise periodization with regular tapering and recovery, when testing and screening can be carried out without confusing overtraining with the normal fatigue of overload training (over-reaching).[7] They failed to induce overtraining by short, near-maximum, high-intensity exercise, suggesting that this is a safe regimen because of the large amounts of rest taken between efforts. This supports our own observation that sprinters and power athletes do not suffer from the overtraining syndrome. There is a drop in the lactate:rating of perceived exertion (**RPE**) ratio with heavy training, but this is not diagnostic of the overtraining syndrome.[30] For a set lactate level the perceived exertion is higher, but this may represent glycogen depletion causing lower lactate levels.

The profile of mood state (**POMS**) questionnaire has been used for many years and is well validated,[2] but as with all questionnaires it is open to misinterpretation by the respondents. The 60 questions have been reduced to 7 while still remaining discriminatory.[31] The score on POMS and other questionnaires can be used to detect staleness in swimmers, but it tends to follow training load closely through the season. The 10 per cent incidence of burn-out in American college swimmers was reduced to zero by daily monitoring with a POMS questionnaire, and reducing training when mood deteriorated and increasing it when mood improved. It is most discriminatory if the mood state fails to improve during tapering. This supports the advice to taper and recover regularly throughout the season as part of the monitoring process. Both performance and mood state have been shown to improve after 5 weeks of physical rest.[16] Low-level exercise has also been shown to speed recovery from the chronic fatigue syndrome.

Central fatigue

At the British Olympic Medical Centre we have shown that overtrained athletes produce a lower peak power in 20-second Wingate sprint tests, and weaker isometric and concentric quadriceps contractions, than do controls who are not overtrained. However, with superimposed tetanic stimulation, the athletes were able to produce the same isometric power as these controls.[33] This suggests that fatigue is central with a failure to activate fast-twitch muscle fibres fully, which fits in with the clinical history of an inability to lift the pace at the end of the race.

The role of amino acids in central fatigue

One important role of some amino acids is to act as precursors for certain brain neurotransmitters. One of these is tryptophan, which is converted in the brain to 5-hydroxytryptamine (**5-HT** or serotonin). There is evidence that tiredness and sleep may, in part, be influenced by the level of 5-HT in the brain; it is possible, therefore, that this neurotransmitter may be involved in central fatigue, that is to say, fatigue originating in the brain.

There are two important additional facts. First, branched chain amino acids (leucine, isoleucine, and valine) are not taken up by the liver but are taken up by muscle where they are used primarily for energy production, their rate of oxidation is increased during exercise.[34] Secondly, both branched chain amino acids and tryptophan enter the brain on the same amino acid carrier. Hence, there is competition between the two types of amino acids for entry into the brain.

A decrease in the level of branched chain amino acids in the blood, due to an increased rate of utilization by muscle, increases the ratio of tryptophan to branched chain amino acids in the bloodstream and favours the entry of tryptophan into the brain. This might result in central fatigue. A further important point is that the blood level of fatty acids may also play an additional role in this type of fatigue. An increase in the plasma fatty acid level above around 1 mM increases the free concentration of tryptophan—and it is probably the free concentration, rather than the total concentration

of tryptophan, that influences the rate of entry of tryptophan into the brain. Hence, an increase in the plasma fatty acid level plus a decrease in that of branched chain amino acids could markedly influence the plasma concentration ratio of free tryptophan to branched chain amino acids. This has been shown to be the case in endurance activity.[35] In rats, endurance exercise produced similar changes in the plasma concentration ratio of free tryptophan to branched chain amino acids. It has also been shown that when this plasma concentration ratio increases, the concentration of 5-HT in the hypothalamus and the brainstem also increases.[36]

In rats, sustained running to the point of fatigue caused an increase in the concentration of tryptophan and in the turnover of 5-HT in the striatal synaptosomes of genetically analbuminaemic rats (**NAR**).[37] This result could explain the fact that the running time in these rats was shortened in comparison with that observed in normal Wistar rats. The reason proposed for this is an increase in plasma free tryptophan levels.

Muscle uses branched chain amino acids for energy formation when muscle glycogen becomes depleted. It is possible that, as the muscle glycogen level approaches depletion, the blood level of fatty acids increases and hence influence the plasma level of free tryptophan.[38] Thus the fatigue caused by the depletion of glycogen in muscle could be due, not to a direct effect of glycogen depletion on the muscle, but to an increase in the level of 5-HT in a specific area of the brain. (Of course, the decrease in the muscle glycogen level will need to change some factor in muscle—possibly the activity of branched chain keto acid dehydrogenase—that will initiate a series of events leading to a change in the 5-HT level in the brain.) Failure of the motor centre in the brain to stimulate muscle contraction would mean that the power output would have to fall. Chronic changes in the levels of 5-HT in both the brain and peripheral nerves may cause physiological and behavioural changes other than fatigue.

Centrally acting 5-hydroxytryptamine and the overtraining syndrome

5-Hydroxytryptamine-containing cells are found in several large clusters in the pons and upper medulla within groups of cells known as the raphe nuclei. Projections from these cells pass rostrally to most areas of the brain via the medial forebrain bundle. The cortex, hippocampus, limbic system, and hypothalamus all receive 5-HT terminals.[39] Projections from the caudal nuclei run to the medulla and spinal cord. With such wide-ranging projections to areas involved in motor and neuroendocrine functions, interpretation of changes in the levels of 5-HT is difficult, but prolonged changes in the level of this neurotransmitter in these areas of the brain could account for the wide-ranging effects of overtraining.

The physiological functions of 5-HT in the brain can be grouped into at least three areas: sleep; motor neurone excitability; and autonomic and endocrine function.

Sleep

Lesions in the raphe nuclei or the administration of *p*-chlorophenylalanine (an inhibitor of 5-HT synthesis) abolish sleep in animals, whereas the microinjection of 5-HT in specific medullary areas of the brain induces sleep. Could this neurotransmitter, therefore, also be involved in the fatigue associated with the overtrained state?

Motor neurone excitability

Descending 5-HT neurones increase motor neurone excitability and, in doing so, increase monosynaptic reflexes and decrease polysynaptic reflexes. Inhibition of polysynaptic reflexes may include those involved in exercise such as running, and may contribute to the decreased maximal work capacity in the overtrained state.

Autonomic and endocrine function

From the medulla oblongata in the brainstem 5-HT neurones project to the hypothalamus which is considered to be the major centre for autonomic, endocrine, and neuronal integration. Rang and Dale[39] observed that 5-HT inhibits the release of factors from the hypothalamus which act to control the rate of release of pituitary hormones. A low rate of gonadotrophin-releasing hormone (**GnRH**) secretion by the hypothalamus would be expected to decrease the rate of release of luteinizing hormone (**LH**) and follicle-stimulating hormone (**FSH**) from the pituitary and hence lower the plasma levels of these hormones. Nash[40] has reported a decrease in the LH release frequency and amplitude after intense exercise in man. This would be expected to lower plasma levels of testosterone. In the female, a decrease in GnRH would be expected to interfere in the complex endocrine system that controls the menstrual cycle, possibly leading to irregular menses or amenorrhoea.[38] Lightman and Everett[41] provide some evidence to suggest that 5-HT plays a role in GnRH rhythmicity—the latter being inhibited by high levels of 5-HT; and if central levels of 5-HT are elevated pharmacologically, then the preovulatory LH surge is lost and amenorrhoea develops. Ulrich *et al.*[42] observed that central regulation of pulsatile FSH and prolactin release appears to involve 5-HT3 receptor mediated processes. Lesions in the ventromedial hypothalamus, which decrease the level of 5-HT, lead to hyperphagia. Hence, an elevation in the level of 5-HT in this area of the brain could explain the loss of appetite in overtrained subjects.

Similar considerations regarding the entry of tryptophan and its conversion pathway to 5-HT apply to peripheral nerves as well as to central nerves.[39] Hence, peripheral 5-HT levels could be elevated in the overtrained state. 5-HT is known to stimulate sympathetic afferent nerves in the heart thereby causing an increase in heart rate, a well-established sign of overtraining. In contrast, 5-HT inhibits the rate of noradrenaline release from vascular sympathetic nerve endings which might explain changes in blood pressure seen in the overtrained state.

Prevention and early detection of overtraining syndrome

Athletes tolerate different levels of training and competition stress. Overtraining for one athlete may be insufficient training for another; moreover, each athlete's tolerance level may change throughout the season. Individual training must be reduced when other stresses, such as examinations, are present. Unfortunately, because athletes are exhausted most of the time, unless they are tapering for a competition, it is difficult for them to tell whether their fatigue is due to overtraining or over-reaching. A persistent rise in early morning heart rate provides evidence that something is wrong.[43] Underperformance is usually noticed too late, and serial measurements of haemoglobin, haematocrit, and creatine kinase do not help. Good diet, full hydration, and rest between training sessions will help athletes to tolerate hard training. Those with a full-time job or other commitments do not recover as quickly as those who can rest after training. Since there are no objective tests to predict which athletes are going to break down during a period of hard training, adequate recovery time has to be allowed for all. Periodization of training should allow this, with particular care taken at times of intensive interval training and hard monotonous training.

Management of chronic fatigue

The treatment of any chronic fatigue syndrome requires a holistic approach. Rest and regeneration strategies are central to recovery. Athletes will not rest, but fortunately their drive to exercise can be channelled to help speed their recovery. They should exercise aerobically sustaining a pulse rate of 120 to 140 beats/min (so they can easily conduct a conversation while exercising) for a few minutes (5 to 10 min) each day, ideally in divided sessions, and slowly build this up over many weeks. Recovery generally takes about 6 to 12 weeks. Many make the mistake of trying to follow a normal training session, suffering from severe fatigue for several days before partially recovering, and then doing it again. Cross-training (in another sport) may be the only way of avoiding the tendency to increase exercise intensity too quickly. The clinician must set a positive but restricted exercise programme. Once a reasonable volume of exercise is achieved (about 1 h per day) training can then be carefully started with sessions incorporating work at or above the onset of blood lactate accumulation (**OBLA**). Before this, it is probably safe to allow occasional sprint/power sessions involving a maximum of 3×10 s of flat-out exercise with at least 3 min of complete rest between bouts.[18]

Regeneration strategies were widely used in the old Eastern bloc countries, although there are no controlled trials of treatment.[25] These involve rest and relaxation with counselling and psychotherapy. Massage and hydrotherapy are used, and nutrition is looked at in detail. Large quantities of vitamins, minerals and dietary supplements are given, although there is no evidence of their effectiveness. Any stresses outside sport are reduced as far as possible.

Athletes are often surprised at the performances they can produce despite 12 weeks of extremely light exercise, and it is then that care must be taken not to increase training too fast. They need to train hard to go faster, but in order to benefit from all their hard work they must rest and recover completely at least once a week.

Exercise, infections, and the immune system

Upper respiratory tract infections occur frequently in athletes after prolonged, exhaustive exercise compared with the normal sedentary population or with non-competing athletes.[44–48] For example, in a study of participants in the Los Angeles marathon who were infection-free before the race, the number who became ill during the week after the race was almost sixfold higher than the control group. A control group of endurance athletes who had undergone a similar level of training but who did not participate in the marathon.[49] A high incidence of infections has also been observed in military personnel undergoing prolonged and repeated intensive training.[50,51] It has been suggested that moderate, regular exercise helps to reduce the level of infection in sedentary individuals but that, in individuals who undertake intensive or excessive training, the incidence of

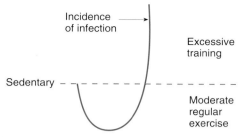

Fig. 1 The incidence of infection in sedentary individuals can be decreased with moderate exercise but increases sharply in individuals who undertake excessive amounts of exercise, or who suffer from overtraining. (Modified from ref. 45, with permission.)

infection can increase sharply: an overall view of this situation has been graphically described by Nieman's 'J-curve' which is emphasized as being descriptive, rather than quantitative (Fig. 1).[45]

Risk factors for upper respiratory tract infection

Weidner[48] critically evaluated 10 epidemiological studies which investigated the incidence of URTI in different sports. The majority of the studies which showed an increased incidence of URTI after physical activity were performed on runners.[48] A longitudinal study of 530 male and female runners suggested that a URTI was more likely to occur with higher training mileage.[52] Similarly, the risk of illness increased in endurance runners when training exceeded 97 km/week.[49] Another study, involving marathon runners, demonstrated that the stress of competition more than doubled the risk of contracting an URTI.[53]

There is a switch from nose to mouth breathing as exercise levels increase bypassing the nasal filter mechanism.[54] This also dries up bronchial secretions and impedes the protective activity of the cilia, which cover the cell surface with mucus.[55,56] The high incidence of infections after prolonged, exhaustive exercise indicates that the immune system function of some athletes may be depressed by the stress of hard training and/or competition (that is to say, immunosuppressed). It is important to determine whether or not overtrained athletes suffer more severe and more prolonged infections, or whether they are simply more prone to URTI.

The immune response to exhaustive exercise

Cells of the immune system are normally present as circulating cells in the blood and lymphoid organs (spleen, lymph nodes), and as scattered cells in virtually all tissues except the central nervous system. When an infectious agent attacks, in the first instance the inflammatory response acts together with the innate (naturally occurring) immune response; this is accompanied by the adaptive (acquired) immune response, involving T (thymus-derived) and B (derived from bone marrow) lymphocytes. There is evidence that the numbers of circulating white blood cells and their subsets, together with plasma cytokine levels, are markedly altered as a result of prolonged, exhaustive exercise. A substantial increase in the numbers of circulating white blood cells after strenuous exercise, mainly due to a large increase in circulating polymorphonuclear neutrophils, was first observed by Larrabee in 1902.[57]

Several publications have demonstrated not only that the total number of white blood cells (**WBC**) in the circulation is substantially increased during the recovery period immediately after a marathon or intensive training session,[45,58] but also that there is a transient increase in circulating lymphocyte numbers at the start of the recovery period. However, the numbers of circulating lymphocytes have generally been observed to decrease below pre-exercise levels within 30 min of cessation of exercise.[45]

It has been suggested that low-intensity exercise is beneficial to the immune system:[59] Nieman *et al.* observed elevated natural killer cell activity and reduced URTI symptoms in mildly obese women undertaking brisk-walking exercise for 15 weeks.[49] An increase in the lymphocyte response to mitogenic stimulation *in vitro* and in the number of natural killer cells and lymphocytes in the blood has been observed in response to moderate, regular exercise.[45,60,61] In contrast, there is considerable evidence that prolonged, exhaustive exercise is associated with adverse effects on immune function.[7,46,59,61-69]

These effects include:

- decreased cytolytic activity of natural killer (NK) cells;

- lower circulating numbers of T lymphocytes for 3 to 4 h after exercise;

- a decrease in the proliferative ability of lymphocytes;

- impaired antibody synthesis;

- decreased immunoglobulin levels in blood and saliva;

- a decreased ratio of CD4 to CD8 T-cells.

T lymphocytes

The numbers of T lymphocytes, as a percentage of the total lymphocytes, are reduced and remain low for several hours after strenuous exercise: in particular, a considerable reduction in the circulating levels of CD4, although not CD8 cells, has been reported compared with normal values.[7,63,66] Natural killer cell (CD16) activity is markedly reduced.[65] Studies on athletes after strenuous exercise have reported either decreased rates of lymphocyte proliferation,[70-72] or no change in proliferation,[73,74] but one study did report an increased rate of lymphocyte proliferation.[75] Nieman *et al.* observed an almost 30 per cent decrease in lymphocyte proliferation which was maintained for more than 3 h after running at around 75 per cent $V\text{O}_2$max on a treadmill for 2.5 h.[76]

Neutrophils

Neutrophils, together with macrophages, are responsible for phagocytosis and are the first cells to respond to such an invasion. Unlike most lymphocytes, neutrophils die within a few days of leaving the bloodstream. Even allowing for the effects of dehydration which could result in a greater density of cells in the blood,[58] the numbers of circulating neutrophils increase dramatically as part of the response to prolonged, strenuous exercise but their function is suppressed.[57,77]

Immunosuppression and glutamine

Glutamine is an important fuel for some cells of the immune system, such as lymphocytes and macrophages, and that it may possess specific immunostimulatory effects.[78,79] Since the total amount of such cells in the average human is very large, possibly more than 1400 g, their fuel requirements could place severe demands on the

Table 1 Some lines of evidence for the high utilization of glutamine in cells

1. The maximal catalytic activity of glutaminase, the key enzyme in the glutamine utilization pathway, is high:

   In freshly isolated lymphocytes and macrophages.[78,80]

2. The rates of utilization of glutamine are high:

   (a) in freshly isolated lymphocytes and macrophages;[78,80]

   (b) in cultured lymphocytes and macrophages, and in T- and B-lymphocyte-derived cell lines.[78,80,81]

3. A high rate of glutamine utilization by lymphocytes *in vitro* maintains unusually high intracellular concentrations of glutamine, glutamate, aspartate, and lactate. Very similar levels of these intermediates are seen in intact lymph nodes removed from anaesthetized rats and frozen rapidly prior to extraction of the tissue.[88]

body as a whole. The immune system must be able to respond instantly, effectively, and specifically to an immune challenge. This response often involves the rapid proliferation of particular clones of the cells or the rapid synthesis and secretion of peptides and proteins. There is evidence glutamine is utilized at a high rate by these cells (Table 1).

In addition, glutamine appears to be used at similar rates by T and B lymphocytes (although lymphocyte subsets have not been specifically studied).[78,80,81] Direct evidence for high rates of utilization would require arteriovenous difference measurements, together with blood flow measurements, to be made across lymphoid organs such as lymph nodes. Even if this could be done, the interpretation of the data might be difficult since it is known that adipose tissue is anatomically associated with lymph nodes[82] and that adipose tissue can release glutamine at a high rate.[83] Indeed, this association may be 'designed' to provide fuel (and perhaps even exert control) over the function of cells within the lymph node.[84] In a study measuring fluxes across the pig spleen before and after surgery it was found that the spleen actually released glutamine and ammonia before surgery.[85] There are two possible explanations: either, *in vivo*, splenocytes in lymph organs use little glutamine, or glutamine is provided by adipose tissue and arteriovenous differences reflect the balance between release from adipose and uptake by immune cells.

Lymphocytes respond to an infection by proliferating to produce enough cells to attack the invading organisms; therefore the DNA content of each lymphocyte must double for each cell cycle and RNA could increase much more. Glutamine provides the nitrogen required for the synthesis of the purine and pyrimidine nucleotides present in DNA and RNA. In macrophages, a considerable amount of mRNA is required for the new peptide and protein synthesis that occurs in response to an infection (for example, cytokine production). In addition, when macrophages attack microorganisms they produce reactive oxygen species which may kill the micro-organism but will also damage the DNA of the macrophages. For the repair of DNA, new nucleotides will be repaired. Thus, it is hypothesized that the high rate of glutamine utilization provides optimal conditions to accommodate changes in the demand for

nucleotide synthesis.[78,79] It provides a dynamic buffer system for the intermediates of the pathway, including intracellular glutamine and aspartate which are essential for the *de novo* synthesis of purine and pyrimidine nucleotides during proliferation. It can also cater for a variation in the production of mRNA in macrophages and lymphocytes, as well as the repair of DNA and RNA damaged by the reactive oxygen species produced by these cells to kill the phagocytosed micro-organisms.[10] This theory is known as branched point sensitivity in metabolic control.[79] To provide for this a continuous, high rate of glutamine utilization is required. *In vitro* experiments on lymphocytes have shown that their proliferative response is dependent upon the concentration of glutamine in the culture medium.[79,86] It is suggested, therefore, that if the concentration of plasma glutamine is decreased *in vivo* below a physiological level, the function of cells of the immune system might be impaired.

Lymphocytes and macrophages use both glucose and glutamine to generate energy, and the rate of glutamine utilization is similar to, or even greater than, that of glucose.[81] However, glutamine is not completely oxidized, but is converted mainly into glutamate, aspartate, and alanine. This partial oxidation is termed 'glutaminolysis'.

A simple reason for the high rates of utilization might be that they provide for the high energy demand. However, if energy generation *per se* was the major reason for the high rates of utilization, it would be expected that more of the carbon of glucose and glutamine would be completely oxidized, rather than glucose being converted mainly to lactate, and some, or most, of the glutamine to glutamate and aspartate. Therefore, two important questions arise:

1. What are the consequences of these high rates of glutamine utilization for the whole organism?

2. Could the demand ever exceed the ability to provide glutamine?

Although several tissues including liver, adipose, and lung can synthesize and release glutamine into the bloodstream, the tissue thought to be quantitatively the most important for glutamine synthesis is muscle,[87] which also stores and releases glutamine (Fig. 2).

The concentration of plasma glutamine is decreased during or after stress such as major trauma, burns,[89] major surgery,[90] sepsis, and starvation:[81,86,91] if the plasma concentration of glutamine is decreased, the immune response might be impaired. Thus, it is of interest that the plasma concentration is decreased in athletes after prolonged, exhaustive exercise such as running a full marathon, and after repeated bouts of intensive training.[92-95] The plasma glutamine concentration varies according to the duration of the exercise (Table 2).

The rate of glutamine release across the plasma membrane, which occurs via a specific transporter, appears to be controlled by various hormones and may be influenced by cytokines. Glutamine synthesis is important for maintaining the store of glutamine in muscle; however, the release from muscle, rather than synthesis, appears to be the key regulatory step controlling the concentration of glutamine in the bloodstream under normal conditions. Muscle not only provides glutamine but helps to regulate the plasma level, via the transporter system in the membrane.[99]

The plasma concentration of glutamine can therefore be con-

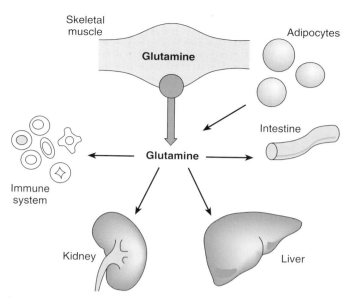

Fig. 2 The release of glutamine by skeletal muscle is considered to be the flux-generating step for the utilization of glutamine by a number of tissues. The arrows indicate the transport of glutamine from skeletal muscle to a number of different tissues. (Modified from ref. 88, with permission.)

Table 3 Plasma amino acid concentrations in untrained, trained, and overtrained subjects

	Plasma glutamine concentrations (μM)		
	Glutamine	Alanine	BCAA*
(1)			
Untrained	664	530	489
Trained	580	346	519
Overtrained	510	350	490
(2)			
Trained			
(Experimental)	608	498	357
(Follow-up)	621	452	473
Overtrained			
(Experimental)	503	438	333
(Follow-up)	535	487	394

* BCAA, branched chain amino acid.
Values are mean ± SEM. Statistical difference between trained and overtrained athletes is indicated by [a]$p <0.01$; [b]$p <0.05$. (1) Includes recreational (untrained) runners; (2) samples taken when 'overtrained' athletes were first diagnosed (experimental) then 6 weeks later (follow-up). (Data from ref. 96.)

sidered to provide a metabolic link between muscle and cells of the immune system. In a study of athletes with the overtraining syndrome, Parry-Billings measured the concentrations of glutamine, alanine, and branched chain amino acids in sedentary controls, trained athletes, and overtrained athletes[96] and found that the plasma concentrations of alanine and branched chain amino acids were similar in trained and overtrained athletes. However, in a later study, the plasma concentration of glutamine were found to be lower in overtrained athletes compared with that in trained athletes, and the concentration in trained subjects lower than that in recreational runners (see Table 3 and ref. 94).

Table 2 Plasma glutamine concentrations in runners undertaking different levels of exercise

Exercise	Plasma glutamine (μM)	
	Pre-exercise	Post-exercise
Marathon race	669 ± 25 $n = 18$	533 ± 29[b] $n = 18$
30-km indoor race	532 ± 23 $n = 6$	503 ± 24 $n = 6$
15-mile training run	699 ± 21 $n = 9$	679 ± 20 $n = 9$
30-km treadmill run	641 ± 17 $n = 12$	694 ± 29 $n = 12$
Sprints (10 x 6 s)	556 ± 21 $n = 10$	616 ± 21[a] $n = 10$
Rowers (5-km ergotest)	663 ± 21 $n = 13$	778 ± 24[b] $n = 13$

Means ± SEM; [a]$p < 0.05$; [b]$p <0.01$
Data from refs 96 and 97, with permission; all samples were measured enzymatically.[98]

Since samples were taken from resting subjects some time after their performance had been impaired, these results suggest that overtraining may have a long-term effect, specifically on plasma glutamine concentrations. Further, following a 6-week recovery period (during which the overtrained subjects either rested completely or undertook only low-intensity training) and despite a significant improvement in exercise performance, the plasma glutamine concentration remained below control values (Table 3). This suggests that immunosuppression due to overtraining may persist for longer than indicated by the impaired physical performance.

The exercise-induced immunosuppression is not specific to any particular type of exercise. Indeed, it has been demonstrated in a variety of athletes, including runners, swimmers, skiers, and ballet dancers. Prolonged exercise, particularly if it is undertaken regularly, can cause a marked decrease in the plasma glutamine level.

Therefore, it is important to investigate whether supplementation of the diet with glutamine or glutamine–peptides or maintenance of glycogen levels in muscle by adequate dietary carbohydrate could prevent immunosuppression in the overtrained state.

The effects of glutamine feeding upon infection incidence

Parenteral glutamine feeding has been undertaken with measurable effects on the immune system have been observed (Table 4).

Recently, glutamine intervention studies have provided some evidence that the incidence of infection in endurance athletes taking two drinks of glutamine (2×5 g) after prolonged exhaustive exercise is reduced compared with those taking a placebo (Tables 5 and 6).[107]

There was a beneficial effect following giving two glutamine drinks to marathon runners after a race, compared with giving a

Table 4 Some beneficial effects of glutamine feeding upon the immune system

Recipients	Clinical situation	Method of feeding	Beneficial effects
Humans	Bone marrow transplant[100,101]	TPN (L-glutamine)	Decreased number of positive microbial cultures
			Decreased number of clinical infections
			Enhanced recovery of circulating lymphocytes total T lymphocytes, CD4 helper, CD8 suppressor
Humans	Colorectal cancer[102]	TPN (Glycyl-glutamine dipeptide)	Enhanced postoperative T-lymphocyte DNA synthesis
Rats	Healthy—suppressed[103] biliary IgA	TPN (L-glutamine)	Increased biliary concentration of IgA normally suppressed by TPN
Rats	Tumour bearing[104]	TPN (Alanyl-glutamine dipeptide)	Increased phagocytic activity of alveolar macrophages
Rats	Sepsis[105]	TPN (Alanyl-glutamine dipeptide)	Increased rate of lymphocyte proliferation and increased number of lymphocytes
Rats	Chemotherapy[106]	Oral	Decreased sepsis defined as decreased white blood cell count plus decreased positive blood cultures

placebo. However, self-reporting by athletes can lead to difficulties in interpretation of what constitutes an infection, although there is support for this method of data collection.[108] Large numbers need to be recruited.

The effects of feeding glutamine upon immune cell function

In one marathon study, 37 runners were given two drinks of glutamine (2×5 g) or placebo (2×5 g malto-dextrin) immediately after and 2 h after a race: lymphocyte proliferation was significantly decreased in the placebo group in samples taken just prior to the second drink, compared with the glutamine group ($p < 0.05$) (L.M. Castell and E.A. Newsholme, unpublished data). In *in vitro* studies, the killing ability of neutrophils was improved by the addition of glutamine to the culture medium.[109] Seventeen marathon runners who volunteered to return the morning after a marathon (at 16 h) were randomly divided into nine who took a glutamine drink and eight for a placebo drink. Unfortunately, five out of the nine in the glutamine group failed to return for sampling (all eight in the placebo group returned). However, numbers of both neutrophils and total leucocytes ($p < 0.001$ and $p < 0.05$, respectively) in blood samples from the glutamine group were closer to normal at 16 h compared with the placebo group.[97] No change was observed in lymphocyte numbers at 16 h. The concentration of the cytokine interleukin-8, which is a chemoattractant for neutrophils, was meas-

Table 5 Incidence of infections reported by athletes during the 7-day period after different types of exercise

	Numbers		Percentage of infections
	Studies	Participants	
Marathons	5	88	46.8 ± 4.8
Ultramarathon	2	40	43.3 ± 4.8
Middle-distance training session	3	41	24.7 ± 4.0
Rowers	4	45	54.5 ± 7.8

Data from 14 studies. Percentage of infections ± SEM. Significant difference betrween combined marathon and ultramarathon studies versus middle-distance studies, $p < 0.01$.

Table 6 Results of questionnaires from a double-blind study on the incidence of infections in runners during the 7-day period following a full or ultramarathon, with two drinks of either glutamine or placebo

	No. of participants	No. without infections	Participants without infections (%)
Glutamine	72	57	80.8 ± 4.2[a]
Placebo	79	31	48.8 ± 7.4[a]

Percentage of infections ± SEM; data taken from 8 studies. Statistical significance between groups denoted by [a]$p < 0.001$.

Table 7 Plasma amino acid concentrations during 24 weeks of military training

Weeks of training	Plasma amino acid concentration (μM)		
	Glutamine	Alanine	BCAA
1	466	309	431
12	484	367	412
24	300**	427*	444

Intensive physical training took place between weeks 12 and 24. Statistical significance between weeks 1 and 24 indicated by *p < 0.02 **p <0.01.

ured in cell-culture medium 2 h after the marathon, and was found to be decreased (p < 0.02) in the glutamine group compared with the placebo group.

Although there is increasing evidence that overtraining leads to a depletion of plasma glutamine,[94,110] a clear mechanism has not yet been established, but the following possibilities should be considered:

1. There may be an imbalance between the rates of glutamine release and uptake leading to a decreased release of glutamine from muscle.

2. An increased use of glutamine by other tissues, including cells of the immune system, may occur.

3. Acidosis may occur.

A persistent decrease in plasma glutamine concentration after prolonged and repeated bouts of exhaustive exercise may be of significance in the immunosuppression which can occur in individuals undergoing a rigorous training regime. In a study of military personnel (M. Parry-Billings, personal communication) a marked decrease in the concentration of plasma glutamine was observed at the end of a 24-week intensive training period (Table 7).

In another study, also on military personnel undergoing a 5-day 'survival' training course, Parry-Billings commented on the magnitude and speed of weight loss (6 to 8 kg in 5 days) and the subsequent symptoms akin to the overtraining syndrome.[96]

Summary

The overtraining syndrome in athletes is a condition of chronic fatigue, underperformance, and an increased vulnerability to infection, leading to recurrent infections. The exact way in which the stress of hard training and competition leads to the observed spectrum of symptoms, is not yet known. Immunological, psychological, endocrinological, and physiological factors all seem to play a part in the failure to recover from exercise.

Prevention requires the careful monitoring of physiological and psychological parameters, and also of the response to training. Careful consideration should be given to appropriate nutrition. Symptoms normally resolve in 6 to 12 weeks, but may continue for longer, or recur, if athletes return to running too soon.

References

1. Budgett R. The overtraining syndrome. *British Medical Journal* 1994; **309**: 465–8.
2. Morgan WP, Brown DR, Fascm Raglin JS, O'Connor PJ, Ellickson KA. Psychological monitoring of overtraining and staleness. *British Journal of Sports Medicine* 1987; **21**: 107–14.
3. Dyment P. Frustrated by chronic fatigue? *Physician and Sportsmedicine* 1993; **21**: 47–54.
4. Fry RW, Morton AR, Keast D. Overtraining syndrome and the chronic fatigue syndrome. *New Zealand Journal of Sports Medicine* 1991; **19**: 48–52.
5. Budgett R. The overtraining syndrome. *British Journal of Sports Medicine* 1990; **24**: 231–6.
6. Morton RH. Modelling training and overtraining. *Journal of Sports Science* 1997; **15**: 335–40.
7. Fry RW, Morton AR, Keast D. Periodisation and the prevention of overtraining. *Canadian Journal of Sports Sciences* 1992; **17**: 241–8.
8. Fry AC, Kraemer WJ. Does short-term near-maximal intensity machine resistance training induce overtraining? *Journal of Strength and Conditioning Research* 1994; **8**: 188–91.
9. Hooper SL, Mackinnon LT, Gordon RD, and Bachmann AW. Markers for monitoring overtraining and recovery. *Medicine and Science in Sports and Exercise* 1995; **27**: 106–12.
10. Derman W, Schwellnus MP, Lambert MI, Emms M, Sinclair-Smith C, Kirby P, Noakes TD. The worn-out athlete: A clinical approach to chronic fatigue in athletes. *Journal of Sports Sciences* 1997; **15**: 341–51.
11. Hooper SL, Mackinnon LT. Monitoring overtraining in athletes. *Sports Medicine* 1995; **20**: 231–7.
12. Holmes G, Kaplan J, Gantz N. Chronic fatigue syndrome: a working case definition. *Annals of Internal Medicine* 1988; **108**: 337–8.
13. Noakes TD. *The lore of running.* Cape Town: Oxford University Press, 1986.
14. Israel S. Zur Problematik des Ubertrainings aus internistischer und leistungsphysiologischer Sicht. *Medecin und Sport* 1976; **16**: 1–12.
15. Lehmann M, Foster C, Keull J. Overtraining in endurance athletes: a brief review. *Medicine and Science in Sports and Exercise* 1993; **25**: 854–62.
16. Koutedakis Y, Budgett R, Faulmann L. Rest in underperforming elite competitors. *British Journal of Sports Medicine* 1990; **24**: 248–52.
17. Kindermann W. Das Ubertraining-Ausdruck einer vegetativen Fehlsteuerung. *Deutsche Zeitschrift fur Sportsmedizin* 1986; **37**: 138–45.
18. Budgett R. The overtraining syndrome. *Coaching Focus* 1995; **28**: 4–6.
19. Coen B, *et al.* Control of training in middle and long distance running by means of the individual anaerobic threshold. *International Journal of Sports Medicine* 1991; **6**: 519–24.
20. Wilson I. The overtraining syndrome. *Coaching Focus* 1995; **28**: 2–3.
21. Costill DL, Flynn MG, Kirway JP, Houmard JA, Mitchell JB, Thomas R, Park SH. Effects of repeated days of intensified training on muscle glycogen and swimming performance. *Medicine and Science in Sports and Exercise* 1988; **20**: 249–54.
22. Noakes TD. *The lore of running* (2nd edn). Cape Town: Oxford University Press, 1992.
23. Morgan WP, Costill DC, Flynn MG, Raglin DS, O'Connor PJ. Mood disturbance following increased training in swimmers. *Medicine and Science in Sports and Exercise* 1988; **20**: 408–14.
24. Flynn MG, Pizza FX, Boone JB, Andres FF, Michaud TA, Rodríguez-Zagás JR. Indices of training stress during competitive running and swimming seasons. *International Journal of Sports Medicine* 1994; **15**: 21–6.

25. Kereszty A. Overtraining. In: Larson L, eds. *Encyclopedia of sports sciences and medicine*. New York: MacMillan, 1971: 218–22.

26. Barron JL, Noakes TD, Levy W, Smith C, Millar RP. Hypothalamic dysfunction in overtrained athletes. *Journal of Clinical Endocrinology and Metabolism* 1985; **60**: 803–6.

27. Lehmann M, Dickhuth HH, Gendrisch E, Lazar W, Thum M, Kaminski R, Aramendi JF, Peterke E, Wieland W, Keul J. Training–overtraining. A prospective experimental study with experienced middle and long distance runners. *International Journal of Sports Medicine* 1991; **12**: 444–52.

28. Lehmann M, Scnee W, Scheu R, Stockhansen W, Bachl N. Decreased nocturnal catecholamine excretion: parameter for an overtraining syndrome in athletes? *International Journal of Sports Medicine* 1992; **13**: 236–42.

29. Morton RH. The quantitative periodisation of athletic training: a model study. *Sports Medicine: Training and Rehabilitation* 1991; **3**: 19–28.

30. Snyder AC. A physiological/psychological indicator of overreaching during intensive training. *International Journal of Sports Medicine* 1993; **14**: 29–32.

31. Raglin JS, Morgan WP. Development of a scale for use in monitoring training-induced distress in athletes. *International Journal of Sports Medicine* 1994; **15**: 84–8.

32. Berglund B, Safstrom H. Psychological monitoring and modulation of training load of world class canoeists. *Medicine and Science in Sports and Exercise* 1994; **26**: 1036–40.

33. Koutedakis Y, Frischknecht R, Vrbová G, Sharp G, Budgett R. Maximal voluntary quadriceps strength patterns in Olympic overtrained athletes. *Medicine and Science in Sports and Exercise* 1995; **27**: 566–72.

34. Wagenmakers AJM, Brookes JH, Coakley JH, Reilley T, Edwards RHT. Exercise-induced activation of the branched-chain 2-oxo acid dehydrogenase in human muscle. *European Journal of Applied Physiology* 1989; **59**: 159–67.

35. Blomstrand E, Hassmen P, Newsholme EA. Administration of branched-chain amino acids during sustained exercise. *European Journal of Applied Physiology* 1991; **63**: 83.

36. Blomstrand E, Perrett D, Parry-Billings M, Newsholme EA. Effect of sustained exercise on plasma amino acid concentrations and on 5-hydroxytryptamine metabolism in six different brain regions in the rat. *Acta Physiologica Scandinavica* 1989; **136**: 473.

37. Yamamoto T, Castell LM, Botella J, *et al.* Changes in the albumin binding of tryptophan during postoperative recovery: a possible link with central fatigue? *Brain Research Bulletin* 1997; **43**: 43–6.

38. Newsholme EA, Leech AR, Duester G. *Keep on running*. Chichester: Wiley, 1994.

39. Rang HP, Dale MM. *Pharmacology*. London: Churchill Livingstone, 1987.

40. Nash HL. Can exercise suppress reproductive hormones in man? *Physician and Sportsmedicine* 1987; **15**: 180–9.

41. Lightman SL, Everett BJ. *Neuroendocrinology*. Oxford: Blackwell Scientific Publications, 1986.

42. Ulrich U, Nowara I, Rossmanith. Serotinergic control of gonadotrophin and prolactin secretion in women. *Clinical Endocrinology*, 1994; **41**: 779–85.

43. Dressendorfer RH, Wade CE, Scaff JH. Increased morning heart rate in runners: a valid sign of overtraining? *Physician and Sportsmedicine* 1985; **13**: 77–86.

44. Linde F. Running and upper respiratory tract infections. *Scandinavian Journal of Sports Science* 1987; **9**: 21–3.

45. Nieman D. Exercise infection and immunity. *International Journal of Sports Medicine* 1994; **15**: S131.

46. Fitzgerald L. Overtraining increases the susceptibility to infection. *International Journal of Sports Medicine* 1991; **12**: 55–8.

47. Brenner IKM, Shek PN, Shepherd RJ. Infection in athletes. *Sports Medicine* 1994; **17**: 69.

48. Weidner TG. Literature review: upper respiratory illness and sport and exercise. *International Journal of Sports Medicine* 1994; **15**: 1–9.

49. Nieman D, Johanssen LM, Lee JW, Arabatzis K. Infectious episodes before and after the Los Angeles marathon. *Journal of Sports Medicine and Physical Fitness* 1990; **30**: 289–96.

50. Lee DJ. Immune responsiveness and risk of illness in US Air Force Academy recruits during basic recruit training. *Aviation, Space, and Environmental Medicine* 1992, June, 517–23.

51. Gray GC, Mitchell BS, Tueller JE, *et al.* Adult pneumonia hospitalizations in the US Navy: rates and risk factors for 6522 admissions 1981–1991. *American Journal of Epidemiology* 1994; **139**: 793–802.

52. Heath GW, Ford ES, Craven TE, Macera CA, Jackson KL, Pate RR. Exercise and the incidence of upper respiratory tract infections. *Medicine and Science in Sports and Exercise* 1991; **23**: 152–7.

53. O'Connor SA, Jones DP, Collins JV, Heath RB, Campbell MJ, Leighton MH. Changes in pulmonary function after naturally acquired respiratory infection in normal persons. *American Review of Respiratory Disease* 1979; **120**: 1087.

54. Niinima V, Cole P, Mintz S, Shephard RJ. The switching point from nasal to oronasal breathing. *Respiration Physiology* 1980; **42**: 61–71.

55. Rylander R. Pulmonary defence mechanism to airborne bacteria. *Acta Physiologica Scandinavica* 1968; **72** (Suppl. 306): 6–85.

56. Müns G, Singer P, Wolf F, Rubinstein I. Impaired nasal mucociliary clearance in long-distance runners. *International Journal of Sports Medicine* 1995; **16**: 209–13.

57. Larrabee RC. Leucocytosis after violent exercise. *Journal of Medical Research* 1902; **2**: 76–82.

58. Haq A, Al-Hussein K, Lee J, Al-Sedairy S. Changes in peripheral blood lymphocyte subsets associated with marathon running. *Medicine and Science in Sports and Exercise* 1993; **25**: 186–90.

59. Fitzgerald L. Exercise and the immune system. *Immunology Today* 1988; **9**: 337–9.

60. Nieman DC, Nehlsen-Cannarella SL, Markhof PA, *et al.* The effects of moderate exercise training on natural killer cells and acute upper respiratory tract infections. *International Journal of Sports Medicine* 1990; **11**: 467–73.

61. Nieman DC. Immune response to heavy exertion. *Journal of Applied Physiology* 1997; **82**: 1385–94.

62. Keast D, Cameron K, Morton AR. Exercise and immune response. *Sports Medicine* 1988; **5**: 248–67.

63. Lewicki R, Tahorzewski H, Majewska E, Nowak Z, Bag Z. Effect of maximal physical exercise on T-lymphocyte subpopulations and on interleukin-1 (IL-1) and interleukin (IL-2) production *in vitro*. *International Journal of Sports Medicine* 1988; **9**: 114–17.

64. Ryan AJ, Brown RL, Frederich EC, Falsetti HL, Burbod RE. Overtraining of athletes; a round table. *Physician and Sportsmedicine* 1983; **11**: 93–110.

65. Pedersen BK. Influence of physiological activity on the cellular immune system: mechanisms of action. *International Journal of Sports Medicine* 1991; **12**: S23.

66. Shinkai S, Shore S, Shek PN, Shepherd RJ. Acute exercise and immune function. *International Journal of Sports Medicine* 1994; **13**: 452–61.

67. Hoffman-Goetz L, Pedersen BK. Exercise and the immune system. *Immunology Today* 1994; **15**: 382.

68. Shepherd RJ, Rhind S, Shek PJ. Exercise and the immune system. *Sports Medicine* 1994; **18**: 340.

69. Castell LM, Poortmans JR, Leclercq R *et al.* Some aspects of the acute phase response after a marathon race, and the effects of glutamine supplementation. *European Journal of Applied Physiology* 1997; **75**: 47–53.

70. Tvede N, Pedersen BK, Hansen FR. Effect of physical exercise on

blood mononuclear cell subpopulations and *in vitro* proliferation responses. *Scandinavian Journal of Immunology* 1989; **29**: 383–9.

71. MacNeil B, Hoffman-Goetz L, Kendall A, *et al.* Lymphocyte proliferation responses after exercise in men; fitness intensity and duration effects. *Journal of Applied Physiology* 1991; **70**: 179–85.

72. Field CJ, Gougeon R, Marliss EB. Circulating mononuclear cell numbers and function during intense exercise and recovery. *Journal of Applied Physiology* 1991; **71**: 1089–97.

73. Green RL, Kaplan SS, Rabin BS, *et al.* Immune function in marathon runners. *Annals of Allergy* 1981; **47**: 73–5.

74. Oshida Y, Yamanouchi K, Hayamizu S, *et al.* Effect of acute physical exercise on lymphocyte subpopulations in trained and untrained subjects. *International Journal of Sports Medicine* 1988; **9**: 137–40.

75. Soppi E, Varjo P, Eskola J, *et al.* Effect of strenuous physical stress on circulating lymphocyte number and function before and after training. *Journal of Clinical and Laboratory Immunology* 1982; **8**: 43–6.

76. Nieman DC, Simandle S, Henson DA, *et al.* Lymphocyte proliferative response to 2.5 hrs of running. *International Journal of Sports Medicine* 1995; **16**: 404–8.

77. Smith JA. Exercise immunology and neutrophils. *International Journal of Sports Medicine* 1997; **18**: 546–55.

78. Ardawi MSM, Newsholme EA. Glutamine metabolism in lymphocytes of the rat. *Biochemical Journal* 1983; **212**: 835.

79. Newsholme EA, Crabtree B, Ardawi MSM. Glutamine metabolism in lymphocytes: its biochemical physiological and clinical importance. *Quarterly Journal of Experimental Physiology* 1985; **70**: 473–89.

80. Ardawi MSM, Newsholme EA. Metabolism in lymphocyte and its importance in the immune response. *Essays in Biochemistry* 1985; **21**: 1–44.

81. Newsholme EA, Newsholme P, Curi R, Challoner E, Ardawi MSM. A role for muscle in the immune system and its importance in surgery, trauma, sepsis and burns. *Nutrition* 1988; **4**: 261–8.

82. Pond C. Interpretation of the organisation of mammalian and adipose tissue: its relationship to the immune system. *Proceedings of the Nutrition Society* 1996; **24**: 393–400.

83. Frayn KN, Khan K, Coppack SW, Elia M. Amino acid metabolism in human subcutaneous adipose tissue *in vivo*. *Clinical Science* 1991; **80**: 471–4.

84. Pond C. Interactions between adipose tissue and the immune system. *Biochemical Society Transactions* 1996; **55**: 111–26.

85. Deutz NEP, Reijven PLM, Athansas G, Soeters PB. Post-operative changes in hepatic intestinal splenic and muscle fluxes of amino acids and ammonia in pigs. *Clinical Science* 1992; **83**: 607–14.

86. Parry-Billings M, Evans J, Calder PC, Newsholme EA. Does glutamine contribute to immunosuppression? *Lancet* 1990; **336**: 523–6.

87. Marliss EB, Aoki TT, Pozefsky T, Most AS, Cahill GF. Muscle and splanchnic glutamine metabolism in postabsorptive and starved men. *Journal of Clinical Investigation* 1971; **50**: 814–17.

88. Opara E. Studies of glutamine metabolism in skeletal muscle and other tissues. University of Oxford: DPhil thesis, 1993.

89. Stinnett JD, Alexander JW, Watanabe C *et al.* Plasma and skeletal muscle amino acids following severe burn injury in patients and experimental animals. *Annals of Surgery* 1981; **195**: 75–92.

90. Powell H, Castell LM, Parry-Billings M, *et al.* Growth hormone suppression and glutamine flux associated with cardiac surgery. *Clinical Physiology* 1994; **14**: 569–80.

91. Calder PC. Glutamine and the immune system. *Clinical Nutrition* 1994; **13**: 2–8.

92. Decombaz J, Reinhardt P, Anantharaman K, von Glutz G, Poortmans J. Biochemical changes in a 100km run: free amino acids urea and creatinine. *European Journal of Applied Physiology* 1979; **41**: 61–72.

93. Brodan V, Kuhn E, Pechar J, Tomkova D. Changes of free amino acids in plasma in healthy subjects induced by physical exercise. *European Journal of Applied Physiology* 1986; **35**: 69–77.

94. Parry-Billings M, Budgett R, Koutedakis Y, *et al.* Plasma amino acid concentrations in the overtraining syndrome: possible effects on the immune system. *Medicine and Science in Sports and Exercise* 1992; **24**: 1353–8.

95. Poortmans JR, Siest G, Galteau MM, Houot O. Distribution of plasma amino acids in humans during submaximal prolonged exercise. *European Journal of Applied Physiology* 1974; **32**: 143–7.

96. Parry-Billings M. Studies of glutamine release from skeletal muscle. University of Oxford: DPhil thesis, 1989.

97. Castell LM. The role of some amino acids in exercise fatigue and immunosuppression. University of Oxford: MSc thesis, 1996.

98. Windmueller HG, Spaeth AE. Uptake and metabolism of plasma glutamine by the small intestine. *Journal of Biological Chemistry* 1974; **249**: 5070–9.

99. Newsholme E and Parry-Billings M. Properties of glutamine release from muscle and its importance for the immune system. *Journal of Parenteral and Enteral Nutrition*, 1990; **14**: 63–7S.

100. Ziegler TR, Young LS, Benfell K, Scheltinga MR, Hortos K, Bye RL, Wilmore DW, Morrow F, Jacobs DO, Smith RJ, Antin JH. Clinical and metabolic efficacy of glutamine supplemented parenteral nutrition after bone marrow transplantation. *Annals of Internal Medicine* 1992; **116**: 821–8.

101. Ziegler TR, Bye RL, Persinger RL, *et al.* Glutamine-enriched parenteral nutrition increases circulating lymphocytes after bone marrow transplantation. *Journal of Parenteral and Enteral Nutrition* 1994; **18**: 17S.

102. O'Riordain MG, Fearon KCH, Ross JA, *et al.* Glutamine-supplemented parenteral nutrition enhances T-lymphocyte response in surgical patients undergoing colorectal resection. *Annals of Surgery* 1994; **220**: 212–21.

103. Burke DJ, Alverdy JA, Aoys E, Moss GS. Glutamine-supplemented total parenteral nutrition improves gut immune function. *Archives of Surgery* 1989; **124**: 1396.

104. Kweon MN, Moriguchi S, Mukai K, Kishino Y. Effect of alanylglutamine-enriched infusion on tumor growth and cellular immune function in rats. *Amino Acids* 1991; **1**: 7.

105. Yoshida S, Hikida S, Tanaka Y, *et al.* Effect of glutamine supplementation on lymphocyte function in septic rats. *Journal of Parenteral and Enteral Nutrition* 1992; **16** (Suppl. 1).

106. Klimberg VS, Nwokedi E, Hutchins LF, *et al.* Glutamine facilitates chemotherapy while reducing toxicity. *Journal of Parenteral and Enteral Nutrition* 1992; **16**: 83–7S.

107. Castell LM, Poortmans J, Newsholme EA. Does glutamine have a role in reducing infections in athletes? *European Journal of Applied Physiology* 1996; **73**: 488–91.

108. Mackinnon LT, Hooper SL. Plasma glutamine and upper respiratory tract infection during intensified training in swimmers. *Medicine and Science in Sports and Exercise* 1996; **28**: 285–90.

109. Ogle CK, Ogle JD, Mao J-X, *et al.* Effect of glutamine on phagocytosis and bacterial killing by normal and pediatric burn patient neutrophils. *Journal of Parenteral and Enteral Nutrition* 1994; **18**: 128–33.

110. Rowbottom DG, Keast D, Goodman C, Morton AR. The haematological, biochemical and immunological profile of athletes suffering from the overtraining syndrome. *European Journal of Applied Physiology* 1995; **70**: 502–9.

3.7 The endocrinology of exercise

Paul J. Jenkins, Trevor A. Howlett, and A. B. Grossman

Introduction

The endocrine system is intimately involved in the homeostasis of an organism affecting particularly:

(1) regulation of energy and metabolism;

(2) maintenance of fluid and electrolyte balance;

(3) stress responses;

(4) reproductive function;

(5) growth and development.

Physical activity affects many, if not all, of these, and it is thus perhaps not surprising that both acute and chronic exercise are now known to be powerful modulators of the endocrine system.[1] With the introduction of radioimmunoassay techniques and the ability to measure circulating levels of hormones, it has become clear that acute exercise affects the release of a large number of hormones, and also that chronic exercise, in addition to altering these acute endocrine responses, may further lead to long-term alterations in endocrine homeostasis. The most important of these is female gonadal dysfunction: with the increasing popularity of exercise, often compounded by the desire to lose weight, these changes are becoming more relevant in endocrine practice. In addition to endocrine responses to exercise, more recently there has been increasing interest in the effects of endocrine manipulation and replacement on exercise capability, both in terms of normal physiology and the potential enhancement of athletic performance.

Exercise type, absolute intensity, and relative intensity

Recreational exercise takes many forms, as do the experimental exercise protocols and the types of subjects used by investigators. Hormonal responses have thus been described in untrained subjects, joggers, amateur or professional competitive runners, rowers, cyclists, swimmers, and dancers (male and female), using a variety of acute stimuli; these include, in the laboratory, step-climbing, bicycle ergometer, and exercise treadmill, and, in the field, competitive and non-competitive events, short runs and marathons, swimming, or other sports, and even military endurance-training programmes. There is, of course, no guarantee that these types of experimental or recreational exercise are in any way equivalent, and indeed the large number of factors known to modify the acute response to exercise would suggest the very opposite. Furthermore, there is also evidence that the neuroendocrinology of recreational exercise is quite different to that seen in élite professional athletes.

A comparison of the intensity of exercise used in different studies can also be difficult. Exercise intensity may be poorly controlled ('20-min vigorous exercise', 'exercise to maximum tolerated capacity', etc.), expressed in terms of absolute workload (in a variety of units), or expressed as a percentage (measured directly or calculated) of the individual subject's maximum work capacity. Work capacity, in turn, may be expressed as either maximum tolerated workload in the particular experimental system or as the measured maximum aerobic capacity ($\dot{V}O_2$max). Since by training a subject may typically increase their $\dot{V}O_2$max by 10 to 15 per cent or more, the choice between expressing the exercise intensity in absolute or relative terms is particularly important. The same absolute work may represent a smaller relative load after training, so that the hormonal response to the same load may alter during training without representing any change in normal endocrine regulatory mechanisms. Most authorities therefore consider that reference should be made to the relative intensity of the exercise stimulus, expressed as $\dot{V}O_2$max, rather than in terms of absolute workload. It should be noted, however, that change in the hormonal response to a given absolute stimulus *per se* represents a hormonal response to training, and might be an important part of the body's mechanism of adaptation to exercise. However, even when the relative exercise intensity is controlled it seems clear that the duration of exercise must represent an important factor; unfortunately, reports in the literature vary widely, citing periods as ranging from 5 min to several hours, or simply 'until exhaustion'.

These inconsistencies in the definition of the exercise stimulus, in addition to the other modifying factors discussed below, may account for many of the apparently contradictory descriptions of the responses of hormonal to acute exercise and chronic exercise training.

Catecholamines

Release of the catecholamines, adrenaline and noradrenaline, from the adrenal medulla is the earliest endocrine response to acute exercise. Indeed, it occurs prior to actual activity with the anticipatory stress of competition being responsible for the 'butterflies', sweaty palms, dry mouth, etc. felt prior to the event. In addition to initiating this state of arousal for a 'fight or flight' response, the release of catecholamines plays a vital role not only in the cardiorespiratory and thermoregulatory responses to exercise, but also in stimulating lipolysis, glycolysis, and hepatic glucose production. Their release is proportional to the intensity of exercise. But, with training, levels are reduced for the same absolute workload, although probably remaining unchanged for the same relative workload.

Growth hormone and insulin-like growth factor-1

Normal physiology

Growth hormone (**GH**) is a 22 kDa pituitary protein that has wide-ranging metabolic and anabolic effects, including effects on growth and development. It is secreted in a pulsatile manner under the control of two hypothalamic hormones, GH-releasing hormone and the inhibitory somatostatin, which themselves are under the influence of a variety of central neurones including cholinergic, γ-amino-butyric acid-controlled (**GABA**) neurones and endogenous opioids. GH secretion is increased by stress, a fall in blood sugar, and fasting, and is enhanced at night, principally during non rapid-eye movement sleep. Growth hormone circulates in the blood bound to a GH-binding protein. Although it has some effects itself, including stimulation of the cartilaginous growth plate, the majority of its metabolic and mitogenic actions are primarily mediated by a family of peptides, the insulin-like growth factors (**IGF**), principally IGF-1. IGF-1, synthesized by the liver, circulates bound to a variety of binding proteins of which eight have currently been characterized, with binding protein-3 being the most important. Thus, the bioactivity of GH depends on an interplay between its local concentration, the binding proteins, the activity of specific proteases that cleave off IGF-1, and IGF-1 receptors.

Effect of exercise

Growth hormone

The pulsatility of GH release means that single measurements need to be interpreted with caution when extrapolating to the effects of exercise. However, based on a large number of studies, it is now clear that GH levels rise in response to acute exercise, with a threshold level reached at approximately 30 per cent of $\dot{V}O_2max$, and also after resistive exercise. Levels can rise up to 50-fold in proportion to the intensity of exercise, beginning after 10 min of 'high intensity' exercise.[2,3] Such responses are generally believed to be exacerbated by anaerobic exercise and hypoxia, although the latter has been questioned in one study.[3] In common with basal release, the GH response to exercise is more pronounced in pubertal than pre-pubertal children.[4]

Interestingly, in addition to the acute stimulation, daytime exercise also appears to affect the nocturnal secretion of GH, with prolonged exercise (greater than 4 h) increasing the proportion of GH secreted in the second half of sleep.[5]

The effect of training on the GH response to acute exercise is uncertain, with conflicting results being reported. Thus, attenuated responses to both the same absolute[6] and relative[7] exercise intensity have been reported, but with no change being reported in another study where females entered an intensive training programme and acted as their own controls.[8] Amplification of GH release was, however, reported in female runners after 1 year of intensive anaerobic training, with an approximate twofold increase in both basal and exercise-stimulated levels.[9]

Since exercise is a simple and safe stimulus to GH release, a number of workers have studied its use as a clinical screening test for GH deficiency. Intensive well-controlled exercise may exclude a GH deficiency (by a response of more than 20 mU/l in 68 per cent of children with short stature, but less well-controlled exercise is unreliable.[10]

There is lack of agreement on the mechanisms responsible for these alterations in GH. The opiate antagonist naloxone has been shown to block the exercise-related rise in GH levels,[11] although others have reported that it has no effect by itself, but potentiates the GH inhibitory actions of the γ-aminobutyric acid (**GABA**)-controlled (GABAergic) neurones.[12] These discrepancies might be explained by the fact that the latter study[12] involved untrained subjects compared to highly trained athletes in the former[11].

IGF-1

It might be expected that, as in normal physiology, the observed exercise-associated rise in GH would be mirrored by a rise in circulating IGF-1. Assays for this peptide have only been available for the last few years, but studies to date have given conflicting results. Cappon et al.[13] reported a small (14 per cent) rise in IGF-1 within 10 min of the onset of high-intensity exercise that persisted for approximately 30 min and which was independent of GH release. However, they measured the 'total bound' rather than 'free' IGF-1, unlike other studies that reported no increase in its level, either during, just after, or in the 24 h following exercise.[14] It is likely that the acute rise reported by Cappon and colleagues[13] might reflect changes in the volume of distribution, known to be decreased with exercise, rather than increased hepatic synthesis and release.

In contrast to these findings, it seems clear that habitual resistance (weight training 2 to 3 times a week) and endurance training is associated with increases in circulating IGF-1 compared to a sedentary lifestyle. A number of cross-sectional studies have reported serum IGF-1 levels to be proportional to the levels of exertion.[14–16] Whether or not this increase in serum IGF-1 is responsible for the changes in body shape and musculature that occurs with habitual exercise is uncertain. Current evidence suggests that it is tissue IGF-1, either taken up from the circulation and/or produced in a paracrine fashion, that is most important. In animal studies, increased IGF-1 immunoactivity has been reported in rat tibialis muscles 4 days after severe acute resistance exercise, shown to result in muscle hypertrophy.[17] Increases in muscle IGF-1 mRNA and protein content have also been reported with chronic training, and these, in part, were independent of GH activity.[18] This GH independence was supported in another study[19] which demonstrated up to 15-fold increases in IGF-1 mRNA in soleus and plantaris muscles in hypophysectomized rats after the distal gastrocnemius tendon had been cut, resulting in compensatory hypertrophy of these muscles. However, no increase in muscle IGF-1 mRNA in response to training was reported in a recent study in humans, despite increases in muscle fibre diameter.[20] Reasons for this discrepancy might include species differences, different protocols used to induce hypertrophy, and age of the subjects.

Taken together, the evidence suggests that the changes in skeletal musculature in response to exercise are probably due, in part, to increases both in systemic IGF-1 and in the GH-independent modulation of muscle IGF-1 gene expression by, as yet, unknown paracrine factors.

Exogenous GH and exercise capability

With the introduction of recombinant human growth hormone (**rGH**), there has been increasing interest in the anabolic effects of this hormone—particularly those on skeletal musculature, both in terms of physiological replacement in GH deficiency and its alleged abuse by athletes.

Growth hormone deficiency

Over the last few years, it has become increasingly clear that patients deficient in GH have an abnormal body composition with: decreased lean mass (approximately 9 per cent); increased fat; decreased extracellular water; and decreased bone density. Although the administration of rGH in physiological doses can reverse many of these changes, its effects on muscle strength and exercise capability are less well defined. Cuneo *et al.*[21] reported a 17 per cent increase in $\dot{V}O_2$max after 6 months' treatment compared to placebo, but they did not assess any improvement in strength. An increase in isometric strength of 18 per cent was recorded after 3 years' treatment with growth hormone by Jorgenson *et al.*,[22] but this reached only 66 per cent of that seen in subjects with normal GH secretion. Beshyah and colleagues reported increased exercise time and muscle strength after 12 but not 6 months' treatment, but they gave no normal values.[23] A similar long-term effect on muscle strength, but not exercise time, has also been reported by Rodriguez-Arnao *et al.*[24] It seems likely that any increase in $\dot{V}O_2$max and exercise time may result more from the effects of GH on erythropoiesis and cardiac function rather than on muscle strength. Several other studies have failed to demonstrate any improvement in muscle strength after a programme of resistance training, despite increases in serum IGF-1 levels to within the normal range and restoration of body composition towards normal.[25,26] Furthermore, rGH appears to have no influence on tissue levels of IGF-1 mRNA.[25] Some of these discrepancies in the effects on muscle strength in GH-deficient adults might be explained by the dosages of GH used. Thus, the two studies that reported positive effects used 0.08 and 0.04 IU/kg bodyweight/day, respectively[22,23] compared with 0.02 IU/kg bodyweight/day in the study showing no effect.[25]

Growth hormone abuse by athletes

Over the last decade or so there have been increasing anecdotal reports of widespread self-administration of GH by athletes, in the belief that it augments performance in both endurance and power sports. However, to date, scientific evidence suggests that such pharmacological doses of GH are without benefit and, indeed, may be associated with significant side-effects. Thus, Yarasheski *et al.* administered rGH or placebo in a double-blind fashion to non-training young men prior to and during a 12-week programme of daily weight training. They observed no difference between the two groups with regard to muscle strength, despite serum GH and IGF-1 levels increasing sixfold and threefold, respectively, in the GH group[27] (Fig. 1). Deyssig *et al.* have also reported the effects of pharmacological doses of GH on muscle strength, but in power athletes already undertaking regular intensive training (8 to 14 h/week). Again, despite the elevation of both serum GH and IGF-1 levels to approximately three times normal levels, there was

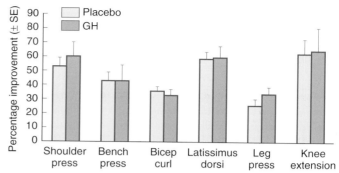

Fig. 1 Percentage improvement in muscle strength with placebo or rGH (40 µg/kg/ day) after 12 weeks' heavy-resistance training in previously untrained men. (Data from Yarasheski *et al.*[27].)

no significant difference in muscle strength between the GH and placebo groups; there was also no change in body composition.[28] Furthermore, patients with acromegaly, a disease characterized by increases in the endogenous secretion of GH (often more than 100-fold), suffer from myopathy despite hypertrophy of their muscle fibres.[29] Overall, therefore, it would appear that exogenous GH, even in pharmacological doses, is of no benefit either in altering body composition or enhancing muscle strength capabilities. Self-administration of such doses is not without potentially serious adverse effects. In the two studies mentioned above, approximately 25 per cent of the subjects receiving GH developed carpel tunnel syndrome and withdrew from the studies.[27,28] A significantly increased morbidity, and indeed mortality, is also seen in patients with acromegaly compared to the normal population in whom GH levels are normal, with hypertension, cardiomyopathy, respiratory disease, diabetes, abnormal lipid metabolism, and osteoarthritis all occurring more commonly. In addition, these patients are also at increased risk of cancer, particularly of the breast and colon. It is probable, therefore, that these pathologies will also occur with prolonged abuse of GH.

One further potential adverse effect of GH administration is that relating to the transmission of prion diseases. It has been reported that due to the high cost of rGH, particularly on the 'black market', some athletes are purchasing the cheaper cadaveric GH, extracted from human pituitary glands. GH produced in this way has been associated with the transmission of the invariably fatal Creutzfeldt–Jacob disease. Its production has thus been banned in most countries, including the United Kingdom, but it remains readily available in Eastern European countries.[30]

Whether the lack of any scientific evidence demonstrating a benefit from the use of GH or knowledge of its ill-effects will deter athletes from GH abuse remains to be seen. In contrast to anabolic steroids, the exogenous administration of GH is currently impossible to prove. However, the sports governing bodies and the International Olympic Committee Medical Commission are well aware of these limitations and are actively engaged in trying to surmount them. Measurements of circulating IGF-1 and IGF-binding protein-3 are unlikely to have the requisite sensitivity or specificity to be of use in the unequivocal proof of GH abuse, but it may be that with the use of sensitive techniques, such as high-performance liquid chromatography (**HPLC**), it will soon be possible to detect subtle differences in the molecular structure that may distinguish endogenous from exogenous GH.

Pituitary–adrenal axis

Normal physiology

Cortisol, the major steroid hormone synthesized and secreted by the adrenal cortex, has multiple physiological actions, including glucose homeostasis, modulation of inflammatory and immune responses, and maintenance of circulating volume. Its secretion is controlled by the anterior pituitary adrenocorticotrophic hormone (**ACTH**), secreted as part of the precursor pro-opiomelanocortin molecule which itself is under the control of hypothalamic corticotrophin-releasing hormone (**CRH**) and, to a lesser extent, arginine vasopressin (**AVP**).

ACTH and cortisol are secreted in a diurnal rhythm, being highest on awakening and declining to very low levels during sleep. Its secretion may be influenced by a variety of central neuronal pathways, including those signalling 'stress', which result in increased secretion.

Acute exercise

As stress is one of the major stimulants to cortisol release, it is perhaps not surprising that its levels rise in response to acute exercise.[31,32] Such rises are proportional to the intensity of exercise, with a critical level of 60 per cent $\dot{V}O_2$max being generally regarded as necessary to induce cortisol release. During low-intensity exercise, the circulating cortisol level falls, probably reflecting both the underlying circadian rhythm and increased removal from the circulation. As might be expected, the increased release of cortisol follows a rise in ACTH, but, interestingly, one study has suggested that this occurs in response to AVP secretion rather than CRH, the circulating levels of which were unaltered after 15 min of exercise at 90 per cent of $\dot{V}O_2$max.[31]

The effect of physical training on the cortisol response to acute exercise remains controversial. Cortisol levels after the same absolute workload may fall, but some well-controlled studies have shown a clear potentiation of the plasma cortisol response to the same relative intensity after training,[7,8] (although this has been disputed). In one study the cortisol response during marathon running was shown to be directly proportional to the degree of fitness of the runners,[33] but other studies of trained athletes have failed to show that cortisol responds at all to intense (although often uncontrolled) exercise.[34]

Chronic exercise

Chronic exercise also results in alterations in the pituitary–adrenal axis, with basal cortisol levels being elevated.[35-38] Levels are higher in amenorrhoeic compared to eumenorrheic athletes[36,39] (see below), but whether this is cause or effect is unclear, particularly as cortisol binding globulin has been reported to be higher in the former group.[35] Basal ACTH levels have not been reported to be raised in any group of athletes,[37,38] but they do rise equally in amenorrhoeic and eumenorrhoeic athletes in response to exercise.[35,38] An increased adrenal response, perhaps resulting from increased adrenal sensitivity, has been reported in amenorrhoeic athletes, but so also has a diminished response.[38] Responses to CRH in chronically trained athletes have been reported to be blunted,[35] a situation similar to patients with functional hypothalamic amenorrhoea,[37] although interpretation is complicated in both these cases by a higher basal cortisol level.

Fluid and electrolyte balance

Normal fluid and electrolyte homeostasis depends principally on the interaction of two hormones—the mineralocorticoid aldosterone (under the control of the renin–angiotensin system) which promotes renal tubular sodium resorption, and the posterior pituitary antidiuretic hormone (**ADH**), also known as arginine vasopressin (**AVP**), which promotes water resorption from the renal collecting ducts. More recently, a third hormone has been shown to be involved, atrial natiuretic peptide (**ANP**), which promotes renal sodium loss.

Exercise, particularly endurance exercise, has been shown to have profound effects on all these interactions. AVP secretion is increased dramatically, both in response to the increased plasma osmolality consequent upon water loss secondary to sweating and in response to the 'stress' of exercise.[31] The latter may be involved in the cortisol response to exercise (see above).

Similarly, ANP secretion also increases,[40] probably secondary to the increased heart rate and atrial distension that accompanies exertion. However, the latter cannot be the sole mechanism as the rise in ANP secretion can be attenuated by progressive rehydration during severe exertion to maintain normal plasma volume.[40]

These physiological responses in AVP and ANP secretion play a vital role in maintaining fluid and electrolyte homeostasis during severe endurance exercise, for example marathon running. It has been estimated that an élite runner loses up to 1.5 litres of fluid during a race, and thus minimizing renal loss and replenishing this fluid are vital to preventing progressive dehydration, hyperosmolality, and cardiovascular collapse.

Interestingly, and paradoxically, there have been a few reports of hypo-osmolar collapse occurring in association with marathons, although the reasons are unclear. A review of these cases has shown that they tend to occur in inexperienced runners a couple of hours after the end of the race. It may be that in response to the exhortations to drink, these submaximal athletes drink large amounts of fluid in excess of that lost by sweating, thus effectively inducing a state of water intoxication, a situation analogous to that seen in some cases of collapse associated with the drug 'Ecstasy'.

Pituitary–gonadal axis

Female

Normal physiology

In normal women the maintenance of regular ovulatory menstrual cycles depends on the pulsatile release of the pituitary gonadotrophins, luteinizing hormone (**LH**), and follicle-stimulating hormone (**FSH**). This itself is dependent upon the synchronous pulsatile secretion of gonadotrophin-releasing hormone (**GnRH**) originating from a group of hypothalamic neurones termed the GnRH pulse generator. The GnRH pulse generator is subject to modulation by numerous central neural mechanisms, including

Table 1 Prevalence (per cent) of menstrual abnormalities in different sports

Sport	Amenorrhoea	Oligomenorrhoea	Amenorrhoea and oligomenorrhoea	Eumenorrhoea
Badminton	0	0	0	100
Cyclists	30	40	70	30
Dancers	27	24	52	48
Gymnasts	71	29	100	0
Hockey	0	17	17	83
Rowers (heavyweight)	0	33	33	66
Rowers (lightweight)	46	21	67	33
Runners	45	20	65	35
Swimmers	0	31	31	69

Reproduced from ref. 45 with permission.

endogenous opioids which are now known to exert a tonic inhibitory effect.[41] The withdrawal of this inhibitory tone midway through the cycle results in the 'LH surge' and consequent ovulation,[42] which is followed by the luteal phase of the cycle, lasting approximately 14 days.

Oestradiol is the principal steroid released by the ovary in response to LH; its level gradually increases during the first half of the cycle, reaches a peak with the LH surge, and declines precipitously thereafter, mirroring the increase in progesterone levels during the luteal phase which precedes menstruation.

Effects of acute exercise

Knowledge of the acute responses of luteinizing hormone and follicle-stimulating hormone to exercise is confused: studies have reported no change, a rise, or a fall. The known pulsatile nature of the secretion of these hormones must account, at least in part, for these discrepancies. One study which assessed LH pulsatility in considerable detail during and after acute exercise reported a significant reduction (by nearly 50 per cent) in LH pulse frequency (but not in pulse amplitude) in the 6 h following exercise.[43] However, this has not been confirmed by other workers; a more recent study has shown no major change in gonadotrophin pulse parameters during acute intense exercise.[44]

The plasma oestradiol level does not appear to change in response to moderate exercise during the follicular phase, although when an athlete becomes exhausted the oestradiol level may rise during the midfollicular phase; oestradiol and progesterone may both rise at all exercise intensities in the midluteal phase. Testosterone, androstenedione, and the adrenal androgen dehydroepiandrosterone-sulphate (**DHEA-S**), all rise during acute exercise, although some or all of this may represent an adrenocortical response.

Effects of chronic exercise

What is much more certain and clinically the more important endocrinological consequence of exercise is the effect on the female reproductive system. Exercise-induced primary or secondary amenorrhoea (**EIA**) is a common finding in the endocrine outpatient clinic, and a detailed exercise history is now mandatory in all women with reproductive dysfunction. The increasing encouragement to participate in recreational and competitive sport together with the propagation that slimness is the 'ideal' has resulted in an increased prevalence of EIA. However, not all athletes are affected equally; the frequency of menstrual irregularities and EIA varies between the sports, being highest in gymnasts and lowest in badminton players (Table 1)—the factors associated with EIA are decreased body-mass index and intensity of training.[45] In prepubertal children, excessive exercise delays the onset of puberty with menarche being shown to occur 3 years later than normal among a group of ballet dancers.[46] Indeed, each year of training leads to a delay of about 5-months in menarche[47] but with a rapid progression on cessation of exercise.

Although amenorrhoea is the final menstrual consequence of excessive exercise, more subtle disturbances precede it resulting from alterations in the activity of the GnRH pulse generator. Several studies have indicated that the initial abnormalities appear to be a reduction in the frequency of LH pulses[48] but with no change,[48] or even elevation,[35] of their amplitude. Such changes may result in anovulatory cycles and infertility. A loss of the sleep-associated changes in LH release has also been reported.[35] Subsequent changes are shortening of the luteal phase which may result in oligoamenorrhoea prior to complete amenorrhoea. Such changes may occur with as little as 3 h exercise per week[49] or a weekly running schedule of 20 miles per week,[48] beginning within a few weeks of commencing exercise.[50] Despite the decrease in LH pulse frequency, the capacity of the pituitary gland to respond to exogenous GnRH appears to be maintained, or even accentuated, in some athletes.[35,48]

Although alterations in the GnRH pulse generator would seem to underlie most of the menstrual irregularities associated with exercise, they are not the only mechanism responsible for impaired gonadal function, as significantly lower oestrogen levels have been recorded in female athletes despite normal episodic LH secretion.[49] Whilst the precise pathogenic mechanisms remain elusive, accumulating evidence suggests the most likely candidates relate to endogenous opioids and/or peripheral metabolic signals.

Pathogenesis of exercise-induced amenorrhoea (EIA)

Opioids There are three separate groups of endogenous opioids—enkephalins, endorphins, and dynorphins. β-Endorphin is synthesized from the ACTH precursor pro-opiomelanocortin and released from the anterior pituitary in parallel with ACTH in response to a wide variety of stimuli, including exercise. Not surprisingly, a number of groups have reported a rise in plasma β-endorphin levels during exercise.[32,51] Met-enkephalin has also been reported to be released in response to acute exercise, but which is almost abolished with increasing training,[51] perhaps reflecting neuroendocrine adaptation to exercise. No consistent change has been seen in plasma levels of the potent opioid peptide, dynorphin, during exercise. Whether chronic exercise is associated with the activation of endogenous opioids is debatable, with only one study reporting elevated basal plasma β-endorphin levels.[52]

The major question, however, is whether these changes in plasma opioids are capable of directly modulating the GnRH pulse generator. Opioid modulation of hypothalamic-releasing hormone secretion may occur, at least in part, at sites which are outside the blood–brain barrier and therefore accessible to the effects of circulating opioids. However, in most cases the absolute levels of plasma opioids achieved are extremely low, and it is unclear whether such levels would be sufficient to stimulate opioid receptors. The release of met-enkephalin may simply reflect activation of the adrenal medulla, a major source of opioid peptides, while β-endorphin is co-released with ACTH. It is perhaps more likely that changes in the activity of opioid pathways within the hypothalamus, and/or elsewhere in the brain, are responsible. Evidence that endogenous opioids (plasma or central) are implicated in EIA was provided by McArthur *et al.* who administered the opioid antagonist naloxone to amenorrhoeic female athletes and noted a prompt restoration of LH and FSH pulsatility.[53] However, several other studies have failed to confirm this effect. This inconsistency may relate to changes in body composition, as we have suggested that opioid-related amenorrhoea will not occur in subjects who have a low percentage of body fat.[54]

Further circumstantial evidence in support of the role of opioids is the upward shift in the circadian rhythm of cortisol levels seen in highly trained athletes, possibly due to an increased release of hypothalamic corticotrophin-releasing hormone (see above). This elevation in cortisol levels is more marked in amenorrhoeic than eumenorrhoeic athletes.[39] Williams *et al.*[55] have shown that CRH inhibits the electrical activity of the GnRH generator in the rhesus monkey, an effect that can be prevented and/or reversed with opiate blockade. Thus, it is conceivable that EIA may, in part, be caused by the activation of central 'stress mechanisms' with the subsequent release of CRH and increased opioidergic inhibition of GnRH release.

Nutritional/metabolic cues The role of nutritional and/or metabolic factors in EIA has long been held to be important; it has variously being ascribed to loss of weight, loss of per cent volume fat, altered lean:fat ratio, decreased calorie intake, and increased energy expenditure. Early work suggested that it was a fall in bodyweight and per cent body fat below a critical level that was a major factor.[56] Certainly, menstrual irregularities are common with a bodyweight of less than 47 kg in the Western world, although this is not inviolate as exercise may result in menstrual dysfunction with no alteration in weight or per cent body fat,[53] and, conversely, cessation of exercise without any change in body characteristics can lead to the resumption of menstrual cycles.[46] However, it is likely that 'metabolic stress' in some form is important, since although the undertaking of regular intensive exercise in previously sedentary subjects rapidly leads to menstrual irregularities, these are exacerbated by concomitant weight loss;[50] a number of studies have shown amenorrhoeic athletes to have decreased bodyweight and/or percentage body fat compared to athletes with normal cycles.[35,48]

We have recently sought to elucidate these metabolic signals by performing a cross-sectional study on a group of élite athletes and professional dancers undertaking chronic severe exercise and who were graded according to menstrual status.[39] Our results showed that, as a group, the subjects showed a low per cent body fat and significantly lower serum LH, FSH, and oestradiol levels, compared to normal population references. When individual factors were correlated independently against menstrual score, there were significant correlations for cortisol, progesterone, insulin, insulin-like growth factor binding protein-1, weight, and body-mass index; percentage body fat did not correlate with menstrual irregularities. However, when a multivariant stepwise discriminant analysis was performed, most of these correlations disappeared and only serum cortisol and IGF-binding protein-1 emerged as significant independent factors. Each of these correlated positively with amenorrhoea ($r = + 0.42$ and $r = + 0.41$, respectively, both $p < 0.05$), and together accounted for the majority of the total variance (Fig. 1). Insulin was negatively correlated with menstrual score, but after removal of the IGF-binding protein-1 factor did not exert an independent effect. IGF-binding protein-1 is thought to modulate both the peripheral acute insulin-like and growth-promoting actions of IGF-1. It is principally secreted by the liver and this is directly regulated by insulin: high insulin levels suppress IGF-binding protein-1 while low concentrations lead to increased secretion. Calorie restriction is associated with an increase in its concentration. Thus, IGF-binding protein-1, either on its own or through its interactions with IGF-1 which itself has been implicated in the regulation of puberty,[57] may be a peripheral signal reflecting metabolic status and available fuel reserves. As such, it might interface between these fuel reserves and reproductive control at a hypothalamic and possibly ovarian level.

In addition, the recently discovered peptide, leptin, might also play a role in the metabolic control of reproduction. This peptide, a product of the obesity (*ob*) gene, is synthesized and secreted by fat cells in response to increasing adiposity. As its levels rise it acts, through negative feedback, as a 'satiety factor' suppressing appetite and controlling energy homeostasis. Although direct evidence is currently lacking, it is also thought to interact with the reproductive axis. *Ob-ob* mice, which are deficient in leptin, have suppressed LH levels and are infertile, abnormalities which are restored by injection of this peptide.[58] Furthermore, in fasted normal mice, in which leptin and LH secretions are suppressed, such replacement will also restore LH secretion.[59]

In conclusion, exercise-induced amenorrhoea may result from a multifactorial combination of activation of the hypothalamo–pituitary–adrenal axis and opioidergic modulation, and changed levels of

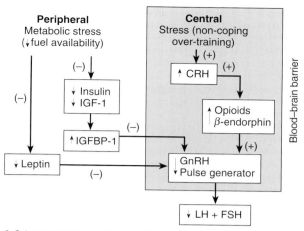

Fig. 2 Schematic representation of putative pathogenic mechanisms of exercise-induced amenorrhoea.

nutritional factors such as leptin and IGF-binding protein-1, both contributing, in varying degrees in different individuals, to the menstrual irregularity (Fig. 2).

Male

Effect of acute exercise

Most studies have shown a rise in testosterone levels with acute exercise,[60-62] which is probably a reflection of a decrease in plasma volume and hepatic clearance rather than an increased production rate since there is no concurrent change in LH secretion. However, longer lasting periods of exercise appear to be associated with a reduction in testosterone levels.

Effect of chronic exercise

Unlike in women, evidence concerning the effects of chronic exercise on the male reproductive axis is conflicting; reduction, no change, or elevation of serum testosterone levels have all been described. A small fall in serum testosterone was reported in men running more than 60 km a week,[63] but it remained within the normal range. This was supported by another study, although the authors found that testosterone levels fell below the normal range in response to a reduction in per cent body fat during the training season,[64] a situation perhaps analogous to exercise-induced amenorrhoea and previously reported in male anorectics.[65] These levels returned to normal on cessation of exercise and restoration of body-weight to normal. However, a number of other studies have failed to record any change in serum testosterone with chronic exercise.[62,66,67] In contrast to this, levels have been reported to increase in weightlifters in response to training, correlating with improvements in strength,[68] although the possibility of exogenous administration would vitiate these studies. Some workers have suggested that there is a reduction in the testosterone to cortisol ratio with very stressful exercise which might reflect the syndrome of over-training, with a consequent alteration in the proportion of anabolic to catabolic hormones.[69,70] However, it is likely that these results are due largely to the increase in cortisol levels which occur with exercise rather than a reduction in testosterone. Regardless of whether there are subtle alterations in the male pituitary–gonadal axis, there

appears to be no effect on reproductive function with no reduction in sperm count or morphology reported in marathon runners.[67]

Similar controversies exist with regard to LH pulsatility. A significant reduction in both the frequency and amplitude of LH pulses in male marathon runners compared to normal controls was reported by MacConnie *et al.*,[60] but with no change in serum testosterone, and no change in the testicular response to human chorionic gonadotrophin (**hCG**). Another study, however, failed to replicate these findings, observing no change in LH pulsatility.[66] These discrepancies might be explained by differences in the amount of training undertaken by the subjects, with a weekly mileage of 80 to 100 miles (129 to 161 km) in the former study compared to 50 (80 km) in the latter, although this still represents very strenuous exercise and is far in excess of that which induces gonadal dysfunction in women.

Insulin

The changes in insulin secretion and glucose metabolism during acute exercise are complex. Plasma insulin levels fall in normal lean individuals, in obese subjects, and in diabetics. This fall in insulin level is, in part, a response to the increased utilization of glucose, and also a result of increased sympatho-adrenomedullary activity at α_2-adrenoceptors. However, there is also an increase in insulin sensitivity due to an rise in insulin receptor number and affinity. These acute effects of exercise on glucose metabolism are maintained by exercise training; despite basal levels of plasma insulin being lower and a less marked fall during exercise, insulin sensitivity is increased and therefore glucose tolerance is unchanged, or even improved. Intensive exercise training may achieve modest improvements in fasting hyperglycaemia and glucose tolerance in type 2 diabetics, and possibly also in type 1 diabetics.

Prolactin

Several groups have reported a small rise in serum prolactin levels with acute exercise in normal controls, including during pregnancy, and in recreational and competitive runners, although it has been suggested that this occurs, at least in normal individuals, only when the lactate inflection point is reached. The effect of training is again uncertain; some investigators have found that the prolactin response occurs only in trained individuals, while others have reported no rise in prolactin in trained runners after a regular daily run, or even during intensive exercise in amenorrhoeic athletes.[34] However, investigations showing a prolactin response in untrained subjects have largely employed male volunteers, whereas those showing no response have used females; in spite of this, the possibility of a sex difference does not seem to have been formally tested.

Thyroid hormones and thyroid-stimulating hormone

Most studies agree that intensive acute exercise causes a rise in plasma thyroxine, free thyroxine index, and free T_4 and T_3, although in one study no change was reported during a marathon run.[33] In addition, isolated studies have reported a fall in either T_4 or T_3. Most workers have found no change in plasma thyroid-stimulating hormone (**TSH**) during acute exercise, although a small fall was noted in one study.[71]

Opioid modulation of the experience of exercise

Several workers have pointed to a link between opioid peptides and the subjective experience of exercise. The release of opioids into plasma during exercise has been suggested to be the physiological basis of what runners recognize as the 'runners high',[72] or what others might consider 'addiction to running'; however, there is little direct experimental evidence to confirm this concept. Changes in plasma β-endorphin levels showed a statistical correlation with changes in feelings of 'pleasantness' in one study; another noted analgesia to a proportion of stimuli after a 6-mile run which was partially blocked by naloxone, as well as increases in psychometric parameters corresponding to 'joy' and 'euphoria' (which were blocked by naloxone) and 'cooperation' and 'conscientiousness' (which were not). We, and others, have also reported that an infusion of naloxone during exercise results in an increase in the perceived effort of exercise.[71]

In summary, there is considerable circumstantial evidence to suggest that changes in central opioids may modulate the perception of the exercise stimulus.

Factors modifying the hormonal response to acute exercise

Changes in many components of the 'exercise stimulus', other than the exercise intensity and degree of training, may modify the hormonal response. Many of these factors remain poorly characterized, and the following list may well be incomplete.

Competition and psychological factors

The adrenocortical response to exercise is clearly enhanced by the psychological 'stress' of competition. Thus, urinary 17-hydroxy-corticosteroids, plasma cortisol, and salivary cortisol all show greater increases during a race than during training. Anticipatory rises of catecholamines, TSH, and LH have also been reported before intensive exercise, again presumably related to psychological factors. Such 'stress' is extremely difficult to quantify and thus control. It is therefore unclear to what extent 'stress' may vary before and after training or in response to different exercise-testing protocols, and thus what effect it may have on the hormonal responses under these circumstances.

Circadian rhythm

The relationship between the circadian rhythm of plasma cortisol and its response to exercise has been studied in detail by Brandenberger et al.[73] The plasma cortisol incremental rise seen during exercise was similar at all times of day when performed during 'quiescent periods' (namely, without any meal-related or other secretory peaks); however, in view of the lower basal values in the evening, the peak value achieved was lower.

Feeding and fasting

The cortisol response to acute exercise also interacts with the meal-related secretory peaks of plasma cortisol.[73] Thus, exercise performed shortly after the midday meal may result in a diminished cortisol response to exercise; conversely, exercise shortly before lunch may attenuate the meal-related cortisol rise. Prolonged fasting potentiates the exercise-induced secretion in plasma cortisol, GH, and prolactin, and a high-fat diet may also increase the GH response.

Menstrual cycle

As mentioned above, the oestradiol and progesterone responses to acute exercise vary during the menstrual cycle, being greater during the luteal phase. Other hormonal responses may also vary: thus, the GH response to bicycle ergometer exercise is much greater in mid-cycle around the time of ovulation. Generally speaking, most workers tend to study exercise during the follicular phase.

Body temperature

Body temperature rises during intense exercise, reaching temperatures as high as 40 °C to 41 °C during marathon running. The cortisol response to marathon running has been noted to be greater in hot than in cool weather. The GH and prolactin responses to passive external body heating are greater than those to exercise producing an equivalent rise in body temperature. This suggests that not only do changes in body temperature represent a major component of the 'exercise stimulus', but also, at least in the case of GH and prolactin, that other components may be exerting the opposite effect. It is unclear to what extent different exercise protocols and exercise training may modify the temperature response to exercise and therefore modulate any hormonal changes.

Other factors

Hypoxia greatly potentiates the GH, cortisol, and insulin responses to acute exercise. The GH response is greater in lean than in obese subjects, and conversely greater in type 1 than type 2 diabetes mellitus where it is normalized by strict control. In view of the complicated nature of the exercise stimulus and the difficulty in controlling for all these factors during training, it is perhaps not surprising that the reported changes in the hormonal responses to acute exercise after training remain controversial.

Conclusions

Exercise has been shown to alter the secretion of many hormones, both acutely and in response to chronic exercise training. However, there remain many contradictions in the literature concerning the responses of individual hormones. Many of these uncertainties probably relate to the complex and variable nature of the exercise stimulus, which remains poorly understood and therefore difficult to measure and thus to compare between studies. The mechanism of the hormonal adaptation to exercise is also poorly understood; the suggestion of a role for endogenous opioids is of great interest, but confirmation of their importance awaits further studies and in particular the advent of long-acting opioid antagonists.

Although the physiological significance of these exercise-induced hormonal changes is now broadly known, often relating to the maintenance of homeostasis, many questions remain unanswered. Is the muscular development produced by exercise related to hormonal changes such as the release of androgens or growth hormone, or is it more dependent on a paracrine action of insulin-like growth factor-I? Similarly, are some female competitors in field events naturally androgynous, or do they become so because of the release of androgens during training, or is it simply due to the administration of 'anabolic' steroids? Does the activation of opioid pathways during exercise allow the athlete to 'break the pain barrier' to achieve a more spectacular performance? The answers to these and other fascinating questions currently remain elusive, but with further physiological and, increasingly, molecular studies, the endocrinology of exercise is being unravelled.

References

1. Howlett TA. Hormonal responses to exercise and training: a short review. *Clinical Endocrinology* 1987; **26**: 723–42.
2. Felsing NE, Brasel JA, Cooper DM. Effect of low and high intensity exercise on circulating growth hormone in men. *Journal of Clinical Endocrinology and Metabolism* 1992; **75**: 157–62.
3. Knudtzon J, Bogsnes A, Norman N. Changes in prolactin and growth hormone levels during hypoxia and exercise. *Hormone and Metabolic Research* 1989; **21**: 453–4.
4. Beshyah SA, Shahi M, Foale R, Johnston DG. Cardiovascular effects of prolonged growth hormone replacement in adults. *Journal of Internal Medicine* 1995; **237**: 35–42.
5. Kern W, Perras B, Wodick R, Fehm HL, Born J. Hormonal secretion during nighttime sleep indicating stress of daytime exercise. *Journal of Applied Physiology* 1995; **79**: 1461–8.
6. Sutton JR, Lazarus L. Growth hormone in exercise: comparison of physiological and pharmacological stimuli. *Journal of Applied Physiology* 1976; **41**: 523–7.
7. Bloom SR, Johnson RH, Park DM, Rennie MJ, Sulaiman WR. Differences in the metabolic and hormonal response to exercise between racing cyclists and untrained individuals. *Journal of Physiology* 1976; **258**: 1–18.
8. Bullen BA, Skrinar GS, Beitins IZ, *et al.* Endurance training effects on plasma hormonal responsiveness and sex hormone excretion. *Journal of Applied Physiology* 1984; **56**: 1453–63.
9. Weltman A, Weltman JY, Schurrer R, Evans WS, Veldhuis JD, Rogol AD. Endurance training amplifies the pulsatile release of growth hormone: effects of training intensity. *Journal of Applied Physiology* 1992; **72**: 2188–96.
10. Lin T, Tucci JR. Provocative tests of growth hormone release: a comparison of results with seven stimuli. *Annals of Internal Medicine* 1974; **80**: 464–9.
11. Moretti C, Fabbri A, Gnessi L, *et al..* Naloxone inhibits exercise-induced release of PRL and GH in athletes. *Clinical Endocrinology* 1983; **18**: 135–8.
12. Coiro V, Volpi R, Maffei ML, *et al.* Opioid modulation of the gamma-aminobutyric acid-controlled inhibition of exercise-stimulated growth hormone and prolactin secretion in normal men. *European Journal of Endocrinology* 1994; **131**: 50–5.
13. Cappon J, Brasel JA, Mohan S, Cooper DM. Effect of brief exercise on circulating insulin-like growth factor I. *Journal of Applied Physiology* 1994; **76**: 2490–6.
14. Kraemer WJ, Aguilera BA, Terada M, *et al.* Responses of IGF-1 to endogenous increases in growth hormone after heavy-resistance exercise. *Journal of Applied Physiology* 1995; **79**: 1310–15.
15. Poehlman ET, Copeland KC. Influence of physical activity on insulin-like growth factor-1 in healthy younger and older men. *Journal of Clinical Endocrinology and Metabolism* 1990; **71**: 1468–73.
16. Hagberg JM, Seals DR, Yerg JE, *et al.* Metabolic responses to exercise in young and older athletes and sedentary men. *Journal of Applied Physiology* 1988; **65**: 900–8.
17. Yan Z, Biggs RB, Booth FW. Insulin-like growth factor immunoreactivity increases in muscle after acute eccentric contractions. *Journal of Applied Physiology* 1993; **74**: 410–14.
18. Zanconato S, Moromisato DY, Moromisato MY, *et al.* Effect of training and growth hormone suppression on insulin-like growth factor I mRNA in young rats. *Journal of Applied Physiology* 1994; **76**: 2204–9.
19. DeVol DL, Rotwein P, Sadow JL, Novakofski J, Bechtel PJ. Activation of insulin-like growth factor gene expression during work-induced skeletal muscle growth. *American Journal of Physiology* 1990; **259**: E89–95.
20. Taaffe DR, Jin IH, Vu TH, Hoffman AR, Marcus R. Lack of effect of recombinant human growth hormone (GH) on muscle morphology and GH-insulin-like growth factor expression in resistance-trained elderly men. *Journal of Clinical Endocrinology and Metabolism* 1996; **81**: 421–5.
21. Cuneo RC, Salomon F, Wiles CM, Hesp R, Sonksen PH. Growth hormone treatment in growth hormone-deficient adults. II. Effects on exercise performance. *Journal of Applied Physiology* 1991; **70**: 695–700.
22. Jorgensen JOL, Thuesen L, Muller J, Ovesen P, Skakkebaek NE, Christiansen JS. Three years of growth hormone treatment in growth hormone-deficient adults: near normalization of body composition and physical performance. *European Journal of Endocrinology* 1994; **130**: 224–8.
23. Beshyah SA, Freemantle C, Shahi M, *et al.* Replacement treatment with biosynthetic human growth hormone in growth hormone-deficient hypopituitary adults. *Clinical Endocrinology* 1995; **42**: 73–84.
24. Rodriguez-Arnao J, Fulcher K, Jabbar A, *et al.* Effects of GH replacement therapy on body composition, quadriceps strength test and aerobic capacity in GH deficient patients. [Abstract] *Journal of Endocrinology* 1996; **148**(Suppl.): 365.
25. Taaffe DR, Pruitt L, Reim J, *et al.* Effect of recombinant human growth hormone on the muscle strength response to resistance exercise in elderly men. *Journal of Clinical Endocrinology and Metabolism* 1994; **79**: 1361–6.
26. Yarasheski KE, Zachwieja JJ, Campbell JA, Bier DM. Effect of growth hormone and resistance exercise on muscle growth and strength in older men. *American Journal of Physiology* 1995; **268**: E268–76.
27. Yarasheski KE, Campbell JA, Smith K, Rennie MJ, Holloszy JO, Bier DM. Effect of growth hormone and resistance exercise on muscle growth in young men. *American Journal of Physiology* 1992; **262**: E261–7.
28. Deyssig R, Frisch H, Blum WF, Waldhor T. Effect of growth hormone treatment on hormonal parameters, body composition and strength in athletes. *Acta Endocrinologica* 1993; **128**: 313–8.
29. Nagulesparen M, Trickey R, Davies MJ, Jenkins JS. Muscle changes in acromegaly. *British Medical Journal* 1976; **2**: 914–15.
30. Deyssig R, Frisch H. Self-administration of cadaveric growth hormone in power athletes. *Lancet* 1993; **341**: 768–9.
31. Wittert GA, Stewart DE, Graves MP, *et al.* Plasma corticotrophin releasing factor and vasopressin responses to exercise in normal man. *Clinical Endocrinology* 1991; **35**: 311–17.
32. Strassman RJ, Appenzeller O, Lewy AJ, Qualls CR, Peake GT. Increase in plasma melatonin, beta-endorphin, and cortisol after a 28.5-mile mountain race: relationship to performance and lack of effect of naltrexone. *Journal of Clinical Endocrinology and Metabolism* 1989; **69**: 540–5.
33. Dessypris AG, Wager G, Fyhrquist F, Makinen T, Welin MG, Lamberg BA. Marathon run: effects on blood cortisol-ACTH, iodothyronines-TSH and vasopressin. *Acta Endocrinologica* 1980; **95**: 151–7.
34. Loucks AB, Horvath SM. Exercise-induced stress responses of amenorrheic and eumenorrheic runners. *Journal of Clinical Endocrinology and Metabolism* 1984; **59**: 1109–20.
35. Loucks AB, Mortola JF, Girton L, Yen SSC. Alterations in the hypothalamic–pituitary–ovarian and the hypothalamic–pituitary–adrenal axes in athletic women. *Journal of Clinical Endocrinology and Metabolism* 1989; **68**: 402–11.

36. Ding J, Sheckter CB, Drinkwater BL, Soules MR, Bremner WJ. High serum cortisol levels in exercise-associated amenorrhea. *Annals of Internal Medicine* 1988; **108**: 530–4.

37. Biller BMK, Federoff HJ, Koenig JI, Klibanski A. Abnormal cortisol secretion and responses to corticotropin-releasing hormone in women with hypothalamic amenorrhea. *Journal of Clinical Endocrinology and Metabolism* 1990; **70**: 311–17.

38. De Souza MJ, Maguire MS, Maresh CM, Kraemer WJ, Rubin KR, Loucks AB. Adrenal activation and the prolactin response to exercise in eumenorrheic and amenorrheic runners. *Journal of Applied Physiology* 1991; **70**: 2378–87.

39. Jenkins PJ, Ibanez-Santos X, Holly J, *et al*. IGFBP-1: a metabolic signal associated with exercise-induced amenorrhoea. *Neuroendocrinology* 1993; **57**: 600–4.

40. Follenius M, Candas V, Bothorel B, Brandenberger G. Effect of rehydration on atrial natriuretic peptide release during exercise in the heat. *Journal of Applied Physiology* 1989; **66**: 2516–21.

41. Jenkins PJ, Grossman A. The control of the gonadotrophin releasing hormone pulse generator in relation to opioid and nutritional cues. *Human Reproduction* 1993; **8**: 154–61.

42. Rossmanith WG, Mortola JF, Yen SSC. Role of endogenous opioid peptides in the initiation of the midcycle luteinizing hormone surge in normal cycling women. *Journal of Clinical Endocrinology and Metabolism* 1988; **67**: 695–700.

43. Cumming DC, Vickovic MM, Wall SR, Fluker MR, Belcastro AN. The effect of acute exercise on pulsatile release of luteinizing hormone in women runners. *American Journal of Obstetrics and Gynecology* 1985; **153**: 482–5.

44. McArthur JW. The effects of submaximal endurance exercise upon LH pulsatility. *Clinical Endocrinology* 1990; **32**: 115–26.

45. Wolman RL, Harries MG. Menstrual abnormalities in elite athletes. *Clinical Sports Medicine* 1989; **1**: 95–100.

46. Warren MP. The effects of exercise on pubertal progression and reproductive function in girls. *Journal of Clinical Endocrinology and Metabolism* 1980; **51**: 1150–7.

47. Frisch RE, Gotz-Welbergen AV, McArthur JW, *et al*. Delayed menarche and amenorrhea of college athletes in relation to age of onset of training. *Journal of the American Medical Association* 1981; **246**: 1559–63.

48. Veldhuis JD, Evans WS, Demers LM, Thorner MO, Wakat D, Rogol AD. Altered neuroendocrine regulation of gonadotropin secretion in women distance runners. *Journal of Clinical Endocrinology and Metabolism* 1985; **61**: 557–63.

49. Pirke KM, Schweiger U, Broocks A, Tuschl RJ, Laessle RG. Luteinizing hormone and follicle stimulating hormone secretion patterns in female athletes with and without menstrual disturbances. *Clinical Endocrinology* 1990; **33**: 345–53.

50. Bullen BA, Skrinar GS, Beitins IZ, von Mering G, Turnbull BA, McArthur JW. Induction of menstrual disorders by strenuous exercise in untrained women. *New England Journal of Medicine* 1985; **312**: 1349–53.

51. Howlett TA, Tomlin S, Ngahfoong L, *et al*. Release of beta endorphin and met-enkephalin during exercise in normal women: response to training. *British Medical Journal* 1984; **288**: 1950–2.

52. Laatikainen T, Virtanen T, Apter D. Plasma immunoreactive beta endorphin in exercise-associated amenorrhea. *American Journal of Obstetrics and Gynecology* 1986; **154**: 94–7.

53. McArthur JW, Bullen BA, Beitins IZ, Pagano M, Badger TM, Klibanski A. Hypothalamic amenorrhea in runners of normal body composition. *Endocrine Research Communications* 1980; **7**: 13–25.

54. Grossman A. Imura H, Shizume K, Yoshida S, eds. *Progress in endocrinology*. Amsterdam: Excerpta Medica, 1988; 441–8.

55. Williams CL, Nishihara M, Thalabard J, Grosser PM, Hotchkiss J, Knobil E. Corticotropin-releasing factor and gonadotropin-releasing hormone pulse generator activity in the rhesus monkey. Electrophysiological studies. *Neuroendocrinology* 1990; **52**: 133–7.

56. Frisch RE, McArthur JW. Menstrual cycles: fatness as a determinant of minimum weight for height necessary for their maintenance or onset. *Science* 1974; **185**: 949–51.

57. Hiney JK, Ojeda SR, Dees WL. Insulin-like growth factor I: a possible metabolic signal involved in the regulation of female puberty. *Neuroendocrinology* 1991; **54**: 420–3.

58. Barash IA, Cheung CC, Weigle DS, *et al*. Leptin is a metabolic signal to the reproductive system. *Endocrinology* 1996; **137**: 3144–7.

59. Ahima RS, Prabakaran D, Mantzoros C, *et al*. Role of leptin in the neuroendocrine response to fasting. *Nature* 1996; **382**: 250–2.

60. MacConnie SE, Barkan A, Lampman RM, Schork MA, Beitins IZ. Decreased hypothalamic gonadotropin-releasing hormone secretion in male marathon runners. *New England Journal of Medicine* 1986; **315**: 411–17.

61. Vogel RB, Books CA, Ketchum C, Zauner CW, Murray FT. Increase of free and total testosterone during submaximal exercise in normal males. *Medicine and Science in Sports and Exercise* 1985; **17**: 119–23.

62. Fellmann N, Coudert J, Jarrige JF, *et al*. Effects of endurance training on the androgenic response to exercise in man. *International Journal of Sports Medicine* 1985; **6**: 215–19.

63. Wheeler GD, Wall SR, Belcastro AN, Cumming DC. Reduced serum testosterone and prolactin levels in male distance runners. *Journal of the American Medical Association* 1984; **252**: 514–16.

64. Strauss RH, Lanese RR, Malarkey WB. Weight loss in amateur wrestlers and its effect on serum testosterone levels. *Journal of the American Medical Association* 1985; **254**: 3337–8.

65. Wheeler MJ, Crisp AH, Hsu LKG, Chen CN. Reproductive hormone changes during weight gain in male anorectics. *Clinical Endocrinology* 1983; **18**: 423–9.

66. Rogol AD, Veldhuis JD, Williams FA, Johnson ML. Pulsatile secretion of gonadotropins and prolactin in male marathon runners. Relation to the endogenous opiate system. *Journal of Andrology* 1984; **5**: 21–7.

67. Bagatell CJ, Bremner WJ. Sperm counts and reproductive hormones in male marathoners and lean controls. *Fertility and Sterility* 1990; **53**: 688–92.

68. Hakkinen K, Pakarinen A, Alen M, Kauhanen H, Komi PV. Neuromuscular and hormonal adaptations in athletes to strength training in two years. *Journal of Applied Physiology* 1988; **65**: 2406–12.

69. Vervoorn C, Quist AM, Vermulst LJM, Erich WBM, de Vries WR, Thijssen JHH. The behaviour of the plasma free testosterone/cortisol ratio during a season of elite rowing training. *International Journal of Sports Medicine* 1991; **12**: 257–63.

70. Adlercreutz H, Harkonen M, Kuoppasalmi K, *et al*. Effect of training on plasma anabolic and catabolic steroid hormones and their response during physical exercise. *International Journal of Sports Medicine* 1986; **7**: 27–8.

71. Grossman A. The role of opioid peptides in the hormonal responses to acute exercise in man. *Clinical Science* 1984; **67**: 483–91.

72. Appenzeller O. What makes us run? *New England Journal of Medicine* 1981; **305**: 578–9.

73. Brandenberger G, Follenius M, Hietter B. Feedback from meal-related peaks determines diurnal changes in cortisol response to exercise. *Journal of Clinical Endocrinology and Metabolism* 1982; **54**: 592–6.

3.8 Exercise and the skeleton

Jane H. Gibson and Jonathan Reeve

Introduction

Many studies have demonstrated higher bone density in young adults who regularly exercise. The relationship between exercise and bone mineral density (**BMD**) is marked in athletes,[1-4] but it has also been demonstrated in the general population in those with high levels of normal daily activity.[5-8] At one time it was expected that the more intense the exercise the greater the bony response, but during the last 10 years it has become clear that, for some young women, intensive athleticism is associated with low BMD.[9-15] Such changes in BMD are linked to profound alterations in the hypothalamic–pituitary–ovarian axis resulting in menstrual irregularity such as oligomenorrhoea and amenorrhoea. Although these conditions were initially thought to be relatively benign, it is now known that the hypo-oestrogenic state is associated with reduced bone density. The vertebral bodies, may be reduced by as much as 25 per cent. Women with menstrual irregularities are more prone to injury[16] and concern has arisen that in the long-term there may be a risk of clinical osteoporosis and fracture. Attention has therefore focused on the causes of athletic amenorrhoea in an effort to find ways of reducing its incidence without reducing athletic performance.

The role of exercise in developing peak bone mass, maintaining bone mineral during the premenopausal years, and then in the prevention of postmenopausal bone loss is complex. For this and other public health reasons, the promotion of moderate regular exercise throughout the population now has high priority, but there is uncertainty about how much exercise is moderate and what type of exercise should be proposed.

Bone metabolism in the general population

Bone mass continues to increase after the closure of the endochondral growth plates and reaches a peak during the second and third decades (Fig. 1). Teegarden *et al.*[17] estimated that by the age of 22.1 ± 2.5 years, 99 per cent of peak bone mineral density (**PBMD**) is attained and by the age of 26.2 ± 3.7 years, 99 per cent of peak bone mineral content (**PBMC**) is achieved. In women, factors contributing to the attainment of PBMC include genetic disposition,[18,19] race,[20] physical activity,[21,22] calcium intake,[23,24] body mass,[17,21,22,25] alcohol, smoking, medications, and underlying disease. Between the ages of 18 and 21 years, after longitudinal growth ceases, the skeleton goes through a period of consolidation during

which it becomes less metabolically active, remodelling driven by osteoclastic resorption reduces and, as a consequence, a moderate amount of additional bone mineral is added to the skeleton by filling in remodelling cavities.[26]

After the mid-twenties there follows a period of relative stability to changes in bone density until the age of 35 to 40 years. From then (until the menopause in women) there is a slow decline from some regions of the skeleton, notably the femoral neck,[27] but not from others.[28] Normally, spinal bone mineral density is stable over this period.

During the perimenopausal and immediate postmenopausal years there is a phase of accelerated bone loss throughout the skeleton which may initially be as high as 8 per cent per year in trabecular bone.[29,30] Ravn *et al.*[31] found that the decrease in BMD of the proximal femur reached values of 9 to 13 per cent in the first 5 years after the menopause. In the spine, bone loss initially averages 3 per cent annually as assessed by dual–energy photon or X–ray absorptiometry, but this rate of loss is attenuated to only about 1 per cent annually some 5 years later.[30] In Japanese women a decrease in spinal BMD of 20 per cent has been found within 10 years of the menopause. Beyond 10 years the rate of spinal bone loss appears to be very low.[32,33] Similarly, in the femur, the rate of loss of bone mineral slows again within 10 years of the menopause to a background

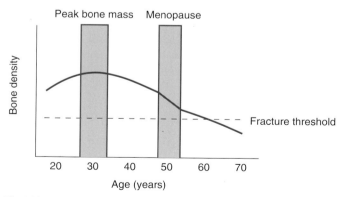

Fig. 1 Variation of bone mineral density with age in women. There is a rapid increase of bone mineral during the first three decades with peak bone mass reached in the middle of the third decade. Bone density remains relatively constant from then until approximately 40 years of age after which there is a slow decline of 0.5–1.0 per cent per year. During the perimenopausal and immediate postmenopausal years there is rapid loss of bone mineral (up to 8 per cent). This loss slows down once again to 0.5–1.0 per cent through to old age.

0.5 to 1.0 per cent[31,33] until old age when it may again start to accelerate in the femur.[34]

Thus, two types of bone loss seem to occur during the lifetime of a woman. First, from the fourth decade onwards there is a very gradual age-related loss of bone mineral which appears to occur in both cortical and trabecular type of bone. The mechanism by which age-related bone loss is mediated is unknown, but it has been likened to the gradual decline in other organs such as muscle mass. Men may suffer from a similar type of bone loss to this first type. Secondly, in women, at the menopause and for 5 to 10 years afterwards, there is an additional accelerated rate of bone loss which is most marked in trabecular bone. Treatment with oestrogen-containing products at the menopause reduces or eliminates this accelerated loss of bone mineral.[29,35] Bone mineral loss is directly linked to falling sex hormone levels (particularly oestrogen) at the menopause.

It follows that for a given rate of postmenopausal bone loss, the higher the initial bone mass at the menopause, the less likely it is that bone density will fall low enough in later years to result in osteoporotic fracture.[36] An understanding of factors contributing to high bone density is therefore important. Kröger *et al.*[37] estimated that perimenopausal women in the lowest quartile of spinal BMD had a 2.9 times greater risk of fracture than those in the highest quartile. The respective risk for femoral fracture was 2.2 times from the lowest to the highest quartile. Similarly, Cummings *et al.*[38] followed more than 8000 women aged 65 years and over for approximately 2 years. Bone densities of all regions of the hip were closely related to the risk of hip fracture. Women in the lowest quartile for femoral neck BMD had an 8.5 times greater risk of fracture than those in the highest quartile. For each standard deviation decrease in femoral neck BMD, the increased fracture risk was 2.6-fold and in the lumbar spine it was 1.6-fold. These findings have been confirmed in a recent meta-analysis of similar studies.[39] Also, Cummings *et al.* suggested that a one SD decrease in femoral neck BMD was associated with an increase in risk of hip fracture equivalent to a 14.5 year increase in age. However, it is now clear that rates of bone loss vary rather unpredictably in postmenopausal women, so that a measurement of BMD made at menopause may not accurately predict risk 10 or 20 years later.[40]

Much interest has naturally centred on factors governing the attainment of maximal potential peak bone density, maintenance of bone density in the premenopausal years, and on the minimization of the postmenopausal loss of bone mineral. Encouraging higher levels of physical activity within the general population might go some way towards reducing the fracture epidemic, particularly in the elderly, but these levels must be achievable by a substantial proportion of those at risk.[41]

The effect of exercise and mechanical forces on bone

Julius Wolff in 1892[42] first suggested that bone responds to mechanical stress to increase strength at areas of high strain. Ground reaction forces during weight-bearing activity are therefore likely to provide a suitable stimulus for bone remodelling. Indeed, immobility due to bedrest, for example spinal cord injury or weightlessness

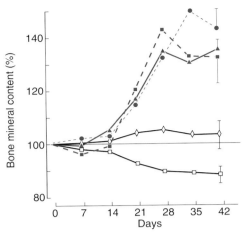

Fig. 2 Percentage change in the bone mineral content at the mid-shaft of a functionally isolated avian ulna over a 6-week experimental period in bones subjected to zero (□), 4 (◇), 36 (■), 360 (▲), or 1800 (●) consecutive cycles a day of an identical loading regimen. The vertical lines for 6-week values indicate standard deviations. The transverse scans were made using a ^{125}I source. (Reproduced from ref. 46 with permission.)

(in space), are all associated with rapid, and sometimes profound, losses in bone mineral.

However, the mechanical strain concept of bone remodelling suggests that mechanical stress applied to bone will stimulate an increase in bone mass at that site even in the absence of ground reaction forces. This is supported by studies of non weight-bearing bones. National-level Finnish squash players had 15.6 per cent greater BMD in the humerus of the playing side compared to the non-playing side,[43] and in tennis players BMD is higher in the dominant arm than the non-dominant side.[44,45] In a study of national-level female rowers and non-rowing athletes, back strength was greater in both flexion and extension in the rowers and bone density of the lumbar spine was correspondingly higher in this group even when adjusted for bodyweight.[14]

The number and weight of loading cycles applied to bone are probably as important as the type of exercise undertaken. Rubin and Lanyon[46] and Lanyon[47] have shown that, in experiments with some animal models, a maximal adaptive response can be engendered by a very small number of cycles of increased strain, no additional benefit was gained by increasing the number of loading cycles (Fig. 2) providing the peak strain achieved was sufficiently high. Frost's 'Mechanostat' theory of bone remodelling requires that a minimum effective strain must be exceeded in order to initiate the modelling process and thus potentiate an increase in bone mass driven by increased bone formation.[48] This suggests that the mechanical adaptability of bone is best suited to respond to dynamic events of short duration and high intensity rather than low-intensity activities repeated over a long period of time. If this applies in humans one might expect higher bone density in those performing short-duration, high-load exercise than in those involved in predominantly aerobic, low-intensity exercise.

There is currently much interest in the cell biology underlying the mechanical adaptability of bone cells. Viewed under the microscope, the mineralized matrix of bone is covered by what appears to be an inactive thin layer of lining cells, derived from previously active bone-forming osteoblasts, which separates the matrix from the bone marrow. Similarly, bones externally are covered by periosteal cells which become rather inactive when growth has ceased. Throughout the bone matrix another class of bone cells is to be found, the osteocytes, which live in lacunae and communicate with one another and with lining cells and periosteal cells by means of dendritic processes extending throughout a fine network of tiny canals (canaliculi.) It is the osteocytes that are thought to sense mechanical forces. The way that most investigators now agree they do this is through the so-called streaming of extracellular fluid, bearing nutrients and signalling molecules. Fluid streaming is greatly promoted by minute deformations of the bone matrix of the order of 0.2 per cent (cortical bone) or 0.5 per cent (trabecular or cancellous bone).[49] These deformations are measured in (non-dimensional) units of strain where one strain represents a deformation of 1 cm horizontally for each centimetre of a bone's vertical length. Bone of course deforms irreversibly when it is deformed by more than 0.4 to 1.0 per cent

There is less agreement, however, on how osteocytes promote bone formation and resorption at selected locations so that bone models itself to achieve the most mechanically efficient distribution of bone mineral both during growth and adulthood. Lanyon and his co-workers have demonstrated that after a rapid, transient increase in the enzyme glucose 6-phosphate dehydrogenase,[50] mechanical stimulation leads to a more prolonged production of prostaglandins, agents that can have effects both to promote bone formation and bone resorption in different circumstances. Inhibition of bone resorption by teams of multinucleate osteoclasts appears to be achievable with repeated deformations of as little as 200 to 400 μstrain (0.02 to 0.04 per cent),[51] whereas strains capable of promoting bone formation need to be 10-fold larger, a target that for major bones in human populations can only be achieved by children and young athletes.

The recruitment of cells that form or resorb bone to bone surfaces targeted for remodelling remains a subject of intensive investigation. Until very recently it was thought that new bone formation invariably followed bone resorption, with osteoclasts and osteoblasts working together in teams.[52] While this is the general rule, for example in the increased remodelling that occurs after a normal menopause, it is now clear that, in some circumstances, lining cells can be transformed back into osteoblasts without the intervention of osteoclasts. This might occur during the initiation of modelling bone 'drifts' induced by intensive mechanical stimulation. In old age, and in some other instances such as after the menopause, osteocytes may be affected by necrosis or apoptosis (programmed cell death).[53] Their disappearance may affect the ability of bone to transduce mechanical forces and to initiate the repair of microscopic cracks. These occur even under normal circumstances in spinal trabeculae and the femoral head and neck from at least middle age onwards and are marked by microcallus under the microscope. The dynamics of bone-cell populations can clearly have a profound effect on the ability of bone cells to fulfil their function. For instance, if oestrogen suppression during athletic amenorrhoea leads to osteocyte apoptosis,[53] there may be a consequent disruption of the signalling pathways responsible for microfracture repair, leading to crack enlargement and the development of a clinical stress fracture.

Young athletes

Cross-sectional studies

Bone mineral densities of the femur, pelvis, tibia, and os calcis have all been shown to be high in athletes undertaking weight-bearing sport[1-4] when compared to sedentary controls. Of all sports, weight-lifting is likely to provide the greatest stimulus to increased bone formation in the spine. Granhed et al.[54] calculated that the load applied to the third lumbar vertebra during a single dead lift during the mens' World Championships in Power Lifting was as high as 36.4 kN. Bone mineral content of the lumbar spine was extremely high in the lifters compared to age- and weight-matched sedentary controls (7.06, SD 0.87 g/cm vs. 5.18, SD 0.88 g/cm). There was also a close correlation between the estimated annual weight lifted and bone mineral content (**BMC**). Similar results were found by Conroy et al.[55] and Virvidakis et al.[56] in élite junior weightlifters. Studies comparing women who lift weights with those who run, swim, or cycle have found that BMD is significantly higher in the lifters compared to sedentary control groups and the other exercisers.[1,57,58]

Bone mineral density of the spine and femur is correlated with muscle strength,[59] although most reports of such relationships concern older non-athletic women. Sinaki and Offord[60] found a significant positive relationship between BMD of the lumbar spine and back extensor strength in postmenopausal women which held true even after adjustment for age. In a large study of 709 and 1080 elderly men and women, respectively, quadriceps strength was found to predict bone density in the proximal femur in men only.[61] However, when age- and weight-adjusted BMD of the femoral neck was analysed, in tertiles of muscle strength and calcium intake, those in the highest tertiles had approximately 5 per cent greater bone density than those in the lowest tertiles. This was true for both men and women. In younger women, femoral neck and spinal BMD have also been found to correlate with both quadriceps and hamstring and trunk extensor strength.[62] Grip strength has been found to correlate well not only with forearm BMD but also with BMD at distal sites in elderly women.[63-65] It is likely that, in this group of women at least, grip strength reflects the habitual level of daily activity, but it should be remembered that such associations do not necessarily imply causality. Because of its relative ease of measurement, grip strength might, in future, prove suitable as a contributing measurement in an overall screening programme to detect those at risk of osteoporosis.

Exercise programmes

Cross-sectional studies on athletes and the general population have demonstrated relationships between bone density and the type and intensity of exercise, but it is possible that these have been the result of selection bias, reflecting a likelihood that those with higher bone density will exercise more intensively. Only prospective, randomized studies of exercise programmes can eliminate this possibility. Extremely intensive weight-bearing training in military recruits has been found to result in marked increases in bone density in the tibia (5.2 to 11.1 per cent) over as little as 14 weeks. However, the drop-out rate due to stress fractures was high at 40 per cent and this type of training is unsuitable for most of the population.[66] A more suitable supervised aerobic exercise and weight-training programme of 35 weeks' duration in previously untrained college women was shown to result in small but significant increases in lumbar BMD with no detectable changes in the femur.[67] In a similar study performed over 2 years, small gains in BMD were found in both spine and femur.[68] Even in previously trained gymnasts, an increase in lumbar BMD has been noted with short-term, increased training programmes.[69] Other short-term studies support the relationship between exercise programmes and beneficial effects on bone density in young adults,[70] but the effect may be short-lived with a return to baseline bone-density levels after only 3 months' detraining.[71]

Bone density and exercise in children and adolescents

The effects of exercise on BMD during the prepubertal and pubertal years may be less marked than in later adolescence. Slemenda and Johnston[4] compared 44 young female skaters and non-skaters aged 10 to 23 years. Bone density was higher in the skaters, but this difference was not apparent until about the age of 15 years. Alternatively, this might have reflected overall levels of commitment to the sport and length of participation at different ages. Kröger et al.[72] found no relationship between bone density or the annual rate of increase of spinal and femoral BMD and levels of sporting activity in 65 Finnish children aged 7 to 20 years. In contrast, Slemenda et al.[21] found a more substantial effect of physical activity in boy twins participating in a study of calcium supplementation than they did for calcium. Grimston et al.[73] were able to demonstrate higher BMD in 13-year-old boys who trained intensively for weight-bearing sports compared to swimmers, but this trend was less evident in the girls. Similarly, in a 15-year longitudinal study of 98 females and 84 males aged between 13 and 27 years, BMD of the lumbar spine at age 27 years was correlated with the amount of weight-bearing activity during the preceding years in males but not in females.[74] Cooper et al.[75] found that BMD in a population-based study of young women was correlated with past and present levels of physical activity.

Menstrual irregularity and bone density in athletes

Normal bone metabolism requires an intact hypothalamic–pituitary–ovarian axis. In women the key hormones are oestrogen and progesterone. Oestrogen prevents bone resorption and decreases remodelling, whereas progesterone promotes bone formation and accelerates remodelling. In the normal hormonal milieu, bone resorption and formation are 'coupled' so that appropriate remodelling can occur as required. In the presence of low levels of oestrogen and progesterone, resorption increases since bone formation is insufficiently increased to compensate, with a net loss of bone mineral. Even asymptomatic disturbances of ovulation, such as anovulation or a short luteal phase, have been associated with bone mineral losses of up to 4 per cent per year.[76] The menstrual cycle in many female athletes is disrupted, and this has now been recognized as having profound effects on bone mineral content.

Incidence of menstrual abnormalities

Short luteal phases, anovulatory cycles, oligomenorrhoea, and amenorrhoea have all been described in athletes. Whereas secondary amenorrhoea occurs in only 5 per cent of the general population it is

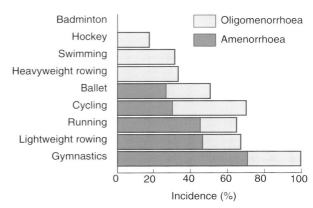

Fig. 3 Incidence of menstrual irregularities in British National Squad athletes from different sports attending the British Olympic Medical Centre. (Reproduced from ref. 77 with permission.)

common in sports in which thinness may be an added advantage to performance, such as running, gymnastics, ice-skating, and dancing. In the Great Britain National squads of these sports in 1988, 50 to 100 per cent of women reported some form of menstrual dysfunction at some time previously (Fig. 3).[77] The incidence may also be high in other sports. Recently, Güler and Hasçelik[78] demonstrated an overall rate of 30 per cent for oligomenorrhoea and amenorrhoea amongst top team-game athletes from a number of different countries. Volleyball players from Czechoslovakia, Belgium, and Sweden had the highest rates at 43 per cent. The term 'athletic amenorrhoea' has now come into use to describe secondary amenorrhoea associated with intense exercise.

Causes of menstrual disturbance

Intensity of training

There is no doubt that the aetiology of athletic amenorrhoea is multifactorial. Increasing intensity of training has been shown in some studies to correlate with an increasing incidence of menstrual dysfunction.[10,78-81] Others have been unable to confirm this relationship,[82] and it is clear that there are other factors correlated with intensity of training which must be accounted for.

Body composition

Amenorrhoeic runners have been found to be lighter and leaner than their eumenorrhoeic peers.[11,79,81-85] It is well known that profound weight loss, as occurs in anorexia nervosa, is associated with amenorrhoea, and it seems likely that low weight or changes in body composition in some way contribute to the development of this disorder in athletes. But, as yet, the exact relationship remains obscure.

Menstrual history

There may be a relationship between age at start of training, age at menarche, and the likelihood of later menstrual irregularity. Güler and Hasçelik[78] found that of the 96 top team-game athletes sampled, those with menstrual dysfunction tended to be younger, had started training at an earlier age, and were more likely to have started training before menarche. In élite speed skaters, those who reported prolonged intermenstrual intervals also had the highest average age at menarche.[86] It has also been shown that women with menstrual irregularity prior to the start of training are more likely to develop irregularity during training.[83,84] This suggests that immaturity of the hypothalamic–pituitary–ovarian axis may make menstrual irregularity more likely at times of psychological or physiological stress.

Nutritional intake

Several recent reports have suggested that the calorie intake of amenorrhoeic athletes may be lower than that of eumenorrhoeic subjects and that restriction of energy intake may be causally related to menstrual dysfunction. Nelson *et al.*[12] used a 3-day dietary record to compare the intakes of 11 amenorrhoeic and 17 eumenorrhoeic highly trained runners. They reported the mean energy intake of amenorrhoeic runners to be 520 kcal/day less than eumenorrhoeics. The difference in calorie intake was highly significant ($p < 0.005$) when expressed as a function of lean body mass. Baer[87] also found lower intakes ($p < 0.05$) in amenorrhoeic runners compared to both eumenorrhoeic runners and controls (1627 ± 75, 1944 ± 45, 1950 ± 56 kcal/day, respectively). Out of a further seven studies on runners, five have shown lower total calorie intakes in the amenorrhoeic athletes, but these differences have not been statistically significant (Table 1).[88-92] In only two studies has calorie intake been shown to be higher in amenorrhoeic athletes than in eumenorrhoeic athletes.[93,94]

Eating disorders

The current literature suggests a high incidence of anorexic or bulimic types of behaviour in some athletes, particularly those competing in events in which low weight conveys an advantage or which

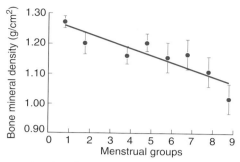

Fig. 4 The regression of vertebral bone density (L1–L4) on menstrual history for 97 active women. The mean ± SE is shown for each of the following groups: (1) R, $n = 21$; (2) R/O, $n = 7$; (3) O/R, $n = 2$; (4) O/O, $n = 5$; (5) R/A, $n = 22$; (6) A/R, $n = 9$; (7) O/A, $n = 10$; (8) A/O, $n = 10$; (9) A/A, $n = 11$. R, regular menstruation; O, oligomenorrhoeic; and A, amenorrhoeic. The pattern is current status/history. (Reproduced from ref. 101 with permission.)

are judged on aesthetic appeal.[88,89,91,92,99,100] Preoccupation with weight and food, a desire to maintain a low bodyweight or body fat and intensive exercise are all hallmarks of anorectic behaviour. Both anorexia and bulimia are associated with menstrual disturbance, and it may be that disordered eating rather than energy intake *per se* is the main contributor to the high incidence of amenorrhoea.

The effects of menstrual irregularity on bone

Menstruation and bone density of non-weight-bearing bones

During the last decade several studies have examined the effect of menstrual irregularity on BMD. Studies on amenorrhoeic runners compared to either eumenorrhoeic runners or sedentary controls have been consistent in showing lumbar BMD to be 10 to 20 per cent lower in those with amenorrhoea.[9-14] In the largest study of its kind, Drinkwater *et al.* demonstrated a linear relationship between vertebral BMD and lifetime menstrual history in 97 active women (Fig. 4).[101] Those who had a long history of oligoamenorrhoea had a mean BMD which was 17 per cent lower than in those who had always had regular periods. A linear relationship between lumbar spine BMD and oestradiol has also been demonstrated by Nelson *et al.*[12] in amenorrhoeic and eumenorrhoeic runners. The linear relationship between degree of menstrual dysfunction and vertebral bone density has been confirmed in our laboratory in national- and international-standard endurance runners. Bone density of the lumbar spine was 15.6 per cent lower in amenorrhoeic runners and 10.1 per cent lower in those who had 4 to 9 menses per year (oligomenorrhoeic) when compared to eumenorrhoeic peers (Fig. 5).[15]

The effect of hypo-oestrogenism may not be as marked in other athletes as in runners. Young *et al.* found a significant but small reduction of only 3.5 per cent in the lumbar spine of ballet dancers with slightly greater reductions of 5 to 6 per cent in the ribs, arms, and skull when compared to non-dancers with regular menstrual cycles.[102] Robinson *et al.* showed that runners had 12 per cent lower lumbar BMD than controls, whereas values in gymnasts were 5.5 per cent higher than controls, despite a similar prevalence of oligoamenorrhoea in the two athletic groups.[103] The gymnasts were

Table 1 Comparison of energy intake between amenorrhoeic (AM) and eumenorrhoeic (EU) athletes

EU (kcal/day)	n	AM (kcal/day)	n	Ref.
Runners				
2490	9	1582*	8	90
2250 ± 141	17	1730 ± 152*	11	12
2489 ± 132	33	2151 ± 236	12	95
1937 ± 383	9	1732 ± 236	6	96
1965 ± 98	14	1623 ± 145	14	10
1715 ± 281	6	1272 ± 136	11	11
1971 ± 145	19	2046 ± 115	12/13	93
1690 ± 227	5	1781 ± 283	8	94
1817 ± 523	38	1832 ± 463	38	97
1944 ± 45	10	1627 ± 75*	10	87
Dancers				
1405 ± 379	19	1116 ± 365*	19	98

Energy intake of female athletes estimated from 1-day to 7-day dietary recall and records.

kcal/day, mean ± SD.

Comparison between women with amenorrhoea and regular menstrual cycles:* $p < 0.05$, ** $p < 0.005$

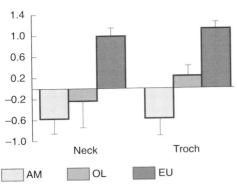

Fig. 5 Bone mineral density of proximal femur in national- and international-standard, middle- and long-distance runners. BMD was compared with the age-matched European reference range (expressed as Z-score, i.e. standard deviations above or below the age-matched mean). In both regions measured, BMD was lower in the groups with menstrual irregularity: AM vs. EU, $p < 0.001$, OL vs. EU, $p < 0.01$. Neck, neck of femur; Troch, trochanteric region; AM, amenorrhoeic ($n = 24$); OL, oligomenorrhoeic ($n = 9$) EU: eumenorrhoeic ($n = 17$). (Reproduced from ref. 15 with permission.)

much stronger generally than the runners or controls, and it is possible that the greater muscular stresses applied to the spine in gymnasts help to offset any reduction in bone mineral due to menstrual dysfunction. Certainly in rowers this seems to be the case. Wolman et al.[14] found that in a group of élite athletes, rowers with prolonged amenorrhoea had higher lumbar bone density than non-rowers, and rowers with or without menstrual dysfunction had significantly greater back strength than amenorrhoeic runners.

Menstruation and bone density of weight-bearing bones

There is less agreement about the effect of amenorrhoea on weight-bearing bones in which the muscular stresses of exercise and the effect of ground reaction forces may offset bone loss. Reduction in femoral shaft BMD in amenorrhoeic active women has been noted by one author,[101] but Wolman et al. found no difference in femoral shaft BMD between amenorrhoeic and eumenorrhoeic runners, rowers, and dancers.[3] Femoral neck, calcaneal, and total leg BMD have also been shown to be well maintained despite amenorrhoea.[85,93,101,102,104] However, in Robinson's study, lower femoral neck BMD was found in a group of 20 runners (of whom 30 per cent were oligoamenorrhoeic) compared with eumenorrhoeic sedentary controls.[103] When analysed according to more detailed menstrual history there was a 17 per cent difference in BMD between those runners who had always had regular menstrual cycles and those who had had prolonged amenorrhoea. Numbers in each group were too small for more detailed analysis. These results are very similar to those obtained for endurance runners in our laboratory. Amenorrhoeic women were 16.5 per cent and 19.5 per cent lower in bone density at femoral neck and trochanteric regions, respectively, when compared with the eumenorrhoeic runners. Reductions for those with prolonged oligomenorrhoea were 12.4 per cent and 11.1 per cent (Fig. 5).[15] This suggests that there may be a linear relationship between the number of yearly menstrual cycles and bone density of other skeletal regions in addition to the spine.

More recently, controversy has arisen as to whether bone density should be expressed according to bodyweight. Most population studies have shown that body mass is a significant independent predictor of bone density: those who are lightest have the lowest bone density. This is of particular relevance in athletes who are, in many sports, lighter than their sedentary peers. Amenorrhoeic athletes tend to be even lighter still. Some authors have therefore analysed their data after adjustment for body mass. Myerson et al.,[104] Robinson et al.,[103] and Young et al.[102] all found that previously noted differences between amenorrhoeic and eumenorrhoeic athletes were eliminated when this method was used. Only Drinkwater et al.[101] found a continuing trend towards reduced lumbar spine BMD even when adjusted for weight. In our analysis of 50 endurance runners, BMD of the lumbar spine and femoral neck were correlated with weight in the 17 amenorrhoeic runners but not in those who were oligomenorrhoeic or eumenorrhoeic. It is possible that, in athletes, weight only becomes a significant predictor of bone density in the presence of very low levels of oestrogen.

Mechanism of reduced bone density in amenorrhoea

Amenorrhoea in athletes is a form of hypothalamic hypogonadism. Pulsatile release of luteinizing hormone (**LH**) and follicle-stimulating hormone (**FSH**) are reduced in amenorrhoeic athletes.[105] Some normally menstruating runners also have reduced LH pulsatility.[105,106] Gonadotrophin-releasing hormone (**GnRH**) stimulation studies have revealed an exaggerated response of the pituitary to exogenous GnRH in amenorrhoeic athletes.[105,107] This implies that **GnRH** production by the hypothalamus is suppressed whilst pituitary function is retained. Reduced LH and FSH pulsatility means that the ovaries do not prepare a follicle for release, ovulation does not occur, and there is no luteal phase. Levels of oestrogen and progesterone may remain at early follicular levels throughout the cycle even if normal menses are present.

Very few investigators have been able to study the changes in bone occurring at the microscopic level in such athletes. However, Warren et al. performed a bone biopsy on a 20-year-old dancer with long-standing anorexia and primary amenorrhoea who suffered a femoral head collapse.[108] She was known to have lumbar BMD which was more than two standard deviations below the normal mean for her age. On microscopy, femoral cortical bone was markedly reduced in thickness and increased in porosity. At the trabecular level, the resorption surfaces were greatly increased although the formation surface was normal. It is unknown whether such changes occur in all amenorrhoeic athletes, the rate at which they might occur, or whether they are reversible with resumption of menses or treatment with appropriate hormones.

Consequences of low bone density in athletes (Table 2)

Stress fractures (Figs 6 and 7)

Lloyd et al. reviewed the medical records of 207 collegiate athletes and found radiographically confirmed fractures (type of fracture not defined) in 9 per cent of regularly menstruating women and 24 per cent of women with irregular or absent menses.[109] In dancers, two papers report a relationship between bone injuries or stress

Table 2 Potential bony consequences of athletic amenorrhoea	
Short-term consequences	**Long-term consequences**
Increased incidence of stress fractures	Failure to achieve maximum potential peak bone mass may predispose to early osteoporosis and fracture after the menopause
Increased incidence of other bony and soft-tissue injuries	
Osteoporotic fractures	
? Susceptibility to scoliosis	
Recurrent injuries interfere with training programme so failure to achieve expected goals	

fractures and amenorrhoea,[110,111] and a survey of 240 female athletes showed a higher incidence of stress fractures in those with fewer than five menses per year (49 per cent) compared to those with ten or more menses per year (29 per cent).[112] Lindberg et al. found that 49 per cent of the amenorrhoeic runners in his study had had stress fractures in the previous year, whereas none of the eumenorrhoeic runners had suffered such injuries.[113] However, two reports found no significant relationship between menstrual history and stress fractures, although both contained small numbers of subjects and so lacked statistical power.[114,115] Recognition of the possibly increased risk of stress fractures in amenorrhoeic women is important because delay in diagnosis can result in full thickness fracture.[116]

It remains controversial whether the increased rate of stress fractures in amenorrhoeic athletes is related to low BMD. Femoral bone density has been shown to be low in young, male military recruits with femoral stress fractures,[117] and Myburgh et al.[118] found that in athletes with similar training habits, those with stress fractures were more likely to have lower femoral neck and spinal bone density, lower dietary calcium intake, current menstrual irregularity, and lower oral contraceptive use. But Carbon et al.[119] assessed élite female runners with and without stress fractures and found no difference in the femoral BMD between the two groups. Others have also described a lack of association between tibial BMD and stress fractures in military recruits.[120] While Kimmel et al. have recently found an association between stress fractures in novice female military recruits and both low ultrasound attenuation in the calcaneus and increasing age.[121] One possibility is that the association between amenorrhoea and stress fractures is due to impaired microfracture

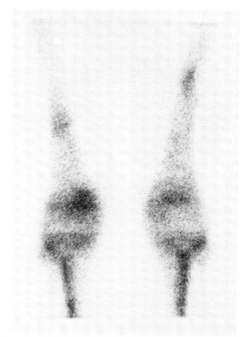

Fig. 6 Technetium-99m methylene diphosphonate bone scan of femurs of a female 10 000 m runner. This athlete had been amenorrhoeic for more than 10 years and had bone mineral density of hip and spine more than two standard deviations below expected for her age. She complained of 'pulled hamstrings' unresponsive to physiotherapy. The bone scan reveals bilateral areas of increased uptake reflecting stress fractures.

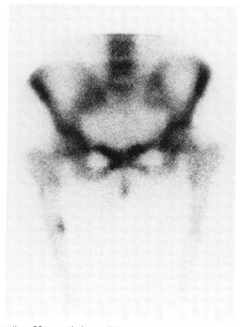

Fig. 7 Technetium-99m methylene diphosphonate bone scan of femurs of a female marathon runner. This athlete had been amenorrhoeic for 6 years and had bone mineral density of hip and spine more than two standard deviations below expected for her age. She complained of medial thigh and groin pain, and the bone scan reveals a stress fracture at the proximal one-third of the right femur.

healing, in the absence of adequate levels of oestrogen. Another possibility is that during amenorrhoea osteocyte function is compromised with an inadequate ostrogenic response to stress.

Musculoskeletal injuries

Stress fractures may not be the only injury to be more prevalent in amenorrhoeic athletes. Participants in a 10 km race who responded to a questionnaire were more likely to have taken time off from training due to any form of musculoskeletal injury if they had irregular menses.[109] In Benson's study of 49 female dancers, those with abnormal menses had more 'bone injuries' (mean = 15.0) than normally menstruating dancers (mean = 5.0) ($p < 0.05$).[110] Additionally, dancers with a low body mass index ($p < 19.0$ kg/m^2) took longer to recover from low-grade musculoskeletal injury (mean = 24.1 days) than those with a higher index (mean = 11.6 days) ($p < 0.05$).

More severe bony injury also occurs in amenorrhoeic athletes. In dancers, scoliosis was found to be more common in those with delayed menarche and in whom anorectic behaviour was more prevalent.[111] Warren et al. later described a 20-year-old ballet dancer with long-standing anorexia nervosa, primary amenorrhoea, and low BMD, who suffered femoral head collapse.[108] Recently we have reported an osteoporotic fracture in the neck of humerus of a 30-year-old marathon runner with a history of anorexia and low bone density.[122]

Long-term consequences

Amenorrhoeic athletes may be at risk of premature osteoporosis and fractures but, as yet, there is little long-term data on the natural history of bone metabolism in this condition. As previously shown, bone mass peaks at approximately 20 to 30 years of age, so athletes should be at their highest BMD during their most athletic years. Eumenorrhoeic athletes have higher peak BMD (PBMD) than the mean for the population. But if amenorrhoeic athletes fail to attain their maximum potential PBMD at this age, it is unknown whether they will be able to 'catch up' later in life. If the lifetime risk of hip fracture is related to peak bone mass, eumenorrhoeic athletes are likely to be at reduced risk of osteoporotic fracture throughout their lifetime, whereas amenorrhoeic athletes may always be at a relative disadvantage.

But BMD may increase when menstruation returns in these athletes. Drinkwater et al. followed nine athletes over a 15.5-month period.[81] Of these, seven had regained menses and two women had remained amenorrhoeic. Lumbar BMD increased by 6.3 per cent in the former amenorrhoeic women whilst decreasing a further 0.3 per cent in those who had remained amenorrhoeic. Small increases in BMD were also seen in the radius. These results are very similar to those of Lindberg et al. who retested seven amenorrhoeic runners at 15 months.[13] Although four recovered menses and showed an improvement of 6.5 per cent in lumbar BMD, the other three remained amenorrhoeic and showed no improvement in BMD.

Some data are available from anorexics with amenorrhoea. Rigotti et al. followed cortical bone density of the radius in non-athletic patients with anorexia nervosa over a median period of 25 months.[123] Only 6 of the 27 women who regained menses (although most gained some weight), took calcium supplements and exercised regularly. There were no significant changes in BMD in women

who regained menses, received oestrogen therapy, or who gained weight to more than 80 per cent of their ideal weight. In addition, there was a high incidence of vertebral compression fractures and non-spine fractures. But weight gain and either oestrogen therapy or return of menses in anorexics has been shown to be associated with improvements in spinal BMD (Bachrach et al.[124]). Studies on recovered anorexics also suggest that total body BMD may return towards normal for their age.[124,125]

These short-term studies suggest that small improvements in BMD may occur in some regions of the skeleton, particularly those that are high in trabecular bone such as the spine, when menstruation returns. However, changes in cortical bone may not occur so rapidly, if at all. It is also unknown whether improvements in trabecular bone are maintained over several years.

There is some evidence from cross-sectional studies of older premenopausal and postmenopausal women that certain gynaecological parameters may have important associations with BMD. A greater number of pregnancies, early menarche, and a greater number of days bleeding have all been correlated with higher radial BMD.[126] In this study, for each decade of menstruation, radial BMD was 2 per cent higher, but there was no association with the length of the menstrual cycle or a previous history of irregularity. This contrasts with findings by Georgiou et al. who found that BMD of the forearm in postmenopausal women had a better linear correlation with the total number of menstrual cycles than with age or years since the menopause.[127] We have compared the BMDs of lumbar spine and proximal femur in premenopausal veteran runners, aged 40 years and over, who have a history of menstrual dysfunction with peers who have always had regular menstruation. Bone density was similar in all femoral regions measured but was lower in the lumbar spine in those with previous menstrual irregularity. Our results suggest that for the femur, continued weight-bearing exercise may be sufficient to offset any bone mineral loss incurred at a younger age, but that there may be long-lasting effects of amenorrhoea on other parts of the skeleton.[128] Only long-term prospective studies of amenorrhoeic athletes will be able to confirm or refute this.

Treatment of reduced bone density in athletes (Table 3)

Drinkwater et al.[81] and Lindberg et al.[13] demonstrated an increase in BMD associated with resumption of menses, but in all cases return of menses was associated with a reduction in training volume or intensity and a concomitant increase in weight. Not all athletes are willing to alter their training habits in order to resume menstruation. For some, menstruation is a nuisance and for others it interferes with performance. In such athletes treatment to prevent further bone mineral loss or to improve low bone density despite amenorrhoea would be of interest. Treatment regimes used in women with secondary amenorrhoea not willing to resume monthly menstruation have included calcium supplementation, recently introduced forms of hormone replacement therapy such as continuous combined regimes, and intranasal calcitonin.

Hormone replacement therapy

De Cree et al. used 2 mg cyproterone acetate and 50 µg ethinyl oestradiol as a combined oral contraceptive in seven amenorrhoeic ath-

Table 3 Therapeutic options in the management of athletic amenorrhoea	
Interventions which have some evidence of efficacy in athletes	Interventions for which evidence of efficacy is awaited in athletes
Reduction of risk factors which predispose to menstrual dysfunction, thus allowing return to normal menstruation	Hormone replacement therapy
	Nasal calcitonin
Calcium supplementation	Oral bisphosphonates
Oral contraceptive pill (not 'mini-pill')	

letes.[129] During 8 months of treatment, BMD in the lumbar spine increased by 9.5 per cent compared with a control group of four athletes in whom BMD increased by only 1.6 per cent. Very little change occurred in either group in the radius. It is difficult to assess the effect of the cyproterone acetate on bone density, indeed the increase may have been solely due to the relatively high dose of oestrogen used. In a study of 15 non-athletic women with primary and secondary amenorrhoea, Haenggi et al. showed increases of 2.5 per cent and 2.9 per cent per year in the lumbar spine and Ward's triangle, respectively, when women were treated with an oral contraceptive containing 0.03 mg ethinyloestradiol and 0.15 mg desogestrel.[130] Non-significant increases in BMD were observed in the femoral neck and tibia, suggesting that the greatest effects occur at sites high in trabecular bone. Similarly, treatment with medroxyprogesterone in physically active women with menstrual cycle disturbances has shown significant improvements in spinal BMD.[131] But treatment with oestrogen and progestins in anorexia nervosa patients with proven low spinal trabecular BMD have given conflicting results. Only those with a bodyweight less than 70 per cent of ideal appeared to derive benefit from treatment, in that further bone loss was prevented compared to controls. The greatest changes were seen in those controls who regained menses in whom there was a 19.4 per cent increase in BMD.[132]

Calcium

Treatment with calcium has been suggested to be weakly effective by Prior et al. in his study of 61 active women but no effect has been shown by others.[131] Baer et al. treated seven adolescent amenorrhoeic runners with 1200 mg calcium carbonate and 400 IU vitamin D daily.[87] During a 12 month period the subjects consumed an average of 2400 mg calcium daily, but BMD of the lumbar spine did not increase and in two subjects it declined further.

Intranasal calcitonin

In non-athletes with menstrual abnormalities, intranasal calcitonin and oestrogen or progesterone replacement have been used. In seven women with primary amenorrhoea who completed 6 months of treatment with either intranasal calcitonin or a combined oestrogen/progesterone therapy, BMD of the lumbar spine increased by 4.1 per cent in the first group and by 9.2 per cent in the latter group.[133]

Bisphosphonates

As yet there are no studies on the effect of the bisphosphonates on low bone density in amenorrhoeic athletes. They are now becoming widely accepted as a treatment of choice for established osteoporosis in postmenopausal women,[134] but their role in hypogonadal bone loss in premenopausal women is still conjectural.

Although some mention was made in these studies on the incidence of side-effects with treatment, no mention was made of the effects of treatment on athletic performance. Side-effects associated with hormone therapy by women who have experienced prolonged amenorrhoea, such as breast tenderness, weight gain, and emotional lability, are unlikely to be tolerated by runners. Calcium in high doses may also cause troublesome gastrointestinal upsets in a minority, which are particularly difficult for runners.

Summary

Effective treatment of reduced bone density in young women seems possible, at least in the short-term, although side-effects may be a particular problem in athletes and may reduce compliance. The long-term effects of treatment are unknown and must await further investigation. A more effective approach to the problem must be in the prevention of athletic amenorrhoea, with prompt assessment and treatment should it occur.

Bone density in perimenopausal and postmenopausal women

A dramatic consequence of the ageing of the population has been the enormous increase in the numbers of osteoporotic fractures. Although undoubtedly vertebral and radial fractures cause considerable morbidity, it is the mortality and cost associated with hip fractures that cause particular concern to the health planners. The mortality rate at one year following fracture is almost 20 per cent, and in those who do survive very few regain their previous level of mobility. Based on past trends in hip fracture rate, it is estimated that the total number of cases (men and women) will rise from about 50 000 in 1985 to almost 120 000 in 2016.[135]

Vertebral fractures are harder to quantify as many are asymptomatic, but Melton et al. suggested that the prevalence may be as high as 26.5 per cent in all women aged over 55 years.[136] A report from the United States, based on 1986 data, estimates that vertebral fractures accounted for 10 per cent of all osteoporosis-related hospital admissions in women over the age of 45 years.[137] In Europe, rates of prevalent deformities in population samples of men and women aged over 50 (mean age approximately 65 years) were in excess of 10 per cent. However, not all vertebral deformities are due to osteoporosis.[138]

The role of exercise in preventing osteoporosis and fracture

The prevention of osteoporosis and its devastating consequences has become a key issue and much effort is being devoted to understanding its aetiology. The incidence of hip fracture is directly related to bone strength, the risk of falling, and the neuromuscular responses to falling. The higher the bone density in early adult life, the lower the risk of fracture in later years. Those women with greater bone density at the menopause are also at lower risk of fracture. Cooper et al. showed that increased daily activity protected against fracture in men and women aged 50 years and over.[139] Muscle power was independently associated with the risk of fracture with a fivefold increase between the lowest and highest fifths of strength, and was significantly related to all measured indices of activity. In a 15-year prospective study of 1419 elderly men and women in Britain, Wickham et al. showed that the relative risk of hip fracture was 5.2 in those who were housebound compared to those with full outdoor activity.[140] Physical activity such as household work, strenuous conditions of employment, and sport during early adult years also appears to protect women from later fracture, regardless of the level of activity at the time of fracture.[141]

A greater understanding of the mechanisms by which bone mass in old age can be improved, and the risks of falling reduced, will help to focus preventive programmes. Regular exercise may be one method of maintaining BMD, preventing the development of osteoporosis, and reducing the rate of falling. However, the amount of exercise required to have a maximal effect is unknown. Nor is it known whether exercise in the elderly is as beneficial as activity in the early adult years.

Cross-sectional studies

Population-based studies of older women have consistently shown higher bone density in those women who are moderately active compared with those who are sedentary.[5-8] For instance, Krall and Dawson-Hughes found higher whole-body BMD in postmenopausal women walking approximately 1 mile per day compared to those walking shorter distances.[19] The rate of bone loss in these active postmenopausal women was also slowed.

Two cross-sectional studies on older 'athletic' women have also shown higher BMD than age-matched non-exercisers. In both studies women were considered athletic if they exercised for at least 1 h, three times a week at the equivalent intensity of a game of tennis. The most significant differences in bone density occurred in the oldest, postmenopausal women in whom bone density was maintained compared to the control groups in whom it declined.[142,143] We have examined the effects of much greater volumes of training in premenopausal middle- and long-distance runners over the age of 40 years. In this study of 50 subjects, athletes trained an average of 7.1 h per week and ran an average of 32.1 miles per week. Bone density of the proximal femur and lumbar spine was very high, regardless of whether training had started at a young age or after the age of 30 years.[128]

Thus regular activity in older women appears to be associated with significant skeletal benefits. However, very intensive exercise in postmenopausal women may not have the same advantages. Michel et al. found that women exercising for more than 5 h per week had quite low lumbar BMD compared with other women who trained less intensively.[144] In a 2-year prospective, follow-up study to this, Michel et al. confirmed that, in females over the age of 50, extreme levels of exercise (greater than 300 min per week) were associated with low bone density.[145] And Nelson et al. found that endurance-trained postmenopausal women (running 22.6 ± 2.4 miles per week) had surprisingly similar lumbar, femoral, and radial BMD to age-matched sedentary women, although, when adjusted for weight, lumbar and radial bone density was higher in the active group.[146] Similar results were found by us in 24 postmenopausal, long-distance runners who ran an average of 30.6 miles per week and trained, on average, for 6.7 h per week.[147] Bone density in these women was no greater than expected for their age, even after adjusting for their lower weight, and indeed was very low in those who trained the most intensively.

Exercise programmes

The evidence for beneficial effects of exercise intervention programmes on bone density in postmenopausal women is conflicting. Most studies have involved small numbers of subjects for a maximum of one year. In some, the type of exercise has been inappropriate to the site of bone measured, for example a weight-bearing exercise study has been accompanied by bone-density measurements at the radius. Other studies have involved women over a wide age range, and this may have obscured any benefits available in the immediate postmenopausal period compared with the very elderly (or vice versa).

Not surprisingly, findings from these studies therefore range from no apparent benefit[148,149] to marked increases in BMD. Dalsky et al. noted an increase in lumbar BMD of 5.2 per cent and 6.1 per cent after 9 and 22 months, respectively, of walking, jogging, and stair-climbing in 55- to 70-year-old women.[150] After 13 months' detraining, BMD had declined to 1.1 per cent above baseline. Chow et al. measured changes in bone mass of the trunk and upper thigh by neutron activation, expressed as the calcium index.[151] After 1 year of aerobics and strength training 16 women, on average 7 years' postmenopausal, had a significant increase in calcium index compared to non-exercising controls. In a 2-year longitudinal study of men and women over the age of 50 years, Michel et al. found a high correlation between increasing exercise levels and bone density in those exercising at moderate levels, but low levels of BMD at extremely high levels of exercise.[145]

Others have shown that BMD may not increase with exercise in older women, but rates of bone loss may be slowed or halted.[70,152-156] This effect may be most marked in those women closest to the menopause.[157]

It therefore remains unclear whether exercise intervention in postmenopausal women is an appropriate form of treatment for established osteoporosis or whether indeed it can be recommended for the maintenance of bone density. Although cross-sectional and population studies support regular physical activity as a means of reducing osteoporosis, the volume and intensity of exercise required is unknown. The effects of exercise on bone remodelling leading to net bone reduction may require the presence of premenopausal levels of sex hormones. Prospective studies of exercise intervention in postmenopausal women both on and off hormone replacement therapy would help to answer this question.

Regular exercise may have other benefits in the elderly population at risk of osteoporotic fracture. Physical activity improves neuromuscular function and can reduce the rate of hip fracture from falling.[140] Indeed, exercise and balance training programmes within the nursing-home setting have shown a 10 to 25 per cent reduction in the rate of falling compared to controls.[158] This alone is compelling evidence for maintaining physical activity in the very elderly.

Calcium intake and bone density in athletes

Bone mass is higher in children and adolescents with a high calcium intake[159,160] and this may result in a greater bone mass in later life.[23] Work on healthy premenopausal women supports a role for dietary calcium in the development of bone, particularly when associated with exercise.[161,162] The synergistic effect of calcium and exercise on bone has also been demonstrated in animal models.

A positive linear relationship between trabecular BMD in the lumbar spine and calcium intake in athletes has been demonstrated by Wolman et al.,[163] a finding that was independent of menstrual status and which has not been shown in other studies.[1,12,73] These differences may be due to methodology, particularly in the assessment of calcium intake or statistical confounding by another risk factor. Alternatively, the relationship between calcium intake and bone mineral content may not be linear. Kanders et al. showed a positive relationship between calcium intake and vertebral BMD in normal healthy eumenorrhoeic women but not above a daily intake of 800 to 1000 mg.[161] The ability of an individual to adapt to a low calcium intake may be genetically determined.[164,165]

A low dietary calcium intake has been reported in many athletes, particularly in amenorrhoeic women.[91,166–171] Low oestrogen levels are associated with decreased intestinal absorption of calcium and increased urinary loss, so dietary calcium requirements may be even higher in amenorrhoeic athletes.[171] Both Marcus et al.[11] and Nelson et al.[12] found that 55 per cent of amenorrhoeic athletes failed to meet the recommended daily allowance (**RDA**) for calcium compared to 35 to 40 per cent of cyclic women. Kaiserauer et al. also noted a lower intake in amenorrhoeic compared to eumenorrhoeic runners (600 mg versus 1200 mg/day, $p < 0.05$).[90] Yet it remains unclear how much of the variance in BMD in amenorrhoeic athletes is due to low calcium intake.

Bone density in male athletes

Cross-sectional studies on young men have confirmed that those who exercise tend to have higher bone density than non-exercisers.[51,173] As described above, those who lift weights have the highest bone density of all.[60–62,174,175] The relationship between activity and BMD may not be true for all sports. A study of 15- to 19-year-old cyclists found lower bone mineral content and bone density in the cyclists compared to sedentary normal subjects.[176] The cyclists had been training on the road for at least 10 h per week for the last 2 years. Smith and Rutherford compared bone densities of a small number of male rowers, triathletes, and sedentary controls.[177] As expected the rowers had significantly higher total body mass and spinal bone density than the controls, but there was no such difference between the triathletes and controls. Testosterone levels were low in the triathletes, and the authors suggest that low

testosterone levels may have negated any beneficial effect of exercise on the skeleton. Certainly, it is known that hypogonadal men are at increased risk of osteoporosis. Low testosterone levels in endurance-trained male athletes may be the male equivalent of athletic amenorrhoea. If this is so, a similar syndrome of paradoxically low bone density may occur in such athletes and this needs further investigation.

Most cross-sectional studies on older men, whether population-based or on athletic groups, have shown a continuing relationship between high levels of exercise and greater BMD.[143,178,179] And in healthy men aged 61 to 84 years markers of physical fitness and strength, such as back strength and maximal oxygen uptake, have been shown to correlate well with axial bone density.[45] Whereas exercise intervention studies in postmenopausal women have often failed to show improvements in BMD, similar studies in men consistently show some benefit.[145,180,181] However, Michel et al. showed that intensive levels of weight-bearing exercise in a small number of men over the age of 65 years may be associated with paradoxically low, lumbar bone density.[144,145]

Conclusions

Regular, moderate physical activity appears to have beneficial effects on bone density at all ages, although exercise intervention programmes in elderly men and women have been unable to demonstrate this benefit. How much and what type of exercise should be recommended is still unknown. High-intensity training has advantages and disadvantages for skeletal metabolism, and questions remain about the long-term effects of menstrual irregularity on bone mineral. As yet, there is very little information on the treatment of athletic amenorrhoea and its long-term effects on bone density.

References

1. Heinrich CH, Going SB, Pamenter RW, Perry CD, Boyden TW, Lohman TG. Bone mineral content of cyclically menstruating female resistance and endurance-trained athletes. *Medicine and Science in Sports and Exercise* 1990; **22**: 558–63.
2. Risser WL, Lee EJ, Leblanc A, Poindexter JMH, Schneider V. Bone density in eumenorrhoeic female college athletes. *Medicine and Science in Sports and Exercise* 1990; **22**: 570–4.
3. Wolman RL, Faulmann L, Clark, Hesp R, Harries MG. Different training patterns and bone mineral density of the femoral shaft in elite, female athletes. *Annals of Rheumatic Diseases* 1991; **50**: 487–9.
4. Slemenda CW, Johnston CC. High intensity activities in young women, site specific bone mass effects among female figure skaters. *Bone and Mineral* 1993; **20**: 125–32.
5. Aloia JF, Vaswani AN, Yeh JK, Cohn SH. Premenopausal bone mass is related to physical activity. *Archives of Internal Medicine* 1988; **148**: 121–3.
6. Zylstra S, Hopkins A, Erk M, Hreshchyshyn MM, Anbar M. Effect of physical activity on lumbar spine and femoral neck bone densities. *International Journal of Sports Medicine* 1989; **10**: 181–6.
7. Jónsson B, Ringsberg K, Josefsson PO, Johnell O, Birch-Jensen M. Effects of physical activity on bone mineral content and muscle strength in women, a cross-sectional study. *Bone* 1992; **13**: 191–5.
8. Zhang J, Feldblum PJ, Fortney JA. Moderate physical activity and bone density among perimenopausal women. *American Journal of Public Health* 1992; **82**: 736–8.

9. Cann CE, Martin MC, Genant HK, Jaffe RB. Decreased spinal mineral content in amenorrhoeic women. *Journal of the American Medical Association* 1984; **251**: 626–9.

10. Drinkwater BL, Nilson K, Chesnut CH, Bremner WJ, Shainholtz S, Southworth MB. Bone mineral content of amenorrhoeic and eumenorrhoeic athletes. *New England Journal of Medicine* 1984; **311**: 277–81.

11. Marcus R, Cann C, Madvig P, *et al*. Menstrual function and bone mass in elite women distance runners. *Annals of Internal Medicine* 1985; **102**: 158–63.

12. Nelson ME, Fisher EC, Catsos PD, Meredith CN, Turksoy RN, Evans JE. Diet and bone status in amenorrhoeic runners. *American Journal of Clinical Nutrition* 1986; **43**: 910–16.

13. Lindberg JS, Powell MR, Hunt MM, Ducey DE, Wade CE. Increased vertebral bone mineral in response to reduced exercise in amenorrhoeic runners. *Western Journal of Medicine* 1987; **146**: 39–42.

14. Wolman RL, Clark P, McNally E, Harries M, Reeve J. Menstrual state and exercise as determinants of spinal trabecular bone density in female athletes. *British Medical Journal* 1990; **301**: 516–18.

15. Wilson JH, Reeve J, Harries MH. Determinants of bone mineral density in female athletes (abstract). *Bone* 1994; **15**: 450

16. Lloyd T, Triantafyllou SJ, Baker ER, *et al*. Women athletes with menstrual irregularity have increased musculoskeletal injuries. *Medicine and Science in Sports and Exercise* 1986; **18**: 374–9.

17. Teegarden D, Proulx WR, Martin BR, *et al*. Peak bone mass in young women. *Journal of Bone and Mineral Research* 1995; **10**: 711–15.

18. Hansen MA, Hassager C, Jensen SB, Christiansen C. Is heritability a risk factor for postmenopausal osteoporosis? *Journal of Bone and Mineral Research* 1992; **7**: 1037–43.

19. Krall EA, Dawson-Hughes B. Heritable and lifestyle determinants of bone mineral density. *Journal of Bone and Mineral Research* 1993; **8**: 1–9.

20. Harris SS, Wood MJ, Dawson-Hughes BD. Bone mineral density of the total body and forearm in premenopausal black and white women. *Bone* 1995; **16**: 311S–315S.

21. Slemenda CW, Reister TK, Hui SL, Miller SL, Christian JC, Johnston CC Jr. Influences on skeletal mineralization in children and adolescents: evidence for varying effects of sexual maturation and physical activity. *Journal of Pediatrics* 1994; **125**: 201–7.

22. Valimaki MJ, Karkkainen M, Lamberg-Allardt C, *et. al*. Exercise, smoking and calcium intake during adolescence and early adulthood as determinants of peak bone mass. *British Medical Journal* 1994; **309**: 230–5.

23. Matkovic V, Kostial K, Simonovic I, Buzina R, Brodarec A, Nordin BEC. Bone status and fracture rates in two regions of Yugoslavia. *American Journal of Clinical Nutrition* 1979; **32**: 540–9.

24. Nieves JW, Golden AL, Siris E, Kelsey E, Linsay R. Teenage and current calcium intake are related to bone mineral density of the hip and forearm in women aged 30–39 years. *American Journal of Epidemiology* 1995; **141**: 342–51.

25. Rice S, Blimkie CJ, Webber CE, Levy D, Martin J, Parker D, Gordon CL. Correlates and determinants of bone mineral content and density in healthy adolescent girls. *Canadian Journal of Physiology and Pharmacology* 1993; **71**: 923–30.

26. Parsons TJ, Prentice A, Smith EA, Cole TJ, Compston E. Bone mineral mass consolidation in young British adults. *Journal of Bone and Mineral Research* 1996; **11**: 264–74.

27. Pearson J, Dequeker J, Reeve J, *et al*. Absorptiometry of the proximal femur: Normal European values standardised with the European spine phantom. *Journal of Bone and Mineral Research* 1995; **10**: 315–24.

28. Dequeker J, Pearson J, Reeve J, *et al*, Dual X-ray absorptiometry: Cross-calibration and normative reference ranges for the spine: results of a European Community Concerted Action. *Bone* 1995; **17**: 247–54.

29. Gotfredson A, Nilas L, Riis BJ, Thomsen K, Xhristianse C. Bone changes occurring spontaneously and caused by oestrogen in early postmenopausal women, a local or generalised phenomenon? *British Medical Journal* 1986; **292**: 1098–100.

30. Reeve J, Pearson J, Mitchell A, *et al*. Evolution of spinal bone loss and biochemical markers of bone remodelling after menopause in normal women. *Calcified Tissue International* 1995; **57**: 105–10.

31. Ravn P, Hetland ML, Overgaard K, Christiansen C. Premenopausal and postmenopausal changes in bone mineral density of the proximal femur measured by dual energy X-ray absorptiometry. *Journal of Bone and Mineral Research* 1994; **9**: 1975–80.

32. Soda M-Y, Mizunuma H, Honjo S-I, Okano H, Ibuki Y, Igarashi M. Pre- and postmenopausal bone mineral density of the spine and proximal femur in Japanese women assessed by dual energy X-ray absorptiometry: a cross-sectional study. *Journal of Bone and Mineral Research* 1993; **8**: 183–9.

33. Greenspan SL, Maitland SL, Myers LA, Krasnow ER, Kido MB. Femoral bone loss progresses with age, a longitudinal study in women over the age of 65 years. *Journal of Bone and Mineral Research* 1994; **9**: 1959–65.

34. Jones G, Nguyen T, Sambrook P, Kelly PJ, Eisman JA. Progressive loss of bone in the femoral neck in elderly people, longitudinal findings from the Dubbo osteoporosis epidemiology study. *British Medical Journal* 1994; **309**: 691–5.

35. Riis BJ, Thomsen K, Strøm V, Christiansen C. The effect of percutaneous and natural progesterone on postmenopausal bone loss. *American Journal of Obstetrics and Gynecology* 1987; **56**: 61–5.

36. Black DM, Cummings SR, Melton LJ. Appendicular bone mineral and a woman's lifetime risk of hip fracture. *Journal of Bone and Mineral Research* 1992; **7**: 639–45.

37. Kröger H, Kotaniemi A, Kröger L, Alhava E. Development of bone mass and bone density of the spine and femoral neck–a prospective study of 65 children and adolescents. *Bone and Mineral* 1993; **23**: 171–82.

38. Cummings S.R, Black DM, Nevitt MC, *et al*. Bone density at various sites for prediction of hip fractures. *Lancet* 1993; **341**: 72–5.

39. Marshall D, Johnell O, Wedel H. Meta-analysis of how well measures of bone mineral density predict occurrence of osteoporotic fractures. *British Medical Journal* 1996; **312**: 1254–9.

40. Hui SL, Slemenda CW, Johnston CC Jr. The contribution of bone loss to postmenopausal osteoporosis. *Osteoporosis International* 1990; **1**: 30–4.

41. Cooper C, Barker DJP. Risk factors for hip fracture. *New England Journal of Medicine* 1995; **332**: 814–15.

42. Wolff JD. In *Das Geretz der Transformation der Knocken*. (Translated by Maquet P. and Furlong R.) 1986 Springer-Verlag, Berlin.

43. Haapasalo H, Kannus P, Sievanen H, Heinonen A, Oja P, Vuori I. Long-term unilateral loading and bone mineral density and content in female squash players. *Calcified Tissue International* 1994; **54**: 249–55.

44. Dalén N, Låftman P, Ohlsén H, Strömberg L. The effect of athletic activity on bone mass in human diaphyseal bone. *Orthopedics* 1985; **8**: 1139–41.

45. Pirnay E, Bodeux M, Crielaard JM, Franchimont P. Bone mineral content and physical activity. *International Journal of Sports Medicine* 1987; **8**: 331–5.

46. Rubin CT, Lanyon LE. Regulation of bone formation by applied dynamic loads. *Journal of Bone and Joint Surgery* 1984; **66A**: 397–402.

47. Lanyon LE. "Why does a mechanism that successfully matches bone strength to bone loading before the menopause fail when oes-

trogen level decline?" In: Compston JE, ed. *Osteoporosis: new perspectives on causes, prevention and treatment*. Royal College of Physicians of London, 1996.

48. Frost H.M. The role of changes in mechanical usage set points in the pathogenesis of osteoporosis. *Journal of Bone and Mineral Research* 1992; **7**: 253–261.

49. Lozupone E, Nico B, Mancini L, Favia A, Lamanna M, Cagiano R. The dynamic of the flow of the interstitial fluid into the osteocyte lacunae and canaliculi of bone cultured *in vitro*. *Bone* 1996; **19** (Suppl. 3): 150S (Abstract).

50. el Haj AJ, Minter SL, Rawlinson SC, Suswillo R, Lanyon LE. Cellular responses to mechanical loading *in vitro*. *Journal of Bone and Mineral Research* 1990; **5**: 923–32.

51. Lanyon LE. Bone loading—the functional determinant of bone architecture and a physiological contributor to the prevention of osteoporosis. In: Smith R, ed. *Osteoporosis*. Royal College of Physicians of London, 1990.

52. Eriksen EF. Normal and pathological remodelling of human trabecular bone: Three dimensional reconstruction of the remodelling sequence in normal and in metabolic bone disease. *Endocrine Reviews* 1986; **7**: 379–407.

53. Tomkinson A, Reeve J, Shaw R, Noble BS. The death of osteocytes via apoptosis accompanies oestrogen withdrawal in human bone. *Journal of Clinical Endocrinology and Metabolism* 1998 (in press).

54. Granhed H, Jonson R, Hansson T. The loads on the lumbar spine during extreme weight lifting. *Spine* 1987; **12**: 146–9.

55. Conroy BP, Kraemer WJ, Maresh CM, *et al.* Bone mineral density in elite junior Olympic weightlifters. *Medicine and Science in Sports and Exercise* 1993; **25**: 1103–9.

56. Virvidakis K, Georgiou E, Korkotsidid A, Ntalles K, Proukakis C. Bone mineral content of junior competitive weight-lifters. *International Journal of Sports Medicine* 1990; **11**: 244–6.

57. Davee AM, Rosen CJ, Adler RA. Exercise patterns and trabecular bone density in college women. *Journal of Bone and Mineral Research* 1990; **5**: 245–50.

58. Heinonen A, Oja P, Kannus P, Sievanen H, Manttari A, Vuori I. Bone mineral density in female athletes in different sports. *Bone and Mineral* 1993; **23**: 1–14.

59. Pocock N, Eisman J, Gwinn T, *et al.* Muscle strength, physical fitness, and weight but not age predict femoral neck bone mass. *Journal of Bone and Mineral Research* 1989; **4**: 441–8.

60. Sinaki M, Offord KP. Physical activity in postmenopausal women: effect on back muscle strength and bone mineral density of the spine. *Archives of Physical Medicine and Rehabilitation* 1988; **69**: 277–80.

61. Nguyen TV, Kelly PJ, Sambrook PN, Gilbert C, Pocock NA, Eisman JAJ. Lifestyle factors and bone density in the elderly; Implications for osteoporosis prevention. *Journal of Bone and Mineral Research* 1994; **9**: 1339–46.

62. Eickoff J, Molczyk L, Galagher JC, De Jong S. Influence of isotonic, isometric and isokinetic muscle strength on bone density of the spine and femur in young women. *Bone and Mineral* 1993; **20**: 201–9.

63. Bevier WC, Wiswell RA, Pyka G, Kozak KC, Newhall KM, Marcus R. Relationship of body composition, muscle strength, and aerobic capacity to bone mineral density in older men and women. *Journal of Bone and Mineral Research* 1989; **4**: 421–32.

64. Kritz-Silverstein D, Barrett-Connor E. Grip strength and bone mineral density in older women. *Journal of Bone and Mineral Research* 1994; **9**: 45–51.

65. Sinaki M, Wahner HW, Offord KP. Relationship between grip strength and related regional bone mineral content. *Archives of Physical Medicine and Rehabilitation* 1989; **70**: 823–6.

66. Margulies JY, Simkin A, Leichter I, *et al.* Effect of intense physical activity on the bone mineral content in the lower limbs of young adults. *Journal of Bone and Joint Surgery* 1986; **68A**: 1090–3.

67. Snow-Harter C, Bouxsein ML, Lewis BT, Carter DR, Marcus R. Effects of resistance and endurance exercise on bone mineral status of young women, a random exercise intervention trial. *Journal of Bone and Mineral Research* 1992; **7**: 761–9.

68. Friedlander AL, Genant HK, Sadowsky S, Byl NN, Glüer C-C. A two-year program of aerobics and weight training enhances bone mineral desnity of young women. *Journal of Bone and Mineral Research* 1995; **10**: 574–85.

69. Nichols DL, Sanborn CF, Bonnick SL, Ben-Ezra V, Gench B, DiMarco NM. The effects of gymnastics training on bone mineral density. *Medicine and Science in Sports and Exercise* 1994; **26**: 1220–5.

70. Bassey EJ, Ramsdale SJ. Weight-bearing exercise and ground reaction forces, a 12-month randomized controlled trial of effects on bone mineral density in healthy postmenopausal women. *Bone* 1995; **16**: 469–76.

71. Vuori I, Heinonen A, Sievanen H, Kannus P, Pasanen M, Oja P. Effects of unilateral strength training and detraining on bone mineral density and content in young women, a study of mechanical loading and deloading on human bones *Calcified Tissue International* 1994; **55**: 59–67.

72. Kröger H, Kotaniemi A, Kröger L, Alhava E. Development of bone mass and bone density of the spine and femoral neck—a prospective study of 65 children and adolescents. *Bone and Mineral* 1993; **23**: 171–82.

73. Grimston SK, Engsberg JR, Kloiber RM, Hanley DA. Menstrual, calcium, and training history, relationship to bone health in female runners. *Clinics in Sports Medicine* 1990; **2**: 119–28.

74. Welten DC, Kemper HCG, Post GB, *et al.* Weight-bearing activity during youth is a more important factor for peak bone mass than calcium intake. *Journal of Bone and Mineral Research* 1994; **9**: 1089–96.

75. Cooper C, Cawley M, Bhalla A, *et al.* Childhood growth, physical activity and peak bone mass in women. *Journal of Bone and Mineral Research* 1995; **10**: 940–7.

76. Prior JC, Vigna YM, Schechter MT, Burgess AE. Spinal bone loss and ovulatory disturbance. *New England Journal of Medicine* 1990; **323**: 1221–7.

77. Wolman RL, Harries MG. Menstrual abnormalities in elite athletes. *Clinical Sports Medicine* 1989; **1**: 95–100.

78. Güler F, Hasçelik Z. Menstrual dysfunction and delayed menarche in top 7 athletes of team games. *Sports Medicine, Training and Rehabilitation* 1993; **4**: 99–106.

79. Feicht CB, Johnson TS, Martin BJ, Sparkes KE, Wagner WW. Secondary amenorrhoea in athletes. *Lancet* 1978; **II**: 1145 (letter).

80. Dale E, Gerlach DH, Wilwhite AL. Menstrual dysfunction in distance runners. *Obstetrics and Gynecology* 1979; **54**: 47–53.

81. Drinkwater BL, Nilson K, Ott S, Chesnut CH. Bone mineral density after resumption of menses in amenorrhoeic athletes. *Journal of the American Medical Association* 1986; **256**: 380–2.

82. Glass AR, Deuster PA, Kyle SB, Yahiro JA, Vigersky RA, Schoomaker EB. Amenorrhoea in Olympic athletes *Fertility and Sterility* 1987; **48**: 740–5.

83. Schwartz B, Cumming DC, Riordan E, Selye M, Yen SSC, Rebar RW. Exercise-associated amenorrhoea; A distinct entity? *American Journal of Obstetrics and Gynecology* 1981; **141**: 662–70.

84. Shangold MM, Levine HS. The effect of marathon training upon menstrual function. *American Journal of Obstetrics and Gynecology* 1982; **143**: 862–9.

85. Harber VJ, Webber CE, Sutton JR, MacDougall JD. The effect of amenorrhoea on calcaneal bone density and total bone turnover in runners. *International Journal of Sports Medicine* 1991; **12**: 505–8.

86. Casey MJ, Foster C, Thompson NN Jones EC Snyder AC. Menstrual function in elite speed skaters. *Sports training, Medicine and Rehabilitation* 1991; **2**: 69–76.

87. Baer JT, Taper LJ, Gwazdauskas FG, *et al*. Diet, hormonal and metabolic factors affecting bone mineral density in adolescent amenorrhoeic and eumenorrhoeic female runners. *Journal of Sports Medicine and Physical Fitness* 1992; **32**: 51–8.

88. Brownell KD, Rodin J, Wilmore JH. Eat, drink, and be worried? *Runner's World* 1988; **Aug 28**: 28–34.

89. Rosen LW, Hough DO. Pathogenic weight-control behaviours of female college gymnasts. *The Physician and Sportsmedicine* 1988; **16**: 141–4.

90. Kaiserauer S, Snyder AC, Sleeper M, Zierath J. Nutritional, physiological, and menstrual status of distance runners. *Medicine and Science in Sports and Exercise* 1989; **21**: 120–5.

91. Rucinski A. Relationship of body image and dietary intake of competitive ice-skaters. *Journal of the American Dietetic Association* 1989; **89**: 98–100.

92. Prussin RA, Harvey PD. Depression, dietary restraint and binge-eating in female runners *Addictive Behaviour* 1991; **16**: 295–301.

93. Snead DB, Weltman A, Weltman JY, *et al*. Reproductive hormones and bone mineral density in women runners. *Journal of Applied Physiology* 1992; **72**: 2149–56.

94. Wilmore JH, Wambsgans KC, Brenner M, *et al*. Is there energy conservation in amenorrhoeic compared with eumenorrhoeic runners? *Journal of Applied Physiology* 1992; **72**: 15–22.

95. Deuster PA, Kyle SB, Moser PB, Vigersky RA, Singh A, Schoomaker EB. Nutritional intakes and status of highly trained amenorrhoeic and eumenorrhoeic runners. *Fertility and Sterility* 1986; **46**: 636–43.

96. Myerson M, Gutin B, Warren MP, *et al*. Resting metabolic rate and energy balance in amenorrhoeic and eumenorrhoeic runners *Medicine and Science in Sports and Exercise* 1991; **23**: 15–22.

97. Watkin VA, Myburgh KH, Noakes TD. Low nutrient intake does not cause the menstrual cycle interval disturbance seen in some ultramarathon runners. *Clinical Journal of Sport Medicine* 1991; **1**: 154–61.

98. Hergenroeder AC, Fiorotto ML, Klish WJ. Body composition in ballet dancers measured by total body electrical conductivity. *Medicine and Science in Sports Exercise* 1991; **23**: 528–33.

99. Weight LM, Noakes TD. Is running an analog of anorexia? A survey of the incidence of eating disorders in female distance runners. *Medicine and Science in Sports and Exercise* 1987; **19**: 213–17.

100. Mulligan K, Butterfield GE. Discrepancies between energy intake and expenditure in physically active women. *British Journal of Nutrition* 1990; **64**: 23–6.

101. Drinkwater BL, Bruemner B, Chesnut CH. Menstrual history as a determinant of current bone density in young athletes. *Journal of the American Medical Association* 1990; **263**: 545–8.

102. Young N, Formica C, Szmukler G, Seeman E. Bone density at weight-bearing and nonweight-bearing sites in ballet dancers, the effects of exercise, hypogonadism, and body weight. *Journal of Clinical Endocrinology and Metabolism* 1994; **78**: 449–54.

103. Robinson TL, Snow-Harter C, Taaffe DR, Gillis D, Shaw J, Marcus R. Gymnasts exhibit higher bone mass than runners despite similar prevalence of amenorrhoea and oligomenorrhoea. *Journal of Bone and Mineral Research* 1995; **10**: 26–34.

104. Myerson M, Gutin B, Warren MP, Wang J, Lichtman S, Pierson RN. Total body bone density in amenorrhoeic runners *Obstetrics and Gynecology* 1992; **79**: 973–8.

105. Loucks AB, Mortola JF, Girton L, Yen SSC. Alterations in the hypothalamic-pituitary-ovarian and the hypothalamic-pituitary-adrenal axes in athletic women. *Journal of Clinical Endocrinology and Metabolism* 1989; **68**: 402–11.

106. Cumming DC, Viekovic MM, Wall SR, Fluker MR. Defects in pulsatile LH release in normally menstruating runners. *Journal of Clinical Endocrinology and Metabolism* 1985; **60**: 810–12.

107. Vedhuis JD, Evans WS, Demers LM, Thorner MA, Wakat D, Rogol A. Altered neuroendocrine regulation of gonadotrophin secretion in women distance runners. *Journal of Clinical Endocrinology and Metabolism* 1985; **61**: 557–63.

108. Warren MP, Shane E, Lee MJ, *et al*. Femoral head collapse associated with anorexia nervosa in a 20-year-old ballet dancer. *Clinical Orthopedics and Related Research* 1990; **251**: 171–6.

109. Lloyd T, Triantafyllou SJ, Baker ER, *et al*. Women athletes with menstrual irregularity have increased musculoskeletal injuries. *Medicine and Science in Sports and Exercise* 1986; **18**: 374–9.

110. Benson JE, Geiger CJ, Eisermann PA, Wardlaw GM. Relationship between nutrient intake, body mass index, menstrual function, and ballet injury. *Journal of the American Dietetic Association* 1989; **89**: 58–63.

111. Warren MP, Brooks-Gunn J, Hamilton LH, Warren LF, Hamilton WG. Scoliosis and fractures in young ballet dancers. *New England Journal of Medicine* 1986; **314**: 1348–53.

112. Barrow GW, Saha S. Menstrual irregularity and stress fractures in collegiate female distance runners. *American Journal of Sports Medicine* 1988; **16**: 209–14.

113. Lindberg JS, Fears WB, Hunt M, Powell MR, Boll D, Wade CE. Exercise-induced amenorrhoea and bone density. *Annals of Internal Medicine* 1984; **101**: 647–8.

114. Frusztajer NT, Dhuper S, Warren MP, Brooks-Gunn J, Fox RP. Nutrition and the incidence of stress fractures in ballet dancers. *American Journal of Clinical Nutrition* 1990; **51**: 779–83.

115. Grimston SK, Engsberg JR, Kloiber RM, Hanley DA. Menstrual, calcium, and training history, relationship to bone health in female runners. *Clinics in Sports Medicine* 1990; **2**: 119–28.

116. Leinberry CF, McShane RB, Stewart WG, Hume EL. A displaced subtrochanteric stress fracture in a young amenorrhoeic athlete. *American Journal of Sports Medicine* 1992; **20**: 484–7.

117. Pouilles JM, Bernard J, Tremollieres F, Louvet JP, Ribot C. Femoral bone density in young male adults with stress fractures. *Bone* 1989; **10**: 105–8.

118. Myburgh KH, Hutchins J, Fataar AB, Hough SF, Noakes TD Low bone density is an aetiological factor for stress fractures in athletes *Annals of Internal Medicine* 1990; **113**: 754–759

119. Carbon R, Sambrook PN, Deakin V, *et al*. Bone density of elite female athletes with stress fractures. *Medical Journal of Australia* 1990; **153**: 373–6.

120. Milgrom C, Giladi M, Simkin A, *et al*. The area moment inertia of the tibia, a risk factor for stress fractures. *Journal of Biomechanics* 1989; **22**: 1243–8.

121. Kimmel DB, Lappe JM, Laurin MJ, Hise L, White M, Stegman MR. Prediction of stress fracture risk during basic training in female soldiers by calcaneal ultrasound. *Journal of Bone and Mineral Research* 1996; **11** (Suppl. 1): S110 (Abstract).

122. Wilson JH, Wolman RL. Osteoporosis and fracture complications in an amenorrhoeic athlete. *British Journal of Rheumatology* 1994; **33**: 480–1.

123. Rigotti NA, Neer RM, Skates SJ, Herzog DB, Nussbaum SR. The clinical course of osteoporosis in anorexia nervosa. *Journal of the American Medical Association* 1991; **265**: 1133–8.

124. Bachrach LK, Katzman DK, Litt IF, Guido D, Marcus R. Recovery from osteopenia in adolescent girls with anorexia nervosa. *Journal of Clinical Endocrinology and Metabolism* 1991; **72**: 602–6.

125. Treasure JL, Russell JFM, Fogelman I, Murby B. Reversible bone loss in anorexia nervosa. *British Medical Journal* 1987; **295**: 474–5.

126. Fox KM, Magaziner J, Sherwin R, *et al*. Reproductive correlates of bone mass in elderly women. *Journal of Bone and Mineral Research* 1993; **8**: 901–8.

127. Georgiou E, Ntalles K, Papageorgiou A, Korkotsidis A, Proukakis

C. Bone mineral loss related to menstrual history. *Acta Orthopedica Scandinavia* 1989; **60**: 192–4.

128. Wilson JH, Harries MG, Reeve J. Bone mineral density in premenopausal veteran female athletes and the influence of menstrual irregularity (abstract). *Clinical Science* 1994; **86**(2): 2p.

129. De Cree C, Lewin R, Ostyn M. Suitability of cyproterone actetate in the treatment of osteoporosis associated with athletic amenorrhoea. *International Journal of Sports Medicine* 1988; **9**: 187–92.

130. Haenggi W, Casez J-P, Birkhaeuser MH, Lippuner K, Jaeger P. Bone mineral density in young women with long-standing amenorrhoea, limited effect of hormone replacement therapy with ethinyoestradiol and desorgestrel. *Osteoporosis International* 1994; **4**: 99–103.

131. Prior JC, Vigna YM, Barr SI, Rexworthy C, Lentle BC. Cyclic medroxyprogesterone treatment increases bone density, a controlled trial in active women with menstrual cycle disturbances. *American Journal of Medicine* 1994; **96**: 521–30.

132. Klibanski A, Biller BMK, Schoenfield DA, Herzog DB, Saxe VC. The effects of estrogen administration on trabecular bone loss in young women with anorexia nervosa. *Journal of Clinical Endocrinology and Metabolism* 1995; **80**: 898–904.

133. Biberoglu K, Yildiz A, Gursoy R, Kandemir O, Bayhan H. Bone mineral content in young women with primary amenorrhoea. In: Christiansen C, Overgaard K, eds. *Osteoporosis 1990: Proceedings of the 3rd International Symposium on Osteoporosis, Copenhagen, Denmark, 14–20 October 1990.* Copenhagen: Osteopress APS, 1990: 712–14.

134. Black DM, Cummings SR, Karpf DB, *et al.* The Fracture Intervention Trial Research Group Randomised trial of effect of alendronate on risk of fracture in women with existing vertebral fractures. *Lancet*; **348**: 1535–41.

135. Kanis JA, Pitt FA. Epidemiology of osteoporosis and osteoporotic fractures. *Bone* 1992; **13**: S7–S15.

136. Melton LJ, Kan SH, Frye MA, Wahner HW, O'Fallon WM, Riggs BL. Epidemiology of vertebral fractures in women. *American Journal of Epidemiology* 1989; **129**: 1000–11.

137. Phillips S, Fox N, Jacobs J, Wright WE. The direct medical costs of osteoporosis for American women aged 45 years or older. *Bone* 1988; **9**: 271–9.

138. O'Neill TW, Felsenberg D, Varlow J, Cooper C, Kanis JA, Silman AJ. The prevalence of vertebral deformity in European men and women: the European Vertebral Osteoporosis Study. *Journal of Bone and Mineral Research* 1996; **11**: 1010–17.

139. Cooper C, Barker DJP, Wickham C. Physical activity, muscle strength, and calcium intake in fracture of the proximal femur in Britain. *British Medical Journal* 1988; **297**: 1443–6.

140. Wickham C, Walsh K, Cooper C, *et al.* Dietary calcium, physical activity and risk of hip fracture, a prospective study. *British Medical Journal* 1989; **299**: 889–92.

141. Åström J, Ahnqvist S, Beertema J, Jónsson B. Physical activity in women sustaining fracture of the neck of the femur. *Journal of Bone and Joint Surgery* 1987; **69B**: 381–3.

142. Jacobson PC, Beaver W, Grubb SA, Taft TN, Talmage RV. Bone density in women, college athletes and older athletic women. *Journal of Orthopaedic Research* 1984; **2**: 328–32.

143. Talmage RV, Stinnett SS, Landwehr JT, Vinvent LM, McCartney WH. Age-related loss of bone mineral density in non-athletic and athletic women. *Bone and Mineral* 1986; **1**: 115–25.

144. Michel BA, Bloch DA, Fries JF. Weight-bearing exercise, over-exercise, and lumbar bone density over age 50 years. *Archives of Internal Medicine* 1989; **149**: 2325–9.

145. Michel BA, Lane NE, Bloch DA, Jones HH, Fries JF. Effect of changes in weight-bearing exercise on lumbar bone mass after age fifty. *Annals of Medicine* 1991; **23**: 397–401.

146. Nelson ME, Meredith CN, Dawson-Hughes B, Evans WJ. Hormone and bone mineral status in endurance-trained and sedentary postmenopausal women. *Journal of Clinical Endocrinology and Metabolism* 1988; **66**: 927–33.

147. Wilson JH, Reeve J, Harries M. The influence of exercise on postmenopausal bone loss *Bone and Mineral* 1994; **25**(Suppl. 2): S28.

148. Blumenthal JA, Emery CF, Madden DJ, *et al.* Effects of exercise training on bone density in older men and women. *Journal of the American Geriatric Society* 1991; **39**: 1065–70.

149. Smidt GL, Lin S-Y, ODwyer KD, Blanpied PR. The effect of high-intensity trunk exercise on bone mineral density of postmenopausal women. *Spine* 1992; **17**: 280–5.

150. Dalsky GP, Stocke KS, Ehsani AA, Slatopolsky E, Lee WC, Birge SJ. Weight-bearing exercise training and lumbar bone mineral content in postmenopausal women. *Annals of Internal Medicine* 1988; **108**: 824–8.

151. Chow R, Harrison JE, Notarius C. Effect of two randomised exercise programmes on bone mass of healthy postmenopausal women. *British Medical Journal* 1987; **295**: 1441–4.

152. Rundgren A, Aniansson A, Ljungberg P, Wetterquist H. Effects of a training programme on mineral content of the heel bone. *Archives of Gerontology and Geriatrics* 1984; **3**: 243–8.

153. Smith EL, Gilligan C, McAdam M, Ensign CP, Smith PE. Deterring bone loss by exercise intervention in premenopausal and postmenopausal women. *Calcified Tissue International* 1989; **44**: 312–21.

154. Rikli RE, McManis BG. Effects of exercise on bone mineral content in postmenopausal women. *Research Quarterly in Exercise and Sport* 1990; **61**: 243–9.

155. Grove KA, Londeree BR. Bone density in postmenopausal women, high impact vs low impact exercise. *Medicine and Science in Sports and Exercise* 1992; **24**: 1190–4.

156. Revel M, Mayoux-Benhamou MA, Rabourdin JP, Bagheri F, Roux C. One year psoas training can prevent lumbar bone loss in postmenopausal women, a randomized controlled trial. *Calcified Tissue International* 1993; **53**: 307–11.

157. Martin D, Notelovitz M. Effects of aerobic training on bone mineral density of postmenopausal women. *Journal of Bone and Mineral Research* 1993; **8**: 931–6.

158. Province MA, Hadley EC, Hornbrook MC, *et al.* The effects of exercise on falls in elderly patients. A preplanned meta-analysis of the FICSIT trials Frailty and Injuries: Cooperative Studies of Intervention Techniques. *Journal of the American Medical Association* 1995; **273**: 1341–7.

159. Chan GM. Dietary calcium and bone mineral status of children and adolescents. *American Journal of Diseases of Childhood* 1991; **145**: 631–4.

160. Sentipal JM, Wardlaw M, Mahan J, Matkovic V. Influence of calcium intake and growth indexes on vertebral bone mineral density in young females. *American Journal of Clinical Nutrition* 1991; **54**: 425–8.

161. Kanders B, Dempster DW, Lindsay R. Interaction of calcium nutrition and physical activity on bone mass in young women. *Journal of Bone and Mineral Research* 1988; **3**: 145–9.

162. Halioua L, Anderson JJB. Lifetime calcium intake and physical activity habits, independent and combined effects on the radial bone of healthy premenopausal Caucasian women. *American Journal of Clinical Nutrition* 1989; **49**: 534–41.

163. Wolman RL, Clark P, McNally E, Harries M, Reeve J. Dietary calcium as a statistical determinant of spinal trabecular bone density in amenorrhoeic and oestrogen-replete athletes. *Bone and Mineral* 1992; **17**: 415–23.

164. Krall EA, Parry P, Lichter JB, Dawson-Hughes B. Vitamin D receptor alleles and rates of bone loss: influences of years since menopause and calcium intake. *Journal of Bone and Mineral Research* 1995; **10**: 978–84.

165. Ferrari S, Rizzoli R, Chevalley T, Slosman D, Eisman JA, Bonjour J-P. Vitamin D receptor gene polymorphisms and change in lumbar spine bone mineral density. *Lancet* 1995; **345**: 423–4.

166. Benson JE, Allemann Y, Theintz GE, Howald H. Eating problems and calorie intake levels in Swiss adolescent athletes. *International Journal of Sports Medicine* 1990; **11**: 249–52.

167. Pate RR, Sargent RG, Baldwin C, Burgess ML. Dietary intake of women runners. *International Journal of Sports Medicine* 1990; **11**: 461–6.

168. Bergen-Cico DK, Short SH. Dietary intakes, energy expenditures, and anthropometric characteristics of adolescent female cross-country runners. *Journal of the American Dietetic Association* 1992; **92**: 611–12.

169. Delistraty DA, Reisman EJ, Snipes MA. Physiological and nutritional profile of young female figure skaters. *Journal of Sports Medicine and Physical Fitness* 1992; **32**: 149–55.

170. Frederick L, Hawkins ST. A comparison of nutrition knowledge and attitudes, dietary practices, and bone densities of postmenopausal women, female college athletes, and non-athletic women. *Journal of the American Dietetic Association* 1992; **92**: 299–305.

171. Stensland SH, Sobal J. Dietary practices of ballet, jazz, and modern dancers. *Journal of the American Dietetic Association* 1992; **92**: 319–24.

172. Nordin BEC, Heaney RP. Calcium supplementation of the diet, justified by present evidence. *British Medical Journal* 1990; **300**: 1056–60.

173. Bernard J, Telmont N, Benazet JF, *et al.* Sports activity and body composition. Study by whole body osteodensitometry of 169 men between 17 and 21 years of age. *Revue Rhumatique Mal Osteoartic* 1991; **58**: 467–70.

174. Karlsson MK, Johnell O, Obrant KJ. Bone mineral density in weight-lifters. *Calcified Tissue International* 1993; **52**: 212–15.

175. Hamdy RC, Anderson JS, Whalen KE, Harvill LM. Regional differences in bone density of young men involved in different exercises. *Medicine and Science in Sports and Exercise* 1994; **26**: 884–8.

176. Rico H, Revilla M, Hernandez ER, Gomez-Castresana F, Villa LF. Bone mineral content and body compostition in postpubertal cyclist boys. *Bone* 1993; **14**: 93–5.

177. Smith R, Rutherford OL. Spine and total body bone mineral density and serum testosterone levels in male athletes. *European Journal of Applied Physiology* 1993; **76**: 330–4.

178. Orwoll ES, Ferar J, Oviatt SK, McClung MR, Huntington K. The relationship of swimming exercise to bone mass in men and women. *Archives of Internal Medicine* 1989; **149**: 2197–200.

179. Cheng S, Suominen H, Heikkinen E. Bone mineral density in relation to anthropometric properties, physical activity and smoking in 75 year old men and women. *Aging* 1993; **5**: 55–62.

180. Blumenthal JA, Emery CF, Madden DJ, *et al.* Effects of exercise training on bone density in older men and women. *Journal of the American Geriatric Society* 1991; **39**: 1065–70.

181. Menkes A, Mazel S, Redmond RA, *et al.* Strength training increases regional bone density and bone remodelling in middle-aged and older men. *Journal of Applied Physiology* 1993; **74**: 2478–84.

4

Acute sports injuries

William D. Stanish

Sports medicine has undergone an enormous rate of growth and expansion over the past decade. This medical discipline has evolved from a background which focused principally on the first aid management of the acute athletic injury. Limited initially in its scope, sports medicine as applied to the acute knee injury, for example, has broadened its scientific base. Current sports medicine literature alerts the practitioner to expanding knowledge in such areas as the pathomechanics of injury, the biology of tissue repair, and contemporary techniques and treatments. Recent studies, prompting outcome analyses of particular injuries (and their therapy), have emphasized the importance of understanding the benefits (and hazards)—both objective and subjective—of specific treatments.

Fundamental principles in the diagnosis and treatment of acute sports injuries

When evaluating the patient with an acute sports injury, basic principles of medicine must be followed. A superficial or cursory physical examination after a careless medical history will invariably invite disaster and a potentially unsatisfactory result.

Principle I

Conduct a complete history and physical examination

Although acknowledged as the very cornerstone to medicine, there is no substitute for completing a medical history and a physical examination of an injured athlete. A hastily conducted physical examination of an acute knee sprain may interpret a collateral ligament disruption as an acute injury, when in fact a chronic laxity pre-existed. Overlooking pre-existing pathology within the wrist, such as an disunited fracture of the scaphoid, leads to confusion and misinformation.

Principle II

Understand the diagnosis

Having made an accurate diagnosis of a particular pathology, it follows that the sports medicine practitioner must understand that pathology. Whereas an acute subluxation of the acromioclavicular joint generally has a benign natural history, an acute anterior dislocation of the shoulder presents an entirely different scenario. A forceful manual relocation of the shoulder to expedite early return to sport, may jeopardize the future health of the athlete.

Principle III

Accurate understanding of the options for treatment

Any intervention, be it a physical modality such as ultrasound or a more invasive surgical procedure, must be weighed against the potential risks, hazards, and complications. A sports medicine surgeon may recommend a reconstructive procedure for a torn anterior cruciate ligament, when in fact that athlete may have been coping (in the face of a torn anterior cruciate ligament) with muscle retraining and functional bracing. Further, some cases of chronic tendinosis are better served with surgical debridement and revascularization than with an ill-designed exercise programme. The natural history of the particular injury must be understood in order to guarantee that the treatment programme will 'do no harm' and could potentially rectify the disorder.

Principle IV

Adequate and accurate follow-up

Science is full of bias and sports medicine is no exception. Critical and thoughtful analysis of a particular injury (and/or treatment) is fundamental to advancing the science. For example, to employ non-steroidal anti-inflammatory medications for an athlete with an acute low back sprain, or to perform a repair of an acute meniscal tear, requires the same meticulous follow-up. Rigorous attention must be directed to follow-up in order to achieve a subjective and objective outcome analysis. Only when this is accomplished can a meaningful comparison of treatment formats be achieved.

The acute knee injury

It was impossible to predict the current explosion of knowledge pertaining to the injured knee. Historically managed with rest and medications, the acute knee sprain is now rehabilitated very aggressively with early motion, functional bracing, and early return to sport. Tears of the meniscus, particularly of an acute nature, can frequently be repaired surgically with impressive results. The long-term dividends when the meniscus is preserved, are obvious. Meniscus transplantation is being explored and may offer a viable alternative for the knee joint in which complete meniscectomy had been necessary.

Acute osteochondral injuries of the knee joint can frequently be repaired with direct respositioning of the detached fragments. Recently, transplantation of chondrocytes has received special attention, as has osteochondral autografting. Both of these techniques offer certain promise but long-term follow-up studies are not yet available.

Injuries to both the posterior cruciate ligament and the posterolateral corner of the knee remain a major problem for those practitioners dealing with complex knee instabilities. An isolated tear of the posterior cruciate ligament can usually be treated without surgery, with emphasis on a programme that resorts to early motion, muscle strengthening, and neuromotor rehabilitation. When injured in conjunction with the lateral collateral ligament or complete posterolateral corner, immediate surgical repair and reconstruction becomes mandatory and is clearly the treatment of choice, but the ability of the athlete to return to full and uncompromised sport after such an injury is unlikely.

Acute knee injuries in the growing athlete offer different challenges. Once regarded as a joint where the epiphyseal plate was the weakest link, current studies have suggested that the anterior cruciate ligament in the growing athlete can be injured with or without a bony avulsion. In many adolescents the anterior cruciate ligament is exactly as seen in the adult. However, unique to the growing athlete is the acute avulsion of the tibal tubercle, with or without extension into the articular surface. Anatomical restoration of the joint is vital to optimize joint function. Acute epiphyseal injuries do occur in the childhood athlete. When displaced, particularly in Salter Harris III, IV, and V types, open reduction, with restoration of the anatomy and stabilization of the fracture, is imperative.

The widespread use of magnetic resonance imaging (MRI) has opened new windows and has presented new challenges in the management of acute knee injury. MRI has revealed bone bruising which has afforded several new problems in our understanding of the natural history of the acute joint injury. When the knee joint is insulted sufficiently to produce a bruise of the osteochondral fabric of the joint, the repair mechanism within the knee must be mobilized to some degree. However, as with a fracture of the tibial plateau, when the bone bruise is large, is on the weight bearing surface, and/or is detached, prognosis is uncertain.

MRI also assists in the follow-up of such procedures as surgical repair of the meniscus and autografting/allografting to the articular surface. The healing patterns within ligament injuries (and their surgical reconstruction) can now be tracked more effectively over time. In many cases MRI obviates the need for second-look arthroscopy which still remains the gold standard in analysing the outcome of knee pathology.

The foot and ankle

Acute injuries to the foot and ankle usually involve the soft tissues, more specifically ligaments and tendons about the foot and ankle. Most tendon and ligament injuries about the foot and ankle heal spontaneously without worrisome residuum. After the inflammation subsides, the process of neuromuscular retraining, strengthening and functional adaption commences.

The acute ankle sprain is extremely common in sports. Historically, the patient with an acute ankle sprain was forcibly immobilized, placed on a non-weight bearing programme, and treated with drugs.

Nowadays, the patient is examined much more carefully and often imaging is used (in some cases CT scans or MRI). Physical examination must include examination and stressing of all the major ligaments, as well as the inferior tibia-fibula syndesmosis, and evaluation of the joint surfaces (including the subtalar joint and talar gutters) is essential to rule out a concomitant osteochondral insult.

Stress radiography can be of significant benefit in understanding the degree of ligament injury, as well as revealing subtle pathologies, such as disruptions of the deltoid ligament and/or complete diastasis of the distal syndesmosis between the tibia and fibula. Current data suggest that ankle joint instability, or persistent subluxation, should be addressed surgically to restore congruency of the joint and reduce the gap between the torn ligaments. Such operations do maximize joint integrity and stability after these injuries and afford a more ideal healing environment. There are several fractures about the foot and ankle in athletes that provide unique challenges for treatment. Jones' fracture, through the diaphysis of the fifth metatarsal, usually heals very slowly. Some sports medicine surgeons dealing with élite athletes tend to operate on these fractures on the premise that non-unions are very common. Conventional wisdom, however, suggests surgery (open or percutaneous fixation) should be reserved for a displaced Jones' fracture, an established disunited fracture or a fracture demonstrating delayed union. Surgery does not speed the healing of fractures biologically but will stabilize the broken fragments and thus optimize rehabilitation.

Basketball players tend to get fractures of the navicular. This is a very severe injury to the foot of an athlete, as the tarsal navicular has a precarious blood supply and tends to displace, disturbing the talar navicular joint. It can be a career-ending trauma, if not dealt with quickly and appropriately. Surgery to reduce and stabilize the fragments is often necessary.

Shoulder

Acute injuries to the shoulder are very common in athletics, but current techniques of analysis and treatment have reduced morbidity considerably. More accurate assessment of the injury is now being achieved and a more precise management programme can thus be designed. For instance, an athlete who suffered an anterior dislocation of the shoulder for the first time would historically be treated with a forceful reduction of the dislocation without adequate radiography (or imaging). Current techniques, which include MRI and CT scanning, offer more effective evaluation of the labrum/biceps complex, the rotator cuff, and the bony tissues (including the greater and lesser tuberosities, allowing improved insight into outcomes; for example, a concomitant rotator cuff tear, with an acute anterior dislocation, changes the prognosis for an older athlete entirely.

Furthermore, an athlete who suffered an anterior dislocation of the shoulder was invariably forcibly immobilized on the premise that the outlook was improved (with splinting) and allowed healing of the Bankart lesion. Recent studies have suggested that prolonged splinting does not improve the prognosis and there is a shift towards early and more aggressive treatment which entails surgical stabilization of the injured soft tissues, followed by more rapid rehabilitation. The same approach is used for injuries of the anterior cruciate ligament and displaced fractures. Those younger individuals suffering an anterior dislocation of the shoulder, resulting in a displaced lift-off of the cartilaginous labrum, may be treated with surgery. This more aggressive approach is still open to debate.

Fractures of the greater or lesser tuberosities, or the glenoid face, require special attention. If displacement is greater than 5 mm, surgical intervention is recommended. CT scanning and MRI provide further insights for the practitioner and usually facilitate decision making.

Injuries to the acromioclavicular joint occur frequently in sports, and can be managed with early motion and pain control. When a complete dislocation of the acromioclavicular joint does occur—Grade IV or Grade V—surgical fixation, with reduction, is necessary. If treated non-operatively, shoulder weakness becomes a common complaint. Clinical examination, combined with stress radiographs, will assist in the evaluation and subsequently the management. Evaluation of the patient after a week following the injury allows a more accurate assessment of the degree of dislocation, as involuntary guarding will have subsided. Grade I, II, and III injuries to the acromioclavicular joint are readily treated with immediate rehabilitation, recognizing that discomfort will usually take 4 to 6 weeks to subside.

Wrist and hand

Acute injuries to the wrist and hand have frequently been underestimated in athletes. A fracture of the scaphoid in the dominant arm can often end the competitive season for a throwing athlete. Prolonged immobilization, for about 20 weeks, has been the traditional treatment for an undisplaced fracture through the waist of the scaphoid. Operative intervention has improved technically to the point that immediate stabilization of a scaphoid fracture can be employed by the sports medicine team but it must be reiterated that open reduction and internal fixation does not enhance the biological prorression towards successful healing; however, reduction and fixation of the fracture does optimize the healing environment and facilitates the rehabilitation process. This is not to suggest that all fractures of the scaphoid should be treated surgically; careful assessment of the personality of the fracture (site and degree of displacement), combined with understanding the needs of the athlete, must be used in the management of this injury.

Summary

Sports medicine has taken conventional medical concepts of the assessment of management of many acute injuries and has advanced the science. Current approaches in the management of shoulder dislocations, acromioclavicular disruptions, and rotator cuff pathology, are byproducts of our experiences with injured athletes. Sports medicine literature has delineated the improved evaluation and treatment of joint injuries with arthroscopy (and arthroscopic surgery). With rare exceptions, acute sports injuries are now better managed with complete and accurate examination, and expeditious restoration of anatomy with early rehabilitation. Outcome analyses invariably demonstrate the value of this approach.

4.2.1 Acute knee injuries: an overview

Robert J. Johnson

The most common injury that ends the careers of athletes probably involves destruction of one or more of the major ligaments of the knee. Injuries to the knee result in more problems for athletic individuals than injuries to any other joint.[1] Therefore the subject of the acute knee injury is all too frequently the focus of attention of the sports medicine community. Fortunately, the majority of acute knee injuries are relatively minor in nature or can be resolved with simple non-surgical therapy and thus result in relatively short periods of disability or reduced activity. Even relatively minor injuries, however, can become a chronic problem. While they may not interfere with the activities of daily living, they can be very frustrating for those athletes who require stressful performance of their knees. Thus, full understanding of the mechanism of injury, the biomechanics of the normal knee, the pathophysiology of the injury and repair process as it applies to the knee, diagnostic procedures, surgical and non-surgical treatment regimens, and rehabilitation principles and methods is vitally important to those who care for the injured athlete's knee. It is the purpose of the authors of this section of the text to discuss the material necessary not only to diagnose and treat the major knee ligament injuries appropriately, but also those lesser injuries which, as far as the athlete is concerned, may be career threatening or only a nuisance for a relatively short period of time.

Acute injuries of the menisci

It has been stated that the most common injuries sustained by athletes involve damage to the menisci.[1,2] Meniscectomy is the most frequently performed orthopaedic operative procedure, accounting for 10 to 20 per cent of all surgery.[1] Before the turn of the century the meniscus was considered to be a functionless remnant of muscle origin.[3] Many surgeons in the early to mid-portion of the present century suggested that the menisci were functionless and when damaged they should be totally removed.[1, 4-9] In fact, Smillie advised that even if damage to the meniscal structure was only suspected, it should be totally removed.[8] It was believed that unless the meniscus was totally excised, a fibrocartilaginous replacement would not form or that the retained portion of a partially resected meniscus would result in degenerative arthritis. In 1948, Fairbank wrote his classic paper on the meniscus in which he implied that the

structure did, in fact, serve a function by sharing in the transmission of load across the joint.[10] It was not until the 1960s and 1970s that several papers were published which clearly showed that removal of the meniscus was not necessarily a benign procedure.[11-16] Innumerable recent studies have confirmed that the meniscus does serve a valuable biomechanical function for the knee.[17-25] Thus, the concept of partial meniscectomy (removal of only the damaged portion of the structure), made possible by the development of practical arthroscopic techniques, became well substantiated as superior to resection of the entire structure.[26-28] Arthroscopic procedures also have allowed the next logical step in the treatment of damaged menisci, that is, the repair of certain lesions rather than their resection (Figs 1,2).[29-35] There can be little doubt that preservation of all components of the torn meniscus is superior to removal, if the healed structure retains the ability to function biomechanically. In the recent past, several investigations have sought to improve the surgeon's ability to retain fragments of torn menisci effectively.[36,37] However, preservation of crushed and deformed fragments of non-functioning menisci certainly does not serve a useful purpose. At the present time there is little evidence that the healed meniscus still serves its original biomechanical purpose, although it appears logical to assume that they do retain this function.[22, 33,37-39] Efforts are being addressed now to devise techniques to replace menisci that require excision.[40-48] Allografting procedures are being performed, and some attempts to implant scaffold devices that encourage the ingrowth of the patient's own cells to produce a viable replacement

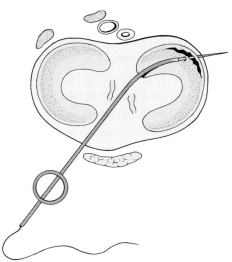

Fig. 1 Meniscal repair. A curved cannula is inserted through the contralateral portal and used for suturing to avoid popliteal vessels and nerve. (Redrawn from ref. 143, with permission.)

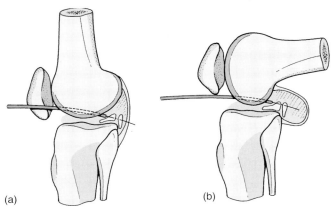

Fig. 2 Meniscal repair. The needle traverses a tear of the medial meniscus in extension (a) to avoid compromise of the meniscus (b). (Redrawn from ref. 143, with permission.)

meniscus are being studied and advocated.[49] However, little evidence exists to suggest that these procedures can successfully restore the function of the meniscus and prevent degenerative changes from occurring. Only time will tell if these measures can result in the restoration of biomechanical functions.

Ligament injuries

Acute injuries of the knee ligament have long been recognized as a major problem for the athlete, but probably no subject in sports medicine has resulted in more controversy and confusion. Like other topics discussed in this section of the text, there has been a very dramatic change in the way that these injuries have been treated over the years. Almost everyone, including athletes and sports fans, realizes that a major injury to the knee ligaments could be the death knell to an athletic career. Hopefully, recent advances in the recognition and treatment of a portion, if not the majority, of these severe injuries can lead to the continuation of athletic careers.

Ligament injuries about the knee were recognized before the turn of the century. Most physicians believed that major ligament injuries should be treated non-operatively, often with prolonged periods of immobilization in casts or splints. Campbell in the first edition of his text (1939) stated that 'operative measures for acute rupture of the lateral ligaments of the knee are seldom, if ever required, as the most extensive ruptures usually undergo repair if properly treated by conservative measures. Repair is indicated in the presence of symptoms of derangement from complete or partial rupture or elongation of long duration'.[4] In 1935 Milch observed that, in his opinion, 'the anterior crucial ligament is not an essential structure as its loss is compatible with relatively normal function of the joint'.[50] Thus the majority of early operative procedures described in the literature discussed reconstruction of ligament injuries that either had been overlooked at the time of injury or deliberately treated by non-operative means. Those individuals perhaps most responsible for the development of opinion tending to treat acute ligament disruptions with surgical repair were Palmer (1938) in Europe and O'Donoghue (1950) in North America.[51,52] After these surgeons and many other investigators demonstrated that labourers and athletes probably were served better by early surgical intervention, the standard treatment for most complete knee

ligament ruptures, especially if more than one was destroyed, was early operative intervention. Various criteria were developed to determine who was a candidate for surgery and who should be non-surgically treated, and certainly no unanimity was established as to which ligament should be repaired and which could be ignored.

Until recently, the majority of knee surgeons believed that only the collateral ligaments and the posterior cruciate ligament were of significant structural and biomechanical importance. With regard to this problem many of the great educators taught that the anterior cruciate ligament was unimportant.[50,53] This coupled with the fact that the vast majority of physicians, including orthopaedic surgeons, could not recognize accurately the presence of a complete tear of the anterior cruciate ligament, led to the feeling that this structure could be ignored or simply cut away if it was found to be torn. Over the past 15 to 20 years no subject of sports orthopaedics has received as much attention as the injured anterior cruciate ligament. Keller reported in February 1996 that 1300 articles concerning the anterior cruciate ligament were published in the world literature between 1990 and 1995.[54] For the last 15 years approximately one-third of the papers submitted for presentation at the conferences of the American Orthopedic Society for Sports Medicine have dealt with subjects relating to the anterior cruciate ligament (D. Brown, personal communication). Clearly, during the same period of time it has become almost universally accepted that the anterior cruciate ligament does contribute to the functional stability of the knee, and that its disruption often leads to devastating problems for the injured athlete. However, there can be no doubt that many patients do function quite satisfactorily without their anterior cruciate ligament .

The natural history of the knee deficient in the anterior cruciate ligament, although intensively studied, is still unknown.[55,56] No one can predict with certainty whether a patient who has sustained an acute disruption of this ligament will function almost normally or develop significant symptoms if the ligament is not successfully surgically repaired or reconstructed. One group of authors has suggested that the majority of patients can recover with non-operative treatment and return successfully to sport and occupational activity with little or no restriction.[57-61] Others have implied that return to vigorous sport and stressful work leads to a high incidence of reinjury events (so-called pivot shift episodes) that require the patients to alter their lifestyles substantially in order to avoid significant degeneration of their knee joints.[62-65] Obviously, various authors have assigned differing degrees of significance to the reinjury events and the pain, swelling, and disability that they cause. Some investigators believe that restriction of activity which requires an athlete to alter his or her level of competition or switch to a less vigorous sport is unimportant, while others feel that such change is of great concern. Some have stated that episodes of reinjury are not likely to lead to further degenerative changes within the knee, while others express concern about the almost inevitable destruction of menisci and, eventually, the articular cartilage if pivot shift events continue to occur. It has been suggested that even unrecognizable dysfunction associated with knees without anterior cruciate ligaments may lead to joint degeneration.[66,67] Depending on the interpretation of these factors and others, various physicians have formed widely divergent opinions as to what constitutes an indication for surgical intervention in the case of the patient with a torn anterior cruciate ligament.

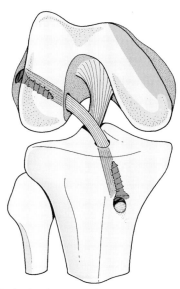

Fig. 3 Bone–patellar tendon–bone procedure for anterior cruciate ligament insufficiency. (Redrawn from ref. 144, with permission.)

Another matter that adds to the confusion in deciding whether or not to operate is that outcome studies reveal a significant number of the surgical interventions performed for injuries of the anterior cruciate ligament do not succeed, and even if they do appear to restore subjectively satisfactory function, they are not capable of preventing degenerative changes later.[63,68,69] Even if patients eventually return to sport following repairs or reconstructions, no one can be certain that they will continue to do well indefinitely. Many methods of treatment are ardently praised by enthusiastic investigators who find that early postoperative results appear to be excellent, only to find later at follow-up that the results have deteriorated. The literature is replete with short-term follow-up studies, but very few long-term results have been published.[63] Results followed for 10 years or more are probably necessary before the orthopaedic community will have a truly accurate assessment of the natural history of repairs or reconstructions of the anterior cruciate ligament.[70] Many procedures including innovative use of prosthetics, allografts, and augmentations have not yet stood the 'test of time'.

The determination of the treatment of choice in the case of the destroyed anterior cruciate ligament is still evolving. At the time of writing, the 'gold standard' for treatment of these individuals with a high-risk lifestyle following injury to the anterior cruciate ligament is probably the complete replacement of the ligament with a bone–patellar tendon–bone autograft (Fig. 3).[71,72] Some believe that the incidence of postoperative parapatellar pain is unacceptably high following this procedure and have advocated alternative procedures.[73] At the present time, the repair of a ruptured anterior cruciate ligament without augmentation has been demonstrated to be an inferior treatment approach.[74–79] Although many papers report satisfactory results following repair with autograft augmentation, this approach seems to be becoming less popular.[74,75,78,80–82] It appears that the use of extra-articular reconstructions in replacing the function of the anterior cruciate ligament has also fallen out of favour.[83] Some investigators still advocate its use in the treatment of young patients with open epiphyses, as an adjunct to intra-articular recon-

struction, and for older sedentary patients with chronic dysfunction of the anterior cruciate ligament. In theory, an allograft reduces the morbidity of the replacement of the ligament, but concerns revolving around the transmission of viral disease and healing problems have not been totally overcome.[84,85] Pure prosthetic replacement devices are unproven as viable alternatives and have been associated with a high risk of failure. Much more research is necessary before the place of allografts and prosthetic ligament augmentation devices in the treatment of knee ligament injuries can be fully established.

There can be little doubt that the occurrence of a truly 'isolated' tear of any ligament is essentially an impossibility, but certainly most surgeons have observed a number of cases where the clinical and even operative evidence indicates that only one structure has sustained severe damage. Perhaps the most dramatic change in approach to the treatment of such injuries is that rendered to those who sustain tears of the medial collateral ligament. Complete tears of this ligament are suspected when valgus stress applied to the fully extended knee reveals a mild increase in laxity and a soft end-point and a dramatic increase in laxity on application of valgus stress at 20 to 30 degrees of flexion. In the 1960s and 1970s most surgeons probably would have treated such injuries with surgical repair in the acute setting. Now many investigators are advocating non-operative treatment and quite rapid rehabilitation.[86,87] Until quite recently, 'isolated' second degree tears of the medial collateral ligament were treated with prolonged casting, but now it has been well documented that these injuries can be treated very satisfactorily with aggressive conservative rehabilitation and return to vigorous activity in 4 to 6 weeks.[86,87]

The posterior cruciate ligament can be disrupted in essentially an 'isolated' fashion. The functional results of such injuries treated without repair or reconstruction appear to be much more satisfactory than those of isolated injury to the anterior cruciate ligament.[88,89] This finding, together with the nearly universal observation that reconstructions and repairs of the posterior cruciate ligament are often unsuccessful, has led to a much more conservative approach in the management of these lesions than for those of the anterior cruciate ligament.[90] Although there are a few advocates of acute repair or reconstruction of 'isolated' injuries of the posterior cruciate ligament, the majority of opinion probably now favours treating them non-surgically.[91,92] Keller *et al.* have recently demonstrated that significant degenerative and functional changes can result even when 'isolated posterior cruciate ligament injuries are treated without surgery'.[93] Thus, as surgical skills and results of reconstructions of the posterior cruciate ligament improve, it is likely that we will see a trend toward an expansion of the indications for surgery to replace this ligament. It appears that the management of injuries to this ligament when coupled with the destruction of other major stabilizers or the posterior lateral components of the knee requires an aggressive surgical approach to avoid disability.[89]

When injured in a relatively isolated fashion, the lateral collateral ligament can be managed conservatively, but care must be taken to avoid overlooking significant damage to the arcuate ligament and the popliteus tendon, for if they are also damaged, non-surgical management may be very disappointing.[94]

The lack of well controlled, randomized, prospective, long-term outcome studies comparing one surgical technique with another has

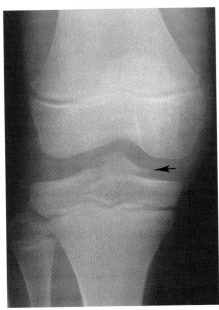

Fig. 4 Avulsion of the tibial spine.

made it almost impossible for anyone seriously using the literature to determine which approach, if any, is superior.[62] Notable exceptions to this statement are articles published by Andersson et al.,[74] Engebretsen et al.,[75] and most recently by Grøntvedt et al.[78] The readers are urged to review the studies in order to understand better the appropriate way to design and perform excellent outcome research. Only when more of such studies become available will information exist that allows us to establish the method of choice for treatment of these knee ligament injuries. Also, the lack of standardization of follow-up methodology has resulted in an inability to compare the relative merits of one treatment regimen with another. Thus, those individuals who treat knee ligament injuries remain frustrated when they assess their own approach to their patients' problems. The surprising lack of knowledge of the detailed biomechanics of the knee has also led to much confusion concerning the treatment methods. Proliferation of information concerning the complexities of knee function will undoubtedly assist in advancing our approaches concerning the proper treatment of knee ligament injuries, but this demands that all those concerned with these matters must critically keep abreast of the explosion of information now occurring and apply these changes to their own practices.

Fractures and dislocations

Fortunately for the athlete, the incidence of fractures about the knee is relatively low in sports activities.[95] However, those mechanisms of injury that result in ligament disruptions in young adults may produce fractures of the epiphyseal plate of the distal femur or proximal tibia in children with open epiphyses or in tibia plateau fractures in older age groups. Ligament injuries may result in avulsions of relatively small fragments of bone from their attachment sites in patients of all age groups. Growing children often tear away the inferior attachment of their anterior cruciate ligaments with a fragment of bone, which on occasions is quite large (Fig. 4). Such fractures are quite rare in adults. Children also more frequently tear

away small fragments of bone with sprains of the medial collateral ligament, most frequently from the proximal end. Tibial tubercle avulsion occurs almost exclusively in children. Avulsions of the fibular head are not uncommon in severe lateral knee injuries in adults. The Segond fracture or lateral capsular avulsion, arising from the inferior attachment of the mid-lateral capsule on to the tibia just anterior to the fibular head, is a relatively common occurrence and is almost always associated with the complete disruption of the anterior cruciate ligament (Fig. 5).[96]

The 'lateral notch sign' described by Warren et al.,[97] probably represents an injury of the lateral femoral condyle (an exaggeration of the normally present linea terminalis) which is occasionally observed in patients with chronic anterior cruciate insufficiency.

Fractures of the patella are more frequently the result of falls and vehicular accidents than sports activities, but the patella is the bone most commonly fractured in sports injuries involving the knee.[95] Osteochondral fractures of the distal femur occasionally occur in association with dislocations of the patella. More severe intra-articular fractures of the femur are very rare. Stress fractures involving the patella do occasionally occur, but stress fractures of the femur and tibia involving the joint surfaces are uncommon. Stress fractures in distance runners are not infrequent, and most often involve the anteromedial tibia, 2.5 to 5.0 cm below the joint, when they occur within the vicinity of the knee.

Several investigators have observed occult fractures of the tibia and femur during investigations of ligamentous injuries of the knee using magnetic resonance imaging (MRI) techniques.[98–103] This is especially true of the lateral femoral condyle and the posterior lateral tibia plateau in patients sustaining ruptures of the anterior cruciate ligament. At the present time the clinical significance of these radiographically indeterminable injuries remains to be defined. Osteochondritis dessicans and osteonecrosis are beyond the scope of this section of the text, and are discussed elsewhere.

The treatment of fractures involving any joint surface demands accurate reduction and maintenance of near perfect position while healing occurs. Thus open reduction and internal fixation of fractures of the patella, distal femur, and tibia plateaus are frequently required. Bone grafts are very often necessary in the management of tibia plateau fractures. The principles of strong fixation and early protected motion, often with prolonged avoidance of weight bearing (tibia plateau fractures), are advocated. The treatment of epiphyseal

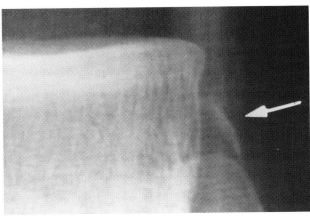

Fig. 5 Segond's fracture (arrow).

injuries also demands special care to avoid damaging the already vulnerable epiphyseal plate. The treating physician must be aware of the potential for total or partial growth arrest and prepare the parents as well as the patient for these eventual complications should they occur.

Avulsion fractures produced by ligament disruptions can often be ignored if they are small, thus requiring no alteration in the treatment that is necessary for the ligament itself. Avulsions of the anterior cruciate ligament, which free large fragments from the tibia plateau, have advocates of open reattachment, but the older literature suggested that minimal to moderately displaced fragments could be treated closed by simple extension of the knee.[104] Present knowledge suggests that this approach is probably incorrect for two reasons. First, in full extension, the intact anterior cruciate ligament is under relatively high strain and thus actually lifts the bony fragment from its bed. Second, fragments of bone and interspersed soft tissue often make the reduction impossible unless the debris is surgically removed. Arthroscopic or open debridement of the bed and fixation of the bone fragments probably provide the best means of treatment in all but the most minimally displaced of this type of fracture.[95]

Knee dislocations occurring in sports events are also quite rare, but these devastating injuries are certainly the epitome of the knee ligament injury. Results from closed treatment with prolonged casting as advocated in the early part of the century were often surprisingly good. Although most authors in recent years have advocated repair, repair with augmentation, or immediate reconstruction for as many of the totally disrupted ligaments as possible in the acute phase of treatment, the presence of contaminated open wounds and other life-threatening injuries frequently make acute surgery impractical.[105-107] In such cases, relatively stable knees often result from prolonged immobilization of the joint, but residual abnormal laxity of at least some of the major ligaments frequently necessitates late reconstructions. Ideally, once the vascularity of the knee has been assured, open repair or primary reconstruction of all the destroyed ligaments should be accomplished. Because of the dire consequences (amputation) of missing significant arterial injury at the level of the knee, Doppler pressure measurement or arteriography should be performed before extensive surgery is undertaken on these knees.[105,108] Delay in surgery until the acute reaction has diminished and the range of motion has returned to nearly normal, as is now advocated for the treatment of 'isolated' or double ligament injuries, is probably impractical in these severely traumatized knees. Thus surgery is best performed after a few days, but within 2 weeks of the original injury if possible. Depending on the success in establishing strong fixation of the various injured structures, the postoperative management of such extensive surgery often requires careful and prolonged immobilization if healing is to be successful.

Dislocation of the proximal tibiofibular joint is rare in sports trauma.[109] When it is recognized early, non-surgical management is usually sufficient. Even in cases of recurrent subluxation or dislocation, surgical reconstruction of the joint is rarely necessary.[110]

Ligament injuries of the knee are frequently associated with fractures of the tibia plateau, femur, and tibial shaft.[111,112] Thus these injuries must be suspected and carefully ruled out whenever there is a major fracture in the vicinity of the knee.

Rehabilitation

Rehabilitation following knee ligament surgery or serious injury is universally accepted as being very important to the final outcome of the treatment.[113,114] However, the performance of such rehabilitation programmes is tempered by one of the most frustrating dilemmas faced by any knee surgeon. On the one hand it is necessary to protect the injured structures (usually ligament repairs, reconstructions, partial or even complete disruptions) so they can heal without further injury. On the other hand there are the numerous problems resulting from immobilizing the joint while healing occurs. The detrimental effects of even short-term immobilization, including periarticular muscle atrophy, articular cartilage damage, capsular arthrofibrosis, weakening of the non-injured bone and ligamentous tissue, and loss of range of motion, have been documented in voluminous literature.[115] The ongoing problem for the knee surgeon is how to compromise between these seemingly diametrically opposed circumstances. As documented in other chapters in this section of the text, there have been dramatic changes with time concerning how various surgeons have managed their patients' rehabilitation. In the early part of this century, prolonged casting (6 to 10 weeks) following major ligament injury, whether operated or treated conservatively, was often the standard. Although it was appreciated that muscle rehabilitation and re-establishment of functional range of motion were necessary, very little detail was provided on how these were to be achieved. By the 1950s and 1960s, emphasis was placed on quadriceps rehabilitation, but again little detail was offered. By the late 1970s, a number of surgeons were beginning to allow motion as early as 2 to 4 weeks following the surgery or injury, but not until the late 1980s were the majority of physicians allowing immediate motion, which now appears to be the standard of care. How such motion is performed (passively administered by a therapist or patient, continuous passive motion, or with active muscle control) is much more variable. Burks et al. sounded a note of caution in the use of continuous passive motion machines when they reported a number of early failures of reconstructions of anterior cruciate ligaments performed in vitro.[116] In contrast, several authors have demonstrated that when properly positioned these machines do not appear to have harmful effects on nearly isometrically positioned grafts of anterior cruciate ligament.[117-119] The advocates of continuous passive motion machines have stated that swelling and pain are minimized in the early postoperative phase, but those who question the cost effectiveness of this treatment point out that there is no difference between groups of patients treated with or without these machines within a few weeks of the surgery.[117]

Quadriceps muscle activity was often advocated in an unlimited fashion as soon as practical after ligament surgery, until several investigators revealed that the quadriceps acts antagonistically to the anterior cruciate ligament between approximately 50 degrees of flexion and full extension.[120-124] In recent years, many surgeons have suggested that isotonic quadriceps loading into full extension be avoided until several months after reconstruction of the anterior cruciate ligament.[125] The use of antishear devices in quadriceps and hamstring cocontractor to reduce the loading on the freshly injured, repaired, or reconstructed anterior cruciate ligament has been advocated, but the effect of these techniques is yet to be proven.[123,126-128] The vast number of different muscle rehabilitation programmes advocated following knee ligament surgery implies that no one method can readily be established as the most appropriate. New techniques such as isokinetic, eccentric, closed kinetic chain, and sports specific training all have their enthusiasts, but the timing and safety of these programmes must be carefully considered if harm to the patient is to be avoided. Early institution of closed kinetic chain activities to rehabilitate the quadriceps 'safely' following reconstruction of the anterior cruciate ligament has been essentially universally accepted.[129,130] Recent studies in our laboratory suggest that squatting activities produce strain within the anterior cruciate ligament at similar levels to that of open kinetic chain activities which are usually deferred until much later in rehabilitation protocols following surgery of these ligaments.[125,131] Advocates of aggressive rehabilitation do not report detrimental effects from early quadriceps activity, but there can be no doubt that repaired, reconstructed, or even injured ligaments are vulnerable to overloading if rehabilitation programmes are too aggressive.[113]

Casting was the most common means of protecting complex knee ligament repairs and reconstructions until the 1980s, when various knee rehabilitation braces became the standard. Cast bracing did have some advocates in the 1970s.[132] In recent years, with stronger graft material and fixation techniques, some surgeons have avoided casts and braces completely in the postoperative management of their patients. In the past, prolonged avoidance of weight bearing for up to 4 months following ligament injury or surgery was often suggested. As recently as 1981, the majority of surgeons questioned by Paulos *et al.* did not allow weight bearing until 8 weeks or longer following repairs or reconstructions of anterior cruciate ligaments[124] Shelbourne and co-authors, and Barber-Westin *et al.* now allow their patients to begin weight bearing, as tolerated, immediately after bone–patellar tendon–bone grafts.[133-135] The trend toward better fixation techniques and reconstruction rather than repair of injured ligaments has made such practices at least technically possible.

As patients increase their activity following knee ligament surgery or injury, the question of whether or not to prescribe a functional knee brace is often considered. Although much anecdotal information concerning their effectiveness exists, very little hard data proving that these devices can shield the injured, repaired, or reconstructed ligaments adequately from stress have been published.[136] Much more investigation using strict scientific principles is necessary before answers concerning the place of functional knee braces in rehabilitation can be established.

The question of when to return an athlete to sport has remained controversial. During the 1950s and 1960s the main criterion for success following ligament surgery appeared to be simply how quickly the athlete could return to sport. In the 1970s and early 1980s a much more conservative approach was advocated as more was learned about the healing properties of repaired and reconstructed ligaments and the potential dangerous effects of early muscle activity. During that time many investigators were not recommending return to full activities for a year or more.[124] In recent years a definite trend toward more rapid rehabilitation and return to full activities has been advocated, as several investigators have reported no deleterious effects in their patient populations when their athletes return to full activities from 4 to 6 months after bone–patellar tendon–bone grafts of their anterior cruciate ligaments (W.G. Clancy, personal communication).[134,135,137] These authors stressed that a bone–patellar tendon–bone graft placed iso-

metrically and firmly fixed can probably tolerate vigorous early rehabilitation and early return to sports, but this same rapid rehabilitation may not be successful with other operative procedures.

There can be no standard recipe for rehabilitation programmes following any knee ligament injury, repair, or reconstruction. The trend toward aggressive advances in weight bearing, range of motion, muscle exercises, and return to functional activities has potential dangers. This is especially true in the case of the cruciate ligaments. It has been well documented in many studies of healing in animal models that normal tensile strength, modulus, stiffness, and maximum stress of repaired or reconstructed anterior cruciate ligaments return slowly and never completely.[138,139] It has also been shown that vigorous quadriceps contractions from 50 degrees of flexion to full extension place significant loads on the injured cruciate ligament.[120-125] It is frequently stated that some tensile loading of healing tissue is probably beneficial (Wolff's law), but no one knows how much is detrimental and how much is safe. It is not known when full muscle rehabilitation and return to activities is safe. Those advocating rapid rehabilitation believe that present fixation methods, accurate placement of the graft at the time of surgery, and the use of stronger graft material make it possible for aggressive rehabilitation to succeed. Initially, the weak link in any repair or reconstruction is the fixation of the repair or graft.[140,141] Modern techniques (interference fit, screw and washer, and other forms of fixation) allow at least some early motion and muscle function, but no one knows how much. Within a few weeks of surgery, fixation of cruciate grafts is no longer the primary concern because of the deterioration of the strength of that portion of the graft, which courses from tunnel to tunnel. At 6 to 8 weeks following surgery, this portion of the reconstruction is at its weakest.[139] It is at this time that those advocating a rapid rehabilitation are markedly advancing the activities of their patients. Also, care must be taken in applying rapid rehabilitation methods to cases where weaker grafts, repaired ligament tissues, and less than ideal surgical techniques have been employed. At the present time our limited knowledge of the healing process, the detailed biomechanics of the knee, and many technical variables which are difficult to control during and following surgery (accurate placement and fixation of the graft, tensioning of the graft and the effects of active and passive motion on healing, and compliance with rehabilitation protocols) make it impossible to develop an ideal, universally appropriate, rehabilitation programme. Care must be taken to base decisions on the development of one's own rehabilitation programme on scientific fact rather than anecdotal statements of how rapidly someone else's patients were able to return to sports. Marketing pressures rather than sound scientific principles may have more to do with the present trend toward rapid return of athletes to sports activities following major ligament surgery. Each surgeon should carefully weigh all the data presently available and be prepared to improve his or her own programmes as the results of long-term, randomized, and controlled studies clearly show than one programme is superior to another.[113] Unfortunately such outcome studies are as yet unavailable.[142]

References

1. Renström P, Johnson RJ. Anatomy and biomechanics of the menisci. *Clinics in Sports Medicine* 1990; **9**: 523–38.

2. Sonne-Holm S, Fledelius I, Ahn N. Results after meniscectomy in 147 athletes. *Acta Orthopaedic Scandinavica* 1980; **51**: 303–9.

3. King D. The function of semilunar cartilages. *Journal of Bone and Joint Surgery* 1936; **18A**: 1068.

4. Campbell WC. *Operative orthopaedics*. St. Louis: CV Mosby Co, 1939: 406, 415.

5. Dandy DJ, Jackson RW. Meniscectomy and chondromalacia of the femoral condyle. *Journal of Bone and Joint Surgery* 1975; **57A**: 1116–19.

6. Dandy DJ, Jackson RW. The diagnosis of problems after meniscectomy. *Journal of Bone and Joint Surgery* 1975; **57B**: 349–52.

7. Quigley TB. Knee injuries incurred in sports. *Journal of the American Medical Association* 1959; **171**: 1666.

8. Smillie JS. *Injuries of the knee joint*. 4th edn. Edinburgh: Churchill Livingstone, 1971: 68.

9. Watson-Jones OR. *Fractures and joint injuries*, Vol. 2. Edinburgh: Livingstone, 1955: 769–73.

10. Fairbank TJ. Knee joint changes after meniscectomy. *Journal of Bone and Joint Surgery* 1948; **30B**: 664–70.

11. Appel H. Late results after meniscectomy in the knee joint. A clinical and roentgenological follow-up. *Acta Orthopaedic Scandinavica* 1970; Suppl. 133: 1–111.

12. Gear MWL. The late result of meniscectomy. *British Journal of Surgery* 1967; **54**: 270–2.

13. Huckel J. Is meniscectomy a benign procedure? *Canadian Journal of Surgery* 1965; **8**: 254–60.

14. Jackson JP. Degenerative changes in the knee after meniscectomy. *British Medical Journal* 1968; **2**: 525.

15. Johnson RJ, Kettelkamp DB, Clark W, Leaverton P. Factors affecting late results after meniscectomy. *Journal of Bone and Joint Surgery* 1974; **56A**: 719–29.

16. Tapper EM, Hoover NW. Late results after meniscectomy. *Journal of Bone and Joint Surgery* 1969; **51A**: 517–26.

17. Ahmed AM, Burke DL. *In vitro* measurement of static pressure distribution in synovial joints: I. Tibial surface of the knee. *Journal of Biomechanical Engineering* 1983; **105**: 216–25.

18. Baratz ME, Rehak DC, Fu FH, Rudert MJ. Peripheral tears of the meniscus. The effect of open versus arthroscopic repair on intra-articular contact stresses in the human knee. *American Journal of Sports Medicine* 1988; **16**: 1–6.

19. Bargar WL, Moreland JR, Markoff KL, Shoemaker SC, Amstutz HC, Grant TT. *In-vivo* stability testing of post-meniscectomy knees. *Clinical Orthopaedics* 1980; **150**: 247–52.

20. Krause WE, Pope MD, Johnson RJ, Wilder DG. Mechanical changes in the knee after meniscectomy. *Journal of Bone and Joint Surgery* 1976; **58A**: 599–604.

21. Kurosawa H, Fukuboyashi T, Hakajima H. Load-bearing mode of the knee: physical behavior of the knee joint with and without menisci. *Clinical Orthopaedics* 1980; **149**: 283–90.

22. Newman AP, Anderson DR, Daniels AU. Mechanics of the healed meniscus in a canine model. *American Journal of Sports Medicine* 1989; **17**: 164–75.

23. Newman AP, Anderson DJ, Daniels AU, Jee KW. The effect of medial meniscectomy and coronal plane angulation on *in vitro* load transmission in the canine stifle joint. *Journal of Orthopaedic Research* 1989; **7(2)**: 281–91.

24. Seedholm BB, Hargreaves DJ. Transmission of the load in the knee joint with special reference to the role of the menisci: II. Experimental results, discussion and conclusions. *English Medicine* 1979; **8**: 220–8.

25. Walker PS, Erkman MH. The role of the menisci in force transmission across the knee. *Clinical Orthopaedics* 1975; **109**: 184–92.

26. Jackson RW. The virtues of partial meniscectomy. *Second International Seminar on Operative Arthroscopy, Maui* 1980; 89–95.

27. Jackson, RW, Dandy DJ. Partial meniscectomy. *Journal of Bone and Joint Surgery* 1976; **58B**: 142.

28. McGinty JB, Lawrence FD, Marwin R. Partial or total meniscectomy. *Journal of Bone and Joint Surgery* 1977; **59A**: 763–6.

29. Cassidy RE, Shauffer AJ. Repair of peripheral meniscus tears. A preliminary report. *American Journal of Sports Medicine* 1981; **9**: 209–14.

30. Eggli S, Wegmüller H, Kosiua J, Huckell C, Jakob RP. Long term results of arthroscopic meniscal repair. *American Journal of Sports Medicine* 1995; **23**: 715–20.

31. DeHaven KE. Peripheral meniscus repair. An alternative to meniscectomy. *Orthopaedic Transactions* 1981; **5**: 399–400.

32. Henning CE. Arthroscopic repair of meniscal tears. *Orthopedics* 1983; **6**: 1130.

33. DeHaven KE *et al*. Open meniscus repair. Technique and two to nine year results. *American Journal of Sports Medicine* 1989; **17**: 773–7.

34. DeHaven KE, Lohrer WA, Lovelock JE. Long term results in open meniscal repair. *American Journal of Sports Medicine* 1995; **23**: 524–30.

35. Wirth CR. Meniscus repair. *Clinical Orthopaedics* 1981; **157**: 153–60.

36. Arnoczky SP *et al*. Meniscal repair using an exogenous fibrin clot. An experimental study in dogs. *Journal of Bone and Joint Surgery* 1988; **70A**: 1209–17.

37. Henning CE, Lynch MA, Yearout KM, Vequist SW, Stallbaumer RJ, Decker KA. Arthroscopic meniscal repair using an exogenous fibrin clot. *Clinical Orthopaedics* 1990; **252**: 64–72.

38. Ferro TD, Gershuni DH, Danzig LA, Hargens AR, Oyama BK, O'Hara R. The mechanical strength of healed tears in canine menisci. *Proceedings of 34th Annual Meeting, Orthopedic Research Society, Atlanta, GA, 1–4 February 1988*. Park Ridge, IL: The Orthopedic Research Society: 146.

39. Krause WR, Burdette WA, Loughran TP. Properties of the normal and repaired canine meniscus. *Proceedings of 35th Annual Meeting, Orthopedic Research Society, Las Vegas, NV, 6–9Feb 1989*. Park Ridge, IL: The Orthopedic Research Society: 207.

40. Arnoczky SP, McDevitt CA, Schmidt MB, Mow VC, Warren RF. The effect of cryopreservation on canine menisci: a biochemical, morphologic, and biomechanical evaluation. *Journal of Orthopaedic Research* 1988; **6(1)**: 1–12.

41. Jackson DW, McDevitt CA, Atwell EA, Arnoczky SP, Simon TM. Meniscal transplantation using fresh and cryopreserved allografts—an experimental study in goats. *Proceedings of 36th Annual Meeting, Orthopedic Research Society, New Orleans, LA, 5–8 February 1990*. Park Ridge, IL: The Orthopedic Research Society: 221.

42. Keating EM, Malinin TI, Belchic G. Meniscal transplantation in goats: an experimental study. *Proceedings of 34th Annual Meeting, Orthopedic Research Society, Atlanta, GA, 1–4 February 1988*. Park Ridge, IL: The Orthopedic Research Society: 147.

43. Milachowski KA, Weismeier K, Wirth CJ. Homologous meniscus transplantation. Experimental and clinical results. *International Orthopaedics* 1989; **13(1)**: 1–11.

44. Milton J *et al*. Transplantation of viable, cryopreserved menisci. *Proceedings of 36th Annual Meeting, Orthopedic Research Society, New Orleans, LA, 5–8 February 1990*. Park Ridge, IL: The Orthopedic Research Society: 220.

45. Minns RJ. The Minns menical knee prosthesis: biomechanical aspects of the surgical procedure and a review of the first 165 cases. *Archives of Orthopaedic and Trauma Surgery* 1989; **108(4)**: 44–8.

46. Stone KR, Rodkey WG, Webber RJ, McKinney L, Steadman JR. Mensical regeneration using copolymeric collagen scaffolds: *in vitro* studies evaluated clinically, histologically, and biochemically. *American Journal of Sports Medicine* 1992; **20**: 104–20.

47. Wojtys EM, Carpenter JE. Meniscal replacement—early experience. *Arthroscopy* 1994; **3**: 337.

48. Zukor DJ *et al.* Allotransplantation of frozen irradiated menisci in rabbits. *Proceedings of 36th Annual Meeting, Orthopedic Research Society, New Orleans, LA, 5–8 February 1990.* Park Ridge, IL: The Orthopedic Research Society: 219.

49. Siegel MG, Roberts CS. Meniscal allografts. *Clinics in Sports Medicine* 1993; **12**: 59–80.

50. Milch H. Injuries to the crucial ligaments. *Archives of Surgery* 1935; **30**: 805.

51. O'Donoghue DH. Surgical treatment of fresh injuries to the major ligaments of the knee. *Journal of Bone and Joint Surgery* 1950; **32A**: 721–38.

52. Palmer I. On the injuries to the ligaments of the knee joint. *Acta Chirurgica Scandinavica* 1938; **53** (Suppl. 8).

53. Hughston JC, Barrett GR. Acute anteromedial instability: long-term results of surgical repair. *Journal of Bone and Joint Surgery* 1983; **65A**: 145–53.

54. Keller RB. Kennedy Lectureship, *American Orthopedic Society for Sports Medicine* Specialty Day, Feb 25, 1996.

55. Johnson RJ. The anterior cruciate: a dilemma in sports medicine. *International Journal of Sports Medicine* 1983; **3**: 71–9.

56. Johnson RJ, Beynnon BD, Nichols CE, Renström PA. Current concepts review: the treatment of injuries of the anterior cruciate ligament. *Jounal of Bone and Joint Surgery* 1992; **74A**: 140–51.

57. Chick RR, Jackson DE. Tears of the anterior cruciate ligament in young athletes. *Journal of Bone and Joint Surgery* 1978; **60A**: 970–3.

58. Giove TP, Miller SJ, Kent BE, Sanford TL, Garrick JG. Non-operative treatment of the torn anterior cruciate ligament. *Journal of Bone and Joint Surgery* 1983; **65A**: 184–92.

59. Hughston JC. Acute knee injuries in athletes. *Clinical Orthopaedics* 1962; **23**: 114.

60. Kennedy JC, Weinbert HW, Wilson AS. The anatomy and function of the anterior cruciate ligament. *Journal of Bone and Joint Surgery* 1974; **56A**: 223–35.

61. McDaniel W, Dameron TB. Untreated ruptures of the anterior cruciate ligament. *Journal of Bone and Joint Surgery* 1980; **62A**: 696–705.

62. Kannus P, Jarvinen M. Conservatively treated tears of the anterior cruciate ligament. Long-term results. *Journal of Bone and Joint Surgery* 1987; **69A**: 1007–12.

63. Johnson RJ, Eriksson E, HŠggmark T, Pope MH. Five to ten year follow-up after reconstruction of the anterior cruciate ligament. *Clinical Orthopaedics* 1984; **183**: 122–40.

64. Hawkins RJ, Misamore GW, Merritt TR. Follow-up of the acute nonoperative isolated anterior cruciate ligament tear. *American Journal of Sports Medicine* 1986; **14**: 205–10.

65. Noyes FR, Mooar PA, Matthews DS, Butler DL. The symptomatic anterior cruciate deficient knee. Part I: The long-term functional disability in athletically active individuals. *Journal of Bone and Joint Surgery* 1983; **65A**: 154–62.

66. Gerber C, Matter P. Biomechanical analysis of the knee after rupture of the anterior cruciate ligament and its primary repair. *Journal of Bone and Joint Surgery* 1983; **65B**: 391–9.

67. Marans JH, Jackson RW, Glossop ND, Young C. Anterior cruciate ligament insufficiency: a dynamic three-dimensional motion analysis. *American Journal of Sports Medicine* 1989; **17**: 325–32.

68. Fried JA, Bergfeld JA, Weiker, G, Andrish JT. Anterior cruciate reconstruction using the Jones-Ellison procedure. *Journal of Bone and Joint Surgery* 1985; **67A**: 1029–33.

69. Daniel DM, Stone ML, Dobson BE, Fithian DC, Rosman DJ, Kaugman KR. Fate of the ACL-injured patient. A prospective outcome study. *American Journal of Sports Medicine* 1994; **22**: 632–43,.

70. Bennedetto KP. Long term results of ACL reconstruction—a two stage follow up study. Presented at the *Combined Congress of the International Arthroscopy Association and The International Society of the Knee, Hong Kong, 29 March, 1995.*

71. Clancy WG Jr, Nelson DA, Reider B, Narechania RG. Anterior cruciate ligament reconstruction using one-third of the patellar ligament, augmented by extra-articular tendon transfers. *Journal of Bone and Joint Surgery* 1982; **64A**: 352–9.

72. O'Brien SJ, Warren RF, Paulos H, Panariello R, Wickiewicz TL. Reconstruction of the chronically insufficient anterior cruciate ligament with the central third of the patellar tendon. *Journal of Bone and Joint Surgery* 1991; **75A**: 278–86.

73. Sachs RA, Daniel DM, Stone ML, Gorfein RF. Patellofemoral problems after ACL reconstruction. *American Journal of Sports Medicine* 1989; **17**: 760–5.

74. Andersson C, Odensten M, Good L, Gillquist J. Surgical or non-surgical treatment of acute rupture of the anterior cruciate ligament. *Journal of Bone and Joint Surgery* 1989; **71A**: 965–74.

75. Engebretsen L, Benum P, Fasting O, Mølster A, Strand T. A prospective randomized study of the surgical techniques for treatment of acute ruptures of the anterior cruciate ligament. *American Journal of Sports Medicine* 1990; **18**: 585–90.

76. Engebretsen L, Renum P, Sundalswall S. Primary suture of the anterior cruciate ligament. A 6 year follow-up of 74 cases. *Acta Orthopaedic Scandinavica* 1989; **60**: 561–4.

77. Feagin JA Jr, Curl WW. Isolated tear of the anterior cruciate ligament: 5 year follow-up study. *American Journal of Sports Medicine* 1976; **4**: 95–100.

78. Grøntvedt T, Engebretsen L, Benum P, Fasting O, Mølster A, Strand T. A prospective randomized study of three operations for acute rupture of the anterior cruciate ligament. *Journal of Bone and Joint Surgery* 1996; **78A**: 159–68.

79. Sandberg R, Balkfors B, Nilsson B, Westlin N. Operative versus non-operative treatment of recent injuries to the knee ligaments. *Journal of Bone and Joint Surgery* 1987; **69A**: 1120–6.

80. Jonsson T, Peterson L, Renstrom R, Althoff B, Myrhage R. Augmentation with longitudinal patellar retinaculum in the repair of an anterior cruciate ligament rupture. *American Journal of Sports Medicine* 1989; **17**: 401–8.

81. Sgaglione NA, Warren RF, Wickiewicz TL, Gold DA, Panariello RA. Primary repair with semitendinosus tendon augmentation of acute anterior cruciate injuries. *American Journal of Sports Medicine* 1990; **18**: 64–73.

82. Straub T, Hunter RE. Acute anterior cruciate ligament repair. *Clinical Orthopaedics* 1987; **227**: 238–50.

83. Pearl AJ, Bergfeld JA, eds. *Extra-articular reconstruction in the anterior cruciate ligament.* Champlain, IL: American Orthopedic Society of Sports Medicine, Human Kinetics Publishers, 1992: 1–55.

84. Jackson *et al.* A comparison of patellar tendon autograft and allograft used for anterior cruciate ligament reconstruction in the goat model. *American Journal of Sports Medicine* 1993; **21**: 176–84.

85. Noyes FR, Barber SD. The effect of an extra articular procedure on allograft reconstructions for chronic ruptures of the anterior cruciate ligament. *Journal of Bone and Joint Surgery* 1991; **73A**: 882–92.

86. Mok WW, Good C. Nonoperative management of acute grade III medial collateral ligament injury of the knee. *Injury* 1989; **20**: 277–80.

87. Clancy WG, Bergfeld J, O'Connor GA, Cox JS. Functional rehabilitation of isolated medial collateral ligament sprains. Knee Symposium, *American Journal of Sports Medicine* 1979; **7**: 206–13.

88. Parolie JM, Bergfeld JA. Long term results of nonoperative treatment of isolated posterior cruciate ligament injuries in the athlete. *American Journal of Sports Medicine* 1986; **14**: 35–8.

89. Torg JS, Barton TM, Pavlov H, Stine R. Natural history of the

posterior cruciate deficient knee. *Clinical Orthopaedics* 1989; **246**: 208–16.

90. Kennedy JC, Galpin RD. The use of the medial head of the gastrocnemius muscle in the posterior cruciate deficient knee. *American Journal of Sports Medicine* 1982; **10**: 63–74.

91. Clancy WG, Shelbourne KD, Zoellner GB, Keene JS, Reider B, Rosenberg TD. Treatment of knee joint instability secondary to rupture of the posterior cruciate ligament. *Journal of Bone and Joint Surgery* 1983; **65A**: 310–22.

92. Hughston JC, Bowden JA, Andrews JR, Norwood LA. Acute tears of the posterior cruciate ligament. Results of operative treatment. *Journal of Bone and Joint Surgery* 1980; **62A**: 438–50.

93. Keller PM, Shelbourne KD, McCarroll JR, Rettig AC. Nonoperatively treated isolated posterior cruciate ligament injuries. *American Journal of Sports Medicine* 1993; **21**: 132–6.

94. Kannus P. Nonoperative treatment of grade II and III sprains of the lateral compartment of the knee. *American Journal of Sports Medicine* 1989; **17**: 83–9.

95. Cohn SL, Sotta RP, Bergfeld JA. Fractures about the knee in sports. *Clinics in Sports Medicine* 1990; **9**: 121–39.

96. Woods GW, Stanley RF, Tillos HS. Lateral capsular sign: X-ray clue to a significant knee instability. *American Journal of Sports Medicine* 1979; **7**: 27–39.

97. Warren RF, Kaplan N, Bach BR Jr. The lateral notch sign of anterior cruciate insufficiency. *American Journal of Knee Surgery* 1988; **1(2)**: 119–24.

98. Graf BK, Cook DA, DeSmet AA, Keene JS. 'Bone bruises' on magnetic resonance imaging evaluation of anterior cruciate ligament injuries. *American Journal of Sports Medicine* 1993; **21**: 220–3.

99. Jackson DW, Jennings LD, Maywood RM, Berger PE. Magnetic resonance imaging of the knee. *American Journal of Sports Medicine* 1988; **16**: 29–38.

100. Lee JK, Yao L. Occult intraosseous fracture: magnetic resonance appearance versus age of injury. *American Journal of Sports Medicine* 1989; **17**: 620–3.

101. Speer KP, Warren RF, Wickiewicz TL, Horowitz L, Henderson L. Observations on the injury mechanism of anterior cruciate ligament tears in skiers. *American Journal of Sports Medicine* 1995; **23**: 72–81.

102. Spindler KP *et al.* Prospective study of osseous, articular, and meniscal lesions in recent anterior cruciate ligament tear by magnetic resonance imaging and arthroscopy. *American Journal of Sports Medicine* 1993; **21**: 551–7.

103. Vellet AD *et al.* Occult posttraumatic osteochondral lesions of the knee: prevalences, classification, and short term sequelae evaluated by MR imaging. *Radiology* 1991; **178**: 271–6.

104. Meyers MH, McKeever FM. Fracture of the intercondylar eminence of the tibia. *Journal of Bone and Joint Surgery* 1959; **41A**: 209–22.

105. Good L, Johnson RJ. The dislocated knee. *Journal of the American Academy of Orthopedic Surgeons* 1995; **3**: 284–92.

106. Kennedy JC. Complete dislocation of the knee joint. *Journal of Bone and Joint Surgery* 1963; **45A**: 889–904.

107. Meyers MH, Moore TM, Harvey JP. Traumatic dislocation of the knee. *Journal of Bone and Joint Surgery* 1975; **57A**: 430–3.

108. McCutchan JD, Gillham NR. Injury to the popliteal artery associated with dislocation of the knee: palpable distal pulses do not negate the requirement for arteriography. *Injury* 1989; **20**: 307–10.

109. Tureo VJ, Spinella AJ. Anterolateral dislocation of the head of the fibula in sports. *American Journal of Sports Medicine* 1985; **13**: 209–15.

110. Weinert CR, Raczka R. Recurrent dislocation of the superior tibiofibular joint. *Journal of Bone and Joint Surgery* 1986: **68A**: 126–8.

111. Delamarter RB, Hohl M, Hopp E. Ligament injuries associated with tibia plateau fractures. *Clinical Orthopaedics* 1990; **250**: 226–33.

112. Templeman DC, Marder RA. Injuries of the knee associated with fractures of the tibial shaft. Detection by examination under anesthesia: a prospective study. *Journal of Bone and Joint Surgery* 1990; **72A**: 1392–5.

113. Johnson RJ, Beynnon BD. Rehabilitation following anterior cruciate ligament reconstruction: what do we really know? *Iowa Orthopedic Journal* 1995; **15**: 19–23.

114. Stanish WD, Lai A. New concepts of rehabilitation following anterior cruciate ligament reconstruction. *Clinics in Sports Medicine* 1993; **12**: 25–58.

115. Johnson RJ. The effect of immobilization on ligaments and ligamentous healing. *Contemporary Orthopaedics* 1980; **2**: 237–41.

116. Burks R, Daniel D, Losse G. The effect of continuous passive motion on anterior cruciate ligament reconstruction stability. *American Journal of Sports Medicine* 1984; **12**: 323–7.

117. Noyes FR, Mangine RE, Barber S. Early knee motion after open and arthroscopic anterior cruciate ligament reconstruction. *American Journal of Sports Medicine* 1987; **15**: 149–60.

118. Reinecke S, Arms S, Renström P, Johnson RJ, Pope MH. Continuous passive motion and its effect on knee ligament strain. In: Johnson B ed. *International Series on Biomechanics: Human Kinetics*, Champaign, IL 1987; **6A**: 111–18.

119. Rosen MA, Jackson DW, Atwell EA. The efficacy of continuous passive motion in the rehabilitation of anterior cruciate ligaemnt reconstruction. *American Journal of Sports Medicine* 1992; **20**: 122–7.

120. Arms SW, Pope MH, Johnson RJ, Fischer RA, Arvidsson I, Ericksson I. The biomechanics of anterior cruciate ligament rehabilitation and reconstruction. *American Journal of Sports Medicine* 1984; **12**: 8–18.

121. Beynnon BD, Fleming BC, Johnson RJ, Nichols CE, Renström PA, Pope MH. Anterior cruciate ligament strain behavior during rehabilitation exercises *in-vivo*. *American Journal of Sports Medicine* 1995; **23**: 24–34.

122. Henning CE, Lynch MA, Glick KR. An *in vivo* strain gauge study of elongation of the anterior cruciate ligament. *American Journal of Sports Medicine* 1985; **13**: 22–6.

123. Maltry JA, Noble PC, Woods GW, Alexander JW, Feldman GW, Tullos HS. External stabilization of the anterior cruciate deficient knee during rehabilitation. *American Journal of Sports Medicine* 1989; **17**: 550–4.

124. Paulos LE, Noyes FR, Grood ES, Butler DL. Knee rehabilitation after anterior cruciate ligament reconstruction and repair. *American Journal of Sports Medicine* 1981; **9**: 140–9.

125. Huegel M, Indelicato PA. Trends in rehabilitation following anterior cruciate ligament reconstruction. *Clinics in Sports Medicine* 1988; **7**: 801–11.

126. Malone T. Clinical use of the Johnson anti-shear device: how and why to use it. *Journal of Orthopaedic and Sports Physical Therapy* 1986; **7**: 304–9.

127. Nisell R, Ericson MO, Nemeth G, Elsholm J. Tibiofemoral joint forces during isokinetic knee extension. *American Journal of Sports Medicine* 1989; **17**: 49–54.

128. Renstrom P, Arms SW, Stanwyck TS, Johnson RJ, Pope MH. Strain within the anterior cruciate ligament during hamstring and quadriceps activity. *American Journal of Sports Medicine* 1986; **14**: 83–7.

129. Lutz GE, Palmitier RA, Chao EYS. Comparison of tibiofemoral joint forces during open kinetic chain and closed kinetic chain exercises. *Journal of Bone and Joint Surgery* 1993; **75A**: 732–9.

130. Yack HJ, Collins CE, Whieldon TJ. Comparison of closed and open kinetic chain exercises in the anterior cruciate ligament deficient knee. *American Journal of Sports Medicine* 1993; **21**: 49–54.

131. Fleming BC *et al.* Anterior cruciate ligament strain during an open and a closed kinetic chain exercise: an *in vivo* study. *Transactions of the 41st meeting of the Orthopedic Research Society, Orlando, FL, 13–16 February 1995*: 631. Orthopaedic Research Society, Palatine, IL.

132. Häggmark T, Eriksson E. Cylinder or mobile cast brace after knee ligament surgery: a clinical analysis and morphologic and enzymatic studies of changes in the quadriceps muscle. *American Journal of Sports Medicine* 1979; **7**: 48–56.

133. Barber-Westin SD, Noyes FR. The effect of rehabilitation and return to activity on anterior–posterior knee displacements after anterior cruciate ligament reconstruction. *American Journal of Sports Medicine* 1993; **21**: 264–76.

134. Shelburne KD, Klootwyk TE, Wilckens JH, De Carlo MS. Ligament stability 2 to 6 years after anterior cruciate ligament reconstruction with autogenous patellar tendon graft and participation in accelerated rehabilitation program. *American Journal of Sports Medicine* 1995; **23**: 575.

135. Shelbourne KO, Nitz P. Accelerated rehabilitation after anterior cruciate ligament reconstruction. *American Journal of Sports Medicine* 1990; **18**: 292–9.

136. Beynnon BD *et al.* The effect of functional braces on strain on the anterior cruciate ligament *in vivo*. *Journal of Bone and Joint Surgery* 1992; **74A**: 1298–311.

137. Glasgow SG, Gabriel JP, Sapega AA, Glasgow MT, Torg JS. The effect of early versus late return to vigorous activity on the outcome of anterior cruciate ligament reconstruction. *American Journal of Sports Medicine* 1993; **21**: 243–8.

138. Paulos LE, Payne FC, Rosenberg TD. Rehabilitation after anterior cruciate ligament surgery. In: Jackson DW, Drez D, eds. *The anterior cruciate deficient knee*. St. Louis: CV Mosby, 1987: 291–314.

139. Butler DL *et al.* Mechanical properties of primate vascularized vs. nonvascularized patellar tendon grafts: changes over time. *Journal of Orthopaedic Research* 1989; **7**: 68–79.

140. Daniel DM. Principles of knee ligament surgery: graft fixation. In: Danel D, Akeson W, O'Connor J, eds. *Knee ligament structure, function, injury and repair*. New York: Raven Press, 1990: 20–6.

141. Kurosaka M, Yoshiya S, Andrish JT. A biomechanical comparison of different surgical techniques of graft fixation in anterior cruciate ligament reconstruction. *American Journal of Sports Medicine* 1987; **15**: 225–9.

142. Noyes FR. ACL autograft vs. allograft: long term results. Presented at American Academy of Orthopedic Surgeons course entitled: *Comprehensive Sports Medicine Course on the Knee and Lower Extremity*. Steamboat Springs, Colorado, 6 Jan, 1995.

143. Rosenberg TP, Paulos LE, Parker RD, Abbott PJ. Arthroscopic knee surgery of the knee. In: Chapman MW, Madison M, eds. *Operative orthopaedics*. Philadelphia: JB Lippincott Co., 1988: 1585–604.

144. Feagin JA, Lambert KL, Cunningham RR. Repair reconstruction of the anterior cruciate ligament. In: Chapman MW, Madison M, eds. *Operative orthopaedics*. Philadelphia: JB Lippincott Co., 1988: 1641–50.

4.2.2 Knee ligament sprains— acute and chronic

William D. Stanish

Introduction

Knee ligament injuries are common in sport. These injuries may occur as a consequence of athletic activity, or secondary to high-energy insults in both industry and on the highways. However, knee ligament damage caused by a violent insult during sport has attracted the most attention.

Since the classic works of O'Donoghue *et al.*,[1] Hughston,[2] and others, much controversy has been created as to the best technique for the medical and surgical management of knee ligament tears. Specifically, treatment of the torn anterior cruciate ligament of the knee has attracted most of the controversy. Unfortunately, most studies on the natural history of knee ligament instabilities are limited by subjective bias, tend to be retrospective in nature, and usually have a relatively short follow-up. In spite of this reality, valuable information can be obtained from the majority of these investigations.

This chapter is designed to place maximum emphasis on the clinical aspects of the medical problem of knee ligament injuries. Each type of knee ligament tear will be profiled to facilitate an understanding of the mechanism of injury, the clinical signs and symptoms, and the options for treatment. Distinctions are drawn between acute ligament tears and the chronically unstable knee. The basic science of knee ligament injury and repair has been included in the text to provide a platform for enhanced clinical interpretation of the ligament injury.

Ligament healing

Healing is a matter of time, but is sometimes also a matter of opportunity. (Hippocrates)

The following discussion will deal specifically with the healing process of ligaments and the factors which influence the rate and degree of success of that process. It is intended that a review of recent experimental and clinical studies will establish a time–strength relationship for healing ligaments. This process will afford a better appreciation of treatment regimens which provide the most opportune conditions for repair. Furthermore, it is expected that by initially presenting the fundamental concepts of soft-tissue healing and then discussing those factors pertaining particularly to ligament healing, newer concepts in treatment will be enhanced.

The healing process in ligaments is generally divided into three phases:

I.   the substrate phase;

II. the proliferative phase; and

III. the remodelling phase.

Phase I

The substrate phase occurs during the first 4 days following injury. This phase involves the vascular response to the insult, haemostasis, and cellular response. Cells, including polymorphonuclear leucocytes, lymphocytes, macrophages, and mast cells (as well as fibroblasts), aggregate at the wound site during this inflammatory process. By the end of this phase, neovascularization has begun at the edges of the wound.

Phase II

The proliferative phase commences approximately 4 days postinjury and continues for 2 to 3 weeks. This period is also termed the

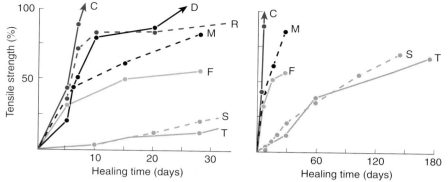

Fig. 1 Relative healing rates for linear incisional wounds in different tissues, the tensile strength being calculated as a percentage of that of the respective intact tissues: C, corpus ventriculi (rat); D, duodenum (rat); R, rumen ventriculi (rat); M, lateral abdominal wall muscle (rabbit); F, fascia (linea alba, rabbit); S, skin (dorsal thoracic, rat); and T, tendon (peroneus brevis, rabbit). (Redrawn from ref. 4, with permission.)

fibroblastic phase to reflect the proliferation of fibroblasts at the site of insult such that they become the dominant cell types. The result of this cellular proliferation is the production of collagen, which in turn relates directly to the rapid return to wound strength which occurs during this time. The quality and type of collagen may differ dramatically from the structure of the virgin ligament.

As stated by previous authors, including Peacock,[3] this phase has important structural features which must be recognized when a tissue, such as ligament, is being considered. Peacock[3] states, 'It has been observed that the rate at which all wounds gain strength is the same during the first 14 to 21 days after wounding.' However, the percentage of normal, unwounded strength that is gained by the wound varies markedly with specific tissues. The tensile strength will also vary according to the degree of trauma, the age of the individual who has been injured, and the presence of other variables such as diabetes, etc. In general, there is an inverse ratio between normal breaking strength of the tissue and the percentage of strength that the wound regains in 14 to 21 days. This suggests that the absolute gain in strength in the early phase of wound healing is related to the chemical events occurring in all tissues. The gain in strength is apparently limited by the rapidity with which these universal events occur.

Figure 1 illustrates the significance of this phenomenon. Although ligament tissue was not specifically represented in this study, the healing rate would be expected to approximate most closely that of tendon. It is apparent that factors which affect the biochemical events of the proliferative phase will also be an important consideration in determining optimum conditions for ligament healing.

Phase III

The remodelling of wound repair differs from the first two phases in that its duration is indistinct and continues for a very lengthy period. Early in the remodelling phase, the number of fibroblasts and the collagen production peak and then begin to decrease gradually. The result is the formation of a collagen scar which undergoes remodelling as the fibres become aligned parallel to the direction of the tension on the scar. There is continued turnover of collagen during this phase and the wound strength continues to increase as the collagen realigns, matures, and shifts from type III collagen (of healing wounds) to the type I collagen of normal tissue. The pre-

valance of type III collagen remains and thus it can be suggested that there is a permanent aberration of structure.

The persistence of this phase is considered to be primarily a product of the mechanical stresses on the wound. It is universally conceded that although this phase is of long duration, the repaired tissue never regains the architecture or strength of the tissue that was present prior to injury. Figure 2 gives a graphical summary of the ligament healing process.

Factors which influence ligament healing

The phases of wound healing are influenced by many factors, the control of which provides the potential for establishing ideal conditions for repair. It should be realized that the induction of so-called 'super healing' is definitely not attainable; however, factors disturbing ligament healing can be controlled.

An injury of the ligament is the initial stimulus to repair. Dunphy[6] suggests that although there can be an optimum stimulus to repair in the clinical setting, the situation following a clean laceration made by a knife affords the environment for ideal repair. Any

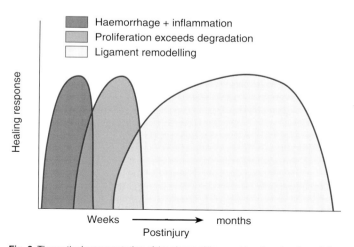

Fig. 2 Theoretical representation of the phase of ligament healing showing relative durations and overlap of stages. Treatment is aimed at optimizing proliferation and remodelling in as short a time as possible. (Redrawn from ref. 5, with permission.)

additional trauma is inhibitory and will disturb wound repair. Johnson[7] makes the point that the use of surgically traumatized animal ligaments, as experimental models, cannot reproduce the traumatically torn ligament in the athlete.

Such injuries are known to demonstrate various degrees of disruption throughout the entire ligamentous unit; thus it is obvious that in the majority of such clinical cases, the healing process of injured ligaments begins under less than ideal conditions.

The degree of damage incurred is also related to the mode of injury. Incomplete ligament tears, although healing by the same pathway as complete disruptions, will not produce as profound a deficit (as a complete disruption) and consequently will probably yield a more functional tissue.

Adequate nutrition and vasculature are essential throughout the healing process.[8,9] Vitamin C (ascorbic acid) is particularly important and a deficiency in this vital substrate can result in a wound with decreased tensile strength, secondary to a prolonged substrate phase, and decreased collagen synthesis. Availability of protein is also important, with protein deficiency resulting in retarded healing. The production of type III collagen is particularly dependent upon an adequate supply of cystine during scar formation.

The detrimental effect produced by poor vascular perfusion is due to a number of factors. Apart from carrying the original inflammatory cells that initiate wound healing, blood supply and oxygen availability to the wound are inherently related. Poor perfusion or a low oxygen concentration will slow the rate of healing and may, in fact, increase the risk of infection. If infection does ensue, wound healing can be significantly impaired. Since all surgical procedures result in some degree of bacterial contamination, the presence of other factors which predispose to poor wound healing must be controlled to reduce the chance of sepsis.

The effects of electrical stimulation on healing rates has been studied for many mesodermal tissues. Stanish *et al.*[10] suggest that the use of electromagnetic stimulation may prove to be a valuable adjunct to the healing of surgically repaired ligaments. The use of electrical muscle stimulation (EMS) during the early periods of healing can result in increased cross-sectional area of the repaired tissue, which consequently provides an improved tensile strength.

Undoubtedly, the factor affecting the healing rate of ligaments which has received the most attention is the issue of wound stressing.[11,12] The stressing of ligaments during healing has been considered in many studies dealing with forced immobilization and scheduling of remobilization.

In essence, it has been established that the primary concern is to protect the wound site during the first two phases of healing so that a certain degree of strength can be regained. It has also been demonstrated that mobilization, or application of stress upon a wound, in the latter phase of healing is essential if maximum repair with respect to biochemical and biomechanical parameters is to be achieved.

Ligament—structure and behaviour

In order to appreciate the healing process of ligaments, it is fundamental to establish their normal biochemical and biomechanical properties.

Ligaments are composed of approximately 60 to 80 per cent of

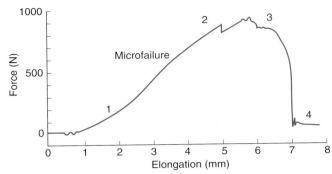

Fig. 3 Nearly 8 mm of joint displacement occurred before the ligament reached complete failure. (Redrawn from ref. 5, with permission.)

water by weight. Collagen accounts for 70 to 90 per cent of the dry mass; and, of this, approximately 90 per cent is type I collagen, with the remainder being type III collagen. Type III collagen is an immature form of collagenous material and reflects the dynamic behaviour in ligaments. There is also an elastin component and small amounts of proteoglycans, as well as a minor cellular component. The collagen content is the most crucial constituent and is responsible for the mechanical properties of ligaments. The strength of collagen is directly related to its structure which consists of both inter- and intramolecular crosslinks.

Failure will occur when the resistance of the fibres or their crosslinks is exceeded. Also of particular importance when considering the ability of a ligament to resist deformation is the crimped pattern in which it is arranged. It is suggested that this microscopic phenomenon provides a buffer which will allow for slight elongation of the ligament, with full return to its natural state when the force is removed. When the limits of this crimp are exceeded, irreversible damage to the ligament may occur.

The biomechanical behaviour of ligaments is most interesting. Ligaments are considered to be viscoelastic and, according to Fung,[13] viscoelasticity is a term used to describe the combined properties of hysteresis, relaxation, and creep. Hysteresis describes the phenomenon by which the stress–strain relationship of a cyclically loaded substance differs during loading and unloading. Relaxation is the characteristic by which the stress in a material decreases in time after the material is suddenly strained and the strain is maintained. Creep is defined as the continued deformation of a body when it is suddenly stressed and the stress is maintained.

According to Frank and co-workers,[14-16] the result of these properties allows for 'some joint displacement with relatively little effort, but provides increasing resistance as deformation increases'.[14] The biochemical structure and the consequential biomechanical properties yield the typical load–deformation curve (Fig. 3).

As soon as injury occurs, the healing process begins. The assessment of the healing properties of ligaments has been the focus of many studies which have analysed the biochemical and biomechanical parameters in animal models. Animal studies have distinct limitations, but they have addressed many aspects of healing under controlled conditions and provide the advantage of postmortem study. By comparison, human studies are rather limited, but they do provide valuable information with respect to the degree of function which can be regained subject to the various treatment regimens.

Danielson,[17] has studied the *in-vitro* maturation of collagen and provided baseline data concerning the rate of collagen production. This study concluded that the strength gains do plateau at approximately 3 months, as illustrated in Fig. 4.

Furthermore, it provides a correlation between the number of reducible crosslinks and the mechanical structure of the fibres. It is conceded that although *in-vitro* maturation occurs in the same pattern as the *in-vivo* process, the rate of maturation in living tissue would be expected to be relatively slower. In fact, this has been verified in a number of *in-vivo* experiments.

The study of living ligaments under controlled conditions has been divided into two categories: non-repaired and repaired ligaments. Non-repaired ligaments are allowed to heal without surgical intervention, and as a result scar tissue forms between the opposed ends of the severed ligaments. Macroscopically, the repair site appears not to change beyond 6 weeks postinjury. However, changes in histochemical and biomechanical parameters may continue for months or even years. Surgically repaired ligaments tend to heal by primary intention due to the close approximation of the severed ends—in other words, the gap has been narrowed. In reality, however, it has been shown that there is indeed scar tissue formation between the opposed ends of the ligament in these repairs.

The results of the surgical repair hastens healing during the early phase of the repair process, and during this time the biomechanical properties will exceed those of the non-repaired ligaments. Following these two groups over the long term demonstrates that there is no difference between the repaired and the non-repaired ligaments. The clinical application of this phenomenon is important. It must be recognized that the surgically repaired ligament will provide superior results under certain circumstances, such as those injuries involving the anterior cruciate ligament of the knee.

Although it is apparent that in the final analysis the mode of

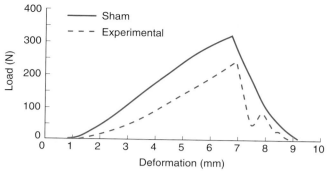

Fig. 5 Biomechanical (structural) results. Typical load–deformation diagrams of experimental and sham ligaments from the same 14-week-old animal. Note that the first millimetre of deformation for these samples represents their 'laxity'. (Redrawn from ref. 15, with permission.)

healing is relatively unimportant, it is convenient to keep the two groups (repaired and non-repaired) separate when evaluating the completeness of the healing process.

In studies detailing untreated ligament injuries, Frank and co-workers discussed many of the measurable parameters for midsubstance insults in the medial collateral ligament in rabbits. Histologically, even after 40 weeks the healing ligaments showed a disorganized matrix, increased fibroblasts, and abnormal crimp. Biochemically, the significant findings are higher levels of type III collagen, increased collagen turnover, and total collagen which approached only 70 per cent of normal tissue. Peak failure stresses were found to be only 60 per cent of normal and this value reached a plateau 14 weeks after injury.

Frank *et al.*[14] made the following definitive statement, subject to their findings regarding untreated injuries of the medial collateral ligament (Fig. 5):

Based on the vast difference between the properties of the medial collateral ligament scar and normal ligament tissue, even at 40 weeks (without treatment), it is probably safe to assume that the scar will never be mechanically normal and its components possibly never the same as the normal medial collateral ligament. (Frank *et al.*[14])

In situations where surgical repair is indicated, it has been determined that a combination of repair, short-term immobilization, and early remobilization provides the environment for optimum healing.

Vailas *et al.*[12] evaluated the healing of surgically repaired medial collateral ligaments in four groups of rats. It was concluded that surgical repair, followed by immobilization for 2 weeks, and then progressive exercise for 6 weeks, yielded the maximum values for all parameters. Although this study ended 12 weeks postoperatively, Vailas *et al.* stated that the regimen described, 'enhanced the healing process by inducing a more rapid return of tissue DNA, collagen synthesis, and separation force to within normal limits' (Fig. 6).

The use of immobilization is an important factor in the healing process, regardless of whether surgical repair or non-repair is employed. Amiel and co-workers,[11,19] have studied the effect of immobilization on collagen turnover. They found that the immobilization of intact collateral ligaments of rabbits resulted in increased collagen turnover, produced decreased stiffness, and inferior mechanical properties compared with controlled ligaments. Earlier work by Noyes[20] on primates indicated that after immobilization for 8

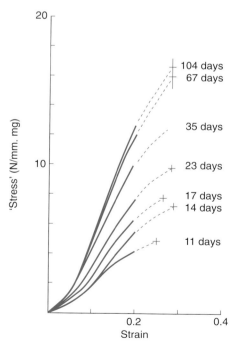

Fig. 4 Stress–strain curves for reconstituted collagen fibrils matured *in vitro* at 37 °C for different time periods after aggregation. (Redrawn from ref. 17, with permission.)

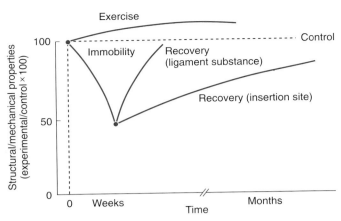

Fig. 6 The relative effects of exercise, immobilization, and remobilization on ligament complexes. (Redrawn from ref. 18, with permission.)

weeks, a decrease of 39 per cent in load to failure could be documented (Fig. 6) Furthermore, Noyes suggested that a 12-month interval after this immobilization was necessary before ligament strength returned to normal. The theoretical curves in Fig. 6 illustrate the relative effects of exercise, immobilization, and remobilization on ligament complexes.[12] Although these studies were performed on perfectly intact ligaments, it is obvious that the deleterious effects caused by prolonged immobilization must be taken into account when attempting to predict healing rates.

Cabaud *et al.*[21] studied the effects of different treatment regimens on acutely injured anterior cruciate ligaments in dogs and monkeys. It was found that monkeys that had suffered a transected anterior cruciate ligament (which was sutured and then immobilized for 6 weeks) were able to achieve a return of approximately 60 per cent of the preinjury strength, even with 4 months of rigorous exercise.

In a separate study[22] it has been shown that, regardless of the type of treatment, all healing ligaments have the same histological appearance at 6 weeks. By 12 weeks there is a trend towards the cell pattern and collagen-fibre orientation resembling that in normal ligaments. An associated return of biomechanical properties has been documented. Exercise has the most beneficial effect on mechanical properties during the 6- to 12-week period postinjury.

Savio Woo *et al.*[18] have studied the long-term results of different treatments in dogs subjected to isolated medial collateral ligament insults. Treatments ranged from non-repair and normal activity to surgical repair and immobilization for 6 weeks. This study, and others, conclude that the optimum treatment for isolated medial collateral ligament disruptions was conservative management with early mobilization. This has corroborated our clinical experience. More importantly, however, were the results which demonstrated that even with this ideal treatment, namely early mobilization, the medial collateral ligament regained only 68 per cent of the mechanical properties of the control ligaments at 48 weeks postinjury (Figs 7 and 8).

Clinical studies differ from controlled studies in that it is difficult to define accurately the degree of injury and completeness of healing achieved. As such, clinical studies cannot provide the definitive data offered by experimental investigations. It should also be recognized that a lower quality of healing may be acceptable to the non-athlete, as opposed to the very active patients who expose their ligaments to greater stress. The theoretical curve in Fig. 9 was obtained by Noyes.[20]

This curve demonstrates that during normal activity the force exerted on the anterior cruciate ligament is about 30 per cent of the force required to rupture the intact ligament. It can be assumed that during the process of repair the ligament can withstand functional activities very early in healing. However, ligament stiffness and joint laxity are also important aspects of overall joint function. Recent data by Savio Woo and others suggests that the level of failure for the anterior cruciate ligament is about 2000 N.

Summary of the ligament healing process

A framework has been provided to understand ligament healing. Clinical and experimental data regarding ligament healing can be summarized as follows.

1. Ligament healing follows the basic phases of soft-tissue healing with the strength of the healed ligament being proportional to the collagen content. An important stimulus to healing is progressive stress loading.

2. In long-term studies, both non-repaired and repaired ligaments are capable of achieving equally successful repair.

3. Early mobilization is considered an essential component to achieve optimum results. It has been shown that remobilization is most beneficial during the 6- to 12-week period postinjury.

4. Maximum mechanical strength regained in the experimental healing models does not exceed 70 per cent of the normal ligament at 48 weeks' follow-up.

5. Human ligament healing follows the same pattern of healing as that seen in most animal models, but it proceeds at a slower rate.

Sprains of the medial collateral ligament of the knee

Introduction

Sprains to the medial collateral ligament complex of the knee are very common. In most surveys, injuries to this ligament are the most frequent of all knee ligament tears. Historically, most medial collateral ligament sprains were treated with forced immobilization, combined with a prolonged programme of non-weight bearing. More recently, a functional approach has been adapted, leading to reduced morbidity and enhanced function.

Basic anatomy

Static

The architecture of the medial collateral ligament of the knee is very interesting (Fig. 10). The ligament is basically constructed of two distinct sheets—the superficial and deep components. These two ligaments take their origin from the medial femoral condyle and insert along the medial aspect of the tibia. The deep layers intimately attach to the medial meniscus, along its vascularized periphery.

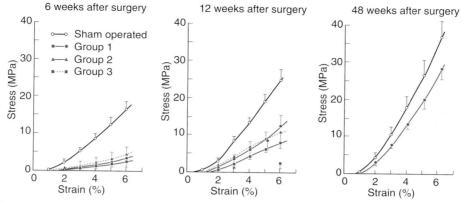

Fig. 7 The mechanical properties of the medial collateral ligament substances from sham-operated controls and experimental knees at 6, 12, and 48 weeks after surgery. (Redrawn from ref. 23, with permission.)

Specifically, the medial collateral ligament merges into the posterior medial capsule and the posterior oblique ligament.

The superficial medial collateral ligament is intimately adjacent to the semimembranosus and underlies the sartorius, gracilis and semitendinosus. The more anterior reflection of the medial collateral ligament is invaginated by the retinaculum and covered by the upper portion of the pes anserinus.

The circulation to the medial collateral ligament is provided by a cascade of vessels[25] essentially originating from the superior medial geniculate artery and the inferior medial geniculate. The vessels serving the medial collateral ligament provide the arterial supply to the peripheral rim of the medial meniscus, which is fundamental to successful meniscal repair.

Dynamic

The medial collateral ligament of the knee is vital to normal knee biomechanics, as it is the primary restraint to valgus forces about the knee. Furthermore, when the knee is externally rotated on the femur, the medial collateral ligament faces this force and thus controls, to a major degree, the efforts of external rotation. Of course, the medial collateral ligament functions in harmony with the posteromedial complex and the cruciate ligaments as secondary restraints.

The medial collateral ligament of the knee is very strong and is able to withstand a force of several hundred Newtons before failing incontinuity or disrupting grossly. The medial collateral ligament complex becomes strained whenever the knee is placed in a forced valgus position (Fig. 11).

If the knee is at 0 degrees (straight), the medial collateral ligament shares this valgus force with the posterior medial structures and the cruciate ligaments. However, once the knee is flexed to 30 degrees, and further to 60 degrees,[26] the medial collateral ligament becomes more responsible for absorbing the valgus stress.

If, or when, the medial collateral ligament fails under valgus load, then the anterior cruciate ligament will next absorb the further challenge of this continuing stress. It is vital to understand that, as the knee fails in valgus, the tibia rotates externally on the femur. Further stress will disrupt the anterior cruciate ligament and insult the articular surfaces of the femur and tibia. This will result in so-called bone bruises or overt tibial plateau fractures.

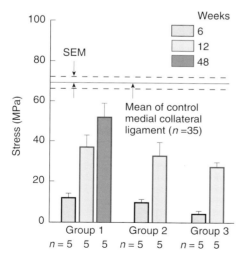

Fig. 8 Tensile strength of medial collateral ligament for all animal groups. The mean ± SEM of 35 sham-operated control medial collateral ligaments are shown. At 13 weeks, significant improvement in tensile strength was seen over that for 6 weeks ($p < 0.01$). All the experimentals had tensile strengths significantly less than those for the intact controls ($p < 0.01$). At 48 weeks, a continuing increase was noticed for the Group I experimentals, but values were still well below that for the controls. (Redrawn from ref. 23, with permission.)

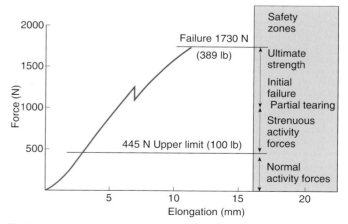

Fig. 9 Hypothetical load–elongation curve for the anterior cruciate ligament–bone unit is shown with the idealized safety zones to be considered in evaluating a ligament replacement. (Redrawn from ref. 20, with permission.)

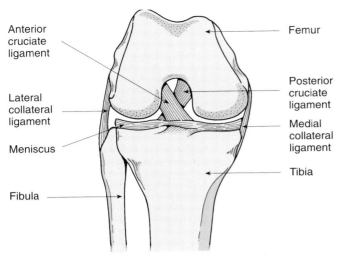

Fig. 10 Medial collateral ligament.

Mechanism of injury to the medial collateral ligament

The most frequent mechanism of injury to the medial collateral ligament complex is a forced valgus injury to the knee.[27] Typically, this trauma occurs when the athlete is hit from the lateral side and the knee is driven medially. Obviously, the injury may occur in any sporting event; however, contact sports such as soccer, rugby, ice-hockey, and football are notorious.

Sprains of the medial collateral ligament follow the traditional classification of ligament injuries and are graded as follows:

- Grade I—a microscopic structural injury to the ligament without gross disruption and which on clinical examination manifests a firm endpoint;

- Grade II—a partial macroscopic disruption of the ligament demonstrating obvious injury on inspection, and although there is an endpoint on stressing, it is softer and less distinct than with Grade I;

- Grade III—a complete gross disruption of the ligament with loss of integrity on stressing and manifesting a loss of the firm endpoint on examination.

The medial collateral ligament may be the sole victim in the valgus/external rotation type of injury. However, it is important to understand that the force may continue after the medial collateral ligament fails (Grade III injury). If the force is not totally dissipated while tearing the medial collateral ligament, then disruption of the anterior cruciate ligament may follow (Fig. 12).

Clinically, this type of injury occurs commonly and results in marked knee instability with a completely disrupted medial collateral ligament and anterior cruciate complex. Peripheral detachment of the medial meniscus, with associated bone bruises, are likely. Far less frequently, a complete knee dislocation may occur if the force is so great that it disrupts the medial collateral ligament, as well as the anterior cruciate and posterior cruciate ligaments. Although such a situation is rare, it is very serious and commonly associated with neurological or vascular insults.

Signs and symptoms of sprains of the medial collateral ligament

As mentioned previously, sprains of the medial collateral ligament are the most common knee ligament sprains. These medial collateral disruptions, or sprains, generally are Grade I or Grade II. As with all ligament sprains which are incomplete (all but Grade III insults) the knee joint remains stable but has distinct clinical manifestations.

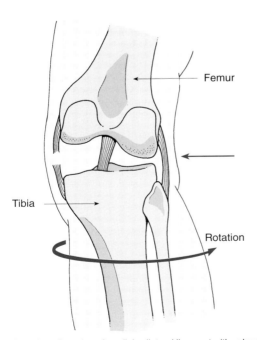

Fig. 11 Complete disruption of medial collateral ligament with valgus force.

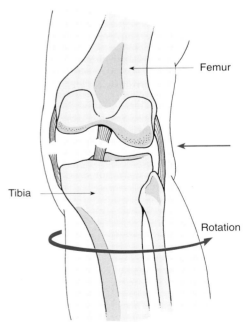

Fig. 12 Complete disruption of medial collateral ligament and anterior cruciate ligament with valgus/external rotation force.

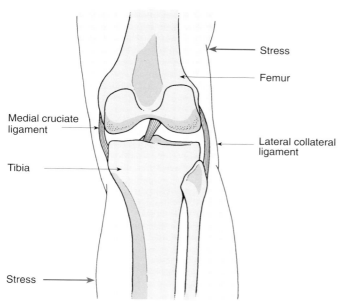

Fig. 13 Examination to stress the medial collateral ligament at 45 degrees of flexion.

Grade I sprains

Typically, the athlete will present with a history of having been struck on the lateral side of the knee with the knee straight (or bent slightly) and the knee fixed. The injury occurs so quickly that the patient/athlete has only a vague recollection of the specifics of the incident. Of course, pain is immediate and, depending on the degree of ligament disruption, may be modest or quite marked. Swelling is usually mild and without a massive haemarthrosis. Usually the athlete will immediately cease sporting activities, but there are exceptions depending on the constitution of the athlete whose pain threshold may be very high! A careful clinical examination is essential.

In the acute phase (day 1 to day 10) the knee is usually held in a position of mild flexion. The bony prominences of the knee are somewhat obscured by the swelling which is evident medially. There may be a mild effusion within the knee joint but, as stated previously, a dramatic haemarthrosis is rare. The knee is warm to the touch; however, the remainder of the knee examination can be unusually normal to palpation.

On physical stressing of the knee, the examiner must isolate the medial collateral ligament and then apply gentle force. This manoeuvre is designed to mimic the mechanism of injury. The physical examination is best conducted with the knee in 45 degrees of flexion, with the heel resting on the examining table.

With a Grade I injury, the medial collateral ligament demonstrates a firm and distinct endpoint to a valgus stress applied at this angle (Fig. 13).

Grade II sprains

A moderate sprain of the medial collateral ligament of the knee is termed a Grade II sprain of the ligament, which results in increased laxity of the joint. However, when a valgus stress test is applied to the knee at 30 to 45 degrees of flexion, the endpoint is softer but is still present. A word of caution is necessary.

It is essential to examine the opposite (normal) knee initially to gain valuable information as to the character and quality of the normal ligaments. Each individual is surprisingly different in the quality of their tissues and their inherent laxity.

With the Grade II sprain, there is usually a more severe degree of ecchymosis and swelling than with the Grade I insult, and the knee joint may demonstrate a significant effusion. Pain is obviously greater than with the more minor Grade I sprain.

Grade III sprains

The severe and complete sprain of the medial collateral ligament of the knee is a serious injury. At the point of complete disruption, the force which is applied to the knee has overwhelmed both the tensile strength of the medial collateral ligament and also associated restraints such as the anterior cruciate ligaments.

The patient/athlete usually has very severe pain, gross swelling of the soft tissues around the knee, and immediate profound disability. Indeed these athletes are unable to finish the game! Remarkably, the knee joint itself may not have a haemarthrosis.

With disruption of the medial collateral ligament and the joint capsule (which is intimate with the medial collateral ligament), the haemarthrosis commonly evacuates itself from the joint, reducing the patient's discomfort. The physical examination demonstrates that the medial collateral ligament is completely torn, with widening of the joint on valgus stressing and a very indistinct endpoint. In order to conduct this examination, in the acute phase, it is critical to have the patient relaxed or sedated. Muscle spasm and apprehension may thwart an effective and satisfactory evaluation.

In more chronic circumstances, with a complete medial collateral ligament tear, the patient will usually demonstrate clinical signs of insufficiency of the medial collateral ligament, as well as the anterior cruciate ligament: this will be discussed in the next section. Pure Grade III instability of the medial collateral ligament, without an associated anterior cruciate ligament tear, is very unusual.[28] Invariably the patient will show medial opening on valgus testing, but will have very little, if any, functional disability.

Clinical mimes

Frequently, injuries to the medial collateral ligament of the knee may be confused with other forms of knee pathology. Patients with dislocations, or subluxations of the patella, commonly present with a history of receiving a valgus force to the knee. Subsequently the knee is swollen on the medial side, and may be irritable to valgus stressing; furthermore, the injury usually occurs in the active population, particularly in young females who are very athletic. Palpation of the joint, performed carefully, will provide helpful clues to differentiate the medial collateral sprain from patella instability.

Other features which are important to remember include:

1. Tenderness will be over the medial retinaculum, adjacent to the patella, rather than over the anatomical course of the medial collateral ligament.

2. The apprehension test applied to the patella will be positive. This test is performed with lateral pressure on the patella (directed laterally) with the knee held passively at 45 degrees of flexion.

3. There is no joint gapping with patella dislocation, in contrast to Grade II and Grade III sprains to the medial collateral ligament.

Tears of the medial meniscus may occur in isolation or in combination with sprains of the medial collateral ligament. Isolated medial meniscus tears are normally a consequence of a low-energy injury such as rotation in a squatting position, in contrast with medial collateral ligament disruptions which demand significant force.

Palpation and stressing of the joint will provide the most valuable information. Joint line tenderness is usual with tears of the medial meniscus but not with disruptions of the medial collateral ligament. With isolated injuries to the medial meniscus there is some, albeit mild, apprehension to valgus stressing of the knee.

Treatment

Grade I tear—medial collateral ligament

Because of the relative stability of the knee joint, extensive clinical experience has dictated that the Grade I injury should be treated conservatively with emphasis on a functional approach.[29] The natural history of this problem is quite predictable. The patient usually suffers a modest degree of discomfort for 1 to 2 weeks, gradually resolving over 4 to 6 weeks. The athlete is able to return to full activities when the knee is painfree. However, the athlete may experience mild discomfort with acute unexpected valgus stress. This is not unusual and may linger for several months. During the acute phase of injury the following measures will prove helpful.

Acute phase—days 1 to 14

1. Apply ice to the knee four times daily for 20 to 30 min each time.

2. Apply a firm elastic wrap to the knee, allowing range of motion within the limits of pain.

3. Use a cane or crutches to allow partial weight-bearing within the limits of pain.

Subacute phase—days 14 to 28

1. Gradually increase the range of motion and weight-bearing.

2. Use progressive strengthening with organized physiotherapy to enhance the strength of the quadriceps and hamstring mechanism. Electrical muscle stimulation may prove helpful during this phase of recovery.

Chronic phase—after 28 days

1. Emphasis is now placed on strength and power training, specifically for the quadriceps and hamstring mechanisms combined with the complimentary muscle groups.

2. Institute sports-specific training, as well as more vigorous controlled challenges such as skipping, running, slalom, and eccentric loading.

3. The intermittent use of a knee brace to control valgus may be helpful to facilitate return to sports.

Grade II sprains of the medial collateral ligament

The treatment plan for medial collateral ligament tears follows the general format described for Grade I disruptions. However, the recovery period will usually be longer—upwards of 3 months before full return to sporting activities. Supportive knee bracing can be used in the latter stages of rehabilitation to support the healing

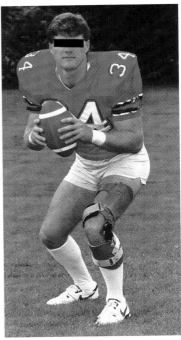

Fig. 14 A knee orthosis to provide valgus stability.

medial collateral ligament. Bracing may also enhance proprioception and allow the athlete enhanced security (Fig. 14). The athlete must continue his or her exercises for many months, as muscle function can be extremely retarded, particularly in chronic injury (when assessed late by the sports medicine practitioner), the older athlete, and the more severe Grade II tears.

Grade III medial collateral ligament sprains

Historically, complete tears of the medial collateral ligament were managed with plaster immobilization for 6 weeks, followed by rigorous and lengthy physiotherapy. The disaster of prolonged immobilization was quite predictable and led to severe muscle atrophy, which was sometimes irreversible. Furthermore, the medial collateral ligament would heal in a lengthened state, not dissimilar from the pretreatment situation. To make matters more complex, the Grade III tear is frequently associated with a complete disruption of the anterior cruciate ligament. The history of this combined instability is very perplexing, commonly leaving the athlete with a chronic knee instability which is most disabling.

Recent advances in our understanding of Grade III tears of the medial collateral ligament can be summarized as follows.

1. If the Grade III tear of the medial collateral ligament occurs in isolation, which is rare, it should be treated with pain control combined with functional bracing and aggressive rehabilitation.

2. The recovery period to full athletic activities can be upwards of 20 weeks after an isolated Grade III sprain.

3. If a medial collateral Grade III injury occurs with a complete disruption of the anterior cruciate ligament, surgical repair with reconstruction of the anterior cruciate ligament is

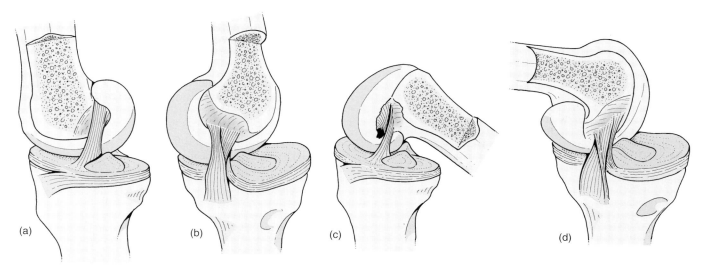

Fig. 15 (a) The anterior cruciate ligament with the knee in full extension; (b) the posterior cruciate ligament with the knee in full extension; (c) the anterior cruciate ligament with the knee in flexion; (d) the posterior cruciate ligament with the knee in flexion (most of the ligament is taut, as a small posterior portion loosens). (Redrawn from ref. 41, with permission.)

commonly necessary in order to reduce morbidity and produce a more complete restoration of function.

Summary

The medial collateral ligament complex of the knee is commonly injured in athletics as a consequence of a valgus/external rotation force. Usually the injury is incomplete and can be treated with early motion and strengthening. Prolonged immobilization can lead to impaired healing and increased morbidity.

The complete Grade III tear of the medial collateral ligament is invariably associated with a partial or complete tear of the anterior cruciate ligament. The combination of complete tears of the anterior cruciate ligament and medial collateral ligament usually demand surgical repair and/or reconstruction in order to restore knee joint stability.

Sprains of the anterior cruciate ligament of the knee

Introduction

Over the past decade injuries to the anterior cruciate ligament have received more attention than any other athletic injury.[30–34] This overwhelming attention has been generated by the high prevalence of anterior cruciate ligament tears in athletes, coupled with the associated morbidity. An athlete with anterior cruciate ligament instability is frequently unable to re-establish the preinjury performance and may never be able to return to sport. Much has been written about the best technique for treating anterior cruciate ligament tears.[30,33,35–38] However, the results have frequently proven disappointing.

The anterior cruciate ligament is the fulcrum for knee stability. Complete disruption of this ligament leaves the athlete with considerable functional instability. Rotatory instability of the knee ensues, exposing the adjacent supporting ligaments and menisci to further degeneration.

Anatomy of the anterior cruciate ligament

The anterior cruciate ligament is located in the centre of the knee joint, intertwined with its partner the posterior cruciate ligament (Fig. 15). These structures are covered with a synovial sheath, except for the posterior aspect of the posterior cruciate ligament which is essentially extrasynovial. The anterior cruciate ligament is approximately 3 cm long and takes its origin from the superior lateral bony extreme of the intercondylar notch. Some fibres at the origin of the anterior cruciate ligament actually roll around the lateral femoral condyle, in the position referred to as 'over the top'.[17,20,21,39,40]

From the bony origin, the anterior cruciate ligament of the knee traverses distally and medially to attach along the interspinous region of the tibia. The insertion of the anterior cruciate ligament of the tibia may cover an area as broad as 3 cm to 5 cm between the tibial spines.

According to Girgis and other workers,[41,42] the anterior cruciate ligament is constructed of two distinct bands, the anteromedial band and the posterolateral band. These portions of the anterior cruciate ligament are intimately attached and are not always readily distinguished on gross inspection. An intermediate band of the anterior cruciate ligament has recently been described.

The nerve supply and circulation of the anterior cruciate ligament have been discussed in the literature.[43] However, from a clinical standpoint it is vital to understand that the network of vessels permeating the anterior cruciate ligament essentially originates from the synovium and the bone–ligament interface. The intraligament blood circulation[44–46] of the anterior cruciate ligament is rather scanty, which parallels the very poor ability of the anterior cruciate ligament to heal itself.

The medial and lateral menisci,[47,48] as well as the posterior cruciate ligament, must be viewed as operating in concert with the anterior cruciate ligament. The mechanics of this intimate arrangement will be discussed in the next section. The anatomy of the anterior cruciate ligament can be summarized as follows:

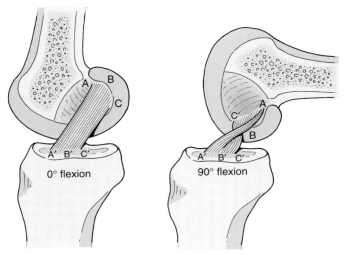

Fig. 16 In flexion there is lengthening of the anteromedial band of the anterior cruciate ligament A' and shortening of the posterolateral aspect of the anterior cruciate ligament C (C'). B (B') represents the intermediate band, which in fact is the transition between the anteromedial and the posterolateral portion. (Redrawn from ref. 41, with permission.)

1. It originates from a broad base on the medial side of the lateral femoral condyle and traverses to insert in the interspinus area of the tibia;

2. It is very strong (withstands a force of 2000 N) and is approximately 3 cm in length;

3. Its blood supply is very meagre, and hence its ability to heal, if injured, is rather poor.

The dynamic anterior cruciate ligament

Major reviews of the biomechanics of the anterior cruciate ligament of the knee have been written. From a clinical standpoint, the basics of behaviour must be understood. The anterior cruciate ligament is the major restraint controlling anterior translation of the tibia on the femur. This translation calls upon secondary restraints to assist the anterior cruciate ligament in this role; specifically the posterior cruciate ligament and the collateral ligaments constrain the anterior movement of the tibial surface as it slides forward on the femoral condyles.[49] Furthermore, the anterior cruciate ligament is able to twist upon itself as the knee moves from complete flexion to full extension (Fig. 16). With the two bands intertwined (anteromedial and posterolateral), a portion of the anterior cruciate ligament remains taut throughout this complete range of motion. The rotation of the femur and tibia is controlled by the anterior cruciate ligament, working in synchrony with the posterior cruciate ligament, collateral ligaments, and menisci.

The anterior cruciate ligament possesses very little inherent elasticity. Application of a force straining it by more than 5 per cent of its resting length, will result in rupture. This rupture may be complete and obvious on gross inspection, or it may be partial, demonstrating failure in continuity. The anterior cruciate ligament is able to resist a force of 1700 N before failure.[50-53] Recent data suggests that the tensile strength of the anterior cruciate ligament is more in the range of 2100 N.

Mechanisms for injury of the anterior cruciate ligament

The anterior cruciate ligament is disrupted as a consequence of a forced valgus stress to the knee. This force, with a blow to the outer aspect of the knee, initially disrupts the medial collateral ligament and then tears the anterior cruciate ligament as the second component of the injury. The third component of the injury complex includes detachment of the medial meniscus and bone contusions about the lateral compartment of the knee. Obviously, this injury is quite common in soccer, American football, and rugby, as tackles from the side are intrinsic to these activities.

Isolated tears of the anterior cruciate ligament, are believed to be relatively rare, and some authors have debated as to whether this injury could occur without associated soft-tissue disruption. They can occur in sports or as a result of an injury in the workplace. The knee is usually fully extended when the insult occurs. With the foot firmly planted, the athlete rotates or changes direction about the fixed foot (Fig. 17). If this unusual stress continues, the femur continues to rotate externally over the tibia at which time the anterior cruciate ligament will disrupt. Eventually, the posterolateral capsule and lateral collateral ligament will also be stretched and injured. In athletics, this is the most common mechanism of injury to the anterior cruciate ligament. Furthermore, the medial and/or lateral meniscus may be damaged during the same manoeuvre.

In combination with the posterior cruciate ligament, the anterior cruciate ligament may be completely disrupted with an insult of hyperextension to the knee. This may occur when the athlete is clipped, which is an illegal technique in most sports.

In summary, the anterior cruciate ligament is most frequently injured in sport as a consequence of a forced external rotation of the femur on the fixed tibia with the knee in full extension. A complete

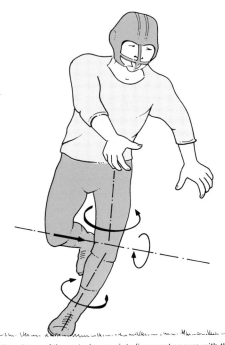

Fig. 17 An isolated tear of the anterior cruciate ligament occurs with the knee in full extension, coupled with forced internal rotation of the tibia on femur.

tear of the anterior cruciate ligament necessitates an insult of high energy (2000 N), which commonly occurs in high-velocity sporting activities. The pathology of the anterior cruciate ligament may be a complete disruption (Grade III sprain) or a more moderate sprain (Grade I or Grade II).

Signs and symptoms of sprains of the anterior cruciate ligament

The athlete suffering an injury of the anterior cruciate ligament has invariably absorbed a blow of significant violence; that is to say, tackled from the side or twisted while skiing. The patient generally has significant, if not severe, pain and usually falls to the ground immediately. When the anterior cruciate ligament is completely disrupted, a snap or pop is frequently audible and can sometimes be heard by the spectators. The athlete is rarely able to continue and retreats to the sidelines with assistance. The knee becomes swollen very rapidly, which suggests active bleeding, in contrast with a simple effusion which usually takes hours to accumulate. As the knee continues to distend with blood, the injured athlete complains of increasing pain compatible with the degree of swelling. Even with a chronic injury, the patient/athlete is frequently able to recollect the specifics of the initial injury because the severity of the pain makes the experience quite indelible.

Occasionally, the athlete will describe a lesser insult with a minor feeling of instability, followed by a further twist to the knee, triggering the snap, followed by acute pain and swelling. This scenario suggests that a partial tear of the anterior cruciate ligament occurred with the first insult which became a complete disruption with the subsequent trauma.

Consistently, an athlete with an injured anterior cruciate ligament will describe the high-energy twist to the knee, provoking a rather sickening feeling of the knee 'going one way and my body going the other'. A direct blow to the knee very rarely, if ever, injures the anterior cruciate ligament. It is usually a trauma secondary to rotation, with or without a collision.

The physical examination of the knee must be performed very carefully. If a haemarthrosis is evident, the examination will be difficult and frequently inconclusive. Aspiration of the knee to remove the haemarthrosis is appropriate. Furthermore, it may be necessary to sedate the patient to examine the extremity adequately. The patient/athlete with muscle spasm or anxiety renders the situation very tense for all concerned. This predicament can be rectified with mild sedation or general anaesthesia. The leg/knee should be unencumbered with bandages or a tourniquet, which may disguise subtle findings. In more chronic cases, inspection for muscle wasting, knee sag, or bony abnormalities is essential.

Palpation is the most important part of the physical examination of the injured knee and may provide the most useful clues to the diagnosis. It must be remembered that the knee has been injured and that movement will provoke pain and anxiety. The examiner can comfort the patient and quell further apprehension by initially examining the uninjured extremity. Palpation of the injured knee should follow a very specific routine.

1. After a complete history has been taken, the patient should point out the area most tender.

2. The examiner should avoid areas of acute tenderness until the

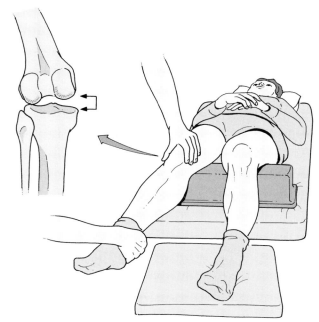

Fig. 18 The valgus stress test: the knee is held at 30 degrees of flexion and the tibia is pulled laterally as the femur is stabilized with the opposite hand. This assesses the integrity of the medial collateral ligament.

final stages of the examination. (Areas of distinct tenderness generally determine the underlying tissue damage.)

3. Palpation of the medial collateral ligament, anteromedial corner, lateral collateral ligament, posterolateral corner, and adjacent retinaculum offers clues as to which structures or combination of structures have been injured.

4. The presence or absence of an effusion or haemarthrosis should be noted. The absence of an effusion does not necessarily mean that a major ligament sprain has not occurred. If there is a tear in the capsule, the haemarthrosis may have escaped to the surrounding tissues.

5. Determining the range of motion of the knee is not helpful at this point, as restricted range of motion is predictable in view of the trauma.

6. The integrity of the medial collateral ligament and the lateral collateral ligament should be examined carefully with the knee at 30 degrees of flexion (Fig. 18). Gently springing the knee into valgus at 30 degrees of flexion will assess the integrity of the medial collateral ligament, and a varus manoeuvre can help determine the status of the lateral collateral ligament.

7. The integrity of the anterior cruciate ligament is analysed using the anterior-drawer manoeuvre, the Lachman test, or the pivot-shift manoeuvre as described below. The anterior-draw manoeuvre is performed at 90 degrees of knee flexion with a gentle pressure behind the tibial plateau, drawing the tibia forward on the femur. This technique must be performed with a progressive pull rather than aggressive tugging because reflex hamstring spasm will limit its value. (NB When the anterior cruciate ligament has been disrupted

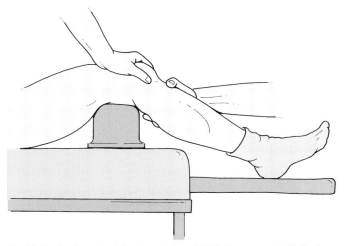

Fig. 19 The Lachman test: the knee is flexed at 30 degrees and, with the femur stabilized, the tibia is drawn forward. The degree of instability is based on the abnormal movement compared with the contralateral extremity.

completely but the collateral ligaments and the menisci are intact, the anterior-draw manoeuvre will frequently be negative.)

The Lachman test is conducted at 30 degrees of flexion with a stress identical to that used in the anterior-draw manoeuvre (Fig. 19). This stress, directed from behind the upper tibia, is designed to slide the tibia forward on the femur. The opposite hand of the examiner stabilizes the femur firmly as the stress is applied to the tibia. A positive test, compared with the opposite knee, is determined by an abnormal excursion of the tibia upon the distal femur. A minimal increase in the anteroposterior movement (less than 10 mm) is considered a mild Grade I instability. A moderate Grade II anterior cruciate ligament instability exists when the excursion is approximately 10 mm to 15 mm, and a major anteroposterior instability (Grade III) offers abnormal movement of greater than 15 mm. With this degree of instability, a very soft endpoint occurs on testing. The specificity of the Lachman manoeuvre[54] in determining the integrity of the anterior cruciate ligament is very high. At least 98 per cent of all complete anterior cruciate ligament disruptions will be obvious on performing the Lachman test. However, tight hamstrings, an anxious patient, or a joint effusion may thwart the accuracy of this examination.

The pivot-shift manoeuvre[55] is difficult to perform properly; however, it is a precise test for determining the quality of the anterior cruciate ligament (Fig. 20). It demands very precise handling of the patient, particularly after the acute injury. The patient must be relaxed and without hamstring spasm to comply with the test.

The pivot-shift stress test is designed to mimic the mechanism of the injury which produces an isolated anterior cruciate tear. The examiner attempts to demonstrate abnormal movement of the lateral tibial plateau on the fixed femur. With the knee in full extension, the examiner stabilizes the femur and then forcibly internally rotates the tibia on the femur. While maintaining this pressure, the examiner then firmly places a valgus stress on the knee while gradually flexing to 30 degrees. Abnormal displacement of the tibia on the femur occurs when the knee is in full extension under valgus load with internal rotation. The tibia then returns to its normal pos-

ition on the femur, as the knee is flexed to 30 degrees. This abnormal excursion on the tibia is seen as an abnormal slide, depending on the degree of instability and the chronicity of the anterior cruciate ligament tear.

This test is most accurate in determining the integrity of the anterior cruciate ligament; however, considerable skill and experience is required when testing knees with instability.

Differential diagnosis

Confusion can occur when the patient/athlete presents with a history of having incurred a high-energy injury to the knee, resulting in immediate pain, swelling, and profound disability. The patient will often state that the knee 'gave way' at the time of the trauma. Other causes of acute knee swelling and pain should be considered.

Patella dislocation/subluxation

Patella dislocation may provoke immediate swelling or haemarthrosis of the knee. During dislocation, the patella may injure the surface of the lateral femoral condyle, resulting in an osteochondral fracture. The resulting haemarthrosis will invariably be fat laden and will frequently recur, even after aspiration. Fat globules are rare

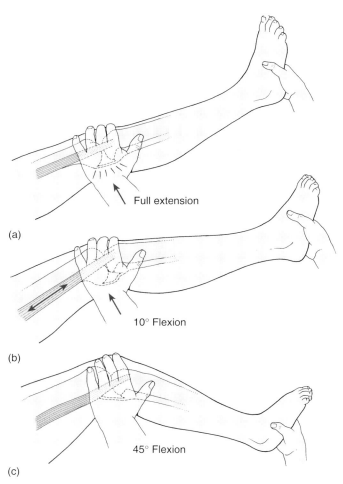

(a) Full extension
(b) 10° Flexion
(c) 45° Flexion

Fig. 20 The pivot-shift phenomenon: the abnormal subluxation of the lateral tibial plateau occurs in full extension with further flexion, the iliotibal band moves posterior and the lateral tibial plateau reduces to its normal anatomical position.

in anterior cruciate disruption, except if an avulsion of the tibial spine has occurred. Furthermore, the haemarthrosis does not generally recur once aspirated from the knee joint.

Injuries of the menisci

Detachment of the menisci from their peripheral rim can provoke an acute haemorrhage into the knee. This injury usually occurs in conjunction with a major insult to the collateral ligaments, but it can exist in isolation. If the physical examination reveals stability of the ligaments, then the meniscal tear, or detachment, as confirmed by the clinical deduction, arthroscopy, or magnetic resonance imaging (**MRI**), may be treated expectantly.

Osteochondral fractures

Acute osteochondral fractures can occur in isolation or in conjunction with an acute ligament sprain. An acute osteochondral fracture, usually of the femur, occurs as a consequence of major trauma and can provoke a major knee haemorrhage. The diagnosis may be difficult from strictly a clinical standpoint and commonly necessitates arthroscopic examination, computed tomographic (**CT**) or MRI assessment. If the fragment is large, the prudent approach necessitates surgery to secure the osteochondral fragment to its bed and allow early movement thereafter.

These clinical mimes all possess the common denominator of:

(1) provocation by major trauma;

(2) immediate pain and incapacity;

(3) rapid accumulation of joint fluid, which is usually blood;

(4) need for examination under anaesthesia, arthroscopic inspection, or specialized radiological examination to delineate the pathology accurately.

Treatment of injuries to the anterior cruciate ligament

The treatment for the disruption of the anterior cruciate ligament is very controversial. However, several features of this perplexing problem are receiving international consensus.

Grade I and Grade II sprains of the anterior cruciate ligament

Mild and moderate sprains of the anterior cruciate ligament may occur alone or in combination with sprains of the collateral ligaments.

Isolated Grade I/Grade II sprains of the anterior cruciate ligament

The history of these injuries is benign. Both these sprains are partial disruptions of the anterior cruciate ligament, leaving the knee intrinsically stable. The treatment protocol is as follows.

1. Establish the diagnosis clinically and be prepared to confirm the diagnosis with examination under anaesthesia, combined with arthroscopy.

2. When the patient has acute pain, the following measures will prove helpful. Aspirate the haemarthrosis and then apply ice packs directly to the knee; follow this with partial weight-bearing, as well as oral analgesia.

3. After 48 h on the above programme, or when the acute episode starts to resolve, support the knee with a wrap or a brace. These measures enhance the confidence of the athlete and facilitate the rehabilitation process.

4. After 1 week, and as the swelling and pain resolve, start the process of increasing the stress to the knee. This part of the rehabilitation programme, which emphasizes strength and power training, should be closely monitored by a trained therapist.

5. As the strength and power of the quadriceps muscle improves, the next phase of rehabilitation is directed towards skill acquisition—running, changing direction, and jumping. Less strenuous skills such as swimming and cycling should be accomplished before a more aggressive programme is adopted.

6. Unrestricted return to sports can occur when the athlete is able to perform all sport-specific skills in a satisfactory fashion, as judged by the therapist, the coach, and in some circumstances the parents.

Even with a partial tear of the anterior cruciate ligament (Grade I or Grade II) the recovery period may be very lengthy, sometimes approaching 20 weeks. Prolonged immobilization after the acute injury, an anxious patient or parent, and/or an inaccurate diagnosis, should always be considered if the rehabilitation process is slow.

Grade I and Grade II sprains of the anterior cruciate ligament, combined with a Grade III sprain of a collateral ligament

When an athlete suffers a complete tear of the medial collateral ligament, for instance, and a partial tear of the anterior cruciate ligament, the knee should be treated in the same fashion as the isolated Grade I/II anterior cruciate ligament sprain.

The collateral ligament will heal, albeit in a lengthened state; however, the history of this injury is benign inasmuch as it should not be treated surgically. Likewise, prolonged immobilization is unnecessary for this injury, as mandatory casting will predictably produce tissue atrophy. This atrophy may be irreversible and recalcitrant to physical therapy.

A complete tear of the lateral collateral ligament, with an incomplete tear of the anterior cruciate ligament, is most uncommon and a thorough physical examination, with or without anaesthesia, should be conducted to confirm the diagnosis.

Grade III complete sprains of the anterior cruciate ligament

A complete tear of the anterior cruciate ligament is a very serious injury and there is international debate regarding ideal treatment. The following is a personal protocol for the treatment of a Grade III anterior cruciate ligament tear.

Isolated Grade III anterior cruciate ligament sprains

Once the diagnosis is established by physical examination and confirmed by examination under anaesthesia, and/or arthroscopy, the athlete is categorized as follows.

1. The immature athlete with open epiphysis is treated non-surgically, according to the treatment protocol advocated for the Grade I/II anterior cruciate ligament sprain. However, if there is an avulsion of the ligament, one would treat this injury surgically using a transarthroscopic approach.

2. The athlete who, regardless of age, wishes to continue participating in sports, is deemed a surgical candidate. Surgery for reconstructing the anterior cruciate ligament generally utilizes a biological graft. This graft can be harvested from the semitendinosis/gracilis, the iliotibial band, or from the patellar tendon. The postoperative programme is identical with the physiotherapy designed for the Grade I/Grade II anterior cruciate ligament sprain. The time to full recovery may be 1 year.

3. The purely recreational athlete with modest sport-related expectations is treated with knee bracing, early weight-bearing, and progressive strengthening. This patient/athlete can return to the sport of choice when he or she personally feels able, on the basis of objective input from the physiotherapist. If such a patient feels that his or her knee disability is profound, surgical reconstruction of the anterior cruciate ligament is the treatment of choice.

There are controversies surrounding the treatment for anterior cruciate sprains.[32,34,56,57]

1. Direct surgical repair of the torn anterior cruciate ligament should not be the sole method of restoring anterior cruciate ligament integrity. If the anterior cruciate ligament is avulsed with a fragment of the tibia or femur, then securing the bony fragment is accepted as a legitimate surgical measure.

2. Knee bracing provides a valuable aid to the patient taking part in a sport with an anterior cruciate ligament tear.[58] Most knee braces will control approximately 40 per cent of the anterior cruciate instability (Fig. 21).

3. Physiotherapy, following reconstruction of the anterior cruciate ligament, is a vital part of the rehabilitation process. Early mobilization with a progressive increase in the stress to the anterior cruciate ligament reconstruction is fundamental. Current difficulties following anterior cruciate reconstructive surgery include arthrofibrosis and osteoarthritis, rather than recurrence of the instability.

Grade III sprains of the anterior cruciate ligament in combination with sprains of the collateral ligaments

Although the anterior cruciate ligament commonly disrupts in isolation, this injury may be accompanied by sprains of the medial collateral ligament, the lateral collateral ligament, and/or the posterior cruciate ligament. When an athlete presents with an acute or chronic complete medial collateral and anterior cruciate ligament disruption, reconstruction of the latter with repair or reconstruction of the former is most appropriate. The medial collateral ligament acts as a major stress shield for the anterior cruciate ligament, which is thus valuable to the reconstruction of the anterior cruciate.

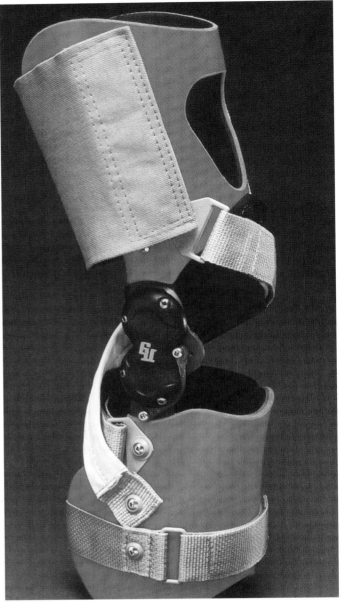

Fig. 21 Custom-made derotation brace designed to control anterior cruciate instability.

In the sedentary individual, functional cast-bracing after the acute injury may be sufficient to facilitate rehabilitation.[59] A knee brace may be required to provide functional stability during more challenging activities.

Complete sprains of the lateral collateral ligament of the knee usually occur with disruption of the anterior cruciate ligament and frequently the posterior cruciate ligament. This circumstance, when possible, requires surgical repair and reconstruction of all structures.

The posterolateral capsule and support structures must be reconstructed to thwart posterolateral instability. However, it must be remembered that the anterior cruciate ligament remains the cornerstone to the knee, and thus usually commands surgical attention if completely disrupted in combination with its neighbours: the medial collateral ligament, lateral collateral ligament, and/or posterior cruciate ligament.[31-34,36,60-69]

Posterior cruciate ligament

As stated previously, the knee is one of the most complex joints within the human body. Considerable demands are placed upon the knee during everyday activities, particularly in view of our bipedal gait. By virtue of its bony construction, the knee is unstable, but it is supported by a number of muscles, ligaments, and cartilages that hold the osseous structures in proper alignment throughout all phases of movement. To reiterate, these structures act as a unit, but their functions can be separated (to a certain degree) during clinical examination.

We shall discuss the posterior cruciate ligament in isolation, but its dependence on the other soft-tissue structures must be remembered.

Anatomy

The posterior cruciate ligament arises from the tibial plateau in a rather narrow attachment in the most posterior aspect of the intra-articular region, essentially in a groove in the posterior aspect of the tibia well below the joint line. From there, it travels upwards, forwards, and medially, and fans out to a wide insertion on the lateral surface of the medial femoral condyle; namely, the medial aspect of the intercondylar notch (Fig. 22).

The average length of the posterior cruciate ligament has been determined to be 38 mm, and its width 13 mm, although it fans out proximally to 32 mm[41] at its insertion on the medial femoral condyle. Most of its blood supply is from the medial geniculate artery, branches of which reach the posterior cruciate ligament via the synovial membrane which surrounds it.[70]

The femoral attachment of the posterior cruciate ligament is in the form of a semicircle; the proximal edge is straight and perpendicular to the long axis of the femur, while the distal edge is convex and lies in the transverse plane. By virtue of the position of its attachments, the posterior cruciate ligament can be separated into two functional units which blend into one another and are not anatomically separable. These are simply called the anterior and posterior portions of the posterior cruciate. Both sections arise from the rather narrow tibial attachment, and as the ligament fans out the anterior portion inserts into the distal convex part of the femoral

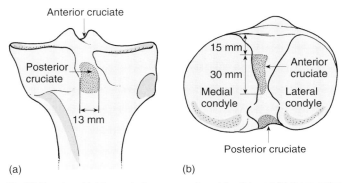

Fig. 22 Drawing of (a) the posterior upper portion of the tibia and (b) the superior surface of the tibia to demonstrate the average measurements and relationships of the tibial attachments of the anterior and posterior cruciate ligaments. (Redrawn from ref. 41, with permission.)

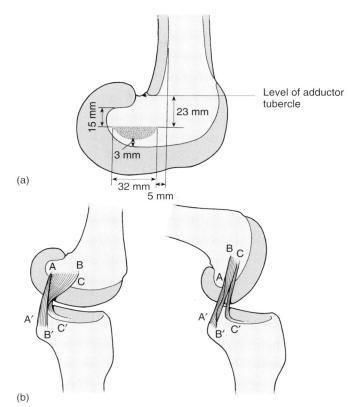

Fig. 23 Structure and attachments of the posterior cruciate ligament. (a) Lateral surface of the medial condyle of the femur showing average measurements and relationships of femoral attachment of posterior cruciate ligament (shaded area). (b) Change in shape and tension of posterior cruciate ligament components in extension and flexion. With flexion there is tightening of the bulk of the ligament, B–B', but less tension on the small band, A–A'. C–C' is the ligament of Humphry attached to the lateral meniscus. (Redrawn from ref. 41, with permission.)

attachment while the much smaller posterior portion extends to the upper limit of the femoral insertion (Fig. 23).

In 70 per cent of knees a band of fibres will extend from the posterior cruciate ligament to the posterior horn of the lateral meniscus; this structure is known as the anterior or posterior meniscofemoral ligament, depending on its relationship to the posterior cruciate ligament as it passes to the meniscus. It is also known as the ligament of Humphrey and/or ligament of Wrisberg. Only rarely will both structures be present in the same knee, but occasionally one may be quite robust and well developed.[71] In these cases, they may actually be strong enough to mask classic findings on clinical examination.

Biomechanics

The posterior cruciate ligament works in concert with the anterior cruciate ligament (and other soft-tissue structures) to stabilize the knee. The bulk of the fibres of the posterior cruciate ligament (chiefly its anterior portion) are taut when the knee is fully flexed and relaxed as the knee is extended, while the majority of the posterior fibres of the anterior cruciate ligament are loose in flexion and taut in full extension[41] (Fig. 24).

The main function of the posterior cruciate ligament is to resist posterior displacement of the tibia on the femur in the flexed knee—

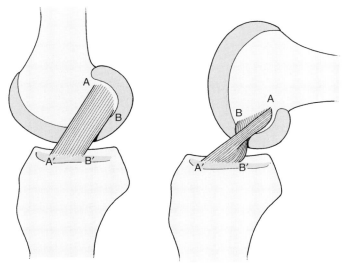

Fig. 24 Drawing presenting changes in shape and relative tension of the anterior (A–A') and posterior portions (B–B') of the anterior cruciate ligament in extension and 90 degrees of flexion. (Redrawn from ref. 41, with permission.)

it provides 95 per cent of the restraining force to this posterior-drawer movement.[71] The posterior cruciate ligament also helps to resist varus and valgus forces, and to a lesser extent helps to prevent internal rotation of the tibia on the femur in the flexed knee.[41] It also appears to assist in the 'screw home' mechanism of internal rotation of the femur on the tibia which locks the knee in full extension, preventing any significant rotation in this position.

Overall, the posterior cruciate ligament is one of the most important, if sometimes underrated, stabilizers of the knee.[72,73] Its tensile strength at the point of failure is normally twice that of the anterior cruciate ligament (average of 3400 N).[74]

Injury to the posterior cruciate ligament

Because of the interdependence of all the knee-supporting structures, isolated posterior cruciate ligament rupture can occur but is unusual. Associated injuries found during surgery for posterior cruciate ligament repair include anterior cruciate ligament tears, medial collateral ligament tears, posterior oblique capsular ligamentous damage, lateral compartment damage, and meniscal tears (usually medial meniscus).[75]

Injury to the posterior cruciate ligament occurs in the flexed knee, as most of the fibres are taut, when the tibia is driven posteriorly on the femur with substantial force. The most common scenario is a motor-vehicle accident, when the tibia strikes the dashboard and is suddenly stopped while the femur continues forward with the inertia of the body. In sports injuries, the posterior cruciate ligament is damaged when the athlete falls on to a flexed knee with the foot plantar-flexed. In this case, force is delivered through the tibial tubercle, causing a shear force on the posterior cruciate ligament. If the foot is dorsiflexed, most of the force is absorbed by the patella, which may be fractured while transferring the energy to the femur, and the posterior cruciate ligament is spared (Fig. 25).

A similar injury may be caused by hyperextension and rotation on a planted foot, where the posterior cruciate ligament ruptures before the anterior cruciate ligament (Fig. 26).[71]

Treatment

Before any course of treatment is introduced, the exact nature of the injury must be understood. A physiological classification of acute versus chronic can be determined from the patient's history and physical examination, but more invasive methods are required to define the tear anatomically; the defect may be in the substance of the posterior cruciate ligament, or a bone fragment may be avulsed from either the femoral or (more commonly) the tibial attachment.[77] In most cases, diagnostic arthroscopy can define the nature of the ligamentous damage and also discover the extent of the associated injuries which commonly occur. This must be performed cautiously as some injuries may escape detection, and during arthrotomy one must be prepared to modify techniques as the local anatomy demands.

Whatever the mechanism of injury, the force required to disrupt the posterior cruciate ligament is considerable. Before the weakest portion of the ligament fails, stretching occurs, resulting in diffuse interstitial damage and overall lengthening of the posterior cruciate ligament. This has been documented for injuries involving bone avulsions,[56] and is probably equally true for rupture through the substance of the ligament. Therefore, any repair should shorten the posterior cruciate ligament to stabilize the knee effectively. Theoretically, this may be done by overlapping the torn ends of the ligament or advancing the avulsed fragment of bone as the repair is performed. Reconstruction with autograft is usually necessary.

If the patient presents in the acute phase, within 2 or 3 days of the injury, immediate primary repair is warranted,[77-79] as this seems to give the best functional results in the long term. Interstitial tears should be repaired first, incorporating the posterior capsule for added support. Complimentary grafting is vital as direct repair alone is unsatisfactory. This will also tend to increase the blood supply to the damaged ligament. If a piece of bone has been avulsed, it should be placed in position (slightly advanced beyond its anatomical position, as mentioned above), and stabilized with a screw or staple (Fig. 27).

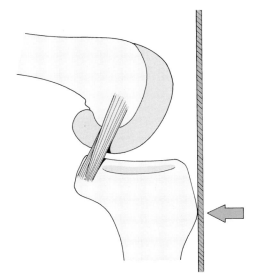

Fig. 25 Injury of the posterior cruciate ligament when the athlete falls on to a flexed knee with the foot plantar-flexed.

The treatment of more chronic injuries is the subject of much controversy. Some authors[78,80,81] have reported good results with conservative treatment in a limited number of patients. This therapy is based on an intensive physiotherapy programme, with the aim of strengthening the quadriceps femoris, gastrocnemius, and hamstring muscles. These act as dynamic stabilizers of the knee, and when strengthened can give good symptomatic relief in patients who place only moderate demands on their knees. The knee does not return to normal with this treatment and will show evidence of instability on examination with a subjective feeling of unsteadiness, particularly on bearing weight on a semiflexed knee. However 50 to 75 per cent of patients will judge the functional result as at least adequate for the activities of daily living, not requiring any further intervention. Some of these patients have been followed for 2 years,[81] and have demonstrated good maintenance of symptomatic relief up to that point. These results, as applicable to a limited num-

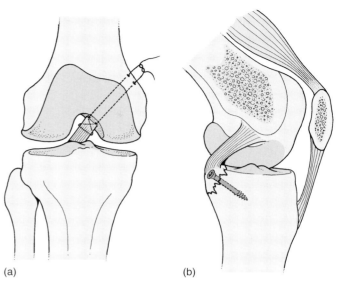

Fig. 27 (a) Reattachment of the posterior cruciate ligament to the medial femoral condyle. (b) Screw reattachment of a bone fragment avulsed with the posterior cruciate ligament from the posterior tibia.

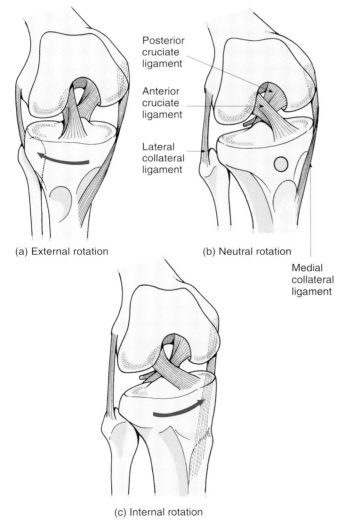

Fig. 26 In addition to their synergistic functions, cruciate and collateral ligaments exercise basic antagonistic functions during rotation. (a) In external rotation it is collateral ligaments that tighten and inhibit excessive rotation by becoming crossed in space. (b) In neutral rotation none of the four ligaments is under unusual tension. (c) In internal rotation collateral ligaments become more vertical and are more lax, while cruciate ligaments become coiled around each other and come under strong tension. (Redrawn from ref. 76, with permission.)

ber of patients, are encouraging, but until long-term follow-up is available, recommendations arising from these reports should be viewed with caution.

However, long-term difficulties do arise in these patients. The abnormal tracking of the knee joint in the absence of the posterior cruciate ligament accelerates degenerative changes in the articular surfaces with resultant early osteoarthritis.[71] The fact that these changes are not seen within the first 1 to 2 years postinjury, but are quite commonly found thereafter, supports the hypothesis that this degeneration is produced by abnormal wear rather than by any damage to the articular surface that was produced at the time of injury. Most recently, MRI imaging of the knee has suggested that both factors may be implicated in producing joint damage.

Competitive athletes and others who place heavy demands on their knee joints cannot accept the disability associated with conservative therapy, and many different operative procedures have been developed in an attempt to recreate a normal or near-normal knee. These procedures are designed mainly to deal with injuries in the chronic phase, although some authors[71] advocate reconstruction in the acute phase since they have found the results of primary repair of interstitial tears to be somewhat inferior.

Free patellar-tendon graft has been used to reconstruct the posterior cruciate ligament with ostensibly excellent results.[71] The midportion of the patellar tendon (some 10 to 12 mm wide), together with both osseous attachments, is harvested and then secured with the knee flexed at 90 degrees. The bone attachments are placed within drill holes, and animal experiments have shown that these will revascularize readily. The alignment of the graft is important; it must lie in the exact line of the original posterior cruciate ligament. Just prior to closure of the arthrotomy, a posterior-drawer stress is placed on the knee in order to ensure static stability. Postoperatively, the patient should have his or her knee immobilized for 7 to 10 days, after which an intensive course of specialized physiotherapy is started. The total recovery time until the knee can be safely subjected to moderate stresses is 5 to 6 months. When this procedure is followed, static stability is usually excellent, and most patients eventually return to their original level of athletic activity.[56]

The free tendon graft, as inserted, is obviously ischaemic. Histological studies have documented a degree of ischaemic necrosis, followed by revascularization, and finally, remodelling.[82]

The strength of the graft actually decreases in the first 3 months or so, during the ischaemic and revascularization phases. Clinically, this may lead to a transient increase in posterior–anterior instability. During the remodelling phase, the graft has the potential to increase its strength in response to its environment. Andrish and Woods augmented their grafts with Dacron in an attempt to protect the reconstruction during the initial stages, when the graft is weakest. However, they observed significant resorption of the biological graft, as well as failure of the synthetic material. Only 4 out of 10 experimental knees maintained the ligament and Dacron graft intact, and in only 2 of those 4 was the tensile strength more than that of the contralateral control knee. This atrophy of the ligament was attributed to stress shielding, and demonstrates the dependence of the graft on external stresses during the remodelling period.

Another procedure for posterior cruciate ligament reconstruction involves the use of the gastrocnemius muscle for the reconstruction.[84,85] The medial head of the gastrocnemius is removed from its femoral attachment, with or without an attached bone block, and directed anteriorly through a hole in the posterior capsule.

A drill hole is made in the medial femoral condyle from just anterior to the origin of the medial collateral ligament to the old site of insertion of the posterior cruciate ligament in the intercondylar notch. The gastrocnemius is pulled through the drill hole, with the bone block (if one is used) lying in a slot cut adjacent to the drill hole. A heavy non-absorbable suture or cancellous screw is used for fixation. In this position, the gastrocnemius acts as a dynamic stabilizer, pulling the femur posteriorly on the tibia as it contracts (Fig. 28). Weight-bearing can begin as soon as the patient is relatively comfortable, and most activities can be resumed within 4 to 6 weeks. Approximately 80 per cent of patients will have good to excellent results,[84,85] with substantially decreased pain and instability.

Iliotibial band, semitendinosis tendon, popliteus tendon, and meniscus have all been used for posterior cruciate ligament reconstruction, although not as successfully as the procedures previously mentioned. Various synthetic replacements have been introduced, but 50 per cent or more are unsuccessful because of breakdown of the implant.[85]

Conventional wisdom suggests the use of autogenous semitendinosis-gracilis grafts or free patellar-tendon grafts are the ideal.

Achilles tendon allografts have also been employed with some success.[86–93]

Summary

In a joint as complex as the knee, it is difficult to separate out an individual structure such as the posterior cruciate ligament for study and treatment. Any method of repair or reconstruction must take into account the interdependence of all the supporting structures of the knee.

Many different operative procedures have been developed over the years for reconstruction of the posterior cruciate ligament. Data

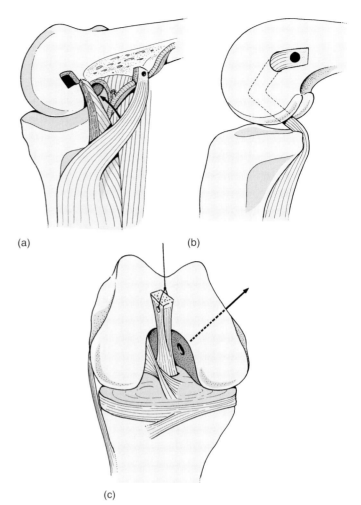

(a)   (b)

(c)

Fig. 28 The transfer of the medial head of the gastrocnemius for posterior cruciate reconstruction employs the posterior entry of the bone plug to sit in the original site of the posterior cruciate origin on the inner aspect of the medial femoral condyle. (Redrawn from ref. 84, with permission.)

for the long-term analysis of these procedures are still pending, but as these become available we shall have a clear idea of the best therapy for posterior cruciate ligament injuries with and without damage to associated structures.

References

1. O'Donoghue DH, *et al*. Repair of the anterior cruciate ligament in dogs. *Journal of Bone and Joint Surgery* 1966; **48A**: 503–19.
2. Hughston JC. The anterior cruciate deficient knee. *American Journal of Sports Medicine* 1983; **11**: 1.
3. Peacock, EE. *Wound repair*. 3rd edn. Philadelphia: WB Saunders, 1984.
4. Schmid-Schonbein GW, Woo SLY, Zweifock BW, eds. *Frontiers in biomechanics*. New York: Springer-Verlag, 1986.
5. Hunter LY, Funk JF, eds. *Rehabilitation of the injured knee*. St Louis: C.V. Mosby, 1984.
6. Dunphy JE. *Wound healing*. New York: Medcom Press, 1974.
7. Johnson RJ. The anterior cruciate ligament problem. *Clinical Orthopaedics and Related Research* 1983; **172**: 14.
8. Bucknall TE, Ellis H. *Wound healing for surgeons*. London: Bailliere Tindall, 1984.
9. O'Donoghue DH. A method for replacement of the anterior cruci-

ate ligament of the knee. *Journal of Bone and Joint Surgery* 1963; **45A**: 905–24.

10. Stanish WD, Rubinovich M, Kozey J, McGillivary G. The use of electricity in ligament and tendon repair. *Physican and Sportsmedicine* 1985; **13**: 109–16.

11. Amiel D, Akeson WH, Harwood FL, Frank CB. Stress deprivation effect on metabolic turnover of the medial collateral ligament collagen. *Clinical Orthopaedics and Related Research* 1983; **172**: 265–70.

12. Vailas AC, *et al.* Physical activity and its influence on the repair process of medial collateral ligaments. *Connective Tissue Research* 1981; **9**: 25–31.

13. Fung YC. *Biomechanics—mechanical properties of living tissues.* New York: Springer-Verlag, 1981.

14. Frank C, Amiel D, Woo SLY, Akeson WH. Normal ligament properties and ligament healing. *Clinical Orthopaedics and Related Research* 1985; **196**: 15–25.

15. Frank C, Woo SL, Amiel D, Harwood F, Gomez M, Akeson WH. Medial collateral ligament healing. *American Journal of Sports Medicine* 1983; **11**: 379–89.

16. Frank C, Amiel D, Akeson WH. Healing of the medial collateral ligament of the knee. *Acta Orthopaedica Scandinavica* 1983; **54**: 917–23.

17. Danielson CC. Mechanical properties of reconstituted collagen fibrils. *Connective Tissue Research* 1983 ; **9**: 219–25.

18. Woo SLY, *et al.* The biomechanical and morphological changes in the medial collateral ligament of the rabbit after immobilization and remobilization. *Journal of Bone and Joint Surgery* 1987; **69A**: 1200–11.

19. Amiel D, Wood SLY, Harwood FL, Akeson WH. The effect of immobilization of collagen turnover in connective tissue: a biochemical–biomechanical correlation. *Acta Orthopaedica Scandinavica* 1982; **53**: 325–32.

20. Noyes FR. Functional properties of knee ligaments and alterations induced by immobilization. *Clinical Orthopaedics and Related Research* 1977; **123**: 210–42.

21. Cabaud HE, Rodkey WG, Feagin JA. Experimental studies of acute anterior cruciate ligament injury and repair. *American Journal of Sports Medicine* 1979; **7**: 18–22.

22. Gomez MA, Woo SL, Inoue M, Amiel D, Harwood F, Kitabayashi L. Medial collateral ligament healing subsequent to different treatment regimens. *Journal of Applied Physiology* 1989; **66**: 245–52.

23. Woo SLY, Inque M, McGurk-Burleson E, Gomez MA. Treatment of the medial collateral ligament injury. *American Journal of Sports Medicine* 1987; **15**: 22–9.

24. Noyes FR, Keller CS, Grood ES, *et al.* Advances in the understanding of knee ligament injury, repair, and rehabilitation. *Medicine and Science in Sports and Exercise* 1984; **16**, No. 5.

25. Arnoczky SP, Warren RF. Microvasculature of the human meniscus. *American Journal of Sports Medicine* 1982; **10**: 90–5.

26. Shaperio MS, Markolf KL, Finerman GAM, Mitchell PW. The effect of section of the medial collateral ligament on force generated on the anterior cruciate ligament. *Journal of Bone and Joint Surgery* 1991; **73A**: 248–56.

27. Fetto JF, Marshall JL. Medial collateral ligament injuries of the knee: a rationale for treatment. *Clinical Orthopaedics and Related Research* 1978; **132**: 206–18.

28. Seering WP, Piziali RL, Nagel DA, Schurman DJ. The function of the primary ligaments in the knee in varus-valgus and axiorotation. *Journal of Biomechanics* 1980; **13**: 785–94.

29. Indelicato PA. The non-operative management of complete tears of the medial collateral ligament of the knee. *Journal of Bone and Joint Surgery* 1983; **65A**: 323–9.

30. Andrews JR, Carson WG, eds. Symposium on the anterior cruci-

ate ligament, Part II. *Orthopaedic Clinics of North America* 1985; **16**: 2.

31. Arnold JA, Coker TP, Heaton LM, Park JP, Harris WD. Natural history of anterior cruciate tears. *American Journal of Sports Medicine* 1979; **7**: 305–13.

32. Balkfors B. The course of knee ligament injuries. *Acta Orthopaedica Scandinavica (Suppl.)* 1982; **198**: 1–99.

33. Clancy WG, Ray JM, Zoltan DJ. Acute third degree anterior cruciate ligament injury. A prospective study of conservative nonoperative treatment and operative treatment with repair and patellar tendon augmentation. *American Journal of Sports Medicine* 1985; **13**: 435–6.

34. Fetto JF, Marshall JL. The natural history and diagnosis of anterior cruciate ligament insufficiency. *Clinical Orthopaedics and Related Research* 1980; **147**: 29–38.

35. Barrett GR, Jiminez WP, Thomas JM. Aggressive rehabilitation protocol following anterior cruciate ligament reconstruction (bone–patella–bone). *Journal of the Mississippi State Medical Association* 1991; **32**: 45–8.

36. Eriksson E. Sports injuries of the knee ligaments. Their diagnosis, treatment, rehabilitation, and prevention. *Medicine and Science in Sports* 1976; **8**: 133–44.

37. Noyes FR, Bassett RW, Grood ES, Butler DL. Arthroscopy in acute traumatic hemarthroses of the knee: incidence of anterior cruciate tears and other injuries. *Journal of Bone and Joint Surgery* 1980; **62A**: 687–95.

38. Odensten M, Lysholm J, Gillquist J. Sutures of fresh ruptures of the anterior cruciate ligament—a five year follow-up. *Acta Orthopaedica Scandinavica* 1984; **55**: 270–2.

39. Daniel D, Akeson W, O'Connor J. *Knee ligaments: structure, function, injury, and repair.* New York: Raven Press, 1990.

40. Slocum DB, Larson RL. Rotatory instability of the knee. Its pathogenesis and clinical test to demonstrate its presence. *Journal of Bone and Joint Surgery* 1968; **50(A)**: 211–25.

41. Girgis FG, Marshall JL, Al Monajen ARS. The cruciate ligaments of the knee: anatomical functional and experimental analysis. *Clinical Orthopaedics and Related Research* 1975; **106**: 216–31.

42. Kennedy JC, Weinberg HW, Wilson AS. The anatomy and function of the anterior cruciate ligament as determined by clinical and morphological studies. *Journal of Bone and Joint Surgery* 1974; **56A**: 223–35.

43. Barrack RL, Skinner HB. The sensory function of knee ligaments. In: Daniel D, Akeson W, O'Connor J, eds. *Knee ligaments: structure, function, injury and repair.* New York: Raven Press, 1990: 95–114.

44. Arnoczky SP. Anatomy of the anterior cruciate ligament. *Clinical Orthopaedics and Related Research* 1983; **172**: 19–25.

45. Arnoczky SP. Blood supply to the anterior cruciate ligament and supporting structures. *Orthopaedic Clinics of North America* 1985; **16**: 15–28.

46. Arnoczky SP, Rubin RM, Marshall JL. Microvasculature of the cruciate ligament and its response to injury. *Journal of Bone and Joint Surgery* 1979; **61A**: 1221–9.

47. Brantigan OC, Voshell AF. The mechanics of ligaments and meniscii of the knee joint. *Journal of Bone and Joint Surgery* 1941; **23**: 44–66.

48. Brantigan OC, Voshell AF. The tibial collateral ligament: its function, its bursae and its relation to the medial meniscus. *Journal of Bone and Joint Surgery* 1943; **25**: 121–31.

49. Woo SLY, Young EP, Kwan MK. Fundamental studies in knee ligament mechanics. In: Daniel D, Akeson W, O'Connor J, eds. *Knee ligaments: structure, function, injury and repair.* New York: Raven Press, 1990: 115–34.

50. Noyes FR, DeLucas JL, Torvik PJ. Biomechanics of anterior cruciate ligament failure: an analysis of strain rate sensitivity and

mechanisms of failure in primates. *Journal of Bone and Joint Surgery* 1974; **56A**: 236–53.

51. Noyes FR, Grood ES. The strength of the anterior cruciate ligament in humans and rhesus monkeys: age related and species related changes. *Journal of Bone and Joint Surgery* 1976; **58A**: 1074–82.

52. Smith JW. The elastic properties of anterior cruciate ligaments of the rabbit. *Journal of Anatomy* 1954; **88**: 369–80.

53. Trent PS, Walker PS, Wolf B. Ligament length patterns, strength, and rotational axes of the knee joint. *Clinical Orthopaedics and Related Research* 1976; **117**: 263–70.

54. Torj JS, Conrad W, Kalen V. Clinical diagnosis of anterior cruciate ligament instability in the athlete. *American Journal of Sports Medicine* 1976; **4**: 84–93.

55. Galway RD, Beaupre A, MacIntosh DL. Pivot shift. A clinical sign of symptomatic anterior cruciate insufficiency. Proceedings of the Canadian Orthopaedic Association. *Journal of Bone and Joint Surgery* 1972; **54B**: 763–4.

56. Clancy WG. Knee ligament injury in sports: the past, present and future. *Medicine and Science in Sports*, 1983; **15**: 9–14.

57. Hirshman HP, Daniel DM, Miyasaka Kenji. The fate of unoperated knee ligament injuries. In: Dale Daniel, *et al.*, eds. *Knee ligaments structure, function, injury and repair*. New York: Raven Press, 1990: 481–503.

58. Marans HG, Jackson RW, Picconin J, Silver RL, Kennedy DK. Functional testing of braces for anterior cruciate ligament-deficient knees. *Canadian Journal of Surgery* 1991; **34**, 167–72.

59. Kannus P, Jarvinen M. conservatively treated tears of the anterior cruciate ligament of the knee. *Journal of Bone and Joint Surgery* 1987.

60. Nisonson B. Anterior cruciate ligament injuries. Conservative versus surgical treatment. *Physician and Sportsmedicine* 1991; **19**: 82–9.

61. Noyes FR, McGinniss GH, Grood ES. The variable functional disability of the anterior cruciate ligament deficient knee. *Orthopedic Clinics of North America* 1985; **16**: 47–67.

62. O'Brien SJ, Warren RF, Pavlov H. Reconstruction of the chronically insufficient anterior cruciate ligament with the central third of the patellar tendon. *Journal of Bone and Joint Surgery* 1991; **73A**: 278–85.

63. Palmer I. On the injuries to the ligaments of the knee joint. A clinical study. *Acta Chirurgica Scandinavica (Suppl.)* 1938; 53.

64. Smillie IS. *Injuries of the knee joint*. 5th edn. Edinburgh: Churchill Livingstone, 1978: 189–253.

65. McKernan DJ, *et al.* Tensile properties of grisilis semi-tendinosis and patellar tendons from the same donor. *Transactions from the 41st Orthopaedic Research Society* 1995; **20**: 39.

66. Bach BR, Jones GT, Sweet FA, Hager CA. Arthroscopy assisted anterior cruciate ligament reconstruction using patellar tendon substitutions. *American Journal of Sports Medicine* 1994; **22**: 758–67.

67. Andersson C, Odensten M, Good L, Gillequist J. Surgical or nonsurgical treatment of acute ruptures of the anterior cruciate ligament: a randomized study with long-term follow-up. *Journal of Bone and Joint Surgery* 1989; **71A**: 965–74.

68. Stanish WD, Lai A. New concepts of rehabilitation following anterior cruciate reconstruction. *Clinics of Sports Medicine* 1993; **12**: 1.

69. Shelbourne KD, Klootwyk T. The miniarthrotomy technique for anterior cruciate ligament reconstruction. *Operative Techniques in Sports Medicine* 1993; **1**: 26–39.

70. Scapinelli R. Studies on the vasculature of the human knee joint. *Acta Anatomica* 1968; **70**: 305–31.

71. Clancy WG, Shelbourne KD, Zoellner GB, Keen JS, Reider B, Rosenberg TD. Treatment of knee joint instability secondary to

rupture of the posterior cruciate ligament. *Journal of Bone and Joint Surgery* 1983; **65A**: 310.

72. Butler DL, Noyes ER, Grood E. Ligamentous restraints to anterior–posterior drawer in the human knee. *Journal of Bone and Joint Surgery* 1980; **62A**: 259–70.

73. Hughson JC, Andrews JR, Cross MJ, Moschi A. classification of knee ligament instabilities, Part 1. *Journal of Bone and Joint Surgery* 1976; **58A**: 159–72.

74. Kennedy JC, Hawkins RJ, Willis RB, Danylchuk KD. Tension studies on human knee ligaments. Yield point, ultimate failure and disruption of the cruciate and tibial collateral ligament. *Journal of Bone and Joint Surgery* 1976; **58A**: 350–5.

75. Loos WC, Fox JM, Blazina ME, Del Pizzo W, Friedman MJ. Acute posterior cruciate ligament injuries. *American Journal of Sports Medicine* 1981; **10**: 150–4.

76. Müller W. *The knee: form, function, and ligamentous reconstruction.* New York: Springer-Verlag, 1983.

77. Bianchi M. Acute tears of the posterior cruciate ligament: clinical study and results of operative treatment in 27 cases. *American Journal of Sports Medicine* 1983; **11**: 308–14.

78. Cross MJ, Powell JF. Long term follow-up of posterior cruciate ligament rupture: a study of 116 cases. *American Journal of Sports Medicine* 1984; **12**: 292–7.

79. Strand T, Molster AO, Engesaeter LB, Raugstad TS, Alho A. Primary repair in posterior cruciate ligament injuries. *Acta Orthopaedica Scandinavica* 1984; **55**: 545–7.

80. Dandy DJ, Pusey RS. The long term results of unrepaired tears of the posterior cruciate ligament. *Journal of Bone and Joint Surgery* 1982; **64B**: 92–5.

81. Tegner Y, Lysholm J, Gillquist J, Oberg B. Two year follow-up of conservative treatment of knee ligament injuries. *Acta Orthopaedica Scandinavica* 1984; **55**: 176–80.

82. Chiroff RT. Experimental replacement of the anterior cruciate ligament. A histological and microradiographic study. *Journal of Bone and Joint Surgery* 1975; **57A**: 1124.

83. Andrish JT, Woods LD. Dacron augmentation in anterior cruciate reconstruction in dogs. *Clinical Orthopaedics and Related Research* 1984; **183**: 298–302.

84. Insall JN, Hood RW. Bone block transfer of the medial head of the gastrocnemius for posterior cruciate insufficiency. *Journal of Bone and Joint Surgery* 1982; **64A**: 691–9.

85. Kennedy JC, Galpin RD. The use of the medial head of the gastrocnemius muscle in the posterior cruciate deficient knee. Indications, techniques, results. *American Journal of Sports Medicine* 1982; **10**: 63–74.

86. Saddler SC, *et al.* Posterior cruciate ligament anatomy and length—tension behaviour of PCL fibers. *American Journal of Knee Surgery* 1996; **9**: 194–9.

87. Noyes FR, Barber-Westin SD. Treatment of complex injuries involving the posterior cruciate and posterolateral ligaments of the knee. *American Journal of Knee Surgery* 1996; **9**: 200–14.

88. Noyes FR, Barber-Westin SD. Surgical restoration to treat chronic deficiency of the posterolateral complex and cruciate ligaments of the knee. *American Journal of Sports Medicine* 1996; **24**: 415–26.

89. Veltri DM, Deng XH, Torzilli PA, Warren RF, Maynard MJ. The role of the cruciate and posterolateral ligaments instability of the knee: a biomechanical study. *American Journal of Sports Medicine* 1995; **23**: 436–43.

90. Noyes FR, Barber-Westin SD. Posterior cruciate ligament allograft reconstruction with or without a ligament augmentation device. *Arthroscopy* 1994; **10**: 371–82.

91. Peterson CA, Warren RF. The management of acute and chronic posterior cruciate ligament injuries. *American Journal of Knee Surgery* 1996; **9**: 172–84.

92. Harner CD, Xerogeanes JW, Livesey GA, *et al.* The human PCL

complex: an interdisciplinary study. *American Journal of Sports Medicine* 1995; **23**: 736–45.

93. Covey DC, Sapega AA. Injuries of the posterior cruciate ligament: current concepts review. *Journal of Bone and Joint Surgery* 1993; **75A**: 1376–86.

Further reading

Jokl P, Kaplan N, Stovell P, Keggi K. Non-operative treatment of severe injuries to the medial and anterior cruciate ligaments of the knee. *Journal of Bone and Joint Surgery* 1984; **66A**: 741–4.

Jarvinen M, Kannus P. The clinical and radiological long term results after primary knee ligament surgery. *Archives of Orthopaedic and Trauma Surgery* 1985; **104**: 1–6.

Lysholm J, Gillquist J. Evaluation of knee ligament surgery results with special emphasis on use of a scoring scale. *American Journal of Sports Medicine* 1982; **10**: 150–4.

McDaniel WJ, Dameron TB. The untreated anterior cruciate ligament rupture. *Clinical Orthopaedics* 1983; **172**: 158–63.

O'Donoghue DH. An analysis of the end results of surgical treatment of major injuries to the ligaments of the knee. *Journal of Bone and Joint Surgery* 1955; **37A**: 1–13.

Feagin, JA, Curl WW. Isolated tear of the anterior cruciate ligament: five year follow-up study. *American Journal of Sports Medicine* 1976; **4**: 95–100.

Satku K, Chew CN, Seow H. Posterior cruciate ligament injuries. *Acta Orthopaedica Scandinavica* 1984; **55**: 26–9.

4.2.3 Acute injuries of the meniscus

Owen H. Brady and Brian J. Hurson

Introduction

The advent of knee arthroscopy has provided orthopaedic surgeons with a greater understanding of knee pathology. This, combined with the increasing awareness of the functional significance of the meniscus[1-7] and the knowledge of the long-term sequelae of meniscectomy,[4,8-11] has led to major changes in the management of meniscal injuries. As a result, the removal of this structure (once merely thought of as 'vestigial fibrocartilage') is avoided at all costs. The meniscus is indeed 'a fibrocartilage of some distinction'.[12]

Embryology

The menisci develop from the proximal tibia. Embryologically, the lower limb bud appears at 4 weeks of gestation.[13] Chondrification of the femur, tibia, and fibula begins at 6 weeks, at which stage the blastema of the knee joint is present. This consists of a continuous structure which has no joint space. However, there are two identifiable chondrogenic layers which sandwich a less dense layer between them. It is this less-dense layer that develops into the menisci and cruciate ligaments. Menisci can be identified at 7 weeks and are well defined by 8 weeks of gestation.[13]

The growth of the menisci proceeds simultaneously with that of the tibia and femur. Growth configuration changes occur in response to alteration in the intra-articular condylar surfaces.[13] Histologically, the collagen fibre alignment alters in response to change in biomechanical function.[1] The longitudinal fibres develop in response to the circumferential stress and the radial fibres develop in response to tension stresses.

Prenatally, the menisci or semilunar cartilages are very cellular and have an abundant blood supply.[13] With growth, there is a gradual decrease in the vascularity of the central area.[6] This avascular area spreads radially.

Anatomy

The menisci are concentric in shape and have a triangular cross-section (Fig. 1). They have a thick, peripherally attached base which tapers centrally towards a thin free apex. Their superior concave surfaces articulate with the femoral condyles throughout all ranges of movement, while their flat inferior surfaces articulate with the tibial plateaus. The menisci cover two-thirds of the articulating surface of the tibia and transmit about 50 per cent of axial load across the joint.[7] They are attached to the intercondylar area of the tibia by tough fibrous anterior and posterior horns. Peripherally, they are attached to the synovial membrane and capsule. The coronary ligament also attaches the circumference of the menisci to the tibia, preventing excessive peripheral displacement. The anterior horns are attached to each other by the transverse ligament (when present).

Medial meniscus

The medial meniscus is semicircular, and is broader posteriorly than anteriorly (Fig. 1). Its anterior horn is attached in front of the origin of the anterior cruciate ligament. The posterior horn is attached between the posterior horn of the lateral meniscus and the origin of the posterior cruciate ligament. At its periphery, the medial meniscus is attached to the deep fibres of the medial collateral ligament (Fig. 2).

Lateral meniscus

The lateral meniscus is more circular in shape (Fig. 1). It makes up four-fifths of a circle and, unlike the medial meniscus, it has the same breadth throughout. It is attached to the tibia anteriorly by its anterior horn, which is situated immediately posterolateral to the origin of the anterior cruciate ligament. The posterior horn is

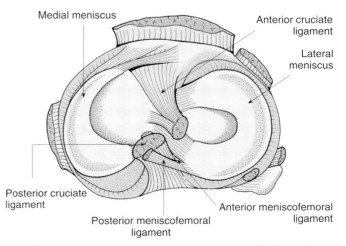

Fig. 1 The tibial plateaus showing the menisci and their relationship to intracapsular ligaments.

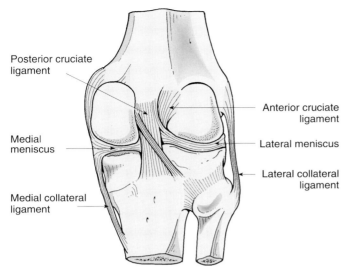

Fig. 2 Posterior view of the knee joint showing the menisci and their relationship to cruciate and collateral ligaments.

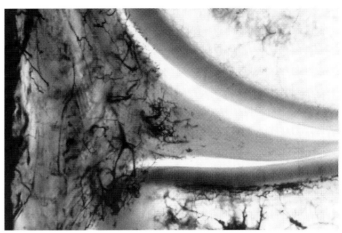

Fig. 3 Frontal section of the medial compartment of the knee, demonstrating perimeniscal capillary plexus penetrating the peripheral border of the medial meniscus. (Reproduced from ref. 15, with permission.)

inserted into the tibia in front of the posterior horn of the medial meniscus. It is also attached to the medial femoral condyle by the anterior and posterior meniscofemoral ligaments—the ligaments of Humphrey and Wrisberg, respectively.[14] (Fig. 1). These run anteromedially in a parallel fashion and are separated only by the posterior cruciate ligament. The lateral meniscus is grooved in its periphery by the tendon of popliteus, whose most medial fibres are inserted to its posterior horn. Here, the coronary ligament is deficient. In contrast with the medial meniscus, the fibular collateral ligament is not attached to its underlying cartilage (Fig. 2).

Blood supply

The blood supply of the menisci is derived from the terminal branches of the superior and inferior medial and lateral geniculate arteries. These vessels supply the connective tissue adjacent to the periphery of the meniscus.[6] Arnoczky and Warren,[15,16] as well as Danzig *et al.*[17] have shown that the collateral branches perforate the outer 20 to 30 per cent of the meniscus[13] (Figs 3 and 4). This leaves an inner 70 to 80 per cent, which is the 'avascular segment'. The central meniscus is more vascular than the superior or inferior surfaces. The anterior and posterior horns are enveloped by synovial tissue, and are therefore more highly vascularized than the middle segment.

Ultrastructure of the menisci

The meniscus is composed of cells surrounded by an extracellular matrix. The basic cell of the meniscus is the fibrochondrocyte. Two distinct types of fibrochondrocyte have been observed,[18] and are identified by their round or oval shape. The meniscal surface fibrochondrocytes are usually oval, while those of the deeper layers tend to be more rounded. Both contain few mitochondria, suggesting that anaerobic glycolysis is their main respiratory pathway.[6]

The extracellular matrix is composed of collagen, proteoglycans, matrix glycoproteins, and elastin. Bullough *et al.*,[3] using polarized light microscopy, showed that the extracellular matrix is composed mainly of circumferentially arranged collagen fibres. These provide

tensile strength and, to a lesser extent, radially arranged cross-links which provide shear strength[1] (Fig. 5). The radially orientated fibres are more densely packed in the meniscal surface layer, which is 30 to 120 mm thick. Collagen makes up about 60 to 70 per cent of the dry weight of the meniscus. Type I collagen makes up about 98 per cent of the total collagen content; the remainder is made up of types II, III, and V. The collagen fibres are arranged in bundles of 50 to 150 μm in diameter.[6]

Proteoglycans are hydrophilic, negatively charged micromolecules held together by collagen fibrils. They provide the meniscus with a high capacity to resist large compressive loads.

However, they do not contribute significantly to its tensile strength. Little is known, as yet, about the types and functions of the matrix glycoproteins. They are thought to be active in the pro-

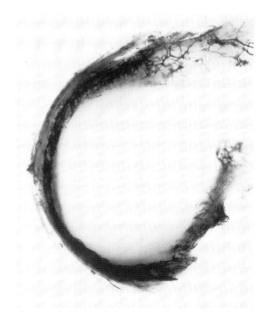

Fig. 4 Superior aspect of the medial meniscus, demonstrating the peripheral vasculature as well as the highly vascular synovial tissues that cover the anterior and posterior horns. (Reproduced from ref. 15, with permission.)

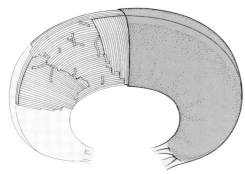

Fig. 5 Ultrastructure of the meniscus. The collagen fibre alignment pattern is seen from the superficial to deep layers of the meniscus. (Adapted from ref. 3, with permission.)

cess of repair and regeneration of the torn meniscus.[6] Elastin acts as a cross-link between collagen fibres. This connective tissue component enables the meniscus to recoil towards its normal anatomical shape when the circumferential stress displacing it has subsided.

Mobility of the menisci

Flexion and extension movements of the knee joint take place above the menisci, that is, between the menisci and femoral condyles. Rotation of the joint takes place below the menisci, that is, between the menisci and tibial plateaus. When the knee joint is extended, the menisci are separated, while in flexion their natural elastic recoil tends to approximate them.

The lateral meniscus is more mobile than the medial meniscus and can move by up to 1 cm. This mobility is due to a combination of factors including the close proximity of its anterior and posterior horns (which allow a greater degree of pivot), the fact that the posterior horn is not attached to the capsule or coronary ligament, and finally, the fact that it is not stabilized by its adjacent collateral ligament, as is the case with the medial meniscus. During flexion, the menisci are displaced posteriorly and are simultaneously internally rotated. During knee extension the menisci are displaced anteriorly and are externally rotated.

Functions of the menisci

Once regarded as useless vestigial organs, the menisci are now known to play an important role in transmission of forces,[3,5,19-21] joint stabilization,[7] shock absorption,[22] nutrition of articular cartilage, and lubrication of the knee joint.[23,24] Considerable clinical evidence indicates that removal of, or damage to, the menisci can have detrimental effects on the knee joint. Fairbank[9] has demonstrated radiographical signs of joint degeneration following meniscectomy. The severity of these changes is related to the amount of meniscal tissue removed.[25,26]

The menisci act as spacers that fill the dead space between the incongruous femoral condyles and tibial plateaus. They resist excessive movements of the tibia on the femur. In the cruciate-deficient knee, the menisci serve as important secondary knee stabilizers.[27]

The arrangement of the collagen bundles within the meniscus appears to be ideal for absorption and translation of vertical compression loads into circumferential stresses. They distribute these forces across the joint by increasing the contact area between the femoral condyles and tibial plateaus. Distribution of the load results

in a decrease in the magnitude of pressure (force per unit area) between the opposing hyaline cartilage surfaces. Thus the irreplaceable hyaline cartilage is protected from excessive damaging pressures. Meniscectomy dramatically alters the pattern of static loading across the knee joint.[28] Several studies have demonstrated higher peak stresses,[29] greater stress concentration,[5,30] and decreased shock-absorbing capabilities[20,31] after total meniscectomy.

Walker and Erkman[7] have shown that the menisci take between 50 and 70 per cent of the total knee load. More specifically, 90 per cent of the load across the knee joint passes through the medial compartment and 50 per cent of this is taken by the medial meniscus. Conversely, 10 per cent of the total load across the knee joint passes through the lateral compartment, of which 70 per cent is taken by the lateral meniscus.

Synovial fluid functions as a joint lubricant as well as a medium through which substances can diffuse. The fibrocartilage, as well as the hyaline cartilage, can thus absorb nutrients and excrete end-products of metabolism.

Meniscal injury mechanisms

When the shear stress within the meniscus exceeds the tissue strength, a tearing injury results. A tear occurs in one of two ways. Either an excessive abnormal force takes place within a normal meniscus, or a normal force takes place within an abnormal or degenerate meniscus. The former causes a vertical-type tear, while the latter causes a horizontal cleavage tear.[32] Vertical tears are more commonly seen in sporting injuries, whereas horizontal cleavage tears occur in patients with degenerative menisci.

As previously stated, the menisci are displaced posteriorly in flexion and anteriorly in extension. With hyperflexion the posterior halves of both menisci are compressed between the posterior aspects of the femoral condyles and tibial plateaus. The medial meniscus is prone to injury when the tibia is externally rotated relative to the femur. The lateral meniscus is more prone to injury when the tibia is internally rotated.

When the femur is internally rotated while the knee is flexed, the posterior horn of the medial meniscus is forced radially towards the intercondylar area by the medial femoral condyle. If the knee is then suddenly extended, the posterior horn may be torn. When the femur is externally rotated while the knee is flexed, the posterior horn of the lateral meniscus is forced radially towards the intercondylar area. If the knee is then suddenly extended, the meniscus is straightened and may be torn.

Medial meniscal injuries are seen up to five times more commonly than lateral meniscal injuries in most sports.[33] This is related to the higher incidence of 'side-on' tackles that apply a valgus strain to the knee. Injury to the medial meniscus also results from its firm attachment to the deep fibres of the medial collateral ligament, which decreases its mobility. Because of the valgus nature of these injuries, there is often a concomitant injury of the medial collateral ligament (Fig. 6).

Baker et al.[33] have shown the predominance of injuries to the medial meniscus compared with the lateral meniscus in a variety of sports: American football, 75 per cent; basketball, 75 per cent; skiing, 78 per cent; and baseball, 90 per cent. The only exception is wrestling, which has an almost equal incidence at 55 per cent.

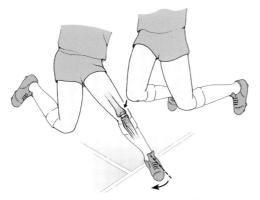

Fig. 6 The side-on tackle applies a valgus knee strain that may cause meniscal injury as well as medial collateral ligament injury.

Pathology—ageing of the meniscus

In youth, the meniscus is white, translucent, and has an abundant blood supply. It is mobile, elastic, and supple. With time, the smoothly contoured, parallel collagen fibres which run concentrically around the meniscus degenerate. The meniscus becomes brittle and yellowish in colour. Its vascularity decreases, and as it loses its translucency it becomes less elastic and supple. With hardening, it becomes more prone to injury. This loss of shear strength is a direct result of an increase in cross-linkage between parallel collagen fibres.[34] Dystrophic calcification, hyaline acellular degeneration, and myxoid degeneration contribute to the ageing process.[35] Progressive fissuring and cleavage tearing ensue. In general, the meniscus of the active child can withstand repeated insult without injury. The meniscus of the elderly is seldom acutely injured because of the relative inactivity that accompanies old age. However, the meniscus of the sportsperson is 'at risk' as this is the stage when it is undergoing degeneration from translucent white to opaque yellow.

Classification of meniscal tears

There are many classifications of meniscal tears. However, all are based on two distinct tear patterns: vertical and horizontal (Fig. 7). Vertical tears may be longitudinal or transverse (radial). Horizontal

tears were originally described by Smillie[32] as horizontal cleavage tears. Flap or oblique tears result from a combination of vertical and horizontal tearing. Tears may occur in association with discoid menisci or cysts of the meniscus.

The majority of sports-related tears are of the vertical type. Tears of the horizontal type are much less common. Flap or oblique tears are sometimes referred to as 'parrot beak tears'.

Vertical longitudinal tears

A vertical longitudinal tear occurs as a result of an excessive force acting upon a normal meniscus. These tears usually occur in young patients, often as a result of significant trauma, and are frequently associated with anterior cruciate ligament injuries. The thin concave edge of the meniscus is most commonly involved. The classic vertical longitudinal tear is the 'bucket handle tear', frequently responsible for the 'locked knee'. It is usually caused by a combination of compression with simultaneous rotation of the femur on a fixed tibia. The longitudinal tear is more common than the transverse tear.

Transverse tears are usually caused by a compression force which attempts to distract and displace the anterior and posterior horns of a meniscus. In so doing, an excessive traction force is applied to the thin concave edge of the meniscus, resulting in a tear of the middle third of the lateral meniscus. The transverse tear originates centrally and runs radially towards its vascular periphery.

Horizontal tears

The horizontal tear most commonly occurs in a degenerate meniscus, and was first termed a horizontal cleavage tear, by Smillie in 1962.[32] It occurs as a result of a normal force acting on an abnormal or degenerate meniscus and is most commonly seen in those over 40 years of age. Smillie[36] has shown that the posterior half of the medial meniscus or the middle segment of the lateral meniscus[35] are most commonly involved. Two out of every three horizontal tears involve the lateral meniscus. In the sportsperson, this type of injury occurs in an already degenerate meniscus. There is a close association with osteoarthritis.[37] Other features associated with meniscal degeneration are chondrocalcinosis[38,39] and cyst formation.[40]

Histological changes seen in the degenerative meniscus are similar to those seen in degenerative injury to the joint hyaline cartilage,[41] that is, fibrochondrocyte necrosis, fibrochondrocyte proliferation, fibrillation, and loss of matrix protein polysaccharide.

It is very difficult to distinguish microscopically between traumatic and degenerative tears. Hough and Webber[41] suggest that gross examination is the easiest and probably the most accurate method of deciding on the actual type of tear.

Ferrer et al.[35] have demonstrated that the extension of the horizontal cleavage type of tear into the parameniscal region would appear to be the cause of cyst formation.

Regeneration

King in 1936 was the first to document that tears limited to the avascular segment of the semilunar cartilage probably never healed.[25] Tears involving the vascularized area of the meniscus cause haemorrhage and clot formation within the torn area. This is followed by migration of fibroblasts and ingrowth of new capillaries. Fibrous healing results which resembles mature fibrocartilage.

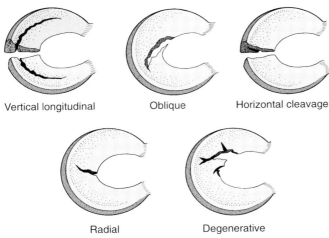

Vertical longitudinal   Oblique   Horizontal cleavage

Radial   Degenerative

Fig. 7 Classification of meniscal tears.

Arnoczky and Warren[16] have shown that regeneration may occur following meniscectomy but this is inconsistent. The new meniscus is composed of fibrous tissue. It is narrower, thinner, and has a smaller surface area than the original. The concave edge is less well defined and no obvious line of cleavage exists between capsule and meniscus. Regeneration may also occur following partial excision of a meniscus, provided that the vascular periphery is involved.

Diagnosis of meniscal injuries

A careful history and thorough physical examination are the most important prerequisites to making a diagnosis of a meniscal injury or, indeed, any knee complaint. Most patients with meniscal tears will present some time following the initial injury and after the acute symptoms have subsided. In obtaining the history of a knee disorder, careful documentation should be made of the nature of the initial injury as well as the time and duration of symptoms. The actual mechanism of injury should be ascertained, that is, whether the injury was a result of a contact or non-contact activity. It is also helpful to determine the position of the extremity at the time of the original injury.

As pain is the predominant complaint, it is important to determine what activities precipitate this pain. The severity of the pain and the functional level that the patient reaches before pain prevents any further activity are noted. Most mechanical knee pain is intermittent in nature. Pain that is constant and persistent, particularly at night, may be caused by the presence of arthritis or, more rarely, a bone tumour.

Presenting complaints

Pain

It is helpful to ask the patient to point to the specific area of knee pain. This is the least confusing method of determining its anatomical location. Pain is the most common presenting complaint in patients with meniscal pathology. It can usually be localized to the medial or lateral side of the knee. It is commonly precipitated by twisting and turning movements, or by forced flexion or extension. In some patients the symptoms are only present during sporting activities, while others experience symptoms during activities of daily living.

Swelling

Knee swelling associated with a meniscal tear is usually mild and increases with activity. The swelling gives rise to stiffness, and a complaint of decreased flexibility. This stiffness must not be confused with 'locking'.

Locking

Locking is a symptom indicating inability to extend the knee fully. It implies displacement of a torn meniscus into the intercondylar notch—usually a bucket handle tear. Forced extension or flexion is associated with further severe pain, either in the medial or lateral joint line. Locking may last for seconds, minutes, hours, or days. It may be relieved spontaneously. Commonly, patients are able to 'wriggle' the knee into extension with perceptible relief of pain.

The presence of a loose body within the knee may cause true locking episodes. Difficulty in extending the knee may also be seen immediately after injury in patients with acute injuries, secondary to the presence of pain and spasm. It may take a number of days to regain full knee extension in patients who have sustained an anterior cruciate ligament injury.

Instability

A patient with a meniscal tear may complain that his or her knee 'gives way'. This 'giving way' is always preceded by pain, that is, the pain causes the 'giving way'. This is in contrast with true instability, which is usually associated with anterior cruciate ligament deficiency. In knees that are anterior cruciate deficient, episodes of instability occur without warning and are followed, rather than preceded, by pain.

History of presenting complaints

An accurate history of the presenting knee complaint should be carefully elicited and documented. Almost all younger patients will be able to recall accurately a history of some type of twisting or overloading episode (e.g. during football, running, racket sport, or basketball). Some patients may continue their activity, while others may find it too painful to bear weight on the affected knee. Most patients will complain of pain and difficulty moving the knee following the initial injury. The difficulty with knee movement is usually pain related, although in a small number of patients this difficulty will be due to true 'locking' secondary to a displaced, torn meniscal fragment.

Patients with an acute meniscal tear usually develop a gradual, mild knee effusion over a period of approximately 12 h. This is in contrast with patients who sustain anterior cruciate ligament injuries, who will almost always develop a large knee effusion immediately following the original injury (haemarthrosis).

A number of patients, usually older people, will present with symptoms suggestive of meniscal pathology, but will not recall a specific twisting or overloading event. Many of these will have developed their symptoms of pain and swelling over weeks or months. Some may recall experiencing their first episode of joint pain while squatting or while ascending from a squatting or sitting position. These patients are commonly between 40 and 60 years old and may demonstrate at least some evidence of degenerative joint disease on radiographs. Patients with overt degenerative arthritis may develop degenerative meniscal tears and suffer symptoms which are indistinguishable from those associated with the underlying arthritis.

Examination

Examination of the knee starts with observation of the patient's gait. Any evidence of antalgic gait, a flexion contracture, or hip or back disease should be carefully noted, remembering that hip or back disease may manifest with knee pain.

Knee examination should be performed with both legs exposed entirely, so that the findings for the affected knee can be adequately compared with those for the normal knee. Alignment of the lower extremity is best judged with the patient standing and walking.

In addition to looking for specific signs of meniscal pathology, a careful search is also made for ligament injuries as well as patella problems. Evidence of bruising, skin abrasions, and localized swelling should be observed. General palpation for swellings, such as a bursa over the tibial tubercle, popliteal cysts, or palpable masses which may represent tumours, should be performed. Examination of the proximal tibiofibular joint is particularly important in patients presenting with lateral knee pain.

Early presentation

Early examination, soon after the initial injury has occurred, usually reveals generalized knee tenderness, mild effusion, and limitation of knee movements. Palpation of the medial or lateral joint line may be associated with marked tenderness. However, the majority of patients will also have tenderness above or below the joint line, indicating some element of either a medial or lateral collateral ligament sprain, thus making it difficult to differentiate between pure ligament sprain and ligament sprain associated with meniscal injury. It is reasonable to direct initial treatment to the sprained ligaments in these patients. Most patients with isolated ligament sprains should be able to return to their sporting activities within 2 to 4 weeks. Those patients who still complain of persistent joint-line pain after this time should be suspected of having a meniscal tear.

Patients presenting with a locked knee following a twisting injury should be suspected of having a bucket handle tear of one of the menisci. The side of the meniscal tear is usually clarified by eliciting joint-line tenderness or by eliciting pain on passive extension. Inability to extend the knee may also be seen in patients who have an acute tear of the anterior cruciate ligament. However, these patients usually present with a large swollen knee (haemarthrosis).

After the acute symptoms have settled, a patient presenting with a meniscal tear will usually have some persistent knee swelling, complain of joint-line pain, and may experience episodes of intermittent locking. More rarely, a patient may have been unable to straighten the knee since the initial twisting injury, that is, have persistent locking.

Clinical signs

Patients with meniscal tears may exhibit one or a number of clinical signs.

Joint-line tenderness

Joint-line tenderness is usually a reliable indicator of meniscal injury. This is more specific if the tenderness is confined to the joint line, the periphery of the meniscus. Tenderness above or below the joint line may indicate the presence of a concomitant collateral ligament sprain, or the presence of degenerative joint disease.

Swelling

Effusions associated with meniscal tears are usually mild. Large chronic effusions are not commonly seen with isolated meniscal tears, and usually indicate the presence of arthritis. The patellar tap sign may not be present in patients with small or mild knee swellings. In these knees, a visible ripple of fluid in the parapatella fossa can be demonstrated by first expressing fluid from one side of the joint and then gently stroking the opposite side with the palm of the hand.

Tibial rotation tests

Tibial rotation tests have been described by McMurray[19] and Apley.[42] They were devised in attempts to differentiate a torn meniscus from other knee pathology. Both aim at trapping or catch-

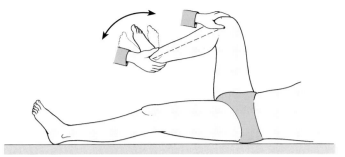

Fig. 8 McMurray's test: the hip is flexed to 90°, the knee is flexed greater than 90°, and the tibia is internally and externally rotated. The joint line is palpated for clicks.

ing the torn meniscus between the femoral condyle and the tibial plateau. A positive rotation test is associated with either a palpable or an audible click which may or may not reproduce the patient's painful symptoms. These tests are helpful when positive, but not when negative, and may be difficult to perform on an acutely painful knee. It is important to perform the rotation test on the opposite knee, as quite frequently similar clicking may also be present. The McMurray manoeuvre[19] is performed by externally rotating the leg with the knee fully flexed (Fig. 8). A varus stress is then applied as the knee is gradually extended. A palpable, audible, or painful click may indicate a tear of the posterior horn of the medial meniscus. The manoeuvre is then repeated with forcible internal rotation, while applying a valgus stress, to elicit posterolateral meniscal clicks.

The Apley grinding test[42] is performed with the patient in the prone position. The examiner rotates the flexed tibia on the femur while exerting downward pressure along the long axis of the tibia. With pressure exerted during rotation, pain may be felt in the region of a torn meniscus.

In addition to the tibial rotation tests, Insall[34] has shown that squatting and duck-walking may reproduce joint-line pain. On occasion, a loose meniscal fragment can be palpated in the area of the coronary ligaments.

Quadricep wasting

Quadricep wasting is a non-specific finding which may reflect knee pathology in general rather than a meniscal tear in particular.

In addition to looking for the foregoing signs, it is important that a careful overall assessment of the knee is performed. The integrity of the medial and lateral collateral, as well as the anterior and posterior cruciate ligaments, should be assessed. Weight-bearing radiographs should exclude the presence of fractures, loose bodies, osteochondral injuries, or arthritis.

Meniscal cysts and associated tears

Meniscal tears may occur in association with cysts of the menisci. These are more commonly seen on the lateral side and are invariably associated with a radial or horizontal cleavage tear of the lateral meniscus. Patients usually present with pain in the lateral joint-line region which persists for a number of hours after activity. Most patients are conscious of a small swelling on the lateral joint line which fluctuates in size. Examination will reveal a tender palpable mass on the lateral joint line. This 'lump' is maximally distended at approximately 30° of flexion. The differential diagnoses are those of a ganglion, an osteophyte in an arthritic knee, or very rarely a small, soft tissue tumour such as a synovial cell sarcoma.

Meniscal cysts have traditionally been treated by total meniscectomy and open removal of the cyst. Currently, these cysts can now be treated effectively by arthroscopic methods. The torn meniscus is excised, allowing decompression of the cyst. The resection will usually require removal of a large segment of the meniscus because of the fragmented multiplane nature of the associated tear. It is not necessary to remove the cyst through a separate skin incision.

Discoid meniscal tears

A discoid meniscus is characterized by a round rather than a crescent shape. About 90 per cent occur on the lateral side of the knee. Symptoms may occur following a tear, causing pain and discomfort, clicking, swelling, or a mechanical block to extension. The majority of patients presenting are under the age of 15 years. Arthroscopic management is recommended for symptomatic tears. Resection of the central portion of the discoid is performed, leaving a rim about the width of a normal meniscus behind. The remaining rim will retriangulate and look much like a normal meniscus in time.[43]

Haemarthrosis

Immediate knee swelling following a twisting injury implies bleeding into the joint—haemarthrosis. In the absence of a fracture, the patient has a 75 to 80 per cent chance of sustaining a tear of the anterior cruciate ligament and a 50 per cent chance of having a peripheral tear of one of the menisci (J.B. Hurson and E. Kessopersadh, personal communication).[44] There is a smaller chance of sustaining a patella dislocation, with tearing of the medial retinaculum. Such patients usually give a very clear history of being aware that the patella was dislocated to the lateral aspect of the joint. The knee in those circumstances would have been in a flexed position. Most patella dislocations reduce spontaneously as the knee is extended.

Examination is difficult in the presence of a large, painful, swollen knee. It is important that the knee be re-examined following aspiration. Aspiration should be performed under sterile conditions using a large-bore needle—16-gauge or preferably a 14-gauge. It may be impossible to aspirate blood and clots through small-bore needles. A local anaesthetic, which may be combined with adrenaline, may be injected prior to aspiration. Special attention to injecting the synovium and capsule is important, as the most painful aspect of the procedure is the stretching of these regions. In the presence of a large effusion, the procedure can be carried out with equal facility from either medial or lateral aspects. Technically, there is no difficulty in aspirating large knee effusions.

The knee should be re-examined following aspiration. Particular attention should be paid to the medial and lateral collateral ligaments, as well as to the anterior and posterior cruciates. A radiograph will rule out any bony injury.

The question of performing an urgent arthroscopy on patients with a haemarthrosis is controversial. We feel that urgent arthroscopy is not usually warranted. The treatment of a painful haemarthrosis involves initial aspiration affording pain relief, followed by further clinical examination. Attention should be directed to regaining range of movement, muscle strength, and resolution of swelling. Any major injury to the medial or lateral collateral ligaments should be treated early. Many patients will rehabilitate and go on to uneventful recovery without any further residual symptoms. Clinical evidence of meniscal tears will become obvious with time. It is appreciated that, at times, this 'wait and see' policy may delay treatment of meniscal tears. This may be of particular importance in some groups of patients such as high-level or professional sportspersons. In these circumstances an arthroscopy may be indicated early during rehabilitation.

In the past, it was felt that urgent arthroscopy was warranted in order to treat anterior cruciate ligament ruptures in the acute phase. However, it is now well documented that reconstruction of acute anterior cruciate ruptures is associated with increased morbidity, particularly in terms of difficulty in restoring range of movement. Therefore it is important to allow return of full range of movement, muscle strength, and resolution of swelling prior to performing an anterior cruciate ligament reconstruction.

Diagnostic adjuvants

The reliability of clinical examination for the diagnosis of meniscal disorders of the knee has ranged from 64 to 85 per cent in previous reports (Table 1).[45-51] In an attempt to improve diagnostic accuracy, some authors recommend the use of diagnostic adjuvants, such as arthrography, computed tomography (CT), and magnetic resonance imaging (MRI).

Arthrography

The diagnostic accuracy of knee arthrography (Table 1) is dependent on the expertise of the radiologist, and ranges from 68 to 97 per cent.[46-54] It is more useful in the diagnosis of medial meniscal pathology. In a minority of patients it fails to demonstrate tears involving the posterior horn of the lateral meniscus. This is due to the greater mobility of the lateral meniscus and the presence of the popliteus tendon. The advantages of arthrography include ready availability to practising physicians, outpatient procedure, and low complication rate.

Magnetic resonance imaging

Because of its remarkable soft-tissue resolution, MRI has become an important diagnostic modality in the evaluation of lesions of the menisci. Its overall accuracy ranges from 65 to 98 per cent (Table 1).[54-59] A negative predictive value for the diagnosis of a torn meniscus is 83 to 97 per cent,[54,58] which means that on 3 to 17 per cent of occasions a negative finding on the MRI study may hide the presence of a torn meniscus. MRI has the advantage of being non-invasive, but has the disadvantages of being expensive and time consuming. Furthermore, it requires that the knee can fully extend. The authors do not advocate the routine use of MRI for the evaluation of meniscal tears. As with all branches of clinical medicine, physicians must match clinical signs and symptoms with MRI findings before instituting surgical treatment, because there is a reported 5.6 per cent prevalance of meniscal tears in the asymptomatic population.[60]

If the clinical history and physical signs suggest symptomatic meniscal pathology, arthroscopy is indicated. MRI is only indicated if a diagnosis is unclear and when it is felt that the treatment of the

Table 1 Diagnostic accuracy of meniscal tears

Investigators	Clinical examination (%)	Arthrography (%)	Arthroscopy (%)	Combined clinical examination (arthrography arthroscopy) (%)	CT scan (%)	MR imaging (%)
Nicholas et al. 1970[50]	80	97				
Casscells 1971[65]			80			
Jackson and Abe 1972[49]	68.5	68.2	95			
De Haven and Collins 1975[46]	72	78	94			
McGinty and Metza 1978[52]		Lateral 72 Medial 84	91 under general anaesthetic 95 under local anaesthetic			
Tegtmeyer et al. 1979[53]		Single Contrast 96.5 Double Contrast 95				
Gillies and Seligson 1979[47]	85	83	68			
Ireland et al. 1980[48]	64	86	92	98.3		
Daniel et al. 1982[45]	72	Medial 89 Lateral 85				
Selesnick et al. 1985[51]	82.6	73.2	94.4	96.8		
Passariello et al. 1985[61]					Medial 89.2 Lateral 96.1	
Manco et al. 1987[56]					92.2	87.5
Silva and Silver 1988[59]			92			65
Polly et al. 1988[57]						Medial 98 Lateral 90
Fischer et al. 1991[54]						Medial 89 Lateral 88
Raunest et al. 1991[58]						78
Kelly et al. 1991[55]						88

patient will be affected by the result. It is important that this modality is used wisely and that unnecessary expense is avoided.[58,61]

Computed tomography

CT scanning has achieved a diagnostic accuracy of 90 per cent (Table 1).[56,62] However, it has the disadvantage of using ionizing radiation. The quality of the image is diminished in the presence of a haemarthrosis.[63]

Arthroscopy

The advent of arthroscopy of the knee over the past 20 years has revolutionized the diagnosis and treatment of meniscal tears. It allows visualization and direct palpation of the various intra-articu-

lar structures. A probe can be used to assess the integrity of the medial and lateral menisci, the anterior cruciate ligament, and the status of the articular surfaces of the femoral condyles, tibial plateaus, and patella, as well as the condition of the synovial lining of the joint. The widespread use of arthroscopy has eliminated the necessity for exploratory arthrotomies and enables meniscal surgery to be performed as an outpatient procedure. This surgery can be performed under general, spinal, or local anaesthesia. It is usually associated with minimal pain, allowing patients to walk immediately following surgery without the necessity for crutches. Rehabilitation is rapid, allowing patients to return to work within days and to sport in 2 to 3 weeks. In addition to the clinical benefits, there are significant economic advantages in terms of containment of hospital costs, reduced absence from work, and early return to sport.

Indications for arthroscopy

Diagnosis and treatment of meniscal tears are the main indications for arthroscopy of the knee. However, not every painful knee requires a diagnostic arthroscopy. Before considering arthroscopy, a careful history should be obtained, a thorough clinical examination should be made, and weight-bearing radiography of the knee should be performed.

Patients presenting with typical symptoms of joint-line pain and swelling, with or without episodes of locking, may be considered for arthroscopy. Patients with positive clinical signs, including joint-line tenderness, effusion, and meniscal catching signs, such as a positive McMurray sign,[19] are the most obvious candidates. Arthroscopy is also considered for those patients who have persistent symptoms suggestive of a meniscal tear, despite the absence of clinical signs. Prudent clinical judgement is paramount. If symptoms are vague and diffuse, the success rate from arthroscopy is similarly reduced. Arthroscopy should not be considered unless there is a reasonable chance of benefit to the patient in terms of either providing more information than was known clinically or a chance of providing treatment. Performing arthroscopy on patients who have little chance of gaining from the procedure only serves to increase their expectations, which in turn will lead to further disappointment.

Historical treatment of meniscal tears

For many years total meniscectomy was the gold standard for any meniscal pathology. Smillie[32] recommended total meniscectomy in preference to partial meniscectomy, irrespective of the type of lesion encountered. He maintained that, following meniscectomy, a new meniscus was regenerated, creating a perfect replica of the excised meniscus. This has subsequently been contested and disproved.[28]

Knowledge of the consequences of total meniscectomy[4,8,9,11] and the functional role of the meniscus in force transmission and shock absorption has led to the principle of preserving as much functional meniscal tissue as possible. In partial meniscectomy, meniscal resection is confined to the loose unstable fragment, such as a displaceable inner edge of a bucket handle tear or the flap in an oblique tear. Following partial meniscectomy, a stable or balanced rim of healthy meniscal tissue is preserved. This intact, balanced, peripheral rim provides joint stability and protects the articular surfaces by its load-bearing functions. Preservation of this peripheral cartilage rim is particularly important in patients who have already had major ligamentous injuries.[64]

Many studies have shown that there is an increased incidence of degenerative change following either partial or total meniscectomy.[4,8,9,23,65-70] Although the long-term results of partial meniscectomy are far superior to that of total meniscectomy,[71,72] the functional results tend to deteriorate with time. Lack of radiographic changes does not necessarily correlate with subjective symptoms and functional outcome.[73] It is therefore important to counsel patients regarding the long-term expectations of partial meniscectomy. This has led to the perceived need to consider repairing torn menisci. Several studies have documented that the peripheral one-third of the meniscus has a vascular supply[15,16] and that tears in that zone have a potential to heal.[25,74,75] The first report of a meniscal repair

was by Annandale in 1885.[76] In 1936, King showed that peripheral tears of a meniscus could heal and that tears confined to the avascular meniscal substance probably never healed.[25] More recent studies have shown that the process of healing is initiated by the formation of a blood clot at the site of the tear.[74] This clot contains fibrin, serum factors, and blood cells. The fibrin forms a scaffolding that anchors the clot to the torn meniscal edges. Meniscal cells at the edge of the tear proliferate and then migrate into the fibrin scaffolding under the influences of growth factor and chemotactic factors, thus resulting in repair. King's findings have been confirmed by Heatley[77] in the rabbit and by Cabaud *et al.*[78] in the dog and monkey. The healing process is not initiated if the tear is limited to the avascular segment of the meniscus.

Vascular injection studies have provided documented evidence of the vascularity of the outer 10 to 30 per cent of the adult human meniscus.[15,79] There is even greater penetration of the vasculature in the skeletally immature individual.[6,13] This documented vascularity of the outer zone of the meniscus has provided the fundamental basis for meniscal suturing. Healing of meniscal tears following suture has been shown to be further enhanced by the application of an exogenous blood clot to the area of meniscal repair.[80] Arnoczky *et al.*[74] demonstrated the role of fibrin clot formation in the healing of meniscal tissue. The recent development of meniscal repair techniques has taken advantage of this healing potential and it is hoped that it will prevent degenerative knee changes which are seen following either total or partial meniscectomy. The rationale behind meniscal repair is to return the knee joint to its original integrity without removal of any meniscal substance. The aim of repair is to reduce opposing, torn, meniscal edges anatomically and to maintain this reduction with sutures until healing is complete.[81]

Current management of meniscal injuries

Although diagnostic adjuvants such as arthrography[48,50,51,53] and MRI[54,56,57,59,63,82] can be helpful in diagnosing meniscal tears, the ultimate treatment decision is always based on the exact type, location, and extent of meniscal tears, which are best determined by direct visualization and palpation at arthroscopy.[46,47,49,83]

Arthroscopic management of the torn meniscus is now standard, and has virtually replaced arthrotomy and open meniscectomy. Arthroscopy affords much better exposure than can be gained by arthrotomy. Tear patterns can be readily appreciated and explored, allowing appropriate management strategies to be planned.

Current management strategies for meniscal tears include partial meniscectomy, meniscal repair, and the most conservative treatment of all, which is to leave the tear alone. Nowadays, it is very rare to resort to total meniscectomy. Decisions as to the best option will depend on clinical evaluation, associated lesions, and the type, location, and extent of the tear, which can best be evaluated at arthroscopy.

The first decision to be made following the diagnosis of a meniscal tear is whether the tear should be treated surgically or left alone. Partial-thickness split tears and full-thickness (10 mm or less) or short (5 mm or less) radial tears that are stable on probing can be left alone. Most commonly, such tears are found incidentally in knees with more extensive pathology, such as tears of the other

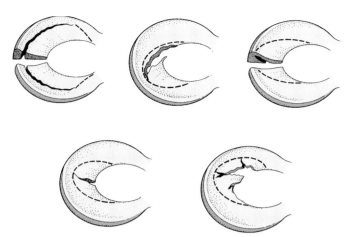

Fig. 9 Partial meniscectomy resection lines.

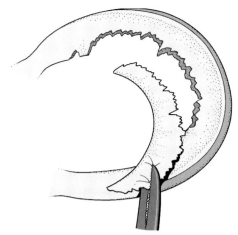

Fig. 10 Partial meniscectomy: removal of the mobile torn fragment *en bloc*.

meniscus, or in association with anterior cruciate ligament tears. Weiss *et al.*[84] followed 52 patients who had partial-thickness or short radial tears. Their average follow-up was over 4 years. They found that only six patients (12 per cent) required subsequent surgical treatment.

Once a torn meniscus is found to require surgical treatment, it is necessary to determine whether or not repair of the tear is feasible. The tear is evaluated for its length, width, and depth. A careful assessment of the quality of the torn meniscus is made, that is, whether or not it has significant alteration of shape. Frequently, tears which have been displaced into the intercondylar notch for some time have shortened and cannot be properly repositioned to the original rim of the torn meniscus. Meniscal tears which have undergone alteration in shape and size are not suitable for repair and should be resected.

Partial meniscectomy

Meniscal tears which are not suitable for repair because they are located within the avascular zone or because of the extent of meniscal substance damage are treated by partial meniscectomy.[85] Short-term outcome studies for arthroscopic partial menisectomy suggest that partial lateral menisectomy in stable knees is comparable with partial medial meniscectomy.[11,86,87] When partial meniscectomy is performed, only the unstable offending segment is removed, leaving behind an intact peripheral rim which maintains stability and protection to opposing articular surfaces (Fig. 9).

Once the decision is made to resect the torn mobile part of the meniscus, it is removed either *en bloc* or piece by piece with a basket forceps or punch (Fig. 10). Following removal of the obviously mobile torn fragment, a further check of the remaining meniscus is made to ensure that the rim is balanced and stable.

Metcalf and co-workers[88,89] have elegantly outlined the classic principles of partial meniscectomy. Only the torn portion of the meniscus that can protrude into the centre of the joint need be excised. They describe an imaginary line that represents the inner margin of a normal meniscus (Fig. 11). Any meniscal fragment that can be pulled past this boundary is likely to become caught between the joint surfaces during weight bearing and cause symptoms. As much meniscal rim as possible is preserved. Patients are advised of the benefits of keeping this rim, and are made aware of the possi-

bility of developing further symptoms some time in the future.[73] In reality, this is more possible then probable.

Partial meniscectomy is now performed almost exclusively through the arthroscope and rarely through a formal arthrotomy. Arthroscopic surgery requires considerable training, in both the identification of the various intra-articular structures and the different surgical techniques. Surgeons who are at the learning phase of arthroscopic surgery are better advised to perform an open partial meniscectomy if they are encountering difficulties with closed techniques.

Meniscal repair

Meniscal suturing has become a common procedure for peripheral meniscal tears. However, arthroscopic suturing carries a risk of neurovascular injury. Tears limited to the outer portion of the meniscus heal best—by virtue of their relatively good supply of blood. The healing rate for a lateral meniscal tear is lower than that of the medial meniscus. This is probably due to the greater mobility of the lateral meniscus as well as the fact that tears near the popliteal hiatus are relatively avascular. Anterior cruciate ligament reconstruction combined with meniscal repair appears to increase the healing rate of the meniscus.[90] Tears suitable for repair are those

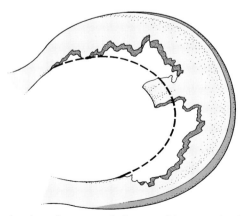

Fig. 11 The imaginary line represents the normal inner margin of the medial meniscus. A torn fragment protruding beyond this line requires resection as it will cause symptoms as it catches in the joint interface.

within the vascular zone[91] (the outer third of the meniscus) that are unstable on probing, are longer than 7 mm, and have not sustained major surgical damage.[85] Retears of a previously repaired meniscus may also be considered for further repair if the meniscus has not undergone alteration in shape and size.[92]

Tears of the posterior segment of the meniscus are the most difficult to suture and often require open arthrotomy. Ishmura et al.[93] report an 80 per cent success rate using fibrin glue.

The 'ideal' patient profile for meniscal repair is a patient less than 30 years of age, with a tear rim width of 3 mm or less, repaired in conjunction with an anterior cruciate ligament reconstruction, at a relatively short time interval after injury.

Despite MRI being a useful adjuvant in diagnosing internal derangement of the knee, it has not proven to be of use in evaluating the meniscus following repair.[94] This is because of the persistence of abnormal MRI signals within scar tissue of the healed meniscus.

Meniscal repair can be performed by open direct suture of tears which are at the very periphery of the meniscus, or by using variously described arthroscopic techniques. Both open and closed techniques have been reported with equally good results.[80,95] Traumatic tears within the vascular zone have healing rates of up to 90 per cent whether the repairs are performed by open or by arthroscopic methods.[64,91,95-100] De Haven's study[85] has indicated that the time from injury to surgery does not alter the rate of healing in isolated meniscal tears. Isolated tears of up to 8-year duration have been successfully repaired. However, acute tears of less than 2-month duration associated with anterior cruciate ligament rupture have significantly greater rates of healing following repair than chronic tears seen after many months.

Henning et al.[80] have reported their indications for meniscal repair. They would consider all medial and lateral tears for repair, except where the repair would replace less than 25 per cent of the missing area. When a tear suitable for repair is seen in a knee that is anterior cruciate ligament deficient, it is recommended that the meniscus be repaired at the time of the anterior cruciate ligament reconstruction.[80,95] If reconstruction is not performed, there is a strong possibility that the meniscal repair will break down.

Rehabilitation following meniscal surgery

Worldwide, opinions vary greatly regarding the use and effect of intra-articular analgesia for pain relief after arthroscopic knee surgery.[101-104] At the completion of the operative procedure, we routinely inject bupivacaine, 0.25 per cent with adrenaline, into the knee joint. This provides early postoperative analgesia, thereby decreasing the necessity for oral analgesia. The skin punctures are closed with a single suture. Adhesive strips can be used instead of sutures. A light compression bandage is applied around the knee and removed after 3 or 4 h.

If partial meniscectomy has been performed, isometric quadriceps exercises are started as soon as the patient is awake in the recovery room. Early, active range of movement is started on the day of surgery. Full weight bearing is allowed as soon after surgery as recovery from the anaesthetic allows. Crutches are not used. All meniscal surgery is performed as an outpatient procedure, that is, the patient is discharged home on the day of surgery. Patients are given a prescription for oral analgesia as well as anti-inflammatory

medication on discharge. They are advised to remove the light compression dressing 3 to 4 h after surgery. Flexion and extension exercises are continued. A full range of knee movement should be restored by 5 to 7 days. We have found that patients regain full range of movement and full quadriceps strength more rapidly if their postoperative exercise programme is monitored by a physical therapist.

Early return to work is encouraged, after 1 or 2 days for patients with sedentary occupations and after 5 to 7 days for patients engaged in heavy manual labour. Sporting activity is allowed when there is a full range of knee motion, 75 per cent quadriceps strength, no pain, and minimal or no residual effusion. This usually takes approximately 2 weeks. Exceptionally, patients who have had a medial bucket-handle tear excised may return to sport within 7 to 10 days.

Postoperative effusions usually resolve over a period of 2 to 3 weeks. Our personal observation has been that effusions in patients who have had lateral meniscal surgery seem to last longer than in those who have had surgery on the medial meniscus.

Rehabilitation programmes following meniscal repair vary. We allow patients to start weight bearing, with crutches, immediately following surgery. Early, full range of movement is encouraged. Crutches are discarded after a few days. Running and contact sports are allowed after 4 to 6 months. Cannon, who uses the modified Henning technique of arthroscopic repair, recommends no weight bearing for 4 weeks and partial weight bearing for a further 4 weeks.[105] Crutches are discarded at 8 weeks, return to straight running is allowed at 5 months, and return to contact sports at 9 months.

Results

A more rational conservative approach to meniscal surgery has evolved over the last few decades as the long-term effects of total meniscectomy have been demonstrated by such workers as Fairbank, Jackson, Dandy, and Johnson. In 1948, Fairbank[9] published a study of 107 cases that were reviewed over a 14-year period after total meniscectomy. He noted radiographic changes in 67 per cent of patients after medial meniscectomy and in 50 per cent of patients after lateral meniscectomy. These changes included formation of an anteroposterior ridge projecting downwards from the margin of the femoral condyle over the old meniscal site, flattening of the marginal half of the femoral articular surface, and narrowing of the joint space. In a 17-year follow-up study, Johnson et al.[68] showed that only 42 per cent of 99 patients had satisfactory results after total meniscectomy. He also noted that meniscectomy may lead to knee instability. These typical long-term results, together with a fuller understanding of the functional significance of the meniscus, led to the concept of partial meniscectomy.

In the mid-1970s Dandy and Jackson[8] compared the results of partial meniscectomy with those of total meniscectomy: 91 per cent of the partial meniscectomy group were asymptomatic after 5 years, while 65 per cent of the total meniscectomy group were asymptomatic. McGinty et al.,[28] in a 5.5-year follow-up study of 128 patients, found that there was no subjective or objective evidence to favour total meniscectomy over partial excision in the management of bucket handle or anterior horn tears. At follow-up, Fairbank radiography changes occurred in 60 per cent of the total meniscectomy group and in only 30 per cent of the partial meniscectomy group. Their results showed that there was a lower postoperative morbidity, a shorter hospital stay, and less time spent on crutches in those patients who had a partial meniscectomy. The major complication rate was 2.6 per cent compared with 14.6 per cent in favour of partial meniscectomy.

Several authors have reported consistently good results following meniscal repair. In a long-term follow-up of 33 repaired menisci, De Haven[85] reported an overall retear rate of 21 per cent. He noted that 14 per cent of acute repairs and 33 per cent of chronic repairs sustained retears. There was a retear rate of 11 per cent in patients with stable knees and 42 per cent in patients with unstable knees. He emphasizes the need for early repair. In a previous study,[65] he had shown that the retear rate in menisci that were repaired with simultaneous anterior cruciate ligament reconstruction was less than 10 per cent.

Hamberg et al.,[98] in an 18-month follow-up study of 50 cases of meniscal repair, showed that there was an 11 per cent incidence of retear in chronically torn menisci and a 9 per cent incidence of new rupture at a different site. There was a 6 per cent incidence of new rupture and no cases of retear in menisci repaired within 2 weeks of being torn.

In a 2- to 10-year follow-up of 71 meniscal repairs, Hanks et al.[95] found that the failure rate of open repair compared with arthroscopic repair was very similar, 11 per cent and 8.8 per cent respectively. The failure in knees that were anterior cruciate ligament deficient was 13 per cent compared with 8 per cent in those that were stable. Cannon and Vittari[106] found a 93 per cent meniscus healing rate in patients who had had a simultaneous anterior cruciate ligament reconstruction. This compared with a 50 per cent success rate in those patients whose anterior cruciate ligament was not reconstructed.

Henning et al.,[80] in a series of 153 arthroscopic meniscal repairs using an exogenous fibrin clot, showed an overall healing rate of 64 per cent; 24 per cent were incompletely healed and 12 per cent had failed. Follow-up was 4 months. In knees that were anterior cruciate ligament deficient, the failure rate was 1.5 per cent if the repair was performed within 2 months of injury. This rose to 20 per cent if the repair was performed more than 2 months after the initial injury. They found that using an exogenous fibrin clot improved their healing rate from 59 to 92 per cent.

Future directions

The use of laser technology in meniscal surgery is still in the developmental stage. Smith and Nance[107] were the first to report on the use of the carbon dioxide laser in arthroscopy. Initially these lasers were large and cumbersome to use and there was concern regarding the by-products of vaporization, namely smoke and carbon ash.[108–110] The ability to deliver laser energy precisely to the areas of pathology is appealing, but this precision may also concentrate the energy, creating the potential for a significant injury to the nearby articular cartilage.[111–114] Recent technological advances have led to the development of mid-range infra-red (IR-B), solid-state lasers such as the neodymium:YAG laser and the holmium:YAG laser.[115–117] These newer lasers are more compact and can be used in an aqueous medium. They cause significantly less injury to the surrounding healthy meniscal tissue. It has been shown that the use of pulsed laser energy can promote a significant stimulation in synthesis of hyaline cartilage matrix.[118] This stimulation of cartilage matrix synthesis may prove to be clinically useful in the future.

Cisa et al.[119] have demonstrated that vascularized synovial flaps sutured into the meniscal defect can induce a reparative response. Similarly, carbon fibre implants have been inserted into meniscal defects. However, they induce a rather exaggerated tissue response resulting in excessive fibrous tissue generation.[75]

Arnoczky and Warren[74] have used an exogenous fibrin clot to effect healing of the meniscal defect that is limited to the avascular segment. They state that the fibrin clot appears to act as a chemotactic and mitogenic stimulus for reparative cells and provides a scaffold for the reparative process. Although the reparative tissue is grossly and histologically different from the normal meniscal tissue, it is morphologically similar to the fibrous tissue seen in the vascular area of the meniscus.[16]

Webber et al.[120] are performing exciting new work in the development of an ideal culture system, which theoretically should allow complete healing of mid-substance tears. Their organ culture model makes it possible rapidly to identify and quantify the factors necessary in effecting meniscal wound repair.

Stone et al.[121] are investigating the use of a collagen-based meniscal prothesis. This acts as an absorbable regeneration template and offers the possibility of inducing regrowth of new menisci.

Probably the most adventurous current experimental work is that of meniscal transplantation. Meniscal transplantation has two main objectives: first, to stabilize the knee joint, and second, to prevent the progression of established degeneration of hyaline articular cartilage. Longer follow-up and further studies are necessary to show whether meniscal transplantation will prove durable and prevent progressive degeneration of articular cartilage in the long term. Van Arkle and de Boer,[122] in a prospective 2- to 5-year follow-up study of 23 patients with cryopreserved meniscal transplants that were not matched for tissue antigens, showed a satisfactory result in 20 patients. Follow-up arthroscopy was performed in 12 patients. The allograft was found attached firmly to the knee capsule in all cases. There were no signs of inflammation or rejection. Arnoczky et al.[123] have studied cellular repopulation of deep-frozen meniscal autografts in the dog. Their results demonstrate the ability of extrinsic cells, which appear to be derived from the synovium, to populate a devitalized meniscus and differentiate into cells that resemble meniscofibrochondrocytes. This repopulation is associated with a remodelling of the collagen orientation in the superficial and subsuperficial layers of the meniscus. The central core of the meniscus remained acellular. They feel that this remodelling of the collagen orientation may make the transplanted meniscus more susceptible to injury, and that long-term studies are required to document fully the biomechanical consequences of this remodelling process.

Jackson et al.[124] were the first to document the fate of transplanted viable chondrocytes in meniscal allografts using the DNA probe technique. They noted the rapid loss of DNA in the transplanted meniscus secondary to cell necrosis. The meniscal allograft subsequently became repopulated rapidly with host cells that started migrating into its substance within a few days, and then modulated themselves into cells resembling fibrochondrocytes. The process occurred prior to revascularization of the allograft, and likewise before the traditional immunological reaction had occurred.

This process may also help to expain why no short-term rejection problems have been observed and why the meniscus would appear to be 'immunologically privileged'.

The early independent results reported by Garrett and Stevenson[125] and by Milahowshi and coworkers[126,127] are encouraging. They have noted an arrest in the progress of degenerative changes in articular cartilage. Meniscal transplantation may be of particular benefit in the knee that is anterior cruciate ligament deficient,[127] as meniscectomy in these patients potentially renders these knees even more unstable.[68,70,128,129] Although no specific complications have been observed, there is shrinkage of transplanted material.[127] Canham and Stanish[130] have shown that a minimum of shrinkage occurs in transplanted tissue-culture-stored allogenic menisci.

Garrett and Stevensen[125] recently reported on a 2.5-year follow-up study of six, fresh, meniscal transplants in the human knee. Four patients were reviewed arthroscopically and found to have healed transplant–rim junctions. No patient required further surgery.

Disease transmission is an ever-present potential hazard. AIDS has now almost reached epidemic proportions with a large number of the population unaware of their HIV status. The use of allografts poses a risk to the recipient. There has been a seroconversion in a patient after a fresh frozen allograft was used during anterior cruciate ligament reconstruction. Sterilization of a graft by irradiation may structurally weaken it, as over 4 Mrad of irradiation may be required for eradication of the virus. Despite rigorous testing of donor allograft material, the potential for disease spread still exists.

References

1. Aspden RM, Yarker YE, Hukins DWL. Collagen orientations in the meniscus of the knee joint. *Journal of Anatomy,* 1985; **140**: 371.
2. Aspden RM. A model for the function and failure of the meniscus. *Engineering in Medicine* 1985; **14**: 119.
3. Bullough PG, Munueral L, Murphy J, Weintein AM. The strength of the menisci of the knee as it relates to their fine structure. *Journal of Bone and Joint Surgery* 1970; **52B**: 564–70.
4. Krause WR, Pope MH, Johnson RJ, Wilder DG. Mechanical changes in the knee after meniscectomy. *Journal of Bone and Joint Surgery* 1976; **58A**: 599–604.
5. Kurosawa H, Fukubayashi T, Nakajima H. Load-bearing mode of the knee joint: physical behaviour of the knee joint with or without menisci. *Clinical Orthopaedics* 1980; **149**: 283.
6. McDevitt CA, Webber RJ. Ultrastructure and biochemistry of meniscal cartilage. *Clinical Orthopaedics* 1991; **252**: 8–18.
7. Walker PS, Erkman MJ. The role of the menisci in force transmission across the knee. *Clinical Orthopaedics* 1975; **109**: 184–92.
8. Dandy DJ, Jackson RW. The diagnosis of problems after meniscectomy. *Journal of Bone and Joint Surgery* 1975; **57B**: 349.
9. Fairbank TJ. Knee joint changes after meniscectomy. *Journal of Bone and Joint Surgery* 1948; **30B**: 664–70.
10. Goodfellow J. Editorials and annotations: he who hesitates is saved. *Journal of Bone and Joint Surgery* 1980; **62B**: 1–2
11. Northmore-Ball MD, Dandy DJ. Longterm results of arthroscopic partial meniscectomy. *Clinical Orthopaedics* 1982; **167**: 34.
12. Ghosh P, Taylor TKF. The knee joint meniscus: a fibrocartilage of some distinction. *Clinical Orthopaedics* 1987; **224**: 52–63.
13. Clark CR, Ogden JA. Development of the menisci of the human knee joint: morphological changes and their potential role in childhood meniscal injury. *Journal of Bone and Joint Surgery* 1983; **65A**: 538–47.
14. Heller L, Langman J. The menisco-femoral ligaments of the human knee. *Journal of Bone and Joint Surgery* 1964; **46B**: 307–13.
15. Arnoczky SP, Warren RF. Microvasculature of the human meniscus. *American Journal of Sports Medicine* 1982; **10**: 90–5.
16. Arnoczky SP, Warren RF. The microvasculature of the meniscus: its response to injury: experimental study in the dog. *American Journal of Sports Medicine* 1983; **11**: 131.
17. Danzig L, Resnick D, Gonsalves M, Akeson WH. Blood supply to the normal and abnormal menisci of the human knee. *Clinical Orthopaedics* 1983; **172**: 271–6.
18. Ghadially FN, Thomas I, Young N, Lalonde JMA. Ultrastructure of rabbit semilunar cartilage. *Journal of Anatomy* 1978; **125**: 499.
19. McMurray TP. The semilunar cartilages. *British Journal of Surgery* 1941; **29**: 407–14.
20. Seedhom BB, Hargreaves DJ. Transmission of the load in the knee joint with special reference to the role of the menisci. *Engineering in Medicine* 1979; **8**: 220.
21. Shrine N. The weight-bearing role of the menisci of the knee. *Journal of Bone and Joint Surgery* 1974; **56B**: 381.
22. King D. The function of semilunar cartilages. *Journal of Bone and Joint Surgery* 1936, **18**: 1069–76.
23. Appel H. Later results after meniscectomy in the knee joint. A clinical and roentogenologic follow-up investigation. *Acta Orthopaedica Scandinavica* 1970; **133** (Suppl.): 1–111.
24. Huckell JR. Is meniscectomy a benign procedure? A long term follow-up study. *Canadian Journal of Surgery* 1965; **8**: 254–60.
25. King D. The healing of semilunar cartilages. *Journal of Bone and Joint Surgery* 1936; **18**: 333–42.
26. Cox JS, Nye CE, Schaefer WW, Woodstein IJ. The degeneration effects of partial and total resection of the medial meniscus in dogs' knees. *Clinical Orthopaedics* 1975; **109**: 178.
27. Fithian DC, Kelly MA, Mow VC. Material properties and structure—function relationships in the menisci. *Clinical Orthopaedics* 1990; **252**: 19–31.
28. McGinty JB, Geuss LF, Marvin RA. Partial or total meniscectomy. A comparative analysis. *Journal of Bone and Joint Surgery* 1977; **59A**: 763–6.
29. Ahmad AM, Burke DL. *In vitro* measurement of static pressure distribution in synovial joints. Part 1: Tibial surface of the knee. *Journal of Biomechanical Engineering* 1983; **105**: 216.
30. Fukubbayashi T, Kurosawa H. The contact area and pressure distribution pattern of the knee. *Acta Orthopaedica Scandinavica* 1980; **51**: 871.
31. Voloshin AS, Wosk J. Shock absorption of the meniscectomized and painful knees. A comparative *in vivo* study. *Journal of Biomedical Engineering* 1983; **5**: 157.
32. Smillie IS. *Injuries of the knee joint,* 3rd edn. London: Churchill Livingstone, 1962.
33. Baker BE, Peckham AC, Pupparo F, Sanborn JC. Review of meniscal injury and associated sports. *American Journal of Sports Medicine* 1985; **13**: 1.
34. Insall JN. *Surgery of the knee.* New York: Churchill Livingstone, 1984: 230
35. Ferrer-Roca O, Vilalta C. Lesions of the meniscus. Part 1: Macroscopic and histologic findings. *Clinical Orthopaedics* 1980; **146**: 289–300.
36. Smillie LS. *Injuries of the knee joint,* 4th edn. London: Churchill Livingstone, 1970.
37. Noble J, Hamblen DL. The pathology of the degenerate meniscus lesion. *Journal of Bone and Joint Surgery* 1975; **57B**: 180–6.
38. Pritzker KPH, Renlund RC, Cheng PT. Which came first: crystals or osteoarthritis? A study of surgically removed femoral heads. *Journal of Rheumatology* 1983; **10**: 38.
39. Sokoloff L, Varma AA. Chondrocalcinosis in surgically resected joints. *Arthritis and Rheumatism* 1988; **31**: 750.

40. Ferrer-Roca O, Vilalta C. Lesions of the meniscus. Part II: Horizontal cleavages and lateral cysts. *Clinical Orthopaedics* 1980; **146**: 301–7.

41. Hough AJ, Webber RJ. Pathology of the meniscus. *Clinical Orthopaedics* 1990; **252**: 32–40.

42. Apley AG. The diagnosis of meniscal injuries: some new clinical methods. *Journal of Bone and Joint Surgery* 1947, **29**: 78–84.

43. Vandermeer RD, Cunningham FK. Arthroscopic treatment of the discoid lateral meniscus: results of long term follow up. *Arthroscopy* 1989; **5**: 101–9.

44. Noyes FR, Bassett RW, Grood ES, Butler DL. Arthroscopy in acute traumatic haemarthrosis of the knee: incidence of anterior cruciate tears and other injuries. *Journal of Bone and Joint Surgery* 1980; **62A**: 687–95.

45. Daniel D, Daniels E, Aronson D. The diagnosis of meniscus pathology. *Clinical Orthopaedics* 1982; **163**: 218–24.

46. De Haven KE, Collins HR. Diagnosis of internal derangements of the knee: the role of arthroscopy. *Journal of Bone and Joint Surgery* 1975; **57A**: 802–10.

47. Gillies H, Seligson D. Precision in the diagnosis of meniscal lesions: a comparison of clinical evaluation, arthrography, and arthroscopy. *Journal of Bone and Joint Surgery* 1979; **61A**: 343–6.

48. Ireland J, Trickey EL, Stoker DJ. Athroscopy and arthrography of the knee: a critical review. *Journal of Bone and Joint Surgery* 1980; **62B**: 3–6.

49. Jackson RW, Abe I. The role of arthroscopy in the management of disorders of the knee: an analysis of 200 consecutive examinations. *Journal of Bone and Joint Surgery* 1972; **54B**: 310–22.

50. Nicholas JA, Freiberger RH, Killoran PJ. Double-contrast arthrography of the knee: its value in the management of two hundred and twenty-five derangements. *Journal of Bone and Joint Surgery* 1970; **52A**: 203–20.

51. Selesnick FH, Noble HB, Bachman DC, Steinberg FL. Internal derangement of the knee: diagnosis by arthrography, arthroscopy, and arthrotomy. *Clinical Orthopaedics* 1985; **198**: 26–30.

52. McGinty JB, Metza RA. Arthroscopy of the knee. Evaluation of an out-patient procedure under local anaesthesia. *Journal of Bone and Joint Surgery* 1978; **60A**: 787.

53. Tegtmeyer CJ, McCue FC, Higgins SM, Ball DW. Arthrography of the knee: a comparative study of the accuracy of single and double contrast techniques. *Radiology* 1979; **132**: 37–41.

54. Fischer SP, Fox JM, Del Pizzo W, Friedman MJ, Snyder SJ, Ferkel RD. Accuracy of diagnosis from magnetic resonance imaging of the knee. *Journal of Bone and Joint Surgery* 1991; **73A**: 2–10.

55. Kelly MA *et al*. MR imaging of the knee: clarification of its role. *Arthroscopy* 1991; **7**: 78–85.

56. Manco LG, Lozman J, Coleman ND, Kavanaugh JH, Bilfield BS, Dougherty J. Noninvasive evaluation of knee meniscal tears: preliminary comparison of MR imaging and CT. *Radiology* 1987; **163**: 727–30.

57. Polly DW, Callaghan JJ, Sikes A, McCabe JM, McMahon K, Savory CG. The accuracy of selective magnetic resonance imaging compared with the findings of arthroscopy of the knee. *Journal of Bone and Joint Surgery* 1988; **70A**: 192–8.

58. Raunest J, Oberle K, Loehnert J, Hoetzinger H. The clinical value of magnetic resonance imaging in the evaluation of meniscal disorders. *Journal of Bone and Joint Surgery* 1991; **73A**: 11–16.

59. Silva I, Silver DM. Tears of the meniscus as revealed by magnetic resonance imaging. *Journal of Bone and Joint Surgery* 1988; **70A**: 199–202.

60. LaPrade RF, Burnett QM, Veenstra MA, Hodgman GC. The prevalance of abnormal magnetic resonance imaging findings in asymptomatic knees. With correlation of magnetic resonance to arthroscopic findings in symptomatic knees. *American Journal of Sports Medicine* 1994; **22**: 739–45.

61. Senghas RE. Indications for magnetic resonance imaging. (Editorial.) *Journal of Bone and Joint Surgery* 1991; **73A**: 1.

62. Passariello R, Trecco F, Paulis P, Masciocchi C, Bonanni G, Zobel BB. Meniscal lesions of the knee joint: CT diagnosis. *Radiology* 1985; **57**: 29–34.

63. Reichier MA, Hartzman S, Duckwiler GR, Bassett LW, Anderson LJ, Gold RH. Meniscal injuries: detection using MR imaging. *Radiology* 1986; **159**: 753–7.

64. De Haven KE. Meniscus repair in the athlete. *Clinical Orthopaedics* 1985; **198**: 31–5.

65. Casscells SW. The torn or degenerated meniscus and its relationship to degeneration of the weight-bearing areas of the femur and tibia. *Clinical Orthopaedics* 1978; **132**: 196–200.

66. Cox JS, Cordell LD. The degenerative effects of medial meniscus tears in dogs' knees. *Clinical Orthopaedics* 1977; **125**: 236–42.

67. Jackson JP. Degenerative changes in the knee after meniscectomy. *British Medical Journal* 1968; **2**: 525–7.

68. Johnson RJ, Kettlekamp DB, Clark W, Leaverton P. Factors affecting late results after meniscectomy. *Journal of Bone and Joint Surgery* 1974; **56A**: 719.

69. Seedhom BB, Dawson D, Wright V. Function of the menisci, preliminary study. *Journal of Bone and Joint Surgery* 1974; **56B**: 381–2.

70. Tapper EM, Hoover NW. Late results after meniscectomy. *Journal of Bone and Joint Surgery* 1969; **51A**: 517–26.

71. Fauno P, Nielsen AB. Arthroscopic partial meniectomy: A long-term follow-up. *Arthroscopy* 1992; **8**: 345–9.

72. Bolano LE, Grana WA. Isolated arthroscopic partial menisectomy. *American Journal of Sports Medicine* 1993; **21**: 432–7.

73. Jaureguito JW, Elliot JS, Lietner T, Dixon LB, Reider B. The effects of arthroscopic partial menisectomy in an otherwise normal knee: a retrospective review of functional, clinical, and radiographic results. *Arthroscopy* 1995; **11**: 29–36.

74. Arnoczky SP, Warren RF, Spivak JM. Meniscal repair using an exogenous fibrin clot: an experimental study in dogs. *Journal of Bone and Joint Surgery* 1988; **70A**: 1209–16.

75. Veth RPH, Den Heeten GJ, Jansen HWB, Nielsen HKL. An experimental study of reconstructive procedures in lesions of the meniscus: use of synovial flaps and carbon fibre implants for artificially made lesions in the meniscus of the rabbit. *Clinical Orthopaedics* 1983; **181**: 250–4.

76. Annandale T. An operation for displaced semilunar cartilage. *British Medical Journal* 1885; **i**: 779.

77. Heatley FW. The meniscus—can it be repaired? An experimental investigation in rabbits. *Journal of Bone and Joint Surgery* 1980; **62B**: 397–402.

78. Cabaud HE, Rodkey WG, Fitzwater JE. Medial meniscus repairs. An experimental and morphologic study. *American Journal of Sports Medicine* 1981; **9**: 129–34.

79. Scapinell R. Studies of the vasculature of the human knee joint. *Acta Anatomica (Basel)* 1968; **70**: 305.

80. Henning CE, Lynch MA, Yearout KM, Vequist SW, Stallbaumer RJ, Decker KA. Arthroscopic meniscal repair using an exogenous fibrin clot. *Clinical Orthopaedics* 1990; **252**: 64–72.

81. Kawai Y, Fukubayashi T, Nishino J. Meniscal suture: an experimental study in the dog. *Clinical Orthopaedics* 1989; **243**: 286–93.

82. Stoller DW, Martin C, Crues JV, Kaplan L, Mink JH. Meniscal tears: pathologic correlation with MR imaging. *Radiology* 1987; **163**: 731–5.

83. Dandy DJ, Jackson RW. The impact of arthroscopy on the management of disorders of the knee. *Journal of Bone and Joint Surgery* 1975; **57B**: 346–8.

84. Weiss CB, Lunberg M, Hamberg, P, De Haven KE, Gillquist J. Non-operative treatment of meniscal tears. *Journal of Bone and Joint Surgery* 1989; **71A**: 811.

85. De Haven KE. Decision-making factors in the treatment of meniscus lesions. *Clinical Orthopaedics* 1990; **252**: 49–54.

86. Northmore-Ball MD, Dandy DJ, Jackson RW. Arthroscopic, open partial, and total meniscectomy: a comparative study. *Journal of Bone and Joint Surgery* 1983; **65B** :400–4.

87. Pellacci F, Verni E, Gagliardi S, Goretti C. Arthroscopic lateral menisectomy in adults with stable knees. A medium-term evaluation of the results and a comparison with similar lesions of the medial meniscus. *Italian Journal of Orthopaedics and Traumatology* 1990; **16**: 9–17.

88. Metcalf RW. Arthroscopic meniscal surgery. In: McGinty JB *et al.*, eds. *Operative arthroscopy*. New York: Raven Press, 1991: 203–36.

89. Metcalf RW, Coward DB, Rosenberg PD. Arthroscopic partial meniscectomy: a five year follow up study. *Orthopaedic Transactions* 1983; **7**: 504.

90. Tenuta JJ, Arciero RA. Arthroscopic evaluation of meniscal repairs: factors that affect healing. *American Journal of Sports Medicine* 1994; **22**: 797–802.

91. De Haven KE. Peripheral meniscal repair: an alternative to meniscectomy. *Journal of Bone and Joint Surgery* 1981; **63B**: 463.

92. De Haven KE, Lohrer WA, Lovelock JE. Long term results of meniscal repair. Presented at the *Combined Congress of the International Arthroscopic Association and the International Society of the Knee, Toronto, May 1991.*

93. Ishmura M, Tamai S, Fujisawa Y. Arthroscopic meniscal repair with fibrin glue. *Arthroscopy* 1991; **7**: 177–81.

94. Hurley JA, Kirk P, and Bronstein R. The usefulness of magnetic resonance imaging in evaluating menisci after meniscal repair. Presented at the *Annual Meeting of the Arthroscopy Association of North America, Boston, Massachusetts, April 1992.*

95. Hanks GA, Gause TM, Sebastianelli WJ, O'Donnell CS, Kalenak A. Repair of peripheral meniscal tears: open versus arthroscopic technique. *Arthroscopy* 1991; **7**: 72–7.

96. Cassidy RE, Shaffer AJ. Repair of peripheral meniscus tears: a preliminary report. *American Journal of Sports Medicine* 1981; **9**: 209–14.

97. Dolan WA, Bhaskar, G. Peripheral meniscus repair: a clinical and pathologic study of 75 cases. *Orthopaedic Translations* 1983; **7**: 503.

98. Hamberg P, Gillquist J, Lysholm J. Suture of new and old peripheral meniscus tears. *Journal of Bone and Joint Surgery* 1983; **65A**: 193–7.

99. Rosenberg TD *et al.* Arthroscopic meniscal repair evaluation with repeat arthroscopy. *Arthroscopy* 1986; **2**: 14.

100. Scott GA, Jolly BJ, Henning CE. Combined posterior incision nd arthroscopic intra-articular repair of the meniscus. *Journal of Bone and Joint Surgery* 1986; **68A**: 847.

101. Solanki DR, Enneking FK, Ivey FM, Scarborough M, Johnston RV. Serum bupivacaine concentrations after intra-articular injection for pain relief after knee arthroscopy. *Arthroscopy* 1992; **8**: 44–7.

102. Boden BP, Fassler S, Cooper S, Marcchetto PA, Moyer RA. Analgesic affect of intra-articular morphine, bupivicaine, and morphine–bubivicaine after arthroscopic knee surgery. *Arthroscopy* 1994; **10**: 104–7

103. Ates Y, Kinik H, Binnet MS, Ates Y, Kanakci N, Kecik Y. Comparison of prilocaine and bubivicaine for post arthroscopic analgesia: a placebo-controlled double-blind trial. *Arthroscopy* 1994; **10**: 108–9.

104. Joshi GP, McCarroll SM, Brady OH, Hurson BJ, Walsh G. Intra-articular morphine for pain relief after anterior cruciate ligament reconstruction. *British Journal of Anaesthesia* 1993; **70**: 87–8.

105. Cannon WD. Arthroscopic meniscal repair. In: McGinty JB *et al.*, eds. *Operative arthroscopy*. New York: Raven Press, 1991; 237–51.

106. Cannon WD, Vittari JM. Arthroscopic meniscal repair results in anterior cruciate ligament reconstructed knee versus isolated repairs in stable knees. Presented at the *Combined Congress of the International Arthroscopic Association and the International Society of the Knee, Toronto, May 1991.*

107. Smith JB, Nance TA. Laser energy in arthroscopic surgery. Presented at the *Annual Meeting of the Arthroscopy Association of North America, Colorado, California, January 1983.*

108. Smith CF, JohansenWE, Vangness CT, Sutter LV, Marshall GJ. The carbon dioxide laser; a potential tool for orthopaedic surgery. *Clinical Orthopaedics* 1989; **242**: 43–50.

109. Whipple T, Caspari E, Meyers J. Synovial response to laser induced carbon ash residue. *Lasers in Surgery and Medicine* 1984; **3**: 291–5.

110. Sisto DJ, Blazina MD, Hirsh LC. The synovial response after CO_2 laser arthroscopy of the knee. *Arthroscopy* 1993; **9**: 574–5.

111. Brillheart AT. The technical problems of laser arthroscopy. Presented at the *Annual Meeting of the Arthroscopy Association of North America, Boston, Massachusetts, April 1992.*

112. Smith CF *et al.* Comparisons of tissue effects of a surgical scalpel, an electrocortery apparatus and a carbon dioxide laser system when used for making incisions into the menisci of New Zealand rabbits. *Lasers in Surgery and Medicine* 1984; **3**: 305.

113. Stein E, Seddlack T, Fabian RL, Nishioka N. Acute and chronic effects of bone abolation with a pulse holmium laser. *Lasers in Surgery and Medicne* 1990; **10**: 384–8.

114. Garino JP, Lotke PA, Seppiga AA, Reilly PJ, Esterhai JL. Osteonecrosis of the knee following laser-assisted arthroscopic surgery: a report of 6 cases. *Arthroscopy* 1995; **11**: 467–74.

115. Trauner K, Nishioka N, Patel D. Pulsed holmium: yttrium–aluminum–garnet (Ho:YAG) laser abalation of fibrocartilage and articular cartilage. *American Journal of Sports Medicine* 1990; **18**: 316–20.

116. Miller DV, O'Brien SJ, Arnoczky SP, Kelly A, Feely SV, Warren RF. The use of contact Nd:YAG laser in arthroscopic surgery: Effects on articular cartilage and meniscal tissue. *Arthroscopy* 1989; **5**: 245–53.

117. Collier MA *et al.* Effects of holmium:YAG laser on equine articular cartilage and subchondral bone adjacent to traumatic lesions: a histopathological assessment. *Arthroscopy* 1993; **9**: 536–45.

118. Spivak JM, Grande DA, Ben-Yishay A, Menche DS, Pitman MI. The effect of low-level Nd-YAG laser energy on adult articular cartilage *in vitro*. *Arthroscopy* 1992; **8**: 36–43.

119. Cisa, J, Basora J, Madarnas P, Ghibely A. Meniscus healing, experimental methods in the rabbit model with a synovial flap. Presented at the *Combined Congress of the International Arthroscopic Association and the International Society of the Knee, Toronto, May 1991.*

120. Webber RJ, York JL, Van Der Schilden JL, Hough AJ. An organ culture model for assaying wound repair of the fibrocartilaginous knee joint meniscus. *American Journal of Sports Medicine* 1989; **17**: 393–400.

121. Stone KR, Rodkey WG, Webber RJ, McKinney L, Steadman JR. Future directions: collagen based prostheses for meniscal regeneration. *Clinical Orthopaedics* 1990; **252**: 129–35.

122. van Arkle ERA, deBoer HH. Human meniscal transplantation: preliminary results at 2 to 5-year follow-up. *Journal of Bone and Joint Surgery* 1995; **77B**: 589–95.

123. Arnoczky SP, DeCarlo EF, O'Brien SJ, Warren RF. Cellular repopulation of deep-stroke frozen meniscal autographs: an experimental study in the dog. *Arthroscopy* 1992; **8**: 428–36.

124. Jackson DW, Whelan J, Simon TM. Cell survival after transplantation of fresh meniscal allograft: DNA probe analysis in a goat model. *American Journal of Sports Medicine* 1993; **21**: 540–50.

125. Garrett JC, Stevenson RN. Meniscal transplantation in the human knee: a preliminary report. *Arthroscopy* 1991; **7**: 57–61.

126. Milahowski KA, Weismeier K, Erhard TW, Remberger K. Transplantation of meniscus: an experimental study in sheep. *Sportverletzung Sportschaden* 1987; 1: 20.
127. Wirth CJ, Kohn D, Milachowski KA. Meniscus transplantation in knee joint instability. Presented at the *Combined Congress of the International Arthroscopy Association and the International Society of the Knee, Toronto, May 1991.*
128. Levy IM, Torzilli PA, Warren RF. The effect of medial meniscectomy on anterior–posterior motion of the knee. *Journal of Bone and Joint Surgery* 1982; **64A**: 883–8.
129. Hsieth HH, Walker PS. Stabilising mechanisms of the loaded and unloaded knee joint. *Journal of Bone and Joint Surgery* 1976; **58A**: 87–93.
130. Canham W, Stanish W. A study of the biological behaviour of the meniscus as a transplant in the medial compartment of a dog's knee. *American Journal of Sports Medicine* 1986; **14**: 376–9.

4.2.4 The patella: its afflictions in relation to athletics

Andrew H. Turtel, Jeffrey Minkoff, and Barry G. Simonson

Introduction

The patellofemoral articulation is among the most complex and least understood articulations in the body. Its disorders, to which have been ascribed the frequently used, though nebulously defined, diagnoses of chondromalacia, maltracking, malalignment, and instability, are among the more commonly seen disorders in young and middle-aged recreational and subélite competitive athletes presenting to sports medicine practices. Conversely, these are more rarely seen in élite amateur and professional populations. This observation does not necessarily imply an absence of developmental and structural disorders of the patellofemoral joint in these athletes. However, it follows as a natural corollary of the doctrine of natural selection that the more severely afflicted athletes are less likely to achieve an élite status. In some instances of more moderate structural handicaps, athletes of élite destiny may override or compensate for their physical disability by virtue of exceptional motor strength and/or technical skills.

Of course, there are the usual exceptions to customary trends. Gymnasts and some dancers are characteristic of athletes whose excellence is predicated upon a measure of joint laxity and flexibility. These performers often achieve an élite status despite their possession of frank patellofemoral instability or even recurrent patellar dislocation.

Parapatellar disorders, such as patellar tendinitis and retinacular inflammation, are quite common among élite athletes. They are particularly prevalent among athletes whose sports require repetitive percussion and/or deceleration in an eccentric format. Basketball and high jumping are prime examples of such sports, and it is from the latter that the name 'high jumper's knee' is derived. Combined physicals have been initiated by the National Basketball Association in recent years. The purpose of these physicals is to pre-evaluate, for all National Basketball Association professional teams, those college players most likely to be drafted. Approximately 100 players are examined each year. Injuries recorded are not for a single playing year but for the span of the player's basketball life. Extensor mechanism problems are the most numerous among all recorded injuries and diagnosis. These problems include chondromalacia with maltracking or alta, patellar tendinitis, patellar fracture, quadriceps tendinitis, and a ruptured patellar tendon. Despite the range and apparent severity of some of the entities listed, no player manifested a degree of disability which precluded competitive play (Hefferon, personal communication).

Despite the common presence of patellar laxity and alta among élite basketball players, patellar tendinitis is frequently the only symptomatic manifestation (versus instability or retropatellar pain) in this group.

A number of patellofemoral disorders are predicated upon chronology. Certain congenital and/or development disorders (for example, dysplasias) are evidenced in the preadolescent period. Osgood–Schlatter's disease and the Sinding-Larsen–Johansson syndrome are manifested in the periadolescent period. Patellar tendinitides are most often seen in younger adults. Distal quadriceps tendinitis and impingements of patella magna are most characteristic of middle-aged athletes. Quadriceps rupture is most commonly observed in the seventh decade. Chondromalacia and manifestations related to maltracking and instability are seen at all ages.

Fractures of the patella are uncommonly observed in the athletic population. Symptoms related to multipartite patellae are usually a consequence of superimposed trauma and are seen in younger athletes. Iatrogenic fractures are created in the process of autogenous bone–patellar tendon–bone harvesting for anterior cruciate ligament reconstructions.

What follows is a detailed discussion of patellofemoral disorders, their presentation, diagnosis, and treatment, and their relationship to athletic participation.

Patella

The patella is a sesamoid bone which develops within the quadriceps muscle–tendon unit. Its development begins during the ninth embryonic week. The shape of its cartilaginous anlage is well defined by birth, but ossification is not initiated until between the ages of 3 and 6 years. The ossification may occur in as many as six separate centres which gradually coalesce. Ossification is usually complete by the start of the second decade.

Patellar morphology

Anthropological studies by Vriese disclosed no apparent racial differences in the morphological dimensions of the patella. Its vertical length varies between 47 and 58 mm, and its width between 51 and 57 mm. Anteroposterior thickness is more variable, with a range of 2 to 3 cm when measured from the subchondral area of the median ridge to the superficial cortex. The chondral surface is also of variable thickness; its central portion is thickest, and, in fact, is the thickest in the body, being rather more than 0.6 cm.

The anterior or extensor surface of the patella is slightly convex and is divisible into three parts. The superior third of this surface is rough. It receives the insertion of the quadriceps tendon, a portion of which continues in the distal direction over the anterior patellar surface to form the deep fascia overlying and adherent to the latter.

The middle third is replete with vascular foramina, and the distal third is incarcerated within the patellar tendon.[1]

The posterior surface of the patella is divisible into superior and inferior portions, comprising roughly 75 per cent and 25 per cent of the surface, respectively. The superior portion is exclusively articular. The inferior portion is dotted with vascular orifices related to the normally adherent infrapatellar fat pad.[1]

The ovoid articular surface comprises two major facets divided by a vertically oriented promontory, the 'median ridge'. The lateral facet is usually wider and the medial facet shows the greatest variability. The latter is subdivided into the medial facet proper and a smaller odd facet segregated by a small vertical ridge which corresponds to the curve of the lateral border of the medial femoral condyle of the fully flexed knee. The medial ridge conforms to the straight medial border of the lateral femoral condyle. Interesting discussions of the patellar facets and their relations are available in the literature.[1-5]

The patella serves two major functions. One is to protect the femoral condyles and the other is to enhance the effectiveness of the extensor apparatus of the knee joint. The latter is accomplished in two ways. The first is by increasing the moment arm of the extensor mechanism and keeping the force being generated centralized. The second is by providing a low-friction articular surface, thereby increasing the efficiency of glide of the extensor apparatus.[6]

Congenital and developmental abnormalities

Several developmental abnormalities of the patellofemoral mechanism either impact upon the efficiency of its functions or may produce symptoms.

Hypoplastic or absent patella

The most dramatic abnormality is absence of the patella. This is an extremely rare condition which is not encountered in the élite athlete by virtue of the performance disability with which it is associated. Absence of the patella is most commonly one component of arthro-onychodysplasia or the nail-patella syndrome. The mechanical disability engendered by a congenitally absent patella is less severe than might be imagined because the associated enlargements of the femoral condyles and tibial tubercle enhance the leverage of a centralized extensor mechanism. However, when absence or hypoplasia of the patella occurs as an isolated entity, there may be a decentralization of the extensor mechanism.[7,8]

Severe lateral dislocation of the extensor mechanism (and patella, if present) is not so rare. The authors have seen at least one such case in which hypoplastic femoral condyles and laterally dislocated hypoplastic patella and extensor mechanism failed to preclude participation as a varsity player on a high-school basketball squad (Fig. 1).

Multipartite patellae

Multipartite patellae, particularly bipartite patellae, are very common. The incidence of bipartite patellae in adolescents has been reported to be between 0.2 and 6 per cent.[9] It is usually evident by 12 years of age. Secondary ossification centres responsible for this entity are most commonly seen superolaterally, but can be seen at

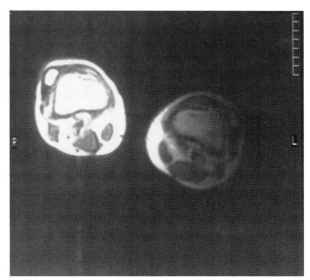

Fig. 1 MRI axial view showing hypoplastic femoral condyles and a congenital dislocated patella.

the distal pole, at the lateral margin, anterocentrally, or anterodistally. The incidence is predominant in males by a 2:1 ratio.[9]

While the bipartite patella has been said to be bilateral in most instances, Rockwood and Green report a unilateral occurrence of 57 per cent.[10] The variance in demographic reports may, in part, be ascribable to a clinical differential between the developmental and post-traumatic varieties. Indeed, the greatest import of the developmental bipartite patella, typically an asymptomatic entity, is its differentiation from an acute fracture of the patella. In the skewed circumstances in which a patient presents with patellar pain, the distinction between entities is often discernible by plain radiography. The fractured patella demonstrates irregular margins of cancellous bone, while the developmental entity is hallmarked by smooth margins of cortical bone (Fig. 2). Bilateral mirror-image lucencies may establish the diagnosis of the developmental form. **MRI**, **CT**, or bone scans can be used for differentiation if necessary.

Osgood–Schlatter's disease

The most frequently encountered symptomatic condition of the patellofemoral mechanism during development is that known as Osgood–Schlatter's disease. Osgood–Schlatter's disease is more frequent in males than in females (3:2 ratio), more predominant on the left side, and bilateral in up to 25 per cent of cases.[11] Characteristically, a periadolescent male between the ages of 11 and 15 years will present with pain and swelling about the tibial tubercle of one or both knees.[12] Pain is frequently exacerbated by impact and decelerating activities such as running, jumping, and cutting. The most commonly described physical findings are exquisite tenderness about an obviously enlarged tibial tubercle with overlying soft-tissue swelling (Fig. 3).

What is of importance, although not commonly reported or appreciated, is that the syndrome (not a disease) is often associated with patella alta and/or instability, tibiofemoral rotational laxity, and tenderness about the medial patellar retinaculum, inferior pole, and/or the patellar tendon. These additional findings may implicate

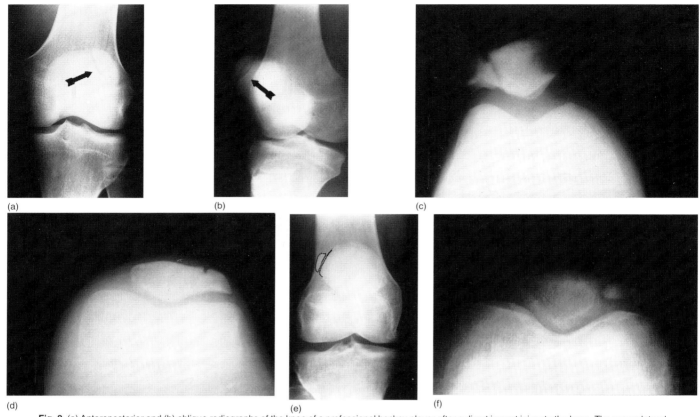

(a)   (b)   (c)

(d)   (e)   (f)

Fig. 2 (a) Anteroposterior and (b) oblique radiographs of the knee of a professional hockey player after a direct impact injury to the knee. The superolateral location of the lucent line (arrow) and its relatively smooth margins leave doubt as to whether this is a fracture or a bipartate patella. Pain severity, effusion, and a bone scan confirmed the suspicion of acute patellar fracture. (c) Axial radiograph demonstrating a patellar fracture. The irregularity of fragment margins should be noted. (d) Axial radiograph in which a bipartite fragment of the lateral facet was incidentally noted. Despite slight irregularity of the fragment margins, the patient manifested no patellar symptoms and denied a history of direct trauma to the patella. (e) Anteroposterior radiograph demonstrating a more traditional bipartite fragment of relatively small size and smoothly marginated (see market lines). (f) Axial radiograph of an obviously fractured patella. The fragment is situated medially and has been sheared from the patella as a consequence of an acute patellar dislocation.

instability of the patella and maltracking as causative agents in an entity which hedges the issue of acquired versus developmental afflictions.

Pursuant to the foregoing paragraph is the commonly provided

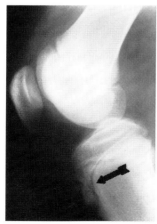

Fig. 3 Lateral radiograph of an adolescent (open epiphyses) male with pain over the tibial tubercle accompanied by severe tenderness and swelling. The irregularity of the tubercular apophysis and the small opacification anterior to it should be noted.

explanation that Osgood–Schlatter's disease is a 'traction apophysitis'.[13] What this means in terms of deducing a mechanism by which this syndrome develops is not altogether clear. In 1903, when Osgood and Schlatter independently described the syndrome which bears their names, they suggested that trauma was the inciting cause.[11]

With respect to the pathogenesis of Osgood–Schlatter's disease, Uhry[14] determined that it is traumatically induced. He indicated that the trauma resulted in a laceration of the interface between the patellar tendon and the tubercle, and in some instances at the cartilaginous plate between the tuberosity and the metaphysis.

During the apophyseal stage (Ib in the classification of Ogden and Southwick (1976), the tuberosity is susceptible to injury (cited in reference 11). Microavulsions can take place throughout the bone and/or cartilage of the secondary ossification centre because they are weaker than the distal fibrous tissue and adjoining bone.[11] La Zerte and Rapp reported that histological sections from the tuberosity defect show the presence of granulation tissue and osteoid, suggesting the presence of a healing fracture (cited in reference 11). Apparently, forceful contractions of the quadriceps by active adolescents can produce these 'fractures' in susceptible tubercles.

According to this explanation, it would not be difficult to assume that dysfunctional patellofemoral mechanisms (for example,

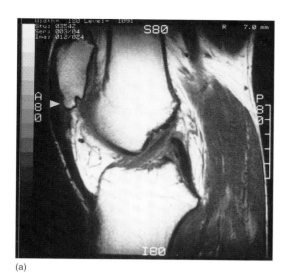 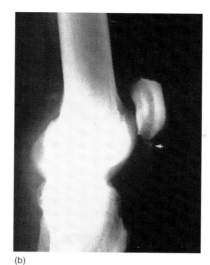 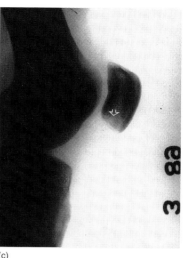

(a) (b) (c)

Fig. 4 (a) Sagittal magnetic resonance (**MR**) image of the knee of a professional basketball player with severe inferior pole pain and tenderness. This appearance is consistent with Stage IVa findings of the Medlar and Lyne classification, in which there is incorporation of calcification by the inferior pole (arrow). (b) Lateral radiograph of the knee of a professional basketball player with minimal inferior pole symptoms. This radiograph demonstrates Stage IVb in the Medlar and Lyne classification, in which the calcific mass is separate from the patella (arrow). (c) Lateral radiograph of the knee of a professional basketball player with no opacities about the inferior pole. Instead, there is a lucent zone (arrow). This player's symptoms were so severe and recalcitrant that surgery, with debridement of the inferior pole, was necessary.

instability and maltracking) played an aetiological role, propagating eccentric tensile forces to the tubercle and thereby producing an indirect traumatic force to the tubercle. Additional credence for these suppositions is provided by the frequent reduction in symptoms produced by bracing, strengthening, and quadriceps-stretching programmes. These hypotheses also explain the cessation of symptoms with apophyseal fusion. Obviously, the exclusive occurrence of this syndrome during early adolescence rules out its interference in the performance of élite athletes other than gymnasts and perhaps the youngest of female élite athletes.

Plain radiography often reveals swelling anterior to the tibial tubercle, thickening of the patellar tendon, and, not infrequently, alta or malposition of the patella on specific lateral and axial views, respectively. In more chronic cases, or in older adolescents, enlargement of the tubercle and opaque densities near the distal insertion of the tendon may be observed. The most obvious radiographic finding, when present, is fragmentation of the tuberosity. It is also the most variable finding.

Only in the most severely symptomatic cases do afflicted adolescents refrain from activities voluntarily. More typically, parental concern is the stimulus for a visit to the paediatrician or orthopaedic surgeon. Treatment is first targeted at the parents by allaying any fears that Osgood–Schlatter's disease is a foreboding condition, despite the pain and the ominous-sounding name. Typically, the parents are assured that it is a self-limiting syndrome, rarely lasting more than 1 to 2 years from its inception. This is a half truth. The truthful half relates to the almost inviolate trend of a reduction in symptoms confined to the tubercle *per se*. However, it should be appreciated that the patella tendon manifestations often associated with this syndrome may regress, persist, or become more predominant with continued growth and development of the adolescent.

Treatment of the child is conducted from among several limited options which include activity moderation, soothing physical therapeutic modalities, brace or compression bandage facsimiles, and

strengthening and stretching exercises for the muscles controlling the knee. The application of extended knee cylinder casts is no longer an option because of its atrophic effects. In the past, recalcitrant cases, or those in which expedient functional return was deemed necessary, were often treated by tubercular excision with a risk of affecting the growth of the subjacent proximal tibial physis. Occasionally, there is a rationale for excising loose tubercular fragments which are producing symptoms. Such surgical exercises should be discouraged until after growth has been completed to avoid growth-plate arrest and the development of recurvatum and/or valgus of the knee.

Patellar tendinitis and Sinding-Larsen–Johansson syndrome

Sinding-Larsen (1921) and Johansson (1922) each described an entity in adolescents in which there is inferior pole tenderness and radiographic fragmentation without any consistent history of trauma.[11] This entity is another in the continuum of chronologically related traction lesions within the patellofemoral apparatus. Its symptomatic focus is at the distal pole of the patella, a predilected site in prepubescents and young adults as opposed to the tubercular locus (Osgood–Schlatter's disease) of adolescents, the quadriceps tendinitides of older adults, or the degenerative quadriceps ruptures of septuagenarians.

Typically, the afflicted patient is between 10 and 13 years of age. The stages of radiographic progression of the disorder have been characterized by Medlar and Lyne (1978) (Fig. 4):[11]

Stage I Normal findings

Stage II Irregular inferior pole calcification

Stage III Coalescence of calcification

Stage IVa Incorporation of calcification by the inferior pole

Stage IVb A calcified mass, separate from the patella

The onset of symptoms (focal pain and swelling) are often attributed to the patient's having participated in repetitive jumping, running, kicking, or other activities responsible for eccentric and decelerative impulse loading of the extensor mechanism. This is consistent with the theory of Curwin and Stanish who suggested that overload occurs in the eccentric phase of quadriceps usage, as when landing from a jump.[15] It is also for this reason that Blazina coined the name 'jumper's knee'.[16] Eccentric contractions of the quadriceps in sports like basketball and volleyball, during the touchdown or landing phase, may cause inflammation of the paratenon and possible degenerative changes in the tendon itself.

Sinding-Larsen–Johansson syndrome and patellar tendinitis are similarly derived from overuse traction formats, albeit at different stages of development. The high-school, college, and adult athletes afflicted with patellae tendinitides entities present with pain and swelling at the distal pole of the patella and the subjacent portion of the patellar tendon. On physical examination, tenderness is most easily elicited by placing the knee in extension, to relax the extensor mechanism, and then palpating the deepest portion of the distal tip of the patella which has been made to stand proud by applying a distally and posteriorly directed force to the superior pole with the opposite hand. There is usually no intra-articular swelling, loss of motion, or symptoms attributable to meniscal pathology (joint-line tenderness).

Pathologically, the entity, represents a partial tear (or tears) of the patellar tendon just distal to the inferior pole.[17] The deep central fibres of the tendon are those most typically involved. Histologically, the involved areas demonstrate mucoid degeneration and fibrinoid necrosis. Plain radiography is usually unremarkable in cases of less than several months duration. In more chronic cases, fibrocartilaginous metaplasia within the tendon may result in a zone of opacification contiguous with the inferior pole.

Blazina *et al.*[17] classified the clinical progression into three phases:

Phase I Pain after activity only

Phase 2 Pain during and after activity

Phase 3 Same as in Phase 2, but performance is diminishing.

Roels *et al.* (1978) suggested a similar progression, but with tendon rupture as the ultimate phase.[11]

Ultrasonography may have some worth in the evaluation of patellar tendinitis. It is non-invasive and may document the presence of oedema, haemorrhage, partial rupture, or calcification which may not be evident on plain radiographs. The usual tendon thickness at the inferior pole (usually less than 5 mm) may be increased to more than 10 mm by oedema or haemorrhage and is calculable by ultrasonography.[18]

Bone scans can be used to demonstrate the uptake of tracer at the inferior or superior poles of the patella, with activity at the bone–tendon interface implying a chronic microfailure-reparative process.[19] Abnormal sonograms and positive bone scans usually indicate a chronic and refractory disease process. Jackson *et al.* (1988) (cited in reference 18) and El Kourey *et al.*[19] revealed the value of MRI in documenting the components of patellar tendinitis including localization of focal lesions and areas of tendon thickening.

The use of these studies for assistance in surgical decision making is, as yet, unclear.

Biomechanical factors that predispose to these conditions include quadriceps weakness, hamstring tightness or contracture, and muscle fatigue. All place increased stress on quadriceps contraction needed to generate force and movement. In addition, it is likely that excessive tibial/femoral axial rotatory laxity and pes planus place excessive demands on the extensor mechanism with untoward results.

The obvious dilemma for the élite athlete afflicted with an inferior pole syndrome who must practice or compete virtually daily throughout a well-defined season, and whose performance is his or her future, is how to keep symptoms minimized while averting a progression in pathology. This is sometimes impossible without sacrificing a portion of the season.

Options for treatment may include each of the four major categories (pharmacological, physiotherapeutic, immobility, and surgical) depending upon the severity, chronicity, and expediency of the case in point. Activity modification (curtailment of impulsion activities) is often necessary for the abatement of any inflammatory stimulus. A more rapid reduction of inflammatory signs and symptoms may be accomplished by physiotherapeutic modalities (ice, ultrasound, phonophoresis, iontophoresis, electrotherapy) and non-steroidal anti-inflammatory drugs (**NSAIDs**). These treatments should not be administered for the purpose of allowing participation (that is to say, merely to mask symptoms while allowing damage to accrue), except under the most limited circumstances when participation in a vital event (for instance, a championship or a career-determining event) must not reasonably be abandoned. Steroidal injections are to be avoided for the same reason, as well as for fear of creating iatrogenic degeneration within the tendon.

Physical therapy is a standard of treatment. It is broken down into three phases: acute, recovery, and maintenance programmes.[20] Apart from the application of modalities, the strengthening of all muscle groups of the extremity must be undertaken, titrating the arcs and loads to levels which do not provoke symptoms during or after the sessions. Eccentric strengthening of the quadriceps must be included in the regimen to help make the extensor mechanism more resistant to (namely to absorb more of the energy of) those impulsion forces which perpetrate the onset of symptoms. Traction effects upon the painful insertion site of the inflamed tendon into the inferior pole may be reduced by maintaining a vigil of quadriceps stretching. In some cases, the implementation of patellar restraining braces may impede symptoms by reducing patellar mobility and recoil, and by diffusing the forces at the inferior pole (Fig. 4). The return to athletics is gradual with sport-specific exercises preceding actual participation. Attempts to return too soon risk recurrence.

Recalcitrant cases (and some with a special need for expedient resolution) may solicit surgical intervention, although such invasive treatment is rarely necessary. When surgery is performed, it is directed at the excision of degenerated or necrotic tendon and any calcified metaplastic tissue. The nature and magnitude of surgical pathology is a function of the duration of the condition. A representative progression may be as follows: degenerated tissue at 3 to 4 months; haemorrhage and cyst formation at 6 to 12 months; and gritty metaplastic cartilage after 1 year. Surgery for this entity may be performed using local anaesthesia. When the local anaesthetic is administered layer by layer, the focus of tenderness can often be identified intraoperatively.

Postoperatively, motion of the knee is initiated immediately. As the acute symptoms subside, quadriceps stretching to prevent 'hitches' in extensor mechanism glide as well as hamstring stretching to inhibit a block to terminal extension are initiated. Once full painless motion is achieved, a slow progression of resistive exercises (see above) is begun. Ultimately, agility, proprioceptive, and pleiometric activities are progressed towards a return to normal athletic function. The foregoing sequence is normally accomplished in a period of 3 to 4 months.

It must be understood that many individuals whose activities induce an inferior pole–patellar tendon pain syndrome have predisposing structural assemblages of their extensor mechanisms. Patellae which are alta, too lax, or too tight, which have excessive static or dynamic Q angles, and which have various malalignments are among the structural formats which may assist activities in the production of tensile injuries to the extensor apparatus. The severity of underlying aberrations in patellofemoral function may determine the need to consider treatments above and beyond those necessary for the tendinitis alone, even to the extent of considering derotational bracing or patellar mechanism realignment.

Élite basketball players are among those athletes who commonly manifest an inferior pole syndrome. They are stereotypically tall with high-riding patellae and elongated tendons subjected to a whipping action by virtue of their jumping and cutting manoeuvres. One of us (JM) has attended only two players who required surgical treatment for severe recalcitrant symptoms in his experience with two professional basketball teams spanning a 15-year period.

Iatrogenic considerations and arthrofibrosis

A greater awareness of the rising incidence of iatrogenically induced inferior pole syndromes developed in the 1980s. It was during this decade that the popularity of bone–patellar tendon–bone substitutes for the anterior cruciate ligament reached a peak. After harvests of the central third of the tendon (Fig. 5), inferior pole syndromes arose with some frequency and often persisted for periods of up to 12 to 18 months' postoperatively. It was not clear whether these symptoms were primarily the result of the patellar fracture, harvesting, the reaction to the tendon defect created, the magnitude of the overall surgery, atrophic effects, the nature of the initiated physical therapy programmes, or other factors. As the decade progressed, the magnitude of surgery was reduced by the advent of arthroscopically assisted reconstruction; motion was started immediately and many of the atrophic effects of the surgery were eliminated. Nevertheless, a reasonable incidence of the syndrome persisted, leaving patellar fracture and tendon harvest-site responses, therapy formats, and generalized inflammatory responses with tardy restoration of patellar glide as probable culprits. The use of allografts, iliotibial band, or pes tendon substitutes resulted in a reduced incidence and severity of inferior pole syndromes. However, some incidence was observed, leaving failure of patellar glide restoration (by virtue of cicatrix about the tendon and fat pad, or captured knee motion by virtue of anisometrically tensioned grafts) and therapy formats as probable sources. In view of these suppositions, it is interesting that autogenous bone–patellar tendon–bone substitute procedures yield an estimated 5 to 10 per cent incidence

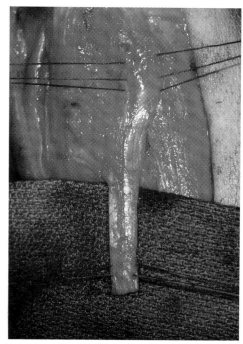

Fig. 5 Patellar tendon autograft with bone from the patella and the tibial tubercle at its respective ends.

of arthrofibrotic responses with curtailments of terminal extension and flexion of the operated knees. A characteristic finding in these cases is pain with activity in terminal extension at the inferior pole of the patella, which often must be alleviated by additional surgery to free patellar glide. Frequent findings include a relative patella baja, patellar tendon fibrosis and adherence to the anterior capsule and fat pad, adhesions in and about the suprapatellar pouch, and degenerative changes of the anterior portions of the femoral condyles (Fig. 6). Unfortunately, after these findings have appeared, even after single or multiple procedures to improve motion or decrease pain, function is rarely completely restored.

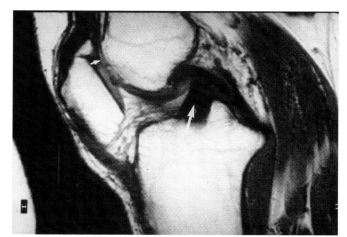

Fig. 6 Sagittal MR image demonstrating a dramatic patella baja. A fluid-containing tissue occupies the interval between the patella and anterior condylar surface of the femur which demonstrates articular irregularity (small arrow). Incidentally noted is the posterior position of the anterior cruciate ligament (large arrow).

That physical therapy can result in iatrogenically induced inferior pole syndromes has become well known in the wake of the rise of strengthening machinery throughout the 1980s. The forces generated by the use of some machine therapy forms can result in micro- or macrotears of the variety described above. Machines with ballistic high-speed and open-chain formats, have been particularly implicated.

Patellar tendon and quadriceps disruption

Disruptive injuries to the extensor mechanism were reported by such ancients as Galen.[21] Nevertheless, quadriceps and patella tendon ruptures are relatively uncommon injuries, relatively more common in males, and relatively specific with respect to the age bracket above and below in which each is likely to occur. Siwek and Rao[21] retrospectively studied 117 patients with patellar tendon or quadriceps ruptures. The results of their study revealed that 80 per cent of patients with patellar tendon ruptures were aged 40 or less, while 88 per cent of those with quadriceps ruptures were more than 40 years of age.

There is a general consensus that extensor mechanism ruptures are more likely to occur as a sequel to pre-existing pathology at or near the site of rupture.[7] Predisposing pathology includes chronic tendinitis, repetitive traumatic microtears, and degenerated tissue (from wear and tear or ageing). Each of these pathologies can be produced by 'overuse' activities and/or by poor structural mechanics. McLaughlin (1949) (cited in reference 22) reported that biopsies were routinely performed on freshly ruptured tendons at the New York Presbyterian Hospital and that microhistological sections repeatedly revealed a decrease in the collagen content of the tendon fibres, fibrotic degeneration, and a marked loss of nuclei. Speed (1950) added that fatty degeneration was often seen at rupture sites in obese patients.[22]

When ruptures of the extensor mechanism occur without a prodrome or history of predisposing pathology or when spontaneous bilateral ruptures occur, an underlying systemic disorder must be considered (Fig. 7).[23,24] Some of the disorders which have been associated with such ruptures are rheumatoid arthritis, systemic lupus erythematosus, gout, chronic renal failure, secondary hyperparathyroidism, diabetes mellitus, and peripheral vascular disease. The use of local and systemic steroids has also been implicated in the production of extensor mechanism ruptures. Nevertheless, Kelly et al.[25] found no correlation with the use of steroid injections in a series (n = 14) of ruptures. Most commonly, tears of the quadriceps occur through the rectus tendon at its insertion into the proximal pole of the patella. Tears may begin several centimetres more proximally, and not infrequently they may extend to the aponeurotic expansions of the vasti (Fig. 8).[22] Sometimes, the rectus tendon will avulse a small piece of bone from the patella. Patellar tendon disruptions are most common at the inferior pole of the patella where associated avulsions of bone fragments may be seen. Mid-substance rupture tears of the quadriceps or patellar tendons are the least common varieties.[26]

Disruptions at the tibial insertion are rare in adults, but do occur in adolescents. In 1990, Chow et al.[27] reported that 150 avulsion fractures of the tibial tubercle had been reported up to 1986. The injury is of concern because it involves the growth plate. Chow et al.

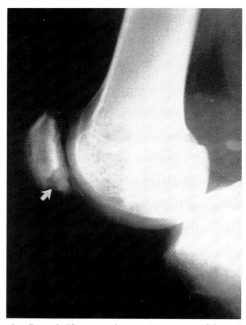

Fig. 7 Lateral radiograph 10 years subsequent to rupture of the patellar tendon from the distal pole in a teenage male under active treatment for leukaemia. It reveals patella alta and irregularity of the inferior pole to which the avulsed tendon was reattached by sutures through drill holes.

reviewed 16 patients after an average follow-up of 3.7 years. They classified the injuries in accordance with the classification of Ogden and Southwick (1976) (Fig. 9). Most cases can be treated conservatively. Of these 16, 12 patients with a combination of type I and type II avulsions could actively extend their knees and required no surgery. Review of their series revealed a male and a left-sided predominance. Only one patient had an appreciated pre-existing condition, which was Osgood–Schlatter's disease. The present authors have experienced two such avulsions over a 15-year period, one in a patient with leukaemia (Fig. 7) and the other with a pre-existing 'jumping' patella, which is a flagrant manifestation of J-sign tracking.

Type II and higher grades of avulsion require internal fixation.

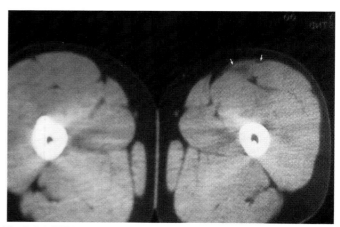

Fig. 8 Axial MR image of the mid-thigh of a college soccer player who sustained a rupture of the rectus muscle (between arrows) several centimetres proximal to the patella.

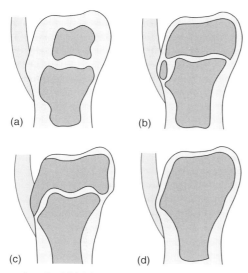

Fig. 9 Stages of proximal tibial development. (a) Cartilaginous stage. (b) Apophyseal stage. (c) Epiphyseal stage. (d) Bony stage. (Redrawn from ref. 25, with permission.)

Chow *et al.*[27] recommend a cancellous screw and tension-band wiring. They reported no late occurrences of genu recurvatum in any of their cases.

Most disruptions are due to indirect trauma. Anzel *et al.* (1959) corroborated this contention, stipulating that the majority of ruptures in their large series were due to indirect trauma.[23] A strong eccentric contraction of the quadriceps muscle with the knee in flexion is the usual indirect traumatic cause. In a classic report, McMaster (1933) contended that without prior degenerative attenuation, the enormous tensile strength of the tendon will preclude rupture.[24] Jobe *et al.* calculated that the force needed to rupture the infrapatellar tendon is about 17.5 times bodyweight. However, it is clear that repetitive microtrauma and systemic conditions may substantially weaken these tendons, lessening the force needed to rupture them.[28]

Patients who have sustained a quadriceps tendon rupture traditionally present with a history of having fallen or stumbled. Pain is often acute and immediate, as is an unsettling sensation of instability within the extremity. The pain may preclude an effective evaluation of knee extension ability. An injection of local anaesthetic may facilitate the physical examination, especially when diagnosis of a rupture is not corroborated by finding a gap in the tendon or by radiographic identification of a patella baja (particularly with a fragment of bone avulsed from its proximal pole). Lesser tears may not preclude an ability to extend the knee completely, making the decision to explore the injury site surgically more difficult.[29] Tardy presentations (after several weeks) are usually more for dysfunction than pain, and any defect in the tendon which may have existed has often become partially or wholly obliterated by collagenous ingrowth (although tenderness usually persists). Apart from the most innocuous of tears, surgical repair is a virtual necessity for restoring adequate knee function, no less athletic function.

Primary suture techniques, passing the sutures through drill holes in the patella, are the most frequently practiced. Ruptures through pathological or degenerated tissue may require reinforcement of the suture repair with such augmentations as Dacron tapes,

fascia lata, pes tendons, or reflected flaps from the quadriceps apparatus itself. If the repair and the tissue appear sound, early passive motion should be initiated, as should submaximal quadriceps setting exercises. Active motion without loading may be initiated within a few weeks in many instances, but weight bearing should be curtailed for at least 6 to 8 weeks to avoid an unwitting transmission of force across the suture line before some tensile strength has developed at the repair site. Naturally, the size of the defect, the quality of the tissues, the expediency of recovery, and the personality of the patient will help to determine the rates of progressing motion and loading. Athletes will generally not defer treatment for a major injury disability and, for this reason, late reconstruction of quadriceps tendons will not be discussed here.

Patients with patellar tendon ruptures also present after having sustained injury as a result of a violent, eccentric, quadriceps mechanism stress, as in basketball rebounding. As with the quadriceps rupture, there is immediate pain, instability, inability to extend the knee, and a defect at the rupture site. There may be a fragment avulsed from the inferior pole and/or alta appearance of the tendon on a plain radiograph. The principles of repair (with or without augmentation) and postoperative management are similar to those described for ruptures of the quadriceps tendon. Undue loading of the patellar mechanism must be avoided for several months at least. Early restoration of range of motion is necessary to avoid contractures within the extensor apparatus and subsequent loss of motion and patellar tendon inflammation.

Anterior knee pain: chondromalacia, instability, and malalignment

The related entities of chondromalacia, patellar instability, and patellar malalignment are among the banes of the practicing orthopaedic surgeon. For the most part, the orthopaedic literature has dealt with each of these entities as if they were primary or isolated pathologies. Fortunately, patellar pathology alone has rarely been a cause for permanent abandonment of participation, once an élite status has been achieved. Among the authors none has witnessed a forced retirement due solely to patellar pathology in a combined professional team experience totalling more than 40 years (including soccer, American football, basketball, and ice hockey). Nevertheless, Hayes *et al.*[30] cite Schneider (1962) in stating that articular cartilage degeneration is a leading cause of restricted sports activity.

Chondromalacia patella, in particular, has been treated as an isolated patellar pathology by many authors (idiopathic chondromalacia).[31] Chondromalacia, which literally means softened cartilage, has inappropriately become a receptacle for all manner of anterior knee pain. Hayes *et al.*[30] state that patellofemoral contact pressures have been implicated in the pathogenesis of articular cartilage degeneration, citing Pfeil (1966) and Ohno (1988) among others. In many instances it is a known consequence of direct trauma to the patella (Fig. 10), infection, postinjury and postoperative atrophic dystrophies, and patellar instability or maltracking syndromes. It is not unreasonable to surmise that the seemingly idiopathic forms are consequent to less evident forms of the entities listed above.

Chondromalacia has been staged in accordance with the degree of damage which is present, but without positive correlations to a

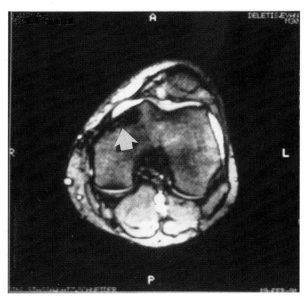

Fig. 10 Axial MR image of the knee of an individual whose flexed knee impacted an immovable object with substantial force. Patellar pain and crepitation followed shortly thereafter, consistent with the development of chondromalacia. A bony defect or 'bone bruise' is noted just medial to the trochlear groove (arrow), attesting to the magnitude of impact.

spectrum of symptom severity and functional disability. The articular surface of the patella has no sensory innervation. Nevertheless, patients with chondromalacia are typically reported to complain of retropatellar pain. Whether this pain derives from the underlying spongiosa or from the adjacent retinacula is a matter of speculation. Many patients are more disturbed by the gritty crepitation experienced while extending the knee than by any associated pain. The flaking and fibrillated articular surface frequently incites the synovium to produce effusions. Fulkerson and Shea[32] rightly indicate that correlations between articular cartilage degeneration (with crepitus) and patellar pain are inconsistent.

Supportive treatments are similar to those described above for other patellar afflictions. NSAIDs may reduce inflammatory sequelae and have superseded the aspirin regimens thought to prevent a progression of chondromalacia.[33] Physical therapy for the institution of modalities, stretching, and strengthening should be initiated empirically. The response to physical therapy is less predictably successful than it is for some patellar entities with a more obvious mechanical basis. Bracing is sometimes a detriment, with the compression increasing the sensation of painful crepitation. In other instances, as when chondromalacia is an accompaniment of patellar instability, bracing may provide a sense of increased stability as well as a reduction in pain or swelling.

Patients with continued pain may respond to a specific taping programme instituted by Jenny McConnell, an Australian physical therapist.[34] If associated maltracking can be identified, specific taping to counteract these mechanical forces has resulted in a 96 per cent success in decreasing patients' symptoms.

When instability or maltracking of the patella is not identifiable as a cause of symptomatic chondromalacia, the role of surgery is limited and its success is unpredictable.

According to Buckwalter et al.[35] loss of large areas of articular cartilage or the presence of full thickness 'holes' will compromise

joint function. However, the issue is how to deal with these entities. Buckwalter et al. point out that articular cartilage injury response has been studied for a quarter of a millennium since Hunter (1743) observed that articular ulcerations are not repaired. They indicate that current research reaffirms Hunter's contention that while cartilage is repaired under certain conditions, for the most part repair attempts fail to restore its normal molecular composition and durability.

Several methods of chondrogenesis, including cartilage shaving, abrasion chondroplasty, articular surface load alteration, gels, and electrostimulation, have been proposed.[36] O'Donoghue[37] and Johnson[38] reported that patellar articular shaving and/or abrasion may relieve symptoms. However, Buckwalter et al. caution that the efficacy of these frequently performed procedures has not been established for parameters, apart from symptomatic relief, that may occur for variable periods.

Historically, most surgery has been preoccupied with smoothing of the chondral surface. In the era prior to that of therapeutic arthroscopy (that is to say, prior to the mid-1970s) an arthrotomy was performed: the patella was released and everted, and a scalpel blade was used to pare damaged facets down to shiny cartilage. Whether the apparent improvements noted in some cases were due to the shaving or to inadvertent realignment from having released the patella or to other factors (retinacular release) is again not clear. The postoperative course was often protracted, restoration of motion was often difficult, and results were often not gratifying. In some instances in which the most severe damage was confined to a limited area of the articular surface, such as the odd facet, facetectomy was performed with some success.[36] In the most flagrant and recalcitrant cases patellectomy was not uncommon. Symptoms were often alleviated, but sometimes were superseded by knee instability due to a reduction in leverage of the extensor mechanism.

The advent of therapeutic arthroscopy, and of power-shaving instrumentation in particular, at the end of the 1970s created a more palatable option to arthrotomy. Using chondral abrasion of varying depth and surface area, as well as selective synovectomy, debridement and chondroplasty could be effected by closed methods on an outpatient basis. Results were better than those with its open counterpart, morbidity was substantially lower, and the initiation of early motion was dramatically expedited. However, whether arthroscopic chondral abrasion or skilled scalpel planing of the softened or fibrillated articular surface were used, controversy pertinent to the principles of these procedures persists.

Although the removal of damaged cartilage may temporarily reduce symptoms and eliminate the likelihood of synovial inflammation by flaking chondral debris, the articular surface is reduced in thickness, accelerating potential exposure of the underlying bone. In their preoccupation with achieving a smooth articular surface, the Chinese have reported success (reduced crepitation and pain) in using silicone plugs to fill articular divets (J.M. Minkoff, personal communication).

Since the advent of arthroscopy, facetectomy has essentially become a procedure of historical interest and the salvation of the patella has become a universal doctrine. For many surgeons who may have considered patellectomy in the past, the Macquet procedure or Fulkerson's modification of tubercle elevation (see below) has become its replacement.[38] Elevation of the tibial tubercle affords greater leverage to the extensor mechanism, and reports of great satisfaction in relieving the signs and symptoms of chondromalacia pervade the literature.[38-42] The good results may be fortuitous, since it has yet to be proved that the manifestations of chondromalacia derive from inadequate extensor leverage. Furthermore, the Macquet operation produces a protuberant and often painful tubercular region as well as other complications (Fig. 11).

Recently, increased interest has been directed towards resurfacing damaged articular surfaces. Chondrocyte transplants have been proposed by several authors and results published.[43] Unfortunately, the procedure is, as yet, unproven, although demand is being driven by unrealistic public expectations and entrepreneurial forces. A recent symposium at the annual meeting of the American Academy of Orthopedic Surgeons attempted to place the procedure in perspective with regard to actual outcomes and cost effectiveness.[44] The general feeling of those on the panel is that the data on autologous chondrocyte transplantation is insufficient, and although approved (in femoral resurfacing) for use by the Federal Drug Administration in the United States of America, no statements have been made with regard to the procedure's efficacy. Presently, this technique must still be viewed as investigational especially for patella resurfacing.

'Maltracking' of the patella is a particularly difficult subject to comprehend and discuss. Its complexities are profound, and the interface of its dynamics has yet to be reasonably elucidated. Maltracking may be represented by abnormal glide patterns attributable to patellar instability. The instability may result in maltracking due to the extremes of patellar laxity, medial and/or lateral, or due to weakness or dysplasia of the extension mechanism. The instability may be manifested in a limited portion of the arc of knee motion

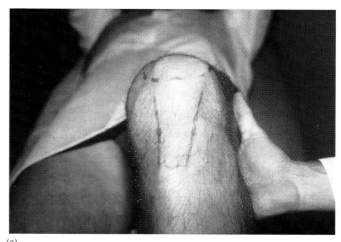

(a)

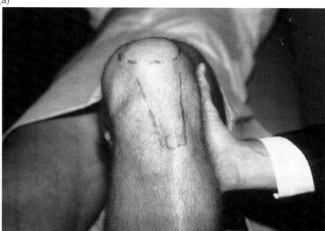

(b)

Fig. 12 Young adult male with patellar symptoms and patellar laxity. Maximally internally and externally rotated photographs of the tibia with the knee flexed are shown. The wide rotational excursion adds to the potential for patellar displacement by altering the angles of pull of the patellar tendon.

(most commonly near the extended position) or through larger portions of the arc. Small or alta patellae, hypoplastic or dysplastic femoral condyles, and rotational laxities of the tibiofemoral articulation are among the additional factors which have been found to contribute to some patellar instabilities (Fig. 12).

Unfortunately, there are no absolute parameters which define the limits of normal versus abnormal. Attempts to define these limits by radiographic indices have been numerous and helpful, but leave large voids in intelligence towards therapeutic planning. For a comprehensive historical review of the values and limitations of radiography in the evaluation of chondromalacia, instability, and the maltracking syndromes, the reader is referred to reference 45 (Table 1).[45]

Maltracking may also be a consequence of fixed malpositioning of the patella at one or many points in the arc of motion. An extreme example of such malpositioning was reported in the section on aplastic and hypoplastic patellae, that is to say a patella and extensor mechanism which resides in a position of permanent lateral dislocation. Individuals with excessive Q angles are virtually assured of some quantity of maltracking (malalignment), the responsibility for which can be shared between malpositioning and instability.

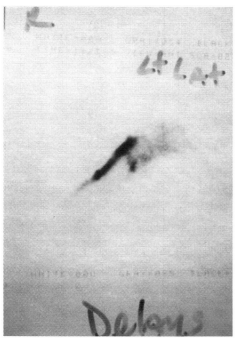

Fig. 11 Bone scan of the knee of a patient with proximal anterior tibial pain 2 years after a Macquet operation. A dramatic uptake is noted over the area of tibial cortical elevation where the patient manifested severe pain and incomplete union. Excision of the elevated section of cortex led to complete resolution of symptoms.

Table 1 Confusion of definitions by pathological, radiological, and clinical criteria

Bentley and Dowd	Chondromalacia is a syndrome comprising irregularity of the patellar undersurface, retropatellar and 'movie sign' pains, and crepitation.
Stougard	Chondromalacia is poorly correlated with anterior knee pain
Bentley and Dowd	Abnormal patellar tracking is a rare cause of chondromalacia
Insall et al.	Malalignment is a frequent finding (excessive Q angles) in patients with chondromalacia
Brattstrom	Recurrent patellar dislocation is often associated with femoropatellar dysplasia seen as a foreshortened lateral femoral condyle on axial radiography
Insall and Salvati	Patella alta exists with a 98% confidence level if the LT:LP ratio is 1.2 or less
Lancourt and Cristini	Greater incidence of patella alta with both instability and chondromalacia
Marks and Bentley	Alta correlated with sex (female) rather than with chondromalacia
Bentley and Dowd	LT:LP ratio mean of 1.25 with subluxation, and normal with chondromalacia
Merchant et al.	Patellar subluxation is 95% assured if the congruence angle is greater than +16°
Laurin et al.	93% of patients with chondromalacia have a patellofemoral index of more than 1.6 (at 20° knee flexion) and 100% of patients with subluxation have an index greater than 1.6
Moller et al.	For both unilateral chondromalacia and unilateral subluxation, side-to-side comparisons of the congruence angle are more important than the raw numbers
Bentley and Dowd	The mean congruence angle of subluxation cases is normal in contrast with the findings of Merchant and of Aglietti and Cerulli who found mean angles of +16° or more
Dowd and Bentley	Patients with instability had increased PT:P ratios and sulcus angles but often normal congruence angles
Sikorski et al.	Abnormal patellar tilts and rotations are observed in chondromalacia at given intervals of the flexion arc
Imai et al.	Malalignment is present when the patella is not centred by 60° of flexion using axial arthrography
Schutzer et al.	The patella is subluxated if the congruence angle exceeds 0° or the patella tilt angle is less than 8° with knee evaluated by CT at 10° of flexion.

Reproduced from ref. 45, with permission.

The indiscriminate use and interchange of verbiage implying the presence of a patellar disorder has added measurably to the confusion on the subject. 'Maltracking' is not 'instability', but may be due to the latter. 'Malalignment' may produce 'maltracking'; either may produce 'chondromalacia' or be associated with 'instability', but need not be. 'Patellar tendinitis' may be produced by repetitive overuse of the extensor mechanism, but it may also be an accompaniment of and partially induced by 'malalignment' and/or 'instability'. Similarly, the term 'subluxation' is frequently misused. It is used by most to imply that the patella has an ability to dislocate partially from the trochlea, but is used by others in referring to a fixed partial dislocation of the patella. In the former instance it should be said that the patella is 'subluxable', while in the latter it should be stated that the patella is permanently 'subluxed' (namely, it manifests a fixed malalignment) (Fig. 13).

With respect to patellar instability (conditions of 'subluxability' and 'dislocatability'), the most flagrant forms may present at a very young age, often in pre- or periadolescent females, and often as part of a syndrome of ubiquitous ligamentous laxity (Fig. 14).[46] Other findings may be associated with this syndrome. Included among them is an alta patella which adds to instability because the patella rests precariously on the anterior femoral surface proximal to the stabilizing trochlear groove. Patella alta is easily identified on clinical examination and by the use of one of several radiographic indices.

When youngsters of lax habitus exhibit a trilogy of femoral anteversion, external tibial torsion (productive of a large Q angle), and pronated feet, an ungainly malalignment is present about the knee (Fig. 15). It is termed the 'malicious malalignment syndrome' by virtue of its pernicious symptoms and its reluctance to respond to non-operative (or even operative) treatment. In some cases, operative treatments have been so bold as to include proximal-femoral, external-derotational osteotomies, sometimes in combination with internal-derotational osteotomies of the proximal end of the tibia. Individuals with severe anatomical disfigurations about the knee are generally incapable of achieving a competitive level of athletic accomplishment.

Traumatic dislocations of the patella are less frequent in patients with seemingly normal patellofemoral and knee joint anatomy than

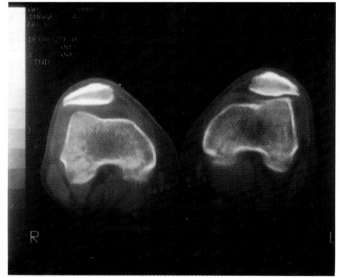

Fig. 13 CT scan showing fixed displacements (malalignments) of the patellae bilaterally.

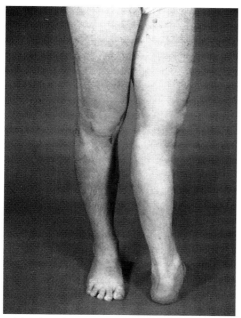

Fig. 14 Loose-jointedness in a male with symptoms of (and prior surgery for) patellar subluxation.

in individuals with obvious anatomical predispositions. Generally, a violent force is required to produce a dislocation. Occasionally, dislocations are medial. However, most commonly they are lateral, having been produced either by a laterally directed blow to the medial side of the patella or by the dynamics of a strong quadriceps contraction acting upon an extending knee with the tibia (and tubercle) in external rotation relative to the femur. Once dislocated, the patella may 'hang up' on the lateral aspect of the lateral wall of the trochlea with the knee partially flexed, or spontaneous reduction

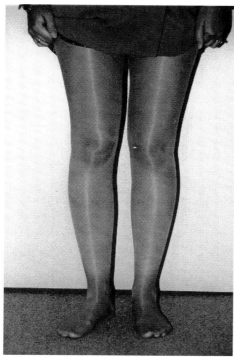

Fig. 15 A relatively benign form of malicious malalignment.

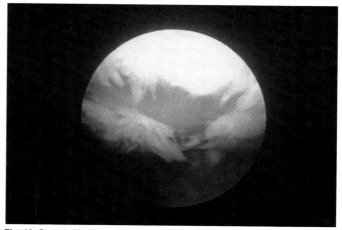

Fig. 16 Chondral fracture of the undersurface of the patella viewed by arthroscopy. (Reproduced from ref. 41, with permission.)

may occur. The greater the angle of knee flexion at which the traumatizing force is applied, the greater is the likelihood that an osteochondral fracture of the patella or femoral condyles will occur because of the more stable seating of the patella within the trochlea at progressive angles of flexion.

If the patella is dislocated upon presentation, reduction is accomplished by extending the knee while coaxing the patella medially over the lateral condylar eminence. Analgesia and/or sedation may be necessary adjuncts to the reduction. When the patella has reduced spontaneously prior to presentation for treatment, the diagnosis is based upon the historical description of the event, the presence of retinacular tenderness, patient apprehension about any manipulation of the patella, and any evidence from the radiographs which must be taken when the diagnosis is known or suspected. Fractures resulting in a splitting of the chondral articular surface may only be appreciated by arthroscopy (Fig. 16). Those representing compressions of the subchondral bone might only be appreciated on an MR image as an area of altered signal which may be expected to resolve over a period of several weeks (Fig. 17). Thereafter, only technetium bone scanning may reveal evidence of its having been present. Plain radiographs may reveal free fragments, most often deriving from the inferior portion of the medial facet of the patella or those emanating from fractures of the femoral condyles.

There is some controversy surrounding the treatment of an acute patellar dislocation. Following an avulsion of bone from the medial aspect of the patella, some surgeons will intervene with excision or replacement of the fragment and repair of the torn medial retinaculum (with a lateral release when necessary to enhance patellofemoral congruence).[47] In the past decade it has been discovered that arthroscopy after acute dislocations may reveal a rent in the medial retinacular tissue; this may then be repaired by arthroscopic suturing techniques, with the aim of preventing potential recurrences attributable to progressive stretching of a retinaculum which had already been torn.[48]

A common procedure among other orthopaedic specialists has been to immobilize the knee in extension for up to 6 weeks before initiating physical therapy toward a restoration of motion.[47] The rationale for this approach is the hope that scarring of the torn tissues will prevent recurrence. This is probably as unlikely to inhibit

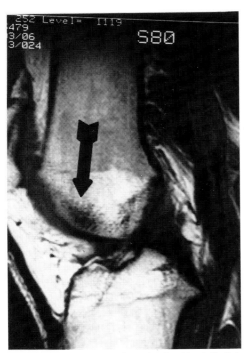

Fig. 17 Sagittal MR image of the knee of a professional basketball player who suffered a hyperextension injury with subsequent anterior knee pain. The 'bone bruise' of the anterior portion of the femoral condyle (arrow), where patellofemoral compression occured, should be noted.

future patellar dislocation as postdislocation immobilization of the shoulder has been in preventing further dislocation of that joint.

Unfortunately, there are no randomized, prospective studies comparing the results of the various treatment options to guide the treating physician. For the élite competitive athlete, temporal considerations may dictate the treatment option selected. Such an individual afflicted in the midst of the season or approaching a critical event can most often be restored to a competitive level by the immediate initiation of physical therapy to reconstitute motion, strength, and agility (as long as no loose fracture fragment is present). Gymnasts, who often fit the description of the hyperlax 'predisposed' individual mentioned above, may dislocate the patella with virtually no symptomatic consequence and require no treatment.

Treatments for malalignments and instability have been varied. Whether thought to be intractable or not, almost all cases deserve trials of non-operative treatment inclusive of anti-inflammatory agents, physical therapy, and bracing. Surgical treatments have been numerous in variety. They have included realignments of proximal patellar mechanisms intended to improve the influence of the pull of the quadriceps muscle and retinacula, distal realignments designed to alter the direction of pull of the patellar tendon, simple retinacular (lateral) releases, and adjunctive procedures such as derotational osteotomies or tendon transfers to the patellar tendon to inhibit the patella, its tendon, or the tibial tubercle from lateral or external displacement. There are no published reports reflecting the relative successes of any of these procedures in an athletic population.

It must be recognized that surgery cannot enlarge a small patella, deepen a hypoplastic trochlea, effectively lower a patella alta, or correct other developmental anatomical factors predisposing to fixed or unstable malalignments. Surgery can release, tighten, or redirect the

pulls of tissues influencing patellar glide, but with little hope of achieving normality rather than merely a beneficial modification. There are many factors to consider. For example, a patella may be too lax, producing pain when it is displaced medially and reproducing a familiar sense of instability upon being displaced laterally (while the knee remains passively extended). Ignoring for the moment the existence of any other influencing factors, does the surgeon release the lateral retinaculum and tighten the medial or tighten both retinacula to different degrees? Are the intended tightenings or releases performed in extension or at the angle of knee flexion at which symptoms are most commonly manifested? What length of release or tightening is optimum to control the symptoms? How can the effects of these procedural titrations be evaluated intraoperatively when the patient is not functioning? Vision may assess passive alignment in a very gross fashion, but affords little ability to assess the functional dynamics of a 'corrected' extensor mechanism (Fig. 18). Furthermore, these surgical procedures are not excisional; they alter the way that the mechanism works, and the alteration may progressively change the dynamics for better or worse for many months following the operation.

Little objective scientific insight regarding the anticipated influences of commonly practiced procedures is available; one study of particular interest should be described. Hayes et al.[30] used pressure-sensitive film to study patellofemoral contact patterns in cadaveric knees subjected to artificially induced quadriceps loading. The effects of several surgical procedures were studied in this way. Results implied that lateral and medial capsular plication produced increased pressures on the medial and lateral facets, respectively, and that the changes were dependent upon the angle of flexion of the knee. However, lateral release did not produce a consistent reduction of peak pressure or alteration in contact area. Alterations of the Q angle may alter contact patterns and create areas of high peak stresses; however, a prediction as to what angle changes might be beneficial or detrimental is not forthcoming. Tibial tubercle ele-

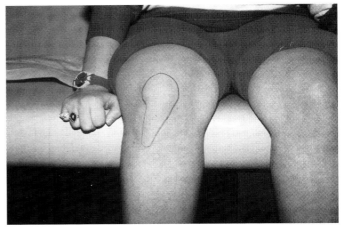

Fig. 18 The knee shown has an alta but centralized appearance. There is an obviously large Q angle. Examination may reveal patellar laxity either medially or laterally. Intraoperative radiography to determine patellar indices is not practised. Therefore the only parameter that can be used to assess dynamic alterations during surgery is gross visual inspection which is unlikely to appreciate mediolateral shifts, tibial rotatory excursions, and patellar tilts occurring at various angles in the passive mode created by general or spinal anaesthesia. Local anaesthesia and/or sensory epidural anaesthesia which retains muscle control and patient perception, to a degree, may be helpful.

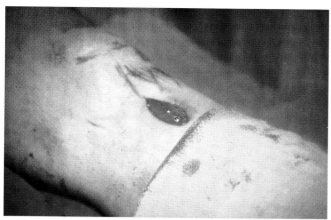

Fig. 19 Tibial tubercle osteotomy.

vations produced modest alterations of contact patterns but no substantial reductions in average or peak contact pressures.

Semidynamic intraoperative monitoring of surgical procedures is possible with the use of 'sensory epidural anaesthesia'. The patient is awake and motor ability is retained but attenuated. Active knee motion assists visual assessments and, on occasion, the patient may provide feedback relative to the sense of function and glide.

In view of the above results, it requires little imagination to realize that a single procedure is unlikely to produce gratifying results for the great variety of dysfunctional patellar entities which present for surgery. Unfortunately, the generally benevolent advent of arthroscopy has had a somewhat questionable influence upon the treatment of these entities. Its simplicity and low morbidity have led to an almost excessive performance of arthroscopic lateral retinacular releases. Early reports of success were high,[49] but reported success rates have diminished substantially. Hayes *et al.*[30] cite Osborne and Fulford (1982) who reported a time-related failure pattern of lateral release for symptomatic patients with chondromalacia. From an early result of pain relief in almost 90 per cent of cases, success dropped to under 40 per cent after 3 years. There are several obvious reasons for this diminution. One is the inability of a simple release to address a complexity of considerations such as those discussed above. Hayes *et al.*[30] assert that, despite the recent popularity of lateral releases for patellar alignment problems and chondral damage, these procedures have been used 'with no particular regard for differences in aetiological mechanisms or locations of the lesions'. A second reason for diminishing success is the not infrequent consequence of making a lax patella even looser by the release of restraining tissue. A third relates to the Q angle, both static and dynamic. When the Q angle is large (for instance greater than 15 to 20 degrees), the resultant forces acting upon the patella will favour lateral displacement even if a lateral release has been performed (as an isolated procedure). If, with flexion of the knee, external rotatory laxity of the tibia permits the Q angle to enlarge even more, then a procedure to reduce this thrust must be considered. A modification of the Trillat procedure, by which the tubercle is osteotomized at its proximal end (to which the patellar tendon is attached) and is rotated medially and transfixed, is often successful for this purpose (Fig. 19).[50-52]

More critical evaluation of clinical patella problems and their curative procedures have been introduced. Fulkerson and Shea[53]

compiled an excellent review whereby patella tilt and subluxation (Schutzer *et al.*[54]) were identified and isolated as clinical entities to determine which procedures best addressed each situation. In short, without the presence of tilt, lateral release was not indicated. Subluxation necessitated a more aggressive distal tubercle transfer.[52] With this more critical evaluation, various reports show that lateral release procedures alone, both open and arthroscopic, have proven more efficacious.[55,56]

The conclusion is that the design and anticipated results of surgery to alter patellar glide should be based upon the specific dysfunctions involved in the individual case. As already indicated, examination provides limited clues. The most commonly used guides to the design of a procedure are derived from the radiographic indices. Most are based upon plain axial radiography with or without arthrography (Fig. 20), and some upon CT axial scans which permit evaluations in an extended position of the knee (less than 20 degrees of flexion) (Fig. 21).

When utilizing plain axial radiography, debate continues as to the proper degree of knee flexion and whether the quadriceps mechanism should be in an active or passive state.[60,61] Teitge *et al.* have described stress radiographs utilizing a force directed in both the medial and lateral directions in conjunction with axial radiographs.[62] They found a reproducible technique where a 4 mm displacement in either direction in a symptomatic knee (in relation to the asymptomatic side) was evidence of patellofemoral instability.

Another interesting technique involves a modification of the above stress radiographs. Rather than direct external forces, lateral rotation of the tibia with the femur held in neutral position allows the tibial tubercle to rotate laterally. Because of the known role of rotational tibiofemoral laxity in the occurrence of patella subluxation and dislocation, this technique, developed by Malghem and Maldague,[63] discloses the effects of the displacing forces seen in the recognized positions of instability.

In another publication, Malghem and Maldague[64] discuss the use of a single, plain radiograph taken from the lateral position to determine proximal trochlear-groove depth. This measurement ascertains depth insufficiency and its relationship to patella dislocation and instability. Utilizing their measurement technique, one is able to determine, at least in the proximal portion of the trochlear groove, an absolute depth of patella tracking. They found that a trochlear depth of less than 5 mm was seen in 90 per cent of the knees that they ultimately operated on for recurrent instability, and conversely in only 20 per cent of their asymptomatic group. They concluded that depths of less than 5 mm greatly increased the risk of patella instability.

Fulkerson and Shea[32,53] imply that malalignment and instability syndromes are classifiable and distinguishable by CT imaging techniques alone, and further that the categories discernible by imaging allow the clinician to anticipate a quantity of associated chondral damage and a definitive treatment plan. They describe five categories of patellar imaging findings (three of which have subtypes). The concept is interesting, but naïve, in assuming that formulaic approaches to patellofemoral conditions are likely to succeed consistently. Most of these studies present the patella in an adynamic state at only one or two angles of flexion (Tables 2, 3, 4, and 5).

Cine CT or MRI have been used in an attempt to reveal patellar displacements at progressing angles of knee flexion, but still in an adynamic fashion.[65]

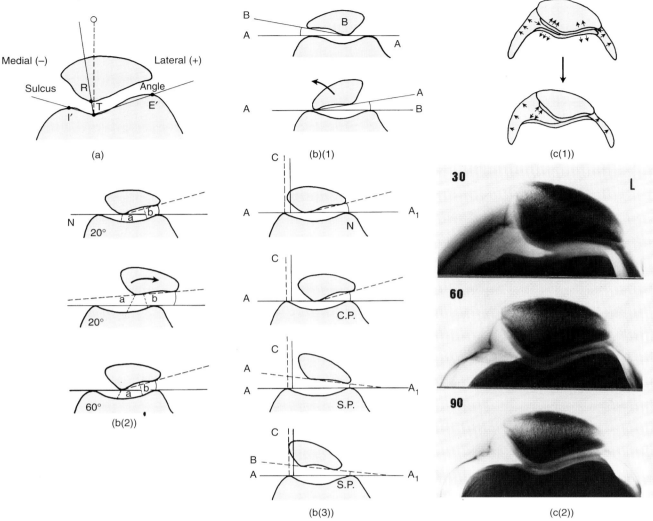

Fig. 20 Examples of axial radiographic techniques used to evaluate the tilt or displacement of the patella. (a) Merchant technique[57]: technique with patient supine and the knee flexed to 45°. Using reference line TO, the congruence angle (OTR) is negative if R is medial to TO and positive if it is lateral to TO. An angle of +16° was determined to be abnormal at the 95th percentile (meaning subluxed) see Tables 2 and 3). (b) Laurin method[58]: supine technique with the knee in 20° of flexion (a more extended angle than that used for all other plain radiographic axial techniques). Three indices are determinable (see Table 4). (b(1)) The lateral patellofemoral angle (LPS): the angle is formed by ABB and is open laterally in most normal knees. (b(2)) The patellofemoral index (PFI): a ratio of medial and lateral patellofemoral interspaces. The ratio is more than 1.6 in most cases of chondromalacia. (b(3)) The lateral patellar displacement (LPD): disorders are based on the relative displacements of the patella from perpendicular line C which rises from the promontory of the lateral wall of the groove. Lateral displacements are seen in a small number of knees with chondromalacia and a greater number of knees with subluxation (versus merely tilt). (c) Axial views in conjunction with arthrography. The best known of these methods is that of Imai *et al.*[59] (c(1)) Imai *et al.* make the point that arthrographic enhancement of axial views helps delineate the chondral surface outline, permitting a distinction between apparent tilt and true tilt. They also make the point that abnormal tilts will disappear at increasing angles of knee flexion, whereas they may persist in knees with subluxation. (c(2)) Axial arthrographic views performed at three angles of knee flexion demonstrate significant tilt at 30° and apparent patellar reduction at 60° and 90°. (Reproduced from ref. 59, with permission.)

These realities make it wise to delay surgery in elective instances until the patient has been seen and studied sufficiently to gain a maximum understanding of the complaints and dynamics.

The above doctrine is equally applicable to the implementation of physical therapy and bracing. There are virtually limitless alterations to the strengthening programmes initiated to gain better control of patellar glide. The quantity of load and the nature of the load (free weight, isokinetics, cam accommodations, elastic resistance, water resistance, arcs through which load is applied, use of concentric versus eccentric loading, repetition patterns, frequency of loading, and speed of loading) can each be varied to accommodate symptoms (Table 6). The situation in which rotational laxity of the tibiofemoral joint exerts a whipping influence upon the patella and its tendon can be taken as an example. Attempted use of isokinetic ballistic machines is often provocative and results in peripatellar pain. It is often possible to overcome this problem by using an antishear bar to curtail tibial displacement in the same fashion in which it is customarily used in patients with instability due to an anterior cruciate ligament deficiency. The same principles apply to bracing considerations for these problems. Whereas standard patellar braces

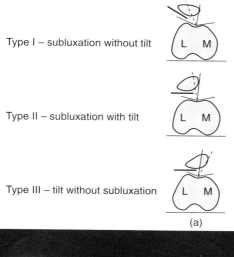

Type I – subluxation without tilt

Type II – subluxation with tilt

Type III – tilt without subluxation

(a)

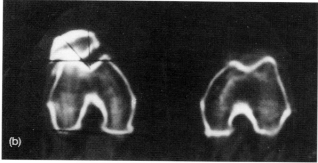

Fig. 21 Schutzer *et al.*[54] ascertained normal and abnormal indices for axial CT imaging with regard to patellar subluxation. In type I, the angle is greater than 0°. In type II, the trochlear is very shallow and the congruence angle is greater than 0°. In type III, the congruence angle is less than 0°. The type of treatment (e.g. lateral release or anteriorization of the tubercle) is based on the severity of the type. (Redrawn from ref. 54, with permission.) (b) Type II (subluxation and tilt) subluxation with osteophyte formation.

may be unsuccessful in controlling symptoms in patellar instability due to a rotational laxity of the tibia upon the femur, derotational braces used for tibiofemoral instabilities are often successful (Fig. 22).

The foregoing information was intended to review highlights and principles of patellofemoral glide and tracking disorders, their treatment, and their relative roles in athletics. Indeed, complete books have been written on the subject of the patella. It is hoped that the reader will at least have been made familiar with the gamut of existing disorders and provided with an insight into the complexities governing their management.

Patellofemoral arthrosis

This condition, with symptoms of pain, stiffness, and swelling in varying proportions, is infrequently encountered among competitive athletes (recreational or otherwise). Osteophytes widen the margins of the patella, creating a patella magna (Fig. 23). Broadening and incongruity of the patella compromise patellar excursion and accentuate pressure at contact points. The result is pain and reduced extensor leverage. The knee lacks full extension and the gait is rather stiff. Stair climbing and descent are often particularly difficult as a result of pain, weakness, and crepitation.

The arthrosis is most commonly manifested about the lateral

portion of the patellofemoral joint, consistent with the lateral vector of force deriving from the physiological valgus common to the knee joint. The lateral facet shows a greater incidence of wear both clinically and at necropsy.[1] Isolated medial patellofemoral arthritis is much less commonly observed.

The diagnosis of patellofemoral arthrosis is usually easily deduced on physical examination by inspecting and/or palpating the irregularly enlarged patella, the crepitation with motion, and the lack of passive full extension. Plain radiographs demonstrate the enlarged irregular perimeter of the patellar on anteroposterior views, and often show projectile promontories extending proximally from the superior margin and/or distally from the inferior margin of the patella. However, the incongruency and enlargements are best observed on axial views, either plain films or CT images. When the arthrosis is incipient, technetium bone scanning may be of value in deducing the presence of arthritic disease.

Non-operative treatment consists of strengthening and stretching the muscles about the knee at levels of loading and in arcs which are non-provocative. NSAIDs may allay symptoms, but their use for the purpose of participation in sports should be construed as being potentially deleterious. Bracing is often counterproductive; the pressure from the brace frequently magnifies the pre-existing perception of stiffness.

For the most part (and depending upon the magnitude and focus of the arthrosis) surgical treatments hold little promise of substantial or protracted relief of symptoms. Arthroscopic abrasion chondroplasty can occasionally restore the eroding articular surface with inconsistent short-lived benefits. Focal painful impingements can sometimes be modified by open and/or arthroscopic cheilotomy or partial facetectomy.

Associated retinacular releases may facilitate glide of the patella. The Macquet operation, the purpose of which is to offset offending patellofemoral loading forces and to enhance the leverage of the extensor mechanism, offers a faint hope of persistently improved mechanics. However, the procedure is accompanied by a protracted recuperative period and a multifaceted potential morbidity.

Reflex sympathetic dystrophy

Reflex sympathetic dystrophy is an entity shrouded in confusion by virtue of its broad array of presenting manifestations, and its frequent resilience to multiform treatment approaches. Its relevance to this chapter is the reported finding by Katz and Hungerford (1987) that 65 per cent of reflex sympathetic dystrophies about the knee originate at the patellofemoral joint.[2]

Reflex sympathetic dystrophy appears to be a relative of the causalgia classically described by Mitchell, Moorehouse, and Keen (1964) of cases reported during the American Civil War.[2] It is commonly known that porotic bone changes are a typical consequence of reflex sympathetic dystrophy. At the beginning of the twentieth century, Sudeck recognized an osteoporosis which could occur in 'younger' individuals and yet not be consequent to disuse (Sudeck's atrophy). It was soon concluded that the mechanism of production was related to the autonomic nervous system.[2] DeTakats (1937) applied the term 'reflex dystrophy' to describe a wide clinical spectrum of reflex sympathetic dystrophy. The classical presentation of which includes a swollen, painfully immobile limb, that is hypersensitive to touch.[65] However, not all presentations are so clearly

Table 2 Comparative congruence angles reported by authors studying normal, chondromalacic, and subluxating patellae

Authors	Mean normal CA	Abnormal 95% limits	Mean CA in chondromalacia	Mean CA in subluxation
Merchant et al.	−6°	+16°	—	+16°a
Aglietti and Cerulli	−9°	—	0°	+17°
Bently and Dowd	—	—	−8.1°	Normalb

CA = congruence angle.
a Within 95% confidence limits.
b Of 33 cases, four were outside the 95th percentile of normal subjects.
Reproduced from ref. 45 with permission.

marked. Homans (1940) discussed less or minor causalgic forms,[2] and Casten and Betcher (1955) recognized three grades of severity of the syndrome.[65] It is contended that reflex sympathetic dystrophy of the tibiofemoral and patellofemoral articulations is more frequent than commonly thought, but the lack of suspicion, particularly in cases at the lower end of the spectrum of overt manifestations, has been a deterrent to its detection.[1] The patellofemoral articulation is predisposed to reflex sympathetic dystrophy on the basis of its subcutaneous location and its consequent vulnerability to concussive trauma. The rich and anastamotic circulation of the patella, subject to the influence of autonomic control, may be an additional predisposing cause.

The autonomic nervous system is involved, to some degree, with any injury, its response generally being proportional to the magnitude of injury.[1] The autonomic disturbance usually abates with progression of the injury repair process. However, for reasons which have not been clearly elucidated, the usual abatement sometimes fails to occur, and the result is reflex sympathetic dystrophy. Onset without trauma has been recognized, most typically in the upper extremities. However, the traumatically induced onset is much more typical. Direct trauma to the patella (as in a direct blow to or a fall onto the knee) is the most frequent inciting cause of reflex sympathetic dystrophy of the patella. Reflex sympathetic dystrophy of the patella and its environs may also result from more insidious traumatic affectations (for example, overloading with weights in quadriceps building or recurrent subluxation).[2]

Table 3 Distinguishing normal patellae from chondromalacia and patellar instability using a variety of plain radiographic indices

Study	Normal patella (mean value)	Chondromalacia	Instability
Congruence angle	−8.1°	−6.48°	−1.8°
Sulcus angle	139°	138°	147°a
Pt:P ratio	1.03b	1.09	1.25a

a Significantly higher than in normal patellae.
b Generally higher in women.
Adapted from ref. 24. Reproduced from ref. 45, with permission.

Theories of the pathogenesis of reflex sympathetic dystrophy have been numerous, but none has been accepted with universal accord. Hungerford and Fulkerson[2] suggest that the most favoured theory is that of Lorente de No (1938) as applied by Livingston (1941). According to this theory the painful stimulus enters the cord through afferent fibres which stimulate the internuncial pool, leading to the spread of the stimulus in multiple directions within the cord; the resulting efferent consequence at the periphery serves to restimulate the afferents, thereby creating a vicious circle. Among the efferent consequences are local circulatory disturbances. The circulatory changes were recognized by Leriche (1923) nearly two decades earlier. He postulated that an initial vasoconstriction was produced by the initiating trauma and that this was superseded by a secondary phase of vasodilatation. The result, in effect, was a simulated inflammatory response (heat and rubor) due to heightened regional vascularization. Increased blood flow was confirmed by later investigators (for example, de Takats (1937)) using objective laboratory apparatus.[2]

The implication of the above discussion is that the vascular alterations of reflex sympathetic dystrophy are associated with a disturb-

Table 4 Percentages of normal and abnormal indices in normal, chondromalacic, and subluxatable patellae using the Laurin method

	LPD (%)a	LPA (%)b	PFI (%)c
Normal	100/0	97/3/0	100/0
Chondromalacia }	70/30	90/10/0	3/97
Subluxation	47/53	0/60/40	0/100

a Lateral patellar displacement: per cent medial to line C/per cent lateral to line cc.
b Lateral patellofemoral angle: open laterally/parallel/open medially.
c Patellofemoral index: 1.6 or less/more than 1.6.
Adapted from ref. 58 with permission.

Table 5 Use of arthroscopy and radiographic indices to distinguish normal chondromalacic, and subluxatable patellae

Group	Presenting symptoms	Q angle in extension (±2.SD)*		Sulcus angles (±2 SD)	Congruence angles (±2 SD)	Insall-Salvati index (±2 SD)	Median angle of alignment on arthroscopy		
		Women	Men				Lateral facet	Median ridge	Medial facet
1. Control (n = 17)	None in the patellofemoral joint	12–16°	7–11°	134–143°	–13° to –6°	0.94–1.10	20°	35°	50°
							All patients with medial facet contact by 45° could centre patella with quadricep contraction		
2. Idiopathic (n = 20)	Retropatellar pain	13–20°	10–15°	136–145°	–8° to –2°	1.07–1.27	20°	35°	50°
							All could centre patellar by isometric quad at 45°		
3. Instability (n = 13)	Sense of instability + apprehension sign	16–24°	12–20°	140–153° (significantly higher)	–11° to +8° (median +4)	1.13–1.44 (significantly higher)	30°	55°	85°
							All with medial facet contact by 85° could centre with quadriceps contraction†		

*Flexion to 30° increased Q angle. External rotation increased Q angle.
†External rotation of tibia had an adverse effect on centring for group 3. Chondromalacia was present in a large percentage of groups 2 and 3.
(Adapted from Sojbjerg JO, *et al.* Arthroscopic determination of patellofemoral malalignment. *Clinical Orthopedics*, 1987; **215**: 243–47, with permission.)

ance of the sympathetic nervous system. Furthermore, recent investigations by Roberts provide evidence that the pain patterns of reflex sympathetic dystrophy may also have a derivation in the sympathetic nervous system disturbances which characterize the syndrome.[66]

Contemporary theories of pathogenesis are reviewed by Omohundro and Payne[66] and are listed chronologically below.

1. Sunderland (1978): nerve injury results in abnormal sympathetic afferent discharges.

2. Devor (1983): spontaneous ectopic discharges may be generated at the nerve injury site where neuroma formation or focal demyelination may occur.

Table 6 Variables to alter in therapy in the presence of pain or difficulty

1. Reduce loads: less weight, negatives, buoyancy (water)

2. Reduce arcs or amplitudes of lift

3. Vary loads in different portions of arcs or amplitudes

4. Reduce repetitions: per set, total, or intervals between

5. Variation of load format: free weight, cam, isokinetic, isometric, concentric, eccentric, others

6. Alter frequencies: less quantity more time per day or week, same quantity less often, other combinations

7. Time of day: low endurance problems work earlier in day, stiffness problems—work after stretching or later in day

8. Modalities: may reduce discomfort to allow more work

9. Drugs: NSAID may reduce inflammatory discomfort

10. Braces: may better control instability for better tolerance

11. Speed: higher speeds are often less painful

12. Biofeedback: may help reduce workout difficulties

13. Special devices: antishear bars, arc blockers, double or single extremity systems, alternating extremity, and other systems

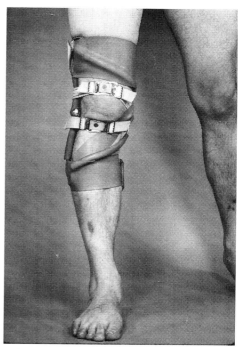

Fig. 22 Derotational braces reduce tibiofemoral rotational laxity and hence reduce displacing pulls upon the patella.

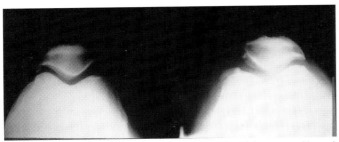

Fig. 23 Axial radiographs of a retired professional hockey defenceman with a unilateral patella magna and no history of patellar fracture.

3. Barasi and Lynn (1983) and Roberts and Elardo (1985): sympathetic discharges result in hypersensitization of the peripheral mechanoreceptors and/or nociceptors.

4. Janig (1985): artificial synapses (ephapses) are created secondary to injury which lead to a shunting of sympathetic efferent to sympathetic efferent stimulation near the site of injury.

Omohundro and Paynecaution stated that none of the theories proposed account for the variety of clinical manifestations expressed in reflex sympathetic dystrophy. They claim that the Roberts theory (1986) is best capable of explaining the clinical features of reflex sympathetic dystrophy. This theory suggests that sympathetic efferent activity may be normal and that the symptoms expressed in reflex sympathetic dystrophy are a function of a reduced threshold in the mechanoreceptors near the injury site. Trauma, activating the C-nociceptive sensory units (for instance, mechanoreceptors), sensitizes the wide dynamic range neurones in the cord, which, in turn, produce spontaneous activity and a lower threshold for firing. Such a mechanism could result in the experience of hypersensitivity (hyperpathia) with a seemingly normal touch or stimulus.[66]

Regardless of the pathogenic theorem accepted, the clinical onset of reflex sympathetic dystrophy is divisible into three types.

1. Pain begins immediately and is out of proportion to the inciting trauma.

2. A typical post-traumatic course and pain level is noted for several days, and then persists or worsens to preclude movement of the knee due to the severity of pain.

3. A typical post-traumatic course is observed with a progressive resolution of symptoms, or even their disappearance. Subsequently, there is a resurgence of pain and an expression of reflex sympathetic dystrophy features.

When reflex sympathetic dystrophy has established itself, there may be evidence of variably expressed symptoms and signs. The *sine qua non* symptom is severe pain. Night pain is quite characteristic. Stiffness, in conjunction with painful motion, is also quite typical. Hyperpathia is a common cardinal feature, as is sensitivity to cold.[66] The often disproportionate severity of symptoms in relation to the initiating trauma, and the known exacerbation of symptoms as a result of emotional stress, have subjected reflex sympathetic dystrophy victims to speculation that their affliction is of a functional rather than organic aetiology. Mayfield and Devine (1945) evaluated

patients with reflex sympathetic dystrophy and determined that, for the most part, they were psychiatrically stable.[2]

Stiffness of the knee, in varying proportions, is the most characteristic physical finding. The parapatellar soft tissues are indurated as well as tender, adding to the painful restriction of motion and stiffness.[2] At different stages, rubor and vascularity of the involved area may predominate, or coldness and a cyanotic appearance may prevail. The various complexes of signs and symptoms associated with reflex sympathetic dystrophy may wane over a period of months or persist as long as a few years. These symptoms and signs are characteristic and alerting, but not pathognomonic. Therefore diagnostic tests are often performed to gain corroboration.

Plain radiographs typically demonstrate a honeycombed microcystic, and osteopenic appearance of the patella (and/or other bones) on axial views. However, this almost (but not quite) pathognomonic appearance does not become apparent until fairly late in the disease.

Bone scans are positive in 49 to 92 per cent of cases in reports reviewed by Omohundro and Payne and they are characterized by an increased uptake. Hungerford and Fulkerson indicate that thermography is reliable and practical in establishing local vascular temperature alterations and in ruling out non-organic disorders. Temperature differentials of 2 °C or more are suggestive of reflex sympathetic dystrophy.[66]

Citing Ficat *et al.* (1973), Hungerford and Fulkerson[2] indicate that intraosseous pressure readings and venography and core biopsies demonstrate stasis and ischaemia in reflex sympathetic dystrophy. Neither these tests nor bone scanning or thermography are unequivocally diagnostic; they are just corroborative.

A potentially therapeutic endeavour—a sympathetic blockade—is the best diagnostic test for establishing the presence of reflex sympathetic dystrophy.[66] Sympathetic blocks can be performed in numerous ways (which will not be described here). If a block (or blocks) is effective in relieving the manifestations of reflex sympathetic dystrophy, the diagnosis is confirmed and a potentially long siege may be averted by a relatively simple and innocuous exercise. Toumey[67] stated that failure of a single block is insufficient evidence that blocks will not work. With the use of long-acting agents and repetitive blocks, the cycle of pain may ultimately be broken. While there is a positive correlation between the results of a sympathetic block and those of sympathectomy (permanent variety), Toumey and others demonstrated an inverse relationship between the latter and the duration of the reflex sympathetic dystrophy syndrome.[1,2,67] Furthermore, sympathectomy may be successful in relieving the sensitivity to cold and any regional cyanosis, but without necessarily relieving the pain.[1]

Relief of pain is the critical aim of treatment for reflex sympathetic dystrophy, for without relieving the pain, initiation of successful physical therapy to restore motion and to reverse atrophic bone and soft-tissue changes would be difficult and delayed at the very least. In addition to the use of blocks to accomplish this end, numerous drug therapy programmes have been proposed. Omohundro and Paynes[66] list the following groups of drugs as being potentially useful:

(1) oral sympatholytic drugs (e.g. prazosin, phenoxybenzamine, propanolol);

(2) anti-inflammatory drugs (prednisolone and non-steroids);

(3) tricyclic drugs (e.g. amitriptyline, desipramine, doxepin, and imipramine);

(4) anticonvulsants (e.g. phenytoin and carbamazepine);

(5) calcium-channel blockers (e.g. nifedipine);

(6) narcotic analgesics—to break the pain cycle, but with care to avoid addiction because of the length of treatment which may be required.

Various combinations of drugs may be helpful, although individually the drugs used may be valueless. Bircher (1967, 1971) reported success in animal models using a combination of Tandearil (anti-inflammatory), Hydergine (co-dergocrine) (vasodilator), and Valium (diazepam), whereas none of these drugs was effective when used alone.[2]

The principal liability of this condition to athletes is the protracted recovery time. Significant functional residual symptoms are essentially nil in most cases. Physical therapy is the mainstay of treatment. Intermittently, continuous passive motion alternated with frequent intervals of active motion within a tolerable arc is suggested. Strength development as an instigator of regional blood flow and as an aid to overcoming stiffness is also important. Hydrotherapy with the performance of resistive exercises in water is gentle and often painlessly effective. In an attempt to break cycles of vascular spasms and to stimulate local circulation, contrast treatments, using alternating applications of heat and cold, have been reported to be of value. Facilitation of range of motion, when severely curtailed, by manipulation under general or regional anaesthesia with or without arthroscopy has been discouraged as being provocative.[1,2] When physical therapy, pharmacological treatments, and other supportive measures fail to bring about a progression of improvement after several months, a continuous epidural block should be performed.[66]

The cardinal concepts are those of early suspicion of reflex sympathetic dystrophy and an aggressive approach to the reduction of pain so that physical therapy can be undertaken to restore function.

Patella magna

Patella magna is traditionally a sequel to prior infection or trauma. Trauma may be represented by fracture or an open patellar operation (rarely performed today) for malalignment or general exploration of the knee (Fig. 24). It is rarely seen prior to middle age, although it may be seen in young adults, and it is a frequent accompaniment of a patellofemoral or more ubiquitous degenerative arthritis of the knee joint. Congenital forms of patella magna have been described,[1] but the overwhelming majority are a consequence of osteophytic broadening of the medial and/or lateral facets. Liabilities of the condition include pain with athletic activities and a reduced leverage of the extensor mechanism by virtue of entrapment and reduced excursion of the oversized patella and its relative incongruence with respect to the trochlear sulcus. Since patella magna is rarely seen in highly competitive athletes, treatments other than physical therapy are rarely considered. Occasionally, and if pain is significant, a miniaturization may be considered, or if symptoms are very focal, a facetectomy at the site of pain may be appropriate.

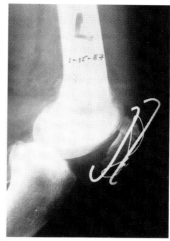

Fig. 24 Splaying of fragments, callus formation, and altered patellar dynamics consequent to patellar fractures frequently result in a secondary patella magna.

Plica syndrome

Three arthroscopically discernible synovial folds are identifiable within a knee: a suprapatellar fold; a medial fold; and an infrapatellar fold (ligamentum mucosum).[68] Asymptomatic plicae have been reported to be presented in between 18.5 and 55 per cent of arthroscopically inspected knees. A direct trauma to the flexed knee can convert an asymptomatic plica (usually the medial and less often the superior) into an enlarged symptomatic plica.[68,69] The trauma, whether an athletic-related contusion or a dashboard injury, produces haemorrhage and synovitis. Eventually hyalinization and fibrotic thickening can produce a hard bowstrung plica, which can erode the medial facet of the patella and the medial femoral condyle.[69] The resulting plica syndrome consists of anteromedial knee pain, pseudolocking, retropatellar crepitation, and often the presence of a tender palpable cord (the plica) in the interval between the medial aspects of the patella and the medial femoral condyle (Fig. 25). Symptomatic plicae are not encountered with great frequency. Broom and Fulkerson[69] reported their presence in 29 of 730 knee arthroscopies performed for anterior knee pain. Little more than half the patients in their series reported a history of the trauma, and about three-quarters of the patients were consistently involved in athletics. As with the arthroscopic lateral release for patellar maltracking, plical excision may be performed to excess. An MRI or CT

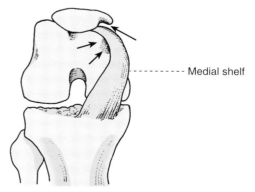

Fig. 25 Medial shelf. (Redrawn from ref. 68, with permission.)

Medial shelf

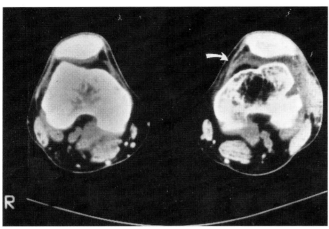

Fig. 26 MRI axial view showing a large medial shelf (arrow) which was confirmed and excised by arthroscopy.

arthrogram may demonstrate the presence of a large plical cord in advance of any surgery considered (Fig. 26). In instances in which plical symptoms are severe, arthroscopic resection can produce dramatic relief.

References

1. Ficat RP, Hungerford DS. *Disorders of the patellofemoral joint.* Baltimore: Williams and Wilkins, 1977.
2. Hungerford DS, Fulkerson JP. *Disorders of the patellofemoral joint.* Baltimore: Williams and Wilkins, 1990: 247–64.
3. Outerbridge RE. Further studies on the etiology of chondromalacia patellae. *Journal of Bone and Joint Surgery* 1964; **46B**: 179–90.
4. Outerbridge RE. The etiology of chondromalacia patella. *Journal of Bone and Joint Surgery* 1961; **43B**: 752.
5. Wiberg G. Roentgenographic and anatomic studies on the femoropatellar joint with special reference to chondromalacia patellae. *Acta Orthopaedica Scandinavica* 1941; **12**: 319.
6. McCarrol JR, O'Donoghue DH, Giana WR. The surgical treatment of chondromalacia of the patella. *Clinical Orthopedics* 1983; **175**: 130.
7. Crenshaw AH, ed. *Campbell's operative orthopedics.* 7th edn. St Louis: CV Mosby, 1987: 2233–6.
8. Stanislavjevic S, Zemenick G, Miller D. Congenital, irreducible, permanent lateral dislocation of the patella. *Clinical Orthopaedics* 1976; **116**: 190–9.
9. Rockwood CA, Wilkins KA, King RE. *Fractures in children.* Philadelphia: JB Lippincott, 1984: 248.
10. Rockwood CA, Green DP. *Fractures in adults.* 2nd edn. Philadelphia: JB Lippincott, 1984: 948.
11. Graf BK, Fujisaki CK, Reider B. Disorders of the patellar tendon. In: Reider B, ed. *Sports medicine: The school-age athlete.* Philadelphia: WB Saunders, 1991:355–64.
12. Osgood RB. Tibial tubercle occurring during adolescence. *Boston Medical Science Journal* 1903; **148**: 114.
13. Jacob RP, Von Gumppenberg S, Engelhorst P. Does Osgood Schlatter's disease influence the position of the patella? *Journal of Bone and Joint Surgery* 1981; **63B**: 579.
14. Uhry E, Jr. Osgood–Schlatter disease. *Archives of Surgery* 1944; **48**: 406.
15. Curwin S, Stanish WD. *Jumper's knee. Tendinitis: its etiology and treatment.* Lexington: DC Heath, 1984.
16. Jackson RW. Etiology of chondromalacia patella. *AAOS Instructional Course Lectures* 1976; **25**: 36.
17. Blazina ME, Kerlan RK, Jobe FW, Canter VS, Carison GJ. Jumper's knee. *Orthopedic Clinics of North America* 1973; **4**: 66.
18. Ray JM, McCombs W, Sternes RA. Basketball and volleyball. In: Reider B, ed. *Sports medicine: the school-age athlete.* Philadelphia: WB Saunders, 1991: 601–31.
19. El-Koury GY, Wira RL, Berbaum KS, *et al.* MR imaging of patellar tendinitis. *Radiology* 1992; **184**: 849–54.
20. Kibler WB, Chandler TJ, Pace BK. Principles of rehabilitation after chronic tendon injuries. *Clinics in Sports Medicine* 1992; **11**: 661–71.
21. Siwek CW, Rao JP. Ruptures of the extensor mechanism of the knee joint. *Journal of Bone and Joint Surgery* 1981; **63A**: 1932.
22. Ramsey RN, Muller GE. Quadriceps tendon rupture: a diagnostic trap. *Clinical Orthopaedics* 1970; **70**: 161.
23. Kamali M. Bilateral traumatic rupture of the infrapatellar tendon. *Clinical Orthopaedics* 1979; **142**: 131–4.
24. Sherlock DA, Hughes A. Bilateral spontaneous concurrent rupture of the patellar tendon in the absence of associated local or systemic disease. *Clinical Orthopaedics* 1988; **237**: 179–83.
25. Kelly DW, Carter VS, Jobe FW, Kerlan RK. Patella and quadriceps tendon ruptures—jumper's knee. *American Journal of Sports Medicine* 1984; **12**: 375–80.
26. Doud GSE, Bentley G. Radiographic assessment in patellar instability and chondromalacia patellae. *Journal of Bone and Joint Surgery* 1986; **68B**: 297–300.
27. Chow SP, Lam JJ, Leong JCY. Fracture of the tibial tubercle in the adolescent. *Journal of Bone and Joint Surgery* 1990; **72B**: 231–4.
28. Goodrich MS, DiFiore RJ, Tippens JK. Bilateral simultaneous rupture of the infrapatellar tendon: a case report and literature review. *Orthopedics* 1983; **6**: 1472–4.
29. Karlsson J, Lundin O, Lossing IW. Partial rupture of the patellar ligament. *American Journal of Sports Medicine* 1991; **19**: 403–8.
30. Hayes WG. Patellofemoral contact pressures and the effects of surgical reconstructive procedures: articular cartilage and knee joint function. In: Ewing JJ, ed. *Basic science and arthroscopy.* New York: Raven Press, 1990: 7–77.
31. Insall J, Falvo KA, Wise DW. Chondromalacia patella. *Journal of Bone and Joint Surgery* 1976; **58A**: 1–8.
32. Fulkerson JP, Shea KP. Mechanical basis for patellofemoral pain and cartilage breakdown; Articular cartilage and knee joint function. In: Ewing JW, ed. *Basic science and arthroscopy.* New York: Raven Press, 1990: 93–102.
33. Chrisman OD, Snook GA. Studies on the protective effect of aspirin against degeneration of human articular cartilage. *Clinical Orthopaedics* 1968, **56**: 77.
34. McConnell J. The management of chondromalacia patellae: A long term solution. *Australian Journal of Physiotherapy* 1986; **33**: 215.
35. Buckwalter JA, Rosenberg LC, Hunzilken BB. Articular cartilage: composition, structure, response to injury and methods of facilitating repair of articular cartilage and knee joint function. In: Ewing JW, ed. *Basic science and arthroscopy.* New York: Raven Press, 1990: 19–26.
36. O'Donoghue RB. Treatment of chondral damage to the patella. *American Journal of Sports Medicine* 1981; **9**: 1.
37. Johnson LL. Arthroscopic abrasion chondroplasty: historical and pathologic perspective: present status. *Arthroscopy* 1986; **2**: 54–69.
38. Macquet P. Advancement of the tibial tuberosity. *Clinical Orthopaedics* 1986; **115**: 22.
39. Macquet P. Mechanics and osteoarthritis of the patellofemoral joint. *Clinical Orthopaedics* 1979; **144**: 70–3.
40. Radin EL. A rational approach to the treatment of patellofemoral pain. *Clinical Orthopaedics* 1979; **144**: 107.
41. Radin EL. Anterior tibial tubercle elevation in the young adult. *Orthopedic Clinics of North America* 1986; **17**: 297–302.

42. Ferguson AB, Brown TD, Fu FH, Rutkowski R. Relief of patello-femoral contact stress by anterior displacement of the tibial tubercle. *Journal of Bone and Joint Surgery* 1979; **61A**: 159.

43. Brittberg M, Lindahl A, Nilsson A, *et al.* Treatment of deep cartilage defects in the knee with autologous chondrocyte transplantation. *New England Journal of Medicine* 1994; **331**: 889–95.

44. American Orthopaedic Society for Sports Medicine. *Specialty Day Symposium.* Atlanta, Georgia, February 1996.

45. Minkoff JM, Fein L. The role of radiography in the evaluation and treatment of common anarthrotic disorders of the patellofemoral joint. *Clinics in Sports Medicine* 1989; **8**: 203–60.

46. Caner D, Sweemam R. Familial joint laxity and recurrent dislocation of the patella. *Journal of Bone and Joint Surgery* 1988, **40B**: 664.

47. Bassett FN. Surgery of the patellofemoral joint: acute dislocation of the patella, osteochondral fractures and injuries to the extensor mechanism of the knee. *AAOS Instructional Course Lectures* 1976; **25**: 46.

48. Cash JD, Hughston JC. Treatment of acute patellar dislocation. *American Journal of Sports Medicine* 1988; **16**: 244.

49. McGinty JB, McCarthy JC. Endoscopic lateral retinacular release: a preliminary report. *Clinical Orthopaedics* 1981; **1**: 120.

50. Brown DE, Alexander AH, Lichtman DA. The Elmslie–Trillat procedure: evaluation in patellar dislocation and subluxation. *American Journal of Sports Medicine* 1984; **12**: 104–9.

51. Cox JS. Evaluation of the Elmslie–Trillat procedure for knee extension realignment. *American Journal of Sports Medicine* 1982; **5**: 303.

52. Fulkerson JP. Anteromedialization of the tibial tuberosity for patellofemoral malalignment. *Clinical Orthopaedics* 1983; **177**: 176–81.

53. Fulkerson JP, Shea KP. Disorders of patellofemoral alignment. *Journal of Joint and Bone Surgery* 1990; **72A**: 1424–9.

54. Schutzer SF, Ramsby GR, Fulkerson JP. Computed tomographic classification of patellofemoral pain patients. *Orthopedic Clinics of North America* 1986; **17**: 235–48.

55. Dzioba RB. Diagnostic arthroscopy and longitudinal open lateral release: a four year follow up study to determine predictors of surgical outcome. *American Journal of Sports Medicine* 1990; **18**: 343–8.

56. Kolowich PA, Paulos LE, Rosenberg TD, *et al.* Lateral release of the patella: Indications and contraindications. *American Journal of Sports Medicine* 1990; **18**: 359–65.

57. Merchant AC, Mercer RL, Jacobsen RH, Cool CR. Roentgeno-graphic analysis of patellofemoral congruence. *Journal of Bone and Joint Surgery* 1974; **56A**: 1391–6.

58. Laurin CA, Dussault R, Levesque HP. The tangential X-ray investigation of the patellofemoral joint: X-ray technique, diagnostic criteria and their interpretation. *Clinical Orthopaedics* 1979; **144**: 16–26.

59. Imai N, Mercer RL, Jacobsen RH, Col CR. Clinical and roentgenologic studies on malalignment disorders of the patellofemoral joint: Classification of patellofemoral alignments using dynamic sky-line view arthrography with special consideration of the mechanism of the malalignment disorders. *Journal of the Orthopaedic Association* 1987; **61**: 1–15.

60. Walker C, Cassar-Pullicino VN, Vaisha R, McCall IW. The patello-femoral joint—a critical appraisal of its geometric assessment utilizing conventional axial radiography and computed arthro-tomography. *British Journal of Radiology* 1993; **66**: 755–61.

61. Masri BA, McCormack RG. The effect of knee flexion and quadriceps contraction on the axial view of the patella. *Clinical Journal of Sport Medicine* 1995; **5**: 9–17.

62. Teitge RA, Warren WF, Des Madryl P, Matelic TM. Stress radiographs of the patellofemoral joint. *Journal of Joint and Bone Surgery* 1996; **78A**: 193–203.

63. Malghem J, Maldague B. Patellofemoral joint: 30 degree axial radiograph with lateral rotation of the leg. *Radiology* 1989; **170**: 566–7.

64. Malghem J, Maldague B. Depth insufficiency of the proximal trochlear groove on lateral radiographs of the knee: relation to patella dislocation. *Radiology* 1989; **170**: 507–10.

65. Shellock FG, Mink JN, Fox JM. Patellofemoral joint: kinematic MR imaging to assess tracking abnormalities. *Radiology* 1988; **168**: 551–3.

66. Omohundro PH, Payne R. Reflex sympathetic dystrophy. Cincinnati, OH: Fellowship Project, unpublished.

67. Toumey JW. Occurrence and management of reflex sympathetic dystrophy. *Journal of Bone and Joint Surgery* 1948; **30A**: 883.

68. Patel D. Plica as a cause of anterior knee pain. *Orthopedic Clinics of North America* 1986; **17**: 273–7.

69. Broom MJ, Fulkerson JP. The plica syndrome: a new perspective. *Orthopedic Clinics of North America* 1986; **17**: 279–81.

4.2.5 Fractures and dislocations

J. Robert Giffin and Jean-Louis Briard

Introduction

As a result of the increasing participation and competitiveness in both organized and unsupervised sporting activities, the number of individuals presenting with acute knee injuries continues to rise. Compared with the incidence of other soft tissue knee trauma, fractures and dislocations about the knee occur infrequently in the sports population.

However, fractures and dislocations about the knee can be devastating to the athlete in terms of rehabilitation and eventual return to sport. Therefore, physicians who deal with athletes must be able to suspect, diagnose, and properly treat these rare injuries. The key to sound management is early recognition and this chapter will address most of the skeletal injuries encountered about the knee.

Dislocations of the knee

Traumatic injury to the lower extremities of athletes occurs frequently in sports. Athletic injuries are the second most common cause of knee dislocation[1] and although this type of knee trauma is uncommon, it can result in disruption of the popliteal artery. Vascular compromise could result in amputation, as the worst possible case scenario, if circulation is not restored within 6 to 8 h.

The primary care physician must conduct a neurovascular examination during their initial assessment of an athlete who has sustained significant trauma to the knee. Recognition of this potential limb-threatening injury by the attending physician will ensure thorough investigation and surgical correction of any associated vascular injuries, thereby reducing the likelihood of a disastrous situation.

Some knee dislocations are never recognized because of spontaneous reduction prior to evaluation by a physician. Patients with multidirectional knee instability may have suffered a dislocation at the time of their injury, thus it is widely accepted that any patient in whom three or more of the major ligaments have been disrupted should be evaluated and treated as having sustained a knee dislocation.

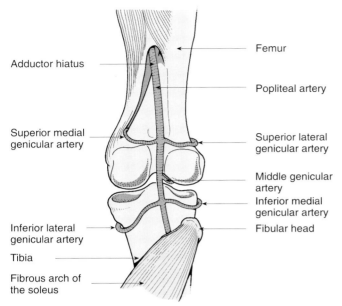

Fig. 1 The popliteal artery is tethered at the adductor hiatus and the fibrous arch of the soleus.

Emergency transportation of the athlete to a hospital with appropriate radiographic facilities and both orthopaedic and vascular consultants is vital to avoid the development of severe sequelae. The potential seriousness of the knee dislocation is not restricted to the circulation, as other crucial anatomical structures may also be injured. Peripheral nerve damage can lead to grave functional sequelae and ligamentous injuries can also result in residual laxity or instability.

Anatomy

The popliteal artery is at risk of injury during knee trauma because it is relatively fixed within the popliteal fossa (Fig. 1). Proximally it is tethered at the adductor magnus hiatus and distally it is tethered at the fibrous arch of the soleus before its division into the anterior and posterior tibial arteries.

Despite its collateral arteries, perfusion of tissues could be insufficient to maintain the viability of the deep leg musculature in the event that the popliteal artery is stretched, transected, or crushed. The neurovascular structures that accompany the artery through the fossa are not as firmly bound and therefore are less likely to be injured. Neurological damage when it occurs is usually caused by traction with stretching the peroneal nerve around the posterior femoral condyle.

Classification

Knee dislocations are classified by the direction in which the tibia is displaced in relation to the femur.[2] There are five major types of dislocation: (1) anterior, (2) posterior, (3) lateral, (4) medial, and (5) rotatory. There are four rotatory subclassifications, each representing an anatomic quadrant: (1) anteromedial, (2) anterolateral, (3) posteromedial, and (4) posterolateral (Fig. 2). The relative incidence of the each type of dislocation varies considerably between published reports, but most authors agree that the anterior dislocation is the most common, followed by the posterior.

The traditional classification by direction does not take into consideration the possibility that a knee may have been dislocated and then spontaneously reduced. Thus, it is useful to classify knee dislocations further in terms of the ligamentous structures involved, as many combinations of cruciate and collateral ligament disruptions are possible. This is best evaluated at the time of injury (if tolerated) or during an examination under anaesthesia. These subclassifications can be very useful in decision making and placement of surgical incisions. Finally, knee dislocations have also been classified by the level of energy sustained (high or low), as well as if they are open or closed, indicating the need for immediate attention.

Mechanism of injury

Trauma caused by high speed vehicles continues to be the most common mechanism of injury involved in knee dislocations. However, as mentioned previously, low velocity dislocations of the knee can also occur on the athletic field.

As demonstrated by Kennedy,[2] hyperextension of the knee

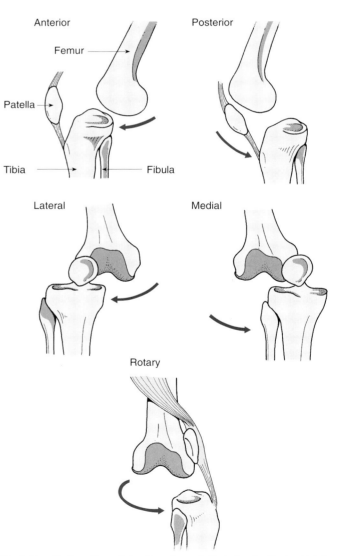

Fig. 2 Classification of knee dislocations. Arrows indicate the direction in which the tibia is displaced on the femur.

greater than 30 degrees from neutral will usually result in rupture of the posterior capsule. The tibia then translates forward on the femur causing the subsequent disruption of the posterior and anterior cruciate ligaments. At 50 degrees of hyperextension the popliteal artery could also be torn and the injury becomes a surgical emergency.

Posterior dislocations usually occur when a force is applied directly to the anterior tibia. The force that is required to produce this translocation of the tibia posteriorly is much larger than the force necessary to cause an anterior dislocation.[1] The posterior displacement of the bone stretches the popliteal artery which may become disrupted just proximal to its trifurcation.

A lateral dislocation occurs with a valgus force that disrupts the medial supporting structures and displaces the tibia laterally on the femur. With a medial dislocation, a varus force damages the lateral ligamentous structures as well as both cruciate ligaments. The extreme rotatory moments that are required most likely occur with high energy accidents.[2]

Although rare, the most common rotatory dislocation occurs in the posterolateral direction. The mechanism of injury involves a sudden rotatory moment that both abducts and internally rotates the tibia in a flexed non-weight-bearing limb.[3] This may cause the femoral condyle to 'buttonhole' through the medial capsule and tibial collateral ligament. If these structures become trapped within the joint, the injury is often irreducible. This is usually evidenced by a transverse groove in the skin at the medial joint line (dimple sign) which becomes more prominent if a reduction is attempted, thus requiring an open reduction.

Associated injuries

Vascular injuries

Dislocations that occur in the anterior or posterior plane are more likely to result in the disruption of popliteal artery flow and the overall calculated risk of vascular injury in all knee dislocations is 32 per cent.[4] Two major types of injury mechanisms have been described. One involves a traction injury to the artery, which commonly occurs with anterior dislocations. The other is a direct contusion of the vessel by the posterior rim of the tibia during a posterior dislocation.[5]

Experiments[6] have shown that traction applied to an artery will rupture the intima and media prior to tearing of the outer elastic advential layer. Such injuries may result in thrombosis of the vessel prior to the initial examination, resulting in absence of distal pulses. However, transmission of a pulse through a non-occlusive intimal tear may give the false impression of an intact popliteal pulse. Furthermore, arterial compromise could manifest itself in a delayed fashion, since a thrombosis may not occur for hours or even days following trauma.

The consequence of thrombosis is an ischaemia of the tissue supplied by the occluded artery. Animal studies have revealed that after 6 to 8 h of ischaemia, irreversible damage occurs. DeBakey and Simeone[7] in a review of arterial injuries during the Second World War found an amputation rate of 72.5 per cent when the popliteal flow was disrupted. Green and Allen[4] demonstrated that in knee dislocations, 86 per cent of the limbs in which the flow of the popliteal artery was not restored within 8 h resulted in amputation.

A diagnosis of vasospasm should never be accepted as the aetiology of diminished perfusion without angiographic confirmation. Even with a compatible angiogram, if the spasm does not respond promptly to appropriate pharmacological agents or if the limb is not well perfused, the vessel should be explored surgically.[8]

Ligament injuries

Knee dislocations result in extensive soft tissue injuries with rupturing of the primary ligaments and stripping of the capsule from the bone. In the vast majority of cases, both the anterior cruciate and the posterior cruciate are ruptured. However, the common belief that both cruciate ligaments must be disrupted in order for a knee to dislocate has been disproved.[9] Complete dislocations have been reported with either the anterior or posterior cruciate ligaments intact. Dislocations occurring purely in the sagittal plane can macroscopically spare the collateral ligaments from injury.

Nerve injuries

The reported incidence of nerve injury with knee dislocations is extremely variable, but has been estimated to be approximately 25 per cent.[5] Although injuries to the tibial nerve have been described, the majority of cases involve the common peroneal nerve associated with medial, lateral, and rotatory dislocations.

Signs and symptoms

The importance of an accurate patient history, diligent observation, and a thorough examination must be emphasized when attempting to achieve the correct diagnosis. The position of the athlete's extremity following the traumatic insult will dictate the order of the assessment process.

If the extremity is in a position of obvious deformity, the circulatory status of the injured limb is evaluated first. In most instances, the dislocation can easily be reduced at the scene by gently applying traction to the limb and pressure on the femur opposite the direction of the deformity. The circulatory status must be assessed again following the reduction of the dislocation and care must be taken never to hyperextend the knee. Lastly, the extremity should be immobilized in slight flexion for transport.

If a deformity of the injured leg is not obvious, careful assessment of the ligamentous stability is indicated with gentle manipulation. The vascular and neurological status should also be evaluated, remembering that sensory disturbances and paralysis could be caused by ischaemia only, not infarction. Severe trauma to the knee must be quickly evaluated and the patient referred to the most appropriate centre because of the high likelihood of major ligamentous disruption or dislocation with associated potential vascular injury.

Imaging

Standard radiographs should be obtained in order to assess the position of the tibia in relation to the femoral condyles and to check for the presence of any associated fractures. Arteriography is currently indicated for all patients with knee dislocations or severe ligamentous instability. Furthermore, arteriography should be performed in the operating room in order to avoid delay of correction of vascular compromise.

The use of arteriography in the management of a patient with a knee dislocation who has normal pulses and no history of ischaemia is more debatable. These patients need not undergo arteriography acutely as long as the status of the patient is closely observed by a vascular surgeon or other experienced personnel and necessary facilities are available to perform an emergency repair if required.[9]

Treatment

Arterial repair

The vascular repair or the use of an intravascular shunt should be of first priority in order to decrease the duration of ischaemia. The most common method of vascular repair is resection of the damaged segment followed by a reverse saphenous interposition graft from the contralateral limb. Rarely is the injury so localized that a direct repair is possible. Injuries to the popliteal vein should be repaired when possible, in order to lower the risk of venous thrombosis and pulmonary embolism.[5] The liberal use of four-compartment fasciotomy as a prophylactic measure for significant ischaemia (greater than 4 h) is recommended.[5,9] Intraoperative angiography should be employed routinely upon completion of the repair to check the integrity of the vascular reconstruction.

Ligament repair/reconstruction

There are three treatment approaches for ligamentous injuries following knee dislocations: (1) non-surgical, (2) acute repair, and (3) delayed reconstruction. The treating orthopaedist must tailor the treatment to the individual needs of the patient. Age, activity level, job requirements, and individual goals all enter the decision-making process.[9] In all cases, the joint must be reduced and maintained in its anatomical position to decrease the risk of arthritis.

Some authors have recommended a delayed surgical repair of all torn ligaments (2 to 3 weeks) unless there is an absolute acute surgical indication, such as irreducibility. Primary repair of bony avulsions of the cruciate ligament has been more successful than repair of insubstancial tears. If delayed reconstruction is planned, the posterior cruciate must be addressed first to maintain the correct position of the joint.

Ideally, adequate strength and range of motion should be obtained prior to reconstruction. More aggressive rehabilitation protocols including an early range of motion exercises in a hinged brace are being advocated by most authors to decrease stiffness. The rehabilition is lengthy and the recovery is never complete.

Prognosis and complications

Vascular complications can be very serious, causing ischaemia which may lead to amputation. Complications may include acute renal tubular necrosis from myoglobinaemia or possible compartment syndrome if a fasciotomy is not performed at the time of the vascular repair. Late complications of ischaemic contracture and ulceration may develop unexpectedly, and nerve palsies that do not recover can be salvaged with tendon transfers.

Few patients who have suffered a knee dislocation will recover normal knee function. Regardless of the type of treatment undertaken, significant rates of stiffness, pain, and instability are generally the rule rather than the exception.[9] Generally stiffness is more of a problem than symptoms of instability. With aggressive rehabilita-

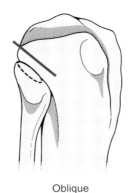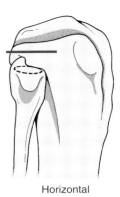

Oblique   Horizontal

Fig. 3 Ogden types of proximal tibiofibular joints, oblique and horizontal.

tion, a large majority of patients will resume their normal activities but only a minority will return to athletics at their previous level.

Dislocation of the proximal tibiofibular joint

Dislocation of the proximal tibiofibular joint is uncommon and recurrent instability is very rare. An awareness of this injury is crucial, as the diagnosis is frequently missed. There have been slightly more than 100 reported cases in the English literature, most of which have been associated with sports-related injuries.[10-14]

Anatomy

The proximal tibiofibular articulation is a diarthrodial joint that is inherently stable. The articular surfaces vary in size, shape, and inclination (Fig. 3). The articular facet of the fibula is on the posteroinferior aspect of the lateral tibial condyle and is bordered anteriorly by the lateral tibial sulcus. The fibular facet is usually elliptical and almost flat. The articular surfaces are covered with hyaline cartilage, surrounded by a synovial membrane and a joint capsule that is distinct from that of the knee. The capsule is thicker anteriorly and is reinforced by both anterior and posterior tibiofibular ligaments, the former being the much stronger of the two. Superior support is provided by the lateral or fibular collateral ligament. The motion of the proximal tibiofibular articulation consists of proximal–distal translation as well as axial rotation and is related to movement occurring in the talocrural joint.[14]

Classification

There are three types of acute traumatic dislocations of the proximal tibiofibular articulation (Fig. 4). (1) The most frequent dislocation occurs in the anterolateral direction (about 90 per cent) secondary to a fall on a flexed and adducted leg, with the foot in an inverted position.[13] (2) Dislocation in the posteromedial direction is the result of either a direct blow (horseback rider's knee) or a twisting injury. This injury is more often associated with peroneal nerve injuries[11,14] and may lead to chronic problems because of difficulty in maintaining reduction. (3) A dislocation in the superior direction does not occur as an isolated lesion and is always associated with a fracture of the tibia or a severe ankle injury.[10]

Lyle[15] described the subluxation as a fourth type of disruption of the proximal tibiofibular joint. These subluxations are chronic in nature and are the result of neglected anterolateral or posteromedial dislocations. The subluxations are often associated with peroneal nerve disturbances and must be differentiated from the idiopathic recurrent dislocations.

Signs and symptoms

Following the trauma the patient can usually describe the mechanism of injury and will state that the joint feels unstable. Clinical presentation can range from the athlete being completely disabled with a limb that is non-weight bearing to just complaining of slight discomfort over the lateral aspect of their knee or ankle.

On examination, the dislocated fibular head is usually prominent and tender to palpation. Soft tissue swelling is mild during the acute stages and mobilization of the ankle may produce knee pain. The fibular head may be hypermobile compared with the contralateral side and peroneal nerve function must be evaluated.

Radiographic findings are often subtle and comparison of the injured side with the normal knee is helpful in determining the diagnosis. Films of an anterior dislocation show that the fibula is laterally displaced and the proximal interosseous span is widened on the anteroposterior view. The lateral view reveals the fibular head is displaced anteriorly and overlapped by the tibia (Fig. 5).

Chronic tibiofibular dislocation

The patient typically presents with a history of derangement in maximum flexion of the knee and has symptoms of clicking and pain over the lateral compartment. The pain, which can radiate distally to the foot, is aggravated by walking and jumping. Clinically it may mimic a lateral meniscal injury, which would be included in the differential diagnosis. However, the diagnosis can be confirmed with the presence of tenderness and swelling directly over the tibiofibular joint. When assessing the mobility of the fibular head, the physician should determine the quality of the joint's end feel and to determine if an anteroposterior drawer sign is present. Radiographs and CT scans may also be employed to demonstrate the dislocation.

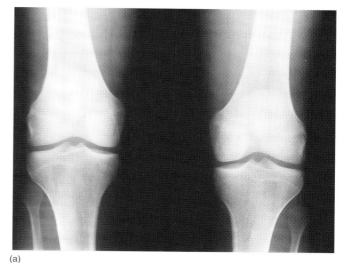

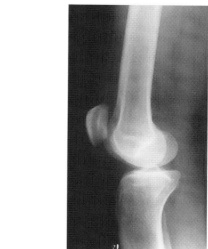

Fig. 5 Anteroposterior (a) and lateral (b) radiographs of a proximal tibiofibular dislocation.

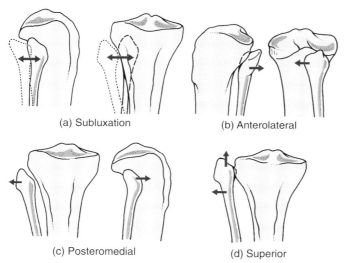

Fig. 4 Ogden classification of disruptions of the proximal tibiofibular joint into subluxations and three types of dislocations—anterolateral, posteromedial, and superior.

(a) Subluxation   (b) Anterolateral

(c) Posteromedial   (d) Superior

Treatment

Acute anterior derangements are nearly always reducible by direct manipulation; however it may be necessary to perform the reduction under general anaesthesia on occasion.[14] The knee is flexed to 90 degrees, the foot inverted, and direct manipulation reduces the fibular head with an audible snap. The knee is strapped and the patient begins progressive weight bearing on crutches over a period of 3 weeks. The presence of an associated ankle injury may require the use of a cast immobilization. If the closed manipulation fails or if the dislocation reoccurs; open reduction is warranted.[16] Ligament reconstruction and fixation with Kirschner's wires may be required. A short leg cast is then applied for a period of 6 weeks.

In chronic cases, the presence of disability or peroneal palsy warrants surgical intervention. Some surgeons prefer to resect the head and neck of the fibula coupled with a careful reconstruction of the periosteal tissue sleeve. Others prefer to perform an arthrodesis of the superior tibiofibular joint and a 2-cm resection of the fibular shaft.

In conclusion, the diagnosis of dislocation of the superior tibio-fibular joint should not be overlooked as a cause of post-traumatic lateral knee pain. Chronic derangement of the proximal tibiofibular articulation may be mistaken for meniscal pathology, lateral ligament tears, or popliteal tendinitis.

Osteochondritis dissecans

Osteochondritis dissecans is a localized injury or condition affecting the articular surface in which a fragment of cartilage and subchondral bone separate partially or completely from the underlying bony matrix. Although this condition occurs relatively infrequently, it is primarily found in the knee, ankle, and elbow.

The aetiology and treatment of osteochondritis dissecans are still a matter of controversy. There is both a juvenile and adult form of this condition. A very favourable prognosis can be expected when treating the young patient prior to the closure of their epiphysis. Intervention in adults is much more aggressive and results of treatment are not uniformly successful.

Aetiology

Various theories regarding the aetiology of osteochondritis dissecans have been proposed (ischaemia, constitutional effects, trauma), but none have been accepted universally or have explained its occurrence adequately. These lesions are most probably caused by several factors that can vary depending on the specific joint involved and the specific area of the joint involved.[17]

Ischaemia

Ischaemia had been a popular theory of early investigators who suggested that obstruction of end arteries to the femoral condyle was a possible cause of osteochondritis dissecans.[17] However, the work of Rogers and Gladstone[18] demonstrated that the distal femur has a network of anastomosing vessels in the subchondral bone. They concluded that ischaemia alone was an unlikely cause of osteochondritis dissecans of the knee. Furthermore, the pathology of the avascular necrosis differs from that of osteochondritis dissecans. In avascular necrosis, fragmentation occurs between necrotic layers of bone; whereas in osteochondritis dissecans, the fragment separates from a completely normal bony matrix.

Constitutional

While there have been multiple reports[19] of familial occurrence suggesting a hereditary factor, the usual presentation of osteochondritis dissecans is not familial in nature.[20] However, multiple epiphyseal dysplasia, with its autosomal dominant or recessive pattern of inheritance, should be considered in the differential diagnosis of patients who have osteochondritis dissecans.[21]

Abnormalities of endochondral ossification of the epiphysis commonly occur in childhood and usually resolve without any long-term sequelae.[22,23] A delayed ossification process may give the radiological appearance of a crater or an accessory epiphysis. The crater is filled with radiolucent hyaline cartilage which may become partially calcified along its deep surface. Compressive forces may shear the edges of the crater and progressively detach the deeper partially calcified portion. This accessory nucleus of bone may separate with subsequent partial reattachment. Further trauma during childhood could result in a complete separation.

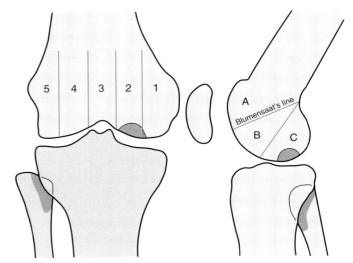

Fig. 6 Radiographic (anatomical) classification.

Trauma

Trauma has been discussed extensively in the literature as a possible aetiological factor in the development of osteochondritis dissecans of the knee. The proximity of the lateral aspect of the medial femoral condyle to the tibial spine, the insertion of the posterior cruciate ligament, and the medial aspect of the patella in full flexion has fostered theories of indirect trauma as the aetiology of osteochondritis dissecans.[19]

Although a direct blow to the knee could create an acute transchondral fracture with radiographic findings similar to osteochondritis dissecans, most patients do not recall any obvious single traumatic event. However, it is common for patients to report a long history of exercise and sports at a young age.[24]

Cahill[25] has insisted on the role of minimal or insignificant trauma in the production of osteochondritis dissecans. He reported that the investigation of the mechanical properties of bone offers substantiated evidence that the initial lesion of osteochondritis dissecans could be a fatigue failure of previously normal subchondral bone. Joint scintigraphy of patients with juvenile osteochondritis dissecans demonstrated a healing pattern typical of fractures, and thus Cahill[26] concluded that juvenile osteochondritis dissecans is a failure of the subchondral bone as a result of cumulative stresses. In summary, the current trend of thought is to recognize a multifactoral cause or several predisposing factors when considering the aetiology of osteochondritis dissecans.

Classification

Radiographic

Numerous anatomical classifications have been described for osteochondritis dissecans in the literature according to the progression of the lesion.[27,28,29] Cahill *et al.*[26] described a useful classification (Fig. 6) in which the anteroposterior radiograph is divided into five segments starting from the medial side (the condyles are bisected with the notch designated as area 3). The lateral radiograph is divided into three segments on the basis of Harding's[30] description: A, anterior to the Blumensaat line (intercondylar notch); B, between the Blumensaat line and a line drawn along the posterior femoral cortex; and C, the condylar area posterior to the femoral cortex line. This classification provides a more precise method for accurately mapping the location and ascertaining the size of the lesion.

Arthroscopic

Arthroscopy provides direct visualization and a technique for manual testing of the integrity of the cartilage. Although arthroscopy is rarely indicated for diagnosis only, lesions can be classified into 5 stages: (1) intact; (2) early separation; (3) partially detached; (4) complete detachment, with salvageable crater and loose bodies; and (5) unsalvageable crater and loose bodies.[28]

Incidence and location

The incidence of osteochondritis dissecans is estimated at between 0.05 and 0.08 per cent of the population.[31] The greatest incidence of the disease occurs in the first half of the second decade of the physiologically active adolescent; though osteochondritis dissecans may affect anyone from 5 to 50 years old. The distribution among sexes is not equal, with males being mainly affected (70 per cent).[19] Anatomic locations have been extensively studied (Fig. 7). The distribution of the lesions in most studies approaches the locations described by Aichroth.[32] Furthermore, osteochondritis dissecans occurs bilaterally 30 per cent of the time.[17]

Hughston *et al.*[29] distinguished between lesions on the most distal weight-bearing aspect of the femoral condyle and those that occurred more posteriorly. They found that a great majority of defects on the lateral condyle were equally distributed between posterior and distal location. Outerbridge[33] reviewed 14 cases of osteochondritis dissecans affecting the posterior area of both the medial and lateral condyles. It has been his experience that the presence of a defect in this posterior location results in a poor prognosis for the patient.

Clinical features

The symptoms of osteochondritis dissecans of the knee will depend on the stage of presentation. Patients who present early in their course will complain of non-specific knee pain which developed insidiously and is aggravated by physical activity. Onset may be acute in nature, especially in older patients, and all age groups may complain of joint effusion. As the lesion progresses, symptoms of

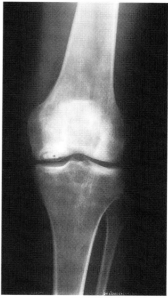

Fig. 8 Osteochondritis dissecans involving the lateral aspect of the medial femoral condyle in a skeletally mature patient.

giving way, painful buckling, catching, or locking may be reported as the lesion becomes unstable or forms a loose body.

Physical examination may reveal quadriceps atrophy, effusion, limitation of femoral passive range of motion, and localized tenderness to palpation directly over the site of the lesion with the knee in a flexed position. Wilson[34] has described a sign in which the pain can be reproduced by first flexing and internally rotating the knee and then extending the leg slowly. The test will be positive if a lesion is located in the common posterolateral site of the medial femoral condyle. A positive sign can be confirmed if the pain is subsequently relieved by externally rotating the tibia.

Imaging studies

Radiographic evaluation

The lesion usually appears as a well-defined area of subchondral bone separated from the remaining femoral condyle by a crescent-shaped radiolucent line. The classic location on the posterolateral medial condyle may not be apparent on a standard anteroposterior view (Fig. 8) and is best visualized using the tunnel view. Although the lateral view is sometimes difficult to read, it does allow an estimation of the size of the defect. Because of the potential variations in the location of an osteochondritis dissecans lesion, if the disorder is suspected, the radiographic examination should include anteroposterior, lateral, oblique, notch, and skyline patellar views.

Scintigraphic evaluation

The role of joint scintigraphy in the diagnosis and treatment of osteochondritis dissecans has been stressed by Cahill[26] and Mesgarzadeh.[35] It allows for differentiation between osteochondritis dissecans and an accessory ossification centre. Technetium polyphosphate uptake is a measure of both osteoblastic activity and regional blood flow.[36] The level of scintigraphic activity in a symptomatic knee indicates the remaining potential for healing of the osteochondritis dissecans fragment. Cahill[26] insists on the value of repeated bone

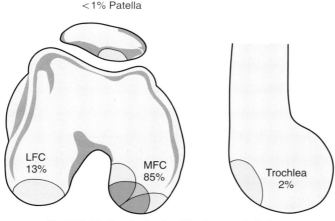

Fig. 7 Distribution of osteochondritis dissecans in the knee.

scintigraphy to assess the progression of the healing and to determine if and when more radical procedures must be done.

Magnetic resonance imaging (MRI) evaluation

More recently MRI has been employed to analyse the mechanical stability of the lesion in osteochondritis dissecans. It provides direct visualization of any displacement of the fragment, the fluid interfaces, and the integrity of the articular surfaces. The findings on the magnetic resonance images closely correlate with the arthroscopic findings[37] and can be utilized to follow the healing response and the degree of revascularization of the lesion.[36]

Prognosis

Once a diagnosis has been established, the prognosis of the patient is dependent upon several variables. The patient's age (epiphysis open or closed), integrity of the articular cartilage, and stability of the lesion are very reliable indicators of clinical outcome. The severity of the athlete's subjective complaints (i.e. catching, buckling, locking) in addition to radiographic findings are good parameters for predicting loosening. The juvenile form of osteochondritis dissecans was previously considered to have an excellent prognosis for healing without complication. However, recent reports have demonstrated that healing does not always occur spontaneously and that loosening or complete detachment of the fragment can occur.[25,31]

Osteochondritis dissecans of the skeletally mature patient may be complicated with mechanical detachment of the lesion. The formation of loose bodies and tibial plateau alteration could possibly diminish the performance of the athlete. Long-term follow-up has shown the development of osteoarthritis in the majority of the patients even though the athletes have remained asymptomatic for an extended interval of time. The osteoarthritis secondary to an osteochondral defect tends to begin a decade earlier than does primary gonarthrosis.[31] Results following surgical procedures are not consistent because of ensuing secondary degeneration, especially in patients who had been diagnosed and treated after skeletal maturity.

Treatment

The object of treatment is to promote healing of the lesion and prevent detachment in an attempt to preserve a smooth articular surface.

The treatment of osteochondritis dissecans can range from observation to surgical intervention which depends primarily on the age of the patient and secondarily on the degree of involvement. Conservative measures may include a trial of orthotics or the use of splints and crutches as symptoms require. The prudent use of physiotherapy may help to maintain the patient's strength and retard atrophy. The aim of surgical treatment is to improve the stability of the fragment by enhancing its blood supply. Numerous surgical techniques have been described including excising the fragment, drilling,[38] crater debridement, grafting,[39,40] and fixation with pins, screws,[41] or bone pegs.[42] The goal is to restore the surface congruity which may require grafting, debridement, or the repositioning of loose bodies.[43,44]

Children who have a symptomatic lesion should be managed initially with limitation of activity until they no longer have symptoms. Good results can be expected with close clinical observation and

serial imaging in about 50 per cent of patients.[24] Cahill[26] suggests that the healing process should be monitored with bone scans. When the scan shows decreased activity, healing is assumed to have taken place. Surgery is only indicated if the lesion remains active and symptomatic for greater than 6 to 12 months. Arthroscopic drilling is the treatment of choice for intact lesions[17,28] and completely separated fragments should be managed in a manner similar to that used in adults.[17]

In older adolescents and adults, the treatment must be more aggressive and the prognosis remains guarded. Indications for operative treatment in the skeletally mature patient include a lesion larger than 1 cm and involvement in a weight-bearing surface.[28] Lesions with intact articular cartilage can be drilled in a retrograde fashion under arthroscopic guidance. Large intact lesions may require grafting, especially when the defects are posterior.[33] Those with early separation should be debrided at their border, drilled, and pinned in place. Partially detached lesions require debridement of the crater, reduction, and fixation. Salvageable loose bodies should be prepared and replaced when possible, especially if they involve a portion of a weight-bearing surface. The use of allografts or osteochondral autografts to restore surface congruity of large intra-articular defects appears to be promising but unproved. Finally, excision should be reserved for small fragments or for lesions that cannot be reconstructed.

Although most of the procedures are performed arthroscopically, open surgery may be required to deal with large lesions and difficult locations. Rehabilitation consists of a programme of early range of motion exercises as well as strengthening of the musculature about the knee. The length of time during which weight-bearing is restricted can range from 2 to 3 weeks to several months dependent upon the procedure performed. The fibrocartilage forming at the base of a crater on a weight-bearing surface must be given sufficient time to mature before being subjected to body force. Grafting may require splinting for 4 to 6 weeks and weight bearing should be restricted until there is radiographic evidence of healing.

Osteochondritis dissecans is best diagnosed and treated before skeletal maturity, and restoration of the articular surface should be attempted whenever possible. However, older patients who have an advanced lesion may be managed with total knee arthroplasty or tibial osteotomy.

Fractures about the knee

Major fractures in adults

Fractures about the knee are relatively rare in athletics and are usually limited to contact and high velocity sports. Associated vascular disruption is again rare, but the potential does exist. Arterial injury is a surgical emergency, therefore immediate recognition and investigation is essential.

Fractures about the knee can be very serious and may terminate an athlete's career. Proper treatment is critical if the athlete is going to be able to return to sport and compete at their previous level. The evaluation of a fracture should include examination of all of the soft tissues and neurovascular structures around the knee. A precise description of the fracture including its displacement and stability must be documented and potential complications addressed. Radiographs and occasionally tomographs or CT scans must be employed to allow for proper description and categorization of the fracture into one of the accepted classification schemes.

The most widely accepted classification scheme of supracondylar fractures was devised by Müller and colleagues.[45] This system is relatively simple to use and identifies three general types of fractures, each with three subtypes (Fig. 9). The Schatzker[46] classification (Fig. 10) for tibial plateau fracture is mainly used in North America, whereas Europeans tend to use Müller's or Dupre's classification schemes.

Fractures of the proximal end of the fibula occur mainly in association with proximal tibial fractures, especially split compression, bicondylar, and subcondylar types. The integrity of the peroneal nerve, anterior tibial artery, biceps tendon, and lateral collateral ligament must be assessed following a proximal fibular fracture to rule out any associated injury to these anatomical structures.

The indications for non-operative and operative treatment depend on many factors, such as fracture displacement or depression, the patient's health and skin condition, associated soft tissue

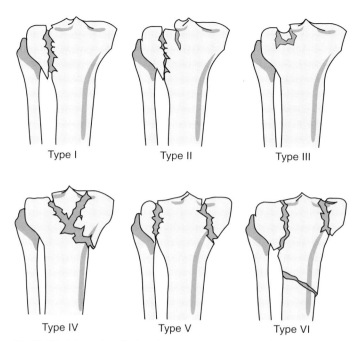

Fig. 10 Schatzker's classification of tibial plateau fractures. Type I, pure cleavage fracture. Type II, cleavage combined with depression. Type III, pure central depression. Type IV, fractures of the medial condyle. Type V, bicondylar fractures. Type VI, tibial plateau fracture with dissociation of the tibial metaphysis and diaphysis.

injuries, additional fractures, and character of the fracture (open or closed). Internal fixation decreases the rehabilitation time of the athlete by facilitating the early return of knee function.

Operative methods for displaced articular fractures emphasize accurate restoration of the articular surface through open reduction and internal fixation. Displaced extra-articular fractures are treated by internal fixation in order to maintain overall limb alignment and to enable early motion. Articular fractures can be treated in special cases with arthroscopy and cannulated screws to lessen the trauma caused during open reduction.[47–49]

Approximately 30 per cent of plateau fractures have associated ligament damage which must always be addressed in any treatment plan.[49,50] Neurovascular status must always be a concern with knee trauma and restoring circulation takes precedence over fracture treatment.

Major fractures in children

The paediatric musculoskeletal system differs from that of adults in a number of significant ways. The bones of a child differ in both architecture and physiology when compared with an adult. A child has a cartilaginous epiphyseal plate that is weaker than bone and ligament.[51] The distal femur is responsible for 70 per cent of the longitudinal growth of the femur and lengthening of the proximal tibia accounts for 60 per cent of the longitudinal growth of the tibia.[52] The high proportion of cartilage in bone during the growing years leads to a unique vulnerability both to trauma and infection of the growth plate. Knee trauma that is overlooked in the presence of a fracture of the femur or tibia could lead to growth arrest. Adolescents who have sustained fractures in their lower limbs that did not initially appear to have epiphyseal plate involvement should nevertheless be evaluated and followed for possible epiphyseal injury

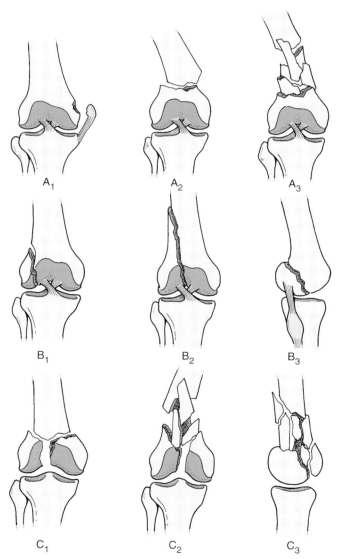

Fig. 9 Müller's classification of supracondylar fractures.

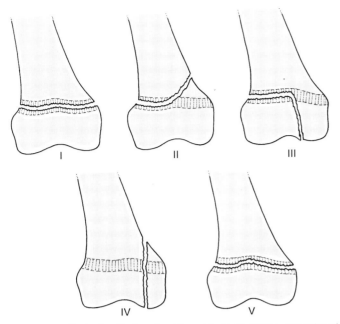

Fig. 11 Salter–Harris classification of epiphyseal fractures. Type I, separation of epiphysis. Type II, fracture-separation of epiphysis. Type III, fracture of part of epiphysis. Type IV, fracture of epiphysis and epiphyseal plate. Type V, crushing of epiphyseal plate.

about the knee that can only be detected after additional growth has taken place.[53]

Ligament injuries are often associated with epiphyseal fractures about the knee.[54] Epiphyseal injury may cause a rapid arrest of growth[55] and the consequent development of serious bony deformity without proper intervention. The Salter–Harris[56] classification of epiphyseal plate injuries (Fig. 11) is based on the following: (1) the mechanism of injury; (2) the relationship of the fracture line to the growing epiphysis; (3) the method of treatment; and (4) the prognosis of the injury with regards to growth disturbances. There is a poor prognosis for growth following a displaced type IV epiphyseal injury unless a perfect surgical reduction is obtained and a type V injury is of great concern because of the crushing of the plate.

Distal femoral epiphysis fractures

The distal femoral epiphysis is the most common fracture site in young athletes. Salter–Harris type II injuries with displacement in the coronal plane occur more frequently, but the hyperextension injury is potentially more serious. The popliteal artery, the lateral peroneal nerve, and other soft tissues are easily injured when the distal end of the femoral shaft is driven posteriorly into the popliteal fossa during a hyperextension epiphyseal fracture.

Stress radiographs may be required to confirm the diagnosis and treatment must be meticulous to avoid complication. The treatment of these injuries is dictated by the fracture type and the amount of displacement. Failure to obtain adequate alignment or loss of the initial reduction can result in angular deformity or growth disturbance.

Proximal tibial epiphysis fractures

Proximal tibial epiphysis fractures are rare since the insertion sites for the collateral ligaments are distal to the growth plate. This type of injury usually occurs as a result of indirect force, with the most common mechanism of injury being a valgus force that produces a Salter–Harris type II fracture and associated greenstick fracture of the fibula.[57] Complications may include limb-length inequality and angular deformity, but these occur less frequently than with distal femoral injuries because of the smaller contribution of the proximal tibial epiphysis to overall limb growth.

Avulsion fractures

Avulsion fractures are the result of excessive stress on specific structures that are firmly anchored to bone. The mechanism of injury and the direction of the traumatic stress can be determined by examining the resultant joint laxity. Avulsion fractures can be observed in many different sites including the lateral capsule, tibial eminence, tibial tubercle, patella, popliteus tendon, collateral ligaments, biceps tendon, and facia lata.

Lateral capsular ligament avulsion fracture (Segond's fracture)

As described by Woods and colleagues,[58] the fleck of bone chipped off the tibia is posterosuperior to Gerdy's tubercle and represents an avulsion of the meniscotibial portion of the middle one-third of the lateral capsular ligament. The lesion is best seen on a routine anteroposterior radiograph just distal to the articular cortex of the lateral tibial condyle. It can vary in size from a faint fleck to several millimetres and be displaced from the tibial plateau anywhere from 1 to 5 mm.

Recognition of this fracture in a traumatized knee provides substantial evidence of a significant injury to the lateral capsule (Fig. 12). This fracture has a very strong association with a rupture of the anterior cruciate ligament and usually presents with a haemarthrosis. Mensical injuries, both medial and lateral, as well as medial collateral ligament tears are also common.[59]

Anterior tibial eminence fracture

Avulsion of the anterior tibial eminence frequently occurs as an isolated lesion but ligaments, menisci, and other soft tissues can also be damaged. These injuries are seen in both adults and adolescents; however, the lesions are most frequently observed in the 8- to 15-year-old athlete involved in bicycling or skiing. The usual mechanism of injury involves excessive tensile force being applied to the anterior

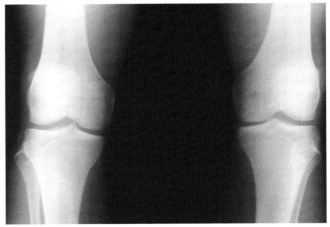

Fig. 12 Anteroposterior radiograph of a Segond's fracture: avulsion of the meniscotibial portion of the middle one-third of lateral capsular ligament. This indicates a severe lateral capsular injury.

cruciate ligament leading to an avulsion of the tibial eminence. Because of the relative joint laxity in children, the femoral condyle may 'knock off' the tibial eminence in some injuries.[60] Meyers and McKeever[61] described a radiographic classification of anterior tibial eminence fractures according to their displacement (Fig. 13).

Anterior tibial eminence fractures should be treated by closed reduction when necessary and immobilization of the knee in extension. Arthroscopy may be utilized to ensure adequate reduction of the fragment. Open or arthroscopic reduction and internal fixation is usually reserved for reduction of a type III fracture. Reduction of these fractures may be prevented by the anterior horn of the medial meniscus or floating of the broken-off fragment. The long-term prognosis of this injury must remain guarded because of persistent laxity of the anterior cruciate ligament.[62]

Fracture of the posterior intercondylar eminence

The posterior intercondylar eminence declines steeply from the tibial spines to the posterior surface of the proximal tibial metaphysis and provides attachment for the posterior cruciate ligament. The

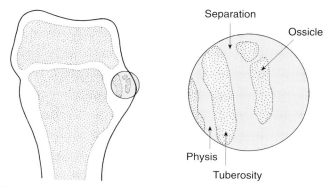

Fig. 14 Ogden–Southwick concept of Osgood–Schlatter's lesion. The primary lesion appears to be an avulsion of ossicles at the insertion of the patellar tendon on the anterior aspect of the developing ossification centre of the tibial tuberosity. This results in callus formation in the intervening area, thus enlarging the anterior portion of the tuberosity. The epiphysis of the tibial tuberosity remains intact.

mechanism of injury involved in a fracture of the posterior intercondylar eminence is forced hyperextension (with a concomitant rupture of the anterior cruciate ligament) or a blow to the anterior proximal end of the tibia. This injury is observed in older adolescents or adults. The patient typically presents with a swollen knee that is painful in flexion and is tender to palpation in the posterior fossa.

The fracture is best visualized by lateral radiography when displacement has taken place. The fracture is best reduced through a posteromedial approach, thereby preserving the medial gastrocnemius head and fixing the broken off fragment with suture, screw, or staple.

The extensor mechanism

The extensor mechanism can fail at multiple locations. Avulsion fractures may occur at the superior pole of the patella, along its medial border, or at the insertion of the patellar ligament on the tibial tuberosity.

Fractures of the tibial tuberosity have been observed in adults but are usually encountered in late adolescence in gymnasts, basketball players, or high jumpers. The injury occurs during a period in which the proximal tibial epiphysis and the secondary ossification centre of the tubercle are undergoing modification. Columnated bone cells are replacing most of the fibrocartilagenous elements making it more susceptible to tensile stress. An avulsion fracture of the tuberosity leaves the germinal cartilage cells exposed on the tubercle.

This situation is completely different from Osgood–Schlatter's disease,[63] which has no epiphyseal involvement. The lesion in Osgood–Schlatter's disease (Fig. 14) is caused by multiple tears at the insertion of the patellar tendon on the most anterior aspect of the tuberosity. On occasion a fragment of bone may be broken off and produce calcification in the midst of the tendon insertion.

It has been hypothesized[64] that Osgood–Schlatter's disease predisposes the athlete to further injury of the extensor mechanism. A few cases have been reported but no firm association has been demonstrated; therefore, patients with Osgood–Schlatter's disease should not to be withheld from athletics.

The mechanism of injury can be forced flexion of the knee against an eccentric quadriceps contraction. Patients present with

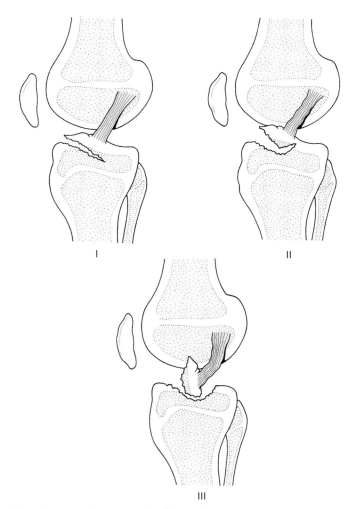

Fig. 13 Meyers and McKeever classification of fractures of the intercondylar eminence of the tibia. Type I, minimal displacement of the broken off fragment. Type II, displacement of the anterior portion of the broken off fragment, producing a beak-like appearance. Type III, complete displacement of the fragment with or without rotation.

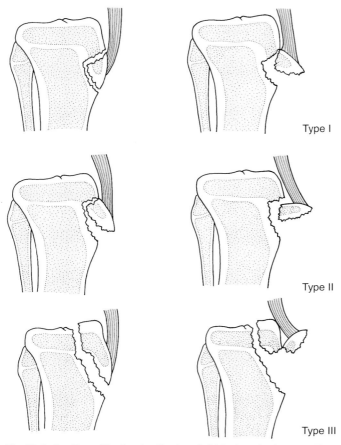

Type I

Type II

Type III

Fig. 15 Ogden–Tross–Murphy classification of tibial tuberosity fractures. Three types of fractures have been described depending on the distance of the fracture from the distal tip of the tubercle. Each type is then divided into two subtypes depending on the severity of displacement and comminution. Type I, the fracture is distal to the normal junction of the ossification centres of the proximal tibia and tuberosity. Type II, the separation occurs anteriorly through the area bridging the ossification centres of the tibial tubercle and the proximal tibial epiphysis. Type III, the separtion extends across the proximal tibial epiphysis into the knee joint.

pain, swelling, and tenderness about the knee. The integrity of the extensor mechanism must be checked. A careful examination of the neurovascular structures must be performed. Radiographic examination including oblique films will allow for proper description of the fracture according to the Ogden–Tross–Murphy classification[64] (Fig. 15).

The Ogden–Tross–Murphy type III injury is a Salter–Harris type III fracture[65] of the proximal tibial epiphysis. Non-displaced fractures should be casted in extension, whereas a displaced fracture requires open reduction and internal fixation (pin, screw, or tension band). Despite the concern of potential growth disturbances, none have been reported in the literature to date. Prominence of the tubercle with local sensitivity and/or patellofemoral pain in the patella alta or baja may occur.

Avulsion of the popliteus tendon

This isolated lesion may be a rare cause of haemarthrosis. The mechanism of injury usually involves a twisting motion that is never well described by the patient. Radiography may reveal a small fragment on the lateral condyle and arthroscopic examination clearly

demonstrates the lesion.[66] The potential benefit of surgical reinsertion of the displaced fragment has yet to be determined.

Avulsion of the collateral ligaments

Although isolated collateral ligament avulsion can occur, more frequently this injury is associated with significant soft tissue trauma. The medial collateral ligament usually breaks off from its proximal attachment. The lateral collateral ligament is pulled off distally usually producing a type I epiphyseal fracture of the proximal fibula. A type III avulsion fracture, in which the fibular styloid is pulled upwards, has also been described. The integrity of the peroneal nerve and anterior tibial artery must be assessed.

Avulsion of the fascia lata

Avulsion of the fascia lata can occur at the level of Gerdy's tubercle. This lesion requires high energy and is usually associated with additional rupturing of other lateral structures. On radiography, the avulsion fragment from Gerdy's tubercle is usually located more anteroinferior than Segond's fracture (Fig. 16).

Osteochondral and chondral fractures

Landells[67] noted that subchondral bone does not develop its structural integrity until skeletal maturity. The adolescent has little calcified cartilage; therefore, tangential forces are directed to the subchondral region, explaining the high incidence of osteochondral fractures in this age group. In adults the articular cartilage tends to tear along the junction of calcified and uncalcified cartilage, which is referred to as the tide mark.[67,68] For this reason, adults are more likely to sustain chondral fractures rather than osteochondral lesions when exposed to similar tangential forces (Fig. 17).

Osteochondral fractures

The majority of osteochondral fractures arise in adolescents. The mechanism of injury usually involves a tangentially directed force that combines both shear and compression. However, the force can be purely compressive in nature as would occur during impaction.[68] The most frequent osteochondral fractures are related to patellar

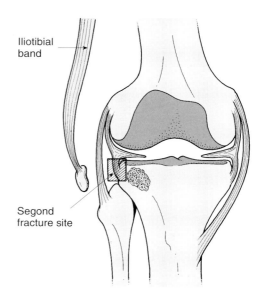

Iliotibial band

Segond fracture site

Fig. 16 Avulsion fracture of the iliotibial band from Gerdy's tubercle. This lesion is usually located more inferiorly and anteriorly than Segond's fracture.

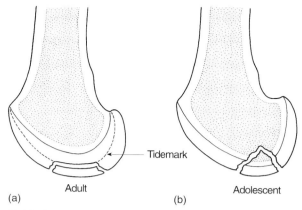

Fig. 17 (a) Adults tend to sustain chondral fractures along the tide mark where the shear forces are dissipated. (b) In adolescents the tangential forces are directed to the subchondral region, explaining the high incidence of osteochondral fractures in this age group.

dislocations. In addition to the patella, most other lesions are located in the lateral [69] condyles.

Clinical presentation is that of an acute injury resulting from a direct blow or twisting motion with the knee in a more or less extended position. Some patients can feel a crack and pain may preclude weight bearing. Swelling occurs within the hour and aspiration of the knee reveals a blood-stained synovial fluid containing fat globules. A displaced fragment may cause locking of the joint.

Radiographs confirm the diagnosis by demonstrating the osteochondral fragment, but several views may be required. The defect may be more difficult to visualize in the early phase. Recently, MRI has allowed a better detection of osteochondral injuries.[70,71] When displaced, surgical treatment is required. Arthroscopy will confirm the diagnosis so that the the location, size, and stability of the lesion can be assessed.

If both cartilagenous and bony portions are intact, reduction and internal fixation should be performed. This could prove to be difficult, if delayed, because of the fibrous tissue formed in the crater. If the bony portion is too small or too fragmented to accommodate an internal fixation, the entire fragment should be excised and the bed debrided. Early rehabilitation should allow a good early result, but long-term prognosis remains unknown.

Chondral fractures

The articular cartilage of the knee is exposed to acute and repetitive trauma from both endogenous and exogenous sources. Chondral fractures represent a failure of the tensile and shock-absorbing capabilities of hyaline cartilage. These lesions can occur in isolation or may be associated with other abnormal mechanics, such as a rupture of the anterior cruciate ligament.

Complete chondral fractures can be stellate craters or present as flaps with a vertical margin.[72,73] Incomplete chondral fractures can form an incomplete flap or a defect not reaching the subchondral bone.[74] Some lesions have an intact surface in which the disruption is of the deep cartilage structure caused by large shear forces. These lesions are both difficult to evaluate and treat. The defects are usually located on the femoral condyles both medially and laterally. They can also be found in the non-meniscal weight-bearing area in extension, as well as more posteriorly in flexion as reported by

Terry[75]. Finally, there has been a report of one case on the lateral tibial plateau.

Most patients are able to recall a specific mechanism of injury involving contact, impaction, or torsion. Others are unable to recall any specific information regarding their injury. Symptoms are usually somewhat non-specific. Pain can be either localized or diffuse. Intermittent pain exacerbated by physical activity is the most common complaint.

Physical examination reveals a picture of mechanical internal derangement, suggestive of a meniscal lesion.[76,77] Signs and symptoms include joint line tenderness, clicking, catching, and sometimes locking. Knee effusion may occur acutely following trauma or be delayed in presentation. Radiographs show no evidence of osseous injury, and arthrography when performed is normal. The diagnosis is frequently delayed and not made prior to surgery. As a result of persistent symptoms or the possibility of a meniscal lesion, the patient finally undergoes an arthroscopic examination.

Terry[75] insists on examining the posterior condyles in deep flexion. In addition to locating and describing the lesion, the rest of the internal structures of the knee should be examined for associated pathology. The following rationale for the treatment of chondral lesions must be kept in mind.

Hyaline cartilage has no capacity for healing. Healing can occur after subchondral bone has been exposed. Injury to the subchondral bone will set up an inflammatory response leading to production of fibrous tissue or fibrocartilage which will never have the qualities of the original hyaline cartilage (endurance, shock-absorbing and gliding properties).

Incomplete lesions will be debrided to avoid abrasion. Complete lesions will be debrided until their margins are stable and adjacent subchondral bone will be slightly abraded or perforated to promote the healing response. The postoperative course is usually longer than after an arthroscopic partial meniscectomy. The prognosis depends on the extent and location of the lesions and any associated pathology. The rehabiliation is lengthy and necessitates enhancing motion and strength.

References

1. Cohn SL, Taylor WC. Vascular problems of the lower extremity in athletes. *Clinics in Sports Medicine* 1990; **9**: 449–70.
2. Kennedy JC. Complete dislocation of the knee joint. *Journal of Bone and Joint Surgery* 1963; **45A**: 889–904.
3. Quinlan AG, Sharrad WJW. Posterolateral dislocation of the knee with capsular interposition. *Journal of Bone and Joint Surgery* 1958; **40A**: 660–3.
4. Green NE, Allen BL. Vascular injuries associated with dislocation of the knee. *Journal of Bone and Joint Surgery* 1977; **59A**: 236–9.
5. Good L, Johnson RJ. The dislocated knee. *Journal of the American Academy of Orthopedic Surgeons* 1995; **3**: 284–92.
6. Rich NM, Spencer FC. Concomitant fractures and nerve trauma. In: *Vascular trauma*. Philadelphia: WB Saunders, 1978: 125–55.
7. DeBakey ME, Simeone FA. Battle injuries of arteries in World War II, an analysis of 2471 cases. *Annals of Surgery* 1946; **123**: 534–79.
8. Cone JB. Vascular injury associated with fracture-dislocations of the lower extremity. *Clinical Orthopaedics and Related Research* 1989; **243**: 30–5.
9. Tornetta, P III. Knee dislocation. In: Levine AM, ed. *Orthopaedic knowledge update: trauma*. Rosemont: American Academy of Orthopedic Surgeons, 1996: 145–52.

10. Crothers OD, Johnson JTH. Isolated acute dislocation of the proximal tibiofibular joint. *Journal of Bone and Joint Surgery* 1973; **55A**: 181–3.

11. Ogden JA. Subluxation and dislocation of the proximal tibiofibular joint. *Journal of Bone and Joint Surgery* 1974; **56A**: 145–54.

12. Parkes JC, Zelko RR. Isolated acute dislocation of the proximal tibiofibular joint. *Journal of Bone and Joint Surgery* 1973; **55A**: 177–80.

13. Safran MR, Fu FH. Uncommon causes of knee pain in the athlete. *Orthopedic Clinics of North America* 1995; **26**: 547–59.

14. Turco VJ, Spinella AJ. Anterolateral dislocation of the head of the fibula in sports. *American Journal of Sports Medicine* 1985; **13**: 209–15.

15. Lyle HHM. Traumatic luxation of the head of the fibula. *Annals of Surgery* 1925; **82**: 635–9.

16. Benazet JP, Saillant G, Cazeneuve JF, Lazennec JY, Roy Camille R. Le traitement chirurgical de l'instabilité chronique de l'articulation peroneo-tibiale supérieure. *Journal de Traumatologie du Sport* 1989; **6**: 97–102.

17. Schenck RC Jr, Goodnight JM. Current concepts review: osteochondritis dissecans. *Journal of Bone and Joint Surgery* 1996; **78A**: 439–56.

18. Rogers WM, Gladstone H. Vascular foramina and arterial supply of the distal end of the femur. *Journal of Bone and Joint Surgery* 1950; **32A**: 867–74.

19. Mubarak SJ, Carroll NC. Juvenile osteochondritis dissecans of the knee. Etiology. *Clinical Orthopaedics and Related Research* 1981; **157**: 200–11.

20. Roy Petrie PW. Aetiology of osteochondritis dissecans. Failure to establish a familial background. *Journal of Bone and Joint Surgery* 1977; **59B**: 366–7.

21. Ribbing S. The hereditary multiple epiphyseal disturbance and its consequences for the aetiogenesis of local malacias—particularly the osteochondrosis dissecans. *Acta Orthopaedica Scandinavica* 1955; **24**: 286–99.

22. Barrie HJ. Osteochondritis dissecans 1887–1987. *Journal of Bone and Joint Surgery* 1987; **69B**: 693–5.

23. Steiner ME, Grana WA. The young athlete's knee: recent advances. *Clinics in Sports Medicine* 1988; **7**: 527–46.

24. Cahill BR. Osetochondritis dissecans of the knee: treatment of juvenile and adult forms. *Journal of the American Academy of Orthopedic Surgeons* 1995; **3**: 237–47.

25. Cahill BR. Treatment of juvenile osteochondritis dissecans and osteochondritis dissecans of the knee. *Clinics in Sports Medicine* 1985; **4**: 367–84.

26. Cahill BR, Phillips MR, Navarro R. The results of conservative management of juvenile osteochondritis dissecans using joint scintigraphy. *American Journal of Sports Medicine* 1989; **17**: 601–6.

27. Chiroff RT, Cook CP. Osteochondritis dissecans. A histologic and microradiographic analysis of surgically excised lesions. *Journal of Trauma* 1975; **15**: 689–96.

28. Guhl JF. Arthroscopic management of osteochondritis dissecans in arthroscopic surgery. In: McGinty JB, ed. *Arthroscopic surgery update*. Rockville: Aspen Systems Corporation, 1985: 63–84.

29. Hughston JC, Hergenroeder PT, Courtenay BG. Osteochondritis dissecans of the femoral condyles. *Journal of Bone and Joint Surgery* 1984; **66A**: 1340–8.

30. Harding WG III. Diagnosis of osteochondritis dissecans of the femoral condyles. The value of the lateral X-ray view. *Clinical Orthopaedics and Related Research* 1983; **123**: 25–6.

31. Linden B. The incidence of osteochondritis dissecans in the condyles of the femur. *Acta Orthopaedica Scandinavica* 1976; **47**: 664–7.

32. Aichroth P. Osteochondritis dissecans of the knee: a clinical survey. *Journal of Bone and Joint Surgery* 1971; **53B**: 440–7.

33. Outerbridge RE. Osteochondritis dissecans of the posterior femoral condyle. *Clinical Orthopaedics and Related Research* 1983; **175**: 121–9.

34. Wilson JN. A diagnostic sign in osteochondritis dissecans of the knee. *Journal of Bone and Joint Surgery* 1967; **49A**: 477–80.

35. Mesgarzadeh M, *et al.* Osteochondritis dissecans: analysis of mechanical stability with radiography, scintigraphy, and MR imaging. *Radiology* 1987; **165**: 775–80.

36. Cahill BR, Berg BC. 99m-Technetium phosphate compound joint scintigraphy in the management of juvenile osteochondritis dissecans of the femoral condyles. *American Journal of Sports Medicine* 1983; **11**: 329–35.

37. Dipaola JD, Nelson DW, Colville MR. Characterizing osteochondral lesions by magnetic resonance imaging. *Arthroscopy* 1991; **7**: 101–4.

38. Bradley J, Dandy DJ. Results of drilling osteochondritis dissecans before skeletal maturity. *Journal of Bone and Joint Surgery* 1989; **71B**: 642–44.

39. Lee CK, Mercurio C. Operative treatment of osteochondritis dissecans *in situ* by retrograde drilling and cancellous bone graft: A preliminary report. *Clinical Orthopaedics and Related Research* 1981; **158**: 129–36.

40. Yamashita F, Sakakida K, Suzu F, Takai S. The transplantation of an autogeneic osteochondral fragment for osteochondritis dissecans of the knee. *Clinical Orthopaedics and Related Research* 1985; **201**: 43–50.

41. Johnson LL, Uitvlugt G, Austin MD, Detrisac DA, Johnson C. Osteochondritis dissecans of the knee. Arthroscopic compression screw fixation. *Arthroscopy* 1990; **6**: 179–89.

42. Gillespie HS, Day B. Bone peg fixation in the treatment of osteochondritis dissecans of the knee joint. *Clinical Orthopaedics and Related Research* 1979; **143**: 125–30.

43. Anderson AF, Lipscomb AB, Coulam C. Antegrade curettement, bone grafting and pinning of osteochondritis dissecans in the skeletally mature knee. *American Journal of Sports Medicine* 1990; **18**: 254–61.

44. Lipscomb PR Jr, Lipscomb PR Sr, Bryan RS. Osteochondritis dissecans of the knee with loose fragments. *Journal of Bone and Joint Surgery* 1978; **60A**: 235–40.

45. Müller ME, Allgöwer M, Schneider R, Willenegger H. *Manual of internal fixation*. 3rd edn. New York: Springer Verlag, 1991.

46. Schatzker J, McBroom R, Bruce D. The tibial plateau fracture: the Toronto experience 1968–1975. *Clinical Orthopaedics and Related Research* 1979; **138**: 94–104.

47. Mast J, Jakob R, Ganz R. *Planning and reduction technique in fracture surgery*. Heidelberg: Springer-Verlag, 1989.

48. Siliski JM, Mahring M, Hofer HP. Supracondylar-intercondylar fractures of the femur. Treatment by internal fixation. *Journal of Bone and Joint Surgery* 1989; **71A**: 95–104.

49. Koval KJ, Helfet DL. Tibial plateau fractures: evaluation and treatment. *Journal of the American Academy of Orthopedic Surgeons* 1995; **3**: 86–94.

50. Delamarter RB, Hohl M, Hopp E Jr. Ligament injuries associated with tibial plateau fractures. *Clinical Orthopaedics and Related Research* 1990; **250**: 226–33.

51. Speer DP, Braun JK. The biomechanical basis of growth plate injuries. *The Physician and Sports Medicine* 1985; **13(7)**: 72–8.

52. Mayer PJ. Lower limb injuries in childhood and adolescence. In: Micheli LJ, ed. *Pediatric and adolescent sports medicine*. Boston: Little Brown, 1984: 80–106.

53. Hresko MT, Kasser JR. Physeal arrest about the knee associated with non-physeal fractures in the lower extremity. *Journal of Bone and Joint Surgery* 1989; **71A**: 698–703.

54. Bertin KC, Goble EM. Ligament injuries associated with physeal fractures about the knee. *Clinical Orthopaedics and Related Research* 1983; **177**: 188–95.

55. Stephens DC, Louis E, Louis DS. Traumatic separation of the

distal femoral epiphyseal cartilage plate. *Journal of Bone and Joint Surgery* 1974; **56A**: 1383–90.

56. Salter RB, Harris WR. Injuries involving the epiphyseal plate. *Journal of Bone and Joint Surgery* 1963; **45A**: 587–622.

57. Edwards PH Jr, Grana WA. Physeal fractures about the knee. *Journal of the American Academy of Orthopaedic Surgeons* 1995; **3**: 63–9.

58. Woods GW, Stanley RF, Tullos HS. Lateral capsular sign: X-ray clue to a significant knee instability. *American Journal of Sports Medicine* 1979; **7**: 27–33.

59. Goldman AB, Pavlov H, Rubinstein D. The segond fracture of the proximal tibia: a small avulsion that reflects major ligamentous damage. *American Journal of Roentgenology* 1988; **151**: 1163–7.

60. Strizak AM, Stoberg AJ. Knee injuries in the skeletally immature athlete. In: Nicholas JA, Hershman EB, eds. *The lower extremity and spine in sports medicine*. St Louis: CV Mosby Company, 1986: 1262–91.

61. Meyers MH, McKeever FM. Fracture of the intercondylar eminence of the tibia. *Journal of Bone and Joint Surgery* 1970; **52A**: 1677–84.

62. Willis RB, Blokker C, Stoll TM, Paterson DC, Galpin RD. Long-term follow-up of anterior tibial eminence fractures. *Journal of Pediatric Orthopedics* 1993; **13**: 361–4.

63. Ogden JA, Southwick WO. Osgood–Schlatter's disease and tibial tuberosity development. *Clinical Orthopaedics and Related Research* 1976; **116**: 180–9.

64. Ogden JA, Tross RB, Murphy MJ. Fractures of the tibial tuberosity in adolescents. *Journal of Bone and Joint Surgery* 1980; **62A**: 205–14.

65. Abrams J, Bennett E, Kumar SJ, Pizzutillo PD. Salter–Harris type III fracture of the proximal fibula. A case report. *American Journal of Sports Medicine* 1986; **14**: 514–16.

66. Gruel JB. Isolated avulsion of the popliteus tendon. *Arthroscopy* 1990; **6**: 94–5.

67. Landells JW. The reactions of injured human articular cartilage. *Journal of Bone and Joint Surgery* 1957; **39B**: 548–62.

68. Kennedy JC, Grainger RW, McGraw RW. Osteochondral fractures of the femoral condyles. *Journal of Bone and Joint Surgery* 1966; **48B**: 436–40.

69. Matthewson MH, Dandy DJ. Osteochondral fractures of the lateral femoral condyle. *Journal of Bone and Joint Surgery* 1978; **60B**: 199–202.

70. Lee JK, Yao L. Occult intraosseous fracture: magnetic resonance appearance versus age of injury. *American Journal of Sports Medicine* 1989; **17**: 620–3.

71. Maywood RM, Jackson DW, Berger P. Athletic injuries to the knee. Evaluation using magnetic resonance imaging. *The Physician and Sports Medicine* 1988; **16(5)**: 81–95.

72. Dzioba RB. The classification and treatment of acute articular cartilage lesions. *Arthroscopy* 1988; **4**: 72–80.

73. Hubbard MJS. Arhroscopic surgery for chondral flaps in the knee. *Journal of Bone and Joint Surgery* 1987; **69B**: 794–6.

74. Johnson-Nurse C, Dandy DJ. Fracture-separation of articular cartilage in the adult knee. *Journal of Bone and Joint Surgery* 1985; **67B**: 42–3.

75. Terry GC, Flandry F, Van Manen JW, Norwood LA. Isolated chondral fractures of the knee. *Clinical Orthopaedics and Related Research* 1988; **234**: 170–7.

76. Gerard Y, Segal P, Henry C. Lesions traumatiques cartilogineuses pures du condyle interne du genou en pratique sportive. *Revue de Chirurgie Orthopedique et Reparatrice de l'Appareil Moteur* 1976; **62**: 245–52.

77. Hopkinson WJ, Mitchell WA, Curl WW. Chondral fractures of the knee. Cause for confusion. *American Journal of Sports Medicine* 1985; **13**: 309–12.

4.3 The shoulder

4.3.1 Introduction

William D. Stanish

Historically, disorders of the shoulder joint were extremely difficult to diagnose and manage. It was always difficult to differentiate, for example, a lesion of the rotator cuff from other sources of shoulder pain such as glenohumeral instability. For example, a young competitive swimmer, would present with signs and symptoms of classical rotator cuff impingement of the shoulder. Frequently, the medical problem was recalcitrant to a conservative non-surgical format of treatment. However, upon more extensive evaluation it would become apparent that the patient was manifesting rotator cuff irritability and tendinitis as a consequence of shoulder instability. Often this shoulder instability was of the multidirectional variety which in most academic circles was regarded as best managed without surgery.

Contemporary radiographic techniques have expanded our understanding of these disorders. The judicious use of shoulder arthroscopy, coupled with CT scanning and MRI, have defined shoulder diseases more precisely. Arthroscopic surgery of the shoulder has fostered major advances in the management of disorders of the shoulder. Arthroscopic surgery of the shoulder has provided an important diagnostic and therapeutic tool which closely parallels the impact of the arthroscope in dealing with disorders of the knee.

Lesions of the superior glenoid labrum have been defined as a direct byproduct of arthroscopy. Information from the skilled arthroscopist has allowed us to gain a more thorough understanding of shoulder biomechanics in health and disease. Injuries to the glenoid labrum may occur as a consequence of an acute traumatic event or may indeed be produced in chronic overuse, for instance with repetitive overhead movements such as those used in baseball, cricket, and javelin. When unresponsive to a non-surgical (conservative) programme of treatment, many of these labral tears can be managed successfully with arthroscopic debridement or, in some situations, with transarthroscopic stabilizations.

Arthroscopic evaluation of the shoulder also affords vital information regarding concomitant pathology of the shoulder such as osteoarthrosis, which is frequently underestimated on the plain radiograph. Furthermore, ailments of the rotator cuff can frequently be determined by arthroscopy. The superior surface is best viewed through the subacromial space and the inferior surface of the cuff can be evaluated from the shoulder portal.

These arthroscopic avenues have provided successful techniques for surgical decompression of the rotator cuff, avoiding the traditional open acromioplasty. Furthermore, the patient suffering with unidirectional shoulder instability may opt for the closed arthroscopic surgical technique. Controversy still surrounds the use of the shoulder scope in these situations (versus traditional techniques); however, it is undeniable that in the future the efficacy of minimally invasive surgery will be acknowledged. With current techniques, the physician is able to achieve a more thorough understanding of the pathomechanics related to disorders of the shoulder. Faced with this improved 'vision' employing MR and CT scanning, the practitioner is able to improve upon the success of a surgical or non-surgical treatment.

MRI evaluation of the rotator cuff is particularly promising. Historically, a complete tear of the rotator cuff was best evaluated using the shoulder arthrogram. This technique remains the gold standard in terms of its specificity and sensitivity. However, ultrasonography and MRI have been deployed to delineate the more difficult clinical problem, which is the partial rotator cuff disruption. Certainly MRI will continue to advance our understanding of soft tissue injuries in and about the shoulder.

CT scanning has continued to enhance our understanding of shoulder pathology, particularly of complex fractures. Four-part fractures of the proximal humerus, and injuries to the bony glenoid face, as well as seemingly trivial fractures of the tuberosities are best evaluated with CT. Plain radiographs frequently underestimate the gravity and complexity of these lesions.

Treatment of instability of the shoulder joint, including frank dislocations and mild subluxations, is one example that has undergone rapid improvement in technique. Practitioners in ancient times had no difficulty in diagnosing an overt shoulder dislocation. In the Greek literature, between BC 450 and AD 100, physicians recognized that shoulder instability; i.e., dislocations, were related to joint laxity. The treatment regimen used would include cauterizing the axillary tissues with a hot iron, thus fibrosing the adjacent fat and fibrous tissues. Hippocrates stated in his explanation of the surgical technique that careful attention to detail must be taken in order to avoid major vessels. Obviously, inherent scarring with this technique would produce a contracture, decreasing the intracapsular volume and thus thwarting the possibility of recurrent dislocations. This form of treatment has been modified through time - thank goodness. The basic premise of these 'primitive techniques' was to decrease the available capsular volume, coupled with a programme of postoperative immobilization. Contemporary treatment for shoulder instability is directed towards obtaining the same goals dictated by the ancient Greeks. The objective was, and is, to decrease the intracapsular volume through a precise inferior capsular shift thus providing a soft tissue buttress in order to stabilize the joint. In the future, laser cautery of the inferior capsular, after trans-arthroscopic plication of the capsule, can be envisaged.

Dislocations of the shoulder joint, which are a very common result of athletic injuries, can also be treated by non-surgical means. After an acute dislocation, some methods have relied on mechanical devices for providing traction and abduction to the upper extremity to reduce the dislocated joint. Other methods were strictly manipulative. Hippocrates described a method resembling a current technique. The classical Hippocratic method would have the patient stand upright, with the axilla resting on a horizontal beam. Traction was applied to the arm by the practitioner, while countertraction was supplied by the patient's body or by an assistant. These techniques for closed reduction of the shoulder are illustrated in wall paintings from the tomb of Ramses II (BC 1200). The Ancient Egyptians actually reduced shoulders which were dislocated, using the Kocher technique.

Open surgical techniques, as mentioned previously, have advanced since the Hippocratic technique of cautery. In 1894 Ricord described the open surgical method for capsular repair. A wide variety of surgical techniques were described in the early part of this century, all purporting to have a better solution for the problem of shoulder instability. These techniques included the Clairmont ligamentous sling for suspension, the Bankart glenoid labrum repair, the Nicola tenodesis of the head of the biceps, the Magnuson and Stack subscapular transfer, Putti-Platt subscapularis suturing, DuToit staple capsulorrhaphy, the coracoid transfer described by Bristow, and more current procedures described by Charles Neer and others. Recent literature has supported arthroscopic stabilization employing either a bone anchor technique, biodegradable tacks, or a cinching with posterior sutures.

The unfortunate athlete presenting with an obvious anterior - unidirectional - shoulder dislocation, acute or chronic, is an apparently simple problem. However, on closer inspection this clinical problem may be more complicated. For example, following the first shoulder dislocation there is no consensus in terms of the appropriate management. Currently, there is a school of thought that suggests early surgery for the first time dislocator (with an obvious Bankart lesion) provides improved results. More conservative caregivers suggest a period of immobilization after the first time dislocation; however, this approach is more steeped in tradition than science. Are there sufficient scientific data to suggest that early surgical stabilization is the ideal treatment for the first time dislocator?

Compelling also is the intriguing issue of the athlete with multidirectional shoulder instability. Usually youthful and with enhanced physiological joint laxity, this patient does very unpredictably with surgical treatment. Thorough analysis of the type and degree of shoulder dysfunction is vital to the successful treatment programme for this individual. For each and every athlete that demonstrates recurrent frank dislocation of the shoulder, there exists a comparable cohort of individuals who suffer with recurrent subluxation of the shoulder without obvious complete dislocations. These patients, unfortunately, behave in a similar fashion to the dislocator inasmuch as the altered joint biomechanics and pathology are identical. Understandably, they too respond rather poorly to a programme of bracing and strengthening and often need surgery.

The work of Codman in 1911 provided major advances in our understanding of shoulder disease. Codman described a rupture of the rotator cuff which, at that point, was an undiscovered clinical entity. Smith, in 1934, observed defects in the supraspinatus tendon, although the frequency and significance of this problem was not appreciated. It was the work of Codman and others that clarified the diagnosis, pathology, and treatment of injuries to the rotator cuff, and to this day few changes to these original observations are needed, although there are refinements in diagnoses and operative techniques. The work of Charles Neer and others over the past decade has refined our understanding of the rotator cuff in health and disease.

The integrated components of the shoulder work with profound precision producing a joint that demonstrates a remarkable range of motion but with stability and power. However, when any component of this linkage fails, such as occurs with a significant disruption of the supraspinatus tendon, deterioration of function rapidly follows. Most experts foster the approach of rapid surgical repair for such a lesion, rather than prolonged and possibly futile physiotherapy. However, dealing with more chronic rotator cuff tendonosis is quite another issue. If, indeed, the rotator cuff is being abraded by an overhanging subacromial spur, then the obvious solution is surgically to remove the spur to alleviate the impingement. The option of open surgery versus arthroscopic decompression exists, and each technique has its advocates. Tendon degeneration may reveal itself in the throwing athlete after years of cricket, baseball, or tennis. Tendonosis, with only a limited chance of healing remains a dilemma in sports medicine.

Since the original reports of Codman, various methods of rotator cuff repair have been devised. Mayer recommended a fascia repair for larger rotator cuff disruptions. Bosworth recommended transplantation of the infraspinatus and supraspinatus into a more proximal defect in the greater tuberosity. Mclaughlin excised the non-viable rotator cuff edges and inserted the healthy edge into a raw bed of bone. Before the work of Neer, complete acromioplasty to decrease the rotator cuff was conducted but this has been superseded by the more contemporary procedure, which includes a partial resection of the acromion to relieve classical impingement. The use of partial acromioplasty in the individual with a large rotator cuff defect offers spurious results. Contemporary literature suggests that meticulous surgery must be employed to repair rotator cuff defects without tension. Arthroscopic debridement, used alone in the individual with a massive cuff tear, does provide some pain relief but does not enhance function.

Advances in our understanding of the shoulder joint in athletics have derived from a greater understanding of biomechanics and more precise imaging techniques. Injuries of overuse and pathology from high velocity forces are usually elucidated with a precise physical examination, augmented with CT and/or MR scanning. The chapters that follow detail the understanding and treatment of shoulder disorders, whether a product of overuse or a single episode of trauma.

Further reading

1. Corpus Hippocrates, In Bick EM. *History and source book of orthopaedic surgery.* New York: Hospital for Joint Diseases, 1933: 13.
2. Brockbank W, Griffiths D. Orthopaedic surgery in the sixteenth and seventeenth centuries. I. Luxations of the shoulder. *Journal of Bone and Joint Surgery*, 1948; **30**: 365.

3. Hussein MK. Kocher's method is 3000 years old. *Journal of Bone and Joint Surgery*, 1968; **50-B**: 669.

4. Ricord: traitement des luxations recidivantes de l'epaule par la suture de la capsule articulaire ou arthrorraphie. *Gazette des Hôpitaux* 1894:49. In: Bick EM. *History and source book of orthopaedic surgery*. New York: Hospital for Joint Diseases, 1933: 179.

5. Clairmont P, Ehrlich H. Ein neues operations-verfahren zur behandlung der habituellen schuterluxation mittels muskelphastick. *Archiv für Klinische Chirurgie*, 1909; **89**: 798.

6. Bankart AB. The pathology and treatment of recurrent dislocation of the shoulder joint. *British Journal of Surgery*, 1938; **26**:23.

7. Nicola J. Recurrent anterior dislocation of the shoulder. A new operation. *Journal of Bone and Joint Surgery*, 1929; **11**: 128.

8. Magnuson PB, Stack JK. Recurrent dislocation of the shoulder. *Journal of the American Medical Association*, 1943; **123**: 889.

9. Osmond-Clarke H. Habitual dislocation of the shoulder. The Putti-Platt operation. *Journal of Bone and Joint Surgery*, 1948; **30-B**: 19.

10. DuToit GT, Roux D. Recurrent dislocation of the shoulder. *Journal of Bone and Joint Surgery*, 1956; **38-A**: 1.

11. Helfet J. Coracoid transplantation for recurring dislocation of the shoulder. The W. Rowley Bristow operation. *Journal of Bone and Joint Surgery*, 1958; **40-B**: 198.

12. Neer CS. Anterior acromioplasty for the chronic impingement syndrome in the shoulder. A preliminary report. *Journal of Bone and Joint Surgery*, 1972; **54A**: 41–50.

13. Codman EA. Complete rupture of the supraspinatus tendon. Operative treatment with report of two successful cases. *Boston Medical and Surgical Journal*, 1911; **164**: 7087.

14. Smith JG. Pathological appearances of seven cases of injury of the shoulder joint with remarks. *London Medical Gazette*, 1834; **14**: 280; (reported in *American Journal of Medical Science*, 1834; **16**: 219–24.)

15. Mayer L. Rupture of the supraspinatus tendon. *Journal of Bone and Joint Surgery*, 1937; **19**: 640–2.

16. Bosworth DM. The supraspinatus syndrome. Symptomatology, pathology, and repair. *Journal of the American Medical Association*, 1941;**117**: 422–38.

17. Mclaughlin HL. Rupture of the rotator cuff. *Journal of Bone and Joint Surgery*, 1962; **44A**: 979–83.

18. Armstrong JR. Excision of the acromion in the treatment of the supraspinatus syndrome. *Journal of Bone and Joint Surgery*, 1949; **31B**: 436–42.

19. Stanish WD, Curwin S. *Tendinitis: its etiology and treatment.*, Lexington, MA: Collamore Press, D.C. Heath and Company, 1984.

20. Riley GP, Harrall RL, Constant CR. Tendon degeneration and chronic shoulder pain: changes in the collagen composition of the human rotator cuff tendons in rotator cuff tendinitis. *Annals of Rheumatic Diseases*, 1994; **53**: 359–66.

21. Paavolainen P, Ahovuo J. Ultrasonography and arthrography in the diagnosis of tears of the rotator cuff. *Journal of Bone and Joint Surgery*, 1994; **76A**: 335–40.

22. Ciero RA, Wheeler JH, Ryan JB, McBride JT. Arthroscopic Bankart repair vs non-operative treatment for acute initial anterior shoulder dislocations. *American Journal of Sports Medicine*, 1994; **22**: 589–94.

23. Montgomery TJ, Yerger B, Savoie FH. Management of rotator cuff tears: a comparison of arthroscopic debridement and surgical repair. *Journal of Shoulder and Elbow Surgery*, 1994; **3**: 70–8.

24. Zvijac JE, Levy HJ, Lemak LJ. Arthroscopic subacromial decompression in the treatment of full thickness rotator cuff tears: a 3-6 year follow-up. *Arthroscopy*, 1994; **10**: 518–23.

25. Lazarus MD, Chansky HA, Misra S, *et al.* Comparison of open and arthroscopic subacromial decompression. *Journal of Shoulder and Elbow Surgery*, 1994; **3**: 1–11.

26. Esser RD. Open reduction and Internal fixation of three and four part fractures of the proximal humerus. *Clinical Orthopaedics*, 1994; **299**: 244–51.

27. deLatt EAT, Visser CPJ, Coene LNJEM, *et al.* Nerve lesions in primary shoulder dislocations and humeral neck fractures: a prospective clinical and EMG study. *Journal of Bone and Joint Surgery*, 1994; **76B**: 381–833.

28. Itoi E, Newman SR, Kuechle DK, *et al.* Dynamic anterior stabilizers of the shoulder with the arm in abduction. *Journal of Bone and Joint Surgery*, 1994; **76B**: 834–6.

29. Gazielly DF, Gleyze P, Montagnom C. Functional and anatomical results after rotator cuff repair. *Clinical Orthopaedics*, 1994; **304**: 43–53.

30. Matsen FA, Arntz CT. Subacromial impingement. In: Rockwood CA, Matsen FA. *The shoulder*. Philadelphia: W.B. Saunders, 1990; Vol. 2: 623–36.

31. Lippitt SB, Matsen FA. Mechanisms of glenohumeral joint stability. *Clinical Orthopaedics*, 1993; **291**: 20–8.

4.3.2 Glenohumeral instability

R. Mitchell Rubinovich

Introduction

The glenohumeral joint is a mixed blessing. On the one hand it has a greater range of movement than any other joint in the human body. On the other, it is more susceptible to dislocation and recurrent instability than any other articulation. This chapter will deal with the problem of shoulder instability in the acute and subsequent forms. Other common problems of the shoulder such as rotator cuff tears or lesions of the acromioclavicular joint, except in those situations where the lesions coexist with shoulder instability, will be considered in other chapters.

The population dealt with in this chapter encompasses all ages. It is not unusual in any sports medicine clinic to see patients in their sixties and seventies. Furthermore, as the interest in physical fitness continues to grow, such individuals will account for a greater percentage of sports injuries.

Historical perspective

Interest in dislocation about the shoulder dates back to antiquity. The Edwin Smith Papyrus describes the treatment of a dislocation in an epileptic patient.[1] A drawing in the tomb of Upuy (1200 BC) depicts what would seem to be the earliest recorded use of the Kocher method of reduction.[2] Hippocratic texts from 400 BC describe not only the diagnosis and treatment of acute dislocations but also the problem of recurrent dislocation and its treatment. Indeed, only in the past few hundred years has the Hippocratic technique of scarring the inferior joint capsule with a hot poker been supplanted by less dramatic methods. Textbooks on medicine from the sixteenth and seventeenth century detail many elaborate contraptions used to reduce a dislocated shoulder, some of which bear an uncanny resemblance to devices used during the Spanish Inquisition (Fig. 1).[3] All this rich history has prompted Rockwood to say that 'nothing is new' regarding this problem. Nevertheless, an attempt will be made to describe some of the newer material.

were seen in 7.4 per cent of patients, with 2.8 per cent involving the axillary nerve. While vascular damage is always mentioned as a complication of shoulder dislocation, it appears to be exceedingly rare. In a 5-year period accounting for 216 dislocations, only one patient, an 85-year-old female with multiple injuries, suffered an injury to the axillary artery.[5] Injuries to the rotator cuff may occur, particularly in the older population. One study quotes an incidence of 57 per cent, documented by arthrography, in middle-aged and elderly patients.[7]

Anatomy and physiology

The shoulder joint, and its cousin the hip, are ball-and-socket joints. The socket of the hip is the acetabulum. Its configuration allows almost complete coverage of the head of the femur, giving the hip enormous stability. The cost of this stability is a very limited range of movement. However, the shoulder has a very shallow socket. The glenoid covers only 25 per cent of the humeral articular surface. This allows a wide range of motion, but sacrifices stability.

The shoulder's stability derives, for the most part, from soft-tissue extensions and reinforcements. These can be roughly divided into static and dynamic stabilizers. The static group includes the labrum, the glenohumeral ligaments, and the joint capsule. Dynamic stabilizers include a superficial layer of muscles, the deltoid and teres major, and the more important deep layer, consisting of the subscapularis, supraspinatus, infraspinatus, and teres minor muscle tendon units.

In the normal scapula the glenoid has a forward inclination of between 2 degrees and 12 degrees. The scapula itself is rotated forward through 45 degrees, thereby giving an overall anterior inclin-

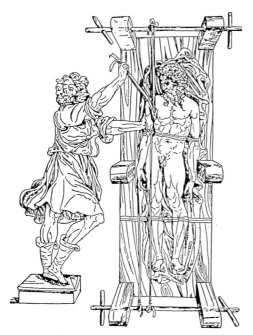

Fig. 1 Using the rack to reduce a dislocated shoulder. (Reproduced from ref. 3, with permission.)

Classification

There are almost as many published classifications of shoulder instability as there are methods of treating the problem. A good classification should possess a rationale in addition to being an encyclopaedic listing of the problem. Current classifications are based on initial presentation pattern, degree of initial trauma, or suspected underlying pathoanatomy. The classification presented here is based on the direction of instability (Table 1). It has the advantage of being easy to remember, so that when faced with a clinical situation the clinician can mentally review all the possibilities and proceed appropriately. Although it may appear to leave out certain situations (for example, posterior voluntary dislocation), these omissions will be explained in subsequent sections.

Epidemiology

The shoulder is the most commonly dislocated joint in the human body. Two prospective epidemiological studies have been conducted, one in Sweden[4] and the other in the United States of America.[5] The findings were remarkably similar. The overall incidence of dislocations is between 12 and 17 per cent per 100 000 per year. When only primary dislocations were included, the rates were almost equal at 11.3 and 12.3 per 100 000 per year. Rowe[6] has pointed out that there are equal numbers of dislocations before and after the age of 45, but there is a distinct bimodal pattern to the distribution with a first peak in the third decade and a second peak between the ages of 60 and 80. The early peak is associated with sports-related injuries. The second peak is in the geriatric population and is related to falls in the home. Anterior dislocations are by far the most common, accounting for 97.2 per cent of all dislocations. Posterior dislocations accounted for 2.8 per cent.[5] It is presumed that the rarer forms of dislocation, such as luxatio erecta, were not seen because of the small sample size. Neurological lesions

Table 1 Classification of glenohumeral instability

I   ANTERIOR
   Acute
      Dislocation
      Subluxation
      Labral instability
   Recurrent
      Subluxation
      Dislocation
   Chronic
   Voluntary or habitual

II POSTERIOR
   Acute
      Subluxation
      Dislocation
   Recurrent
      Subluxation
      Dislocation
   Chronic

III INFERIOR
   Luxatio erecta
   Subluxation
      Traumatic
      Atraumatic

IV MULTIDIRECTIONAL

ation to the glenohumeral joint.[8] This gives the shoulder significantly greater stability posteriorly than anteriorly. The glenoid labrum is attached circumferentially to the glenoid. It deepens the glenoid cavity and allows attachment of the glenohumeral ligaments and the long head of the biceps. It is more developed anteriorly and thus contributes more to anterior than to posterior stability.[9]

There are three glenohumeral ligaments. The superior and middle glenohumeral ligaments are most involved in stability with the arm at 0 degrees to 90 degrees of abduction.[10] The inferior glenohumeral ligament originates from the anteroinferior, inferior, and posteroinferior rim of the glenoid labrum. This ligament is the most important static stabilizer of the shoulder.[11] In selective cutting experiments in cadavers, the shoulder could not be dislocated until the entire inferior glenohumeral ligament was incised including its posterior attachment.[8]

The deltoid and supraspinatus work in concert to inhibit inferior movement of the humeral head. The subscapularis acts to rotate the humeral head inwards and thereby resist anterior subluxation. It is of note that with the shoulder abducted and externally rotated (a position of inherent instability), the tendon of the subscapulis rotates superiorly so that it can no longer function (actively or passively) to resist minor subluxation.[8]

Shoulder stability is also enhanced by two mechanical properties. These are the vacuum[12] and concavity-compression effects.[13] The vacuum effect can best be appreciated by thinking of a plunger in a syringe. With the syringe tightly capped it is impossible to withdraw the plunger. Once the syringe is uncapped or vented, the plunger moves easily. The normal shoulder has less than 1 cm^3 of free fluid. The intra-articular pressure is slightly negative. Without free fluid to fill the gaps, attempted displacement of the humeral head increases the negative intra-articular pressure thereby increasing stability. This effect can be demonstrated by inferiorly subluxating a lax shoulder. The soft tissue in the subacromial area is sucked inwards, creating the so-called Sulcus sign (see the section on Multidirectional instability). Furthermore, various authors have demonstrated the increased laxity of the shoulder created by allowing air into the glenohumeral space.[12] This has significance when assessing a joint arthroscopically for instability.[14] Joint effusions and unsealed capsular defects can negate the vacuum effect. This helps us to understand post-traumatic inferior subluxation (see the section on Inferior instability).

To understand concavity-compression, think of a ball rolling on a table-top. Pressure on the ball will do little to resist its sliding along the flat surface. If, however, the ball lies in a concavity or hollow, displacement will be resisted by both the depth of the concavity and the force pushing the ball into the concavity. Erosion of bone or labral tears decrease the depth of the glenoid concavity. Similarly, weakness of shoulder musculature will decrease the compression of the humeral head into the glenoid. Glenohumeral instability will be increased by either.

Orthopaedic literature is filled with speculation as to the 'essential' pathological lesion in shoulder instability. The first mention of this concept was by Bankart in 1938, when he described the lesion that still bears his name.[15] This lesion is essentially an avulsion of the anterior glenoid labrum and its attached glenohumeral ligaments. The capsule and ligaments can now strip off the anterior neck of the glenoid, forming a pouch into which the humeral head

can recurrently dislocate. The labrum develops as a separate structure embryologically, which would explain why it is possible to tear the anterior capsule through a plane between the glenoid and labrum.[16] Alternatively, the head can dislocate anterior to the labrum through the capsule and glenohumeral ligaments, which would result in stretching of the anterior capsule. This redundant tissue would then allow for recurrent dislocations on the basis of incompetent ligamentous restraints. Whether the head is going anterior or posterior to the labrum is not really that important. Recognizing the incompetence of the anterior static stabilizers of the shoulder is much more to the point.

Once the anterior capsule has failed, several bony changes may take place secondarily. These are important to recognize for the following reasons: first, in difficult diagnostic situations they may be important clues as to the existence of instability and its predominant direction; second, the erosion of bone on the humerus or glenoid may compound the problem of an already unstable joint.

There are two important radiological signs of anterior instability. The Hill–Sachs lesion was described in 1940.[17] This is a posterior impaction fracture of the humeral head caused by impingement on the anterior glenoid rim. It can be found in almost all cases of recurrent anterior dislocations if it is sought with appropriate radiological views (see the section on Diagnosis).[18] When large, a Hill–Sachs lesion may articulate with the glenoid in the abducted externally rotated position and contribute to recurrent episodes of instability. Injury to the anterior glenoid can occur by avulsion or erosion. In an anterior dislocation with a Bankart lesion, bone may be pulled off with the labrum. This may involve only small flakes of bone, or alternatively significant portions of the articular surface. Recurrent instability may cause the formation of bony deposits anterior to the glenoid, marking areas of injury and bleeding.

The glenoid may also be eroded by recurrent episodes of instability. Each time the head slides forward over the rim the bone is progressively scuffed. This may lead to alarming amounts of bone loss in long-standing recurrent cases, occasionally requiring bone grafting to restore sufficient bony stability.

Lesions to posterior shoulder anatomy are much less well defined. Reverse Bankart lesions are not common. The static ligamentous stabilizers are less important and the muscular support is less developed than anteriorly. The common thread in most cases of posterior recurrent instability is a redundant posterior capsule.[9]

One bony lesion should be mentioned here. McLaughlin[19] has described a second form of impaction fracture seen anteriorly. This usually occurs in posterior dislocations either acutely or in cases of persistent posterior dislocations which are commonly missed. Like the Hill–Sachs lesion it may also contribute to instability by articulating with the glenoid.

Diagnostic tests

Diagnostic tests are divided into radiological and invasive procedures, with the latter including examination under anaesthesia and diagnostic arthroscopy.

Radiographic tests

The standard trauma series for the shoulder should include a true anteroposterior view, a trans-scapular lateral view (Neer's), and an axillary view of the shoulder.[20] When all three views are obtained

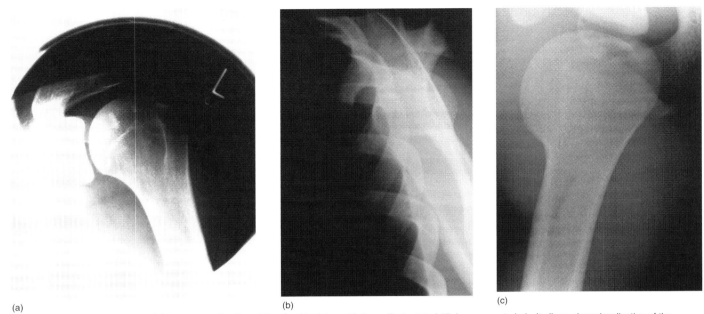

(a)　(b)　(c)

Fig. 2 The trauma series. (a) Anteroposterior view of the shoulder taken with the patient rotated 45 degrees posteriorly. It allows clear visualization of the joint space and the relationship between the humeral head and the glenoid. (b) The trans-scapular lateral (Neer's) view. The acromion, coracoid process, and body of the scapula are clearly seen. The glenoid fossa, while not actually visualized, is at the junction of the Y formed by the three bony elements. The humeral head lies directly over the junction. (c) The axillary view. Again, the acromion and coracoid process are clearly seen. The glenoid articular surface can also be seen, as can its relationship to the humeral head. The three views together constitute a full trauma series and all should be obtained routinely.

and interpreted correctly, it is unlikely that any significant pathology will be missed.

The anteroposterior view of the shoulder should be made at 90 degrees to the surface of the glenoid (Fig. 2(a)–(c)). Because the scapula is rotated forward 35 to 40 degrees, it is necessary to rotate the patient's affected side posteriorly to match this inclination. A small amount of inferior angulation will also help to clear the clavicle and allow better visualization. Attention should be paid to the greater tuberosity as 10 per cent of all anterior dislocations will have an associated fracture to this structure.[16]

The trans-scapular view was described by Neer (Fig. 3).[21] This can be obtained with the patient sitting or supine and does not require the arm to be moved or removed from a sling. The patient is rotated 45 degrees forward on the affected side. The cassette is placed anterior to the shoulder and the X-ray beam is projected along the body from posterior to anterior. The view obtained will show the coracoid and acromion processes, marking the anterior and posterior aspects of the shoulder, respectively. The body of the scapula is projected as a vertical line inferior to the junction of the coracoid and the acromion. Although not actually seen in this view, the glenoid fossa is situated at the junction of this Y (Fig. 4). The humeral head should be superimposed over the Y junction in the glenoid fossa. While clearly showing instances of anterior dislocation, this view may be quite misleading if the humeral head is posteriorly dislocated. This demonstrates the necessity of the third component of the trauma series, the axillary view.

The axillary view is often omitted because it is believed that it is too painful to perform in the trauma situation. This is not true. The patient is placed supine and the shoulder is abducted only far enough to position the X-ray tube between the hip and the arm. This is often only 20 to 30 degrees (Fig. 5). The arm can be sup-

ported on a table or by an intravenous pole placed beside the patient. The cassette is placed above the acromion and the film exposed. This view is essential to verify the true position of the humeral head and must not be deleted.

Further views of the shoulder are useful in patients suspected of having recurrent instability.

The anteroposterior view of the shoulder in full internal rotation may reveal the presence of a Hill–Sachs lesion evident as a depres-

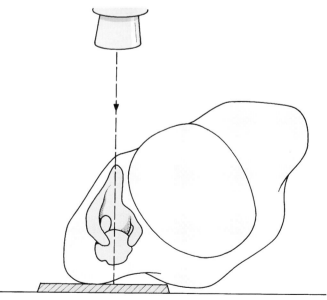

Fig. 3 The trans-scapular lateral view. The X-ray beam passes along the axis of the body of the scapula.

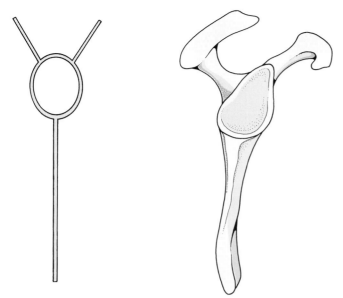

Fig. 4 The scapula as seen on the trans-scapular (Neer's) view. The coracoid process, acromion, and body of the scapula intersect at the glenoid fossa forming a Y junction. While the glenoid cannot be seen on this view, its position will be known from the other three bony landmarks.

sion or linear density at the superolateral margin of the humeral head.

The Stryker notch view is an even more sensitive technique for picking up Hill–Sachs defects. The patient lies supine with the arm forward flexed 100 degrees. The elbow may be flexed and the hand placed beside the patient's head to help position the arm. The X-ray tube is then angled 45 degrees cephalad (Fig. 6(b)). The lesion will be demonstrated as a circular bite laterally on the humeral head adjacent to the articular surface. In cases of recurrent anterior dislocation this view will show a Hill–Sachs lesion in more than 90 per cent of patients.[18] It is therefore very useful where the diagnosis is unclear. A similar view, the craniocaudal, can be taken with the arm at the patient's side. The patient is supine in the anatomical position

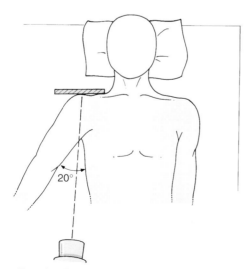

Fig. 5 The axillary view. The arm only needs to be abducted 20 degrees to obtain an adequate view.

and the tube is angled 45 degrees caudal (Fig. 6(c)). While this view has the advantage of not having to move the patient's arm, it is slightly less sensitive to the presence of Hill–Sachs lesions.[18]

The West Point prone axillary view gives the best detail of the anterior glenoid. The patient is placed prone with the arm abducted and the elbow flexed over the edge of a supporting table. The X-ray beam is directed from inferior to superior through the axilla and angled 25 degrees anteriorly from the horizontal (Fig. 6(a)). This gives excellent detail of the anterior glenoid rim. Lesions in this area will be present in 10 per cent of patients with anterior instability.[16] The lesion may vary from small flake fractures and bony deposits (the so-called bony Bankart lesion) to true fractures of the anterior glenoid.

If a diagnosis is still in doubt, various stress films can be taken in the hope of catching the humeral head in a subluxated position. Posterior instability can often be difficult to identify. The cephalo-scapular projection can be useful in this situation. The patient flexes forward 45 degrees at the waist and rests the elbow on a table in front of him or her (Fig. 6(d)). Leaning on the elbow exerts posterior pressure on the humeral head, subluxating it over the posterior glenoid rim. The X-ray beam is projected horizontal to the floor. This view allows clear visualization of the humeral head while displacing the shadows of the acromion and coracoid processes. The clavicle still overlaps the joint, but is usually quite radiolucent and only partially visible.[22]

Another stress view is the Stripp axial.[23] The patient sits on a stool, with their back against a solid object, allowing him or her to lean posteriorly. The arm is forward flexed about 40 degrees and the X-ray cassette is placed superior to the shoulder joint (Fig. 6(e)). An angled foam sponge may be used here to help keep the cassette level to the ground. The X-ray beam is then projected upwards parallel to the vertical. Since the patient is leaning backwards, the beam is able to clear the hip and buttocks. This angle generates a clear view of the relationship between the humeral head and the glenoid. This view can be employed as a stress film for patients who feel that they can reproduce their instability by actively contracting their muscle or by passively pushing on the humeral head.

Arthrography of the shoulder is of some academic interest in unstable shoulders, but its use as a diagnostic tool is limited. The normal volume of the intact glenohumeral joint is 15 to 18 cm^3.[16] Low-volume shoulders are associated with contracture of the capsule, as seen in conditions such as adhesive capsulitis. A volume in excess of 20 cm^3 is associated with paralytic conditions of the shoulder (as in syringomyelia) and with recurrent shoulder instability. This fact in itself would not make arthrography meaningful. However, up to 30 per cent of acute dislocations can be shown to have ruptures of the rotator cuff.[16] This percentage climbs significantly when only patients over 50 years of age are considered. While most of these ruptures heal spontaneously (or at least are not clinically significant), suggestions are that any patient over the age of 40 who does not progress after reduction should have an early arthrogram (preferably within 4 weeks) to identify lesions of the rotator cuff.[24]

While plain arthrography is of limited use in shoulder instability, arthrotomography can be very helpful. Here, a small amount of dye is injected into the shoulder, followed by 10 cm^3 of room air. Tomographic cuts of the glenoid are then carried out in a modified axillary projection.[25] The resulting radiograph shows the profiled

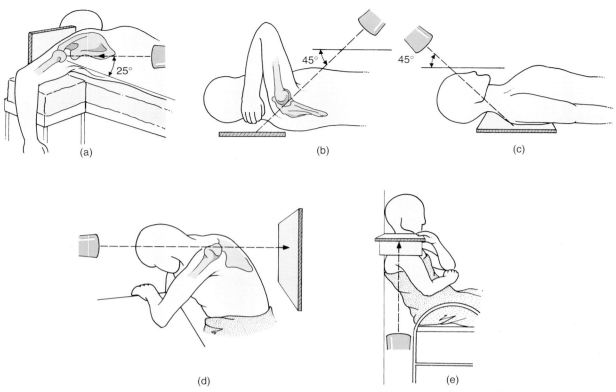

Fig. 6 Instability views. In cases where the presence or direction of instability is in question, various views may be obtained to look for stigmata of recurrent dislocation, or to catch the humeral head in a subluxated position. (a) The West Point axillary view: this view gives excellent detail of the anterior glenoid rim. (b) The Stryker notch view: this is the most sensitive view for demonstration of a Hill–Sachs lesion. (c) The craniocaudal view (also used for demonstration of Hill–Sachs lesions): while not as sensitive as the Stryker view, the patient does not have to position his or her arm overhead. (d) The cephaloscapular view: the patient leans forward on his or her elbow, applying a posterior stress to the glenohumeral joint. In cases of recurrent posterior subluxation, the humeral head may slide over the posterior glenoid lip, establishing the diagnosis. (e) The Stripp axial view: this view clearly demonstrates the direction of the instability.

glenoid in an inferosuperior projection, clearly revealing the anterior and posterior labrum (Fig. 7). When this technique is used, lesions of the labrum can be delineated very accurately. In one study comparing preoperative arthrotomography with intraoperative findings, a positive correlation was found in 16 out of 17 patients.

Arthrotomography may also be useful in picking up patients with lesions of the glenoid labrum, but who do not have anatomical instabilities. These patients, described as having 'functional instability,'[25] would otherwise be completely undetected (see below under Labral disorders).

The latest addition to diagnostic visualization techniques has been magnetic resonance imaging (**MRI**). This exciting new technique offers superior visualization and definition of the soft tissue in and around the shoulder without requiring the injection of radio-opaque material into the joint. MRI can easily visualize Hill–Sachs lesions and erosions of the bony glenoid.[26] This alone would not make the technique attractive. However, it is possible to use MRI to visualize lesions of the labrum, including Bankart lesions, stripping of the anterior glenoid neck,[27] tears of the glenohumeral ligaments, and attenuation or atrophy of the subscapularis tendon.[28] The latter lesion cannot be seen by any other means. In addition, MRI is superior to arthrography in identifying tears of the rotator cuff.[29] However, current cost and availability make universal access to MRI impossible. The clinically relevant information available through

MRI is also available through conventional radiographic techniques.

Surgical invasive tests

If, after thorough radiological assessment (as well as a carefully conducted history and physical examination), the diagnosis is still in doubt, an examination under anaesthesia can be carried out. A great deal of clinical experience is required to be able to distinguish true pathological instability from variations of the normal shoulder. Palpation of an anaesthetized shoulder (with complete muscle relaxation) is quite different from palpation of a shoulder in the standard clinical situation. Anyone planning to use examination under anaesthetic as a diagnostic test should take every opportunity to examine normal shoulders of patients anaesthetized for other procedures in order to build up an accurate perspective of normal.

With the patient anaesthetized in the supine position the shoulder is abducted between 70 degrees and 100 degrees. The examiner holds the patient's arm tucked between his hip and his elbow, allowing both hands to be free to manipulate the shoulder. The humerus is grasped proximally near its neck. The humeral head is then gently levered anteriorly, posteriorly, or inferiorly, feeling carefully for a clunk as the head slips over the glenoid rim. While any amount of anterior slide may be considered pathological, up to 50 per cent posterior slide is within normal limits.[30] Even more credence can be

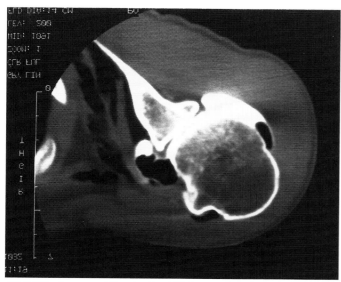

Fig. 7 CT arthrogram of the shoulder. This is an axillary cut showing both the humeral head and the scapula. The glenohumeral articular surface is clearly seen. The labrum is seen at the anterior and posterior margins of the glenoid as dark triangular wedges. They are outlined on their deep surface by the bony glenoid and superficially by dye injected into the joint. Both are normal. Dye passing into the substance of the labrum would signify a tear.

attributed to findings on the symptomatic shoulder when they are absent from the contralateral normal shoulder.[31] Norris[11] has added a further dimension to examination under anaesthetic. He advocates the use of a neurorest for the head and a C-arm fluoroscopy unit to allow direct visual confirmation of any palpated instability.

The final diagnostic tool is the arthroscope. Interest in and use of this instrument regarding the shoulder has flourished in recent years.

Arthroscopy will certainly give a clear view of the interior of the shoulder joint. It can recognize bony lesions. The Hill–Sachs lesion is easily seen from a posterior portal, although care must be taken not to confuse the normally present bare area on the back of the humeral head with a pathological impaction fracture. The articular surface of the humerus and glenoid can also be evaluated for chondromalacia. The glenoid labrum can be seen circumferentially, and its attachment verified both visually and by probing with an arthroscopic hook. Tears of the labrum not involving attachment of the glenohumeral ligaments, but causing functional instability, can also be identified. The glenohumeral ligaments can be seen, as can the superior edge of the subscapularis tendon. Another useful aspect of arthroscopy is its capability to identify tears of the rotator cuff, either complete or partial.

Although it may seem that all this information would make the diagnosis of instability very straightforward, this is not the case. First, the arthroscopist must develop a catalogue of normal anatomy. Despite our growing expertise, such a catalogue is not readily available, and the arthroscopist must often develop it through extensive experience. Seeing the lesion is easy. Deciding whether it represents true pathology is not.

Secondly, while clues to the direction of one instability may be present, other instabilities may have left no evidence. For example, while an isolated erosion of the anterior glenoid labrum would lead one to suspect anterior instability, the associated inferior dislocation

of a multidirectional instability may have left no intra-articular stigmata. Overdependence on arthroscopic findings would therefore lead the surgeon to overlook a very important component of the patient's problem.

Finally, with the shoulder in position for an arthroscopic examination and using skin traction to distract the joint, it is often difficult to assess the degree or even direction of instability. A recent experimental study showed that the introduction of room air into an otherwise stable cadaver shoulder caused the shoulder to subluxate without any division of muscle or ligament.[32] The author surmises that the shoulder was partially stabilized by negative intra-articular pressure. Thus information obtained from the shoulder after the introduction of irrigating cannula and arthroscopic equipment should be treated with caution.

Summary

In summary, the acute shoulder must be evaluated using a three-view trauma series. Additional information can be added in suspected cases of recurrent instability using selected instability views. While arthrography can be helpful in certain situations (particularly in older patients with dislocations), the arthrotomogram is generally more useful. MRI (when available) gives the most information without the use of invasive techniques. Examination under anaesthesia (when used by experienced examiners) is helpful in difficult cases, particularly cases of multidirectional instability. Arthroscopy, while potentially a powerful tool, needs to be interpreted cautiously and by an experienced eye.

Acute anterior dislocation

As the shoulder is the most commonly dislocated joint, and anterior dislocation is the most common, the patient with an anteriorly dislocated shoulder is seen frequently in most emergency rooms. Although diagnosis and treatment appear to be straightforward several pitfalls await the unwary. This section will help familiarize readers with this common clinical situation and point out some of the traps.

Presentation

There are three common mechanisms of injury:

(1) a fall on the outstretched hand;

(2) a blow against the anterior arm forcing it into extension while it is abducted and externally rotated; or

(3) a blow from behind directly on to the posterior aspect of the humeral head.

The first usually occurs as an attempt to cushion a fall. The last two are more common in sports-related injuries as an athlete tries to block an object in front of him (for example, in basketball) or tries to tackle another athlete who is running by (for example, in football or rugby). The injury is often quite painful. The patient presents to the emergency room clutching the elbow and forearm in an attempt to support and stabilize the limb. The history must include not only current injury, but also any antecedent injury or surgery.

Physical examination

Once the patient is undressed the deformity is visibly obvious even in muscular individuals. From the front, there is a squaring off of the shoulder. This is caused by medial displacement of the humeral head. The deltoid muscle, which usually drapes over this round prominence, now falls directly downwards over the tip of the acromion. There is often a visible fullness in the vicinity of the coracoid process. In addition, the arm will appear longer, owing to inferior displacement of the humerus. This will be most easily recognized by comparing the relative level of the two elbows. From behind, the shoulder will also appear square, with the posterior glenoid rim tenting outward against the supraspinatus and infraspinatus.

The arm itself will be held slightly abducted and internally rotated. Further internal rotation is painful, and the patient will be unable to touch the opposite shoulder.

Palpation of the shoulder will help to define the relationship of the various bony prominences more closely. A thorough examination of all bones and joints around the shoulder must also be undertaken to look for associated fractures and injuries.

The next step is a thorough neurovascular examination. The lower portions of the brachial plexus can be fully assessed by a motor and sensory examination of the hand and forearm. The upper plexus becomes more difficult to assess since motor function about a dislocated shoulder cannot be tested accurately. Therefore, sensory examination is extremely important. Two areas of special interest are the autonomous sensory area of the axillary nerve, over the lateral deltoid, and the lateral aspect of the proximal forearm innervated by the terminal sensory branch of the musculocutaneous nerve. Documentation of sensory examination is mandatory before any attempts at reduction are carried out. This has both medical and legal implications. Medically, if a nerve lesion is evident only post-reduction, more aggressive investigation and treatment will be warranted than when the patient presents with an established deficit. Legally, a patient who has a neurological deficit postreduction, and who did not have documentation of this injury prereduction, may well assume that the neurological lesion was caused by the reduction and not the injury. While most authors emphasize this point, Goss[33] has stated that 'sensory exam for axillary nerve lesions is completely unreliable'. He recommends electromyographic (EMG) evaluation for suspected lesions. Unfortunately, this is not possible until 3 weeks after the injury. Other investigators have shown denervation potentials in patients with normal sensory examinations.[34] Despite this spectre of unreliability, a thorough documented examination is still highly desirable.

The vascular status of the limb can be assessed by pulses, colour, and capillary refill. Although vascular injury is rare, any patient who demonstrates signs of vascular compromise warrants a full investigation including arteriography.[8]

Radiography

A complete trauma series should be carried out before an attempt at reduction is made. The exception to this rule is the patient who presents to the physician shortly after suffering the dislocation. This most commonly occurs at a sporting event when the on-field physician examines an athlete. In this situation, a gentle reduction may be carried out before spasm and swelling make it more difficult. However, the clinician should be experienced and feel relatively

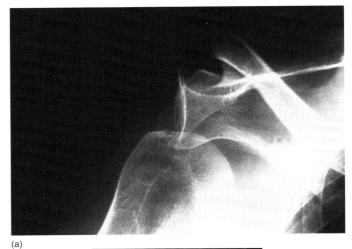

(a)

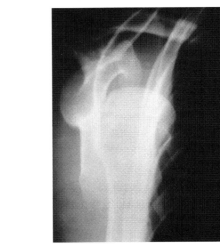

(b)

Fig. 8 Anterior dislocation. (a) Anteroposterior view showing typical subglenoid position of the humeral head. The glenoid fossa is vacant. (b) Trans-scapular (Neer's) view of an anterior dislocation in the subcoracoid position. (This is not the same shoulder as in (a).) With the head dislocated, the glenoid becomes visible. The position of the head under the hooked silhouette of the coracoid process identifies the anterior nature of the dislocation.

comfortable with the diagnosis. There have been instances where an athlete was referred for care after multiple attempts to reduce the shoulder in the dressing room had failed. The athlete did not have a shoulder dislocation, but rather a third-degree acromioclavicular dislocation. Prereduction radiographs are particularly useful in older individuals where fractures of the humeral shaft, often undisplaced and undiagnosed, may complicate management.

The anteroposterior radiograph will show the humeral head displaced medially, overlapping the glenoid neck and lying either in the subcoracoid or subglenoid position (Fig. 8(a)). The dislocation itself is often distracting, and therefore a careful search for associated pathology is sometimes neglected. Special attention must be paid to the greater tuberosity, the surgical neck of the humerus, and the glenoid. It should be remembered that these fractures may be undisplaced and subtle.

The trans-scapular lateral will confirm the anterior nature of the dislocation (Fig. 8(b)). While the anteroposterior view often shows a typical configuration, a definite diagnosis of anterior displacement cannot be made unless two views 90 degrees to each other are compared.

The axillary view, while not essential in the diagnosis of anterior dislocation, should be made routinely. As will be discussed later in the section on Posterior instability, the most common cause of a missed posterior dislocation is the omission of the axillary view. This view should be obtained in all trauma series.

Once the shoulder has been reduced, postreduction films are mandatory. An anteroposterior and Neer's view will be sufficient. It is essential to prove that the head is actually in the glenoid fossa before the patient leaves the emergency room. If the patient returns for a follow-up visit with the shoulder dislocated, it will be difficult to prove that the dislocation occurred while the arm was immobilized unless all the documentation is available.

Reduction

While there are numerous ways of reducing a shoulder, several important principles apply in all situations.

1. Spasm of the muscle around the joint is the opposing force to reduction. Once the muscle is relaxed, reduction will be easy (except in unusual circumstances).

2. Spasm is fuelled by pain and augmented by the stretch reflex. Any time that striated muscle is elongated suddenly the involuntary reaction is contraction of the muscle and increased spasm.

3. Spasm can be broken by fatiguing the muscle and by medication.

If reduction is attempted by using brute force, regardless of how much stronger than the patient the doctor is, the attempt is doomed to failure. It is essential to a successful reduction that the anatomical relationships are restored without causing further damage to bone or soft tissue. While the audible and palpable clunk of the shoulder popping back into place may seem satisfying, the ideal reduction occurs so gently that only re-examination of the patient and subsequent radiographs reveal that a successful reduction has indeed taken place.

The easiest way to fatigue skeletal muscle is with traction. This can be accomplished either by attaching a weight to the patient's arm and letting it dangle, or by attaching one's own bodyweight and leaning away. The present author calls this 'water skiing.' Grabbing and pulling simply means that the doctor's muscle fatigues as quickly as the patient's, resulting in a deadlock. However, leaning away from the patient allows gravity to do the work.

The reduction is best carried out under conscious sedation. This means that the patient is relaxed and relatively pain-free, while still maintaining all their protective reflexes. A combination of narcotics and benzodiazepines is most effective. These are generally administered intravenously as this allows for rapid onset of action and easier titration of dose. The author prefers a shorter acting medication in this situation since the patient is usually very comfortable postreduction and does not need continuing analgesia. Short-acting medications also allow the earlier discharge of the patient. My personal preference is a combination of meperidine (pethidine) and midazolam. The meperidine is administered first. The midozolam is then given in small incremental doses until the desired degree of sedation is reached. The patient must be carefully monitored during the procedure for adverse effects such as hypertension or respiratory suppression. There must be the necessary equipment for resuscitation of the patient available during the procedure. Both classes of medications are reversible (naloxone for narcotics and flumazenil for benzodiazepines) and these agents should also be available.

All reduction techniques are based on traction, leverage, and rotation, either alone or in combination. All can be used effectively, but each has inherent risks. These risks must be understood when deciding on a technique.

As mentioned earlier, traction reduces spasm. It also helps distract the humeral head from the glenoid. If the head is wedged under the glenoid or if a Hill–Sachs fracture has occurred, traction may avoid further damage to bony structures. It also allows reduction of the joint while keeping the delicate articular cartilage away from the edge of the glenoid. However, indiscriminate traction (and countertraction applied over a small surface area) may injure vascular and neurological structures in the axilla.

Leverage over a fulcrum is a powerful reduction tool. However, it can be quite dangerous if the bones are not disengaged first. For example, if the glenoid edge hooks the posterior aspect of the humeral head, leverage may cause a fracture of the anatomical neck, reducing the shaft into the glenoid while leaving the articular surface dislocated (Fig. 9).

Rotation shares the same danger as leverage. It also exposes the humeral shaft to rotational torque, a situation that can easily result in a spiral fracture of the shaft. Osteoporotic individuals are particularly susceptible to this latter complication. A further problem with rotation is the possibility of increased stripping of the capsular structures causing further soft-tissue damage. At least one author has suggested that rotational techniques may increase the risk of recurrent dislocation.[35] With all this in mind, let us review some of the reduction methods in common use.

The Hippocratic technique is one of the oldest and most widely known methods (Fig. 10). The patient lies supine and the physician places his unshoed heel in the patient's axilla. (It is unclear whether Hippocrates meant to place the heel against the chest wall or directly into the axilla.) The arm is then pulled inferiorly and abducted about 45 degrees. Once distracted, the arm is adducted and the heel is used to help lever the head around the inferior glenoid and back into the joint. Several problems exist with this technique. Control of the amount of traction is difficult. Due to the operator's position it is hard to maintain traction for the 5 to 10 min often necessary to fatigue the muscles fully. The countertraction provided by the heel is dangerously close to the neurovascular structures of the axilla, and is applied over too small a surface area. Therefore this technique is not recommended.

Milch has described a technique using pure leverage.[36] While palpating the humeral head in the axilla, the arm is slowly abducted. A firm upward and lateral pressure is constantly applied to the head. When fully abducted the arm is externally rotated and traction applied. The head can now be pushed into the glenoid by manual pressure. The danger in this technique is that the humerus and glenoid are not distracted before they are moved, allowing for the possibility of articular surface damage.

The Kocher manoeuvre is a similar technique, using leverage.[36] With traction applied to the elbow, the arm is externally rotated to about 60 degrees. The elbow is then adducted across the chest. Finally, the arm is internally rotated allowing the head to reduce.

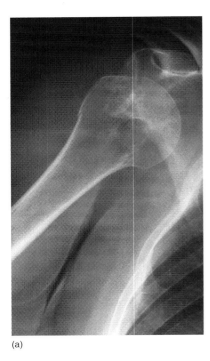
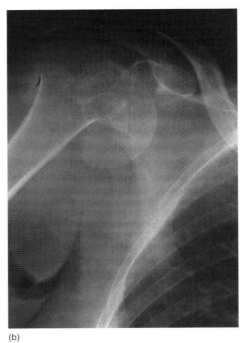

(a)   (b)

Fig. 9 Anterior dislocation associated with a fracture of the surgical neck. (a) While the dislocation is obvious, the surgical neck fracture is not. It is best seen as a break in the cortex laterally. It was missed at presentation in the emergency room. (b) The same patient after an attempted closed reduction. The fracture has displaced leaving the humeral head in a subcoracoid position, while the humeral shaft was reduced into the glenoid fossa. The patient required open reduction and internal fixation.

The acronym TEAM has been applied to this manoeuvre (traction, external rotation, adduction, and medial rotation). As with Milch's technique, leverage on the undistracted humerus can be dangerous. It has the further disadvantage of using rotation in two different directions.

Hanging methods use traction as the sole mechanical tool. Countertraction is achieved either by the patient's own weight or through a large flat surface applied to the patient. Therefore they are relatively safe.

The classic hanging technique was described by Stimson (Fig. 11). The patient lies prone on a stretcher with a pad anterior to the affected shoulder and pectoral region. The arm dangles downward in a forward flexed position. A weight (4.5 kg or 10 lb) is attached to the wrist and allowed to hang freely. (Having the patient grasp the weight would cause muscle contraction and oppose complete relaxation.) The operator checks the patient's axilla from time to time, and as the head descends attempts to push it gently into the glenoid fossa.[34] Alternatively, a supraclavicular block can be used and the

patient positioned without weights. The patient's relaxed arm will act as the distracting force.[37] The advantage of the Stimson technique is that it allows a controlled gentle reduction comfortably, and with little risk. However, it is time consuming and requires the patient to be prone, thus making it difficult to monitor ventilation. Nevertheless, it is probably the technique of choice for the inexperienced operator.

One further traction method deserves mention. The so-called Eskimo technique was shown to a physician in Greenland by native hunters. It was subsequently taught to non-medical staff in outlying

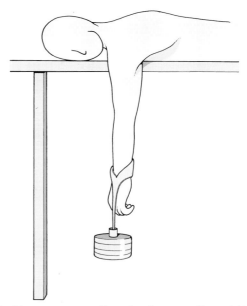

Fig. 11 The Stimson manoeuvre. The patient lies prone with a weight attached to the wrist. The technique is easy to perform and comfortable for the patient. However, it is time consuming.

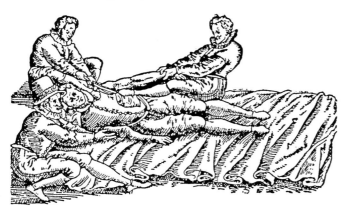

Fig. 10 A seventeenth century woodcut demonstrating the Hippocratic technique of shoulder reduction. (Reprinted from ref. 3, with permission.)

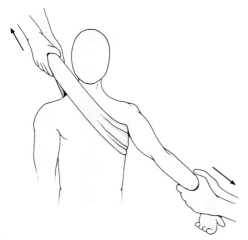

Fig. 12 The traction–countertraction reduction. This is the safest and most effective method of reducing an anterior dislocation. If an assistant is unavailable to apply countertraction, the sheet around the patient's body can be attached to the stretcher.

emergency rooms and resulted in a success rate of 74 per cent when used by inexperienced operators.[38] The patient lies laterally on the floor, with the affected side up. Two people grasp the wrist and bring the arm slowly to 90 degrees of abduction, applying enough upward force to suspend the other shoulder several centimetres from the ground. If the shoulder does not reduce in a few minutes, manual pressure is applied to the axilla as in Stimson's method. Although inelegant and requiring two people to apply traction, this technique does have a certain appeal, not least of which is its application in a setting where an experienced surgeon is unavailable. However, it is impractical for older patients and others who might have difficulty in lying on the floor.

The author's preference is for the traction–countertraction technique (Fig. 12). The patient lies supine on a stretcher. A sheet is wrapped around the chest and axilla on the affected side. It is then attached to the stretcher on the other side of the patient, or wrapped around the waist of an assistant. The elbow is flexed, allowing the operator to grip the patient's forearm. This gives a handle to pull on and helps control rotation of the humerus. The arm is abducted 45 degrees. The operator now leans back slowly, maintaining steady traction on the arm. Once fully distracted, gentle pressure in the axilla will aid its reduction. The technique uses pure traction with a broad area of countertraction. Furthermore, if properly placed, the countertraction will be against the chest wall and not the delicate axillary contents. The operator maintains rotational control and can speak to the patient, thus adding a little 'verbal anaesthesia'. The patient is supine and therefore both comfortable and accessible.

If several attempts using at least two reduction methods have failed with the patient fully relaxed, a reduction under general anaesthesia will be required. Factors which may lead to a reduction under general anaesthesia include an impacted fracture of the humeral head (locking it into place), an obese or muscular individual (making manipulation difficult), or an exceptionally nervous patient who is unable to relax. In addition, soft tissues may be trapped in the glenohumeral joint, blocking concentric reduction. A further indication for reduction under general anaesthesia is a fracture of the humeral shaft. In this situation it is often impossible to manipulate the shoulder without further displacement of the fracture, and the complete muscle relaxation afforded by general anaesthesia is recommended. In any event, the principle of a gentle atraumatic reduction still applies and must be adhered to in order to avoid iatrogenic injury to the shoulder.

Open reduction

Open reduction of the shoulder is indicated in the following circumstances:

1. Failure of closed reduction under general anaesthesia. The head will often be found buttonholed through the capsule. Entrapment of the long head of the biceps may also block reduction.

2. Fractures of the greater tuberosity which do not reduce anatomically along with the head. Any displacement of over 1 cm should be considered non-anatomical. Not only will the bony fragment impinge on abduction of the shoulder, but there will certainly be an associated tear of the rotator cuff that will need repair.

3. Fractures of the glenoid compromising more than 30 per cent of the articular surface. This will require internal fixation at the time of surgery.

Postreduction

Once reduced, the shoulder should be immobilized, adducted to the body, and internally rotated. It can be held in position by a commercially available shoulder immobilizer which is easy to apply, comfortable to wear, and relatively inexpensive. Several models are available. Alternatively, a Velpeau sling can be made from materials found in most emergency rooms. The arm is placed in a triangular bandage in the reduced position. The sling is then strapped to the patient's body by wrapping several 15 cm (6 inch) elastic bandages around the chest and affected arm. This keeps the arm at the side and impedes external rotation of the humerus. The thorny question of how long the patient's shoulder should be immobilized will be dealt with in the section on Recurrent dislocation. As mentioned earlier, a postreduction anteroposterior and trans-scapular lateral radiograph are taken to verify the reduction.

Complications

The major complications to watch for in acute anterior dislocations are redislocation, associated fractures, tears of the rotator cuff, neurological injury, and vascular damage. Recurrent dislocation is more common in the young and decreases with age. The inverse is true for all other complications. Recurrence is sufficiently important that it merits its own section and will be dealt with later in this chapter.

The Hill–Sachs lesion, a posterior impaction fracture of the humeral head, has been reported in 10 to 55 per cent of anterior dislocations (Fig. 13).[16] This rises to nearly 100 per cent of patients with recurrent episodes.[18] It does not require specific treatment, but does give important clues as to diagnosis and prognosis. As special views may be required to see the lesion, it may be overlooked in the

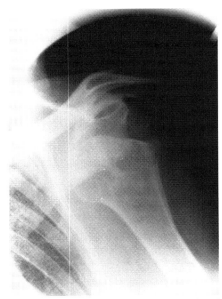

Fig. 13 Anteroposterior view demonstrating an anterior dislocation and a large Hill–Sachs lesion. The latter is a posterior inpaction fracture of the humeral head caused by impingement of the anterior glenoid lip against the dislocated humeral head. It is seen as a crescentic lucency at the superolateral margin of the humeral head.

acute situation. Fractures of the greater tuberosity occur in approximately 10 per cent of acute dislocations.[16] They are best seen on the anteroposterior view (Fig. 14). With reduction of the glenohumeral joint the majority reduce spontaneously. Any displacement of more than 1 cm merits open reduction and internal fixation. If left dis-

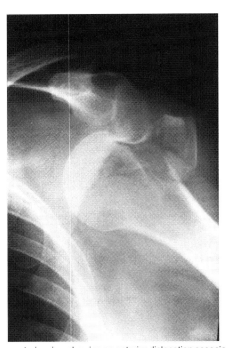

Fig. 14 Anteroposterior view showing an anterior dislocation associated with a displaced fracture of the greater tuberosity. Fractures of the tuberosity occur in approximately 10 per cent of anterior dislocations and should be looked for carefully.

placed, the fragment will impinge on the underface of the acromion, blocking full abduction. Late repair is more difficult and the results may be poor. These fractures are usually associated with tears of the rotator cuff and neglect may lead to rotator cuff insufficiency. If the tuberosity reduces anatomically, the shoulder can be treated as an uncomplicated dislocation without fear of redisplacement. Fractures of the humeral shaft and surgical neck are not uncommon, but are beyond the scope of this chapter.

Fractures of the glenoid rim will be present in 10 to 20 per cent of acute dislocations.[8] For the most part these are small flakes of bone that accompany an avulsed glenoid labrum—the so-called bony Barkart lesion. If small, they are insignificant and require no specific treatment. Fractures of 30 per cent or more of the articular surface will lead to inherent bony instability, and therefore indicate the need for acute open reduction and internal fixation. If left unattended, they will lead to difficult reconstructive situations requiring bone grafting.

Tears of the rotator cuff occur in between 30 and 50 per cent of patients with anterior dislocations.[7,16] The clinician must be vigilant for this injury as the dislocation may make diagnosis difficult. While it is possible to demonstrate the lesion arthrographically in a very high percentage of patients, the incidence of long-term insufficiency drops to only 5 per cent.[16] This would imply that with reduction of the shoulder, the cuff has the ability to heal. Rowe *et al.*[39] have pointed out the potential cleavage plane between the subscapularis and the supraspinatus tendons. It may be here that the rotator cuff tears, allowing it to heal on its own, but this is only conjecture. While acute repair of the rotator cuff is unnecessary, any patient with demonstrated insufficiency who has associated pain and functional disability should be considered for delayed surgery. Such repair is definitely easier before atrophy, and therefore before retraction of the edges makes anatomical suturing impossible. Hence, arthrography is indicated after 4 to 6 weeks in patients who are not progressing in their postreduction course of treatment.

Brachial plexus injuries, if carefully looked for, will be found in approximately 5 per cent of patients. The majority are infraclavicular and incomplete, with full recovery expected. Isolated lesions of the axillary nerve will be found in 5 to 10 per cent of the patients.[7] This usually occurs as a traction neuropraxia with the humeral head trapping the axillary nerve in the quadrilateral space. As Goss[33] has pointed out, sensory examination is not totally reliable and EMG examination may be needed in suspected cases. This examination will look for denervation potentials in the deltoid muscle, but will not be positive until at least 3-weeks postinjury. The majority of these lesions are transient and recovery should be expected without treatment.[8] Axillary nerve lesions may occur in conjunction with tears of the rotator cuff making the latter diagnosis difficult. The presence of an axillary nerve lesion (particularly in an older individual) should make one suspect a concurrent cuff tear.

Vascular injury with anterior dislocation occurs but is very uncommon. It may be associated with multiple injuries or high-velocity trauma. Despite the low incidence, the clinician must always be vigilant for vascular compromise, as any delay in recognition and treatment will lead to disastrous end results. Any patient displaying signs of vascular injury—including decreased pulses, expanding haematomas, or pallor of the arm—should be evaluated aggressively, with inclusion of an arteriogram if deemed necessary.

Recurrent anterior dislocation

Recurrent subluxation

Before discussing recurrent anterior dislocation, it is necessary to introduce one further concept: recurrent subluxation. This was first described by Blazina and Satzman in 1969, and defined further by Rowe.[40] The patient is usually a young active athlete who recalls an episode of forced extension and rotation with the arm abducted. The patient's chief complaint is recurrent episodes of weakness or giving way in the shoulder with overhead activities, such as throwing or serving in tennis. Often the patient describes a complete lack of strength—hence the name 'dead arm syndrome'.[40] The symptoms may have been initiated by an episode of frank dislocation, but usually the patient denies any such episodes. Approximately 50 per cent of these patients are unaware that the shoulder is unstable.[41] The remaining 50 per cent will describe a sensation of the shoulder slipping out of place followed by spontaneous reduction. Such patients are never able to demonstrate the instability voluntarily, but are usually aware of the position causing the sensation (namely, abduction and external rotation).

On physical examination the patient will have a full range of motion, no tenderness, and no signs of rotator cuff insufficiency. The apprehension sign will be universally positive. To perform this test, abduct the patient's arm between 90 and 120 degrees. While standing behind the patient, externally rotate the arm and apply gentle pressure to the back of the humeral head. A reproduction of the patient's symptomatology, or a feeling that the shoulder is about the pop out, is taken as a positive test. The patient may resist external rotation or flex the shoulder by leaning the body forward, also indicating a positive test. Examination of the opposite shoulder is helpful as a comparison. Another useful test can be carried out with the patient supine on an examining table. This manoeuvre is described in the section on Examination under anaesthesia. While actual subluxation may be difficult to detect in the conscious subject, the patient may experience the symptomatology signifying a positive test.

The XRAY series for instability may provide clues to diagnosis. The West Point view may show changes of the anterior glenoid—either fuzziness of the rim or actual soft-tissue calcification. The Stryker notch view may show a Hill–Sachs defect even in patients who have not had a frank dislocation.[31] The most important factor for accurate diagnosis is awareness of the syndrome and an index of suspicion. Once the syndrome is recognized, treatment proceeds as with recurrent dislocation.

Recurrence rate

Many factors appear to affect the rate of recurrence in acute anterior dislocation. One, which is universally accepted, is age at first dislocation. All authors agree that the younger the patient, the greater the likelihood of later recurrence. Rowe's classic paper of 1956 stated that for patients under the age of 20 the recurrence rate was 94 per cent, between the ages of 20 and 40 it fell to 74 per cent, and after the age of 40 only 14 per cent recurred.[6] This trend has been subsequently corroborated by many authors, although most find rates lower than those reported by Rowe. The reason for this age distribution remains a subject of debate. Some authors attempt to explain it on the basis of associated pathology. When tears of the

rotator cuff or posterior capsule occur, the shoulder may dislocate in a way which spares the anterior capsular structure. If the superior or posterior lesions heal, there will be no residual Bankart lesion or anterior capsular redundancy. Such tears may be more likely in older individuals who are known to have incipient weakening of the cuff on an age-related basis. Other authors suggest that as younger patients are more active in sports, they are more likely to be exposed to traumatic events predisposing them to recurrent episodes.

The mechanism of injury has also been implicated in the recurrence rate. Bankart[15] believed that abduction external rotation injuries caused a dislocation through a tear in the anterior capsule. He believed that this tear would heal and therefore have a lower recurrence rate. A direct blow posteriorly would tear the glenoid labrum off the glenoid (that is to say, a Bankart lesion), which would not heal, thereby leading to recurrent dislocation. However, Rowe's study shows no correlation between mechanism and recurrence.[42]

I believe that patients who have dislocated at an early age have a particular anatomical predisposition to instability. This could be due to insufficient strength of capsular material, or perhaps improper attachment of the glenoid labrum. Most people are exposed to a certain number of traumatic episodes during their youth. Some with an anatomical predisposition will dislocate, thereby creating a cohort prone to subsequent instability. Those of 'heartier stock' who do not dislocate in their youth may dislocate later in life when normal anatomy is eventually exposed to an overpowering traumatic event. In this situation, the shoulder will heal with little propensity for redislocation. The theory would allow for a spectrum of predisposition with those at one extreme dislocating younger, intermediate types dislocating later, and a stable type which would dislocate only much later in life, perhaps after the normal attrition of ageing leads to weakening of surrounding tissues.

Many authors have attempted to reduce redislocation rates by immobilization immediately after the primary injury. Earlier authors suggested an immobilization period of 6 weeks, particularly in the young, basing this on the projected healing time of soft tissues. Subsequent studies by several authors have failed to show this to be effective.[33,40,43] Hovelius[44] has shown no change in redislocation rates with up to 4 weeks of immobilization.

Despite a lack of statistical evidence, most authors still suggest a 3-week period of immobilization for patients under the age of 30, and a 1-week period of immobilization for older patients. The patient must be informed from the outset of the high redislocation rate, regardless of immediate therapy.

Certainly bony lesions appear to influence the recurrence rate. In patients with fractures of the greater tuberosity the rate fell to between 3 and 7 per cent,[33,40] while fracture of the surgical neck was not associated with any recurrence.[33] The Hill–Sachs lesion was not found to influence the redislocation rate in younger patients, but in patients over the age of 23 the recurrence rate was significantly higher.[44]

Treatment options

When the patient presents with episodes of recurrent dislocations, several options are available. First, the patient may wish to accept the instability. While most patients who have two or more redislocations can expect to continue dislocating without treatment, one prospective study showed that 20 per cent of patients with two or more redislocations during the first 2-years' postprimary dislocation had no further dislocations in the subsequent 3 years.[44]

No study has conclusively shown that stabilizing a recurrently unstable shoulder would change the incidence of late degeneration. Indeed, two studies have shown an equal incidence of degeneration in untreated and surgically stabilized patients.[45,46] Furthermore, the severity of the arthritis was not related to the number of recurrences.[45]

Conservative measures can be instituted. Some authors believe that strengthening exercises would be of benefit for recurrent dislocation.[8] They suggest exercises for both internal and external rotators in order to improve dynamic stability of the shoulder. Other authors disagree.[30] As stated previously (in the section on Anatomy), the subscapularis muscle, a prime dynamic stabilizer, is superior to the shoulder with the arm abducted and externally rotated. Consequently, in the shoulder's most vulnerable position, the subscapularis would be useless in preventing dislocation. Furthermore, when the arm is abducted and externally rotated, those muscles that would be most useful in preventing dislocation are neurogenically inhibited to allow full range of motion at the shoulder. Nevertheless, for patients unwilling to accept their instability, but who are not yet ready for surgery, a temporizing course of physiotherapy and strengthening exercises seems to be reasonable.

Bracing is also available. These braces, which are used almost exclusively during sporting activities, attempt to block abduction and external rotation by means of a harness. The brace straps around the patient's chest, with a second strap encircling the arm just distal to the axilla. While they may be effective in preventing dislocation, they place a dangerous fulcrum over the humerus against which a fracture can occur. They should be used with caution, particularly in contact sports.

The third and final option is surgical correction of the instability. When should surgery by advised? There are no absolute indications for stabilization. Although recurrent dislocation is associated with an increased risk of late degenerative arthritis, this risk is not related to the number of recurrences, nor is it reduced by surgical correction. Surgery does not guarantee a return to normal stability since the overall rate of redislocation postoperatively is approximately 10 per cent.[16] The prime indication for surgery is the patient's dissatisfaction with the status quo, coupled with his or her acceptance of the surgical risks involved.

Some authors, including Jobe,[2] have concluded that in the young competitive athlete—particularly when a throwing shoulder is involved—primary repair is indicated with the first dislocation. Although this may seem radical, statistics do lead to this conclusion. Early repair is also recommended for patients whose occupation or sport may expose them to severe bodily harm if their shoulder should dislocate at a potentially dangerous moment. This applies to people working on roofs and ladders, or particularly in sports such as long-distance, open-water swimming.

Surgery

Once a surgical course is selected, the physician is faced with choosing from literally hundreds of procedures and their variations. Although the choice may seem endless, there are certain principles involved which can be evaluated to help determine the most appropriate one. Generally speaking, all operations for recurrent instability approach the problem via one of three mechanisms.

1. They may block external rotation, thereby avoiding the position of vulnerability.

2. They may try to maintain stability by buttressing the front of the joint with bone or soft tissue.

3. They may attempt to identify the specific pathology and reconstruct the normal anatomy.

In addition, any of these procedures may involve the use of metal fixation implants.

Current thinking is that restriction of motion is not only unnecessary but undesirable, and is often listed as a postoperative complication. Buttressing operations are often performed extra-articularly, thereby not allowing full intra-articular evaluation (a factor associated with increased recurrence rates). Metal staples and screws have the disadvantage of breaking and migrating, and can impinge on the articular surface. This may result in severe degenerative changes postoperatively.[45] Consequently, the ideal operation would:

(1) identify and correct pathological anatomy without metal implants or designed restriction of movement;

(2) have a low recurrence rate;

(3) not be associated with major complications;

(4) permit visualization of the joint and be relatively easy to perform.

While many procedures do not achieve all the prerequisites of the perfect operation, most have been performed over the decades with surprisingly similar success rates. Perhaps the original Hippocratic technique of hot-poker scarification merits a second look!

The actual surgical techniques are not discussed in this chapter. However, some of the currently popular procedures will be outlined to make it easier for physicians to relate to patients who have undergone previous surgical repairs.

The Magnusen–Stack operation is a transfer of the subscapularis tendon distally on the humerus lateral to the biceps tendon. It is designed to cause an internal rotation contracture and to provide an anterior sling to prevent inferior movement of the head. Because of its goal and because it utilizes a large metallic staple, this procedure is not recommended. Once popular, it is now rarely used. A radiograph showing a staple in the humerus distal to the joint usually signifies a previous Magnusen–Stack repair.

The Putti–Platt procedure is an operation that first detaches the subscapularis tendon near its insertion on the humerus. The joint is then opened and the stump of the tendon on the lesser tuberosity is sutured to the glenoid labrum. This provides an intra-articular reinforcement to the anterior capsule. It can be combined with reattachment of the glenoid labrum. This procedure addresses most requirements. Unfortunately, it may also lead to an internal rotation contracture of the shoulder by shortening the excursion of the subscapularis. This operation has frequently been performed in the past with excellent results, but is no longer common (particularly in throwing athletes) because of the potential restriction in range of movement. Nevertheless, it remains an excellent choice for non-throwing individuals.

The Eden–Hybinette procedure is a buttressing operation that attaches an anterior bone block to the glenoid. It is fraught with many problems, not least of which is the screw fixation necessary to hold the graft. The bone may be resorbed and may migrate or impinge on the humeral head. For these reasons it has been supplanted by other techniques.

Another buttress-type operation is the Bristow repair. Here the tip of the coracoid is detached with the short head of the biceps and the coracobrachialis. The bone is then transferred to the glenoid neck and screwed on via a split in the subscapularis tendon. Not only is the bone block present as a buttress, but the attached muscles are intended to work as an anterior sling, stabilizing the front of the joint as the arm is brought up into abduction and external rotation. While the operation is still popular, it has fallen into disrepute in recent years for several reasons. The musculocutaneous nerve pierces the coracobrachialis just distal to its attachment to the coracoid. The nerve is at risk during transfer. The muscles moved are important flexors of the shoulder and may not function as effectively from their new location. There is no way of addressing any associated intra-articular pathology with this procedure. Finally, there is the problem of metallic screws.

The Dutoit procedure uses a large metal staple placed through a longitudinal split in the subscapularis to reattach the capsule to the anterior glenoid neck. Although quick, this procedure offers no visualization of the intra-articular structures. Malposition and migration of Dutoit staples can produce shoulder arthrosis. Thus it has been widely condemned.

The Bankart repair, as popularized by Rowe, is the 'gold standard' against which most other techniques are measured. The actual procedure may be of interest.[40]

Basically, the subscapularis is detached and the shoulder opened via a T-shaped incision. The glenoid and labrum are visualized, and if a detachment is noted it is reattached with interrupted sutures via drill holes in the glenoid rim. The procedure fulfils most of the prerequisites but is very difficult to perform. Rowe, himself, claims an average operative time of 2.75 h. This is well beyond the average of 1 to 1.5 h, even in the hands of a very experienced surgeon. However, it is designed to allow early range of movement and little, if any, restriction in external rotation. The procedure has been simplified by the recent advent of suture anchors. These are small metallic devices which are barbed on one end. A drill hole is made in the bone and the anchor is impacted into it. The barbs fold down as they pass through the drill hole and then spring open, anchoring the device in the bone. A suture is attached to the anchor before it is seated.[47,48]

The author's procedure of choice is a technique described by Neer: the capsular shift (Fig. 15).[21] Here the subscapularis is detached and the capsule is opened in a T-shaped fashion. The shoulder is inspected and, if necessary, intra-articular work is performed. The capsule is closed by shifting the lower portion of the 'T' upwards and laterally. The upper flap is then moved laterally and inferiorly, double vesting the repair. Placement of the flaps is made with the shoulder in neutral rotation so as to avoid an internal rotation contracture. The main advantage is that it not only complies with all the prerequisites, but also allows obliteration of inferior capsule redundancy. It can be performed in a similar fashion through a posterior capsulotomy, making it adaptable to cases of posterior instability. It is also the procedure of choice for multidirectional instability (see later). Finally, the operation is easier to perform than a classic Bankart procedure (1 h as opposed to 2 h).

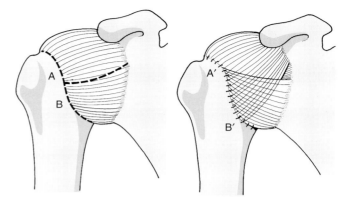

Fig. 15 Neer's capsular shift procedure. The capsule is opened in a T-shaped fashion. The capsule is then closed by shifting the inferior half upwards from A to A′ and the superior half downwards from B to B′.

Postoperatively, the patient is immobilized in a sling identical with that used in the acute situation. The duration of immobilization must be tailored to the patient and to the operation. Procedures that rely on an internal rotation contracture often keep the patient in a sling for up to 6 weeks. Most other techniques suggest beginning movement at or near the 3-week mark. In the throwing athlete, where any loss of external rotation may compromise function, earlier mobilization is the rule.

Postoperative complications fall into five major categories. The first are general postoperative complications such as haematoma and/or infection. As in all surgical procedures, the incidence of these complications can be reduced by meticulous technique.

The second is recurrence. According to various authors, the recurrence rate may range from 0 to 10 per cent. The actual rate probably lies closer to the higher figure.

The third complication is neurovascular injury. The musculocutaneous nerve is particularly at risk where it passes through the coracobrachialis. The nerve can be injured in procedures which release the tendon, or by overzealous retraction. The axillary artery is inferior to the humeral neck and is surprisingly close to the surgical field. Fortunately, injury to this large vessel and the accompanying brachial plexus is exceedingly rare.

The fourth complication is restriction of movement. This is generally related to the specifics of the technique and the length of postoperative immobilization. Most patients who complain of limitation of movement can regain significant amounts of range by means of aggressive physiotherapy if the problem is recognized early.

The final complication is late arthrosis or degenerative change. While some degree of degeneration may be inherent in the recurrently unstable shoulder, much is related to surgical errors causing the shoulder to be overly tight, or to misplacement or migration of metallic implants.

Arthroscopy
Arthroscopic repair techniques are also available. These fall into two major categories: stapling and transglenoid suturing.

In stapling techniques the glenoid rim is abraded to expose bleeding bone. The glenohumeral ligaments are identified and transferred medially and superiorly, reducing any pathological laxity. The ligaments are then reattached to the glenoid neck with a staple, either metallic or, more recently, biodegradable.

In transglenoid techniques, the ligament is first tagged with multiple sutures using an arthroscopic suture passer. A pin is then drilled through the glenoid neck from the front to the back and the sutures are passed down the drill hole. They are then tied subcutaneously over the posterior surface of the scapula. A sports medicine surgeon finds any technique which allows the performance of surgery without major skin incisions seductively attractive. However, experience has shown that caution must be exercised before committing to arthroscopic stabilization. Some prerequisites are necessary.

First, the surgeon must have mastered diagnostic arthroscopy of the shoulder. Before he can repair the shoulder, he must be able to see and recognize the pathology. In addition to the usual operative complications already described, he must add those peculiar to arthroscopic surgery, including puncture of vital structures by errant portals, injuries to the brachial plexus by improper positioning of the patient, and soft-tissue dissection by irrigating fluids. Furthermore, it seems that, even in the best hands, arthroscopic stabilization has a higher rate of recurrence than open procedures. Hawkins[49] has reported a recurrence rate of 16 per cent. However, Rubinovich and Coughlin (unpublished data) and other series have reported significantly higher rates of recurrence ranging from 30 to 44 per cent.[50,51] While it may be premature to abandon arthroscopic stabilization, caution must be exercised in patient selection. Some advantages are offered by arthroscopic procedures. Fewer assistants are required. The surgery is performed on an outpatient basis. Cosmesis is somewhat better. Whether these benefits outweigh the potential risk of recurrence has to be decided by the patient and the surgeon.

Summary

The personal approach of the author to the patient with recurrent instability is as follows: first, establish a diagnosis by history, physical examination, and radiographs. If the patient is functionally impaired and fully understands the risks of surgery, surgical stabilization is then undertaken. Patients unwilling to undergo surgery are sent for rehabilitative exercises. Braces are rarely used and are avoided in contact sports. The author's surgical procedure of choice is the capsular shift. On occasion, arthroscopic stapling is performed, but this procedure is generally restricted to low-demand individuals who are concerned about cosmesis and who understand the increased risk of recurrence with this form of stabilization.

Acute posterior dislocation

Posterior dislocation of the shoulder is extremely uncommon.[52] The incidence in reported series varies from 1.5 to 3.7 per cent. Due to its rarity and because of the difficulty in interpreting standard radiographic films, many acute dislocations are missed at initial presentation only to be picked up later as chronic dislocations. This is unfortunate, as late treatment is more difficult and generally associated with a poorer outcome. It is also easy to avoid if the clinician follows a few simple rules.

Presentation

As with anterior dislocation, the patient will present with pain and decreased movement about the shoulder. The mechanism of injury is often a fall on the outstretched hand with the shoulder flexed, adducted, and internally rotated. A direct blow anteriorly may dislocate the shoulder, but this is less common since it is resisted by both the anterior tilt of the glenoid and the surrounding prominences of the coracoid and acromion. Other situations which should alert the physician to a possible posterior dislocation are seizures and electrical injury. These events cause forcible contraction of the shoulder musculature with the stronger anterior muscles forcing the shoulder out posteriorly. Multiple trauma should also alert the physician, as should alcohol-related injuries which always seem to result in unusual phenomena.

Physical examination

Physical examination will show a patient holding the arm internally rotated and slightly flexed. The anterior shoulder may lack its usual fullness, and the acromion and coracoid processes will seem overly prominent. Attempts at external rotation will be painful. The most striking feature will be the inability to rotate the humerus externally. Another feature is the patient's inability to supinate the hand with the shoulder forward flexed.[41]

Radiography

The anteroposterior view of the shoulder may be misleading. The humeral head does not fully dislocate from the glenoid, but usually lies in full internal rotation with a varying amount of articular surface remaining in the glenoid (Fig. 16(a)). The demarcation between that portion of the humeral head in the glenoid and that portion dislocated is often marked by an impaction fracture of the humeral head (Fig. 17). Again, this fracture may not be evident on the anteroposterior view. Marked internal rotation of the humerus and a slight overlap of the head in the glenoid may be the only signs noted.

The trans-scapular lateral view may also show only subtle findings. The head is posteriorly displaced, but only marginally (Fig. 16(b)). As the glenoid position is only inferred on this projection, the dislocation may be missed entirely.

The key diagnostic clue is the axillary view. This point cannot be overemphasized. The common thread linking all missed posterior dislocation cases is the omission of this one radiograph. Not only does this projection clearly show the dislocation, but it also delineates the presence and size of any impaction fracture (Fig. 18).

Reduction

Reduction of the posterior dislocation is made difficult by the impaction fracture and is compounded by the unfamiliarity of most physicians with this entity. Unless the humerus can be gently disengaged from the posterior lip of the glenoid, reduction will be either impossible or disastrous, resulting in a shearing off of the articular surface through the impaction fracture.

Once the patient is suitably relaxed, as with an anterior reduction, a manoeuvre combining elements of flexion, adduction, and lateral traction is carried out. The latter is necessary to disengage the head from the glenoid and is effected by pushing against the inside of the humerus high on the shaft near the axilla. Once disengaged, the head can be reduced by external rotation. Should closed reduction be unsuccessful under intravenous sedation, an attempt under general anaesthesia will be needed. As with anterior

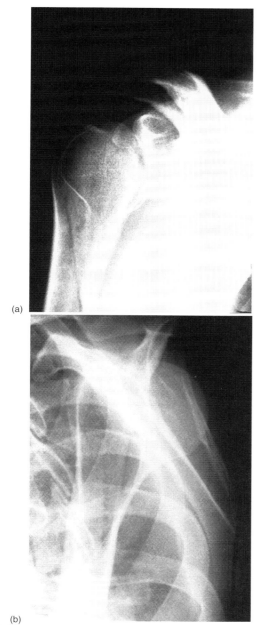

(a)

(b)

Fig. 16 Posterior dislocation. (a) The anteroposterior view showing very subtle signs of a posterior dislocation. The joint space is obliterated and there is slight overlap of the glenoid and the humeral head. This gives the articular surface of the glenoid a sclerotic appearance. In addition, the humeral head is internally rotated, foreshortening the neck and causing the lateral aspect of the head to appear radiolucent. (b) The trans-scapular (Neer's) view of the same shoulder. The articular surface is directed posteriorly, demonstrating the dislocation and its direction, but the head remains superimposed over the area of the glenoid fossa. While detectable, the dislocation could easily be overlooked. The subtle nature of the posterior dislocation seen on the radiograph underlines the need for the axillary view in a trauma series.

dislocations, a gentle hand will be rewarded with fewer complications and better long-term results.

Postreduction

After reduction the shoulder is assessed for stability. If stable, it is immobilized in moderate external rotation for a period of 4 to 6

weeks. This may be shortened for older individuals. If there is no impaction fracture, a situation said to be rare,[53] recurrent instability will be low. In the usual instance, namely cases with impaction fractures, the prognosis is related to the size of the fracture. Since posterior dislocation is so rare, there are few studies of actual recurrence rates. However, one such study found recurrences in 9 out of 24 patients.[20] As with anterior instability, age plays an important role with younger patients more likely to suffer recurrences. Operative repair with specific reference to the treatment of the impaction fracture will be dealt with in the section on Chronic dislocation.

Posterior subluxation

Recurrent posterior subluxation is much more common than posterior dislocation of the shoulder.[53,54] The humeral head slips posteriorly over the glenoid rim and spontaneously reduces, a situation analogous to recurrent anterior subluxation. Most commonly, the patient presents complaining primarily of pain rather than instability.[54] The disability is usually mild, rarely interfering with activities of daily living (although occasionally it is severe enough to interfere with sports, particularly in the dominant arm of a throwing athlete). There may be a history of an antecedent event, but this is rare. Most patients present with an insidious onset of symptoms perhaps related to various overuse phenomena.

Presentation

The posterior subluxators fall into several categories based on physical examination. The first are those patients who can actively demonstrate their instability by contraction of muscles or positioning of the arm. This usually includes a combination of forward flexion, adduction, and internal rotation. These patients are not to be confused with patients who can actively dislocate anteriorly. The latter group often have underlying emotional or psychiatric problems. This issue will be taken up later in the section on habitual and wilful voluntary dislocation.

The next group of patients are those who cannot reproduce their symptoms at will, but who can be subluxated by the examiner. Again, flexion, adduction, and internal rotation accompanied by axial load may reproduce the subluxation. Most patients subluxate between 70 degrees and 110 degrees of forward flexion. Beyond this point the shoulder reduces spontaneously, perhaps owing to the winding up of the capsule and tightening of posterior structures. The final and most difficult group of patients are those in whom the subluxation cannot be demonstrated on clinical examination. This group may well be confused with anterior subluxators, as symptoms occur in both conditions with the arm forward-flexed.

Any patient who is diagnosed as having posterior instability must be carefully evaluated for associated multidirectional instability, since correction of one component alone may fail to reduce symptoms and may even exacerbate the problem. Once again, this will be dealt with in a subsequent section.

Radiographs of the shoulder should include anteroposterior, lateral, and axillary projections. These are used mainly to rule out any other pathology since radiographic findings are usually absent. Recurrent subluxation rarely progress to frank posterior dislocation and so will not lead to impaction fractures of the head.[20] Up to 20 per cent of such patients may have calcification of the posterior

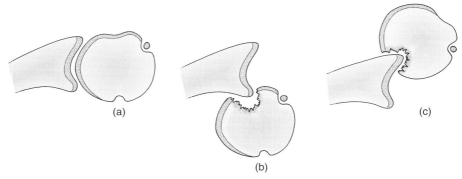

Fig. 17 Impaction fractures of the humeral head: (a) reduced position of the glenohumeral joint; (b) posterior dislocation with an anterior impaction fracture or McLaughlin lesion; (c) anterior dislocation with a posterior impaction fracture or Hill–Sachs lesion.

capsule, or even small flake fractures of the posterior glenoid rim,[17] but these are generally small and often missed. CT scanning is much more sensitive to their presence. A CT scan is also helpful in assessing the orientation of the glenoid relative to the body. As discussed in the section on Diagnostic techniques, stress films are very useful, particularly in patients who can actively or passively subluxate their shoulder (Fig. 19(a)(b)).

When all other tests prove negative, examination under anaesthesia can be helpful. It should be re-emphasized that up to 50 per cent posterior glide of the humeral head is within the normal range.[11]

Initial treatment

Initial treatment should always be conservative, as most patients will respond to an aggressive programme of strengthening exercises.[17] These include strengthening of the rotator cuff musculature along with the deltoid and stabilizers of the scapula. Only when an extended trial of conservative management fails should the patient be considered for surgical repair. Remember that demonstrable instability *per se* is not an indication for correction. The patient must also have significant functional disability to warrant intervention.

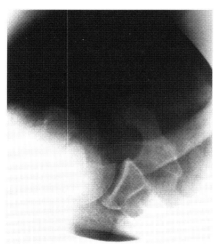

Fig. 18 McLaughlin lesion. An axillary view of the shoulder in the reduced position. A large defect is noted anteriorly in the humeral head, adjacent to its articular surface. This is an impaction fracture caused by the posterior lip of the glenoid while the shoulder is posteriorly dislocated.

The pathoanatomy of posterior instability is less well defined than its anterior counterpart. Reverse Bankart lesions are rare. The capsule is not reinforced by specific named ligaments, and the function of the posterior musculature is less important to stability than at the anterior aspect of the shoulder. The prime posterior stabilizer is the anterior inclination of the glenoid articular surface. Perhaps because of this lack of specific pathology, surgical repairs are less reliable than for anterior instability. This difficulty is compounded by the relative infrequency of the problem and the inexperience of most surgeons in correcting it.

Surgical techniques generally consist of bony operations, soft-tissue operations, or a combination of both. The posterior glenoid osteotomy is carried out by first detaching the external rotators from the humeral head. The neck of the glenoid is cut partially through with an osteotome and then levered forward, increasing the anterior inclination of its surface. It is propped open using a bone graft from the posterior acromion or the iliac crest. This procedure is technically demanding and care must be taken to avoid completely cutting across the neck or cracking the osteotomy into the glenoid articular surface. It is recommended for those patients in whom the primary deficit is felt to be relative retroversion of the glenoid.

A second bony correction can be carried out by taking a block of bone from the posterior iliac crest and attaching it to the posterior glenoid neck in such a way that it overhangs the humeral head thus providing a buttress against subluxation (Fig. 20). This technique has been used with good, though certainly not universal, success. One patient who incorporated the graft radiologically presented 3 years after surgery with recurrent symptoms. On examination, the humeral head could be seen sliding laterally over the graft before it subluxated out posteriorly.

Soft-tissue procedures have also been described. These are generally procedures which either overlap or shift a redundant posterior capsule. They also have a high rate of recurrence, in part related to the poor quality of the tissue normally found at the back of the shoulder.

Summary

Posterior subluxation is the most common form of posterior instability of the shoulder. While many patients can easily demonstrate their instability, difficult cases may need specialized radiography or even examination under anaesthesia before a diagnosis can be made. Strengthening exercises are often curative and should

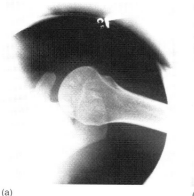

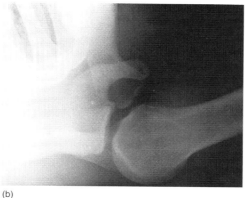

(a)

(b)

Fig. 19 Posterior subluxation. Modified axillary views of a patient able to subluxate his shoulder voluntarily by positioning his arm and contracting his muscles. (a) Reduced position: note the anterior attitude of the articular surface, and the close proximity of the head to the coracoid process. (b) Subluxated: the articular surface is now posterior to the glenoid and the greater tuberosity appears to lie in the glenoid fossa. The space between the coracoid process and humeral head is increased owing to the posterior translation of the head.

be attempted before any surgical procedure is undertaken. Repair is only for patients with functional disability. Failure of operative techniques with the resultant recurrence of subluxation is much more common in posterior than anterior repairs.

Chronic dislocation

For the purposes of the following discussion a shoulder will be considered chronically dislocated after a period of 3 weeks. This arbitrary cut-off point is used as there is no general consensus available in the literature. The common presenting complaint is lack of range of motion, with pain only on attempted movement.[55] The most common cause of a missed posterior dislocation is the omission of an axillary radiograph, whereas the most common cause of a missed anterior dislocation is the lack of any radiographs. Many of these patients are referred late after being treated for varying amounts of time as frozen shoulders. Treatment of the dislocation must be individualized and considered in relation to the patient's symptoms, age, and disability.

Presentation

The physician must be alert to the diagnosis in any patient with chronic limitation in range of shoulder movement. A history of seizure, electroshock therapy, multiple trauma, or alcoholism should raise suspicion. In addition, the elderly always seem to be at risk of neglect of acute problems.

Rowe and Zarins[56] have suggested simple tests designed to identify the unreduced shoulder.

1.   Flex both elbows to 90 degrees: this manoeuvre will show the

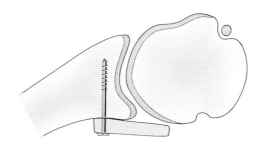

Fig. 20 Posterior bone-block procedure for recurrent posterior instability. The rectangular graft is taken from the iliac crest or the posterior acromion and attached to the posterior glenoid. By slightly overlapping the head of the humerus it acts as a buttress against posterior translation.

rotational limitation characteristic of chronic dislocation. Patients dislocated posteriorly will have marked internal rotation deformities. This deformity is further demonstrated by flexing the shoulder forward and asking the patient to turn the palm upwards. While the forearms will supinate, the internal rotation deformity of the humerus keeps the palm facing medially. The patient dislocated anteriorly will be locked in external rotation. This is even more disabling than an internal rotation contracture as the patient will be unable to bring the hand to their head for grooming or eating, or to their back for personal hygiene.

2.   Observe the patient from above. Comparison of the contralateral shoulder will demonstrate a fullness anteriorly or posteriorly depending on the direction of the dislocation. This may be made more dramatic by the disuse atrophy of the shoulder girdle which often accompanies the chronic deformity.

3.   Palpate the angle of the scapula as the shoulder is manipulated. As the humeral head is usually locked against the glenoid, the scapula will be felt to move in unison with the humerus.

4.   Radiography: a full trauma series is indicated with particular emphasis on the axillary view. The most probable cause of a missed dislocation is an incomplete or absent radiological investigation at the time of the original injury. Although stated at the outset, this point merits repetition.

Examination of the patient must also include a complete neurological assessment. The axillary nerve may have been damaged at the time of injury or by continued pressure placed on it by the dislocated head. Injuries to the median and ulnar nerve have also been reported.

Treatment

Treatment is dependent on the patient's needs. The age of the dislocation must be established. In shoulders dislocated for more than 6 months the viability of the articular cartilage is questionable and total joint arthroplasty has to be considered.

Posterior dislocations are usually complicated by the presence of a posterior impaction fracture. The presence and size of such fractures will determine the therapeutic course and can be assessed by axillary views or CT scanning.

The following recommendations can be made with regard to treatment.

1. For defects less than 20 per cent of the articular surface, an attempt at gentle closed reduction should be made, followed by open reduction if unsuccessful. Undue force is absolutely contraindicated in the closed reduction. Damage to vascular structures can lead to disastrous complications. In addition, the bone will be osteoporotic and easily fractured. Postreduction, some authors suggest transarticular fixation with screws and pins.[55] However, Rowe and Zarins[56] suggest that the arm be immobilized at the patient's side with the humerus in slight extension for 4 to 6 weeks. This modification simplifies care and does not seem to affect the outcome adversely.

2. For defects between 20 and 40 per cent, open reduction and transfer of the subscapularis tendon into the defect is advised. This technique was described by McLaughlin in 1952.[19]

3. For defects greater than 40 per cent of the articular surface, or for any dislocations older than 6 months, an arthroplasty is indicated. If the glenoid is intact a hemiarthroplasty will suffice. Otherwise total shoulder arthroplasty will be required.

Patients with untreated anterior dislocation can be managed similarly. In the anterior dislocation, however, the main complicating factor is erosion of the anterior glenoid rim. This may require reconstruction by a total shoulder arthroplasty, with or without bone grafting.[57] A concomitant tear of the rotator cuff may also be present, requiring repair at the time of reduction. While recurrence of posterior instability is rare, reconstruction of anterior capsular structures may be required to combat recurrent anterior instability.[57]

Those who refuse treatment may still obtain reasonable results. Rowe and Zarins[56] reported eight shoulders treated in this way with one good, four fair, and three poor results. However, the same study demonstrated superior results in patients receiving active care.

Summary

An ounce of prevention is worth a pound of cure. Almost all chronic dislocations can be avoided through proper radiographic evaluation. Once established, the problem will tax even the most experienced surgeon. Proper treatment demands careful assessment of the patient's needs and a skilled pair of hands.

Multidirectional instability

While awareness of shoulder instability dates back to the time of the Pharaohs,[1] Neer and Foster, in 1980, were the first to recognize multidirectional instability.[58] Although not as common as anterior instability alone, it is by no means rare. Missing a patient with multidirectional instability and treating them for a unidirectional instability is a frequent cause of surgical failure.[21,54] Inferior subluxation is the hallmark of multidirectional instability.[11]

Presentation

The patient with multidirectional instability may present primarily with an anterior or posterior pattern of recurrent instability. There may be an antecedent history of trauma or repetitive overuse injuries. The latter is common in sports requiring extreme flexibility such as gymnastics or swimming. In addition, patients often manifest signs of inherent ligamentous laxity in joints other than the shoulder. Genetic disorders which cause systemic ligamentous laxity, such as the Ehlers–Danlos syndrome, should alert the physician to the possibility of multidirectional instability. As well as the usual manifestations of instability, the patient may complain of a dull ache in the arm when it hangs at the side or with overhead use. Carrying heavy objects may be uncomfortable. Patients with multidirectional instability sometimes describe vague intermittent paraesthesiae, leading the observer to suspect emotional or psychiatric disorders.[21]

Physical examination

The cardinal feature of multidirectional instability is inferior laxity. This can be documented by producing a positive sulcus sign. The patient sits with the arm comfortable at their side and the shoulder completely relaxed. The examiner grasps the elbow and pulls downwards using steady, firm pressure. A dimple or gap will form at the edge of the acromion process in affected individuals. This dimple is caused by the inferior subluxation of the humeral head and resultant negative pressure in the subacromial space. Multidirectional instability can occur as anteroinferior, posteroinferior, or a combined anterior, posterior, and inferior instability.

Treatment

The initial management of multidirectional instability should be conservative. Neer[21] recommends repeated examinations over a 1-year period combined with an aggressive strengthening programme before any consideration of surgery. The patient's emotional stability, motivation, and actual disability should be carefully evaluated during this period. Once a surgical approach has been chosen, the procedure must be able to deal with the combined elements on an individual patient basis. Neer's capsular shift operation has been designed with this aim in mind.[58] It can be performed from an anterior approach to correct anteroinferior instability, or from behind for posteroinferior instability. For tridirectional instability a combined anterior and posterior approach can be used.

Surgical repairs may fail for the following reasons.

1. The surgery is instituted for the wrong pathology. The identification of multidirectional instability does not imply that it is causing the patient's symptoms. The complaints may be vague and non-specific. Associated skeletal pathology, including rotator-cuff tendinitis or acromioclavicular arthritis, may be the primary cause of symptoms. Correction of multidirectional instability without addressing the primary pathology will result in continuing symptoms.

2. The surgery corrects one element of the instability while failing to correct instability in another direction.

3. The surgery corrects one element of the instability and either increases another element of the instability or forces the shoulder to remain subluxated in a secondary direction. For example, a patient with combined anterior, posterior, and inferior multidirectional instability who undergoes a

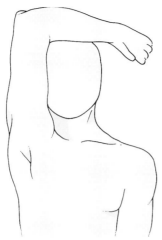

Fig. 21 Luxatio erecta. The classic hyperabducted position of the arm in an inferior dislocation of the shoulder.

Putti–Platt repair may develop an internal rotation contracture forcing the head to remain posteriorly subluxated.

Summary

The patient with multidirectional instability presents a diagnostic and therapeutic challenge. The physician must identify all the components of the instability, decide which patients require surgery, and then address all demonstrable pathology. An error at any one stage may result in failure.

Inferior instability

Luxatio erecta

Direct inferior dislocation of the shoulder, luxatio erecta, is exceedingly rare and must be differentiated from inferior subluxation. The latter is commonly seen after shoulder injury. In luxatio erecta the humeral head dislocates directly inferiorly, lodging in a completely inverted position relative to its normal anatomy. The head is directed downwards and the humeral shaft upwards. The incidence of such a dislocation is so small that it has not been calculated in the literature. It can occur at any age and has a marked predisposition for men, with 92 per cent of all recorded cases occurring in males.[59] The mechanism of injury is hyperabduction of the arm. The humerus comes into contact with the acromion as the arm is fully elevated, and with continued abduction this bony prominence acts as a fulcrum, levering the humeral head out of the glenoid. The patient presents with the arm fully abducted, the elbow flexed, and the hand and forearm resting on the patient's head (Fig. 21).

Pre- and postreduction radiographs are important since luxatio erecta has a very high incidence of associated injury including fractures about the shoulder.[60] Reduction is usually easy using a traction–countertraction technique. With the patient supine, a sheet is passed over the top of the affected side to keep the patient from sliding upwards. The shoulder is hyperabducted gently and pulled upwards. Reduction with an audible click signifies that the head has returned to the glenoid and the arm can be brought to the side.

Mallon *et al.*[59] have suggested the use of fluoroscopy to ensure that the head has been reduced prior to lowering the arm. This may be useful but is not mandatory. Fractures of the tuberosity are common but are usually reduced anatomically. Other fractures reported include the acromion, the glenoid, the body of the scapula, and osteochondral fractures of the humeral head. Neurological injury is very common. A literature search of 80 patients revealed an overall incidence of 59 per cent,[59] with the axillary nerve being most commonly involved. Spontaneous resolution over a period of months is to be expected. Injury to the rotator cuff is also possible, and postreduction evaluation and follow-up are necessary. Vascular injury, while not common, is more likely to occur in luxatio erecta than in any other dislocation. As stated in previous sections, any suspicion of vascular compromise should be evaluated immediately by clinical examination, Doppler studies, and, if necessary, an arteriogram. Postreduction immobilization is suggested for 4 weeks, although the literature does not report a single case of recurrence.

Inferior subluxation

Inferior subluxation is a clinical entity totally unrelated to luxatio erecta. The patient has usually sustained a trauma to the shoulder, either bony or soft tissue, and presents over a period of days to weeks with gradual inferior drooping of the shoulder. On occasion, this may be seen in the emergency room at the time of the initial trauma. A sulcus sign may develop and radiography will reveal the humeral head partially subluxated from the glenoid fossa in an inferior direction. There is never a component of anterior or posterior displacement. This situation is distinct from the patient with multidirectional instability who may show inferior subluxation, but only with stress downwards on the arm. The incidence of inferior subluxation postfracture may be as high as 10 to 20 per cent.[61] It may also occur in patients with neurological lesions (axillary and others) about the shoulder. It has been suggested that the aetiology is an inhibition of shoulder musculature by pain or paralysis, although solid documentation is lacking. The natural history of the condition is spontaneous reduction and recovery over a period of weeks to months, depending on the underlying associated pathology. However, it should be noted that in the non-traumatic situation, inferior subluxation has been associated with more ominous pathology including Pancoast's tumour of the lung.[62] A careful history should easily exclude the latter.

Labral disorders

Labral disorders can occur alone or in combination with instability of the shoulder. The former presents with painful clicking or locking of the shoulder, often with overhead activities. Physical examination may demonstrate the painful click with manipulation of the shoulder. Diagnosis can be confirmed by a CT arthrography, by MRI (with or without intra-articular gadolinium), or by arthroscopy. Care must be taken to differentiate these patients from those who have glenohumeral instability with associated labral lesions. If the shoulder is stable when examined under anaesthesia, arthroscopic debridement may be an easy and effective means of treatment.[63,64] If the shoulder is unstable, arthroscopic debridement has a high failure rate[65,66] and may even increase pre-existing instability.[67] Stable lesions are usually located in the superior labral margin, while those associated with instability are usually located anteroinferiorly.[64,68]

Habitual and voluntary dislocation

An undefined percentage of patients presenting with glenohumeral instability will be able to demonstrate their instability voluntarily during clinical examination. Subsequent care of these patients can be simplified by dividing them into several subgroups.

The habitual or wilful dislocator

This group of patients can usually dislocate or subluxate their shoulder anteriorly. The dislocation and subsequent reduction are painless and cause the patient little consternation. Approximately 50 per cent will be shown to have psychiatric or emotional problems.[33] This subset has been shown to have a much lower incidence of the usual pathological lesions associated with recurrent anterior instability.[69] Careful assessment of the patient's emotional stability and motivation are important. Surgical results in this group are universally poor. A determined patient will be able to undo almost anything that can be done to stabilize the joint. Also, narcotic addicts sometimes develop the ability to dislocate their shoulder in the hope of receiving intravenous medication. Patients who present repeatedly to the emergency room with dislocations should be evaluated carefully for stigmata of drug dependency.

Voluntary anterior dislocators

The subgroup may be difficult to differentiate from the wilful dislocator without a full psychiatric evaluation. However, once defined, this group will respond well to physiotherapy. Those who fail in conservative treatment should be considered as surgical candidates and can be expected to have results similar to the general population.[33]

Voluntary posterior subluxation

This subgroup is distinct from the anterior voluntary stability group. Patients with recurrent posterior subluxation are able to demonstrate their instability by muscular contraction or by positioning of the arm. They should not be considered emotionally unstable, and treatment can proceed as discussed in the section on Recurrent posterior subluxation.

References

1. Rockwood CA, Green DP. *Fractures.* Philadelphia: JB Lippincot, 1975.
2. Jobe FW. Unstable shoulders in the athlete. *American Academy of Orthopedic Surgeons Instructional Course Lectures* 1985; **34**: 228–31.
3. Brockbank W, Griffiths DL. Orthopedic surgery in the sixteenth and seventeenth centuries. *Journal of Bone and Joint Surgery* 1948; **30B**: 365–75.
4. Kroner K, Lind T, Jensen J. The epidemiology of shoulder dislocations. *Archives of Orthopedic and Trauma Surgery* 1989; **108**: 288–90.
5. Simonet WT, Melton LJ III, Cofield RH, Ilstrup DM. Incidence of anterior dislocation in Olmstead County, Minnesota. *Clinical Orthopedics and Related Research* 1984; **186**: 186–91.
6. Rowe CR. Prognosis in dislocation of the shoulder. *Journal of Bone and Joint Surgery* 1956; **38A**: 957–77.
7. Johnson JR, Bayley JLL. Early complications of acute anterior dislocation of the shoulder in the middle-aged and elderly patient. *Injury* 13: 431–4.
8. Daulton SE, Snyder SJ. Glenohumeral instability. *Baillière's Clinical Rheumatology* 1989; **3**: 511–34.
9. Hawkins RJ, Bell RM. Posterior instability of the shoulder. *American Academy of Orthopedic Surgeons Instructional Course Lectures* 1989; **38**: 211–15.
10. O'Brien SJ, Warren RF, Schwartz E. Anterior shoulder instability. *Orthopedic Clinics of North America* 1987; **18**: 395–408.
11. Norris TR. Diagnostic techniques for shoulder instability. *American Academy of Orthopedic Surgeons Instructional Course Lectures* 1985; **34**: 239–57.
12. Gibb TD, Sidles JA, Harryman DT, McQuade KJ, Matsen FA. The effect of capsular venting on glenohumeral laxity. *Clinical Orthopaedics and Related Research* 1991; **268**: 120–7.
13. Matsen FA, Harrymon DT, Sidles JA. Mechanics of glenohumeral instability. *Clinics in Sports Medicine* 1991; **10**: 783–8.
14. Pagnani MJ, Deng XH, Warren RF, Torzilli PA, Altchech DW. Effect of lesions of the superior portion of the glenoid labrum on the glenohumeral translation. *Journal of Bone and Joint Surgery* 1995; **77A**: 1003–10.
15. Bankart ASB. The pathology and treatment of recurrent dislocation of the shoulder joint. *British Journal of Surgery* 1938; **26**: 23–9.
16. Tullos HS, Bennett JB, Brayly WG. Acute shoulder dislocations; factors influencing diagnosis and treatment. *American Academy of Orthopedics Surgery Instructional Course Lectures* 1984; **33**: 364–85.
17. Hill HA, Sachs MD. The grooved defect of the humeral head. A frequently seen unrecognized complication of dislocation of the shoulder joint. *Radiology* 1940; **35**: 690–700.
18. Rozing PM, De Bakker HM, Obermann WR. Radiographic views in recurrent anterior shoulder dislocation. *Acta Orthopaedica Scandinavica* 1986; **57**: 228–30.
19. McLaughlin HL. Posterior dislocation of the shoulder. *Journal of Bone and Joint Surgery* 1952; **34A**: 584–90.
20. Schwartz E, Warren RF, O'Brien SJ, Fronek J. Posterior shoulder instability. *Orthopedic Clinics of North America* 1987; **18**: 409–19.
21. Neer CS II. Involuntary inferior and multi-directional instability of the shoulder; etiology, recognition and treatment. *American Academy of Orthopedic Surgeons Instructional Course Lectures* 1985; **34**: 232–8.
22. Oppenheim WL, Dawson EG, Quinlan C, Graham SA. The cephaloscapular projection. *Clinical Orthopedics and Related Research* 1985; **195**: 191–3.
23. Horsfield D, Stutley J. The unstable shoulder—a problem solved. *Radiography* 1988; **54**: 74–6.
24. Hawkins RJ, Bell RH, Hawkins RH, Koppert GJ. Anterior dislocation of the shoulder in the older patient. *Clinical Orthopedics and Related Research* 1986; **206**: 192–5.
25. Pappas AM, Goss TP, Kleinman PK. Symptomatic shoulder instability due to lesions of the glenoid labrum. *American Journal of Sports Medicine* 1983; **11**: 279–88.
26. Seeger LL. Magnetic resonance imaging of the shoulder. *Clinical Orthopedics and Related Research* 1989; **244**: 48–59.
27. Tsai JC, Zlatkin MB. Magnetic resonance imaging of the shoulder. *Radiologic Clinics of North America* 1990; **28**: 279–91.
28. Holt RG, Helms CA, Steinbach L, Neumann C, Munk PL, Genant HK. Magnetic resonance imaging of the shoulder; rational and current applications. *Skeletal Radiology* 1990; **19**: 5–14.
29. Habibian A, Stauffer A, Resnick D, Reicher MA, Rafii M, Kellerhouse L, Zlatkin MB, Newman C, Sartoris DJ. Comparison of conventional and computed arthrotomography with MRI imaging in the evaluation of the shoulder. *Journal of Computer Assisted Tomography* 1989; **13**: 968–75.

30. Johnson PH. Recurrent subluxation of the shoulder. *Journal of the Arkansas Medical Society* 1988; **84**: 335–7.

31. Hastings DE, Coughlin LP. Recurrent subluxation of the glenohumeral joint. *American Journal of Sports Medicine* 1981; **9**: 352–5.

32. Kumar VP, Balasubramanian P. The role of atmospheric pressure in stabilizing the shoulder. *Journal of Bone and Joint Surgery* 1985; **67B**: 720–1.

33. Goss TP. Anterior glenohumeral instability. *Orthopedics* 1988; **11**: 87–95.

34. Cofield RH, Kavanagh BF, Frassica FJ. Anterior shoulder instability. *American Academy of Orthopedic Surgeons Instructional Course Lectures* 1985; **34**: 210–27.

35. Plummer D, Clinton J. The external rotation method for reduction of acute shoulder dislocation. *Emergency Medicine Clinics of North America* 1989; **7**: 165–75.

36. Beattie TF, Steedman DJ, McGowan A, Robertson CE. A comparison of the Kocher and Milch techniques for acute anterior dislocations of the shoulder. *Injury* 1986; **17**: 349–52.

37. Rollinson PD. Reduction of shoulder dislocations by the hanging method. *South African Medical Journal* 1988; **73**: 106–7.

38. Poulsen SR. Reduction of acute shoulder dislocations using the Eskimo technique: a study of 23 consecutive cases. *Journal of Trauma* 1988; **28**: 1382–3.

39. Rowe CR, Southmayd WW, Patel D. The Bankart procedure—a long term end result study. *Journal of Bone and Joint Surgery* 1978; **60A**: 1–16.

40. Rowe CR. Acute and recurrent anterior dislocations of the shoulder. *Orthopedic Clinics of North America* 1980; **11**: 253–70.

41. Zarins B, Rowe C. Current concepts in the diagnosis and treatment of shoulder instability in athletes. *Medicine and Science in Sports and Exercise* 1984; **16**: 444–8.

42. Rowe CR. Recurrent anterior transient subluxation of the shoulder. *Orthopedic Clinics of North America* 1988; **19**: 767–72.

43. Kiviluoto O, Pasila M, Jaroma H, Sundholm A. Immobilization after primary dislocation of the shoulder. *Acta Orthopaedica Scandinavica*, 1980; **51**: 915–19.

44. Hovelius L. Anterior dislocation of the shoulder in teenagers and young adults. *Journal of Bone and Joint Surgery* 1987; **69A**: 393–9.

45. Samilson RL, Prieto V. Dislocation arthropathy of shoulder. *Journal of Bone and Joint Surgery* 1983; **65A**: 456–60.

46. Sutro CJ, Sutro W. Delayed complications of treated reduced recurrent anterior dislocations of the humeral head in young adults. *Bulletins of the Hospital for Joint Diseases* 1982; **42**: 187–216.

47. Levine WN, Richmond JC, Donaldson WR. Use of the suture anchor in open Bankart reconstruction. *American Journal of Sports Medicine* 1994; **22**: 723–6.

48. Richmond JC, Donaldson WR, Fu F, Harner CD. Modification of the Bankart reconstruction with a suture anchor. *American Journal of Sports Medicine* 1991; **19**: 343–6.

49. Hawkins RJ. Arthroscopic stapling repair of shoulder instability: A retrospective study of 50 cases. *Journal of Arthroscopic and Related Surgery* 1989; **5**: 122–8.

50. Green MR, Christensen KP. Arthroscopic Bankart procedure: two to five year follow-up with clinical correlation to severity of glenoid labral lesion. *American Journal of Sports Medicine* 1995; **23**: 276–81.

51. Walch G, Boileau P, Levigne C, Mandrino A, Negret P, Donell S. Arthroscopic stabilization of recurrent anterior shoulder dislocation: results of 59 cases. *Arthroscopy* 1995; **11**: 173–9.

52. May VR. Posterior dislocation of the shoulder. Habitual, traumatic and obstetrical. *Orthopedic Clinics of North America* 1980; **11**: 271–85.

53. Hawkins RJ, McCormack RG. Posterior shoulder instability. *Orthopedics* 1988; **11**: 101–7.

54. Fronek J, Warren RF, Bowen M. Posterior subluxation of the glenohumeral joint. *Journal of Bone and Joint Surgery* 1989; **71A**: 205–16.

55. Neviaser TJ. Old unreduced dislocations of the shoulder. *Orthopedic Clinics of North America* 1980; **11**: 287–94.

56. Rowe CR, Zarins B. Chronic unreduced dislocations of the shoulder. *Journal of Bone and Joint Surgery* 1982; **64A**: 494–505.

57. Hawkins RJ. Unrecognized dislocation of the shoulder. *American Academy of Orthopedic Surgeons Instructional Course Lectures* 1985; **34**: 258–63.

58. Neer CS II, Foster CR. Inferior capsular shift for involuntary inferior and multi-directional instability of the shoulder. *Journal of Bone and Joint Surgery* 1980; **62A**: 897–908.

59. Mallon WJ, Bassett FH III, Goldrev RD. Luxatio erecta: the inferior glenohumeral dislocation. *Journal of Orthopedic Trauma* 1990; **4**: 19–24.

60. Saxema K, Stavas J. Inferior glenohumeral dislocation. *Annals of Emergency Medicine* 1983; **12**: 718–20.

61. Yosipovitch Z, Goldberg I. Inferior subluxation of the humeral head after injury to the joint. *Journal of Bone and Joint Surgery* 1989; **71A**: 751–3.

62. Lev-Toaff AS, Karasick D, Rao VM. Drooping shoulder—nontraumatic cause of glenohumeral subluxation. *Skeletal Radiology* 1984; **12**: 34–6.

63. Terry GC, Friedman SJ, Uhl TL. Arthroscopically treated tears of the glenoid labrum. *American Journal of Sports Medicine* 1994; **22**: 504–12.

64. Scarpinato DF, Bramhall JP, Andrews JR. Arthroscopic management of the throwing athlete's shoulder: Indications, techniques and results. *Clinics of Sports Medicine* 1991; **10**: 913–27.

65. Andrew JR, Kupferman SP, Dillnon CJ. Labral tears in throwing and racquet sports. *Clinics in Sports Medicine* 1991; **10**: 901–11.

66. Payne L. Tears of the glenoid labrum. *Orthopaedic Review* 1994; **23**: 557–83.

67. Altcheck DW, Russell WF, Wickiewicz TL, Ortiz G. Arthroscopic labral debridement. *American Journal of Sports Medicine* 1992; **20**: 702–6.

68. Glasgon SG, Bruce RA, Yacobucci GN, Torg JS. Arthroscopic resection of glenoid labral tears in the athlete: a report of 29 cases. *Arthroscopy* 1992; **8**: 48–54.

69. Rosaaen BJ, De Lisa JA. Voluntary shoulder dislocation: case study. *Archives of Physical Medicine and Rehabilitation* 1983; **64**: 326–8.

4.3.3 Injuries of the rotator cuff

Mario M. Berkowitz, Mark K. Bowen, and Russell F. Warren

Introduction

The shoulder plays an important role in the performance of nearly all athletic activities. There are many popular sports in which repetitive overhead motion is critical. This activity is well tolerated by most participants; however, in some the stresses are extreme and the repetition may result in injury. Pain and dysfunction may result and limit effective participation. Shoulder disability in the athlete is frequently related to injury to, or to alterations in the function of, the rotator cuff.

Rotator cuff injury in the general population has been attributed to attritional degeneration that usually occurs over several years. The impingement syndrome has been implicated and the continuum of the pathological process has been well described.[1,2] Rotator cuff tears frequently represent the end result of this process and most commonly occur after the fifth or sixth decades. The cuff often tears following minimal trauma in an area weakened by the degenerative process.

Rotator cuff injuries in the athlete appear to result from several different pathological processes. They are commonly seen in sports requiring repetitive overhead motions such as swimming, baseball, volleyball, and tennis. The repetitive, forceful overhead motions that take place injure the rotator cuff by creating high loads within the tendon. Cuff injury may be related to overuse with fatigue, collagen failure with progressive attrition of the tendon(s), and to instability.

The role of glenohumeral instability in rotator cuff injury has received increased attention recently.[3,4] When the static restraints of the bony and capsuloligamentous anatomy of the glenohumeral joint are exceeded, the rotator cuff may be subjected to high eccentric loads. Less commonly, an acute macrotraumatic injury may be the mechanism of cuff disruption. Impingement, or mechanical compression, in the athlete is now felt to occur more commonly as a secondary condition related to tendon fatigue, failure due to high loads, or increased glenohumeral translations that occur with instability and associated posterior capsular contracture (Suzuki *et al.* 1996, unpublished data). In some young patients coracoacromial arch anatomy plays some pathological role, but it is much less frequent than in patients over the age of 40.

Anatomy

The rotator cuff comprises four muscles (supraspinatus, infraspinatus, teres minor, and subscapularis), whose musculotendinous insertions envelope the humeral head. The insertion of the supraspinatus contains an area of relative risk for injury due to its blood supply (Fig. 1). In 1939, Lindblom and Palmer[5] demonstrated that there are areas of decreased vascularity near the insertion of the supraspinatus tendon. Moseley and Goldie[7] described this as a 'critical zone' or watershed area where vessels in the muscle belly anastomose with those from the insertion. Rothman and Parke[8] showed that this area is hypovascular relative to the remainder of the cuff and suggested that it was prone to degeneration. In 1970, Rathburn and MacNab,[9] using microangiographic techniques, observed that this avascular zone is constant and precedes the development of degenerative changes. They concluded that arm position affects the vascularity of the cuff, with adduction leading to 'wringing out' the blood vessels by compression. The actual importance of this vascular anatomy appears to relate to tendon healing following injury, rather than representing an area of susceptibility to injury.

Rotator cuff function

Motion of the shoulder is the result of complex bony relationships and muscle interactions. The shoulder comprises three joints (the

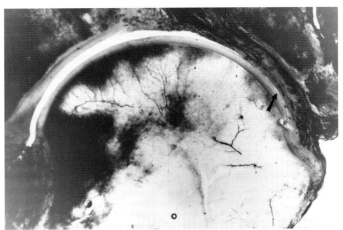

Fig. 1 Injection study of the humeral head and rotator cuff demonstrates the area of decreased vascularity in the tendinous insertion. (Reproduced from ref. 6 with permission.)

sternoclavicular, acromioclavicular, and glenohumeral) and one articulation (the scapulothoracic). While each muscle of the rotator cuff has a specific function in shoulder movement, it appears that the primary function of the entire cuff is to stabilize the glenohumeral joint. The rotator cuff performs this role by generating a joint compressive load with muscle contraction. Poppen and Walker[10] studied the forces at the glenohumeral joint and estimated that the joint reaction force of the 90-degree abducted unweighted arm approached bodyweight. They further analysed rotator cuff function, and observed that the subscapularis and infraspinatus have small lever arms and act at nearly 90 degrees to the glenoid face. The supraspinatus has a slightly larger lever arm, and acts at approximately 80 degrees to the glenoid. They concluded that since these muscles act nearly perpendicular to the glenoid with small lever arms, they function primarily as joint compressors, with the supraspinatus playing a small additional role as an arm abductor.[10] We have also noted that the infraspinatus has a small, but distinct, function as an abductor as well.

The cuff appears to function by creating a stable fulcrum through which the deltoid can act to achieve arm elevation. If rotator cuff function becomes impaired for whatever reason, upward displacement of the humeral head may occur and the normal fulcrum of the head on the glenoid is lost. With superior translation, impingement of the humeral head and the rotator cuff occurs under the acromion. Altchek *et al.*[11] and Paletta *et al.*[12] used radiographic techniques to document the superior migration of the humeral head that occurs in patients with stage II and stage III impingement. We have recently found that superior migration of the humeral head will also occur with fatigue induced by repetitive loading on the Cybex machine (Wickiewicz and Warren, unpublished data).

The most critical function of the shoulder is to elevate the position of the hand. This occurs by way of movement of the scapula on the thorax as well as rotations at the glenohumeral joint. This interaction has been studied extensively by several investigators.[13–16] Poppen and Walker[16] conducted a radiographic analysis of shoulder abduction and found an overall ratio of glenohumeral to scapulothoracic motion of 2:1. In the first 20 degrees of elevation the ratio is approximately 4:1; above this the contribution of the glenohumeral and scapulothoracic motions are almost equal 5:4. We have noted that this ratio is altered in cuff disease, with an increased component from the scapulothoracic region occuring as the arm is elevated (Paletta *et al.*)[12]

Rotator cuff biomechanics: throwing

Overhead motion is an integral part of many sports and is best exemplified by the act of throwing which has been described as occurring in five phases: wind-up, cocking, acceleration, deceleration, and follow-through. Throwing involves a transfer of energy from the body to the arm and the object being propelled. Part of this kinetic energy is absorbed by the rotator cuff. This is seen to the greatest extent during the follow-through phase of throwing where the cuff muscles act eccentrically to decelerate the arm and contain the humeral head on the glenoid surface. At this point the rotator cuff tendons are subjected to high-tensile and compressive forces. The distraction force during follow-through is about 80 per cent of bodyweight. Dillman *et al.*[17] have shown that during the throwing motion, the angular velocity of the arm is 7150 degrees per second as it moves from maximal external rotation to internal rotation. The force of anterior glenohumeral translation at the fully cocked position is calculated at approximately 40 per cent of bodyweight.

The wind-up phase is mostly attributed to activity of the deltoid, while the cocking phase is concluded by activation of the subscapularis and pectoralis major.[18] During the cocking phase, a torque of 17 000 kg/cm is generated. In a skilled athlete the cuff remains relatively quiet during arm acceleration. However, it may be quite active when technique and training are suboptimal. During follow-through the supraspinatus, infraspinatus, and teres minor become active to aid in decelerating the humeral head.

Rotator cuff in athletes

The rotator cuff in the athlete whose chosen sport involves overhead movements is subjected to high repetitive loads. Cuff injury may range from fatigue to primary collagen failure. Aetiologies that have been implicated in rotator cuff injury include overuse, glenohumeral joint instability, acute trauma, and mechanical compression from 'impingement' of the subacromial type (Fig. 2). More commonly it appears that the impingement is intrinsic, as described by Jobe[18] with strain occuring in the supraspinatus and infraspinatus as the arm is positioned at 90 degrees of elevation and 90 degrees of external rotation. In addition to throwing sports, other sports with a

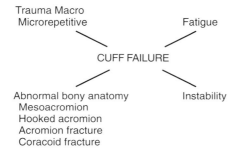

Fig. 2 Diagram demonstrating the many different possible aetiologies of rotator cuff failure.

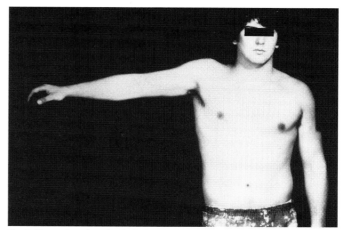

Fig. 3 Young American football player who presented with marked weakness of shoulder abduction 2 weeks after an anterior dislocation. Arthrography revealed a large rotator cuff tear.

high incidence of shoulder pain and dysfunction include tennis, volleyball, swimming, and water polo. Overuse and fatigue due to eccentric loading of the cuff commonly occur in athletes participating in these sports. Of additional interest is the high incidence of suprascapular nerve palsy recently observed in volleyball players.[19]

Competitive swimmers maintain rigorous training schedules, swimming 7 to 20 km/day. Swimmers complete a stroke every 0.6 s and travel through the water at up to 1.9 m/s.[20] Rotator cuff overload and 'tendinitis' are frequently seen, as is associated glenohumeral joint instability and labral damage. Whether instability occurs primarily or becomes more prominent with cuff fatigue and failure is not clear. It is apparent that alterations in glenohumeral joint function lead to mechanical impingement of the cuff and consequent pain. Despite the high incidence of shoulder pain in swimmers, progression to a complete rotator cuff tear is infrequent, although it will occur in some patients.

Similar mechanisms of cuff injury occur in tennis players. In contrast with throwing sports and swimming, tennis is frequently played by an age group with a higher risk of cuff degeneration. It is not uncommon to see tennis players in their forties and fifties with a history of shoulder pain who have progressed to a complete rotator cuff tear.

Although cuff injury in athletes is most frequently the result of microtraumatic overuse, an acute macrotraumatic episode may also be seen as a cause of rotator cuff contusion or disruption. An acute traumatic injury to the cuff may occur in the setting of an anterior shoulder dislocation. This has been referred to as the 'posterior mechanism' of anterior shoulder instability,[21,22] and is explained by the relative weakness of the rotator cuff, caused by attrition, compared with the anterior capsular structures. While this has been seen most frequently in the older athlete, we have treated younger athletes who have sustained a cuff tear with traumatic anterior dislocation. It has also occurred during a game of American football, where a player dislocated his shoulder making a tackle (Fig. 3). Blevins *et al.* recently reported on the senior author's experience (R.F.W.) of this injury in 10 contact athletes (9 professional American-football players) who presented with signs of acute rotator cuff dysfunction following a direct blow to the shoulder.[23]

Surgically verified pathology included rotator cuff contusion, partial-thickness tears, and full thickness tears. The majority of these athletes (9 out of 10) returned to play professional football within 4 months of surgery. These excellent results contrast with the low rate of return to sports of throwers with rotator cuff injury who where treated by acromioplasty and cuff repair. This is probably due to the different mechanism of injury (acute macrotrauma versus repetitive microtrauma) and instability, as well as to the different demands placed on the shoulder in contact versus throwing sports. We have also treated a number of skiers (of various ages) who presented with either a partial or a complete cuff tear following a fall. In most, dislocation did not occur, but rather the mechanism was one of compression as the forces were absorbed by the elbow or hand.

It is important to appreciate that an anterior dislocation associated with an avulsion fracture of the greater tuberosity will generally heal without weakness or recurrent instability providing the tuberosity is well reduced. Impingement, like pain, may persist in patients with a small undisplaced fracture. However, an unrecognized or untreated cuff disruption following a traumatic episode has a poor prognosis for return of function. We recommend that individuals over 40 of age who have persistent pain and weakness after an anterior dislocation be evaluated aggressively for cuff and nerve injury.

Magnetic resonance imaging (**MRI**) is excellent for determining the type and extent of cuff injury. In the rare case where a rotator cuff tear occurs with a nerve injury, we recommend early surgery to repair the rotator cuff and observation of the nerve injury.

Rotator cuff impingement

In an athlete whose sport involves overhead motion, rotator cuff impingement may occur primarily, but more commonly it develops secondary to tendon overload or glenohumeral instability. The classic impingement syndrome, which is well described by Neer,[1,2] is implicated uncommonly in the patient under 30 years of age. Primary impingement is most likely to occur during the cocking phase of the throwing motion as the cuff passes beneath the coracoacromial arch. Bony anatomy may play some role by predisposing to the impingement process; however, irregularities of the coracoacromial arch generally develop as a result of abnormal forces placed on the bone. Variations in acromial anatomy, such as a hooked acromion or os acromiale, may limit the available subacromial space. Bigliani *et al.* observed three different acromial shapes and correlated the presence of a hooked acromion with rotator cuff tears.[24] However, these findings are felt to be developmental and not aetiological. Nevertheless, the study correctly emphasizes that the space beneath the coracoacromial arch may be compromised by anteroinferior acromial osteophyte, arthrotic/hypertrophic changes at the acromioclavicular joint, coracoacromial ligament thickening, and proliferative subacromial bursitis, or by prominence of the greater tuberosity. Rotator cuff tears that occur with primary impingement are associated with mechanical compression, and may be observed on either side of the cuff, although more commonly on the articular side.

While impingement may precede the development of a tear in an 'overhead' athlete, it is more likely that repetitive high loading of the cuff tendons with increased glenohumeral translation during throwing causes the gradual failure of tendon fibres. This may lead to a cycle of inflammation, fatigue, and cuff failure. While tendinitis is a commonly used diagnostic term, inflammation probably plays only a small role in the later stages of cuff injury where collagen degeneration appears to be the primary pathological process.

Cuff dysfunction may result in diminished effective control of the humeral head on the glenoid. This has the potential to stress the cuff further, as continued activity is associated with greater translations and strain of the cuff tendons. Weakness of the cuff results in superior translation of the humeral head, reducing the available space under the coracoacromial arch and encroaching on that necessary for smooth passage of the rotator cuff.[11,12] Thus, in addition to tendon failure, there is also mechanical impingement. Although the impingement process does not generally progress to a complete tear in the young athlete, partial tears are not unusual and a college or professional athlete who continues forceful throwing may complete a tear. Rotator cuff tears due to tendon overload are most frequently seen to develop on the articular side of the cuff.

Instability and cuff injury

The shoulder maintains a uniquely delicate balance between mobility and stability. Static and dynamic factors interact to limit translations of the humeral head on the glenoid. The critical dynamic role of the rotator cuff in providing joint compression has been discussed. The most important components of the static stabilizers are the glenohumeral ligaments. The various ligaments function in a load-sharing manner, and their relative roles vary with arm position, rotation, and direction of applied stress. Excessive translation may occur with injury or failure of the dynamic containment mechanism, or with capsuloligamentous injury. It remains unclear which factor is most critical to glenohumeral stability. It is likely that the static and dynamic restraints function synergistically with varying roles depending on the demands and position of the shoulder. Excessive translation due to failure of static constraints may cause cuff injury by direct mechanical compression or through the increased loads on the cuff that occur during distraction or shear of the humeral head on the glenoid. Tendon failure related to underlying instability is referred to as secondary tensile overload. In simple terms, increased strain is produced in the rotator cuff as it works to limit excessive translation and maintain stability. Recently, Jobe[18] has referred to the articular side cuff failure seen in the supraspinatus of the throwing athlete as internal impingement.[18] This cuff injury is generally secondary to instability. It is noted that when the arm is placed into the position of 90 degrees of elevation with maximal external rotation, the tendon of the supraspinatus lies on the posterosuperior edge of the glenoid and creates strain injury at that site. Excess anterior translation, as with anterior subluxation, will increase the likelihood of injury. In addition, it should be noted that with maximum external rotation there should be a coupled posterior translation of the humeral head on the glenoid. This would have a protective effect on the supraspinatus tendon. Stretching of the posterior inferior glenohumeral ligaments will result in a loss of this coupled motion and cuff injury may result.

Anterior subluxation is the most frequent instability observed in athletes; however, posterior and multidirectional instability are also seen and may represent a group with an underlying predisposition. Throwers are commonly noted to have increased external rotation with a corresponding loss of internal rotation. Increased tension in the posterior capsule may play some role. Harryman *et al.*[25] have shown that tightening of the posterior capsule causes increased anterior translation with arm abduction and flexion. Thus the development of tight posterior structures may increase anterior shear forces in a thrower.

Review of the senior author's experience (R.F.W.) with partial-thickness rotator cuff tears in athletes supports the concept that underlying instability may be the primary pathology (Payne *et al.* 1997).[26] In athletes with increased anterior translation and a normal-appearing subacromial space, arthroscopic tear debridement yielded only 38 per cent satisfactory results and a 25 per cent return to sports. The results in athletes with increased anterior translation and an inflamed subacromial bursa were somewhat better, with 58 per cent satisfactory results and a 50 per cent return to sports. Presently, to improve these results, we will decrease the anterior translation by tightening the anterior capsule.

An athlete with recurrent anterior subluxation may present with the classic description of 'dead arm' symptoms, such as sudden sharp pain and weakness after the arm is abducted and externally rotated as in throwing. These patients frequently have a past history of macrotrauma to the shoulder. Patients with microinstability as the underlying cause of rotator cuff pathology most commonly present with pain related to a specific overhead activity. A sense of movement or looseness of the shoulder may also be described. Characteristic findings on physical examination include a positive impingement sign, posterior shoulder pain, and a relocation test that eliminates the pain. At times, it may be difficult to distinguish between pain with forward elevation (impingement) and pain with apprehension (subluxation). Patients with greater degrees of instability (subluxation) will note apprehension with the arm placed at 90/90. This is also relieved by posterior pressure on the humeral head during the relocation test.

Diagnosis of rotator cuff injuries

History

In the evaluation of athletes with shoulder problems, pain is the most frequent presenting complaint. They may also have complaints as vague as a loss of pitching speed, power, or endurance. Instability other than recurrent dislocation is not usually appreciated by patients. Pain may occur superiorly, but more frequently it is posteriorly localized with the arm at 90 degrees. The pain may radiate down the arm to the area of the deltoid insertion. The pain is generally increased with overhead motion, particularly with the inciting activity. It is helpful to determine at what point in the throwing cycle that pain occurs. Pain during the cocking phase suggests that anterior subluxation may be taking place. Pain on follow-through with the arm flexed, adducted, and internally rotated raises concern over the possibility of posterior instability. Pain at night is quite common in older patients with rotator cuff tears. In younger athletes, pain is mainly experienced during or after activity. Pain frequently diminishes with a period of rest; but without proper rehabilitation it will recur with activity.

A history of trauma to the shoulder can be divided into recurrent microtrauma or macrotrauma, depending on an analysis of the insult to the shoulder. When the onset of symptoms is related to a clear traumatic event it is useful to ascertain the mechanism and the position of the arm at the time of injury. A microtraumatic aetiology is further investigated for details of training, overuse, and technique.

Differential diagnosis

Several pathological processes may present with similar symptoms to those seen with rotator cuff injuries, including neurological conditions such as cervical radiculopathy and brachial plexus or suprascapular nerve injuries. A careful physical examination and an arthrogram or magnetic resonance imaging (MRI) as well as electrodiagnostic studies will often provide sufficient information to clarify the diagnosis. Recurrent glenohumeral subluxation (anterior, posterior, or multidirectional) may cause symptoms that mimic those seen with injury to the rotator cuff. Similarly, it may be difficult to distinguish injuries to the labrum, superior labral anterior posterior lesions (**SLAP** lesions), or abnormalities of the biceps tendon. Examination under anaesthesia may be necessary to detect occult instability. Also, MRI and/or arthroscopic inspection will aid in clarifying the diagnosis. Arthroscopy is currently the best method to confirm internal impingement, since contact of the undersurface of the tendon on the posterosuperior glenoid can be directly visualized. Arthroscopy is also the best way to rule out the presence of a SLAP lesion, which is common in throwers. Recently, with improved MRI techniques we have detected 86 per cent of SLAP lesions preoperatively.[27]

Examination

Examination of the shoulder should begin with an inspection for symmetry, atrophy, and deformities. Infraspinatus atrophy may occur with suprascapular nerve palsy or a large rotator cuff tear. The supraspinatus is more difficult to evaluate for atrophy as it is covered by the trapezius muscle. A rupture of the biceps tendon produces a characteristic bulge in the upper arm with contraction. It is useful to observe patients from behind while they elevate their arms as this may bring out subtle cuff dysfunction as the scapula raises excessively creating what we have called the 'shrug sign' (R.F.W.).

Palpation should begin medially at the sternoclavicular joint and proceed laterally to include the clavicle, the acromioclavicular joint, and the bicipital groove. The greater tuberosity and supraspinatus are palpable just distal to the anterolateral aspect of the acromion with the arm hanging. Tenderness of the acromioclavicular joint is the most reliable indicator of active pathology in the joint. Tenderness in the area of the biceps is not unusual and may be related to mechanical impingement or, rarely, to tensile injury to the biceps tendon. Interpretation of tenderness in this area may be difficult as it may occur in the absence of pathology if palpation is too vigorous.

Range of motion is recorded and compared with the contralateral shoulder. For any deficits in active motion, passive motion should also be evaluated. Motions tested include forward elevation, internal and external rotation at 0 degrees and 90 degrees of abduction. Many athletes, particularly throwers, demonstrate an asymmetrical range of motion, and typically have increased external rotation and a loss of internal rotation. It is not unusual to observe what appears to be a symmetrical increased range of motion in some athletes, particularly swimmers. While joint laxity may contribute to success in their sport, it may also increase their susceptibility to injury.

Muscle strength testing is performed in an attempt to assess the function of individual muscles as well as the cervical nerve roots and brachial plexus. Of particular interest to the evaluation of the rotator cuff is testing forward elevation, external and internal rotation, and biceps strength. Injured tendons will frequently produce pain with eccentric loading.

Stability testing is performed in both the sitting and supine position. The humeral head is manually translated in the anterior and posterior direction on the glenoid using the 'load–shift' manoeuvres as previously reported.[23,28] Inferior instability is evaluated with the 'sulcus sign' test. We grade anterior and posterior translation as follows: 1+, increased translation; 2+, humeral head jumps over the glenoid edge with a grind; 3+, humeral head locks out over the glenoid. Inferior translation or the 'sulcus sign' is graded by the number of millimetres of inferior displacement with respect to the lateral edge of the acromion (1+, < 1 cm; 2+, 1 to 2 cm; 3+, > 2 cm). Apprehension in abduction and external rotation is a sensitive test for anterior subluxation. The relocation test may also be positive. In this test a posteriorly directed force applied while the arm is abducted and maximally externally rotated eliminates previously demonstrated apprehension and/or pain. Some pain may be the result of rotator cuff injury or labral tears. In addition, pain and/or crepitation produced on stressing the shoulder should be noted as it may indicate the presence of a labral injury. Apprehension related to posterior instability with the arm adducted and flexed is less frequent, and is usually present only after an acute instability episode.

There are several 'special tests' that are useful in evaluating the rotator cuff. The impingement sign is positive when pain is produced near terminal forward elevation. Impingement pain may also be elicited with the abduction test by abducting to 90 degrees and internally rotating the arm. The impingement test is performed by injecting approximately 10 ml of a local anaesthetic into the subacromial space. The test is considered positive if the impingement sign is eliminated. While this test can be very useful in localizing the source of pain, it may contribute to confusion over the diagnosis as it may be positive in a patient with impingement secondary to anterior instability of the shoulder. The Speed and Yergusson test may be helpful in localizing pain to the biceps tendon. Injection in the area of the bicipital groove can, at times, provide useful diagnostic information.

SLAP lesions are difficult to prove on examination, but we have found the O'Brien manoeuvre useful. This test is performed with the arm adducted at 90 degrees and internally rotated. Resisted elevation is painful with a SLAP lesion as the superior labrum is compressed. If the arm is supinated the pain is absent.

Diagnostic tests

In the majority of young athletes plain radiographs will be normal. We use an instability series which includes an anteroposterior view in internal and external rotation, a West Point view, and a Stryker notch view.[29] Possible radiographic findings include a Bankart lesion, glenoid erosions, a Hill–Sachs lesion, a Bennett lesion, or ossification abnormalities of the acromion. A coracoacromial arch or outlet view is performed as a trans-scapular lateral of the scapula with the beam tilted caudally approximately 10 degrees. Classic findings of advanced rotator cuff disease include subacromial spurs, acromial hooking, decreased acromiohumeral distance, and sclerosis or cystic changes in the undersurface of the acromion and/or

greater tuberosity. These radiographic findings are uncommon in a young athlete.

Ultrasonography has been used effectively in many centres as a non-invasive method for confirming the presence of a rotator cuff tear.[30–32] However, it has proved to be highly examiner-dependent in terms of sensitivity and specificity, particularly in the diagnosis of incomplete tears.

Arthrography has been the traditional gold-standard with a high sensitivity for detecting full-thickness rotator cuff tears.[33] It has the disadvantage of being an invasive procedure, but may provide other potentially useful information regarding capsule volume and, when combined with a computed tomogram (CT) scan, an excellent view of the glenoid labrum. Visualization of incomplete rotator cuff tears is unreliable but can be improved with double-contrast techniques.[34,35]

MRI is being used increasingly, although several studies have assigned a fairly high sensitivity and specificity to its use,[36–40] one has to be careful not to overestimate the degree of rotator cuff pathology. Large tears of the supraspinatus with retraction could be readily visualized; however, poor quality scans were frequently misinterpreted for partial-thickness tears.[41] Newer technology in software design and surface coils has greatly improved the diagnostic accuracy. MRI can prove invaluable in the diagnostic process, especially in the setting of less-common clinical situations such as partial-thickness cuff tears with labral injury. The advantages of MRI are that it is non-invasive, provides an assessment of location and size of tear, quality, and retraction of tissue, and may delineate other areas of shoulder pathology such as labral tears and SLAP lesions.

In a recent review, held at our institution, to assess prospectively the accuracy of unenhanced MRI of 103 labral tears with arthroscopic confirmation, the sensitivity for a SLAP lesion was 86 per cent, for anterior labral tears 100 per cent, and for posterior labral injury 74 per cent. The specificity was about 95 per cent for each. Presently, we routinely use MRI in the evaluation of cuff disease in the athlete, as we find that this aids prognosis and management.[27]

The role of arthroscopy in the diagnosis and treatment of rotator cuff injuries has increased exponentially during the last two decades. The use of the arthroscope for the primary diagnosis of cuff pathology may prove superfluous. However, arthroscopic examination has become invaluable in the definite diagnosis of other lesions which may coexist with rotator cuff disease. Glenoid labral injury or detachments (SLAP lesions), capsular and glenohumeral ligament complex attenuation, biceps tendon subluxation, focal glenohumeral articular surface cartilage injury, and intra-articular synovitis all may prove difficult or impossible to diagnose with clinical accuracy.[42] Articular and bursal partial-thickness tears of the cuff are easily identified. Evaluation of the subacromial space and coracoacromial ligament may also provide diagnostic information.

As MRI has improved, diagnostic arthroscopy for shoulder pain has become infrequently used. Generally, it is performed for a specific diagnosis with a specific treatment in mind.

Determining cuff tear size

Determination of the size of a rotator cuff tear clinically may be difficult despite a careful physical examination and modern radiographical techniques. A helpful clinical finding is the presence of a significant deficit in external rotation strength. In the absence of limiting pain, such weakness is usually consistent with a large tear involving the infraspinatus in addition to the supraspinatus. MRI provides a clear representation of rotator cuff anatomy and, with improved software, tear size and quality of the tissue remaining have been accurately predicted.

Treatment considerations

Treatment of rotator cuff injuries and symptoms referrable to the rotator cuff is preventive, non-operative, or operative, and may encompass one or all of these modalities. In addition to making an accurate diagnosis it is critical to assess the sport(s), level of participation, and demands placed on the athlete's shoulder. Incorporation of this knowledge will contribute to the development of the most effective treatment programme.

Non-surgical management

Clearly, the most successful treatment for the rotator cuff is prevention, best achieved with an intensive upper and lower extremity conditioning programme and sound technique. Carefully developed off-season and preseason programmes are essential. Several elements are critical: overall body strength and conditioning; upper and lower extremity flexibility; shoulder and rotator cuff strengthening; and an analysis of technique. Fatigue and overuse are probably involved in most rotator cuff injuries. A properly designed programme will produce benefits in endurance and prevention of injury, while inappropriate exercises may actually predispose to injury. Rotation contractures are common in athletes participating in throwing sports and may cause subtle muscular compensations. Stretching is performed to achieve as full and symmetrical a range of motion as possible. The rotator cuff may be strengthened using surgical tubing, isokinetic machines, or free weights. Because the rotator cuff in an 'overhead' athlete functions critically in an eccentric manner, we emphasize exercises that work the rotator cuff eccentrically. The periscapular muscles, including the latissimus dorsi, the rhomboids, the serratus anterior, and the trapezius, create a stable platform for the shoulder joint and are also emphasized in the strengthening programme.

Once a rotator cuff injury is established, the majority will respond to rest, avoidance of painful positions and activities, and a rehabilitation programme that emphasizes stretching and eccentric with concentric strengthening for control of the humeral head and the scapula. The initial phase of therapy is directed at treating the 'tendinitis' with rest, ice, non-steroidal anti-inflammatory medication (NSAIDs), and, infrequently, injection of corticosteroids. Stretching designed to address contractures or limitations of motion is also started early. We are careful not to push stretching to positions of impingement.

As with our preventive therapies, the primary treatment goal is to restore health and strength to the rotator cuff. This may benefit patients who have experienced primary tensile failure of the rotator cuff as well as those with subtle instabilities. Once pain is well controlled and range of motion is restored, strengthening and more sport-specific exercises can progress. The emphasis of the strengthening phase is to improve power, endurance, timing, and muscular control of the arm. Rotator cuff strengthening with internal and external rotation exercises using Theraband scapulothoracic stabilizers (including the serratus anterior, rhomboids, latissimus dorsi,

and trapezius) are also included in the strengthening programme. Trunk and lower extremity exercises are not neglected in the total rehabilitation programme. As symptoms are eliminated and strength improves, activities that develop coordination and propioception are added. Finally, return to overhead sporting activities is begun. Coaching in this phase is critical since a poor throwing technique will lead to the recurrence of pain. Technical problems such as opening too soon, overstriding, and poor foot placement must be addressed by sound coaching.

Surgical management: rotator cuff tears

As discussed earlier, the most predictable and gratifying results in the management of rotator cuff injuries occur with non-operative treatment. While surgical intervention may give excellent results (depending on the underlying pathology), return to overhead sports following any operative procedure is more unpredictable.

Primary tensile failure of the rotator cuff will most probably respond to a non-operative programme such as that outlined above. Surgical intervention in the form of examination under anaesthesia and arthroscopy may be useful diagnostically as well as therapeutically. Debridement of partial cuff tearing may have a therapeutic effect; however, response is more probably related to postoperative rehabilitation than to debridement of failed rotator cuff tissue.

Arthroscopic debridement of the torn rotator cuff in conjunction with arthroscopically assisted subacromial decompression has been applied in a variety of clinical settings. Andrews *et al.* managed 36 patients with partial supraspinatus tears with arthroscopic debridement.[43] They reported an 85 per cent rate of good or excellent results with return to preoperative activity levels. Snyder *et al.* observed a similar outcome in 31 cases.[44] They noted no significant effect of subacromial decompression on the results, and concluded that acromioplasty should be reserved for bursal side partial-thickness tears.

Arthroscopic decompression and debridement has also been used for full-thickness tears of various sizes, with variable results. Gartsman found a 28 per cent failure rate requiring revisional open repair for the treatment of full-thickness tears.[45] However, Levy *et al.* reported an 84 per cent rate of satisfactory results in similar cases.[46] The authors noted that smaller width tears had a better outcome using this technique. Ogilvie-Harris and Demaziere prospectively compared two matched groups of patients with full-thickness tears 1 to 4 cm in width, one treated with arthroscopic decompression and debridement, and the other with open decompression and repair.[47,48] At 2 and 5 years, pain relief, range of motion, and patient satisfaction was similar for both groups. Patients with open repair had better strength and functional capacity. The authors thus recommend debridement for lower demand patients.[47]

Debridement of so-called 'massive' cuff tears has been pursued in both an open and arthroscopic fashion. These tears are often very wide ($\geq$ 5 to 10 cm) with chronically fixed retraction. Rockwood and co-authors recently reported the results of open acromioplasty, subacromial decompression, and debridement of 53 cuff defects wider than 5 cm that could not be adequately mobilized for repair.[49] At minimum 3-year follow-up, 83 per cent had achieved satisfactory pain relief and functional capacity.

The results of purely arthroscopic subacromial decompression and cuff debridement for massive tears have been variable. Burkhart reported 100 per cent pain relief with strength preservation in 10 patients with normal preoperative strength and range of motion.[50] Olsewski and Depew found a 77 per cent rate of satisfactory outcome, mostly in sedentary patients, where pain was the main preoperative symptom.[51] Ellman *et al.* prospectively compared the results of 40 patients with a minimum of 2 years' follow-up.[52] They found a 90 per cent satisfactory outcome in low-demand patients with tear widths of 1 to 2 cm. Larger, 'repairable' tears (2 to 4 cm) correlated with only a 50 per cent rate of satisfactory outcome, while 86 per cent of patients with massive tears had excellent pain relief and were satisfied subjectively with the result. Strength and range of motion were not restored.[35,52] We have previously reported that acromioplasty without cuff repair gave inferior results to cuff repair.

If rotator cuff failure presents as a complete tear, operative repair should be considered for best results in most patients, and particularly in athletes who wish to perform at their usual level. An older athlete might manage by modifying his or her activities; however, pain is frequently a persisting complaint.[53] In the athletic population with an overuse injury the tear is frequently small. When there is a history of significant trauma to the shoulder, a large avulsion-type tear from the insertion site may be encountered. In the older athlete the impingement process may have led to tendon degeneration and a large tear. Despite excellent surgical reconstructive techniques, predicting the success of return to sports participation following rotator cuff repair is difficult.[35,54-56] Results are dependent on the quality of the remaining cuff, tissue retraction, and the adequacy of the repair. Care must be taken not to overtighten the cuff as this may also predispose to failure.

Inspection of the extent and quality of both normal and abnormal portions of the rotator cuff during arthroscopy can prove invaluable for the intra-operative decision-making process. Often, the appropriate surgical plan can only be finalized after obtaining the information gained at arthroscopic examination.

In the case of rotator cuff tears, tear size, thickness, contour, retraction, and mobility, as well as tissue and bone quality are critical in determining the optimal surgical approach and repair plan. If the surgeon wishes to retain the options of a fully arthroscopic or arthroscopically assisted intervention, arthroscopic examination is the only modality that can reliably evaluate all these factors without open exploration.

While impingement has been addressed arthroscopically for some time, increasingly we are applying arthroscopic techniques to the treatment of the rotator cuff tears. Historically, full-thickness cuff tears have been surgically managed with open subacromial decompression, anterior acromioplasty, and direct repair.[57] Codman is credited with the first such repair in 1909.[58] Reviews of patients treated with open, cuff repair techniques have found some variability in results. While Neer reported 91 per cent excellent or satisfactory results,[59] other authors describe pain relief in only 58 to 85 per cent of cases.[60-64] Factors such as tear size, degree of retraction, tissue quality, chronicity, and enrolment in 'Workman's Compensation programs' in the United States have been found to correlate with outcome. Cofield combined the overall results of multiple, open repair series and found an 87 per cent average rate of pain relief, while patient satisfaction averaged 77 per cent.[65]

Arthroscopy has also been successfully applied to the treatment of cuff tears. Modes of intervention may be divided into three realms: fully arthroscopic repair; arthroscopically assisted 'mini-open' repair; and arthroscopic debridement.

Fully arthroscopic repair, with arthroscopic subacromial decompression followed by tear mobilization and fixation with arthroscopically placed, soft-tissue fixation devices such as suture anchors or staples, is presently in the developmental phase (Fig. 4). Johnson has reported on 31 cuff tears treated with arthroscopic repair using a metallic staple, placed under arthroscopic visualization, to fix the reduced tear.[66] Tear size was 4 cm or less, and up to four staples were placed. Routine staple removal following recovery was recommended as a second open procedure. Follow-up arthroscopy on 29 patients at a mean of 4.7 months postrepair demonstrated complete healing in 20 (69 per cent). Of 15 patients who returned for the minimum 2-year follow-up, 14 had good or excellent motion and strength. The author subsequently recommends this technique for 1 to 2-cm wide mobile tears.[66]

Snyder has reported a repair technique using suture anchors and a 'Suture Shuttle Relay' passed through an arthroscopic suture-punch to insert sutures through the tear edges. These sutures then draw the tear edge laterally and fix it to a bony trough created at the humeral articular margin.[67] (Fig. 4) No patient series have, as yet, been published.

Baylis and Wolf recently reported the outcome of 54 full-thickness tears managed with arthroscopically placed sutures and suture-anchors.[68] A 1-year, minimum follow-up revealed an 85 per cent rate of good to excellent results. Arthroscopic evaluation at 5 months postrepair revealed a 70 per cent healing rate in 23 cases.[68]

Arthroscopically assisted 'mini-open' cuff repair is rapidly gaining in popularity.[66,67,69-74] This technique involves arthroscopic subacromial decompression followed by splitting of the deltoid for a distance of 3 to 4 cm laterally over the actual tear to facilitate repair[74] (Fig. 5). Care must be taken to avoid an excessively distal deltoid split, which can endanger the axillary nerve. This technique preserves the anterior deltoid insertion on the acromion, which diminishes the risk of deltoid repair failure inherent in a 'fully-open' approach[75] and may hasten postoperative recovery.[67,69,70-76] Disadvantages include those related to the more-limited exposure: large tears (≥ 3 to 5 cm in width) and tears of the subscapularis or teres minor are difficult to fully visualize, mobilize, and repair.

The results of 'mini-open' repair were first reported by Levy *et al.* in 1990.[71] Of 25 patients followed for a minimum of 1 year, 84 per cent had good or excellent objective clinical results, while 96 per cent were subjectively satisfied. All patients with 'small or moderate' sized tears had a satisfactory clinical result.[71] Multiple reports have since confirmed between 85 and 95 per cent rates of satisfactory clinical and functional outcome.[69,70,72-74,76] These series also agree that the most significant factor affecting results is tear size. Liu and Baker recently retrospectively compared the results of 'fully-open' versus 'mini-open' techniques.[73] They report similar functional results in both groups, but note a more rapid return to full activity in the arthroscopically assisted repairs. Tears less than 1 cm in width had a uniformly excellent outcome in both groups. Tears between 1 and 3 cm in width had a better outcome if treated with a 'mini-open' technique, while tears from 3 to 5 cm in width fared better in the 'fully-open' group.[76]

Blevins *et al.* recently reviewed our institutional experience of 64 patients who underwent 'mini-open' repair.[77] Of these, 61 had full-

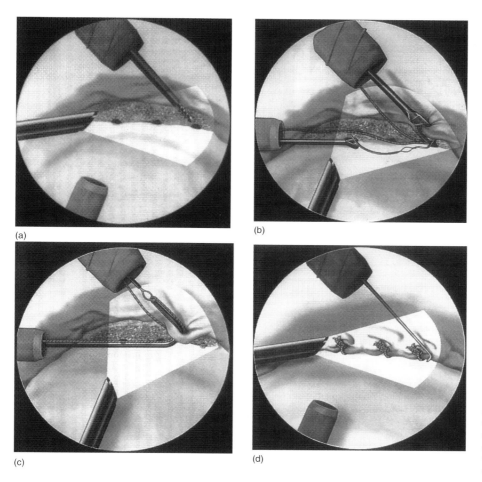

Fig. 4 Fully arthroscopic rotator cuff repair. Arthroscopic view of the rotator cuff tear edge and greater trocanter bony bed. (a) Drilling holes for placing the suture anchors. (b) Suture passing through the tear edges, with a suture punch. (c) Retrieval of suture with a 'suture shuttle relay'. (d) Final result after arthroscopic knot-tying technique.

thickness, and 3 had more than 50 per cent partial-thickness tears. At minimum follow-up of 1 year (mean 29.9 months), a statistically significant improvement in the study cohort's active-extremity elevation, pain, and functional capacity was noted. Clinically detectable cuff weakness was noted in 22 per cent of patients postoperatively versus 83 per cent preoperatively. In all, 89 per cent

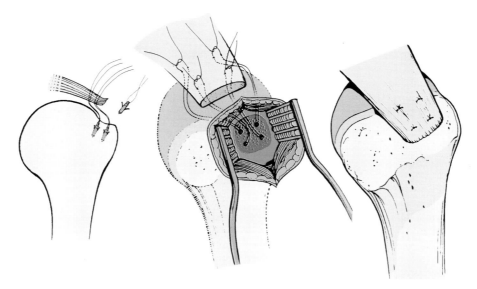

Fig. 5 Arthroscopically assisted 'mini-open' rotator cuff repair. A deltoid splitting approach is used, incorporating the lateral arthroscopy portal. A bony bed has been prepared at the greater tuberosity. Placement of suture anchors in medial and lateral rows.

of patients were subjectively satisfied with their result. No correlation was found between tear size and final Hospital for Special Surgery Shoulder Score.[77]

Indications for rotator cuff arthroscopy

When surgical intervention for cuff dysfunction is deemed appropriate the decision to incorporate arthroscopy in the surgical plan is based on the character of the cuff pathology, the aetiology and duration of the disorder, the patient's physiological profile, and coexistent shoulder pathology.

Given the previously outlined applications of arthroscopy for cuff disease, we incorporate arthroscopy in our surgical plan if:

(1) the exact preoperative clinical diagnosis remains unclear,

(2) coexistent non-cuff pathology amenable to arthroscopic diagnosis or treatment (e.g. SLAP or Bankart lesions, intra-articular loose bodies or synovitis, etc.) is present or suspected on preoperative evaluation, or

(3) the rotator cuff pathology is deemed likely to be amenable to fully arthroscopic or 'mini-open' treatment.

We presently perform glenohumeral and subacromial arthroscopy on the vast majority of patients undergoing surgical procedures for rotator cuff pathology.

Surgical technique

We routinely use interscalene block anaesthesia for shoulder procedures.

Patients are placed on the operating table in the 'beach chair' position. The shoulder is then carefully examined under anaesthesia, passive range of motion and glenohumeral stability are documented.

The upper extremity is prepared and draped in sterile fashion, and shoulder arthroscopic portals established, by principles previously reported.[66,78,79] This is followed by a complete methodical examination of the glenohumeral joint. An attempt is made to document if anterior capsular laxity or redundancy exist. The status of the glenoid and humeral head articular cartilage is noted.

The arm is then placed in the 'rotator cuff position': approximately 45 degrees of forward flexion, 30 to 60 degrees of abduction, and variable external rotation. This relaxes tension on the supra- and infraspinatus portion of the cuff to allow better visualization. The cuff undersurface is carefully inspected and probed. If no tear is present, and outlet impingement is the preoperative diagnosis, all coexistent intra-articular pathology is addressed and subacromial decompression performed if the findings in the subacromial space are diagnostic. The surgeon should see degenerative changes in the superficial cuff and coracoacromial ligament.

While the arthroscope remains in the glenohumeral joint, the size, thickness, tissue quality, and mobility of any cuff tearing is assessed using probes and grasping instruments placed through the anterior and lateral subacromial portals. The lateral portal is established 2 cm lateral to the lateral border of the acromion, and roughly midway between the anterior border and midportion of the acromion. This location is optimized to provide both access to the cuff tear for probing and potential 'mini-open' repair, as well as for subacromial decompression and anterior acromioplasty. A blunt probe is passed through this portal, and on to the bursal surface of the cuff. If a full-thickness tear is present, the probe will pass easily through the tear into the joint. If a partial-thickness tear is present, probing the bursal surface gives the surgeon a sense of tear thickness and remaining tissue quality.

Full-thickness tear edges are debrided to stable tissue with a 4.5-mm, motorized, full-radius resector. Only then may a tear be fully assessed for retraction and mobility. A tear is considered mobile if, with the arm held in neutral rotation at the side of the trunk, the edge of the tear can be grasped with arthroscopic forceps and reduced to the anatomical tendon insertion site.

If a partial-thickness, articular-surface rotator cuff tear is present, the depth and tissue quality are assessed following debridement of any loose, frayed fragments. Tears of less than 30 per cent thickness, with good remaining tissue quality, are debrided to stable tissue using a full-radius resector. Tears of 30 to 50 per cent thickness, that are 1 cm or less in width, in non-athletes, are also debrided to stable tissue. These tears in athletes (particularly in throwing sports) are of concern—they may progress to larger, complete tears—and are repaired via arthroscopically placed sutures. Partial-thickness tears of more than 50 per cent thickness and more than 1 cm in width are similarly repaired arthroscopically or in 'mini-open' fashion in all patients(Figs 4 and 5, respectively).

If a partial-thickness, articular surface cuff tear is of indeterminate depth on probing, a monofilament marking suture is passed through the tear via the lateral subacromial portal. The intra-articular end of the suture is grasped and drawn out through the anterior portal. The two external ends are then clamped and retracted while intra-articular work is completed. During subsequent subacromial arthroscopy, the suture localizes the bursal-surface portion of the tear, which can then be assessed for tissue quality and thickness.

If 'mini-open' cuff repair is contemplated, the eventual bone-bed insertion site for the tear may be prepared with the full-radius resector. All remaining soft tissue and debris is removed from the cortical bone bordered by the articular surface medially, the greater tuberosity laterally, the biceps tendon anteriorly, and the remaining cuff insertion posteriorly. Care is taken to preserve cortical integrity to allow purchase for suture anchors (Fig. 5).

Arthroscopically assisted subacromial decompression is undertaken prior to cuff repair, or as a primary procedure in cases of isolated outlet impingement. Decompression provides three benefits: it reduces the main mechanical source of attritional cuff wear; diminishes shear and compression stress on the repair site; and improves arthroscopic visualization.

Following subacromial decompression, the bursal surface of the rotator cuff is assessed. If the bursa is thickened excessively as often seems the case in throwers it is debrided to expose the rotator cuff. Complete cuff examination can be achieved with rotation and abduction/adduction of the humeral head. Previously placed, partial-tear marking sutures are visualized and the bursal-side cuff surface probed in these areas to rule out occult full-thickness lesions.

Partial-thickness, bursal-sided cuff tears may be present. These are lightly debrided with a shaver or repaired with arthroscopic or 'mini-open' techniques if greater than 30 to 50 per cent of the thickness.

Full-thickness tears generally require repair. Small width (1 to 2 cm), mobile tears are fixed with a fully arthroscopic technique, including abrasion of the anatomical tendon insertion site, placement of one or two suture anchors, and arthroscopic suture-tying techniques (Fig. 4).

Larger tears are characterized through preoperative and arthroscopic evaluation as 'mobile', 'fixed retraction/repairable', or 'fixed retraction/irreparable'. Mobility is assessed as discussed previously with tissue-grasping forceps or retention sutures placed in the cuff through the lateral subacromial portal (Fig. 6). Irreparable is defined as marked tendon retraction to the glenoid, poor remaining cuff-tissue quality, and MRI evidence of marked cuff muscle atrophy.

Mobile tears are treated with 'mini-open' repair. Using an arthroscopic suture-punch placed in the lateral portal (Fig. 6), multiple retention sutures are placed in stout tissue along the debrided edge of the tear. The lateral subacromial portal incision is extended either longitudinal or transversely, exposing the underlying deltoid fascia. The deltoid is then split in line with its fibres directly over the tear (Fig. 5). Care is taken to avoid splitting the deltoid more than 4 cm distal to the lateral border of the acromion to protect the axillary nerve, a self-retaining retractor is useful in maintaining deltoid retraction. The acromioplasty may be confirmed with finger palpation. The rotator cuff tear is exposed and assessed via humeral rotation. Tear mobility may be maximized with blunt intra- and extra-articular dissection using a small elevator.

Two rows of suture anchors are placed in the previously prepared humeral bone bed: one row lies just lateral to the articular surface margin, while the second row lies just medial to the crest of the greater tuberosity. The goal is to create a broad tendon insertion

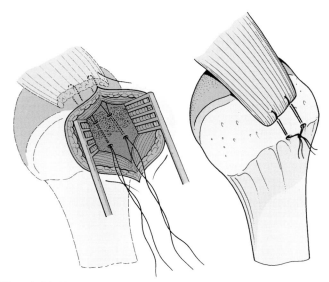

Fig. 7 A deltoid splitting approach is used, incorporating the lateral arthroscopy portal. A bleeding bony bed has been prepared at the greater tuberosity. Sutures placed arthroscopically using a suture punch are secured through drill holes and are tied over a bony bridge.

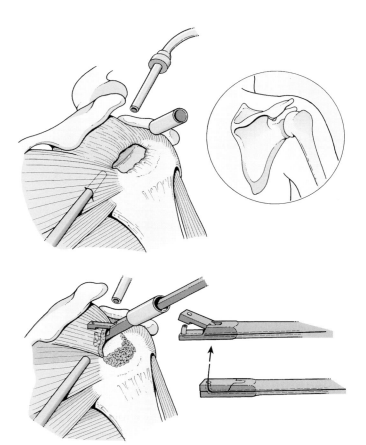

Fig. 6 Arthroscopic-assisted repair of the rotator cuff requires excellent fluid inflow and visualization of the subacromial space. Special suture-passing instruments are used to place sutures in the torn rotator cuff.

rather than the edge inserted in a trough. The site of each anchor is spaced by at least 1 cm of cortical bone to prevent excess stress-riser formation and failure. This requirement determines the number of anchors used (Fig. 5).

Alternatively, if the cortical bone quality cannot support suture anchors, lateral suture tunnels are made in the greater tuberosity using awls and a tenaculum clamp (Fig. 7).

If suture anchors are used, the cuff edge is reduced to the medial edge of the greater tuberosity, and the medial anchor sutures are then passed directly cephalad through the cuff in a vertical mattress fashion. These are not tied at this point. The lateral anchor sutures are then passed through the cuff edge, again in a vertical mattress fashion, and tied with the arm in neutral rotation at the side of the trunk. The medial anchor sutures are then tied. This results in a doubly-reinforced section of the cuff tendon approximated to a bony surface to maximize healing.

Tears classified as 'fixed-retraction/irreparable' are usually massive in size (width, > 5 cm; area > 15 to 20 cm) with retraction to the edge of the glenoid. They are treated with arthroscopic debridement and minimal subacromial decompression, with preservation of the anterior portion of the coracoacromial ligament and its attachment to the acromion. Removal of the coracoacromial ligament and standard acromioplasty on these patients with cuff deficiency may result in anterior superior instability.

If arthroscopic or 'mini-open' repair is contemplated, all coexistent problems, such as labral tears, SLAP lesions, loose bodies, etc. are treated arthroscopically prior to proceeding. If significant anterior or multidirectional instability is present, the rotator cuff lesion is repaired prior to capsular shift, as closure of the tear defect may significantly alter the mechanics of the instability pattern. Repair of the cuff after capsular shift may constrain the joint excessively.

When preoperative evaluation and/or arthroscopic examination evidenced a tear classified as 'fixed-retraction/repairable', we proceed with an open reconstruction. We explore the rotator cuff through a superior approach (Fig. 8). The deltoid is detached along

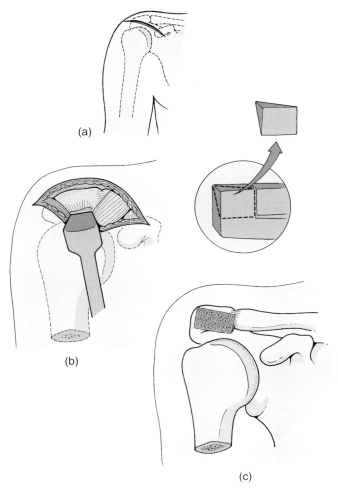

(a)

(b)

(c)

Fig. 8 We explore the rotator cuff through a superior approach. (a) The deltoid is detached along the anterior aspect of the acromion only, from the anterolateral corner to the acromioclavicular joint. (b) A 3-cm longitudinal split is extended along the deltoid fibres from the corner. (c) An anterior acromioplasty is then performed. (Redrawn from ref. 56, with permission.)

the cuff in a vertical mattress fashion (Fig. 5). These are not tied at this point. The lateral anchor sutures are then passed through the cuff edge, again in a vertical mattress fashion, and tied with the arm in neutral rotation at the side of the trunk. The medial anchor sutures are then tied. This results in a doubly reinforced section of the cuff tendon approximated to a bony surface to maximize healing. The biceps is not tenodesed unless it is grossly disrupted. Repair of the anterior deltoid is crucial and should be though drill holes in the acromion.

Large tears, although unusual in the younger athlete, are more common in the older athlete and often present a more challenging and technical problem. This type of patient is represented by the 60-year-old tennis player who plays several days a week and has noticed a loss of power. Plain radiographs may document proximal migration of the humeral head and sclerotic changes in the undersurface of the acromion as well as in the greater tuberosity [80] consistent with a massive rotator cuff tear. In such situations when pain is reasonably controlled, activity modification and rehabilitation may be the most prudent approach. If surgery is attempted for massive cuff tears, aggressive mobilization of the tissue is critical. This requires release of the capsule deep to the cuff as well as incising the coracohumeral ligament. Pain relief is of value; however, return of strength and function is largely dependent on the quality of the tissue and the performance of the repair. In these difficult reconstructions, cuff debridement may be considered if the patient's rehabilitation potential is poor; however, functional results are frequently poor and continued participation in an overhead sport is unlikely.

Our postoperative rehabilitation for rotator cuff repairs is guided by our findings at the time of surgery. For large rotator cuff tears we may use a splint that holds the arm in approximately 20 degrees of abduction if the repair was difficult due to tissue retraction. This allows the tendon to heal without tension and in a favourable position with regard to the vascularity of the supraspinatus tendon.[9] In general, tendon attachment takes 6 weeks, following which further healing continues to take place. Passive and active–assisted motion,

the anterior aspect of the acromion only, from the anterolateral corner to the acromioclavicular joint. A 3-cm longitudinal split is extended along the deltoid fibres from the corner. The first step is an acromioplasty to remove the source of impingement and also to provide for sufficient visualization of the rotator cuff tissue. Once the rotator cuff is adequately identified, it is assessed by size, tissue quality, and mobility of the cuff tissue using probes and grasping instruments. A tear less than 2 cm in length is small, 2 to 5 cm is moderate, and more than 5 cm is large.

A broad elevator is used to release tissue both intra- and extra-articularly in order to mobilize the rotator cuff tissues sufficiently (Fig. 9). This is critical to allow the rotator cuff to be repaired without tension and with the arm at the side. We prepare a broad, bleeding bony surface at the greater tuberosity as a bed for the tendon repair. The type of repair performed is dictated by the size and anatomy of the tear (Figs 10, 11, and 12). Using the principles mentioned above, two rows of suture anchors are placed in the previously prepared, humeral bone bed. If suture anchors are used, the cuff is reduced to the medial edge of the greater tuberosity, and the medial anchor sutures are then passed directly cephalad through

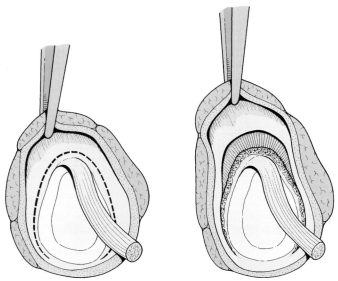

Fig. 9 It is often necessary to perform an intra-articular release of the capsule and rotator cuff, particularly when the rotator cuff is large or retracted. (Redrawn from ref. 56, with permission.)

including pendulum exercises and forward flexion, are begun immediatetely postoperatively, followed by isometrics and progressive strengthening. The pace of therapy is guided by the size of the tear, the quality of the tissue, and judgement on the security of the repair, which we propose is registered immediately postoperative.

In patients with small to moderate tears, postoperative pendulum exercises are started on day 1 and we begin the use of a pulley for overhead elevation at approximately 1 week. Passive motion is thus continued for 6 weeks postoperatively, following which active-assisted motion is permitted. Rotator cuff strengthening exercises with Theraband rubber tubing are begun at 6 weeks. Isotonic exercises at the side are begun at about 8 weeks, and progress to 90 degrees of abduction at 12 weeks. Patients with difficult large tears are splinted for 6 weeks, but assisted elevation is performed daily. The major cause of failure following cuff repair is the use of excessive weight during the first 3 months. It is better to work on motion and use light strengthening exercises with Theraband while tendon healing progresses.[81] Gentle swimming may be started in the third month. In general, throwing and other overhead activities such as serving should be avoided until 6 months. Return to throwing

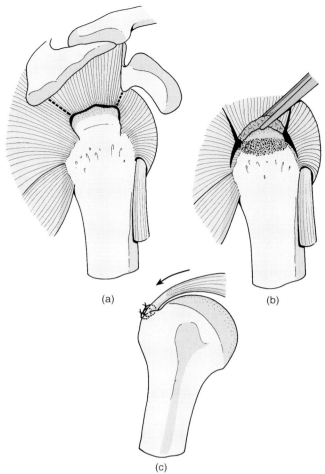

Fig. 11 (a) Moderately sized tears (2–5 cm) frequently require extensive dissection on both sides of the rotator cuff to achieve sufficient length of the cuff tissue; (b) relaxing incisions parallel to the cuff fibres towards the spine of the scapula and the coracoid may be required to advance retracted tissue; (c) the tendon is secured to a bony surface with non-absorbable sutures. (Redrawn from ref. 56, with permission.)

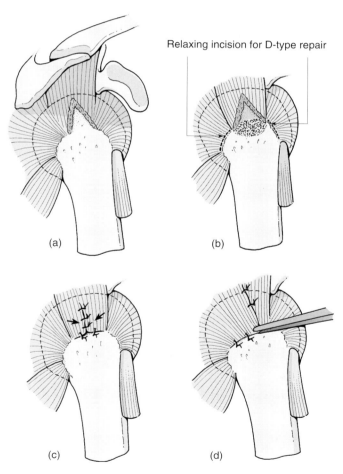

Relaxing incision for D-type repair

Fig. 10 (a) Smaller tears less than 2 cm often form a V-shape as supraspinatus retracts; (b) preparation of a broad, bleeding bony bed for reattachment of the tendon; (c) a V-shaped tear may be converted to a Y-shape and advanced laterally, with repair to bone; (d) if a V-shaped tear is difficult to close, one edge may be advanced to fill the defect. (Redrawn from ref. 56, with permission.)

involves a gradual progression, controlling the variables of distance, speed, and number of throws. These are increased over an approximately 3-month period, making only one change at a time. Pool therapy during the second to sixth week has been quite useful to aid patients in an assisted range of motion programme. It seems to allow patients to achieve greater degrees of motion with less discomfort and apprehension.

Surgical management: impingement

Primary impingement in the young athlete is unusual, and is more likely to occur secondary to instability or cuff failure with resulting loss of downward displacement of the humeral head. Similarly, a primary anatomical abnormality of the coracoacromial arch is rare. Eccentric overload of the rotator cuff is probably the most common inciting cause in the 'overhead' athlete. The mainstay of management is a well-designed rehabilitation programme. Occasionally, conservative treatment fails and a decompressive procedure is considered. A decompression is indicated when symptoms continue despite therapy and work-up reveals a rotator cuff tear, or clear

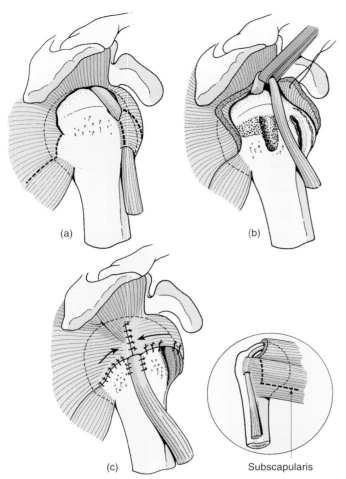

Subscapularis

Fig. 12 (a) Large retracted tears of the rotator cuff may require more extensive mobilization of the cuff tissues, including a superior transfer of the upper subscapularis tendon and/or mobilization of the infraspinatus and teres minor; (b) repositioning the biceps tendon into a more posteriorly positioned groove to aid in closure of the defect; (c) superior advancement of infraspinatus and subscapularis to the biceps tendon. (Redrawn from ref. 56, with permission.)

matic, allowing earlier rehabilitation, and comparable success rates to that of open procedures in patients with isolated impingement.[45,84-88] It also allows for an intra-articular examination of the glenohumeral joint, and assessment for signs of occult instability. The results of arthroscopic decompression are rewarding in terms of pain relief; however, its impact on athletes has not been as favourable. Ellman[89] reported good to excellent results in 88 per cent of his patients without comment on their activity level. Altchek et al.[84] reported an 83 per cent good to excellent rate in patients with stage II impingement, and 76 per cent of athletic patients returned to full participation in sports. However 55 per cent of throwers and swimmers had significant residual symptoms, and 83 per cent of these had inferior labral tears at arthroscopy. Fly et al.[90] noted that 77 per cent of athletes less than 40-years-old returned to overhead sports following arthroscopic subacromial decompression; however, many were unable to return to their previous level of participation. They also noted a high failure rate associated with labral pathology. Failures in each of these studies can probably be attributed to errors in diagnosis or inconsistent removal of acromial bone. Although we are not aware of any large, prospective-randomized series with long-term follow-up comparing these two procedures, our current experience with a large number of arthroscopic acromioplasties leads us to conclude, as reported by Altchek et al., that the functional results of arthroscopic decompression duplicate that of open procedures, with substantially less perioperative morbidity.[84] On occasion changes consistent with impingement will be seen in throwers without obvious bone deformity (Hook). In this situation a soft tissue debridement alone may be all that is necessary.

Following arthroscopic subacromial decompression, rehabilitation is begun on the initial postoperative day. Rehabilitation goals include elimination of pain and restoration of range of motion, normal strength, and function in desired sports. We begin with passive stretching and strengthening exercise and progress to a resisted programme as tolerated.

Surgical management: instability

The diagnosis of shoulder instability in an athlete with shoulder pain and loss of function is frequently difficult. The player frequently gives a history characteristic of a pattern of overuse with findings that are consistent with rotator cuff pathology. It is unusual for an overhead athlete to describe a sensation of instability, rather pain, often posteriorly, will be their main complaint. A physical examination noting apprehension and a positive relocation test is suggestive of the diagnosis of anterior subluxation. Anterior and posterior glenohumeral instability is examined using the 'load--shift'[35] manoeuvres. Inferior instability is evaluated with the 'sulcus sign' test. The mainstay of management of the athlete with glenohumeral joint instability and secondary rotator cuff injury (either tensile failure or internal impingement) is an aggressive rehabilitation programme. Emphasis is on stretching and strengthening of the internal and external rotators and periscapular muscles.

If non-operative treatments fail and surgery is required, the underlying pathology of the instability should be addressed directly. As discussed earlier, subacromial decompression, both open and arthroscopic, has not produced satisfactory results in the majority of athletes. It is unclear what role, if any, arthroscopic decompression

impingement signs are seen in the absence of detectable instability. We combine all subacromial decompressions with a careful examination under anaesthesia and arthroscopy to confirm that a subtle instability is not present.

Open acromioplasty has a well-documented history of good results in the non-athletic population. Neer first described anterior acromioplasty with subacromial bursectomy and coracoacromial ligament resection ('open decompression') in 1972, reporting satisfactory results in 15 out of 16 cases.[1] Rockwood and other authors have confirmed a 70 to 90 per cent rate of pain relief with preservation of function using an open surgical approach. High-demand 'overhead' athletes represent a greater challenge to our diagnostic and surgical skills. Tibone et al. reported on young patients who underwent anterior acromioplasty for stage II impingement: only 43 per cent returned to sports, with fewer returning to overhead throwing.[82,83] These results may reflect untreated subtle instabilities in some of their patients, many of whom were athletes engaged in sports involving competitive throwing.

Arthroscopic decompression with anterior acromioplasty is now a well-developed technique with the advantage of being less trau-

has in this population of patients. It would be a significant advantage if we could define a population of athletes with underlying subluxation who might still benefit from decompression rather than undergoing more extensive shoulder stabilization surgery. If instability is not clearly present, the capsule and labrum are competent, and cuff degeneration is observed, a soft tissue decompression and cuff debridement may provide symptomatic relief when combined with a repeat of the rehabilitation programme.

At the time of surgery a careful examination under anaesthesia using the previously described manoeuvres is performed to note mild degrees of instability. If the humeral head can be loaded on the edge of the glenoid in a thrower this is often all that is noted, yet the relocation manoeuvre will be positive preoperatively. While performing a complete methodical examination of the glenohumeral joint the anterior glenoid labrum is identified and probed to access fraying, midsubstance split tears, or Bankart lesions. The superior, middle, and inferior glenohumeral ligament are identified and probed to access tissue quality and continuity. The anterior band is followed out to the humeral neck with internal rotation of the arm to rule out a humeral side avulsion injury.[91] The tendon of the subscapularis is inspected from the medial glenoid neck to its insertion on the lesser tuberosity. The arm is internally and externally rotated to verify whether the subscapularis tendon and anterior glenohumeral ligament take up tension in external rotation. An attempt is made to pass the arthroscope easily along the anterior glenoid rim into the anterior axillary pouch, the so-called 'drive-through test', which indicates anterior capsular laxity or redundancy. A Hill–Sachs defect is sought in patients with evidence of glenohumeral instability.

If a Bankart lesion is observed, effort is directed towards repairing this pathological lesion. This can be achieved either by arthroscopic techniques using one of several different fixation methods (Fig. 13) or by using motion-sparing, open stabilization techniques. Regardless of the repair method, in the high-demand 'overhead' athlete it is important not to overtighten the capsule or advance the subscapularis tendon. In open reconstructive surgery, exposure of the capsule is achieved either by splitting the subscapularis muscle or partially incising the upper half of the tendon just medial to its insertion. If the subscapularis is released, considerable care is taken in its repair in order to avoid shortening the tendon. A transverse incision in the capsule allows exposure of the Bankart lesion, if present, thus avoiding the shortening that a vertical incision would create. The capsulolabral repair can then be performed from the inside out, and the capsule can also be tensioned in the superior direction. Tension is set with the arm abducted to 60 degrees with 30 to 40 degrees of external rotation. This approach minimizes shortening of the capsule in the medial–lateral direction and maintains the critical range of motion.

When anterior instability is due to capsular insufficiency and not a Bankart lesion, or when multidirectional instability is detected by the presence of a 'sulcus sign', a capsular shift procedure is indicated. Arthroscopic techniques for releasing the capsule and shifting it medially and superiorly exist; however, they are more technically demanding and may provide less predictable results. An open capsular shift is preferred and performed either lateral or medially at the glenoid[92] (Fig. 14). Based on the presence or absence of a Bankart lesion the shift may be medial (T-plasty) or lateral (Neer). More recently we have used a radio-frequency probe

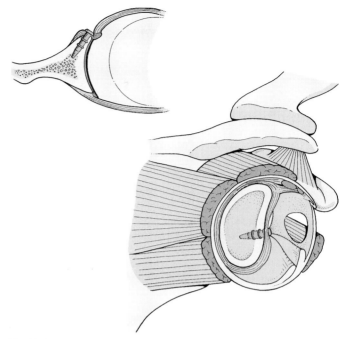

Fig. 13 Arthroscopic Bankart repair with an absorbable cannulated fixation device. Following preparation of the anterior glenoid, the capsulolabral detachment is secured to the glenoid using one or more Suretacs®.

(orater) to shrink the collagen a small amount to decrease glenohumeral translation. We and others have found that heat will disrupt collagen cross-links resulting in collagen shortening. At 67°C an optimal shortening of 15 per cent was achieved with less strength loss than higher temperatures. To date we have performed this on 20 patients with mild subluxation in swimmers and throwers. Short-term results at 6 to 12 months are encouraging with two failures to date due to recurrent trauma in contact sports.

Postoperative rehabilitation in an 'overhead' athlete is begun immediately. The pace of progression of the rehabilitation depends on the technique used and the quality of the repair achieved. Passive elevation, internal rotation, and external rotation to the limits of the repair is allowed. At 4 weeks external rotation is increased and

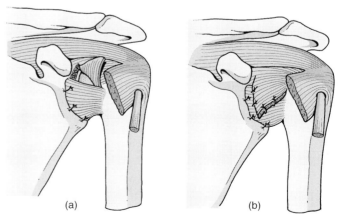

Fig. 14 Illustration depicting T-plasty capsular shift performed at the glenoid side involving a superior shift of the inferior capsular flap (a) and an inferior shift of the superior flap (b). (Redrawn from ref. 92 with permission.)

internal and external rotation strengthening is commenced. Stretching is progressed in a thrower with the aim of achieving a full external rotation 6 weeks after surgery.

Conclusions

Many athletic activities require shoulder motions that place a high degree of stress on the rotator cuff. Shoulder complaints in the athlete are frequently referred to rotator cuff dysfunction or injury. Rotator cuff failure may occur as the result of one or a combination of different potential aetiological processes. In addition to tensile failure of the rotator cuff from overload, glenohumeral instability is frequently recognized as a contributing factor to cuff injury. An accurate diagnosis is critical to the successful treatment of these athletes. A well-designed shoulder and total-body rehabilitation programme remains the mainstay of treatment for the majority of the pathologies encountered. Surgical interventions should correct specific pathologies, be well designed with minimal trauma, and allow early restoration of shoulder motion.

References

1. Neer CSI. Anterior acromioplasty for the chronic impingement syndrome in the shoulder. A preliminary report. *Journal of Bone and Joint Surgery* 1972; **54A**: 41.
2. Neer CSI. Impingement lesions. *Clinical Orthopaedics and Related Research* 1983; **173**: 70–7.
3. Warren RF. Subluxation of the shoulder in athletes. *Clinics in Sports Medicine* 1983; **2**: 339–54.
4. Jobe FW, Kvitne RS. Shoulder pain in the overhand or throwing athlete. The relationship of anterior instability and rotator cuff impingement. *Orthopaedic Review* 1989; **18**: 963–75.
5. Lindblom K, Palmer F. Rupture of the tendon aponeurosis of the shoulder joint—the so-called supraspinatus rupture. *Acta Chirurgica Scandinavica* 1939; **82**: 133.
6. Arnoczky SP, Altchek DW, O'Brien SJ. Anatomy of the shoulder. In: McGinty JB, ed. *Operative arthroscopy*. New York: Raven Press, 1991: 425.
7. Mosley HF, Goldie I. The arterial patterns of the rotator cuff of the shoulder. *Journal of Bone and Joint Surgery* 1963; **45B**: 780.
8. Rothman RH, Parke WW. The vascular anatomy of the rotator cuff. *Clinical Orthopaedics and Related Research* 1965; **41**: 176.
9. Rathbun JB, MacNab I. The microvascular pattern of the rotator cuff. *Journal of Bone and Joint Surgery* 1970; **52B**: 540.
10. Poppen NK, Walker PS. Forces at the glenohumeral joint in abduction. *Journal of Bone and Joint Surgery* 1978; **58A**: 165.
11. Altchek DW, Schwartz E, Warren RF. Radiologic measurement of superior migration of the humeral head in impingement syndrome. Annual Meeting of the American Shoulder and Elbow Surgeons, New Orleans, LA, 1990. *Journal of Shoulder and Elbow Surgery* 1996; **5**: 186–93.
12. Paletta GA, Warner JP, Warren RF. Biplanar X-ray evaluation of the shoulder in patients with instability and rotator cuff tear. Annual Meeting of the Shoulder and Elbow Surgeons, Anaheim, CA, 1991. *Journal of Shoulder and Elbow Surgery* (in press)
13. Doddy SG, Waterland JC, Freedman L. Scapulohumeral goniometer. *Archives of Physical Medicine and Rehabilitation* 1970; **51**: 711.
14. Freedman L, Munroe RH. Abduction of the arm in scapular plane: scapular and glenohumeral movements. *Journal of Bone and Joint Surgery* 1966; **18A**: 1503.
15. Inman VT, Saunders JR, Abbott LC. Observations on the function of the shoulder joint. *Journal of Bone and Joint Surgery* 1944; **26A**: 1.
16. Poppen NK, Walker PS. Normal and abnormal motion of the shoulder. *Journal of Bone and Joint Surgery* 1976; **58A**: 195.
17. Dillman CJ, Fleisig GS, Andrews JR. Biomechanics of pitching with emphasis upon shoulder kinematics. *Journal of Orthopedics and Sports Physiotherapy* 1993; **18**: 402–8.
18. Jobe CM. Posterior superior glenoid impingement: expanded spectrum. *Journal of Arthroscopy and Related Surgery* 1995; **11**: 530–6.
19. Ferretti A, Cerullo G, Russo G. Suprascapular neuropathy in volleyball players. *Journal of Bone and Joint Surgery* 1987; **69A**: 260–3.
20. Counsilman JE. Forces in swimming two types of crawl stroke. *Research Quarterly* 1955; **26**: 127.
21. McLaughlin HL. Dislocation of the shoulder with tuberosity fracture. *Journal of Bone and Joint Surgery* 1963; **43A**: 1615.
22. Craig EV. The posterior mechanism of acute anterior shoulder dislocations. *Clinical Orthopaedics and Related Research* 1984; **190**: 212.
23. Blevins FT, Altchek DW. Arthroscopic subacromial decompression for impingement. In: Parisien JS, ed. *Current techniques in arthroscopy*. Philadelphia: Current Medicine, 1994: 51.
24. Bigliani LV, Morrison SD, April EW. The morphology of the acromion and its relationship to rotator cuff tears. *Orthopaedic Transactions* 1986; **10**: 228.
25. Harryman DT, Sidles JA, Clark JM, McQuade KJ, Gibb TD, Matsen FA. Translation of the humeral head on the glenoid with passive glenohumeral motion. *Journal of Bone and Joint Surgery* 1990; **72**: 1334–43.
26. Payne LZ, Altchek DW, Craig EV, Warren RF. Arthroscopic treatment of partial rotator cuff tears in young athletes—a preliminary report. *American Journal of Sports Medicine* 1997; **25**: 299–305.
27. Potter HG, Gusmer PB, Schate JA, *et al.* Labral injuries: accuracy of detection with unenhanced MR imaging of the shoulder. *Radiology* 1996; **2**: 519–24.
28. Field LD, Warren RF, O'Brien SJ, *et al.* Isolated closure of rotator interval defects for shoulder instability. *American Journal of Sports Medicine* 1995; **23**: 557
29. Pavlov H, Warren RF, Weiss CB Jr, Dines DM. The roentgenographic evaluation of anterior shoulder instability. *Clinical Orthopaedics and Related Research* 1985; **184**: 153–8.
30. Harcke HT, Grissom LE, Finkelstein MS. Evaluation of the musculoskeletal system with sonography. *American Journal of Roentgenology* 1968; **150**: 1253–61.
31. Mack LA, Kilcoyne RS, Matsen FA III. Sonographic evaluation of rotator cuff. *Radiology* 1984; **153**: 23.
32. Middleton WD, Reinus WR, Tatty WU, Melson CL, Murphy WA. Ultrasonic evaluation of the rotator cuff and biceps tendon. *Journal of Bone and Joint Surgery* 1986; **68A**: 440.
33. Goldman AB, Gelhman B. The double-contrast shoulder arthrogram. A review of 158 studies. *Radiology* 1978; **127**: 655–63.
34. Mink JH, Harris E, Rappaport M. Rotator cuff tears: evaluation using double-contrast shoulder arthrography. *Radiology* 1985; **157**: 621–3.
35. Ellman H. Diagnosis and treatment of incomplete rotator cuff tears. *Clinical Orthopaedics and Related Research* 1990; **254**: 64–74.
36. Evancho AM, Evancho AM, Stiles RG, Fajman WA, Flower SP, Macha T, Brunner MC, Fleming L. MR imaging diagnosis of rotator cuff tears. *American Journal of Roentgenology* 1988; **151**: 751–4.
37. Iannotti JP, Zlatkin MB, Esterhai JL, Kressel HY, Dalinka NK, Spnidler KP. Magnetic resonance imaging of the shoulder. *Journal of Bone and Joint Surgery* 1991; **73A**: 17–29.
38. Kieft GJ, Bloem JL, Rozing PM, Obermann WR. Rotator cuff impingement syndrome: MR imaging. *Radiology* 1988; **166**: 211–14.

39. Kneeland JB, Middleton WD, Carrera GF, Zeuge RC, Jesmanowicz A, Froncisz W, Hyde JS. MR imaging of the shoulder: diagnosis of rotator cuff tears. *American Journal of Roentgenology* 1987; **149**: 333–7.

40. Zlatkin MB, Iannotti JP, Roberts MC, Esterhai JL, Dalinka MK, Kressel HY, Schwartz JS, Lenkinski RE. Rotator cuff disease: diagnostic performance of MR imaging. *Radiology* 1989; **172**: 223–9.

41. Seeger LI, Gold RH, Bassett IW, Ellman H. Shoulder impingement syndrome: MR findings in 53 shoulders. *American Journal of Roentgenology* 1988; **150**: 343.

42. Kibler WB. Specificity and sensitivity of the anterior slide test in throwing athletes with superior glenoid labral tears. *Arthroscopy* 1995; **11**: 296.

43. Andrews JR, Broussard TS, Carson WG. Arthroscopy of the shoulder in the management of partial tears of the rotator cuff: preliminary report. *Journal of Arthroscopy* 1985; **1**: 117.

44. Snyder SJ, Pachelli AF, DelPizzo W, *et al*. Partial thickness rotator cuff tears: results of arthroscopic treatment. *Arthroscopy* 1991; **7**: 1.

45. Gartsman GM. Arthroscopic acromioplasty for lesions of the rotator cuff. *Journal of Bone and Joint Surgery* 1990; **72A**: 169.

46. Levy HJ, Gardner RD, Lemak LJ. Arthroscopic subacromial decompression in the treatment of full-thickness rotator cuff tears. *Arthroscopy* 1991; **7**: 8.

47. Ogilvie-Harris DJ, Demaziere A. Arthroscopic debridement versus open repair for rotator cuff tears. A prospective cohort study. *Journal of Bone and Joint Surgery* 1993; **75B**: 416.

48. Ogilvie-Harris DJ, Wiley AM. Arthroscopic surgery of the shoulder. *Journal of Bone and Joint Surgery* 1986; **68B**: 201.

49. Rockwood CA, Williams GR, Burkhead WZ. Debridement of degenerative irreparable lesions of the rotator cuff. *Journal of Bone and Joint Surgery* 1995; **77A**: 857.

50. Burkhart SS. Arthroscopic treatment of massive rotator cuff tears. Clinical results and biomechanical rationale. *Clinical Orthopaedics and Related Research* 1991; **267**: 45.

51. Olsewski JM, Depew AD. Arthroscopic subacromial decompression and rotator cuff debridement for stage II and stage III impingement. *Arthroscopy* 1994; **10**: 61.

52. Ellman H, Kay SP, Wirth M. Arthroscopic treatment of full-thickness rotator cuff tears: 2–7 year follow-up study. *Arthroscopy* 1993; **9**: 195.

53. Hawkins RH, Misamore GW, Hobeika PE. Surgery of full-thickness rotator-cuff tears. *Journal of Bone and Joint Surgery* 1985; **67A**: 1349.

54. Ellman H, Hanker G, Bayer M. Repair of the rotator cuff. End-result study of factors influencing reconstruction. *Journal of Bone and Joint Surgery* 1986; **68A**: 1136.

55. Kimmel J, Bigliani LB, McCann PD, Wolfe I. Repair of rotator cuff tears in tennis players. Annual Meeting of the American Academy of Orthopaedic Surgeons, New Orleans, LA, 1990. *American Journal of Sports Medicine* 1992; **29**: 112–7.

56. Warren RF. Surgical considerations for rotator cuff tears in athletes. In: Jackson DW, ed. *Shoulder surgery in the athlete*. Rockville, MD: Aspen, 1985: 73.

57. Neer CS, Foster CR. Inferior capsular shift for involuntary inferior and multidirectional instability of the shoulder. *Journal of Bone and Joint Surgery* 1980; **62A**: 897.

58. Codman EA. Complete rupture of the supraspinatus tendon. Operative treatment with report of two successful cases. *Boston Journal of Medical Surgery* 1911; **164**: 708.

59. Neer CS, *et al*. Tears of the rotator cuff: long-term results of anterior acromioplasty and repair. *Presented at the American Shoulder and Elbow Surgeons Fourth Meeting. Atlanta, GA, February 1988.*

60. Debeyre J, Patte D, Emelik E. Repair of ruptures of the rotator cuff with a note on advancement of the supraspinatus muscle. *Journal of Bone and Joint Surgery* 1965; **47B**: 36.

61. Godsil RD Jr, Linscheid RL. Intratendinous defects of the rotator cuff. *Clinical Orthopaedics* 1970; **69**: 181.

62. Heikel HVA. Rupture of the rotator cuff of the shoulder. Experiences of surgical management. *Acta Orthopaedica Scandinavica* 1968; **39**: 477.

63. Peterson CJ. Long term results of rotator cuff repair. In: Bayley I, Kessel L, eds. *Shoulder surgery*. Berlin: Springer-Verlag, 1982: 64.

64. Samilson RL, Binder WF. Symptomatic full thickness tears of the rotator cuff: an analysis of 292 shoulders in 276 patients. *Orthopedic Clinics of North America* 1975; **6**: 449.

65. Cofield RH. Current concepts review: rotator cuff disease of the shoulder. *Journal of Bone and Joint Surgery* 1985; **67A**: 974.

66. Johnson L. *Diagnostic and surgical arthroscopy of the shoulder*. St Louis: Mosby Year Book, 1993.

67. Snyder SJ. Evaluation and treatment of the rotator cuff. *Orthopedic Clinics of North America* 1993; **24**: 173.

68. Baylis RW, Wolf EM. Arthroscopic rotator cuff repair: clinical and arthroscopic second-look assessment. *Presented at the Annual Meeting of the Arthroscopy Association of North America, San Francisco, CA, May 1995.*

69. Beach WR, Caspari RB. Arthroscopic management of rotator cuff disease. *Orthopedics* 1993; **16**: 1007.

70. Hawkins RJ, Bokor DJ. Clinical evaluation of shoulder problems. In: Rockwood CA Jr, Matsen FA III, eds. *The shoulder*. Philadelphia: WB Saunders, 1990: 168.

71. Levy HJ, Uribe JW, Delandy LG. Arthroscopically assisted rotator cuff repair: preliminary results. *Arthroscopy* 1990; **6**: 55.

72. Liu SH. Arthroscopically-assisted rotator cuff repair. *Journal of Bone and Joint Surgery* 1994; **76B**: 592.

73. Liu SH, Baker CL. Arthroscopically assisted rotator cuff repair: correlation of functional results with integrity of the cuff. *Arthroscopy* 1994; **10**: 54.

74. Paulos LE, Kody MH. Arthroscopy enhanced 'mini-approach' to rotator cuff repair. *American Journal of Sports Medicine* 1994; **22**: 19.

75. Groh GI, Simoni M, Rolla P, Rockwood CA. Loss of the deltoid after shoulder operations: an operative disaster. *Journal of Shoulder and Elbow Surgery* 1994; **3**: 243.

76. Baker CL, Liu SH. Comparison of open and arthroscopically assisted rotator cuff repairs. *American Journal of Sports Medicine* 1995; **23**: 99.

77. Blevins FT, Warren RF, Altchek DW, *et al*. Arthroscopically assisted rotator cuff repair: results using a mini-open deltoid approach. *Arthroscopy* 1996; **12**: 50.

78. Altchek DW, Warren RF, Skyhar MJ. Shoulder arthroscopy. In: Rockwood CA, Matsen FA, eds. *The shoulder*. Philadelphia: WB Saunders, 1990: 258.

79. Wantabe M, Takeda S, Ikeuchi H. *Atlas of arthroscopy*. 3rd edn. New York: Igaku-Shoin, 1978.

80. Umans H, Berkowitz M, Pavlov H, Warren RF. Correlation of radiographic findings at the acromio-tuberosity interval and glenohumeral articulation on this 'Activie Abduction View' and conventional views with rotator cuff status and cartilage wear at arthroscopy. *Abstract submitted at the American Roentgen Ray Society 1997 Annual Meeting.*

81. Gore DR, Murray MP, Sepic SB, Gardiner GM. Shoulder-muscle rotator cuff tears. *Journal of Bone and Joint Surgery* 1986; **68A**: 266.

82. Tibone JE, Elrod B, Jobe FW, Kerlan RK, Carter VS, Shields CL Jr, Lombardo SJ, Yocum L. Surgical treatment of tears of the rotator cuff in athletes. *Journal of Bone and Joint Surgery* 1986; **68A**: 887.

83. Tibone JE, Jobe FW, Kerlan RK, Carter VS, Shields CL Jr, Lombardo SJ, Yocum L. Shoulder impingement syndrome in athletes treated by an anterior acromioplasty. *Clinical Orthopaedics and Related Research* 1985; **198**: 134.

84. Altchek DW, Warren RF, Wickiewicz TL, Skyhar MJ, Ortis G, Schwartz E. Arthroscopic acromioplasty. *Journal of Bone and Joint Surgery* 1990; **72A**: 1198–207.

85. Esch JC, Ozerkis LR, Helgager JA, Kane N, Lilliott N. Arthroscopic subacromial decompression: results according to degree of rotator cuff tear. *Arthroscopy* 1988; **4**: 241.

86. Hawkins RJ, *et al.* An analysis of failed arthroscopic decompression. *Arthroscopy* 1991; **7**: 315.

87. Lazarus MD, Chansky HA, Misra S, *et al.* Comparison of open and arthroscopic subacromial decompression. *Journal of Shoulder and Elbow Surgery* 1994; **3**: 1.

88. Paulos LE, Franklin JL. Arthroscopic shoulder decompression: development and application: a five year experience. *American Journal of Sports Medicine* 1990; **18**: 235.

89. Ellman H. Arthroscopic subacromial decompression: analysis of 1–3 year results. *Arthroscopy* 1987; **3**: 173.

90. Fly WR, Tibone JE, Glousman RE, Jobe FW, Yocum LA. Arthroscopic subacromial decompression in athletes less than 40 years old. *Orthopaedic Transactions* 1990; **14**: 250.

91. Wolf EM, Cheng JC, Dickson K. Humeral avulsion of glenohumeral ligaments as a cause of anterior shoulder instability. *Arthroscopy* 1995; **5**: 600.

92. Altchek DW, Warren RF, Skyhar MJ, Ortiz G. T-plasty modification of the Bankart procedure for multidirectional instability of the anterior and inferior types. *Journal of Bone and Joint Surgery* 1991; **73A**: 105–12.

4.3.4 Injuries of the acromioclavicular joint

Catherine M. Coady and Jay S. Cox

Introduction

Injuries to the acromioclavicular joint are commonly encountered in the athletic population, especially in those participating in sports associated with high-impact collisions or falls such as ice hockey, skiing, wrestling, football, and equestrian events. Athletes in their second and third decade of life are more commonly affected,[1] and males are injured more than females (4:1 to 10:1).[1,2] Sprains (subluxations) of the acromioclavicular joint are more common than complete dislocations.

Over the years, considerable debate has arisen as to the appropriate treatment of athletes sustaining acromioclavicular joint dislocations. A review of the literature reveals that there is very little consensus regarding treatment and the indications for surgery. Numerous treatments, both surgical and non-surgical, have been advocated to restore normal anatomy and function after dislocation. Recent studies comparing the operative to non-operative treatment of acromioclavicular dislocations have demonstrated that the latter yields as good as, if not better, outcome than surgical treatment. These outcome studies challenge the orthopaedic dogma that all dislocated joints should be reduced anatomically to achieve a satisfactory functional result. There are, however, proponents for surgical intervention in the young active population and for those employed in heavy labour. There are few orthopaedic injuries where the recommended treatment varies so greatly between authors.

The effective treatment of injuries to the acromioclavicular joint requires knowledge of the relevant anatomy and pathology, accurate identification of the injury type, understanding of the natural history, as well as knowledge of the available treatment options.

Anatomy and pathology

The acromioclavicular joint is a diarthrodial joint between the lateral end of the clavicle and the medial acromion. A partial or complete intra-articular cartilagenous disc may be present within the joint.[3] Marked degeneration occurs in the disc until it is essentially non-functional by the fourth decade of life.[4] The primary stabilizers of the acromioclavicular joint are the superior and inferior acromioclavicular ligaments which provide horizontal stability, and the coracoclavicular ligaments which confer vertical stability (Fig. 1). The aponeurosis of the trapezius and deltoid merge with the superior acromioclavicular ligament, thereby providing support and stability to the acromioclavicular joint and making it stronger than the inferior acromioclavicular ligament. The majority of the support is provided by the coracoclavicular ligament which serves to anchor the lateral end of the clavicle to the acromion process. The coracoclavicular ligament spans between the clavicle and coracoid process and consists of two components: the medial, cone-shaped conoid ligament; and the more lateral trapezoid ligament. The conoid portion arises on the posteromedial aspect of the coracoid and inserts on the posteromedial aspect of the clavicle. It prevents posterior subluxation of the clavicle. The trapezoid portion originates on the anterolateral aspect of the coracoid and inserts on the anterior portion of the clavicle. It functions to prevent anterior clavicular subluxation. The average length of the coracoclavicular ligament is 1.3 cm.[5]

The acromioclavicular joint allows for a gliding motion between the clavicle and the acromion and contributes to the rotation of the scapula on the clavicle with abduction of the shoulder. Inman *et al.*[6] showed that the total range of motion of the acromioclavicular joint

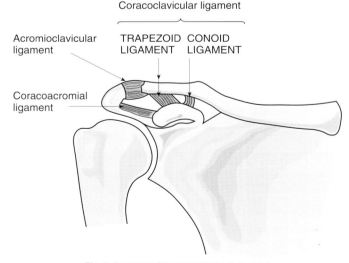

Fig. 1 Anatomy of the acromioclavicular joint

to be about 20 degrees, occurring both in the first 30 degrees of abduction and after 135 degrees of arm elevation.

Rosenorn and Pederson[7] demonstrated the importance of the integrity of the coracoclavicular ligament in their anatomical studies of the acromioclavicular joint. They found that if the acromioclavicular joint and surrounding capsule were disrupted, there was 0.5 to 1 cm of displacement. If the coracoclavicular ligament was also severed, the resultant displacement was typically 1.5 to 2.5 cm of superior displacement. Fukuda et al.[8] found that at large displacements, the conoid ligament provides the primary restraint to superior displacement and that the acromioclavicular ligament acts as a primary constraint for posterior displacement of the clavicle. However, Urist[3] had previously concluded that complete separation can occur without rupture of the coracoclavicular ligament. He stated that when the distance between the coracoid and clavicle is increased, the coracoclavicular ligament may be stretched but not necessarily torn. Rockwood et al.[1] repeated the anatomical studies of Urist, and found that when the acromioclavicular ligament and/or the trapezius and deltoid muscles are injured the clavicle can be dislocated from the acromion in a horizontal plane with only slight upward displacement in the vertical direction. When the conoid and trapezoid ligaments are detached, the lateral clavicle can only then be completely dislocated in the vertical plane. Following acute disruption to the joint, the articular surfaces of the joint and interarticular disc may be severely traumatized. In addition, there may be associated fractures of the clavicle, acromion, or coracoid process.

There is a continuum of soft tissue injuries with an acute acromioclavicular dislocation; here, the following structures usually give way in the sequence: (1) the intra-articular disc and acromioclavicular ligament; (2) the lateral end of the clavicle is stripped out from its inferior periosteum; (3) the coracoclavicular ligament and clavipectoral fascia are torn; and (4) with severe trauma, there is complete dislocation of the joint with disruption of the deltoid and trapezius muscle attachments.

Mechanism of injury

The superficial position of the acromioclavicular joint makes it vulnerable to a variety of disruptive forces. Injuries to the acromioclavicular joint typically occur as a result of a sudden, direct downward force applied to the superolateral aspect of the acromion, for example when a hockey player falls and strikes the apex of his shoulder. Nielsen[9] found that 70 per cent of acromioclavicular joint injuries are the result of a direct injury. The direct force causes the scapula to depress, pulling the clavicle through the coracoclavicular ligament. If the impact is forceful enough, the clavicle pushes against the first rib which, in turn, produces a counterforce, this prevents further displacement causing injury to the acromioclavicular and, possibly, the coracoclavicular ligaments, as well as the insertions of the trapezius and deltoid muscles. The severity of the injury is determined by the magnitude of the applied force. Glick et al.[10] described two other mechanisms of acromioclavicular joint injuries as a result of indirect forces. One mechanism occurs when the athlete sustains a direct blow from behind with the ipsilateral arm fixed on the ground, this drives the clavicle forward and away from the acromion. Another cause of an indirect injury arises when the athlete falls on their outstretched hand or elbow while the arm is in a position of abduction and slight flexion, this results in a backward and outward force on the acromion.

Diagnosis

Typically, the athlete will present soon after an acute injury and with their arm splinted to their side. A complete history should be obtained from the patient, including details of the following: mechanism of the injury; severity of the force sustained; degree of pain and disability; time since the injury; previous injuries; arm dominance; occupation; and sporting activities.

Most movements are restricted secondary to pain. Depending on the severity of the injury, the involved acromioclavicular joint may be swollen and ecchymosis may be present. The contour of the shoulder should be noted, as well as deformity at the acromioclavicular joint. In general, the shoulder droops in an inferior direction and the clavicle remains in its anatomical position. Palpation of the dislocated acromioclavicular joint will reveal tenderness and/or soft-tissue deficiency. Although rare, a complete examination of the brachial plexus and surrounding vasculature should be performed to rule out any possible trauma. Finally, the examination should include a careful analysis of the surrounding structures which may reveal an associated fracture of the acromion, clavicle, or coracoid, with other soft-tissue injury.

Classification

In 1963, Tossy et al.[11] classified acromioclavicular injuries into the three well-known grades of sprain, subluxation, and dislocation. In this classification scheme, a type I injury or sprain is a partial tear of the acromioclavicular ligament. The distal clavicle is not displaced and the coracoclavicular ligament is intact. A type II injury or subluxation describes a rupture of the acromioclavicular ligament with a partial tear of the coracoclavicular ligament. Displacement of the clavicle is less than the full width of the clavicle on the acromion. A type III injury, or dislocation, occurs when the acromioclavicular and the coracoclavicular ligaments are severed resulting in a complete displacement of the distal clavicle in relation to the acromion, greater than the width of the clavicle. Rockwood et al.[1] proposed a more comprehensive classification to describe acromiclavicular joint injuries (Fig. 2). He further subclassified the type III injuries to encompass a variety of injury patterns of the more severely dislocated acromioclavicular joints. In this classification scheme, type I and II injuries remain as previously described. Type III disruptions involve a complete rupture of the acromioclavicular and coracoclavicular ligaments with displacement of the full width of the clavicle. However, the deltoid and trapezius aponeuroses over the distal clavicle remain intact. A type IV injury is one where there is a posterior dislocation of the clavicle. With this injury pattern the distal clavicle is displaced posteriorly through the muscle aponeurosis. The clavicle may not be reducible in a closed fashion as it may be buttonholed through the muscle fibres. A type V injury occurs when there is a type III pattern with a complete rupture of the deltoid and trapezius musculature. The distal clavicle is covered only by skin and subcutaneous tissue (Fig. 3). A type VI injury is a very rare pattern, whereby there is a complete dislocation of the clavicle at the sternoclavicular and acromioclavicular joints and the distal clavicle becomes trapped under the coracoid. This occurs from a very severe direct force to the superior surface of the distal clavicle along

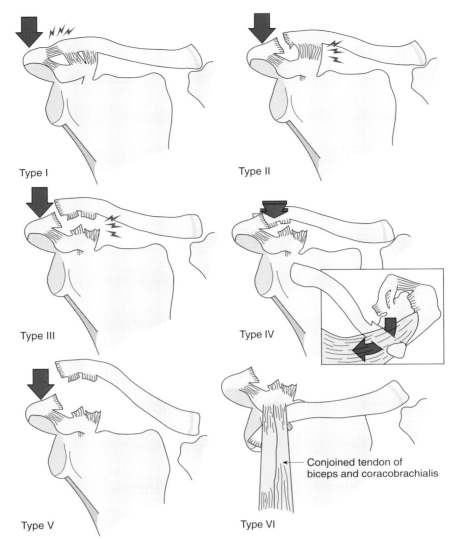

Fig. 2 Classification of acromioclavicular joint injuries. (Top left) In the type I injury a mild force applied to the point of the shoulder does not disrupt either the acromioclavicular or the coracoclavicular ligaments. (Top right) A moderate to heavy force applied to the point of the shoulder will disrupt the acromioclavicular ligaments, but the coracoclavicular ligaments remain intact. (Centre left) When a severe force is applied to the point of the shoulder both the acromioclavicular and the coracoclavicular ligaments are disrupted. (Centre right) In a type IV injury not only are the ligaments disrupted but the distal end of the clavicle is also displaced posteriorly into or through the trapezius muscle. (Bottom left) A violent force applied to the point of the shoulder not only ruptures the acromioclavicular and coracoclavicular ligaments but also disrupts the muscle attachments and creates a major separation between the clavicle and the acromion. (Bottom right) This is an inferior dislocation of the distal clavicle in which the clavicle is inferior to the coracoid process and posterior to the biceps and coracobrachialis tendons. The acromioclavicular and coracoclavicular ligaments are also disrupted. (From ref. 1, with permission.)

with abduction of the arm and retraction of the scapula. It typically occurs in high-energy injuries such as motor vehicle or motorcycle accidents.

Radiographic assessment

Radiographs are an important adjunct in the assessment of athletes presenting with acromioclavicular joint disruptions. In addition to the clinical findings, diagnosis and classification of an acromioclavicular injury are confimed with roentgenograms. The routine view is an anteroposterior view, preferably with the patient sitting or standing and with no support of the injured extremity. The views should be taken with the X-ray beam at an upward tilt of 10 to 15 degrees, as described by Zanca[12], this yields a true anteropos-

terior view of the acromioclavicular joint. In a normal anteroposterior view of the acromioclavicular joint, the distal clavicle and acromion may be superimposed on the spine of the scapula. However, this may obscure the joint and small fractures may be overlooked.

Stress views of the acromioclavicular joint may be important in revealing an occult dislocation in a patient presenting with what appears to be a type II injury. Further instability may be detected at the acromioclavicular joint by suspending 10 to 15 lb (4.5 to 6.8 kg) weights to both wrists and obtaining an AP view of both shoulders, this allows comparison of the injured with the uninjured joint. The patient should be instructed not to hoist the weights as this will lead to a tendency to lift the extremity involuntarily, thereby diminishing the true amount of acromioclavicular separation. A transaxillary lateral view is also important in assessing the anteroposterior displacement of the clavicle.

Radiographic assessment of a type I injury will reveal no change in relation to the opposite uninjured extremity. A radiograph of a type II injury will depict the distal end of the clavicle being displaced superiorly in relation to the acromion, but less than the full width of the clavicle. In a type III injury, there is complete acromioclavicular dislocation with the distal end of the clavicle displaced above the superior edge of the acromion. It is important to note that the inferior displacement of the scapula caused by the pull of gravity on the arm, and not by the superior displacement of the clavicle, is the reason for the increased coracoclavicular distance and resulting clinical and radiographic appearance in acromioclavicular joint dislocations (Fig. 4). An axillary lateral view is essential in a type IV injury to show posterior clavicular displacement. A type V injury pattern reveals gross inferior displacement of the scapula to the clavicle. Type VI injuries show subcoracoid displacment of the clavicle. Radiographs are also invaluable in evaluating the presence of any other significant pathology, such as a fractured clavicle or coranoid, which may alter the treatment plan.

Treatment

The treatment of acromioclavicular joint injuries varies according to the severity or grade of the injury. The management of injuries to the acromioclavicular joint may range from skilful neglect to the use of slings, braces, harnesses, or surgery. Most authors agree on the conservative management of acute type I and II sprains. In addition, many concur that the displacement and functional impairment resulting from types IV, V, and VI acromioclavicular dislocations are too great and should be surgically reconstructed.[1,13-15] However, the treatment of type III injuries is the subject of great debate in the literature.

Type I injuries

Type I sprains are the most common injury encountered. The joint is stable and there is either no or minimal loss of motion of the shoulder joint. The treatment of acute type I injuries is symptomatic. These measures include ice packs, rest, and anti-inflammatory medication. Active physiotherapy-assisted range of motion is initiated early in treatment, followed by isometric strengthening. Once

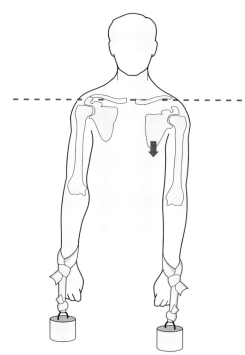

Fig. 4 Schematic drawing of a patient with a complete type III acromioclavicular dislocation. The major deformity seen in this injury is a downward displacement of the scapula and upper extremity—not an upward elevation of the clavicle.

full motion and strength have returned, the athlete may return to sporting activities.

Type II injuries

Treatment of type II subluxations is also symptomatic. Most authors agree that the patients should be treated with a sling for comfort for 7 to 14 days, followed by a gradual rehabilitation programme. Ice, rest, and anti-inflammatory agents are recommended in the initial management of these injuries. However, the deformity present within the joint is permanent. Others have recommended using adhesive strappings, splints,[16] pressure pads, or harnesses such as the Kenny–Howard sling[17] to reduce the dislocation. The main complication arising from these devices is skin irritation, which may necessitate their discontinuation. The use of these devices to reduce the dislocation and maintain the reduction is not always rewarding; compliance is low for athletes wearing a harness for the recommended 6 weeks. In the athlete treated with a simple sling for comfort, gentle range of motion exercises followed by strengthening exercises may be initiated when the pain subsides. The acromioclavicular joint should be protected from further injury, thus heavy lifting and contact sports should be avoided for at least 6 weeks to avoid aggravating or reinjuring the acromioclavicular joint. The length of treatment depends on the symptoms and the level of competition. Athletes may return to sports as soon as they have a full range of motion, normal strength, and are free of pain, this generally takes between 2 and 4 weeks.

Full functional recovery is the norm for type I and II injuries. Unfortunately, a potential complication of type I and II injuries is post-traumatic arthritis in the acromioclavicular joint secondary to

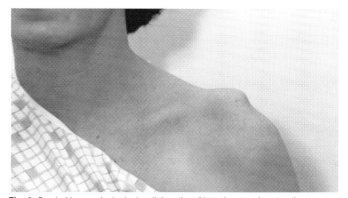

Fig. 3 Grade V acromioclavicular dislocation. Note the prominent, subcutaneous position of the clavicle.

internal derangement of the joint itself. Many patients may continue to have symptoms and may show progressive degeneration within the joint. Significant discomfort may develop in patients who stress their acromioclavicular joint during work or with sporting activities. Cox[18] was surprised to find that many patients with type I and II injuries had a greater number of residual symptoms than expected (36 per cent and 48 per cent, respectively). If progressive pain, weakness, or limitation of motion persist, an excision of the distal end of the clavicle may be necessary.

Type III injuries

The treatment of type III injuries has been and remains very controversial. Essentially, there are some authors who advocate surgery and others that propose closed methods of treatment. Moreover, there is disagreement as to which type of treatment yields the best results. There have been well over 30 different operative and non-operative methods described in the literature.[1,3] The current trend appears to be towards a more conservative approach. In the early 1970s, Powers and Bach[19] polled orthopaedic chairmen regarding their treatment of acromioclavicular dislocations, these authors found that 91.5 per cent advocated operative treatment of type III injuries and that their preferred fixation method was across the acromioclavicular joint (61 per cent). More recently, Cox[20] revisited this issue and surveyed orthopaedic residency chairmen and orthopaedic surgeons active in sports medicine, this survey substantiated the shift towards non-operative treatment. He found that chairmen preferred a more conservative approach (72.2 per cent) as did team physicians (86 per cent). When surgery was required, both team physicians (96.4 per cent) and chairmen (72.3 per cent) preferred coracoclavicular fixation with either tape or suturing as their chosen method.

Historically, the treatment of acromioclavicular joint dislocation was mainly surgical, and all attempts were made to attain and maintain an anatomical reduction of the acromioclavicular joint. The rationale for operative intervention was to give the patient the best chance to obtain normal shoulder function by restoring normal anatomy. More recently, several authors have challenged this notion[10,19,21-29] reporting that non-operative treatment yields as good, if not better, results than surgical treatment. Glick et al.[10] examined 35 athletes including 19 pro-football players with old unreduced acromioclavicular dislocations and found that none of the athletes were disabled. He concluded that an anatomical reduction was not a prerequisite for satisfactory function. Dias et al.[21] investigated 44 patients treated non-operatively and found that 20 patients had no discomfort, 22 had mild discomfort, and 2 had moderate symptoms. A retrospective review performed by Galpin et al.[22] of type III injuries revealed that non-operative patients took less time to become pain-free (2.8 months versus 4.5 months) and that they also had less time away from sports (1.7 months versus 2.2 months). Bannister et al.[23] performed a randomized controlled study of patients sustaining type III injuries in which 27 patients were treated with coracoclavicular screws and 33 were treated non-operatively with a sling for 2 weeks. At one year, 88 per cent of the non-operative group and 77 per cent of the operative group had good or excellent results. At 4 years, 59 per cent of the non-operative group had a perfect result, and the remainder had a good or excellent result. For the operative group, 60 per cent had a perfect

result, 24 per cent had a good or excellent result, and 16 per cent had a fair result.

The proponents of surgical acromioclavicular joint reconstruction report that not all patients treated conservatively do well. Dawe[30] reported in his paper of 30 patients treated conservatively that 50 per cent experienced sufficient discomfort to force them to change jobs or give up contact sports. Reports in the literature of conservative management reveal a 10 to 20 per cent incidence of painful sequelae which may be due to meniscal damage, persistent instability, or the development of arthritis.[22,25,31,32] The study of Taft et al.[27], with a follow-up of 9.5 years, shows the important difference in the frequency of post-traumatic arthritis between anatomically reduced and unreduced acromioclavicular dislocations (25 per cent vs 43 per cent). The surgical proponents state that these findings are a strong argument for operative treatment with a low complication rate. Krueger-Franke et al.[33] examined competitive and recreational athletes with acromioclavicular joint disruptions treated operatively and found a 90 per cent good or excellent result. In their study of 15 patients treated operatively for type III dislocations, Roper and Levack[34] found that all patients denied pain or discomfort at rest and with strenuous activity. Their strength and range of motion were normal compared to the uninjured side. Stam and Dawson[35] found that their group of patients treated with coracoclavicular fixation using Dacron tape recovered their shoulder function quicker than patients treated conservatively. Weinstein et al.[36] examined 44 patients with type III injuries who were treated surgically by coracoclavicular fixation with heavy non-absorbable suture and found that 96 per cent early repairs and 77 per cent late repairs had satisfactory results. They noted a trend towards an early return to sports and heavy labour in the early repair group. They concluded that surgical reconstruction for acromioclavicular dislocation provides reliable results, including the use of the arm for sports or repetitive work.

Another facet that must be seriously considered in the athlete sustaining an acromioclavicular dislocation is the potential for loss of strength and endurance in the involved extremity. Glick[10] noted that 8 of his 35 patients had residual weakness which he attributed to the lack of a proper rehabilitation programme. Rehabilitation of the injured musculature is an extremely important aspect of treatment.[18] The therapy should include an early, active exercise programme with attention focused on the deltoid and trapezius muscles. It had long been suspected that failure to reduce and stabilize a complete dislocation would result in the loss of shoulder strength. Studies have shown that residual shoulder weakness following type III injury is no greater in patients treated non-operatively than in patients treated surgically.[37-39] However, many authors, including those who advocate conservative management, agree that individuals requiring high levels of shoulder strength for work or athletes involved with repetitive endurance activities, such as swimming or throwing, may need to be considered for an acute reconstruction[1,25,33,39-43] Surgical reconstruction in these individuals is felt to result in a shoulder with more endurance that will stand up to repetitive stresses and heavy loads.

Non-operative treatment

A variety of shoulder-taping methods and harnesses designed to reduce the acromioclavicular disruption have been advocated. It is easy to reduce the acromioclavicular joint, but difficult to maintain the reduction for 6 weeks when treated non-operatively. These methods require optimal patient compliance, but are associated with skin-pressure problems and ulceration as well as a failure to maintain the reduction. The majority of treating physicians recommend 'skilful neglect', prescribing a simple sling for the patient's comfort. Analgesics and/or anti-inflammatories may be prescribed initially for pain control. Once the pain subsides, a progressive rehabilitation programme is initiated which concentrates on regaining motion and strength in the affected shoulder. The athlete should not return to their sport until they have a painless range of motion and until full strength has been restored, which typically takes 8 to 12 weeks. Participants in contact sports will require a longer time interval to avoid reinjuring the acromioclavicular joint. The patient should be aware that they will have a residual deformity; however, few find it cosmetically disturbing. Little correlation has been found between clinical appearance, radiographic results, and the incidence of significant pain and disability. If athletes complain of pain or disability, they may require a delayed reconstructive procedure.

Several authors[2,18,23] have advocated symptomatic treatment for athletes, allowing them a rapid return to competition. They emphasize early and agggressive strengthening and range of motion of the shoulder.

Operative treatment

When conservative management fails, or a patient is deemed not to be a candidate for closed treatment, operative reconstruction can be undertaken. The goals of operative intervention are: to attain and maintain an anatomical reduction of the acromioclavicular joint; provide relief from pain; and to restore normal function and strength. These goals can be attained surgically by reducing the acromioclavicular joint, by repairing and/or reconstructing the ligaments that provide stability, and by restoring the function of the musculature. With a reconstruction, the reduction of the joint must be maintained and protected until the repaired or reconstructed ligaments heal sufficiently to take over the burden of function safely. A very important fact in the success or failure of operative procedure is the management of the soft tissues. A multitude of surgical procedures have been devised for dislocations of the acromioclavicular joint. The six general principles of surgical repair include: (1) reduction of the distal clavicle and maintenance of reduction of the coracoclavicular or acromioclavicular joint; (2) repair of the coracoclavicular ligament, if possible; (3) repair of the acromioclavicular ligament, if possible; (4) debridement of the acromioclavicular joint; (5) excision of the distal clavicle if there is existing articular cartilage changes in the acromioclavicular joint or if the distal clavicle is damaged; and (6) repair of the deltoid and trapezius muscle aponeuroses. The currently recommended operative procedures for acute acromioclavicular dislocation include: acromioclavicular repair; coracoclavicular repair; and primary distal clavicle excision with joint debridement (Fig. 5).

Acromioclavicular repair, fixation, reconstruction

A variety of fixation methods have been used to stabilize the dislocated acromioclavicular joint including smooth pins,[44] Steinman pins,[45] screws, suture wires, plates,[46,47] or a combination of these methods. The major problems with smooth wires have been breakage and migration, thus most authors recommend the use of threaded Steinman pins. Along with pin fixation, repair or recon-

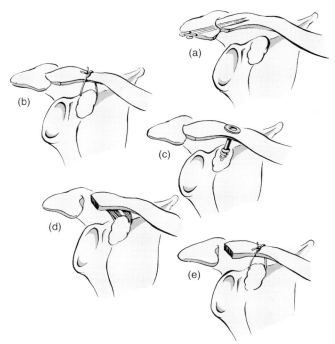

Fig. 5 Various operative procedures for injuries to the acromioclavicular joint. (a) Steinmann pins across the acromioclavicular joint. (b) Suture between the clavicle and the coracoid process. (c) A lag screw between the clavicle and the coracoid process. (d) Resection of the distal clavicle when the coracoclavicular ligaments are intact. (e) Resection of the distal clavicle with suture, fascia, or ligament between the clavicle and the coracoid process when the coracoclavicular ligaments are missing. (Redrawn from ref. 1, with permission.)

struction of the acromioclavicular or coracoclavicular ligaments may be performed.[33,35] Neviaser[48] augments his pin fixation with transference of the coracoacromial ligament. With the pins in place, most authors recommend motion of less than 40 degrees of elevation and gentle isometrics. Pins are removed 6 to 8 weeks later, after which range of motion and strengthening exercises are allowed.

Coracoclavicular repair, fixation, reconstruction

In 1949, Bosworth[5] first described the placement of a coracoclavicular screw to maintain reduction. This technique involved inserting a distally threaded screw from the distal clavicle into the base of the coracoid process. There have been several modifications of Bosworth's original technique involving the primary repair of the coracoclavicular ligament or transference of the coracoacromial ligament in addition to coracoclavicular fixation.[49-51] Coracoclavicular fixation devices depend on an intact coracoid process. Other variations in fixation techniques of the coracoid to the clavicle have been described which include the use of wire,[50,52] suture,[36] or synthetic graft.[35,53,54] Loop fixation using synthetic graft material, such as Dacron or Goretex, encircling the clavicle and coracoid has been reported with good success. Rehabilitation following synthetic grafts is faster, with range of motion exercises started when the pain subsides. Isometrics are initiated immediately and progress to isotonic exercises. Generally, heavy lifting and contact athletics are not to be resumed until 8 weeks after surgery.

Complications pertaining to coracoclavicular fixation include clavicular erosion, as a result of pressure necrosis with wire- and graft-loop fixation,[54] and screw pullout.

Comparisons of acromioclavicular and coracoclavicular repairs have yielded mixed results. Lancaster *et al.*[55] found a higher failure rate with coracoclavicular fixation, but noted a higher minor complication rate with acromioclavicular fixation. Others have demonstrated improved results with coracoclavicular fixation, especially loop fixation. Taft *et al.*[27] found that patients with acromioclavicular fixation had a higher incidence of post-traumatic arthritis than those managed with a coracoclavicular screw.

Excision of the distal end of the clavicle

Primary resection of the distal clavicle in the acute type III injury is usually indicated for fracture or arthritis involving the acromioclavicular joint. The recommended technique involves resection of the distal clavicle lateral to the coracoclavicular ligament. Powers and Bach[19] showed that less than 1 per cent of orthopaedic surgeons favoured immediate excision. The study by Cox[20] revealed that only 34 per cent of team physicians and 22 per cent of orthopaedic chairmen advocated primary excision of the distal clavicle at the time of surgery. In 1977, Browne *et al.*[56] reported that excision of the distal clavicle in the surgical treatment of acromioclavicular dislocations offered no significant improvement over coracoclavicular fixation alone. In 1972, Weaver and Dunn[43] described a method of treating acute and chronic dislocations whereby the distal clavicle is resected with transfer of the coracoacromial ligaments to the intramedullary shaft of the distal clavicle. This procedure has since been modified with the inclusion of coraclavicular fixation to protect the ligament reconstruction. The rationale for including resection of the distal clavicle is to prevent late acromioclavicular arthritis and osteolysis of the distal clavicle.

Certainly, the method of treatment must be selected to meet the needs of each patient. One cannot assume that all acromioclavicular joint dislocations are alike and that similar results will be obtained with one treatment regime. Age, occupation, athletic activity, and the wishes of the patient must all be considered. In most patients, it is reasonable to begin treatment with short periods of immobilization in a sling until they are free of pain and to instigate early rehabilitation of the shoulder for range of motion and strengthening. Young athletes and labourers engaged in heavy work may benefit from an acute reconstruction. If the patient remains symptomatic months after the injury despite physiotherapy, then a delayed reconstructive procedure may be necessary. Although there are few studies looking at the delayed treatment of acromioclavicular dislocations, it appears that in patients ultimately requiring surgical reconstruction the results are inferior compared with those treated acutely.[36,57] Weinstein *et al.*[36] noted a trend toward better results in patients undergoing early repair versus late reconstruction (96 per cent versus 77 per cent).

A variety of complications have been reported with both operative and non-operative methods of treatment (Table 1).

Type IV injuries

In a type IV pattern there is severe posterior diplacement of the clavicle which may become embedded within the trapezius muscle. This type of injury will lead to impaired shoulder function if left in its dislocated position. Most authors agree that this requires operative anatomical reduction and fixation with either acromioclavicular or coracoclavicular fixation.

Table 1 Complications of treatment in acromioclavicular injuries

Non-operative	Operative
Deformity	Wound infection/haematoma
Degenerative arthritis	Scar
Chronic instability	Traumatic arthritis
Calcification of soft tissue	Fixation failure
Skin irritation/ulceration	Inadequate reduction/fixation
Joint stiffness	Iatrogenic fracture
Muscle atrophy/weakness	Residual deformity
	Loss of motion
	2nd procedure to remove hardware
	Anaesthetic risk

Type V injuries

In type V injuries, there is gross displacement of the acromioclavicular joint with associated significant damage to the deltoid and trapezius muscles and fascia. It is incompatible with normal shoulder function if left unreduced. This pattern of injury requires stable fixation because all the restraints have been damaged. If the clavicle cannot be anatomically reduced, or if there is damage to its articular surface, an excisional arthroplasty may be performed.

Type VI injuries

Type VI injuries are very rare. Attempts at closed reduction are usually unsuccessful. Rockwood *et al.*[1] recommend an extra-articular technique with coracoclavicular lag screw, repair of the ligament, and imbrication of the deltoid and trapezius fascia over the top of the clavicle.

It should be noted that patients with type IV, V, and VI injuries rehabilitate much slower due to the severity of the initial injury.

Chronic acromioclavicular joint dislocations and arthritis

The injured acromioclavicular joint may be a source of considerable pain and crepitus. Pain in the region of the joint that worsens with direct compression suggests the diagnosis. If the symptoms can be relieved by infiltration of the acromioclavicular joint with a local anaesthetic, surgical excision of the lateral 1 to 1.5 cm of the clavicle may be beneficial.

Taft *et al.*[27] reported an increased frequency of post-traumatic arthritis between anatomically reduced and unreduced acromioclavicular dislocations (15 per cent vs 45 per cent). However, only 29 per cent of those who had demonstrable post-traumatic osteoarthitis were sufficiently disabled by pain to require excision of the distal clavicle. No correlation between the presence or amount of degenerative changes in the acromioclavicular joint and degree of pain could be found.

Some patients treated non-operatively for complete acromioclavicular dislocations go on to develop instability, persistent pain, and crepitus. Athletes with chronic acromioclavicular instability may develop significant symptoms that limit their ability to perform activities of daily living and sports. The incidence of symptoms is not necessarily related to radiographic appearance. In chronically dislocated acromioclavicular joints, the Weaver and Dunn technique, as well as modifications of this method, have been used. Mulier *et al.*[13] found that 90 per cent of patients requiring a reconstructive procedure after failed conservative management had a good to excellent result. They felt that a high percentage of excellent results can be expected as long as the procedure is performed correctly, with the removal of no more than 1 cm of the clavicle and joint capsule and repair of muscle attachments. For chronic type III injuries, Dewar and Barrington[58] advocate the use of a dynamic muscle transfer to hold the clavicle down. This technique involves the transfer of the coracoid process to the clavicle. However, caution is advised with the use of this procedure because of the potential injury to the musculocutaneous nerve and because the clavicle may piston with stressful activity.

Conclusions

Acromioclavicular joint injuries in athletes are common. The majority of injuries are minor sprains which heal uneventfully. The treatment modalities for sports-related acromioclavicular dislocations are generally agreed upon, with the exception of type III injuries. It is important to distinguish between partial and complete injuries as this diagnosis affects both treatment and outcome. Type I and II injuries are treated symptomatically, with the knowledge that degenerative arthritis may develop in the acromioclavicular joint. The current trend in uncomplicated type III injuries is a nonoperative approach. If the athlete develops subsequent problems, a delayed reconstruction may be undertaken. In athletes involved in heavy lifting or prolonged overhead activities, surgery may be considered acutely. Type IV, V, and VI injuries are generally treated operatively. With these injuries, there is more soft tissue and bony disruption, thus the patients typically rehabilitate much slower. Stable, chronic, and painful acromioclavicular injuries can be treated by distal clavicle excision with good results. In chronically dislocated acromioclavicular joints, a coracoclavicular reconstruction, using either a dynamic muscle transfer or a transfer of the acromioclavicular ligament, is advocated.

No matter what form of treatment is chosen, the ultimate goal is to restore painless function to the injured acromioclavicular joint in order to return the athlete safely and expeditiously back to their sport.

References

1. Rockwood CA Jr, Williams GR, Young DC. Injuries to the acromioclavicular joint. In: Rockwood CA Jr, Green DP, Bucholz RW, eds. *Fractures in adults.* 3rd edn. Philadelphia: JB Lippincott, 1991: 1181–251.
2. Dias JJ, Gregg PJ. Acromioclavicular joint injuries in sport: recommendations for treatment. *Sports Medicine* 1991; 11: 125–32.
3. Urist MR. Complete dislocations of the acromioclavicular joint. *Journal of Bone and Joint Surgery* 1946; 28: 813–37.
4. DePalma AF. The role of the disks of the sternoclavicular and the acromioclavicular joints. *Clinical Orthopaedics and Related Research* 1959; 13: 222–32.
5. Bosworth M. Complete acromioclavicular dislocation. *New England Journal of Medicine* 1949; 241: 221–5.
6. Inmann VT, Saunders JB, Abbott LC. Observations on the function of the shoulder joint. *Journal of Bone and Joint Surgery* 1944; 26: 1–30.
7. Rosenørn M, Pedersen EB. The significance of the coracoclavicular ligament in experimental dislocation of the acromioclavicular joint. *Acta Orthopaedica Scandinavica* 1974; 45: 346–58.
8. Fukuda K, Craig EV, An K, Cofield RH, Chao EY. Biomechanical study of the ligamentous system of the acromioclavicular joint. *Journal of Bone and Joint Surgery* 1986; 68A: 434–9.
9. Nielsen WB. Injury to the acromio-clavicualr joint. *Journal of Bone and Joint Surgery* 1963; 45B:207.
10. Glick JM, Milburn LJ, Haggerty JF, Nishimoto D. Dislocated acromioclavicular joint: follow-up study of 35 unreduced acromioclavicular dislocations. *American Journal of Sports Medicine* 1977; 5: 264–70.
11. Tossy JD, Mead NC, Sigmond HM. Acromioclavicular separations: useful and practical classification for treatment. *Clinical Orthopaedics and Related Research* 1963; 28: 111–19.
12. Zanca P. Shoulder pain: involvement of the acromioclavicular joint (analysis of 1,000 cases). *American Journal of Radiology* 1971; 112: 493–505.
13. Mulier T, Stuyck J, Fabry G. Conservative treatment of acromioclavicular dislocation evaluation of functional and radiological results after six years follow-up. *Acta Orthopaedica Belgica* 1993; 59: 255–61.
14. Sondergard-Petersen P, Mikkelsen P. Posterior acromioclavicular dislocation. *Journal of Bone and Joint Surgery* 1982; 64B: 52–3.
15. Hastings DE, Horne JG. Anterior dislocation of the acromioclavicular joint. *Injury* 1978; 10: 285–8.
16. Anzel SH, Streitz WL. Acute acromioclavicular injuries. A report of nineteen cases treated non-operatively employing dynamic splint immobilization. *Clinical Orthopaedics and Related Research* 1974; 103: 143–9.
17. Allman FL. Fractures and ligamentous injuries of the clavicle and its articulation. *Journal of Bone and Joint Surgery* 1987; 69A: 924–7.
18. Cox J. The fate of the acromioclavicular joint in athletic injuries. *American Journal of Sports Medicine* 1981; 9: 50–3.
19. Powers JA, Bach PJ. Acromioclavicular separations: closed or open treatment. *Clinical Orthopaedics and Related Research* 1974; 104: 213–23.
20. Cox, JS. Current method of treatment of acromioclavicular joint dislocations. *Orthopedics* 1992; 15: 1041–4.
21. Dias JJ, Steingold RF, Richardson RA, Tesfayohannes B, Gregg PJ. The conservative treatment of acromioclavicular dislocation: review after five years. *Journal of Bone and Joint Surgery* 1987; 69B: 719–22.
22. Galpin RD, Hawkins RJ, Grainger RW. A comparitive analysis of operative versus nonoperative treatment of grade III acromioclavicular separations. *Clinical Orthopaedics and Related Research* 1985; 193: 150–5.
23. Bannister GC, Wallace WA, Stableforth PG, Hutson MA. The management of acute acromioclavicular dislocation: a randomised prospective controlled trial. *Journal of Bone and Joint Surgery* 1989; 71B: 848–50.
24. Rosenørn M, Pedersen EB. A comparison between conservative and operative treatment of acute acromioclavicular dislocation. *Acta Orthopaedica Scandinavica* 1974; 45: 50–9.
25. Larsen E, Bjerg-Nielsen A, Christensen P. Conservative or surgical treatment of acromioclavicular dislocation: a prospective, controlled, randomized study. *Journal of Bone and Joint Surgery* 1986; 68A: 552–5.
26. Imatani RJ, Hanlon JJ, Cady GW. Acute, complete acromioclavicular separation. *Journal of Bone and Joint Surgery* 1975; 57A: 328–31.

27. Taft TN, Wilson FC, Oglesby JW. Dislocation of the acromioclavicular joint: an end-result study. *Journal of Bone and Joint Surgery* 1987; 69A: 1045–51.

28. Bjerneld H, Hovelius L, Thorling J. Acromio-clavicular separations treated conservatively: a 5 year follow-up study. *Acta Orthopaedica Scandinavica* 1983; 54: 743–5.

29. Jacobs B, Wade PA. Acromioclavicular joint injury: an end result study. *Journal of Bone and Joint Surgery* 1966; 48A: 475–86.

30. Dawe CJ. Acromioclavicular joint injuries. *Journal of Bone and Joint Surgery* 1980; 62B: 269.

31. Urist MR. Complete dislocations of the acromioclavicular joint. Follow-up notes on articles previously published in the Journal. *Journal of Bone and Joint Surgery* 1963; 45A: 1750–3.

32. Kennedy JC, Cameron H. Complete dislocation of the acromioclavicular joint. *Journal of Bone and Joint Surgery* 1954; 36B: 202–8.

33. Krueger-Franke M, Siebert CH, Rosemeyer B. Surgical treatment of dislocations of the acromioclavicular joint in the athlete. *British Journal of Sports Medicine* 1993; 27: 121–4.

34. Roper BA, Levack B. The surgical treatment of acromioclavicular dislocations *Journal of Bone and Joint Surgery* 1982; 64B: 597–9.

35. Stam L, Dawson I. Complete acromioclavicular dislocations: treatment with a Dacron ligament. *Injury* 1991; 22: 173–6.

36. Weinstein DM, McCann PD, McIlveen SJ, Flatow EL, Bigliani LU. Surgical treatment of complete acromioclavicular dislocations. *American Journal of Sports Medicine* 1995; 23: 324–31.

37. Walsh WM, Peterson DA, Shelton G, Neumann RD. Shoulder strength following acromioclavicular injury. *American Journal of Sports Medicine* 1985; 13: 153–7.

38. MacDonald PB, Alexander MJ, Frejuk J, Johnson GE. Comprehensive functional analysis of shoulders following complete acromioclavicular separation. *American Journal of Sports Medicine* 1988; 16: 475–80.

39. Wojtys EM, Nelson G. Conservative treatment of grade III acromioclavicular dislocations. *Clinical Orthopaedics and Related Research* 1991; 268: 112–19.

40. Neer CS. *Shoulder reconstruction.* Philadelphia: WB Saunders Company, 1990.

41. Sage FP, Salvatore JE. Injuries of acromioclavicular joint: study of results in 96 patients. *Southern Medical Journal* 1963; 56: 486–95.

42. Smith MJ, Stewart MJ. Acute acromioclavicular joint separations. A 20-year study. *American Journal of Sports Medicine* 1979; 7: 357–60.

43. Weaver JK, Dunn HK. Treatment of acromioclavicular injuries, especially complete acromioclavicular separation. *Journal of Bone and Joint Surgery* 1972; 54A: 1187–94.

44. Lizaur A, Marco L. Acute dislocation of the acromioclavicular joint: traumatic anatomy and the importance of deltoid and trapezius. *Journal of Bone and Joint Surgery* 1994; 76B: 602–6.

45. Phemister DB. The treatment of dislocation of the acromioclavicular joint by open reduction and threaded-wire fixation. *Journal of Bone and Joint Surgery* 1942; 24A: 166–8.

46. Habernek H, Weinstabl R, Schmid L, Fialka C. A crook plate for treatment of acromioclavicular joint separation: indication, technique, and results after one year. *Journal of Trauma* 1993; 35: 893–901.

47. Sim E, Schwarz N, Hocker K, Berzlanovich A. Repair of complete acromioclavicular separations using the acromioclavicular-hook plate. *Clinical Orthopaedics and Related Research* 1995; 314: 134–42.

48. Neviaser JS. Acromioclavicular dislocation treated by transference of the coraco-acromial ligament. *Clinical Orthopaedics and Related Research* 1968; 58: 57–68.

49. Copeland S, Kessel L. Disruption of the acromioclavicular joint: surgical anatomy and biological reconstruction. *Injury* 1980; 11: 208–14.

50. Ejeskar A. Coracoclavicular wiring for acromioclavicular joint dislocation: A ten year follow-up study. *Acta Orthopaedica Scandinavica* 1974; 45: 652–61.

51. Weitzman G. Treatment of acute acromioclavicular joint dislocation by a modified Bosworth method. *Journal of Bone and Joint Surgery* 1967; 49A: 1167–78.

52. Bearden JM, Hughston JC, Whatley GS. Acromioclavicular dislocation: method of treatment. *American Journal of Sports Medicine* 1973; 1: 5–17.

53. Morrison DS, Lemos MJ. Acromioclavicular separation: reconstruction using synthetic loop augmentation. *American Journal of Sports Medicine* 1995; 23 : 105–10.

54. Dahl E. Follow up after coracoclavicular ligament prosthesis for acromioclavicular joint dislocation. *Acta Chirurgica Scandinavica* 1981; 506: 96.

55. Lancaster S, Horowitz M. Alonso J. Complete acromioclavicular separations : a comparison of operative methods. *Clinical Orthopaedics and Related Research* 1987; 216: 80–8.

56. Browne JE, Stanley RF, Tullos MS. Acromioclavicular joint dislocations: comparative results following operative treatment with and without primary distal clavisectomy. *American Journal of Sports Medicine* 1977; 5: 258–63.

57. Bannister GD, Wallace WA, Stableforth PG, Hutson MA. A classification of acute acromioclavicular dislocation: a clinical, radiological and anatomical study. *Injury* 1992; 23: 194–6.

58. Dewar FP, Barrington TW. The treatment of chronic acromioclavicular dislocation. *Journal of Bone and Joint Surgery* 1965; 47B: 32–5.

4.3.5 Shoulder rehabilitation: principles and clinical specifics

Terry R. Malone

Introduction

The shoulder is the most mobile, and thus the least constrained, major joint in the human body. Stability is provided through a combination of active and passive structures. No other joint is so dependent upon musculature for stability and control. The inherent dichotomy of stability and mobility requires the rehabilitative specialist to approach patients with shoulder pathologies with care and precision. In this chapter we shall attempt to provide general principles of rehabilitation based upon anatomy and pathology in relation to the functional demands of the shoulder. Other chapters in this textbook address specific pathologies (rotator cuff, shoulder instability, and injuries of the acromioclavicular joint), and thus we shall not attempt to be all-encompassing but rather eclectic in providing clinical insight to the rehabilitation challenges presented by the shoulder complex.

Anatomy

The shoulder complex must be considered as a whole, as single structures cannot be appreciated without recognizing the impact provided by each component of the 'complex'. Additionally, many

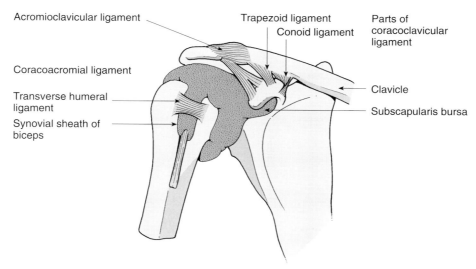

Fig. 1 Orientation of the glenohumeral joint and ligamentous/bony orientation. (Redrawn from ref. 9, with permission.)

compensatory patterns/positions are seen in athletes/workers which may have evolved to allow better performance of specific athletic or work activities (for example, tennis serve, throwing, typing, etc.). The importance in interpreting these alterations has been described by numerous authors.[1,2] Clinical recognition of these alterations requires awareness of the inter-relatedness and linkage of the shoulder in activity.

Skeletal anatomy

Three bony structures (clavicle, scapula, and humerus) comprise the shoulder skeleton. Unfortunately, many individuals do not recognize that these inter-related structures function as a single entity through the three synovial joints (sternoclavicular, acromioclavicular, and glenohumeral) and one physiological joint (scapulothoracic) to allow the multiple synchronous actions seen in the upper extremity. Many movements seen during shoulder function are provided through the contribution of each individual joint rather than action at the glenohumeral joint alone. Failure to realize these distinct contributions allows the patient to fall into the 'robbing Peter to pay Paul' sequence. Clinician awareness is critical, as the pattern of the musculofascial structures which 'bind' the shoulder to the trunk may be altered, thus resulting in structural or functional alteration in upper-extremity activities.

The clavicle is anchored to the trunk at the sternoclavicular joint, which has two synovial cavities separated by a fibrocartilaginous disc.[3,4] This joint functions primarily as a 'saddle', allowing rotation but with other displacements. The acromioclavicular joint provides a gliding action and does not overly constrain the scapula.[3] The clavicle acts as a strut (yard-arm) or crankshaft to enable greater functioning of the shoulder complex.[5]

The scapula is a complex triangular structure which provides sites for muscular/ligamentous attachment and bony articulation. Interestingly, its axial/appendicular orientation is completely controlled by musculature or fascial constraint. Clinicians frequently forget the enormous neuromuscular demands of shoulder function, and thus do not recognize the need for a stable base (proximal control) for normal distal activity.[6] The glenoid fossa is deepened by the fibrocartilaginous labrum; this increases the limited articulation and is extremely important in the high demands of athletic participation.[7,8]

The proximal humerus includes the humeral head with the greater and lesser tuberosities, as well as the proximal body or shaft. Examination of the glenohumeral joint demonstrates the inherent lack of stability and the resultant demands placed on neuromuscular control (Fig. 1).

Stability

The stability of the shoulder complex can be divided into passive and active components. Inherent passive stabilizers include numerous fibrous structures, but their contributions vary with composition and joint position. Individual variation in composition is obvious and dictates the level of laxity seen with direct measures. Joint position is critical, as the ability of a structure to control movement must be correlated to fibre alignment/orientation. An example of this is the need for patients to be urged to work on increasing rotation at multiple areas or points of flexion rather than working only within the extremes of the range of motion.

The use of the arthroscope allowed a much greater appreciation of the shoulder complex to emerge during the 1980s and 1990s.[10,11] Shoulder ligamentous restraints are frequently described by location and orientation. The glenohumeral ligaments are divided into superior, middle, and inferior (Fig. 2), with each portion exhibiting different levels of tension throughout the range of motion. O'Brien et al.[10] have demonstrated the importance of viewing the capsule in total rather than addressing only specific portions. The function of these structures has been stated beautifully by Terry et al.: 'The static restraints of the scapulohumeral joint provide stability for the humeral head in the glenoid cavity, limit extremes of motion of the glenohumeral joint, and guide positioning of the humerus during normal shoulder movement'.[11] It should also be noted that these structures work in a complementary fashion with the glenoid labrum. Many of the problems related to throwing can be attributed not only to the tremendous demands but also to the concept of mechanical links. We frequently talk of lower-extremity patterns being dominated by closed kinetic chain activities while the upper extremity functions very much in an open pattern. This places extreme demands on musculature, as the greatest muscular activity is present during deceleration (Fig. 3).[12,13]

Active stabilizers

Hughston describes the functionality of the complex as being almost completely dependent on the 'synergism of musculotendinous units'. The scapula is supported and anchored to the scapula by six muscles, while nine muscles provide the free movements seen at the glenohumeral joint. The complex inter-relationships of the musculature have been described eloquently by Hollinshead,[3] Kent,[14] and Perry.[15] Hollinshead describes the glenohumeral actions as being best delineated as the short muscles acting to retain the humerus in its proper orientation, with the longer muscle responsible for the freedom of movement of the humerus upon the glenoid. Complex force couples are required for normal patterns of movement with minimal changes requiring major adaptive responses which may predispose the individual to future injury and/or degeneration. Because of the complex synergistic relationships, it is often difficult to determine whether a muscle is acting as a prime mover or a stabilizer, thus preventing undesired proximal movement which would alter length-to-tension ratios. We believe that the supraspinatus is the key to shoulder rehabilitation, and is also the muscle most frequently unable to perform the 'fine tuning' required for formal athletic activities. The maintenance of the humeral head in the 'centred position' on the glenoid is an absolute requirement for normal shoulder function. Additionally, the external rotators are quite synergistic with the supraspinatus and require attention during most rehabilitative programmes. The importance of the musculature is displayed vividly by the early inferior subluxation which occurs in a flaccid shoulder or a shoulder inhibited by an effusion: there is a loss of proprioceptive feedback following injury to capsular structures, and a normalization of this neural mechanism should not be overlooked.[16] Neural activity (drive, recruitment, synchronization) has a direct relationship with musculature, and thus they are interwoven and both demand attention during the rehabilitation process.

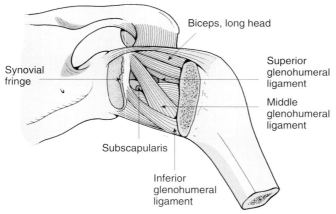

Fig. 2 The anterior glenohumeral ligamentous/capsular structures seen from a posterior exposure looking forward. (Redrawn from ref. 9, with permission.)

Biceps, long head
Superior glenohumeral ligament
Middle glenohumeral ligament
Synovial fringe
Subscapularis
Inferior glenohumeral ligament

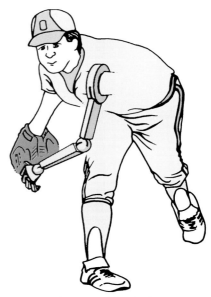

Fig. 3 The open kinetic chain pattern of function is seen in the upper extremity. (Reproduced from ref. 2, with permission.)

Special evaluation of the athletic shoulder

General evaluation of the shoulder complex has been presented by numerous authors.[17-21] The throwing shoulder requires additional evaluation because of the enormous stresses presented and the adaptations seen in the musculoskeletal system. The throwing athletes typically demonstrate a large increase in external rotation with a corresponding loss of internal rotation when the throwing shoulder is compared with the normal shoulder. This relative increase is even further enhanced after the athlete has warmed up—primarily, it appears to be an adaptation to allow a greater distance for acceleration, thus allowing the throwing athlete to achieve a greater velocity. A second compensatory change is the hypertrophy of the upper-extremity musculature of the throwing shoulder. Possibly associated with this finding is the characteristic drooping or depression of the dominant shoulder.[22] Subtle postural and mechanical anomalies are thus the rule rather than the exception when evaluating the throwing shoulder. Clinicians would do well to realize the 'normalcy' of these changes and their implications, including alteration of length-to-tension ratios, and the need for these adaptive responses if an athlete is to be successful following rehabilitation.

A functional evaluation of the shoulder is probably one of the most important facets of the total evaluation scheme which frequently is not utilized by many clinicians. It is imperative to determine when the chief complaint appears during a specific action, as well as determining its severity and reproducibility. As stated previously, it is sometimes difficult to determine whether a muscle is acting as a prime mover or as a stabilizer, but adding information as to where in the range of motion and what action is being performed may allow the clinician to determine whether the muscle is acting as a stabilizer (isometric or eccentric muscle activation) or as a prime mover (concentric contraction). This information is imperative for a proper structuring of the rehabilitation sequence. It is not enough for the clinician to determine that the shoulder pops or catches;

Table 1	Functional sequence of pain
Level 1	Pain after specific activity
Level 2	Pain during and after specific activities, but not affecting performance
Level 3	Pain during and after specific activity, and affecting performance of such activity
Level 4	Pain with activities of daily living
Level 5	Pain at rest

rather, specific information as to when the pop or catch occurs, whether it occurs consistently or inconsistently, and whether there is pain associated with this action gives much information that is both relevant and important.

Principles of shoulder rehabilitation

The following principles are presented to allow development of a well-structured and sequenced rehabilitation scheme.

Principle 1: let pain be the guide

Pain must be recognized as the controlling factor in our rehabilitation sequence, because motion-specific or action-specific pain requires the modification or elimination of that activity. Pain is frequently a sign of inflammation to a specific structure, or impingement on a specific structure through a specific movement. The use of a functional classification scheme of pain for patient progression (Table 1) is recommended.

A functional classification pattern allows the patients to communicate what is happening during their rehabilitation in relation to activities, and also allows them to become aware of their progression. It is imperative that the patients become active participants within the rehabilitation sequence and take 'ownership' of their specific problem. As previously stated, inflammation may play a predominant role and thus must be controlled by minimizing continued or secondary insult (elimination of offending exercise), pharmacological intervention (steroidal or non-steroidal anti-inflammatory drugs), or cryotherapy modalities. Severe pain may also necessitate the use of pain modulation techniques, including manual therapy techniques (oscillations), transcutaneous neuromuscular stimulation (**TENS**), high-voltage, microamperage stimulation (**MENS**), and/or other physical therapy, pain modulation techniques/modalities. A guiding/over-riding pattern is that the rehabilitation programme must reach the cause of the problem rather than treating the symptoms presented. Pain control must be followed by an appropriate intervention/rehabilitation programme.

Principle 2: exercise must be performed in a painfree/available range of motion

Muscles are absolutely critical to the control of the upper extremity. Since the shoulder is dependent upon musculature for its functional stability, rehabilitation protocols must address early strengthening within the available range of motion provided by specific problems. An example is the use of isometric exercises at multiple angles in those patients whose pathology dictates the restriction of the range of motion. As soon as isometric exercise is painfree, partial range of motion isotonic activities can be performed, as well as what may be called isodynamic actions involving the use of surgical tubing (Fig. 4).

It is important to note that exercises of this type (using surgical tubing) can be performed with an emphasis on concentric or eccentric muscle activation. We attempt to determine the type of lesion (cause of problem) and address it by matching the muscular demand to functional activity. An example of this process is the use of early activities, below 60 degrees of abduction and forward-flexion with minimal external rotation, performed as soon as tolerated by patients with anteroinferior shoulder dislocations. We have found the use of surgical tubing to be very helpful as well as being a very portable means of exercise. We also attempt to ensure that the patient is provided with a means of performing the exercises requested, and have found the **BREG** shoulder therapy kit to be extremely useful. This collapsible therapy kit comprises a collapsible bar, a rope-and-pulley set, and multiple 'surgical tubing' sets with different resistances (Fig. 5). Patients must be aware of remaining in a controlled pattern of exercise when using tubing, as muscular control is the goal and uncontrolled actions can be counterproductive leading to inflammation or continued alteration in muscle activation. This is commonly seen during external rotation movements if one end of the tubing is fixed, which means that the end of the range of motion experiences the greatest loads. We modify this problem by having the patient hold the tubing in both hands and allowing them to adjust the tension by moving the other (uninvolved) hand, this has the effect of decreasing or increasing the tension as desired.

Principle 3: increase range of motion at multiple planes

Clinicians frequently attempt to increase rotation only at the extremes of the range of motion. In order to recognize the rotational components and their effect on the multiple structures of the shoulder capsule, it is very helpful to work on internal and external rotation at different portions of forward-flexion or abduction. With athletes it is also imperative to work on rotation in functional positions. We frequently view throwing as involving overhead activity when, in fact, the glenohumeral actions occur from 70 to 100 degrees of abduction.[23]

Specificity of range of motion would thus dictate that internal/external rotation work is performed with the arm in a 70- to 100-degree abduction position, thus mimicking the throwing position (Fig. 6).

A combination of Principles 1 and 3 is involved in the treatment of the patient with adhesive capsulitis. Clinicians frequently use thermotherapy modalities applied over the shoulder when the area of maximal involvement is in the inferior fold of the shoulder capsule. Thus clinicians should apply their modality to the axilla, but may also wish to apply a similar modality over the shoulder for generalized relaxation. This is particularly true if these patients have been treated previously, and they may question the treatment if they

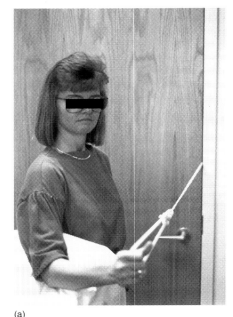

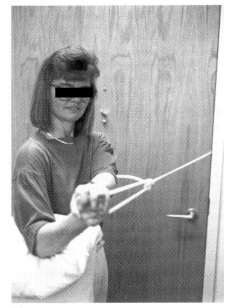

(a)

(b)

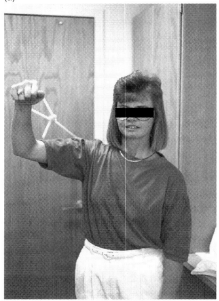

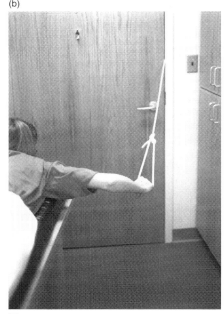

(c)

(d)

Fig. 4 The use of surgical tubing is extremely flexible: (a) external rotation in a standing position with the humerus slightly forward-flexed and abducted, a position found to be more comfortable for many patients with impingement syndrome when strengthening the external rotators. (b) Subjects can emphasize the eccentric component by stretching the tubing with the contralateral extremity and then slowing allowing a return, thus eccentrically controlling the movement. (c) Specific positioning and speed can be included during the workout by working on a throwing pattern, as well as incorporating a plyometric (stretch–contraction or stretch–shortening cycle) using surgical tubing. (d) Strengthening in a sport-specific position is extremely critical for rotational strength and endurance as demonstrated in the freestyle swimming position (the athlete can work on both internal and external rotation in this position). A similar example of this process is for patients to work from 20 to 30 degrees of abduction in combination with slight forward-flexion into what is referred to as the 'scapular plane position', and for them to move only to approximately 60 degrees, thus staying in a very comfortable part of the range of motion. Any impingement symptoms are minimized and functional strengthening is allowed; this is a plane of motion frequently used.

are not receiving similar patterns or at least a consistency of application!

Principle 4: strengthen proximal musculature

Proximal stability is required for normal upper-extremity function. Clinicians must address any weakness of the scapular stabilizers, as well as recognizing the important role that upward rotation plays in allowing enhanced functional athletic activities (Fig. 7).

Clinicians must also address the endurance needs of the patient involved in activity that requires repetitive or continued positioning (swimming, typing, overhead work, etc.) as well as addressing the absolute maximum effort demanded of athletes in events such as pitching or tackling in power-dominated sports.

Principle 5: strengthen individual muscles

The ability of the practitioner to isolate and thus provide appropriate strengthening of an individual muscle is paramount. Teaching the patient to avoid compensatory muscular action or abnormal substitutions is absolutely vital to long-term success.

In addition, individual muscles must be strengthened at a variety of length-to-tension ratios since their activity may demand different levels of performance/activation, as well as requiring different functions (eccentric versus concentric or stabilizing) throughout the range of motion. It is also important for the clinician to apply appropriate resistance, but mixing and matching the effort required is frequently useful. An example of this is to use a variety of sets and repetition combinations to 'bombard' the neuromuscular system

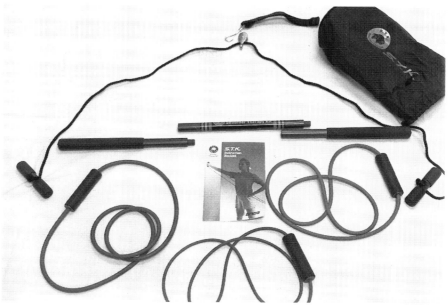

Fig. 5 The BREG shoulder therapy kit: this kit comprises a collapsible bar, an overhead pulley with mounting apparatus for door positioning, three different thicknesses of surgical tubing, an instructional booklet, and a canvas bag in which all these materials can be stored and transported.

with differing demands, thus emphasizing motor learning throughout the rehabilitation sequence. An example is to use not only isotonic (concentric and eccentric) activities, but also to supplement these with isodynamic (surgical tubing) and isokinetic movements during the rehabilitation progression. Another interesting factor is the use of speed-controlled, eccentric activity, which is available with the newer, active-isokinetic dynamometers. These activities can be performed against the motorized equipment which may actually give a different demand and message to the neural system than those seen with the eccentric activity performed isotonically. This is an assumption, but it may be quite helpful in allowing a variety of demands to be placed on the neuromuscular system. One of the advantages of the use of isokinetic equipment is that it allows the patient to work in isolated rotational patterns, but it does not allow them to substitute inappropriate movements or demand that

they attempt to perform at an uncomfortable level. Isokinetic exercise which is performed concentrically is extremely safe and is completely dependent upon the forces applied by the individual. We have much less information and experience with eccentric dynamometry (controlled patterns), but the use of these devices is increasing with excellent clinical results. Some of these devices allow both an active eccentric mode (that is to say, the machine pushes as long as the minimum force required of the patient is present) and resistance against the passive movement mode—a situation that is very comfortable and allows additional exercise applications.

Principle 6: strengthen muscles in groups—within functional patterns

Once the clinician has ensured that proximal stability and adequate strength are established in individual muscles, the patient must be

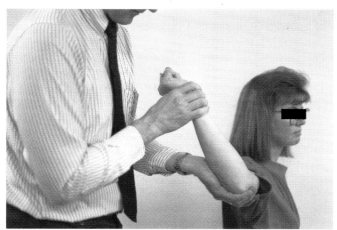

Fig. 6 Stretching should be performed within a specific range of motion which is demanded by the activity—external rotation stretching performed by a thrower in a 90-degree glenohumeral abduction position. (The increased external rotation seen in most throwers should be noted.)

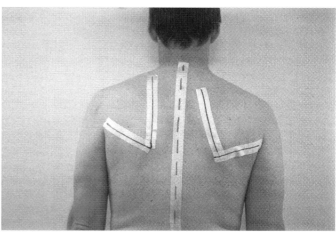

Fig. 7 The slightly upwardly rotated position of the dominant (throwing) extremity which may be an adaptation to allow greater acceleration and thus more effective throwing. The depression (lower rest position) of the dominant shoulder should also be noted.

progressed into functional patterns. Strengthening in patterns has been espoused very strongly by the proponents of proprioceptive neuromuscular facilitation.[24] An interesting expression is the functionalization of individual muscular strength. This is a very apt description of this phase of the rehabilitation process, as the patient works in diagonal patterns which are much more appropriate and require neuromuscular coordination of rotation and fine movements distally with proximal stability.

Principle 7: don't beat a dead horse

If no response is seen in the first 6 to 8 weeks, it is unlikely that a significant turnaround or response will occur. It has been the author's experience that most patients with shoulder injuries will respond relatively quickly (4 weeks or less) if conservative management is going to be successful. Our protocols typically are designed to demonstrate improvement and progression within this 6-week period. This approach has allowed us to minimize the abuse of patients presenting with a primary lesion or those with an underlying condition. In the latter, for instance, a previous cuff lesion may be related to an insufficiency of the supraspinatus muscle to keep the humeral head correctly positioned, this lesion may have healed but now presents as a lengthened structure which is unable to create enough force to balance functional actions at the shoulder. The observation of a timed response has been supported by Morrison *et al.*; they reported that if no change was observed in patients with impingement conditions within 6 weeks of conservative treatment, then they rarely saw improvements after this time.[25]

Principle 8: functional rehabilitation— functional progression

Once the patient has proceeded through the rehabilitation sequence and has moved through the various levels of pain, the culmination of these activities should be a functional progression. Functional progressions are designed to allow the individual to return to their activities of choice through specific adaptations to imposed demands.[21,26] During this phase of rehabilitation, attention is directed to specific activities such that rehabilitation addresses velocity, level of resistance, type of contraction, and endurance required for a specific performance. An example is the progression of the tennis player from controlled ground strokes to controlled overheads, with a slow progression on to a flat serve prior to the initiation of either a slice or twist serve. The progression allowed must not only proceed according to the reaction of the patient as he or she attempts to perform the activity properly, but also to the response of the tissue the following day (that is to say, both the immediate response as well as the residual response seen the next day should be monitored). The rehabilitation/functional progression must be designed with intermediate as well as with long-term aims in mind.

We conclude this chapter with a variety of case studies demonstrating the application of these principles, and with examples of how modification of the exercise sequence is required to fit the individual needs of the specific patient.

Case study 1

A 17-year-old, white male, interscholastic swimmer presented with shoulder pain of 6 months' duration. The pain had worsened dramatically over the last 3 weeks, with a decrease in his ability to per-

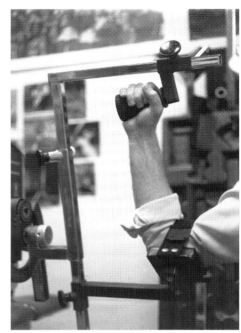

Fig. 8 Isokinetic evaluation—test position of internal/external rotators.

form. Pain was now present during normal daily activities, but the symptoms were greatly exacerbated during swimming. He was most symptomatic with freestyle, which, unfortunately, was his primary competitive stroke. Upon questioning, this patient related that his routine had recently changed to include the use of hand paddles for 2500 to 3000 m daily. Interestingly, this coincided with the increase in his symptoms. This individual had sought medical attention approximately 3 months earlier; he had been placed on a strengthening routine and an attempt was made to decrease his swimming with the use of a kickboard over a 3- to 4-week period. Unfortunately, the strengthening routine implemented included primarily those activities which increased internal rotation strength and were performed in non-swimming oriented positions. He had also used the kickboard in an extended position (arms in front of the body), which would not improve but rather maintain the symptoms associated with this condition. Examination of his present routine also revealed two daily workouts of approximately 5000 to 6000 m each, with approximately 1200 to 1300 m being accomplished with the use of hand paddles. It is our experience that the use of hand paddles will greatly increase swimming shoulder problems, as rotation is the least well controlled of the movements and thus the most demanding.

Initial plan

This athlete was exhibiting level 5 to level 4 pain, since he was experiencing pain with activities of daily living and minimal pain at rest. Isokinetic evaluation of his internal/external rotators revealed that the external rotators were only capable of generating approximately 40 per cent of the internal rotators in a concentric pattern (Fig. 8). Falkel and Murphy[21] have reported similar findings in the evaluation of swimmers with shoulder pain. Our initial management thus centred on the following modalities.

1.   Controlling inflammation (oral anti-inflammatory drugs).

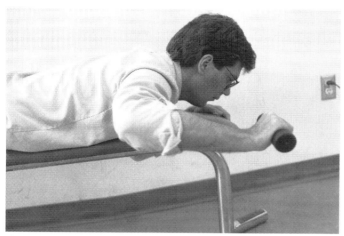

Fig. 9 Prone weight-training positions for strengthening the external rotators (see also Fig. 4(d) on the use of surgical tubing). This position is ideal for the swimmer but would not be as applicable to the thrower, i.e. the thrower would exercise in an upright standing position.

2. Maintaining aerobic base by using a kickboard placed under the abdomen, and discontinuing hand paddles.

3. Modifying strength training to emphasize external rotation in multiple angles of abduction and forward-flexion and swimming position patterns (Fig. 9).

4. Using modalities to decrease impingement types of problems at the suprahumeral space (moist heat and ultrasound)—these were applied with the arm in an abducted and slightly forward-flexed position to minimize vascular problems (Fig. 10).[21,27]

5. Altering swimming practice to emphasize quality of stroke rather than quantity—thus allowing only a few hundred metres to be performed using the shoulder, but emphasizing quality during that time-frame. It is our opinion that coaches have too often emphasized distance, and thus quantity rather than quality of stroke. This has led to Olympic swimmers actually being survivors rather than the best trained. The

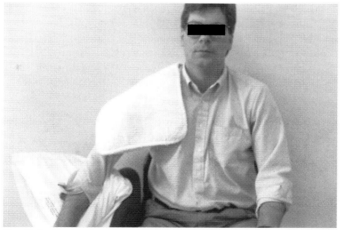

Fig. 10 Positioning of the upper extremity during the application of modalities to minimize vascular compromise.

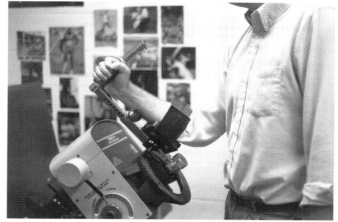

Fig. 11 Modified base position for internal/external rotation to minimize vascular compromise.

only swimmers able to survive these exhausting workouts were those who were fortunate in having a very large suprahumeral space and excellent external rotator/ supraspinatus musculature.

6. After workouts, ice massage to the suprahumeral area was performed for 10 to 12 min.

After 10 days of this treatment strategy, increasing endurance was emphasized in the subject's external/internal rotator strengthening sequence. A total of 20 to 50 repetitions were being performed, and he was able to increase from two to three sets up to four to five sets utilizing the modified base position at a velocity of approximately 240 degrees/s (Fig. 11). This position helps to minimize the vascular compromise which may be present, as well as providing greater space to the suprahumeral area. This athlete used this routine for approximately 3 weeks, and was also using pull cords and surgical tubing in a swim-simulated stroke position to work again on endurance as well as the specific strengthening needed for the external/internal rotation component. He was allowed to increase his swimming as symptoms permitted, and was swimming approximately 3000 m each day with relatively minimal symptoms. Over the next 3 weeks, he increased this to where he was able to swim 5000 m daily and has continued at that level with no return of symptoms. After 6 weeks of modified workouts, his isokinetic strength assessment revealed that his external rotators were now 55 per cent of his internal rotators as measured concentrically.

This case presentation highlights the integration of sports-specific rehabilitation with appropriate medical management in the presentation of a young swimmer with shoulder pain. The actual aetiology of this problem is frequently thought to be an impingement or supraspinatus tendinitis. The actual entity is not as important as the appropriate management of symptoms and attention to the causative factors. Too often, medical practitioners will either tell the swimmer to stop swimming or only address the pain. The pain that is present is a signal to the clinician to find and address the cause of the patient's pain. Previous intervention had been unsuccessful, as the causative factors had not been addressed (external rotational weakness, supraspinatus weakness, use of hand paddles, and use of a kickboard with the shoulders in an extended position).

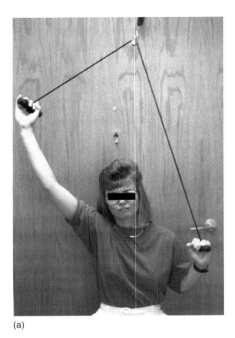

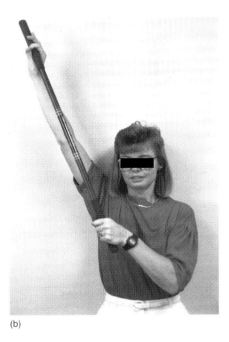

(a)   (b)

Fig. 12 (a) Assistive pulleys which allow the person to perform active movement when possible, assisted if necessary. (b) The use of a BREG stick to assist in abduction. It may often be helpful to supinate rather than using the pronated position.

One of the areas in sports medicine which demands further attention is the integration of medical and coaching expertise in the formulation of training programmes. Swimming is one of the areas where this is easily seen but not easily achieved.

Case study 2

A 62-year-old, white man was self-referred to the clinic for evaluation of right shoulder pain. He reported that 10 days previously, while attempting to start his lawnmower, he experienced an acute onset of pain when the starter 'caught' as he was attempting to pull on the starter cord. He continued to have pain both during the day and at night (Level 5—pain at rest). Examination revealed an inability to abduct the arm actively, and the drop arm test was positive. An arthrogram was performed which demonstrated a complete thickness tear, and the patient chose to have surgical intervention. A separation of approximately 1 cm in the superior rotator cuff was repaired. Postoperative management began with sling immobilization for 4 weeks. During this period, he was allowed to forward-flex and abduct assistively, using the opposite hand to support the weight of the affected arm (designed to minimize distraction forces—this is a modified pendulum exercise). Additional recommendations during the early part of postoperative management included supporting and propping the arm with pillows when writing or sitting. This is particularly important if the person is going to be in an automobile for long periods.

We frequently instruct the patient in self-oscillation techniques, but again they must be performed without distraction forces during the initial weeks. Typically, between the third and fourth week of their postoperative course, patients are allowed to begin more active/assistive patterns. These can be accomplished using a stick, dowel rod, cane, tennis racket, golf club, etc., or assistive pulley patterns (Fig. 12). The use of water, when available, is preferable, as buoyancy allows fairly rapid redevelopment of neuromuscular co-ordination and minimizes the development of disassociation seen with scapular and glenohumeral actions. The normal two-to-one ratio of glenohumeral-to-scapulothoracic contributions to abduction are not present following rotator-cuff repairs. Patients will have great difficulty moving in normal patterns, and will attempt to maintain the glenohumeral position and move primarily through the scapulothoracic joint. Water appears to be a very good medium to minimize a continuation of this adaptive or compensatory movement pattern. At approximately 6 weeks after the operation, the patient is allowed to begin a more aggressive active programme, and weights are often attached to the wrist rather than held in the hand (Fig. 13). This helps to minimize the formation or maintenance of abnormal movement patterns or compressive activities frequently seen with these patients.

The primary function of the supraspinatus may be to position the head of the humerus properly during shoulder movement. These actions may be extremely demanding, and therefore any lack of neural control leads to abnormal force–couple relationships and abnormal shoulder function. A very interesting finding in these patients is the difficulty in moving from a concentric contraction into an eccentric or lowering muscle activation pattern. These patients frequently say: 'It hurts the most when I try to lower the arm after I have raised it'. We believe that this is related to the transfer of increased stress to the tendon as the contribution of the contractile element of the muscle is decreased. Thus it is very important to work on both concentric and eccentric activities, but these must be done lower in the range of motion rather than in the more demanding side-arm positions. Another technique which is frequently used is to teach the patient self-mobilization/distraction patterns at 8 to 10 weeks after the operation (Fig. 14). This may be quite helpful in those patients who have a chronic rather than a traumatic development of shoulder dysfunction, but it is most important in those patients tending to have impingement problems associated with rotator-cuff lesions. Surgical tubing is used in these patients, as both concentric and eccentric activities can be per-

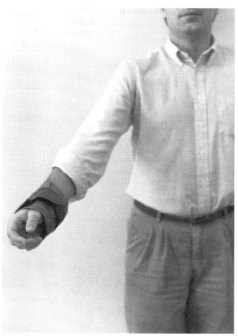

Fig. 13 It is often helpful to suspend the weight rather than allowing the patient to grasp it, thus minimizing abnormal muscular patterns. The scapular plane positioning (functional pattern) should be noted.

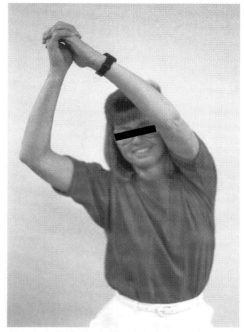

Fig. 15 Teaching the individual to 'roll' assistively from a forward-flexed position into external rotation and abduction as he or she returns from the forward-flexed position. The term to describe this to the patient may be to 'roll out and down' or 'roll out and over' as the arm is lowered.

formed and little equipment is required. The clinician is reminded of the caveat of making the tubing resistance adjustable to avoid too great a stress at the extreme range of motion. One additional, active-assistive technique which is very helpful in regaining full abduction patterns is for the patient to forward-flex with the hands interlocked and, rather than returning in a forward-flexion pattern, to rotate the

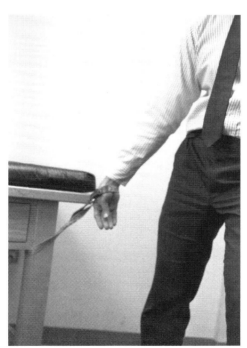

Fig. 14 Self-mobilization/distraction patterns utilizing a belt and a stabilizing object.

extremity into an abduction pattern and controllably lower through that range with the assistance of the opposite extremity (Fig. 15). This seems to be quite useful and helpful for many patients.

We attempt to educate our patients who have had a rotator-cuff repair into a 3-month, 6-month, 1-year sequence. We tell them that it will be 3 months before they begin to have functional ranges and control of those ranges, while at 6 months they will know how much range and control they can achieve. The most sobering information for them is that between 6 months and 1 year they will gain an additional 10 to 15 per cent of strength, and therefore it will be a year before they will know how well they will be able to do.

This case study presents many common-sense activities that can be provided following rotator-cuff injury and repair. One of the important factors is to warn patients (and the general public) of the danger of starting motors with a pull cord, as we find this to be a fairly common mechanism of injury. The patient described in this case study did not wish to wait to see if he would be able to tolerate the limitations presented by his injury using a conservative approach to treatment, but many individuals should be allowed an opportunity to determine what would be their own natural course. In this case, it was his dominant extremity, and he was a very active individual and wished to have the best possible result. At 6 months he had essentially a full range of motion, and was swimming three times each week. At his 1-year assessment, he was asymptomatic and doing extremely well.

Case study 3

A 42-year-old university professor came to the clinic complaining of pain and stiffness in his left shoulder. Examination revealed the classic pattern seen with adhesive capsulitis: marked loss of abduction, external rotation, internal rotation, and forward-flexion. It is

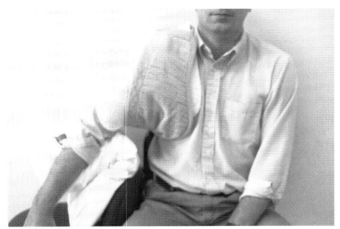

Fig. 16 In adhesive capsulitis, the application of moist heat should be superior and inferior to the glenohumeral joint, thus reaching the axillary fold.

our experience that the loss of the rotations is pathognomonic of this condition. He is also diabetic, which we have frequently seen to be related to this condition. He could not relate any acute episode of onset, but rather complained of a slow progression over 3 to 4 months.

As he preferred not to have an injection, he was provided with oral anti-inflammatory medication and a conservative management approach which included a supervised exercise sequence three times weekly to supplement his thrice daily independent programme. He was instructed in self-mobilization techniques (Fig. 14), moist heat was applied over and to the axilla in an attempt to reach the inferior capsular recess (Fig. 16), and an assistive passive–active programme was utilized for forward-flexion, abduction, and external rotation. These activities included a wall stretch (facing and away from the side) and using a door-frame for external rotation patterns. He also worked at multiple levels of rotation at different levels of forward-flexion and abduction.

His supervised therapy sequence included ultrasound to the inferior fold/axilla, moist heat (as previously described), mobilization (inferior glide, glides in abduction, and rotational patterns), and stretching routines. After 1 month, the patient had achieved a very marked increase in his abduction (120 degrees combined glenohumeral and scapulothoracic actions) and was able actively to forward-flex approximately 140 degrees. He was also using the forward-flexion roll into abduction sequence quite effectively (Fig. 15). His external rotation had improved from 5 to 10 degrees to approximately 35 to 40 degrees. He was placed on a maintenance/supervised physical training sequence once a week for the next month, and continued using his thrice-daily programme independently. His clinical progress reached a plateau, but his functional level continued to show a gradual improvement over the next few months.

This case study demonstrates the usual onset of adhesive capsulitis of the shoulder. It has an insidious onset, women present earlier than men (as their activities of daily living demand greater activities of the hand behind the back), and it has an apparent link to other disease processes (diabetes, etc.). It is imperative to educate these patients in the proper control of their condition, and to make them aware that this problem may arise in the future. There is debate as to

how aggressively this entity should be treated, but we have found conservative measures to be helpful in the majority of cases, particularly as they begin to regain range of motion in the later stages.

Conclusions

The great mobility and lack of inherent stability at the shoulder make it a very challenging complex for the rehabilitation specialist. We have recommended that the clinician becomes aware of the functional sequence of pain and uses this as a guide to the rehabilitation process. A series of principles interlinks the total process, with the final ones being those of functional rehabilitation leading to return to the desired activity. Clinicians must learn to examine the specific actions required and the type of contraction imposed on the shoulder complex during shoulder activities. During rehabilitation, concentric activity alone is frequently utilized when, in reality, eccentric activity is symptomatic and required (see Chapter 4.4.4). Finally, the aim of the rehabilitation process must be function, and patients must become responsible for their ultimate return to the functional state.

References

1. Kibler B. Scapular position in throwing athletes. Presented to the *American Orthopedic Society for Sports Medicine*, Traverse City, MI, 1989; and Kibler WB. Role of the scapula in the overhead throwing motion. *Contemporary Orthopaedics* 1991; **22**: 525–32.
2. Kegerreis S, Jenkins L. In: Malone TR, ed. *Sports injury management. Vol. 2, Throwing injuries.* Baltimore: Williams & Wilkins, 1989.
3. Hollinshead WH. Functional anatomy of the limbs and back, 3rd edn. Philadelphia: WB Saunders, 1969.
4. Gould JA. *Orthopaedic and sports physical therapy*, 2nd edn. St Louis: CV Mosby, 1990; 3rd edn., 1997.
5. Hughston JC. Functional anatomy of the shoulder. In: Zarins B, Andrews, JR, Carson WG, eds. *Injuries to the throwing arm.* Philadelphia: WB Saunders, 1985: 43–50.
6. Soderberg GL. *Kinesiology: application to pathological motion.* Baltimore: Williams & Wilkins, 1986.
7. Bost FC. the pathological changes in recurrent dislocation of the shoulder. *Journal of Bone and Joint Surgery* 1942; **26**: 595–613.
8. Saha AK. Mechanics of elevation of the glenohumeral joint. Its application in rehabilitation. *Acta Orthopaedica Scandinavica* 1973; **44**: 667–78.
9. *Grant's atlas of anatomy*, 7th edn. Baltimore: Williams & Wilkins, 1978.
10. O'Brien SJ, Neves MC, Arnoczky SP, *et al.* The anatomy and histology of the inferior glenohumeral complex of the shoulder. *American Journal of Sports Medicine* 1990; **18**: 449–56.
11. Terry GC, Hammon D, France P, Norwood LA. The stabilizing function of passive shoulder restraints. *American Journal of Sports Medicine* 1991; **19**: 26–34.
12. Jobe FW, Tibone JE, Perry J, Moynes D. An EMG analysis of the throwing shoulder in throwing and pitching: a second report. *American Journal of Sports Medicine* 1984; **12**: 218–20.
13. Jobe FW, Tibone, JE, Perry J, Moynes D. An EMG analysis of the throwing shoulder in throwing and pitching: a second report. *American Journal of Sports Medicine*, 1984; 12: 218–20.
14. Kent BE. Functional anatomy of the shoulder complex. *Physical Therapy*, 1971; **51**: 867–87.
15. Perry J. Shoulder anatomy in biomechanics. In: *Clinics in sports medicine—injuries to the shoulder in the athlete.* Philadelphia: WB Saunders, 1983: 247–70.

16. Smith EL, Brunolli J. Shoulder kinesthesia after anterior gleno-humeral joint dislocation. *Physical Therapy* 1989; **69**: 106–12.
17. Davies, GJ, Gould JA, Larson RL. Functional examination of the shoulder girdle. *Physician in Sports Medicine* 1981; **9**: 82–102.
18. Hoppenfeld S. *Physical examination of the spine and extremities.* New York: Appleton-Century-Crofts, 1976.
19. Magee DJ. *Orthopaedic physical assessment.* Philadelphia: WB Saunders, 1987.
20. Malone TR. Elements of a standardized shoulder examination. In: Andrews JR, Wilk KE, eds. *The athlete's shoulder.* New York: Churchill Livingstone, 1994: 39–44.
21. Falkel JE, Murphy TC. In: Malone TR, ed. *Sports injury management—shoulder injuries.* Baltimore: Williams & Wilkins, 1988.
22. Priest JD, Nagel DA. Tennis shoulder. *American Journal of Sports Medicine* 1976; **4**: 213–42.
23. Atwater AE. Biomechanics of overarm throwing movements and of throwing injuries. *Exercise and Sports Science Review* 1979; **7**: 43.
24. Voss DA, Ionta MK, Meyers VJ. *Proprioceptive neuromuscular facilitation: patterns and techniques*, 3rd edn. Philadelphia: Harper & Row, 1985.
25. Morrison DS, Frogameni A, Woodworth P. Conservative manage-ment for subacromial impingement of the shoulder. *Journal of Shoulder and Elbow Surgery* 1994; Jan/Feb: s–12 (Abstract).
26. Kegerreis ST. The construction and implementation of functional progression as a component of athletic rehabilitation. *Journal of Orthopaedic and Sports Physical Therapy* 1983; 4: 14.
27. Rathburn JB, MacNab I. The microvascular pattern of the rotator cuff. *Journal of Bone and Joint Surgery* 1970; **52B**: 540–53.

Bibliography

Readers are urged to review the following references for specific rehabilitation information

Texts

Andrews JR, Wilk KE, eds. *The athlete's shoulder.* New York: Churchill Livingstone, 1994.

Donatelli RA, ed. *Physical therapy of the shoulder*, 2nd edn. New York: Churchill Livingstone, 1991.

Kelly MJ, Clark WA, eds. *Orthopedic therapy of the shoulder.* Philadelphia: JB Lippincott, 1995.

Special issues of *The Journal of Orthopaedic and Sports Physical Therapy: Current shoulder issues*—Part 1 (Vol. 18; No. 1, July 1993) and Part 2 (Vol. 18; No. 2, August 1993)

4.4 The ankle

4.4.1 Acute and overuse ankle injuries

J. E. Taunton, D. Robertson Lloyd-Smith, and Peter A. Fricker

Ankle injuries are extremely common: they occur in acute and chronic overuse situations. In this chapter we review the epidemiology and anatomy of ankle injuries. Overuse and acute injuries will be discussed, together with their mimics. Details of diagnosis and management will be included and the role of shoes, orthotics, taping, and braces in the prevention and management of ankle injuries will also be discussed.

Epidemiology

Ankle injuries are the single most common sporting injury, resulting in the greatest time lost from practice and games. Garrick[1] has performed some of the most extensive studies of the epidemiology of ankle injuries. He evaluated the injuries from four American high schools during the 1973 to 1974 and 1974 to 1975 school years. He identified 3049 students participating in 19 sports with a total of 1197 injuries. The three most common sites were the thigh, knee, and ankle, representing, respectively, 14.6 per cent, 14.5 per cent, and 14.1 per cent of all injuries. The most common injury was the ankle ligament sprain which represented 11.8 per cent of all injuries. A total of 161 ankle injuries were observed, of which 83.9 per cent were ligament sprains, 6.2 per cent were muscle strains, 2.5 per cent were lacerations, and 2.5 per cent were fractures. The only identifiable difference between the males and females was in the strain injury. This was believed to be related to male-dominated American football where 90 per cent of the musculotendinous strains occurred.

Injuries to the lateral ankle complex are extremely common and, in fact, Garrick's[2] early epidemiological study showed that they account for 38 to 45 per cent of all injuries. An earlier study of West Point cadets reported inversion sprains to be the most common injury, with an incidence of 33 per cent.[3] Garrick[2] had also found that 85 per cent of ankle injuries were sprains, with 85 per cent of these being inversion sprains. Chapman[4] and Balduini and Tetzlaff[5] have indicated that eversion sprains account for 6 per cent of ankle sprains with syndemosis injuries comprising 10 per cent of ankle injuries. Garrick[2] reported that one-sixth of all time lost in sport is a result of ankle sprains.

The sports most commonly resulting in ankle injuries were basketball, American football, soccer, and cross-country running for males; for females they were cross-country running, basketball, badminton, and gymnastics. Basketball resulted in an injury rate of 13.1 per cent ankle injuries per season for the males, and 11.4 per cent for the females. The rates for American football were 10.9 per cent, and those for cross-country running were 7.8 per cent for males and 11.5 per cent for females.

Garrick also evaluated 11 141 sports injuries sustained from 1980 to 1984 inclusive. Figure skating, basketball, and soccer produced the greatest number of ankle injuries. Ankle sprains were the most common injuries seen in basketball and soccer, whereas other overuse injuries (often associated with excessive boot pressure) were most common in figure skating. A significant number of ankle injuries were also reported in gymnastics and ballet. In gymnastics, the most common cause of injury was repetitive forced dorsiflexion of the ankle from 'landing short' in practice, producing anterior impingement injuries. In ballet, dancing in a hyperplantar flexed position resulted in posterior impingement injuries including os trigonum stress.

Overuse ankle injuries are commonly seen in our clinic at the University of British Columbia, Clement et al.[6] reported a retrospective survey of the clinical records of 1650 runners seen over a 3-year period. The lower leg and foot accounted for 46.7 per cent of the total injuries. The most common individual injuries in the ankle region were distal tibial stress fractures, tibialis posterior tendinitis, and peroneal tendinitis. These injuries accounted for 2.6 per cent, 2.5 per cent, and 1.9 per cent, respectively, of all injuries documented. Aetiological factors fell into five categories: training errors; lack of strength or flexibility; biomechanical and anatomical factors; poor running shoes; and poor training surfaces.

We have recently updated this study with a clinical study of 4175 runners seen over a 4-year period (1985 to 1988).[7] These athletes were grouped as recreational, marathon, and middle-distance competitive runners. The pattern of injuries had changed in the time between the two studies with a higher proportion of knee injuries and a relatively lower frequency of lower leg, ankle, and foot injuries. Much of this change appears to be attributable to footwear improvements. Bony stress injuries were more common among the middle-distance runners, possibly because of more intense training. The highest proportion of ankle overuse injuries were reported from cycling, ice skating, ballet, and running with added speed and interval sessions. In addition, this group carried out more of their training using spikes and racing flats with lower shock-attenuation and stability.

Walter et al.[8] reported that 22 per cent of all running-related injuries affected the foot and ankle. Marti et al.[9] reported a higher incidence of foot and ankle injuries in their studies of runners. They found that 40 per cent of the total injuries were to the foot and ankle, with some 15 per cent being lateral ankle ligament sprains. Macintyre *et al.*[7] found that only 2.1 per cent of the total injuries were ankle sprains. Garrick and Requa,[10] in their investigation of a large series of ankle injuries over 7 years, found that 27.6 per cent were due to overuse, with the highest proportion being from cycling, ice skating, ballet, and running.

Stress fractures are now commonly seen in sports medicine clinics. We analysed 320 athletes with bone scan-positive stress fractures seen over a period of 3.5 years.[11] The most common site of stress fracture was the tibia (49.1 per cent), followed by the tarsals (25.3 per cent), metatarsals (8.8 per cent), femur (7.2 per cent), and fibula (6.6 per cent). Tarsal stress fractures were seen in older athletes, and a history of trauma was significantly more common in injuries to the tarsal bones. Tarsal stress fractures also took the longest time to diagnosis (16.2 weeks) and to recovery (17.3 weeks). The average time to diagnosis for all stress fractures was 13.4 weeks and the average time to full recovery was 12.8 weeks. Pronated feet were most commonly found in tibial stress fractures and tarsal bone fractures, and cavus feet were most frequently seen with metatarsal and femoral stress fractures. Running was by far the most common activity involved, providing 221 of the 320 cases, with aerobic fitness classes the next most common, accounting for 25 cases.

Anatomical considerations

The ankle joint is a ginglymus or hinge joint. Dorsiflexion and plantar flexion occur at the ankle joint and the range of motion varies from 50 to 90 degrees. The ankle joint comprises the distal tibia and fibula which form the mortise for the articulation with the talus. The transverse axis of the ankle joint is slightly oblique.[12] The mortise itself is formed by the articular facet of the distal tibia and its extension the medial malleolus, plus the articular facet of the fibula with its extension, the lateral malleolus, which is longer than the medial malleolus. The wedge-shaped talus is wider anteriorly, which results in maximum stability in dorsiflexion but vulnerability to injury in plantar flexion. Weight-bearing transfer of force occurs from the talus to the foot. The talus is positioned on the anterior two-thirds of the calcaneus. The anterior head of the talus is rounded and articulates with the tarsal navicular. The navicular also articulates with the medial column of the foot which comprises the three cuneiforms and the first three metatarsals. The calcaneus articulates with the cuboid and the fourth and fifth metatarsals to comprise the lateral column of the foot.

The ankle joint has a capsule which Akesson described as being thin both anteriorly and posteriorly.[13] The capsule is reinforced by both medial and lateral collateral ligaments. The lateral ligament complex comprises the anterior talofibular ligament, the calcaneofibular ligament, and the posterior talofibular ligament. The strong medial ligament is also known as the deltoid ligament and can be divided into the anterior tibiotalar, tibionavicular, tibiocalcaneal, and posterior tibiotalar ligaments.

The ankle mortise is stabilized by very strong anterior and posterior tibiofibular ligaments. These are supported by the inferior transverse and interosseus ligaments forming the distal tibiofibular syndesmosis.

The subtalar joint is the site of the bulk of the inversion and eversion movements of the foot. This joint is supported by lateral, medial, and posterior talocalcaneal ligaments. There is also an interosseus talocalcaneal ligament within the sinus tarsi.

The functional anatomy of the ankle ligaments is summarized by Gray.[12] Briefly, the deltoid ligament is so strong that a bony avulsion fracture usually occurs with ankle eversion before significant ligament damage is sustained. The middle portion of the deltoid ligament, in combination with the calcaneal fibular ligament, control ankle eversion and inversion. The anterior and posterior aspects of the deltoid ligament limit plantar flexion and dorsiflexion of the foot. In addition, ankle abduction is limited by the anterior fibres. The posterior talofibular ligament of the lateral complex assists the calcaneal fibular ligaments in controlling posterior displacement of the foot. Anterior displacement is controlled primarily by the anterior talofibular ligaments. The anterior talofibular ligament also limits plantar flexion.

Ankle movement is a result of muscle actions that have origins from the distal end of the femur, the tibia, and the fibula, and which are applied to the foot. Dorsiflexion of the ankle is accomplished by the muscles of the anterior tibial compartment. These muscles are the tibialis anterior, extensor digitorum longus, and extensor hallucis longus. The last two muscles also extend (dorsiflex) the toes. This muscle compartment is innervated by the deep peroneal nerve. Plantar flexion of the foot and ankle is effected by the muscles of the superficial calf compartment: the gastrocnemius and soleus. Their insertion is by a common tendon, the Achilles tendon, attached to the posterior calcaneus. There is a retrocalcaneal bursa which separates this tendon from the calcaneus proximal to its insertion. These muscles are supplied by the tibial nerve. The deep posterior calf compartment has three muscles which act upon the foot and the ankle. The tibialis posterior acts as an inverter and plantar flexor of the foot. Its tendon travels in a tunnel over the posterior aspect of the medial malleolus and is held in place with the tendons of flexor digitorum longus and flexor hallucis longus by the flexor retinaculum, thus forming the tarsal tunnel. Also travelling in this tunnel is the tibial nerve which partially innervates the deep posterior compartment. The medial malleolus can be a site of nerve entrapment. The nerve then divides into the medial and lateral plantar nerves after it passes deep into the abductor hallucis muscle. The popliteus is the fourth muscle of the deep posterior compartment and is proximal within this compartment.

The lateral compartment of the lower leg everts the foot. This compartment is innervated by the superficial peroneal nerve and comprises the peroneus longus and peroneus brevis muscles. Their tendons travel in the posterior groove of the lateral malleolus and are held in place by the superior peroneal retinaculum. The peroneus brevis inserts into the tubercle on the base of the fifth metatarsal bone and the peroneus longus passes through a groove on the plantar aspect of the cuboid bone to insert into the base of the first metatarsal and on to the medial cuneiform.

The sensory nerve supply to the anterior aspect of the lower leg, ankle, and foot is shown in Fig. 1. The vascular supply to the ankle is derived from the malleolar branches of the anterior tibial and peroneal arteries.

Biomechanics of the ankle

The action at the ankle is primarily that of dorsiflexion and plantar flexion, with inversion and eversion being primarily a function of

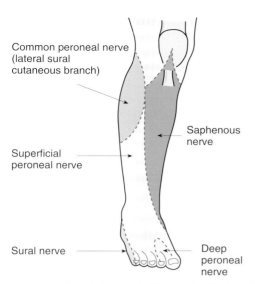

Common peroneal nerve
(lateral sural
cutaneous branch)

Saphenous
nerve

Superficial
peroneal nerve

Sural nerve

Deep
peroneal
nerve

Fig. 1 Sensory supply to the anterior aspect of the lower leg. (Redrawn from ref. 77 with permission.)

the subtalar joint. A discussion of the biomechanics of the ankle must include those of the foot, particularly when considering the gait cycle. A knowledge of normal and abnormal gait is important in understanding overuse injuries in particular. A full discussion of the biomechanics is beyond the scope of this chapter, however. The reader is referred to the literature.[14–16]

Nuber[17] pointed out that the obliquity of the ankle's motion permits dorsiflexion and plantar flexion together with other motions of the foot. Lateral deviation and pronation are associated with dorsiflexion of the ankle, while medial deviation and supination accompany plantar flexion. In reality, pronation is a complex motion of the ankle, subtalar joint, and midtarsal joints producing dorsiflexion, eversion, and abduction of the foot.

During running, the gait cycle is that of a stance (or support) phase alternating with a swing phase. Slocum and James[18] were among the first in the orthopaedic literature to describe the biomechanics of running and to point out the differences from walking. They divided the stance phase into foot contact, midsupport (or full weight bearing until plantar flexion starts), and finally toe-off. Mann[19] has studied, in detail, the function of the ankle during running. He has shown that the foot is dorsiflexed some 10 degrees at heel strike, and then continues to dorsiflex through half the stance phase to a total of 20 degrees. During toe-off there is a rapid plantar flexion to approximately 25 degrees. This cycle is repeated through some 1000 footstrikes per mile (675 per kilometre).

Mann et al.[20] performed an electromyographic study of the actions of the muscles during running. They showed that the tibialis anterior muscle is active at heel strike and continues to be active throughout the first half of the stance phase, primarily contracting concentrically. The anterior group is active during 75 per cent of the swing phase associated with dorsiflexion. The gastrocnemius and deep calf muscles function during the first 60 per cent of the stance phase and the last 25 per cent of the swing phase. The gastrocnemius functions eccentrically in the early part of the stance phase contributing to ankle stability. Mann believes there is minimal contribution of the deep calf muscles at toe-off, with the gastrocnemius

terminating their activity with the beginning of ankle plantar flexion. The peroneal muscles contract during the midsupport phase of stance and stop firing just prior to toe-off.

As the foot descends at the end of the swing phase, it is in a supinated position. It then pronates through midstance to supinate prior to toe-off. Pronation of the foot after heel strike, associated with ankle dorsiflexion, is an important component of shock absorption. This action occurs in combination with knee flexion and hip extension and absorbs the ground reactive force of some 2 to 2.5 times bodyweight with each heel strike. The complex action of pronation also enables the foot to adapt to the surface upon which it is walking or running. Resupination of the foot prior to toe-off is vital to ensure a rigid lever for propulsion. Associated with pronation of the foot is internal tibial rotation. This early portion of the stance phase is also the beginning of knee flexion and hip extension. Knee extension and further hip extension occurs during supination in the last half of the stance phase. The supinated or pes cavus foot which does not pronate sufficiently results in poor shock absorption. The restricted subtalar motion in the cavus foot transfers more stress of rotation to the ankle joint. In contrast, excessive pronation results in greater ankle dorsiflexion, subtalar eversion, and forefoot abduction. In addition, there is excessive internal tibial rotation which can result in tibial stress syndrome and patellofemoral pain syndrome. Toe-off is also less effective in the pronated foot as the foot is not locked, and this can produce excessive strain on the plantar fascia.

Injury prevention

As stated, ankle inversion injuries are extremely common and result in a considerable loss of time from training and competition. Preventive measures include exercise programmes, adhesive taping, bracing, and shoe modifications. A number of interventions are attempted each year by university, national, and professional teams in an attempt to minimize ankle injuries.

Exercise programmes

An ankle injury prevention programme has been developed by Dale Ohman, Head Coach of the Men's Varsity Volleyball Team at the University of British Columbia.[21] In response to a large number of ankle inversion injuries in one season he developed a very practical programme which requires 10 min of explanation and demonstration plus practice during the first week of training. Thereafter, 5 min per practice session is required to implement and maintain the programme. The essential elements are flexibility and balance drills for proprioception training, with some strengthening components.

There are four specific exercises in his programme. The first requires the athlete to balance on one leg while bending forward with the head up and the back horizontal. The arms are spread out to the side, parallel to the floor. The other leg is held extended at the hip and parallel to the floor. The athlete balances for 20 s initially and progresses to 30 s on each leg; the standing (support) leg is alternated in each training session. These features are similar for the remaining three exercises. The second exercise requires the athlete to balance on one foot, and then to side-bend at the hip with the free leg parallel to the floor and the arms perpendicular to the floor. In the third exercise the athlete balances on one leg, leaning backwards on a slightly bent knee with the free leg raised in front parallel to the floor. Both arms are held out sideways and parallel to the floor. In the fourth exercise the athlete balances on the same hand and foot. The free arm is raised perpendicular to the floor and the free leg is abducted as high as possible. Since this programme was introduced, there has been a significant reduction in the number and severity of ankle sprains.

Gastrocnemius and soleus muscle stretching and specific ankle inversion, eversion, and dorsiflexion exercises can be added to this (essentially balance) programme to provide a comprehensive preventive programme.

Proprioceptive training on a wobble board, used as a balance board, is also useful. The exercise programme can employ simple resistance devices such as surgical tubing or a bicycle inner tube. A programme of exercises progressing to three sets of 20 repetitions is effective and develops strength and endurance.

Bauenhauer et al.[22] have recently reported on a prospective study of ankle injury risk factors. This is followed in the same publication with a test–retest reliability report of the ankle injury risk factors. This group examined intrinsic risk factors and found that generalized joint laxity, anatomical measurements of foot and ankle alignment, and ankle ligament stability were not found to be significant risk factors leading to ankle injury in 145 college-aged athletes monitored throughout a season. In addition, it was found that a history of a previous mild ankle sprain did not increase the risk of a subsequent ankle inversion. A significant risk factor was a muscle strength imbalance when calculated as an elevated eversion to inversion strength ratio (more than 1.0). In addition, ankles with a greater plantar-flexion strength and a further strength imbalance, as calculated by a smaller dorsiflexion to plantar-flexion ratio, also had a higher incidence of inversion sprains. The authors suggest altering the strength deficits and imbalances before a sport season and following the changes in the incidence of ankle injury. The test–retest reliability of all measures assessed over a 1-year period had a high correlation coefficient.

Taping and bracing

Garrick and Requa[23] and Emerick[24] have documented the effectiveness of ankle taping in the prevention of ankle sprains. Fumich et al.[25] took these studies a step further by evaluating the role of taping the ankle in neutral inversion and in inversion with plantar flexion—the most vulnerable position. Their taping system yielded good control in both positions. A major problem with taping is the known loss of effectiveness after approximately 20 min of exercise.[25,26] This may be a result of loss of skin adhesion or mechanical failure of the tape, or both.

Bunch et al.[27] utilized the ankle support, made of a polyurethane footform to which an inversion torque was applied, to study the effective control of taping, cloth wrapping, and five different lace-on braces. In addition, they studied the loss of control after 350 inversion cycles. They found that initially adhesive tape offered the best support, with a 25 per cent advantage over the two best lace-on braces and a 75 per cent improvement over cloth wraps and two lace-on braces. There was a significant difference between the control offered by the lace-on braces studied, with the Mikros 9 inch and Swedo-O types being the best. After 350 inversion cycles over a 20-min period, there was no significant difference in the control offered by adhesive taping and the two best braces. They utilized a low-cut Oxford style shoe in this study to reduce the potential additional control of a high-cut shoe. The tape lost 21 per cent effectiveness over the 20-min inversion stress period. The taping technique used 3.8 cm (1.5 inch) tape with the Gibney basketweave and heel-lock method. It was interesting to note that in the preliminary laboratory studies over one-third of the control was lost as a result of inexperienced ankle taping.

More recently, Rovere et al.[28] reported on a 6-year retrospective comparison of ankle taping and a laced ankle stabilizer in the prevention of ankle injuries in collegiate football. During the study period the athletes used high-cut or low-cut boots. Ankle taping was found to be much less effective in preventing ankle injuries and reinjuries than the stabilizer. The cost of a pair of the ankle-stabilizing, lace-on braces was US$32, and they used two pairs per player for the season. The cost of the tape was US$400. Interestingly, the best combination to prevent injuries was a low-cut shoe with the ankle stabilizers. No significant difference was noted between the high-cut shoe with a stabilizer and the low-cut shoe with tape.

The use of an Air-Stirrup in the prevention and treatment of ankle inversion sprains has recently come into favour. Kimura et al.[29] studied subtalar ankle inversion on a specifically designed inversion platform, with and without an Air-Stirrup ankle-training brace, using high-speed cinematographic techniques. Significant control of ankle inversion was seen in the 18 subjects. A mean reduction of ankle inversion of 9.8 degrees was seen. Gross et al.[30] compared the Air-Stirrup and ankle taping in providing ankle support before and after exercise. A total of 22 ankles were randomly treated with either tape or the Air-Stirrup, and then the subjects exercised for 10 min on a 5 m × 10 m figure-of-eight course followed by 20 toe raises on a 15.25 cm step. The ankles were then tested on the Cybex II goniometer measuring three trials of maximum inversion and eversion. The results indicated that both treatment conditions significantly reduced ankle motion, but the Air-Stirrup produced a significantly greater restriction of range of motion, particularly eversion, than taping in pre-exercise testing. Postexercise analysis again showed a significant loss of control with taping but not with the Air-Stirrup.

An ankle brace (Don Joy ankle ligament protector), described as a semirigid orthosis, has been compared with adhesive ankle taping before, during, and after a 3-h volleyball practice.[31] In this study 14 ankles were treated with both methods of support. Maximal losses in taping restriction were noted for both inversion and eversion of the ankle at 20 min into exercise. The orthosis (ankle brace) lost restriction on eversion after 3 hours, but showed no loss of restriction of inversion over this period. Neither support system had a significant effect on jumping ability.

Another interesting brace has been evaluated by the USA Army Research Institute of Environmental Medicine. Amoroso et al.[32] reported on the impact of an outside-the-boot ankle brace on sprains associated with military airborne training. They found that the incidence of inversion ankle sprains was significantly reduced by the use of this outside-the-boot ankle brace. Overall, 5.1 per cent of the non-braced group and 4.3 per cent of the braced group experienced at least one ankle inversion injury. This brace is now available to the public and has a role for use with ice skates and other firm sports boots.

Sitter and Horodyski[33] have recently critically analysed four studies that investigated the effectiveness of prophylactic ankle stabilizers. They summarized these studies by pointing out methodological limitations, but agreed that the ankle stabilizers are effective in reducing the incidence of acute ankle sprains. However, they felt that the effects of stabilizers on ankle sprain severity is still unclear due to varying results. The authors stated that ankle stabilizers do not increase the risk of knee injuries.

Pienkowski et al.[34] have reported on a randomized prospective study utilizing ankle stabilizers. Their objectives were:

(1) to determine if four basketball-related activities were affected by the use of three designs of ankle braces (Universal, Kallassy, and Air-Stirrup ankle training braces);

(2) to determine whether specific braces were better for specific athletic activities; and

(3) to determine whether athlete performance changes with the use of the brace.

They studied 12 high-school basketball players participating in a vertical jump, standing long jump, cone run, and an 18.3 m shuttle run. The results showed that these braces did not affect athletic performance and no brace affected athletic performance in one specific activity more than another brace. Hence, fear of a reduction in athlete performance should not be a reason to avoid wearing ankle stabilizing braces.

Gehlsen et al.[35] compared protective tape wrap and three ankle braces (Active Ankle, Active Innovation Inc., Louisville, KY; Air-Stirrup, Aircast Inc., Summit, NJ; and the Swede-O-Universal, North Brook, MN) in relation to ankle joint strength (plantar flexion and dorsiflexion isokinetic), total work, and range of motion (**ROM**). The results of their investigation showed a significant reduction in force production, total work, and ROM. The Active Ankle and Air Stirrup braces permitted close to full ROM, whereas the tape and Swede-O-Universal braces consistently reduced ROM. There was no significant difference in the dorsiflexion torque, but plantar-flexion torques were reduced with the least change noted in the Active Ankle brace. The authors suggested that an athlete should possibly select a different ankle protective brace depending on the activity situation and the need for ankle ROM and ankle strength.

A 2-year randomized clinical study reported from the West Point Military Academy by Sitler et al.[36] illustrated a significant reduction in the frequency of ankle sprains, but not their severity, with the use of a semirigid ankle stabilizer. Non-braced athletes had three times the injury rate of the braced group. The study included 1601 subjects playing intramural basketball. All athletes used the same type of high-top basketball shoe and the Aircast Sports-stirrup (Aircast Inc., Summit, NJ) was the ankle stabilizer used in the study.

Surve et al.[37], similarly reported a reduction, this time fivefold, in the incidence of recurrent ankle sprains in soccer players using the semirigid orthosis (Sport-Stirrup, Aircast Inc., Summit, NJ). Interestingly, however, there was no difference, when using the orthosis, in the incidence of ankle sprains in those groups with no previous ankle sprains. In both of these studies the authors recorded knee injuries as well as ankle injuries. There was no difference between the ankle-stabilized group and the control group in the incidence of knee injuries. This is an important finding, counter to the concept of the transmission of forces to a higher joint with joint bracing.

Anderson[38] completed her master's thesis with an evaluation of the subtalar stabilizer (**STS**) ankle brace. The brace system is attached by Velcro straps to a semirigid orthotic designed to keep the ankle and subtalar joint in neutral. The orthotic can be modified with a deeper heel seat to offer more control. This study examined the effects of the STS brace controlling an inversion sprain in 30 subjects. The brace was found:

(1) to significantly restrict the degree of calcaneal inversion range of motion during an unexpected inversion drop;

(2) to significantly lengthen the time of inversion thereby decreasing the rate at which the calcaneus inverts during a sudden inversion drop;

(3) to maintain this support significantly following sprinting and lateral movement exercise; and

(4) to provide equal restriction for both males and females.

The STS brace, described above, has been utilized for both men's and women's national field hockey teams with good clinical results in reducing ankle inversion sprains. This system has been particularly useful for athletes with generalized ligament laxity, excessive foot pronation, and a history of recurrent ankle inversion sprains.

The authors are not aware of any long-term prospective and retrospective comparison of stirrup-type, ankle taping, or lace-on braces.

Orthotics

A number of reports have documented the effectiveness of soft and semirigid orthotics in reducing foot and ankle injuries.[6,39,40]

Taunton et al.,[41] using a triplanar electrogoniometer, investigated the effectiveness of semirigid orthotics in reducing pronation in a group of endurance runners. They demonstrated a decrease in calcaneal eversion during the support phase of running. They also noted a significant difference in the response of the right and left legs in many subjects, suggesting the need for 'custom' orthotics for each foot.

Bates et al.[42] had previously reported a reduction in the period of pronation and the maximum extent of pronation with the use of orthotics. Smith et al.[43] utilized high-speed cinematography to evaluate pronation control of soft and semirigid orthotics. The maximum velocity of calcaneal eversion was significantly reduced by both orthotics, but the maximum amount of calcaneal eversion was only significantly reduced with the semirigid orthotics. McKenzie[44] stated that as soft orthotics are clinically effective, controlling the velocity of eversion may be more important than controlling the degree or amplitude of eversion.

Orthotics are designed to achieve biomechanical control, and with the pronated foot this means neutralizing the subtalar point and maintaining the longitudinal arch. In mild degrees of pronation a motion-control shoe or soft orthotic may be sufficient. For more severe pronation, semirigid devices are made from varying grades and thicknesses of plastics. With sports involving rapid lateral changes of direction, we limit the rearfoot posting to 4 degrees to prevent inversion sprains. We measure the degree of subtalar varus,[39,45] subtract 3 degrees, which we have found can be well tolerated, and then post half this value. In addition, we measure the additional forefoot varus and then subtract the tolerable level of 2 to 3 degrees and post an additional half of this value to the forefoot. If there is a significant degree of tibial varum (over 5 degrees), we take this into consideration in the rearfoot posting. As mentioned, caution is used to prevent overcorrection which can result in inversion ankle sprains and lateral knee and leg pains (including iliotibial-band friction syndrome and peroneal tendinitis). While waiting for an orthotic to be constructed, foot pronation can often be controlled with low dye arch taping.

As previously described, the cavus foot suffers from decreased motion of the subtalar joint and hence insufficient pronation and poor shock absorption. Orthotics for the cavus foot are most effective if they are made of a soft material with good shock-absorptive properties and flexibility. Heel lifts to unload the tight gastrocnemius and soleus muscles can be employed. The cavus foot often has a subtalar varus and forefoot valgus. The forefoot is treated with a lateral or valgus post and the rearfoot varus with a modest rearfoot varus medial post. The cavus foot is often associated with a fixed or partially fixed plantar-flexed first ray. This can be similarly treated with a posting under the second to the fifth metatarsal heads. The thickness of the posting or padding should be equal to the degree of plantar flexion of the first ray. Lutter[46] used a flexible longitudinal orthotic with a lateral heel lift.

Shoes

Garrick and Requa[10] completed a prospective study of ankle inversion sprains in intramural basketball players. As previously discussed, they reported a lower incidence of ankle injuries among those players with prophylactic adhesive taping compared with those without any taping. They also found that the risk of ankle injury was lowered in patients wearing high-cut shoes alone. The best combination for reducing ankle injuries[28] was high-cut shoes and ankle taping. This was not seen in a retrospective study of American football ankle injuries[28] where it was found that the combination allowing the fewest ankle injuries was low-cut shoes with a lace-up ankle stabilizer. The low-cut shoe with an ankle stabilizer was better in reducing ankle injuries than the high-cut shoe with a stabilizer. The poorest combination in their study was the high-cut shoe with tape. They felt that it was easier to tighten the lace-up brace when wearing a low-cut shoe, and this may explain their surprising data on shoe type and injury. A review of the newer, supposedly more stable, high-cut shoes being produced would be useful. The relationship of this footwear to the prevention of ankle injury needs to be determined, together with the possible benefits of simultaneous ankle taping or bracing.

Overuse injuries have been attributed, at least in part, to foot type, particularly of either excessive pronation or supination. We now see shoes specifically designed for these two extremes. McKenzie et al.[40] and, more recently, Moore and Taunton[47] have detailed new design features in athletic shoes.

Excessive pronation is partially controlled by the 'motion control' shoes produced by the reputable shoe manufacturers. Such shoes have a straighter last with board-lasting rather than slip-lasting. Straight-lasted shoes reduce pronation, whereas curve-lasted shoes promote pronation and hence are more suitable for the rigid pes cavus (supinated) foot. With board-lasting offering more torsional rigidity, the upper material of the shoe is attached to the firm fibreboard inner sole. In contrast, with slip-lasting the upper is stitched in a 'moccasin' fashion down the middle of the sole, with no firm inner sole, and is then attached to the premoulded middle-sole portion. The 'motion control' shoe also possesses a high-density thermoplastic heel counter which may be reinforced externally by additional material. The stable heel counter is the key to the control of calcaneal eversion. Additional support can be added by medial strapping in the form of leather cradles in the midfoot. The midsole is constructed over shock-absorptive ethylene vinyl acetate (**EVA**) of various densities (or hardnesses, as measured by a durometer); more recently, shoe manufacturers have returned to the more durable polyurethane for the midsole, sacrificing some shock absorption but gaining more durability and stability. Shock absorption is maintained by the inclusion of rearfoot (and often forefoot) air pockets, pillars, or gels. In some shoes more medial pronation control has been attempted by additional higher density EVA medially in the dual-density concept of midsole construction. We have seen more iliotibial-band friction injuries as a result of the lateral side collapsing in these shoes where there was an extreme difference in the medial–lateral densities of the EVA.

The width and shape of the sole and rearfoot can also modify motion control. Very wide heel flares were used in the early 'motion control' shoes, which controlled ankle motion but permitted rapid calcaneal eversion upon heel strike with more internal tibial torsion and reportedly more patellofemoral pain. Nigg[16] has shown that initial pronation can be reduced by a medial support applied more to the posterior side of the medial arch with a round heel shape ('negative heel flare') on the lateral and posterior sides of the heel. Frederick et al.[48] have shown that the best combination of rearfoot control and cushioning occurred in a shoe with a thicker midsole, with a durometer reading of 35, and a rearfoot flare with a reading of 15. With motion-control shoes the challenge is to achieve a balance between torsional (pronation and supination) control and shock absorption. The latter is often compromised in the attempt to gain more pronation control.

The cavus foot needs more shock absorption and features to accentuate pronation. Hence, a curved last with slip-lasting construction is best. The midsole should have a softer EVA with durometer readings in the range of 25 to 30 and a narrower heel flare. A higher heel-lift and an additional shock-absorption insole made of Neoprene, or possibly the newer viscoelastic materials Akton or Zekon, are useful. The air soles in the rearfoot, and particularly the forefoot, as seen in Nike shoes, are also attractive features for the cavus foot. Nigg[16] has shown that initial pronation can be significantly increased by using more flare on the lateral and/or posterior side of the heel. In addition, pronation is increased by relatively hard sole material laterally and softer material medially. He has also shown that the geometry of the shoe influenced the ankle and foot alignment on take-off. Excessive supination during take-off was reduced by a lateral wedge in the forefoot.

More recently, biomechanical research has been applied to achieve more ankle stability for tennis, basketball, volleyball, and aerobic shoes.[16] Aerobic shoes require the combination of forefoot shock absorption with lateral ankle support. Soccer and the various other football boots offer some ankle support, but have poor pronation-control features. Garrick[2] identified that fewer ankle sprains occurred with the multicleated moulded-sole boot as compared to boots with fewer cleats such as the 6-cleated soccer boot. Provision of removable insoles, a feature in some hockey skates and hiking boots, makes it much easier to employ a soft or semirigid orthotic to suit the wearer.

Rule changes

Ankle injuries in volleyball frequently result by inversion from landing on an opponent's foot. It has been suggested that the creation of a safety zone (no landing zone) under the net would decrease the high incidence of ankle injuries in this sport.[49] Analogous scenarios may exist in other sports.

Technique training

Although awaiting research confirmation, emphasis on a 2-foot landing in training, thereby decreasing the exposure of one ankle to injury, makes sense. This may also reduce acute knee injuries.

Paediatric ankle problems

Trott[50] reported that 12.1 per cent of all adolescent injuries seen were in the foot and ankle. Micheli[51] and Beauchamp[52] have published excellent reports on the common paediatric foot and ankle injuries. They relate these injuries to congenital and growth factors and to specific acquired traumatic and overuse injuries. Ankle injuries and dysfunction related to congenital factors include pes cavus foot, equinus contracture, club foot (talipes equinovarus), excessive internal tibial torsion, excessive external tibial torsion, and subtalar coalition.

The pes cavus foot, club foot, and excessive internal tibial torsion foot all tend to supinate with subsequent inversion injuries. Maximizing dorsiflexion with calf stretching, an orthotic with a forefoot valgus post, a more flexible shoe, and external ankle support (taping or brace) are management recommendations.

Equinus contracture and excessive external tibial torsion can result in excessive pronation. Calf stretching and orthotics usually are sufficient to control the increased pronation. When equinus is more severe, occasionally night splinting or casting in dorsiflexion, and rarely Achilles tendon lengthening may be required.[52]

The club foot (or talipes equinovarus) is unstable laterally and is vulnerable to inversion sprains of the ankle and recurrent injury to the anterior talofibular ligament. Protective ankle taping is recommended for the club foot with minor degrees of varus positioning.

Subtalar coalition, by either a bony or fibrous bridge between two tarsal bones, can produce ankle and foot pain. Clinically, subtalar motion is markedly reduced and the affected child often has a spastic, pronated pes planus foot. Peroneal spasm can be seen with subtalar motion testing. The diagnosis is made with oblique radiography of the foot, but a CT scan may be required to identify the coalition accurately. A flattened talar dome is an associated finding. Treatment ranges from semirigid orthotics, to cast immobilization from 4 to 6 weeks to reduce the pain and spasm, to surgical division of the coalition, and other procedures as necessary.

Foot and ankle complaints can be seen with variance of lower extremity alignment. One example is that of persistent femoral neck anteversion with internal femoral rotation, which is associated with excessive external tibial torsion and excessive foot pronation. This complex has been termed the miserable malalignment syndrome by James et al.[39] Similarly, persistent genu valgum can produce excessive foot pronation with resultant medial ankle pain. In the develop-

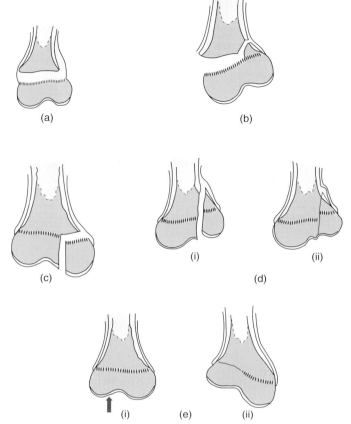

Fig. 2 The Salter–Harris classification of ankle fractures. (a) Type I epiphyseal-plate injury: separation of the epiphysis. (b) Type II epiphyseal-plate injury: fracture-separation of the epiphysis. (c) Type III epiphyseal-plate injury: fracture of part of the epiphysis. (d) Type IV epiphyseal-plate injury (i): fracture of the epiphysis and epiphyseal plate; (ii) bone union and premature closure. (e) (i) Epiphyseal-plate injury: crushing of the epiphyseal plate; (ii) premature closure. (Redrawn from ref. 53 with permission.)

ing child, physiological genu valgum occurs at 3 to 4 years, with a more neutral knee alignment developing by the age of 6 to 7 years.

The ankle is similar to the metatarsals, knees, hips, and elbows. During growth, osteochondritis dissecans can be seen in the talus; although its aetiology is uncertain, repetitive microtrauma may be a factor. Management is initially conservative, provided that there is an adequate remaining growth period. The use of a functional cast for 6 to 8 weeks with maintenance of fitness by cycling or swimming is often enough to provide for resolution of the problem. If pain persists, especially with episodes of catching or locking, a CT scan is indicated to look for a loose fragment within the ankle joint. An unstable fragment is best managed by transarthroscopic fixation followed by continuous passive-motion therapy over 6 to 12 weeks.

Epiphyseal ankle injury is common with inversion or rotation. Salter and Harris[53] have classified these injuries (I–V, Fig. 2) and outlined management with the emphasis on proper reduction. The most common fractures are Salter I and II fractures of the fibula. This pattern suggests the epiphysis, not the ligament, is the weak link in children. Often the radiographic findings are normal or minimal, requiring comparison with the opposite leg. A correct diagnosis may reflect a high index of suspicion and bony not

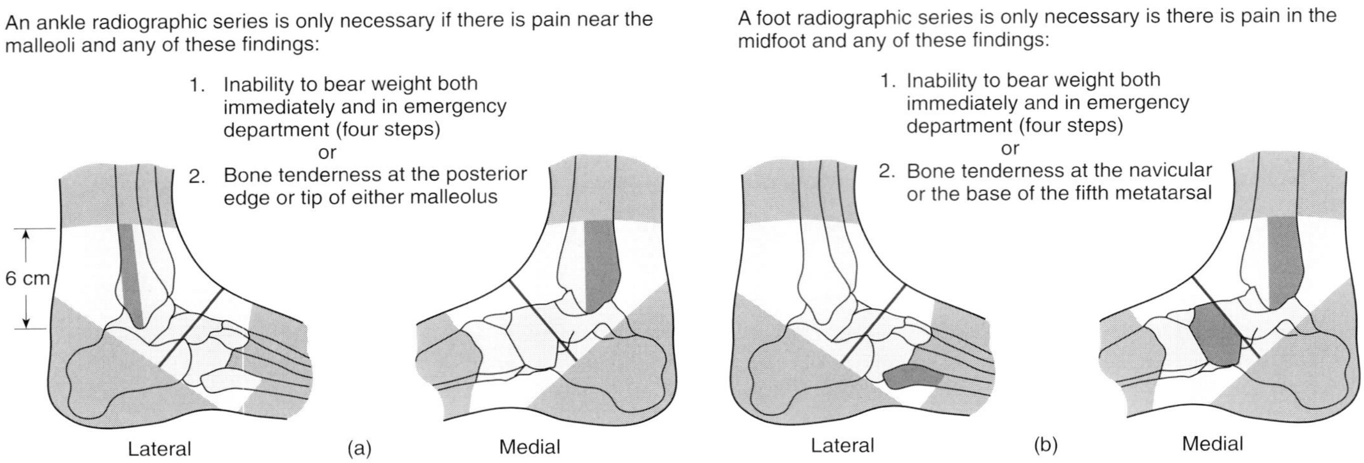

An ankle radiographic series is only necessary if there is pain near the malleoli and any of these findings:

1. Inability to bear weight both immediately and in emergency department (four steps) or
2. Bone tenderness at the posterior edge or tip of either malleolus

A foot radiographic series is only necessary is there is pain in the midfoot and any of these findings:

1. Inability to bear weight both immediately and in emergency department (four steps) or
2. Bone tenderness at the navicular or the base of the fifth metatarsal

6 cm

Lateral   (a)   Medial   Lateral   (b)   Medial

Fig. 3 (a) Refined clinical decision rule for ankle radiographic series in ankle injury patients. (b) Refined clinical decision rule for foot radiographic series in ankle injury patients. (From ref. 54 with permission.)

ligamentous tenderness. Salter I fractures are managed with cast immobolization for 3 weeks; Salter II fractures with closed reduced and 6 weeks of immobilization (3 non-weight bearing, 3 weight-bearing). Growth abnormalities are unusual.

Salter III and IV fractures, if not managed properly, can lead to premature epiphyseal closure or malalignment. Good reduction is essential, and open reduction and internal fixation may be necessary. A unique fracture seen in the adolescent with closing epiphyses is the Salter III or Tillaux fracture. The medial aspect of the distal tibial epiphysis is closed and, with an external rotation force, the inferior tibiofibular ligament avulses the anterolateral quadrant of the ankle complex. Reduction is achieved by internally rotating the foot, but open reduction and internal fixation avoiding the epiphyseal plate, are mandatory for any displacement over 2 mm.

Although uncommon, Salter type V is notable due to the crush injury and almost inevitable premature growth arrest. Treatment involves non-weight bearing for 3 weeks to allow optimal recovery.

Acute injuries

With the high incidence of acute ankle injuries, a physician is frequently presented with an athlete with a painful swollen ankle and the task of differentiating between a fracture or ligament injury. Most often, a radiograph is ordered to err on the side of caution. Recently, the Ottawa Rules (Fig. 3) have developed a set of clinical criteria for ordering radiographs for ankle/foot injuries.[54] These rules are highly sensitive for diagnosing fractures and can reduce the use of radiographs by 30 per cent for the ankle and by 34 per cent for the foot.

Ankle fractures

Chandler[55] presents a clear outline of the management of ankle fractures based on the Danis–Weber classification. This classification system is related to the fracture morphology (with emphasis on the fibula) and divides the fractures into types A, B, and C according to the three zones of the fibula (Fig. 4) A type A fracture is below the level of the tibiotalar joint, and often disrupts the talofibular articulation and, in many cases, is associated with medial ligament disruption. Simple non-displaced type A fibular fractures can be

managed with 6 weeks of cast immobilization or functional bracing, with weight bearing permitted in the last 3 weeks. After this time, aggressive rehabilitation is recommended with the emphasis on ankle strength, flexibility, and balance–proprioceptive exercises.

Stuart *et al.*[56] presented a prospective randomized study on the use of the Aircast Air-Stirrup compared to plaster-cast treatment with below-knee walking casts in the management of 40 cases of stable lateral malleolar fractures. These fractures were the result of supination eversion injuries. All patients were weight bearing as soon as possible. There was no difference in the time to union; however, the authors reported that the group treated in the Air-Stirrup experienced a significant improvement in early comfort, postfracture swelling, range of ankle motion at union, and time to full rehabilitation. At 3-months postfracture the Air-Stirrup group contained a significantly greater number of subjects that were at full range of motion, painfree, and back to full activities.

Displaced fractures in the athlete are best managed with open reduction and internal fixation allowing early rehabilitation. Chandler[55] states that a low transverse fracture of the type A variety can be managed with a tension-band technique or an intramedullary fixation of the fibula. Medial soft-tissue damage may also need to be repaired. A type B fracture of the ankle is at the tibiotalar joint and involves partial disruption of the tibiofibular syndesmosis. In addition to initial radiography with anteroposterior, lateral, and oblique views of the mortise, these more complex fractures are more fully evaluated by CT scans. Type B fractures usually require surgery. With these fractures Chandler[55] advised a medial incision for joint debridement of chondral or osteochondral talar loose bodies and deep medial ligament repair before fracture fixation. The type C fracture is defined as being proximal to the tibiofibular syndesmosis with disruption of the syndesmosis and the interosseous ligament to the level of the fibular fracture. There is often extensive ligamentous damage. These, together with pilon distal tibial fractures, are amongst the most severe ankle fractures and have the poorest prognosis. Internal fixation techniques are similar to those for the type B fracture. The mortise is initially stabilized by medial exploration and lateral plate fixation. The medial ligament repair and medial bony stabilization of the fracture are completed with a single cortical

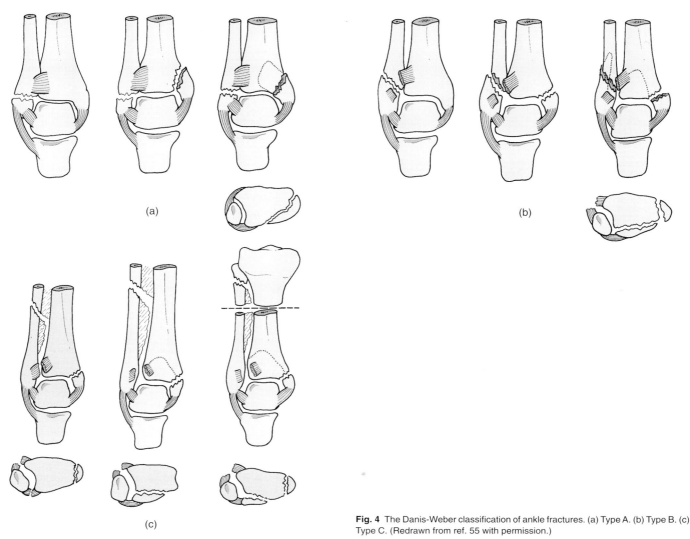

(a)

(b)

(c)

Fig. 4 The Danis-Weber classification of ankle fractures. (a) Type A. (b) Type B. (c) Type C. (Redrawn from ref. 55 with permission.)

screw. Stabilization of the distal tibiofibular syndesmosis is achieved if the screw is placed above the level of the fibular sulcus of the tibia. Chandler[55] advised removal of this screw at 6 to 8 weeks, before weight bearing takes place.

Following internal fixation, these fractures are supported in a posterior splint and a U-splint. Initially, elevation of the leg is needed for 2 weeks. Early ankle and toe dorsiflexion exercises are commenced on the first postoperative day. Non weight-bearing mobility with the aid of crutches is started on the second postoperative day. At the sixth week weight bearing is permitted, with a return to sports at about the end of the third or fourth month after surgery. Pool running and stationary cycling to maintain cardiovascular fitness can possibly be resumed after satisfactory wound closure at 3 weeks. As previously mentioned, full strength, flexibility, and balance must be regained prior to returning to sport. In addition, sport-specific skills must be performed before practices are allowed. For a basketball or soccer player this should involve backward running and 'crossover' and 'cutting drills' with repeated changes of direction. If there has been extensive soft-tissue damage and repair, an external brace or splint is advisable for the first year until full ligamentous healing has taken place.

Ankle sprains

As discussed, ankle inversion sprains are the most common sports injuries. The majority of ankle sprains are of the inversion variety, occurring when one ankle is plantar flexed and the foot is supinated, which is the position of least bony stability for the ankle with support achieved by ligament and musculotendinous function. In this position the peroneal muscles and anterior talofibular ligament are the prime stabilizers of the joint, and McConkey[57] emphasizes that in this position the axis of the anterior talofibular ligament is much closer to the long axis of the fibula. In addition, in the plantar-fixed position the tension in the anterior talofibular ligament maximally increases as the attachment sites of the ligament from the fibula and talus separate. This results from the location of the centre of rotation of the ankle at a point anterior and inferior to the lateral malleolar origin of the ligament.

As well as these functional anatomical considerations, other aetiological factors have been outlined for inversion ankle sprains. Walsh and Blackburn[58] discussed the roles of uneven playing surfaces, poor shoes with inadequate heel counters, and conditions of increased shoe–surface reactive forces such as newly polished floors and artificial turf. Other factors involved are poor peroneal muscle strength, inadequate gastrocnemius–soleus flexibility, and poor balance and proprioception. The pes cavus foot and ankle, with increased forefoot valgus, is at greater risk of injury since the forefoot makes early contact medially (at the first metatarsal head) and not laterally. Athletes with generalized ligament laxity (subtalar, talar, and midtarsal laxity) are also more at risk of inversion sprains.

Classification and diagnosis

Ankle inversion sprains are usually classified from grade I to grade III. Grade I sprains are mild in nature with little swelling, mild tenderness, slight pain on inversion stress, and only mild loss of function. The ankle is stable to an anterior drawer test or radiographic examination for 'talar tilt' with only minor ligament damage. From grade I to grade III ankle sprains there is a progression of injury, first to the anterior talofibular ligament (grade I), then additional involvement of the calcaneus fibular ligament (grade II), and with more severe inversion stress (grade III) including the posterior talofibular ligament.

Although grade I sprains are primarily to the anterior talofibular ligament, with greater degrees of force and more rotational stress the injury may involve the distal tibiofibular syndesmosis or subtalar ligaments. Grade II sprains are of moderate degree with more functional loss and diffuse swelling. Walking and hopping are difficult. Grade III sprains are severe with complete lateral ligament complex rupture, consequent instability, and marked functional impairment. Walking is impossible, and, of course, there is marked swelling and tenderness. The active range of motion of the ankle is markedly reduced and there is gross instability.

Ankle stability is assessed clinically with the anterior drawer test. This is a sensitive indicator of the stability of the anterior talofibular ligament in particular. The anterior drawer test is performed with the ankle in the neutral position and is compared with the non-injured ankle. Laurin and Mathieu[59] have evaluated the anterior drawer test of up to 4 mm with the ankle in the neutral position, and this is reduced with the ankle in the plantar-flexed position. A visible and palpable drawer, which is not reduced by plantar flexion and is greater than the non-injured ankle, indicates complete anterior talofibular ligament rupture.

Clinical diagnosis is aided by radiography to rule out fracture, avulsion injury to bone, osteochondral injury, or syndesmosis separation. Controversy still exists regarding the value of 'talar tilt'; an inversion stress to the ankle, 5 to 10 degrees greater than the non-injured side, is considered abnormal. A positive 'talar tilt' is indicative of significant, if not complete, rupture of the anterior talofibular ligament, which is the major restraint on inversion.

Treatment

Plaster casting is almost a thing of the past in our clinic with the use of the Air-Stirrup. Rehabilitation follows a three-phase plan: phase I, over the first 48 to 72 h, is instituted to limit the extent of the injury, phase II is designed to regain strength and full range of motion of the ankle, and phase III is for the restoration of proprioception, agility, speed, and endurance. Postexercise ice applications continue throughout the programme and return to sport is not permitted until the athlete has regained full range of ankle motion, full strength, and balance, with minimal tenderness, pain, or swelling. In addition, the athlete must be able to perform agility drills, sport-specific jumping, and change of direction drills. Postinjury drills of strength, flexibility, and balance, together with protective taping or bracing, are advised for the remainder of the competitive season. Treatment of grade I and grade II ankle sprains has changed considerably in the past decade with the development of the Air-Stirrup plus the concept of early mobilization including relative rest, ice, compression, and elevation (**RICE**). Many grade III sprains also do well managed non-operatively, but the reinjury rate may be increased compared with those undergoing early repair.

The effects of intermittent compression on oedema in acute ankle sprains was studied by Rucinski et al.[60] They compared the effects of compression wrap, intermittent compression pump, and elevation on postinjury oedema. Interestingly, they found that only elevation consistently reduced the oedema. Both elastic wrap and intermittent compression actually increased the amount of oedema. Ice is still considered to be an important adjunct to elevation. Cryo-cuff ankle therapy using the Jobst pump (Jobst Cryo/Temp system) or Cryo-Cuff (Aircast) has been shown to be very effective in the early treatment of acute ankle sprains.

Eiff et al.[61] investigated early mobilization as compared to immobilization in the treatment of lateral ankle strains—82 patients with grade I and II sprains were seen in a military medical centre. Half of the patients were randomly assigned to the immobilization group—immobilization was for 10 days followed by weight bearing and rehabilitation. The other half of the patients were randomly assigned to early immobilization with an elastic wrap for 2 days and a functional brace for 8 days. At 2 days, weight bearing and rehabilitation exercises started. At 3 weeks, 87 per cent of the immobilization group had pain in contrast to 57 per cent of the mobilization group. At 6 weeks, most were asymptomatic, but one-third had a balance defect. In long-term follow-up at 1 year, only one patient in each group was still symptomatic and three patients in each group had resprained the ankle. It was interesting to note that by 10 days, 54 per cent of the early mobilization group returned to full work duties compared with only 13 per cent of the immobilization group. Hence, both yielded excellent results, but early mobilization allowed a faster return to full work duties.

McConkey[57] reviewed the literature on surgical and non-surgical management of severe ankle sprains. He summarized the indications for surgery of severe grade III ankle sprains as follows:

(1) young, high-level competitive athletes and workers requiring near-normal ankle function for safety and high-risk sports such as volleyball or basketball;

(2) patients with an associated lesion such as a displaced or large osteochondral fracture, peroneal tendon dislocation, or distal syndesmosis disruption;

(3) patients with an ankle joint dislocation.

Physiotherapy plays a very strong role in the management of grade I and grade II injuries. In particular, electrotherapy with ultrasound, short-wave diathermy, and interferential therapy (and perhaps laser therapy for those with experience in this technique) combine well with strength, power, and proprioceptive drills to promote early activity and functional recovery.

Lane[62] has recently described a very successful ankle treatment programme for 26 patients who had suffered radiographically confirmed grade III ankle sprains. The programme consisted of a

Table 1 Hindfoot motion from neutral to supination after a left ankle sprain

Bone	Right	Motion	Left
Tibia–talus	4.5 deg	Plantar flexion	13.0 deg
	4.6 deg	Inversion	10.4 deg
	12.8 deg	Internal rotation	22.7 deg
Talus–calcaneus	7.2 deg	Plantar flexion	10.4 deg
	8.7 deg	Inversion	11.7 deg
	4.7 deg	Internal rotation	3.3 deg

3-week period using an ankle–foot orthosis at all times, except during physical therapy, with immediate weight bearing as tolerated. Patients received physiotherapy, consisting of isometric exercises, whirlpool, electric stimulation, ultrasound, and Jobst compression, daily for a week and then three times per week. After 3 to 5 weeks the ankle–foot orthosis was replaced with a lace-up brace, and range of motion exercises, strengthening exercises, and stationary cycling were introduced. After 5 to 7 weeks, agility drills using the lace-up brace were added along with proprioceptive exercises with a balance board. After 7 weeks, the athlete was introduced to sport-specific drills. The ankle was taped, or the lace-up brace was used, for 6 to 12 months. With this programme 96 per cent of patients returned to activity without restriction after 10 weeks.

Reinjury following a significant ankle sprain is common, with reports of as many as 40 per cent reoccurences in patients who had been treated by early protected mobilization, plaster immobilization, or surgical repair.[63] Jackson et al.[3] saw an 8 per cent reinjury rate at 6 months for all grades of ankle sprains managed non-operatively. The causes of resprains seem primarily to result from inadequate proprioceptive retraining, lack of peroneal strength, and residual lateral ligament laxity. Freeman[63] believes that the feeling of instability is largely due to proprioception loss. McConkey[57] adds other potential sources of functional ankle instability including adhesion formation and ossicle impingement at the talofibular junction, and anteroposterior or rotational instability, rather than varus instability of the talus in the mortise with subtalar joint laxity. The majority of athletes with recurrent sprains are controlled well with strength and proprioception drills together with one of the better ankle braces (either lace-on or stirrup type). A small percentage of athletes with recurrent instability require late ankle reconstruction.

The control of instability by conservative or operative means is very important in the prevention of secondary osteoarthritis and impingement osteophytes, with the possible development of loose fragments. More recent approaches to the spectrum of ligament injury on the lateral side of the foot and ankle from inversion describe the importance of involvement of soft-tissue injury across the subtalar joint (Table 1). This is relevant in planning surgical repair if required.[64,65]

Associated injuries

Associated injuries must always be sought with acute ankle sprains. Such injuries include osteochondral lesions to the talus, peroneal tendon dislocation, tibialis posterior tendon injury, disruption of the distal tibiofibular syndesmosis, and nerve traction injury (particularly of the peroneal nerve). McConkey[57] adds occult and/or unusual fractures which result from excessive inversion stress, including avulsion fracture by the peroneus brevis at the base of the fifth metatarsus, fracture separation of the distal fibular epiphysis in children, capsular avulsion fracture from the lateral calcaneocuboid joint, navicular compression fracture, and fracture of the neck or body of the talus. Forced eversion with dorsiflexion and compression can produce a lateral-process fracture of the talus which is often not seen on initial radiography examination. Bone scans with follow-up CT scans are often required in the presence of persistent disability and tenderness inferior to the lateral malleolus. Fracture fragments may require internal fixation or removal. More frequent osteochondral fractures are seen with a combination of ankle inversion, plantar flexion, and internal rotation of the foot, and the majority of these are to the posterior medial corner of the talus. Less frequently, lateral talar surface lesions are seen with talar shear against the fibula on inversion and subluxation of the ankle. Usually talar dome fractures are seen as a result of a combination of ankle inversion, plantar flexion, and internal rotation of the foot. Avascular necrosis can be a consequence of medial talar fractures, and may or may not be visible on a radiograph. Early diagnosis requires a bone scan or subsequent CT scan. The stability of an osteochondral talar fracture dictates its management. Thompson and Loomer[66] have shown that lateral dome fractures are usually unstable and should be treated with arthroscopic excision of the fragment. Many fractures of the medial corner and dome of the talus are stable and can be treated non-operatively in an orthotic ankle brace. Unstable fractures, particularly if they have undergone avascular necrosis, require arthroscopic excision and perhaps drilling of the underlying defect. Shearer[67] investigated stage 5 osteochondral lesions of the talus (**OLT**). These lesions consist of a radiolucent defect and make up 77 per cent of the total number of talar lesions seen postankle injury. On long-term follow-up of those conservatively managed, he identified a significant reduction in pain on running and walking over time. Pain at rest over time was decreased, but not statistically significant. Activity level increased but was not statistically significant. Good or excellent results were rated in 53 per cent of cases, with 18 per cent fair and 29 per cent poor results. Interestingly, lateral lesions seemed to do better than medial lesions. This appears to be contradict the literature on general OLT. Juveniles (age of diagnosis less than 20 years) did worse than adults. There was no significant change in lesion size over time, although the trend was for the lesions to increase in size. Stage 5 OLT do seem to lead to degenerative changes (generally minor), but there does not appear to be a relationship between these degenerative changes and the clinical result, at least at 39-months follow-up.

Peroneal tendon subluxations can be seen with forced ankle inversion and even more frequently with forced dorsiflexion, as in a forward fall while skiing. With such an injury the peroneal retinaculum is torn from its fibular attachment and is best managed by acute surgical repair. Radiography may show a small avulsion fragment some 2 to 3 cm above the tip of the fibula. Clinically, the tenderness and maximal swelling is located posterior to the lateral malleolus, with additional tenderness along the peroneal muscles and tendons. With resisted eversion, particularly with the foot in plantar flexion, tendon subluxation can be identified. A less frequent peroneal tendon injury in sport is a longitudinal tear of the peroneal longus or brevis.[68] The physical findings include persistent lateral ankle swelling, popping, and pain posterior to the fibula. The treatment is primary repair which is done under local anaesthesia with excellent results.

Stanish et al.[69] have described injuries to the tibialis posterior tendon associated with ankle injuries. They discussed subluxation of the tibialis posterior tendon as a result of severe ankle sprain, particularly in an athlete with a shallow tibial bony trough for the tendon. This dislocation can lead to a sensation of ankle instability on forceful toe-off, because at toe-off the posterior tibial muscle-—tendon unit acts as the prime dynamic stabilizer of the ankle and the prime inverter and supporter of the arch. In addition, medial ankle instability, secondary to a severe eversion injury, may lead to chronic tibialis posterior tendon dislocation with tendinitis and eventual tendon rupture. This requires tendon repair, tendon anastomosis, or even free tendon transplant followed by orthotic foot support. Also, the success of tendon repair has been recently correlated more to MRI than intraoperative grading of tendon degeneration.[70] Rupture of the posterior tibialis tendon, in sport, has also been identified.[71] Early recognition and treatment, before the collapse of the longitudinal arch, enhances postoperative function. MRI is helpful in making the diagnosis.

Distal syndesmosis injuries can be seen with grade III ankle inversion sprains and also with forced eversion with external rotation or abduction. The eversion injury progressively ruptures the syndesmosis ligaments and interosseous membranes, then fractures the fibula as a spiral or transverse fracture, and eventually, as the talus shifts further, ruptures the deltoid ligament. Other mechanisms of syndesmotic injury include inversion and internal rotation, eversion and external rotation with plantar flexion. Diffuse swelling is seen, with maximal local tenderness over the distal syndesmosis (rather than over the anterior talofibular ligament). Midleg and distal compression of the tibia and fibula should be performed by the examiner (the squeeze test), and is painful.[71] Also, external rotation of the foot is particularly painful (the external rotation stress test).[72] A talar shift and/or fibular fracture should be sought on radiographs, but may not be present if only a partial syndesmosis sprain has occurred. Late radiographic evidence of this injury is calcification of the distal interosseous membrane.[73,74] Complete disruptions of the syndesmosis require surgical reduction and internal fixation to prevent recurrent instability and chronic pain. A prime reason for accurate diagnosis is the warning to the athlete (and the coach) that the recovery is prolonged even for a partial sprain.

An uncommon and possibly underdiagnosed ankle injury is isolated rupture of the deltoid ligament.[75] The mechanism is eversion. The patient stands with more pes planus on the injured side, medial ankle swelling tenderness, and laxity of the deltoid ligament on the valgus stress test, which can be confirmed radiographically, with the stress test demonstrating talar tilt without talar shift or widening of ankle mortise. Treatment includes a non-weight-bearing cast for 6 weeks followed by motion-control shoes, orthotic with varus wedge, and an ankle brace.

The diagnosis of cuboid subluxation should be considered with persistent lateral midfoot pain following inversion.[76] It can accompany a lateral ligament sprain and becomes clinically evident after the ankle pain subsides. The treatment includes the usual steps of conservative management plus manual therapy and local support-taping and/or orthotic.

Finally, upon initial clinical examination of the acutely injured ankle, peripheral nerve involvement should be excluded. Grade III ankle sprains have a high incidence of traction injuries to both the peroneal and posterior tibial nerves. Naturally, this can result in prolonged inversion, eversion, and postinjury plantar-flexion weakness. Less frequently, peroneal nerve injuries are seen with milder degrees of inversion ankle sprains.

Schamberger[77] has comprehensively reviewed nerve injuries about the foot and ankle. In brief, inversion supination forces stretch the sural and common peroneal nerves, often with compression of the posterior tibial nerve in the tarsal tunnel. Eversion pronation forces stretch the tibialis posterior nerve with lateral compression forces to the sural nerve. In addition, a stretching (traction) force can be applied to the superficial branch of the common peroneal nerve with excessive plantar flexion of the ankle. On physical examination, a positive Tinel sign can often be elicited, and diagnosis can be confirmed by local anaesthetic nerve blocks and by electromyography and nerve conduction studies.

Although not truly an associated injury, the term anterolateral impingement of the ankle has been proposed to describe postinjury persistent anterolateral pain, sensation of weakness, and instability in an ankle with stable ligaments, slowing return to sport.[78] When arthroscopy was performed after 2 years of symptoms, the findings included hypertrophic synovium and chondromalacia of the talus. There was ultimately improvement in symptoms. An algorithm for the assessment and treatment of post-traumatic chronic ankle pain is depicted in Fig. 5.

Overuse injuries

Stress fractures

Stress fracture commonly affects the ankle, and in a series of 320 athletes with this injury the tibia was involved in 49.1 per cent, the tarsals in 25.3 per cent, and the fibula in 6.6 per cent.[11] Many of these injuries were sited at the ankle joint. Runners are by far the most affected group of patients, and biomechanical factors play an important part in the aetiology of such lesions, emphasizing the fact that stress fractures are overuse in origin. Matheson et al.[11] found that pronated feet were particularly associated with tibial stress fractures and tarsal bone fractures.

The presentation of a stress fracture is typically that of a gradual onset of pain accompanied by tenderness, which is quite easily localized to a particular site such as the lateral malleolus. Pain is associated with activity and is relieved by rest. With progression of the stress fracture, pain develops earlier with activity, takes longer to settle with rest, and it is painful to hop. Eventually, constant pain develops and activity is prevented. There is normally little swelling (if any) to be found and no evidence of bruising or trophic changes of the skin. Vascular and neurological signs are not associated with isolated stress fractures.

The examiner should take note of biomechanical factors such as excessive pronation of the foot and enquire as to recent increases in activity, particularly on hard surfaces. Attention to footwear may reveal inappropriate shoes which lack, 'motion control' (if required) and shock-absorption properties, as discussed earlier in this chapter.

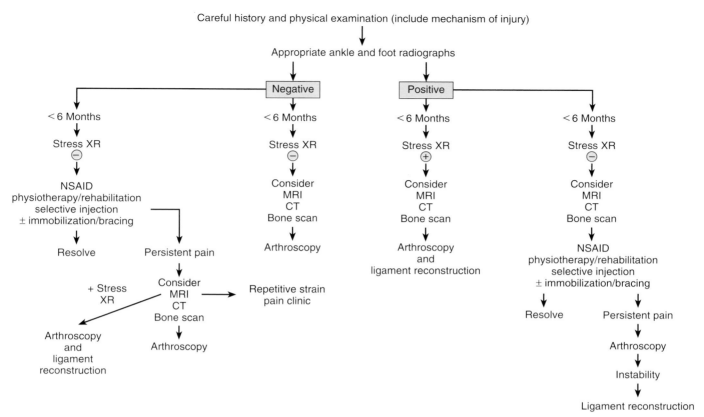

Fig. 5 Treatment of chronic ankle pain. (From ref. 82 with permission.)

The diagnosis of stress fracture is supported by the observation of an area of increased isotope uptake on a technetium-99 bone scan at the site of bone pain and tenderness. Radiographs are typically negative for up to 3 weeks after development of the lesion, but a CT scan may be useful in defining the architecture of the bone and the lesion itself when a positive bone scan has been returned. This is particularly valuable in stress fractures which have a risk of completion and non-union (namely navicular, femoral neck).

Management includes active rest (modifying exercise to limit painful activities and substituting swimming, cycling, and weight training to maintain cardiovascular fitness and strength) with a programme of rehabilitation which grades a return to full sporting activity over a period of 6 to 8 weeks. Typically, non weight-bearing exercise is encouraged until painfree for 2 weeks, and then small increments in weight-bearing activity at weekly intervals are permitted. The diminution in local bone pain, tenderness, and pain when hopping is used as a guide to these gradual increases in the programme. Physiotherapy modalities which may be of use include pulsed magnetic-field therapy and electrical stimulation via superfical (skin-mounted) electrodes. An Aircast ankle stirrup is particularly useful in stress fractures about the ankle, particularly where early mobilization and weight bearing is being encouraged. The Aircast should be worn at least until initial recovery, and for a period thereafter to facilitate return to sport. Biomechanical factors such as excessive pronation and length discrepancy should be attended to, and the fitting of correctly prescribed orthotic devices is recommended together with the provision of appropriate footwear.

Shelboure *et al.*[79] presented a series of six cases of stress frac-

tures of the medial malleolus. Of these, three patients with fracture lines shown on radiographs were treated with open reduction and internal fixation using two 4.0 cancellous screws. The other three cases had normal radiographs with hot bone scans and were managed with an Aircast brace. These patients were permitted unlimited ambulation in the Aircast brace and progressed to full participation in 6 to 8 weeks. Similarly, the surgically treated cases progressed to running activities by 6 weeks and full sports participation by 8 weeks.

Although stress fractures typically present as overuse injuries and therefore are gradual in onset, a stress fracture may occasionally be manifested via acute injuries such as inversion sprains or trauma to the ankle or foot. Navicular, proximal shaft of the fifth metatarsus, and talar fractures may present in this way, and the physician must remember to consider these diagnoses and investigate accordingly.

A stress fracture of the talus is notorious for presenting in an insidious fashion and is often unaccompanied by impressive local tenderness. There may be some effusion of the ankle and some limitation of range of movement, but many patients continue to weight bear, albeit in some discomfort for some time after the onset of symptoms. Typically, hopping is painful and this should alert the clinician to the diagnosis. When the bone scan is positive and a CT scan is recommended, remember that a CT scan may be negative in a talar stress fractures of traumatic origin.[11]

Management depends upon the severity of the lesion, and may range from reduced weight-bearing activities in an Aircast stirrup to ankle protection in a non weight-bearing cast for up to 8 weeks.

Pain when hopping, used as a guide to the reintroduction of weight-bearing activities after an initial rest period, complimented with cycling, swimming, or 'pool running' has been used to maintain fitness. Any lesion affecting the articular cartilage must be reviewed by an orthopaedic surgeon.

Similarly, stress fractures of the tarsal navicular can present as ankle problems. They may present in an acute fashion associated with an ankle sprain or with a more typical history of gradually increasing pain, tenderness, and disability associated with activity. Technetium-99 bone scanning and CT scanning are recommended, with appropriate aggressive management instituted immediately.

Tendinitis

Overuse of the ankle, in running, jumping, and dancing for example, often produces tendinitis of the main functional stabilizers and strong plantar flexors of the ankle. The posterior tibial tendon and the tendons of the peroneal muscles are particularly affected in this respect.

As discussed earlier in this chapter, the posterior tibial tendon is a strong supporter for the medial arch of the foot and is active as a plantar flexor and a controller of pronation during gait. It also works eccentrically with its muscle in landing to absorb shock. The tendon extends along the distal third of the medial tibial margin and inserts on to the medial tarsal navicular surface, with variable attachments to adjacent tarsal bones. It passes behind the medial malleolus and is enclosed in a synovial sheath in this part of its course, where it lies deep to the flexor retinaculum.

Tendinitis is typically of gradual onset and is precipitated by increased or high levels of activity, with limited periods of rest or recovery. The pain is localized to the medial tibial margin or to the tendon adjacent to the medial malleolus. Often there is swelling of the distal tendon and sheath, and pain may be reproduced by resisted plantar flexion and inversion of the foot and ankle.

Biomechanical factors play a significant role in the aetiology of this condition and relief is often rapid once appropriate orthotics have been fitted. Overpronation is perhaps the most important fault in this respect. Attention to footwear is recommended, and sport shoes which control pronation and provide for shock absorption, particularly in basketball and netball, should be considered essential.

Treatment consists of the modification of painful activity until the symptoms and signs subside, regular applications of ice, physiotherapy which employs electrotherapeutic modalities to reduce inflammation, and an exercise programme to stretch and strengthen the posterior tibial muscle and tendon, particularly utilizing an eccentric phase.[69] Non-steroidal anti-inflammatory medication can be very useful, and in recalcitrant cases the judicious administration of a local corticosteroid injection may be helpful, taking extreme care not to inject into the tendon. A rest from jumping and running for 10 days is advised after a corticosteroid injection to minimize the risk of a corticosteroid-associated tendon rupture.

Posterior tibial tendinitis should be distinguished from the medial tibial stress syndrome (shin-splints), the deep calf compartment pressure syndrome, and stress fracture (of the tibial shaft, the medial malleolus, and the tarsal navicular bone). Technetium-99 bone scanning and/or compartment pressure studies may be indicated here.

The tendons of the peroneus longus and brevis provide functional lateral stability of the ankle as everters and plantar flexors of the foot. Although they are more commonly injured in acute inversion sprains, overuse through jumping, running, and dancing may occasionally induce tendinitis or tenosynovitis, typically at the lateral malleolus where the tendons pass deep to the superior and inferior retinacula and curve around the malleolus to insert at their respective sites on the medial cuneiform and metatarsals. Repetitive friction through their common tendon sheath and around the 'pulley' of the malleolus, produces pain of gradual onset with associated local tenderness and swelling of the sheath. Forced plantar flexion and eversion may reproduce the pain.

The treatment of tendinitis in this situation is the same as for posterior tendinitis, with local applications of ice, physiotherapy, and exercises for the tendon(s) and the occasional injection of a corticosteroid along the tendon(s) or within the sheath. Occasionally, a heel-raise provides relief, and a gradual return to sport in appropriate footwear should be possible over 6 to 8 weeks.

The differential diagnosis of peroneal tendinitis or tenosynovitis includes injury to the ligaments of the ankle, bony injury to the fibular tibula, and disruption of structures such as the peroneal retinacula.

Impingement syndrome
Footballer's ankle
Footballer's ankle is a condition whereby repeated microtrauma to the margins of the anterior ankle joint, through repetitive forceful plantar flexion and dorsiflexion, produces traction osteophytes at the capsular ligament attachments and subsequent formation of loose bodies within the joint. The condition is not a true osteoarthritis as the articular cartilage is spared. Any sport which involves this repeated ankle movement can produce such a condition, and soccer, basketball, triple jumping, long jumping, and dance are all well-known causes of footballer's ankle.

Symptoms are usually of gradual onset, with diffuse anterior ankle joint pain; occasionally swelling is noted after activity. There is often local tenderness, and pain can be reproduced by forced ankle plantar flexion or dorsiflexion which stretches the ligament and impinges the ligament attachments, respectively. Plain radiography demonstrates the osteophytes at the joint margins and loose bodies may be seen.

Management depends upon symptoms, as the only definitive treatment is surgical excision of osteophytes with or without removal of loose bodies. If possible, limitation of painful activity should be recommended, and soccer players should be encouraged not to slide on the plantar-flexed foot or kick with the dorsum of the foot when moving the ball forwards. Kicking with the medial surface of the foot is preferred. Anti-inflammatory medication, physiotherapy with electrotherapeutic modalities, ice applications, and occasionally local injection of a corticosteroid can settle the inflammation but should not be seen as curative.

Os trigonum and talar spur (posterior process)
In the normal development of the talus, a posterior process may appear, or may present, as a separate ossicle, the os trigonum. This occurs in approximately 10 per cent of the population.

Impingement of the ossicle or posterior process can result from forced plantar flexion of the ankle and produce a deep pain posterior to the ankle joint, localized deep to the Achilles tendon. This is particularly common amongst ballet dancers, jumpers, and fast bowlers in cricket. Tenderness is usual and forceful plantar flexion reproduces the pain. There may be a little swelling, but usually no bruising, and the Achilles tendon is typically unaffected. Plain radiographs demonstrate the ossicle or talar process and a bone scan may show increased isotope uptake, particularly if there has been disruption of the fibrous union between the os trigonum and the talus, or a fracture of the posterior talar process.

Management consists of initial rest from painful activity, ice applications, anti-inflammatory medication, electrotherapy, and a gradual return to activity as symptoms permit. Occasionally a local injection of a corticosteroid may be indicated which provides relief in most cases. If symptoms persist, surgical excision of the offending ossicle or spur yields good results.[80]

Bursitis at the malleoli

A problem common amongst ice skaters and ice hockey players is bursitis over the lateral or medial malleolus. Wearing tight boots for long periods produces a combination of compression and friction about the malleolus, which results in the development of a painful, tender, and swollen bursa. The diagnosis is simple and no investigations are necessary.

Malleolar bursitis responds quickly to adjustment of footwear to minimize pressure and friction, perhaps with the addition of an orthotic device to correct an underlying biomechanical fault, such as excessive foot pronation, supported by regular applications of ice, non-steroidal anti-inflammatory medication, and physiotherapy. If necessary, a local injection of a corticosteroid may be helpful. Persistent cases may require surgical excision of the offending bursa.

References

1. Garrick JG. Epidemiology of foot and ankle injuries. In: Shepard RJ, Taunton JE, eds. *Medicine and sport science*, Vol. 23 *Foot and ankle in sport and exercise*. Basel: Karger, 1987: 1–7.
2. Garrick JG. Epidemiologic perspective. *Clinics in Sports Medicine* 1982; **1**: 13–18.
3. Jackson D, Ashley, RL, Powell J. Ankle sprains in young athletes. *Clinical Orthopaedics* 1974; **101**: 201–14.
4. Chapman MW. Sprains of the ankle. *AAOS instructional course lecture*. Chicago: American Academy of Orthopedic Surgeons, 1975; **24**: 294–308.
5. Balduini FC, Tetzlaff J. Historical perspectives for injuries of the ligaments of the ankle. *Clinics in Sports Medicine* 1982; **1**: 3–12.
6. Clement DB, Taunton JE, Smart GU, McNicol KL. A survey of overuse running injuries. *Physician and Sportsmedicine* 1981; **9**: 47–58.
7. Macintyre JG, Taunton JE, Clement DB, Lloyd Smith DR, McKenzie DC, Morrell RW. Running injuries: a clinical study of 4173 cases. *Canadian Journal of Sports Medicine* 1989; **1**: 7–11.
8. Walter SD, *et al.* Training habits and injury experience in distance runners: age and sex related factors. *Physician and Sportsmedicine* 1988; **16**: 101–13.
9. Marti B, Vader JD, Minder CE, Abelin T. On the epidemiology of running injuries. *American Journal of Sports Medicine* 1988; **16**: 285–94.
10. Garrick JG, Requa RK. Role of external support in the prevention of ankle sprains. *Medicine and Science in Sports* 1973; **5**: 200–3.
11. Matheson GO, Clement DB, McKenzie DC, Taunton JE, Lloyd-Smith DR, Macintyre JG. Stress fractures in athletes. A study of 320 cases. *American Journal of Sports Medicine* 1987; **15**: 46–58.
12. Gray H. *Anatomy of the human body*. 28th edn. Philadelphia: Lea and Febiger, 1966.
13. Akesson EJ. Anatomy of foot and ankle. In: Shepard RJ, Taunton JE, eds. *Medicine and sport science*, Vol. 23 *Foot and ankle in sport and exercise*. Basel: Karger, 1987: 8–21.
14. Cavanagh PR, Lafortune MA. Ground reaction forces in distance running. *Journal of Biomechanics* 1980; **13**: 397–406.
15. Procter P, Berne N, Paul JP. Ankle joint biomechanics. In: Morechi A, Fidelus K, Kedzier K, Wit, eds. *Biomechanics* V11-A. Baltimore, MD: University Park Press, 1981: 52–6.
16. Nigg BM. Biomechanical analysis of ankle and foot movement. In: Shephard RJ, Taunton JE, eds. *Medicine and sport science*, Vol. 23 *Foot and ankle in sport and exercise*. Basel: Karger, 1987: 22–9.
17. Nuber GO. Biomechanics of the foot and ankle during gait. *Clinics in Sports Medicine* 1988; **7**: 127–42.
18. Slocum DB, James SL. Biomechanics of running. *Journal of the American Medical Association* 1958; **205**: 97–104.
19. Mann RA. Biomechanics of running. In: *AAOS symposium on the foot and leg in running sports*. St Louis: CV Mosby, 1982: 30–44.
20. Mann RA, Moran GJ, Dougherty SC. Comparative electromyelography of the lower extremity in jogging, running and sprinting. *American Journal of Sport Medicine* 1986: **14**: 501.
21. Ohman D. Injury prevention program for the ankle. *SportsAider* 1989; **6**: 1–5.
22. Bauenhauer JF, Alosa DM, Beynnon B. A prospective study of ankle injury risk factors. *American Journal of Sport Medicine* 1995; **23**: 564–70.
23. Garrick JG, Requa RK. The epidemiology of foot and ankle injuries in sports. *Clinics in Sports Medicine* 1988; **7**: 29–36.
24. Emerick CE. Ankle taping: prevention of injury or waste of time? *Athletic Training* 1979; **188**: 149–150.
25. Fumich RM, Ellison AE, Guerin GJ, Grace DD. The measured effect of taping on combined foot and ankle motion before and after exercise. *American Journal of Sports Medicine* 1981; **9**: 165–70.
26. Rarick GL, Bigley GK, Ralph MR. The measurable support of the ankle joint by conventional methods of taping. *Journal of Bone and Joint Surgery* 1962; **44A**: 1183–90.
27. Bunch RP, Bednarski K, Holland D, Macinanti BA. Ankle joint support: a comparison of reusable lace-on braces with taping and wrapping. *Physician and Sportsmedicine* 1985; **13**: 59–62.
28. Rovere GD, Clarke TJ, Yates CS, Burley K. Retrospective comparison of taping and ankle stabilizers in preventing ankle injuries. *American Journal of Sports Medicine* 1988; **16**: 228–33.
29. Kimura IF, Nawoczenski DA, Epler M, Owen MG. Effect of the air stirrup in controlling ankle inversion stress. *Journal of Orthopaedic Sports Physical Therapy* 1987; **9**: 190–3.
30. Gross MT, Bradshaw MK, Ventry LC, Weller KH. Comparison of support by ankle taping and semi-rigid orthosis. *Journal of Orthopaedic Sports Physical Therapy* 1987; **9**: 33–9.
31. Greene TA, Hillman SK. Comparison of support provided by a semi-rigid orthosis and adhesive ankle taping before, during, and after exercise. *American Journal of Sports Medicine* 1990; **18**: 498–506.
32. Amoroso PJ, Ryan JB, Bickby BT, Taylor DC, Leitschub P, Jones BH. Impact of the outside-the-boot ankle brace on sprains associated with military airborne training. *Report T95–1 US Army Medical Research and Development Command*, Natick, MA, October 1994.
33. Sitter MR, Horodyski MB. Effectiveness of prophylactic ankle stabilizers for prevention of ankle injuries. *Sports Medicine* 1995; **20**: 53–7.
34. Pienkowski D, McMorrow M, Shapiro R, Caborn DN, Stagton J. The effect of ankle stabilizers on athletic performance. *American Journal of Sports Medicine* 1995; **23**: 757–62.

35. Gehlsen GM, Pearson D, Bahamonde R. Ankle joint strength, total work and ROM: comparison between prophylactic devices. *Athletic Training* 1991; **26**: 62–5.

36. Sitler M, Ryan J, Wheeler B, *et al.* The efficacy of a semirigid ankle stabilizer to reduce acute ankle injuries in basketball: A randomized clinical study at West Point. *American Journal of Sports Medicine* 1994; **22**: 454–61.

37. Surve I, Schwellnus MP, Noakes T, Lombard C. A fivefold reduction in the incidence of recurrent ankle sprains in soccer players using the sport–stirrup orthosis. *American Journal of Sports Medicine* 1994; **22**: 601–6.

38. Anderson D. The role of external non-rigid ankle bracing in the prevention of inversion injuries. MPE thesis, University of British Columbia, Vancouver, 1992.

39. James SL, Bates BT, Ostering LR. Injuries to runners. *American Journal of Sports Medicine* 1978; **6**: 40–50.

40. McKenzie DC, Clement DB, Taunton JE. Running shoes, orthotics and injuries. *Sports Medicine* 1985; **2**: 334–7.

41. Taunton JE, Clement DB, Smart GW, Wiley JP, McNicol KL. A triplanar electrogoniometer investigation of running mechanics in runners with compensatory overpronation. *Canadian Journal of Applied Sport Science* 1985; **10**: 104–15.

42. Bates BT, Osternig LR, Mason B, James SL. Foot orthotic devices to modify selected aspects of lower extremity mechanics. *American Journal of Sports Medicine* 1979; **7**: 338–42.

43. Smith L, Clarke T, Hamill C, Santopietro F. The effects of soft and semi-rigid orthoses upon rearfoot movement in running. *Medicine and Science in Sport and Exercise* 1983; **15**: 171.

44. McKenzie DC. The role of the shoe and orthotic. In: Shephard RJ, Taunton, JE, eds. *Medicine and sport science*, Vol. 23 *Foot and ankle in sport and exercise*. Basel: Karger, 1987: 30–8.

45. Brody D. Running injuries. *Ciba Foundation Symposium*. Basel: CIBA, 1980; **32**: 1–36.

46. Lutter LD. Cavus foot in runners. *Foot and Ankle* 1981; **1**: 225–8.

47. Moore PH, Taunton JE. Medically based athletic footwear. Design and selection. *New Zealand Journal of Sports Medicine* 1991; **19**: 22–5.

48. Frederick CC, Clarke TC, Hamill CL. The effect of running shoe design on shock absorption. In: Frederick EC, ed. *Sport shoes and playing surfaces*. Champaign, IL: Human Kinetics, 1984: 190–8.

49. Bahr R, Karlsen R, Lian O, Ourebo RV. Incidence and mechanisms of acute ankle inversion injuries in volleyball: a respective cohort study. *American Journal of Sports Medicine* 1994; **22**: 595–600.

50. Trott AW. Foot and ankle problems in adolescents: sport aspects. *American Academy of Orthopaedic Surgeons Symposium on Foot and Ankle*. St Louis: CV Mosby, 1979: 47.

51. Micheli LJ. Overuse in children's sports: the growth factor. *Orthopaedic Clinics of North America* 1983; **14**: 337–60.

52. Beauchamp R. Pediatric foot and ankle problems. In: Shepard RJ, Taunton JE, eds. *Medicine and sport science*, Vol 23 *Foot and ankle in sport and exercise*. Basel: Karger, 1987: 128–44.

53. Salter RB, Harris WR. Injuries involving the epiphyseal plate. *Journal of Bone and Joint Surgery* 1963; **45**: 587–622.

54. Stiell IG, Greenberg GH, McKnight RD, *et al.* Decision rules for the use of radiography in acute ankle injuries; refinement and prospective validation. *Journal of the American Medical Association* 1993; **269**: 1127–32.

55. Chandler RW. Management of complex ankle fractures in athletes. *Clinics in Sports Medicine* 1988; **7**: 127–42.

56. Stuart PR, Brumby C, Smith SR. Comparative study of functional bracing and plaster cast treatment of stable lateral malleolar fractures. *Injury* 1989; **20**: 317–20.

57. McConkey JP. Ankle sprains, consequences and mimics. In: Shephard RJ, Taunton JE, eds. *Medicine and sport science*, Vol. 23 *Foot and ankle in sport and exercise*. Basel: Karger, 1987: 39–55.

58. Walsh M, Blackburn T. Prevention of ankle sprains. *American Journal of Sports Medicine* 1977; **5**: 243–5.

59. Laurin C, Mathieu J. Sagital mobility of the normal ankle. *Clinical Orthopaedics* 1975; **108**: 99–104.

60. Rucinski TJ, Hooker DN, Prentice WE, Shields EW, Cote-Murray DJ. The effects of intermittent compression on edema in post acute ankle sprains. *Journal of Orthopaedic Sports Physical Therapy* 1991; **14**: 65–9.

61. Eiff MP, Smith AT, Smith GE. Early mobilization versus immobilization in the treatment of lateral ankle sprains. *American Journal of Sports Medicine* 1994; **22**: 83–8.

62. Lane SC. Severe ankle sprains. Treatment with an ankle foot orthosis. *Physician and Sportsmedicine* 1990; **18**: 43–51.

63. Freeman MAR. Treatment of ruptures of the lateral ligaments of the ankle. *Journal of Bone and Joint Surgery* 1965; **47B**: 661–84.

64. Gould N. Repair of lateral ligament of ankle. *Foot and Ankle* 1987; **8**: 55–8.

65. Gould N, Seligson D, Gassman J. Early and late repair of lateral ligaments of the ankle. *Foot and Ankle* 1989; **1**: 84–9.

66. Thompson JP, Loomer RL. Osteochondral lesions of the talus in a sports medicine-clinic. *American Journal of Sports Medicine* 1984; **12**: 460–3.

67. Shearer C. Long term follow-up on Stage 5 osteochondral lesions of the talus. MSc thesis, School of Human Kinetics, University of British Columbia, Vancouver, 1996.

68. Bassett FH III, Speer KP. Longitudinal rupture of the peroneal tendons. *American Journal of Sports Medicine* 1993; **21**: 354–7.

69. Stanish WD, Ratson G, Curwin S. Tendinopathies about the foot and ankle. In: Shephard RJ, Taunton JE, eds. *Medicine and sport science*, Vol. 23 *Foot and ankle in sport and exercise*. Basel: Karger, 1987: 80–98.

70. Conti S, Michelson J, Jahss M. Clinical significance of magnetic resonance imaging in preoperative planning for reconstruction of posterior tibial tendon ruptures. *Foot and Ankle* 1992; **13**: 208–14.

71. Woods L, Leach RE. Posterior tibial tendon rupture in athletic people. *American Journal of Sports Medicine* 1991; **19**: 495–8.

72. Hopkinson WJ, St Pierre P, Ryan JB, Wheeler JM. Syndesmosis sprains of the ankle. *Foot and Ankle* 1990; **10**: 325–30.

73. Boytin MJ, Fischer DA, Neumann L. Syndesmotic ankle sprains. *American Journal of Sports Medicine* 1991; **19**: 294–8.

74. Taylor DC, Bassett FH III. Syndesmosis ankle sprains: diagnosing the injury and aiding recovery. *Physician and Sportsmedicine* 1993; **21**: 39–46.

75. McConkey JP, Lloyd-Smith DR, Li D. Complete rupture of the deltoid ligament of the ankle. *Clinical Journal of Sports Medicine* 1991; **1**: 133–7.

76. Marshall P, Hamilton WG. Cuboid subluxation in ballet dancers. *American Journal of Sports Medicine* 1992; **20**: 169–75.

77. Schamberger W. Nerve injuries around the foot and ankle. In: Shephard RJ, Taunton JE, eds. *Medicine and sport science*, Vol. 23 *Foot and ankle in sport and exercise*. Basel: Karger, 1987: 105–20.

78. Ferkel RD, Karzel RP, DelPizzo W. Arthoscopic treatment of anterolateral impingement of the ankle. *American Journal of Sports Medicine* 1991; **19**: 440–6.

79. Shelbourne KD, Fischer D, Rettig AC, McCarroll JR. Stress fractures of the medial malleolus. *American Journal of Sports Medicine* 1988; **16**: 60–3.

80. Fricker PA, Williams JGP. Surgery to the os trigonum and talar spur in sportsmen. *British Journal of Sports Medicine* 1978; **13**: 55–7.

81. Johnson KA, Teasdall RD. Sprained ankles as they relate to the basketball player. *Clinics in Sports Medicine* 1993; **12**: 363–71.

82. Jaivin JS, Ferkel RD. Arthroscopy of the foot and ankle. *Clinics in Sports Medicine* 1994; **13**: 761–83.

4.4.2 The acute ankle sprain

Angus M. McBryde

Introduction

In competitive or recreational activity, for example basketball, acute ankle sprains are the single most frequent specific injuries.[1-4] The lateral ligament complex of the ankle is the most frequently injured single musculoskeletal structure in the body (Fig. 1).[5] Sprains comprise 85 per cent of ankle injuries, occurring in athletes in virtually all sports at all levels of competition and affecting both males and females.[6,7] Of all time lost 25 per cent is attributed to ankle sprain.[8]

An estimated 30 per cent of milder (grade I and grade II) sprains and perhaps 15 per cent of more severe sprains never enter the health-care system. Most of these acute ankle sprains not seen by a practitioner are recurrent acute sprains. Acute sprains occur primarily in persons between the ages of 10 and 35.

Ankle sprains (not strains)[9] are secondary only to back sprains and strains as a cause of disability. In the United States of America alone 20.7 million restricted-activity days occur per year; 5.8 million work and school days are lost; and 500 000 bed-disability days are lost to ankle sprains.[10]

Foot and ankle injuries comprise up to 25 per cent of sports injuries.[8,11,12] Of these injuries, 9.7 per cent involve the ankle alone. Youth soccer (12- to 17-year-olds), for instance, produced an overall 23.1 per cent incidence of ankle injuries, with the percentage rising with the increasing age of the players.[13] In athletes, the ankle of the dominant leg is more frequently sprained. As expected, acute recurrent sprains leave the athlete with more symptoms, greater functional instability, and a greater negative effect on performance.[14]

Primary-care physicians such as family physicians, paediatricians, and emergency-room physicians, plus physician assistants, nurse practitioners, physical therapists, athletic trainers—all are called on to see and treat the acute ankle sprain in all its severities.[15] Orthopaedic surgeons see, at some point in treatment, an estimated 60 per cent of ankle sprains that are formally seen by any practitioner.

The primary-care practitioner can handle 90 per cent of all ankle sprains. But the problem arises with: (1) the need to recognize and select the more severe 10 per cent of cases; and (2) the universal need to diagnose adequately and treat the remaining 90 per cent. A detailed history and physical examination is clearly necessary for the more severe 10 per cent of ankle sprains. This is supplemented by stress radiographs or other studies which are frequently necessary to determine whether more aggressive treatment with implied referral is indicated. At this point in the decision-making process a suboptimal diagnosis is frequently made, with a resultant insufficient acute treatment and rehabilitation programme. Even when the need for referral is recognized, many are 'late referrals', namely after 3 weeks. In essence, the frequency of ankle sprain has caused a casual attitude in treatment.[9]

All these factors, that is to say self-treatment, numerous caregivers, injury frequency, late referrals, etc., cause major difficulties in any study of ankle sprain. Therefore it becomes difficult to select, digest, study, and then quantitate specifically or standardize the injury patterns, diagnosis, management, and rehabilitation.

The history is indispensable to the subsequent diagnosis, treatment, and rehabilitation of an acute ankle sprain. It points up the typical musculoskeletal and usually sports-related injury. Ankle sprain is both a sports-specific injury, for example soccer, and a sports-generic injury, for instance any leg-based sport. Both documented and undocumented histories indicate this fact. Most ankle sprains occur with an agility move while in the immediate pre- or postload phase, namely just prior to or after landing from a jump. The dominant leg is more frequently injured.[16] Other acute sprains occur when the foot is planted on a non-level surface which throws the foot and ankle into supination. There are pre-existing tendencies due to previous injury, increased height and weight,[6] and inherent joint laxity. Other performance factors also predispose to injury, namely conditioning, selective muscle group strength (posterior tibial) or weakness (peroneals), and shoe and/or orthosis ankle protection or modification of foot plant. Competition risk exceeds that of trauma.[17]

More importance should be attached to the history, the physical examination, the accuracy of diagnosis, the treatment, and the rehabilitation of acute ankle sprains.[15]

Anatomy and mechanics of the ankle joint

The ankle (talocrural joint) is a complex hinge joint which is also a mortise joint. There is an inherent stability in its interlocking configuration. The joint and the talus are wider anteriorly with the talus congruently fitting into the tibia-fibula mortise (Fig. 2). Dorsiflexion bony stability is maximum as the talus locks into this mortise. Plantar-flexion stability therefore relies more on ligamentous integrity. This decreased bony stability in plantar flexion is particularly evident on the medial side since the longer lateral malleolus offers a better buttress for the ankle and subtalar joint in all positions. Thus the bony anatomy partially determines that plantar flexion and inversion is the most vulnerable direction for injury.

The lateral collateral ligament complex binds the talus and calcaneus to the fibula (Fig. 3). The anterior talofibular ligament is the

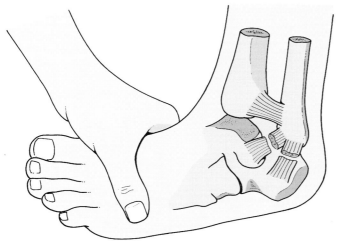

Fig. 1 Injury of the anterior talofibular ligament (ATFL) and the calcaneofibular ligament (CFL) is a most common injury.

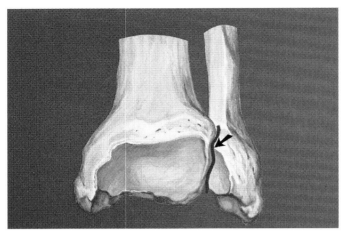

Fig. 2 With weight bearing the talus locks into its tibiofibular bed and there is 40 per cent more stability. Integrity of the opposing articular cartilage at the tibia–fibula junction (arrow) must be maintained. A grade IV sprain can compromise this integrity.

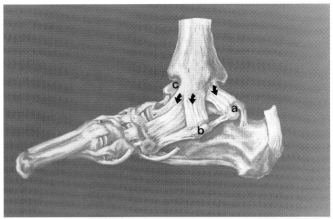

Fig. 4 The medial ankle, hindfoot, and midfoot ligamentous complex. Grade IV ankle sprains involve the deltoid ligament (arrows) and the syndesmosis. A grade I-IV ankle sprain can involve other medial structures: (a) posterior medial and posterior lateral talar processes; (b) sustentaculum tali; (c) the talar dome.

weakest ligament and has a high strain rate prerupture.[18] This correlates with its physiological function of allowing increased ankle plantar flexion and internal rotation.[19] The anterior talofibular ligament checks the forward subluxation of the talus in a sagittal plane. It becomes parallel to the tibia and fibula with full plantar flexion as its lateral talar neck distal attachment moves beneath the lateral malleolus.

The calcaneofibular ligament is extracapsular (Fig. 3). It runs obliquely to insert on the posterior lateral aspect of the os calcis. It is perpendicular to the horizontal axis of the posterior subtalar joint. Thus the calcaneofibular ligament acts as a stabilizer of the subtalar joint as well as the ankle joint as it bridges both joints. It is a primary ankle stabilizer with dorsiflexion and gives major increased support. It prevents talar tilt primarily with straight inversion. The calcaneofibular ligament is four times stronger than the anterior talofibular ligament. A tear often includes a tear of the peroneal tendon sheath, a companion structure in proximity which is always connected.

The posterior talofibular ligament (Fig. 2) is the strongest liga-

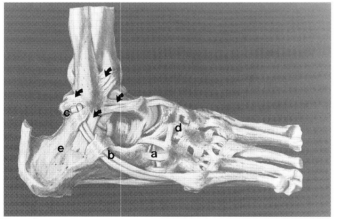

Fig. 3 The lateral ankle hindfoot and midfoot ligamentous complex. A grade I-III ankle sprain primarily involves the calcaneofibular, anterior and posterior talofibular, and anterior tibiofibular ligaments (arrows). Its differential diagnosis can include: (a) calcaneocuboid sprain; (b) peroneal tendon partial tear; (c) subtalar sprain; (d) midfoot ligament sprain; and (e) stress fracture of the os calcis.

ment and runs from the distal fibular to the lateral talar tubercle or posterior to the lateral articular surface of the posterior subtalar joint. An isolated tear promotes only slightly increased hyperextension, but when coupled with anterior talofibular ligament and calcaneofibular ligament tears it promotes major instability[20] including potential instability of the subtalar joint.[21] That potential instability involves the lateral talocalcaneal ligament which protects the subtalar joint and merges with the anterior talofibular and calcaneofibular ligaments.

A range of 20 to 30 degrees of dorsiflexion is available, depending on sport-specific needs, with the mean value for loaded dorsiflexion being 32.5 degrees,[22] although this is a low estimate and a difficult measurement to make biomechanically. The average full range of passive extension is 21 degrees and the average full range of flexion is 23 degrees.[23] When the ankle moves from plantar flexion toward dorsiflexion, initial internal rotation of the talus changes during the last 10 degrees to external rotation towards a neutral position.[24]

The ankle is not a uniaxial joint. There are small but definite adaptive rotations and limited pronation in the ankle joint in the plantar-flexion phase. This helps allow accommodation for non-level ground without losing push-off.[24] Rotation is normally only 12 degrees in the ankle joint but increases with anterior talofibular ligament injury.[25,26] Midfoot joints contribute substantially to transverse axis rotation in 30 degrees of plantar flexion.[24] The articular surface becomes extremely important when loaded, as it decreases that rotation. It affects 30 per cent of stability in rotation and 100 per cent in inversion.[27]

There is a large angle between the calcaneofibular and anterior talofibular ligaments where there is meagre specific ligamentous support. This may result in reduced resistance to inversion since neither the anterior talofibular ligament nor the calcaneofibular ligament offers maximum protection at neutral position within that angle/arc of 10 to 30 degrees of plantar flexion.

The deltoid ligament stabilizes the medial aspect of the ankle (Fig. 4). The tibionavicular, tibiocalcaneal, and anterior and posterior tibiotalar ligaments constitute the superficial portion. The deep portion consists of the transverse tibiotalar ligament which runs anteriorly and posteriorly from the medial malleolus to the talus. The deltoid ligament limits eversion and external rotation. It fans out to a wide insertion on the medial aspect of the talus and calcaneus.

The anterior and posterior talofibular ligaments (Fig. 3), together with the interosseous membrane, anchor the fibula to the tibia. The posterior tibiofibular ligament melds with the inferior transverse (tibiofibular) ligament. Both the posterior and anterior tibiofibular ligaments permit ankle rotation during running and walking gaits.

Little is known about the kinaesthetic information regarding joint position, function, and speed.[28] There is no consistent relationship between lack of functional muscle coordination and mechanical instability. A delayed peroneal proprioceptive response to a quick inversion stress reduces protection and predisposes to injury. Thus a stabilometric type of examination becomes therapeutically pertinent.

In essence, the ankle joint has no single ligament that is dominant in stability. The direction of applied forces, the position of the ankle, the load and velocity on the ankle, the eccentric strength of the extrinsic muscles, and the muscle reaction time all help to determine which stabilizers are most important and where the injury will or will not occur.[29,30]

Mechanism of injury

Of all acute ankle sprains 85 per cent follow excess inversion and plantar flexion; 15 per cent follow excess dorsiflexion and eversion. Slight internal rotation accompanies the usual inversion and plantar-flexion injury. often a plantar-fixed (cleated or studded) shoe allows the body to rotate over that fixed point and the classic injury occurs. When the foot is plantar fixed, and particularly when the triceps surae does not eccentrically decelerate the tibia, there is even more predisposition to lateral ankle ligament disruption.

The inversion, plantar-flexion, and internal-rotation injury can also be described as supination/inversion with external rotation of the tibia on the fixed foot. The anterior capsule ruptures first, followed by the anterior talofibular ligament,[31] the anterior tibiofibular ligament,[32] and the calcaneofibular ligament. If total lateral disruption occurs, the posterior talofibular ligament also tears. The deep anterior deltoid ligament fibres can tear at the extreme of internal rotation and plantar flexion.[31]

Of all anterior talofibular ligament injuries 40 per cent will be accompanied by calcaneofibular ligament injury. Except for the rare, pure-inversion injury with the ankle in neutral position, the calcaneofibular ligament remains intact until the anterior talofibular ligament is torn.[31] The 'blunt ridge'[18] situated at the midportion of the anterior talofibular ligament tents the ligament and predisposes to rupture at that point. The lateral articular facet of the talus and its sunken neck make this blunt ridge an 'anatomical exostosis.'

With children, inversion injuries in that immature skeleton may cause the distal fibular epiphysis to be injured without or occasionally with ligament injury. This is usually a Salter–Harris type II injury.[33] The mechanism of injury also puts stress on an occasionally present accessory fibular epiphysis and can cause an avulsion.

Lateral ligamentous injury with an associated fibular or lateral malleolar fracture can occur in the same way as medial collateral ligament injuries associated with tibial plateau fractures at the knee.[34] Although concomitant rupture with fracture is uncommon, the more aggressive and early mobilization techniques currently used make it important to recognize these associated ligamentous injuries.

History

Initial evaluation of the acute ankle sprain requires a precise history. Appropriate questions must be asked.

1. When did it happen? Was it during recreation or competition? How long before presentation? What were the surface characteristics, for example non-level, cement, sand, etc.? Sports-specific injury tendencies are often present. For instance, running in European cross-country events with non-level surfaces promotes inversion injuries.

2. How did it occur? Was the foot planted? Was it full weight bearing? Was it at foot strike or push-off? Was another person involved? Did someone fall on it? Was an object involved? Associated injuries with ankle sprain are more likely to occur with contact sports, for example American football, rugby, or a soccer collision.

3. How did the foot move? Was the stress twisting or angular? Did the body twist to the right or to the left? Did the foot stay planted at the moment of injury? What were the shoe characteristics? Orthosis? Taping? If the body rotated to the left at the time of a right ankle sprain a severe sprain with possible syndesmosis/interosseous injury should be suspected.

4. How rapidly did the ankle swell? Was it iced and elevated immediately? Was compression applied? If so, what type? The basic principles of treatment, when applied immediately, minimize both the postinjury appearance and the residual functional disability. When an equinus posture, dependence, and heat are used, the sprain at 72 h may seem deceptively severe. Less localized and more diffuse soft-tissue swelling may indicate a more severe injury with the global spread of haemorrhage.

5. What was felt or heard? Was there a 'pop', 'crack', or 'snap'? Was there immediate acute pain? Weakness? Tingling? The subjective sensation at the time of injury can suggest medial, lateral, or interosseous ligament rupture, talar dome fracture, an acute peroneal dislocation, or sural or peroneal nerve stretch, all in the absence of tibial and/or fibular bony injury.

6. Was it possible to bear weight? Was it possible to continue to play? Did weight bearing cause pain? Was there a sensation of instability? Was the ankle 'wobbly' and did it 'give way'? Could you weight bear with a stick or cane? It is unlikely that a more severe grade II or grade III sprain, with or without an additional injury, could permit effective weight bearing effectively. Grade I injuries do allow weight bearing. Continued (intra-articular only) ankle haemarthrosis or subtalar haemarthrosis effectively prevent weight bearing and can indicate intra-articular chondral or osteochondral injury.

7. Was walking, running, or jumping possible? Could agility moves, namely lateral moves, cutting, deceleration be

performed? A grade I injury often permits agility moves with sturdy taping or bracing and supportive footwear.

8. Where was the initial tenderness? Medial? Lateral? Posterior? Leg? Lateral tenderness alone suggests a single-ligament grade I or mild grade II injury. Global tenderness suggests a more severe grade II or a grade III injury. Tenderness over the distal fibula epiphysis or anterior tibia fibula interval or midfoot suggests an associated injury.

9. Was there previous injury? How was it treated? How long ago? How many times previously had the ankle been sprained? Had the ankle returned to 'normal'? Had surgery been performed previously? Recurrent acute sprain suggests inadequate rehabilitation/strength, an unstable ankle, a residual proprioceptive deficit, an associated undiagnosed injury, faulty mechanics, or inappropriate footwear. This type of patient should be followed with full sports-specific return and with a monitored rehabilitation programme. Ankle instability detected on examination could be chronic and not acute in the presence of recurrent acute sprain.

The history, when conducted properly, gives factual information which can be used for: (1) grading the injury; (2) determining treatment; (3) rehabilitation; (4) prognosis; and (5) prevention of subsequent injury.

Examination and diagnostic studies

Physical examination includes inspection, palpation, range of motion assessment of stability, and specific testing for associated injury. Swelling, pain, and disability correlate with the degree of injury unless vigorously and immediately treated with rest, ice, compression, elevation (**RICE**), and protection. As noted earlier, the immediate history in the initial postsprain moments remain most helpful in further diagnosis and the determination of stability.

Local tenderness laterally at the 4, 6, and 8 o'clock positions (looking at the lateral malleolus) gives immediate information about the three lateral ligaments. A positive drawer test in plantar flexion implies anterior talofibular ligament disruption. In a positive test the talus will move forward 4 mm or more than the uninjured ankle. There may be simple absence of a firm endpoint. A positive anterior drawer test in the neutral position suggests that the calcaneofibular ligament and the posterior talofibular ligament have been injured—otherwise, the test would be negative. The deltoid ligament functions as the centre of rotation. With this in mind, the examiner should guide the ankle to a slight internally rotated direction, thereby making the anterior drawer test more reliable.[35]

The talar-tilt test should be attempted during examination by forcefully and smoothly inverting and everting the hindfoot (by holding the os calcis) and comparing it with the contralateral ankle. Radiography may be needed to confirm the positive tilt test by bilateral anteroposterior talar-tilt stress films (Fig. 5).

Midfoot and other ligamentous instabilities, namely subtalar, midfoot, and even tarsal–metatarsal, can confuse the 'ankle sprain' picture. Specific tenderness found with careful palpation along with motion pain in the hindfoot, midfoot, and forefoot suggests something other than a talocrural joint injury. Heel impaction pain suggests ankle or subtalar haemarthrosis and the need for further

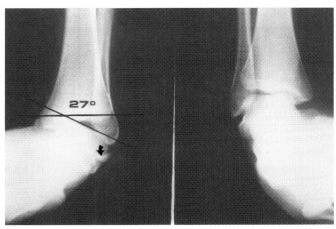

Fig. 5 Talar-tilt stress radiography is reliable and reproducible in trained hands. A measurement of 27 degrees is clearly abnormal (more than 15 degrees above normal) and indicates CFL tear and significant lateral instability. The avulsed fibular attachment of the CFL (arrow) should be noted.

investigation and clinical correlation, for example possible radiographic talar-tilt stress or dye studies.

A major injury (severe pain out of proportion to clinical findings) coupled with a mildly positive drawer test suggests lateral talocalcaneal ligament and subtalar joint injury. The 'squeeze test' with proximal third compression of the tibia and fibula produces distal pain when the syndesmosis is interrupted and interosseous ligament damage has occurred.[36] Ankle injection with local anaesthetic and steroid is often performed, but is not recommended. Local block with anaesthetic alone can be used for differential diagnosis, including trauma to the interosseous membrane, subtalar joint, or calcaneocuboid joint. Injection also allows a better stress test. Specific examiner consistency and repeated use of the differential block optimizes interpretation.

Although the primary examination is physical,[37,38] anteroposterior, lateral, and mortise radiographs are mandatory when there is any significant injury. In the immature skeleton with suspected distal epiphyseal injury, contralateral comparison views should be taken. In addition, lateral stress views and talar-tilt views are indicated if the ankle injury is clearly grade II or questionably grade III with major instability.[39,40] A talar tilt of 15 or 5 degrees more than the opposite ankle on anteroposterior stress projection indicates probable anterior talofibular ligament and calcaneofibular ligament injury. Management decisions for the acute or chronic ankle sprain should not be based on the radiographic talar-tilt test alone.[41] Anteroposterior talar-tilt stress views for varus and anterior instability[42,43] are more helpful than the sagittal stress views. In addition, small flake fractures of the talar dome (osteochondral fractures) may show only on anterior talar-tilt stress films.[44] A forward movement of the talus (beneath the tibia) by 4 mm, as seen on the lateral sagittal stress film, with the anterior drawer test is significant. Although not widely used, quantitative stress methods such as graded stress radiography, where practical, can increase accuracy[42,45] and can be performed regardless of the time of injury. Tenography and arthrography can be used effectively separately.[46] When used together, there is a 100 per cent positive predictive value for calcaneofibular ligament tear.[47]

Arthrography after the first 24 h[18] is usually unsuccessful since clotting occurs and possible abnormal dye distribution is thwarted. Arthrography has both its proponents[18,34,48] and opponents.[49,50] Likewise, tenography or even stress tenography have their proponents[47,51] and opponents. Stress tenography may pick up more double-ligament ruptures, but may also give more false-positives.[52] In some centres, neither tenography nor arthrography is carried out.[15]

Bone scans can help to localize an injury as early as 72 h. Distal tibiofibular and interosseous injury can be picked up on a bone scan for up to 10 weeks.

Magnetic resonance imaging (**MRI**) is beneficial for in-depth differential diagnoses. MRI can delineate injuries which may coexist with ankle sprain as well as document the ligamentous damage itself (Fig. 6). However, its current use is primarily indicated in selective non-resolved ankle sprains and in those failing to respond to a current rehabilitation programme.[53] As MRI is becoming widely available and more reliable, it is replacing many of the imaging techniques now being used.

Types of injury

Clinical testing and radiographic stability patterns of the ankle are helpful with diagnosis and grading.[9] There are numerous classification systems.[54(56] Classifying acute ankle sprains is important primarily for prognosis and not for treatment.[57]

A grade I injury is a partial tear of the anterior talofibular ligament.[58] Only local tenderness is present. This is a 'single ligament' injury. Heel and toe walking is satisfactory. There is no significant subjective or objective instability. A full range of motion is permitted and there is definite but minimal weight-bearing pain. In all, 30 per cent of all ankle sprains meet these criteria.

A grade II injury implies complete anterior talofibular ligament disruption. The drawer test is positive. Moderate decreased range of motion, pain, swelling, and minimally positive talar tilt of less than 15 degrees can be present. The calcaneofibular ligament is horizontal and out of harm's way in plantar flexion. However, it may be injured with a grade II injury. This would be a 'double-ligament' injury. A double-ligament injury always involves a talocalcaneal ligament insult.[43] A total of 40 per cent of all ankle sprains meet these criteria. This is the ankle sprain most common in dancers.[59]

A grade III injury implies damage to three ligaments (anterior and posterior talofibular ligaments and the calcaneofibular ligament) plus varus instability. Both functional treatment and operative repair allow stabilization of this unstable joint. The patient presents in a non weight-bearing status with significant pain and swelling. Anterior and lateral instability is present on examination, and the range of voluntarily and involuntarily motion is reduced. Talar tilt greater than 15 degrees is present. Only 15 per cent of all ankle sprains meet these criteria.

A grade IV injury is an eversion, external rotation, with/without dorsiflexion injury. In successive order, superficial and deep deltoid ligaments, the anterior and posterior tibiofibular ligaments, and the interosseous membrane can all be involved. This can be a more significant injury, frequently with a delayed (2 to 4 months) return to sport compared to the more common lateral sprain.[60,61] There is minimal swelling and pain with isolated anterior tibiofibular ligament sprain. In contrast, posterior tibiofibular ligament injury associated with severe pain is frequently accompanied by a partial, or near complete, interosseous tear.[62] All ankle sprains with medial findings are grade IV in type. Indoor soccer players incur ligamentous diastasis without fracture as a grade IV injury. The tibiofibular diastasis occurring with a grade IV sprain warrants confirmation by stress radiography under anaesthesia. These stress radiographs can show widening and indicate the need for surgery.[36] There may be a radiographic and even a clinical plastic deformation or bend in the tibia or fibula. In all, 15 per cent of all ankle sprains meet these grade IV injury criteria.

Open sprains are quite rare and need immediate irrigation and bridement.[63]

Differential diagnosis and associated injuries

There are numerous acute injuries which may be overlooked or disguised at the time of initial presentation with an injured ankle.[64] Many of these diagnoses are established late and with difficulty.[65] This is especially important with the now universal functional treatment of ankle sprains including aggressive mobilization, early weight bearing, and protected usage. Practitioners (including orthopaedists) must have a high index of suspicion for occult injury in addition to acute ankle sprain. Unrecognized associated injuries may or may not heal, creating the possibility of a new source for chronic ankle impairment.

1. Calcaneocuboid ligament sprain

This is a foot sprain. Appropriate anteroposterior and lateral radiographs of the foot must be ordered. A bony fleck is often seen on the anteroposterior view adjacent to the cuboid laterally.

2. Subtalar joint sprain[55,66]

Type I
Forced supination of the hindfoot with plantar flexion can tear the anterior talofibular ligament with calcaneofibular ligament and lateral capsule ligament tear.

Type II
Forced supination of the hindfoot with plantar flexion resulting in an anterior talofibular ligament tear with talocalcaneal ligament tear.

Type III
Forced supination with dorsiflexion of the ankle can rupture the calcaneofibular ligament, cervical ligament, and interosseous talocalcaneal ligament. Global ligament damage with severe ankle and subtalar sprain occurs with maximum inversion in a neutral ankle position.

3. Sinus tarsi syndrome

Lateral fat-pad necrosis causes anterior lateral ankle pain postinjury. This scarring can usually be controlled by icing, ultrasound, and non-steroidal anti-inflammatory drugs.

4. Synovial pinch

The synovium can hypertrophy with 'pinching' or impingement at the anterior lateral ankle joint line, primarily with dorsiflexion.

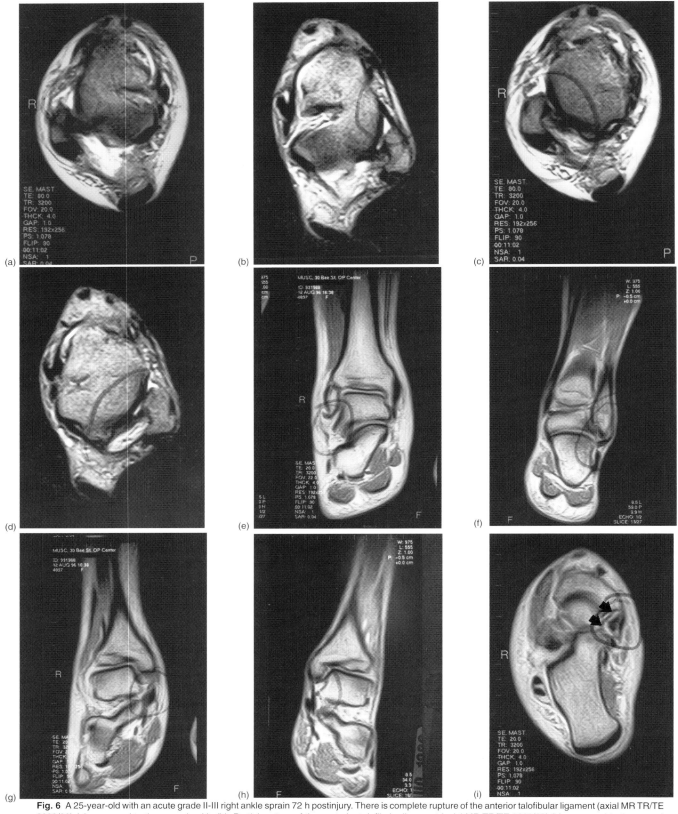

Fig. 6 A 25-year-old with an acute grade II-III right ankle sprain 72 h postinjury. There is complete rupture of the anterior talofibular ligament (axial MR TR/TE 3200/80) (a) compared to the normal ankle (b). Partial rupture of the posterior talofibular ligament (axial MR TR/TE 3200/80) (c) compared to the normal ankle (d). Complete rupture of the calcaneofibular ligament (coronal TR/TE 3200/20) (e) compared to the normal ankle (f). Rupture of the deltoid ligament (coronal TR/TE 3200/20) (g) compared to the normal ankle (h). (i) The spring ligament (calcaneonavicular ligament; axial TR/TE 3200–20) remains intact with this sprain.

5. Meniscoid lesion

Soft-tissue entrapment occurs as a sequelae to acute ankle sprain. Either a synovial fold and/or a piece of the torn anterior talofibular ligament becomes fixed in position and impinges between the lateral malleolus and the lateral talus.[67,68]

6. Anterior capsular impingement

Capsular ligamentous tissue can become shaggy and be caught or impinged at the anterior ankle joint. Arthroscopic removal may be necessary and is successful.

Items 3 to 6 are entities overlapping in aetiology and regional anatomy. Both the arthroscope and MRI have enabled categorization of these lesions. More aggressive and universal functional treatment of acute ankle sprains, particularly recurrent acute ankle sprains, may have increased their incidence.

7. Os calcis anterior process fracture with avulsion of the bifurcate ligament ('beak fracture')

Inversion and internal rotation can cause this injury. Radiography confirms the fracture. Rocking the hindfoot in the medial lateral plane with signs of local tenderness should call attention to the possibility of this diagnosis.

8. Compression fracture of the anterior calcaneal articular facet

Local tenderness and computed tomography (**CT**), MRI, or polytomography may be necessary to detail this injury.

9. Common peroneal nerve injury,[42,69] superficial peroneal nerve, or sural nerve injury

Stretch neuropraxia occurs prior to rupture of the epineurium since connective tissue is strong and will stretch. However, myelin and axoplasm have only a 6 per cent elongation before neuropraxia/axonotmesis occur.[69] Sensory hypoaesthesia or hyperaesthesia in the involved sensory distribution is usually present. Late reflex dystrophy and slow proprioceptive return can accompany this injury.

10. Talar dome fractures (transchondral or osteochondral)[70]

Initial radiographs may appear negative. Repeat radiographs or MRI are often necessary for diagnosis. Osteochondritic lesions can create diagnostic confusion.

11. Lateral talar process fracture with or without lateral talocalcaneal ligament injury[71,72]

This is a common injury seen on the anteroposterior ankle radiographs. The size of the avulsed fragment is variable. The fracture line is vertical. Closed treatment is used.

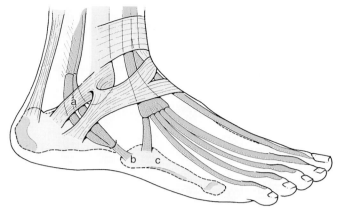

Fig. 7 Tears of the lateral retinaculum and tears of the peroneal tenosynovium occur with CFL tears. This allows tenography and arthrography to help with differential diagnosis (a). The fifth metatarsal is often fractured with supination inversion injuries. The avulsion fractures of the base of the fifth metatarsal (b) or fractures of the proximal diaphysis (c) can occur with or without ankle sprain.

12. Posterior impingement, posterior lateral process fracture (tubercle fracture) or os trigonum fracture/separation[72,73]

This area has the most variable anatomy in the hindfoot. Close radiographic examination and occasional CT or linear tomography scan plus the clinical picture is necessary for diagnosis (Fig. 6(a)(b)).

13. Tibiotalar ligament posteromedial process avulsion

This talar fracture is much less common than a posterolateral process injury. Bilateral CT scanning may be necessary for accurate diagnosis.

14. Peroneal tendon subluxation

Usually radiographs will show a small bone chip. Eversion and dorsiflexion allow the tendon attachment to the fibula to separate, often with a vertical fleck of periosteum and bone. Immobilization for 3 weeks can obviate recurrent subluxation and the need for early or late lateral repair and/or bony buttress.

15. Fracture of the base of 5th metatarsal (Fig. 7)

Avulsion fractures or more distal fractures at the proximal diaphysis can easily be seen on both anteroposterior lateral and oblique views of the foot. However, clinical tenderness without verification by radiography often occurs with an acute or stress fracture. This clinical picture warrants radiographic re-examination in 10 to 14 days. Even with minimal late symptoms there can be delayed or nonunion of the unrecognized fracture. A high index of suspicion is necessary.

16. Inferior tibiofibular ligament injury[62,74]

This is an adult injury that occurs with or without associated bony injury.

17. Interosseous ligament injury (syndesmotic sprain)[75][78]

The anterior tibiofibular ligament is often torn with a grade II ankle sprain. When a grade IV sprain occurs with forced dorsiflexion and external rotation the posterior tibiofibular ligament injury together with interosseous injury can occur. High fibula tenderness suggests an associated 'Maissoneuve' fracture. Mortise views (20 degrees internal rotation oblique) can confirm widening. Surgery with a transmortise syndesmotic screw may be necessary. These injuries are only seen in 1 to 2 per cent of all ankle sprains.

18. Stress fracture of the ankle or hindfoot (Fig. 7(c))

There will have been symptoms prior to the injury. A good history, and a high index of suspicion, is necessary to recognize this repetitive stress problem at presentation.

19. Distal fibula epiphyseal injury in children (Fig. 7(a))[34]

Local anterior and posterior physeal area tenderness make this a potential diagnosis even when radiographs are negative. Many adolescents with major 'sprains' will present with a type I or type II Salter–Harris epiphyseal plate injury rather than the ligamentous injury characteristic of the mature skeleton.[79]

20. Stenosing peroneal tenosynovitis (Fig. 7)[80]

Tenosynovial post-traumatic fracture scarring and inflammation occasionally requires tenosynovectomy.

21. Avulsion fracture of the lateral malleolus (Fig. 7)[81]

An anterior talofibular ligament tear can avulse an anterior lateral chip of fibula bone. A substantial 4 to 6 mm fragment can be avulsed at the fibular attachment of the calcaneofibular ligament.

22. Fracture of the lateral malleolus (Fig. 7)[48]

This injury, which is common, may require surgical intervention.

Treatment

General principles

Ideal treatment for the acute ankle sprain has evolved and is still evolving.[43,82] The pneumatic compression brace and other orthoses (Figs 8(a), (b))[83–86] are successful with early protected mobilization[87] and promote less post-traumatic atrophy and stiffness.[88,89] Thus, a quicker, more efficient, and competent return to sports is achieved. It is apparent that an early, intense postinjury programme can avoid a longer, later, more formal and usually more expensive rehabilitation programme.[49,90] This ideal treatment cannot be achieved in all patients. For some, immobilization, namely in a short-leg cast, permits the patient to remain in the workplace and can be considered appropriate treatment in many cases. Thus, treat-

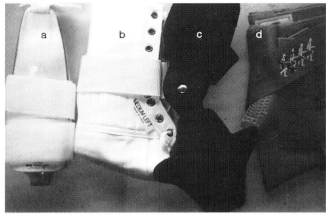

Fig. 8 Ankle braces and supports of many types can be helpful. The pneumatic compression brace (a) is a cornerstone of the functional treatment of ankle sprain. The variably flexible (with or without lateral firm buttresses) lace brace (b) competes with taping for late postinjury protection and prevention. The hinge brace (c) is used less often, but is appropriate for protection even though inversion/eversion mobility is more rigidly controlled than with the other braces. Elastic braces (d) of several types provide less rigid and more dynamic support. (From ref. 64; reprinted by permission of WB Saunders Co.)

ment for the employed person with a routine ankle sprain can differ considerably from that for an élite or lower level competitive athlete participating at a high school, college, professional or even 'mid career' level. The earlier, more aggressive programme for the athlete requires more initial resources, namely additional time, a facilitating environment, trainer/therapy personnel, etc. This early, aggressive, and time-intensive treatment/rehabilitation results in prompt weight bearing, quicker strength regain, earlier return to competition, and reduced later treatment requirements.[32,87,90–92] Early mobilization with this functional treatment must be accompanied by protective ankle support (Fig. 8(c)).[64,90,93,94] Full rehabilitation may take as long as 20 weeks.[7,95]

From Broström's experience in 1976 when all but 3 per cent of acutely operated ankle sprains became normal, there had been a trend towards the primary repair of sprains with proven anterior talofibular ligament and calcaneofibular ligament tears.[96] These observations and the fact that the surgical treatment of acute ankle sprains is successful with minimally increased temporary morbidity is not debated.[37,42,50,97,98] However, there seems to be no concomitant advantage in primary operative repair.[15,51,81,87,99,100–102] The clear trend and sense of the late 1990s is towards non-operative treatment of the sprained ankle. Although there is continuing debate, the aggressive non-operative approach is less expensive and makes surgery unnecessary.[42,45,93,103,104] Even in the series which used a more aggressive non-operative approach, only 12 per cent were surgically repaired.[32]

Certain authors have felt, and still feel, that a grade III sprain with a double-ligament tear needs surgical repair[8,21,45,74,81,89,97,105–107] in selected athletes, namely the highly competitive athlete including the performing artist.[73]

It has been shown that ligamentous tissue is largely retained even with recurrent sprains.[108,109] This fact implies the equally successful results with later reconstruction which have now been verified.[40,42,48] This chronic reconstruction, when coupled with better protective devices, reduces the necessity for primary acute surgery and argues for functional treatment only.[4,37,44,86,103] Surgical repair in children has been reported and can be successful, but in keeping with the current philosophy it is generally unnecessary.[110]

To summarize, current thinking and consensus in the late 1990s is that functional treatment or management is indicated for essentially all grade I, II, and III ankle sprains, with surgery reserved only for isolated highly competitive athletes with proven gross instability/significant subluxation or if there is documented bone or cartilage injury.

A severe eversion grade IV sprain involving the interosseous membrane requires 3 to 6 weeks of cast immobilization. Tibiofibular diastasis, when present and proven radiographically, warrants transtibiofibular fixation in the form of a syndesmotic screw.[44] Heterotopic ossification can occur in up to 50 per cent of interosseous injuries, but does not require surgical excision of the ossification unless frank synostosis is present.[111]

Specific treatment principles

Many algorithms and specific protocols have been suggested.[15,53,112–114] All encourage a systematic approach and are appropriate. By consensus, there are three phases to the treatment and rehabilitation of an acute ankle sprain.

Phase I is cryotherapy with protected range of motion and weight bearing to tolerance. Compression and elevation enhance venous and lymphatic return and help control oedema. A pneumatic-type splint is integral to this early functional treatment (Fig. 8(a)).[84]

Phase II is continuing cryotherapy, isometric strengthening, gradually increasing range of motion, proprioceptive work, and proceeding from full linear stress to early agility work. Phases I and II (disability phases) are estimated to take 8 days for grade I and 15 days for grade II injuries.[115]

Phase III is continued strengthening, including the eccentric mode, flexibility, and proprioceptive work followed by progressive sports-specific return to competitive or full recreational function.

Many modalities are used for the treatment of acute ankle sprains. Ultrasound, ice, and heat delivered in appropriate ways have legitimate therapeutic benefits.[32,116,117] High-voltage pulse stimulation does not enhance ankle sprain treatment.[118] Cryotherapy with ice or an ice substitute[119] is essential for initial care and later rehabilitation. Ice is effective for analgesic purposes.[32] Ice increases the painfree range of motion, decreases muscle fatigue, increases blood flow, and reduces oedema and inflammation. An increase in blood flow to the skin can occur if ice is left on for too long. A significant cooling of the muscle in thin athletes with less than 1 cm of fat occurs within 10 min to a maximum depth of approximately 2 cm into the muscle (or presumably ligament in the case of an ankle sprain). Athletes with more than 2 cm of fat require 20 to 30 min. Cryotherapy (direct and not simple cold application)[119] tends to deliver cold in the range of 3 to 10 °C. Cryokinetics is a combination of ice and exercise. This combination, when coupled with early range of motion and early weight bearing, constitutes functional treatment. Heat should be in the form of contrast baths (alternating with ice) or used alone following ice and elevation.

Non-steroidal anti-inflammatory drugs have a minor treatment role with their mild anti-inflammatory and analgesic properties.[120] Treatment for 1 to 4 days during the acute phase is sufficient.

Rehabilitation of an acute ankle sprain

The aim of postsprain ankle rehabilitation is to restore function and to regain maximum strength in both concentric and eccentric modes.[91,121] The muscles involved are the triceps surae, posterior tibial, peroneal, and anterior tibial. There also needs to be a maximum painfree range of motion and at least 15 degrees of dorsiflexion. This implies that isometry of rehabilitation in the ankle is important just as it is in the knee. The heel cord needs to be supple to permit adequate dorsiflexion, a normal running gait, and to prevent secondary injury. Resolution of any ankle effusion is necessary before rehabilitation is complete.[41]

Proprioception allows the athlete to have a sense of movement and a sense of the position of the ankle (or any part) in space. The importance of proprioception is not adequately understood. Only 2 to 3 per cent of emergency-room physicians and only 25 per cent of orthopaedists have a grasp of, and utilize, the appropriate proprioceptive principles.[15] The necessity for proprioceptive recovery is often ignored in rehabilitation.[72] 'Figure-of-eight' exercises, one-legged stands, tilt boards, and other agility efforts accelerate, promote, and allow testing to define proprioceptive return.[60,95] A full return of flexion can be achieved with such proprioceptive normalizers.[122]

Occasionally an ankle–foot orthosis or even a double upright brace can be used for ambulatory function in working individuals. These selected individuals might need protection postoperatively, or with a major grade III sprain with the need for a prolonged protective range of motion and weight bearing. They are more likely to be recreational athletes without access to aggressive functional treatment who require normal ankle stability during work.

A final note on the athlete's rehabilitation is that he or she should not be allowed to exceed the prescribed protocol. Excessive zeal can be self-defeating and injurious to the athlete, and can even delay return to recreation or competition.

Rehabilitation by any protocol must be systematic and graduated. A functional, optimal progression of a baseball player with a significant grade II–III ankle sprain and a properly supervised and aggressive functional treatment programme might include:

- partial weight bearing at 2 to 5 days;

- full weight bearing at 4 to 7 days;

- walking limp-free slowly at 7 to 10 days;

- linear, slow atraumatic running at 10 to 14 days;

- linear speed work at 14 to 17 days;

- careful cutting, 'figure-of-eight', and lateral moves at half speed at 15 to 21 days;

- agility drills at full speed at 20 to 25 days;

- sport-specific protected practice with sport-specific return near the preinjury level of function at no earlier than 3 weeks.

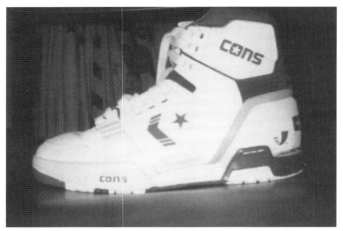

Fig. 9 High-top shoes of an 'off-the-shelf' or specified type can provide additional support. The higher hind uppers coupled, when necessary, with strong heel counters and an in-shoe orthosis provide significant ongoing stability.

Prevention of acute ankle sprains

Training of the ankle is fundamental to injury prevention. Maximum strength is the cornerstone of prevention. This strength can be developed by numerous isometric, concentric, and eccentric methods. Numerous types of equipment are available and range from low-cost to expensive 'high-tech' devices. Benefit will occur with appropriate supervision and programme prescription.

Appropriate footwear enhances stability of the ankle position and facilitates decreased inversion/ankle motion through muscle action. There is some question as to whether the more sophisticated modern athletic shoe increases or in some way masks or absorbs some of the required proprioceptive sensations. High-top shoes (Fig. 9) help reduce inversion ankle injuries.[7] There seems to be no difference in protection between standard high-top shoes, such as modified basketball shoes, and standard lightweight infantry boots.[6] Semirigid custom-made orthoses can assist in an aggressive rehabilitation and prevention programme (Fig. 10). Ankle/foot semirigid orthoses provide increased functional stability input by preloading the ankle and its articular surfaces.[123] Rigid orthoses are rarely indicated.

Ankle taping is generally positive. Elastic ankle guards are of no significant help.[102] The disadvantages of taping are that it decreases performance for certain high-level sports participants, encourages disuse and decreased strength of the ankle-supporting musculature, and decreases subtalar joint motion. Taping, although better than certain 'ankle guards', quickly becomes ineffective[23,124] and is also expensive.[125] In addition, it theoretically preloads other joints, namely the forefoot, and predisposes to turf toe and metatarsalgia.[126] Semirigid ankle orthoses (stirrup type) seem selectively to reduce the incidence of recurrent sprain.[127] There are a number of studies comparing laced ankle stabilizers to taping, etc.[124] Low-topped shoes and laced ankle stabilizers were found to be best in one study.[58] Others[128] found taping better, with 30 to 50 per cent decreased range of motion but loss of effectiveness at 1 h.[99] Neither causes significant interference with performance, although vertical jump and sprinting are measurably altered.[113]

Functional stability and dynamic postural control are critical (ankle disc coordination training) and must not be subordinated to

mechanical support such as orthoses.[129] The latter is supplemental and mainly temporary. Both have a place in the overall treatment programme.

Ankles with previous sprains are twice as likely to be sprained as an ankle with no prior ankle sprain history.[6] Preventive taping or laced stabilizers are recommended particularly in high-risk athletes, for instance soccer players. Recurrent sprains induce an inversion lever. Since relatively weak peroneals allow the heel to plant in mild varus,[80] a protective orthosis as well as a full strength training and agility programme is necessary to prevent an acute sprain in an ankle with a previous sprain.

Mechanical instability can be measured and predisposes to recurrent sprains. Functional instability also causes acute recurrent sprain and is less easily measured. Proprioceptive defects cause this functional instability, and involve prolonged muscular reaction time, weakness, and measurable agility deficit. Although Isakov *et al.*[130] found a normal muscle reaction time with recurrent sprain, subsequent research suggests there is a deficit. Karlson reported

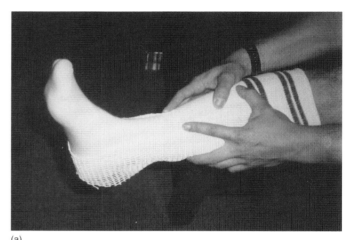

(a)

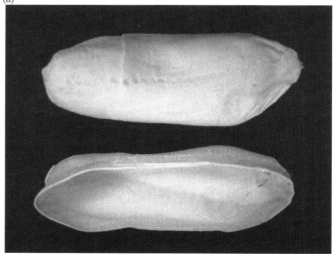

(b)

Fig. 10 (a) Individually customized 'in-house' but easily fabricated and cheap, orthoplast semirigid supports provide excellent and early protection and support. (b) Customized semirigid foot orthoses made from plaster moulds are often indicated postrehabilitation, namely with forefoot valgus and medial post, to help prevent recurrent inversion sprain of the ankle.

prolonged muscle reaction times with mechanical instability. Konradsen and Ravn[131] found similar deficits with functional instability regardless of mechanical instability. Lynch *et al.*[132] found a decreased muscle reaction time (loss of protective reflex) with 20 degrees of plantar flexion compared to neutral.

Fridén *et al.*[133] used stabilometry techniques which suggest significant postsprain agility improvement with functional treatment and a pneumatic brace. Leanderson *et al.*[134,135] noted similar, postural postsprain deficits which improved with coordination, strengthening, and balance board activities.

Prevention of both acute ankle sprain and acute recurrent ankle sprain depends on inherent anatomical stability, strength of supporting muscle groups, muscle reaction time, and additional orthotic and footwear support.

Fatigue after activities as well as simple 'lack of sleep' fatigue can cause local predisposition to sprain. Logical sleep habits adequately meeting individual sleep requirements are desirable.

Since higher values of $W + H^2$, where W is weight and H is height, causes higher lateral ankle sprain morbidity, a normal weight is both desirable and preventive.[6]

Conclusions

The acute ankle sprain is treated by a wide range of medical personnel who deal with recreational and competitive athletic injuries. Many associated and secondary injuries are often unrecognized. Much of the morbidity of pain, instability, and impaired performance are due to untreated, or inadequately treated, ankle sprains.

All practitioners involved in treating sports injuries should have, or should develop, a reasonable protocol for the severe ankle sprain. This protocol includes early diagnosis, aggressive protected and ongoing weight bearing, and functional treatment. This should be done by the patient at home or in a formal physical-therapy setting. Although functional treatment is generally indicated, surgery may be necessary for selected élite athletes and performers.

There should be a clear and conclusive termination point for rehabilitation, at which time the sports can be safely resumed.

With the above points in mind, the ankle is a reasonably forgiving joint: (1) if the appropriate diagnosis is made;[65,101] (2) if treatment is not necessarily shortened or compromised; (3) if adequate rehabilitation is required before return to competition or full use; and (4) if continued protection is used, if indicated. Acute ankle sprain maintains its importance in sports medicine. Continued and increased recognition of the importance of acute ankle sprain is central to proper prevention, diagnosis, treatment, and rehabilitation.

References

1. Henry JH, Lareau B, Neigut D. The injury rate in professional football. *American Journal of Sports Medicine* 1982; **10**: 16–18.
2. Colliander E, Eriksson E, Herkel M, Sköld P. Injuries in Swedish elite basketball. *Orthopedics* 1986; **9**: 225–7.
3. Zelisko AJ, Noble HB, Porter M. A comparison of men's and women's professional basketball injuries. *American Journal of Sports Medicine* 1982; **10**: 297–9.
4. Kannus P, Renström P. Treatment for acute tears of the lateral ligaments of the ankle. *Journal of Bone and Joint Surgery* 1991; **73-A**: 305–23.
5. Garrick JG. The frequency of injury, mechanism of injury, and epidemiology of ankle sprains. *American Journal of Sports Medicine* 1977; **5**: 241–2.
6. Milgrom C, *et al.* Risk factors for lateral ankle sprain: a prospective study among military recruits. *Foot and Ankle* 1991; **12**: 26–30.
7. DeHaven KE, Allman FL, Cos JS, Fowler PJ, Henning CE. Symposium: ankle sprains in athletes. *Contemporary Orthopaedics* 1979; **Feb.**: 56–78.
8. Boruta PM, Bishop JO, Braly WG, Tullos HS. Acute lateral ankle ligament injuries: A literature review. *Foot and Ankle* 1990; **11**: 107–13.
9. Calliet R. *Injuries to the ankle. Foot and ankle pain.* Philadelphia: FA Davis Company, 1968: 117–25.
10. Holbrook TL, *et al.* The frequency of occurrence, impact and cost of selected musculoskeletal conditions in the United States. *American Academy of Orthopaedic Surgeons* 1984, 101.
11. Garrick JG, Requa RU. Epidemiology of foot and ankle injuries in sports. *Clinical Sports Medicine* 1988; **7**: 29–36.
12. Ekstrand J, Tropp H. The incidence of ankle sprains in soccer. *Foot and Ankle* 1990; **11**: 41–4.
13. Schmidt-Olsen S, Jørgensen U, Kaalund S, Sørensen J. Injuries among young soccer players. *American Journal of Sports Medicine* 1991; **19**: 273–5.
14. Yeung MS, Chan K-M, So CH, Yuan WY. An epidemiological survey on ankle sprain. *British Journal of Sports Medicine* 1994; **28**: 112–16.
15. Kay DB. The sprained ankle: current therapy. *Foot and Ankle* 1985; **6**: 22–8.
16. Ekstrand J, Gilquist J. Soccer injuries and their mechanisms: a prospective study. *Medicine and Science in Sports and Exercise* 1983; **15**: 267–70.
17. Bahr R, Karlsen R, Øystein L. Incidence and mechanisms of acute ankle inversion injuries in volleyball. A retrospective cohort study. *American Journal of Sports Medicine* 1994; **22**: 595–600.
18. Kelikian H, Kelikian AS. *Disruption of the fibular collateral ligament. Disorders of the ankle.* Philadelphia: WB Saunders, 1988: 437–95.
19. Attarian DE, DeVito DP, Garrett W Jr. A biomechanical study of human ankle ligaments and autogenous reconstructive grafts. *Surgical Rounds for Orthopaedics* 1987; **April**: 24–7.
20. Leonard MH. Injuries of the lateral ligaments of the ankle. A clinical and experimental study. *Journal of Bone and Joint Surgery* 1949; **31-A**: 373–7.
21. Anderson ME. Reconstruction of the lateral ligaments of the ankle using the plantaris tendon. *Journal of Bone and Joint Surgery* 1985; **67-A**: 930–4.
22. Lindsjö U, Danckwardt-Lillieström G, Sahlstedt B. Measurement of the motion range in the loaded ankle. *Clinical Orthopaedics and Related Research* 1985; **Oct.**: 68–71.
23. Sammarco J. Biomechanics of the ankle. I. Surface velocity and instant center of rotation in the sagittal plane. *American Journal of Sports Medicine* 1977; **5**: 231–4.
24. Lundberg A, Goldie I, Kalin B, Selvik G. Kinematics of the ankle/foot complex: plantarflexion and dorsiflexion. *Foot and Ankle* 1989; **9**: 194–200.
25. McCullough CJ, Burge PD. Rotatory stability of the load-bearing ankle. *Journal of Bone and Joint Surgery* 1980; **62-B**: 460–4.
26. Shoji H, Ambrosia RD, Parlaska R. Biomechanics of the ankle. II. Horizontal rotation and ligamentous injury states. *American Journal of Sports Medicine* 1977; **5**: 235–7.
27. Stormont DM, Morrey BF, An KN, Cass JR. Stability of the loaded ankle. Relation between articular restraint and primary and secondary static restraints. *American Journal of Sports Medicine* 1985; **85**: 295–300.
28. Burgess PR, Wei JY, Clark FJ, Simon J. Signaling of kinesthetic information by peripheral sensory receptors. *Annual Review of Neuroscience* 1982; **5**: 171–87.

29. Bulucu C, Thomas KA, Halvorson TL, Cook SD. Biomechanical evaluation of the anterior drawer test: the contribution of the lateral ankle ligaments. *Foot and Ankle* 1991; **11**: 389–93.

30. Nigg BM, Skarvan G, French CB, Yeadon MR. Elongation and forces of ankle ligaments in a physiological range of motion. *Foot and Ankle* 1990; **11**: 30–40.

31. Dias LS. The lateral ankle sprain: an experimental study. *Journal of Trauma* 1979; **19**: 266–9.

32. Cox JS. Surgical and nonsurgical treatment of acute ankle sprains. *Clinical Orthopaedics* 1985; **188**: 88–96.

33. Ogden JA. *Skeletal injury in the child*. Philadelphia: WB Saunders, 1990: 853–6.

34. Whitelaw GP, Sawka MW, Wetzler M, Segal D, Miller J. Unrecognized injuries of the lateral ligaments associated with lateral malleolar fractures of the ankle. *Journal of Bone and Joint Surgery* 1989; **71-A**: 1396–9.

35. van Dijk CN. *On diagnostic strategies in patients with severe ankle sprain*. Amsterdam: Rodopi, 1994.

36. Hopkinson WJ, St Pierre P, Ryan JB. Syndesmosis sprains of the ankle. *Foot and Ankle* 1990; **10**: 325–30.

37. Henry JH. Lateral ligament tears of ankle. One to six years follow-up study of 202 ankles. *Orthopaedic Review* 1983; **XII**: 31–9.

38. Auletta AG, Conway WF, Hayes CW, Guisto DF, Gervin AS. Indications for radiography in patients with acute ankle injuries: role of the physical examination. *American Journal of Radiology* 1991; **157**: 789–91.

39. Anonymous. X-rays under pressure reveal hidden injury to ankle. *Medical World News* 1967; **Oct.**: 50–1.

40. Brand RL, Collins MF, Templeton T. Surgical repair of ruptured lateral ankle ligaments. *American Journal of Sports Medicine* 1981; **9**: 40–4.

41. Petrik J, Amendola A, Rampersaud R, *et al.* The effects of an isolated ankle effusion on H-reflex amplitude, viscoelasticity and postural control of the ankle. *Meeting of American Orthopaedic Society for Sports Medicine*, Feb. 25 1996, Atlanta.

42. Rijke AM, Jones B, Vierhout PA. Injury to the lateral ankle ligaments of athletes. *American Journal of Sports Medicine* 1988; **16**: 256–9.

43. Staples OS. Ruptures of the fibular collateral ligaments of the ankle. *Journal of Bone and Joint Surgery* 1975; **67-A**: 101–7.

44. Bergfeld JA, Cox JS, Drez D Jr, Raemy H, Weiker GG. Symposium: management of acute ankle sprains. *Contemporary Orthopaedics* 1986; **13**: 83–116.

45. Rijke AM. Lateral ankle sprains. Graded stress radiography for accurate diagnosis. *The Physician and Sportsmedicine* 1991; **19**: 107–18.

46. Ehrensperger J. Arthrography of the ankle joint in injuries of the fibular ligament system in children and adolescents. *Zeitschrift für Kinderchirurgie* 1985; **40**: 71–5.

47. Bleichrodt RP, Kingma LM, Binnendijk LM, Klein JP. Injuries of the lateral ankle ligaments: classification with tenography and arthrography. *Radiology* 1989; **173**: 347–9.

48. Lassiter TE, Malone TR, Garrett WE Jr. Injury to the lateral ligaments of the ankle. *Orthopedic Clinics of North America* 1980; **20**: 629–40.

49. Drez D, Young JC, Waldman D, Shackleton R, Parker W. Non-operative treatment of double lateral ligament tears of the ankle. *American Journal of Sports Medicine* 1982; **10**: 197–200.

50. Ruth CJ. The surgical treatment of injuries of the fibular collateral ligaments of the ankle. *Journal of Bone and Joint Surgery* 1961; **43-A**: 229–39.

51. Evans GA, Hardcastle P, Frenyo AD. Acute rupture of the lateral ligament of the ankle. *Journal of Bone and Joint Surgery* 1984; **66-B**: 209–12.

52. Evans GA, Frenyo SD. The stress-tenogram in the diagnosis of ruptures of the lateral ligament of the ankle. *Journal of Bone and Joint Surgery* 1979; **61-B**: 347–51.

53. Edelman B. MRI plus clinical exam most sensitive to chronic pain after ankle sprain. *Orthopedics Today* 1991; **11**: 14–15.

54. Jahss MH. *Disorders of the foot and ankle*. Volume III, 2nd edn. Philadelphia: WB Saunders, 1991: 2408–10.

55. Trevino SG, Davis P, Hecht PJ. Management of acute and chronic lateral ligament injuries of the ankle. *Foot and Ankle Injuries in Sports* 1994; **25**: 1–16.

56. Davis, P, Trevino SG. Ankle Injuries. In: Baxter DE, ed. *The foot and ankle in sport*. Chicago: Mosby, 1994: 147–69.

57. Moseley JB, Chimenti BT. Foot and ankle injuries in the professional athlete. In: Baxter DE, ed. *The foot and ankle in sport*. Chicago: Mosby, 1994: 321–7.

58. Rovere GD, Clarke TJ, Yates CS, Burley K. Retrospective comparison of taping and ankle stabilizers in preventing ankle injuries. *American Journal of Sports Medicine* 1988; **16**: 228–33.

59. Hamilton WG. Foot and ankle injuries in dancers. *Clinics in Sports Medicine* 1988; **7**: 143–73.

60. Ryan AJ, Cox JS, Inniss B, Rice LE, Woodward EP. Round table discussion: ankle sprains. *The Physician and Sportsmedicine* 1986; **14**: 101–18.

61. Roberts CS, DeMaio M, Larkin JJ, Paine R. Eversion ankle sprains. *Sports Medicine Rehabilitation Series* 1995; **18**: 299–304.

62. Colville MR, Marder RA, Boyle JJ, Zarins B. Isolated injury of the distal tibiofibular ligaments: a clinical and experimental report. *American Journal of Sports Medicine*, 1990; **118**: 196–200.

63. White J. Rare open ankle sprain sidelines Weiss. *The Physician and Sportsmedicine* 1991; **19**: 47–8.

64. McBryde AM. Disorders of the ankle and foot. In: Grana WA, Kalenak A, eds. *Clinical sports medicine*. Philadelphia: WB Saunders, 1991: 466–89.

65. Grana WA. Chronic pain persisting after ankle sprain. *Journal of Musculoskeletal Medicine* 1990; **June**: 35–49.

66. Meyer JM, Garcia J, Hoffmeyer P, Fritschy D. The subtalar sprain. A roentgenographic study. *Clinical Orthopaedics and Related Research* 1988; **Jan.**: 169–73.

67. McCarroll JR, Schrader JW, Shelbourne KD, Rettig AC, Bisesi MA. Meniscoid lesions of the ankle in soccer players. *American Journal of Sports Medicine* 1987; **15**: 255–7.

68. Bassett FH, Gates HS, Billys JB, Morris HB, Nikolaou PK. Talar impingement by the anterior–inferior tibiofibular ligament. *Journal of Bone and Joint Surgery* 1990; **72-A**: 55–9.

69. Nitz AJ, Dobner JJ, Kersey D. Nerve injury and grades II and III ankle sprains. *American Journal of Sports Medicine* 1985; **13**: 177–82.

70. Alexander AH, Barrack RL. Arthroscopic technique in talar dome fractures. *Surgical Rounds for Orthopaedics* 1990; **Jan.**: 27–35.

71. Amis JA, Gangl PM, Graham CE. Inversion ankle injuries: an accurate diagnosis requires a high level of suspicion. Poster presentation to the *Annual meeting of the American Association of Orthopaedic Surgeons*, Cincinnati, 1991.

72. Arendt E. Inversion injuries to the ankle. *Surgical Rounds for Orthopaedics* 1989; **June**: 15–22.

73. Bergfeld JA, Fu F, Garrick J, Hamilton W, Weiker G. Musculoskeletal problems of dance and gymnastics. Presented at *The annual symposium of the American Orthopaedic Society for Sports Medicine*, Palm Springs, 1988.

74. McMaster JH. Tibiofibular synostosis: a cause of ankle disability. *Journal of Bone and Joint Surgery* 1975; **S7-A**: 1035.

75. Marymount JV, Lynch MA, Henning CE. Acute ligamentous diastasis of the ankle without fracture. Evaluation of radionuclide imaging. *American Journal of Sports Medicine* 1986; **14**: 407–9.

76. Lieber L, Gross M. Frank ligamentous diastasis of the ankle. *Orthopaedic Grand Rounds* 1985; **2**: 10–15.

77. Manderson EL. The uncommon sprain. Ligamentous diastasis of

the ankle without fracture or bony deformity. *Orthopaedic Review* 1986; **XV**: 77–81.

78. Hopkinson WJ, St Pierre P, Ryan JF, Wheeler JH. Syndesmosis sprains of the ankle. *Foot and Ankle* 1990; **10**: 325–30.

79. Letts RM. The hidden adolescent ankle fracture. *Journal of Pediatric Orthopedics* 1982; **2**: 161–4.

80. Andersen E. Stenosing peroneal tenosynovitis symptomatically simulating ankle instability. *American Journal of Sports Medicine* 1987; **15**: 258–9.

81. Brand RL. Operative management of ligamentous injuries. In: Torg JS, Welsh RP, Shephard RJ, eds. *Current therapy in sports medicine*, Vol. 2. Toronto: BC Decker, 1990: 239–41.

82. Moseley HF. Traumatic disorders of the ankle and foot. In: Walton JH, ed. *Clinical symposia*. Summit, NJ: Ciba Pharmaceutical, 1965; **17**: 3–30.

83. Carne P. Nonsurgical treatment of ankle sprains using the modified Sarmiento brace. *American Journal of Sports Medicine* 1989; **17**: 256–7.

84. Kimura IF, Nawoczenski DA, Epler M, Owen MG. Effect of the AirStirrup in controlling ankle inversion stress. *Journal of Orthopaedic and Sports Physical Therapy* 1987; **8**: 190–3.

85. Lane SE. Severe ankle sprains. Treatment with ankle–foot orthosis. *The Physician and Sportsmedicine* 1990: **18**: 43–51.

86. Fritschy D, Junet C, Bonvin JC. Functional treatment of severe ankle sprain. *Journal de Traumatologie du Sport* 1987: **4**: 131–6.

87. Konradsen L, Holmer P, Sondergaard L. Early mobilizing treatment for grade III ankle ligament injuries. *Foot and Ankle* 1991; **12**: 69–73.

88. Neumann H, O'Shea P, Nielson J, Climstein M. A physiological comparison of the short-leg walking cast and an ankle–foot orthosis walker following six weeks of immobilization. *Orthopedics* 1989; **12**: 1429–34.

89. Baxter DE. Traumatic injuries to the soft tissues of the foot and ankle. In: Mann R, ed. *Surgery of the foot*, 5th edn. St Louis: Mosby, 1986: 456–501.

90. van den Hoogenband CR, van Moppes FI, Coumans PF, Stapert JWJL, Geep JM. Study on clinical diagnosis and treatment of lateral ligament lesion of the ankle joint: a prospective clinical randomized trial. *International Journal of Sports Medicine* 1984; **5** (Suppl.): 159–61.

91. Rettig AC, Kraft DE. Treat ankle sprains fast-it pays. *Your Patient and Fitness* 1991; **4**: 6–9.

92. Renström P, Kannus P. Management of ankle sprains. *Operative Techniques in Sports Medicine* 1994; **2**: 1–12.

93. Linde F, Hvass I, Jürgensen U, Madsen F. Early mobilizing treatment in lateral ankle sprains: course and risk factors for chronic painful or function-limiting ankle. *Scandinavian Journal of Rehabilitation Medicine* 1986; **18**: 17–21.

94. Raemy H, Jakob RP. Functional treatment of fresh tibular ligament lesions using the aircast splint. *Swiss Journal of Sports Medicine* 1983; **31**: 1–5.

95. Vegso JJ. Non-operative management of ankle injuries. In: Torg JS, Welsh RP, Shephard RJ, eds. *Current therapies in sports medicine-2*. Toronto: BC Decker, 1990: 234–9.

96. Prins JG. Diagnosis and treatment of injury to the lateral ligament of the ankle. *Acta Chirurgica Scandinavica* 1978; **Suppl. 486**: 1–152.

97. Korkala O, Rusanen M, Jokipii P, Kytömaa J, Avikainen V. A prospective study of the treatment of severe tears of the lateral ligament of the ankle. *International Orthopaedics* 1987; **11**: 13–17.

98. Jaskulka R, Fischer G, Schedl R. Injuries of the lateral ligaments of the ankle joint. Operative treatment and long-term results. *Archives of Orthopaedic and Traumatic Surgery* 1988; **107**: 217–21.

99. Myburgh KH, Vaughan CL, Isaacs SK. The effects of ankle guards and taping on joint motion before, during and after a squash match. *American Journal of Sports Medicine* 1984; **12**: 441–6.

100. Sommer HM, Arza D. Functional treatment of recent ruptures of the fibular ligament of the ankle. *International Orthopaedics* 1988; **13**: 69–73.

101. Bassett FH. The treatment of ankle and foot sports injuries. In: Schneider RC, Kennedy JC, Plant ML, eds. *Sports injuries: mechanisms, prevention and treatment*. Baltimore, MD: Williams and Wilkins, 1985: 788–96.

102. Ciullo JV, Jackson DW. Track and field. In: Schneider RC, Kennedy JC, Plant ML, eds. *Sports injuries: mechanisms, prevention and treatment*. Baltimore, MD: Williams and Wilkins, 1985: 212–46.

103. Renström P. Sports traumatology today. A review of common current sports injury problems. *Annales Chirurgiae et Gynaecologiae* 1991; **80**: 81–93.

104. Schaap GR, deKeizer G, Marti K. Inversion trauma of the ankle. *Archives of Orthopaedic and Trauma Surgery* 1989; **108**: 273–5.

105. Peterson L. Ankle ligament injuries and operative treatment principles. *Annales Chirurgiae et Gynaecologiae* 1991; **80**: 168–76.

106. Leach RE, Schepsi A. Ligamentous injuries. In: Yablon IG, Segal D, Leach RE, eds. *Ankle injuries*. New York: Churchill Livingstone, 1983: 193–230.

107. Cass JR, Morrey BF, Katoh Y, Chao EYS. Ankle instability: comparison of primary repair and delayed reconstruction after long-term follow-up study. *Clinical Orthopaedics* 1985; **198**: 110–17.

108. Broström L, Sundelin P. Sprained ankles. IV. Histologic changes in recent and 'chronic' ligament ruptures. *Acta Chirurgica Scandinavica* 1966; **132**: 248–53.

109. Gould N, Seligson D, Gassman J. Early and late repair of lateral ligament of the ankle. *Foot and Ankle* 1980; **1**: 84–9.

110. Vahvanen V, Westerlund M, Kajanti M. Sprained ankle in children. A clinical follow-up study of 90 children treated conservatively and by surgery. *Annales Chirurgiae et Gynaecologiae* 1983; **72**: 71–5.

111. Speir KP, Warren RF, Wall DJ. Update on football injuries. *Mediguide to Orthopaedics* 1991; **10**: 1–6.

112. Larkin J, Brage M. Ankle, hindfoot and midfoot injuries. In: Reider B, ed. *Sports medicine. The school-age athlete*. Philadelphia: WB Saunders, 1991: 365–79.

113. Brage ME. Ankle, hindfoot and midfoot injuries. In: Reider B, ed. *Sports medicine: the school-age athlete*, 2nd edn. Philadelphia: WB Saunders Company, 1996: 403.

114. Litt JCB. The sprained ankle: diagnosis and management of lateral ligament injuries. *Australian Physician* 1992; **32**: 447–56.

115. Jackson DW, Ashley RL, Powell JW. Ankle sprains in young athletes. Relation of severity and disability. *Clinical Orthopaedics* 1974; **101**: 201–15.

116. Lehman JE. *Therapeutic heat and cold rehabilitation*, 3rd edn. Baltimore, MD: Williams and Wilkins, 1982.

117. Halvorson GA. Therapeutic heat and cold for athletic injuries. *The Physician and Sportsmedicine* 1990; **18**: 87–94.

118. Michlovitz S, Smith W, Watkins M. Ice and high voltage pulsed stimulation in treatment of acute lateral ankle sprains. *Journal of Orthopaedic and Sports Physical Therapy* 1988; **9**: 301–4.

119. Hocutt JR, Jaffe R, Rylander CR, Beebe JK. Cryotherapy in ankle sprains. *American Journal of Sports Medicine* 1982; **10**: 316–19.

120. Fredberg U, Hansen PA, Skinhøj A. Ibuprofen in the treatment of acute ankle joint injuries. *American Journal of Sports Medicine* 1989; **17**: 564–6.

121. Hunter S. Rehabilitation of ankle injuries. In: Prentice WE, ed. *Rehabilitation techniques in sports medicine*. St Louis: Times Mirror/Mosby, 1990: 331–8.

122. Garrick JG. A practical approach to rehabilitation illustrated by treatment of ankle injury. *American Journal of Sports Medicine* 1987; **15**: 258–9.

123. Thonnard JL, Bragard D, Willems PA, Plaghki L. Stability of the braced ankle: a biomechanical investigation. *American Journal of Sports Medicine* 1996; **24**: 356–61.

124. Bunch RP, Bednarski K, Holland D, Macinati R. Ankle joint support: a comparison of reusable lace-on braces with taping and wrapping. *The Physician and Sportsmedicine* 1985; **13**: 59–62.

125. Burks RT, Bean BG, Marcus R, Barker H. Analysis of athletic performance with prophylactic ankle devices. *American Journal of Sports Medicine* 1991; **19**: 104–6.

126. Carmines DV, Nunley JA, McElhancy JH. Effects of ankle taping on the motion and loading pattern of the foot for walking subjects. *Journal of Orthopaedic Research* 1988; **6**: 223–9.

127. Surve I, Schwellnus MP, Noakes T, Lombard C. A fivefold reduction in the incidence of recurrent ankle sprains in soccer players using the sport-stirrup orthosis. *American Journal of Sports Medicine* 1994; **22**: 601–6.

128. Garrick JG, Requa R. Role of external support in the prevention of ankle sprains. *Medicine and Science in Sports* 1973; **5**: 200–3.

129. Tropp H, Askling C, Gillquist J. Prevention of ankle sprains. *American Journal of Sports Medicine* 1985; **13**: 259–62.

130. Isakov E, Mizrahi, J, Solzi P, Susak Z, Lotem M. Response of the peroneal muscles to sudden inversion of the ankle during standing. *International Journal of Sport Biomechanics* 1986; **2**: 100–9.

131. Konradsen L, Ravn JB. Prolonged peroneal reaction time in ankle instability. *International Journal of Sports Medicine* 1991; **122**: 290–2.

132. Lynch SA, Eklund U, Gottlieb D, Renstrom AFH, Beynnon B. Electromyographic latency changes in the ankle musculature during inversion movements. *American Journal of Sports Medicine* 1996; **24**: 362–9.

133. Fridén T, Zätterström R, Lindstrand A, Moritz U. A stabilometric technique for evaluation of lower limb instabilities. *American Journal of Sports Medicine* 1989; **17**: 118–22.

134. Leanderson J, Wykman A, Eriksson E. Ankle sprain and postural sway in basketball players. *Knee Surgery, Sports Traumatology, Arthroscopy* 1993; **1**: 203–5.

135. Leanderson J, Eriksson E, Nilsso C, Wykman A. A prospective study of the influence of an ankle sprain on proprioception in the ankle joint. *American Journal of Sports Medicine* 1996; **24**: 370–4.

4.4.3 Tendon/ligament basic science

*Barry W. Oakes**

Introduction

In musculoskeletal practice it is important to develop clinical skills and to establish an accurate diagnosis with anatomical precision to manage a patient optimally. Management regimes are based on both the previous practical experience of the clinician and of others (based on the world literature) as well as information based on experimentation. Recent basic science and clinical reviews are given in refs 1–7.

This chapter will review briefly recent basic science information in relation to the structure and biomechanics of tendons and liga-

* The assistance of W. Cole and D. Chan (Department of Orthopaedics, Royal Children's Hospital, Melbourne) with the discussion on collagen typing of normal human anterior cruciate ligament and anterior cruciate ligament grafts is gratefully acknowledged as is the help of K. Shino with the discussion of human anterior cruciate ligament allografts

ments as well as discussing mechanisms of injury to ligaments/tendons and their repair response before attempting to relate this to practical patient management. A discussion of the remodelling of human anterior cruciate ligament auto- and allografts as well as goat anterior cruciate ligament–patellar tendon autografts is presented. Also recent data on the repair of the sectioned goat anterior cruciate ligament is presented which demonstrates that the injured anterior cruciate ligament has full healing potential contrary to current surgical opinion.

Ligaments and tendon

Structure and biomechanics of ligaments and tendons

There are subtle differences between ligament and tendon morphology,[8] but for the sake of this discussion they will be treated as very similar tissues. The fibroblasts of mature tendons lie in longitudinal rows and are flat elongated cells squeezed laterally between the collagen fibrils. Recently, McNeilly and colleagues[9] have demonstrated (using confocal microscopy coupled with fluorescent dye cellular labelling techniques) that tendon fibroblasts communicate with one another via an extensive 3-dimensional network of long cell processes and gap junctions between the collagen matrix (see Fig. 1). This new information indicates the possibility of intercellular 'talk' between cells similar to that of osteocytes, and hence these tendon cells may be able to sense and co-ordinate a response to mechanical load or lack of load.

Mature adult ligaments and tendons are composed of large-diameter type I collagen fibrils (150 nm or more in diameter) tightly packed together in a rope-like configuration, with a small amount of

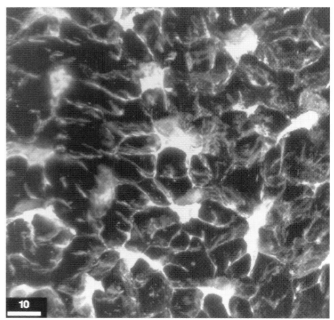

Fig. 1 Confocal microscope image of fluorescent membrane labelled cryosections of a rat digital flexor tendon. The cell bodies are brightly fluorescent and show a network of fluorescent lateral cell processes meeting those of adjacent cells. (Reproduced from ref. 9 with permission and with acknowledgement to Dr Michael Benjamin, University of Cardiff.)

type III collagen dispersed in an aqueous gel containing small amounts of proteoglycan and elastic fibres (Figs 2 and 3). The outstanding feature of both these unique load-bearing tissues is the collagen 'crimp' which is a planar wave pattern found extending in phase across the width of all tendons and ligaments (Fig. 4).[10] This collagen 'crimp' appears to be built into the tertiary stucture of the collagen molecule and is probably maintained *in vivo* by inter- and intramolecular collagen crosslinks as well as a strategically placed elastic fibre network. The 'crimp' may help to attenuate muscle loading forces at the tendoperiosteal junction as well as the musculotendinous junction.

Viidik[1] has recently reviewed the basic biomechanics of ligaments and tendons and the reader is referred to his text for a more

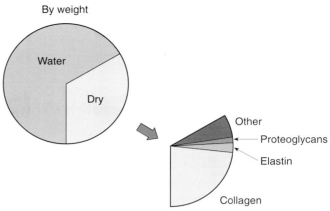

Fig. 3 Approximate dry weight amounts of main tendon/ligament components. Collagen forms the main protein component with smaller amounts of elastin and proteoglycans.

detailed examination of structure–function relationships. The basic function of tendons and ligaments is to transmit force with 'reasonable safety margins'.[1] The longitudinal array of collagen fibrils converts externally applied axial loads to internal lateral compression which results in interfibril friction and heat generation. This heat generation may be responsible for central fibroblast death in thick tendons which has recently been described as exercise-induced hyperthermia.[11] Peak intratendinous core temperatures ranging from 43 to 45 °C have been recorded in racehorse tendons. Temperatures greater than 42.5 °C are known to cause fibroblast death *in vitro*. This is a novel concept, but may gain credibility over time.

Also of interest is the notion that the muscle–tendon unit can act as a spring and the tendon can recoil after being eccentrically stretched, for example during a hopping kangaroo's landing phase. During this landing phase the tendon stretch of the Achilles tendon is stored as elastic energy which is then converted to add extra lift for the animal during the concentric phase of the hop, hence leading to energy conservation.[12,13] Indeed, in the slowly hopping wallaby, strain energy storage in tendons and ligaments accounts for 33 per cent of the negative and positive work that is done whilst the feet are on the ground![14]

Ligament and tendon injury can be closely correlated with the load–deformation (strain) curve.[15,16] This curve can be divided into three regions (Fig. 5).

1. The 'toe' region, or initial concave region, represents the normal physiological range of ligament/tendon strain up to about 3 to 4 per cent of its initial length and is due to the flattening of the collagen 'crimp'. Repeated cycling within this 'toe' region or 'physiological strain range' of 3 to 4 per cent (which may approach 10 per cent in cruciate ligaments due to the intrinsic macrospiral of collagen cruciate fibre bundles) can normally occur without irreversible macroscopic or molecular damage to the tissue.

2. The second part of the load–deformation curve is the linear region, where pathological irreversible ligament/tendon elongation can occur due to partial rupture of intermolecular crosslinks. As the load is increased further, intra- and intermolecular crosslinks are disrupted until macroscopic

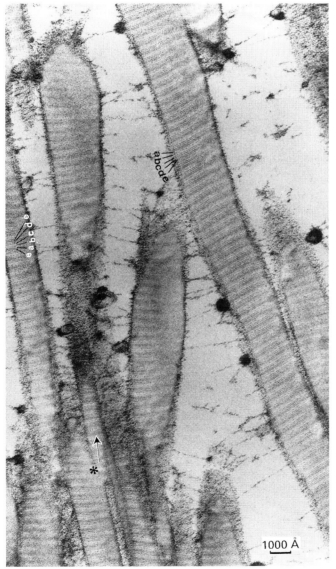

Fig. 2 Adult rat anterior cruciate ligament collagen fixed with Ruthenium red after treatment with elastase at pH 8.8 for 12 h. Typical regular banding periodicity (labelled) and linking filaments, probably hyaluronate, link the fibrils between the c and d bands. The fibre marked with the asterisk appears to be dividing into a smaller fibril. Proteoglycan granules are attached to the fibrils in the region of the c and d bands. 98 000 ×

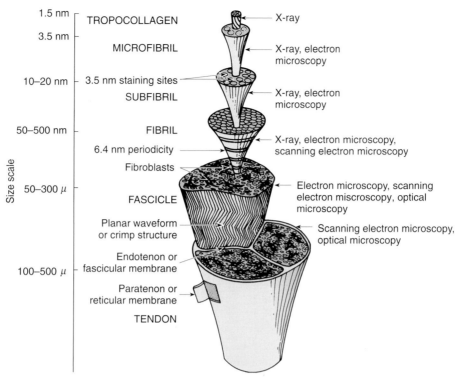

Fig. 4 Structural organization of tendons and ligaments. Note planar 'crimp' seen at the light-microscopic level. (Modified from ref. 18, with permission.)

failure is evident clinically. Electron microscopic studies[17] have shown that the collagen fibrils are elongated in this phase, that the periodicity increases from 67 to 68 nm to

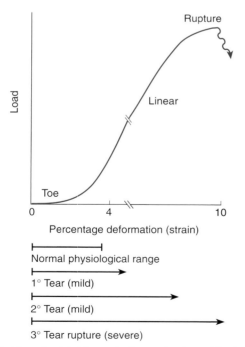

Fig. 5 Load–deformation (strain) curve for ligament/tendon and the clinical correlation with the grading of the injury. The 'toe' region of the curve is entirely within the normal physiological range and that greater than about 4 per cent strain causes tissue damage.

72 nm, and that the banding pattern may become disjointed across the fibrils indicating intrafibril damage by molecular slippage under shear strain.[18] With continued loading into the third region, the banding pattern is completely lost. This suggests that these damaged fibrils can still bear load and may represent a form of work hardening. In mature tendon, ruptured collagen-fibril ends can be observed. Elegant X-ray diffraction and electron microscopic studies coupled with accurate fast- and slow-loading studies of both rat tail and human finger tendons has confirmed that initial damage to the fibril is an intrafibrillar sliding process which occurs only a few milliseconds before macroscopic fibre slippage and failure.[19]

The early part of the linear region corresponds to mild or grade 1 ligament tears (0 to 50 per cent fibre disruption) and the latter part to grade 2 tears (50 to 80 per cent fibre disruption) where there is obvious clinical laxity on stress testing.

There is always some pain associated with grade 1 and 2 injuries after the initial trauma and usually the athlete cannot continue with a grade 2 injury. The severity of the pain is a 'rough' guide to the clinical severity of the injury.

3.   The curve flattens in the third region, and the 'yield' or failure point is reached at 10 to 20 per cent strain dependent upon ligament/tendon fibre bundle macro-organization.

In this region complete ligament tendon rupture occurs at 'maximal breaking load'; this is the dangerous grade 3 ligament rupture on clinical testing. It is 'dangerous' because the athlete experiences severe momentary pain when the trauma is applied and then little pain, the athlete (and often inexperienced examiners) erroneously believe that the injury is trivial and treat it as such with disastrous consequences (see Fig. 5).

Tendons and ligaments behave as non-linear elastic materials. Viscous and plastic behaviour become obvious when cyclical loading–unloading protocols are used during tensile testing in the laboratory. The laboratory testing protocols can be similar to the cyclical loading imposed on tendons and ligaments during running. During such cyclical testing the load–strain curves initially have a large hysteresis loop but as the cycles progress with time this hysteresis loop is lost, it is thought to be due to water being squeezed from the tissue and concurrently aligning the collagen fibrils along the axis of loading. This 'preconditioning' cycling could be thought of as an important part of the warm-up procedure in athletes and is reversible during the non-running period as water and proteoglycans redistribute amongst the non-loaded fibrils. If cycling is stopped, when cycle-testing a specimen of tendon in the laboratory, two further protocols can be used: keeping the stress constant by slowly increasing the strain results in a creep phenomenon. If the strain or deformation is kept constant by increasing the load slowly, stress–relaxation of the tissue occurs (see Viidik[1] and Fig. 10.10 therein).

An enormous amount of work has been performed on the biomechanical properties of human knee ligaments, with the anterior cruciate ligament dominating research because of its key role in maintaining anteroposterior stability of the knee. Rotational injury to the knee with the foot fixed as well as hyperextension of the knee appear to be the two key mechanisms involved in anterior cruciate ligament disruption. Forces of the order of 2000 N are required to disrupt the anterior cruciate ligament and are even higher for the posterior cruciate ligament. Direct falls on to the tibia, or collisions with opponents, such that a posterior displacement force of the tibia on the femur occurs, appears to be a common mechanism for posterior cruciate ligament injury. Collateral ligament injury involves both excessive varus, valgus, or rotational forces. The ligament–bone junction with its special fibrocartilage transition zone is a common region of clinical failure. Recent experimental work in animals indicates that ligament midsubstance strain is much lower than at the insertion sites, which appears to be due to a differing collagen–fibre crimp amplitude and angle. This higher strain at the insertion sites together with ligament insertion geometry could be an explanation for the preferential failure of some ligament insertion sites; especially the femoral attachment of the medial collateral ligament of the knee which has an almost 90 degree insertion into the region of the medial femoral epicondyle compared with its tibial periosteal insertion.

Ligament/tendon insertion to bone

Benjamin and his colleagues[5-7,20,21] have recently studied extensively tendon–bone junctions where the fibrocartilage interface or enthesis exists between the tendon and the bone. They suggest that the width of this unique fibrocartilage interface is dependent upon the relative degree of movement occurring between the tendon and its bone attachment (see Fig. 32). They further suggest that the enthesis prevents collagen fibres bending and perhaps undergoing shear-

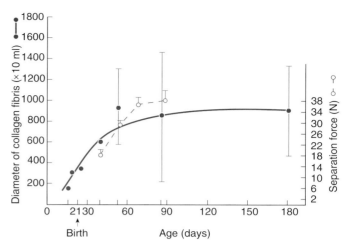

Fig. 6 Increase in diameter of collagen fibrils (full curve through mean diameters with bar representing the largest and smallest fibrils) and tensile strength (broken curve with triangles) with age in the growing rat anterior cruciate ligament. Both curves reach a plateau at about 90 days postconception or about 70 days after birth.

ing, fraying, and failure at this junctional region. These authors have found that the thickest fibrocartilage interface is located in the very mobile Achilles tendon and a lesser thickness of this interface in tendons such as tibialis anterior, posterior, and very little in the long flexor tendons.[22] Interestingly, they observed longitudinal tendon splits in the Achilles tendon with some evidence of repair and also transverse tears at the bone–tendon junction which were filled with fat cells and no repair tissue.[23]

Correlation of collagen-fibril size with mechanical properties of tissues

Parry *et al.*[24] have completed detailed quantitative morphometric ultrastructural analyses of collagen fibrils from a large number of collagen-containing tissues in various species. They came to a number of conclusions that can be summarized as follows:

1. Type 1 oriented tissues such as ligament and tendon have a bimodal distribution of collagen fibril diameters at maturity.

2. The ultimate tensile strength and mechanical properties of connective tissues are positively correlated with the 'mass average diameter' of collagen fibrils. In the context of response of ligaments to exercise, they also concluded that the collagen-fibril diameter distribution is closely correlated with the magnitude and duration of loading of tissues (Fig. 6).

Variation of collagen-fibril diameter with age and correlation with the tensile strength of the anterior cruciate ligament

Oakes[25] measured collagen fibrils in rats of various ages, from 14 days fetal to 2-year-old senile adult rats. The mean diameter and the range of fibres from the largest to the smallest for each time

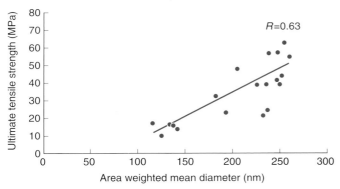

Fig. 7 Area weighted-mean collagen-fibril diameter (nm) across the full width of a rabbit patellar tendon versus patellar tendon ultimate tensile strength. The good correlation (r = 0.63) should be noted, indicating an important relationship between mean collagen-fibril size and the tensile properties of tendons.

interval were plotted against age and this is shown in Fig. 6. The mean fibril diameter begins to plateau at about 7 weeks after birth. Also plotted on this figure is the separation force required to rupture the anterior cruciate ligament in the rat with age. Special grips were used in this study to obviate epiphyseal separation and 70 per cent of the failures occurred within the anterior cruciate ligament. It can be seen that the two curves closely coincide, indicating a close correlation between the size of the collagen fibrils and the ultimate tensile strength of the anterior cruciate ligament as has been suggested by Parry *et al.*[24] This rapid increase in collagen-fibril size over 6 weeks in the growing rat is not seen during normal ligament tissue repair or remodelling.[25-27]

Recent work by Shadwick[28,29] has also elegantly demonstrated a clear correlation between collagen-fibril diameter and the tensile strength of tendons. He determined that the tensile strength of pig flexor tendons was greater than that of extensor tendons, and that this greater flexor tendon tensile strength was correlated with a population of larger diameter collagen fibrils not present in the weaker extensor tendons. Also, very recent studies by Singleton, Oakes, and Haut[30] using the adult rabbit patellar tendon have demonstrated a high correlation between the area weighted-mean collagen-fibril diameter (this method adjusts for the varying numbers of large and small fibrils within a tendon) and both modulus (r = 0.79) and ultimate tensile strength (r = 0.63) (Figs 7 and 8).

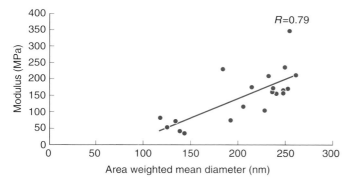

Fig. 8 Area weighted-mean collagen-fibril diameter (nm) across the full width of a rabbit patellar tendon versus patellar tendon modulus. The excellent correlation (r = 0.79) should be noted, indicating that mean fibril diameter and material properties are closely related.

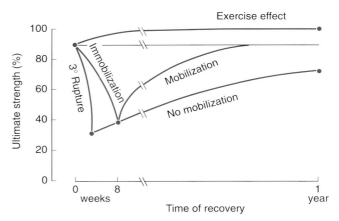

Fig. 9 Effects of immobilization, mobilization, and exercise on recovery of the ligament ultimate tensile strength. The loss in ligament tensile strength after a relatively short period of immobilization (about 8 weeks) requires many months to recover—with no mobilization it may take up to 1 year. The effect of exercise on ligament ultimate tensile strength is small. (Modified from ref. 32, with permission.)

The effects of immobilization on the synovial joints and their capsule

Akeson *et al.*[31] have reviewed their work and that of others on this important topic. There is articular cartilage atrophy with proteoglycan loss and an associated fibrofatty connective tissue, that is synovial derived, which adheres to the articular cartilage. Ligament insertion sites are weakened, and the ligament itself has increased compliance with reduced load to failure due to the loss of collagen mass which may occur with only 8 to12 weeks' immobilization but which may take up to 1 year to recover after mobilization.[32] Capsular changes include loss of water, due to the loss of glycosaminoglycan and hyaluronic acid, which leads to joint stiffness. Clearly joint immobilization is to be avoided, if possible, to prevent the above changes from occurring which take many months to recover (Fig. 9).

Effect of immobilization on ligament tensile strength

The most important study in this context is that conducted by Noyes *et al.*[33] This study used the anterior cruciate ligament of monkeys as part of a **NASA** study performed at that time to examine the effects of prolonged unloading of ligaments in astronauts. They demonstrated clearly that 8 weeks' lower limb cast immobilization led to a substantial loss of ligament tensile strength which took 9 months to recover even with a 'reconditioning' programme. The predominant mode of failure in these experiments was ligament failure as against avulsion fracture failure. The latter was more predominant in the immobilized group due to resorption of Haversian bone at the ligament attachment, but after 5 months of reconditioning femoral avulsion fractures did not occur. It should be noted that there was no surgery, just simple immobilization.

Another important study with direct implications for clinical practice is that of Amiel *et al.*[34] Although this work was done in rabbits, in the context of the previous work by Noyes it is very relevant. The time frames for the changes in ligament tensile strength are similar and hence are probably relevant to clinical orthopaedics.

Amiel *et al.* were able to show that 12 weeks' immobilization of the medial collateral ligament in the growing rabbit led to profound atrophy, such that there was a decrease of approximately 30 per cent in collagen mass as a result of increased collagen degradation. Remarkably, most of this atrophy occurred during weeks 9 to 12 of immobilization. Again, there was no trauma or surgery to the medial collateral ligament in this study.

Hence, it appears from the two studies mentioned above that prolonged immobilization, that is to say 6 to 12 weeks without trauma, can itself lead to profound atrophy of both collateral and cruciate ligaments of the knee joint and that recovery may require at least many months, even a year. This time frame must be kept in mind when managing patients after prolonged knee immobilization and advising them when they can best return to full competitive sport.

Amiel *et al.*[35] have also shown that there is a close relationship between joint stiffness induced by immobilization and a decrease of total gylcosaminoglycan in the periarticular connective tissues. They demonstrated alleviation of this joint stiffness in a rabbit model using intra-articular hyaluronate.

Apart from the original classic work of Noyes *et al.*[33] in which the effects of immobilization on the anterior cruciate ligament of the primate were examined, there have been few investigations into the cause of the decreased strength and elastic stiffness of the anterior cruciate ligament in response to immobilization. Tipton *et al.*,[36] using light microscopy, reported that collagen fibre bundles were decreased in number and size in dogs, suggesting this was the cause of the decreased cross-sectional area seen in immobilized medial collateral rabbit ligaments.[32] The explanation for the decreased strength and elastic stiffness in these immobilized ligaments may also be found at the collagen–fibril level. Binkley and Peat[37] reported a decrease in the number of small-diameter fibrils after 6 weeks' immobilization of the rat medial collateral ligament.

Effect of mobilization (exercise) on ligament tensile strength

There have been a large number of studies investigating this very question and there are several literature reviews available.[15,38–40]

Normal ligaments

The results in experimental animals generally indicate an increase in bone–ligament–bone preparation strength as a response to endurance-type exercise. However, some workers have reported no change in ligament or tendon strength, and this may reflect different exercise regimens, methods of testing, or species differences.

The observation[39–42] that ligament strength depends on physical activity prompted an ultrastructural investigation of the mechanism of this increase in tensile strength within ligaments. Increased collagen content was found in the ligaments of exercised dogs and this correlated with increased cross-sectional area and larger fibre bundles. This accounts for the increased ligament tensile strength, but whether this increased collagen was due to deposition of collagen on existing fibres or due to the synthesis of new fibres had not been investigated. Larsen and Parker[43] had already shown that both the anterior and posterior cruciate ligaments in young male Wistar rats

showed a significant strength increase ($p < 0.05$) after a 4-week intensive-exercise programme.

Oakes and co-workers[25,26] measured the collagen-fibril populations in anterior and posterior cruciate ligaments of young rats subjected to an intensive 1-month exercise programme. This study was performed in an attempt to explain the increased tensile strength found in these ligaments with the intensive endurance-exercise programme, and to detemine if this could be explained at the level of the collagen fibril which is the fundamental tensile unit of ligament.

In this experiment, five pubescent rats (30-day-old) were exposed to a 4-week exercise programme of alternating days of swimming and treadmill running. At the conclusion of the exercise programme the rats were running for 60 to 80 min at 26 m/min on a 10 per cent treadmill gradient, and on alternate days swimming for 60 min with a 3 per cent bodyweight load attached to their tails. The controls were five caged rats of similar age and commencing bodyweightsAfter 30 days the exercise and control rats underwent total body perfusion fixation, after which the anterior and posterior cruciate ligaments were removed and prepared for electron microscopy. Analysis of ultrathin transverse sections cut through collagen fibrils of the exercised anterior cruciate ligaments revealed: (1) a larger number of fibrils per unit area examined (29 per cent increase, $p < 0.05$) compared to the non-exercised caged controls; (2) a fall in mean fibril diameter from 9.66 ± 0.3 nm in the control anterior cruciate ligaments to 8.30 ± 0.3 nm in the exercised anterior cruciate ligaments ($p < 0.05$); (3) as a consequence of (1) and (2) the major cross-sectional area of collagen fibrils was found in the 11.25 nm diameter group in the exercised anterior cruciate ligaments and in the 15 nm diameter group in the controls. However, total collagen fibril cross-section per unit area examined was approximately the same in both the exercised and the non-exercised control anterior cruciate ligaments. Similar changes occurred in the exercised and control posterior cruciate ligaments. These results are shown in Figs 10, 11, and 12. In the exercised posterior cruciate ligaments, the collagen content per microgram of DNA was almost double that of the control, suggesting that the posterior cruciate ligament was loaded more than the anterior cruciate ligament with this exercise regime. The conclusion from this study is that both anterior and posterior cruciate ligament 'fibroblasts' deposit tropocollagen as smaller diameter fibrils when subjected to an intense programme of intermittent loading (exercise) for 1 month, rather than the expected accretion and increase in size of the pre-existing larger diameter collagen fibrils. Very similar ultrastructural observations have been made for collagen fibrils of flexor tendons in exercised mice.[44]

The mechanism of the change to a smaller diameter collagen-fibril population is of interest, and may be related to a change in the type of glycosaminoglycans and hence proteoglycans synthesized by ligament fibroblasts in response to the intermittent loading of exercise. It is well recognized, since the original work of Toole and Lowther,[45] that glycosaminoglycans have an effect on determining collagen-fibril size *in vitro* and this has been confirmed *in vivo* by Parry *et al.*,[46] Merrilies and[47] Flint a change in collagen-fibril diameters between the compression and tension regions of the flexor digitorum profundus tendon as it turns 90 degrees around the talus. Amiel *et al.*[8] have shown that rabbit cruciate ligaments contain more

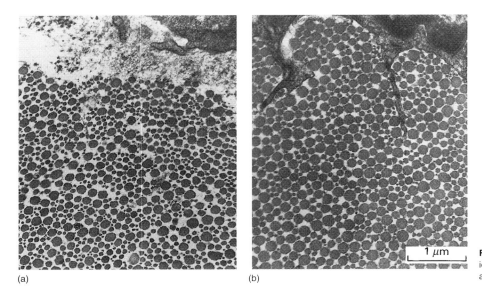

Fig. 10 Transverse sections through exercised anterior cruciate ligament (a) and non-exercised control anterior cruciate ligament (b). Both 21 600 ×

glycosaminoglycans than the patellar tendon, and hence it is likely that glycosaminoglycans also play an important role in determining collagen-fibril populations in cruciate ligaments.

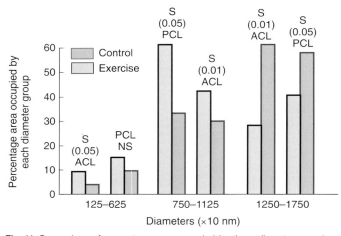

Fig. 11 Comparison of percentage area occupied by three diameter groupings used for statistical analysis for exercised and control anterior and posterior cruciate ligament (ACL and PCL, respectively).

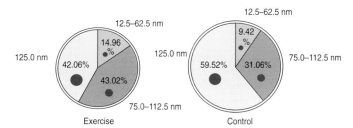

Fig. 12 Comparison of percentage area occupied by the three diameter groupings used for statistical analysis in the exercised and control posterior cruciate ligaments.

Surgically repaired ligaments

Tipton *et al.*[36] demonstrated a significant increase in the strength of surgically repaired medial collateral ligaments of dogs which were exercised for 6 weeks after 6 weeks of cast immobilization. However, they emphasized that 12 weeks after surgery (6 weeks of immobilization and 6 weeks of exercise training) the repair was only approximately 60 per cent of that for normal dogs, and results suggested that 15 to 18 weeks at least of exercise training may be required before a return to 'normal' tensile strength is achieved. Similar observations have been made by Piper and Whiteside[48] using the medial collateral ligament of dogs. They observed that mobilized medial collateral ligament repairs were stronger and stretched out less, that is to say less valgus laxity than medial collateral ligament repairs managed by casting and delayed mobilization. This conclusion is supported by the work of Woo *et al.*[32]

Some insight into the biological mechanisms involved in the repair response with exercise has come from the elegant work of Vailas *et al.*[49] By using [3H]proline pulse-labelling to measure collagen synthesis in rat medial collateral ligament surgical repairs and coupling this with DNA analyses and tensile testing of repaired ligaments subjected to exercise and non-exercise regimens, they were able to show that exercise commencing 2 weeks after surgical repair enhanced the repair and remodelling phase by inducing a more rapid return of cellularity, collagen synthesis, and ligament tensile strength to within normal limits. Further, Woo *et al.*[32] have elegantly demonstrated almost complete return (98 per cent) of structural properties of the transected canine femoral–medial collateral ligament–tibial complex at 12 weeks post-transection without immobilization. Canines immobilized for 6 weeks and the femoral–medial collateral ligament–tibial complex tested at 12 weeks had mean loads to failure 54 per cent that of the control. However, the tensile strength of the medial collateral ligament was only 62 per cent of controls at 48 weeks. This apparent paradox in the non-immobilized dogs was explained by the approximate doubling in cross-sectional area of the healing medial collateral ligament (and hence increased collagen deposition) during the early phases of healing. This repair collagen was most likely with small-diameter fibrils and would account for the poor strain performance of the medial collateral ligament scar collagen and would be similar to the lower curves shown in Figs 9 and 38.

Woo et al.[32] examined the effects of prolonged immobilization and then mobilization on the rabbit medial collateral ligament. Both the structural properties of the femoral–medial collateral ligament–tibial complex and the material properties of the medial collateral ligament were examined. After imobilization, there were significant reductions in the ultimate load and energy-absorbing capabilities of the bone–ligament–bone complex. The medial collateral ligament became less stiff with immobilization and the femoral and tibial insertion sites showed increased osteoclastic activity, bone resorption, and disruption of the normal bone attachment to the medial collateral ligament. With mobilization, the ultimate load and energy-absorbing capabilities improved but did not return to normal. The stress–strain characteristics of the medial collateral ligament returned to normal; this indicates that the material properties of the collagen of the medial collateral ligament in the rabbit return relatively quickly after remobilization, but that the ligament–bone-junction strength return to normal may take many months as represented by the Woo–Akeson–Amiel curves (see Fig. 9).[32]

The detailed biological cellular mechanisms involved in this enhancement and remodelling of the repair are not understood, but they may involve prostaglandin and cyclic-AMP synthesis by fibroblasts subjected to repeated mechanical deformation by exercise.

Amiel et al.[50] have shown that maximal collagen deposition and turnover occurs during the first 3 to 6 weeks after injury in the rabbit. Chaudhuri et al.[51] used a Fourier domain directional filtering technique to determine collagen-fibril orientation in repairing ligaments. The results indicated that ligament collagen-fibril reorientation does occur in the longitudinal axis of the ligament during remodelling. It has also been shown that collagen remodelling of the repairing rabbit medial collateral ligament appears to be encouraged by early immobilization but after 3 weeks' collagen alignment and remodelling appears to be favoured by mobilization.[52,53]

Oakes and co-workers have just completed an interesting study on repair in the goat anterior cruciate ligament.[54] It has almost become an axiom amongst surgeons that the anterior cruciate ligament does not repair after injury. This seems to be the case with complete anterior cruciate ligament rupture;[55] however, the repair of partial tears of the anterior cruciate ligament (grade I and II) has not been examined long-term in large animals. To test the healing of the partially torn anterior cruciate ligament, we transected the posterolateral bundle of the anterior cruciate ligament in 11 adult female goats and tested the ligaments at 12, 24, and 52 weeks and 3 years after surgery. As early as 12 weeks after surgery translucent fibrous tissue covered the wound. The differences in anteroposterior laxity between right and left knees measured at 45 degrees and 90 degrees of flexion were not significantly different at each period. Results of Instron testing of the posterolateral bundle revealed the normalized changes in load-relaxation and Young's modulus were not significantly different at each period, but the ultimate tensile strength and stiffness at 3 years were significantly higher than at 12 weeks ($p < 0.05$). Failure started at the repair site for the 12-week group, but at 24 and 52 weeks the failure occurred throughout the ligament. At 3 years, the specimens failed with bony avulsion, indicating the repaired tissue was not the weakest link of the bone–ligament–bone complex. (See Figs 13 and 14.)

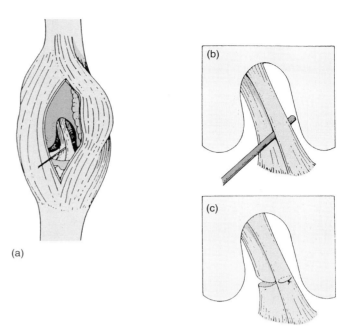

Fig. 13 The operative procedure for the hemitransection injury to the anterior cruciate ligament. A medial arthrotomy was performed and the patella was displaced laterally; a probe was inserted to separate the anteromedial and posterolateral bundles (a and b). c, The posterolateral bundle was completely severed, leaving the anteromedial bundle intact as an internal splint, and a black silk suture was placed on the anteromedial bundle opposite the cut level as a marker of the incision site. (Reproduced from ref. 54, with permission.)

This study shows that, under favourable conditions, partial anterior cruciate ligament injuries are capable of adequate repair. What is more important, the high ultimate tensile strength and stiffness of the 3-year repaired tissue indicate that full structural repair of such an artificial transection injury may be possible.[54]

With this basic biological knowledge there is now a rationale for the use of 'early controlled mobilization' of patients with ligament trauma. The use of a limited motion cast with an adjustable double-action hinge for the knee joint is now accepted in clinical practice and enhances more rapid repair and remodelling as well as preserving quadriceps muscle bulk. Patients are now usually mobilized early in a limited motion cast at 3 weeks rather than the previously empirical time of 6 weeks' immobilization.

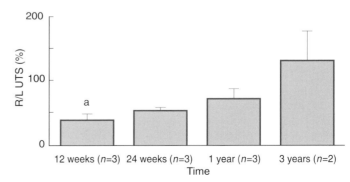

Fig. 14 The mean and standard deviations of normalized percentage ultimate tensile strength for the posterolateral bundles of hemisected anterior cruciate ligaments at intervals after surgery. a, Significantly different from 3-year results. (Reproduced from ref. 54, with permission.)

Collagen-fibril populations in human knee ligaments and grafts

Human anterior cruciate ligament autograft quantitative collagen-fibril studies

In order to gain some biological insight into collagen repair and remodelling mechanisms within human cruciate ligament grafts, biopsies were obtained from autogenous anterior cruciate ligament grafts from patients subsequently requiring arthroscopic intervention because of stiffness, meniscal and/or articular cartilage problems, or removal of prominent staples used for fixation. Most of the anterior cruciate ligament grafts were from the central one-third of the patellar tendon as a free graft ($n = 39$) or in some left attached distally ($n = 8$), and in others the hamstrings ($n = 9$, graft age 10 months to 6 years) or the iliotibial tract was used ($n = 15$, graft age 10 months to 6 years). These biopsies represented approximately 20 per cent of the total free grafts performed over the 3 years of this study. The clinical anterior cruciate ligament stability of the biopsy group differed little from the remainder. All had a grade II to III pivot shift (jerk) preoperatively (10 to 15 mm anterior drawer neutral), eliminated postoperatively in 87 per cent of patients (0.5 mm anterior drawer neutral). Subsequent clinical review at 3 years showed an increase in anterior drawer neutral with a return in 20 per cent of a grade I pivot shift.

A total of 48 biopsies have been quantitatively analysed for collagen-fibril diameter populations in patients aged 19 to 42 years. This data was compared with collagen-fibril populations obtained from biopsies of cadaver anterior cruciate ligaments ($n = 5$) and also biopsies of anterior cruciate ligaments from young (< 30 years, $n = 10$) and old patients (> 30 years, $n = 6$) who had sustained a recent tear. Biopsies were also obtained from normal patellar tendons at operation ($n = 7$) and also from cadavers ($n = 3$) (Fig. 10). Other surgeons, both national and international, have provided 18 anterior cruciate ligament graft biopsies.[56,57]

The results (Figs 11, 12) from the collagen-fibril diameter morphometric analysis in all the anterior cruciate ligament grafts clearly indicated a predominance of small-diameter collagen fibrils. Absence of a 'regular crimping' of collagen fibrils was observed by both light and electron microscopy, as was a less-ordered parallel arrangement of fibrils. In most biopsies capillaries were present and most fibroblasts appeared viable.

Collagen typing of normal human anterior cruciate ligament and anterior cruciate ligament grafts[58]

Recent biochemical analyses of human patellar tendon autografts *in situ* for 2 to 10 years indicates a large amount of type III as well as type V collagen. This confirmed our suspicion that morphologically a large amount of collagen in these remodelled grafts at this age may be type III and not type I as is normally found in the patellar tendon and adult anterior cruciate ligament.[57]

We have examined and quantitated the types of collagen in the normal anterior cruciate ligament and in anterior cruciate ligament grafts using quantitative SDS gel densitometry of cyanagen bromide peptides[58] derived from the tissue in question.

Tissue was obtained from:

* 10 acute ruptured anterior cruciate ligaments (< 1-week-old);

* 10 normal anterior cruciate ligaments;

* 9 autogenous patellar tendon grafts (age 3 months to 2 years).

The normal anterior cruciate ligament contained a mean type I collagen content of 71.13 per cent $\pm$ 9.77 (SD, $n = 10$) and type III content of 28.1 per cent $\pm$ 10.18 (SD, $n = 10$). The acute anterior cruciate ligament ruptures had a similar type I and III collagen content as did the patellar tendon grafts which aged from 3 months to 2 years.

The high content of type III collagen in the normal human anterior cruciate ligament (28.1 per cent) is surprising and was similar to that found in the patellar tendon autografts and the acute anterior cruciate ligament ruptures. This is much higher than that reported by Amiel *et al.*[8] for the normal rabbit anterior cruciate ligament. They suggest the high type III content may reflect a wide variety of force vectors to which the rabbit anterior cruciate ligament is subjected. This is novel and unpublished data for the human anterior cruciate ligament and may indicate previous injury to the 'normal' anterior cruciate ligament tissue (Fig. 15).[57]

Before discussing the biopsy data it is of interest to compare the collagen profiles for the patellar tendon with the normal anterior cruciate ligament. It can be seen that the profiles are different, in that the distribution in the patellar tendon is skewed to the right with a small number of large fibrils not present in the normal anterior cruciate ligament (Fig. 16). Recent elegant work by Butler *et al.*[59] has shown that the patellar tendon is significantly stronger than the human anterior cruciate ligament, posterior cruciate ligament, and lateral collateral ligament from the same knee in terms of maximum stress, linear modulus, and energy density to maximum strength. The larger fibrils observed in the patellar tendon and not found in the anterior cruciate ligament are an obvious explanation for the stronger biomechanical properties.

The biopsies from the grafts were obtained from patients with a good-to-fair rating in terms of a moderate anterior drawer (0 to 5 mm) and correction of the pivot shift, but both these tests of anterior cruciate ligament integrity showed an increasing laxity of the anterior cruciate ligament at the 3-year clinical review. The length of time the grafts were *in vivo* prior to biopsy varied from 6 months to 9 years. The collagen-fibril population did not alter that much for the older grafts (namely > 3 years) which is not what was hoped for or expected but is in keeping with the observation clinically that the anterior cruciate ligament grafts 'stretched out' postoperatively.

The most striking feature of all the biopsies from the autografts, irrespective of whether they were 'free grafts', Jones' grafts, fascia lata, hamstring grafts and independent of the surgeon, was the invariable prevalence of small-diameter fibrils in amongst a few larger fibrils which probably were the original large-diameter patellar fibrils. The packing of the small fibrils in the grafts was not as tight as is usually observed in the normal patellar tendon. (Compare Figs 15(a) and 5(c); Fig. 17 arrows 1 and 2.)

It appears from the quantitative collagen-fibril observations in this study using a non-isometric surgical procedure that the large-

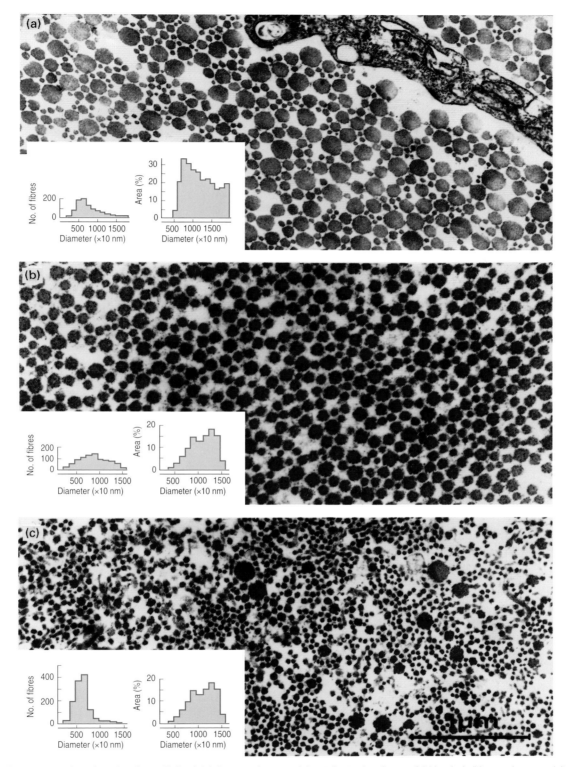

Fig. 15 Transverse sections through collagen fibrils of: (a) the normal young adult patellar tendon, (mean of 6 biopsies); (b) normal young adult anterior cruciate ligament (mean of 6 biopsies); (c) Jones' free graft (mean of 9 biopsies). Magnification 34 100 ×. The insets show on the left, the number of fibrils versus diameter; on the right, percentage area occupied/diameter group. The preponderance of small-diameter fibrils in the graft (c), and large fibrils in the patellar tendon (a) which are not seen in the 'normal' anterior cruciate ligament (b) should be noted.

diameter fibrils of the original graft are removed and almost entirely replaced by smaller less well-packed and oriented fibrils than the larger diameter fibrils found in the normal patellar tendon. The smaller diameter fibrils are probably recently synthesized because

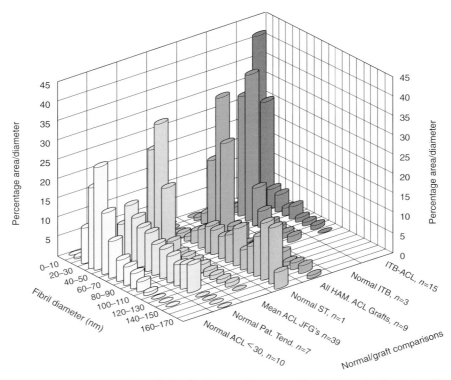

Fig. 16 Summary and comparison histograms of collagen-fibril profiles for normal tissues used for anterior cruciate ligament grafting (patellar tendon (*n* = 7), iliotibial band (*n* = 3), semitendinosus (*n* = 1)) with anterior cruciate ligament autografts derived from the same tissues expressed as per cent area per diameter group. Large-diameter fibrils > 100 nm are found predominantly in the hamstring semitendinusus and to a lesser extent in the normal patellar tendon. The iliotibial band has a profile not unlike that of the normal anterior cruciate ligament. All the autografts (patellar tendon free anterior cruciate ligament grafts (*n* = 39), hamstring anterior cruciate ligament grafts (*n* = 9), and iliotibial band anterior cruciate ligament grafts (*n* = 15)) have predominantly small-diameter fibrils. (Reproduced from ref. 56, with permission.)

they are of smaller diameter than those found in the original patellar tendon.

Is gentle mechanical loading in the anterior cruciate ligament grafts an important stimulus to fibroblast proliferation and collagen deposition? Inadequate mechanical stimulus may occur especially if grafts are non-isometric and are 'stretched out' by the patient before they have adequate tensile strength. A lax anterior cruciate ligament graft may not induce sufficient mechanical loading on graft fibroblasts to alter the glycosaminoglycan:collagen biosynthesis ratios to favour large-diameter fibril formation. Certainly in this study there was anterior cruciate ligament graft laxity which increased postoperatively. This would lend credence to the above notion. However, the use of continuous passive motion in grafted primates does not increase the strength of grafts.

Another more likely possibility is that the 'replacement fibroblasts' in the anterior cruciate ligament grafts are derived from stem cells from the synovium (and synovial perivascular cells) which are known to synthesize hyaluronate, which, in turn, favours small-diameter fibril formation.[46]

The strong correlation of small-diameter fibrils with a lower tensile strength has been observed by Parry *et al.*[24] and Shadwick,[29] and the observations in this study would confirm this and correlates with the observations of Clancy *et al.*[60] and Arnoczky *et al.*[61]

The recent observations by Amiel *et al.*[62] indicate that collagenase may play a role in the remodelling of anterior cruciate ligament tears/grafts.

The conclusion from this study is that the predominance of the small-diameter collagen fibrils (< 7.5 nm) and their poor packing and alignment in all the anterior cruciate ligament grafts irrespective of the type of graft, their age, and the surgeon may explain the clinical and experimental evidence of a decreased tensile strength in such grafts compared with the normal anterior cruciate ligament. It appears that in the adult, the 'replacement fibroblasts' in the remodelled anterior cruciate ligament graft cannot re-form the large-diameter regularly crimped and tightly packed fibrils seen in the normal anterior cruciate ligament even after 9 years which was the oldest graft analysed.

The origin of the 'replacement' fibroblasts which remodel the anterior cruciate ligament grafts is not yet known. It is the author's hunch that they will not come from the actual graft itself, although some of these cells may survive due to diffusion. However, the bulk of the stem cells involved in the remodelling process is probably derived from the surounding synovium and its vasculature.

Human anterior cruciate ligament allografts[63-66]

Recent further studies of biopsies obtained from anterior cruciate ligament human allografts utilizing fresh-frozen Achilles or tibialis anterior tendons ranging in age from 3 to 54 months indicated a similar predominance of small-diameter collagen fibrils.[56,63-65]

Human anterior cruciate ligament allograft specimens were studied as above for the autografts with quantitative collagen-fibril

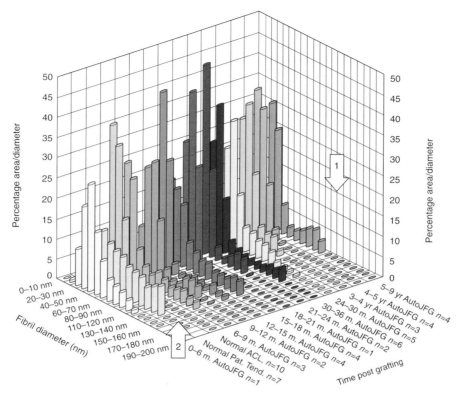

Fig. 17 Summary histograms of all human anterior cruciate ligament–patellar tendon autografts ($n = 39$) versus time compared with the young anterior cruciate ligament ($n = 10$) and normal young patellar tendon ($n = 7$) expressed as percentage area per diameter group. The presence of large fibrils (> 100 nm) in the older 5- to 9-year-old grafts (arrow 1) and the rapid loss of < 100 nm fibrils in the 0- to 6-month postgraft group (arrow 2) which are present in the donor patellar tendon (to the left of arrow 2) should be noted. (Reproduced from ref. 56, with permission.)

analyses[56,57] and were compared with anterior cruciate ligament autografts. The allograft specimens were procured at the time of second-look arthroscopy from the superficial region of the midzone of anterior cruciate ligament grafts after synovial clearage. The grafts used for the anterior cruciate ligament reconstruction were usually from fresh-frozen allogeneic Achilles or tibialis posterior or anterior tendons and were implanted 3 to 96 months prior to biopsy.

A total of 38 patients who had undergone allograft anterior cruciate ligament reconstruction from 3 to 96 months previously and whose anteroposterior stability had been adequately restored were randomly selected. The restored stability of the involved knees was carefully confirmed with both Lachman and pivot shift signs and an objective quantitative knee instability testing apparatus. All these patients were subjected to second-look arthroscopy as a part of the procedure to remove hardware installed for graft fixation. In all, 35 graft biopsies were obtained from this patient group. Their ages ranged from 15 to 37 years at the time of reconstruction.

Anterior cruciate ligament reconstruction technique

A fresh-frozen allograft, 8 to 9 mm in diameter, consisting of part of the Achilles tendon, the tibialis anterior or posterior, peroneal or other thick flexor tendons without any bone attached to their ends were used as an anterior cruciate ligament substitute. The tendons were fixed into drill holes made into the anatomical anterior cruciate ligament attachment sites of the femur and the tibia with sutures, buttons, or staples. Postoperatively, the knee was immobilized for 2

to 5 weeks, then full weight-bearing allowed at 2 to 3 months, jogging recommended at 5 to 6 months, and full activiy allowed at 9 to 12 months.

The normal tissues used were compared with the normal anterior cruciate ligament and the anterior cruciate ligament allografts.

Normal tissues used

The reconstituted Achilles tendon demonstrated a large number of fibrils in the 90 to 140 nm range (40 per cent of total cross-sectional area) together with small-diameter fibrils 30 to 80 nm. The reconstituted tibialis anterior tendon showed more larger diameter fibrils and fewer smaller fibrils than the Achilles tendon. The large fibrils constituted about 80 per cent of the total fibril cross-sectional area. In contrast, the normal anterior cruciate ligament has about 85 per cent of its total cross-sectional area composed of fibrils less than 100 nm in diameter, but there are a small number of large fibrils which account for about 15 per cent of its total cross-sectional area.

Allograft results versus time (Fig. 18)

- *By 3 months* ($n = 2$) there was a predominance of small-diameter fibrils which accounted for more than 85 per cent of the total cross-sectional area of these biopsies with a 'tail' of larger fibrils making the fibril distribution bimodal in shape.

- *At 6 months* ($n = 5$) the fibril distribution was now unimodal with most (apprximately 90 per cent) of the fibril cross-

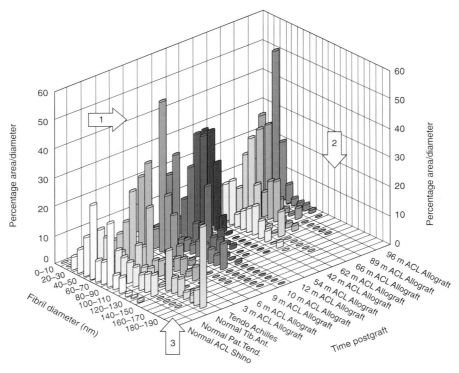

Fig. 18 Summary histograms of all human anterior cruciate ligament allografts versus time postgrafting compared with the normal young anterior cruciate ligament, nomal patellar tendon, and reconstituted tibialis anterior and Achilles tendons expressed as per cent area per diameter group. The early preponderance of the small fibrils at 3 months postgraft (arrow 1) and their persistence even at 96 months postgraft in the majority of biopsies examined should be noted. Some large fibrils are present (arrow 2) at 96 months, but the majority of the large fibrils present in the donor tissues are removed (to the right of arrow 3). (Reproduced from ref. 56, with permission.)

sectional area in the less than 100 nm diameter group. Fibrils larger than 100 nm were obviously fewer than in the 3-month specimens.

- *By 12 months* (n = 12) almost all the cross-sectional area resided in the less than 100 nm diameter fibrils and there was almost complete absence of the large (> 100 nm) fibrils.

This profile persisted in the 13- to 96-month-old allografts. However, there were two exceptions, where one 12-month-old and one 54-month-old anterior cruciate ligament allograft biopsy specimens had significant numbers of large-diameter fibrils in contrast to the earlier observations. In these two specimens the large-diameter fibrils (> 100 nm) accounted for 40 per cent of the total cross-sectional area of the collagen fibrils. However, the large-diameter fibrils in these exceptional grafts were smaller in size and more irregular on their surface than those in the allografts prior to implantation, suggesting perhaps a 'collagenase sculpting' of their exposed surface fibrils.

Parry and colleagues[24] were the first to describe the bimodal distribution of the collagen fibrils in adult mature tendon collagen which is subjected to high tensile loads. The reconstituted (treated by freezing and thawing) human allografts (Achilles and tibiales tendons) and the normal anterior cruciate ligament in this study are also shown to have a bimodal distribution of small- and large-diameter fibrils similar to that described by Parry and colleagues in a large range of other tissues.

Most biopsies of anterior cruciate ligament allografts also dem-

onstrated a bimodal distribution of large and small fibrils similar to the 'normal reconstituted' tendons up until about 6 months after implantation. However, after this time the distribution became more unimodal such that there was an increasing predominance of small-diameter fibrils with a concomitant and progressive loss of the larger 'host tendon' fibrils. It is these larger fibrils in the 'normal' tendon which are responsible for a large percentage of the tendon collagen cross-sectional area and also responsible for the very high tensile strength that these tendons exhibit, which is probably due to the high density of intermolecular collagen crosslinks. These observations suggest that most of the original large-diameter fibrils in the anterior cruciate ligament allografts are replaced by newly synthesized, smaller diameter collagen fibrils (or undergo disaggregation, see below). The loss of the large-diameter fibrils from the 6 months (or older) allografts and the predominance of the small-diameter fibrils seen in this study provide the most likely explanation for the dramatic reduction in tensile strength of anterior cruciate ligament allografts and hence the increased anteroposterior laxity observed in an animal study.[66]

These observations parallel those described above for anterior cruciate ligament autografts, which also demonstrated the loss of large-diameter collagen fibrils of patellar tendon origin within 6 months following implantation. It could be concluded therefore that the remodelling process has a similar time frame in both anterior cruciate ligament tendon allografts and patellar tendon–anterior cruciate ligament autografts. It further suggests that similar mechanisms of collagen degradation and neosythesis may be occurring by the invading synovial cells which repopulate the anterior cruciate ligament graft almost immediately after surgery.

A valid criticism of these studies could be that all the biopsies were obtained from the superficial region of the grafts and that this may not be representative of the bulk of the collagen of the graft. However, in the previous autograft study the biopsies were usually obtained from the middle of the autografts and the observations were no different from those in this allograft study. This suggests that the superficial region from which the biopsies were taken in this study is representative of the collagen within the graft.

Awaiting the appearence of large fibrils with close packing (perhaps under a Wolff's law tensile stimulus) as seen in normal ligament and tendon is probably futile. Currently, there is no evidence that large-diameter fibrils will eventually be formed and become a large proportion of the long-term anterior cruciate ligament grafts, or even that the 'packing' of the small-diameter fibrils becomes closer within these grafts. If denser collagen-fibril packing could be achieved this could possibly enhance the collagen-fibril cross-sectional area which, in turn, could possibly increase the tensile strength of the graft by increased interfibril interactions as already discussed. The explanation for denser packing of fibrils not seen in allo- or autografts may be due to an increased synthesis of small proteoglycans and particularly hyaluronan preventing large collagen-fibril formation.[67]

It should be also mentioned that the conclusions drawn in this discussion are based on the assumption that large collagen fibrils of the allograft tendons do not undergo a process of disaggregation into smaller fibrils similar to that described by glycerol treatment of mature collagen fibrils which is reversible.[68] This is a possibility which must be seriously considered, but that is very difficult to verify experimentally without rigorous immunoelectron microscopy.

The remodelling of collagen in tendon auto-, allo-, and xenografts has been elegantly quantified by the work of Klein et al.[69] They noticed that at 3 months the xenografts lost 99 per cent, allografts lost 63 per cent, and autografts 54 per cent of their original collagen, thus demonstrating a clear antigenic influence on collagen turnover which was substantial even in the autografts at 3 months. The remodelling of collagen during medial ligament repair in the rabbit has also been shown to be prolonged, in that the collagen concentration takes many months to approach normal levels,[70] and appears to be a similar process in larger animals.[71]

The observations and conclusions in this auto/allograft review throw into question the current time frames for rehabilitation. It is generally concluded by most knee surgeons that the graft tissue will eventually 'mature', given enough time, and that graft tensile strength will also increase with time, especially if the athlete waits for up to 1 year for graft maturation. The observations in this study do not support this notion that graft tensile strength will gradually increase with time nor do experimental results. However, collagen crosslink maturation could be very important in these grafts and may be a mechanism for restoring graft tensile strength even when the collagen fibrils remain of small diameter. Recent observations by Butler et al.[72] that anterior cruciate ligament autografts and allografts using the patellar tendon were only about 30 per cent the strength of the normal anterior cruciate ligament at 12 months post-implantation, strongly supports the quantitative fibril observations oulined in this human auto/allograft study.

Goat anterior cruciate ligament–patellar tendon autograft collagen remodelling—quantitative collagen-fibril analyses over 3 years[56,74]

The aim of this study was to quantify, in detail, the collagen-fibril remodelling process in adult goat patellar tendon–anterior cruciate ligament autografts over a 3-year time frame.

In this study, 11 mature female adult goats were used. They were anaesthetized and via a central arthrotomy the middle one-third of the right patellar tendon was harvested. A 'V'-shaped patellar bone component removed by a handsaw was left attached at the femoral end. The tibial end was also left attached. The anterior cruciate ligament was removed and fixed for 'time 0' quantitative collagen-fibril analyses. The lateral femoral condyle was exposed and the posterolateral capsule was opened above the lateral femoral condyle from within the intercondylar notch. A Gigli saw was introduced into the notch, and the posteromedial corner of the lateral femoral condyle was grooved to allow for isometricity of the anterior cruciate ligament graft and also to create a suitable vascular bone bed for anterior cruciate ligament graft attachment. The patellar tendon–anterior cruciate ligament graft was then routed via a drill hole or slot in the tibia under the anterior horn of the medial meniscus through the intercondylar notch and posterolateral capsule 'over the top', and lodged within the groove created by the Gigli saw. The patellar bone was stapled under a periosteal flap to the lateral femoral condyle.

At 6 weeks ($n = 3$), 12 weeks ($n = 2$), 24 weeks ($n = 2$), 52 weeks ($n = 3$), and 3 years ($n = 1$) goats were culled and the anterior cruciate ligament grafts obtained and prepared for quantitative ultrastructural collagen-fibril analyses.

The normal anterior cruciate ligament ($t = 0$, $n = 5$) and anterior cruciate ligament–patellar tendon grafts ($n = 11$) were divided into thirds, and 1 mm thick sections cut from the femoral, middle, and tibial thirds. This section was then cut into a strip and four sections obtained: two were deemed 'superficial' and contained a synovial surface and two were deemed 'deep'. From each section two ultrastructural thin sections were analysed systematically on copper 400 mesh grids. Systematic random sampling was performed such that about 10 per cent of the grid spaces were measured. The tissue sections sampled were photographed for later quantitative ultrastructural collagen-fibril analyses. The patellar tendon was sampled in the central region and two blocks per tendon were analysed as above ($n = 3$). The collagen-fibril profiles were directly quantitated from electron micrograph negatives taken at a 20 000 magnification using a specifically designed software program for automated computerized image analysis within a constant sized inclusion grid. A calibration grid was included at each sitting to accurately determine magnifications. The ASCII data files were imported into the Framework 3 database, and the frequency of fibrils within 20 diameter size classes and the per cent area occupied for each diameter group of fibrils were automatically calculated as a mean (Fig. 19). Statistical analyses were performed using the Kolomorogov–Smirnov nonparametric method.

The results of the study were as follows:

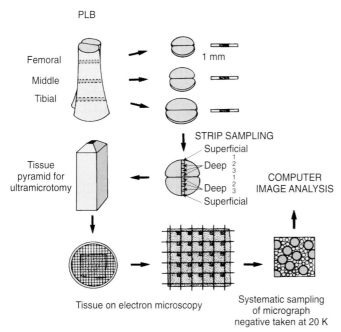

Fig. 19 Shows methodology for sampling the goat anterior cruciate ligament and also tissue blocking and electron microscopic grid random-sampling technique.

The major observation was the complete loss of the large-diameter fibrils at 1 year from the superficial regions of the graft. There was also a concomitant increase in the number of small-diameter fibrils in the deep region at 52 weeks not seen in the superficial regions. Plots of the ratio of large-diameter fibrils (> 100 nm) to small-diameter fibrils (< 100 nm) demonstrated that the major fall in the ratio is seen in the superficial region, reflecting the complete removal of the large-diameter fibrils in the superficial regions of the grafts at 52 weeks (see Figs 21(a–e), 22, and 23).

The collagen-fibril profile for each time group was compared to the control anterior cruciate ligament and patellar tendon with Kolomogorov–Smirnov analyses. Differences were found between the patellar tendon collagen profile and the anterior cruciate ligament grafts with the 12-, 24-, and 52-week groups ($p = 0.005$, 0.07, and 0.1, respectively). All the grafts except the 6-week group contained mainly small fibrils (< 100 nm). The large fibrils were not repopulated in the 1-year grafts, but in the one graft studied at 3 years small numbers of large fibrils (> 100 nm) were present. A positive correlation ($r = 0.6$, $p = 0.07$) was found between the per cent of fibrils larger than 100 nm in diameter with Young's modulus of the grafts which was tested in a separate study.

This study has determined the anatomical regions of the anterior

- *Normal adult goat anterior cruciate ligament*, t = 0

  The distribution was clearly bimodal with a large number of small fibrils less than 100 nm in diameter and a group of larger fibrils more than 100 nm in diameter. A small number of large fibrils (> 100 nm) contributed about 45 per cent of the total collagen-fibril area; these large fibrils seen in the adult goat anterior cruciate ligament are not seen in the normal adult human anterior cruciate ligament.

- *Normal adult goat patellar tendon*, t = 0

  The collagen-fibril distribution was quite different compared to the anterior cruciate ligament with a more unimodal distribution. There were less small-diameter fibrils and more larger diameter fibrils (> 100 nm) than the anterior cruciate ligament. These latter large fibrils contributed 65 per cent of the total collagen-fibril area (Fig. 20).

- *Patellar tendon–anterior cruciate ligament graft tibial region versus femoral region* (Fig. 21)

  At 6 weeks there was a large increase in the number of small-diameter collagen fibrils (< 100 nm) which was greatest at the tibial end. This number of small-diameter fibrils was increased at both ends of the graft at 52 weeks. There was a loss of the large-diameter fibrils (> 100 nm) which could be seen at 6 weeks, and at 52 weeks only a few large fibrils remained at the femoral region. This is reflected if one plots the ratio of large (> 100 nm) to small (< 100 nm) fibrils (see Fig. 22).

- *Patellar tendon–anterior cruciate ligament graft superficial region versus deep region*

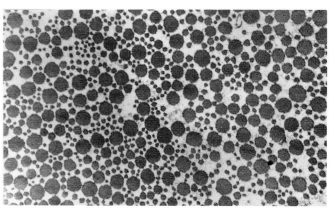

Normal goat patellar tendon

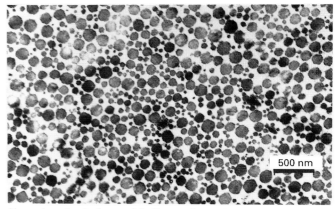

Normal goat anterior cruciate ligament

Fig. 20 Electron micrographs of normal (a) adult goat anterior cruciate ligament and (b) adult goat patellar tendon.

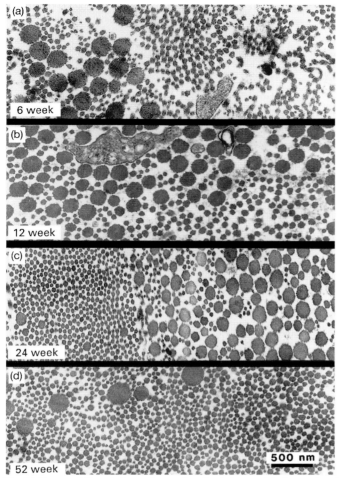

Fig. 21 Representative electron micrographs of anterior cruciate ligament and patellar tendon autografts: (a) at 6 weeks, (b) at 12 weeks, (c) at 24 weeks, and (d) at 48 weeks postgrafting. The progressive loss of the large-diameter fibrils at $t = 0$ (see Fig. 20(b)) and the accumulation of the small-diameter fibrils with increasing graft age should be noted.

cruciate ligament graft which undergo remodelling and found that this process continues for up to 3 years after grafting. This remodelling process changes the collagen-fibril profile of the original patellar tendon to one containing a greater proportion of small-diameter fibrils. The remodelling process occurs from 'without–in' and is more vigorous in the tibial region of the graft. This would be consistent with synovial revascularization of the graft. The rapid depletion of the large fibrils in the grafts at 12 weeks is also consistent with the dramatic decrease in the mechanical and material properties of such grafts (Fig. 24). This collagen-fibril study in the goat also parallels that in the human anterior cruciate ligament–patellar tendon grafts and appears to be a useful model to follow collagen remodelling in anterior cruciate ligament grafts.

A 3-year biomechanical and viscoelastic study of patellar tendon autografts for anterior cruciate ligament reconstruction[74]

Of 27 adult female goats tested, four served as controls and the others received an autograft to the right knee with each left knee

serving as an additional control. The animals with grafts were tested at 0 week ($n = 4$), 6 weeks ($n = 4$), 12 weeks ($n = 4$), 24 weeks ($n = 3$), 1 year ($n = 5$), and 3 years ($n = 3$) after surgery. The anteroposterior laxity of the knee joint, load–relaxation, and structural and mechanical properties of the graft were tested.

The anteroposterior laxity was significantly greater than that of the controls for all groups except at 3 years. Load–relaxation was greater than that of the control anterior cruciate ligaments, but in the 1- and 3-year grafts load–relaxation was less than that of the patellar tendons with 5 min of sustained loading. Between 12 and 52 weeks, the stiffness and the modulus of the grafts were 44 per cent and 49 per cent those of the control ligaments, respectively; the modulus was 37 and 46 per cent that of the control anterior cruciate ligaments and patellar tendons, respectively (Figs 25 and 26). The persistent inferior mechanical performance at 3 years suggests that anterior cruciate ligament grafts in the goat may never attain normal anterior cruciate ligament strength.

A 3-year study of collagen type and crosslinks for anterior cruciate ligament–patellar tendon autografts in a goat model

The collagen matrix provides the tensile strength of ligaments. Previous animal studies have shown that anterior cruciate ligament–patellar tendon autografts contain mainly small-diameter collagen fibrils (< 100 nm) at 1 year postsurgery. The long-term collagen type and biochemical changes are not clear.

This study examined goat anterior cruciate ligament–patellar tendon autografts up to 3 years postsurgery for collagen type and hydroxypyridinium crosslink density.

A total of 22 mature female goats received an anterior cruciate ligament–patellar tendon autograft to the right knee and were tested at 6 weeks ($n = 5$), 12 weeks ($n = 4$), 24 weeks ($n = 5$), 1 year ($n = 5$), and 3 years ($n = 3$). Of these, two in each group were assigned for collagen typing and hydroxypyridinium crosslink density analyses. A further two normal animals served as controls for collagen typing and hydroxypyridinium crosslink density analyses.

Type III collagen analyses with SDS gel electrophoresis showed an increase from 6 to 24 weeks followed by a subsequent decrease. At 3 years, the grafts contained similar amounts of type III collagen as the control anterior cruciate ligament, but it was differently distributed as demonstrated by immunofluorescent labelling of the grafts with specific type III collagen antibodies.

The hydroxypyridinium crosslink density was low in the 6-, 12-, and 24-week groups, but increased in the 1- and 3-year groups. The mean hydroxypyridinium crosslink density in the grafts was similar to the two control anterior cruciate ligaments at less than 24 weeks, but at 1 and 3 years the hydroxypyridinium crosslink density was increased ($p < 0.09$). The hydroxypyridinium crosslink density of the left anterior cruciate ligament of the unoperated goats was higher than the two controls, which could be due to the change in loading to the left knee in these animals (Fig. 27). A negative correlation was found between the per cent type III collagen and Young's modulus, but this was not significant.

A significant positive correlation ($p = 0.01$) was found between the hydroxypyridinium crosslink density and Young's modulus in both the anterior cruciate ligament grafts ($r = 0.8$) and controls ($r =$

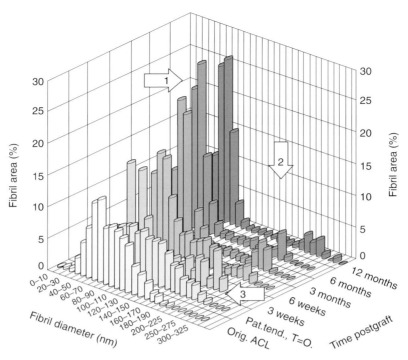

Fig. 22 Three-dimensional histograms of normal goat patellar tendon, anterior cruciate ligament, and anterior cruciate ligament autografts expressed as per cent area covered by the collagen fibrils versus age and fibril diameter. Again there is progressive loss of the large-diameter fibrils and the rapid replacement of these large fibrils (arrow 3) as early as 6 weeks after grafting with a predominance of small fibrils at 12 months postgrafting (arrow 1). The lack of large fibrils at 12 months postgrafting (arrow 2) should be noted.

0.7). The grafts and control anterior cruciate ligaments had comparable mean hydroxypyridinium crosslink densities but different Young's moduli, which implies hydroxypyridinium crosslink density is not the only determinant for material strength.[76] Other factors

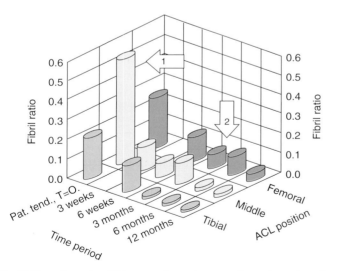

Fig. 23 Three-dimensional histograms of normal goat patellar tendon and anterior cruciate ligament–patellar tendon autografts at $t = 0$, 3, 6,12, 24, and 48 weeks in relation to the femoral middle and tibial regions of the anterior cruciate ligament autografts. Vertical axis is the ratio of large fibrils (> 100 nm) to small fibrils (< 100 nm). Large fibrils are lost from the tibial end of the graft as early as 6 weeks postgrafting, but some large fibrils still remain at the femoral end of the graft at 48 weeks (at approximately 12 months, arrow 2). The predominace of large fibrils in the original patellar tendon used as the donor graft (arrow 1) should be noted.

such as collagen–fibril size, density of packing, and orientation may affect Young's modulus. However, the good correlation on regression analysis suggests the hydroxypyridinium crosslink density may be an indicator for material strength. A previous study of medial collateral ligament scars in rabbits has also demonstrated a positive relationship between hydroxypyridinium crosslink density and failure stress of ligament scar.[77]

These two similar observations in different species and different tissues indicates that hydroxypyridinium crosslink density is one of the determinants for the tensile strength of ligament repair and graft remodelling.

Clinical and ultrastructural observations on Achilles tendon injuries

In this section I will attempt to relate the three phases of healing of soft tissues with that seen in Achilles tendon injuries. Achilles tendon injuries can be classified as described above for ligament injury, namely grades 1 to 3, with the latter being complete rupture. Several patient histories will be used to illustrate these three phases of healing and attempted repair.

Grade-3 complete rupture

Patient profile

An Australian Rules football rover, aged 26, accelerating to avoid an opponent. Clinical signs were a palpable defect in the Achilles tendon and a positive Thompson's sign.

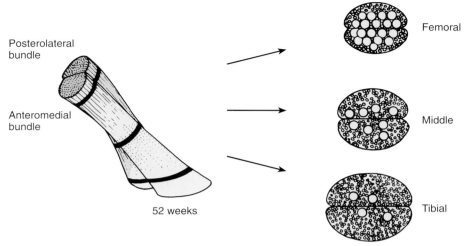

Fig. 24 Summary diagram of goat anterior cruciate ligament graft fibril profiles 12 months after grafting. The preponderence of small fibrils at the tibial end of the graft and some large fibrils remaining in the femoral end of the graft 12 months after grafting should be noted.

A biopsy taken during surgical repair

With this injury there is both collagen bundle failure as well as vascular disruption, and hence bleeding is a feature of these injuries when seen at an early surgical repair. This trauma to the tendon initiates the acute inflammatory phase and hence microscopically there is massive red cell extravasation, fibrin clot formation, as well as collagen-fibril disruption. The damaged tendon becomes oedematous and polymorphonuclear monocytes migrate into this area and release their lysosomal contents. Macrophages also move into the rupture site and commence phagocytosis of damaged cells and tissue. This phase lasts from 0 to 72 h or more and is followed by the repair phase (Fig. 28).

Grade-2 tear

Patient profile

An Australian Rules football ruckman with a 6 months' painful thickened Achilles tendon.

Operation

Excision of paratenon and tendon incision to remove damaged, haemorrhagic, and necrotic regions. Biopsy taken for light- (Fig. 29) and electron microscopy.

Light microscopy demonstrated a thickened paratenon and an oedematous thickened tendon. Ultrastructurally, many fibroblasts had a dilated rough endoplasmic reticulum and prominent nucleoli, indicative of increased collagen synthesis. Apart from the many free red cells, the other feature was the prevalence of many small-diameter collagen fibrils not aligned or closely packed (18 to 20 nm diameter) in amongst the older, larger pre-existing fibrils ranging from 80 to 150 nm diameter. Polymorphonuclear monocytes and macrophages were not common at this stage, perhaps reflecting the slowness of repair in this unique tissue.

This biopsy demonstrated the features of the repair phase which follows the acute inflammatory phase and lasts from 72 h to 4 to 6 weeks. In this patient the repair phase had been perpetuated because of continued activity, a common problem with these athletes

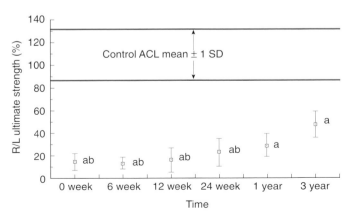

Fig. 25 Anterior cruciate ligament graft ultimate tensile strength (mean ± SD) of the right side (R) expressed as a percentage of that for the left side (L) for control anterior cruciate ligament and grafts at different times after surgery. Symbols 'a' and 'b' indicate values that are significantly different from the control and 3-year groups, respectively ($p < 0.05$). (Reproduced from ref. 74, with permission.)

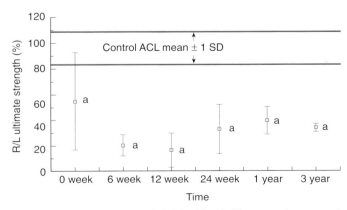

Fig. 26 Young's modulus (mean ± SD) of the right side (R) expressed as a percentage of that of the left side (L) for control anterior cruciate ligament and anterior cruciate ligament grafts at different time intervals after surgery. Symbols 'a' and 'b' indicate values that are significantly different from the control and 3-year groups, respectively ($p < 0.05$). (Reproduced from ref. 54, with permission.)

because when they run the Achilles tendon pain usually subsides and then returns on 'cool-down' often with a vengeance. In other patients, where there was less florid tendinitis and the tendon was clinically painful but not obviously enlarged, discrete areas of increased cellularity were seen in the tendon in the form of free red cells, cell debris, and viable fibroblasts which were surrounded by both large- and many small-diameter collagen fibrils. These areas were almost 'walled-off' from the densely packed collagen of the rest of the tendon by a fibrin precipitate. These discrete areas are probably due to collagen-fibril ruptures or 'microtears' corresponding to the early part of region 2 of the load–deformation curve.

There is, as yet, no evidence that the use of massage or 'deep friction' enhances this repair phase.[78]

Grade-1 injury

Patient profile

A runner, aged 25, with a painful tender lump in the Achilles tendon for 18 months. A biopsy was obtained at open operation.

The lump at operation was firmer than the rest of the tendon and was slightly darker in colour. On light microscopy of the biopsy taken from the nodule the changes in the collagen bundles were very subtle. There was less regular 'crimping' of the collagen bundles and they were not as tightly packed. However, the cause of this less-regular collagen crimp was obvious in that between large-diameter fibrils there were many small-diameter fibrils less well orientated longitudinally. These tendons were interpreted as being in the remodelling phase as there was no increased fibroblast numbers in the nodules and no inflammatory cells were observed (Fig. 30).

The mechanism of acute complete rupture in young athletes 'powering-off' during sprinting indicates that the gastrocnemius–soleus complex can generate sufficient force to rupture the tendon. However, tendon strength usually exceeds that of its muscle by a factor of two, and hence rupture is unusual. The mechanisms involved in partial grade 1 and 2 tears in the Achilles tendon are not as obvious. Viidik[79] has shown that rat tendons *in vitro* undergo increasing deformation or 'plasticity' if cycled to loads less than

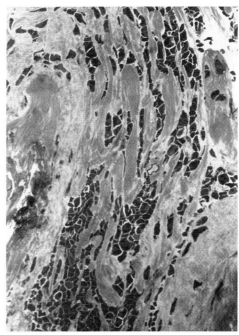

Fig. 28 Light micrograph of acute Achilles tendon rupture at 1 week postinjury showing red cell extravasation together with many polymorphs and macrophages. Epon–Araldite, Azure A–methylene blue.

one-tenth of their failure load, and that strain (or deformation) occurs prior to the linear part of the load–strain curve (Fig. 31). Similar observations have been made both *in vivo* and *in vitro* for rat knee joint ligaments.[80] It is possible that in distance runners a simi-

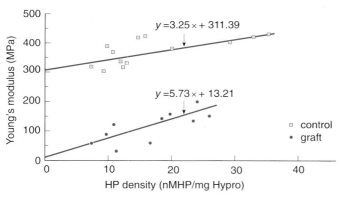

Fig. 27 The relationship between hydroxypyridinium crosslink density and Young's modulus of the anterior cruciate ligament autografts (*r* = 0.8) and control anterior cruciate ligaments (*r* = 0.7). A significant positive corrrelation is shown for both tissues. Linear regression lines predict the Young's moduli of anterior cruciate ligament autografts and anterior cruciate ligament controls from hydroxypyridinium crosslink density are also shown. HP, hydroxypyridinium; nMHP/mg Hypro, nM hydroxypyridinium/mg hydroxproline. (Reproduced from ref. 75, with permission.)

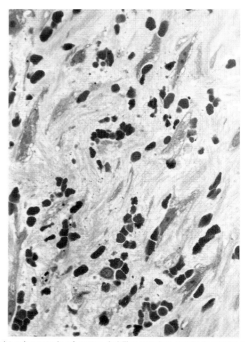

Fig. 29 Light micrograph of acute Achilles tendon grade-2 partial tear after 6 months of pain and swelling. The tendon is oedematous and very cellular, and the fibroblasts are dilated with enlarged rough endoplasmic reticulum indicative of active collagen synthesis. Epon–Araldite, Azure A–methylene blue.

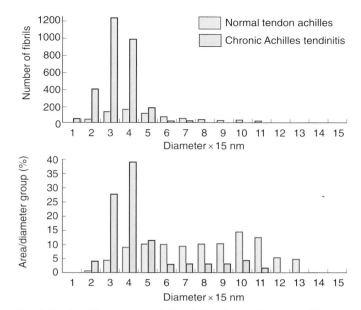

Fig. 30 Number of fibrils versus fibril diameter in patients with chronic Achilles tendinitis and expressed as per cent area occupied for each diameter group versus diameter. The preponderance of small-diameter fibrils in 'repairing' chronic Achilles tendinitis should be noted. The large normal fibrils are not replaced.

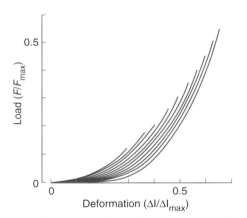

Fig. 31 The effect of 'fatigue failure' or 'plasticity' of load–strain curves with repeated loadings of a tendon to successively higher loads (the curve of the next loading is shifted to the right) within the 'toe' region of the curve and before the linear part of the curve. This effect may be operating in chronic human Achilles tendinitis, especially in those athletes with a small cross-sectional area tendon. (Adapted from ref. 79, with permission.)

lar fatigue plasticity and elongation occurs in the tendon and that this causes the microruptures and repair nodules already described.

The notion that some distance-running athletes may not have an Achilles tendon of sufficient cross-sectional area to sustain the repetitive tendon loading without injury has been investigated by Engstrom et al.[81] In an elegant study they used ultrasound to measure the cross-sectional area of the human Achilles tendon in vivo, and validated this technique as a reliable method to measure the Achilles tendon cross-sectional area using cadaver Achilles tendons.

Here, two groups of distance athletes with and without grade I Achilles tendinitis who were matched for age, weight, and running distance, had their Achilles tendon cross-sectional area measured using the previously validated ultrasound technique. They demonstrated that athletes with grade 1 type Achilles tendinitis had about a 30 per cent decrease in the cross-sectional areas of their Achilles tendons ($p < 0.05$) (see Fig. 33). This indicates that a major mechanism in this type of common injury may simply be fatigue creep failure of Achilles tendon collagen as shown in Fig. 31. Komi et al.[82,83] have develped an in-vivo buckle tranducer which they placed around the Achilles tendon in a number of subjects. Direct force measurments were made on several subjects who were involved in slow walking, sprinting, jumping, and hopping after calibration of the transducer. During running and jumping, forces close to the previously estimated ultimate tensile strength of the tendon were recorded, indicating that fatigue creep in a small cross-sectional tendon is a possible mechanism of injury without the need to invoke other lower limb biomechanical pathology as has been suggested by Clement et al.[84] and Williams.[85]

Basic biomechanics of tissue injury

Muscle–tendon–bone injury

The basic causes of intrinsic muscle injury are still not entirely clear, but have been attributed to inadequate muscle length and strength (for example 'tight' hamstrings, especially in adolescent boys), muscle fatigue, as well as inadequate muscle skills. It is also clear that most muscle injuries occur in the lower limb and most involve the 'two-joint muscles' the hamstrings and the rectus femoris, probably because of the complex reflexes involved in simultaneous co-contraction and co-relaxation involved with these two muscle groups.[86] A recent review of current knowledge of muscle strain injuries is given by Garrett.[87]

Both concentric and eccentric muscle–tendon unit loading can cause muscle–tendon–bone junction injury. The use of eccentric muscle loading to cause increased muscle hypertrophy, as opposed to the use of more conventional concentric loading, has led to the phenomenon of eccentric muscle soreness which is now known to be due, in part, to muscle sarcomere disruption at the Z lines.[88] Eccentric muscle–tendon–bone load can generate more force than concentric contractions and may be the mechanism by which the patellar tendon and its attachments lead to tendoperiosteal partial disruptions at both the superior and inferior poles of the patellar. Studies by Chun et al.[89] demonstrated the inferomedial collagen fibre bundles of the human patellar tendon when subjected to mechanical analysis fail at loads which are much less than the lateral fibre bundles. The biological reasons for this are not clear at the moment, but it helps to explain the prevalence of inferomedial tenderness which is such a common cause of anteromedial knee pain or 'jumper's knee'.

The bone–tendon junction, or enthesis, is one of the commonest sites for tissue injury as is seen with the classic infrapatellar tendinitis which is so refractory to treatment. Benjamin et al.[7] have suggested that the zone of fibrocartilage at the enthesis minimizes local stress concentrations and appears to be characteristic of tendons and ligaments where there is a great change in angle between the tendon or ligament and bone during movement. It is of interest that

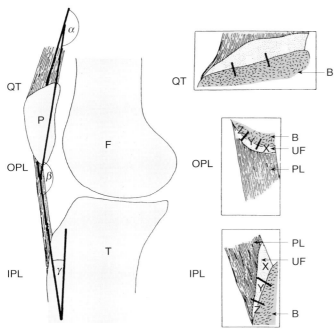

Fig. 32 The attachment zones studied are the insertion of the quadriceps (QT), the origin (OPL), and the insertion (IPL) of the patellar ligament. The angles between the long axis of tendon or ligament and bone are α, β, and γ. The change in these angles is quite large during knee motion. The subdivision of each attachment site into regions X,Y, Z and the major differences in the quantities and distribution of uncalcified fibrocartilage (UF) are illustrated diagrammatically in the drawings to the right of the figure. B, bone; F, femur; P, patellar ligament; T, tibia. (Reproduced from ref. 20, with permission.)

the enthesis which gives the most problems in the clinic (the inferior patellar pole and the patellar tendon) is the one with the least thickness of fibrocartilage (Fig. 32).[20] It is possible that a major mechanism of failure at this enthesis may be due to collagen-fibril shear at this critical highly loaded and very mobile enthesis.

Muscle–tendon junction

Failure at this junctional region is common clinically. There is an increased folding of the terminal end of the last muscle sarcomere, which has important mechanical implications for reducing the stress at this critical junctional region. With muscle injury at this junctional site it is probable that this complex sarcomere muscle membrane infolding to increase the surface area, and hence substantially decrease the stress, is probably not reproduced following repair and may be an explanation for the occurrence of 'retears' at this junction in athletes with previous injury and repair to this region. An excellent, recent, detailed comprehensive review is given by Noonan and Garrett.[90]

Tendon injury

Tendon injury in sport is not uncommon because of the large loads applied. Komi[82,83] has measured the high forces generated in the human Achilles tendon with the surgical introduction of a calibrated buckle transducer for short periods of time. Forces up to 4000 N were recorded in the Achilles tendon with toe running, indicating that it is not surprising that with repetitive loadings of

these magnitudes microfatigue failure could occur with long-distance running, especially in a tendon of small cross-sectional area (Fig. 33).[81] Recent studies by Hasselman *et al.*[91] indicate that the proximal tendon of the rectus femoris, which extends well distal into the muscle belly, can tear at this muscle–tendon junction and can appear as a midmuscle belly haematoma.

Recently, Wilson and Goodship[11] have demonstrated a rise in the core temperature of the equine superficial digital flexor tendon under galloping conditions to a mean peak temperature of 43.3 °C and a maximum of 45.4 °C in one animal. They suggest these core temperatures, or central tendon hyperthermia, are not survivable by tendon fibroblasts and may explain the central lesions seen in the equine superficial digital flexor tendon and also in the human Achilles tendon.

Spontaneous tendon rupture

Spontaneous tendon rupture is uncommon in the young athlete and usually occurs in the older sportsman, for example the long head of the biceps, and then is usually associated with degenerative pathology of the collagen fibrils although the biochemical detail has not been delineated.

Ligament/tendon repair

Acute inflammatory phase (see Figs 34 to 39)

The gap in the ligament/tendon is filled immediately with erthrocytes and inflammatory cells, especially polymorphonuclear leukocytes. Within 24 h monocytes and macrophages are the predominant cells and these actively engage in the phagocytosis of debris and necrotic cells. They are gradually replaced by fibroblasts, which may be from either intrinsic or extrinsic sources, and commence the initial deposition of the type III collagen scar. At this stage, the collagen concentration may be normal or slightly decreased but the total mass of ligament collagen scar is increased.

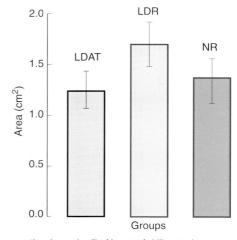

Fig. 33 Cross-sectional area (cm²) of human Achilles tendons measured by ultrasound for two running groups matched for age, weight, and distance compared with a sedentary control group (NR). LDAT, runners with grade I Achilles tendinitis; LDR, runners without Achilles tendinitis. The smaller cross-sectional area of the Achilles tendons in the LDAT group ($p < 0.05$) should be noted. (Reproduced with the permission of Professor A.W. Parker.)

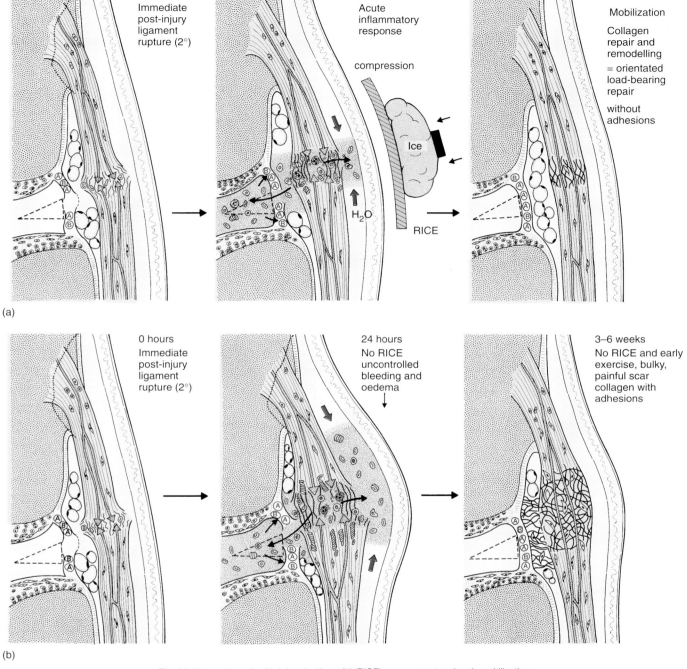

Fig. 34 Ligament repair with (a) and without (b) 'RICE' management and early mobilization.

Glycosaminoglycan content, water, fibronectin, and DNA content are increased (Figs 36 and 37).

Proliferation

Fibroblasts predominate. Water content remains increased and collagen content increases and peaks during this phase (3 to 6 weeks). Type I collagen now begins to predominate and glycosaminoglycan concentration remains high. The increasing amount of scar collagen and reducible crosslink profile has been correlated with the increas-ing tensile strength of the ligament matrix. Recent quantitative collagen-fibril orientation studies indicate that early mobilization of a ligament at this stage (within the first 3 weeks) may be detrimental to collagen orientation. After this time frame there is experimental evidence that mobilization increases the tensile strength of the repair and probably enhances this phase and the next phase of remodelling and maturation.[32,49,93]

With this basic biological knowledge there is now a rationale for the use of 'early controlled mobilization' of patients with ligament

MUSCLE INJURY

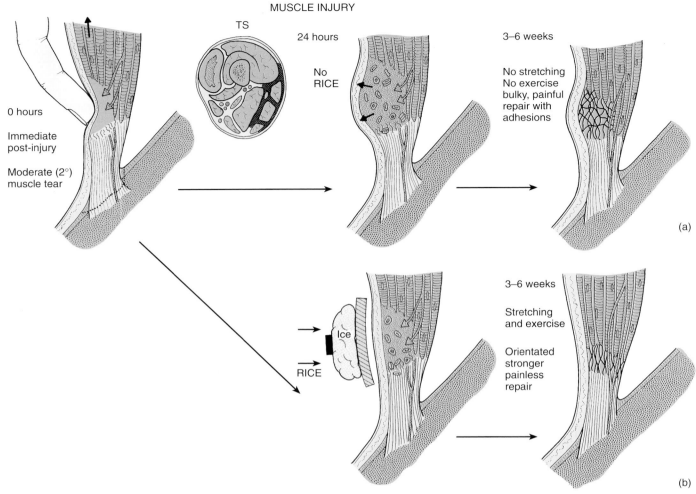

Fig. 35 Muscle repair at the muscle–tendon junction with and without 'RICE' and mobilization.

trauma. The use of a limited motion cast with an adjustable double-action hinge for the knee joint is now accepted and enhances more rapid repair and remodelling as well as preserving quadriceps muscle bulk. Patients are now usually mobilized in a limited motion cast at 3 weeks rather than the previously empirical time of 6 weeks.

Remodelling and maturation (6 weeks to 12 months)

There is a decreasing cell number and hence decreased collagen and glycosaminoglycan synthesis. Water content returns to normal and

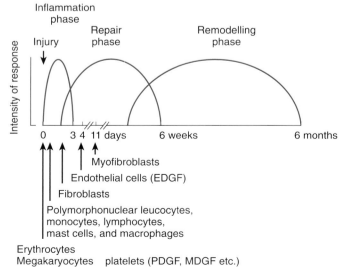

Fig. 36 The three phases of healing and the cells involved.

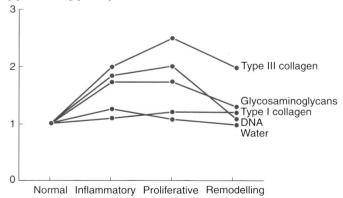

Fig. 37 Ligament repair during the phases of healing and the 'normalized' content of type I and III collagen, water, DNA, and glycosaminoglycans. (Reproduced from ref. 25, with permission.)

collagen concentration returns to slightly below normal, but total collagen content remains slightly increased. With further remodelling there is a trend for scar parameters to return to normal, but the matrix in the ligament scar region continues to mature slowly over months or even years. Scar collagen matrix and adjacent 'normal' matrix may actually shorten the repair region, perhaps by the interaction of ligament/tendon fibroblasts with their surrounding collagen matrix.[94] Collagen-fibril alignment in the longitudinal axis of the ligament occurs even though small-diameter fibrils are involved (see Fig. 38).

Occasionally, calcium apatite crystals will be deposited in the damaged tissues; the classic site for this to occur is in the rotator cuff supraspinatus attachment to the greater tuberosity of the humerus.

Achilles tendon and infrapatellar tendon injuries, especially partial tears, present a dilemma for the clinician in that they are aften intractable to management—although Stanish et al.[95] claim good clinical results from graded eccentric loading regimes for patellar tendinitis. The author has examined Achilles tendon biopsies of patients with chronic localized tears and more generalized thickened tender chronic Achilles tendons. The feature which characterized the pathology ultrastructurally was the persistence of small-diameter collagen fibrils. The large fibrils of the original tendon do not appear to be replaced in either a repairing tendon or ligament (see Fig. 30).

Anterior cruciate ligament injuries appear to be unique in that the chondrocyte-like cells in this special ligament apparently have a limited capacity to proliferate and synthesize a new collagen matrix, and hence repair appears to be limited. Collagenase release may also affect the effectiveness of the repair process.[62]

However, Ng et al.[54] have just completed a long-term biomechanical study of the repair of the goat anterior cruciate ligament after injury. The results are very interesting. To test the healing capacity of the partially torn anterior cruciate ligament, the posterolateral bundle in 11 adult female goats was completely transected. The repairing ligaments were tested at 12, 24, 52 weeks, and 3 years after surgery. As early as 12 weeks after surgery a translucent fibrous tissue covered the transected posterolateral bundle. The differences in the anteroposterior laxity between right and left knees measured at 45 degrees and 90 degrees of flexion were not significantly different at each time period. Results of Instron testing of the posterolateral bundle revealed normalized changes in load–relaxation and Young's modulus were also not significantly different at each time period, but the ultimate tensile strength and stiffness at 3 years were

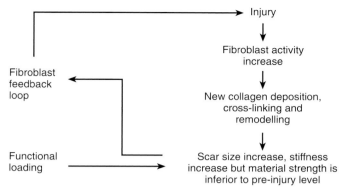

Fig. 39 The hypothetical feedback loop mechanism of the control of collagen deposition during ligament repair. (Reproduced from ref. 74, with permission.)

significantly higher than at 12 weeks ($p < 0.05$). Failure started at the repair site for the 12-week group, but at 24 and 52 weeks the failure occurred through the ligament. At 3 years, the posterolateral bundle specimens failed by bony avulsion, indicating that the repaired tissue was not the weakest link of the bone–ligament–bone complex.

This study shows that under the favourable biological conditions of this experiment, partial anterior cruciate ligament injuries in the goat are capable of adequate repair. What is more important, the high ultimate tensile strength and stiffness of the 3-year repaired tissue indicate that full structural repair of such an injury by artificial transection is possible (see Figs 13, 14, and 39).

References

1. Viidik A. Tendons and ligaments. In: Comper W, ed. *Extracellular matrix*. Amsterdam: Harwood Academic Publishers, 1996; **1**: 303–27.
2. Archambault JM, Wiley JP, Bray RC. Exercise loading of tendons and the development of overuse injuries. A review of the current literature. *Sports Medicine* 1995; **20**: 77–9.
3. Jackson DW, Arnoczky SP, Frank CB, Woo SL-Y, Simon TM, eds. *The anterior cruciate ligament. Current and future concepts.* New York: Raven Press, 1993.
4. Daniel DM, Akeson WH, O'Connor JJ. *Knee ligaments. Structure, function, injury and repair.* New York: Raven Press, 1990.
5. Benjamin M, Qin S, Ralphs JR. Fibrocartilage associated with human tendons and their pulleys. *Journal of Anatomy* 1995; **187**: 625–33.
6. Benjamin M, Raphs JR. Development and functional anatomy of tendons and ligaments. In: Gordon SL, Blair SJ, Fine LJ, eds. *Repetitive motion disorders of the upper extremity*. Rosemont: American Academy of Orthopaedic Surgeons, 1995: 185–203.
7. Benjamin M, Evans EJ, Copp L. The histology of tendon attachments in man. *Journal of Anatomy* 1986; **149**: 89–100.
8. Amiel D, Frank C, Harwood F, Fronek J, Akeson W. Tendons and ligaments: a morphological and biochemical comparison. *Journal of Orthopaedic Research* 1984; **1**: 257–65.
9. McNeilly CM, Banes AJ, Benjamin M, Ralphs JR. Tendon cells *in vivo* form a three dimensional network of cell processes linked by gap junctions. *Journal of Anatomy* 1996; **189**: 593–600.
10. Diamant J, Keller A, Baer E, Litt M, Arridge RGC. Collagen: ultrastructure and its relation to mechanical properties as a function of ageing. *Proceedings of the Royal Society of London (Biol.)* 1972; **180**: 293–315.

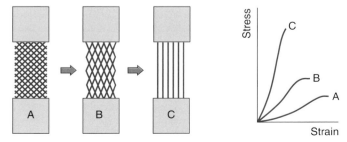

Fig. 38 The effect of collagen repair with identical fibrils but different geometry and the corresponding load–strain response to tensile testing. (Modified from ref. 92, with permission.)

11. Wilson AM, Goodship AE. Exercise induced hyperthermia as a possible mechanism for tendon degeneration. *Journal of Biomechanics* 1994; **27**: 899–905.

12. Proske U, Morgan D. Tendon stiffness: methods of measurement and significance for the control of movement. A review. *Journal of Biomechanics* 1987; **20**: 75–82.

13. Morgan DL, Proske U, Warren D. Measurements of muscle stiffness and the mechanism of elastic storage of energy in hopping kangaroos. *Journal of Physiology, London* 1978; **282**: 253–61.

14. Ker RF, Dimery NJ, Alexander R McN. The role of tendon elasticity in hopping in a wallaby. *Journal Zoology London (A)* 1986; **208**: 417–28.

15. Butler DL, Grood ES, Noyes FR, Zernicke RF. In: Hutton RS, ed. *Exercise and sports sciences reviews.* Franklin Institute Press, 1979; **6**: 125–81.

16. Oakes BW. Acute soft tissue injuries—nature and management. *Australian Family Physician* 1981; **10**: Suppl. 1–16.

17. Viidik A, Ekholm R. Light and electron microscopic studies of collagen fibres under strain. *Zeitschrift für Anatomie und Entwicklungsgeschichte* 1968; **127**: 154–64.

18. Kastelic J, Baer E. Deformation in tendon collagen. In: Vincent J, Currey J, eds. *The mechanical properties of biological molecules.* 1980: 397–435.

19. Knorzer E, Folkhard W, Geercken W, *et al.* New aspects of the aetiology of tendon rupture. An analysis of time-resolved dynamic-mechanical measurements. *Archives of Orthopaedic Trauma Surgery* 1986; **105**: 113–20.

20. Evans EJ, Benjamin M, Pemberton DJ. Fibrocartilage in the attachment zones of the quadriceps tendon and patellar ligament of man. *Journal of Anatomy* 1990; **171**: 155–62.

21. Benjamin M, Evans EJ. Fibrocartilage. A review. *Journal of Anatomy* 1990; **171**: 1–15.

22. Frowen P, Benjamin M. Variations in the quantity of uncalcified fibrocartilage at the insertions of the extrinsic calf muscles in the foot. *Journal of Anatomy* 1995; **186**: 417–21.

23. Rufai A, Ralphs JR, Benjamin M. Structure and histopathology of the insertional region of the human Achilles tendon. *Journal of Orthopaedic Research* 1995; **13**: 585–93.

24. Parry DAD, Barnes GRG, Craig AS. A comparison of the size distribution of collagen fibrils in connective tissues as a function of age and a possible relation between fibril size and distribution and mechanical properties. *Proceedings of the Royal Society of London, Ser. B* 1978; **203**: 305–21.

25. Oakes BW. Ultrastructural studies on knee joint ligaments: Quantitation of collagen fibre populations in exercised and control rat cruciate ligaments and in human anterior cruciate ligament grafts. In: Buckwalter J, Woo SL-Y, eds. *Injury and repair of the musculoskeletal tissues.* Illinois: American Academy of Orthopaedic Surgeons 1988; Section 2: 66–82.

26. Oakes BW, Parker AW, Norman J. Changes in collagen fibre populations in young rat cruciate ligaments in response to an intensive one month's exercise program. In: Russo P, Gass G, eds. *Human adaption.* Department of Biological Sciences, Cumberland College of Health Sciences, 1981: 223–30.

27. Matthew C, Moore MJ, Campbell L. A quantitative ultrastructural study of collagen fibril formation in the healing extensor digitorum longus tendon of the rat. *Journal of Hand Surgery* 1987; **12B**: 313–20.

28. Shadwick RE. The role of collagen crosslinks in the age related changes in mechanical properties of digital tendons. *Proceedings of the North American Congress of Biomechanics* 1986; **1**: 137–8.

29. Shadwick RE. Elastic energy storage in tendons: mechanical differences related to function and age. *Journal of Applied Physiology* 1990; **68**: 1033–40.

30. Singleton C, Oakes BW, Haut R. Honours thesis dissertation, Monash University, 1996.

31. Akeson WH, Amiel D, Abel MF, *et al.* Effects of immobilization on joints. *Clinical Orthopaedics and Related Research* 1987; **219**: 28–37.

32. Woo SL-Y, Gomez MA, Sites TJ, Newton PO, Orlando CA, Akeson WH. The biomechanical and morphological changes in the medial collateral ligament of the rabbit after immobilization and remobilization. *Journal of Bone and Joint Surgery* 1987; **69A**: 1200–11.

33. Noyes FR, Torvic PJ, Hyde WB, De Lucas JL. Biomechanics of ligament failure. 2 An analysis of immobilization, exercise and reconditioning effects in primates. *Journal of Bone and Joint Surgery* 1974; **56A**: 1406–18.

34. Amiel D, Akeson WH, Harwood FL, Frank CB. Stress deprivation effect on the metabolic turnover of the medial collateral ligament collagen: a comparison between nine and 12–week immobilization. *Clinical Orthopaedics and Related Research* 1983; **172**: 265–70.

35. Amiel D, Frey C, Woo SL-Y, Harwood F, Akeson W. Value of hyaluronic acid in the prevention of contracture formation. *Clinical Orthopaedics and Related Research* 1985; **196**: 306–11.

36. Tipton CM, James SL, Mergner W, Tcheng TK. Influence of exercise on the strength of the medial collateral knee ligament of dogs. *American Journal of Physiology* 1970; **218**: 894–902.

37. Binkley JM, Peat M. The effects of immobilization on the ultrastructure and mechanical properties of the medial collateral ligament of rats. *Clinical Orthopaedics and Related Research* 1986; **203**: 301–8.

38. Tipton CM, Vailas AC. Bone and connective tissue adaptions to physical activity. *Proceedings International Conference on Exercise, Fitness and Health. Toronto, 1988.* Champaign, IL: Human Kinetics, 1989: 331–44.

39. Tipton CM, Vailas AC, Matthes RD. Experimental studies on the influences of physical activity on ligaments, tendons and joints: A brief review. *Acta Medica Scandinavica* 1986; **711** (Suppl.): 157–68.

40. Parker AW, Larsen N. Changes in the strength of bone and ligament in response to training. In: Russo P, Gass G, eds. *Human adaption.* Department of Biological Sciences, Cumberland College of Health Sciences, 1981: 209–21.

41. Tipton CM, Matthes RD, Maynard JA, Carey RA. The influence of physical activity on ligaments and tendons. *Medicine and Science in Sports* 1975; **7**: 165–75.

42. Cabaud HE, Feagin JF, Rodkey WG. Acute anterior cruciate ligament injury and augmented repair: experimental studies. *American Journal of Sports Medicine* 1980; **8**: 79–86.

43. Larsen N, Parker AW. Sports medicine: medical and scientific aspects of elitism in sport. Vol. 8. Howell ML, Parker AW, eds. *Proceedings of the Australian Sports Medicine Federation* 1982; 63–73.

44. Michna M. Morphometric analysis of loading-induced changes in collagen-fibril populations in young tendons. *Cell and Tissue Research* 1984; **236**: 465–70.

45. Toole BP, Lowther DA. The effect of chondroitin sulphate–protein on the formation of collagen fibrils *in vitro. Biochemical Journal* 1968; **109**: 857–66.

46. Parry DAD, Flint MH, Gillard GC, Craig AS. A role for glycosaminoglycans in the development of collagen fibrils. *FEBS Letters* 1982; **149**: 1–7.

47. Merrilies MJ, Flint MH. Ultrastructural study of the tension and pressure zones in a rabbit flexor tendon. *American Journal of Anatomy* 1980; **157**: 87–106.

48. Piper TL, Whiteside LA. Early mobilization after knee ligament repair in dogs: an experimental study. *Clinical Orthopaedics and Related Research* 1980; **50**: 277–82.

49. Vailas AC, Tipton CM, Matthes RD, Gart M. Physical activity

and its influence on the repair process of medial collateral ligaments. *Connective Tissue Research* 1981; **9**: 25–31.

50. Amiel D, Frank CB, Harwood FL, Akeson WH, Kleiner JB. Collagen alteration in medial collateral ligament healing in a rabbit model. *Connective Tissue Research* 1987; **16**: 357–66.

51. Chaudhuri S, Nguyen H, Rangayyan RM, Walsh S, Frank CB. A Fourier domain directional filtering method for analysis of collagen alignment in ligaments. *IEEE Transactions of Biomedical Engineering* 1987; **34**: 509–18.

52. MacFarlane BJ, Edwards P, Frank CB, Rangayyan RM, Liu Z-Q. Quantification of collagen remodelling in healing nonimmobilized and immobilized ligaments. *Transactions of the Orthopaedic Research Society* 1989; **14**: 300.

53. Frank C, MacFarlane B, Edwards P, Rangayyan R, Liu Z-Q, Walsh S, Bray R. A quantitative analysis of matrix alignment in ligament scars: a comparison of movement versus immobilization in an immature rabbit model. *Journal of Orthopaedic Research* 1991; **9**: 219–27.

54. Ng GY, Oakes BW, Deacon OD, McLean ID, Lampard D. The long-term biomechanical and viscoelastic performance of repairing anterior cruciate ligament after hemitransection injury in a goat model. *American Journal Sports Medicine* 1996; **24**: 109–17.

55. Grontvedt T, *et al.* A prospective randomized study of three operations for acute rupture of the anterior cruciate ligament. *Journal of Bone and Joint Surgery* 1996; **78-A**: 159–68.

56. Oakes BW. Collagen ultrastructure in the normal ACL and in ACL graft. In: Jackson D., *et al.*, eds. *The anterior cruciate ligament: current and future concepts.* New York: Raven Press, 1993: 209–17.

57. Deacon OW, McLean ID, Oakes BW, Cole WG, Chan D, Knight M. Ultrastructural and collagen typing analyses of autogenous ACL grafts—an update. *Proceedings of the International Knee Society,* May, 1991, Toronto.

58. Chan D, Cole W. *Analytical Biochemistry* 1984; **139**: 322–8.

59. Butler DL, Kay MD, Stouffer DC. Comparison of material properties in fascicle–bone units from human patellar tendon and knee ligaments. *Journal of Biomechanics* 1985; **18**: 1–8.

60. Clancy WG, Narechania RG, Rosenberg TD, Gmeiner JG, Wisnefske DD, Lange TA. Anterior and posterior cruciate reconstruction in Rhesus monkeys: an histological microangiographic and biochemical analysis. *Journal of Bone and Joint Surgery* 1981; **63A**: 1270–84.

61. Arnoczky SP, Warren RF, Ashlock MA. Replacement of the anterior cruciate ligament by an allograft. *Journal of Bone and Joint Surgery* 1986; **63A**: 376–85.

62. Amiel D, Ishizue KK, Harwood FL, Kitayashi L, Akeson W. Injury of the anterior cruciate ligament: the role of collagenase in ligament degeneration. *Journal of Orthopaedic Research* 1989; **7**: 486–93.

63. Shino K, Oakes BW, Inoue M, Horibe S, Nakata K, Ono, K. Human ACL allograft: collagen fibril populations studied as a function of age of the graft. *Transactions of the Annual Meeting of the Orthopaedic Research Society* 1990; **15**: 520.

64. Shino K, Oakes BW, Inoue M, Horibe S, Nakata. K. Human ACL allografts. An electronmicroscopic analysis of collagen fibril populations. *Proceedings of International Society of the Knee,* May 1991, Toronto.

65. Shino K, Oakes BW, Horibe S, Nakata K, Nakamura, N. Human anterior cruciate ligament allografts. An electron microscopic analysis on collagen fibril populations. *American Journal of Sports Medicine* 1995; **23**: 203–9.

66. Shino K, Kawasaki T, Hirose H, Gotoh I, Inoue M, Ono K. Replacement of the anterior cruciate ligament by an allograft. *Journal of Bone and Joint Surgery* 1984; **66B**: 672–81.

67. Scott JE. Proteoglycan: collagen interactions and subfibrillar structure in collagen fibrils. Implications in the development and ageing of connective tissues. *Journal of Anatomy* 1990; **169**: 23–35.

68. Leonardi L, Ruggeri A, Roveri N, Bigi A, Reale E. Light microscopy, electron microscopy and X-ray diffraction analysis of glycerinated collagen fibrils. *Journal of Ultrastructure Research* 1983; **85**: 228–37.

69. Klein L, Lunseth PA, Aadalen R. Comparison of functional and non-functional tendon grafts. Isotopic turnover and mass. *Journal of Bone and Joint Surgery* 1972; **54A**: 1745–53.

70. Frank C, Woo SL-Y, Amiel D, Gomez MA, Harwood FL, Akeson WH. Medial collateral ligament healing: a multidisciplinary assessment in rabbits. *American Journal of Sports Medicine* 1983; **11**: 379–89.

71. Woo SL-Y, Inoue M, McGurk-Burleson E, Gomez MA. Treatment of the medial collateral ligament injury. II: Structure and function of canine knees in response to differing treatment regimes. *American Journal of Sports Medicine* 1987; **15**: 22–9.

72. Butler DL, Grood ES, Noyes FR, *et al.* Mechanical properties of primate vascularized vs. nonvascularized patellar tendon grafts; changes over time. *Journal of Orthopaedic Research* 1987; **7**: 68–79.

73. Oakes BW, Knight M, McLean ID, Deacon OW. Goat ACL autograft remodeling—quantitative collagen fibrils analyses over 1 year. *Transactions of the Combined Meeting of the Orthopaedic Research Societies of USA, Japan and Canada.* Banff, Alberta, Canada, October 1991: 60.

74. Ng GY, Oakes BW, Deacon OD, McLean ID, Lampard D. Biomechanics of patellar tendon autograft for reconstruction of anterior cruciate ligament in the goat. *Journal of Orthopaedic Research* 1995; **13**: 602–8.

75. Ng YF, Oakes BW, Deacon OD, McLean ID, Eyre DR. Long-term study of the biochemistry and biomechanics of anterior cruciate ligament–patellar tendon autografts in goats. *Journal of Orthopaedic Research* 1996; **14**: 851–6.

76. Ng GY, Oakes BW, Deacon OD, McLean ID, Eyre DR. A three year correlation study of hydroxypyridinium cross-link density with Young's modulus of ACL–PT autograft in goats. *Transactions of the Combined Orthopaedic Research Societies Meeting, USA, Canada, and Japan.* San Diego, USA, 1995: 98.

77. Frank CB, Eyre DR, Shrive NG. Hydroxypyridinium cross-link deficiency in ligament scar. *Transactions of the Orthopaedic Research Society* 1994; **19**: 13.

78. Walker J. Deep transverse frictions in ligament healing. *Journal of Orthopaedic and Sports Physical Therapy* 1984; **6**: 89–94.

79. Viidik A. Functional properties of connective tissues. *International Review of Connective Tissue Research* 1973; **6**: 127–215.

80. Weisman G, Pope MH, Johnson RJ. Cyclical loading in knee ligament injuries. *American Journal of Sports Medicine* 1980; **8**: 24–30.

81. Engstrom CM, Hampson BA, Williams J, Parker AW. Muscle–tendon relations in runners. (Abstract) *Proceedings of the Australian Sports Medicine Federation National Conference.* Ballarat, 1985: 56.

82. Komi PV, Salonen M, Jarvinen M, Kokko O. *In vivo* registration of achilles tendon forces in man. Methodological development. *International Journal of Sports Medicine* 1987; **8**: 3–8.

83. Komi PV. Neuromuscular factors related to physical performance. In: Russo P, Balnave R, eds. Muscle and nerve, factors affecting performance. *Proceedings of the 6th Biennial Conference, Cumberland College of Health Sciences,* 1987

84. Clement DB, Taunton JE, Smart GW. Achilles tendinitis and peritendinitis: aetiology and treatment. *American Journal of Sports Medicine* 1984; **12**: 179–84.

85. Williams JGP. Achilles tendon lesions in sport. *Sports Medicine* 1986; **3**: 114–35.

86. Oakes BW. Hamstring injuries. *Australian Family Physician* 1984; **13**: 587–91.

87. Garrett WE. Muscle strain injuries. *American Journal of Sports Medicine* 1996; **24**: S-2–S-8.

88. Friden J, Sjostrom M, Ekblom, B. Myofibrillar damage following intense eccentric exercise in man. *International Journal of Sports Medicine* 1983; **4**: 170–6.

89. Chun KJ, Butler DB, Bukovec MJ, *et al*. Spatial variation in material properties in fascicle–bone units from human patellar tendon. *Transactions of the Orthopaedic Research Society* 1989; **14**: 214.

90. Noonan TJ, Garrett WE. Injuries at the myotendinous junction. *Clinics in Sports Medicine* 1992, **11**: 783–806.

91. Hasselman CT, Best TM, Hughes C, Martinez S, Garrett WE. An explanation for the various rectus femoris strain injuries using previously undescribed muscle architecture. *American Journal of Sports Medicine* 1995; **23**: 493–9.

92. Viidik A. Interdependence between structure and function. In: Viidik A, Vuust J, eds. *Biology of collagen*. London: Academic Press, 1980: 257–80.

93. Hart DP, Danhers LE. Healing of the medial collateral ligament in rats. *Journal of Bone and Joint Surgery* 1987; **69A**: 1194–9.

94. Danhers LE, Banes AJ, Burridge KW. The relationship of actin to ligament contraction. *Clinical Orthopaedics and Related Research* 1986; **210**: 246–51.

95. Stanish W, Rubinovich RM, Curwin S. Eccentric exercise in chronic Achilles tendinitis. *Clinical Orthopaedics and Related Research* 1986; **208**: 65–8.

4.4.4 The aetiology and treatment of tendinitis

Sandra L. Curwin

Introduction

The treatment of tendinitis is a challenge. Insidious onset, slow healing, and unknown pathology make it difficult to devise a scientific treatment plan. Little is known about the physiology of tendon itself, since most research involves ligament injuries and their recovery, yet tendon injuries are more common clinically. Tendons transmit the forces generated by muscles to bony attachments, and are found at the ends of virtually all muscles. Most tendons are small in cross-sectional area, but are tremendously strong—perhaps half as strong as steel. It is said that they are rarely loaded to greater than 25 per cent of their maximum strength. Why, then, are tendons injured at all? Accidents such as severing flexor tendons in the hand may be difficult to avoid, but the recovery pattern and treatment strategy for such injuries is fairly well defined. Far more common, clinically, is the gradual onset of pain and tenderness that eventually alerts the athlete to a lesser tendon injury—tendinitis. There is no clearly defined starting point for this injury, and so the stage of healing and state of the tissue can never be known with certainty by the clinician. Small wonder that this 'simple' overuse injury can cause prolonged disability for the competitive athlete, and a dilemma for both athletes and care providers. How seriously injured is the tendon? What is its mechanical state? Is it safe for the athlete to continue participating in sports? What is the nature of the tendon injury, is it healing? How can mobility and strength be best maintained without hindering healing? Do tendons adapt physiologically to their environment, and if so, how fast? Can tendons respond to changes in loading? How? What type of, and how much exercise is beneficial? When should it be started? Can exercise be used to prevent tendinitis? There are no definitive answers to many of these questions, but there are many opinions.

The purpose of this chapter is to describe the physiology and mechanics of normal and injured tendon, and to show how we can use our knowledge of tendon behaviour to successfully treat tendinitis. However, this knowledge alone will not bring success in treating difficult cases of tendinitis. In such cases, a keen understanding of anatomy, joint mechanics, and movement patterns is also required for a differential diagnosis. Understanding the mechanics of movement exposes the cause of, and thus the solution to, the problem. A treatment plan can then be tailored to the patient, and improvement or resolution of symptoms should occur in 6 to 8 weeks, often with little direct surgical intervention by the clinician.

Structure and function

Structure of the tendon and its components

Tendons and ligaments are 'dense, parallel-fibred connective tissues'. In some respects, they resemble each other: both are composed of cells (fibroblasts) and matrix (proteoglycans and water), and unlike most other tissues, their properties are determined not by their cell content but by their extracellular components. However, many differences exist between ligaments and tendons; indeed, the fine-structure details of tendons themselves may vary among species and even between different tendons in the same animal.[1–3]

Tendon junctions with muscle and bone

Tendons are found interspersed between muscle and bone. Both ends of the muscle have a tendinous insertion that is similar in composition but different in gross morphology. The distal tendon is usually much larger and better developed and is rope-like in structure, while at the proximal end of the muscle the tendon comprises much shorter, smaller fibres and often has a fleshy attachment that blends directly into bone. The bone–tendon junction shows a gradual transition from tendon to fibrocartilage to mineralized fibrocartilage to bone (see Fig. 1).[4]

The myotendinous junction is a layered region of infoldings connecting the actin filament of a terminal sarcomere to tendon collagen fibres.[5,6] The infoldings increase the surface area, resulting in junctions that are loaded in shear, where force is largely parallel to

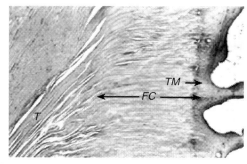

Fig. 1 Light microscopy picture of the bone–tendon junction, showing the transition from tendon (*T*) to fibrocartilage (*FC*) to mineralized fibrocartilage (*TM*) to bone (*B*). (Reprinted from ref. 4 with permission.)

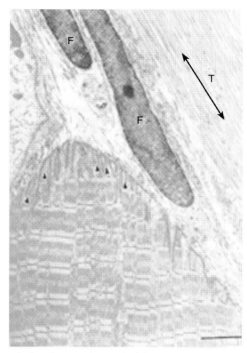

Fig. 2 Transmission electron micrograph of the muscle–tendon junction, illustrating the infoldings of the muscle cell membrane (arrowheads) and loose connective tissue containing fibroblasts (F) near the cell surface. Dense tendon material (T) runs nearby at an oblique angle to the muscle fibre. Bar = 3.0 µm. (Reprinted from ref. 6, with permission.)

the membrane surface.[5] The geometry and configuration of these attachments is illustrated in Fig. 2.

Tissue components

Tendons are composed primarily of collagen and other proteins, glycosaminoglycans, elastin, glycolipids, cells (fibroblasts), and water.[7-9]. Extracellular elements of the tendon are synthesized inside the fibroblasts, where a variety of influences can alter the amount and type of each component.[10] Collagen is actually a family of molecules divided into two major groups: the fibre-forming collagens (types I, II, III, V, XI) and other collagen types which do not form regular fibres (IV, VI, VII, VIII, IX, X, XII, XIII).[11] Different tissues contain different types of collagen, and this partially determines the organization and mechanical behaviour of these tissues. For example, type II collagen is typically found only in cartilage, skin contains a large amount of type III collagen, and the collagen in tendons is mainly type I. Type I collagen is the major load-bearing component in dense connective tissues such as ligament and tendon,[12] and comprises 70 per cent to 80 per cent of their dry weight after all water is removed. These tissues can be used to explore the mechanical properties of this collagen.

Connective tissues, including tendon, also contain a so-called ground substance, a mixture of water and glycosaminoglycan (GAG) compounds that surrounds the collagen fibrils. The ground substance provides frictional adherence between collagen fibrils, yet also provides lubrication and spacing so that fibrils can slide past one another.[7,13] The GAGs, double sugar-type molecules, form only about 1 per cent of the tissue dry weight, but are important because they bind water, which forms 65 per cent to 75 per cent of the total weight of the tendon. GAGs may combine with each other to form long chains, or with a protein core to form proteoglycans.[8,14] Tendon and cartilage proteoglycans are similar in composition, but differ greatly in size. Proteoglycans found in cartilage, or areas of tendon subjected to compression, are much larger than those found throughout most tendons.[14] It seems that proteoglycans play a role in directing and limiting the organization of collagen into fibrils.[9,14,15] Generally, tissues with large amounts of GAGs or proteoglycans contain small-diameter collagen fibrils, and have lower tensile strengths.

Crosslinks

Unlike most proteins, which are 'processed' inside the cells that produce them and remain largely unchanged after leaving the cell, collagen undergoes a number of extracellular modifications that contribute to its function. These changes include crosslinking between molecules and organization into a fibrillar structure that gives collagen its unique load-bearing properties.[16,17] Crosslinking between and within collagen molecules prevents their enzymatic, mechanical, or chemical breakdown, and helps direct the organization of collagen molecules into fibrillar structures.[18] Intramolecular, or reducible, crosslinks are formed within the cell between adjacent amino-acid strands of the triple-helical molecule, and are basically enzyme-facilitated chemical rearrangements of adjacent amino acids. Intermolecular crosslinks form slowly outside the cell, link two or more adjacent molecules, and give the tendon its ability to withstand high levels of tensile force.[11,19] A defect in the number or quality of crosslinks can lead to flaws in connective-tissue mechanical behaviour. In genetic disorders, such as some forms of the Ehler–Danlos syndrome,[20] decreased crosslinking results in weaker tissues that elongate readily when force is applied. The reverse, increased crosslinking, is more likely to occur in diabetic patients, resulting in stiffer tissues that require more force to stretch.[21] This may explain why adhesive capsulitis is up to ten times more prevalent in diabetic patients compared with age-matched control subjects. Similar crosslinking changes take place in joint capsules during immobilization, leading to decreased joint range of motion and increased resistance to movement.[22-25]

Collagen fibrils

Collagen molecules continue to aggregate after leaving the fibroblast,[10,26] but the exact nature of their organization is uncertain. The organization probably varies among tissues. Collagen molecules (tropocollagen) first assemble in groups of five (microfibrils), the molecules overlapped in a head-to-tail fashion dictated by crosslinking ability and by the type and amount of GAGs already present.[3,7,15] Each microfibril is about 4 nm wide. A variable number of microfibrils associate to form collagen fibrils ranging from 30 to 400 nm in diameter, it is at these levels that intermolecular crosslinking occurs.[7,9,22] The molecules become capable of resisting load only after assembling into fibrillar structures.[27] Tissue strength is closely correlated with collagen content, but this collagen must be organized and crosslinked before it can function as a load-bearing unit.[25] The ground substance modifies the organization of collagen in the tissue, both directing and somehow limiting fibril organization.[7,8,9,15] New microfibrils may be added to existing nearby fibrils, thus increasing their size, or they may associate to form new fibrils which are typically much smaller in diameter than the older

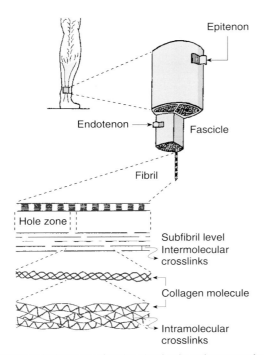

Fig. 3 The hierarchial structure of tendon, showing the various stages from tendon to molecule, and illustrating the location of the intramolecular and intermolecular crosslinks. (Redrawn from ref. 29, with permission.)

fibrils.[13,26] Fibroblasts, squeezed between the growing fibrils, end up as columns of flattened, spindle-shaped cells with thin cytoplasmic processes extending among the fibrils. The strongest tendons contain large numbers of large diameter fibrils. These are generally the oldest fibrils, which also contain the largest numbers of mature crosslinks.[13,27] The space between fibrils is usually too large to allow crosslinking between the collagen molecules of adjacent fibrils, although this may sometimes occur during immobilization.[23,24] The interfibrillar matrix (ground substance) probably plays the greatest role in adhesion between collagen fibrils.[12] Groups of fibrils are surrounded by a loose connective-tissue sheath called the endotenon, which also encloses the nerves, lymphatics, and blood vessels supplying the tendon, to form a fascicle (secondary bundle).[3,28] Fascicles are considered to be the smallest functional load-bearing units within the tendon, and individual fascicles are associated with discrete groups of muscle fibres (or motor units) at muscle–tendon junctions.[5,6] Several fascicles may form a larger group (tertiary bundle) also surrounded by endotenon, while enveloping all the secondary bundles and their endotenon coverings is another sheath, the epitenon. The sheaths may be differentiated by their location and also by their collagen type content. The endotenon contains more type III collagen, organized as small diameter fibrils, while the epitenon, which is largely type I, contains larger diameter fibrils.[3] An additional double-layered sheath of areolar tissue, the peritenon or paratenon, is loosely attached to the outer surface of the epitenon. The peritenon may become a synovial fluid-filled sheath, the tenosynovium, in tendons that are subjected to friction. A simplified version of the hierarchical organization of the tendon is illustrated in Fig. 3.[29] There is some evidence to suggest that the organization may vary from place to place within the tendon, which may explain why there is no universally accepted model of tendon organization.

Mechanical behaviour of the tendon—principles

The organization of the tendon determines its mechanical behaviour. The ground substance 'shrinks' the resting tendon, causing it to have a slightly crimped, or wavelike, appearance.[1,2] The crimp can be straightened easily by the application of a load, but the tendon will immediately recover its original resting length if the load is removed. Little force is required to straighten the crimp, while length changes rapidly—the 'toe' region in the force–elongation curve (see Fig. 4). As the crimped fibrils lose their wavelike appearance, little or no physical deformation of the collagen fibrils themselves takes place.[1,3]

Force application beyond the toe region (2 per cent to 4 per cent elongation) directly loads the collagen fibrils, and there is a linear relationship between applied force and tissue deformation.[30,31] Collagen fibrils dictate the mechanical behaviour of this part of the stress–strain curve, so differences in the slope of the linear region may be interpreted to reflect differences in collagen concentration (or type) and/or crosslinking. As loading continues, sliding between molecules occurs, then slipping between fibrils, and finally gross disruption of the collagen fibrils/fibres themselves.[30,32] As the first fibrils rupture, the force curve plateaus, then drops off rapidly as the remaining fibrils successively fail. Mechanical failure usually occurs at about 8 to 10 per cent elongation from the starting length.[33] Increased crosslinking reduces intrafibrillar slipping among and between collagen molecules.

Tendinitis probably results from repeated loading into the higher linear region of the stress–strain curve. Although the tendon may appear to be physically intact, the collapse of lateral cohesion between collagen fibrils may cause a reduction in tensile strength greater than that suggested by the number of torn fibrils or fibres observed on tissue examination.[31] This is analogous to injuries to the anterior cruciate ligament where the ligament may appear visually near-normal, but is incompetent mechanically. Such tendon damage can occur not only during tissue loading but also during rapid unloading, perhaps as a result of shearing within the tendon.[30] This may help to explain why both sudden or unexpected force application and release are often associated with tendinitis.

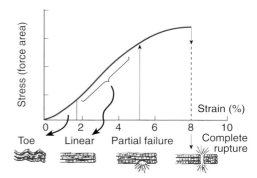

Fig. 4 Stress–strain curve for tendon loaded to failure, showing the regions of the stress–strain curve and the physical states of the tendon. The collagen fibrils, crimped in their resting state, straighten as force is applied, then the collagen fibres are stretched in the linear region of the curve. The slope of the linear region depends on the concentration, organization, and crosslinking of the collagen molecules. At the end of the linear region, some fibres rupture, the remainder will rapidly fail if load continues to be applied.

The breaking strength of the tendon, that is to say the magnitude of the force applied when the tendon ruptures, has historically been used to assess the tensile strength of the tendon,[1] but it probably has little relevance to clinical cases of tendinitis. Tendons rarely rupture under normal loading conditions unless previously injured or diseased,[34] presumably they are seldom loaded *in vivo* to the maximum levels used to rupture tendons in laboratory testing.[2] The tendon probably functions in the toe and linear regions under physiological loading conditions, suggesting that the slope of the linear portion of the curve ($\Delta F/\Delta L$), the stiffness, may be a better indicator of the tendon's *in vivo* mechanical behaviour.[33] Understanding the physical changes occurring in the linear region of the stress–strain curve may be more important in explaining the tissue damage that occurs during tendinitis than is a knowledge of the maximum load the tendon can tolerate before breaking.[35]

The functional mechanical behaviour of tendon, in the normal anatomical setting, can be influenced by a number of factors:

- size
- length
- amount and type of collagen concentration
- amount and type of crosslinks.

While all these factors can affect the force–elongation curve, only changes in the composition of the tendon itself will alter the stress–strain curve, since it is independent of both size and length. Size-dependent features are referred to as the structural properties of the tendon,[1] while features related to tendon composition are called material properties. Changes in either structural or material properties (or both) can affect a tendon's functional mechanical ability, but reflect inherently different methods of adaptation. An increase in tendon size or length can mean simply the production of more tendon by the existing cellular components (like muscle hypertrophy), while a change in collagen concentration or type, or different crosslinking patterns, suggests a more fundamental change in the synthetic pattern of the cell or a change in extracellular processing events such as crosslinking.

Mechanical behaviour of tendon—results of testing and indirect calculations

It has been estimated that the tensile strength of a tendon is about four times the maximum force produced by its attached muscle, and that tendons *in vivo* are rarely stressed to more than 25 per cent of their maximum physiological strength.[2] Estimates of tendon strength have usually been extrapolated from *in vitro* testing, because it is difficult to obtain direct measures of *in vivo* stress–strain behaviour. Studies using transducers implanted on animal tendons showed that tendons were only strained within the toe region of the stress–strain curve during normal daily activities such as walking and trotting.[36] These data make it difficult to see why tendons would be injured during activities, with such a large margin between physiological and maximum loading. Could it be that physiological animal loads are not representative of the loads to which humans are willing to subject their tendons during athletic activities?

Table 1 Forces on tendon during activities		
Activity	**Tendon**	**Force (N)**
Running (slow)	Achilles	4000–5000
Running (fast)	Achilles	8000–9000
Walking	Achilles	1000–3000
Push-off	Achilles	4000
Running (fast)	Patellar	7500–9000
Walking	Patellar	500
Kicking	Patellar	5000
Jumping (take-off)	Patellar	2500
Jumping (landing)	Patellar	8000

Data on human tendon loading have usually been acquired through indirect calculations based on biomechanical models. Barfred estimated maximum Achilles tendon forces of about 4340 N in a person who, while running, suddenly changed direction and ruptured his Achilles tendon, an ordinary push-off (change from backward to forward motion) produced about 2000 N.[37] Data obtained from the *in vitro* testing of human tendons have shown maximum tensile strengths of about 4000 N, so Barfred's data suggests that tendons may be loaded maximally during activities.[17] This author has estimated Achilles tendon forces from 2000 to 5000 N in activities such as running and jumping, and other force estimates suggest that tendons may often be loaded to more than 4000 N during athletic activities (see Table 1).[38] The direct measurement of human tendon forces is rare. However, one example is provided by Gregor and Komi, who placed buckle transducers on the Achilles tendon of volunteers (including themselves!) and recorded forces in the range of 5000 to 6000 N during cycling and running,[39] again suggesting that tendons can be subjected to large loads under daily conditions. Confusion about whether tendons are exposed to potentially damaging forces during activity may arise from the definition of what is considered to be 'physiological loading'. Forces experienced during walking and light exercise (physiological activities for most people) may only be 20 to 30 per cent of those observed during vigorous exercises, yet the latter are physiological for most athletes. From these data, we might even gather that tendons are actually injured far less often than could be expected given their frequent exposure to potentially damaging loads.

Effects of exercise and disuse

The effects of disuse and immobilization on tissues such as muscle, ligament, joint capsule, and tendon have been well established.[22-24,40-46] All musculoskeletal tissues atrophy under conditions of decreased load. In tendon, both collagen and crosslink concentration decline, and the tissues become weaker both structurally and materially.[25] These findings have led to the use of early motion and gradual stress application to treat many hard- and soft-tissue injuries.[47-51]

Normal and healing tendons adapt to increased loads either structurally, by becoming larger and hypertrophying as does muscle,

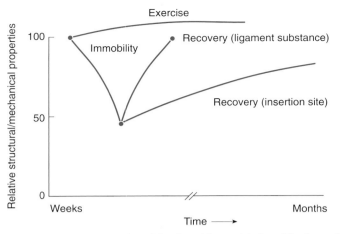

Fig. 5 Regional responses of medial collateral ligament to immobilization and exercise. The insertion sites recover much more slowly than the midsubstance of the ligament. If tendon behaves in the same way, this may help to explain why chronic tendinitis so often occurs at tendon junctions with muscle or bone. (Redrawn from ref. 60, with permission.)

or by changing their material properties to become stronger per unit area.[52,53] Almost all musculoskeletal tissues respond to increased load with an increase in tensile strength.[1,52,53] Muscle rapidly hypertrophies under increased load conditions, and may also increase its connective tissue content.[54] Other connective tissues behave in a similar fashion.[55-59] Different regions of ligaments respond differently to immobilization and recovery (Fig. 5).[60] Junctional areas of ligaments respond more rapidly to immobilization than the midsubstance, but recover more slowly. If tendons behave in the same way, it may help to explain why tendinitis often occurs at bone–tendon junctions.

Activities such as running and jumping can stress tendons to large percentages of the theoretical maximum for mammalian tendon (see Table 1).[38,61] The association of tendinitis or tendon rupture with particular sports, such as badminton (Achilles tendon rupture), implies that the high demands placed on tissues during movements in sports and dance may cause injury.[61-66] The incidence of tendon injuries after sudden increases in the amount of training, or when training is resumed unchanged after a period of inactivity, suggests that the tendon is being subjected to loads which exceed its tensile strength and thus damage the tendon.

Some athletes, though, appear to develop tendinitis while training at the same level of intensity (same magnitude of loading). It is hard to imagine why loads previously well tolerated by the tendon should now produce an injury. Such occurrences suggest that the relationship between training intensity, load, and tendon physiology is more complex than previously thought. Perhaps not all types of exercise have the same effect on tendon? There is evidence to suggest that the amount and pattern of crosslinking in chicken Achilles tendon may be increased with chronically increased loads, but decreased by an intermittent, strenuous running programme, even though the latter would be expected to load the Achilles tendon and has often been used experimentally as a model of increased tendon loading (see Fig. 6).[67,68] There may be other factors capable of inducing changes in the tendon such that previously safe levels of loading are now capable of damaging the tendon, or time itself may be a major influence. Recent animal studies suggest that even low-

force physiological loads are capable of inducing tendinitis if repeated over a prolonged period.[69,70]

Tendon injury

The injured tendon

The most basic principle in the aetiology of tendinitis seems to be that the tendon is exposed to forces which cause damage to the tendon.[61,63,71] Either the forces are too large for the tendon to safely withstand, or the tendon has changed so that 'normal' forces are now causing injury. There are two possible solutions: (1) reduce the force applied to the tendon; or (2) change the tendon or its environment so that the same forces are not harmful. The nature of the actual damage may depend upon the type of force (compressive versus tensile) as well as its magnitude and pattern of application, and each of these factors must be evaluated.

Type of force

Tendon may be subjected to compressive, tensile, or shear force, but is best suited to withstand tensile forces. If abnormal compressive forces are applied to a tendon, it may develop a so-called 'extrinsic' tendinitis.[47,71] The compression may come from an article worn by the patient, for example, tight laces in a high-top shoe or skate may cause tenosynovitis of the extensor tendons at the ankle joint, or the patient's own anatomical variants may be responsible.[71] A large acromion process may cause pressure on the supraspinatus tendon, leading to shoulder impingement syndrome, or a tight tensor fascia lata may contribute to iliotibial-band friction syndrome. Retinacula at the wrist can cause various forms of tenosynovitis, usually in combination with repeated use during occupational or recreational activities.[62] These cases of tendinitis are best treated by the early removal of the external cause, or by changing the anatomical environment through joint mobilization, flexibility exercises, or other appropriate exercise interventions.

Tendinitis may also result from changes or inadequacies within the tendon, the so-called 'intrinsic' forms of tendinitis. In such

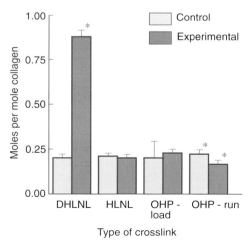

Fig. 6 Intermolecular crosslinking in chicken Achilles tendon after 8 weeks of increased mechanical loading. Both immature (DHLNL) and mature (OHP) crosslinks are increased. This contrasts with strenuous running exercise, where OHP crosslinks are decreased after 8 weeks. * indicates significant difference from control group ($p < 0.05$)

cases, there are no readily identifiable external causes, and tendinitis is attributed to a change in tendon structure.[63] It should be recognized, however, that factors outside the tendon almost always induce the change, except in rare cases involving genetic abnormalities or diseases affecting connective tissue structure.[10,20] The tendon is simply not strong enough to tolerate the tensile loads to which it is subjected. There are two possible solutions: (1) remove or reduce the tensile forces; or (2) cause the tendon to become stronger. Frequently, the loading pattern is within normal limits for such a patient, and force reduction is not a viable long-term solution.[47] There are many athletes and dancers who suffer from chronic tendon pain because they are unable, or unwilling, to reduce the forces applied to their injured tendons.[61,65] This creates a situation where the tendon must be modified to match its environment via an appropriate, strength training programme.

Iliotibial-band friction syndrome (ITBFS)— a simple example of extrinsic tendinitis

Tightness in the tensor fascia lata and/or iliotibial band can give rise to ITBFS, causing pain either at the greater trochanter or the lateral condyle of the femur. External factors such as worn running shoes, leg-length discrepancy, uneven running surfaces, or an increase in running distance may be causing or contributing to the problem. The Ober test will reveal any tightness in the iliotibial band. Differential diagnosis includes abductor tendinitis (an intrinsic tendinitis) and referred pain from the hip or lumbar spine. Treatment consists of removing any external factors and prescribing an appropriate stretching programme for the athlete (see Fig. 7).[72] Ice, modalities, and non-steroidal anti-inflammatory drugs (**NSAIDs**) may be used for the relief of symptoms and reduction of

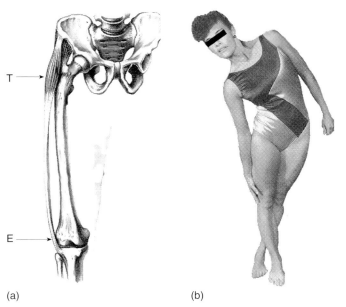

(a)   (b)

Fig. 7 (A) Iliotibial-band friction syndrome can occur at either the greater trochanter (T) or lateral epicondyle of the femur (E) as the tight tensor fascia lata/iliotibial band is stretched over these structures. (B) The solution is to increase the length of the muscle–tendon structure via controlled flexibility exercises. Here the athlete supports her weight on the affected limb, crosses the other limb in front, then leans her upper body toward the unaffected side (Redrawn from refs 71 and 72, with permission.)

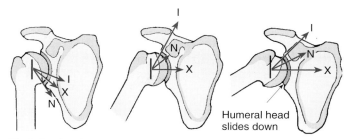

Fig. 8 Resultant force vectors in neutral (N), internal rotation (I), and external rotation (X) for the range of glenohumeral abduction of 0–60 degrees. If the humerus is unable to glide down, or the arm is held in internal rotation during abduction, impingement will result. (Redrawn from ref. 74, with permission.)

inflammation, injection of an anti-inflammatory agent may be necessary in a few cases.

Shoulder impingement syndrome—a complex example of extrinsic tendinitis

Impingement of the supraspinatus tendon, or that of the long head of the biceps brachii, is caused by a reduction in the space between the greater tuberosity of the humerus and the inferior surface of the acromion. The tendons are compressed as the upper limb is moved into flexion or abduction.[73] The solution is to increase the space between the humerus and the acromion, but achieving this goal is difficult and complicated. At the risk of oversimplifying a subject, about which whole chapters exist in other parts of this text, one can divide shoulder impingement into two very broad categories. The first category includes patients whose impingement is related to hypomobility at the glenohumeral joint due to shrinking of the joint capsule. Normally, as the humerus is elevated, the head of the humerus glides downward on the glenoid articular surface, maintaining a subacromial space for the supraspinatus tendon. Tightening of the capsule of the glenohumeral joint pulls the head of the humerus higher on the glenoid and decreases inferior gliding during elevation. This causes compression of the tendon against the undersurface of the acromion. The compression is aggravated by an accompanying reduction in lateral rotation at the glenohumeral joint, which redirects the forces during elevation so that the resultant vector is directed upward toward compression (Fig. 8).[74] This type of impingement will usually appear fairly early in elevation (69 to 90 degrees) and elevation above 120 degrees may be difficult or impossible due to the limitation of motion. There may be no painful arc *per se*, as pain may begin at a particular point in the range of motion, then remain constant or increase. Rotator cuff pathology is inevitable if overhead movements are continued. Most patients fall into Neer's Stage II or III impingement classification and may have experienced previous episodes of shoulder pain in their youth.[73] As a consequence of their severe limitation of glenohumeral range of motion, patients with adhesive capsulitis will frequently develop shoulder impingement, this usually occurs as patients begin to move their upper limb once the acute, painful phase of the capsulitis has subsided.[75] Since the capsule is tight and normal, glenohumeral movement is impossible, repeated attempts to move the arm overhead will probably compress the rotator cuff and eventually cause pathology in these patients. Many patients adapt by changing their

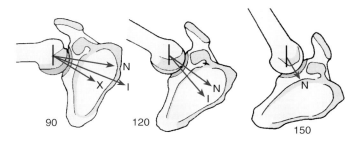

Fig. 9 Force vectors about the glenohumeral joint during progressive abduction from 90–150 degrees in neutral (N), internal rotation (I), and external rotation (X). Failure of the rotator cuff to compress the humeral head against the glenoid or to prevent excessive upward motion of the humerus may result in impingement. (Redrawn from ref. 74, with permission.)

environment so that less elevation of the upper limb is required for functional activities.

Glenohumeral hypomobility is easily diagnosed by assessing the passive joint movement of the affected side and comparing this with the contralateral normal limb, or by the clinician's judgement of the amount of passive glide at the glenohumeral joint if both shoulders are affected.[76] Successful treatment depends on restoring normal mobility to the glenohumeral joint via passive joint mobilization and capsular stretching, followed by strengthening and functional exercises to ensure normal scapulohumeral rhythm.[77] It is essential that treatment be supervised by a skilled physical therapist, since treatment is uncomfortable and must be progressed frequently. Symptoms may easily take 12 weeks, or even longer, to resolve in patients with long-standing impingement related to hypomobility, so patience is required of both the patient and the clinician. Initially, progress is usually rapid, but as mobility nears normal, improvement plateaus. Patients can usually carry out their own treatment at home by this point and it is no longer necessary for the therapist to treat them on a regular basis. Patients who have undergone surgery to decompress the tendon before receiving the appropriate non-surgical therapy will usually require more intervention by the therapist, but the treatment approach is basically the same.

The second broad category of shoulder impingement is that of patients with glenohumeral hypermobility. This may range from simple joint laxity to the patient with multidirectional instability. Generally, these patients are younger and their symptoms will appear higher in the arc of elevation. Range of motion is often normal, and a painful arc is present. Impingement tests are positive, and one or more signs of shoulder hypermobility may be present (apprehension sign, sulcus sign, etc.) (Fig. 9).[72]

Patients with hypermobile glenohumeral joints may develop tendinitis in several ways. One explanation may be overuse of the rotator cuff muscles to keep the head of the humerus properly positioned on the glenoid. A lack of inadequate passive stabilization via capsule and ligaments places increased demands on the rotator cuff. As the rotator cuff fatigues it can no longer provide dynamic stabilization of the head of the humerus on the glenoid during elevation. The force vector of the deltoid muscle is no longer balanced by the rotator cuff, resulting in upward migration of the humeral head. The supraspinatus and/or biceps are compressed against the acromion. Several other factors that may contribute to shoulder tendinitis in the presence of hypermobility are outlined in Table 2. The

reader is encouraged to consult other sources within the text for a more thorough description of the causes and treatment of rotator cuff tendinitis.

The overuse injury—intrinsic tendinitis

This is probably the most familiar description of chronic tendinitis. An otherwise normal tendon is subjected chronically to relatively large loads, perhaps extending into the linear region of the stress–strain curve.[52] The overuse theory holds that this causes partial rupture (microscopic failure) of some of the fibrils within the tendon, or slippage between fibrils, and leads to tendon injury.[78] Such injuries have been likened to the stress fractures that occur in bones subjected to chronic load.[63] The injury is thought to be the result of fatigue of the structure, just as metal beams will fatigue with repeated loading. Individual loads may be within the physiological range, but are repeated so often that recovery cannot occur and the

Table 2 Factors related to shoulder tendinitis	
Factor	**Suggested relationship**
Cervical facet or disc problem	Referred pain mimics tendinitis
Cervicothoracic junction or upper thoracic spine limitation of motion	No sidebending of spine during arm elevation, increased demand for motion at glenohumeral joint
Lack of scapular motion	Increased demand for motion at glenohumeral joint to acheive overhead hand position
Weak scapular prime movers	Inadequate stabilization of proximal attachment of rotator cuff, can lead to overuse or increased GH motion
Rotator cuff weakness or imbalance	Inadequate stabilization of humerus on glenoid, allows upward draft of humerus during elevation
Glenohumeral hypermobility	Overuse of rotator cuff muscles to stabilize humeral head; often secondary to other causes
Overuse syndrome	Repeated overhead movements (as in swimming, throwing) cause impingement beneath coracromial arch
Tight latissimus dorsi	Lack of lateral rotation with arm in overhead position may contribute to impingement
Nerve or nerve root dysfunction	Weakness of one of rotator cuff muscles results in force directed upward through unopposed force vector due to deltoid activity
Glenohumeral hypomobility	Humeral head unable to glide downward during elevation, compresses rotator cuff against acromion

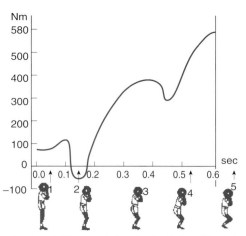

Fig. 10 Resultant knee joint moments from the beginning of the jerk motion until 0.04 s after patellar tendon rupture. The failure occurred at the change from downward to upward motion. (Redrawn from ref. 85, with permission.)

Stress distribution within the tendon

It is generally assumed that force applied to a tendon is distributed symmetrically across the tendon cross-sectional area and throughout its length. However, changes in cross-sectional area along a tendon will cause more stress at some levels. There is also evidence to suggest that tendons are not uniform in composition throughout their length, meaning that some regions may deform more than others in response to the same load.[33,86,87] This can lead to concentrations of stress or strain within the tendon, so that one part of the tendon is actually being subjected to excessive loading while other regions are not. Should the overloaded regions mechanically fail, then the rest of the tendon will be placed at higher risk.

Variations in loading within the tendon may also be related to motor control. Tendon fascicles are associated with discrete motor units, and are probably most heavily loaded when those motor units are active.[88] Not every motor unit within a muscle fires during each activation of the muscle. Slow movement or maintenance of posture requires the use of small motor units composed of slow-twitch muscle fibres, the tendon fascicles associated with these motor units are therefore regularly loaded during daily activities and may be assumed to be 'stronger'. Very rapid loading, or conditions requiring unaccustomed force production, may cause the firing of fast motor units which are seldom used at lower force levels. Presumably, the tendon fascicles associated with these seldom-used motor units have not been exposed to the same loading history as other fascicles within the tendon. Is it possible that these tendon fascicles may actually be weaker as a result of little or no loading during daily activities, and are more easily injured when a sudden demand on the muscle for rapid force production is made? This theory has been used to explain the muscle soreness and damage closely associated with eccentric muscle contraction, could it apply to tendon as well?[84] If so, it suggests that different types of loading may be important in the recovery from, or prevention of, tendon injuries. Whether the explanation is purely mechanical or also involves a neural element, it seems very possible that there are asymmetries in the pattern of loading and fascicle strength within the tendon.[88]

Role of eccentric muscle activation

Force increases as the velocity of active muscle lengthening increases, while the opposite is true during concentric (shortening) muscle activations.[89-91] This may help to explain the frequent connection between eccentric loading and tendon injury.[47,83] The tendon is exposed to larger loads during eccentric loading, especially if the movement occurs rapidly.[38,47,89,90] This is exactly the situation which occurs in landing from or preparing for a jump (patellar tendinitis),[61,92] midstance during running[38] or during a *demie plié* in ballet[65] (Achilles tendinitis), and when hitting a backhand in tennis (lateral epicondylitis).[93] Nearly all shortening activations of muscle–tendon units are preceded by lengthening while the muscle is active. This activation pattern stretches the muscle–tendon unit (**MTU**), creating a passive force in the muscle due to the elongation of its elastic elements, and providing elastic energy if the muscle is allowed to immediately shorten after being lengthened.[89-91] This storage of elastic energy allows the muscle to do more work at less metabolic cost. Unfortunately, it also results in maximum force and maximum elongation being simultaneously applied to the tendon, which may cause damage. Figure 11 shows the forces on the Achilles

structure fatigues. This concept is supported by animal studies.[69,70] Since tendon structure recovers with rest, even after loading into the linear region, time is probably an important element in producing these injuries. This is the type of tendinitis which seems to develop very gradually and is often related to high training levels, such as distance running.[47,63,65] It may be appropriate to consider this as another form of overtraining, and it can be helpful to use this analogy when explaining the disorder to athletes, since most are familiar with situations where high intensities of training result in no improvement, or even a decline, in performance.[79-81]

It is not only high-level athletes, however, who are afflicted with this type of tendinitis, although this group does account for most of the eponyms used, such as tennis elbow and jumper's knee. Many older individuals involved in recreational sports also suffer, as well as non-athletes involved in repetitive loading activities.[82]

Sudden loading/excessive force

The tendon may also be damaged by loading patterns other than chronic ones. Sudden force application, particularly involving lengthening (eccentric) muscle contractions, may lead to muscle or tendon injury.[64,83,84] A sudden maximum muscle activation results in a larger-than-normal force being very rapidly applied to the tendon, causing partial or complete rupture. The filming of a competitive weightlifter performing a lift during which his patellar tendon ruptured (see Fig. 10) showed that the injury occurred as the lifter changed from downward to upward motion, that is to say at the end of the eccentric phase.[85] The force on the patellar tendon was estimated at about 14.5 kN, over 17 times bodyweight!

Sudden force application can cause more damage than a gradual force increase to the same level of loading, and the sudden removal of a given force level is also more likely to cause disruption than a gradual reduction of the same force. The reasons for this are not entirely known, although it appears to involve a disruption of the relationship between the collagen fibrils and their surrounding matrix.[30,31] It appears, however, that the combination of maximum force production, sudden reversal of movement from eccentric to concentric loading, and rapid application and/or release of force are stressful or damaging to the tendon.

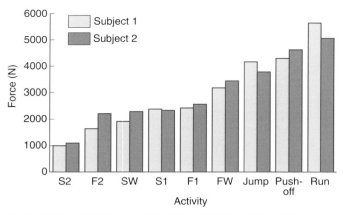

Fig. 11 Achilles tendon forces estimated from kinematic and force platform measurements for two subjects performing a variety of activities: S2—slow drop, weight supported on both feet, into dorsiflexion over the edge of a step; F2—fast drop over a step; SW—slow drop with added weight; S1 and F1—slow and fast drops with weight on one foot; Jump—landing phase of a jump from 0.6 m; Push-off—changeover from backward to forward motion; Run—stance phase of running. There is a progressive increase in load with the various exercises, although there is some variability between the two subjects; running produces the largest Achilles tendon forces in both.

tendon of different activities and exercises.[38] When the kinematics of these activities are examined, in nearly all cases maximum force production and maximum muscle–tendon length coincide, this occurs at the point where the muscle changes from eccentric (lengthening) to concentric (shortening) activation.

Other factors playing a role in tendinitis

Endocrine

It is often difficult to determine why patients have developed tendinitis when no apparent change in loading or training has occurred, and when there have been no examples of sudden, unexpected force application (although this may have happened but went unnoticed by the patient). Perhaps there are other factors which cause tendons to become symptomatic? If these systemic factors act gradually on the tendon, then their effect would only be observed after a considerable time period. Endocrine responses to stress, such as increased glucocorticoid and catecholamine release, may have negative effects on connective tissue,[94-96] increasing turnover and thus resulting in decreased crosslinking.[97,98] Hormones can influence connective tissues such as tendon, but no relationship has yet been demonstrated in cases of tendinitis. It is interesting to speculate, however, that an endocrine response to chronic levels of overtraining[95,96,99] may be, at least partially, responsible for some spontaneous cases of tendinitis. This influence has been suggested for lateral epicondylitis (lack of oestrogen),[93] and the relationship between chronic steroid administration and tendon rupture is well known.[100,101] Only after all other external influences have been eliminated as potential causes, however, should these systemic factors be considered as possible primary causes, it is more likely that they are contributing to, rather than causing, the tendinitis.

Compressive loading

The tensile strength of the tendon may gradually decline over time if it is subjected to chronic compressive loads, or if turnover is

increased markedly, resulting in less mature crosslinking.[102] Less collagen, a change from type I to type II collagen, fewer collagen crosslinks, and more ground substance all result in decreased tissue tensile strength, and these changes all take place in tendons that are subjected to compressive, rather than tensile, loading.[6,7] Compressive loading may also result in regions of decreased blood flow in tendon, as has been demonstrated for supraspinatus tendinitis.[103] Compression, and the changes it causes in tendon composition and mechanical behaviour, is a large factor in rotator cuff tendinitis, and this may suggest a role for loading the supraspinatus tendon with tensile forces during rehabilitation to induce the formation of 'correct' new tendon tissue.[47] Such tensile loading would be expected to induce a change in tendon composition if applied gradually, such that collagen content and crosslinking actually were increased.

Nutritional

The adequate amounts of amino acids supplied by a normal healthy diet are required for all protein synthesis, and this, of course, includes collagen. Co-factors such as vitamin A, vitamin C, and copper are known to be important in collagen synthesis and crosslinking,[10] and iron deficiency can have a negative influence on healing.[104] There is also some evidence to suggest that collagen synthesis is more severely affected than some other proteins during fasting,[98] which may have implications for athletes involved in sports that emphasize a slender build, such as gymnastics and ballet. The nutritional influences on chronic tendinitis remain largely unexplored.

Referred pain

This is a frequently unrecognized cause of tendinitis-like pain, and is due to peripherally located (somatic referred) pain resulting from the irritation of spinal structures such as the zygapophyseal joint capsule, intervertebral disc, or a ligament.[105] It is frequently seen in cases of tennis elbow, where degenerative changes in the cervical spine cause symptoms which exactly mimic those of tennis elbow.[93] This may not be a common cause of tendon pain in the athletic population, but the clinician should be very suspicious if a 'tendinitis' fails to respond to treatment, and one should always conduct a screening examination of the spine in parallel with a peripheral examination, especially if the patient falls into the appropriate age category for degenerative spinal changes. If decreased spinal range of motion or local joint signs are observed, these should be treated before treatment of the peripheral problem is considered separately.

Tendon healing

Much is known about the healing of severed tendons. This work comes from models where the tendon has been divided, surgically or accidentally, and the severed ends re-opposed and held in place via immobilization or suture.[106-109] These models have told us about tendon healing under these conditions, particularly the timing of the biochemical and mechanical changes that take place in the healing tendon. Within days, the initial inflammatory stage triggers an increase in GAG synthesis which is rapidly followed by collagen synthesis, such that the healing wound can be subjected to low levels of force within a matter of days.[110,111] We know that the application of some force (but not too much!) is ideal in encouraging the new

Table 3 Principles governing clinical intervention during tendon healing

	Stage of healing Inflammatory	Fibroblastic/proliferation	Remodelling/maturation
Time (days)	0–6	5–21	20 days onward
Suggested therapy	Rest, ice Anti-inflammatory modalities Decreased tension	Gradual introduction of stress Modalities to increase collagen synthesis	Progressive stress on tissue
Physiological rationale	Prevent prolonged inflammation Prevent disruption of new blood vessels Promote ground substance synthesis	Increase collagen amount Increase fibril size and alignment	Increase collagen crosslinking (ligaments and tendons) Decrease collagen crosslinking (joint capsule) Increase fibril size
Main aims	Avoid new tissue disruption	Prevent excessive muscle and joint atrophy	Optimize new tissue healing

collagen fibrils to align with the direction of force application, and that healing tissues that are subjected to loading are almost always stronger than unloaded tissues, whether this be skin, ligament, or tendon.[112,113] The application of these principles in plastic surgery has led to the design of early motion programmes after tendon repair, and a rehabilitation programme which is truly based on scientific principles. The basic principles are outlined in Table 3.

Confusion exists when it comes to applying this information to tendinitis. Just what is tendinitis? Does tendinitis follow the same healing pattern described for complete lacerations? Little is known about the inflammatory response to the types of mechanical trauma that produce chronic tendinitis. Any injury which involves the tendon or its associated sheaths may be referred to as tendinitis, but a plethora of other terms also exists: tendinosis (degeneration of the tendon without inflammation), tenosynovitis (inflammation of the sheath surrounding the tendon), paratenonitis, peritendinitis. Some authors argue that, with cases of chronic tendinitis which developed very gradually and never appeared to have an acute stage, there is no associated inflammation of the tendon or the tendon sheath, only degeneration within the tendon itself, and so the condition should be called tendinosis.[63,71] This conclusion is based primarily on observations of human tissue obtained during surgical procedures aimed at relieving chronic tendinitis. These observations probably represent the late, fibrotic stage of tendinitis, and do not eliminate the possibility of the earlier presence of inflammation. Sudden tendon rupture without prior symptoms has also been attributed to tendinosis, since areas of degenerative change can be seen in these tendons during surgery which are thought to precede the actual tendon rupture.

One of the major difficulties in scientifically evaluating chronic tendinitis has been the lack of a suitable animal model. Most animal models have used partial laceration or chemical injection to induce a tendon injury and may not be as closely representative of naturally occurring injuries. Racehorses frequently injure tendons, and, indeed, are responsible for much of what we now know about chronic tendinitis,[113,114] but, because of the expense, they cannot be used by most researchers, and, as is true for human tendinitis, the amount (time and/or magnitude) of loading responsible for the tendinitis is unknown.

An animal model is available that appears to simulate the type of overloading which often leads to human tendon dysfunction.[69,70] The ankle joints of anaesthetized rabbits were repeatedly flexed and extended for 2 hours per day while the triceps surae muscle was electrically stimulated. After 4 weeks of exercise, palpation of the exercised tendons showed that all had irregular thickening, with nodules present a short distance from the tendon's insertion into the calcaneus. Light microscopy showed degenerative changes in the tendon and thickening of the tendon sheath (paratenon).[69] Blood flow was increased (about twofold) to both the paratenon and the tendon.[70] Cellular changes suggestive of an inflammatory response were found in the tendon sheath, with degenerative changes in the central portion of the tendon. This model is the first to produce tendon dysfunction through reproducible loading.

The findings from human surgical and postmortem specimens, and from animal studies, suggest that most of the inflammatory changes take place in the paratenon and are accompanied (preceded? followed?) by areas of focal degeneration within the tendon.[69] These findings also suggest that injury to the tendon structure does not occur in isolation, and that it would be uncommon for tendon degeneration to occur without accompanying inflammatory changes. In other words, it should be possible to have paratenonitis without tendinosis (as can occur with extrinsic tendinitis), but not tendinosis without some inflammation of the tendon sheath at some point.

It is unlikely that tendon damage takes place without symptoms being present. Patients may not complain of pain serious enough to prevent them from participating in activities they consider enjoyable (or unavoidable), but careful questioning will often reveal that symptoms were/are present during activities that load the tendon, or that a more acute episode did take place earlier. The clinical signs of tenderness with palpation and pain on loading may be interpreted to reflect the presence of an inflammatory response.[115] The

Table 4 Classification of tendon disorders based on pain and function

Intensity	Level	Pain	Function
Mild	1	None	Normal
	2	With extreme exertion only, not intense	Normal
	3	With moderate exertion, remains 1–2 h after acitivity stops	Slightly decreased or normal
Moderate	4	With any athletic activity, progressively increases, remains 4–6 h after activity stops	Significantly decreased
Severe	5	Starts immediately with any activity loading tendon, rapidly increases, last 12–24 h	Markedly decreased, or prevented by pain, or modified by drugs
	6	During some daily activities as well as sports	Athletics impossible, some daily activities may also be impossible

response, while mostly in the tendon sheath, reflects and accompanies the structural damage to the tendon. The exact relationship is not yet known.

Clinically, it is usually impossible to determine the exact portion of the tendon that is the source of pain. Palpation involves both the tendon and its sheath, and muscle contraction will apply force to an inflamed sheath as well as a damaged tendon. We can, perhaps, define tendinitis as a syndrome of pain and tenderness localized over an area of tendon, aggravated by activities that require activation of the particular muscle–tendon unit thereby applying tensile force to the tendon, or by other outside forces applied to the tendon. The syndrome can include inflammation of the tendon sheath, as in tenosynovitis and tenovaginitis, as well as actual inflammation of the tendon substance itself, and is either caused or followed by degenerative changes in tendon structure. Since it is unlikely that pathological changes can be determined for most patients, it may be helpful to use a classification system based on pain and function, which can be determined clinically, even though the exact relationship between symptoms and pathology remains unknown. Such a system is presented in Table 4.[47]

Treating the injured tendon

General principles for treating tendinitis

There are many principles, physiological and mechanical, that should be considered when treating chronic tendinitis, most have been touched upon earlier in this chapter. Here are some of the most important guidelines for treating all forms of tendinitis:

1.   Identify and remove all negative external forces/factors.
In the case of extrinsic tendinitis, the outside force is usually pressure on the tendon. Identification and removal of the source of pressure is the fundamental treatment for this form of tendinitis, and is imperative if further tendon damage is to be avoided.[57] All other forms of treatment, although helpful in relieving symptoms or restoring range of motion, can only be considered temporary or adjunctive. *Eliminating the cause is the fundamental treatment.*

Not only extrinsic forms of tendinitis are affected by outside forces. External factors may be contributing to, or even causing, intrinsic tendinitis; for example, Achilles or posterior tibial tendinitis that can be caused by excessive foot pronation. This can cause the medial side of the Achilles tendon, or the tibialis posterior muscle–tendon unit, to be overstretched. The anatomical configuration of the Achilles tendon, whereby it twists during descent, may also play a role in Achilles tendinitis.[34]

Probably the single most common contributing factor in almost all cases of chronic tendinitis is a lack of flexibility of the involved muscle–tendon unit. For this reason, a thorough and specific stretching programme is nearly always an essential part of the rehabilitation strategy.

2.   Estimate the phase of healing (stage of tendinitis).
This is a very imprecise process, and requires clinical judgement based on the examiner's clinical experience to be truly successful. Table 4 can be used as a guide for those unfamiliar with treating chronic tendinitis. Generally, the more severe the symptoms, the more closely the choice and timing of loading should resemble that used for an acute-onset tendon injury. Treatment should also progress as it would for an acute injury.

3.   Determine the appropriate focus for initial treatment.
This involves matching treatment with the stage of healing. Most cases of chronic tendinitis should be in the remodelling phase of healing, where force application is the most effective treatment. More severe cases may have to be initially treated with relative rest (reduced loading), ice, and modalities for a short period of time, perhaps 10 to 14 days. This treatment should be followed by gradual stress increase, as is the case for an acute tendon injury or repair.

4.   Institute an appropriate tensile-loading programme.
The healing tendon must be loaded if collagen synthesis, alignment, and maturation via crosslinking is to be ideal. The more acute or severe the injury, the lower the force that should be applied. Passive movement produces very little tensile force, is safe immediately after injury, and is known to have beneficial mechanical effects on tendon. Gentle stretching would be the next step, followed by increased force while stretching, and then active exercise.

5.   Control pain and inflammation.
While the appropriate use of loading during healing should ensure that mechanical disruption and re-injury, provoking an inflammatory response, do not occur, there are cases where additional help may be required to reduce a prolonged inflammatory response. In such cases, drugs, ice, and modalities can be used as adjuncts to treatment.

Specific forms of treatment
Modalities
Physical therapists employ a wide variety of modalities in treating soft-tissue disorders, including: ultrasound; laser; ice; heat; pulsed

electromagnetic current; electromagnetic field therapy; high-voltage galvanic stimulation; acupuncture; interferential current; etc. Most are proposed to 'decrease inflammation and promote healing'. Unfortunately, there is only limited evidence, as yet, to support many of these claims.

Ultrasound is one of the most commonly used modalities. Generally, pulsed ultrasound is recommended for acute injuries, to avoid a thermal effect, and continuous ultrasound is used for more long-standing injuries.[116-118] While there have been reports of no influence on healing tendon, studies have shown that ultrasound increases collagen synthesis by fibroblasts,[119] speeds wound healing,[116,117] and results in increased tensile strength in healing tendons.[120] Ultrasound has little or no effect on inflammation.[121] None of the experimental models used in these studies simulated the clinical situation of chronic tendinitis, so one can only assume that the chronically injured tendon will heal in a manner similar to the severed tendon. Given that one of the explanations for chronic tendinitis is 'failed healing response',[63] it is uncertain whether this assumption will always be true. Ultrasound probably has its most important effects when the synthetic activity of the fibroblasts is maximum, namely the proliferative stage of healing, but because of the long-standing nature of chronic injuries, it may actually be most widely used clinically during the remodelling stage. It would be interesting to see whether ultrasound increases the synthesis of collagen during all stages of healing, especially during remodelling, when the cellular synthesis rate has declined. Stimulation of synthetic activity appears to be ultrasound's most likely means of 'promoting healing', and would, in effect, prolong the proliferative phase of healing. Given the timing of the normal healing response, with the relatively short duration of enhanced cellular synthetic activity, there would seem to be little indication for using ultrasound for periods beyond 2 to 3 weeks at the most.

Another modality widely used in Europe and Canada is laser treatment.[122] Like ultrasound, laser therapy has been shown to increase fibroblast synthesis of GAGs and collagen, and to speed superficial wound healing, but, unlike ultrasound, it has also been shown to decrease inflammation.[122] The use of lasers in non-superficial cases such as chronic tendinitis remains speculative; there is, as yet, no clinical or scientific evidence to support its use for treating deeper tissues like tendon or to suggest its superiority to ultrasound. Given the wide variety of laser types and dosages, much more research is needed on the effects of this modality.

Electrical stimulation has also been demonstrated to have a positive influence on tendon healing.[123,124] Again, results were obtained from acute tendon healing models and may not necessarily represent chronic tendon injuries. Both direct electrical stimulation[123,124] and indirect current via electromagnetic field induction[125] seem to augment tendon healing. Pulsed electromagnetic fields can treat both deep and superficial tissues, and cover larger areas than ultrasound or laser.[126] Questions about timing and dosage remain unclear, but it seems that this treatment needs to be prolonged, for several hours per day, to have an influence on tissue, since clinical use for shorter periods has not shown the same positive effects.[126]

One of the most widely used modalities for all soft-tissue injuries is ice. Its use is recommended immediately after injury to prevent excessive soft-tissue swelling, and it is thought to act mainly by decreasing the activity of inflammatory mediators and decreasing the overall metabolic rate of the injured tissue.[127] Another important effect of ice is analgesia, which allows the use of appropriate forms of exercise, such as passive motion, that otherwise might be uncomfortable for the patient. The use of ice with chronic injuries is less clear, although it can be used for its analgesic effect, and may help offset inflammatory changes induced by mechanical injury to the tendon during exercise.[128]

The use of modalities, although widespread, remains largely speculative in the treatment of chronic soft-tissue injuries. Most scientific studies suggest that increased synthetic activity by fibroblasts is the major effect of most modalities, except ice and, perhaps, laser. Clinicians should always keep in mind that this synthetic activity is mainly part of the proliferative phase of healing, and that mechanical forces are also required during remodelling if the newly synthesized collagen is to assemble and crosslink into a structure capable of withstanding tensile loading. The effects of modalities on chronic injuries remains largely unexplored, and well-designed clinical trials are needed to determine their efficacy in the clinical setting.

Drugs

The most potent anti-inflammatory drugs are the corticosteroids, which are sometimes used, via local injection, to treat chronic tendinitis. The negative effects of systemic corticosteroid use are well known,[100] but the effects of local injection are less clear. Both negative and no effects have been reported,[129,130] however, it is now generally agreed that injection into the tendon substance should be avoided.[131] This is due to both the effects of the drug (which decreases collagen synthesis), the mechanical disruption caused by the needle, and the irritant effect of the solvent in which the drug is dissolved. Given the potent anti-inflammatory effect, and the fact that most inflammatory changes occur in the paratenon, injection into the tendon sheath paratenon may be indicated if inflammation is marked or prolonged.[130,131] If the tendon has been injected, tensile force should be reduced for 10 to 14 days afterwards, and the tendon treated as if it has suffered an acute injury, that is to say by ice, rest, modalities, followed by progressive loading starting at about 2 weeks. Repeated steroid injections into a tendon are almost certain to result in substantial mechanical disruption and should be avoided.[129]

Non-steroidal anti-inflammatory drugs (NSAIDs) are also widely used in the treatment of acute soft-tissue injuries, but less so for chronic injuries such as tendinitis. They are thought to limit inflammation by inhibiting prostaglandin synthesis, although other mechanisms are also involved[132]. Unlike corticosteroids, they do not inhibit fibroblast or macrophage activity. While there is some evidence to show that the prophylactic use of indomethacin may reduce subsequent muscle injury, most clinical studies have been poorly designed, and it is impossible to conclude whether or not the use of NSAIDs has a beneficial effect on postinjury recovery.[133,134] Since acetaminophen has only an analgesic effect, and patients may not distinguish between aspirin and acetaminophen, it is important to find out exactly what drugs the patient is taking, since many of these agents may be self-administered and an anti-inflammatory action may be assumed when none is actually present.

Time after injury (Days)	Treatment	Function
Table 5 Example of exercise treatment programme for acute tendinitis		
6–12	Stretch Achilles tendon (calf stretches) for 2–3 minutes at least twice daily to point of mild discomfort, not pain. Ice afterward	Normal walking pace without discomfort
12–21	Continue stretches, add gentle toe raises with weight evenly distributed on both feet or shifted to unaffected side so that mild discomfort felt in Achilles tendon. Ice afterward	Normal walking without discomfort; ascend/descend stairs
21–42	Shift weight progressively to affected side and increase speed of movement. Ice afterward	Increased speed of walking until pace reached just before symptoms provoked
> 42	Resume training at 25% preinjury level. Progress weight 10–20% each session if no symptoms provoked except in last one-third of exercise session	Resume normal training schedule when preinjury weight level achieved

Some patients may also be self-administering another class of drugs known to affect connective tissues, namely anabolic steroids. While the exact effects of these agents are unknown due to difficulties in determining use and dosage, there is both scientific and anecdotal evidence to suggest that anabolic steroid users are more likely to develop a tendon injury.[135] The effect of anabolic steroids on the healing of these injuries is unknown. Clinicians should be alert to the possibility of anabolic steroids, since their use by young males has become widespread.[136]

Surgery

There is little place for surgery in the treatment of chronic tendinitis unless the tendon ruptures and the gap at the site of injury needs to be approximated. Some authors advocate the removal of scar tissue and repair of the injured tendon, but it is unlikely that it is the surgery, rather than the postoperative healing response and carefully progressed treatment, which causes the improvement in the patient's condition. Almost all cases of chronic tendinitis can be successfully treated without surgery.

Exercise in the treatment of tendinitis

Treating acute tendon injuries using exercise

The guide to treating the severed tendon has been well established and was summarized in Table 3. The main aims are to prevent tissue disruption while minimizing the negative effects of disuse on other parts of the musculoskeletal and cardiorespiratory systems. The recovering tendon is subjected to progressively increasing forces to enhance collagen fibril alignment, improve tensile strength further, encourage continued fibroblast synthetic activity, and prevent adhesions between the healing tendon and adjacent tissues. Table 3 provides a framework on which to base all tendon injury rehabilitation, and can be readily applied to cases of tendinitis where the exact time of injury is known.

Example—Achilles tendon injury in a bodybuilder

E.S. injured his Achilles tendon 5 days ago while performing toe raises. He was unable to continue exercising without producing pain that increased with successive repetitions, so he stopped and applied ice immediately. He was advised to discontinue exercising for 6 weeks, then resume training, but questionned this advice because of his past experience with similar injuries. At initial examination, he reported that he experienced some discomfort (3/10) on rapid walking or while ascending and descending stairs. This discomfort increased to pain (7/10) if he attempted to jog or perform toe raises. Based on these observations, we concluded that E.S. had experienced a moderate to severe tendon injury (Level 4 or 5; based on functional limitations) which could be safely loaded at low levels and progressed according to symptoms. If E.S. followed the advice not to exercise for 6 weeks, it was likely that his symptoms would recur as soon as he resumed training. He was advised to reduce activity for the next 6 weeks since he probably had experienced failure of some portion of the tendon, but that an appropriate, progressive exercise programme should allow him to resume training at about 25 per cent of his preinjury training intensity without a recurrence of symptoms.

Treatment

E.S. followed the treatment schedule outlined in Table 5, with a general warm-up prior to exercise, he maintained his normal training regime for the opposite lower limb and upper body.

Outcome

E.S. was able to resume training at 6 weeks without incident. It took him another 3 weeks to return to his preinjury training level. His 'treatment' was entirely self-directed. He saw a physical therapist 5 days after injury, and again shortly after resuming training.

Special note

Because E.S. is a bodybuilder, it was important to determine whether he had had previous injuries of this nature, and whether he used/uses anabolic steroids. Neither was true in this case, which improved the chances of a positive outcome in a relatively short time.

Treating chronic tendinitis using exercise

In contrast to the relative simplicity of the acute tendon injury, where the onset of the tissue damage is known and the phase of healing can be estimated, when dealing with chronic tendinitis the date of the initial injury may be uncertain and it is difficult to guess where in the healing process the tendon lies. There are no accurate means of assessing human soft-tissue injuries such as tendinitis—although several techniques such as ultrasound, magnetic resonance imaging, and thermography show promise—so even with acute tendinitis we cannot be certain about the degree of injury, but at least we can estimate the stage of healing.

Since our understanding of chronic tendinitis is inadequate, we are forced to make some assumptions on which to base treatment. These assumptions are summarized in Table 6. At worst, these assumptions will make our treatment more conservative than necessary, however, if we progress treatment according to the patient's symptoms and response to the previous treatment, we will rapidly reach the appropriate loading level. It is difficult to retreat if this level is overreached, and a marked worsening of symptoms can undermine the patient's confidence in the clinician and the treatment programme.

The failure of many patients' tendinitis to respond to conventional non-surgical treatment, and a growing appreciation for tendon physiology and mechanics, suggests that a modality-centred approach to the treatment of chronic tendinitis is inadequate. Modalities and drugs should not be abandoned altogether, but they should not form the basis of a treatment strategy for chronic tendin-

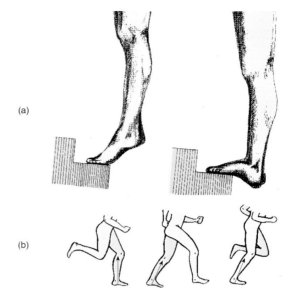

Fig. 12 (a) The Achilles tendon is loaded specifically by standing with the weight supported on the forefoot, then allowing the heels to drop downward over the edge of the support. Light hand support is sometimes required for balance. Loading can be increased by allowing the bodyweight to fall, stopping the descent and immediately return to the starting position ('drop and stop') or by shifting bodyweight to the affected side and/or adding weight to the upper body. (b) While running produces large forces on the Achilles tendon, these cannot be controlled and progressed like a specific exercise. It is best to regard these activities as monitors of success rather than loading strategies.

itis. At best, this will afford a temporary relief of symptoms, and at worst creates dependency on the clinician. An understanding of the ability of tendon to adapt to increased loads, and the belief that chronic tendon injuries are the result of tensile loads exceeding the tendon's mechanical strength, suggests that exercise should be the cornerstone of treatment.

Basic principles of exercise

For any exercise programme to succeed, whether its aim is to strengthen muscle or tendon, basic exercise principles must be followed. For the treatment of chronic tendinitis, these are most important:

1. Specificity of training

Training must be both anatomically and motor specific. In other words, the correct muscle–tendon unit must be loaded, and it must be loaded in a way that produces controlled tensile loading. The exercise should, eventually, closely simulate the pattern of loading during functional activity in the type of loading (tensile; eccentric) and the magnitude and speed of loading. Specificity is achieved by simulating the movement pattern associated with maximal tendon forces, namely a lengthening of the active MTU followed by shortening contraction. The initial magnitude and speed of loading are based on the estimated stage of healing. The more acute the injury, the lower the force, and the slower the eccentric loading. The affected tendon must be subjected to specific, controlled tensile loading, not just a generalized exercise involving use of the affected MTU. For example, the Achilles tendon is loaded by having the patient stand at the edge of a step and then dropping his or her heels downward, rather than running (see Fig. 12). This specific exercise is aimed at countering the potentially negative effects associated

Table 6 Assumptions governing treatment of chronic tendinitis

Assumption	Clinical implications
All cases of tendinitis are acute	Chronic tendinitis cases may initially be 'underloaded'
	Treatment must be continually progressed according to symptoms
Chronic tendinitis follows the same healing pattern as acute tendon injuries	Research findings related to acute tendon injuries will also apply to chronic tendinitis
Inflammation reflects tendon damage	Pain, tenderness, and function can be used to indirectly monitor tendon damage or recovery
The effects of exercise and disuse will be the same for chronic tendinitis as for normal and repaired tendons, and ligaments	Exercise can be used to successfully treat chronic tendinitis

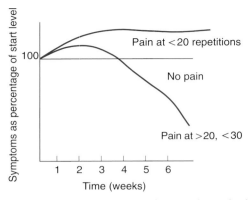

Fig. 13 Symptom intensity with different levels of therapeutic exercise. If pain is felt too early (< 20 reps) the condition usually is made worse, if no pain is felt, symptoms remain static. When the appropriate loading level is achieved (pain between 20 and 30 repetitions) patients should experience a marked decrease in symptoms within 6 to 8 weeks.

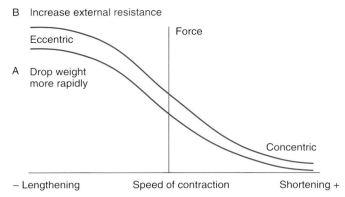

Fig. 14 Force increases with speed during eccentric activation, but decreases as the velocity of concentric shortening increases. To increase the load on the tendon, the patient should perform the exercise more rapidly, emphasizing the downward eccentric phase, or the external load on the limb should be increased. Only one of these variables should be changed within a given session.

with stressful training (for example, hormonal) with the positive effects of exercise on the MTU (increased strength).

2.   Maximal loading
Maximal loading is essential to induce adaptation in musculoskeletal tissues. In the case of an injured tendon, maximal loading can be defined as the force the tendon can withstand without further injury. The patient's symptoms are assumed to reflect potential tendon damage. Clinically, the maximum load is determined by the tendon's tolerance, which is judged by the patient's pain level during exercise. It has been determined empirically that the patient should experience some pain between the 20th and 30th repetition of the specific loading movement.[34] Pain before this (less than 20 repetitions) is usually accompanied by an overall worsening of the patient's condition and is assumed to indicate overloading. Patients who experience no pain or discomfort during the 30 repetitions, yet who have symptoms during functional activities, will usually see no change, suggesting that the loading stimulus is inadequate to induce a change in the tendon. (Fig. 13)

3.   Progression of loading
As the tendon becomes stronger, loading must be progressed so that maximal loads continue to be applied and the tissue will continue to have a stimulus for adaptation. This progress can be made by increasing the speed of movement or by increasing the magnitude of the tensile force by changing the external resistance (see Fig. 14).

The overall progression of loading is determined by the patient's symptoms, as described above, so that a maximum load is always applied (see Fig. 15). As soon as 30 repetitions can be performed without discomfort, the tensile force is increased.

Eccentric exercise programme
The principles outlined above have been incorporated into an 'eccentric exercise programme' for treating chronic tendinitis.[47] The principles can be applied to any injured tendon, following the guidelines in Fig. 15. The overall programme has five steps, which are performed in the order listed, and summarized in Fig. 16:

1.   Warm-up
A generalized exercise such as cycling or light jogging is used to increase body temperature and increase circulation. This exercise is not intended to load the tendon and should be comfortable.

2.   Flexibility
As noted earlier, lack of flexibility is a common finding in chronic tendinitis. It is recommended that the patient perform at least two 30-second static stretches of the involved MTU and its antagonist. More stretching may be done if this is felt to be a major factor in causing the patient's symptoms, that is to say the patient's range of motion is restricted by muscle shortening. Since two-joint muscles are most often involved, it is important that range of motion be examined at both joints simultaneously.

3.   Specific exercise
This is undertaken following the guidelines set out in Fig. 15, based on the principles outlined above. It is suggested that three sets of 10 repetitions be performed, with a brief rest, and sometimes a stretch, between each set. The patient should feel a reproduction of his or

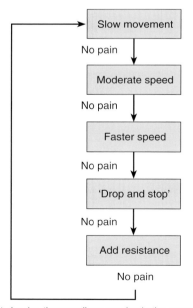

Fig. 15 Flowchart showing the overall progression in the eccentric exercise programme. As soon as 30 pain-free repetitions can be performed, the load is increased. Generally, this is most conveniently achieved by having the patient increase the speed of the movement. Once maximum speed is reached, return to a slow, controlled movement with increased resistance.

```
Steps in the 'EEP'

1. General warm-up
2. Stretch affected muscle–tendon
3. 3 sets of 10 repetitions of specific
   loading activity
4. Repeat stretch
5. Ice tender area
```

Fig. 16 The eccentric exercise programme follows the same sequence as that described in Fig. 15, with the stretching and loading exercises adapted to the affected muscle–tendon unit.

her symptoms after 20 repetitions. If pain is felt earlier, reduce the speed of movement, or decrease the load; if no pain is experienced, increase either the speed or the load (not both). If this is the first exercise session, and the initial level of loading is being determined, the intensity of exercise may be increased and the 30 repetitions repeated until the appropriate level of intensity is reached.

4. Repeat flexibility exercises

5. Apply ice

Ice is applied for 10 to 15 min to the affected (painful to palpation) area. It is hoped that this will help prevent any inflammatory response provoked by microscopic damage to the tendon that might occur during the exercise.

Since this programme is designed for patients with chronic tendinitis, most people are able to participate in athletic activity, but find participation painful (Level 2/3) and/or their performance impaired (Level 4/5). Note that these patients do not need to cease participating in sports unless they are unable to perform. The best course is that patients change nothing about their activity except adding the exercise programme, this makes it much easier to assess the effect of the exercise on the tendon. A decrease in physical activity is almost always accompanied by a parallel decrease in symptoms, and this makes the success of the exercise (or any other treatment) difficult to assess since multiple factors are changing. It is generally best to make only one change at a time and evaluate its effect before moving on to the next intervention. The exercises are performed daily, with continuous progression following the flowchart in Fig. 15, until symptoms are no longer present during functional activity. By this time, the patient should be fully recovered, in that he or she can perform all functional activities without pain. These patients can often be successfully treated with a thorough explanation of the exercise programme, independent performance of the exercise programme, and periodic rechecks in person or by telephone, most will be asymptomatic in 6 to 8 weeks. Telephone rechecks are convenient and inexpensive, and allow the clinician to monitor the level of exercise and functional performance. If no change has occurred, or non-compliance is suspected, an appointment can be made to review the exercise programme.

Programme progression can be monitored in several ways: (1) objectively, via the amount of force applied to the affected limb and/or the speed of movement; (2) subjectively, via the patient's report of pain after specific exercises or activities; and (3) functionally, via the patient's ability to successfully perform those activities considered normal for him or her (for example, basketball lay-up, 1 h of tennis, a 5-mile run, etc.). Strength testing should not be performed until treatment is completed and the patient is asymptomatic. The maximum force levels generated during such testing, especially isokinetic eccentric testing, may damage the healing tendon. While programme progression and success is based almost entirely on a subjective assessment of symptoms by the patient, there is evidence that strength deficits may exist in some tendinitis patients after symptoms have disappeared.[137] This suggests that continued strength training and testing may be appropriate in the latter stages of treatment of chronic tendinitis as a means of preventing its recurrence.

For patients with severe or constant pain (Level 5/6), modification of activity will probably be necessary. Many will have already reduced their activity level, in fact this reduction in performance is the most likely reason for patients seeking professional attention. This level of pain may be interpreted as reflecting a process of acute tendinitis, even though symptoms may have been present for weeks or months, and treatment should begin at a very low level of loading intensity: ice; gentle stretching; passive movement; modalities to stimulate collagen synthesis; etc. Treatment is changed as healing progresses, so that by 2 weeks, more vigorous exercise can usually be introduced as the patient's symptoms will have subsided.

For patients who have curtailed their functional activities, the stage between ending a formal therapeutic programme and resuming full activity creates a delicate balancing act for the patient and clinician. For patients who continued sports participation throughout treatment, this is not a problem. Patients with more severe tendinitis, who have limited their functional activities, must adopt a gradual approach to resuming activity. There are no rules to guide reintroduction to activity, but the patient should be asymptomatic during non-athletic activities and should be performing the eccentric exercise rapidly. Athletic involvement can be started at about 25 per cent of the preinjury level (duration or intensity, depending on the sport and movement), and should be done on alternate days to avoid muscle soreness and to allow evaluation of the tendon's response to training. Assuming that few or no symptoms are produced, progression can be made in approximately 10 to 20 per cent increments, monitoring symptoms, until full training has been resumed. This should take about 8 weeks, making the entire treatment period for a patient with severe tendinitis about 10 to 12 weeks. If pain recurs, or increases in intensity, the patient should return to the previous training level.

Example—lateral epicondylitis in a tennis and squash player

B.L., a 44-year-old male executive, is also a recreational 'A' level tennis and squash player. He presented complaining of pain in the region of his right lateral elbow; this had been a feature for approximately 6 months since he did a considerable amount of remodelling work on his house. The problem had worsened in the past 6 to 8 weeks, so that he now felt his playing was negatively affected. This led him to seek professional advice. He experienced similar elbow pain 3 years ago, which was successfully treated with a cortisone injection and modality-based physical therapy. He was reluctant to have a second injection.

Examination

Examination revealed pain on palpation of the lateral epicondyle and pain with resisted wrist extension. Range of motion of the cervical spine, shoulders, and wrists was within normal limits. Right wrist flexion, with full elbow extension, was moderately restricted

Table 7	Example of exercise programme for chronic tendinitis	
Week	**Treatment**	**Function**
1	Forearm supported on table, 5 lb (2.3 kg) weight (with handle) held in hand, drop slowly into flexion, return to extension	Pain with tennis, squash, performance level 75%
2	Drop 5 lb (2.3 kg) rapidly	Decreased pain, performance level 75% (Level 4)
3	Increase weight to 6.5 lb (2.9 kg)	Decreased pain, performance level 90% (Level 3)
4	Increase weight to 8 lb (3.6 kg)	Decreased pain, performance level 90% (Level 3)
5	Hang weight (2 lb) (0.9 kg) from racquet face, perform eccentric exercise while gripping racquet	Pain after activity, performance level 100% (Level 2)
6	Increase suspended weight to 4 lb (1.8 kg)	No pain with activity, performance level normal (Level 1)

(L = 80 degrees, R = 45 degrees) and produced slight pain (3/10) in the upper lateral forearm. When tested in elbow flexion, wrist flexion increased to 70 degrees.

Assessment

Moderate chronic lateral epicondylitis (Level 3) was precipitated by the excessive use of hand tools and maintained by tennis and squash playing. He felt his performance was about 75 per cent of his normal level of participation.

Treatment

The overall treatment schedule employed is outlined in Table 7. Warm-up, flexibility exercises for the wrist extensors before and after exercise, and ice after exercise were used at each treatment session. The patient was seen for initial evaluation and explanation of the programme, he made four telephone check-ins, and was seen for a final evaluation prior to discontinuing treatment.

Outcome

Objective

- resisted wrist extension with an 8 lb (3.6 kg) weight suspended from a squash racket face, 30 reps pain-free;

- wrist flexion 70 degrees (R), 80 degrees (L); tested with elbow in full extension;

- slightly tender to palpation right lateral epicondyle[†].

Functional

- no reports of limitations in athletic activity.

[†] This area may remain tender long after the patient has fully recovered. This seems to be a peculiarity of lateral epicondylitis.

Success or failure of the programme

When we initially developed the eccentric exercise programme, we monitored over 200 chronic tendinitis patients treated using the programme, and found that most had minimal or no symptoms after 6 weeks (see Fig. 17).[47] These patients had all been treated previously with modality-based therapies, some several times. Similar improvements have been noted by others using eccentric loading slightly different from that suggested in this programme.[137] Most patients will require at least 6 weeks of treatment, a few will experience complete resolution in 2 to 3 weeks, and a very few others will need to continue for 12 to 16 weeks. Modalities can be employed if desired, especially if the patient's symptoms are acute or prolonged and the physiotherapist suspects that the synthetic activity of the tendon is decreased, but these should not be the only treatment used. A similar rationale can be used by the physician to decide on the use of NSAIDs if the inflammatory phase is prolonged.

If the eccentric exercise is unsuccessful in treating the patient's tendinitis, a number of explanations are possible. A slight increase in symptoms at the beginning of the programme should not be viewed with alarm, in fact, it can be considered confirmation that this is a load-related problem. This increase should be temporary. Simply, slightly reduce the magnitude of loading, have the patient avoid performing the exercise programme immediately before or after athletic activity, and encourage the use of ice after exercise. For exercise treatment to be successful, symptoms must be related to tensile loading, usually during eccentric muscle activation (symptoms may not be provoked by concentric or isometric testing). The most common reason for lack of success is incorrect programme progression, the patient is either started at too high a level (and gets worse) or is not progressed to the next level of intensity (and stays the same). A progressive increase in symptoms indicates that an inappropriate level of loading has been chosen, or the patient is doing the exercise incorrectly. Depending on the level of symptoms, the tendinitis may now need to be treated as an acute injury. Little ground is lost if the patient is well educated as to the meaning of increased symptoms, or the therapist immediately adjusts the treatment intensity.

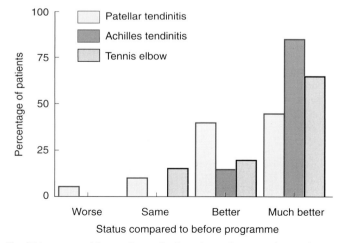

Fig. 17 Improvement in symptoms after 6 weeks on the eccentric exercise programme. Most patients will experience a marked reduction in symptoms by this time, some will require a longer period. These 200 patients performed their exercise programmes in a near-independent fashion with occasional rechecks by the physical therapist and physician.

Should 2 weeks of patient-directed, or 1 week of clinician-directed (two to three treatments) pass without any improvement, the clinician should thoroughly re-evaluate the patient. If he or she remains convinced that tensile loading is the cause (and the solution), the loading programme will need to be adjusted. It is possible that the patient does not have tendinitis, or there may be unrecognized external factors that are causing or perpetuating the problem. A thorough check of spinal and peripheral joint range of motion (active, passive, and accessory), alignment, flexibility, and resisted movements is required in a search for one or more manoeuvres that will reproduce the patient's symptoms—the so-called 'comparable sign'. Such a sign, or signs, can be invaluable in evaluating patient response to treatment. As a rule, if abnormal joint signs are found, these should be treated first. Readers are encouraged to consult other sources for more information about the detailed examination and treatment of the spine and extremities.[138-140] Failure to respond to treatment after the elimination of possible outside factors should make the clinician suspicious about systemic disease, overtraining, or hormonal or nutritional imbalance. Fortunately, these alternative explanations for tendinitis-like symptoms are not common in athletes.

Summary

Chronic tendinitis remains a clinical dilemma. The best treatment is not always possible or recognized, or the patient may fail to follow the appropriate treatment strategy because of functional demands. An ideal treatment will both resolve the current symptoms and prevent their return, and should be based on good science and common sense. The use of exercise to treat chronic tendinitis relies on both of these—the science of tendon adaptation to increased stress and the common sense of patient participation based on their ability to perform. It is not suggested that exercise alone will solve all cases of tendinitis. A careful analysis and systematic elimination of many other factors is often involved. Once these influences have been removed, a knowledge of the adaptation of tendon in response to tensile loading can be used to successfully treat almost all tendon injuries.

References

1. Butler DL, Grood ES, Noyes FR, Zernicke RF. Biomechanics of ligaments and tendons. *Exercise and Sport Science Reviews* 1978; **6**: 125–82.
2. Elliott DH. Structure and function of mammalian tendon. *Biological Reviews of the Cambridge Philosophical Society*, 1965; **40**: 392–421.
3. Kastelic J, Galseki A, Baer E. The multicomposite structure of tendon. *Connective Tissue Research* 1978; **6**: 11–23.
4. Cooper RR, Misol S. Tendon and ligament insertion. A light and electron microscope study. *Journal of Bone and Joint Surgery*, 1970; **52A**: 1–12.
5. Trotter JA, *et al.* A morphometric analysis of the muscle–tendon junction. *Anatomical Record*, 1985; **213**: 26–32.
6. Tidball JG. Myotendinous junction injury in relation to junction structure and molecular composition. *Exercise and Sport Sciences Reviews*, 1991; **19**: 419–46.
7. Flint MH. Interrelationships of muco-polysaccharides and collagen in connective tissue remodelling. *Journal of Embryology and Experimental Morphology*, 1972; **27**: 481–95.
8. Gillard GC *et al.* A comparison of the glycosaminoglycans of weight-bearing and nonweight-bearing human dermis. *Journal of Investigative Dermatology*, 1977; **69**: 257–61.
9. Scott JE, Hughes EW. Proteoglycan–collagen relationships in developing chick and bovine tendons: influence of the physiological environment. *Connective Tissue Research*, 1986; **14**: 267–78.
10. Prockop D, Guzman NA. Collagen diseases and the biosynthesis of collagen. *Hospital Practice;* 1977; **12**: 61–8.
11. Eyre DR. The collagens of the musculoskeletal soft tissues. In: Leadbetter WB, Buckwalter JA, Gordon SL, eds. *Sport-induced inflammation*. Park Ridge: American Academy of Orthopedic Surgeons, 1990; 161–70.
12. Evans JH, Barbenel JC. Structure and mechanical properties of tendon related to function. *Equine Veterinary Journal* 1975; **7**: 1–8.
13. Scott JE. The periphery of the developing collagen fibril: Quantitative relationships with dermatan sulphate and other surface-associated species. *Biochemical Journal* 1984; **218**: 229–33.
14. Koob TJ, Vogel KG. Proteoglycan synthesis in organ cultures from different regions of bovine tendon subjected to different mechanical forces. *Biochemical Journal* 1987; **246**: 589–98.
15. Vogel KG, Trotter JA. The effect of proteoglycans on the morphology of collagen fibrils formed *in vitro*. *Collagen and Related Research* 1987; **7**: 105–14.
16. Viidik A. Tensile properties of Achilles tendon systems in trained and untrained rabbits. *Acta Orthopaedica Scandinavica* 1969; **40**: 261–72.
17. Harkness RD. Mechanical properties of collagenous tissues. In: Gold BS, ed. *Treatise on collagen, Vol. 2 Biology of collagen Part A*. London: Academic Press, 1968; 247–310.
18. Bailey AJ, Robins SP, Balian G. Biological significance of the intermolecular crosslinks of collagen. *Nature* 1974; **251**: 105–9.
19. Hardy MA. The biology of scar formation. *Physical Therapy* 1989; 69: 1014–24.
20. Ihme A *et al.* Ehler–Danlos syndrome type VI: Collagen type specificity of defective lysyl hydroxylation in various tissues. *Journal of Investigative Dermatology* 1984; **83**: 161–5.
21. Monnier VM *et al.* Relation between complications of type I diabetes mellitus and collagen-linked fluorescence. *New England Journal of Medicine* 1986; **314**: 403–8.
22. Akeson WH, Amiel D, Abel MF, Garfin SR, Woo SL-Y. Effects of immobilization on joints. *Clinical Orthopedics and Related Research* 1987; **219**: 28–37.
23. Amiel D *et al.* The effect of immobilization on the types of collagen synthesized in periarticular connective tissue. *Connective Tissue Research* 1980; **8**: 27–35.
24. Amiel D, Woo SL-Y, Harwood FL, Akeson WH. The effect of immobilization on collagen turnover in connective tissue: a biochemical–biomechanical correlation. *Acta Orthopaedica Scandinavica* 1982; **53**: 325.
25. Postacchini F, DeMartino C. Regeneration of rabbit calcaneal tendon: maturation of collagen and elastic fibres following partial tenotomy. *Connective Tissue Research* 1980; **8**: 41–7.
26. Michna H. Morphometric analysis of loading-induced changes in collagen–fibril populations in young tendons. *Cell and Tissue Research* 1984; **236**: 465–70.
27. Doillon CJ *et al.* Collagen fibre formation in repair tissue: development of strength and toughness. *Collagen and Related Research* 1985; **5**: 481–95.
28. Edwards DAW. The blood supply and lymphatic drainage of tendons. *Anatomy* 1946; **80**: 147–52.
29. Enoka RM. *Neuromechanical basis of kinesiology*. Champaign, IL: Human Kinetics, 1994.
30. Knorzer E. *et al.* New aspects of the etiology of tendon rupture: An analysis of time-resolved dynamic–mechanical measurements

using synchotron radiation. *Archives of Orthopaedic and Trauma Surgery* 1986; **105**: 113–20.

31. Mosler E. *et al.* Stress-induced molecular re-arrangement in tendon collagen. *Journal of Molecular Biology* 1985; **182**: 589–96.

32. Steven FS, Minns RJ, Finlay JB. Evidence for the local denaturation of collagen fibril during the mechanical rupture of human tendons. *Injury* 1975; 6: 317–19.

33. Butler DL, Grood ES, Noyes FR, Zernicke RF, Barckett K. Effects of structure and strain measurement technique on the material properties of young human tendons and fascia. *Journal of Biomechanics* 1984; **17**: 579–96.

34. Barfred T. Experimental rupture of the Achilles tendon: comparison of various types of experimental rupture in rats. *Acta Orthopaedica Scandinavica* 1971; **42**: 528–43.

35. Woo SL-Y, Gomez MA, Sites TJ, Newton PO, Orlando CA, Akeson WH. The biomechanical and morphological changes in the medial collateral ligament of the rabbit after immobilization and remobilization. *Journal of Bone and Joint Surgery* 1987; **69A**: 1200–11.

36. Barnes GRG, Pinder DN. In vivo tendon tension and bone strain measurement and correlation. *Journal of Biomechanics* 1974; **7**: 35–42.

37. Barfred T. Kinesiological comments on subcutaneous ruptures of the Achilles tendon. *Acta Orthopaedica Scandinavica* 1971; **42**: 397–405.

38. Curwin SL. Force and length changes of the gastrocnemius and soleus muscle–tendon units during a therapeutic exercise programme and three selected activities. MSc thesis, Dalhousie University, 1984.

39. Gregor RJ, Komi PV, Jarvinen M. Achilles tendon forces during cycling. *International Journal of Sports Medicine* 1987; **8**(Suppl.): 9–14.

40. Booth FW. Effect of limb immobilization on skeletal muscle. *Journal of Applied Physiology* 1982; **52**: 1113–18.

41. Booth FW, Gould EW. Effects of training and disuse on connective tissue. *Exercise and Sport Sciences Reviews* 1975; **3**: 83–107.

42. Jozsa L, Kannus P, Thoring J, Reffy A, Jarvinen M, Kvist M. The effect of tenotomy and immobilization on intramuscular connective tissue. A morphometric and microscopic study in rat calf muscles. *Journal of Bone and Joint Surgery* 1990; **72B**: 293–7.

43. Klein L, Sawson MH, Heiple KG. Turnover of collagen in the adult rat after denervation. *Journal of Bone and Joint Surgery* 1977; **59A**: 1065–7.

44. Noyes FR, Torvik PJ, Hyde WB, DeLucas JL. Biomechanics of ligament failure. II An analysis of immobilization, exercise, and reconditioning effects in primates. *Journal of Bone and Joint Surgery* 1974; **56A**: 1406–18.

45. Vailas AC, Deluna DM, Lewis LL, Curwin SL, Roy RR, Alford EK. Adaptation of bone and tendon to prolonged hindlimb suspension in rats. *Journal of Applied Physiology* 1988; **65**: 373–8.

46. Zuckerman J, Stull GA. Ligamentous separation force in rats as influenced by training, detraining and cage restriction. *Medicine and Science in Sports* 1973; **5**: 44–9.

47. Curwin SL, Stanish WD. *Tendinitis: its etiology and treatment.* Lexington, MA: Collamore Press, DC Heath, 1984.

48. Hitchcock TF, *et al.* The effect of immediate constrained motion on the strength of flexor tendon repairs in chickens. *Journal of Hand Surgery* 1987; **12A**: 590–5.

49. Karpakka J, Vaananen K, Virtanen P, Savolainen J, Orava S, Takala TES. The effects of remobilization and exercise on collagen biosynthesis in rat tendon. *Acta Physiologica Scandinavica* 1990; **139**: 139–45.

50. Curwin SL, Vailas AC, Wood J. Immature tendon adaptation to strenuous exercise. *Journal of Applied Physiology* 1988; **65**: 2297–301.

51. Matsuda JJ, *et al.* Structural and mechanical adaptation of immature bone to strenuous exercise. *Journal of Applied Physiology* 1986; **60**: 2028–34.

52. Silver IA, Rossdale PD. A clinical and experimental study of tendon injury, healing and treatment in the horse. *Equine Veterinary Journal* 1983; **Suppl. 1**: 1–43.

53. Becker H, Diegelman RF. The influence of tension on intrinsic tendon fibroplasia. *Orthopaedic Reviews* 1984; **13**: 65–71.

54. Blanchard O, *et al.* Tendon adaptation to different long-term stresses and collagen reticulation in soleus muscle. *Connective Tissue Research* 1985; **13**: 261–7.

55. Woo SL-Y, Rittel MA, Amiel D, *et al.* The biomechanical and biochemical properties of swine tendons—long-term effects of exercise on the digital extensors. *Connective Tissue Research* 1980; **7**: 177–83.

56. Elliott DH, Crawford GNC. The thickness and collagen content of tendon relative to the strength and cross-sectional area of muscle. *Proceedings of the Royal Society of London Series B* 1965; **162**: 137–46.

57. Tipton CM, Matthes RD, Maynard JA, Carey RA. The influence of physical activity on ligaments and tendons. *Medicine and Science in Sports* 1975; **7**: 165–75.

58. Vailas AC, *et al.* Adaptation of rat knee meniscus to prolonged exercise. *Journal of Applied Physiology* 1986; **60**: 1031–4.

59. Kiiskinen A. Physical training and connective tissues in young mice: physical properties of Achilles tendons and long bones. *Growth* 1977; **41**: 123–37.

60. Woo SLY, *et al.* The biomechanical and morphological changes in the medial collateral ligament of the rabbit after immbolization and remobilization. *Journal of Bone and Joint Surgery* 1987; **69A**: 1200–11.

61. Alexander R McN, Vernon A. The dimensions of knee and ankle muscles and the forces they exert. *Journal of Human Movement Studies* 1975; **1**: 115–23.

62. Blazina M. Jumper's knee. *Orthopedic Clinics of North America* 1973; **2**: 665–73.

63. Clancy WG. Tendon trauma and overuse injuries. In: Leadbetter WB, Buckwalter JA, Gordon SL, eds. *Sports-induced inflammation.* Park Ridge: American Academy of Orthopedic Surgeons, 1990; 609–18.

64. Colosimo AJ, *et al.* Jumper's knee. Diagnosis and treatment. *Orthopaedic Reviews* 1990; **19**: 139–49.

65. Fernandez-Palazzi F, Rivas S, Mujica P. Achilles tendinitis in ballet dancers. *Clinical Orthopaedics and Related Research* 1990; **257**: 257–61.

66. Jorgensen U, Winge S. Injuries in badminton. *Sports Medicine* 1990; **10**: 59–64.

67. Vailas AC, *et al.* Patellar matrix changes associated with aging and voluntary exercise. *Journal of Applied Physiology* 1985; **58**: 1572–6.

68. Wood TO, Cooke PH, Goodship AE. The effect of exercise and anabolic steroids on the mechanical properties and crimp morphology of the rat tendon. *American Journal of Sports Medicine* 1988; **16**: 153–8.

69. Backman C, Boquist L, Friden J, Lorentzon R, Toolanen G. Chronic Achilles paratenonitis with tendinosis: an experimental model in the rabbit. *Journal of Orthopaedic Research* 1990; **8**: 541–7.

70. Backman C, Friden J, Widmark A. Blood flow in chronic Achilles tendinosis. Radioactive microsphere study in rabbits. *Acta Orthopaedica Scandinavica* 1991; **62**: 386–7.

71. Reid D. *Sports injury assessment and rehabilitation.* New York: Churchill Livingstone, 1992.

72. Alexander RM. *The human machine.* New York: Columbia University Press, 1992.

73. Neer CS II. Impingement lesions. *Clinical Orthopedics and Related Research* 1983; **173**: 70–7.

74. Poppen N, Walker P. Forces at the glenohumeral joint in abduction. *Clinical Orthopedics and Related Research* 1978; **135**: 165–70.

75. Neviaser JS. Adhesive capsulitis and the stiff and painful shoulder. *Orthopedic Clinics of North America* 1980; 11: 327–31.

76. Lee D. *A workbook of manual therapy techniques for the upper extremity.* Delta, BC: DOPC, 1989.

77. Malone TR. Shoulder rehabilitation: principles and clinical specifics. In: Harries M, Williams C, Stanish WD, Micheli LJ, eds. *Oxford textbook of sports medicine.* 1st edn. Oxford: Oxford University Press 1994; 460–70.

78. Fackleman BE. The nature of tendon damage and its repair. *Equine Veterinary Journal* 1973; **5**: 141–9.

79. Bonen A, Keizer HA. Pituitary, ovarian and adrenal hormone responses to marathon running. *International Journal of Sports Medicine* 1987; 8(Suppl. 3): 161–7.

80. Bosenberg AT, *et al.* Strenuous exercise causes systemic endotoxemia. *Journal of Applied Physiology* 1988; **65**: 106–8.

81. Vailas AC, Morgan WP, Vailas JC. Physiologic and cellular basis of overtraining. In: Leadbetter WB, Buckwalter JA, Gordon SL, eds. *Sports-induced inflammation.* Park Ridge: American Academy of Orthopedic Surgeons, 1990; 677–86.

82. Matheson GO, Macintyre JG, Taunton JE, Clement DB, Lloyd-Smith R. Musculoskeletal injuries associated with physical activity in older adults. *Medicine and Science in Sports and Exercise* 1989; 21: 379–85.

83. Stanish WD, Rubinovich RM, Curwin SL. Eccentric exercise in chronic tendinitis. *Clinical Orthopaedics and Related Research* 1986; **208**: 65–8.

84. Stauber WT. Eccentric action of muscles: Physiology, injury and adaptation. *Exercise and Sport Sciences Reviews* 1989; **17**: 157–85.

85. Zernicke RF, Garhammer J, Jobe FW. Human patellar tendon rupture. *Journal of Bone and Joint Surgery* 1977; **59A**: 179–83.

86. Curwin SL, Roy RR, Vailas AC. Regional and age variations in growing tendon. *Journal of Morphology* 1994; **221**: 309–20.

87. Kain CC, *et al.* Regional differences in matrix formation in the healing flexor tendon. *Clinical Orthopaedics and Related Research* 1988; **229**: 308–12.

88. Tidball JG. Myotendinous junction: Morphological changes and mechanical failure associated with muscle cell atrophy. *Experimental and Molecular Pathology* 1984; **40**: 1–12.

89. Komi PV. Measurement of the force–velocity relationship in human muscle under concentric and eccentric contractions. *Medicine in Sport* 1973; **8**: 224–9.

90. Komi PV. Neuromuscular performance: factors influencing force and speed production. *Scandinavian Journal of Sports Science* 1979; **1**: 2–15.

91. Bosco C, Komi PV. Potentiation of the mechanical behaviour of the human skeletal muscle through pre-stretching. *Acta Physiologica Scandinavica* 1982; **14**: 543–50.

92. Alexander RM. *The human machine.* New York: Columbia University Press, 1992.

93. Nirschl RP. The etiology and treatment of tennis elbow. *Journal of Sports Medicine* 1974; **2**: 308–19.

94. Horswill CA, *et al.* Excretion of 3-methyl-histidine and hydroxyproline following acute weight-training exercise. *International Journal of Sports Medicine* 1988; **9**: 245–8.

95. Alen M, *et al.* Responses of serum androgenic–anabolic and catabolic hormones to prolonged strength training. *International Journal of Sports Medicine* 1988; **9**: 229–33.

96. Kjaer M. Epinephrine and some other hormonal responses to exercise in man: with special reference to physical training. *International Journal of Sports Medicine* 1989; **10**: 2–15.

97. Newman RA, Cutroneo KR. Glucocorticoids selectively decrease the synthesis of hydroxylated collagen peptides. *Molecular Pharmacology* 1978; **14**: 185–98.

98. Oxlund H, Manthorpe R. The biomechanical properties of tendon and skin as influenced by long-term glucocorticoid treatment and food restriction. *Biorheology* 1982; **19**: 631–46.

99. Davis JM, *et al.* Stress hormone response to exercise in elite female distance runners. *International Journal of Sports Medicine* 1987; 8(Suppl. 2): 132–5.

100. Agarwal S, *et al.* Tendinitis and tendon ruptures in successful renal transplant recipients. *Clinical Orthopaedics and Related Research* 1990; **252**: 270–5.

101. Murison MS, *et al.* Tendinitis—a common complication after renal transplantation. *Transplantation* 1990; **48**: 587–9.

102. Gillard GC, Reilly HC, Bell-Booth PG, Flint MH. The influence of mechanical forces on the glycosaminoglycan content of the rabbit flexor digitorum profundus tendon. *Connective Tissue Research* 1979; **7**: 37–47.

103. Rathbun JB, MacNab I. The micro-vascular pattern of the rotator cuff. *Journal of Bone and Joint Surgery* 1970; **52B**: 540–53.

104. Andrews FJ, *et al.* Effect of nutritional iron deficiency on acute and chronic inflammation. *Annals of the Rheumatic Diseases* 1987; **46**: 859–65.

105. McCall IW, Park WM, O'Brien JP. Induced pain referred from posterior lumbar elements in normal subjects. *Spine* 1979; **4**: 441–6.

106. Abrahamsson S-O, Lundborg G, Lohmander LS. Tendon healing *in vivo.* An experimental model. *Scandinavian Journal of Reconstructive Surgery* 1989; **23**: 199–205.

107. Morcos MB, Aswad A. Histological studies of the effects of ultrasonic therapy on surgically split flexor tendons. *Equine Veterinary Journal* 1978; **10**: 267.

108. Nistor L. Surgical and non-surgical treatment of Achilles tendon rupture. *Journal of Bone and Joint Surgery* 1981; **63**: 394–9.

109. Steiner M. Biomechanics of tendon healing. *Journal of Biomechanics* 1982; **15**: 951–8.

110. Enwemeka CS, Spielholz NI, Nelson AJ. The effect of early functional activities on experimentally tenotomized Achilles tendons in rats. *American Journal of Physical Medicine and Rehabilitation* 1988; **67**: 264–9.

111. Enwemeka CS. Inflammation, cellularity and fibrillogenesis in regenerating tendon: implications for tendon rehabilitation. *Physical Therapy* 1989; **69**: 816–25.

112. Watkins P, Auer JA, Gay S, *et al.* Healing of surgically created defects in the equine superficial digital flexor tendon: collagen-type transformation and tissue morphologic reorganization. *American Journal of Veterinary Research* 1985; **46**: 2091–6.

113. Watkins JP, *et al.* Healing of surgically created defects in the equine superficial digital flexor tendon: effects of pulsing electromagnetic field therapy on collagen-type transformation and tissue morphologic reorganization. *American Journal of Veterinary Research* 1985; **46**: 2097–103.

114. Hitchcock TF, *et al.* New technique for producing uniform partial lacerations of tendons. *Journal of Orthopaedic Research* 1989; **7**: 451–5.

115. Hargreaves KM. Mechanisms of pain sensation resulting from inflammation. In: Leadbetter WB, Buckwalter JA, Gordon SL, eds. *Sports-induced inflammation,* Park Ridge: American Academy of Orthopedic Surgeons, 1990; 383–92.

116. Dyson M, Suckling J. Stimulation of tissue repair by ultrasound: a survey of the mechanisms involved. *Physiotherapy* 1978; **64**: 105–8.

117. Dyson M, *et al.* The stimulation of tissue regeneration by means of ultrasound. *Clinical Science* 1968; **35**: 273–85.

118. Frieder S, *et al.* A pilot study: the therapeutic effect of ultrasound following partial rupture of the Achilles tendon in male rats. *Journal of Orthopedic and Sports Physical Therapy* 1988; **10**: 39–46.

119. Harvey W, Dyson M, Pond JB, Grahame R. The stimulation of protein synthesis in fibroblasts by therapeutic ultrasound. *Rheumatology and Rehabilitation* 1975; **14**: 237.

120. Enwemeka CS. The effects of therapeutic ultrasound on tendon healing. A biomechanical study. *American Journal of Physical Medicine and Rehabilitation* 1989; **68**: 283–7.

121. Snow CJ, Johnson KA. Effect of therapeutic ultrasound on acute inflammation. *Physiotherapy Canada* 1988; **40**: 162–7.

122. Basford JR. Low-energy laser therapy. In: Leadbetter WB, Buckwalter JA, Gordon SL, eds. *Sports-induced inflammation*. Park Ridge: American Academy of Orthopedic Surgeons, 1990; 499–508.

123. Nessler JP, Mass DP. Direct-current electrical stimulation of tendon healing *in vivo*. *Clinical Orthopaedics and Related Research* 1987; **217**: 303–12.

124. Stanish WD, *et al.* The use of electricity on ligament and tendon repair. *Physician and Sports Medicine* 1985; **13**: 109–16.

125. Frank C, *et al.* Electromagnetic stimulation of ligament healing in rabbits. *Clinical Orthopaedics and Related Research* 1983; **175**: 263–72.

126. Binder A, *et al.* Pulsed electromagnetic field therapy of persistent rotator cuff tendinitis: a double-blind controlled assessment. *Lancet* 1984; **i**: 695–8.

127. Knight KL. Effects of hypothermia on inflammation and swelling. *Athletic Training* 1976; **11**: 7–10.

128. Barnes L. Cryotherapy: putting injury on ice. *Physician and Sports Medicine* 1979; **7**: 130–6.

129. Kennedy JC, Willis RB. The effects of local steroid injections on tendons: a biomechanical and microscopic correlative study. *American Journal of Sports Medicine* 1976; **4**: 11–21.

130. Da Cruz DJ, *et al.* Achilles paratendonitis: an evaluation of steroid injection. *British Journal of Sports Medicine* 1988; **22**: 64–5.

131. Leadbetter WB. Corticosteroid injection therapy in sports injuries. In: Leadbetter WB, Buckwalter JA, Gordon SL, eds. *Sports-induced inflammation*. Park Ridge: American Academy of Orthopedic Surgeons, 1990; 527–45.

132. Abramson SB. Nonsteroidal anti-inflammatory drugs: mechanisms of action and therapeutic considerations. In: Leadbetter WB, Buckwalter JA, Gordon SL, eds. *Sports-induced inflammation*. Park Ridge: American Academy of Orthopedic Surgeons, 1990; 421–30.

133. Almekinders LC, Gilbert JA. Healing of experimental muscle strains and the effects of nonsteroidal anti-inflammatory medication. *American Journal of Sports Medicine* 1987; **15**: 357–61.

134. Salminen A, Kihlstrom M, Protective effect of indomethacin against exercise-induced injuries in mouse skeletal muscle fibres. *International Journal of Sports Medicine* 1987; **8**: 46–9.

135. Michna JH. Tendon injuries induced by exercise and anabolic steroids in experimental mice. *International Orthopedics* 1987; **11**: 157–62.

136. Haupt HA. The role of anabolic steroids as modifiers of sports-induced inflammation. In: Leadbetter WB, Buckwalter JA, Gordon SL, eds. *Sports-induced inflammation*. Park Ridge: American Academy of Orthopedic Surgeons, 1990; 449–54.

137. Jensen K, DiFabio RP. Evaluation of eccentric exercise in treatment of patellar tendinitis. *Physical Therapy* 1989; **69**: 211–16.

138. Magee DJ. *Orthopedic physical assessment*. Philadelphia, W.B. Saunders, 1992.

139. Grieve GP, ed. *Modern manual therapy of the vertebral column*. London: Churchill Livingstone, 1986.

140. Wadsworth CT. *Manual examination and treatment of the spine and extremities*. Baltimore: Williams and Wilkins, 1988.

5

Chronic and overuse sports injuries

5.1 An introduction to chronic overuse injuries

Per A.F.H. Renström

Introduction

Most people in society are engaged in sports activities and physical exercise of some kind. These activities invoke a variety of stress responses in the human body, of which many, including improved cardiovascular function, altered body composition, improved muscular strength, increased physical stamina, and a sense of well being or fitness, are beneficial.[1] However, sports also have damaging effects such as overuse injuries.

The term 'overuse injury', as we know it today, originates from a paper by Slocum and James on running injuries, published in 1968.[2] However, examples of overuse injuries first appeared in the literature in 1855 when Breithaupt reported on stress fractures of the metatarsal bone. Runge described the tennis elbow syndrome in 1873, and Albert described Achilles tendinitis in 1893.

Overuse injuries are increasingly common in relation to sports activities, constituting at least 50 to 60 per cent of all sports injuries, but the true incidence is not known. They are related to extrinsic factors such as training errors, poorly instrumented sporting equipment, unsuitable environmental conditions, and intrinsic factors such as malalignments and muscle imbalance.

Overuse injuries constitute a large diagnostic and therapeutic problem because the symptoms are often diffuse and uncharacteristic. Chronic overuse injuries have an insidious development and unpredictable recovery as the healing response varies. Many overuse injuries may not be primarily inflammatory responses at the cellular level but rather degenerative changes with resulting biomechanical failure of tissue matrix integrity. The degree of degeneration decides the rate and outcome of the treatment. Despite early recognition of these injuries, our understanding of them is still very limited, and little scientific evidence concerning their diagnosis and treatment is available. Therefore, the diagnosis is often based on the examining physician's clinical experience in sports medicine. The treatment should be based on specific diagnosis and scientific background, but is still often performed by trial and error. Thus, overuse conditions provide a challenge to sports medicine physicians.

Aetiology of overuse syndromes

Overuse of a tissue is based on repetitive motion without an increase in resistance, whereas overload is characterized by excessive rapid increase in resistance. Overuse injuries in athletes are generally due to repetitive microtrauma of the musculoskeletal system. Factors implicated in overuse injuries can be classified as extrinsic or intrinsic.

Extrinsic factors

A number of activities are implicated with overuse injuries in sports: one is associated with endurance training, which is part of most sports, and another is associated with repetitive performances requiring skill, technique, and/or power, as in gymnastics, high jump, and weightlifting. Overuse syndromes appear to occur about three times more frequently in the former group than in the latter group.[3]

Many overuse injuries are associated with repetitive pounding activities such as running and jumping. A runner weighing 75 kg absorbs a total of 220 000 kg on each foot per 1.6 km assuming a shock absorption of 250 per cent of body weight at ground contact.[4] Running injuries are generally associated with the stance phase portion of the running cycle. At a pace of 1.6 km per 7 min, stance time is approximately 0.2 s, which translates into approximately 5100 contacts per hour of running.[5] These huge repetitive forces suggest that even small biomechanical abnormalities and deviations can result in a significant concentration of stress and load on the human tissue and result in an overuse injury.

Extrinsic factors are present in 60 to 80 per cent of reported injuries to runners.[6-8] The most common causes are changes in running activities such as increased distance, increased intensity, or excessive hill work (Table 1). Leadbetter[10] has called this the principle of transition, which he defines as 'sports injury is most likely to occur when the athlete experiences any change in mode or use of the involved part'. Transition risk is rate dependent. Examples of this are a novice runner who has started to run or an athlete returning to running after an injury. Harvey[6] found that 80 per cent of the athletes visiting his clinic had only recently taken up the sport, or had markedly increased their training intensity a few days to 2 weeks prior to the onset of symptoms. Occasionally, an athlete had started participating in a second sport or another activity which had similar biomechanics, providing added stress which initiated the injury. Adult athletes can develop overuse injuries after 2 years of regular daily training during which both the amount and intensity progressively increase.[3]

Table 1 Extrinsic factors related to injuries in sports
Excessive load on the body
Type of movement
Speed of movement
Number of repetitions
Footwear
Surface
Training errors
Excessive distance
Changes in mode of progression
High intensity
Hill work
Poor technique
Monotonous or asymmetric training
Fatigue
Unsuitable environmental conditions
Dark
Heat/cold
Humidity
Altitude
Wind
Poor equipment
Ineffective rules

Reproduced from ref. 9, with permission.

Running downhill can produce problems in the knee joint. During such activity, there is an increased knee flexion, extensor movement, and patellar femoral forces, increased power absorption, and increased eccentric contraction of the knee extensors.[11] The main body weight is behind the knee joint, which produces increased loads on the extensor muscles resulting in increased risk of fatigue and hence decreased capacity to protect the knee. Downhill running can produce and increase the symptoms from patellofemoral pain and iliotibial band friction syndromes.

The types and conditions of the sports surface used may be of importance. There is a much higher force at first contact for running on asphalt compared with running on grass or sand.[12] The incidence of injuries associated with running on hard surfaces is much greater than that associated with running on wood chips, soft dirt, or a composite surface. Running on uneven or artificial surfaces and on slippery roads can also cause overuse injuries. Running on a banked surface or a cambered road in one direction will probably cause abnormal stress on one side of the body, resulting in a short–long syndrome, with increased secondary pronation on the inner leg, and possibly injuries such as iliotibial band friction syndrome or trochanteric bursitis.

Overuse injuries are more common in soccer played on artificial turf than on grass or gravel.[12,13] Both adolescent and adult tennis players may sustain more overuse injuries, such as medial tibial stress syndrome, Achilles tendinitis, and plantar fasciitis, on fast surfaces with high friction than on slower and more yielding clay courts.

Inadequate or worn shoes can cause increased stress and overuse. It is not acceptable to wear tennis, basketball, or soccer shoes during regular running programmes as they do not have the appropriate features to protect a runner from injuries.

Poorly instrumented sporting equipment can cause overuse injuries, particularly if used in combination with poor technique. Oversized tennis rackets absorb vibration better from tennis balls that are hit off-centre along the vertical axis.[14] The material, size, stringing, and grip size of the racket may all be important factors in the development of tennis overuse injuries. Studies suggest that players should use a light, middle-sized, or oversized racket, with a gut stringing of about 22.7 to 25 kg, and play on slow courts with light balls in order to prevent lateral epicondylitis or at least avoid making the injury worse.

Unsuitable environmental conditions may play a role. Cold and hot environments may influence the metabolic rates and vascular supply of the soft tissues, thus limiting their ability to work efficiently for any length of time.[15]

Rules may also be a factor in preventing overuse syndromes, particularly in young athletes. Thus in junior baseball in the United States, the number of pitches that a player can make per season is limited to prevent the occurrence of the condition known as Little Leaguer's elbow.

Intrinsic factors

Intrinsic predisposing factors may be present in 40 per cent of athletes with running injuries, but only in 10 per cent are they the only demonstrable factor.[16] The most common intrinsic factors related to overuse injuries are given in Table 2.[17]

Malalignments of various types are the most important and common intrinsic factor. The majority of malalignment problems are minor and subtle, and can be corrected with applied external forces.[18] James et al.[7] found that increased pronation was present in about 60 per cent of a group of injured runners. However, it is not known what percentage of uninjured runners have increased pronation. The constraints of pronation are the shape of the subtalar joints, the ligamentous support, and, to a lesser degree, the muscle support (Fig. 1).[4] Maximum muscle participation of the tibialis

Table 2 Intrinsic factors related to injuries in sports
Malalignments
Foot hyperpronation/hypopronation
Pes planus/cavus
Forefoot varus/valgus
Hindfoot varus/valgus
Tibia vara
Genu valgum/varum
Patella alta/baja
Femoral neck anteversion
Leg length discrepancy
Muscle weakness/imbalance
Decreased flexibility
Joint laxity and instability
Female gender
Youth/old age
Overweight
Predisposing diseases

Reproduced from ref. 9, with permission.

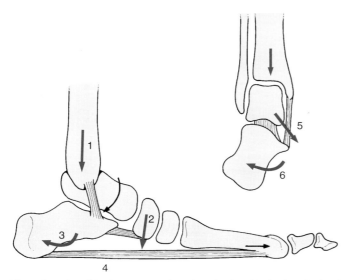

Fig. 1 Pronation of the foot is a complicated mechanism. The load on the foot is from the tibia (1) down towards the talus, which is gliding forward (2) and medially (5). The calcaneus is moving forward–downward (3) and is rotated down into the valgus (6). The plantar aponeurosis (4) is stretched out. There is increased tension in the insertions.

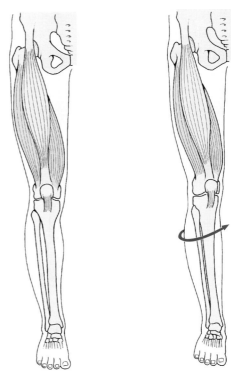

Fig. 2 Excessive pronation of the foot results in compensatory mechanisms of the lower extremities such as internal rotation of the tibia. Left, a normal leg; right, a compensatory internal rotation of the tibia. (Redrawn from Peterson L, Renström P. *Injuries in sports*. London: Martin Dunitz, 1985, with permission.)

anterior, the tibialis posterior, and the soleus is not enough to control excessive eversion forces.

During walking, there is approximately 6° to 8° of subtalar joint motion in normal individuals. The pronation that occurs at the time of ground contact is not an active event. It is the result of loading the body weight on to the foot. With increased pronation, there is an increase of 10° to 12° of subtalar joint motion.

During running, approximately 80 per cent of people have heel initial contact at distance running speeds, while the other 20 per cent have midfoot initial contact.[5] Therefore, running should be differentiated from sprinting, which is characterized by such factors as increased velocity, decreased shock absorption in early stance, and initial contact with the toe. Maximum pronation is usually reached after 40 per cent of the stance phase portion. The foot gradually levels over into supination at around 60 per cent to prepare for push-off.

Some increased pronation of the foot is often physiological, but excessive pronation is potentially harmful. Compensatory hyperpronation may occur for anatomical reasons, such as a tibia vara of 10° or more, forefoot varus, leg length discrepancy, or ligamentous laxity, or because of muscular weakness or tightness in the gastrocnemius and soleus muscles. Excessive pronation will have secondary effects on the lower extremities such as an increased compensatory internal rotation of the tibia resulting in lower leg and knee problems (Fig. 2). The degree of subtalar eversion, and therefore pronation, determines the degree of compensatory internal tibia rotation. This increased rotation of the tibia may also give more proximal effects through the femur and pelvis. In other words the lower extremity should be regarded as a functional unit when carrying out clinical examinations.

Excessive pronation will predispose for injuries on the medial aspects of the lower extremities. An increased pronation is associated with injuries such as medial tibial stress syndrome, tibialis posterior tendinitis, Achilles bursitis or tendinitis, plantar fasciitis,

patellofemoral disorders, iliotibial band friction syndrome, and lower-extremity stress fractures. It must be pointed out that specific anatomical abnormalities and abnormal biomechanics of the lower extremity are not correlated with specific injuries on a predictable basis.[19]

Cavus feet (Fig. 3) are also associated with overuse injuries. James *et al.*[7] found that cavus feet were present in about 20 per cent of their injured group of runners. Athletes with cavus feet have decreased motion at the subtalar and midtarsal joints with resulting

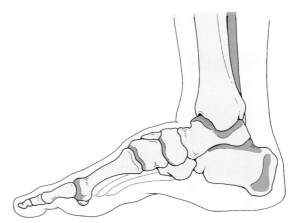

Fig. 3 The cavus foot is a foot which is very inelastic with a very rigid midfoot resulting in increased loads on the anterior and posterior part of the foot. (Redrawn from Peterson L, Renström P. *Injuries in sports*. London: Martin Dunitz, 1985, with permission.)

decreased flexibility of the foot. At foot strike the heel remains in varus, the longitudinal arch is maintained, and the foot does not unlock.[20] There is decreased internal rotation of the tibia and the lower extremity, which means that the tibia remains in external rotation, and the net result is increased stress since the arch continues to be rigid through the midstance phase of running.[8] With this lack of compensatory internal tibia rotation, stress is passed through the lateral foot and knee resulting in injuries of the lateral side of the lower extremity, such as the iliotibial band friction syndrome, trochanteric bursitis, stress fractures, Achilles tendinitis, muscle strain, and metatarsalgia.

Many athletes have a mild genu varum. A lower leg varus alignment of more than 8° to 10° is considered non-physiological and results in compensatory functional foot pronation. There is a low incidence of injury if the total varus is less than 8°, but a marked incidence of running-related injuries if the varus alignment is more than 18°.[21]

An athlete can have a combination of malalignments. Athletes with the so-called miserable malalignment syndrome (Fig. 4), including femoral neck anteversion with internal rotation of the hip and genu varum with or without hyperextension, squinting patella, excessive Q-angle, tibial varum, functional equinus, and compensatory foot pronation, have an increased risk for overuse injuries. A miserable malalignment syndrome may cause such problems with running on a regular basis that it is feasible to recommend that some people with this syndrome should not run long distances.

Leg length discrepancy is commonly discussed with respect to overuse injuries. Leg length discrepancy can be secondary to a difference in leg length, but this condition is quite uncommon. This malalignment is usually functional, and is caused by such activities as running on cambered roads. Leg length discrepancy can give secondary effects such as pelvic tilt to the short side, functional lumbar scoliosis, increased abduction of the hip, excessive pronation, increased knee valgus, and outward rotation of the hip.[22] Leg length discrepancy has been suggested to be a factor in the development of injuries such as iliotibial band friction syndrome, trochanteric bursitis, low back pain, and stress fractures. From an orthopaedic viewpoint, discrepancies of less than 13 mm are cosmetic in most people. However, in top-level athletes a discrepancy of more than 5 to 10 mm may be symptomatic and should then be treated.

The significance of muscle imbalance as an injury-causing factor is a matter of debate. Muscle imbalance means that there is an asymmetry between the agonist and antagonist muscles in one extremity, asymmetry between the extremities, or a difference from the anticipated normal value.[23] An athlete with over 10 per cent difference in quadriceps or hamstring strength between the right and left sides is believed to be at a greater risk of muscular tendon injury. Also, an athlete who has a ratio of hamstring to quadriceps strength in one leg of 60 per cent or less is believed to have a propensity for sustaining muscle injury.[24] In a study of an American football team, hamstring injuries were found in 6.7 per cent of players with a recurrence rate of 13 per cent. Muscle imbalance was found, but after correction the occurrence and recurrence of these injuries disappeared.[25]

Muscle weakness due to scarring and fibrosis from previous injury or surgery may predispose to recurrent injury because the scar tissue is not as strong or elastic as the other components of the muscular tendinous unit. Athletes with a previous joint injury have persistent and long-lasting deficits in muscular strength, power, and endurance in the extremity. The affected joints may be at a greater danger of reinjury than uninjured joints. However, some studies have not found any direct relationship between muscle weakness and injury.[23]

Decreased flexibility and joint laxity may contribute to overuse injuries. Joint instability after anterior cruciate ligament injuries in the knee joint, for example, may result in serious long-term consequences such as post-traumatic osteoarthritis.

Gender may be a factor as there seems to be a higher incidence of overuse injuries among women.[26] The reason for this may be that women have a weaker musculoskeletal system, 25 per cent less muscle mass per body weight, less bone, a wider pelvis, and more mobile joints than men. Menstrual irregularities, which are much more common among female athletes than among non-athletes, constitute a risk factor for certain overuse injuries. There is an increased incidence of stress fractures among amenorrhoeic athletes compared with menorrhoeic athletes in the same sport.[27] A prolonged hypo-oestrogenic state may result in a loss of bone mass and therefore may increase the risk of osteoporotic acute fractures.

Young as well as old age may be a predisposing factor for injuries. During the growth spurt which occurs in most girls at about 12 years of age and in boys at about 14 years, there is a great imbalance between muscle strength, tightness, joint mobility, and co-ordination. In this phase, there is an increased risk of both acute and chronic overuse injuries such as traction apophysitis of the tibial tubercle (Osgood–Schlatter's syndrome) or of joint injury in young pitchers (Little Leaguer's elbow). In gymnastics, intensive training over a long period of time may produce hypermobility of the spinal column and other joints, and the end result may be earlier osteoarthritis.[28] However, this is controversial.

Stanitski[29] considered that factors that lead to injuries in ado-

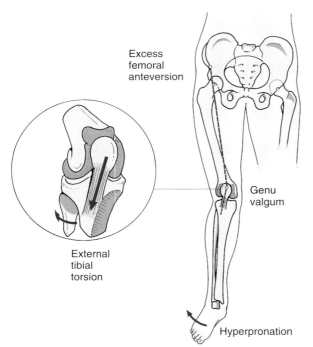

Fig. 4 Malalignment syndrome. (Redrawn from Grana W, Kalenak A. *Clinical sports medicine*. Eastbourne: W. B. Saunders, with permission.)

Excess femoral anteversion

External tibial torsion

Genu valgum

Hyperpronation

lescent athletes include the athlete's own psychobiology, inappropriate equipment, the sports environment (such as playing surfaces), training and coaching errors, and parental influences. Most sport-related injuries in children are minor and self-limiting. The appropriate aims of children and most sports must remain enjoyment with acquisition of sports-specific skills and thereby prevention of overuse injuries.

With ageing, various functions of the body gradually deteriorate. However, active elderly people do better than those who are inactive. Aged persons have a reduced ability to adapt to environmental stress and a loss of tissue homeostasis.[10] Elderly runners have less physical disability, maintain a better functional capacity, and have fewer visits to the physician per year.[30] In elderly athletes, sports injuries are more frequently overuse-related than acute, with the most common injuries found in the muscles and tendons of the lower leg.[31]

Overweight may be a factor in producing overuse symptoms. The development of knee and hip symptoms from osteoarthritis is associated with overweight. Physical activity may further accelerate the osteoarthritic process.[32] Weight reduction in severely obese individuals often leads to a significant relief of their musculoskeletal symptoms.[33]

Predisposing diseases may make athletes more prone to injury. A patient with diabetes who has a low blood sugar level may lose his concentration or co-ordination. Children with Perthes' disease may lose the rotatory function of their knee and may secondarily develop overuse symptoms.

Frequency and type of overuse injuries

The actual incidence of overuse injuries is unknown, since frequently they do not require the athlete to visit a physician. The majority of injuries seen in sports medicine clinics are overuse injuries. The most extensive investigation of overuse injuries has been presented by Orava.[3] He found that in Finland, top-level athletes aged 20 to 29 years and recreational athletes aged 30 to 49 years most frequently visited sports medicine clinics for treatment of overuse injuries, with 15 per cent of the injured athletes being female.

Overuse injuries occur in most sports and often develop when athletes try to advance their training too rapidly. They generally occur in repetitive pounding activities such as long-distance running or in overhead activities such as throwing. Injuries in 'gliding' sports such as cross-country skiing and swimming are not as common and the injury patterns are different from those in running. In Orava's study of the injured individuals, 86.5 per cent participated in endurance sports.[3] Endurance activities increase the incidence of overuse injuries: 91 per cent of ultraendurance triathlete competitors sustained at least one soft tissue overuse injury during the previous year of training.[34]

Most overuse injuries involve the lower extremities. The most frequent locations in Orava's study[3] were the knee (28 per cent), ankle, foot, and heel (21 per cent), and lower leg and shin (17 per cent). In a large survey of 4173 runners, the knee was involved in 40 to 42 per cent of the injuries depending on distance and gender.[35] The lower leg (11 per cent in men and 30 per cent in women) and

foot (10 per cent and 27 per cent) were the most commonly injured regions, followed by the upper leg (3 per cent and 10 per cent), hip (5 per cent and 11 per cent), and low back (2 per cent and 5 per cent). The area of the body most frequently involved in ultraendurance athletes was the back, and the most common pattern was to have multiple areas involved.

The most common structures involved are the muscles and fascias (27 per cent), tendon and muscle insertion (22 per cent), joint surfaces (17 per cent), tendons and tendon sheaths (15 per cent), and bursas, bones, and nerves (21 per cent).[3]

Patellofemoral pain syndrome was diagnosed in one patient out of four (24 per cent in men and 30 per cent in women) with a running injury.[35] Iliotibial band friction syndrome and plantar fasciitis were the second (7 per cent and 8 per cent) and third (5 per cent and 4 per cent) most common injuries. Achilles tendinitis constituted 5 per cent (men) and 3 per cent (women) of the total number of injuries, which is a reduction in frequency compared with reports from 1981.[36] This reduction in Achilles tendon disorders correlates well with the introduction of appropriate, motion control, running shoes having heel wedging of more than 12 mm and increased rear foot support.[8] In addition, an appreciation of the importance of gastrocnemius–soleus flexibility and the need to develop a pattern of warm-up and cool-down activities involving stretching has contributed to the reduced incidence of this disorder.

The injury data in the literature have shown an alarming rise in the incidence of knee pain in runners—from 18 to 50 per cent of injuries in 13 years.[8,35] 6MacIntyre et al.[35] believed that an imbalance or insufficiency in the quadriceps–hamstring muscle groups, or lower extremity malalignment with subsequent abnormal patellofemoral tracking, contributed significantly to knee pain in their patients. According to McKenzie et al.,[8] errors in training judgment with excessive loading, particularly in runners with compromised biomechanical features, represent the primary aetiological factor for this increase in the incidence of knee pain.

The elderly seem to have an increased incidence of overuse injuries. Kannus et al.[37] found that 70 per cent of injuries in a group of injured elderly athletes were overuse injuries compared with 41 per cent in a younger population. In both groups, the knee joint was most frequently affected; 36 per cent in young athletes and 21 per cent in the elderly. Shoulder injuries were present in 18 per cent of the elderly athletes and Achilles tendon injuries were present in 20 per cent, which was significantly more common than among young athletes. Matheson et al.[38] compared young athletes with relatively senior athletes and found that the frequency of tendinitis was similar in both age groups while metatarsal, plantar fasciitis, and meniscal injuries were more common in the older population. Patellofemoral pain syndrome, stress fractures, and periostitis were more common in the younger population. In the older population, the prevalence of osteoarthritis was 2.5 times higher than the frequency of osteoarthritis as the source of activity-related pain. Injuries in elderly athletes occur more frequently in endurance sports, are more frequently overuse related, and are more often degenerative in nature.

Diagnostic principles

The diagnosis of overuse injuries is based on clinical experience and limited science. Therefore the diagnosis is often a challenge.

A correct history of these injuries is of greater importance than for other injuries because it forms the main basis on which diagnosis is made. The clinician must explore in depth the history of the athlete's complaints and the duration and nature of onset of most problems. The pain-causing situations should be analysed, as well as any swelling, locking, or popping. It is important to analyse the patient's training programme, eliciting information, for example, on changes in distance and intensity, number of workouts, type of strengthening or stretching exercises, equipment, location for activities, and competitions. The shoes that the athlete has been wearing and whether there is any specific abnormal pattern of shoe wear should be discussed. Use of orthotics should be discussed, as well as the type of surface or turf on which training has occurred. Nutritional aspects may be of importance. The physician should be aware of the demands and biomechanics of the sport involved in order to be able to analyse how the injury occurred and to determine whether excessive loads are present to cause this injury. In most cases the doctor should be able to suspect the diagnosis accurately from the history.

Physical examination of a leg injury should be thorough; it should include the entire lower extremity and back and be carried out with the patient in standing, sitting, prone, lying, and supine positions. In the standing position, it is possible to examine the back and the overall alignment of the whole lower extremity. The patient should also be observed while walking. In the sitting position, the patient's knee alignment can be evaluated as well as ankle stability and foot configurations. In the supine position, the range of motion of the hip and knee joints can be evaluated. In the prone position, the Achilles tendon, the heel–leg alignment, the subtalar motion, and the sole can be carefully examined. Examination of the functional anatomy with the suspicion of a biomechanical imbalance is the basis for the diagnosis and management of overuse injuries. With a basic understanding of the biomechanics of the extremities and of the stresses which occur during physical activity, most overuse problems can be managed properly.

Radiological examination can sometimes be valuable, and the indications of conventional radiography include suspicion of degenerative changes in a joint, loose intra-articular bodies, and stress fractures (2 to 3 weeks after the onset of symptoms). Special views can sometimes be indicated in, for example, patella and shoulder injuries. According to Merchant et al.,[39] axial patella views at 45° evaluate the congruence angle which indicates a patella subluxation. Axial views at 30° indicate different malformations of the patella and trochlea. Subacromial space views of the shoulder show the Bigliani types of the acromion, which can be helpful in establishing indications for subacromial decompressive surgery. Stress radiographs demonstrating chronic joint instability in the ankle, knee, and elbow can sometimes be of value.

Magnetic resonance imaging (**MRI**) is a non-invasive imaging technique that provides excellent soft tissue contrasts in multiple planes without exposure to ionizing radiation. The MRI technique has been used in sports medicine mainly in the shoulder and knee joints. It provides an excellent non-invasive method for identifying the type, site, and extent of rotator cuff overuse injuries and impingement problems. MRI is also commonly used in the diagnosis of knee pathology with improved accuracy in evaluating meniscus and ligament tears. It is not as accurate in the diagnosis of articular cartilage lesions or the detection of loose bodies. MRI is increasingly used in evaluating tendon pathology, but more research

is needed. It allows the tendons to be identified easily because of the large differences in the relaxation properties of hydrogen in the water molecules in various tissues and fat. The disadvantages of MRI include patient positioning (claustrophobia) and contraindications of metal artefacts such as clips or cardiac pacemakers. MRI will continue to develop and will become the tool of choice as it gradually improves in accuracy, when it can be used for functional evaluation, and when it becomes affordable. MR arthrogram (MRA) is today the diagnostic tool of choice for labrum injuries etc. in the shoulder. MRI spectroscopy has potential for the non-invasive measurement of important metabolites in muscle and therefore opens new possibilities.

CT is used in the diagnosis of ankle and elbow joint overuse injuries. With this technique, it is possible to evaluate the position and frequency of loose bodies and osteophytes. CT of the patella, when properly performed, allows precise reproducible imaging of patellofemoral relationships and reveals normal alignment, excessive lateral tilt, and subluxation of the patella. CT arthrograms are accurate in identifying labrum tears in the shoulder joint, as well as synovial plicae in the knee joint.

Ultrasound evaluation has been shown to be valuable in the diagnosis of Baker cysts, jumper's knee, medial meniscus lesions, and meniscal cysts in the knee. However, diagnosis of lateral meniscus lesions with ultrasound appears to have limitations. Ultrasound is also used to evaluate tendon pathology including Achilles, patella, and rotator cuff tendons with good accuracy. This technique requires special experience for evaluation.

Bone scans, especially triple phase bone scans, allow accurate evaluation of stress reactions in the bone. A bone scan is positive 2 to 8 days after the onset of stress fracture symptoms. A bone scan may also show a diffuse uptake in medial tibial stress syndromes.

The development of the arthroscopy during the last 20 years has meant a revolution in the diagnosis of different joint problems, particularly the knee joint. Experience from knee arthroscopy has been carried over to most of the joints in the body, particularly the shoulder, ankle, wrist, and elbow joints.

Overuse injuries constitute a major diagnostic problem because the symptoms are often diffuse and uncharacteristic. The diagnosis of an overuse injury rests with the identification of not only the affected tissue but also the underlying predisposing conditions. An accurate diagnosis is necessary for a successful treatment. Appropriate diagnosis followed by adequate treatment is required in order to improve or eliminate most of these conditions.

Principles of treatment of overuse injuries

When treating overuse injuries, it is important to consider not only the symptoms but also the cause. Therefore it is important to distinguish the primary and secondary problems.

Treatment of the cause of the injury—the primary problem

1. Training routines should be analysed and changed if necessary. The athlete should only participate in the sport within the limits of pain. For runners, this can include a decrease in the training distance or a change in the stride and pace. A change of surface to a

soft, less sloping surface with minimal curves can be effective for a runner.

2. Malalignments should be corrected if possible. As there are individual combined malalignments, different approaches are available. Sometimes referral to an expert is recommended. Foot orthotics are often used to correct malalignments. Orthotic devices have a significant effect on the amount of maximum pronation, time to maximum pronation, maximum pronation velocity, period of pronation, and movement or rear-foot angle in the first 10° of foot contact.[40] It is important not to overcorrect; it is more reasonable to undercorrect, and the exact rear-foot and forefoot posting necessary to attain a neutral subtalar joint is rarely provided. One possible approach is to post the subtalar position to a maximum of 4° varus as this provides adequate control and minimizes the possibility of initiating a lateral ligament sprain of the ankle.[8] The use of orthotics is still controversial, and there are failures with this type of treatment. Failures may occur because the orthotic devices have not been adjusted or changed as needed from time to time. Athletes with new orthotics seem to adjust to the new situation within a few weeks (N. Naumann and P.A.F.H. Renström, personal communication). Although there are no prospective randomized studies available showing the effect of the use of orthotics, vast experience is available in sports medicine concerning the value of orthotics in compensating and neutralizing different malalignment positions. Sperryn and Rostan[41] followed 50 runners for whom orthotic devices had been prescribed. After 3.5 years, 64 per cent of the runners had relief of symptoms, but only 54 per cent were still using the orthotic device. This indicates that care should be taken to identify athletes with syndromes that will benefit from the use of these devices.

3. Shoes are of great importance in reducing the large impact forces. This shock absorption can be increased by heel confinement.[42] A good shoe is also a stable shoe, giving motion control with a well-fitted heel counter. Modern running shoes are effective and give a maximum point of pronation during the stance phase, which occurs significantly later with bare feet than with the shoe. Shoes should be flexible in the forefoot, or they can cause forefoot overuse problems during push-off. In summary, the shoes should provide cushioning, support, and friction.

4. If the athlete has tight muscles and joints or muscular imbalance, stretching exercises are indicated. If the athlete is excessively flexible, strengthening exercises are indicated.

5. Braces and taping can be used when joint instability is present.

6. Surgical correction of a specific malalignment, such as a patella lateral tilt, can sometimes be indicated.

Treatment of the symptoms

General principles

1. When treating overuse injuries, it is important to have an exact diagnosis before specific treatment is initiated.

2. The treatment of overuse injuries depends on the healing process. The different stages of healing determine the different modes of treatment. An injured tissue such as a tendon, during the first 48 h, demonstrates an inflammatory response characterized by increased vessel permeability leading to swelling in the adjacent area. The weeks following the initial phase are known as the proliferative phase, in which new collagen and mature cross-links are formed. This is followed by a formative phase involving tissue remodelling which can continue for a year. There is, however, little inflammatory reaction in the tendon itself. Most of the changes are characterized by degeneration, which is a change of the tissue from a higher to lower or less functional form. Contributing causes are inadequate oxygen supply, decreased nutrition, hormonal change, chronic inflammation, and ageing. The tendon degenerative process is characterized by fibril disruption, collagen fibril splitting, and fragmentation and loss of collagen molecular orientation.[10] The amount of degeneration usually decides the rate and success of recovery. Tendon strength is a direct function not only of the number and size of collagen fibres but also of their orientation. These fibres respond favourably to tension and motion, and therefore it is important to stimulate protected motion as soon as possible and at the latest during the proliferative phase, that is, in the third week after the injury.[15]

3. The pain experienced is related to the amount of tissue injury. The history of pain can therefore be used as a guide for treatment. The pain can be graded as follows:

Grade 1

- pain only after activity
- duration of symptoms less than 2 weeks

Grade 2

- pain during and after activity
- no significant functional disability
- duration of symptoms more than 2 weeks

Grade 3

- pain during and after activity
- significant functional activity
- duration of symptoms greater than 6 weeks

Grade 4

- constant pain
- complete functional disability
- unable to train and compete
- impending tissue failure

4. The treatment should be individualized. Patient compliance is the single largest factor determining the success or failure of treatment.

5. The treatment should start as early as possible. When overuse injuries have become chronic, they are very difficult to treat.

6. Treatment of overuse injuries is difficult. Early motion and exercises are usually required to stimulate the healing process. However, long experience is required to balance the need for rest against the need for motion. If the injury becomes resistant to therapy, early consultation with more experienced colleagues is advised.

7. It is important to adopt a multidisciplinary approach to these injuries. Teamwork, including the physician, the physiotherapist,

the trainer, the coach, and sometimes the family, is often preferred in developing a suitable treatment and rehabilitation programme.

Treatment of the symptoms—a basic treatment programme

1. Pain and swelling in a joint, for example, will cause muscle inhibition resulting in muscle wasting and weakness. The initial treatment of pain, swelling, and inflammation is of great importance and may include rest, avoidance of weight bearing, elevation, ice, and compression bandaging and protection. Ice treatment is useful during the first 48 h. Ice relieves pain by the direct effect of cold on pain reception and nerve fibre transmission and by a secondary decrease in swelling and inflammation. Ice reduces the chemical activity and therefore can reduce the inflammatory response. The injured part should be protected and rehabilitated in parallel with the healing process. The injured tissue should be activated but protected from significant stress which may incur further damage. Therefore activities should be carried out below the pain threshold. The pain is directly related to the amount of tissue damage.[10] During the period of vulnerability a physiotherapist or trainer should guide the exercise programme.

2. Heat is effective 48 h after the acute phase and in chronic phases as it increases the extensibility of the collagen in connective tissue, decreases joint stiffness, relieves muscle spasm, and gives pain relief. Local heat can be applied in different ways. Heat retainers or neoprene sleeves are valuable tools in both prevention and rehabilitation of muscle and tendon injuries as they can also be applied during activity. Heat can also be applied by other modalities such as high voltage galvanic stimulation, infrared lamps, diathermy, and paraffin baths. Ultrasound is extensively used in addition to electrical stimulation. Application of moist heat by hydrocolater, whirlpool, or thermophore pads may be effective. Laser treatment may be employed.

3. Anti-inflammatory medication may be used for the treatment of overuse injuries, but medical modalities do not affect healing. They are often effective against pain and stiffness, but the athlete should be aware that these medications may mask the symptoms.

4. Exercise is the key to a successful treatment programme of overuse injuries. Immobilization should be avoided as it may result in the loss of ground substances found in collagenous connective tissue, which will result in poor reorientation of the collagen fibres and a reduction in the tensile strength. Joint immobilization will also result in muscle wasting and weakness, joint stiffness, and diminished proprioception. Injured tissues should be protected from significant stress, which may incur further damage, but mobilization should start as early as possible. Repeated exercise will increase the mechanical and structural properties of the tissue. It is important to start an exercise programme very carefully with a gradual increase of the load within the limits of pain. Restoration of the mechanical properties often requires prolonged treatment and guidance by experienced physiotherapists or trainers.

5. Corticosteroid injections should generally be avoided in overuse injuries as they will cause a decrease in metabolic activity and there is a risk of necrosis. Corticosteroids should not be injected into tendons or ligaments; tendon ruptures have been reported secondary to injections of corticosteroids into tendons. However, corticosteroid injections can sometimes be used for specific indications such as chronic conditions at tendon insertion sites or in bursas. However, they should only be used after other non-surgical treatments including rest and exercise have failed. They should not be used before a competition or if an infection is present. If indicated, no more than three injections spaced weeks apart should be given. A corticosteroid injection should be combined with a period of rest and reduced physical activity for 5 to 10 days.

6. Braces and tape can often be used successfully to reduce the load and weight bearing in the injured area.

7. Surgery should be avoided until conservative therapy has failed. Excision of scar and degenerative tissue secondary to a failed healing response in tendons and muscles has often given good results for lateral epicondylitis and in chronic partial tears of tendons such as the Achilles, the adductor longus, or rotator cuff. The rehabilitation period following this type of surgery may be rather long, but the overall results are good. Arthroscopic surgery of the knee joint has proved to be an extremely effective treatment, allowing an early return to sport. The arthroscope can be used in the shoulder to carry out subacromial decompression, repair tears in the labrum and the rotator cuff, and to evaluate instability. Elbow arthroscopy allows removal of loose bodies. Ankle arthroscopy is an effective surgical procedure in patients with synovitis and transchondral defects of the talus. The benefits and long-term results are less predictable in the arthroscopic treatment of ankle osteophytes and arthrosis.

Training programme

Strength training

Strength training should start cautiously as early as possible. The aim of strengthening exercises is recovery of muscle wasting and strength, and the enhancement of recruitment and firing rates of the motor units.[43] Tendon strength is a function of number, size, and orientation of the collagen fibres. They respond favourably to tension and motion.

Careful isometric exercises may be used initially and should be carried out without load. Gradually increasing loads can then be applied. In the early stages it is often enough to use the athlete's injured limb as the load. Isometric contractions can be facilitated with electrical muscle stimulation to avoid persistent pain, weakness, and immobilization. Strength improvement by isometric exercises is limited to the joint angle used during the exercise. When isometric exercises can be carried out without pain at multiple joint angles, active dynamic motion exercises of the injured area and gradual increase in strength training may start. Dynamic exercise correlates better with improved functional performance.

Eccentric exercises can be effective in the treatment of chronic overuse injuries. The tendon is subjected to larger loads which maximize the force production and minimizes time delays and energy expenditure.[44] Eccentric exercises should be avoided early when pain, inhibition, and patient confidence are factors of importance. There is a risk of overloading the tissue. Treatment regimens for chronic overuse injuries have been used by Curwin and Stanish[45] with good clinical results. They have used pain as a regulator for the exercise programme. In chronic overuse injuries, it is sometimes possible to break through a therapy-resistant chronic condition by allowing the athlete to exercise above the pain threshold.

When carrying out strength training, the specificity of the training should be kept in mind. Muscle exercises in different positions will affect the neural factors. These must be trained before the full effect of the muscle training programme can be achieved. The initial strength gain is caused by neural activation and not by muscle hypertrophy.

Flexibility training

It is important to combine strength training with flexibility training. The aim is to restore adequate flexibility on a regional basis together with specific strength and movement.[46] An ideal state of flexibility in the athlete would heighten the sensory feedback mechanism with the advantage of increased proprioceptive accuracy and sensitivity. Studies of the biomechanical effects of stretching show that it will result in greater flexibility and increased length of the muscle–tendon unit.[47] Stress relaxation results in decreased stiffness due to changes in viscoelastic properties. Prolonged stretching leads to decreased stress within a muscle for a given length change with the end result being decreased muscle stiffness. Controlled clinical studies of the effects of stretching are lacking.

There are different methods of flexibility training including ballistic stretching, slow static stretching and contract–relax stretching. The most widely used method in the treatment of overuse injuries is slow static stretching. Contract–relax stretching is based on the proprioceptive neuromuscular facilitation technique and is widely used by physiotherapists. As heat increases the extensibility of the collagen, stretching should be carried out not only during warm-up but also after the training session when the athlete is warm.

Proprioceptive training

Specific exercises that require balance, weight shift, stimulation of antigravity reflexes, and co-ordination appear to facilitate proprioceptive feedback mechanism. Closed kinetic chain exercises as well as specific functional rehabilitation improve the proprioception. Proprioceptive training of ankle functional instability using ankle discs gave maximum results after 10 weeks of training.[15] This type of exercise is more important than strength training for chronic ankle problems.

Sports-specific training

Sports-simulated exercises of the non-injured body parts should be carried out as early as possible following an injury. It is often possible to perform non-gravity exercises by cycling or swimming if other treatments fail. Rowing, cross-country skiing, or roller skiing are other useful alternatives. Pool running is effective in maintaining cardiovascular and muscular fitness. General conditioning is helpful, not only as stimulation but also for increasing the circulation in the injured areas.

Different types of chronic overuse injuries

Overuse injuries occur in most body tissues. The most common sites are in the muscle–tendon units, but problems also occur in other soft tissues such as bursas, fascia, and nerves, as well as in the bones and joints.

Injuries to the muscle–tendon units

Injuries may occur at any point in the muscle–tendon unit—within the muscle belly, within the tendon, at the muscle–tendon junction, or at the origin or insertion of the muscle or tendon into the bone (Fig. 5). Failure will occur at the weakest point within the unit. The

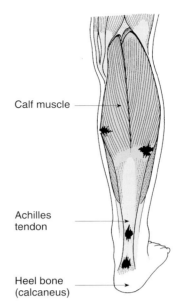

Calf muscle

Achilles tendon

Heel bone (calcaneus)

Fig. 5 Muscle tendon injuries can occur at different locations. (Redrawn from Peterson L, Renström P. *Injuries in sports*. London: Martin Dunitz, 1985, with permission.)

location and severity of the injury are influenced by the athlete's age.

Avulsion fractures through the apophyseal plate or traction and fragmentation of the bone at the attachment site are most likely to occur in young athletes and adolescents. After 25 to 30 years of age, there is progressive degeneration of the collagen fibres, particularly within the tendon, making the tendon itself a weak area and more susceptible to both traumatic and overuse injuries. The muscle is susceptible to injury in all age groups, although muscle injuries seem to be more common in the elderly.[18,31]

Muscle overuse injuries

Muscle strain

Garrett[48] has shown that partial and complete overload injuries to the muscle exhibit disruption of muscle fibres near the muscle–tendon junctions. Healing of partial injuries is characterized by an initial inflammatory response followed by a healing phase marked by fibrosis. Treatment of these strains follows the general principles already mentioned, and the prognosis is good. Chronic conditions may occur, but are not common.

Muscle contusion injuries are characterized by intra- or intermuscular haematomas. The intermuscular injuries heal well with rapid recovery, but intramuscular injuries often heal with fibrosis. In the repair process, there is not only a regeneration of muscle fibres but also a competitive simultaneous production of granulation tissue. An inelastic fibrotic scar tissue localized in the muscle may develop. The healed muscle consequently includes areas of varying elasticity which often result in chronic overuse problems. Pain during or after muscle activity may be experienced by soccer players, for example, in the muscles of their kicking leg. Frequent stretching and strength exercises are necessary as prevention and treatment.

Muscle soreness

Muscle exercise commonly results in injury to fibres in the active muscles, particularly when the exercise is relatively intense, is of long duration, and/or includes eccentric contraction.[49] Friden *et al.*[50] have suggested that myofibrillar lesions are a direct result of mechanical tearing of the z-band, which is the weak link in the myofibrillar contraction chain during high muscle tension. These tears may result in the formation of protein components which, by osmosis, results in oedema and soreness. The precise mechanism underlying these injuries is not well known. This soreness caused by overuse seldom becomes chronic.

Chronic compartment syndrome

The lower leg is the location for chronic compartment syndromes usually caused by muscle hypertrophy as a result of repeated exercise. In the presence of appropriate clinical findings, one or more of the following intramuscular pressure criteria is diagnostic of chronic compartment syndrome of the leg: (i) a pre-exercise pressure of more than 15 mmHg, (ii) a 1-min postexercise pressure of about 30 mmHg, and (iii) a 5-min postexercise pressure of about 20 mmHg.[51] The treatment for this syndrome is specific, with alteration of the training programme, orthosis, medication, and sometimes decompression. Other causes of pain such as stress fractures or medial tibial stress syndrome should be ruled out.

Tendon overuse injuries

The tensile force applied to the tendon is resisted primarily by the collagen, which is characterized by high mechanical strength but poor elasticity. According to Curwin and Stanish,[45] overuse in a tendon means that it has been strained repeatedly until it is unable to withstand further loading, at which point damage occurs. Repeated overload with increasing strain in the tendon will cause the cross-links within the collagen fibres to break. The shearing force will then cause the collagen fibrils to slide, resulting in an injury to the tendon at the microscopic level.

In its resting state, a tendon has a wavy configuration which disappears on 4 per cent stretching. At 4 to 8 per cent strain, the collagen fibres will slide past one another as the cross-links start to break. There is now an inflammatory reaction in the tendon. At 8 to 10 per cent strain, the tendons begin to fail and resist less force as more cross-links are broken. The weakest fibres rupture and the tendon loses its composite structure at the molecular level.[45]

Tendon injury is primarily associated with degeneration in over 90 per cent. There is, however, some development of sports-induced soft tissue inflammation which includes spontaneous resolution, regeneration, or chronic inflammatory response.[52] The chronic inflammatory conditions are associated with persistent structural alterations. They are characterized by either a failure to develop adequate scar tissue restoration or an excessive fibroproductive scar response. Nomenclature for tendon injuries is based on the fact that degeneration characterizes tendon pathology. Tendinosis is intratendinous degeneration due to an atrophic response/abortive healing. The current classification is peritendinitis, peritendinitis with tendinosis, partial rupture and tendinosis, and complete rupture.

Chronic Achilles tendon injuries

Chronic Achilles tendon problems are very common in athletes and are often secondary to malalignment. The most common malalignment is excessive pronation, which results in a compensatory internal rotation of the tibia. This hyperpronation results in a whipping action resulting in an increased stress within the Achilles ten-

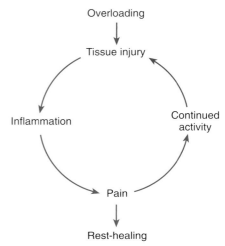

Fig. 6 The pain cycle.

don.[53] Furthermore the Achilles tendon rotates in its distal 15 cm, resulting in a sawing action during walking and running.

In 1982, Clancy[54] suggested two potential causes for chronic Achilles tendon injury: (i) repeated loading of the muscular tendinous unit leads to fatigue of the muscle and shortening and decreased flexibility which may result in passive increased loading of the tendon during the state of relaxation; and (ii) repetitive active loading of the muscular tendinous unit leads to collagen failure.

Peritendinitis Peritendinitis, which in other locations is called tenosynovitis or tenovaginitis, is an inflammation of the sheath or paratendon surrounding the tendon that is caused by tissue friction or by external mechanical irritation.

The diagnosis of chronic peritendinitis is made by a typical history characterized by a gradual onset of pain. There is usually a diffuse tenderness and swelling of the tendon. The so-called pain cycle (Fig. 6) is typical of peritendinitis. Pain disappears during warming up, allowing the athlete to go on with his activities. The athlete develops pain after activity but not enough to prevent performance the following day. When the pain no longer disappears during the warm-up, the injury is chronic. Pain is a sign of injury, and the pain cycle should be interrupted by rest and treatment of the injury.

Tendinosis and partial chronic tear Tendinosis is a degenerative condition in the tendon without inflammation, characterized by fibrinoid degeneration, cartilage metaplasia, and sometimes calcification, which is often seen in the elderly. A chronic partial tear is a symptomatic degeneration of the tendon with vascular disruption and an inflammatory repair response.

Chronic peritendinitis should be differentiated from partial tendon tears. These injuries include a history of sudden onset of pain and are characterized clinically by a distinct palpable tenderness which in most cases is combined with a localized swelling. The diagnosis should be made by the history and clinical examination. Soft tissue radiography can be valuable. An oedema of more than 10 cm decreasing the Kagers triangle is indicative of a partial tear (L. Irstam, personal communication). Ultrasound is helpful, but its use requires experience. MRI is the diagnostic method of choice. If these injuries are not adequately treated initially, delayed healing will occur and they will become chronic and more difficult to treat, often requiring late surgical intervention. It is not known why there is delayed healing or non-healing in these chronic injuries. The picture is very similar to a non-union in fractures.

Explanations for the delayed healing observed in these chronic tendon lesions include the following:

(1) diminished vascularity with subsequent decreased cellularity due to attritional cell death;

(2) failure of reparative cells to penetrate an area of tendon injury, a finding supported by biopsies in younger patients with chronic tendon injury which have failed to demonstrate any cellular activity other than a more metabolically active tenocyte;

(3) accelerated ageing of the tenocyte;

(4) age-dependent changes in the matrix with adverse tendon biomechanical properties[52] (this type of reaction can occur in Achilles and rotator cuff tendons).

Conservative therapy will often give unsatisfactory results. In a group of athletes with Achilles tendon partial tears verified by bursography, Allenmark *et al.*[55] found that even after 10 years, 74 per cent still had severe clinical problems which made physical activity impossible. Surgical treatment with excision of the scar tissue gives good results in more than 80 per cent of cases.

Insertional tendon injuries This type of injury, which is an overuse injury in the tendon insertion into bone, is not very common in adults. In adolescents it is recognized as calcaneal apophysitis (Sever–Haglund's disease) when there is pain at the insertion of the Achilles tendon into the calcaneus, or as Osgood–Schlatter's disease when there is pain at the tendon insertion at the tibial tuberosity.

Chronic patella tendon injuries

Chronic patella tendon injuries follow the same principles as Achilles tendon overuse injuries. The chronic tears are almost always located on the undersurface of the tendon where it inserts into the patella. These injuries can be secondary to impingement between the tendon and the patella lower inferior pole.

Shoulder tendon injuries

Rotator cuff and biceps tendon injuries are common in throwers and in older squash players. The rotator cuff tendons show early degenerative changes and have poor vascularity. Therefore they are difficult to treat and have a long healing and rehabilitation period. These shoulder tendon injuries are often associated with shoulder instability and impingement in the younger athlete.

Overuse injuries in joints

The joint most susceptible to overuse injuries is the knee. It is a major power absorber of negative work as twice as much work is done by the knee during running, for example, as is done by the ankle and hip joints.

Knee overuse injuries

Intra-articular injuries

Intra-articular pathology of the knee is often experienced in team sports and individual sports such as skiing, but is less common in running. Collision or twisting trauma is usually involved, but there may also be repetitive minor trauma in which a degenerative meniscus is damaged. Other injuries that can occur are osteochondritis dissecans and unusual disorders such as the plica syndrome. Articular cartilage lesions can cause long-lasting problems in athletes. Arthroscopic surgery is often used to treat intra-articular injuries, generally with good results.

Patellofemoral disorders

The patellofemoral syndrome is the most common problem in running. This pain syndrome is often associated with pain in downhill running, and with getting up after squatting or sitting for a prolonged time. Patellofemoral disorders are usually associated with some malalignment such as the increased Q-angle secondary to genu valgum, femoral neck anteversion, and external tibial torsion. Muscle imbalance with a tight retinaculum, poor vastus medialis tone, and tight quadriceps muscles can occur. Individuals with patella malalignment should be identified. If this condition is present it is important to separate patella subluxation from patella tilt. Patella subluxation may lead to problems of extensor mechanism instability, increased risk of dislocation, apprehension, and some risk of articular cartilage damage. Abnormal patella tilt may create a pattern of increased lateral loading.

These injuries can often be managed conservatively by control of pain and inflammation. The quadriceps, should be subjected to progressive exertion. Patella brace or taping, orthotic foot control, and motion-controlled shoes, with gradual return to sports are helpful. Surgery may be indicated if conservative treatment fails, but a mechanical disorder must be present.

Iliotibial band friction syndrome

The iliotibial band friction syndrome is quite common and is known as runner's knee; it usually occurs in runners who have been running for less than 4 years and regularly run more than 14 km per week.

At 30° of knee flexion, which is often the case in downhill running, the iliotibial band glides over the lateral knee condyle. In downhill running, there is an excessive stride causing an increased compression of the iliotibial band against the lateral condyle. Structural abnormalities, such as a prominent lateral condyle, a tight iliotibial band, or an excessive genu varum, can also cause this problem, as can foot abnormalities such as excessive pronation, heel varus, cavus feet, and forefoot pronation. Excessive pronation will result in compensatory increased internal rotation of the tibia which draws the insertion site of the iliotibial band at Gerdy's tubercle anteriomedially, resulting in increased tightness. Leg length discrepancy is also associated with this syndrome.

As always, it is important to treat the cause of the injury and therefore the use of a corrective training regime is often effective. Orthotics and good shoes may also be used. If conservative therapy will not help, surgical incision of the posterior iliotibial band, 2 cm proximal of the condyle, is effective.

Hip joint arthritis

Degenerative arthritis of the hip joints is common in the elderly. There is no increased incidence in athletes, and overuse is probably not an important aetiological factor. Intensive running activities for more than 30 to 40 years did not result in an increased incidence of hip arthritis.[56]

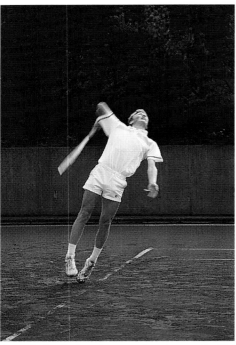

Fig. 7 A pitcher and a tennis player have a major valgus overload in their pitch or serve.

Shoulder overuse injuries

Athletes who throw are at risk because of the repetitive, high velocity, chronic, mechanical stress placed on their shoulders. According to Jobe and Bradely,[57] there is a progressive continuum of shoulder pathology: overuse leads to microtrauma which leads to instability, subluxation, and impingement, which may result in rotator cuff tears. The impingement syndrome without instability is common in throwers and swimmers.

The most pervasive disorder in the young athlete today is due to shoulder instability. Primary shoulder instability can be caused by chronic labral microtrauma and can result in secondary impingement problems. Undetected instability should be ruled out in any athlete with impingement findings. Arthroscopy is the most accurate diagnostic tool for shoulder instability. By understanding the delicate balance between mobility and stability within a normal shoulder, the clinician is better able to understand the aetiology and biomechanics of the problem and can design an optimal treatment programme.

Elbow overuse injuries

Overuse injuries in the elbow are quite common in baseball and other throwing sports, gymnastics, power events, and squash (Fig. 7).

During the cocking and acceleration phases, the pitcher's elbow is subjected to valgus overload which results in medial tension, lateral compression, and extension overload. The muscles in the vicinity of the elbow do not protect against overloading, particularly valgus loads, and therefore the main focus is on static stability. Medial tension can cause a medial epicondylitis. In young pitchers this tension causes traction and apophysitis, resulting in Little Leaguer's elbow. If valgus instability has occurred by attenuation of the anterior oblique ligament, the ulnar nerve may be secondarily injured by repeated mechanical stretching, friction, and compression, resulting in ulnar neuritis. The lateral compression of the radial head against the capitellum may cause osteochondritis dissecans and loose bodies in the elbow. The extension overload often seen in the tennis serve and in boxing may result in impingement posteriorly and cause and osteophytes on the posteromedial aspect of the olecranon.

The valgus motion can be combined with pronation and will then cause lateral overload with lateral epicondylitis as a result. Medial epicondylitis can be caused by a twisted serve in tennis or by a heavy topspin on forehand. This injury must be carefully treated as the recovery and healing time is lengthy. These injuries should be treated according to the general principles discussed earlier with early motion. Elbow muscle counterforce braces may be effective. Arthroscopy is indicated if there is a suspicion of osteochondritis dissecans, loose bodies, or osteophytes.

Overuse syndromes in other soft tissues

Bursitis

Direct trauma to the elbow, the patella, or the knee may result in acute bursitis within an already distended bursa or lead to development of an adventitious bursa or haemobursa (Fig. 8). If the haematoma is not absorbed or evacuated in the acute phase, chronic bursitis will result as calcification and free bodies, and adhesions often form and cause irritation. These injuries can be prevented by appropriate protective equipment and padding.

Friction bursitis can occur in the subacromial bursa in the shoulder, the retrocalcaneal bursa, or subcutaneous bursa around the Achilles tendon.

Trochanteric bursitis frequently occurs after intensive running on banked roads, resulting in a functional leg length discrepancy. This type of bursitis has a tendency to become chronic and can be very difficult to treat. Therefore early treatment with a correction of training errors and malalignment should be considered. In addition to infection, chemical products from degenerative tendon tissue can cause bursitis.

The treatment of bursitis generally involves rest, local decompression with aspiration, protection, and anti-inflammatory medication. In a long-lasting chronic bursitis, surgical excision may be considered.

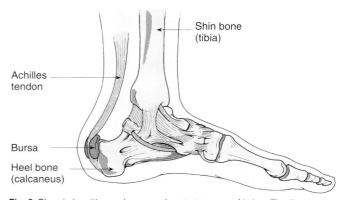

Fig. 8 Chronic bursitis can be secondary to trauma or friction. The figure shows inflammation of the deep bursa located anterior of the attachment and the distal part of the Achilles tendon to the calcaneus. (Redrawn from Peterson L, Renström P. *Injuries in sports*. London: Martin Dunitz, 1985, with permission.)

Nerve injuries

Nerve entrapment syndromes

Nerve entrapment syndromes are not very common, but may develop from overuse as a result of swelling in the surrounding soft tissues secondary to trauma or malalignment. The most common injury is the carpal tunnel syndrome in the wrist. The ulnar nerve may be entrapped at the level of the wrist and cause problems for the cyclist. Entrapment of the posterior interosseus nerve in the forearm is experienced occasionally by tennis players. Soccer players may experience entrapment of nerves such as the genitofemoral, the ilioinguinal, and the cutaneous femoris lateralis within the groin region. Medial and lateral plantar nerves may be entrapped. The tarsal tunnel syndrome may be seen in runners.

Neuromas

The Morton's neuroma or interdigital neuroma can produce pain in the toe area, particularly in runners. Typically, pain is experienced during running but is often relieved after running, particularly if the shoes are removed.

Neuritis

The ulnar nerve may be injured by repeated mechanical stretching and friction, secondary to the large tensile forces generated during throwing. Ulnar neuritis may develop in an unstable elbow secondary to an attenuated ulnar collateral ligament.

The treatment of nerve injuries includes rest and anti-inflammatory medication. Orthotic treatment may be indicated in nerve entrapments of the foot. Sometimes surgery is necessary.

Overuse injuries in bones

Stress fractures

Stress fractures can occur in normal bone during normal situations. There is no single aetiology, but muscle fatigue and biomechanical imbalance are believed to be associated with stress fractures. Skeletal asymmetry, leg length discrepancy, variations of gait, excessive running (over 100 km/week), running on hard sloping surfaces, or prior injury can also predispose to this condition. Women have a decreased bone density and a wider pelvis, resulting in different running patterns, which may predispose to stress fractures. Menstrual disturbances are a factor.

Stress fractures can occur in most bones. In runners, 44 to 50 per cent occur in the tibia, 16 to 24 per cent in the fibula, 16 to 20 per cent in the metatarsals, 6 to 8 per cent in the femur, 6 per cent in the pelvis, and 4 per cent in other bones. These fractures are bilateral in 25 per cent, multiple in 8 to 12 per cent, but do not occur in the same location twice. These stress fractures are diagnosed by a history of pain during activity and by distinct tenderness on palpation. The fracture is verified by a radionuclide bone scanning, which provides the diagnosis 2 to 8 days after onset of symptoms. Because of continual remodelling of the bone, the bone scan can be positive for up to a year.

Sports activities can often be continued within the limits of discomfort. If running can be carried out during the healing phase, it should be done on soft surfaces. Some specific fractures need special management. If a femoral neck fracture does not become pain free in initial walking or running with or without crutches, surgery is indicated to avoid a full fracture and avascular necrosis. Special attention should also be paid to navicular stress fractures, anterior

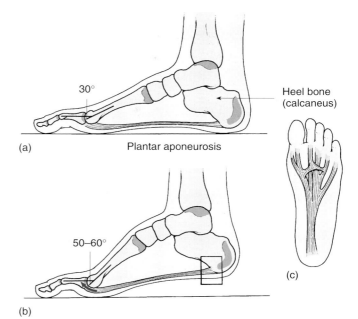

Fig. 9 Plantar fasciitis. (a) The foot and the plantar aponeurosis (fascial) shows the whole foot loaded against the surface. (b) The plantar aponeurosis is stretched during take-off. The marked area indicates the seat of inflammation at the origin of the plantar aponeurosis and the calcaneus. (c) The plantar aponeurosis seen from underneath (Redrawn from Peterson L, Renström P. *Injuries in sports*. London: Martin Dunitz, 1985, with permission.)

tibial stress fractures, and proximal fifth metatarsal stress fractures as these often show delayed healing if not treated properly. They often require early surgery in athletes.

Occult bone lesions

MRI can confirm bone bruises, stress fractures, tibia fractures, femoral fractures, and osteochondral lesions. These occult bone lesions may be responsible for pain and discomfort, but are not evident on routine radiographs. The sensitivity and specificity of these lesions are not yet recognized or correlated with a specific diagnosis. However, it is known that they are present in 60 to 70 per cent of acute anterior cruciate ligament injuries. In patients with continuous pain after an initial trauma, these lesions should be suspected.

Overuse problems of specific injury sites

Foot problems

The forefoot can be the site of many overuse problems. They are often localized in the skin and soft tissues, and appear as blisters, corns, etc. Examples of other common overuse injuries are hammer toes, black toenails, metatarsalgia, or sesamoiditis.

In the midfoot the longitudinal arch can often be high and stiff, and be related to arch pain, peroneal tendinitis, and midtarsal joint problems.

Plantar fasciitis is a major problem in the hindfoot. Painful heel pad, stress fractures in the calcaneus, and entrapment of nerves are not uncommon. Most of these injuries are treated using orthotics and shoes. Plantar fasciitis is an inflammatory reaction which is the result of a fatigue failure of the plantar fascia (Fig. 9). It can be caused by hyperpronation at midstance and is due to inward rotation of the foot and a pull on the medial fascia.[4] The cavus foot produces problems because of its inflexibility. Treatment consists of rest, heat, stretching, and sometimes crutches. Orthotics which unload the injured area are often indicated and helpful. Rigid orthotics should not be used in the cavus foot.

Lower leg pain

Medial tibial stress syndrome is a painful condition with the pain localized in the medial area of the tibia. This may be due to involvement of the tibialis posterior tendon and muscle secondary to increased pronation.[19] There is a greater angular displacement in the subtalar joint in patients with medial tibial stress syndromes than in controls.[58] Stress changes may also occur at the attachment of the soleus muscle. Biomechanically, the soleus is eccentrically stressed with heel eversion. These problems are treated with rest, stretching, and orthotics with varying results. Compartment syndromes and stress fractures can also cause lower leg pain.

Groin pain

Hip and groin pain are common in sports. Groin pain constitutes around 5 per cent of all injuries in soccer.[59] Groin pain is usually caused by overuse injuries in the adductor muscles and tendons, particularly the adductor longus. Sometimes muscles and tendons from the rectus abdomini, rectus femoris, and iliopsoas may cause the pain. Hernia is probably a more common cause of groin pain than recognized.

Intra-articular hip problems may occur in sports, although they are rare. Dancers can have early phases of arthritic changes. Intra-articular abdominal problems, genital infections, inflammatory conditions of the sacroiliac joint, osteitis pubis, nerve entrapments, pelvic stress fractures, and other conditions may give pain syndromes similar to those caused by conventional groin overuse injury syndromes.

Spine overuse injuries

Lower back pain is a common problem in many sports. It may be caused by overuse of the lower back muscles or by imbalance of the back muscles in relation to other muscle groups. Other causes of back problems are sciatica, spondylolysis, and stress fractures. Gymnasts, riders, and rowers may develop intervertebral joint changes in the lumbar spine.[28,60] Wrestlers can demonstrate low back pain[61] as well as cervical spine changes. Overuse injuries in the back region can be avoided with a general and well-balanced exercise programme.

Back pain in athletes must be taken seriously and assumed to be a significant problem until proved otherwise. If the athlete is out of competition for more than 10 days, a full and comprehensive evaluation is indicated.[1]

Conclusions

Overuse injuries are becoming more common in sports because of the increasing number of people in training and recreational activities, with higher intensity at all levels of competition. Overuse injuries constitute a problem for all types of athletes. The injuries may become chronic if intensive training is continued. If this occurs, the injuries are very difficult to treat and unfortunately have forced many athletes into early retirement from their main sport.

Most overuse injuries are caused by extrinsic factors, but intrinsic factors are also common. Malalignments, including excessive pronation and cavus feet, result in secondary compensatory changes in the lower extremity and, therefore, must be regarded as a functional unit. However, specific anatomic abnormalities and abnormal biomechanics of the lower extremity are not correlated with specific injuries on a predictable basis. Leg length discrepancy, poor flexibility, and muscle weakness and imbalance may be other important aetiological factors. Acquired or secondary factors such as kinetic chain dysfunctions are more common than previously acknowledged. Many overuse injuries in running, for example, are manifestations of dysfunction of the kinetic chain, particularly in athletes with recurrent and previous injuries.

The importance of finding a specific diagnosis and identifying kinetic chain dysfunctions in order to secure a successful treatment cannot be overemphasized.

Most of these injuries can heal with conservative regimens, but this requires co-operation between the doctor and a compliant patient. Team work with other specialist physicians and physiotherapists is often needed. These injuries do not cause problems in everyday life, but the physician must understand the importance of the athlete's wish to continue his or her activities and attempt to understand the injury from the athlete's point of view.

There is a need for more investigation of the basic biomechanics of soft tissues and how tissues react to trauma. All musculoskeletal injuries are defined by the reparative response of the cell matrix. The distinction of macrotraumatic (acute) and microtraumatic (clinical overuse) injury patterns is implied by the pathological evidence. More research is needed to study the aetiology, diagnosis, and treatment of these increasingly common injuries. Studies of changes in collagen as a function of events mediated by free radicals secondary to disuse or ischaemia–reperfusion should be encouraged.[62] Overuse injuries are unnecessary and can usually be prevented.

References

1. Weiker GG. Evaluation and treatment of common spine and trunk problems. *Clinics in Sports Medicine* 1989; **8**: 399.
2. Slocum DB, James SL. Biomechanics of running. *Journal of the American Medical Association* 1968; **205**: 720–8.
3. Orava S. Exertion injuries due to sports and physical exercise. A clinical and statistical study of nontraumatic overuse injuries of the musculoskeletal system of athletes and keep-fit athletes. Thesis, University of Oulu, Finland, 1980.
4. Mann RA, Baxter DE, Lutter LD. Running Symposium. *Foot and Ankle* 1981; **1**: 190–224.
5. Cavanagh PR, Kram R. Stride length in distance running. *Medicine and Science in Sports and Exercise* 1990; **21**: 467–79.
6. Harvey JS. Overuse syndromes in young athletes. *Clinics in Sports Medicine* 1983; **2**: 595–607.
7. James SL, Bates BT, Osternig LR. Injuries to runners. *American Journal of Sports Medicine* 1978; **6**: 40–50.
8. McKenzie DC, Clement DB, Taunton JE. Running shoes, orthotics and injuries. *Sports Medicine* 1985; **2**: 324–7.
9. Renström P, Kannus P. Prevention of sports injuries. In: Krauss RH, ed. *Sports medicine*. Philadelphia: W.B. Saunders, 1991.
10. Leadbetter, W. Cell-matrix response in tendon injury. *Clinics in Sports Medicine* 1992; **11**(3): 533–78.
11. Ounpu S. *The biomechanics of running*. Instructional Course 322. Anaheim, Ca: American Society of Sports Medicine, 1991.
12. Nigg B. Causes of injuries: extrinsic factors. In: Dirix A, Knuttgen

HG, Tittel K, eds. *The Olympic book of sports medicine.* Oxford: Blackwell, 1988: 363–75.

13. Renström P, Edberg B, Olofson B, Peterson L, Svennang J. Faktorer med betydelse for skador i football. (Factors of importance for injuries in soccer.) In: *Fotbollsspel pa konstgras.* Stockholm: Statens Naturvardsverk (State Board of Nature and Recreation), 1977.

14. Elliott BC, Blaksby BA, Ellis R. Vibration and rebound velocity characteristics of conventional and oversized tennis rackets. *Research Quarterly on Exercise and Sports* 1980; **51**: 608–15.

15. Teitz C. Overuse injuries. In: Teitz C, ed. *Scientific foundation of sports medicine.* Oxford: Blackwell, 1990: 295–328.

16. Lysholm J, Wilander J. Injuries in runners. *American Journal of Sports Medicine* 1987; **15**: 168–71.

17. Renström P, Johnson RJ. Overuse injuries in sports. A review. *Sports Medicine* 1985; **2**: 316–33.

18. Stanish W. Overuse injuries in athletes: a prospective study. *Medicine and Science in Sports and Exercise* 1989; **16**: 1–7.

19. James, SL, Jones DC. Biomechanical aspects of distance running injuries. In: Cavanagh P, ed. *Biomechanics of distance running.* Champaign, IL: Human Kinetics, 1990: 249–69.

20. Lutter LD. Cavus foot in runners. *Foot and Ankle* 1981; **1**: 225–8.

21. Ross CF, Schuster RO. A preliminary report in predicting injuries in distance runners. *Podiatric Sports Medicine* 1983; **73**: 275–7.

22. Lorentzon R. Causes of injuries: intrinsic factors. In: Dirix A, Knuttgen HG, Tittel K, eds. *The Olympic book of sports medicine.* Oxford: Blackwell, 1988: 376–90.

23. Grace TG. Muscle imbalance and extremity injury. A perplexing relationship. *Sports Medicine* 1985; **2**: 77–82.

24. Safran M, Seaber A, Garnett W. Warm-up and muscular injury prevention. An update. *Sports Medicine* 1989; **8**: 239–49.

25. Heiser TM, Weber J, Sullivan G, Clare P, Jacobs RR. Prophylaxis and management of hamstring muscle injuries in intercollegiate football players. *American Journal of Sports Medicine* 1984; **12**: 368–70.

26. Kannus P, Nittymaki S, Jarvinen M. Sports injuries in women: a one-year prospective follow-up study at an outpatient sports clinic. *British Journal of Sports Medicine* 1987; **21**: 37–9

27. Marcus R, Cann C, Madvig P. Menstrual function and bone mass in elite women distance runners. *Annals of Internal Medicine* 1985; **102**: 158–63.

28. Sward L. The back of the young top athlete; symptoms, muscle strength, mobility, anthropometric and radiological findings. Thesis, University of Göteborg, Sweden, 1990.

29. Stanitski CL. Common injuries in preadolescent and adolescent athletes. Recommendations for prevention. *Sports Medicine* 1989; **7**: 32–41.

30. Lane NE, Block DA, Wood PD. Aging, long distance running and the development of musculoskeletal disability. A controlled study. *American Journal of Medicine* 1987; **82**: 772–80.

31. Peterson L, Renström P. Varldsmasterskap for veteraner—en medicinsk utmaning. (Championships for veterans—a medical challenge.) *Läkartidningen Sweden* 1980; **77**: 3618.

32. Felson DT, Anderson JJ, Naimvk A, Walker AM, Meenan RF. Obesity and knee osteoarthritis. The Framingham Study. *Annals of Internal Medicine* 1988; **109**: 18–24.

33. McGoey BV, Deitel M, Saplys RJF, Likman ME. Effect of weight loss on musculoskeletal pain in the morbidly obese. *Journal of Bone and Joint Surgery* 1990; **72B**: 322–3.

34. O'Toole M, Hiller DB, Smith R, Sisk T. Overuse injuries in ultra-endurance tri-athletes. *American Journal of Sports Medicine* 1989; **17**: 514–18.

35. MacIntyre JG, Taunton JE, Clement DB, Lloyd-Smith DR, McKenzie DC, Morrell RW. Running injuries. A clinical study of 4173 cases. *Clinical Journal of Sports Medicine* 1991; **1**: 81–7.

36. Clement DV, Taunton JE, Smart GE, McNicol KL. A survey of overuse running injuries. *Physician and Sports Medicine* 1981; **9**: 47–58.

37. Kannus P, Nittymaki S, Jarvinen M, Lehto M. Sports injuries in elderly athletes: A three-year prospective, controlled study. *Age and Ageing* 1990; **18**: 263–70.

38. Matheson GO, MacIntyre JG, Taunton JE, Clement DB, Lloyd-Smith R. Musculoskeletal injuries associated with physical activity in older adults. *Medicine and Science in Sports and Exercise* 1989; **21**: 379–85.

39. Merchant AC, Mercer RL, Jacobson RH. Roentgenographic analysis of patellofemoral congruence. *Journal of Bone and Joint Surgery* 1974; **56A**: 1391–6.

40. Bates BT, Osternig LR, Mason BR, James SL. Foot orthotic devices to modify selected aspects of lower extremity mechanics. *American Journal of Sports Medicine* 1979; **7**: 338–42.

41. Sperryn PN, Rostan L. Podiatry and sport physician. In: Bachl H, Prokop L, Suchert E, eds. *Current topics in sports medicine.* Baltimore: Urban, Schwarzenberg, 1984: 930–40.

42. Jorgensson U, Ekstrand J. Significance of heel pad confinement for the shock absorption at heel strike. *International Journal of Sports Medicine* 1988; **9**: 468–73.

43. Dillingham MF. Strength training. *Physical Medicine and Rehabilitation* 1987; **1(4)**: 555–68.

44. Komi PV. Physiological and biomechanical correlates of muscle function: effects of muscle structure and stretch–shortening cycle on force and speed. *Exercise and Sport Sciences Reviews* 1984; **12**: 81–121.

45. Curwin S, Stanish WD. *Tendinitis: its etiology and treatment.* Lexington, MA: The Collamore Press—DC Heath and Company, 1984.

46. Saal JS. Flexibility training. *Physical Medicine and Rehabilitation* 1987; **1(4)**: 537–54.

47. Taylor DC, Dalton JD, Seaber AV, Garret WE. Viscoelastic properties of muscle–tendon units. *American Journal of Sports Medicine* 1990; **18**: 300.

48. Garrett WE. Muscle strain injuries: clinical and basic aspects. *Medicine and Science in Sports and Exercise* 1990; **22**: 436.

49. Armstrong RB. Initial events in exercise-induced muscular injury. *Medicine and Science in Sports and Exercise* 1990; **22**: 429.

50. Friden J, Sjöstrom M, Ekblom B. Myofibrillar damage following intense eccentric exercise in man. *International Journal of Sports Medicine* 1983; **4**: 170.

51. Pedowitz RA, Hargens AR, Mubarak SJ, Gershuni DH. Modified criteria for the objective diagnosis of chronic compartment syndrome of the leg. *American Orthopedic Society for Sports* 1990; **18**: 35.

52. Leadbetter WB, Buckwalter JA, Gordon SL. Sports-induced inflammation. *American Orthopedic Society for Sports Medicine Symposium.* Rosemont, IL: American Academy of Orthopedic Surgery, 1990.

53. Clement DB, Taunton JE, Smart GW. Achilles tendinitis and peritendinitis: etiology and treatment. *American Journal of Sports Medicine* 1984; **12**: 179–84.

54. Clancy WG. Tendinitis and plantar fascitis in runners. In: D'Ambrosia R, Drez D, eds. *Prevention and treatment of running injuries.* Thorofare, NJ: Charles B. Slack, 1982: 77–88.

55. Allenmark C, Renström P, Peterson L, Irstam L. Ten-year follow-ups of verified partial Achilles tendon ruptures. *Proceedings of the American Orthopedic Society for Sports Medicine Meeting, New Orleans.* Chicago, IL: American Orthopedic Society for Sports Medicine, 1990.

56. Konradsen L, Hansen EM, Sondergaard L. Long distance running and osteoarthrosis. *American Journal of Sports Medicine* 1990; **18**: 379.

57. Jobe FW, Bradely JP. The diagnosis and nonoperative treatment of shoulder injuries in athletes. *Clinics in Sports Medicine* 1989; **8**: 419.

58. Viitasalo JR, Kvist M. Some biomechanical aspects of the foot and ankle in athletes with and without shin splints. *American Journal of Sports Medicine* 1983; **11**: 125–30.

59. Renström P, Peterson L. Groin injuries in athletes. *British Journal of Sports Medicine* 1980; **14**: 30.

60. Jackson DW, Wiltse LL, Dingeman R, Hayes M. Stress reactions involving the pars intaricularis in young athletes. *American Journal of Sports Medicine* 1981; **9**: 304–12.

61. Granhed H, Morelli B. Low back pain among retired wrestlers and heavyweight lifters. *American Journal of Sports Medicine* 1988; **16**: 520–3.

62. Gordon GA Stress reactions in connective tissues: a molecular hypothesis. *Medical Hypotheses* 1991; **36**: 289–94.

5.2 Stress fractures

GianCarlo Puddu, Guglielmo Cerullo, Alberto Selvanetti, and Fosco De Paulis

Introduction

Stress fractures are an overloaded pathology due to repetitive exogenous or endogenous microtrauma and/or the application of a few heavy loads whose effects exceed the biological capacities of functional adjustment with resulting partial or complete bone collapse.[1]. Two types of stress fracture are classically distinguished: type I 'fatigue fractures' as defined above,[2,3] and type II 'insufficiency fractures',[2,4] in which normal repetitive loads cause fractures in bones which are less resistant as a result of pathological conditions such as osteoporosis, osteoarthrosis, osteomalacia, Paget's disease, or bone tumours. In this chapter we consider type I fractures.

The first report of stress fractures in the literature appeared in 1855 when the Prussian Army physician Breithaupt described the syndrome of a painful swollen foot associated with marching.[5] In 1897 Stechow published the first radiographic report of this condition in the metatarsal bones (Deutschlander's fracture).[6] However, in the last few years an increasing number of reports describing stress fractures in runners and other sports persons have appeared in the sports medicine and orthopaedic literature, probably because of the increased number of players participating in sports and the improvement of diagnostic techniques such as bone scintigraphy, computed tomography (CT), and magnetic resonance imaging (MRI).

Stress fractures comprise 10 per cent of sports injuries,[3,7] and are particularly common in the weight-bearing sports.

Biomechanical and histological aspects

Stress fractures in athletes are due to the inability of healthy bone to withstand chronic submaximal repetitive mechanical stress or a sudden increase in loads during sports activities.

Bone is a dynamic tissue which, according to Wolf's law, can adapt to load variations (compressive, distractive, rotational and shearing forces) to ensure an equal stress distribution. This adjustment occurs through continual structural remodelling depending on load characteristics (intensity, volume, time of application) and begins with prevalence of osteoclastic activity with consequent weakening of the bone. Osteoblastic activity increases to balance the reabsorption and to supply the required resistance to the bone. If the stress is not eliminated or reduced during this process, plastic deformation can occur in the bone with the possibility of a stress fracture.[8-11] Jones et al.[12] called this process 'stress reactions' and divided it into five stages:

Grade 0 (normal remodelling) is characterized by a thin new periosteal bone, not visible on radiographs, which is clinically asymptomatic. However, the bone scan reveals a small linear area of increased uptake.

Grade 1 (mild stress reaction) is also present as a cortical rearrangement (tunnelling). The subject complains of local pain exacerbated by activity. Tenderness is absent, radiographs are negative, and the bone is intact. However, the bone scan is positive.

Grade 2 (moderate stress reaction) is where cortical reabsorption prevails on periosteal reaction. Pain and tenderness are present, and some indistinct signs may be visible on radiographs. The bone scan is positive and the bone should be intact.

Grade 3 (severe stress reaction) is where periosteal reaction and cortical tunnelling are extensive, and pain persists at rest. Radiographs show cortical thickening and the bone scan is positive.

Grade 4 (stress fracture) is characterized by a bone biopsy with necrotic areas, trabecular microfractures, and granulation tissue. Weight bearing is sometimes impossible because of the pain. Radiographs show the fracture and early signs of callus formation. Scintigraphy is positive.

Aetiology and pathogenesis

Two theories have been proposed to explain stress fractures. According to the overload theory,[13] rhythmic and repetitive contractile activity of the muscles produces stresses at their osseous insertions which reduce the mechanical resistance of the bone. This theory can explain stress fractures of the chest and upper body which are non-weight-bearing areas. According to muscle fatigue theory,[14-17] progressive exhaustion during sports activity makes the muscle less effective as a 'shock absorber'. Abnormal load distribution occurs with stress concentration in restricted areas. This mechanism is applicable to stress fractures in weight-bearing activities.

Other factors associated with stress fractures are as follows.[7,12,18]

Genetic factors Large series which reveal predisposing genetic factors have not been reported in the literature. However there is some anecdotal evidence regarding monozygotic twins submitted to the same stresses.[19]

Race Stress fractures are less frequent in black people, possibly because of their higher bone density.[9,20,21]

Somatotype The risk of stress fracture is higher in large subjects and those whose morphology is inadequate for the required performance.[22-24]

Sex Women are more at risk than men (from 3.5:1 to 10:1).[20,25,26] This difference is probably due to their lower percentage of lean mass and lighter skeletal structure, disadvantageous morphotype for running (large pelvis, coxa vara, genu valgum, lower height, shorter step), anorexia nervosa, and menstrual disorders.[27-32] It has been shown that the oral contraceptive pill reduces the risk of stress fracture in long-distance runners.[33]

Age The risk increases with age, with a peak between 18 and 28 years old when lamellar cortical bone gradually transforms into adult osteonic bone.[34,35] Greenstick fractures are more common in subjects aged less than 16 years.[36]

Physical fitness Stress fractures occur more frequently in sedentary subjects who have just begun sports activity or in athletes who have returned to sport after prolonged inactivity.[37]

Training errors The history of athletes with stress fractures frequently reveals a sudden increase in loads during training, particularly if the subject is not in good physical condition.

Equipment Footwear which is too small or too worn can increase the risk of fracture because the capacity to absorb stresses is reduced.[18] Combat boots are often inadequately designed to absorb stresses from the ground.[38]

Playing surface Running or walking on a hard surface such as cement or asphalt can increase the risk of stress fractures.

Anatomical abnormalities Structural and/or postural abnormalities, such as malalignment or leg length discrepancy, excessive femoral anteversion, flat foot, varus forefoot, and pronation, can result in a non-physiological load distribution.[39]

Clinical, diagnostic, and therapeutic aspects

History

The characteristic history is a dull aching localized pain with insidious onset and progressive worsening with activity. The patient often reports some recent changes in training such as increasing duration or distance, a harder playing surface, or new footwear. In some cases, such as ballet dancers, onset is acute.

Clinical examination

In most cases clinical examination is non-specific or negative, particularly if the area is surrounded by soft tissues. However, tenderness, swelling, and percussion tenderness localized to the fracture site may be noted. If a long time has elapsed since the onset of symptoms, callus may be present. For stress fractures of the femoral shaft, the fulcrum test significantly aids in the early diagnosis and follow-up treatment.[40]

Plain radiographs

In 70 per cent of cases radiographs are negative in the early stages of the pathological changes, and no more than 50 per cent are positive in the later stages.[36] Although radiology is not very sensitive to stress fractures, its usefulness can be increased by using radiographs in two planes, oblique views, high magnifications, and tomograms.

A period from 2 to 12 weeks, depending on the site of the fracture, is required before a stress fracture can be visualized by radiography.[41] Characteristic signs are the local periosteal reaction with addition of new bone (evident after 6 weeks)[30] and endosteal sclerosis. In cancellous bone, early lesions are of the compressive type. Sometimes they are visible on radiographs after 24 h. The classic aspect of a stress fracture is a radiotransparent line which interrupts the cortical continuity (Fig. 1).[42,43]

Bone scanning

Phosphate labelled with technetium-99m is incorporated in osteoblasts and a 'hot spot' appears in areas of bone stress reaction. Scintigraphy is less specific than radiology but is much more sensitive to stress fractures. It can give positive results 6 to 72 h after the onset of pain.[18,44] The most sensitive technique is the triple-phase bone scan which can date the lesion, distinguish partial from complete fractures, and distinguish stress fractures from 'shin splints'.[45] It is useful to perform anteroposterior, lateral, and oblique scans, and to compare them with the contralateral scan.

In the early stages (grade 1) bone scans show a slightly increased uptake over a poorly defined area which becomes progressively more obvious (grade 2) with well-defined margins. Initially only one cortex is involved (grade 3); eventually the other cortex is incorporated (grade 4). Diagnosis of stress fracture is only possible in the last two stages.[46,47] Bone scanning can also be used to monitor the healing process which is demonstrated by a progressive return to normal uptake.[48]

False-positive scans are sometimes obtained for muscle strains, bone cysts, osteoid osteoma, sickle-cell disease, and osteomyelitis. In some cases, when cortical reabsorption dominates over osteoblastic activity, scintigraphy is temporarily negative.[49,50] However, a bone scan may reveal areas of increased uptake in asymptomatic patients.

Computed tomography

Because of its high definition, image clarity, and axial vision, CT reveals stress lesions more effectively than traditional tomography, particularly in specific sites such as the lumbar spine, and provides useful information for differential diagnosis (Fig. 2).

Magnetic resonance imaging

MRI provides a very sensitive method for monitoring variations accompanying stress fractures. It is more precise than scintigraphy and radiography since it shows the exact site of the lesions and can give good chronology of the pathology, as the signal's characteristics

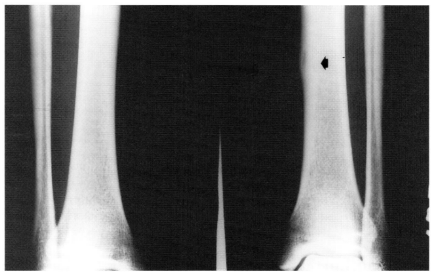

Fig. 1 Classic aspect of a stress fracture on a radiograph: a radiotransparent line interrupts the cortical continuity. The local periosteal reaction, with apposition of new bone, is also evident.

change with the passage of time from the onset of symptoms. A high intensity area surrounding a band at low intensity is seen on T_2-weighted images during the first 3 weeks. Oedema and haemorrhage resolve within 3 weeks but low intensity signals still remain on T_1-weighted images.

Stress fracture is characterized by a line in the cortex, at very low signal intensity, with a surrounding area of bone at reduced intensity on T_1-weighted images. The intensity of the signal on T_2-weighted images is increased to an extent depending on the asso-

ciated pathology (oedema, haemorrhage, medullar fibrosis, and periosteal and endosteal reaction).

MRI also provides useful information for differential diagnosis (osteoid osteoma, Garre's osteomyelitis, osteogenic sarcoma, ischaemic necrosis, and intraosseous occult fractures). In acute injuries it may differentiate strains or ligamentous injuries.[51-54]

General principles of treatment

Conservative treatment of stress fractures is generally successful. The athlete must suspend activity in his or her sport, but other exercises (cycling, swimming, upper-body ergometrics) are encouraged to limit deconditioning. Avoidance of all activities that involve impact loading is mandatory in stress fractures of the lower limbs. Weight bearing can be maintained if it is not painful. When pain is present at rest, it may be necessary to immobilize the limb in plaster or splints. Analgesics or non-steroidal anti-inflammatory drugs can be used to relieve pain. Ice massage is helpful.

When the athlete has been free of pain for 2 or 3 weeks, percussion tenderness is negative, full weight bearing is normal (in stress fractures of the lower limb), and plain radiographs show bone healing, the athlete can gradually return to sport, using pain as a criterion for monitoring effective recovery.

It is necessary to identify the presence of the risk factors discussed previously. Surgical treatment is indicated when there is a high risk that the fracture will not consolidate or in the presence of a non-union.

Upper limbs

Coracoid process

Stress fractures of the coracoid process typically occur in trapshooters and are due to the repetitive percussive action of the butt of the rifle and the cyclic contraction of the coracoid muscles.[55] The athlete complains of an ache in the anterior shoulder while shooting and also at rest if the pathology progresses. Physical examination reveals (i) local tenderness of the coracoid process, (ii) pain on

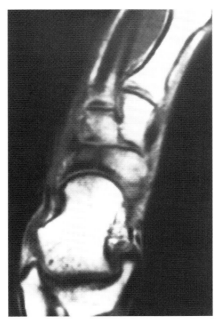

Fig. 2 Stress fracture of the tarsal navicular: CT shows the line of fracture, which interrupts the anterior and posterior cortex, with endosteal sclerosis. The patient had negative radiographs and a positive bone scan. When he returned to sports activity (hurdling) after 2 months of treatment with pulsating magnetic fields, he inverted the impact foot while running. Two months later he developed a stress fracture of the contralateral scaphoid.

resisted adduction and flexion of the shoulder, with (iii) negative signs for rotary cuff pathology or instability.

Plain radiographs are negative but the axillary view reveals the fracture at the base or the middle third of the coracoid process (in rare cases).[56] Treatment is based on avoidance of shooting and painful movements of the shoulder for 2 to 3 months.

Acromion

Stress fractures of the acromion are very rare in athletes. Two cases have been reported in the literature, one in an American football offensive lineman and the other in a professional jay alai player. Treatment consisted of 5 to 6 weeks of avoiding weightlifting and contact sports.[57]

Humerus

Stress fractures of the humerus have been described in young throwing athletes and participants in racket sports who have immature bone and muscle.[58,59] These fractures rarely occur in athletes who have been involved in sport for many years and have developed muscle and cortical hypertrophy. The causes of this injury are the high acceleration forces on the humeral shaft.

The athlete complains of pain during throwing or at the end of the game or training session. Clinical examination reveals local tenderness on deep palpation of the humeral shaft but movement of the shoulder and elbow is painless. Radiographs may be negative but bone scans are positive.

Treatment is based on curtailment or alteration of throwing sports. If the athlete does not rest, the fracture may become complete with dislocation of fragments and the necessity for surgical treatment.

Olecranon

Stress fractures of the olecranon in throwing athletes or gymnasts are due to the repetitive tension generated by the triceps brachii tendon (avulsion-type fracture).[8,60,61] Pain is present during activity and in maximal flexion or extension. Because of the high risk of delayed union or non-union of this fracture it is best treated by immobilization.[62,63] If the fracture is complete, surgical fixation is preferred.

In some cases, when the fracture occurs at the distal end of the olecranon, pain may persist during activity even after healing. In this case surgical excision may be indicated.

Ulna

Stress fractures of the ulnar shaft have been called 'lifting fractures' because they were initially described in farmers involved in digging or lifting heavy objects with a pitchfork. These fractures are occasionally reported in volleyball and tennis players, body-builders, and softball pitchers.[64-68] Two cases have been described in the non-dominant arm of professional tennis players using double-handed backhand stroke.[69] Pain is referred during activity and there is local tenderness in the forearm. Radiographs are usually negative in the early stages but scintigraphy confirms the diagnosis. Rest from athletics for 4 to 6 weeks is generally sufficient to restore normal condition.

Radius

Only two cases of stress fracture of the radius (one was bilateral) have been reported in the literature. They were described in a sailor after training for 'field gun running' and in a female high-level tennis player.[36,70] The treatment of the first patient consisted of 6 weeks of rest which resulted in a good outcome; however, it was 8 months before the tennis player could hit a tennis ball comfortably, but the diagnosis was made over 5 months after the onset of symptoms.

Carpal scaphoid

Stress fracture in the carpal scaphoid has been reported in gymnasts and shot-putters and is due to the forced dorsal flexion that crushes the navicular against the radial styloid.[71,72] The onset is usually insidious, but the symptoms may worsen such that the athlete cannot continue his or her sport. Palpation over the snuffbox generates pain. The same effect is produced by radial deviation and hyperextension. Oblique radiographs can show the fracture in the middle third of the bone,[73,74] and there is an intense uptake in bone scans. CT is also useful.[75] A thumb spica is recommended for 2 to 4 months, followed by intensive rehabilitation.

Metacarpals

Only two cases of stress fracture of the metacarpals have been reported, both in tennis players who held the racket incorrectly.[76,77] They developed a stress fracture at the base of the second metacarpal which healed after 1 month's rest from sport.

Thoracic cage

Sternum

Keating[78] reported stress fracture of the sternum in a wrestler presenting with chest pain approximately a week after performing a hyperextension trunk-stretching exercise. Examination revealed tenderness and a slight palpable prominence 2 cm distal to the sternum angle. A lateral radiograph showed a stress fracture, which was confirmed by a hot spot on the bone scan. The wrestler was allowed to resume his sport 2 months after diagnosis.

Ribs

First rib

Stress fractures of the first rib have been reported in baseball, tennis, American football, and basketball players.[79,80] The fracture generally occurs at the level of the subclavian groove, which is the thinnest part of the rib and is exposed to the strong action of the scalenii, serratus anterior, and intercostal muscles. There may be insidious or acute onset of pain at the base of the neck, sometimes extending under the scapula or towards the pectoral area. Pain may increase during deep breathing. Clinical examination shows an area of local tenderness and pain on resisted shoulder lifting. The diagnosis is confirmed by radiography and bone scan. Occasionally this fracture is complicated by non-union (Fig. 3).

Other ribs

Stress fractures of the other ribs have been described in rowers, gymnasts, golfers, tennis players, and in a female swimmer.[81-84] They usually occur in the posterolateral area, where the serratus anterior muscle exerts a strong bending moment during scapular

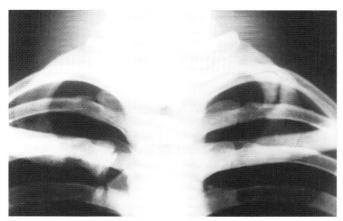

Fig. 3 Non-union of a stress fracture of the left first rib. The injury was revealed in a 25-year-old basketball player during the routine preseason examination. No treatment was necessary.

motion. The athlete complains of a chest pain which is exacerbated by deep breathing, activity, and local palpation. Differential diagnosis between muscle strain and fracture is required, but radiographs and bone scans provide confirmation. Rest from athletic activity for 4 to 8 weeks is sufficient for healing to take place.

Lumbar spine

The lumbar spine is subjected to considerable stress during the maintenance of certain postures in ballet and the performance of various athletic movements. Stress fractures of the lumbar vertebral arch are relatively common, with the site of the injury depending on the direction in which stress is applied. Fractures of the lamina, the pedicles, and the articular processes have been described,[85-87] but injuries of the pars interarticularis are most frequent.[88]

Spondylolysis is a loss of continuity of the pars interarticularis (or isthmus) of the vertebra; it most frequently involves L5, though it can also be found at L4 and, rarely, more proximally.

Spondylolisthesis involves relative anterior slipping of one vertebra over those below. This may be associated with spondylolysis.

Of the five forms of spondylolysis and spondylolisthesis classified by Wiltse *et al.*[89] we shall deal only with those most frequently found in young people and athletes, i.e. dysplastic (type I) and isthmic (type II).

Epidemiology

The incidence of spondylolysis in the general population is 5 per cent,[90] but this figure may be higher among athletes.[91] According to one survey,[92] the incidence in young gymnasts is 11 per cent (four times higher than the 2.3 per cent reported in the general female population) and 6 per cent also suffer from spndylolisthesis.[93] The incidence in adult linemen (American football) is 24 per cent compared with 6.4 per cent in white men and 2.8 per cent in black men.[94]

The incidence of spondylolysis and spondylolisthesis increases from about the age of 5 to 6 years to about the age of 20 and then remains steady; as regards sex and race, it is lowest among black women (1.1 per cent) and highest among white men (6.4 per cent). The incidence reaches 54 per cent in certain Eskimo tribes.[95]

The dislocation starts at about the age of 8 years in girls and about the age of 12 in boys and increases with age, particularly during the adolescent growth spurt (10 to 15 years of age). Girls are more often symptomatic and require surgical stabilization of the lesion more frequently.

Aetiology

Congenital anomalies of the sacrum and spina bifida are associated with spondylolysis and/or lumbosacral instability. However, spondylolysis and spondylolisthesis have never been found at birth or in subjects who have never walked.[96] The possibility of genetic predisposition may explain why cases of spondylolysis are sometimes found among relatives of patients suffering from this pathology.

Lack of continuity of the pars interarticularis is considered to be a stress fracture. It is unilateral in 20 to 25 per cent of cases, and is caused, in predisposed subjects, by repeated forced cyclical movements involving flexion–extension of the lumbar spine, implying functional overloading.[95,97] This initiates a concentration of high shear forces at the isthmus level which increase in movements involving both extension and lateral inclination and/or rotation of the spine.

Athletes most likely to be affected by these pathological changes are those involved in the following activities: gymnastics, weightlifting, wrestling, American football (collisions of linemen produced in the 'three point' position; with a lumbosacral hyperextension), soccer, mountain skiing, handball, judo, swimming, diving, basketball, rugby, parachuting, track and field athletics (pole vaulting, javelin throwing, hurdling), tennis, baseball (pitcher), ballet, lacrosse, karate, and rowing. The following factors may predispose to the condition: lumbar hyperlordosis, high body weight, and a strong paravertebral musculature opposed by a relative deficit of abdominal muscles.

Clinical description

Symptoms are usually absent in children, particularly if they do not practise sport. Discomfort arises at the onset of the adolescent growth spurt. However, the lesion is usually only noticed incidently following radiography. A typical example is an athlete practising one of the sports listed above who has had months of lumbar pain with insidious onset caused and/or exacerbated by physical activity (particularly repeated flexion and extension and/or rotation of the lumbar spine), occasionally extending to the gluteus and the thigh. The symptoms may be temporarily relieved by resting from sport, but if the activity is continued the pain becomes more frequent and intense, sometimes interfering with athletic practice and even with normal daily activities. There is not usually a history of serious trauma, although sometimes the onset of symptoms is acute and may coincide with a minor injury.[98]

Objective examination may be negative in spondylolysis or first- or second-degree spondylolisthesis; sometimes the only evidence available is tightened hamstrings (present in 80 per cent of symptomatic patients). In more advanced spondylolisthesis, the muscular contracture may prevent full flexion of the thigh on the pelvis so that the patient walks in small steps, with the pelvis rotating at each step ('pelvic waddle'). Children run or walk on the tips of their toes with knees semiflexed.

When the lumbar region is palpated, particularly if the patient is symptomatic, tenderness and spasms of the paravertebral muscles may be present at the level of the vertebral defect and the surrounding segments.

The pain is induced and increased by the following movements of the trunk: anterior flexion (if the contraction of the hamstrings is intense, the patient cannot touch the floor with his palms), contralateral rotation and inclination ipsilateral to the injury, and extension while weight bearing (if the defect is bilateral) or on the corresponding leg (if unilateral). In gymnasts and dancers the pain can be induced by making them adopt the arabesque position. In both cases the patient will feel pain when resting in a contralateral single lift position if the injury is unilateral.[99] Straight leg raising is reduced when hamstrings are very contracted.

In the more advanced (third and fourth) degrees of spondylolisthesis, examination of the posture reveals flattening of the lumbar lordosis, a 'step-off' or depression that can be felt on the middle line over the spinous process of the lumbar vertebra which is the site of the injury, a short trunk with a low chest, a transverse transumbilical groove, flared ilia, and flattened buttocks.

Lumbar scoliosis is more often found accompanying spondylolisthesis (particularly the dysplastic type), in women, and in cases of severe slippage. It is secondary to muscular spasm and disappears in asymptomatic periods. Idiopathic structural dorsal or dorsolumbar scoliosis is reported in a third of all cases of spondylolisthesis.[95]

Plain radiographs

Anteroposterior, lateral, and oblique projections (sometimes augmented by tomograms) are used to examine a spondylolysis. In a relatively advanced spondylolysis, the anteroposterior view shows 'décalage' of the alignment of the spinal processes above the lysis resulting from the advancement of the contralateral superior articular process; the differential diagnosis includes osteoid osteoma and it is thus necessary to look for the nidus.[100] The lateral view may occasionally reveal the lysis, but this is better shown by an oblique projection with the typical 'decapitated dog' or 'Scottie dog' image; if the injury is recent the gap will be narrow with irregular margins, but if it is chronic the borders of the injury will be blunt and smooth (Fig. 4).

In examining a case of spondylolisthesis, oblique projections are useful only in those cases of first-degree slip.[101] When L5–S1 spondylolisthesis is advanced, the overlapping of the lumbosacral body over the sacrum may produce the image of an 'inverted Napoleon's hat' on the anteroposterior projection and the isthmic lysis may appear as an interruption of bone continuity just below the pedicle. In the lateral projection under load, lysis or lengthening of the isthmus is seen and the degree of subluxation of the vertebra can be measured in terms of tangential slip (four degrees according to Wiltse's classification[102]; Table 1) and sagittal rotation of the L5 vertebra over the sacrum (Fig. 5). As the slip progresses the following changes can occur: anterior and posterior rounding of the sacral promontory, a wedge-shaped aspect of the L5 body (lumbar index), a vertical position of the sacrum, an increase in lumbar lordosis, and, in adults suffering from first- and second-degree spondylolisthesis, a reduction of the L5–S1 intervertebral space and sclerosis of the anterior margin of the sacrum.

Lateral weight-bearing views at the highest degree of flexion and extension are also useful for evaluating the degree of translatory instability of the unstable vertebra. Radiographs also allow investigation of associated anomalies, such as spina bifida and congenital aplasia of the proximal part of the sacrum or of the superior articular facets. In dysplastic spondylolisthesis the pedicles and pars interarticularis appear lengthened, and in the lateral projection the whole vertebra slips anteriorly and thus produces lysis of the isthmus or the lamina, which favours further anterior slippage of the vertebral body.

Bone scintigraphy

Bone scintigraphy is useful in symptomatic patients with negative radiographs. This can reveal a stress reaction of the pars interarticularis which cannot be visualized radiographically or, when the radiographs show a stress fracture of the isthmus, it can be used to estimate the age of the injury and classify the activity.

In fact, in an asymptomatic patient with negative radiographs and a positive bone scan, preventive treatment may stop the development of the process. When the radiographs show spondylolysis and the bone scan is normal, the injury is a pseudoarthrosis which has been present for about 6 to 12 months and which cannot

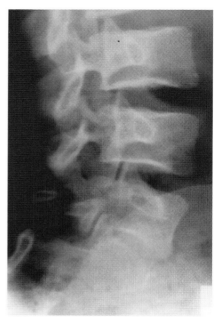

Fig. 4 Spondylolysis: an oblique radiograph shows the typical 'decapitated dog' image. The blunt smooth borders of the injury indicate that it is chronic.

Table 1 Wiltse's classification of spondylolisthesis (percentage of slip of the upper displaced vertebra upon the lower)	
First degree	< 25%
Second degree	25%–50%
Third degree	50%–75%
Fourth degree	> 75%

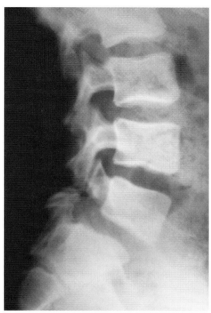

Fig. 5 Second-degree spondylolisthesis in a 24-year-old pole-vaulter occasionally suffering from lumbar pain. The pathology did not influence his sports career.

'heal'.[103–105] Hence there is no point in performing scintigraphy on those patients who have been symptomatic for more than a year unless tumours or osseous infections are suspected.[95]

Computed tomography

CT is useful in adults to visualize the isthmus and to establish the degree of slippage, spinal stenosis, and radicular compression.

Myelography

Myelography is indicated where an osseous neoplasia or discitis is suspected or in those cases with clinical signs of cauda equina syndrome.

Treatment of spondylolysis

If the injury is acute (recent onset of symptoms, normal radiographs, and positive bone scan), recovery may be promoted by immobilizing with plaster (corset or single-leg pantaloon body cast) or thoracolumbosacral orthosis for at least 3 months. In addition, it is vital to avoid activities which may challenge the lumbosacral spine. The efficacy of the treatment is monitored by disappearance of pain and decreasing scintigraphic activity. Sports may be resumed 3 months after the removal of the plaster, provided that the patient remains asymptomatic and that scintigraphy is normal.

The athlete follows a programme of stretching exercises for the paravertebral muscles and hamstrings as well as abdominal and hamstring strengthening exercises avoiding hyperextension of the lumbar spine. The functional demands are gradually increased. It may be necessary to forbid training with weights in the upright position. If the bone scan is positive and radiographs show a recent fracture, the symptomatic patient may be treated as described even if the radiological evidence of recovery of the injury is less clear.

When the injury to the isthmus is chronic (positive radiography and negative scintigraphy), the treatment is symptomatic, including analgesics and temporary rest from athletic activity. The patient may be confined to bed or immobilized in plaster for a short time, and must start a gradual programme of exercises to strengthen the abdominal muscles and to stretch the hamstrings and back muscles. It is sometimes necessary to resort to surgical stabilization of spondylolysis in those rare patients who are refractory to conservative treatment. This may allow a return to sport after about a year.

When spondylolysis is diagnosed in a child, it is necessary to carry out clinical and radiological checks at least every 6 months until the skeleton is fully developed to ensure early recognition of the initial signs of a progression of slippage. Sporting activity need not be severely limited in the child or adolescent with asymptomatic lysis, but the patient must be informed of the possible consequences of participating in high-risk sports. The risk of the development of spondylolisthesis in a child suffering from spondylolysis increases between the ages of 10 and 15 years, particularly if he or she participates in sport, and if recurring episodes of lumbar pain with a dysplastic spondylolisthesis are present. A worsening of the condition is rare after the age of 20 and has never been documented during pregnancy.[95]

Treatment of spondylolisthesis

In first-degree asymptomatic spondylolisthesis the patient must be informed of the possibility of an evolution of the pathology although specific sporting activities need not be curtailed. Clinical and radiographical checks should be performed every 6 to 12 months, and exercises to correct muscular imbalance should be prescribed. When a 'silent' spondylolisthesis exceeds the first degree, sport involving a high risk of physical contact and trauma to the back should be discouraged.

In symptomatic spondylolisthesis, long-term conservative measures are ineffective in over 50 per cent of cases, particularly if the slippage is second degree or above. Patients with slippage of 25 per cent or more and an early degenerative discopathy are more likely to suffer from acute relapsing episodes and to require surgical treatment as adults.[106] Competitive athletes suffering from spondylolisthesis have severe functional limitations and often must change or interrupt their athletic careers.[107]

In first- and second-degree symptomatic spondylolisthesis, surgery is indicated when no result is obtained by reducing physical activity, applying a corset, and maintaining muscular tone. Surgery is also indicated in third- and fourth-degree spondylolisthesis when pain is refractory to conservative treatment or when there are neurological manifestations. A bilateral arthrodesis is generally carried out. If there is radiological evidence of a consolidated osseous fusion (80 to 100 per cent of patients undergoing surgery), a gradual return to sports activity is allowed.[95]

It follows from the above discussion that an early diagnosis of isthmic overload pathology is very important. It might be useful to screen predisposed patients participating in sports at high risk in this respect so that injuries can be identified at an early stage and suitable treatment prescribed.

Sacrum

Only one case of stress fracture of the sacrum has been reported in the literature.[108] It was described in a 40-year-old man who was running 80 km weekly and occurred in the upper portion of the right sacral wing. Treatment consisted of 7 weeks of rest and the patient subsequently resumed intensive training.

Lower limbs

Pelvis

Stress fractures of the pelvis occur most frequently in joggers, long-distance runners, and military recruits.[109] They generally occur in the pubic ramus where it joins the ischium near the symphysis and comprise 1.25 per cent of stress fractures in endurance runners.[110]

It is believed that these fractures are the result of repeated tensions produced in this area during a prolonged race by the rhythmic contraction of the adductors and the obturator muscles. They are more frequent in women, probably because their racing technique is different and/or because of the different geometry of the female pelvis. They can be bilateral and may be complicated by an avulsion fracture at the level of adductor insertion.[109]

Pelvic stress fractures must be considered and suspected when a runner complains of characteristic pain in the buttock or thigh during or after training, which increases if training is continued until the runner has to slow down and starts limping.[111] It is important to enquire whether there has been a sudden change in the running distances, a variation in the racing technique, or a change of training site. There is marked pain when pressure is exerted in the region of the inferior pubic ramus near the symphysis. Upright posture with weight bearing on the limb on the side of the injury is uncomfortable and painful (positive standing sign).[112] Slight pain may limit movements of the hip in abduction and/or external rotation. Differential diagnosis includes insertional tendinopathy of the adductors, muscular strain of the adductors, pubic osteitis, trochanteric bursitis, degenerative pathology of the hip, pain in the lumbosacral spine, tendinopathy, or muscular strain of the hamstrings.

Radiographs are positive 2 to 3 weeks after the fracture, but if a long period elapses before they are carried out, the frequently exuberant aspect of the callus may suggest osteosarcoma. For a further evaluation it is better to combine the usual anteroposterior view with two further projections of the patient horizontal and the X-ray beam inclined at 45° to the longitudinal axis of the body in the cephalic–caudal and caudal–cephalic directions. Tomograms may also be useful. An early bone scan is recommended and is very useful in the 'preradiographic' stage of the injury that may be complicated by delayed union and recurrence; the sclerosis surrounding the margins of the fracture indicates non-union, which recovers on resting.

Treatment requires a period of abstinence from sport, and all activities causing pain are forbidden for 8 to 12 weeks. Crutches are sometimes required for about 4 to 5 weeks, particularly when there is pain under load. Stretching exercises are allowed if they can be tolerated. A gradual return to sport is allowed only if the patient is completely asymptomatic and radiographs show no signs of delayed union or non-union.

Femoral neck

Fracture of the femoral neck is the typical 'insufficiency' fracture which affects elderly people and which can also be found as a stress fracture in long-distance runners, dancers, military recruits, hurdlers, football players, and cross-country skiers. During walking the proximal femur is subject to loads up to six times the body weight with high compressive loads on the concave side of the femoral neck and tensile loads on the convex side. Thus loading increases substantially during running.[113]

This type of fracture must be considered when the athlete, usually a runner who has recently intensified his training programme and/or started to run on a different surface, complains of a pain in the groin extending to the anterior thigh and sometimes to the knee, which starts on weight bearing during or immediately after physical activity and is temporarily relieved by rest and functional unloading of the limb. However, if physical training continues, pain starts earlier and intensifies, eventually becoming constant, preventing training, and sometimes causing a limp.[114] In some cases the pain starts at night and, in the absence of symptoms, the athlete may present to the doctor when the fracture is already complete and displaced. Antalgic gait and discomfort when standing on the foot of the fractured limb (positive standing sign) are observed. Palpation of the groin region above the hip joint is painful. Sometimes this area appears swollen, there is pain in the area of the injury because of percussion or compression of the heel or the great trochanter, and a slight antalgic limitation of the highest degrees of articular excursion (particularly in flexion and internal rotation).[115] Differential diagnosis includes strain of the iliopsoas or the adductor muscles, hernia of the groin, pubic osteitis, bursitis, or synovitis.

Plain radiographs of a femoral neck fracture may be negative during the first 2 to 6 weeks after the onset of symptoms; if the fracture is suspected clinically it may be useful to perform a bone scintigraphy which will allow early discovery of a hot spot in the area of the femoral neck. If this is the case, serialized radiographs can be taken to check the radiological evolution of the injury. Anteroposterior, lateral, and oblique radiographs of the hip are obtained and compared with those of the contralateral hip (fractures are frequently bilateral). Tomograms may be necessary. There are many radiographic classifications of femoral neck fractures.[28,116,117] From a therapeutic viewpoint 'subradiographic' cases, where the clinical picture and scintigraphy suggest a fracture although plain radiographs are still negative (conservative treatment by avoidance of weight bearing until symptoms disappear and scintigraphy becomes normal), must be distinguished from those in which the radiographs show unmistakable signs of stress fracture. In the latter case we adopt the Devas classification which distinguishes two kinds of femoral neck stress fracture.[116]

Compression fractures

Compression fractures are more frequent in young athletes[118] and are located at the cortex of the lower medial margin of the femoral neck. Initially they appear radiographically as a rather opaque area which, if loading continues, becomes more sclerotic; sometimes a small central 'crack' appears whose margins in time become thicker. In the more advanced stages of recovery, the anteroposterior tomogram shows gradual healing of the injury until the smooth aspect of the concave margin of the neck is re-established. This type of fracture seldom displaces, unless stress continues.

If, after diagnosis, radiographs do not show the fracture, treatment is conservative and the patient must be restricted until he or she becomes asymptomatic and active and passive motion of the hip is completely regained and no longer painful. At this point the patient may be allowed to walk with crutches, first non-weight-bearing for about 6 weeks and then partially loaded. When full weight bearing is asymptomatic the patient may abandon one crutch and start swimming/walking in water. He or she may also use a bicycle, gradually abandon the other crutch, and increase the walking distance on soft ground. At all times the guidelines for treatment must be the absence of pain and/or limping and the gradual recovery of the fracture as shown by serial radiography. Finally, the patient is allowed to run, avoiding hard surfaces, first on alternate days for short distances interrupted by walking, and then for longer distances.

If initial radiographs show a fracture of the cortex, it is advisable to admit the patient to hospital and, occasionally, apply skeletal traction. If radiographs show deepening and/or widening of the fracture, internal fixation must be carried out, allowing unloaded walking with crutches from the first day after the operation. A gradual rehabilitation programme is carried out for another 3 months during which participation in contact sports is forbidden.

Distraction-type fracture

Distraction-type fractures occur most frequently in elderly people and military men. Onset is at the superior margin of the femoral neck with interruption of continuity of the cortex (it is seen radiographically in the appropriate anteroposterior view if it is not hidden by the great trochanter) which, if not recognized early, can evolve towards a complete and displaced fracture. If untreated, complications are likely, including aseptic necrosis of the femoral head, delayed union, non-union, and in varus consolidation. Initial radiographs sometimes show a rather large break. A fracture at this site must be considered a surgical emergency. Early diagnosis is essential because the consequences of a delay in starting treatment may have disastrous effects on the athlete's career.[119]

An undisplaced fracture of the femoral neck due to distraction can require the patient to be confined to bed until passive movements of the hip no longer cause pain and radiographs show evidence of the formation of endosteal callus.[120] At this point unloaded walking with crutches is allowed, progressing to partial weight bearing when the callus has filled the fracture gap. Walking without crutches can be started when the fracture is entirely consolidated. If the patient refuses bed rest or if radiographic monitoring during conservative treatment indicates widening of the fracture site, internal osteosynthesis will be necessary.

Surgical reduction and internal fixation are mandatory for displaced fractures. Following surgery, it may be useful to evaluate the vascularization of the femoral head by means of scintigraphy.

Femoral shaft

Stress fractures of the femoral shaft are less frequent than those in the femoral neck and have been reported in runners, hurdlers, skiers, and baseball and basketball players.[121,122] These fractures generally occur in the proximal third of the diaphysis (usually in the subtrochanteric area) because the degree of compressed strain to which the medial side of the loaded femoral diaphysis is subject gradually decreases in a proximal–distal direction and increases in the subtrochanteric region. Moreover, the distractive strains acting on the lateral cortex of the diaphysis are further reduced by the vastus lateralis and the iliotibial tract.[113,123]

The athlete complains of a deep-seated diffuse pain in the groin and/or the thigh or knee, depending on the site of the fracture. The pain increases during or after physical activity, but is not usually intense enough to cause limping. There is no acute trauma; in runners the history sometimes reveals a recent increase in the intensity of training and/or a change in running surface. Examination reveals a widespread pain in the thigh, and palpation sometimes produces pain in the injured region; the range of motion of the hip and knee is normal. The fulcrum test significantly aids in early diagnosis.[40] Tendinitis and muscular injury are the most common initial diagnoses.

According to Provost and Morris,[124] stress fractures of the femoral shafts can be classified radiographically into three groups depending on the site of the injury.

Group I Oblique fracture of the medial cortex of the proximal third of the diaphysis with periosteal reaction and sclerosis. The bone scan shows a medial increased uptake focus in the subtrochanteric region. Its development into a displaced fracture is rare. Treatment consists of bed rest until the patient becomes asymptomatic, followed by gradual restoration of the load, swimming, cycling and, if the athlete remains asymptomatic, running after 6 to 8 weeks.

Group II Oblique spiral displaced fracture of the middle third of the diaphysis. Because of its rapid development, the interval between the onset of symptoms and the diagnosis is often very short (a few days to 1 or 2 weeks). In these cases it is advisable to admit patients to hospital and apply skeletal traction. Unloaded walking with crutches is begun, and partial weight bearing is allowed later depending on the outcome of the radiographs used to monitor rehabilitation. Surgery may be necessary.

Group III Supracondylar transverse fracture of the distal third of the epiphysis which may or may not be displaced. If this fracture is not suspected initially, it may not be diagnosed until it has become completely displaced and osteosynthesis will be necessary. If early diagnosis is made, the patient must be immobilized and load bearing initially forbidden to avoid a complete fracture.

Conservative treatment (temporary cessation of specific sporting activities, bed rest, or crutches) and limitation of contact and jumping sports for 8 to 12 weeks with a gradual return to training after 8 to 14 weeks is usually sufficient for undisplaced stress fractures of the femoral shaft.

Patella

Although initially described as a complication in arthroplasty of the knee, stress fracture of the patella has been observed in healthy subjects as the result of functional overload.[125,126] It is an avulsion fracture characterized by anterior knee pain which increases when extending the leg. The patella is painful when palpated or struck, and is sometimes inflamed.

Radiography may show a transverse fracture subject to the risk of displacement due to the traction exercised by the quadriceps; if the fracture is not displaced it may be necessary to immobilize the patient, whereas if it is displaced it is necessary to reduce and fix it. Alternatively, there may be a vertical fracture, generally of the lateral facet, which may require excision of the fragment if it is displaced or there is non-union.

Tibia

Plateau

Stress fracture may occur in the medial plateau as this bears most of the body weight in the stance phase in the absence of axial alterations.[127,128] Onset is painful and gradual. Pain is in the anteriomedial tibial area just below the medial compartment above the metaphysis and is inclined to increase during activity. This pain is worsened by load and alleviated by rest. The area of the lesion is painful under finger pressure and is sometimes oedematous. There are no signs of meniscal and/or capsuloligamentous pathology. The knee is not swollen.

Differential diagnosis includes injuries of the medial collateral ligament at the tibial insertion level with tendinitis, and/or bursitis of the pes anserinus. In the first case the common valgus stress tests are positive; in the second case pain is felt more posteriorly. However, radiographs and bone scintigraphy are necessary.

Radiographs become positive about 3 weeks after the onset of symptoms and show an area of sclerosis 2 to 3 mm thick (related to the endosteal callus) under and parallel to the internal tibial plateau. The periosteal callus is rarely visible.

A period of rest from sport is usually sufficient (an average of 1 month); if walking is painful or the patient limps, crutches may be advisable. Complications are rare.

Shaft

About 50 per cent of stress fractures in athletes (runners, dancers, baseball players, and swimmers) are in the tibial shaft.[18] The predisposing factors seem to be a narrow tibia,[129] a higher degree of external rotation of the hip,[24] and pronated foot. In the pronated foot an increase of the tibial torsion is produced when the foot is laid down during running. Sometimes the runner's history reveals too much training on steep or sloping ground (the different ways in which the feet are laid down on inclined surfaces require different leg muscle action to maintain balance). Fractures may occur at any point on the shaft but are more frequent between the middle third and distal third of the posteromedial tibial cortex. They are frequently (15 to 46 per cent) multiple and/or bilateral.[130,131] However, in young runners occurrence is most common in the proximal third.

A typical case is that of the runner who, after intensifying training and/or changing to hard or inclined running surfaces, feels a dull aching pain in the anteromedial or posterolateral region of the tibia when he or she stops training. The pain increases with further training on subsequent days. Rest from athletic activity for a few days temporarily relieves the symptoms, but they reappear when training is started again. Despite repeated temporary breaks from athletic activity, onset of pain occurs earlier, and the pain itself becomes more intense, and eventually running becomes difficult or even impossible. Pain continues for longer periods after training is stopped, and is felt even during normal daily activities and, eventually, at rest.

The site of the fracture is particularly painful when palpated under finger pressure. The region is seldom oedematous and the callus is palpable only in the chronic phase. Sometimes pain in the region of the injury can only be induced by striking the tibia. The contralateral tibia should always be examined to determine whether there is a bilateral fracture. Radiographs (anteroposterior, lateral,

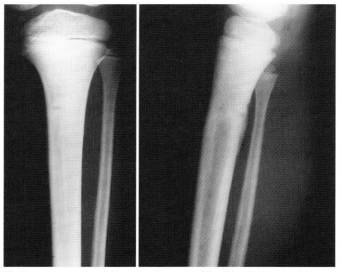

Fig. 6 Anteroposterior and lateral radiographs of the tibia of a 14-year-old soccer player. Stress fractures typically occur at this level (posteromedial aspect of the proximal third of the shaft) at this age and heal after a month of athletic rest.

and oblique projections augmented by tomograms if necessary) show fracture of the proximal third, the presence of an endosteal callus,[132] and, in fractures at the junction of the middle third with the distal third, a periosteal callus with a thickening of the cortex along the posteromedial tibial margin (Figs 1 and 6).[36] Sometimes callus formation causes tibiofibular synostosis.[133]

Differential diagnosis includes entrapment of the popliteal artery, shin splints, posteromedial tibial stress syndrome (osseous reaction to stress which is preradiographic but apparent on scintigraphy), and compartment syndrome (symptoms are independent of the application of loads, the possible presence of muscular hernia, a delayed local paraesthesia and/or dysaesthesia, negative radiographs and scintigraphs, but compartment pressure measurements should be made before, during, and after stress).

Treatment requires a temporary suspension of specific sports and all activities in which heavy loads are applied to the lower limbs. If walking is painful, a period of non-weight-bearing is necessary and a functional brace (Aircast type) may be required.[134] If the patient is asymptomatic at rest and radiographs indicate satisfactory improvement of the injury, a gradual rehabilitation programme is started, involving low frequency activity gradually increasing in intensity provided that the patient remains asymptomatic. Swimming and cycling are useful for this purpose. At this point it can be useful to wear viscoelastic insoles which improve shock absorption. Provided that the patient is asymptomatic, a gradual return to sport is allowed after 4 to 8 weeks (sometimes 3 months in distal tibial fractures).

Particular mention must be made of fractures of the middle third of the anteromedial tibial cortex which occur in activities involving jumping (basketball, figure-skating, volleyball, football, and ballet), but may also be seen in long-distance runners.[135-139] These fractures are caused by repeated tension to which this region is physiologically subject because of its own anatomical curve that is exaggerated by the movements involved in jumping.

In lateral and oblique radiographs (and tomograms) this fracture generally appears as a radiotransparent horizontal wedge or

V-shaped defect open in the front with its peak pointing into the anterior cortex of the middle third of the tibial crest ('sawtooth aspect' or 'dreaded back line'), sometimes surrounded by a sclerotic hypertrophic cortex and/or osteoporotic reabsorption areas. Owing to its subcutaneous position it is sometimes possible to feel a painful swelling. Because of the pathomechanics of the fracture and the poor vascular supply to this area, this injury is often complicated, particularly when it is not protected from further stress, and non-union or complete fracture may result.[140,141] Scintigraphy is useful to define the degree of activity of the injury.

When this fracture is diagnosed, it is necessary to immobilize the patient using a non-weight-bearing or partially unloaded splint or plaster for at least 6 months to encourage consolidation. If radiography shows no evidence of recovery after 4 to 6 months, bone grafting should be considered.[138] Since such a procedure may seem too lengthy, particularly for an athlete, a valid alternative is to consider surgical treatment initially to facilitate an early return to sport.[136]

Medial malleolus

Stress fracture of the medial malleolus has been reported in long-distance runners, footballers, and basketball players. It appears to be due to repeated overloads experienced by the ankle during running when, at the moment when the heel hits the ground (heel strike), the talus rotates internally, bumping against the internal malleolus and thus transmitting the torsion to the tibial diaphysis.[142,143]

In the absence of a specific acute trauma, this condition manifests itself as a medial pain in the ankle with insidious onset and increasing severity. It is worsened by running and jumping, and is temporarily alleviated by rest, but if tension continues athletic activity is restricted and walking may be painful.

Objectively the ankle appears inflamed and the medial malleolus is painful under finger pressure; sometimes there is painful movement with dorsiflexion. Radiographs in two projections augmented by tomograms show an endosteal callus or a vertical fracture at the junction between the medial malleolus and the tibial diaphysis which may propagate superomedially towards the distal metaphysis of the tibia (Fig. 7). If radiographs are negative, bone scans may reveal a subradiographic stage.

When radiographs show the fracture, surgical osteosynthesis is indicated followed by immobilization in plaster and early start of range of movement exercises. After 2 to 3 weeks a splint is applied. The athlete is usually ready to resume sport after 8 weeks.

If radiographs are negative and scintigraphy is positive, a functional splint is prescribed for 6 to 8 weeks until the patient becomes asymptomatic. Weight bearing is allowed if it is not painful, but running and jumping are forbidden. This is followed by jogging on flat ground with gradually increasing distances until the athlete is completely recovered and no longer feels pain.

Fibula

Stress fractures of the fibula are most frequent in the lower part, 4 to 7 cm above the lateral malleolus. They are due to repeated strains caused by eversion of the foot and/or the action of the calf muscles which, pushing the fibula towards the tibia, produce high tension on the distal fibula.[144] These fractures have been observed in runners, gymnasts, ballet dancers, and ice skaters.[145] They are often associated with a pronated foot.

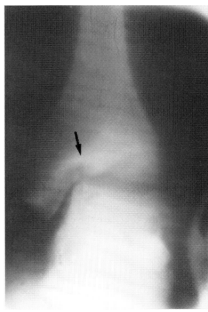

Fig. 7 Stress fracture of the tibial malleolus (arrow) in a 27-year-old long-distance runner revealed by an anteroposterior tomogram.

Clinically, there is an insidious onset of pain in the lateral region of the ankle, which may even give rise to discomfort in walking. Locally there is tenderness and swelling. It is necessary to look for possible subluxation of the peroneal tendons. Radiographs may be positive only 2 or 3 weeks after the onset of symptoms (callus of the posterolateral margin).[146] Thus, if a fracture is suspected, a bone scan would be useful. Rest from athletic activity is sufficient (swimming, cycling, and walking are allowed if they do not cause pain). Running and jumping must be avoided for 3 to 4 weeks, and stretching the calf and the peroneal muscles is important to avoid stiffness or instability of the ankle. If walking is painful, it is necessary to resort to plaster or partial weight bearing for 2 to 3 weeks. The athlete may return to his sport in 6 to 8 weeks.

Stress fractures of the proximal third of the fibula are less frequent. They are usually reported in jumpers and parachutists, and one has been found in an aerobic dancer.[147-149] They are probably due to the combined effects of compression loads, traction strains of the biceps muscle, shear forces, and/or the cyclic activity of the flexor hallucis longus, soleus, tibialis posterior, and peroneus longus muscles.[150] Pain is experienced under effort extending to the lateral proximal region of the leg and sometimes even posteriorly. The differential diagnosis includes entrapment of the peroneal nerve, compartment syndrome, and insertional tendinopathy of femoral biceps. Radiographs may show a periosteal callus on the side of the peroneal neck and scintigraphy is positive. Conservative treatment is sufficient and recovery usually occurs in about 6 weeks.

Talus

Stress fracture of the talus is rare and usually occurs in runners, both novice and expert.[151] It is assumed that the injury is the result of a fulcrum effect which occurs at the neck of the talus when, at heel strike, the subtalar joint is strained in valgus with resulting plantar flexion and internal rotation of the talus head. It is often

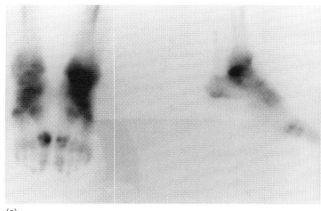

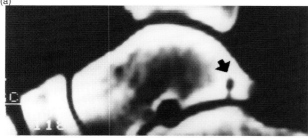

Fig. 8 Stress fracture of the talus in a 22-year-old triple jumper. Radiographs were negative. The bone scan revealed a hot spot at the anke (a), but only a CT scan in sagittal reconstruction (b) showed the exact location of the injury (arrow).

associated with a pronated foot. The athlete suffers from pain in the dorsal aspect of the foot which increases on running. There may be an antalgic limp, pain, and oedema at the site of the injury.

Radiographs show a callus, or a crack in the cortex, at the neck of the talus, parallel to the talonavicular joint, but this is not generally observed until 2 to 3 weeks after the onset of symptoms. This fracture can occur at the posterior apophysis (Fig. 8).

Healing is promoted by immobilization with a weight-bearing cast. Recurrence can be avoided by applying an orthosis inside the footwear. In some cases with positive scintigraphy and negative radiography, CT reveals areas of cancellous bone reabsorption which have been described in the knee as 'occult fracture' (Fig. 9).[152]

Calcaneus

Stress fracture of the calcaneus is characteristically reported in military recruits. It is produced by rigid footwear and by the particular style of the parade march, particularly in subjects in poor physical condition.[153,154] Sometimes it is bilateral. It is rarer in athletes and is manifested as heel pain. After an insidious onset, the pain rapidly becomes so severe that it causes limping or compels the patient to use crutches. The pain spreads to the back of the foot and increases under finger pressure on the medial and lateral facets in an area halfway between the malleolus and the posterior tuberosity of the heel. The 'heel squeeze test' is positive.[155,156]

Differential diagnosis must include pathology of the subtalar joint, plantar fasciitis (in this case pain is more severe on the plantar and medial facet of the heel), entrapment of the plantar nerve, retrocalcaneal bursitis (which has a characteristic scintigram),[157] and Achilles tendinitis. The bone scan is positive at an early stage, and radiographs (axial, lateral, and dorsoplantar) taken 7 to 30 days from

the onset of symptoms may show an endosteal callus perpendicular to the longitudinal axis of the heel between the posterior facet of the subtalar joint and the tuberosity of the heel.[158]

Symptoms generally regress in 3 to 4 weeks with temporary suspension of sport activity and the use of a heel pad and an absorption insole to protect the site of the fracture from excessive shocks during walking. Provided that the athlete is asymptomatic, he or she is usually able to return to sport within 6 to 8 weeks.

Tarsal navicular

Stress fractures of the tarsal navicular are typically reported in athletes practising activities requiring an explosive force in which sprints and jumps are the main athletic movements (basketball, volleyball, triple jump, high jump, long jump, sprinting, hurdling, middle-distance running, ballet, American football, soccer, and figure-skating), but also in long-distance runners, particularly if they use the forefoot in the footstrike.[156,159-163]

Early recognition of the fracture is important because of the severe complications characterizing its development. However, diagnosis is frequently delayed (on average 7.2 months from the onset of symptoms) because of the initially vague symptoms and the frequent lack of fracture signs in routine radiographs.[164] It is a vertical fracture which occurs on the sagittal plane in the middle third of the navicular, at relatively low vascularity, starting on the dorsal surface. Sometimes the foot shows biomechanical alterations that change the normal distribution of loads and/or concentrate them on the navicular (short first metatarsus and/or long second metatarsus, adducted metatarsus, reduced dorsiflexion of the ankle, and/or limited subtalar motion).[164] The shape of the plantar arch does not appear to be a determinant, but an excessive inclination of the foot in the support phase overloads the talonavicular joint.[165] This is also true in the equinus positions of the foot (figure-skating).[137]

Symptoms occur insidiously without acute trauma. There is vague soreness or cramping in the medial dorsal region of the mid-

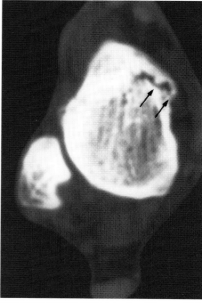

Fig. 9 Intraosseous occult fracture of the talus in a 27-year-old discus thrower. CT shows an area of bone reabsorption with integrity of the cortex.

foot or in the area of the internal side of the longitudinal arch that becomes worse on physical activity and is alleviated by rest, and reappears as soon as sport is taken up again. In the advanced stages training becomes difficult and sometimes even walking is uncomfortable.

Deep palpation of the dorsal aspect of the foot and/or the longitudinal medal arch is painful, but the greatest pain is felt in the area above the navicular; oedema is sometimes present and walking on the toes is uneasy and painful, particularly when resting on the injured foot. Examination of the range of motion often shows reduced dorsiflexion of the ankle and/or lack of mobility in the sub-talar joint.

If a fracture of the navicular is suspected, weight-bearing anteroposterior, lateral, and oblique radiographs must be obtained, possibly augmented with a coned-down anteroposterior projection, and, if necessary, with tomograms. However, navicular fractures frequently do not show up in routine views because the partial fracture deepens for about 5 mm in the dorsal surface of the bone and, even with projections centred on the navicular, it is not clearly seen.

When routine radiographs suggest a fracture of the navicular, they show mechanical alterations often associated with this injury. The anteroposterior view may show a short first metatarsal, abducted metatarsus, fracture of the last four metatarsals, sclerosis of the proximal articular navicular surface, or narrowing of the medial side of the interarticular talnavicular space. The lateral view may show plantar slippage of cuneiform and metatarsals with respect to the talus and the navicular, with consequent malalignment of the dorsal surfaces of the talonavicular and cuneiform–navicular joints. Further findings are talar beaks and accessory ossicles.[166] The bone scan of both feet (frontal, medial, and/or lateral plantar projections) shows increased uptake in the navicular at the site of the injury.

Pavlov's tomographic technique[166] is used for radiographic visualization of stress fractures of the navicular. This technique places the bone in its own true anatomical anteroposterior position. To do this, the forefoot is kept raised and the whole foot is slightly supinated until, under fluoroscopic control, the navicular is no longer completely visible in the medial-lateral direction (at this point the X-ray beam is tangent to the talonavicular joint). The injury then appears linear and sagittal at the middle third of the bone. If the fracture is partial, it is limited to the first 5 mm of the dorsal surface and the proximal articular facet is involved; extension to the distal articular facet is less frequent and a transverse fracture is the least common injury. A deeper tomographic view allows us to establish whether the fracture is limited to the dorsal surface of the navicular or whether it extends through the bone and also involves the plantar surface (complete fracture). CT may also be useful for diagnostic purposes (Fig. 2).

Because of late diagnosis and the relative avascularity of the central third of the navicular, this fracture may develop into a complete fracture which is sometimes displaced (particularly if the athlete continues to train regardless of pain) or complicated by delayed union, non-union, or refracture.[167]

According to Torg et al.[168] and to Khan et al.,[169] treatment should be differentiated as follows.

1. Non-complicated partial fracture and undisplaced complete fracture: non-weight-bearing plaster for 6 to 8 weeks, allowing subsequent weight bearing and a gradual return to sport only if the patient remains asymptomatic and there is radiographic demonstration of union of the fracture. Once the cast is removed, rehabilitation starts with restoration of the motion of the ankle and the application of orthotic devices to footwear for the gradual introduction of weight bearing.

2. Displaced complete fracture: treatment as above or, alternatively, surgical reduction and fixation followed by non-weight-bearing immobilization in plaster for 6 weeks.

3. Fracture complicated by delayed union or non-union: curettage and inlaid bone grafting with internal fixation of unstable fragments (without attempting reduction because in general there is already a fibrous union). Any sclerotic fragments found must not be removed but must be fixed. After the operation, a non-weight-bearing cast must be applied for 6 to 8 weeks. Recovery is monitored by radiographs (sometimes 3 to 6 months are necessary).

4. Partial fracture complicated by a small transverse dorsal fracture: the dorsal fragment may have to be removed.

5. Complete fracture complicated by a widespread transverse dorsal fracture: recovery takes place by immobilization.

Dorsal talar beaks must be removed during surgery.

Metatarsals

Stress fractures of the metatarsal bones were first described in military recruits and were caused by marching. They have been reported in long-distance runners and ballet dancers in particular.[156,170,171] They usually involve the second and third metatarsals. Because of its larger diameter and relatively short length, the first metatarsal is more resistant to bending stress, while the second and third metatarsals are weaker and their heads experience the greatest strain in the propulsive stage of running. Moreover, shearing forces are concentrated at the second metatarsal level.[172] In younger athletes stress fractures are most frequently found in the second metatarsal because of the greater mobility of the first metatarsal associated with excessive inclination of the foot.

The patient feels pain in the dorsal surface of the forefoot which increases with physical activity and is alleviated by rest. Tenderness is felt on palpation of the area of the fractured metatarsal and on passive dorsiflexion of the toe. Swelling is often present and in more advanced cases callus is palpable. Radiographs are positive 10 to 14 days after the onset of symptoms if the first metatarsal is involved but are delayed further for the others.

Fracture of the first metatarsal usually occurs in the proximal metaphysis, and this is seen radiographically as a linear band of sclerosis perpendicular to the direction of application of the load. Fractures of the other metatarsal bones are generally located at the diaphysis or the neck and appear as breaks in the cortex progressively surrounded by a periosteal reaction which reaches its peak with the formation of the callus (Fig. 10).[173] Scintigraphy is useful in preradiographic cases and confirms those in which there is some doubt.

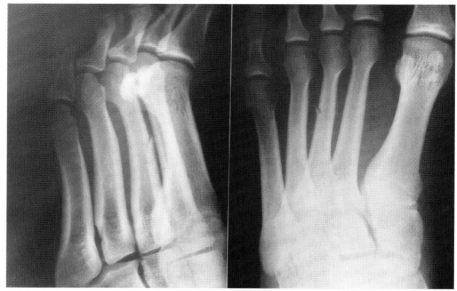

Fig. 10 Stress fracture of the third metatarsal in a long-distance runner. When radiographs show lateral and medial breaks in the cortex, as in this case, it may be necessary to apply a well-moulded weight-bearing cast for 4 to 6 weeks to facilitate the healing process.

Treatment is conservative, involving temporary abstinence from all activities which cause pain. It may be useful to insert an orthosis inside the shoe to reduce strains on the site of the injury (for instance, a 'dome' metatarsal pad applied just proximally to the head of the metatarsal). Rigid shoes are suggested, and swimming and cycling are allowed. Recovery takes place in 4 to 6 weeks. If pain persists it is necessary to apply a well-moulded weight-bearing cast for 4 to 6 weeks.

Female ballet dancers are predisposed to stress fracture of the proximal part of the base of the second metatarsal, involving the medial and volar surface of the second metatarsal–tarsal joint (Lisfranc's joint), which is the most rigid of the five.[174,175] At this level, the three cuneiform bones provide an osseous niche to receive the base of the second metatarsal, which articulates proximally at the bottom of the niche with the second cuneiform, more posteriorly with respect to the other two, and medially and laterally with respect to the first and third cuneiform bones that form the wall of this pocket. Therefore the second metatarsal, anchored to the base, is less mobile; this explains why it tends to fracture just distally, at the base of the second metatarsal bone, when subjected to prolonged and repeated strain.

Factors predisposing to this stress fracture are Greek foot with a short first metatarsal, cavus foot, amenorrhoea, eating disorders (anorexia), and plantar dislocation of the metatarsals due to anterior impingement of the ankle. This fracture must be considered in a female ballet dancer who feels pain on the dorsal aspect of the foot, with an insidious onset which increases on jumping and taking up the *en pointe* position, when the foot is maximally plantar flexed and weight bearing is on the plantar face and on the tip of the distal phalanx of the first two toes.

Tenderness is most obvious on the dorsal aspect of the foot at the first intermetatarsal space around and/or near the proximal part of the second metatarsal. Radiographs (anteroposterior, lateral, and two oblique views, augmented by a dorsoplantar tomogram or magnification) typically show an oblique fracture of the proximal part of

the base of the second metatarsal. If the radiographs are negative and clinical suspicion remains, scintigraphy may reveal a hot spot at the site of the injury.

If an early diagnosis is made, immobilization for 6 to 8 weeks in a non-weight-bearing cast is sufficient. If the patient is asymptomatic and radiographs show recovery, he or she must undertake a programme of rehabilitation consisting of range of motion and flexibility exercises, strengthening of the ankle (initially without weight bearing), swimming, and long-distance walking, which is gradually increased with partial weight bearing. When symptoms continue for many months and the fracture develops into non-union, it is necessary to resort to surgical excision of the necrotic fragment or bone grafting.

Fatigue fractures of the proximal portion of the fifth metatarsal within 1.5 cm distal of the tuberosity where the peroneus brevis muscle is inserted (Jones' fracture) are found in basketball, American football, soccer, and baseball players, and in long-distance runners. The site of the fracture corresponds to the area distally located at the point at which the fifth metatarsal is joined to the fourth metatarsal and the cuboid bone. It is often associated with varus forefoot so that when the foot hits the ground, distraction forces which may eventually produce a stress fracture of the more lateral metatarsal are concentrated on its external part along the base of the fifth metatarsal.[168,176]

Clinically, the athlete feels a vague pain over the fifth metatarsal area or lateral forefoot–midfoot area which increases in intensity insidiously or suddenly, sometimes after an acute trauma, and which may inhibit sporting activity. There is tenderness over the proximal third of the fifth metatarsal. In the initial stage of the injury radiographs (anteroposterior, lateral, and oblique views, augmented by tomograms and magnification) may be negative, and thus it is necessary to use scintigraphy which shows a hot spot at the site of the injury. Complications associated with this fracture are delayed union, non-union, and refracture, probably because of sclerotic obliteration of the medullary channel.[177]

Torg *et al.*[177] have outlined the principles of the basic treatment and the clinical and radiographic classification of this injury.

Acute fracture

There is no previous fracture, although the subject may have had mild symptoms of pain and/or discomfort; there may be an absence of intramedullar sclerosis, a narrow line of fracture with clear margins, and a minimum cortex hypertrophy or slight periosteal reaction. The injury begins in the lateral cortex and develops into a complete fracture, or it may be a fracture which has taken place in an area already abnormally strained. Treatment requires immobilization in a non-weight-bearing case for 6 to 8 weeks.[178] Sometimes clinical recovery may require 20 weeks. If the fracture is displaced, it must be reduced and fixed with a screw.

Delayed union

In delayed union there is pre-existing trauma and/or fracture, a wide transcortical line of fracture with areas of bone reabsorption, a periosteal reaction with cortical hypertrophy, and a moderate degree of intramedullar sclerosis. Conservative treatment may be efficacious but takes rather a long time (an average of 22 weeks), and is generally not acceptable to highly motivated athletes. Therefore surgical treatment is necessary, which consists either of curettage of the sclerotic medullary channel to re-establish its permeability, followed by an inlay tibial bone graft and then immobilization in a non-weight-bearing cast for 6 weeks,[177] or else percutaneous fixation with an intramedullary screw, followed by immobilization with a non-weight-bearing or slipper cast for 2 weeks and then gradual weight bearing with shoes such as tennis shoes with semi-rigid steel soles.[38]

The technique involving osteosynthesis with a screw allows return to sport in about 7 to 14 weeks. It is sometimes necessary to wear shoes with an orthotic device protecting the lateral margin of the foot at the level of the base of the fifth metatarsal to reduce pressure on the head of the screw. Complications due to this technique are fracture of the screw or its dislocation outside the medullary channel, or a screw which is too long.

Non-union

This is characterized by recurrent traumas and symptoms, a large fracture line, a periosteal reaction with cortical hypertrophy, bone reabsorption, and, in particular, complete sclerotic obliteration of the medullary channel. Treatment is exclusively surgical by means of one of the techniques described above. Sport may be taken up again when the patient is asymptomatic and radiographs show a solid union of the fracture and recanalization of the medullary channel without sclerosis.

Great toe

Stress fracture of the proximal phalanx has been described in athletes (fencers, sprinters, and football players) with the hallux valgus deformity.[179] It is probably an avulsion fracture at the level of the insertion area of the collateral ligament caused by the numerous stresses on the great toe from the tendons of the adductor muscles. The effect is mainly evident during positions (tiptoe) or exercises (sprint on place) that exacerbate pain more than any others. In other cases, stress fractures of the proximal phalanx have been ascribed to the numerous stresses present during dorsal hyperflexion and rota-

tion of the great toe in the propulsive and 'toe-off' phase of running, which are more intense on the medial side of the toe.[180,181]

There may be tenderness and swelling at the level of the dorsomedial aspect of the interphalangeal joint, which manifests as a reduced range of motion. Plain radiographs, which may be negative during the first 2 weeks, typically show an oblique dorsomedial fracture, with more or less sclerotic borders, near the interphalangeal joint or extended to its proximal articular surface. It is sometimes visualized as an intra-articular loose body. When radiographs are negative or ambiguous, a bone scan is useful.

It is sufficient to suspend sports activities temporarily, to tape the great toe, or to use shoes with rigid soles. In the case of osteochondral fractures it may be necessary to remove the sclerotic loose body. When the hallux valgus deformity resists conservative treatment, corrective osteotomy of the first metatarsal is indicated.

Great toe sesamoids

Stress fractures of the great toe sesamoid have been reported in runners (spring and long-distance), dancers, basketball players, tennis players, and figure-skaters.[156,174,182,183] They are more frequent in the medial sesamoid, probably because it is located immediately under the head of the first metatarsal. These are traction-type fractures which are due to high repetitive tensile forces at the level of the plantar surface of the first metatarsophalangeal joint, which is often forced into dorsiflexion during body elevation in the propulsive phase of the gait preceding toe-off from the ground. This pathology can occur when the first metatarsal is malaligned.

The onset is insidious, manifesting as medial plantar pain at the level of the first metatarsophalangeal joint which is exacerbated by activity and relieved with rest. The plantar surface of this joint can appear oedematous and painful; there is often a painful limitation of active and passive dorsiflexion which is attributed to synovitis of the first metatarsophalangeal joint.

Differential diagnosis includes sesamoiditis, hallucis tendinitis, metatarsalgia, isolated synovitis or arthrosis of the first metatarsophalangeal joint (in this case radiographs show intra-articular space reduction and bone spurs), sesamoid osteochondritis (more frequent in lateral ossiculum), acute fracture or non-union, and entrapment neuropathies (with a positive Tinel sign).[184] Intra-articular injection with anaesthetic helps to differentiate the extra-articular pathology.

Radiographs are obtained in anteroposterior, lateral, oblique, and axial views with a dorsiflexed great toe, but it is difficult to distinguish a stress fracture from a bipartite sesamoid. Bone scans are useful because the bipartite sesamoid is 'cold'.

If this fracture is untreated, it can evolve into delayed union or non-union. Athletic rest and foam-padding orthosis are indicated. In the case of severe pain a walking cast may be useful. If symptoms persist, surgical excision of the sesamoid may be indicated, whereas bone grafting is better in non-union.

References

1. McBryde AM. Stress fractures in athletes. *American Journal of Sports Medicine* 1975; **3**: 212–17.
2. Devas MB. *Stress fractures.* Edinburgh: Churchill Livingstone, 1975.
3. McBryde AM. Stress fractures in runners. *Clinics in Sports Medicine* 1985; **4**: 737–52.

4. Goergen TG, Venn-Watson EA, Rossman DJ, Resnick D, Gerber K. Tarsal navicular stress fractures in runners. *American Journal of Roentgenology* 1981; **136**: 201–3.

5. Briethaupt MDS. Zur Pathologie des menschlichen Fusses. *Medizinische Zeitung* 1855; **24**: 169–71, 175–7.

6. Stechow AW. Fussödom und Röntgenstrahlen. *Deutsch Militaerische Aerztliche Zeitung* 1897; **26**: 465.

7. Hulkko A, Orava S. Stress fractures in athletes. *International Journal of Sports Medicine* 1987; **8**: 221–6.

8. Hulkko A, Orava S, Nikula P. Stress fractures of the olecranon in javelin throwers. *International Journal of Sports Medicine* 1986; **7**: 210–13.

9. Burr DB, Milgrom C, Boyd RD, Higgins WL, Robin G, Radin EL. Experimental stress fractures of the tibia. Biological and mechanical aetiology in rabbits. *Journal of Bone and Joint Surgery* 1990; **72B**: 370–5.

10. Johnson LC, Stradford HT, Geis RW, Dineen JR, Kerley E. Histiogenesis of stress fractures. *Journal of Bone and Joint Surgery* 1963; **45A**: 1542.

11. Li G, Zhang S, Chen G, Chen H, Wang A. Radiographic and histologic analyses of stress fracture in rabbit tibias. *American Journal of Sports Medicine* 1985; **13**: 285–94.

12. Jones BH, Harris JM, Vinh TN, Rubin C. Exercise-induced stress fractures and stress reactions of bone: epidemiology, etiology and classification. In: Pandolf KB, ed. *Exercise and Sport Sciences Reviews. American College of Sports Medicine Series*, vol. 17. Baltimore: Williams and Wilkins, 1989: 379–422.

13. Stanitski CL, McMaster JH, Scranton PE. On the nature of stress fractures. *American Journal of Sports Medicine* 1978; **6**: 391–6.

14. Baker J, Frankel VH, Burstein A. Fatigue fractures: biomechanical considerations. *Journal of Bone and Joint Surgery* 1972; **54A**: 1345–6.

15. Blickenstaff LD, Morris JM. Fatigue fracture of the femoral neck. *Journal of Bone and Joint Surgery* 1966; **48A**: 1031–47.

16. Clement DB. Tibial stress syndrome in athletes. *American Journal of Sports Medicine* 1974; **2**: 81–5.

17. Frankel VH. Editorial comment. *American Journal of Sports Medicine* 1978; **6**: 396.

18. Matheson GO, Clement DB, McKenzie DC, Taunton JE, Lloyd-Smith DR, MacIntyre JG. Stress fractures in athletes. A study of 320 cases. *American Journal of Sports Medicine* 1987; **15**: 46–58.

19. Singer A, Ben-Yehuda O, Ben-Ezra Z, Zaltzman S. Multiple identical stress fractures in monozygotic twins. Case report. *Journal of Bone and Joint Surgery* 1990; **72A**: 444–5.

20. Brudvig TJS, Gudger RD, Obermeyer L. Stress fractures in 195 trainees: a one-year study of incidence as related to age, sex and race. *Military Medicine* 1983; **148**: 666–7.

21. Trutter M, Broman GE, Peterson RR. Densities of white and negro skeletons. *Journal of Bone and Joint Surgery* 1960; **42A**: 50–8.

22. Lysens RJ, Ostyn MS, Auweele YV, Lefevre J, Vuylsteke M, Renson L. The accident-prone and overuse-prone profiles of the young athlete. *American Journal of Sports Medicine* 1989; **17**: 612–19.

23. Taimela S, Kujala UM, Osterman K. Stress injury proneness: a prospective study during a physical training program. *International Journal of Sports Medicine* 1990; **11**: 162–5.

24. Giladi M, Milgrom C, Simkin A, Danon Y. Stress fractures. Identifiable risk factors. *American Journal of Sports Medicine* 1991; **19**: 647–52.

25. Protzman RR. Physiologic performance of women compared to men: observations of cadets at the United States Military Academy. *American Journal of Sports Medicine* 1979; **7**: 191–4.

26. Reinker KA, Ozburne S. A comparison of male and female orthopaedic pathology in basic training. *Military Medicine* 1979; **144**: 532–6.

27. Cook SD, Harding AF, Thomas KA, Morgtan EL, Schnurpfeil KM, Haddad RJ. Trabecular bone density and menstrual function in women runners. *American Journal of Sports Medicine* 1987; **15**: 503–7.

28. Drinkwater BL, Nilson K, Chesnut CH III, Bremner WJ, Shainholtz S, Southworth MB. Bone mineral content of amenorrheic and eumenorrheic athletes. *New England Journal of Medicine* 1984; **311**: 277–81.

29. Highet R. Athletic amenorrhoea. An update on aetiology, complications and management. *Sports Medicine* 1989; **7**: 82–108.

30. Markey KL. Stress fractures. *Clinics in Sports Medicine* 1987; **6**: 405–25.

31. Warren MP, Brooks-Gunn J, Hamilton LH, Warren LF, Hamilton WG. Scoliosis and fractures in young ballet dancers: relation to delayed menarche and secondary amenorrhea. *New England Journal of Medicine* 1986; **316**: 1348–53.

32. Bennell KL *et al.* Risk factors for stress fractures in female track-and-field athletes: a retrospective analysis. *Clinical Journal of Sport Medicine* 1995; **5**: 229–35.

33. Barrow GW, Saha S. Menstrual irregularity and stress fractures in collegiate female distance runners. *American Journal of Sports Medicine* 1988; **16**: 209–16.

34. Evans FG, Riolo ML. Relations between the fatigue life and histology of adult human cortical bone. *Journal of Bone and Joint Surgery* 1970; **52A**: 1579–86.

35. Worthen BM, Yanklowitz BAD. The pathophysiology and treatment of stress fractures in military personnel. *Journal of the American Podiatric Association* 1978; **68**: 317–25.

36. Hershman EB, Mailly T. Stress fractures. *Clinics in Sports Medicine* 1990; **9**: 183–241.

37. Belkin SC. Stress fractures in athletes. *Orthopedic Clinics of North America* 1980; **11**: 735–42.

38. De Moya RG. A biomedical comparison of the running shoe and the combat boot. *Military Medicine* 1983; **148**: 666–7.

39. James SL, Bates BR, Osternig LR. Injuries to runners. *American Journal of Sports Medicine* 1978; **6**: 40–50.

40. Johnson AW, Weiss CB Jr, Wheeler DL. Stress fractures of the femoral shaft in athletes—more common than expected. A new clinical test. *American Journal of Sports Medicine* 1994; **22**: 248–56.

41. Wilcox JR, Moniot AL, Green JP. Bone scanning in the evaluation of exercise-related stress injuries. *Radiology* 1977; **123**: 699–703.

42. Keats TD. *Radiology of muscoloskeletal stress injury.* Chicago: Year Book, 1990.

43. Pavlov H, Torg JS. *The running athlete: roentgenographs and remedies.* Chicago: Year Book, 1987.

44. Matin P. The appearance of bone scans following fractures, including immediate and long-term studies. *Journal of Nuclear Medicine* 1979; **20**: 1227–31.

45. Martire JR. The role of nuclear medicine bone scan in evaluating pain in athletic injuries. *Clinics in Sports Medicine* 1987; **6**: 13–37.

46. Milgrom C. *et al.* Multiple stress fractures: a longitudinal study of a soldier with 13 lesions. *Clinical Orthopaedics and Related Research* 1985; **192**: 174–9.

47. Zwas ST, Elkanovitch R, Frank G. Interpretation and classification of bone scintigraphic findings in stress fractures. *Journal of Nuclear Medicine* 1987; **28**: 452–7.

48. Roub LW, Gumermann LW, Hanley EN Jr, Clark MW, Goodman M, Herbert DL. Bone stress: a radionuclide imaging perspective. *Radiology* 1979; **132**: 431–8.

49. Milgrome C *et al.* Negative bone scan in impeding tibial stress fractures. A report of three cases. *American Journal of Sports Medicine* 1984; **12**: 488–91.

50. Keene JS, Lash EG. Negative bone scan in a femoral neck stress fracture. A case report. *American Journal of Sports Medicine* 1992; **20**: 234–7.

51. Lee JK, Yao L. Stress fractures: MR imaging. *Radiology* 1988; **169**: 217–20.

52. Mink JH, Deutsch AL. Occult cartilage and bone injuries of the knee: detection, classification and assessment with MR imaging. *Radiology* 1989; **170**: 823–9.

53. Stafford SA, Rosenthal DI, Gebhardt MC, Brady TJ, Scott JA. MRI in stress fracture. *American Journal of Roentgenology* 1986; **147**: 553–6.

54. Fredericson M, Bergman AG, Hoffman KL, Dillingham MS. Tibial stress reaction in runners. Correlation of clinical symptoms and scintigrafy with a new magnetic resonance imaging grading system. *American Journal of Sports Medicine* 1995; **23**: 472–81.

55. Boyer DW Jr. Trapshooter's shoulder: stress fractures of the coracoid process. Case report. *Journal of Bone and Joint Surgery* 1975; **57A**: 562.

56. Sandrock AR. Another sports fatigue fracture: stress fracture of the coracoid process of the scapula. *Radiology* 1975; **117**: 274.

57. Waard WG, Bergfeld JA, Carson WG. Stress fractures of the base of the acromial process. *American Journal of Sports Medicine* 1994; **22**: 146–7.

58. Allen ME. Stress fracture of the humerus. A case study. *American Journal of Sports Medicine* 1984; **12**: 244–5.

59. Rettig AC, Beltz HF. Stress fracture in the humerus in an adolescent tennis tournament player. *American Journal of Sports Medicine* 1985; **13**: 55–8.

60. De Haven HE, Evarts CM. Throwing injuries of the elbow in athletes. *Orthopedic Clinics of North America* 1973; **4**: 801–3.

61. Miller JE. Javelin thrower's elbow. *Journal of Bone and Joint Surgery* 1960; **42B**: 788–92.

62. Torg JS, Moyer RA. Non-union of a stress fracture through the olecranon epiphyseal plate observed in an adolescent baseball pitcher. A case report. *Journal of Bone and Joint Surgery* 1977; **59A**: 264–5.

63. Wilkerson RD, Johns JC. Nonunion of an olecranon stress fracture in an adolescent gymnast. A case report. *American Journal of Sports Medicine* 1990; **18**: 432–4.

64. Hamilton KH. Stress fracture of the diaphysis of the ulna in a body builder. *American Journal of Sports Medicine* 1984; **12**: 405–6.

65. Iwaya T, Takatori I. Lateral longitudinal stress fractures of the patella. Report of three cases. *Journal of Pediatric Orthopedics* 1985; **5**: 73–5.

66. Mutoh Y, Mori T, Suzuki Y, Sugiura Y. Stress fractures of the ulna in athletes. *American Journal of Sports Medicine* 1982; **10**: 365–7.

67. Orava S. Stress fractures. *British Journal of Sports Medicine* 1980; **14**: 40–4.

68. Rettig AC. Stress fracture of the ulna in an adolescent tournament tennis player. *American Journal of Sports Medicine* 1983; **11**: 103–6.

69. Bollen SR, Robinson DG, Chricton KJ, Cross MJ. Stress fractures of the ulna in tennis players using a double-handed backhand stroke. *American Journal of Sports Medicine* 1993; **21**: 751–2.

70. Loosli AR, Leslie M. Stress fractures of the distal radius. A case report. *American Journal of Sports Medicine* 1991; **19**: 523–4.

71. Hanks GA, Kalenak A, Bowman L, Sebastianelli WJ. Stress fractures of the carpal scaphoid: a report of four cases. *Journal of Bone and Joint Surgery* 1989; **71A**: 938–41.

72. Manzione M, Pizzutillo PD. Stress fracture of the scaphoid waist. A case report. *American Journal of Sports Medicine* 1981; **9**: 268–9.

73. Recht MP, Burk L Jr, Dalinka MK. Radiology of wrist and hand injuries in athletes. *Clinics in Sports Medicine* 1987; **71A**: 938–41.

74. Tehranzadeh J, Davenport J, Pais MJ. Schaphoid fracture: evaluation with flexion–extension tomography. *Radiology* 1990; **176**: 167–70.

75. Biondetti PR, Vannier MW, Gilula LA, Knapp P. Wrist coronal and transaxial CT scanning. *Radiology* 1987; **163**: 148–51.

76. Murakami Y. Stress fracture of the metacarpal in an adolescent tennis player. *American Journal of Sports Medicine* 1988; **16**: 419–20.

77. Waninger KN, Lombardo JA. Stress fracture of index metacarpal in an adolescent tennis player. *Clinical Journal of Sport Medicine* 1995; **5**: 63–6.

78. Keating TM. Stress fracture of the sternum in a wrestler. *American Journal of Sports Medicine* 1987; **15**: 92–3.

79. Barrett GR, Shelton WR, Miles JW. First rib fractures in football players. A case report and literature review. *American Journal of Sports Medicine* 1988; **16**: 674–6.

80. Lankenner PA Jr, Micheli LJ. Stress fracture of the first rib. A case report. *Journal of Bone and Joint Surgery* 1985; **67A**: 159–60.

81. Holden DL, Jackson DW. Stress fractures of the ribs in female rowers. *American Journal of Sports Medicine* 1985; **13**: 342–8.

82. Lord MJ, Ha KI, Song KS. Stress fractures of the ribs in golfers. *American Journal of Sports Medicine* 1996; **24**: 118–22.

83. Taimela S, Kujala UM, Orava S. Two consecutive rib stress fractures in a female competitive swimmer. *Clinical Journal of Sport Medicine* 1995; **5**: 254–7.

84. McKenzie DC. Stress fracture of the rib in an elite oarsman. *International Journal of Sports Medicine* 1989; **10**: 220–2.

85. Abel MA. Jogger's fractures and other stress fractures on the lumber sacral spine. *Skeletal Radiology* 1985; **13**: 221–7.

86. Ireland ML, Micheli LJ. Bilateral stress fracture of the lumbar pedicles in a ballet dancer. A case report. *Journal of Bone and Joint Surgery* 1987; **69A**: 140–2.

87. Omar MM, Levinsohn EM. An unusual fracture of the vertebral articular process in a skier. *Journal of Trauma* 1979; **19**: 212–13.

88. Lamy C, Bazergui A, Kraus H, Farfan JE. The strength of the neural arch and etiology of spondylolysis. *Orthopedic Clinics of North America* 1975; **6**: 215–31.

89. Wiltse LL, Newman PH, MacNab I. Classification of spondylolysis and spondylolisthesis. *Clinical Orthopaedics and Related Research* 1976; **117**: 23–9.

90. McCarroll JR, Miller JM, Ritter MA. Lumbar spondylolysis and spondyloisthesis in college football players. A prospective study. *American Journal of Sports Medicine* 1986; **14**: 404–6.

91. Alexander MJL. Biomechanical aspects of lumbar spine in athletes. *Canadian Journal of Applied Sport Sciences* 1985; **10**: 1–10.

92. Jackson DW, Wiltse LL, Cirincione RJ. Spondylolysis in the female gymnast. *Clinical Orthopaedics and Related Research* 1976; **117**: 68–73.

93. Rossi F, Dragoni S. Lisi istmiche lombari e sport. Rilievi radiologici e considerazioni statistiche. *La Radiologia Medica* 1994; **87**: 397–400.

94. Roche MB, Rowe GG. The incidence of separate neural arch and coincident bone variations. *Journal of Bone and Joint Surgery* 1952; **34A**: 491–4.

95. Hensinger RN. Spondylolysis and spondylolisthesis in children and adolescents. *Journal of Bone and Joint Surgery* 1989; **71A**: 1098–1107.

96. Rosenberg NJ, Bargar WL, Friedman B. The incidence of spondylolysis and spondylolisthesis in non ambulatory patients. *Spine* 1981; **6**: 35–8.

97. Walsh WM, Huurman WW, Shelton GL. Overuse injuries of the knee and spine in girl gymnastics. *Orthopedic Clinics of North America* 1985; **16**: 329–50.

98. Eyres KS, Salam A. Unilateral traumatic spondylolysis in tennis players. *Clinical Sports Medicine* 1989; **1**: 211–16.

99. Weiker GG. Evaluation and treatment of common spine and trunk problems. *Clinics in Sports Medicine* 1989; **8**: 399–417.

100. Maldague B, Malghem J. Aspect radio-dynamiques de la spondylolyse lombaire. *Acta Orthopaedica Belgica* 1981; **47**: 441–57.

101. Milbauer D, Patel S. Roentgenographic examination of the spine. In: Nicholas JA, Hershman EB, eds. *The lower extremity and spine in sports medicine.* St Louis: C.V. Mosby, 1986: 1205–7.

102. Wiltse LL, Winter RB. Terminology and measurement of spondylolisthesis. *Journal of Bone and Joint Surgery* 1983; **65A**: 768–72.

103. Ciullo JV, Jackson DW. Pars interarticularis stress reaction, spondylosysis and spondylolisthesis in gymnasts. *Clinics in Sports Medicine* 1985; **4**: 95–110.

104. Hutson ES, Wastie ML. Bone scintigraphy in the assessment of spondylolysis in patients attending a sports injury clinic. *Clinical Radiology* 1988; **39**: 269–72.

105. Wiltse LL, Widell EH Jr, Jackson DW. Fatigue fracture: the basic lesion in isthmic spondylolisthesis. *Journal of Bone and Joint Surgery* 1975; **57S**: 17–22.

106. Saraste H. Long-term clinical and radiological follow-up of spondylolysis and spondylolisthesis. *Journal of Pediatric Orthopedics* 1987; **7**: 631–8.

107. Karpakka J, Takala T, Orava S. The long-term consequences of spondylolysis or spondylolisthesis on athletic activities. *Clinical Sports Medicine* 1989; **1**: 89–93.

108. Schils J, Hauzeur JP. Stress fracture of the sacrum. *American Journal of Sports Medicine* 1992; **20**: 769–70.

109. Pavlov H, Nelson TL, Warren RF, Torg JS, Burstein AH. Stress fractures of the pubic ramus. A report of twelve cases. *Journal of Bone and Joint Surgery* 1982; **64A**: 1020–5.

110. Latshaw RF, Kantner TR, Kalenak A, Baum S, Corcoran JJ Jr. A pelvic stress fracture in a female jogger. *American Journal of Sports Medicine* 1981; **9**: 54–6.

111. Selakovich W, Love L. Stress fractures of the pubic ramus. *Journal of Bone and Joint Surgery* 1954; **36A**: 573–6.

112. Noakes TD, Smith JA, Lindenberg G, Willis CE. Pelvic stress fractures in long distance runners. *American Journal of Sports Medicine* 1985; **13**: 120–3.

113. Oh I, Harris WH. Proximal strain distribution in the loaded femur. An *in vitro* comparison of the distributions in the intact femur and after insertion of different hip-replacements femoral components. *Journal of Bone and Joint Surgery* 1978; **60A**: 75–85.

114. Hajek MR, Noble HB. Stress fractures of the femoral neck in joggers: case reports and review of the literature. *American Journal of Sports Medicine* 1982; **10**: 112–16.

115. Lombardo SJ, Benson DW. Stress fractures of the femur in runners. *American Journal of Sports Medicine* 1982; **10**: 219–27.

116. Devas MB. Stress fractures of the femoral neck. *Journal of Bone and Joint Surgery* 1965; **47B**: 728–38.

117. Fullerton LR, Snowdy HA. Femoral neck stress fractures. *American Journal of Sports Medicine* 1988; **16**: 365–77.

118. Kaltsas D. Stress fractures of the femoral neck in young adults. *Journal of Bone and Joint Surgery* 1981; **63B**: 33–7.

119. Johansson C, Ekenman I, Tornkvist H, Eriksson E. Stress fractures of the femoral neck in athletes: the consequence of a delay in diagnosis. *American Journal of Sports Medicine* 1990; **18**: 524–8.

120. Aro H, Dahlstrom HA. Conservative management of distraction-type stress fractures of the femoral neck. *Journal of Bone and Joint Surgery* 1986; **66B**: 65–7.

121. Hershman EB, Lombardo J, Bergfeld JA. Femoral shaft stress fractures in athletes. *Clinics in Sports Medicine* 1990; **9**: 111–19.

122. Sullivan D, Warren RF, Pavlov H, Kelman G. Stress fractures in 51 runners. *Clinical Orthopaedics and Related Research* 1984; **187**: 188–92.

123. Butler JE, Brown SL, McConnell BG. Subtrochanteric stress fractures in runners. *American Journal of Sports Medicine* 1982; **10**: 228–32.

124. Provost RA, Morris JM. Fatigue fractures of the femoral shaft. *Journal of Bone and Joint Surgery* 1969; **51A**: 487–98.

125. Devas MB. Stress fractures of the patella. *Journal of Bone and Joint Surgery* 1960; **42B**: 71–4.

126. Teitz CC, Harrington RM. Patellar stress fracture. *American Journal of Sports Medicine* 1992; **20**: 761–5.

127. Cahil BR. Stress fracture of the proximal tibial epiphysis. A case report. *American Journal of Sports Medicine* 1977; **5**: 186–7.

128. Engber WD. Stress fractures of the medial tibial plateau. *Journal of Bone and Joint Surgery* 1977; **59A**: 767–9.

129. Giladi M *et al.* Stress fractures and tibial bone width. A risk factor. *Journal of Bone and Joint Surgery* 1987; **69B**: 326–9.

130. Blatz DJ. Bilateral femoral and tibial shaft stress fractures in a runner. *American Journal of Sports Medicine* 1981; **9**: 322–5.

131. Donati RB, Echo BS, Powell CE. Bilateral tibial stress fractures in a six-year-old male. A case report. *American Journal of Sports Medicine* 1990; **18**: 323–5.

132. Daffner RH, Martinez S, Gehweiler JA, Harrelson JM. Stress fractures of the proximal tibia in runners. *Radiology* 1982; **142**: 63–5.

133. Henry JH, Anderson AJ, Claybourn Cothren C. Tibiofibular synostosis in professional basket ball players. *American Journal of Sports Medicine* 1993; **21**: 619–22.

134. Dickson TB Jr, Kichline PD. Functional management of stress fractures in female athletes using a pneumatic leg brace. *American Journal of Sports Medicine* 1987; **15**: 86–9.

135. Blank S. Transverse tibial stress fractures. A special problem. *American Journal of Sports Medicine* 1987; **15**: 97–602.

136. Green NE, Rogers RA, Lipscomb AB. Nonunions of stress fractures of the tibia. *American Journal of Sports Medicine* 1985; **13**: 171–6.

137. Pecina M, Bojanic I, Dubravcic S. Stress fractures in figure skaters. *American Journal of Sports Medicine* 1990; **18**: 277–9.

138. Rettig AC, Shelbourne KD, McCarroll JR, Bisesi M, Watts J. The natural history and treatment of delayed union and non-union stress fractures of the anterior cortex of the tibia. *American Journal of Sports Medicine* 1988; **16**: 250–55.

139. Beals RK, Cook RD. Stress fractures of the anterior tibial diaphysis. *Orthopedics* 1991; **14**: 869–75.

140. Brahms MA, Fumich RM, Ippolita VD. Atypical stress fracture of tibia in a professional athlete. *American Journal of Sports Medicine* 1980; **8**: 131–2.

141. Orava S, Sulkko A. Delayed unions and nonunions of stress fractures in athletes. *American Journal of Sports Medicine* 1988; **16**: 378–82.

142. Rettig AC, Shelbourne KD, Beltz HF, Robertson DW, Arfken P. Radiographic evaluation of foot and ankle injuries in the athlete. *Clinics in Sports Medicine* 1987; **6**: 905–19.

143. Shelbourne KD, Fisher DA, Rettig AC, McCarroll JR. Stress fractures of the medial melleolus. *American Journal of Sports Medicine* 1988; **16**: 60–3.

144. Devas MB, Sweetnam R. Stress fractures of the fibula. A review of 50 cases in athletes. *Journal of Bone and Joint Surgery* 1956; **38B**: 818–29.

145. Ingersoll CF. Ice skater's fracture. *Radiology* 1943; **50**: 469–79.

146. Castillo M, Tehranzadeh J, Morillo G. Atypical healed stress fracture of the fibula masquerading as chronic osteomyelitis. A case report of magnetic resonance distinction. *American Journal of Sports Medicine* 1988; **16**: 185–8.

147. Daffner RH. Stress fractures. Current concepts. *Skeletal Radiology* 1978; **2**: 221–9.

148. Symeonides PP. High stress fractures of the fibula. *Journal of Bone and Joint Surgery* 1980; **62B**: 192–3.

149. Strudwick WJ, Goodman SB. Proximal fibular stress fracture in an aerobic dancer. A case report. *American Journal of Sports Medicine* 1992; **20**: 481–2.

150. Blair WF, Hanley SR. Stress fracture of the proximal fibula. *American Journal of Sports Medicine* 1980; **8**: 212–13.

151. Hontas MJ, Haddad RJ, Schlesinger LC. Conditions of the talus in

the runner. *American Journal of Sports Medicine* 1986; **14**: 586–90.

152. Apple JS, Martinez S, Allen NB, Caldwell DS, Rice JR. Occult fractures of the knee: tomographic evaluation. *Radiology* 1983; **148**: 383–7.

153. Hopson CN, Perry DR. Stress fractures of the calcaneus in women Marine recruits. *Clinical Orthopaedics and Related Research* 1977; **28**: 159–62.

154. Leabhart JW. Stress fractures of the calcaneus. *Journal of Bone and Joint Surgery* 1959; **41A**: 1284–90.

155. Dalby RD. Stress fractures of the os calcis. *Journal of the American Medical Association* 1967; **200**: 131–2.

156. Davis AW, Alexander IJ. Problematic fractures and dislocations in the foot and ankle of athletes. *Clinics in Sports Medicine* 1990; **9**: 163–81.

157. Rupani MD, Molder LE, Espinola DA. Three phases of radionuclide bone imaging in sports medicine. *Radiology* 1985; **156**: 187–96.

158. Pilgaard S. Stress fracture of the os calcis. *Acta Orthopaedica Scandinavica* 1968; **39**: 270–2.

159. Campbell G, Warnekros W. Tarsal stress fracture in a long-distance runner. A case report. *Journal of the American Podiatric Association* 1983; **72**: 532–5.

160. Fitch KD, Blackwell JB, Gilmour WN. Operation for non-union of stress fracture of the tarsal navicular. *Journal of Bone and Joint Surgery* 1989; **71B**: 105–10.

161. Hulkko A, Orava S, Petokallio P, Tultaoura I, Walden M. Stress fracture of the navicular bone: nine cases in athletes. *Acta Orthopaedica Scandinavica* 1988; **56**: 303–5.

162. Towne LC, Blazina ME, Cozen LN. Fatigue fracture of the tarsal navicular. *Journal of Bone and Joint Surgery* 1970; **52A**: 376–8.

163. Orava S, Karpakka J, Hulkko A, Takala T. Stress avulsion fracture of the tarsal navicular. An uncommon sports-related overuse injury. *American Journal of Sports Medicine* 1991; **19**: 392–5.

164. Torg JS *et al.* Stress fractures of the tarsal navicular. A retrospective review of twenty-one cases. *Journal of Bone and Joint Surgery* 1982; **64A**: 700–12.

165. Ting A *et al.* Stress fractures of the tarsal navicular in long-distance runners. *Clinics in Sports Medicine* 1988; **7**: 89–101.

166. Pavlov H, Torg JS, Freiberger RH. Tarsal navicular stress fractures: radiographic evaluation. *Radiology* 1983; **148**: 641–5.

167. Coughlin L, Kwok D, Oliver J. Fracture dislocation of the tarsal navicular. A case report. *American Journal of Sports Medicine* 1987; **15**: 614–15.

168. Torg JS, Pavlov H, Torg E. Overuse injuries in sport: the foot. *Clinics in Sports Medicine* 1987; **6**: 291–320.

169. Khan KM, Fuller PJ, Brukner PD, Kearney C, Burry HC. Outcome of conservative and surgical management of navicular stress fracture in athletes. Eighty-six cases proven with computerized tomography. *American Journal of Sports Medicine* 1992; **20**: 657–66.

170. Drez D Jr, Young JC, Johnston RD, Parker WD. Metatarsal stress fractures. *American Journal of Sports Medicine* 1980; **8**: 123–5.

171. Kadel NJ, Teitz CC, Kronmal RA. Stress fractures in ballet dancers. *American Journal of Sports Medicine* 1992; **20**: 445–9.

172. Gross TS, Bunch RP. A mechanical model of metatarsal stress fracture during distance running. *American Journal of Sports Medicine* 1989; **17**: 669–74.

173. Levy JM. Stress fractures of the first metatarsal. *American Journal of Roentgenology* 1978; **139**: 679–81.

174. Hamilton WG. Foot and ankle injuries in dancers. *Clinics in Sports Medicine* 1988; **7**: 143–73.

175. Micheli LJ, Sohn RS, Soloman R. Stress fractures of the second metatarsal involving Lisfranc's joint in ballet dancers: a new overuse of the foot. *Journal of Bone and Joint Surgery* 1985; **67A**: 1372–5.

176. Santopietro FJ. Foot and foot-related injuries in the young athlete. *Clinics in Sports Medicine* 1988; **7**: 563–89.

177. Torg JS, Balduini FC, Zelko RR, Pavlov H, Peff TC, Das M. Fractures of the base of fifth metatarsal distal to the tuberosity. Classification and guidelines for non-surgical and surgical management. *Journal of Bone and Joint Surgery* 1984; **66A**: 209–14.

178. Zogby RG, Baker BE. A review of non operative treatment of Jones' fracture. *American Journal of Sports Medicine* 1987; **15**: 304–7.

179. Yokoe K, Taketomo M. Stress fracture of the proximal phalanx of the great toe. A report of three cases. *American Journal of Sports Medicine* 1986; **14**: 240–2.

180. Jones P. Fatigue failure osteochondral fracture of the proximal phalanx of the great toe. *American Journal of Sports Medicine* 1987; **156**: 616–18.

181. Orava S, Weitz H, Hulkko A, Karpakka J, Takata T. Intra-articular stress fracture of the proximal phalanx of the great toe in athletes. *Clinical Sports Medicine* 1989; **1**: 105–7.

182. McBryde AM, Anderson RB. Sesamoid foot problems in the athlete. *Clinics in Sports Medicine* 1988; **7**: 51–60.

183. Van Hall ME, Keene JS, Lange TA, Clancy WG Jr. Stress fractures of the great toe sesamoids. *American Journal of Sports Medicine* 1982; **10**: 122–8.

184. Chillag K, Grana WA. Medial sesamoid stress fracture. *Orthopedics* 1985; **8**: 819–21.

5.3 Chronic exertional compartment syndrome

Michael J. Dunbar, William D. Stanish, and Nancy E. Vincent

Introduction

The athlete is susceptible to two forms of compartment syndrome: acute or chronic. The acute form presents as a well-described pattern of signs and symptoms and is most often related to an antecedent history of extremity trauma. Acute compartment syndrome is a true surgical emergency and must be dealt with in a prompt surgical fashion to limit irreversible neuromuscular dysfunction.

Chronic compartment syndrome results from repetitive or exertional activities and subsequently is often referred to as chronic exertional compartment syndrome. The term 'chronic exertional compartment syndrome' will be used in this chapter. With the population becoming increasingly involved in sports and recreational activity, the pathological entity of chronic exertional compartment syndrome is being increasingly recognized. Although the pathophysiology of acute and chronic compartment syndrome is similar, the clinical presentation and functional outcome are vastly different.

Chronic exertional compartment syndrome is most often non-emergent due to its reversible course. Despite its reversible nature, this syndrome is responsible for considerable morbidity and limitation of activity in the athlete. Furthermore, the diagnosis is not easily established and requires an in-depth knowledge of anatomy and physiology coupled with a high degree of clinical suspicion. This is of the utmost importance as undiagnosed chronic exertional compartment syndrome can prevent athletes from achieving their full potential. Unfortunately, athletes limited in their activity because of persistent complaints of debilitating pain despite obvious objective findings, as may well be the case in chronic exertional compartment syndrome, are not uncommonly dismissed as malingerers.

Chronic exertional compartment syndrome is the most common form of compartment syndrome in athletes. This coupled with the difficulty in confirming the diagnosis has prompted the thrust of this chapter to concentrate on chronic exertional compartment syndrome with specific references to acute compartment syndrome for the purpose of illustrating common pathophysiological principles.

This chapter will place particular emphasis on the pathophysiology of chronic exertional compartment syndrome, as it is the belief of the authors that only through an in-depth understanding of the pathophysiology can the subtleties of this disorder be appreciated.

Nomenclature

Unfortunately, a myriad of terms have been applied to chronic exertional compartment syndrome which has led to confusion. The syndrome was first described by Horn[1] and Hughes[2] who used the term 'march gangrene' to describe the condition seen in new army recruits who were forced to endure long marches. Others followed with such terms as anterior tibial stress syndrome, medial tibial stress syndrome, shin splints, marked synovitis, calf hypertension, exercise myopathy, exercise ischaemia, march myositis, ischaemic myositis, and chronic exercise-related compartment syndrome (Table 1). The term chronic exertional compartment syndrome is preferable as it is descriptive with respect to pathophysiology yet generalized with respect to anatomical location.

Definition

A compartment syndrome is a condition in which increased pressure in a limited space compromises the circulation and function of the tissues within that space.[3] More specifically, chronic exertional

Table 1 Synonyms for chronic exertional compartment syndrome commonly found in the literature

Anterior tibial stress syndrome

Medial tibial stress syndrome

Shin splints

Marked synovitis

Calf hypertension

Exercise myopathy

Exercise ischaemia

March myositis

Ischaemic myositis

Chronic exercise-related compartment syndrome

Table 2	Essential features of chronic exertional compartment syndrome

Limiting myofascial compartment

Increased intracompartmental pressure

Decreased tissue perfusion

Abnormal neuromuscular function

compartment syndrome may be defined as an activity-related, reversible, myofascial intracompartmental-pressure increase resulting in decreased tissue perfusion and abnormalities of neuromuscular function. The essence of the pathophysiology of chronic exertional compartment syndrome is contained within the definition. To this end, it is useful to distill the salient points of the definition to use as a conceptual model in understanding the basic pathophysiology. Again, such an understanding is paramount for an adequate appreciation of this syndrome. The essential features of these definitions are listed in Table 2.

Pathophysiology

Myofascial compartment

Overview

Muscle groups within the body are generally arranged into compartments bound by a relatively non-yielding envelope of fascia, usually with an osseous border. This is particularly true of the extremities and axial skeleton. This strong, enveloping fascia limits volume increases within a muscle compartment. Consequently, an increase in volume within a compartment results in an increase in pressure within the same compartment. Why one athlete is symptomatic with chronic exertional compartment syndrome at a given level of activity and another is asymptomatic for the same level of activity is poorly understood. This may relate to anatomical differences in compartmental fascias.

Fascia

The compartmental fascia of patients suffering from chronic exertional compartment syndrome may be abnormal. Turnipseed *et al.* observed an increase in thickness and structural stiffness of compartmental fascia in patients diagnosed with chronic exertional compartment syndrome compared to asymptomatic volunteers.[4] This increase in fascial thickness was noted to be greatest in areas where dense myofascial scarring had occurred, such as in areas of repetitive trauma.

    The importance of fascial thickness and stiffness in the pathophysiology of chronic exertional compartment syndrome lies in their relationship to intracompartmental volume and pressure. According to Turnipseed *et al.*, an increase in intracompartmental volume in the face of thick and stiff fascia results in a linear increase in pressure. Simply put, there appears to be a linear relationship between intracompartmental volume and pressure under these circumstances.

Hernias

Fascial hernias have been found to occur at a significantly higher rate in patients diagnosed with chronic exertional compartment

syndrome.[5] The incidence of fascial defects in patients with this syndrome is reported to be in the range of 20 to 60 per cent.[6–8] This is particularly true of the anterior and lateral tibial compartment, as the superficial peroneal nerve pierces the fascia on the anterolateral aspect of the lower leg at the junction of the middle and distal third of the tibia. This is represented schematically in Fig. 1. Entrapment of the superficial peroneal nerve at this level can result in a well-described syndrome that presents in a similar fashion to chronic exertional compartment syndrome.[9–11] This entrapment neuropathy is frequently misdiagnosed as chronic exertional compartment syndrome. The significance of the increased incidence of anterior tibial compartment fascial hernias in athletes with chronic exertional compartment syndrome of the same compartment is unknown.

Location

Any compartment is susceptible to compartment syndrome, however, certain compartments in the athlete show a predilection toward chronic exertional compartment syndrome, most cases of which occur in the lower leg. This may be a function of the dependent nature of the lower leg during activity. Figure 2 illustrates the cross-sectional anatomy of the lower leg with its four major compartments, as well as the contents of each. The four compartments are the anterior, peroneal (or lateral), deep posterior, and superficial posterior. Some authors propose the existence of a fifth separate compartment in some individuals around the posterior tibial muscle.[21] The predominant site for chronic exertional compartment syndrome in the lower leg is the anterior compartment. This syndrome has also been reported in the deep posterior tibial compartment, the peroneal compartment, superficial posterior tibial compartment, deep posterior tibial muscle compartment, anterior and posterior thigh, forearm, foot, and paraspinal muscles.

Increased intracompartmental pressure

Overview

Normal resting compartment pressure is between 0 and 8 mmHg.[12,13] Exercise results in an increase in muscle volume in the

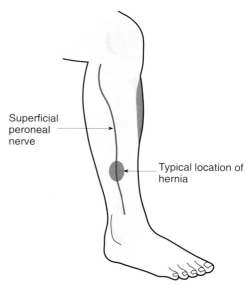

Fig. 1 Anatomical location of fascial hernia associated with the superficial peroneal nerve.

Superficial peroneal nerve

Typical location of hernia

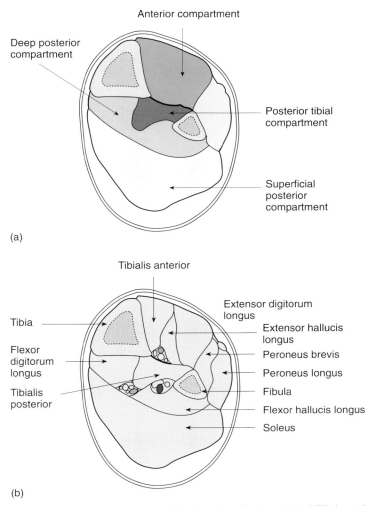

Fig. 2 (a) Cross-sectional anatomy of the four major compartments of the lower leg with the postulated fifth (posterior tibial) compartment. (b) Cross-sectional anatomy of the muscular contents of the compartments of the lower leg.

magnitude of 8 to 20 per cent.[14,15] This increase in volume, in the face of a minimally yielding envelope of fascia, results in increased pressure within the compartment. A correlation between intracompartmental volume and pressure has been established, in the presence of abnormally stiff fascia,[4] as mentioned above. Here, small changes in compartment muscle volume can cause linear increases in pressure.

Muscle relaxation

Exercising skeletal muscle behaves in a similar fashion to cardiac muscle, in that skeletal muscle is perfused during muscle relaxation.[16] Hence, increased intracompartmental pressure elevated sufficiently to interfere with tissue (muscle) perfusion would have the most significant effect during muscle relaxation. The muscle relaxation pressure, therefore, probably plays the key role in the pathophysiology of chronic exertional compartment syndrome. Increased muscle relaxation pressures in the order of 35 to 55 mmHg in patients with chronic exertional compartment syndrome have been correlated to decreased muscle blood flow.[17] The concept of muscle relaxation pressure is particularly important when considering the diagnostic methods for measuring intracompartmental pressure.

Failure to measure this pressure during the appropriate phase of cycle may result in spurious data.

Intracompartmental vessels

Increased intracompartmental pressure translates to increased pressure on intracompartmental vessels. The Law of LaPlace ($T = Pr$) can be used to mathematically describe the pressure equilibrium of vessels where T is the transmural wall tension, P is pressure, and r is the vessel radius. Transmural wall tension (T) represents the net distending force within a vessel. Subsequently, the pressure term (P) represents the equilibrium between pressure inside the vessel $P(\mathrm{I})$ and pressure outside the vessel $P(\mathrm{O})$ with $P = P(\mathrm{I}) - P(\mathrm{O})$. The Law of LaPlace can be rewritten as follows[18] and is simplified diagramatically in Fig. 3:

$$T = [P(\mathrm{I}) - P(\mathrm{O})] \times r.$$

Transmural wall tension in a vessel is directly related to the difference between internal and external pressures. Therefore, as the pressure outside the vessel approaches the pressure inside the vessel $[P(\mathrm{O}) = P(\mathrm{I})]$, the transmural wall tension (T) approaches zero. Due to the fact that the venous system is a capacitance system with thin

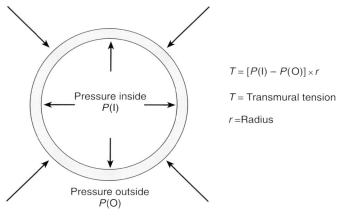

$$T = [P(I) - P(O)] \times r$$

T = Transmural tension

r = Radius

Fig. 3 Schematic representation of the factors involved in determining the net distension force (transmural tension) as derived from the Law of LaPlace.

walls, the outside pressure will be transmitted to the blood inside the vessel as the transmural wall tension approaches zero. The net result is that a local increase in intracompartmental pressure will result in an increase in venous pressure. This concept is illustrated in Fig. 4.

Decreased tissue perfusion

Decreased arteriovenous gradient

An increase in local venous pressure can be deleterious because of its relationship to perfusion as described by the Hagen–Poisseulle equation:[19]

$$Q = \Delta P \frac{\pi r^4}{8\mu L}$$

Here, Q = blood flow, ΔP = change in pressure, r = radius, μ = viscosity of the fluid, and L = length. The term $\pi r^4/8\mu L$ may be

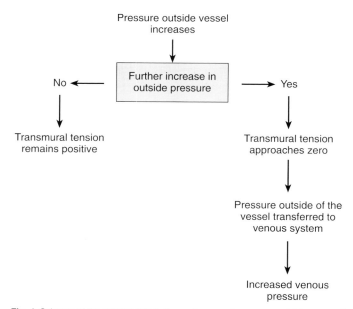

Fig. 4 Schema of the relationship between increased pressure outside a vessel and increased venous pressure.

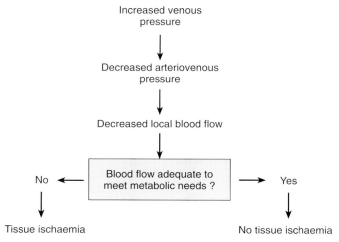

Fig. 5 Schema of the relationship between increased venous pressure and tissue ischaemia.

simplified to K and assumed constant for the sake of argument. The change in pressure (ΔP) can be defined as arterial pressure (Pa) minus venous pressure (Pv), which is referred to as the arteriovenous pressure gradient. The resultant equation then becomes:

$$Q = (Pa - Pv)K.$$

It follows that as venous pressure (Pv) increases, local blood flow (Q) will decrease because of the decrease in the arteriovenous pressure gradient. Local blood flow may decrease to the point that it no longer meets the metabolic demands of the exercising tissue thus resulting in ischaemia.[18] Figure 5 provides an overview of this pathological chain of events.

It is important to note that compartmental pressures great enough to cause symptoms are rarely higher than systolic blood pressure. Subsequently, pulses distal to an involved compartment are generally preserved. The presence or absence of a distal pulse is therefore a poor indicator of a compartment syndrome.[20]

Return to pre-exercise pressures

When activity is stopped, volume and pressure within the involved compartment gradually return to pre-exercise levels. In a compartment unaffected with chronic exertional compartment syndrome, the change in pressure back to pre-exercise levels is almost instantaneous. A prolongation of increased intracompartmental pressure post-exercise is felt to be suggestive of chronic exertional compartment syndrome.

Abnormal neuromuscular function

Pathogenesis

Abnormalities in neuromuscular function within the involved compartment manifest as pain, weakness, and dysaesthesia. The pathogenesis of pain associated with chronic exertional compartment syndrome remains poorly understood, but the dominant theory implies an ischaemic genesis; the ischaemia being related to insufficient blood flow to meet metabolic needs. Certainly, the pain associated with chronic exertional compartment syndrome has been related in nature to that of vascular ischaemic claudication as seen in peripheral vascular disease,[4] and the rapid subsidence of symptoms upon cessation of activity is suggestive of an ischaemic factor.

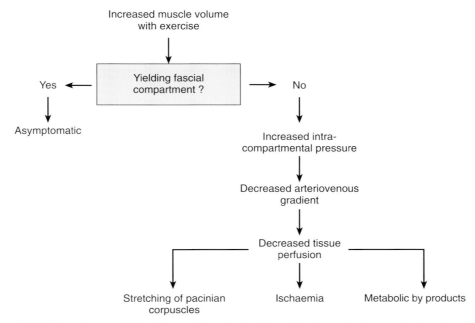

Fig. 6 Schematic representation of the possible pathophysiology of chronic exertional compartment syndrome.

Experimental models of compartment syndrome have demonstrated reduced blood flow to muscles.[18,21-24]

Despite experimental models and intuitive reasoning, evidence of ischaemic injury has not been demonstrated on muscle biopsy in patients with chronic exertional compartment syndrome. Hayes *et al.* did demonstrate reversible compartment ischaemia using thallous chloride scintigraphy;[44] however, the presence of chronic exertional compartment syndrome in their study group was not well defined, leaving the significance of these results in question. Amendola *et al.* using methoxy-isobutyl-isonitrile (nuclear medicine imaging) in a prospective double-blind study were unable to demonstrate consistent ischaemic changes at peak exercise in symptomatic patients.[25] Phosphorus nuclear magnetic resonance spectroscopy has been employed by Balduini *et al.*[26] in a recent clinical study. They concluded that ischaemia does occur in chronic exertional compartment syndrome, but they reasoned that it is transient, uncommon, and unlikely to occur at intracompartmental pressures less than 160 mmHg.

Other factors may account for the pain of chronic exertional compartment syndrome. Muscle oedema and swelling may stretch sensory pacinian corpuscles in fascia and periosteum, causing pain.[4] The metabolic by-products of altered muscle metabolism, secondary to reduced local blood flow, may directly cause pain as well.[22,27] It may be that all of the above mechanisms play a role in the pathogenesis of chronic exertional compartment syndrome pain (Fig. 6).

Neurological abnormalities

Neurological abnormalities may also occur within an involved compartment. Increased intracompartmental pressure can decrease nutrient blood flow to the nerve which may result in weakness of the neuromuscular unit. Dysaesthesiae can also result from this mechanism, usually resulting in a sensory change distal to the compartment through which the involved nerve passes. In this respect, knowledge of anatomy can assist in the diagnosis of chronic exer-

tional compartment syndrome by correlating clinical findings to known anatomical relationships. For example, the deep peroneal nerve courses through the anterior tibial compartment, supplying sensation to the first web space. Clinical findings of paraesthesia in the first web space therefore indicate anterior tibial compartment involvement. Additional examples can be found in Table 3.

Diagnosis

History

Symptoms

The hallmark feature of chronic exertional compartment syndrome is pain in the involved compartment brought on by activity. Typically, the athlete will describe a dull, aching or crampy type pain, although the pain may be sharp in nature. The pain can be localized to an exact compartment and the patient usually experiences symptoms within the entire boundary of the compartment. This is true of the anterior tibial compartment in particular. In the case of the deep tibial compartment, the pain tends to occur over the posteromedial border of the tibia, usually over the middle third of the tibia, and may radiate down to the ankle. Weakness of the musculature and dysaesthesias of the sensory nerve within the involved compartment may also be a component of the athletes' complaints. The pain is relieved with rest, but relief is not immediate upon cessation of exercise. As the syndrome becomes progressively more severe, more time is required for resolution of symptoms. Generally, the athlete is completely asymptomatic the next day until the activity is resumed.

Provoking factors

The amount of activity required to produce symptoms varies from athlete to athlete, but is usually consistent for the individual athlete. Typically, 10 to 30 min of sustained activity is required to reproduce

Table 3 Neuromuscular contents of the compartments of the lower extremity with associated dysaesthesia pattern

Compartment	Muscles	Nerve	Symptoms
Anterior	Tibialis anterior Extensor hallucis longus Extensor digitorum longus	Deep peroneal	Dysaesthesia 1st web space
Lateral	Peroneus longus Peroneus brevis	Superficial peroneal	Dysaesthesia dorsum of foot
Deep posterior	Flexor hallucis longus Flexor digitorum longus	Tibial	Dysaesthesia medial or plantar aspect of the foot
Superficial posterior	Gastrocnemius Soleus Plantaris	Sural	Rare to have dysaesthesia
Posterior tibial	Posterior tibial	None	—

the symptoms. A change in training routine, or an increase in intensity of activity, is often associated with the development of symptoms[28] and can occur in individuals with either low or high levels of fitness.[31] This is particularly frustrating when symptoms develop *de novo* in the élite athlete. Certain repetitive loading sports such as running, soccer, and cycle racing have a higher incidence of chronic exertional compartment syndrome.[30]

Athletic performance is adversely affected by the symptoms of chronic exertional compartment syndrome,[29] which force athletes to modify or reduce their activities or to perform with pain. The continuation of activity, despite painful symptoms, is referred to as 'pushing through' and this has been known to lead to acute compartment syndromes. If the athlete continues to train at the same or an increasing level, then symptoms become progressively worse in the majority of cases.[29] A voluntary forced hiatus from activity in an effort to alleviate painful symptoms is often begrudgingly embarked upon by the athlete.

Location

Chronic exertional compartment syndrome occurs most often in the anterior compartment of the lower leg, followed in frequency by the deep posterior compartment of the lower leg.[21,30] This syndrome has also been described in the lateral[8,31] and superficial compartments of the lower leg as well as in the anterior and posterior thigh, the forearm,[32-34] the feet,[35] and the paraspinal muscles.[36] Symptoms are usually bilateral, in the order of 75 to 95 per cent.[37] Athletes presenting with unilateral complaints should be directly questioned regarding symptoms in the contralateral compartment. Chronic exertional compartment syndrome can occur concurrently in more than one compartment in the same extremity.

Physical examination

At rest

The physical examination for chronic exertional compartment syndrome is most often unrewarding in the rested athlete. Typically, the patient will present in a rested state and will subsequently be completely asymptomatic during the examination. A directed physical examination of the compartment involved, as elicited by the history,

will be unremarkable. The exception is the greater propensity for fascial hernias to occur in the anterior tibial compartment of those suffering from chronic exertional compartment syndrome, as mentioned previously. The presence of physical findings in the rested athlete should lead the examiner to entertain a different diagnosis, for example pain on palpation along the tibia proper is more suggestive of a stress fracture or periostitis.

During activity

In order for the physical examination to demonstrate objective findings, the athlete should be examined either during the activity that reproduces the symptoms or immediately postactivity; a fullness or tightness may then be appreciated in the involved compartment. Passive stretching of the muscles within the compartment should exacerbate the pain. For example, passive plantar flexion of the great toe (extensor hallucis longus) would cause pain in a pathological anterior compartment. Weakness may be present in the involved muscle group. Occasionally, decreased sensation in the distribution supplied by a sensory nerve traversing the involved compartment can be identified. To illustrate, an athlete with chronic exertional compartment syndrome of the anterior tibial compartment may present with a fullness in the anterior compartment, exacerbation of pain on passive dorsiflexion of the great toe, weakness of the extensor hallucis longus muscle, and decreased sensation in the first web space.

Diagnostic tests

Intracompartmental pressure studies

Athletes suspected of having chronic exertional compartment syndrome should have the diagnosis confirmed by measuring intramuscular compartment pressures in the involved compartment. Considerable debate exists in the literature as to the most appropriate way to document these pressures and numerous methods and protocols have been proposed. In order for a diagnostic test to be useful in the clinical setting, it must be standardized and reproducible so that test measures can be correlated to clinical outcomes.

Several monitoring techniques have been described, these

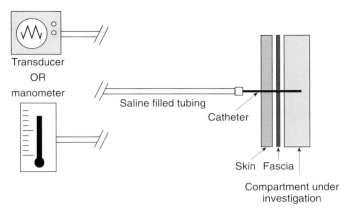

Fig. 7 Schema of the basic components of an intracompartmental pressure monitoring device.

include the slit catheter,[38] wick catheter,[23] microcapillary infusion,[39] microtip pressure method,[40] and needle manometer.[41] Although details of each method are beyond the scope of this chapter, suffice it to say that each device involves the insertion of a needle-type device into the compartment under investigation. The inserted cannula is hooked to a manometer or transducer which gives a pressure reading (Fig. 7). All of the aforementioned devices were initially devised for the measurement of static compartment pressure.

Dynamic measurement of intracompartmental pressure during exercise is advocated for the same reasons that the physical examination should be performed on exercising patients.[42] To reiterate, since chronic exertional compartment syndrome has a dynamic pathophysiology, pathological increases in intracompartmental pressure may only be demonstrable in the exercising athlete. To this end, many investigators recommend pre-exercise, dynamic (during-exercise), and postexercise intracompartmental pressure studies. Rorabeck recommends that patients with symptoms of chronic exertional compartment syndrome may benefit from surgical treatment if they have postexercise pressures higher than those of pre-exercise, or if the postexercise pressure remains greater than 15 mmHg for more than 15 min after the cessation of exercise.[42]

The two systems that are most amenable to dynamic pressure recording are the wick and slit catheter methods. The slit catheter system has been extensively reported in recent literature and appears to be the method of choice.[5,28,42] Furthermore, the slit catheter system is easy to use and reliable.

Dynamic compartment pressure measurement is subject to a wide fluctuation of pressure readings depending on the phase of the muscle contraction cycle. More specifically, pressure readings can be taken within the compartment during muscle contraction and muscle relaxation. The mean muscle pressure, the average of muscle relaxation and contraction pressures, has also been studied. Patients with chronic exertional compartment syndrome have demonstrated a significant increase in pressure during muscle contraction, relaxation, and in the mean muscle pressure.[17,39,40] Unfortunately, dynamic measures of pressure are influenced by the muscular force of contraction and the depth of insertion of the needle.[7,43] For these reasons, Pedowitz *et al.* recommend the static measurement of pressure in athletes pre-exercise, 1 min postexercise, and 5 min postexercise.[5] The compartment involved should be placed in a consistent and relaxed position to standardize readings and limit the

influence of muscle tension and position on pressure readings. The usefulness of the pressure readings is limited by uncertainties in the depth of the needle when attempting to locate a deep compartment. Also, more than one compartment may be symptomatic, but only one can readily be studied at a time.

Despite the lack of consensus regarding the most appropriate way to measure and correlate compartment pressures, several features appear to be consistent. Pressures should be measured in athletes who are exercised to the point of reproducing their symptoms. Whichever regime is chosen, it should be standardized and reproducible in the hands of the investigator. A delay in return of postexercise pressures to pre-exercise levels is important regardless of the method used. Finally, pressure readings must be interpreted in the face of a thorough history and physical examination.

Investigations to rule out other pathologies that may present with symptoms similar to those of chronic exertional compartment syndrome are essential (see 'Differential diagnosis' below).

Plain radiographs

The value of plain radiography in ruling out conditions other than chronic exertional compartment syndrome should not be underestimated. The plain radiograph of the involved anatomy reveals a plethora of useful data; for instance, the absence of bone tumours can be established and stress fractures may also be revealed, although not necessarily so. However, there are no identifiable plain radiographic changes associated with chronic exertional compartment syndrome.

⁹⁹ᵐTc-Pyrophosphonate bone scan

The bone scan is useful in that, although not specific, it is very sensitive for both bony pathology and pathology of the bone–soft tissue interface. To this end, it is a useful tool for screening out stress fractures and periostitis. A stress fracture shows as a focal area of bone with increased uptake that correlates with a painful bony area on palpation. Periostitis will present in a similar fashion to a stress fracture on plain bone scan with the exception that the area of involvement will be more extensive; for example, shin splints (periostitis) show as an increased area of uptake along the tibial ridge. Like plain radiographs, there are no identifiable changes on bone scan associated with chronic exertional compartment syndrome.

Nerve conduction studies

Nerve conduction studies are useful in circumstances where the distinction between chronic exertional compartment syndrome and nerve dysfunction is ambiguous. This is especially true when paraesthesias and numbness are present at rest. The classic site of nerve entrapment, namely the superficial peroneal nerve, may mimic chronic exertional compartment syndrome of the anterior or lateral tibial compartment. Nerve conduction studies can be useful for distinguishing between these entities. However, care must be taken in interpreting the results as chronic exertional compartment syndrome may produce latent changes in nerves travelling through an involved compartment.

Others

In an effort to produce a non-invasive diagnostic tool for chronic exertional compartment syndrome, several investigative tools have been studied including magnetic resonance imaging,[25] nuclear magnetic resonance spectroscopy,[26] and thallous chloride scintigraphy.[44] Although these tests are promising in their preliminary results, the

Table 4 Differential diagnoses for chronic exertional compartment syndrome

Stress fracture

Periostitis

Nerve entrapment

Infection (osteomyelitis)

Tumours of bone and soft tissue

Vascular claudication

Deep vein thrombosis

definitive studies have yet to be done. At this time, the routine use of these modalities as part of the diagnostic battery for chronic exertional compartment syndrome can not be recommended.

Differential diagnosis

Several disease processes may present in a similar fashion to chronic exertional compartment syndrome and may, in fact, be confused with it. This is evident from two recent studies where only approximately one-third of patients referred to clinical investigators with a tentative diagnosis of chronic exertional compartment syndrome were confirmed as having the disorder.[5,45] Although the diagnostic criteria for chronic exertional compartment syndrome in these studies were not without subjectivity, they nevertheless illustrate the importance of a sound knowledge of the differential diagnoses, in addition tendonitis, stress fracture, periostitis, nerve entrapment, infection, tumours of bone and soft tissue, deep vein thrombosis, and vascular claudication. These have been summarized in Table 4.

Management

Overview

Chronic exertional compartment syndrome, unlike acute compartment syndrome, can be treated on an elective basis. Acute compartment syndrome is a true surgical emergency and must be treated in a expedient manner to limit irreversible neuromuscular dysfunction.

In keeping with the controversies surrounding the diagnosis of chronic exertional compartment syndrome, there is also debate regarding the treatment of choice. A dichotomy exists with some authors favouring a trial of non-operative measures,[46,47] while others are adamant that non-surgical treatments are of no value.[30] There is a general consensus that fasciotomy is useful in the management of chronic exertional compartment syndrome.

Limitation of activities

Athletes with chronic exertional compartment syndrome can always modify their activity to avoid reproduction of their symptoms. This is easily accomplished because most sufferers have a good understanding of the type, magnitude, and duration of activities that reproduce their symptoms. Another option is to continue the activity at a symptomatic level and push through the pain and discomfort. The difficulty arises when individuals wish to continue at their current level of activity; such is the case with competitive athletes. Certainly, there is a selection bias for desire to continue activity in those patients presenting to a physician with complaints of chronic exertional compartment syndrome. Athletes who are willing to modify their activity will often do so on their own cognizance and therefore will never present to the clinician.

Non-surgical modalities

Non-operative methods of treatment that have been recommended for chronic exertional compartment syndrome include stretching, physiotherapy, adequate fluid hydration, non-steroidal anti-inflammatory drugs, and, in the case of lower extremity chronic exertional compartment syndrome, changing of footwear.[20] There are no definitive studies to conclude that these methods of treatment are effective in allowing the athlete to return to full, symptom-free activity. However, in the athlete who can afford the time investment, a trial of these modalities over a 6-month period may be worthwhile. The alternative is surgical intervention or cessation of the activity that reproduces symptoms.

Surgical intervention

Surgical intervention for the treatment of chronic exertional compartment syndrome in the form of fasciotomies has proven beneficial.[27,29,48,49] Athletes undergoing fasciotomies have been reported to return to premorbid activity;[20] indeed, some athletes were able to exceed their premorbid activity level.[20] The indication for fasciotomy is generally the failure of a 3- to 6-month course of non-operative treatment in an individual who wishes to continue at a level of activity that would otherwise create limiting symptoms of chronic exertional compartment syndrome.

Fasciotomies for chronic exertional compartment syndrome should result in division of the complete fascial extent of the involved compartment. The fascia is the limiting factor in this condition with little, if any, restrictive role attributable to the skin. Surgically, fascial division can be performed with minimal skin incisions and results in a full return to activity.

Failure of operative intervention

Failure to provide relief of symptoms with fasciotomy may be the result of several factors. These include inadequate fascial release, misdiagnosis of chronic exertional compartment syndrome, inappropriate rehabilitation, development of restricting scar tissue, and the presence of disease in an additional compartment. The existence of a possible fifth compartment in the lower leg that may be involved in the failure of operative intervention has been increasingly recognized (Fig. 2(a)).[21] In some individuals, the posterior tibialis muscle may have its own fascial compartment, and failure to release this for deep posterior compartment symptoms may result in persistence of complaints.

Rehabilitation

A critical aspect of surgical intervention for chronic exertional compartment syndrome is postoperative treatment. The patient should be started on immediate range of motion exercises of the joints above and below the operated area. Activity is progressed to as tolerated, with early activity encouraged. Generally, the athlete will return to full activity by 6 to 12 months. The thrust of this aggressive rehabilitation is to prevent or limit the development of non-yielding fascial scar tissue that may decrease or negate the effectiveness of the surgical intervention.

Summary

Chronic exertional compartment syndrome is a painful, activity-limiting disorder that can affect any athlete, especially those participating in the running sports. The diagnosis of this syndrome is impeded by the lack of physical findings in the resting athlete and a significant number of alternative diagnoses that may present in a similar fashion. A thorough knowledge of anatomy and pathophysiology is necessary to make an accurate diagnosis.

The underlying pathophysiology is debated. One popular theory postulates that exercise-induced muscle swelling within a non-yielding fascial compartment results in increased intracompartmental pressure. This increased intracompartmental pressure decreases tissue perfusion, probably resulting in painful ischaemia; as a consequence, athletes are often forced to limit their activity.

There are no specific physical findings in the rested athlete. Even the symptomatic athlete manifests few clinical signs. The diagnosis is best made with pre- and postexercise intracompartmental pressure readings. The specific diagnostic algorithm for pressure measurements is disputed. However, it seems that a delay in return of postexercise pressure to pre-exercise levels is helpful in establishing the diagnosis.

Treatment for chronic exertional compartment syndrome is debated with respect to the role of non-operative treatment. Some authors favour a 3- to 6-month course of stretching, physiotherapy, etc., but others suggest that non-operative treatment is ineffective. Surgical fasciotomy relieves symptoms and allows the athlete to return to premorbid levels of activity. Aggressive rehabilitation is needed in the immediate postoperative period to ensure high success rates.

References

1. Horn CE. Acute ischemia of the anterior tibial muscle and the long extensor muscles of the toes. *Journal of Bone and Joint Surgery* 1945; **27**: 615–22.
2. Hughes JR. Ischemic necrosis of the anterior tibial muscle due to fatigue. *Journal of Bone and Joint Surgery* 1948; **30-B**: 581–94.
3. Matsen FA. *Compartment syndromes.* New York: Grune and Stratton, 1980.
4. Turnipseed WD, Hurschler C, Vanderby R Jr. The effects of elevated compartment pressure on tibial arteriovenous flow and relationship of mechanical and biomechanical characteristics of fascia to genesis of chronic anterior compartment syndrome. *Journal of Vascular Surgery* 1995; **21**: 810–17.
5. Pedowitz RA, Hargens AR, Mubarak SJ, Gershuni DH. Modified criteria for the objective diagnosis of chronic compartment syndrome of the leg. *American Journal of Sports Medicine* 1990; **18**: 35–40.
6. Fronek J. Management of chronic exertional compartment syndrome of the lower extremity. *Clinical Orthopaedics* 1987; **220**: 217–27.
7. Mubarak SJ, Hargens AR. *Compartment syndrome and Volkmann's contracture.* Philadelphia: WB Saunders, 1981.
8. Reneman RS. *The anterior and lateral compartment syndrome of the leg.* The Hague: Mouton, 1968.
9. Lowdon IMR. Superficial peroneal nerve entrapment. A case report. *Journal of Bone and Joint Surgery* 1985; **67-B**: 58–9.
10. McAuliffe TB, Fiddian NJ, Browett JP. Entrapment neuropathy of the superficial peroneal nerve. A bilateral case. *Journal of Bone and Joint Surgery* 1985; **67-B**: 62–3.
11. Styf J. Entrapment of the superficial peroneal nerve. Diagnosis and results of decompression. *Journal of Bone and Joint Surgery* 1989; **71-B**: 131–5.
12. Lee BY, Brancato RF, Park IH, Shaw WW. Management of compartment syndrome. *American Journal of Surgery* 1984; **148**: 383–8.
13. Whiteside TE, Haney TC, Morimoto K, Harada H. Tissue pressure measurements as a determinant for the need of fasciotomy. *Clinical Orthopaedics and Related Research* 1975; **113**: 43–51.
14. Puranen J, Alavaikko A. Intracompartmental pressure increase on exertion in patients with chronic compartment syndrome in the leg. *Journal of Bone and Joint Surgery* 1981; **63-A**: 1034–9.
15. Rorabeck CH, MacNab I. The pathophysiology of the anterior tibial compartment syndrome. *Clinical Orthopaedics and Related Research* 1975; **113**: 52–7.
16. Folkow B, Gaskell P, Waaler BA. Blood flow through limb muscles during sustained contractions. *Acta Physiologica Scandinavica* 1970; **80**: 61–72.
17. Styf J. Intramuscular pressure and muscle blood flow during exercise in chronic compartment syndrome. *Journal of Bone and Joint Surgery* 1987; **69-B**: 301–5.
18. Black KP, Taylor DE. Current concepts in the treatment of common compartment syndromes in athletes. *Sports Medicine* 1993; **15**: 408–18.
19. Chien S, Lee MM. Blood flow in small tubes. In: Renkin EM, Michel CC, eds. *Handbook of physiology.* Section 2: The cardiovascular system. Vol. IV. The microcirculation. Bethesda, MD: American Physiologic Society, 1984.
20. Hutchinson RH, Ireland ML. Common compartment syndromes in athletes. Treatment and rehabilitation. *Sports Medicine* 1994; **17**: 200–8.
21. Davey JR, Rorabeck CH, Fowler PJ. The tibialis posterior muscle compartment: an unrecognized cause of exertional compartment syndrome. *American Journal of Sports Medicine* 1984; **12**: 391–7.
22. Baumann JU, Sutherland DH, Hanggi A. Intramuscular pressure during walking: An experimental study using the wick catheter technique. *Clinical Orthopaedics and Related Research* 1979; **145**: 292–9.
23. Mubarak SJ, Hargens AR, Owen CA, Garetto LP, Akeson WH. The wick catheter technique for measurement of intracompartmental pressure: A new research and clinical tool. *Journal of Bone and Joint Surgery* 1976; **58-A**: 1016–20.
24. Qvarfordt P, Christenson JT, Eklöf B, Ohlin P, Saltin B. Intramuscular pressure, muscle blood flow, and skeletal muscle metabolism in chronic anterior tibial compartment syndrome. *Clinical Orthopaedics and Related Research* 1983; **179**: 284–90.
25. Amendola A, Rorabeck CH, Vellett D, Vezina W, Rutt B, Nott L. The use of magnetic resonance imaging in exertional compartment syndromes. *American Journal of Sports Medicine* 1990; **18**: 29–34.
26. Balduini FC, Shento DW, O'Connor KH, Heppenstall RB. Chronic exertional compartment syndrome: correlation of compartment pressure and muscle ischemia using 31P NMR spectroscopy. *Clinics in Sports Medicine* 1993; **12**: 151–65.
27. Rorabeck CH, Bourne RB, Fowler PJ. The surgical treatment of exertional compartment syndrome in athletes. *Journal of Bone and Joint Surgery* 1983; **65-A**: 1245–51.
28. Eislele SA, Sammarco GJ. Chronic exertional compartment syndromes. In: Heckman JD, ed. *Instructional course lectures.* Parkridge: American Academy of Orthopedic Surgeons, 1993; **42**: 213–17.
29. Detmer DE, Sharpe K, Sufit RL, Girdley FM. Chronic compartment syndrome: diagnosis, management and outcomes. *American Journal of Sports Medicine* 1985; **13**: 162–70.
30. Martens MA, Moeyersoons JP. Acute and effort-related compartment syndrome in sports. *Sports Medicine* 1990; **9**: 62–8.

31. Blasier D, Barry RJ, Weaver T. Forced march-induced peroneal compartment syndrome: A report of two cases. *Clinical Orthopaedics and Related Research* 1992; **284**: 189–92.

32. Wasilewski SA, Asdourian PL. Bilateral chronic exertional compartment syndromes of forearm in an adolescent athlete: case report and review of the literature. *American Journal of Sports Medicine* 1991; **19**: 665–7.

33. Tompkins DG. Exercise myopathy of the extensor carpi ulnaris muscle: Report of a case. *Journal of Bone and Joint Surgery* 1973; **59-A**: 407–8.

34. Imbriglia JE, Boland DM. An exercise induced compartment syndrome of the dorsal forearm: A case report. *Journal of Hand Surgery* 1984; **9**: 142–3.

35. Lokiec F, Siev-Ner I, Pritsch M. Brief reports: Chronic compartment syndromes of both feet. *Journal of Bone and Joint Surgery* 1991; **73-B**: 178–9.

36. Konno S, Kikuchi S, Nagaosa Y. The relationship between intramuscular pressure of the paraspinal muscles and low back pain. *Spine* 1994; **19**: 2186–9.

37. Jones DC, James SL. Overuse injuries of the lower extremity: Shin splints, iliotibial band friction syndrome, and exertional compartment syndromes. *Clinics in Sports Medicine* 1987; **6**: 273–90.

38. Rorabeck CH, Castle GS, Hardie R, Logan J. Compartmental pressure measurements: An experimental investigation using the slit catheter. *Journal of Trauma* 1981; **21**: 446–9.

39. Styf JR, Korner LM. Microcapillary infusion technique for measurement of intracompartmental pressure during exercise. *Clinical Orthopaedics and Related Research* 1986; **207**: 253–62.

40. McDermott AGP, Marble AE, Yabsley RH, Phillips MB. Monitoring dynamic anterior compartment pressures during exercise: A new technique using the STIC catheter. *American Journal of Sports Medicine* 1982; **10**: 83–9.

41. Brace RA, Guyton AC, Taylor AE. Re-evaluation of the needle method for measuring interstitial fluid pressure. *American Journal of Physiology* 1975; **229**: 603–7.

42. Rorabeck CH. Diagnosis and management of compartment syndromes. In: Heckman JD, ed. *Instructional course lectures*. Parkridge: American Academy of Orthopedic Surgeons, 1989; **38**: 466–72.

43. Sejersted OM, Hargens AR, Kardel KR, Blom P, Jensen O, Hermansen L. Intramuscular fluid pressure during isometric contraction of human skeletal muscle. *Journal of Applied Physiology* 1984; **56**: 287–95.

44. Hayes AA, Bower GD, Pitstock KL. Chronic (exertional) compartment syndrome of the legs diagnosed with thallous chloride scintigraphy. *Journal of Nuclear Medicine* 1995; **36**: 1618–24.

45. Styf J. Diagnosis of exercise-induced pain in the anterior aspect of the lower leg. *American Journal of Sports Medicine* 1988; **16**: 165–9.

46. Rorabeck CH, Fowler PJ, Nott L. The results of fasciotomy in the management of chronic exertional compartment syndrome. *American Journal of Sports Medicine* 1988; **16**: 224–7.

47. Black KP, Shultz TK, Cheung NL. Compartment syndromes in athletes. *Clinics in Sports Medicine* 1990; **9**: 471–87.

48. Schepsis AA, *et al.* Surgical management of exertional compartment syndrome of the lower leg: Long term followup. *American Journal of Sports Medicine* 1993; **21**: 811–17.

49. Styf JR, Korner LM. Chronic anterior compartment syndrome of the leg: Results of treatment by fasciotomy. *Journal of Bone and Joint Surgery* 1986; **68-A**: 1338–47.

5.4 Overuse injuries of the knee

William D. Stanish and Robert M. Wood

Introduction

The knee joint is commonly afflicted with overuse injuries. The knee may be predisposed to injury in circumstances where its architectural design is abnormal, for example genu valgum, patella alta, etc. If the knee joint is morphologically normal, it may become injured when challenged beyond its capacity, as may occur when a jogger increases his or her mileage too quickly. In this chapter we review problems of overuse related to the knee joint and then offer some proposals for managing these difficulties.

Anatomy of the knee

With a unique design, it is convenient to describe the human knee as two condylar joints between the corresponding condyles of the femur and the tibia. Furthermore, a joint exists between the patella and the trochlea of the femur. The condylar joints are separated by two fibrocartilage menisci between the corresponding articular surfaces (Fig. 1). The plateau of the tibia possesses two separate articular facets. The medial facet lies completely on the superior surface of the condyle, but the lateral facet curves backwards over the posterior aspect of the tibial condyle. This bevelled margin allows withdrawal of the lateral meniscus on flexion. The femoral condyles are separated posteriorly by a deep notch, but fuse anteriorly into a trochlear groove for articulation with the patella. The lateral ridge of the trochlea is very prominent. Viewing the condyles laterally, it can be seen that they are cam-shaped, that is to say flatter at the end of the femur and more highly curved at the free posterior margin. The articular surface of the medial condyle is narrower, longer, and more curved than that of the lateral condyle. This is important in the passive rotation that occurs when extending the knee.[1,2]

The articular surface of the patella is divided by a vertical ridge into a lateral and medial surface; this medial surface is further divided by a second vertical ridge into two smaller areas. The lateral articular surface of the patella is in contact with the lateral condyle of the femur in all directions of flexion. In extension, the area next to it lies on the trochlea, and the most medial of the three articular surfaces of the patella is not in articulation with the femur. In flexion, this surface glides into articulation with the medial condyle and the middle of the three surfaces lies in the intercondylar notch of the femur.[3]

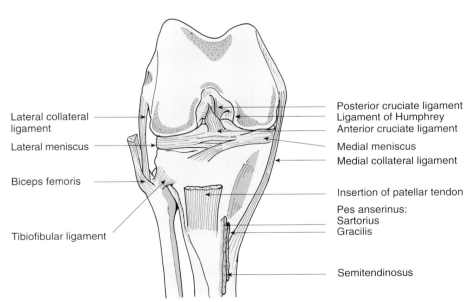

Lateral collateral ligament

Lateral meniscus

Biceps femoris

Tibiofibular ligament

Posterior cruciate ligament
Ligament of Humphrey
Anterior cruciate ligament

Medial meniscus
Medial collateral ligament

Insertion of patellar tendon

Pes anserinus:
Sartorius
Gracilis

Semitendinosus

Fig. 1 The anterior view of the knee. The two menisci separate the femur from tibia.

The capsule which surrounds the knee joint is usually thin and in some areas is deficient. It is attached to the femur above the intercondylar fossa, to the margins of the femoral condyles, to the margins of the patella, and to the patellar tendon, as well as to the margins of the tibial condyles. The patellar tendon and patella serve as a capsule to the anterior aspect of the joint. As the capsule extends from the femur to the tibia, it is attached to the outer aspects of the menisci. That part of the capsule between the tibia and the menisci is known as the coronary ligaments. Medially, the capsule is fused with the medial collateral ligament. Laterally, a strong thickening of the capsule extends from the lateral epicondyle to the head of the fibula. This lies deep to the lateral ligament and forms part of the origin of the popliteus tendon. On both sides, the capsule is strengthened by aponeurotic expansions of the vastus muscles and overlying fascia. These fascial–aponeurotic sheets are known as the medial and lateral retinaculum of the patella.[4] The capsule is reinforced by four main ligaments: the patella retinacula; the medial collateral ligament; the lateral collateral ligament; and the oblique popliteal ligaments.

The patella retinacula extends from the patella to the lower margins of the condyles of the tibia; these are fibrous expansions from the quadriceps tendon and from the lower margins of the vastus medialis and lateralis.[4] In front of the collateral ligaments, they blend with the capsule; anteriorly they are attached to the margins of the ligaments and patella below the patellar attachment of the capsule.

The medial collateral ligament is attached to the epicondyle of the femur below the adductor tubercle and to the subcutaneous surface of the tibia, roughly a hand's breadth below the knee. The anterior margin of this ligament lies free except at its attached extremities. This part of the ligament is not attached to the medial meniscus and, in fact, is separated from it by a small bursa. The posterior margins of the medial collateral ligament converge to insert into the medial meniscus. Over the condyle of the tibia the ligament is separated from bone by the forward extension of the semimembranosus tendon in the intervening bursa. From its tibial attachment, the ligament slopes slightly back as it passes up to be inserted behind the axis of flexion of the medial femoral condyle. The medial collateral ligament is drawn taut by full extension of the knee.[1,2]

The lateral collateral ligament is attached to the lateral epicondyle of the femur in continuity with the short external lateral ligament (Fig. 2). It slopes down and back to the head of the fibula. It lies free from the capsule and lateral meniscus, being separated from the meniscus by the popliteus tendon. Like the medial collateral ligament, it is attached just behind the axis of flexion of the femoral condyle and is drawn taut by full extension of the knee.[1,2]

The oblique popliteal ligament is a thick rounded band of great strength, perforated by the middle genicular vessels. It is an expansion of the insertion of the semimembranosus as it slopes up to the popliteal surface of the femur. The oblique nature of this ligament limits external rotation in the locked position of the knee.[1]

A structure which is closely related to the capsule but functionally distinct from it is the patellar tendon. It lies in a smooth area, slightly oblique on the tibial tuberosity. The patella retinacula, fibrous extensions from the tendon of the quadriceps femoris, are inserted into the edges of the patella and ligaments of the patella, as well as into the inferior borders of the tibial condyles. Several bursae

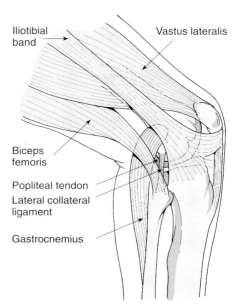

Fig. 2 The lateral collateral ligament of the knee. It bridges the lateral femoral condyle and the proximal fibula in proximity to the popliteal tendon and the biceps femoris.

lie in close association with the ligaments and the patella, notably the superficial and deep infrapatellar bursae.[5,6]

Some intra-articular structures are relevant with respect to both the static and dynamic anatomy of the knee. The cruciate ligaments are two very strong ligaments which lie within the capsule of the knee, but outside the synovial membrane. The anterior cruciate ligament attaches to the anterior part of the tibial plateau, in front of the tibial spine, and extends superiorly and posteriorly to a smooth insertion on the lateral femoral condyle, well back in the intercondylar notch. The posterior cruciate ligament attaches to the posterior part of the head of the tibia between the condyles and passes anteriorly and superiorly medial to the anterior cruciate ligament. It is attached to a smooth impression on the medial femoral condyle, well forward in the intercondylar notch. The cruciate ligaments are essential to the anteroposterior stability of the knee joint. The posterior cruciate ligament is the main stabilizing factor preventing the femur from sliding backwards off the tibial plateau in a weight-bearing flexed knee. The anterior cruciate prevents forward displacement of the tibia on the femoral surface. This ligament also limits extension of the lateral condyle of the femur and causes medial rotation of the femur in the act of fully extending the knee (Fig. 3).[1,7,8]

The menisci are kidney-shaped cartilages composed of dense fibrous tissues. Each meniscus lies on the superior surface of its respective femoral condyle. They are avascular except at their attachments. The medial meniscus is fixed at its anterior and posterior horns by fibrous tissue invested in the tibia. The lateral meniscus is likewise attached to the tibia and both its horns (Fig. 4). The circumference of the meniscus is attached by a very lax capsule to the articular margins of the femur and the tibia, except beneath the popliteal tendon. Here there is a gap in the capsule through which the popliteal tendon and bursae migrate.

The popliteal tendon lies between the capsule and the synovial membrane. This tendon does not lie free within the cavity of the

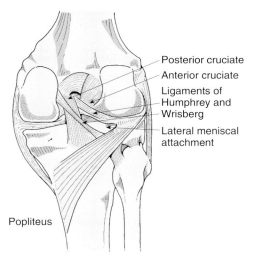

Fig. 3 The posterior cruciate ligament attaches to the posterior part of the proximal tibia and passes anteriorly and superior to the anterior cruciate ligament.

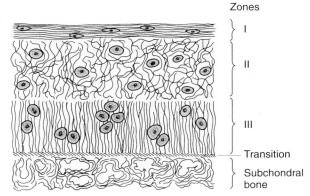

Fig. 5 Normal articular cartilage. The three zones in transition to subchondral bone.

knee joint but is firmly adherent to the capsule. The adherence of this tendon makes a prominent ridge on the internal surface of the capsule. The ridge is invested with the synovial membrane of the joint cavity, both above and below the lateral meniscus. The bare popliteal tendon is in contact with the bare lateral meniscus between the upper and lower synovial reflections. The tendon may even be attached to the lateral meniscus, but this is rare.[9-11]

Since the knee is a condylar joint, its movements are complex. The shapes and curvatures of the articular surfaces are such that hinge movements are combined with gliding and rolling, coupled with rotation about a vertical axis. With the knee extended, the axis of rotation extends from the head of the femur to the medial intercondylar tubercle of the tibia. Hence the lateral condyle swings around this vertical axis through the medial condyle.[12,13]

When the knee is flexed with the leg remaining fixed, the thigh rotates laterally during the first part of flexion and the femur rolls backward on the tibia. Conversely, when the knee is extended the thigh rotates medially during the final part of extension. This is known as the locking or screw-home mechanism and is attributed to the vastus medialis. This action makes the articular surfaces more congruent and puts the joint in a position of maximum stability.

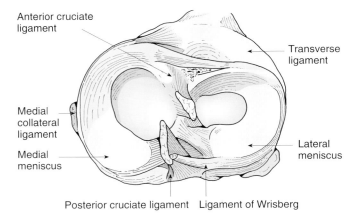

Fig. 4 The medial and lateral menisci are composed of fibrocartilage and are fixed with anterior and posterior horns.

The popliteus muscle initiates flexion of the knee by unscrewing the locked knee joint.[2,12,14]

When the thigh is fixed and the leg is free to move, the tibia rotates on the femur. Since medial rotation of the tibia is equivalent to lateral rotation of the femur, it can be deduced that, in this case, initiation of flexion of the knee is accompanied by medial rotation of the leg and the terminal part of extension of the knee is accompanied by lateral rotation of the leg.[1,12,14]

Before describing changes observed in the articular surface in various overuse injuries of the knee, the histology of normal cartilage must be considered.

Histology of articular cartilage

Articular cartilage is a composite material consisting of a cellular and an extracellular component. The chondrocytes compose the cellular component, while the extracellular component consists of an intricate arrangement of mucopolysaccharide ground substance and collagen fibres.[15] Three zones which differ in relative size and composition have been identified within articular cartilage (Fig. 5).

Zone I, which is the outermost layer, forms a thin tough skin over the surface of the articular cartilage. In this zone the collagen fibres have a definite orientation, lying parallel and presenting a relatively smooth surface. Also, the collagen fibres in this zone are rather small.[16,17] Zone II, which lies immediately deep to zone I, presents a more disorganized arrangement of collagen. In this zone the collagen fibres tend to be coiled, presenting large open spaces in the meshwork which are filled with ground substance.[16,17] Zone III, which is the deepest zone, consists of large cellular fibres which are radially oriented and arranged more densely, or closer together, than zone II collagen fibres.

The different arrangement of the collagen fibres in each of the three zones allows each zone to take a different responsibility. The circumferentially arranged fibres in zone I present a low diffusion effect upon compression, while the more randomly oriented collagen fibres of zone II act as an area of energy storage. The fibres of zone III serve as an attachment between the articular cartilage and the underlying subchondral bone.[16,17]

These fibres also present a geometric pattern which provides resistance to the shearing forces of articulation. The three layers also differ with respect to chondrocyte activity—those in zone I

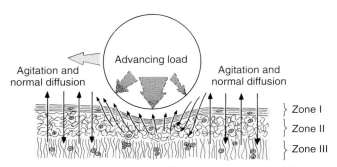

Fig. 6 Joint lubrication and cartilage nutrition are maintained by the ability of lubricants and nutrients to permeate articular cartilage.

tend to be relatively inactive, while chondrocytes in the deeper layers are more active.

Joint lubrication and cartilage nutrition are maintained by the ability of lubricants and nutrients to permeate articular cartilage, a property attributed to the ultrastructure and biochemical composition of the cartilage. With ageing, the mechanism by which articular cartilage obtains its nutrients changes slightly. In the child, nutrition of the cartilage is achieved by diffusion of nutrients from within the joint and from subchondral bone into the articular cartilage (Fig. 6).[17] After maturity, nutrition is dependent solely upon diffusion from superficial to deep layers. Studies have shown that the permeability of the articular cartilage tends to change with the compressive load imposed.[18]

During periods of non-compression, fluids are able to penetrate the cartilage by simple diffusion. However, when stresses are placed on the cartilage, several changes take place. First, the collagen fibres of the middle zone (zone II) form a densely oriented structure; in other words, the fibres become more densely packed together. Second, compressing the proteoglycan component of the ground substance tends to increase its density. Both these changes have the effect of decreasing the permeability of the articular cartilage. When a stress is placed on the articular cartilage, fluid extrudes from it, and when the stress is removed the fluid is resorbed by the cartilage. This phenomenon is important in the maintenance of joint lubrication.[17]

The integrity of articular cartilage is essential to the normal functioning of each and every joint, and any alteration in either the biochemical composition of the ground substance or the collagen architecture will have undesirable effects on articular cartilage function, with respect to permeability, lubrication, and biomechanical function.

Chondromalacia patella

Chondromalacia patella is a condition which affects young healthy individuals. Invariably these patients complain of pain about the patella, and, in fact, manifest degenerative changes to the articular cartilage of the patella. As a distinct entity, it was first described by Budlinger in 1906. Although much has been written about this condition, it continues to pose a major problem to the practitioner in terms of both diagnosis and treatment.

The most notable problem is differentiating chondromalacia patella from other conditions of the knee such as disorders of the meniscus. There appears to be no single sign which is pathognomonic of either condition. Several points must be established in

dealing with chondromalacia patella. .[17] First, the aetiology of chondromalacia patella is multifactorial and frequently related to malalignment of the lower extremity. This results in abnormal stresses to the patella. The ultimate effect of this abnormal stress is damage to the articular surface. Second, other possible causes of anterior knee pain must be eliminated before chondromalacia patella is diagnosed. Third, conservative non-surgical treatment is indicated in most circumstances.

Pathology

Chondromalacia patella is a pathological finding of cartilage on the posterior aspect of the patella.

The most common lesion is fibrillation of the articular cartilage at the junction of the medial and odd facets. This fibrillation may spread to involve most of the medial facet. Histologically, chondromalacia patella is characterized by maintenance of the superficial zone of articular cartilage with the initial changes occurring primarily in the deeper zones. The main changes observed include specific alterations of the mucopolysaccharide ground substance and loss of the normal energy-storing capacity of the middle zone. These changes result in the application of abnormal forces to the underlying subchondral bone and subsequent fissuring, with fibrillation occurring throughout the layers of articular cartilage. In severe cases, all layers of articular cartilage may erode to the subchondral bone (Fig. 7).[19]

Goodfellow *et al.*[19] have differentiated between changes in the articular cartilage, which are commonly seen in older subjects, and the alterations seen in the adolescent with chondromalacia patella. Surface degeneration with superficial fibrillation is the characteristic change seen in the articular cartilage of old individuals. It is described as changes involving the superficial layer with eventual involvement of all layers, including the subchondral bone. These changes are also seen in youth in areas such as the medial articular margin of the odd facet of the patella. This is usually a region of non-contact, and since cyclical loading is necessary for normal articular cartilage nutrition, the area will be nutritionally deficient, resulting in degenerative changes. These degenerative changes may lead to osteoarthritis.

Chondromalacia patella in the adolescent involves degeneration of the articular cartilage and allegedly does not progress to osteo-

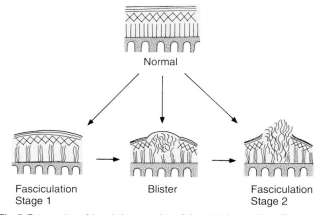

Fig. 7 Progression of basal degeneration of the articular cartilage.(Reproduced from ref. 19, with permission.)

arthritis. This allegation is controversial. Stage I of degeneration is known as blistering and involves a normal gross appearance of the articular cartilage. However, some softening of the cartilage occurs and the normal architecture of zone III is disrupted. The superficial and deeper layers remain relatively intact. Alterations in the ground substance are seen histologically, with loss of normal staining characteristics and chondrocyte proliferation. The superficial layer of articular cartilage may eventually be involved, with disruption of the tangentially oriented collagen fibres which present a rough, uneven, and deeply fissured surface.[17]

There has been difficulty in explaining the development of pain from pathological conditions such as those already described, because articular cartilage is devoid of the nerve fibres mediating pain and usually at this stage there is no evidence of synovial reaction. When the overlying articular cartilage has lost some of its ability to absorb energy, the subchondral bone is subjected to abnormal forces. These forces on the subchondral bone can explain the pain observed, since it is richly endowed in pain fibres. It has been suggested by Darracott and Vernon-Roberts[20] that the initial changes with chondromalacia patella occur in the subchondral bone and are characterized by chondrocyte hyperplasia with vascularization and advancing ossification into the deeper zone of the articular cartilage. This process is accompanied by new bone formation and either focal or diffuse osteoporosis. This process is thought to precede changes within the articular cartilage and may be secondary to an alteration of blood supply in the subchondral bone. Involvement of the subchondral bone in such a fashion seems consistent with the theory of pain production and may well have merit in understanding the aetiology of this condition.

Factors in the aetiology

There are numerous aetiological factors of chondromalacia patella. These include direct trauma to the knee, incongruency of the patellofemoral joint, internal derangements of the knee, recurrent subluxation of the patella, malrotation of the tibia on the femur, malalignments of the extensor mechanism, or extended periods of immobilization following surgery.

Direct trauma to the knee has been implicated as the major aetiological factor in the pathogenesis of chondromalacia patella. In 1986, Chrisman[21] confirmed the previous hypothesis that mechanical trauma can lead to degradation of articular cartilage. Using a weighted pendulum, a blow was delivered to the normal articular cartilage. Within two hours a fourfold increase in the concentration of free arachidonic acid in the cartilage was found using gas chromatography. Arachidonic acid is an unsaturated fatty acid which is essential for human nutrition, and is a major component of the bipolar phospholipid cell membranes. When released, it is a precursor for local hormones and chemotactic factors such as prostaglandins. Prostaglandin E_2 is the major prostaglandin released under these circumstances and, by its activation of cAMP, deterioration of articular cartilage may ensue due to the release of catheptic proteases. These enzymes are exuded into the cartilage matrix where they split the protein links attaching chondroitin sulphates to major components of the cartilage matrix. The loss of matrix leads to the softening, and possibly the fibrillation, of articular cartilage seen in chondromalacia patella.

A discussion of the aetiological factors of chondromalacia mala-

cia patella would be incomplete without mention of lower-extremity malalignment. Rotational and angular malalignments of the lower extremity have a significant influence on patellofemoral joint mechanics. Persistent anteversion through the femoral neck frequently remains unrecognized and is often associated with a series of compensatory growth disturbances throughout the limb.

James and co-workers[17,22] have described an alignment abnormality in active young individuals which is known as the 'miserable malalignment'. These patients show significantly increased internal rotation of the hip while in the extended position. Examination in individuals who are standing with the feet parallel reveals bilateral squinting of the patella and apparent genu varum, and often an associated recurvatum. More distally there is tibia varum and the foot presents a compensatory pronation. Very frequently this anterior knee pain, once initiated, is extremely difficult to manage.

Presentation of chondromalacia patella

The hallmark of chondromalacia patella is anterior knee pain. The symptoms appear in two groups of patients.[23] The first group involves the somewhat inactive teenage female. In this group the symptoms are triggered by prolonged periods of sitting with the knees flexed, for example in an automobile or in a classroom. The patient's symptoms may be alleviated by walking for a short time. The second group of patients with symptomatic chondromalacia patella comprises the highly active person in their late teenage years or early twenties. Symptoms in this group of people are aggravated by activity, in particular those activities which involve stresses on the knee joint in flexion and twisting. In both groups ascending stairs or hills causes exacerbation of the condition, as does deep knee-bending exercises such as squats. The pain itself is always experienced in the retropatellar area and is described by the patients as aching. Roughly one-third of the cases are bilateral. A sensation of catching, grating, or even false locking is commonly described by patients, and these may be accompanied by a feeling of instability or giving way. Most patients will give a history of a rather insidious onset of pain without a major trauma. The pain may occur with activity, but more commonly it will occur with a period of rest following vigorous activity.

Physical examination

It must be stressed that the physical examination of a patient having chondromalacia patella must include the entire lower extremity. A comprehensive examination of the lower extremity must be divided into four phases: standing, sitting, supine, and evaluation while prone. Inspection and palpation are the major diagnostic tests, combined with more specific techniques to complete the comprehensive examination of the lower extremity.[24]

Standing examination

In this examination the patient stands upright, facing the examiner, with the feet held slightly apart and aligned directly towards the examiner. The patient should be wearing running shorts or comparable clothing so that the entire lower extremity can be viewed by the examiner. General alignment of the lower extremity is first observed with attention directed to mechanical malalignment such as genu varum or valgum deformities. Next, the angle of the lower tibia to the floor is measured. An angle of 10 degrees or more demands excessive subtalar joint pronation to offer a plantar grade foot. The

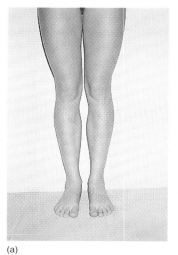
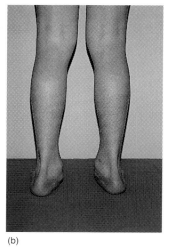

(a)   (b)

Fig. 8 A patient with 'miserable malalignment', characterized by femoral anteversion, squinting patellae, genu varum, patella alta, increased Q-angle, external tibia rotation, tibia varum, and compensatory pronation of the feet. (Reproduced from ref. 17, with permission.)

excessively pronated foot is accompanied by a compensatory internal rotation of the tibia. Commonly, this increased amount of rotation triggers stress through the peripatellar tissues of the knee.[17,22,24] The status of the foot, particularly as it relates to excessive pronation, is then determined by first stabilizing the subtalar joint in the neutral position. This is accomplished by palpating the talar head between the thumb and index finger over the anterior aspect of the ankle, while the patient transfers the weight to the lateral border of the foot and the medial aspect of the heel is lifted from the floor. The position in which the talar head is palpated equally on the medial and lateral aspects of the ankle is considered to be the neutral position of the subtalar joint, and is the optimal position for normal, lower-extremity weight bearing.[17,22,24]

An individual with the foot in excessive pronation will have an increased internal tibia rotation. This will result in prolonged and increased forces absorbed by the soft tissues of the knee (Fig. 8).[24]

Noting the position of the patellae, with the feet pointing directly ahead, will help detect rotational malalignments. The so-called 'squinting patellae', where both patellae point medially, is a sign of increased femoral torsion or excessive femoral anteversion. A close observation of the gait pattern of the patient will be valuable in detecting rotational abnormalities.

The standing examination should also include viewing the lower extremity from the lateral aspects. This is the best position for observing flexion contractures or genu recurvatum.

Sitting examination

This part of the physical examination concentrates on the patellofemoral joint and is performed while the patient is seated on a normal examining table with their legs hanging freely at 90 degrees of flexion.

The position of the patella, as it sits over the distal aspect of the femur, is first evaluated. The normal patella sinks deeply into the patellofemoral sulcus at 90 degrees of flexion.[24] A patient with patella alta will demonstrate a protuberant patella which appears to point towards the ceiling. Patella alta and patella infera (baja) have

been associated with numerous patellofemoral disorders and these conditions should be sought in patients with patellofemoral complaints.[24,25]

Next, the alignment of the patella and the patella tendon is assessed. As the knee is flexed, the patella derotates and decreases the quadriceps angle as the patella tendon orients itself in the same longitudinal axis as the anterior crest of the tibia. The 'grasshopper-eye' patella is one sign of abnormal patellar tracking. This is a lateral tilting of the patella and can be easily seen as the knee is flexed to 90 degrees. Patella tracking is further evaluated by palpating the patella as the knee is passively flexed and extended. The tracking should be smooth, longitudinal, and accompanied by only small amounts of rotation. Any abrupt or sudden movements of the patella should be considered abnormal.[24]

Finally, the sitting examination should be concluded by palpation of the patella for crepitus as the knee is actively flexed and extended. The presence of crepitus does not always correlate with pain or the degree of patellar involvement since there may be minimal pain with marked crepitus and vice versa.

Supine examination

This part of the examination is important in determining the mobility of the patella. The quadriceps angle can also be measured at this time.

Patella mobility is tested with the knee in full extension and at 30 to 40 degrees of flexion. Most patellae demonstrate a moderate amount of lateral mobility in full extension; however, instability of the patella must be suspected if the patella displaces more than half its width in this position. At 30 degrees of flexion there should be little or no lateral mobility of the patella. If the patient has a grossly unstable patella, it may be possible to sublux it over the lateral femoral condyle. This will often cause apprehension in the patient, as the same sensation is felt with episodes of giving way.[24,26]

All borders of the patella should be palpated for tenderness. Facets can be examined by displacing the patella medially and laterally with the knee extended and palpating the border of the medial and lateral facets. This will elicit varying degrees of tenderness with chondromalacia.

The final component of the supine examination involves compressing the patella against the femoral condyles while the patient is tensing the quadriceps. Once again, varying degrees of discomfort will be reported and this is often accompanied by crepitus in the presence of chondromalacia patella.

Prone examination

The examination of the lower extremity and patellofemoral joint is concluded with the patient in the prone position with the feet extended beyond the end of the examining table. Hip motion is measured with the knee in 90 degrees of flexion, while preventing the pelvis from tilting. Most adults will have more external than internal rotation; however, a discrepancy of over 30 degrees may be considered normal.[24]

Next, measurements are taken to determine the leg–heel and heel–forefoot alignment. These measurements must be taken with the subtalar joint in the neutral position. The neutral position is achieved by applying pressure beneath the fourth metatarsal head and dorsiflexing the ankle until resistance is met. The foot is then inverted and everted to the point at which the foot appears to fall off to one side. This point in the arc of motion is the neutral position of the subtalar joint.[24]

With the subtalar joint held in its neutral position, leg–heel alignment can be evaluated as follows. A line is drawn along the longitudinal axis of the distal portion of the posterior leg and a second line drawn over the longitudinal axis of the posterior portion of the calcaneus. A normal value for leg–heel alignment is 2 to 3 degrees of varus.[24]

The heel–forefoot alignment is then assessed, once again with the foot held in the neutral position. This is determined by noting the relationship of the tranverse plane of the forefoot at the metatarsal head in relation to the vertical axis of the heel. Normally the transverse of the forefoot should be perpendicular to the vertical aspect of the heel. If the plane of the forefoot of the metatarsal head is such that the medial side of the foot rises above a perpendicular plane to the heel, the forefoot is supinated (varus). However, if the medial side of the foot falls below the perpendicular plane of the heel, the foot is in pronation (valgus). A flat or severely pronated foot often has forefoot supination and subtalar varus, while the varus foot often has plantar flexed first ray and subtalar varus.[24]

Treatment

It is generally agreed that the patellofemoral pain syndrome, more specifically chondromalacia patella, should be managed initially by conservative measures. Several authors, including DeHaven et al.[27] in a prospective study of chondromalacia patella, have demonstrated that a non-surgical programme was successful in 82 per cent of patients. Furthermore, 66 per cent of conservatively treated patients were able to return to unrestricted athletic activities. Only 8 per cent required surgical intervention. Most authorities considered rest, quadriceps strengthening, and medication to be important ingredients of any conservative programme.

Non-surgical treatment

Before commencing a treatment programme for managing patello-femoral pain, the physician must take the necessary time to educate the patient about the condition. He or she must be reassured that the condition is not serious but that reduction of painful activities for a period may be necessary. The nature of the patellofemoral programme and the specific treatments must be explained. These practices can prove to be time-consuming: however, they are essential in maximizing patient cooperation and compliance.

Acute pain must be managed by restriction of activities associated with increased patellofemoral pressure such as weight bearing with a flexed knee. The value of immobilization of the knee is outweighed by its harm in causing muscle atrophy and weakness, and possibly interfering with the nutrition of the joint cartilage.[28]

Mild or moderate pain can generally be managed by relatively minor modifications of activities. In most cases only activities which cause knee pain in each individual should be avoided, whereas all other activities are permitted and, in fact, encouraged. If the patient must sit for long periods of time, they must be informed that sitting with the knee in relaxed extension will reduce pain afterwards. Swimming can be substituted for jogging as a means of promoting physical fitness.[28,29]

Strengthening the quadriceps muscle group is the most important part of the conservative management of chondromalacia patella. Atrophy and weakness of the quadriceps almost always accompanies

disorders of the patellofemoral joint, and, although the mechanism is not completely clear, quadriceps strengthening helps alleviate patellofemoral pain. It has been suggested that quadriceps strengthening may be related to alteration of the contact surfaces of the patella within the trochlea, thereby relieving pain.[28,30]

Although several exercise programmes have been suggested for quadriceps rehabilitation, isometric and progressive resistance exercises performed with the knee in full extension have been found to be the most useful. The programme may be altered according to the severity of the pain in each individual. Patients with severe pain should be prescribed an isometric exercise regime consisting of maximum isometric quadriceps recruitment for 5 s with the leg in the fully extended position. This exercise should be repeated at least 50 to 100 times per day. When this exercise can be performed in a pain-free fashion, progressive resistive exercises may be instituted. Straight-leg raising exercises, with weights around the ankles, have proved to be effective in further increasing the strength of the quadriceps group. The maximum weight can be lifted through 10 repetitions to an angle of 45 degrees at the hip, and is used initially for a maximum of 30 to 40 repetitions a day. The weight can be increased to 20 to 30 lbs (9 to 13.6 kg) as strength increases. It must be emphasized that these exercises must be performed with the knee in the fully extended position. Even short arc (less than 30 degrees) knee flexion has been shown to be detrimental in some circumstances.[28]

When the exercise programme is followed, a gradual return to full activities is usually possible after 4 weeks. Some patients will find it necessary to be reminded to continue a maintenance programme of periodic quadriceps exercises to prevent recurrent patellofemoral pain.

Aspirin and other non-steroidal anti-inflammatory drugs are currently the only medications used in the management of chondromalacia patella. Although Chrisman[21] demonstrated that aspirin did not promote matrix healing with established cartilage defects, there is some rationale for the use of aspirin in patellofemoral disorders. Aspirin or other anti-inflammatory drugs are chiefly used as a means of reducing the synovitis that follows cartilage destruction in chondromalacia patella, and possibly as a means of preventing a further breakdown of articular cartilage. A dose of 600 mg four times a day is recommended in the patient who does not respond to rest and quadriceps muscle strengthening. Intra-articular steroid injections should be reserved for those unique circumstances where synovitis is the major component.

Other conservative measures, such as knee bracing which provides support for the knee or prevents lateral subluxation of the patella, have been utilized with varying degrees of success. Orthotics within shoes have provided useful correction in runners with excessive foot pronation. Gruber suggests that conservative treatment for chondromalacia patella should be abandoned if there is no improvement after 3 months, or if the symptoms worsen after 1 month.[31]

However, the physician should be alert to the patient who has a very low pain threshold.

Surgical treatment of chondromalacia patella

In less than one-third of patients with chondromalacia patella, the pain associated with the condition is so severe and disabling that operative treatment is considered. Several operative procedures have been suggested and varying degrees of success have been recorded. Operative procedures used in treating chondromalacia patella fall into the following categories:

(1) arthroscopic debridement of articular surface;

(2) patellofemoral realignment procedures;

(3) procedures to reduce patellofemoral joint pressure;

(4) salvage procedures.

It is of the utmost importance to determine the aetiology of the patient's symptoms prior to initiating surgical treatment. For example, the patient with anterior knee pain secondary to chronic overuse and with normal patellofemoral alignment would not benefit from a patellofemoral realignment procedure.

Debridement of the patella, performed in a transarthroscopic fashion, has resulted in varying degrees of success. This procedure has been performed extensively by Wiles et al.[32] with satisfactory results. However, Bentley[33] reports only a 25 per cent success rate in over 60 patients.

Historically, the most encouraging procedure was devised by Insall et al.[34] in which, following a lateral release of the retinaculum, the medial and lateral components of the quadriceps expansion are brought together to medialize the patella. These authors reported a very high success rate.

Hughston and Walsh[35] have taken a different approach to the operative treatment of chondromalacia patella. They emphasize the importance of a proximal realignment of the patella by advancement of the vastus medialis. They report a 71 per cent success rate over a 15-year period. An alternative approach to realignment has been to transpose the patellar tendon medially, coupled with a lateral release of the quadriceps retinaculum. However, it is clear that the scientific explanation for the success of some of these operations remains rather vague.

Several procedures have been devised with the idea of decreasing the pressures exerted across the patellofemoral joint. Of particular note is the Maquet[36] tibial tubercle elevation. This procedure proposes that anterior displacement of the tibial tubercle will decrease the compressive forces acting across the patellofemoral joint. According to Maquet's original calculations, the tibial tubercle must be elevated 2 cm in order to achieve a patellofemoral force reduction of 50 per cent. More recent studies, however, indicate that the tibial tubercle needs to be elevated just 1 cm to achieve the desired goal.[37] The Maquet procedure is not without complications. Skin breakdown directly over the tibial tubercle and fractures of the tibia have been seen in association with this procedure.

The patient with incapacitating anterior knee pain refractory to conservative and other surgical measures may be a candidate for patellar resurfacing arthroplasty[38] or even patellectomy. These salvage procedures must be done with extreme caution, however, as their results are unpredictable.

In general, surgery for chondromalacia patella must be approached in a very cautious fashion.

Iliotibial-band friction syndrome

Iliotibial-band friction syndrome is an overuse injury frequently affecting individuals participating in endurance athletic activities. This syndrome, which commonly manifests itself as a poorly local-

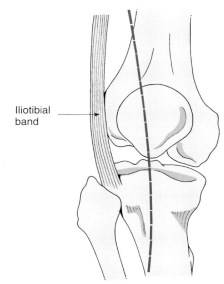

Fig. 9 The iliotibial band is the thickened strip of fascia lata that passes distally over the lateral femoral condyle to insert into Gerdy's tubercle. The alignment of the femur and tibia is denoted by the dotted line.

ized pain over the lateral femoral condyle, has rarely been described in the literature. Once seen almost exclusively in long-distance runners, it is now being recognized in other marathon-type athletes such as cyclists.

In terms of anatomy, the iliotibial band is a thickened strip of fascia lata that receives part of the insertion of the tensor fascia lata and the gluteus maximus (Fig. 9). It passes distally down the lateral aspect of the thigh in continuity with the lateral intermuscular septum and inserts into Gerdy's tubercle on the lateral tibial condyle. When the knee is in full extension the iliotibial band lies anterior to the line of flexion of the knee. Since the iliotibial band is free of bony attachments between the lateral femoral epicondyle and Gerdy's tubercle, it is free to move posterior to this axis upon flexion of the knee (Fig. 10). This posterior translocation of the iliotibial band typically occurs when the knee is at 30 degrees of flexion. It is postulated that this movement against the lateral femoral condyle leads to inflammation of the iliotibial band, resulting in the discomfort associated with this friction syndrome.[39]

Sutker et al.[41] report that the iliotibial-band friction syndrome is

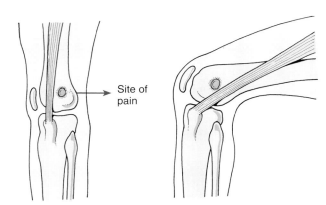

Fig. 10 The iliotibial band moves behind the lateral femoral condyle on flexion of the knee and returns to the anterior position in extension.

an overuse injury which most commonly affects males between 20 and 40 years of age who have been running 20 to 40 miles (32 to 34 km) per week for at least 3 years. A common physical finding in these men was a varus alignment of the knee. Sutker *et al.* also found that it was predominantly a unilateral disease.

The pain associated with iliotibial-band friction syndrome occurs on the outer aspect of the knee, in close relationship to the lateral femoral condyle. In a paper describing iliotibial-band friction syndrome in 16 military trainees, Renne[40] noted that the patients were first seen because of a limp and pain on the lateral aspect of the knee when walking or running. The symptoms commonly occur after a long run or hike, with the pain worsening with increased distance. The pain usually worsens when walking up or down stairs and hills. Any activity which causes excessive compression between the iliotibial band and the lateral femoral condyle may cause or aggravate symptoms. This may occur, for example, in the runner who increases his/her length of stride or the cyclist who rides with the seat excessively high.[40-42]

Both Renne[40] and Sutker *et al.*[41] reported the following physical findings. All patients had focal tenderness at a point over the lateral femoral epicondyle, approximately 3 cm proximal to the knee joint. The pain was reproduced by having the person support their whole bodyweight on the affected leg, with the knee held in 30 degrees of flexion, gradually rocking over the top of the weight-bearing extremity. This manoeuvre is known to bring the iliotibial band into prominence. A full range of motion of the hip and knee is present. In a select group of patients, a peculiar 'creak' is felt while palpating the lateral femoral condyle during flexion and extension of the knee. Renne described this sensation as resembling rubbing a finger over a wet balloon.

Tenderness or effusion of the knee, ligament laxity, swelling, and a positive McMurray's test are all absent. Varus stressing of the knee does not predictably trigger discomfort. The functional examination reveals that the patients could jog in place, hop, squat, and rise without significant discomfort.[40-42]

As mentioned earlier, the knee alignment of individuals presenting with iliotibial-band friction syndrome is neutral or varus; it is extremely uncommon for a patient with genu valgum to present with this particular syndrome, presumably because less stress is put on the iliotibial band in that particular alignment.

In Renne's study of 16 military trainees who were diagnosed as having the iliotibial-band friction syndrome,[40] the radiographs of the symptomatic knees could not be distinguished from those of age-matched controls. No degenerative changes or prominent osteophytes were observed. Sutker *et al.*[41] report that three of the runners in their study had arthrograms which were within normal limits.

In the treatment of an athlete with iliotibial-band friction syndrome, it must be stressed that this disorder is an overuse injury. Perhaps the most valuable component of the treatment regime for this condition is reduction of the stress to the knee. The patient should also be told to avoid conditions which make the symptoms worse, such as running up or down hills. Shortening the running stride may also be helpful; however, this has not been proved.[40-42]

In addition to reducing the athletic stress, oral non-steroidal anti-inflammatory medications have proved to be useful in the reduction of inflammation associated with this syndrome. With per-

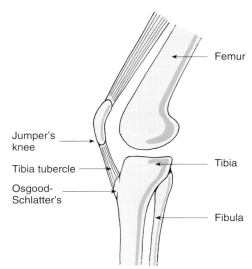

Fig. 11 The site of maximum tenderness in jumper's knee in contrast to Osgood–Schlatter's disease.

sistence of the symptoms, steroid injections may be given at 2-week intervals until the pain disappears.[40] Renne found that, with these measures, all the patients were able to complete the remaining 3 months of military training. Lateral shoe orthotics have also been shown to be effective in relieving the symptoms of this condition.[40,42]

If the treatment format described above is unsuccessful, a period of total rest (4 to 6 weeks) is recommended. Surgery remains the very last resort. Surgical options include percutaneous or open release of iliotibial-band fibres at the area where the iliotibial band migrates over the lateral femoral condyle. Holmes has effectively used a technique which involves excising an elliptical piece from the posterior aspect of the iliotibial band off the lateral femoral condyle.[39]

Patellar tendinitis

Patellar tendinitis, or 'jumper's knee', refers to a clinical syndrome frequently seen in athletes who participate in sports which usually involve jumping, thus placing excessive stress on the extensor apparatus of the knee. Generally, the pathology associated with jumpers' knee is triggered by incessant jumping, sometimes with single-foot landings. Volleyball players, basketball players, and high jumpers will frequently present with symptoms consistent with patellar tendinitis.

The actual pathology associated with jumpers' knee is localized at the level of the bone–tendon junction, thus suggesting that jumper's knee is an overload lesion comparable with other insertional tendinopathies (Fig. 11).

The normal junction between bone and tendon shows four distinct zones: namely, tendon, fibrocartilage, mineralized fibrocartilage, and bone (see Chapter 4.4.4). A well-demarcated borderline, the 'blue line' separates the fibrocartilage from the mineralized fibrocartilage; none of the zones has a thickness exceeding 2 mm. In jumpers' knee, or patellar tendinitis, the 'blue line' is absent, the fibrocartilage is much thicker than normal, and pseudocysts can be present at the borderline between the mineralized fibrocartilage and bone.[44] Patellar tendinitis is characterized by the insidious onset of aching in the knee centred over the infrapatellar region, usually localized to the inferior pole of the patella. A study[44] of volleyball players presenting with symptoms of jumpers' knee showed that 65 per cent had pain over the inferior pole of the patella, 25 per cent had discomfort over the superior pole, and 10 per cent had pain at the site of the insertion of the patellar tendon into the tibial tuberosity. In mild cases, pain was predominantly felt during, and more frequently after, athletic activity. Day-to-day activities such as climbing and descending stairs can frequently aggravate the pain. The aching type of discomfort usually disappears after a period of rest ranging from a few hours to several days depending on the severity of the symptoms. Some patients may report swelling of the knee, but upon further questioning it appears that they are describing a feeling of fullness in the area of the lesion. Rarely, the onset of pain may be related to a discrete injury during a take off or landing, followed by the development of persistent aching in the knee. Less frequently, the onset of pain can be attributed to a direct blow to the knee such as being kicked or falling on hard ground.[45]

If untreated, the symptoms experienced by the patient may progress to become more frequent and disabling. As it worsens, the condition leads to persistent discomfort which completely disrupts athletic activity. In these cases, pain may be present even when the patient walks, causing a disturbed gait and decrease in the excursion of the knee joint. The discomfort may be relieved when the patient lies in a supine position with the knee fully extended. The pain may also occur after prolonged sitting, so that the individual feels compelled to extend the knee.

If the patient is permitted to continue with intense athletic activity, a catastrophic circumstance may occur with complete rupture of the tendinous attachment to the involved pole. This is rare.

The diagnosis of patellar tendinitis can be established on the basis of physical examination by demonstrating exquisite tenderness upon palpation at the inferior/superior pole of the patella or at the insertion of the patellar tendon to the tibial tuberosity. At times, a cystic fluctuation may be present in that area. However, a generalized effusion of the knee is rather unusual. Signs of injury of the meniscus and ligaments are absent.

Certain anatomical abnormalities such as patellar hypermobility, patella alta, Osgood–Schlatter's disease, or genu recurvatum may be present; however, their role in the pathological process of patellar tendinitis is not yet understood.[45]

In evaluating the patient radiographically, plain radiographs of the knee including tangential views are appropriate. The radiographs may be reported as normal initially, or lucency at the involved pole of the patella may be observed. Adolescents and teenagers should show irregular centres of ossification in the involved poles or a periosteal reaction at the anterior surface of the patella in the involved area.[45] Elongation of the involved pole, occasionally with a stress fracture at the junction of the main portion of the patella, has also been observed. Other alterations observed in radiographs of patients with patellar tendinitis include fatigue fractures of the inferior pole of the patella, calcification of the involved tendon, and patella alta. A complete avulsion of the inferior pole of the patella has been seen, but exclusively in the endstage of this condition.

Recently, the ultrasound computed tomographic (CT), and magnetic resonance imaging (MRI) findings associated with patellar tendinitis have been described in the literature.[47,48]

Tendon enlargement and reduced echogenicity were seen consistently on ultrasound visualization of affected tendons. CT findings include tendon enlargement and reduced attenuation of the central portion of the tendon. MRI images of affected tendons in patellar tendinitis showed increased signal intensity on T_1, T_2, and proton-density weighted images and increased anteroposterior (AP) diameter of the tendon proximally (greater than 7 mm). In addition, the margins of affected tendons were indistinct, especially posterior to the thickened segment. Jumpers' knee can be classified according to symptoms into four stages.[45,46]

Stage I

The individual manifesting the early phases of patellar tendinitis, who has pain only after activity, can be treated with mild restriction of activity, non-steroidal anti-inflammatory agents, and ice massage. In most instances, the symptoms will disappear and remain quiescent after the medication is terminated. In other cases, the symptoms will disappear while on medication, only to reappear when those same medications are discontinued. Local corticosteroid injections are not recommended for the individual with stage I patellar tendinitis. Some symptoms may be alleviated with the use of a long, elastic knee support or a horseshoe type of orthotic inserted around the patella. This can be fabricated from felt, which is readily available.

Stage II

These patients should use the same treatment modalities as the individual with less pain. They should use moist heat. If the aching becomes more intense and the athlete is becoming impaired in his or her performance, a low-dose corticosteroid injection may be employed. The athlete should be made aware of the potential hazard of corticosteroid injections. A programme of repeated injections of cortisone should not be condoned.

Stage III

These patients suffer with pain which is present before, during, and after athletic performance. These individuals should be advised to curtail their athletic activities, while being placed on an aggressive exercise programme to strengthen their patellar tendon. This has been well described by Stanish and Curwin.[49]

It should be noted that, even for those individuals with stage I or stage II patellar tendinitis, an aggressive exercise programme is an essential component of rehabilitation once the initial inflammatory phase has been controlled.

Stage IV

In most cases, a complete rupture of the patellar tendon is treated surgically. After a brief period of immobilization the patient is gradually started on a progressive exercise programme, finally terminating with an eccentric loading programme to the tendons. It is generally accepted that it will be 6 to 12 months before the athlete can return to aggressive ballistic activities. The surgical procedures have been described by many authors including Blazina et al.[45]

Excision of the degenerative portion of the involved tendon has been described by some workers, while others have suggested that a resection of the involved pole of the patella may prove successful.

Medial compartment overload

Introduction

Osteoarthritis is a degenerative disease of synovial joints. Although the initial changes in an osteoarthritic joint are still the subject of speculation, several consistent observations have been made. Freeman and Meachian[50] have suggested that the initial lesion is in the cartilage fibre framework of the articular surface, causing an abnormally wide separation of the fibres, a deterioration in the mechanical strength of the matrix, and thus an increased susceptibility to further structural damage during use of the knee joint. A second hypothesis[50-52] considers the importance of proteoglycan in giving cartilage its unique properties and protecting the collagen fibre framework from damage during joint use. A change in proteoglycan synthesis by chondrocytes occurs in the early stages of experimentally induced osteoarthritis in dogs, and is accompanied by an ultrastructural deterioration in the collagen framework of the articular cartilage.[53] Another hypothesis suggests that the initial event may be an enzymatic degradation of the collagen in the articular cartilage by collagenase activity, or enzymatic degradation of the proteoglycan resulting in loss of its protective effect against collagen framework damage. The common factor in all theories of the initiation of osteoarthritis is change in the collagen framework of articular cartilage.[54]

When a person with normally aligned extremities stands on both legs, the line of weight bearing travels from the centre of the femoral head to the centre of the knee and through the centre of the ankle.[55]

In patients with abnormally aligned lower extremities, however, the line of force is very different. In a patient with genu varum the weight-bearing line will pass through the medial tibial plateau (Fig. 12), while in a patient with genu valgum the weight-bearing line will pass through the lateral tibial plateau. During normal walking, a force of approximately three times bodyweight is transmitted through the knee, with the largest portion of this force being borne on the medial side of the knee.[56] Other activities, such as running or climbing stairs, increase the force transmitted through the knee to approximately four to five times bodyweight.[56] Therefore it should not be surprising that individuals who are involved in regular vigorous physical activity tend to have knee problems, particularly medial knee problems. This so-called medial compartment overload may result in several disease processes, the most important of which is osteoarthritis.

Of all the joints, the knee best illustrates the biomechanical contribution to osteoarthritis and its progression. The enormous stresses which are put on the knee joint during physical activities evoke a response by the musculoskeletal system, resulting in osteoarthritis. Any pre-existing problems to the knee joint which produce increased articular surface stress result in a predictable osteoarthritis of the knee. These problems include meniscal tears, instability secondary to ligament disruption, irregularity of the articular surface secondary to a tibial plateau fracture, and angular deformities following fractures to the femur or tibia.[57]

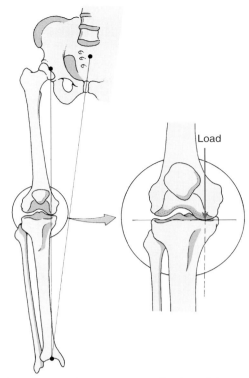

Fig. 12 A knee demonstrating genu varum resulting in medial compartment overload.

Pain, usually with activity, is virtually always a presenting complaint of a patient with osteoarthritis of the knee. The patient may also complain of stiffness in the morning and after sitting for a prolonged period. This stiffness tends to lessen with activity but returns later in the day.[58]

The history obtained from the patient is extremely important in determining the extent of the problem and the mode of therapy which should be employed. The most important piece of information, which must be extracted, is whether or not there is pain with activity. The physician must determine, with the help of the patient, if there is pain with weight bearing, the location of the pain, and the specific limitations.

Some patients will have osteoarthritis, but will demonstrate extremely mild symptoms. Frequently, there is no history of an initiating cause such as trauma. Many patients will describe intermittent difficulty with the knee that has gradually worsened over a period of years. The patient/athlete may also describe an apparent increase in deformity of the lower extremities.

Physical examination of the osteoarthritic knee should be directed towards demonstrating the location and degree of articular cartilage degeneration. Initially, any patient presenting with a lower extremity problem should be carefully observed standing, walking, and then running on the spot. Males, who are more prone to varus deformity of the knee, tend to have more medial compartment osteoarthritis than females, because varus alignment tends to overload the medial compartment of the knee. The range of motion of the knee should be noted. Care should be taken in differentiating mechanical disturbance of the knee seen with loose bodies or meniscal damage. The knee should be checked for injuries to ligaments, particularly the anterior and posterior cruciate ligaments. Osteo-arthritis can occur as a consequence of long-standing knee instabil-ity. Finally, examination of the osteoarthritic knee should include an examination of the hip and ankle. A neurological examination and examination of the vascular tree should be routine.

In the radiographic analysis to delineate medial compartment osteoarthritis, plain radiographs of the knee should be augmented with weight-bearing radiographs. For a more in-depth analysis, CT scanning may be helpful and confirmatory in determining the pres-ence of ligament and/or meniscal disturbance.

The treatment of osteoarthritis of the knee depends strongly on the severity of the symptoms, the structural abnormalities present, and associated factors such as the age of the patient and concomitant medical difficulties.[57] Most patients should initially be treated with a non-surgical programme consisting of exercise modification. Intra-articular cortical steroid injections should be used cautiously to control the inflammatory component of the osteoarthritis. Emphasis should be placed on isometric exercises designed to increase the strength of the surrounding musculature. Those exer-cises specific for quadriceps strengthening are similar to those pre-viously described for patients with chondromalacia patella.

One treatment which is frequently overlooked by the practi-tioner is the importance of weight loss by the athlete. Usually this tactic is fundamental to the more mature athlete. As mentioned pre-viously, the knee receives a compressive force during weight bearing which approximates three times bodyweight, depending on the pos-ition of the knee. It follows that if a patient/athlete looses 1 kg of bodyweight, the force transmitted through the knee joint may be decreased by as much as 3 kg. The patient must understand that increased stress on the knee joint means increasing pain.

Another non-surgical technique for the treatment of medial compartment osteoarthritis of the knee is the use of lateral heel wedges in shoes. Shoe orthotics, although cumbersome, are effect-ive in relieving symptoms of medial compartment osteoarthritis.

Surgical intervention in medial compartment overload, with sec-ondary osteoarthritis, is reserved for those patients who are refrac-tory to non-surgical measures and are in considerable pain. Some examples of surgical procedures which may be performed are debridement, high tibial osteotomy, hemiarthroplasty, and if all else fails, complete knee arthroplasty.

Osteochondritis dissecans

Introduction

Osteochondritis dissecans is a condition in which part of the articu-lar surface of a joint separates due to a plane of cleavage through the subchondral bone. This condition is found most commonly in the knee, most specifically in the medial femoral condyle. However, it may occur in other joints such as the hip, ankle, and elbow.

In almost 75 per cent of cases the patient suffering with this condition is a young athletic male. The symptoms are usually uni-lateral. The literature reveals that there are two different clinical subsets which frequently present with osteochondritis dissecans:

(1) the child, or younger adolescent (5 to 15 years of age) who demonstrates open growth plates;

(2) the older adolescent or adult (15 to 50 years of age).

Theories

The most widely accepted theories regarding the aetiology of osteo-chondritis dissecans are trauma and ischaemia.

Trauma was first suggested as a cause for osteochondritis dis-secans by Paget[58] and König.[59]

König believed that trauma caused necrosis to part of the under-lying bone and this was followed by a dissecting inflammation which caused the fragment of bone and articular cartilage to separate from the underlying bone. In 1933, Fairbanks[60] published a paper which strongly supported the theory that trauma plays at least a part in triggering osteochondritis dissecans. Fairbanks suggested that the tibial spine could impinge against the medial femoral condyle dur-ing rotational strains (applied to the tibia or femur) and thus would cause a fracture through the subchondral bone. The articular sur-face could remain intact for a time, depending on the stress to the knee. If, in fact, the knee continued to be used in its normal fashion, repeated movement could provoke a non-union and the fracture would eventually extend through the articular surface.[61]

Direct trauma to the knee has always been proposed in the aeti-ology of osteochrondritis dissecans. The medial articular facet of the patella has been shown to contact the classic site of osteochon-dritis dissecans when the knee is fully flexed. In an experimental study in dogs, Rebhein[62] produced lesions, caused by repeated minor trauma to the anterior aspect of the knee, which histologically and radiographically resembled those of osteochondritis disse-cans.[61]

Many researchers have suggested ischaemia as a major factor in the development of osteoarthritis dissecans. The theory presented is that obstruction of end arteries to the femoral condyle, at the site of involvement, could precipitate a separation between the cartilage and the bone. Everything from fat emboli to bacterial infection has been proposed to cause such vascular obstruction.[63]

Enneking[65] compared the blood supply of subchondral bone to that of bowel mesentery with its end-arterial arcade and found that terminal branches of vessels to subchondral bone anastomose poorly with their neighbours. Therefore, infarction will result in the necrosis of a wedge-shaped piece of bone immediately beneath the articular cartilage. A zone of granulation tissue is formed between the viable bone and the necrotic wedge, as in the growth of vascular buds, and mesenchymal cells initiate resorption of the necrotic bone. The intact overlying articular cartilage usually holds the wedge in place; however, additional trauma may cause fracture of the articular cartilage and loosening of the wedge. The articular car-tilage will remain intact since its nutrient supply is the synovial fluid, but the subchondral bone will undergo necrosis because of the loss of blood supply.[63]

Recently, biomechanical studies[64] have shown that repeated vig-orous exercise involving extreme knee flexion produces rapidly changing strain patterns in the distal femur. This may be respon-sible for the local subchondral bone collapse seen in osteochondritis dissecans.

Symptomatology

The symptoms of osteochondritis dissecans are often poorly local-ized and non-specific. Patients usually report pain, but of varying degrees. Not infrequently stiffness and possible knee swelling is evi-dent. As the condition progresses, a sensation of catching, locking, or giving way may be described. The symptoms more commonly exacerbate with exertion and if a loose body is formed in the joint, symptoms will become more specific.[63]

Physical examination

Physical examination may reveal quadriceps atrophy. Rarely, an effusion may be obvious. The involved femoral condyle, usually medial, is frequently tender to palpation when the knee is flexed. The loose body may be palpated, but this is extremely rare. The patient may walk with the tibia externally rotated in order to avoid impinging the tibial eminence with the lateral aspect of the medial femoral condyle. Flexing the knee to 90 degrees while internally rotating the tibia will usually result in pain elicited at 30 degrees of flexion—this is known as a positive Wilson test.[66] This pain is relieved by externally rotating the tibia.

Radiographic evaluation

Radiographic examination of the affected knee will reveal a well-circumscribed area of subchondral bone, sometimes separated from the remaining femoral condyle by a crescent-shaped radiolucent line.[63] An intercondylar notch or a view of the intercondylar notch—a tunnel view—is often the most useful radiography, as the classic location of the lesion is the lateral aspect of the medial femoral condyle. Harding[67] reports that the defect of osteochondritis dissecans is commonly located in this subarticular bone of the medial femoral condyle between two radiographic lines. One line extends anteriorly from the density of the roof of the intercondylar notch, and the other extends distally from the posterior cortex of the distal femoral diaphysis. Osteochondritis dissecans may also involve the articular surface of the patella.

Treatment of osteochondritis dissecans

The treatment of osteochondritis dissecans depends on the skeletal maturity of the patient and the stage of the lesion. When the individual is skeletally immature the knee has a greater capacity for healing. Thus the non-displaced osteochondritis dissecans lesion in patients under 15 years of age can be treated with reduced activity, immobilization, and observation for up to 16 weeks.[68]

Aggressive surgery, such as drilling or pinning the osteochondritic defect is reserved for partially or completely separated fragments, or for those lesions which do not completely heal after the generally prescribed 16 weeks of immobilization. Although cannulated screws have been used most extensively for fragment fixation, comparable results have been observed with Herbert screws and tibial cortical-bone peg fixation. Absorbable pin (poly(p-dioxanone)) fixation has also been used with some success, but long-term results for this treatment method are not yet available.[69]

Patients in whom absorbable pins are used are saved the possible morbidity associated with a second operative procedure for hardware removal. The function of drilling the bone in a child who does not respond quickly to immobilization is merely to speed the revascularization and to reduce the period of morbidity. Most cases do extremely well regardless of the treatment protocol. Unfortunately, the story is quite different for adults with osteochondritis dissecans.

Linden[70] evaluated 67 joints in 58 patients with an average follow-up of 33 years. None of these patients had loose fragments replaced or internal fixation of any kind. Linden concluded that children did well and generally had no secondary degenerative changes or complications. In contrast, adults often had pain, instability, and decreased range of motion. Osteoarthritis of the affected knee eventually appeared in 100 per cent of patients who developed osteochondritis dissecans after closure of the physis.

Arthroscopic surgery is an invaluable tool in the diagnosis and treatment of osteochondritis dissecans. With the aid of an arthroscope, the lesion may be visualized, drilled, curetted, or pinned. Loose bodies can be removed with minimal morbidity. Guhl[71] classifies lesions by location, percentage of weight-bearing surface, and the degree of separation. The treatment chosen depends on these factors.

Operative treatment is indicated in a symptomatic adult knee with a lesion greater than 1 cm and involvement of the weight-bearing surface. Lesions with intact articular cartilage are drilled, while those which involve early separation of a fragment are drilled and may be pinned in place. Postoperative therapy is individualized and depends on the extent and the severity of the original lesion. Those patients with intact lesions may bear weight immediately, while those with loose bodies or detached fragments can begin weight bearing when the lesions are stable.

The younger patient with osteochondritis dissecans involving a significant portion of the weight-bearing surface of the femoral condyle poses a serious therapeutic dilemma, particularly if the segment is completely separated and cannot be replaced. These patients are not candidates for knee arthroplasty, and other modes of treatment have also proved quite ineffective. Gross[72] has done some work with fresh osteochondral allografts in this condition, and has reported excellent results in patients who had osteoarthritis, post-traumatic osteoarthritis, and osteonecrosis. Osteotomy of the tibia or femur is potentially quite a useful tool in the treatment of osteochondritis dissecans; this may have some effect in unloading the overloaded medial compartment, thereby decreasing the pressure on the osteochondritic lesion.

Recently, work has been carried out on treating cartilaginous and osteocartilaginous defects in the knee with autologous chondrocyte transplantation. A Swedish group has reported impressive results after transplanting cultured autologous chondrocytes into areas of deep cartilage defects in femoral condyles. On follow-up arthroscopy, the transplanted areas were not only macroscopically similar to surrounding healthy cartilage, but biopsy specimens taken from the transplanted area were microscopically similar to the surrounding cartilage.[73]

Clanton and DeLee[63] have devised the following summary for the treatment of osteochondritis dissecans. In the first instance it is essential to differentiate between childhood and adult forms. The symptomatic child is initially treated by decreasing activity. Multiple epiphyseal dysplasia and irregular ossification must be ruled out, and then arthroscopy is indicated. This permits a direct visualization of the lesion and drilling of the soft, but intact, articular cartilage. Flap fragments are reattached with pins after the base is curetted under arthroscopic control. Loose bodies are treated in the same fashion as in the adult.

The treatment of the symptomatic adult is more aggressive and is based upon the radiographic and arthroscopic appearance of the lesion. Soft, but intact, cartilage is drilled via the arthroscope. The arthroscope also allows drilling, curettage, and peg stabilization of separated but undisplaced fragments. Loose bodies in non-weight-bearing areas are removed during arthroscopy and the crater is debrided to offer a bleeding surface. Any larger loose bodies consisting of articular cartilage and bone must be reattached, particularly if a weight-bearing area of the femoral condyle is involved—this usually requires an arthrotomy. Cancellous bone graft is used in the base of the crater when there is a need to support a loose segment and for elevation in restoring joint congruity. Osteotomy, or the use of an allograft, is considered when the defect remains after surgical debridement and is followed by non-weight-bearing ambulation coupled with continuous passive motion.

Conclusion

Osteochondritis dissecans can be very perplexing, particularly when the joint surface damage is extensive. Surgery is reserved as a last resort, but may be necessary in the very severe case.

References

1. Last RJ. *Anatomy: regional and applied.* 7th edn. New York: Churchill Livingstone, 1984.
2. Kaplan EB. Some aspects of functional anatomy of the human knee joint. *Clinical Orthopaedics* 1962; **23**: 18–29.
3. Hungerford DS, Perry M. Biomechanics of the patellofemoral joint. *Clinical Orthopaedics* 1979; **144**: 9–15.
4. Turek SL. *Orthopaedics—principles and their applications.* Philadelphia: JB Lippincott, 1984.
5. Teider B, Marshall JL, Koslin B, Girgis FG. The anterior aspect of the knee joint. *Journal of Bone and Joint Surgery* 1981; **63A**: 351–6.
6. Fulkerson JP, Hungerford DS. *Disorders of the patellofemoral joint.* Baltimore: Williams and Wilkins, 1990.
7. Girgis FG, Marshall JL, Al Monajem ARS. The cruciate ligaments of the knee joint: anatomical, functional, and experimental analysis. *Clinical Orthopaedics* 1975; **106**: 216–31.
8. Odensten M, Gilliquist J. Functional anatomy of the anterior cruciate ligament and a rationale for reconstruction. *Journal of Bone and Joint Surgery* 1985; **67A**: 257–61.
9. Smillie IS. *Injuries of the knee joint.* Edinburgh: Livingstone, 1970.
10. Last RJ. The popliteus muscle and the lateral meniscus. *Journal of Bone and Joint Surgery* 1950; **32B**: 93–9.
11. Cohn AK, Mains DB. Popliteal hiatus of the lateral meniscus. *American Journal of Sports Medicine* 1979; **7**: 221–6.
12. O'Rahilly R, Gardiner ED, Gray DJ. *Anatomy. A regional study of human structure.* Philadelphia: WB Saunders, 1986.
13. Shaw JA, Eng M, Murray DG. The longitudinal axis of the knee and the role of cruciate ligaments in controlling transverse rotation. *Journal of Bone and Joint Surgery* 1974; **56A**: 1603.
14. Barnett CH. Locking at the knee joint. *Journal of Anatomy* 1953; **87**: 91–5.
15. McCall J. In: Wright V, ed. *Lubrication and wear in joints.* Philadelphia: JB Lippincott, 1969.
16. Weiss C, Rosenberg L, Helfet AJ. An ultrastructural study of normal adult human cartilage. *Journal of Bone and Joint Surgery* 1968; **50A**: 663–74.
17. James SL. Chondromalacia of the patella in the adolescent. In: Kennedy JC, ed. *The injured adolescent knee.* Baltimore: Williams and Wilkins, 1979.
18. Mansour JM, Mow VC. The permeability of articular cartilage under compressive strain and at high pressures. *Journal of Bone and Joint Surgery* 1976; **58A**: 509–10.
19. Goodfellow J, Hungerford DS, Woods C. Patellofemoral joint

mechanics and pathology. Chondromalacia patella. *Journal of Bone and Joint Surgery* 1976; **58B**: 291–9.
20. Darracott J, Vernon-Roberts B. The bony changes in chondromalacia patellae. *Rheumatology and Physical Medicine* 1971; **11**: 175–9.
21. Chrisman OD. The role of articular cartilage in patellofemoral pain. *Orthopedic Clinics of North America* 1986; **17**: 231–4.
22. James SL, Bates BT, Ostering LR. Injuries to runners. American Journal of Sports Medicine 1978; 6: 40–50.
23. Bentley G, Dowd G. Current concepts of etiology and treatment of chondromalacia patellae. *Clinical Orthopaedics* 1984; **189**: 209–27.
24. Carson W, James SL, Singer KM, Winternitz WW. Patellofemoral disorders: physical and radiographic evaluation. *Clinical Orthopedics* 1984; **185**: 165–77.
25. Hughston JC. Subluxation of the patella. *Journal of Bone and Joint Surgery* 1968; **50A**: 1003.
26. Dimon JH. Apprehension test for subluxation of the patella. *Clinical Orthopedics* 1974; **103**: 39.
27. DeHaven KE, Dolan WA, Mayer PJ. Chondromalacia patellae in athletes. Clinical presentation and conservative management. *American Journal of Sports Medicine* 1979; **7**: 5–11.
28. Fisher RL. Conservative treatment of patellofemoral pain. *Orthopedic Clinics of North America* 1986; **17**: 269–72.
29. Smillie JS. *Diseases of the knee joint.* London: Churchill Livingstone, 1974.
30. Radin EL. A rational approach to the treatment of patellofemoral pain. *Clinical Orthopedics* 1979; **144**: 107–9.
31. Gruber MA. The conservative treatment of chondromalacia patella. *Orthopedic Clinics of North America* 1979; **10**: 105–15.
32. Wiles P, Andrews PS, Bremmer RA. Chondromalacia of the patellae: a study of the latest results of excision of the articular cartilage. *Journal of Bone and Joint Surgery* 1960; **42B**: 65.
33. Bentley G. The surgical treatment of chondromalacia patellae. *Journal of Bone and Joint Surgery* 1978; **60B**: 74.
34. Insall J, Falvo D, Wise D. Chondromalacia patella. A prospective study. *Journal of Bone and Joint Surgery* 1976; **58A**: 1–8.
35. Hughston JC, Walsh WM. Proximal and distal reconstruction of the extensor mechanism for patellar subluxation. *Clinical Orthopedics* 1979; **144**: 36.
36. Maquet P. Biomechanical treatment of osteoarthritis of the knee. In: Maquet P, ed. *Biomechanics of the knee.* 5th edn. New York: Springer, 1984; 139.
37. Koshino T. Changes in patellofemoral compressive force after anterior or anteromedial displacement of tibial tuberosity for chondromalacia patellae. *Clinical Orthopaedics and Related Research* 1991; May(266): 133–8.
38. Harrington KD. Long-term results for the Mckeever patellar resurfacing prosthesis used as a salvage procedure for severe chondromalacia patellae. *Clinical Orthopaedics and Related Research* 1992; Jun(279): 201–13.
39. Holmes JC, Pruitt AL, Whalen NJ. Iliotibial band syndrome in cyclists. *American Journal of Sports Medicine* 1993; **21**: 419–24.
40. Renne JW. The iliotibial band friction syndrome. *Journal of Bone and Joint Surgery* 1975; **57A**: 1110–11.
41. Sutker AN, Jackson DW, Pagliano JW. Iliotibial band syndrome in distance runners. *Physicians and Sports Medicine* 1981; **9**.
42. Noble CA. Iliotibial band fricion syndrome in runners. *American Journal of Sports Medicine* 1980; **8**: 232–4.
43. Ferretti A, Appolito E, Mariani PP, Puddu G. Jumper's knee. *American Journal of Sports Medicine* 1983; **11**: 58–62.
44. Ferretti A, Papandrea P, Conteduea F. Knee injuries in volleyball. *Sports Medicine* 1990; **10**: 132–8.
45. Blazina ME, Karlan RK, Jobe FW. Jumper's knee. *Orthopedic Clinics of North America* **4**: 665–73.

46. Roels J, Martens M, Mulier JC, Burssens A. Patellar tendinitis (jumper's knee). *American Journal of Sports Medicine* 1978; **6**: 362–8.

47. Davies SG, Baudouin CJ, King FB, Perry JD. Ultrasound, computed tomography and magnetic resonance imaging in patellar tendinitis. *Clinical Radiology* 1991; **43**: 52–6.

48. el-Khoury GY, Wira RL, Berbaum KS, Pope TL Jr, Mona JU. MR imaging in patellar tendinitis. *Radiology* 1992; **184**: 849–54.

49. Stanish WD, Curwin S. *Tendinitis: its etiology and treatment*. Lexington MA: Collamore Press, 1984.

50. Freeman MAR, Meachian G. Aging and degeneration. In: Freeman MAR, ed. *Adult articular cartilage*. 2nd edn. Tunbridge Wells: Pitman Medical, 1979; 487–543.

51. Muir IHM. Biochemistry. In: Freeman MAR, ed. *Adult articular cartilage*. 2nd edn. Tunbridge Wells: Pitman Medical, 1979; 145–214.

52. Marondas A. Physicochemical properties of articular cartilage. In: Freeman MAR, ed. *Adult articular cartilage*. 2nd edn. Tunbridge Wells: Pitman Medical, 1979; 215–90.

53. Mcdevitt CA, Muir H. Biochemical changes in the cartilage of the knees in experimental and natural osteoarthritis in the dog. *Journal of Bone and Joint Surgery* 1976: **58B**: 94–101.

54. Meachian G, Brooke G. The pathology of osteoarthritis. In: Moskowitz RWD, Howell DS, Goldberg VM, Mankin HJ, eds. *Osteoarthritis, diagnosis and management*. Philadelphia: WB Saunders, 1984.

55. Maquet PJG. *Biomechanics of the knee*. New York: Springer-Verlag, 1976.

56. Morrison JB. *The forces transmitted by the human knee joint*. Thesis, University of Strathclyde, Glasgow, 1967.

57. Kettefkamp DB, Colyer RA. Osteoarthritis of the knee. In: Moskowitz RW, Howell DS, Goldberg VM, Mankin HJ, eds. *Osteoarthritis, diagnosis and management*. Philadelphia: WB Saunders, 1984.

58. Paget J. On the production of some of the loose bodies in joints. *St. Bartholomew's Hospital* 1870; **6**: 1.

59. König F. Verber freie Korper in den Gelentren. *Deutsche Zeitschrift fur Chirurgie* 1887–8; **27**: 90.

60. Fairbanks HAT. Osteochondritis dissecans. *British Journal of Surgery* 1933; **21**: 67.

61. Green JP. Osteochondritis dissecans of the knee. *Journal of Bone and Joint Surgery* 1966; **48B**: 82.

62. Rebhein F. Die Entstehung der Osteochondritis dissecans. *Archiv fur klinische Chirurgie* 1950; **256**: 69.

63. Clanton TO, DeLee JC. Osteochondritis dissecans. History, pathophysiology and current treatment concepts. *Clinical Orthopaedics* 1982; **167**: 50.

64. Nambu T, Gasser B, Schneider E, Bandi W, Perren SM. Deformation of the distal femur: a contribution towards the pathogenesis of osteochondrosis dissecans in the knee joint. *Journal of Biomechanics* 1991; **24**: 421–33.

65. Enneking WF. *Clinical musculoskeletal pathology*. Gainesville, FL: Shorter, 1977; 147.

66. Wilson JN. A diagnostic sign in osteochondritis dissecans. *Journal of Bone and Joint Surgery* 1967; **49A**: 477.

67. Harding WG III. Diagnosis of osteochondritis dissecans of the femoral condyles: the value of the lateral X-ray view. *Clinical Orthopaedics* 1977; **123**: 25.

68. Smillie IS. Treatment of osteochondritis dissecans. *Journal of Bone and Joint Surgery* 1957; **39B**: 248.

69. Rey Zuniga JJ, Sagastibelza J, Lopez Blasco JJ, Martinez Grande M. Arthroscopic use of the Herbert screw in osteochondritis dissecans of the knee. *Arthroscopy* 1993; **9**: 668–70.

70. Linden B. Osteochondritis dissecans of the femoral condyles. *Journal of Bone and Joint Surgery* 1977; **59A**: 769.

71. Guhl JF. Arthroscopic treatment of osteochondritis dissecans. *Clinical Orthopaedics and Related Research*, 1982; **167**: 65–74.

72. Gross AE. *Course on rehabilitation of articular joints by biological resurfacing*. St. Louis, MO; November 1979.

73. Brittberg M, Lindahl A, Nilsson A, Ohlsson C, Isaksson O, Peterson L. Treatment of deep cartilage defects in the knee with autologous chondrocyte transplantation. *New England Journal of Medicine* 1994; **331**: 889–95.

5.5 Overuse injuries of the foot and ankle

M.P. Schwellnus, Wayne Derman, and T.D. Noakes

Introduction

Our approach to the diagnosis of injuries to the foot and ankle is initially to establish whether the injury is acute or chronic in nature. If the injury is chronic then it is important to establish whether the injury is due to repetitive chronic trauma or chronic overuse, or if it results from an acute traumatic incident which has caused persistent foot or ankle pain. Chronic foot and ankle pain that persists after an acute traumatic incident can be due to a number of clinical conditions which are listed in Table 1. These conditions are not strictly overuse injuries and will therefore not be discussed further in this chapter.

Chronic overuse injuries of the foot and ankle present with a symptom, usually pain, that is of gradual onset. The duration of the symptom is variable and can be present for days or weeks. In these injuries it is important to establish the anatomical site of the pain early on as this provides a valuable clue to the possible aetiology of the injury.

Pain in the foot and ankle region can be in the area of the heel, the midfoot, or the forefoot. Heel pain can be posterior, plantar, medial, lateral, or diffuse while midfoot pain can be medial, central, or lateral. Forefoot pain is either predominantly dorsal or plantar.

Table 2 lists the clinical conditions associated with pain in these areas. This list is not exhaustive, but provides a basis from which to establish a working diagnosis. Some of the more common conditions that are listed in Table 2 will be discussed. Systemic and other causes of chronic foot and ankle pain are also reviewed.

Table 1 Differential diagnosis of chronic ankle pain after an acute ankle injury

1. Chronic ligamentous instability with synovitis
2. Osteochondral fractures
3. Anterolateral impingement syndrome
4. Sinus tarsi syndrome
5. Subluxing peroneal tendons
6. Osteoarthritis of the ankle joint
7. Tibiofibular ligament sprain

Heel pain

Posterior heel pain

Achilles tendon lesions

Achilles tendon lesions can present with posterior heel pain. A detailed discussion of the classification, clinical presentation, and the management of these lesions is beyond the scope of this chapter.

Haglund's syndrome

Introduction

Haglund's syndrome was first described in 1928, and is characterized by posterior heel pain and a painful swelling (so-called 'pump bump') or thickening of tissue at the insertion of the Achilles tendon into the calcaneus.[1]

Incidence

This syndrome is described in all age groups of either sex and is not related to the amount of daily activity.

Aetiology and pathology

The presumed aetiology is constant irritation of the posterior calcaneal tissues due to rigid, low-backed shoes. This causes an irritation with resultant bony changes which can be detected on radiographs. Other causes of posterior heel pain with swelling are retrocalcaneal bursitis, Achilles tendinitis, and Reiter's syndrome. These syndromes can be distinguished from Haglund's syndrome on the basis of the clinical presentation and radiographic findings.

Clinical presentation

The patient presents with symptoms of posterior heel pain and the development of a tender swelling. On examination, the tender palpable swelling is present at the site of insertion of the Achilles tendon into the calcaneus.

Radiological features

The following radiological features are characteristic of this syndrome:[1]

(1) loss of the lucent retrocalcaneal recess between the Achilles tendon and the bursal projection;

(2) associated Achilles tendinitis (Achilles tendon wider than 9 mm and 2 cm above the bursal projection);

(3) cortically intact but prominent bursal projection;

(4) a positive parallel pitch line (a radiological measurement allowing the degree of bursal projection to be calculated).[1]

Table 2 Differential diagnosis of common overuse injuries in the foot	
1. Heel pain:	
Posterior heel pain:	Achilles tendon lesions
	Haglund's syndrome
	Posterior impingement syndrome
	Calcaneal apophysitis
Plantar heel pain:	Plantar fasciitis
	Calcaneal spur formation
	Calcaneal periostitis
	Calcaneal nerve entrapment
	Fat-pad syndrome
Medial heel pain:	Tarsal tunnel syndrome
	Medial plantar entrapment
	Tibialis posterior tendinitis
Lateral heel pain:	Lateral plantar nerve entrapment
	Peroneal tendinitis
	Sinus tarsi syndrome
	Sural nerve entrapment
Diffuse heel pain:	Calcaneal stress fracture
	Tarsal coalition
2. Midfoot pain:	
Medial midfoot pain	Plantar fasciitis
	Tibialis posterior tendinitis
	Navicular stress fracture
Central midfoot pain	Extensor tendinitis
	Tarsal coalition
	Anterolateral impingement syndrome
	Tarsal coalition
Lateral midfoot pain	Cuboid stress fracture
	Peroneal tendinitis
	Cuboid subluxation
	Stress fracture of the 5th metatarsal
	Iselin's disease
3. Forefoot pain:	
Dorsal:	Extensor tendinitis
	Navicular stress fractures
	Metatarsal stress fractures
	Common peroneal nerve entrapment
Plantar:	Metatarsal stress fractures
	Interdigital neuroma
	Sesamoid injury

Management

Initial management is conservative with:

(1) shoe modification, including the prescription of a corrective orthotic to control excessive ankle pronation;

(2) heel lift;

(3) corticosteroid injection (care must be taken not to inject into or near the Achilles tendon).

Surgical excision of the bursal projection can be considered if conservative measures fail.

Posterior impingement syndrome

Posterior impingement syndrome, also known as the os trigonum syndrome, talar compression syndrome, or the posterior tibiotalar impingement syndrome, refers to a condition in which there is mechanical impingement of either soft tissue or an accessory bone (os trigonum) between the tibia and the talus in extreme plantar flexion of the ankle.[2,3]

The pathology of the condition is related to the mechanical irritation during repetitive, forced, extreme ankle plantar flexion, of:

(1) soft tissues (posteroinferior tibiofibular ligament, tibial slip ligament, flexor hallucis longus tendon, posterior tibial nerve);

(2) a prominent posterior talar tubercle;

(3) a tibial labrum on the posterior lip of the tibia; or

(4) the os trigonum.

The posterior tubercle of the talus, which arises from a separate ossification centre, can remain as accessory bone separate from the main bone in 3 to 13 per cent of cases. This accessory bone is the os trigonum.[2,3]

Patients, usually ballet dancers or gymnasts, present with posterolateral heel or ankle pain during extreme plantar flexion. Other diagnostic features of the condition are:[2,3]

(1) pain in the posterolateral aspect of the ankle joint;

(2) stiffness of the ankle joint, in particular limitation of plantar flexion;

(3) posterior heel swelling;

(4) acute pain on forced plantar flexion of the ankle joint;

(5) a sudden endpoint to forced plantar flexion of the ankle joint;

(6) a palpable, tender os trigonum;

(7) pain on active flexion and extension of the great toe if the flexor hallucis longus is impinged.

A useful clinical diagnostic test for this condition is to inject a local anaesthetic into the region. If symptoms are relieved without changing the maximum ankle-joint range of motion, the diagnosis can be confirmed. The presence of an os trigonum or a prominent posterior talar tubercle can be confirmed by radiographs which should include a lateral view in maximum plantar flexion.

Management of this condition is initially conservative and should include rest, non-steroidal anti-inflammatory medication, and local infiltration of the region with corticosteroids. Failed conservative treatment is an indication for ankle arthroscopy. In cases where the impingement is bony (os trigonum, prominent posterior talar tubercle), surgical removal of the bone produces a successful result.[2]

Calcaneal apophysitis (Sever's disease)

In children, a number of overuse injuries of the lower limb, including the foot and ankle, have been described in relation to growth plates. These are usually traction injuries where tendons attach to growth plates (apophyses). Traumatic calcaneal apophysitis is an injury that usually occurs in the 8- to 13-year-old age group and is the result of excessive traction of the Achilles tendon on the calcaneal apophysis. Patients present with posterior heel pain with or without a lump. It is characteristic that lateral pressure and not direct pressure elicits pain in the area.[4] Biomechanical abnormalities that may be associated with this condition are:

- tight gastrocnemius–soleus muscle
- excessive internal femoral rotation
- rearfoot valgus
- forefoot varus.

Radiographs may show non-specific sclerosis and fragmentation.

In general, management of this injury aims to reduce the load on the tendon by restricting activity, altering lower limb biomechanics if necessary, and treating the symptoms. Specific conservative measures consists of heel elevation, Achilles tendon stretching, antipronation shoes or orthotics, activity restriction (which can be for up to 4 to 6 weeks), and local or systemic anti-inflammatory treatment.

Plantar heel pain

Injuries of the plantar fascia and attachments
Anatomy
The plantar fascia is a thick band of longitudinally arranged fibres which originate from the tuberosity of the calcaneus. The fascia is also known as the plantar aponeurosis and consists of thinner medial and lateral portions, and a thick central portion.[5,6] Distally, the thick central portion divides into five slips (one for each digit). The distal slips insert into the sides of the flexor tendon sheaths of each toe.[7]

The tuberosity and adjacent regions of the calcaneus also serve as important sites of attachment for several other muscles deep to the plantar fascia. These structures help to maintain the integrity of the long arch of the foot. These muscles are the abductor hallucis (medial tuberosity), flexor digitorum brevis (medial tuberosity), and the abductor digiti minimi (lateral aspect of the tuberosity).[8]

Deeper to this muscle layer, the quadratus plantae muscle originates from two heads (medial and lateral) just distal to the tuberosity. The long plantar ligament also arises distal to the tuberosity and inserts onto the inferior aspect of the cuboid and the bases of the third, fourth, and fifth metatarsal heads.[7]

Biomechanics and pathology
The plantar fascia spans the calcaneocuboid, the talonavicular, the tarsometatarsal, and the metatarsophalangeal joints. Dorsiflexion of the toes (either by muscle action or by passive stretch as in excessive weight bearing) increases the tension in the plantar fascia. This is most marked when the big toe dorsiflexes.[9] Eversion of the calcaneus as a result of excessive rearfoot pronation, a cavus foot, and inflexibility of the Achilles tendon have all been suggested as causes for increased tension in the plantar fascia throughout the stance phase of the gait cycle.[7,10] These tensile forces are highest in the plantar fascia during the stance phase and the push-off phase of the running cycle.

Recurrent mechanical loading of the connective tissue of the plantar fascia and its attachments will cause microtrauma and result in chronic inflammation. Inflammation as a result of trauma to the plantar fascia itself is true plantar fasciitis. However, persistent application of forces to the attachments can result in injury to the periosteum (calcaneal periostitis) and the continuous repair and remodelling can lead to fibrosis and later ossification at the ligamentous periosteal junction (calcaneal spur formation). Three separate syndromes can therefore be distinguished on the basis of the structures involved. These are:

- plantar fasciitis
- calcaneal periostitis, and
- calcaneal spur formation.

It has been hypothesized that spur formation also occurs in other structures that attach to the calcaneus in the region of the tuberosity, including the flexor digitorum brevis muscle, the quadratus plantae muscle, the abductor hallucis muscle, and the long plantar ligament.[6,11] This is supported by the observation that in 50 per cent of cases the spur is not always formed at the site of the plantar fascia origin.[12]

Clinical presentation
The classical clinical presentations of these three overuse injuries are similar, and generally differ only with respect to the site of pain location. Pain located over the medial calcaneal tuberosity would be typical of calcaneal periostitis (in the absence of a spur) or a calcaneal spur. Pain if located in the region distal to the tuberosity or on the medial longitudinal arch, is consistent with true plantar fasciitis. These syndromes may occur in combination because the mechanism of the injury is similar.

The characteristics of the pain are described below.[1,5–7,10,13–15]

1. A low-grade pain of gradual onset is present which subsequently follows the classical progression of pain associated with an overuse injury.

2. Pain is experienced that is aggravated by weight bearing (in running particularly during the push-off phase of the gait cycle).

3. It is worse in the morning upon rising or after a prolonged period of sitting (reason not known).

4. Heel tenderness is present on examination (anteromedial 92 per cent, central 7 per cent, combination 1 per cent).

5. Pain is precipitated by passive dorsiflexion of the metatarsophalangeal joints.

6. It can be accompanied by a decreased range of motion of the first toe.

7. It is common in the elderly and obese population (related to connective tissue changes with age and the increased loading, respectively).

8. A fascial granuloma can sometimes be felt on the medial border of the fascia.

9. Pain is present which is not associated with severe swelling.

A full clinical examination including a biomechanical evaluation should be performed to identify causes of excessive tension in the plantar fascia and its attachments. Rearfoot valgus is a common biomechanical factor associated with these injuries. The clinical examination should therefore include an inspection of the athlete's footwear. It has also been stated that a limitation of ankle dorsiflexion due to inflexibility of the gastrocnemius–soleus complex as well as weakness of the posterior calf muscles may also predispose to this condition and these should be identified and corrected.[16,17]

Differential diagnosis

The clinical presentation of a chronic plantar fascial injury must be distinguished from that of an acute rupture of the plantar fascia.[15,18] In an acute rupture of the plantar fascia, the athlete may have a history of chronic pain over the plantar fascia for some time and then experience sudden severe pain accompanied by a snapping sensation under the foot during sports participation.[19] Further distinguishing features would be the rapid onset of swelling in the region distal to the calcaneal tuberosity (the medial longitudinal arch becomes convex rather concave after a rupture) and a palpable defect in the plantar fascia.[15,19] Previous multiple steroid injections into the site have been reported in 33 per cent of cases of ruptured plantar fascia.[18]

Injuries to the plantar fascia must also be distinguished from a number of conditions causing subcalcaneal heel pain, including the fat-pad syndrome, nerve entrapments around the foot, apophysitis, bursitis, and stress fractures.[6] It is also important to exclude systemic diseases that can be associated with heel pain such as Reiter's syndrome, ankylosing spondylitis, psoriatic arthritis,[8] gout, and rheumatoid arthritis.[15] A feature of systemic diseases is that they often cause bilateral disease. Finally, in an athlete presenting with heel pain, nerve root compression of the S1 vertebra must be excluded.

Special investigations

Routine roentgenograms of the heel may be performed to exclude other injuries, tumours, or arthrosis.[6] It must be emphasized that the heel spur is present in only about 50 per cent of patients presenting with chronic plantar fascia pain and that a heel spur is found in about 15 per cent of asymptomatic adults.[20] A bone scan is occasionally requested when a stress fracture of the calcaneus is suspected. However, a positive bone scan (blood pool and delayed images) has been reported in patients with plantar fascial injuries.[6]

Management

The principles of management of chronic plantar fascia injuries are:

(1) to reduce the pain;

(2) to decrease the load on the plantar fascia and its attachments;

(3) to assist healing; and

(4) to prevent recurrence of the injury.

Pain can be reduced by decreasing activity or with complete rest. Ice, anti-inflammatory medication, with or without analgesics, may also be useful.[5,6] Runners should also be advised to avoid hard running surfaces, hill running, and speed training as these forms of activity would increase the tension in the plantar fascia. Alternative forms of exercise, such as swimming and cycling, can be encouraged during the rehabilitation phase. Stretching of the gastrocnemius–soleus complex should be encouraged. Resistance exercise has also been advocated in the recovery phase of plantar fascial injuries.[14] Physiotherapeutic modalities, such as ultrasound, are not consistently effective and few controlled studies have been conducted to establish their effectiveness.[15]

Cortisone injections into the area are commonly administered, but this should be done with caution as the risk of acute rupture of the plantar fascia may be increased.[18]

The tension applied to the plantar fascia can be reduced by altering training (as described above), strapping, and by the use of orthotics. A specific strapping technique has been described (Low dye strapping technique).[1] This technique apparently stabilizes the head of the first metatarsal during plantar flexion and decreases pronation.[15]

A variety of orthotic devices have been described for the treatment of chronic plantar fascia injuries.[6] These include:

- a heel lift with or without a hole to reduce pressure at the painful area;

- arch supports;

- full-length, custom-made orthotics;

- antipronation running shoes.

Advice regarding orthotics and referral to a sports podiatrist is important in the management of these injuries.

Tension night splints with the ankle in 5 degrees dorsiflexion have been successful in difficult cases.[5,6] Since conservative treatment is reported to be effective in 92 to 96 per cent of cases,[6] surgical management for this condition is therefore indicated in less than 10 per cent of injuries. The indication is a persistent injury (lasting for longer than 1 year) that has not responded to conservative treatment.[15] In one series, surgical release of the plantar fascia relieved symptoms in all patients.[21] Others report less dramatic results after surgical treatment; 50 to 60 per cent obtaining prompt and permanent relief.[7] A number of surgical techniques have been described,[6] and most involve a plantar fasciotomy with resection of the osseous spur.[7] There is a need for controlled clinical trials comparing conservative and surgical treatments for this condition.

Guidelines for return to full activity

The ability to withstand full passive dorsiflexion of the toes and ankle without reproducing the pain indicates functional progression. The athlete can then be encouraged to start a walking programme followed by a gradual introduction of running, but avoiding hill running, speedwork, and hard surfaces.

Calcaneal nerve entrapment

Anatomy

The calcaneal nerve is the last of the three branches of the posterior tibial nerve (Fig. 1). It has also been suggested that this nerve arises from the plantar nerves. It consists of an anterior and a posterior branch which supply sensory fibres to the skin over the heel. The

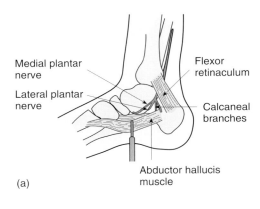

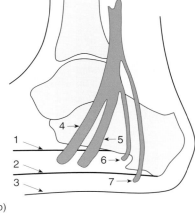

Fig. 1 (a) Anatomy of the posterior tibial nerve. (b) Relationships of the subcalcaneal nerves to various calcaneal structures. (1) Long plantar ligament. (2) Plantar fascia. (3) Skin. (4) Medial plantar nerve. (5) Lateral plantar nerve. (6) Nerve to abductor digiti quinti. (7) Medial calcaneal nerve.

main (medial) branch lies between the deep fascia of the proximal part of the abductor hallucis muscle and the medial anterior corner of the calcaneal tuberosity.

Clinical features

It is often difficult to distinguish this nerve-entrapment syndrome from chronic plantar fascia injuries. Patients present with intense pain in the heel when running or walking. The pain does not respond to conservative treatment. The nature of the pain is that of intense sharp pain on heelstrike.[22] Continuous low-grade pain and early morning pain are less common. It can be distinguished from chronic plantar fascia injuries by the following features:

(1) associated decreased sensation over the heel;

(2) painless dorsiflexion of the toe;

(3) pain on heelstrike rather than toe-off;

(4) intense tenderness over the medial anterior part of the heel pad rather than the plantar fascia attachments;

(5) pain on stretching of the abductor hallucis muscle, and shortening of the flexors of the foot.[22]

Management

Surgical decompression has been used successfully in the treatment of this condition.[22]

Fat-pad syndrome

Anatomy and pathology

This condition is also known as the 'bruised heel syndrome', or the 'painful heel pad'.[6] The fat pad of the heel consists of fibrous septa in which fat globules are distributed. This anatomical arrangement allows for effective force distribution over the area and acts as a natural shock absorber.[8] It has been estimated that 20 to 25 per cent of the contact force at heel strike is absorbed by the fat pad.[6] Age-related deterioration in the capacity for shock absorption occurs due to changes in the properties of elastic tissue.

In the fat-pad syndrome there is subcutaneous fat pad bruising, and occasionally associated tissue necrosis. Pain originates from both free nerve endings and Pacinian corpuscles which have been identified in the fat pad.

Clinical presentation and management

Patients present with diffuse heel pain on the plantar surface of the heel. This may be precipitated by excessive loading in jumping sports such as tennis, long jump, and hurdles. Tenderness can be elicited over the heel, particularly on the posterior aspect of the heel, directly over the fat pad.[6]

Management is conservative and is aimed at decreasing the forces applied to the heel. Symptomatic treatment will consist of local anti-inflammatory modalities and systemic non-steroidal anti-inflammatory medication. Restriction of jumping and running activities may be necessary and soft, heel pads may be beneficial. Adequate shock-absorbing footwear may prevent recurrent injuries. A decrease in walking or running speed with shorter strides is also advised.[6]

Medial heel pain

Tarsal tunnel syndrome

Introduction

Recently, entrapment of the sensory nerves of the foot has been described by several groups.[6,8,22–24] In most cases the pathology is related to entrapment with compression along the course of the nerve. The compression can result from:

(1) congenital abnormalities in structures through which the nerve passes;

(2) trauma to the nerve or surrounding tissues resulting in inflammation and scarring;

(3) forces applied to the nerve or surrounding structures during movements such as running;

(4) external forces such as tight-fitting shoes.

General symptoms and signs of nerve entrapment syndromes in the foot are:

(1) tenderness at the site of entrapment;

(2) pain peripheral to the site of entrapment;

(3) a positive Tinel's sign (reproduction of the symptoms on percussion of the nerve);

(4) sensory changes in the distribution of the nerve (tingling, numbness);

(5) pain described as 'burning', or a 'sharp' pain;

(6) nocturnal pain presumed to be a result of venostasis and engorgement.

One of the causes of medial heel pain can be entrapment of the posterior tibial nerve, giving rise to the 'tarsal tunnel syndrome'. Branches of the posterior tibial nerve can also be involved and these conditions will also be discussed.

Anatomy of the posterior tibial nerve

The tarsal tunnel is a fibro-osseus tunnel formed by a floor—consisting of the talus, calcaneus, tibialis posterior muscle, flexor digitorum longus muscle, and the flexor hallucis longus muscle—and a roof, consisting of the flexor retinaculum. The distal end of the tarsal tunnel is narrow and blends with the superficial and the deep fascia of the abductor hallucis muscle.[25]

The posterior tibial nerve runs deep to the soleus muscle in the posterior compartment. It exits the posterior compartment and passes deep to the flexor retinaculum between the medial malleolus and the calcaneus. It lies posterior to the posterior tibial artery and anterior to the flexor hallucis longus muscle. Posteroinferior to the medial malleolus, it divides into three nerves: the calcaneal nerve; medial plantar nerve; and the lateral plantar nerves (Fig. 1).[22,24,26]

Clinical features

Entrapment of the posterior tibial nerve along its course through the tarsal tunnel gives rise to the 'tarsal tunnel syndrome'. The site of entrapment is the fibro-osseus tunnel behind the medial malleolus. Causes of entrapment of this nerve in athletes are severe rearfoot valgus, chronic flexor tenosynovitis, post-traumatic scarring, and inflammatory collagen vascular disease. Less commonly, tumours, varicose veins, and an enlarged venous plexus can be responsible for the nerve entrapment in the tarsal tunnel.[4,24,26,27] The aetiology of this condition in runners has also been related to repetitive indirect trauma to the heel and from poorly fitting running shoes.[23,28]

This condition presents as pain, initially insidious in onset, localized to the plantar aspect of the foot, sometimes also in the region of the metatarsals or radiating up the lower leg.[8,25] Pain may sometimes develop only during running and be absent when walking. Tenderness is present along the tarsal tunnel with pain radiating into the leg and foot on palpation. Numbness and tingling in the plantar area can also be important symptoms.[12] Radiographs may reveal an os trigonum which compresses the tibial nerve.[12] Nerve conduction tests and electromyography may be of diagnostic value.[26,28]

Management

Conservative management should generally be attempted initially, namely restricting activity, treating inflammation if suspected, correcting shoes, and prescribing antipronation orthotics.[26-28] If these measures fail, surgical decompression can be considered.[24] However, surgical decompression should be considered with caution as the outcome is variable.[29]

Medial plantar nerve entrapment

Anatomy

The medial plantar nerve is one of the three branches of the posterior tibial nerve (Fig. 1). It passes deep to the abductor hallucis muscle and runs anteriorly between this muscle and the flexor digitorum brevis muscle. The nerve runs in close proximity to the calcaneonavicular ligament and joint. It supplies sensation to the plantar surface of the medial three toes, as well as motor branches to a number of small muscles of the foot.

Clinical features

Compression of the medial plantar nerve will produce sensory changes to the medial plantar aspect of the foot. This can be elicited clinically by pressure on the site of entrapment (calcaneonavicular joint) resulting in sensory signs in the distribution of the nerve.[12] Recently acquired orthotics may sometimes cause this condition.[24,27]

Management

Surgical decompression is required if conservative treatment consisting of rest, anti-inflammatory medication, and modification of abnormal biomechanics, fails.

Tibialis posterior tendinitis

In patients with tibialis posterior tendinitis, the typical symptoms and signs of paratendinitis are elicited in the area of the flexor retinaculum on the medial aspect of the foot. This injury may be associated with excessive rearfoot valgus (pronation) which results in increased tension in the tendon. Management is aimed at correcting the biomechanical abnormality as well as treating the inflammation.[4]

Lateral heel pain

Lateral plantar nerve entrapment

Anatomy

The lateral plantar nerve is one of the three branches of the tibial nerve (Fig. 1). It passes through fibrous openings between the abductor hallucis and quadratus plantae muscles in close proximity to the medial tubercle of the calcaneus.[8] Inflammation of the origin of the plantar fascia or calcaneal spur formation can result in compression of this nerve. The lateral plantar nerve supplies sensation to the lateral (fourth and fifth toes) plantar surface of the foot. Entrapment of a branch of the lateral plantar nerve innervating the abductor digiti quinti muscle has recently also been implicated in chronic medial calcaneal pain.[6,27]

Clinical features

The clinical features are similar to those that generally apply to entrapment neuropathies as discussed under Tarsal tunnel syndrome. Compression of the entrapment site (medial calcaneal tuberosity) elicits sensory change in the distribution of the nerve and is an important diagnostic sign.

Management

Conservative management is the same as for chronic plantar fascia injuries and includes rest, non-steroidal anti-inflammatory drugs, heel cups, calf-muscle stretching programmes, orthotics, and corticosteroid injections.[27] Surgical decompression may be required, and many forms of surgical treatment have recently been described.[6]

Peroneal tendinitis

Inflammation of the peroneal tendons (longus and brevis) or the sheaths (paratendinitis) can cause lateral heel pain in the athlete. The site of inflammation is around the peroneus longus or brevis tendons as they pass posterior to the lateral malleolus. Predisposing factors to this injury in athletes are:[4]

(1) excessive rearfoot varus (supination);

(2) previous ankle ligament sprains;

(3) absence of os peroneum (an accessory bone that decreases friction in the tendon);

(4) plantar-flexed first metatarsal (forced dorsiflexion increases the tension in the tendon).

Management of this injury is conservative by altering training, correcting excessive supination, and treating symptoms. Surgery is indicated in cases of failed conservative treatment.

Sinus tarsi syndrome

Definition
The sinus tarsi syndrome can be defined as a clinical syndrome of diffuse lateral foot pain presenting in athletes either after acute ankle sprains or as an injury of gradual onset. It was first described in the late 1950s and is now well recognized as a cause of chronic lateral foot pain.

Anatomy
The sinus tarsi is the lateral extension of the tarsal canal which is made up of the sulci of the talus and the calcaneus.[30] It runs an oblique course posteromedially and anterolaterally, and is bounded by the anterolateral surface of the talar body, the inferolateral surface of the talar neck, and the anterosuperior surface of the calcaneus. It contains several important structures, in particular, the talocalcaneal (interosseus) and the cervical ligaments. The talocalcaneal ligament maintains the alignment between the talus and the calcaneus, becoming lax with pronation and taut with supination. The cervical ligament prevents rearfoot valgus. Severing these ligaments causes subtalar joint instability.

Aetiology and pathology
The precise aetiology and pathology of sinus tarsi syndrome is not known. It has been suggested that the cause is damage to the structures within the sinus tarsi, in particular the ligaments, either as a result of an acute lateral ankle ligament sprain with forced inversion, or repetitive damage from excessive subtalar joint pronation.[4,30,31] Other postulated causes for the syndrome are synovial hypertrophy, entrapment of a branch of the peroneal nerve, and exostosis associated with degenerative joint disease.[30]

Diagnosis
The patient usually presents with the following clinical signs:[30,31]

1. Chronic lateral ankle pain is of gradual onset, or follows an acute lateral ligament sprain.

2. Pain may be more severe in the early morning but improves with exercise.

3. Pain is aggravated by movements of the ankle which require forced eversion (running around a corner, or on a cambered road).

4. There is marked tenderness over the opening of the sinus tarsi.

5. Subtalar instability may be present.

6. Sensory changes, including a positive Tinel's sign, may be elicited with forceful forefoot supination.

The most reliable clinical diagnostic test is infiltration of the sinus tarsi with local anaesthetic which should abolish the pain.

Radiographic findings are normal and an arthrogram may demonstrate loss of integrity of capsuloligamentous structures of the ankle.[30]

Management
The management of this condition is conservative and a number of treatment modalities have been advocated, but none of these has been studied in well-conducted clinical trials. The following conservative treatment modalities can be used:[30,31]

(1) relative rest, ice, non-steroidal anti-inflammatory drugs;

(2) correction of abnormal foot biomechanics, most commonly excessive subtalar joint pronation;

(3) rehabilitation involving strength and proprioceptive training;

(4) local infiltration of the sinus tarsi with corticosteroids.

Sural nerve entrapment

Anatomy
The sural nerve has its origin in the popliteal fossa from a branch of the common peroneal nerve (peroneal communicating branch of the common peroneal nerve) and a branch of the tibial nerve (medial sural cutaneous nerve). It supplies the skin on the lateral and posterior part of the distal third of the leg. Of importance is that the nerve enters the foot posterior to the lateral malleolus and supplies sensation to the lateral margin of the foot and the lateral side of the fifth toe. It is vulnerable to entrapment posterior to the lateral malleolus and at the styloid process of the fifth metatarsal.[23] Recurrent lateral ankle sprains may lead to fibrosis and subsequent entrapment of this nerve.[27]

Clinical features
The clinical features of sural nerve entrapment are numbness and paresthesia over the lateral forefoot and toe areas. This may be caused by minor trauma, tight-fitting shoes, or a bony injury to the base of the fifth metatarsal.

Management
Surgical decompression may be required if conservative measures, consisting of footwear modification and anti-inflammatory treatment, fail.

Diffuse heel pain

Calcaneal stress fracture

Clinical presentation and diagnosis
The patient will present with heel pain associated with increased activity in the period before the onset of pain. The following presenting features are important:[32,33]

1. The symptoms are of gradual onset.

2. The pain is vague and not confined to one area of the heel.

3. There is exquisite tenderness to palpation on the inferior surface and on both sides of the heel.

4. The pain is aggravated when weight is distributed only on the heel (heel standing) and is relieved when standing on the toes.

5. Non-weight bearing ankle movement is relatively painless.

6. Running is impossible.

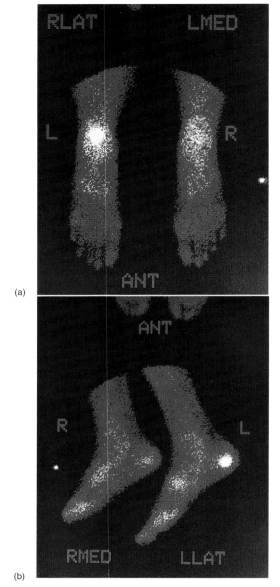

(a)

(b)

Fig. 2 Delayed technetium-phosphate bone scan images of the (a) anterior and (b) lateral aspects of both feet in a runner presenting with diffuse left heel pain. Increased uptake of the left calcaneus is demonstrated, confirming the diagnosis of a left calcaneal stress fracture.

Plain radiographs may show a subtle area of increased density, but the diagnosis of a calcaneal stress fracture, and other stress fractures of the tarsal bones, has to be confirmed by bone scan (Fig. 2) or computed tomography scan.[33]

Management

Conservative management consisting of reduced weight bearing activity, including the avoidance of running for 6 weeks from the onset of pain, shock-absorbing footwear, and general measures to improve bone healing (calcium supplementation and correction of abnormal hormonal status if necessary) is usually adequate. In some cases, immobilization by cast or brace has been advocated.[33]

Tarsal coalition

Definition

Tarsal coalition refers to the fusion of two or more tarsal bones.[4] The fusion can be fibrous, cartilagenous, or osseous.

Aetiology

The aetiology is not always clear, but it may be congenital (autosomal dominant with incomplete penetrance) or as a result of previous trauma.

Incidence

The incidence is around 1 per cent of the population, is more common in males, and is often bilateral. The condition commonly presents for the first time in adolescence.

Pathology

The common coalitions seen in tarsal bones are:

- calcaneonavicular (most common)
- calcaneocuboid
- talocalcaneal
- talonavicular
- mixed.

Clinical presentation

The clinical presentation varies and can be:

(1) intermittent ankle pain aggravated by sports activity;

(2) limitation of supination;

(3) pain and swelling aggravated by pronation or supination;

(4) peroneal spasm causing the foot to lock in pronation (often related to jumping).

Diagnosis

Radiographs may not show the coalition in standard anteroposterior views, but the following radiological signs may be noted:

(1) narrowed posterior talocalcaneal facet joint;

(2) flattened lateral talar process;

(3) irregularity of the medial aspect of the talus;

(4) talar beaking.

A 45-degree oblique view showing a calcaneonavicular bar is diagnostic of calcaneonavicular coalition. Tomograms or computerized tomography, which is the technique of choice, are necessary to confirm the diagnosis of talocoalition.

Management

Conservative management is generally the treatment of choice. In the acute stage, the aim is to relax the peroneal spasm and limit extremes of movement (supination or pronation). This is achieved by a plaster cast in the neutral position for 3 to 6 weeks followed by supportive orthotics to limit extremes of motion. Surgery is indicated for failed conservative treatment, persistent pain, spasm, and deformity. Excision of the bar is moderately successful. Asymptomatic coalition, which is sometimes diagnosed on routine radiographs, is also managed conservatively.

Midfoot pain

Clinically, midfoot pain can present as medial, central, or lateral pain.

Medial midfoot pain

Plantar fasciitis

Plantar fascial injuries have already been discussed under Injuries of the plantar fascia and attachments.

Tibialis posterior tendinitis

Tibialis posterior tendinitis can also present as medial midfoot pain if the inflammation is at the site of insertion of the tendon. This condition has already been mentioned under Tibialis posterior tendinitis.

Navicular stress fracture

Introduction

Until recently, navicular stress fractures were considered uncommon. However, a recent prospective study has shown that this injury now accounts for a large percentage of lower limb stress fractures in athletes.[34]

Clinical presentation

This is an important injury to consider in any patient presenting with medial arch or dorsal foot pain.[35] The patient presents with pain and swelling along the dorsum and the medial arch of the foot which is precipitated or aggravated by activity. Tenderness can be elicited over the talonavicular joint area, and the dorsum of the navicular, the so-called 'N' spot.[36]

These fractures are usually not visible on routine radiographs of the foot.[35] Computed tomography is a very accurate diagnostic investigation for this injury. An anteroposterior tomogram and a technetium bone scan can also be diagnostic (Fig. 3).[35]

Management

There is a risk of non-union in this condition, and therefore the management is more aggressive than in stress fractures of the other tarsal bones or bones of the lower leg.[36] The management is aimed at reducing the load through the navicular. This is best accomplished by:[36]

(1) a non-weight bearing cast for 6 weeks;

(2) rehabilitation for 6 weeks after cast removal with monitoring of pain;

(3) a gradual return to full sporting activity;

(4) correction of abnormal foot biomechanics, if necessary.

It must be noted that radiological evidence of healing lags behind clinical healing. Therefore, the athlete is usually able to return to activity despite a lack of radiological signs of callus formation provided the symptoms have resolved.[32]

Central midfoot pain

Extensor tendinitis

All the extensor tendons, but commonly the extensor hallucis longus, can be involved. The injury can be caused by ill-fitting

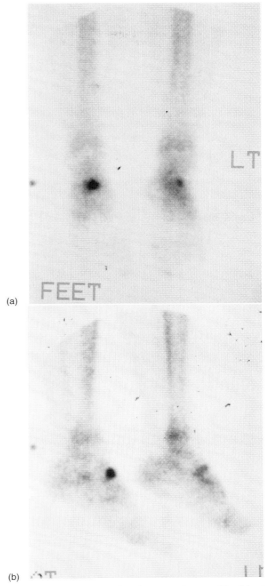

Fig. 3 Delayed technetium-phosphate bone scan images of the (a) anterior and (b) lateral aspects of both feet in a sprinter presenting with medial midfoot pain and tenderness over the 'N' spot. Increased uptake in the region of the right navicular is demonstrated, confirming the diagnosis of a right navicular stress fracture.

shoes, trauma, or excessive hill training. The condition is diagnosed by tenderness on palpation over the dorsum of the foot with the pain aggravated by dorsiflexion of the toes. Crepitus may be elicited. Management is conservative and includes restricting activity, altering training, and adjusting footwear to decrease irritation of the tendon. Surgery may be necessary in chronic cases that are resistant to conservative treatment.

Anterolateral impingement syndrome

Anterolateral impingement syndrome refers to a condition where soft tissues or bony structures in the lateral gutter are traumatized either during an acute inversion ankle 'sprain', or as a result of repeated minor inversion ankle sprains. The term anterolateral quarter compression syndrome was first coined in the early 1950s and a 'meniscoid' band, consisting of a mass of hyalinized connective tissue between the talus and the fibula was identified as the source of chronic pain after an inversion ankle sprain.

More recently, the pathology of this condition has been described in a large series of patients who presented with chronic pain after an ankle sprain.[37] At surgery, the findings in this series showed the following:

(1) hypertrophied and inflamed synovium (100 per cent of cases);

(2) adhesive bands of scar tissue in the lateral gutter (64 per cent of patients);

(3) chondromalacia of the anterolateral talar dome (51 per cent of cases);

(4) a 'meniscoid' type lesion in 13 per cent of cases.

It has also been suggested that chronic capsular irritation can progress to osteophyte formation on the distal talus which, with repeated dorsiflexion, causes abutment between the anterior tibia and the neck of the talus.

Clinical features of the anterolateral impingement syndrome are:[37–40]

(1) history of either an acute severe inversion ankle sprain or of repeated minor inversion ankle sprains;

(2) chronic pain after the ankle sprain, usually in the anterolateral aspect of the ankle joint;

(3) pain that is aggravated by forced dorsiflexion (toe-off during gait);

(4) tenderness on palpation of the anterolateral gutter of the ankle;

(5) presence of a palpable osteophyte;

(6) occasionally, muscle weakness and a sensation of giving way.

Plain radiographs are normal in 50 per cent of patients. Osteophyte formation can be demonstrated on lateral radiographs. Magnetic resonance imaging (**MRI**) shows thickening of the synovium in 30 per cent of cases and may be helpful in the diagnosis of the condition.

Conservative management is the initial treatment of choice and can consist of heel elevation, non-steroidal anti-inflammatory medication, immobilization, and corticosteroid injections. Failed conservative treatment is an indication for arthroscopic removal of the scar tissue.[37–39]

Tarsal coalition
Tarsal coalition, which has been discussed above, can also present as central midfoot pain.

Lateral midfoot pain

Cuboid stress fracture
A stress fracture of the cuboid bone can present as lateral midfoot pain of gradual onset. Patients will present pain severe enough to prevent vigorous physical activity, especially running. Clinical examination reveals tenderness over the area of the cuboid and lateral foot pain on weight bearing, in particular jumping. Radiographs are usually unhelpful in confirming the diagnosis, and a technetium bone scan will show an area of intense uptake in the lateral foot region on the delayed film. An MRI scan or a CT scan is often required to localize the pathology to the cuboid bone, and so confirm the diagnosis of a cuboid stress fracture.

Optimum treatment of this condition has not been well researched. We recommend that athletes be non-weight bearing (either in a cast or a leg walker brace) for 3 weeks, after which the clinical condition can be reviewed. A further 3-week period of immobilization may be required. Factors that affect bone healing (dietary calcium intake, hormonal status) should also be opitimized during the treatment period. A rehabilitation programme and gradual return to sports should be guided by pain over the cuboid, as radiological resolution lags behind clinical progress.

Peroneal tendinitis
Tendinitis of the peroneal tendons can also present as lateral midfoot pain. This condition has already been discussed under Peroneal tendinitis.

Cuboid subluxation
Definition
The cuboid syndrome has been defined as a dorsomedial subluxation of the cuboid bone due to excessive traction of the peroneus longus muscle.[35] Plantar subluxations of the cuboid have also been described.[41]

Aetiology and pathology
The presumed aetiology of this condition is either (1) a sudden excessive contraction of the peroneus longus, or (2) repetitive contraction of the peroneus longus muscle. The pathology is that of dorsomedial subluxation of the cuboid bone and there may be disruption of the intertarsal ligaments when the cuboid is forcefully rotated.[41]

Diagnosis
Clinically, patients may present with a history of an inversion sprain followed by chronic lateral foot pain. Tenderness may be present on palpation of the cuboid, which is often relieved on manual reduction of the subluxed cuboid.[41]

Management
Management of this condition is by manipulation of the cuboid to correct its alignment. The techniques for correcting plantar and dorsal subluxation of the cuboid have been described.[41] Following manipulation, the patient undergoes a rehabilitation programme.

Stress fracture of the fifth metatarsal
The stress fracture of the fifth metatarsal (Jones' fracture) is a unique metatarsal stress fracture as it requires specific and more vigorous management compared with the management of other metatarsal stress fractures. This fracture is complicated by high rates of delayed and non-union. The site of the fracture and the time before initiation of treatment are important factors that influence management and the occurrence of complications, and therefore prognosis. Fractures at the tuberosity of the fifth metatarsal and acute fractures have a better prognosis than distal (more than 1.5 cm from the tuberosity) and chronic fractures. Acute proximal fractures can be managed by cast immobilization for 6 to 8 weeks. Distal acute fractures can also be managed with cast immobilization (6 to 8 weeks), whereas more chronic fractures require internal fixation (intramedullary screw) or bone grafting, or both.[1,32,33]

Traction apophysitis of the base of the fifth metatarsal (Iselin's disease)

This is an overload injury caused by traction of the peroneus brevis tendon. It occurs in children between 10 and 14 years of age. The presentation is that of pain on the side of the foot aggravated by running and wearing shoes. Tenderness can be elicited over the base of the fifth metatarsal and is aggravated by resisted eversion. Management is conservative with restriction of activity, symptomatic treatment, stretching and strengthening exercises. Strapping may also be of value.

Forefoot pain

Dorsal forefoot pain

Extensor tendinitis

Tendinitis of the extensor tendons can also present as dorsal forefoot pain. This condition has already been discussed under Extensor tendinitis.

Navicular stress fractures

Stress fractures of the navicular can occasionally present as dorsal forefoot pain. This condition has been discussed under Navicular stress fracture.

Metatarsal stress fractures

These fractures are usually found in military recruits, ballet dancers, and distance runners.[3] The following are clinical signs of metatarsal stress fractures:

(1) gradual onset of pain in the forefoot area associated with activity;

(2) inability to run because of the pain;

(3) point tenderness over the affected metatarsal;

(4) swelling over the affected area sometimes present.

Standard radiographs are not very helpful and a triple-phase technetium bone scan is usually required to confirm the diagnosis (Fig. 4). Conservative management consisting of non-weight bearing activity, symptomatic treatment, and attendance to factors that can influence bone healing (calcium intake, hormonal status, and systemic abnormalities) is sufficient. Rest is usually required for 6 to 8 weeks, after which activity can be increased gradually.

Common peroneal nerve entrapment

Anatomy and pathology

The common peroneal nerve divides into the deep and the superficial peroneal nerves. The deep peroneal nerve runs in the anterior compartment and passes distally deep to the extensor retinaculum with the anterior tibial artery. It ends by dividing into medial and lateral branches. It supplies sensation to a small area of the dorsum of the foot between the first and second toes. This nerve is exposed to trauma at the tarsometatarsal joint.[23] It can also occur in athletes with previous lateral ankle ligament injuries and is also sometimes associated with osteophytes on the talus.[12] It has been described in runners, soccer players, skiers, and dancers.[27]

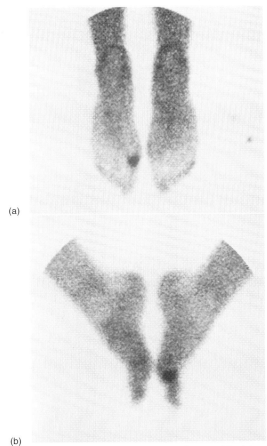

(a)

(b)

Fig. 4 Delayed technetium-phosphate bone scan images of the (a) anterior and (b) lateral aspects of both feet in a ballet dancer presenting with dorsal right-forefoot pain and tenderness over the first metatarsal on the right. Increased uptake in the region of the head of the first metatarsal is demonstrated, confirming the diagnosis of a right first-metatarsal stress fracture.

Clinical features

The clinical presentation is that of pain on the dorsum of the foot, with radiation of pain to the web space between the first and second toes.

Management

Surgical decompression is required if conservative treatment modalities, such as loosening shoe laces, altering the footwear, and local corticosteroid infiltrations, fail.[27]

Plantar forefoot pain

Metatarsal stress fractures

Metatarsal stress fractures can present as plantar forefoot pain. This condition has already been discussed under Metatarsal stress fractures.

Interdigital (Morton's) neuroma

Introduction

Interdigital (Morton's) neuroma, as described by Morton in 1876, is not a true neuroma but rather a perineural fibrosis of the interdigital nerves.[41] Interdigital neuromas in athletes (in particular runners) are thought to result from repetitive trauma to plantar interdigital nerves. This condition has also recently been observed in patients using stair-climbing machines on a regular basis.[43]

Pathology

The possible mechanisms of injury are:[23,24,28,42]

(1) compression of the interdigital nerve against the transverse metatarsal ligament in repetitive dorsiflexion of the toes;

(2) increased stretching with repetitive hyperextension of the metatarsophalangeal joint;

(3) tight-fitting and high-heeled shoes causing compression;

(4) alterations in blood supply (prolonged standing and tight footwear);

(5) excessive pronation.

Clinical features

Patients present with progressive pain and paresthesia in the toes while running. Pain is often relieved by walking barefoot. The space between the third and fourth metatarsals is the most common site of trauma to the interdigital nerves. The diagnosis is confirmed on physical examination by reproduction of symptoms when the foot is either compressed (medial to lateral), or by eliciting pain on direct pressure of the plantar aspect between the metatarsal heads. Usually the neuroma can be rubbed across the underlying structures, reproducing the pain.

Management

The management of interdigital neuroma is initially conservative. The following measures can be used in treatment:[23,24,27,28]

(1) instructing the athlete to loosen shoe laces;

(2) reducing activity;

(3) wearing wider fitting, thicker soled, shock-absorbing shoes;

(4) non-steroidal anti-inflammatory medication and corticosteroid infiltration of the area;

(5) prescribing, if necessary, metatarsal support proximal to the pinched nerve.

Surgical management by excision of the neuroma or decompression of the nerve may be necessary if conservative treatment fails.[23,24,27,42]

Sesamoid injury

Injuries to the sesamoid bones in the foot have also been referred to as sesamoiditis and stress fractures. The medial and lateral sesamoid bones are contained within the tendons of the flexor hallucis brevis muscle and lie under the head of the first metatarsal. These bones increase the mechanical advantage of the flexor hallucis brevis tendons. They are also weight bearing and are therefore subjected to repetitive mechanical loading.

Injury to the sesamoids can occur as a result of impact loading or excessive traction on the flexor hallucis brevis tendons during sprinting. The patient will present with pain under the first metatarsal head. The site is tender, and often the pain can be aggravated

Table 3 Systemic and other causes of chronic foot and ankle pain

1. **Seronegative spondylarthropathies**
   Reiter's syndrome
   Ankylosing spondylitis
   Psoriatic arthritis
   Beçhet's syndrome

2. **Metabolic abnormalities**
   Gout
   Pseudogout
   Osteoporosis
   Osteomalacia

3. **Tumours**
   Glomus tumour of the heel pad
   Simple and aneurysmal cysts
   Osteoid osteoma
   Osteoblastoma
   Chondromyxoid fibroma
   Chondrosarcoma

4. **Arthritides**
   Rheumatoid arthritis
   Juvenile rheumatoid arthritis
   Osteoarthritis

5. **Neuropathies**
   Lumbar spine pathology
   Diabetes mellitus
   Alcoholism
   Reflex sympathetic dystrophy

6. **Other conditions**
   Sarcoidosis
   Paget's disease
   Sickle cell anaemia
   Arteriosclerosis (arch claudication)

by active plantar flexion of the big toe. Radiographic examination is often unhelpful, but may show fractures or fragmentation and possibly avascular necrosis of the sesamoids. Technetium bone scans can differentiate sesamoiditis from a stress fracture. CT scans can help determine whether the stress fracture has been followed by the development of avascular necrosis of the sesamoid.

Management is conservative initially and success has been achieved with the use of orthotics.[44] Other conservative measures include restricting activity, anti-inflammatory medication, and steroid injection. Surgery can be considered for failed conservative treatment and cases with non-union of fractures, avascular necrosis, and persistent pain.

Systemic and other causes of chronic foot and ankle pain

Any athlete presenting with chronic foot or ankle pain may also suffer from a number of systemic conditions and other rare conditions that may cause local pathology. Some of these conditions are listed in Table 3.

References

1. Torg JS, Pavlov H, Torg E. Overuse injuries in sport: the foot. *Clinics in Sport* 1987; **6**: 291–320.
2. Marotta JJ, Micheli LJ. Os trigonum impingement in dancers. *American Journal of Sports Medicine* 1992; **20**: 533–6.
3. Quirk R. Common foot and ankle injuries in dance. *Orthopaedic Clinics of North America* 1994; **25**: 123–33.
4. Santopietro FJ. Foot and foot-related injuries in the young athlete. *Clinics in Sports Medicine* 1988; **7**: 563–88.
5. Batt ME, Tanji JL. Management options for plantar fasciitis. *The Physician and Sportsmedicine* 1995; **23**: 77–86.
6. Karr SD. Subcalcaneal heel pain. *Orthopaedic Clinics of North America* 1994; **25**: 161–75.
7. Kosmahl EM, Kosmahl HE. Painful plantar heel, plantar fasciitis, and calcaneal spur: Etiology and treatment. *Journal of Orthopaedic and Sports Physical Therapy* 1987; **9**: 17–24.
8. Doxey GE. Calcaneal pain: A review of various disorders. *Journal of Orthopaedic and Sports Physical Therapy* 1987; **9**: 25–32.
9. Kotwick JE. Biomechanics of the foot and ankle. *Clinical Sports Medicine* 1982; **1**: 19–35.
10. Warren BL. Plantar fasciites in runners. Treatment and prevention. *Sports Medicine* 1990; **10**: 338–45.
11. McCarthy DJ, Gorecki GE. The anatomical basis of inferior calcaneal lesions. *Journal of the American Podiatry Association* 1979; **69**: 527–36.
12. Murphy PC, Baxter DE. Nerve entrapment of the foot and ankle in runners. *Clinics in Sports Medicine* 1985; **4**: 753–63.
13. Baxter DE. The heel in sport. *Clinics in Sports Medicine* 1994; **13**: 683–93.
14. Chandler TJ, Kibler WB. A biomechanical approach to the prevention, treatment and rehabilitation of plantar fasciitis. *Sports Medicine* 1993; **15**: 344–52.
15. Tanner SM, Harvey JS. How we manage plantar fasciitis. *The Physician and Sportsmedicine* 1988; **16**: 39–47.
16. Kibler WB, Goldberg C, Chandler TJ. Functional biomechanical deficits in running athletes with plantar fasciitis. *The American Journal of Sports Medicine* 1991; **19**: 66–71.
17. Krisoff WB, Ferris WB. Runner's injuries. *The Physican and Sportsmedicine* 1979; **7**: 55–61.
18. Leach R, Jones R, Silva T. Rupture of the plantar fascia in athletes. *Journal of Bone and Joint Surgery* (Am) 1978; **60**: 537–9.
19. Kruse RJ, McCoy RL, Erickson T. Diagnosing plantar fascia rupture. *The Physician and Sportsmedicine* 1995; **23**: 65–9.
20. Leach RE, Jones R, Salter DK. Results of surgery in athletes with plantar fasciitis. *Foot and Ankle* 1986; **7**: 156–61.
21. Clancy WG. Runner's injuries. Part Two: Evaluation and treatment of specific injuries. *American Journal of Sports Medicine* 1980; **8**: 287.
22. Henricson AS, Westlin NE. Chronic calcaneal pain in athletes: Entrapment of the calcaneal nerve? *American Journal of Sports Medicine* 1984; **12**: 152–4.
23. Sammarco GJ. Soft tissue conditions on athletes' feet. *Clinics in Sports Medicine* 1982; **1**: 149–55.
24. Schon LC. Nerve entrapment, neuropathy, and nerve dysfunction in athletes. *Orthopaedic Clinics of North America* 1994; **25**: 47–59.
25. Jackson DL, Haglund B. Tarsal tunnel syndrome in athletes. Case reports and literature review. *American Journal of Sports Medicine* 1991; **19**: 61–5.
26. Jackson DL, Haglund BL. Tarsal tunnel syndrome in runners. *Sports Medicine* 1992; **13**: 146–9.
27. Pecina M, Bojanic I, Markiewitz AD. Nerve entrapment syndromes in athletes. *Clinical Journal of Sport Medicine* 1993; **3**: 36–42.
28. Lorei MP, Hershman EB. Peripheral nerve injuries in athletes. *Sports Medicine* 1993; **16**: 130–47.
29. Pfeiffer WH, Cracchiolo A. Clinical results after tarsal tunnel decompression. *Journal of Bone and Joint Surgery* 1994; **76A**: 1222–30.
30. Shear MS, Baitch SP, Shear DB. Sinus tarsi syndrome: The importance of biomechanically-based evaluation and treatment. *Archives of Physical Medicine and Rehabilitation* 1993; **74**: 777–81.
31. Brukner P, Khan K. Ankle pain. In: *Clinical sports medicine.* Sydney: McGraw-Hill, 1994: 455–62.
32. Alfred RH, Bergfeld JA. Diagnosis and management of stress fractures of the foot. *The Physician and Sportsmedicine* 1987; **15**: 83–9.
33. Eisele SA, Sammarco GJ. Fatigue fractures of the foot and ankle in the athlete. *Journal of Bone and Joint Surgery* 1993; **75A**: 290–98.
34. Bennel KL, Malcolm SA, Thomas SA. The incidence and distribution of stress fractures in competitive track and field athletes—a twelve-month prospective study. *American Journal of Sports Medicine* 1996; **24**: 211–17.
35. Khan KM, Brukner PD, Kearney C, Fuller PJ, Bradshaw CJ, Kiss ZS. Tarsal navicular stress fracture in athletes. *Sports Medicine* 1994; **17**: 65–76.
36. Khan KM, Fuller PJ, Brukner PD, Kearney C, Burry HC. Outcome of conservative and surgical management of navicular stress fracture in athletes. *American Journal of Sports Medicine* 1992; **20**: 657–65.
37. Ferkel RD, Karzel RP, Del Pizzo W, Friedman MJ, Fisher SP. Athroscopic treatment of anterolateral impingement of the ankle. *American Journal of Sports Medicine* 1991; **19**: 440–6.
38. Jaivin JS, Ferkel RD. Arthroscopy of the foot and ankle. *Clinics in Sports Medicine* 1994; **13**: 761–83.
39. McDermott EP. Basketball injuries of the foot and ankle. *Clinics in Sports Medicine* 1993; **12**: 373–93.
40. Grana WA. Chronic pain after ankle sprain. *The Physican and Sportsmedicine* 1995; **23**: 67–75.
41. Mooney M, Maffey-Ward L. Cuboid plantar and dorsal subluxations: Assessment and treatment. *Journal of Orthopaedic and Sports Physical Therapy* 1994; **20**: 220–6.
42. Kay DB. Forefoot pain in the athlete. *Clinics in Sports Medicine* 1994; **13**: 785–91.
43. Vereschagin KS, Firtch WL, Hoffman MA. Transient paresthesia in stair-climbers' feet. *The Physician and Sportsmedicine* 1993; **21**: 63–9.
44. Axe MJ, Ray RL. Orthotic treatment of sesamoid pain. *American Journal of Sports Medicine* 1988; **16**: 411–16.

5.6 Overuse injuries of the spine

Lyle J. Micheli and Craig M. Mintzer

Introduction

Spine-related complaints account for approximately 10 per cent of athletic medical problems.[1,2] High-performance athletes have been reported to have a significant risk for back pain during their career.[3] Certain sports in particular, such as gymnastics, dance, American football, rowing, and weightlifting, result in a higher incidence of spine problems in their participants. The body motion of athletes in these higher-risk sports consists of repetitive flexion, extension, and rotation of the spine.[2-20]

While specific injuries to the spine are relatively uncommon in sports, back pain is a relatively common complaint shared by both athletes and non-athletes. The physician dealing with an athletically active individual complaining of back pain must be aware that the pattern of injury and the significance of back pain in an athlete is quite different from that in a non-athlete. The aetiology and subsequent diagnoses are often different from those seen in the general population.[21] Failure to appreciate the difference between the pattern of diagnosis and the structures injured in the athlete in contrast with the general population can result in misdiagnosis, delay in proper diagnosis, and delay in appropriate treatment. This has a serious impact not only on athletic performance but also on the future potential for healing in a number of these injuries.

As with injuries at any site, two very different mechanisms, or occasionally a combination of the two, may be responsible for complaints of pain in the spinal region. Acute traumatic injuries to the spine are the result of direct blows, twists, or sudden applications of force. Many of these acute injuries, including traumatic fractures, dislocations, and destabilizing soft-tissue injuries, are medical emergencies. Overuse injuries, which are the result of repetitive activity and subsequent microtrauma, are much more specific to training.

The onset of pain can occur during sports participation or training. The mechanism of injury is usually a combination of the repetitive flexion, extension, and rotation of the spine that occurs in training and in competition. Most commonly, the pattern of pain will be one of slow gradual onset. Often the athlete cannot recall exactly when the pain was first experienced. Typically, the pain increases in severity and duration in association with progressive training. Occasionally, an injury which ultimately is diagnosed to be an overuse injury may have an acute onset caused, for instance, by a particular twist or fall. With subsequent diagnostic assessment and evaluation, it becomes evident that the pathology of the injured structure is the result of a slowly progressive change with the acute episode superimposed on this long-standing injury.[22]

Spine anatomy and biomechanics

The spine consists of 7 cervical vertebrae, 12 thoracic vertebrae, and 5 lumbar vertebrae perched upon the sacrum and pelvis. The structure and function of each segment of the spine is specific to demands placed upon it anatomically and physiologically. The vertebrae of the neck have demands for both range of motion and structural integrity. The occiput–C1 articulation accounts for 50 per cent of flexion and extension in the cervical spine. The C1–C2 articulation accounts for 50 per cent of rotation in the cervical spine. Due to biomechanical considerations, the majority of repetitive mechanical activity and stress in the cervical spine is concentrated at the C5–C6 and C6–C7 disc and joint levels. Progressive anatomical and degenerative changes involving the discs and facet joints occur most often at these levels. The majority of the 'overuse injuries' of the cervical spine are the result of these degenerative changes with secondary bony overgrowth and impingement of the neural foramina. Impingement occurs to the exiting nerve roots, but occasionally frank myelopathy due to compression of the spinal cord itself may occur. This should always be considered in the differential diagnosis of neck pain in the older athlete.

Overuse injuries of the thoracic spine are relatively rare, and this is undoubtedly related to the structure and function of the thoracic spine. The 12 vertebral bodies in the thoracic region are rigidly supported by ribs from T1–T10, and the orientation of the facet joints adds to stability. Each osseous segment increases in size from cranial to cephalad, forming a protective bony ring around the neural tube. There is a normal posterior angulation, or kyphus, of the thoracic spine which varies between 20 degrees and 40 degrees. It is noteworthy that, while direct injury to the structures of the thoracic spine from repetitive overuse activities in sports is rare, the structural anatomy and subsequent rigidity of the thoracic spine can indirectly contribute to the occurrence of overuse injuries in both the cervical and lumbar spine.

As an example, a significant flattening in the angulation or kyphus of the thoracic spine with a subsequent 'flat-back' alignment of the spine may result in a relative hypolordosis of the lumbar spine with an apparent increase in the mechanical forces at the high lumbar and thoracolumbar junction. We have observed that repetitive overuse injuries at the thoracolumbar junction, called by some authors 'atypical Scheuermann's disease', is invariably associated with a hypokyphosis of the thoracic spine and hypolordosis of the lumbar spine.[23,24] In contrast, increased postural thoracic kyphosis is often associated with a relative forward head thrust and hyperlordosis of the cervical spine. This is frequently associated with chronic strain of the posterior cervical and cervicothoracic muscles seen in athletes involved in sports such as tennis or swimming. There also appears to be an association between the thoracic kyphus and the development of long-term degenerative changes at the lower cervical spine. These are clinical observations.

The five bony elements of the lumbar spine are joined to the pelvis at the sacrum. In contrast to the cervical spine, the more proximal elements of the lumbar spine contribute relatively less to the flexion, extension, and rotation of the lumbar spine. Major components of lumbar motion, as well as the concentration of relative stresses in the lumbar spine, occur near the base from the L3–L4 juncture through L5–S1. This, in turn, is reflected in the pattern of degenerative changes seen from repetitive activity in the lumbar spine. Failure of both the anterior elements of the spine, especially the disc and surrounding plates, and the posterior elements of the lumbar spine (in particular the pars interarticularis), occur near the base of the spine. The most common level is the L5–S1 followed sequentially by L4–L5 and L3–L4.[25]

There is growing evidence that overuse stress to the posterior elements concentrates primarily at the pars interarticularis. Cadaver and histological studies, as well as computer analog research, have suggested that the incidence of posterior element failure is overwhelmingly at the pars interarticularis.[26,27] Pedicle overuse injury, while rare, has been reported in the literature.[15,22]

Several studies have suggested that the duration and intensity of training is directly related to lumbar spine failure in young athletes.[8,28–30] Unfortunately, we are still not in a position to give coaches, athletes, and parents an accurate statement of how much training is enough and how much is 'too much' for a given sport or a child at a given age.[31,32]

As with overuse injuries in general, a number of risk factors for overuse injury of the lumbar spine can be identified in the development of injury (Table 1). These risk factors include training, in particular its duration and intensity as well as its rate of progression, muscle–tendon imbalances about the spine, and anatomical factors such as pre-existent lumbar lordosis. One study of spine injuries in young athletes in Scandinavia suggested that lumbosacral inclination was the one major factor which could be related to the mani-

festation of back pain.[31] In sports in which there is an element of impact, such as gymnastics, the impact characteristics of the surface may be a contributing factor in the occurrence of injury. While studies of risk factors for overuse injuries in running sports have been performed, to date these factors have not yet been analysed in overuse back injuries. The type of footwear and its ability to dissipate force is also a cofactor in injuries. Recently, gender has been identified as a factor in sports-related injuries such as anterior cruciate ligament tears in female basketball and soccer participants.[33–35] Gender factors also appear to play a role in the development of back pain in industrial populations. Many of the cases of back pain in athletes have been identified in young female gymnasts.[30] Pre-existent cultural conditions which include extended periods of sedentary activity, such as sitting in school, riding in cars or buses, or sitting in front of computer modules, are undoubtedly a factor.[36] A spine which has been deconditioned by these activities and is then put into short intense periods of flexion, extension, and rotation may be at additional risk of overuse injury. Finally, the level of skeletal maturation may play an important role in the occurrence of overuse injury. Studies of young Italian weightlifters, gymnasts, interior linemen in American football, and children in general have strongly suggested that there is an increased risk of overuse injury, particular of the posterior elements of the spine, when repetitive stresses are applied to the growing spine.[3,4,6,37,38] As is becoming increasingly evident in many sports throughout the world, intense high-level training is being applied to younger and younger athletes in such sports as gymnastics, figure skating, tennis, and more traditional team sports such as hockey, soccer, field lacrosse, and field hockey.[39]

Studies of spondylolysis have strongly supported the concept that this is an acquired condition, although a congenital predisposition may exist. In a study of 143 non-ambulatory institutionalized patients over 10 years of age Rosenberg et al.[40] found no cases of spondylolysis. Other studies have suggested a genetic predisposition to this condition, such as in the Inuit population of northern Canada.[41,42]

The majority of spine complaints in the athletically active patient are secondary to chronic overuse injuries resulting in repetitive microtrauma to the thoracolumbar spine.[29] Many of these complaints have an insidious onset and are often classified as 'chronic back strain' thereby delaying the diagnosis and definitive treatment. While repetitive microtrauma and discogenic pain make up the majority of the diagnoses in this category, the more serious problems of metabolic, neoplastic, and infectious aetiologies must be entertained with persistent symptoms, despite the fact that the pain began in association with sport (Tables 2 and 3).

Stress reaction of the pars interarticularis and spondylolysis in the young athlete

Mechanical injury to the pars interarticularis is one of the most frequently encountered anatomical lesions of the spine diagnosed in the young athletic population.[21,43] It has frequently been described as a stress fracture resulting in a bony defect in the pars interarticularis at one or both sides of a given vertebral level.[42–45] The instability and subsequent micro or macro motion created by this lesion

Table 1 Overuse injury risk factors

Training error

Muscle–tendon imbalance

Anatomical malalignment

Footwear

Playing surface

Associated disease state

Nutritional factors

Cultural deconditioning

results in pain, particularly when activities increase the stress placed across the posterior elements of the spine.

Epidemiology

Studies have shown that approximately 6 per cent of adults in the general population have evidence of spondylolysis[37,46,47] and that the mean age of the symptomatic population is between 15 and 16 years of age. More recent studies have demonstrated that spondylolysis is increasingly being diagnosed in younger patients, between 5 and 10 years of age.[48] The increase in diagnosis at this young age may be secondary to the increased participation by chil-

Table 2 Differential diagnosis of spine pathology in athletes less than 20 years of age

Developmental

Scoliosis

Kyphosis

Spondylolisthesis

Spondylolysis

Acquired

Acute

Musculotendinous sprain/strain

Stress fracture

    Spondylolysis

    Vertebral endplate fractures

Fractures

    Ring apophysis fracture

    Transverse processes

    Spinous processes

    Compression fracture

Herniated nucleus pulposus

Infection

    Disc space

    Vertebral osteomyelitis

Chronic

Musculotendinous sprain/strain

Stress fracture

    Spondylolysis

    Vertebral endplate fractures

Spondylarthropathy

Neoplasm

    Osteoblastoma

    Osteoid osteoma

    Metastatic neoplasm

Infection

Table 3 Differential diagnosis of spine pathology in athletes more than 20 years of age

Acute

Musculotendinous sprain/strain

Stress fracture

    Spondylolysis

Fractures

    Transverse processes

    Spinous processes

    Compression fracture of vertebral body

Discogenic pain—acute herniated nucleus pulposus

Infection

Chronic

Musculotendinous sprain/strain

Stress fracture

    Spondylolysis

    Lumbar pedicle fracture

Mechanical

    Facet hypertrophy

    Spinal stenosis

    Herniated nucleus pulposus—degenerative disc disease

Infection

Spondylarthropathy—Reiter's syndrome, ankylosing spondylitis

Metastatic or primary neoplasm

Referred pain

    Intra-abdominal

    Retroperitoneal

    Pelvic

dren in more strenuous and highly organized sporting activities early in life. It has been found that 85 per cent of the lesions occur at the L5 vertebral level.[49] Although pars defects have never been identified in the newborn infant, a genetic predisposition to these lesions has been documented in multiple studies.[12,24–27,40–52] There is considerable variation of incidence between races, with an incidence of 2 per cent in black subjects and as high as 50 per cent in some Inuit communities.[45,51] In the athletic population, this lesion is found much more frequently in athletes who sustain repetitive traumatic stresses on the lumbar spine, as seen in blocking and sled training in American football, or in those who perform specific repetitive lumbar motions, for example in ballet dancing, competitive diving, pole vaulting, hurdling, gymnastics, and most recently fast bowlers in cricket.[3,6,8,11,19,28,53,54]

Pathogenesis

Defects of the pars interarticularis have generally been classified into dysplastic, isthmic (traumatic), and degenerative types. The pathogenesis of this lesion in athletes is believed to be due to repetitive microtrauma and resultant stress fractures of the posterior elements of the spine rather than a congenital condition.[41-45,53] Biomechanical studies have demonstrated that shear stresses across the pars interarticularis are increased when the spine is extended and accentuated with lateral flexion manoeuvres from a hyperlordotic posture.[26,41,53] Similar to other fatigue fractures, routine radiographs of the spine may not be diagnostic early in the course of the stress fractures. The diagnosis of a stress fracture of the pars interarticularis may be confirmed by bone scan.[55] The bone scan, and in particular the computer-enchanced **SPECT** (single-photon emission computed tomography) bone scan, can also help in differentiating an acute from a chronic spondylolysis.[56] These lesions rarely develop an exuberant periosteal reaction and the radiographic evidence of the lesion can persist even in the stable asymptomatic state.

The history of onset of pain is very important in the diagnosis of spondylolysis. In many instances, the onset of symptoms coincides closely with the adolescent growth spurt. The pain usually has an insidious onset and athletes complain of a dull backache which is exacerbated by activity. With continued activity the pain increases in severity and begins to occur with activities of daily living. The symptoms are often relieved by rest. Rarely, there may be radicular symptoms that do not migrate past the knee. A history of repetitive strenuous activity involving flexion/extension and rotation of the spine can almost always be elicited.

On physical examination, 80 per cent of patients are noted to have relatively tight hamstrings.[57] Subtle changes in hamstring flexibility may be noted in hyperflexible athletes such as gymnasts and dancers. In acute spondylolysis palpation usually elicits tenderness that is localized at the involved vertebral level. Pain is usually reproduced by the provocative manoeuvre of having the patient extend the lumbar spine against resistance. Active hyperextension of the lumbar spine while in a one-legged stance specifically stresses the ipsilateral pars and provokes pain.

The diagnostic work-up consists initially of anteroposterior, lateral, and oblique radiographic views of the lumbosacral spine to assess the integrity of the posterior elements. The defect can best be seen as a narrow gap with irregular edges in the pars interarticularis (Fig. 1). Reactive sclerosis as demonstrated by a contralateral dense pedicle may be seen opposite the lesion in unilateral cases. Radiographic changes may not be apparent initially, and radioisotope bone scans are very useful in the prompt confirmation of the diagnosis.[55] SPECT has also been useful in further localizing spondylotic defects.[46,56] When the diagnosis is indeterminate, computed tomographic (**CT**) scanning can be used to assess the integrity of the pars interarticularis (Fig. 2). The diagnosis of osteoid osteoma, facet arthropathy, and infection should be ruled out in the initial work-up when the bone scan is noted to positive. Spondylolysis in the athletic population is generally a mechanically stable lesion, and the usual problem for the patient is the potential for activity-related pain rather than spine instability. Since the isthmic spondylolysis seen in athletes is thought to be a stress fracture of the posterior elements, the current recommended initial management consists of a restriction of activities and immobilization of the lumbar spine with a rigid polypropylene antilordotic lumbosacral brace (Fig. 3).

A brace with 0 to 15 per cent lumbar flexion acts to flatten the lumbar lordosis while immobilizing the spine, relieves the pain, and

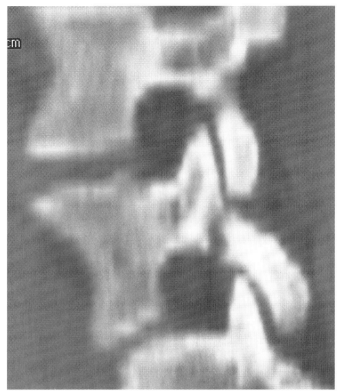

Fig. 1 Axial computed tomographic scan demonstrating the pars defect found in spondylolysis.

should promote healing of the lesion. After a brace has been fitted, the patient wears it for 23 out of 24 h a day for 6 months. Concurrently, physical therapy intervention focuses on abdominal strengthening. Pelvic tilts, antilordotic and lower-extremity flexibility exercises are also prescribed. Most patients are able to resume limited activities to maintain their aerobic fitness and muscle strength when they become pain-free in the brace at 6 to 8 weeks. A progressive decrease of hamstring tightness has been suggested as an indicator of the success of a treatment programme. Bone scans are a useful adjunct to the clinical examination for following the

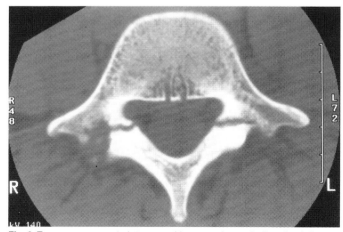

Fig. 2 Transverse computed tomographic scan demonstrating the lytic pars defect.

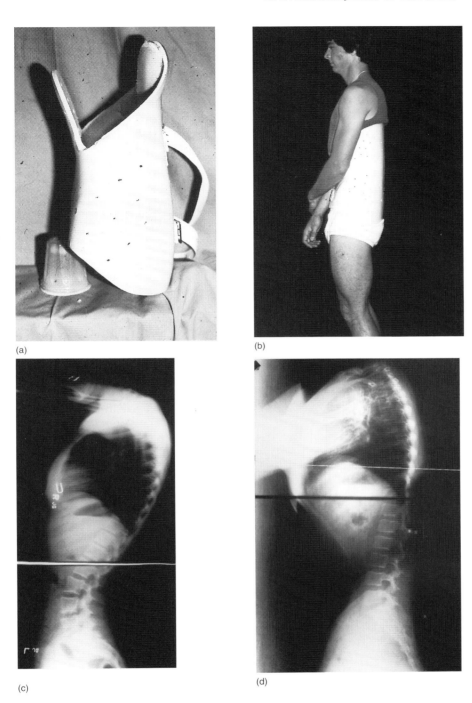

Fig. 3 An antilordotic thermoplastic brace (a) can be used as part of the treatment regimen of young athletes with back pain. (b) A lateral radiograph of the lumbar spine (c) before and (d) after application of a 0 degrees Boston brace.

status of the lesion, since the uptake decreases with either healing or quietening of the inflammation at the defect.

In a prepubescent or pubescent athlete with this lesion, every attempt should be made to achieve union. A focal CT scan of the involved level can accurately assess the status of progressive healing. In young adults with established non-unions, brace treatment can be reduced in those patients with an initially negative bone scan who become asymptomatic after wearing the brace for 4 to 6 weeks. After treatment, patients usually require 4 to 6 months to wean themselves from full-time brace wear as they gradually increase their activities. In one reported series, 32 per cent of patients treated in

this manner healed their lesion and overall 88 per cent were able to resume sports activities that were previously painful, even though some of these lesions had not healed by radiographic criteria.[58] In patients who are asymptomatic, despite an apparent non-union of the lesion, full return to activities including contact sports is allowed. The clinical status of the patient takes precedence over radiographic examination in the follow-up of these lesions.

Athletes who are unable to be weaned from their brace without a recurrence of their symptoms may require surgery. A posterolateral transverse process fusion is the classic form of treatment, although direct osteosynthesis of the lesion has been described.[25,59-61]

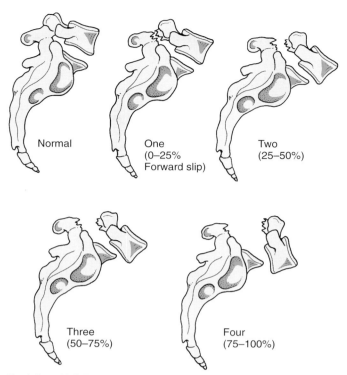

Fig. 4 Spondylolisthesis is graded into four degrees of severity based upon the extent of forward slippage.

After surgery, the patient is immobilized in a cast or brace for 6 months and sports activities are not allowed until 12 months following fusion. Return to contact sports must be individualized after lumbar fusion.[62,63]

Cost containment

Serial radiographs are unnecessary in the follow-up of spondylolytic defects. After an initial screening radiographic series of the lumbar spine, a physician may want to confirm the diagnosis with a SPECT scan. Patients can then be followed clinically over the next several months of brace wear. When patients are being weaned from their brace, or brace wear is being terminated, a single-level CT scan of the lesion is used to assess the status of healing. After an initial evaluation, physical therapy may be readily instituted at home with monthly follow-up. In certain cases where bony union has not been attained despite bracing, transcutaneous electrical stimulation may offer the potential for further healing.

Spondylolisthesis

Spondylolisthesis occurs as one vertebral body slips forward on an adjacent vertebral body (Fig. 4). The aetiologies for this slippage are:

(I)   spondylolysis with macro or micro trauma;

(II)   degenerative changes;

(III) congenital abnormalities; or

(IV) pathological lesions in the bone.

The development of spondylolisthesis is multifactorial and is often associated with females who have the congenital form of spondylolysis. This form of spondylolysis, which features malformed or dystrophic posterior elements, has a much higher incidence of slippage than the isthmic type seen in the athletic population. It is most frequently noted in non-athletic females during their adolescent growth spurt between 10 and 15 years of age. The L5–S1 vertebral level is involved in 85 to 90 per cent of cases. Studies have suggested that there is a genetic predisposition to spondylolisthesis, with reported rates of 27 per cent to 69 per cent in close relatives.[64] The incidence of high-grade spondylolisthesis (more than 75 per cent slippage) is much higher in females than in males.[51,52] The progression of a lytic spondylolysis to spondylolisthesis in adulthood has been reported, but is exceedingly rare.[52]

These patients may give a history similar to that elicited with spondylolysis; although, in some instances, presentation may be with tight hamstrings rather than pain. Sometimes the patient presents with an abnormal gait, abnormal posture or appearance of the trunk, a history of trauma, or rarely a change in bowel or bladder habits. Severe grades of spondylolisthesis with a palpable step-off are rare in the athletic population, and the associated pain and loss of flexibility preclude most athletic participation. The physical examination consists of observation of the patient's stance and profile. Hips and knees may be flexed (with the pelvis tilted) in severe cases of slippage.

Standing anteroposterior (**AP**) and lateral radiographs of the patient demonstrate the abnormality. Spondylolisthesis most often occurs at the lumbosacral junction. When it occurs at L4 it is usually associated with sacralization of L5. The percentage of slip is the ratio of the distance between the posterior aspect of the sacrum and L5 divided by the width of the L5 vertebral body. Grade I slips are less than 25 per cent, grade II 25 to 50 per cent, grade III 51 to 75 per cent, and grade IV 76 to 100 per cent (Fig. 4).

Most authors agree that patients with asymptomatic grade I slips need no athletic restrictions and may be able to participate in contact sports as long as they remain symptom-free. Sport restriction with grade II slips has been debated, but, as yet, no consensus exists. A recent study demonstrated minimum increase in slippage with unrestricted competitive sports competition.[65] Patients with minimal symptoms are treated with sports activity modifications and a conservative programme of physical therapy emphasizing antilordotic exercises, hamstring stretching, and abdominal strengthening. Brace management with a rigid, antilordotic, polypropylene lumbosacral orthosis is carried out for 2 to 6 months in those patients who fail initial conservative treatment (activity modification and physical therapy.) Antilordotic, abdominal strengthening, and hamstring stretching exercises are continued while the patient is still in the brace. Patients may resume their activities in a brace when they become asymptomatic.[25,58] Children and adolescents should have close follow-up until skeletal maturity, with lateral radiographs obtained once a year to guard against progression.

Surgical management is reserved for those patients with progression of slippage and for those children who demonstrate failure of conservative treatment over a 6 to 12-month period. Grade I and II slips can be treated with posterior *in-situ* fusion between L5 and S1.[25,59,66,67] Resolution of symptoms usually accompanies a successful fusion. Higher grades should have their fusion extended from L4 to S1. Nerve-root decompression may need to be performed if there is neurological compromise. Reduction and instrumentation of high-grade slips is controversial.[68,69] Contact sports may be contraindicated after lumbar fusion.[62]

Scheuermann's disease

Some adolescents will compensate for tight lumbodorsal fascia and hamstrings by developing a roundback deformity. This postural deformity is usually transient with no structural abnormalities demonstrated on radiographic examination. This postural deformity corrects with passive extension. Scheuermann's disease, however, is a structural entity that presents with a kyphotic deformity.[24] There are multiple theories as to the aetiology of Scheuermann's disease including necrosis of the ring apophysis, osteochondrosis, juvenile osteoporosis, and mechanical factors such as tight hamstrings. The radiographic criteria for Scheuermann's disease are met when three or more adjacent vertebral bodies are wedged more than 5 degrees.[70,71] An associated non-progressive scoliosis of 10 to 20 degrees is common. Classic Scheuermann's disease, or juvenile thoracic kyphosis, is usually painless and rarely seen in its true form in the athletic population.[23,24] Patients present with a roundback deformity which they cannot reverse with forced hyperextension. Many of these patients have a relatively flat lumbar spine with tight lumbar fascia, hip flexors, and hamstrings. In contrast, 'atypical' or lumbar Scheuermann's disease presents with irregular vertebral endplates at the thoracolumbar junction and is seen more frequently in the athletic population. This form of disease is painful and is associated with activities that produce repetitive microtrauma to the thoracolumbar spine.

Thoracic Scheuermann's disease usually presents without a distinct traumatic history and with deformity rather than pain. The apex of the kyphosis is located between T7 and T9. The reported incidence in the general population ranges from 0.4 per cent to 10 per cent.[72] Radiographic evidence is usually absent until 10 years of age. The radiographic picture which is diagnostic includes irregular vertebral endplates, Schmorl's nodes, narrowed disc spaces, and anterior wedging of three consecutive vertebral bodies.[71] Treatment, if symptomatic or cosmetically unacceptable, initially addresses the tight lumbodorsal fascia and hamstrings with flexibility exercises. Abdominal strengthening exercises are added to this programme. Progressive thoracic kyphosis above 50 degrees in a skeletally immature athlete is an indication for 18 h/day treatment with a Milwaukee or modified Boston brace. Further progression beyond 70 degrees may be an indication for spinal fusion and instrumentation. These patients are then restricted from sports activities, except swimming, 1-year postoperatively. Contact sports and gymnastics are not allowed after surgery, but patients can eventually return to light non-contact activities.[62]

Apophyseal microtrauma, atypical Scheuermann's disease

In young athletes a radiographic picture which resembles the wedged vertebrae and irregular endplates seen in thoracic Scheuermann's disease sometimes occurs in the midthoracic to the midlumbar spine.[23] Unlike typical Scheuermann's disease, the natural history of this process is less well understood. This is most commonly seen in adolescent athletes with repetitive flexion/extension

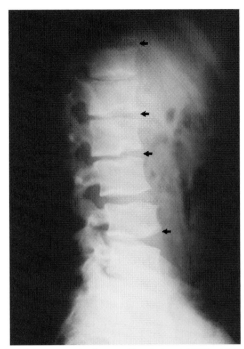

Fig. 5 Atypical Scheuermann's disease with anterior vertebral wedging and irregularity of the vertebral endplates.

of the spine such as rowers and gymnasts participating in very rigorous training programmes. This has been referred to as 'atypical' or lumbar Scheuermann's disease since it appears to be the result of repetitive microtrauma in athletes and does not meet all the radiographic criteria of true Scheuermann's disease (Fig. 5). The peak age is between 15 and 17 years and there is a 2:1 male predominance.

Repetitive flexion and extension of the thoracolumbar junction results in multiple micro growth-plate fractures and secondary bony deformation of the vertebra. Apophyseal fragments at the anterior margin of the vertebral body may be avulsed, resulting in Schmorl's node formation and irregular vertebral endplates (Fig. 5). One recent study demonstrated a high incidence of radiographic abnormalities at the thoracolumbar junction in competitive athletes, especially in wrestlers and female gymnasts.[39] This entity has also been reported to involve the sacrum.[73]

The history is usually significant, with complaints of transient pain at the thoracolumbar junction followed by complaints of moderately severe pain accentuated by activities and relieved by rest. Radicular complaints are rare. These patients are consistently noted to have tight lumbodorsal fascia and hamstrings and relative thoracic hypokyphosis and lumbar hyperlordosis (flatbacks). Neurological examination is unremarkable. Radiographs reveal multiple irregularities of the vertebral endplates, signs of chronic vertebral endplate wedging, and subsequent changes in the disc space.

The hallmark of treatment is rest and avoidance of the inciting activity. Persistent symptoms may be managed with non-steroidal anti-inflammatory drugs (**NSAIDs**). A bracing regimen may be instituted using a semirigid thermoplastic brace with 15 degrees of lumbar lordosis to immobilize the patient until remodelling is seen on plain radiographs.[74] Patients may return to sports while they are

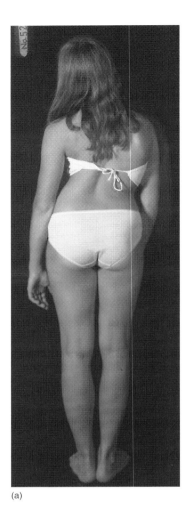

(a)

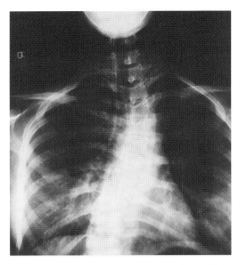

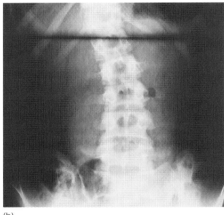

(b)

Fig. 6 (a) A child with scoliosis and secondary spinal asymmetry; (b) a standing coronal radiograph of the spine demonstrating the spinal curvature.

braced, and at the same time are prescribed a flexibility programme. No restrictions are placed on the patients when they are weaned from their brace as long as they have maintained their previous level of fitness. Surgical intervention is rarely indicated in these patients.

Scoliosis

Preparticipation sports screening is an important avenue for evaluating the young athlete for scoliosis.[75,76] Idiopathic scoliosis does not cause pain and does not functionally impair the athlete. Congenital scoliosis has associated renal and cardiac anomalies that should be thoroughly excluded before the young athlete is allowed to participate in sports. Patients with congenital anomalies of the cervical spine and cervicothoracic junction should be advised not to participate in contact sports. This area is very controversial.

Diagnosis

In the skeletally immature child, curves are usually noted by the child's parents, coach, or school nurse as an asymmetry in the child's shoulders or thoracic spine which is accentuated by forward bending or shoulder protraction. These patients should be referred to an orthopaedic surgeon for a full evaluation (Fig. 6).

Management

If a scoliosis curve is noted to progress rapidly or reaches 25 to 30 degrees in the skeletally immature child, a corrective bracing programme is initiated to control the progression of the curve. Patients generally wear the brace for at least 18 h per day and are allowed to participate in sports activities in or out of the brace without restrictions. An active strengthening and flexibility programme is encouraged during brace wear. When growth is complete and the athlete is weaned out of the brace, there are no restrictions placed on patients with residual idiopathic scoliosis. Patients whose curves progress beyond 50 degrees have a high incidence of progression and require anterior and/or posterior spinal fusion. Since the fusion involves significant motion segments of the thoracic and lumbar spine with subsequent loss of mobility, contact sports, gymnastics, and diving sports are usually contraindicated following this treatment.[62] A recent German study concluded that if there are less than three free lumbar segments after fusion then all sports with axial and rotationary burdens should be avoided as there is increased loading on the few remaining segments.[77]

Painful scoliosis may also be the presenting physical finding associated with disc herniations, osteoid osteomas, osteoblastomas, spondylolisthesis, infections, and intraspinal tumours in the child. A painful scoliosis should always raise suspicion in the evaluation of a child with back pain.

Discogenic back pain in the adult athlete

Compression of a nerve root along its anatomical course causes radicular pain. In under 40-year-old athletes, the most common cause of radicular pain is a herniated disc. This condition is rare in the prepubescent child, but the incidence increases from adolescence to adulthood.[78-80] The association between participation in specific sports and an increase in the incidence of disc herniation has not been established. On the contrary, sports participation has been found to be protective when compared with the general population, perhaps this is secondary to the improved fitness achieved by the athlete.[81]

Radicular pain can occur in the cervical or lumbar spine in the nerve root distribution of the particular compressed root. In the lumbar spine, sharp sciatic pain radiating from the buttock and extending below the knee in the distribution of the affected nerve root are the classic symptoms. Initially, symptoms are typically exacerbated by increased activity and the pain may eventually become a dull ache in the buttock or hip region. Subtle signs noted by the athlete or the practitioner are slight symmetrical decreases in hamstring flexibility, paravertebral spasm, scoliosis, and changes in running patterns. Physical examination typically reveals positive straight-leg raising and occasionally sensory and motor changes in the involved nerve root distribution. At present, the diagnostic study of choice is magnetic resonance imaging (**MRI**) (Fig. 7). The MRI results must be coordinated with the physical examination as there is a high incidence of asymptomatic disc pathology.[82,83] In cases where the differential diagnosis includes both disc derangement and spondylolysis, CT scanning can be useful.

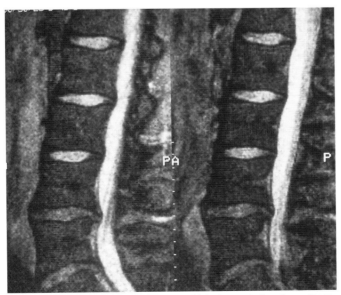

Fig. 7 MRI of the lumbar spine of a young athlete demonstrating disc prolapse.

Management

Conservative therapy remains the primary mode of treatment in these patients. NSAIDs and a relative period of rest for 3 to 5 days usually result in improvement in symptoms. Traction, braces, corsets, and manipulations may be used to help relieve symptoms and improve function. Physical therapy to restore strength and motion to the spine and peripelvic musculature can also be useful. The primary goal of treatment is to allow the spine a period of 'relative rest' during which the damaged disc undergoes healing. During this period of 'relative rest', we sometimes use a semirigid thermoplastic orthotic to protect the back as modified traning is resumed.[2,32,74]

Only 5 to 10 per cent of patients with discogenic pain will eventually require further intervention. Treatment modalities using epidural steroids, percutaneous discectomy, and disc excision have been described.[83-88] The majority of athletes are able to return to activity after successful disc surgery.[89-91] It is not known whether participation in vigorous contact sports following discectomy accelerates degenerative changes.

Referred back pain

Adult athletes may complain of low-back pain which may initially be attributed to a sports injury, but is actually due to another aetiology. Other aetiologies include neoplastic or infectious processes, intra-abdominal, retroperitoneal, or pelvic sources. A history of night pain, fatigue, or recent weight loss should initiate a complete diagnostic evaluation.

Mechanical back pain

In the athletic population, mechanical back pain is generally a diagnosis of exclusion. The symptoms are frequently non-specific and include low-back pain that is exacerbated by activity and relieved by rest. Some authors have suggested that this mechanical pain syndrome is secondary to overuse or stretch injuries to the soft tissues, ligaments, joint capsules, and the facets themselves.[1,92]

Diagnosis

Excessive athletic activity with poor conditioning and training methods, insufficient stretching, and improper technique are commonly noted in the history. Physical examination is rather unremarkable. Plain radiographs and bone scans are normal. Patients with a predisposition to these injuries are noted to have weak abdominal muscles and tight lumbodorsal fascia, hip flexors, and hamstrings. In young athletes, there is usually an 'extension contracture' of the lumbar spine, with loss of foward flexion and tight hamstrings. The site of pain may be hypermobile facet joints.

Management

Acutely, these patients respond well to a programme of rest and modification of activities. Non-steroidal anti-inflammatory drugs (NSAIDs) may be helpful during the acute phase. Hydrotherapy, ultrasound, and electrical stimulation to break up paraspinal spasm are useful adjuncts. Some authors have suggested that injection of steroid and local anaesthetic into the facet joint relieves the symptoms in the majority of patients.[1,93] After the acute phase of pain an individualized rehabilitation and stretching programme must be prescribed for the athlete. Suggestions must be made to the athlete for modifications in technique and training schedules to prevent recurrence of the injury.[94] Persistent pain, despite a careful attempt at conservative therapy, necessitates a more complete diagnostic work-up.

Athletic rehabilitation of the spine

Low-back pain is a very common musculoskeletal ailment in the general population and generates an enormous expense in health care and loss of productivity. In the general population, 50 per cent of patients recover in 2 weeks and 90 per cent are pain-free after 3 months. However, 7 per cent of patients have pain for more than 6 months, and these patients account for 85 to 90 per cent of the compensation for low-back pain.[95,96]

In the athletic population, the rehabilitation of spinal injuries presents the clinician with a complex therapeutic challenge. Few of these patients eventually require surgical intervention. Most of them are not sufficiently debilitated from their injuries to refrain from normal daily activities, yet their athletic performance and enjoyment is significantly restricted. Their motivation to return to sport is high. The ultimate goal for the physician is to return the patient safely to the repetitive demands of athletics in a pain-free state as quickly as possible without exacerbating the problems. In the case of spinal rehabilitation, clear initial goals must be set regarding the time course of immobilization and rehabilitation for each problem. A clear understanding of the natural history of specific problems and the expected time course of rehabilitation is essential for the patient to avoid the psychological pitfalls of a chronic back injury.

Many clinicians stress the role of exercise as a mainstay in the treatment of lumbar spine problems.[94,97] It has been postulated that exercise decreases pain by increasing endorphin levels. A decreased incidence of back pain and injury recurrence has been clearly associated with increased fitness levels.[98,99] Additionally, exercise has important effects on skeletal mineralization.[100] For this reason, we emphasize the maintenance of aerobic cardiovascular fitness in the prevention and rehabilitation of lumbar spine problems. Thermoplastic, antilordotic, thoracolumbar spine braces, such as the Boston brace, have previously been mentioned in a number of therapeutic programmes.[74] These lightweight braces have allowed patients to resume light sports activities while wearing the brace. However, it must be emphasized that all brace prescriptions are accompanied by a physical therapy programme designed to strengthen the abdominal musculature and increase flexibility of the spine and hips. An excellent description of a complete set of spine flexibility and strengthening exercises is outlined by Torg et al.[101]

References

1. Spencer GW, Jackson DW. Back injuries in the athlete. *Clinics in Sports Medicine* 1983; **2**: 191–216.
2. Gerbino PG, Micheli LJ. Low back injuries in the young athlete. *Sports medicine and arthroscopy review.* Philadelphia: Lippincott–Raven, 1996.
3. Ferguson RH, McMaster JF, Stanitski CL. Low back pain in college football lineman. *American Journal of Sports Medicine* 1974; **2**: 63–9.
4. Aggrawal ND, Kaur R, Kumar S, Mathur DN. A study of changes in the spine in weight lifters and other athletes. *British Journal of Sports Medicine* 1979; **13**: 58–61.
5. Brady TA, Cahill BR, Bodnar LM. Weight training-related injuries in the high school athlete. *American Journal of Sports Medicine* 1982; **10**: 1–5.
6. Ciullo JV, Jackson DW. Pars interarticularis stress reaction, spondylolysis, and spondylolisthesis in gymnasts. *Clinics in Sports Medicine* 1985; **4**: 95–110.
7. Garrick JG, Requa RK. Epidemiology of women's gymnastics injuries. *American Journal of Sports Medicine* 1980; **8**: 261–4.
8. Goldberg MA. Gymnastics injuries. *Orthopedic Clinics of North America* 1980; **11**: 717–24.
9. Granhed H, Jonson R, Hansson T. The loads on the lumbar spine during extreme weight lifting. *Spine* 1987; **12**: 146–9.
10. Granhed H, Morelli B. Low back pain among retired wrestlers and heavyweight lifters. *American Journal of Sports Medicine* 1988; **16**: 530–5.
11. Hall SJ. Mechanical contribution to lumbar stress injuries in female gymnasts. *Medicine and Science in Sports and Exercise* 1986; **18**: 599–602.
12. Hensinger RN. Back pain in children. In: Bradford DS, Hensinger RM, eds. *The pediatric spine.* New York: Thieme, 1985; 41–60.
13. Howell DW. Musculoskeletal profile and incidence of musculoskeletal injuries in lightweight women rowers. *American Journal of Sports Medicine* 1984; **12**: 278–81.
14. Hresko MT, Micheli LJ. Sports medicine and the lumbar spine. In: Floman Y, ed. *Disorders of the lumbar spine.* Rockville, MD: Aspen, 1990; 879–94.
15. Ireland ML, Micheli LJ. Bilateral stress fracture in the lumbar pedicle in a ballet dancer. *Journal of Bone and Joint Surgery* 1987; **69A**: 140–2.
16. Jackson DW, Wiltse LL, Cirincione RJ. Spondylolysis in the female gymnast. *Clinical Orthopaedics and Related Research* 1976; **117**: 68–73.
17. McCarroll JR, Miller JM, Ritter MA. Lumbar spondylolysis and spondylolisthesis in college football players. *American Journal of Sports Medicine* 1986; **14**: 404–6.
18. Micheli LJ. Back injuries in gymnastics. *Clinics in Sports Medicine* 1985; **4**: 85–93.
19. Semon RL, Spengler D. Significance of lumbar spondylolysis in college football players. *Spine* 1981; **6**: 172–4.
20. Techakapuch S. Rupture of the lumbar cartilage plate into the spinal canal in an adolescent. A case report. *Journal of Bone and Joint Surgery* 1981; **63A**: 481–2.
21. Micheli LJ, Wood R. Back pain in young athletes. *Archives of Pediatric and Adolescent Medicine* 1995; **149**: 15–18.
22. Maxwell KM, Newcomb CE. Bilateral traumatic L4 pedicular fractures in a healthy male athlete. A case report. *Spine* 1993; **18**: 407–9.
23. Hensinger RN. Back pain and vertebral changes simulating Scheuermann's disease. *Orthopaedic Transactions* 1982; **6**: 1–6.
24. Micheli LJ. Low back pain in the adolescent: differential diagnosis. *American Journal of Sports Medicine* 1979; **7**: 362–4.
25. Bradford DS. Spondylolysis and spondylolisthesis in children and adolescents: current concepts in management. In: Bradford DS, Hensinger RM, eds. *The pediatric spine.* New York: Thieme, 1985; 403–23.
26. Cyron BM, Hutton WC. The fatigue strength of the lumbar in spondylolysis. *Journal of Bone and Joint Surgery* 1984; **60B**: 234–8.
27. Schneiderman, GA, McLain, RF, Hambly, MF, Nielsen, SL. The pars defect as a pain source. A histologic study. *Spine* 1995; **20**: 1761–4.
28. Goldstein JD, Berger PE, Windler GE, Jackson DW. Spine injuries in gymnasts and swimmers. An epidemiologic investigation. *American Journal of Sports Medicine* 1991; **19**: 463–8.
29. Jacchia GE, Butler UP, Innocenti M, Capone A. Low back pain in

athletes: pathogenetic mechanisms and therapy. *Chirurgia Delgi Organi di Movimento* 1994; **79**: 47–53.

30. Konermann W, Sell S. The spine—a problem area in high performance artistic gymnastics. A retrospective analysis of 24 former artistic gymnasts of the German A team. *Sportverletzung Sportschaden* 1992; **6**: 156–60.

31. Sward L. The thoracolumbar spine in young elite athletes. Current concepts on effects of physical training. *Sports Medicine* 1992; **12**: 357–64.

32. Gerbino PG, Micheli LJ. Back injuries in the young athlete. *Clinics in Sports Medicine* 1995; **14**: 571–90.

33. Ireland ML. Special concerns of the female athlete. In: Fu FH, Stone DA, eds. *Sports injuries: mechanism, prevention, and treatment*. 2nd edn. Baltimore: Williams and Wilkins, 1994; 153–87.

34. Ireland ML, Wall C. Epidemiology and comparison of knee injuries in elite male and female United States basketball athletes. *Medicine and Science in Sports and Exercise* 1990; **22** (Suppl. 2): S82.

35. Hutchinson MR, Ireland ML. Knee injuries in female athletes. *Sports Medicine* 1995 **19**: 288–302.

36. Salminen JJ, Oksanen A, Maki P, Pentti J, Kujala UM. Leisure time physical activity in the young. Correlation with low-back pain, spine mobility and trunk muscle strength in 15 year old school children. *International Journal of Sports Medicine* 1993; **14**: 406–10.

37. Baker DR, McHolic W. Spondylolysis and spondylolisthesis in children. *Journal of Bone and Joint Surgery* 1956; **38A**: 933–4.

38. Ikata T, Morita T, Katoh S, Tachibana K, Maoka H. Lesions of the lumbar posterior end plate in children and adolescents. An MRI study. *Journal of Bone and Joint Surgery* 1995; **77B**: 951–5.

39. Sward L, Hellstrom M, Jacobson D, Karlsson L. Vertebral ring apophysis injury in athletes. Is the etiology different in the thoracic and lumbar spine? *American Journal of Sports Medicine* 1993; **21**: 841–5.

40. Rosenberg NJ, Bargar WL, Friedman B. The incidence of spondylolysis and spondylolisthesis in non-ambulatory patients. *Spine* 1981; **6**: 35–8.

41. Troup JDG. Mechanical factors in spondylolisthesis and spondylolysis. *Clinical Orthopaedics and Related Research* 1976; **147**: 59–67.

42. Iltse LL. The aetiology of spondylolisthesis. *Journal of Bone and Joint Surgery* 1962; **44A**: 539–60.

43. Pizzutillo PD. Spinal considerations in the young athlete. *Instructional Course Lectures* 1993; **42**: 463–72.

44. Jackson DW. Low back pain in young athletes: evaluation of stress reaction and discogenic problems. *American Journal of Sports Medicine* 1979; **7**: 364–6.

45. Wiltse LL, Widell EH, Jackson DW. Fatigue fracture: the basic lesion in isthmic spondylolisthesis. *Journal of Bone and Joint Surgery* 1975; **57A**: 17–22.

46. Collier BD, Johnson RP, Carrera GF, Meyer GA, Schwab JP, Fiatley TJ, Isitman AT, Hellman RS, Zielonka JS, Knobel J. Painful spondylolysis or spondylolisthesis studies by radiography and single photon emission computed tomography. *Radiology* 1985; **154**: 207–11.

47. Morita T, Okata T, Katoh S, Miyake R. Lumbar spondylolysis in children and adolescents. *Journal of Bone and Joint Surgery* 1995; **77B**: 620–5.

48. Stinson JT. Spondylolysis and spondylolisthesis in the athlete. *Clinics in Sports Medicine* 1993; **12**: 517–28.

49. Blanda J, Bethem D, Moats W, Lew M. Defects of pars interarticularis in athletes: a protocol for nonoperative treatment. *Journal of Spinal Disorders*, 1993; **6**: 406–11.

50. Frederickson BE, Baker D, McHolick WJ, Yuan HA, Lubicky JP. The natural history of spondylolysis and spondylolisthesis. *Journal of Bone and Joint Surgery* 1984; **66A**: 669–707.

51. Pizzutillo PD. Spondylolisthesis: etiology and natural history. In: Bradford DS, Hensinger RM, eds. *The pediatric spine*. New York: Thieme, 1985; 395–402.

52. Winne-Davies R, Scott JHS. Inheritance and spondylolisthesis: a radiographic family survey. *Journal of Bone and Joint Surgery* 1979; **61B**: 301–5.

53. Hardcastle PH. Repair of spondylolysis in young fast bowlers. *Journal of Bone and Joint Surgery* 1993; **75B**: 398–402.

54. Hardcastle P, Annear P, Foster DH, *et al.* Spinal abnormalities in young fast bowlers. *Journal of Bone and Joint Surgery* 1992; **74B**: 421–5.

55. Papanicolaou N, Wilkinson RH, Emans JB, Treves S, Micheli LJ. Bone scintigraphy and radiography in young athletes with low back pain. *American Journal of Roentogenology* 1985; **145**: 1039–44.

56. Lusins JO, Elting JJ, Cicoria AD, Goldsmith SJ. SPECT evaluation of lumbar spondylolysis and spondylolisthesis. *Spine* 1994; **19**: 608–12.

57. Phalen GS, Dickson JA. Spondylolysis and tight hamstrings. *Journal of Bone and Joint Surgery* 1961; **43A**: 505–12.

58. Micheli LJ, Steiner ME. Treatment of symptomatic spondylolysis and spondylolisthesis with the modified Boston brace. *Spine* 1985; **10**: 937–43.

59. Bradford DS, Iza J. Repair of the defect in spondylolysis or minimal degrees of spondylolisthesis by segmental fixation and bone grafting: *Spine* 1985; **10**: 673–9.

60. Buck JE. Direct repair of the defect in spondylolisthesis. *Journal of Bone and Joint Surgery* 1970; **52B**: 432–43.

61. Burning K, Fredensborg N. Osteosynthesis of spondylolysis. *Acta Orthopaedica Scandinavica* 1973; **44**: 91.

62. Micheli LJ. Sports following spinal surgery in the young athlete. *Clinical Orthopaedics and Related Research* 1985; **198**: 152–7.

63. Wright A, Ferree B, Tromanhauser S. Spinal fusion in the athlete. *Clinics in Sports Medicine* 1993; **12**: 599–602.

64. Hensinger RN. Spondylolysis and spondylolisthesis in children and adolescents. *Journal of Bone and Joint Surgery* 1989; **71A**: 1098–107.

65. Muschik M, Hahnel H, Robinson PN, Perka C, Muschik C. Competitive sports and the progression of spondylolisthesis. *Journal of Pedatrics* 1996; **16**: 364–9.

66. Bradford DS. Treatment of severe spondylolisthesis: a combined approach for reduction and stabilization. *Spine* 1979; **4**: 423–9.

67. Hensinger RN, Lang JR, MacEwen GD. Surgical management of spondylolisthesis in children and adolescents. *Spine* 1976; **1**: 207–16.

68. Boxall D, Bradford DS, Winter RB. Management of severe spondylolisthesis in children and adolescents. *Journal of Bone and Joint Surgery* 1979; **61A**: 479–95.

69. Burkus JK, Lonstein JE, Winter RB. Longterm evaluation of adolescents treated operatively for spondylolisthesis. A comparison of *in situ* arthrodesis only with *in situ* arthrodesis and reduction followed by immobilization in a cast. *Journal of Bone and Joint Surgery* 1992; **74A**: 693–704.

70. Bradford DS, Moe J, Montalvo JF, Winter RB. Scheuermann's kyphosis and roundback deformity. *Journal of Bone and Joint Surgery* 1974; **56A**: 740–58.

71. Sorenson HK. *Scheuermann's juvenile kyphosis*. Copenhagen: Munksgaard, 1964.

72. Murray PM, Weinstein SL, Spratt KF. The natural history and long term follow-up of Scheuermann kyphosis. *Journal of Bone and Joint Surgery* 1993; **75A**: 238–45.

73. Biedert RM, Friederich NF, Grul C. Sacral osseous destruction in a female gymnast: unusual manifestation of Scheuermann's Disease. *Knee Surgery, Sports Traumatology, Arthroscopy* 1993; **1**: 110–12.

74. Micheli LJ, Hall JE, Miller ME. Use of modified Boston brace for back injuries in athletes. *American Journal of Sports Medicine* 1980; **8**: 351–6.

75. Lonstein JE. Natural history and school screening for scoliosis. *Orthopedic Clinics of North America* 1988; **19**: 227–37.

76. Micheli LJ. Preparticipation evaluation for sports competition: musculoskeletal assessment of the young athlete. In: Kelley VC, ed. *Practice of pediatrics*. Philadelphia: Harper and Row, 1984; 1–9.

77. von Strempel A, Scholz M, Daentzer M. Sports capacity of patients with scoliosis. *Sportverletzung Sportschaden* 1993; **7**: 58–62.

78. DeOrio JK, Bianco AJ. Lumbar disc excision in children and adolescents. *Journal of Bone and Joint Surgery* 1982; **64A**: 991–5.

79. Garrido E. Humphreys RP, Hendrick EB, Hoffman JH. Lumbar disc disease in children. *Neurosurgery* 1978; **2**: 22–6.

80. Kurihara A, Kataoka O. Lumbar disc herniation in children and adolescents. A review of 70 operated cases and their minimum 5 year follow-up studies. *Spine* 1980; **5**: 443–51.

81. Mundt DJ, Kelsey, JL, Golden, AL, *et al.* An epidemiologic study on weight lifting as possible risk factors for herniated lumbar and cervical discs. The Northeast Collaborative Group on Low back pain. *American Journal of Sports Medicine* 1993; **21**: 854–60.

82. Boden SD, Davis DO, Dina TS. Abnormal magnetic resonance scans of the lumbar spine in asymptomatic subjects: A prospective investigation. *Journal of Bone and Joint Surgery* 1990; **72A**: 403–8.

83. Healy JF, Haly BB, Wong WH, Olson EM. Cervical and lumbar MRI in asymptomatic older male lifelong athletes: frequency of degenerative findings. *Journal of Computer Assisted Tomography* 1996; **20**: 107–12.

84. Brown FW. Epidurals—management of discogenic pain using epidural and intrathecal steroids. *Clinical Orthopaedics and Related Research* 1977; **129**: 72–8.

85. Day AL, Friedman WA, Indelicato PA. Observations on the treatment of lumbar disc disease in college football players. *American Journal of Sports Medicine* 1987; **15**: 72–5.

86. Green P, Burke A, Weiss C, Langan P. The role of epidural cortisone injection in the treatment of discogenic low back pain. *Clinical Orthopaedics and Related Research* 1980; **153**: 121–5.

87. Jackson DW, Rettig A, Wiltse LL. Epidural cortisone injection in the young athletic adult. *American Journal of Sports Medicine* 1980; **8**: 239–43.

88. Nordby EJ. Chymopapain in intradiscal therapy. *Journal of Bone and Joint Surgery* 1983; **65A**: 1350–3.

89. Matsunaga S, Sakou T, Taketomi E, Ijiri K. Comparison of operative results of lumbar disc herniation in manual laborers and athletes. *Spine* 1993; **18**: 2222–6.

90. Sakou T, Masuda A, Yone K, Nakagawa M. Percutaneous discectomy in athletes. *Spine* 1993; **18**: 2218–21.

91. Kahanovitz N. Surgical disc excision. *Clinics in Sports Medicine* 1993; **12**: 579–85.

92. Jackson DW, Wiltse LL. Low back pain in young athletes. *Physician and Sports Medicine* 1974; **2**: 53–60.

93. Fairbank JCT, Park WM, McCall IW, O'Brien JP. Apophyseal injection of local anesthetic as a diagnostic aid in primary low back syndromes. *Spine* 1981; **6**: 598–605.

94. Gallagher RM, Williams RA, Skelly J, Haugh LD. Workers' compensation and return to work in low back pain. *Pain* 1995; **61**: 299–307.

95. Webster BS, Snook SH. The cost of 1989 workers' compensation low back pain claims. *Spine* 1994; **19**: 1111–16.

96. Jackson CP, Brown MD. Analysis of current approaches and a practical guide to the prescription of exercise. *Clinical Orthopaedics and Related Research* 1983; **179**: 46–54.

97. Jackson CP, Brown MD. Is there a role for exercise in the treatment of patients with low back pain? *Clinical Orthopaedics and Related Research* 1983; **179**: 39–46.

98. Cady LD Jr, Thomas PC, Karwasky RJ. Program for increasing health and physical fitness of fire fighters. *Journal of Occupational Medicine* 1985; **27**: 110–14.

99. Cohen B, Millett PJ, Mist B, Laskey MA, Rushton N. Effect of exercise training programme on bone mineral density in novice college rowers. *British Journal of Sports Medicine* 1995; **29**: 85–8.

100. Hopkins TJ, White AA. Rehabilitation of athletes following spine injury. *Clinics in Sports Medicine* 1993; **12**: 603–19.

101. Torg JS, Vegso JJ, Torg E. The low back. In: Hurley R, ed. *Rehabilitation of athletic injuries: an atlas of therapeutic exercise.* Chicago: Year Book Medical Publisher, 1987.

6

Considerations for unique groups

6.1 Introduction

Lyle J. Micheli

Athletically active individuals or individuals of all ages and backgrounds participating in organized exercise activities can benefit from safe and injury-free exercise. The health benefits of sports and exercise have received traditional support in the medical community and have recently been supported by scientific investigation. The particular benefits to growing children, elderly individuals, whether male or female, and disabled people cannot be overemphasized. In each of these groups, exercise and organized sports can provide important physical and psychological benefits for participants. It is imperative in these groups, in particular, that careful study of sports activities be done with an eye towards the prevention of unnecessary injury, as well as rapid diagnosis, treatment, and rehabilitation when injuries do occur.

Exercise has been demonstrated to be extremely important for the normal growth and development of children. Increasingly, with the growing complexities of urbanized societies, the only exercise many children may get will be in the organized sports or exercise setting. In North America, the growth of organized sports for children and adolescents has continued apace. While a relatively recent phenomenon, with the organization of sports beginning with baseball soon after the end of the Second World War, the rapid growth of organized participation in sports as diverse as soccer, ice hockey, gymnastics, figure skating, and baseball, as well as gridiron football, is evident in nearly every community in North America. In Europe, club sports are increasingly being enriched by the addition of youth and children's sports teams. This is certainly the trend in much of Europe and Asia with athletics, rugby, and soccer as well as other sports benefiting from this development.

The organization of sports participation for children and adolescents can provide opportunities for the prevention of injury. The organized sports setting allows for a careful assessment of mechanisms of injury and, in particular, techniques which may contribute to injury. Steps can then be taken to eliminate or modify playing techniques which increase the risk of injury.

In addition to the well-recognized risk factors for both acute and overuse injury seen in the adult, children have an additional risk for injury because of their more vulnerable growth cartilage at the physeal plates, joint surfaces, and at the sites of major muscle and tendon insertions. In addition, the child is subject to the growth process. Evidence is accumulating to show that growth, and, in particular, the adolescent growth spurt, presents an increased risk of musculoskeletal injury to the child and, in particular, to the child participating in repetitive training activities in sport. Finally, the inconsistency and variability of coaching and training for this age group may well be an additional risk factor for injury. The development of coaching education and certification for youth sports coaches should receive high priority for injury prevention. In addition, the growth and maturation of every young élite athlete should be guarded against harmful training regimens.

While some critics of organized sports for children have suggested that we should return to informal exercise and sports for this age group it is doubtful that this will occur, given recent social and economic trends in both developed and developing countries. Admittedly, overuse injuries from repetitive training are usually seen in organized sports; they rarely occur in the free play, physical education, or informal sports setting. However, the growing social and economic constraints on informal sports and exercise, as well as the concerns for the physical safety of children, will most probably increase the trend toward organized children's sports. It is therefore important for all of us who care about safe and effective sports participation by children and adolescents to ensure that a systematic assessment of risk factors for injury, as well as the institution of preventive techniques, be initiated for this age group.

One of the most recent developments in this trend towards organized sports for children is a report generated by a special committee of the International Federation of Sports Medicine, with the support of the World Health Organization, which met in Hong Kong in January, 1997. This committee called for an organized effort by physicians, parents, coaches, and sports governing bodies to ensure the safety of organized sports for children. In particular, the committee called upon the sports governing bodies to ensure safe and ethical instruction in children's sports by trained or certified coaches.

While there is a general consensus and recognition that physical exercise has many benefits for the growing child or adolescent, it is only very recently that scientific evidence has demonstrated that the continuation of regular exercise and sporting activities are extremely beneficial and may even be lifesaving for the geriatric population. As Dr Menard notes in his comprehensive review, 'the structural and physiological changes associated with an inactive lifestyle may be the greatest health threat facing our aging population' (Chapter 6.4).

It has been known for many years that ageing is associated with progressive decreases in strength, aerobic capacity, and lean muscle mass. It has been recently documented, however, that many of these observed changes are not an inevitable result of ageing, but may frequently be due to the physical inactivity of the aged population, particularly in urbanized and industrialized societies. As Evans and colleagues have determined, men and women in their seventh, eighth, and even ninth decades can show a significant increase in strength and lean body mass in response to a properly designed strength-training programme. This, in turn, results in marked functional improvements. Geriatricians have determined that falling is often the pivotal event which can result in serious injury, loss of ambulation, and institutionalization of the geriatric individual. A geriatric man or woman who was previously independent, living on their own at home or with friends or family, may be rendered bedridden, institutionalized in a nursing home or tertiary care facility, or even subject to early death as a result of a simple fall. While falling can be multifactorial in this population, a number of studies have recently suggested that basic physical weakness may be a major contributor to this event.

The psychological benefits of sports and exercise for the elderly rival the physical and functional improvements achieved. In our own state of Massachusetts, a public health initiative that sponsors organized walking clubs at the community level has reaped immeasurable benefits for this population. These observations suggest that organized sport, walking, and dance activities can be as essential to geriatric care as medication, food, and shelter.

While the benefits of organized sports and sports medicine are being increasingly recognized for children, adolescents, and our geriatric population, the systematic promotion of sports and exercise for the disabled person is a relatively recent phenomenon. The great impetus to the development of therapeutic sports and exercise has come from two very different avenues: paediatric medicine and military medicine. The needs of children with physical disabilities resulting from hereditary or drug-induced defects, cerebral palsy, or certain other childhood-acquired diseases, such as poliomyelitis, received early attention. The Crippled Children Services of the United States were formed in the 1930s. However, the active development and promotion of sports for disabled children is a relatively recent development. Needless to say, this goes well beyond merely assisting the child to obtain the functional level of 'community ambulator'.

A major impetus in the United States to the comprehensive approach to the disabled child's well being was Public Law 94–142, the Education for All Handicapped Children's Act, passed in 1975. As a result of this law and its interpretations, the disabled child has the right to be assessed by an 'individualized education program committee' in order to implement the 'free appropriate education guarantee', which was secured by law.

The implementation of this wide-reaching law popularized the development of a special committee consisting of physical therapists, occupational therapists, speech pathologists, nurses, social workers, and psychologists, as well as physicians, to provide a multifaceted approach to meet the needs of the disabled child. Not only would the musculoskeletal problems of the disabled person be addressed, but also the physical and cognitive problems, including traditional education, physical education, and sports.

The most recent addition to the care team for the disabled child has been the physical educator, sports coach, or dance teacher with specific skills and an interest in sports and fitness programmes for the disabled population. These programmes go one step beyond pure physical therapy. While many of the games and dance movements may incorporate therapeutic exercises or patterns, the structure is indeed that of a game or sport, and as such, requires the special skills of the sport specialist. Needless to say, as injuries were systematically incurred in these 'new games' for these special-needs children, the need for specialized sports medicine training and understanding has also grown.

Changes in the care of disabled military veterans has also paralleled the developments in the care of the disabled child. Dramatic improvements were made in prosthetic and orthotic design and in the development of rehabilitative services and programmes for the patient with spinal cord injury and the amputee. While the initial primary goal of rehabilitation, was, once again, to obtain the level of 'community ambulator', it was soon recognized that disabled servicemen had many other emotional and social needs, including the need for regular and competitive sports. Initially, organized sports activities were barely tolerated, as they all too often resulted in broken prostheses or damaged wheelchairs.

One of the pioneer efforts in the incorporation of sports and systematic exercise into rehabilitation took place at the Veteran's Administration Hospital in Boulder, Colorado, with the development of disabled skiing and riding programmes for the amputee. This programme, in turn, was actively expanded to the civilian population, including paediatric patients with acquired or congenital amputations.

Technical advances and the design of wheelchairs, prosthetics, outrigger skis, and special weight-training machines have now made sports a mechanical possibility for the disabled person. Additionally, special-needs coaches, teachers, and the athletes themselves have collaborated to devise appropriate rules and technique modifications.

Therapeutic exercises aimed at improving the range of motion and developing strength or coordination of a child or disabled adult in a more traditional venue, the hospital or outpatient physical therapy unit, have sometimes been perceived as laborious, potentially painful, or 'boring'. The same exercises, when incorporated into a competitive sport, dance programme, or 'workout session' in a fitness centre, may become a challenge to be mastered or a source of active enjoyment to be pursued by the participants.

Much of the impetus for this new development of specific sports programmes for disabled people has come from the disabled themselves. The development of special ski equipment, lightweight pylons for canoeing or kayaking, and lightweight, low-friction wheelchairs made from thermoplastics and aluminum are a few examples of equipment designed from client demand.

It is imperative that physicians dealing with the child, geriatric, or disabled athlete provide a maximally supportive approach to their special needs as well as their incurred injuries. In our general population, the sports medicine discipline has evolved from an environment in which all too many physicians suggested that an athlete should avoid further sports injuries by ceasing sports participation. It can be detrimental to the social, physical, and emotional growth of the child, the health maintenance of the older adult, or the overall 'rehabilitation' of the disabled person if a restrictive approach is used following the occurrence of an overuse or acute traumatic sports injury. The physician must bring an open mind to sports participation in this setting. He or she must be prepared to learn the details of the physical demands of the given sports and their potential for injury, and make every effort to cooperate with the participants and the coaches in the prevention or early recognition of injuries sustained in this extremely important sports setting.

We are pleased, indeed, to have a separate chapter devoted to the special issue of the female athlete in this second edition of the *Oxford textbook of sports medicine.*

The rapid growth of our knowledge in this area in recent years has served as an impetus for this separate review. Dr Lebrun has achieved a particularly comprehensive and labour-intensive review of this topic in Chapter 6.3.1. Her emphasis upon not only the physiological but also the sociological and historical problems encountered by female athletes provides an excellent perspective for both the management of athletes preparing for competition or in the midst of competition, but it also gives clear directions for ongoing research in this area. Her own pioneering work on the study of the 'female athlete triad' is well known throughout the world.

Whilst her work demonstrates the recent and rapid advances in our understanding of the exercising female, it is clear that there is an all too little systematic study on the volume or intensity of training as it relates to pathological/ endocrinological changes in the exercising female, or the increased risk of injury as volume of training increases. It is to be hoped that future studies of female athletes will include not only a careful assessment of physiological parameters, body composition measures, and anatomical sites of injury, but also a careful measure of the relative volume of training or changes in volume and intensity of training.

In summary, much research remains to be done in the study of sports and exercise activity for these 'special groups'. In particular, careful assessment of injury risk must be made in these settings so that the maximal health benefits of these sports may be attained without sustaining unnecessary injury. Initial clinical observations have, in general, given strong impetus to the further exploration of ways in which sports and exercise can be incorporated into the education and care of these athletes. Coaches, physical educators, and sports medicine specialists must coordinate their efforts to ensure the maximal benefit of safe sports participation without unnecessary risks.

6.2 The growing athlete

J.C. Hyndman

Introduction

The participation of children in sport is accepted as an important component in the development of healthy, well-rounded adults. Traditionally, participation in sport is believed to be important not only in the establishment of a healthy, physical lifestyle but also in the overall development of healthy attitudes with respect to work, competition, preparation, and fair play, all of which are ultimately beneficial to the individual and society at large. However, many paradoxes are evident when the problems of the paediatric athlete are addressed, and health-care professionals must be well aware of these when attending to the needs of these children.

Even a cursory perusal of both the print and electronic media demonstrates the increasing role that sport plays in our society. The influence of sports permeates virtually all aspects of our culture including fashion, lifestyles, and even national goals. Increasing professionalism and globalization of sport all contribute to the tremendous impact that modern high-level participation in sport has upon our young people. Of course, similar influences are exerted upon coaches, administrators, and parents. Consequently, planning in the management of children's sports is all too frequently carried out with the high-level élite athlete as the model. As a result of this top-down planning many inappropriate decisions are made with respect to training, administration, and the management of children's injuries. However, young children form the largest group participating in sports, and a bottom-up planning process would probably be more appropriate if a positive result is to be achieved.

Considerable confusion exists with respect to the correct approach that the health-care professional should adopt in dealing with children. Fundamental to establishing the most appropriate course is a clear definition of what constitutes paediatric sport. The paediatric athlete is a youngster who is still growing. The definition of a child in terms of the concept of 'still growing' is so simple that it is often forgotten or confused with other ill-defined terms such as adolescence. The phenomenon of growth is neither age nor size related, and the cessation of growth varies very considerably with sex and genetic background. According to this definition a child differs from an adult by the presence of growth plates which are necessary for longitudinal growth (Fig. 1).

Apart from secondary sexual characteristics, the existence of growth plates in bones is the only absolute difference between the anatomical structures of children and adults. This absolute difference in structure is clearly implicated in the different injury patterns observed in children compared with adults (Fig. 2).

Principles developed in the treatment of the élite adult athlete are not necessarily transferable to the problems of the growing athlete. No scientific data purported to be obtained from children should be acceptable, unless they are clearly defined as dealing with

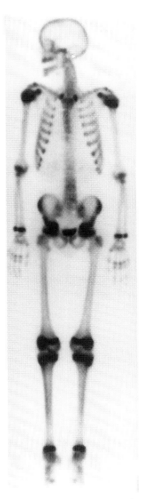

Fig. 1 High-resolution technetium bone scans clearly show the different metabolic activity reflective both of the growth plates present in children and of the importance of growth in determining this absolute difference of the child's skeleton.

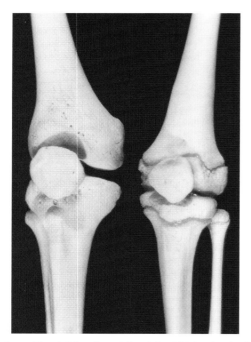

Fig. 2 The knee of the skeleton of an adult and of a child showing clearly the difference between children and adults.

that population which is still growing and in whom growth plates are present. Failure to make this simple observation leads to further misunderstandings and confusion in dealing with the problems of the growing athlete.

The presence of growth plates in bone results in definable biomechanical differences from the mature bone of adults. This essential difference frequently leads to a different expression of injury when the body is subjected to a similar trauma. Generally, this results in more frequent bone injuries compared with the soft-tissue injuries that are so common in adults (Fig. 3).

Indeed, even within different age groups of growing children the expression of bone injury may be predicated on the variability of growth velocity. For example, fractures of the distal radial epiphyseal plate occur more frequently in older children than in younger and slower growing children where these fractures more frequently involve the shaft of the bone and not the growth plate.[1] Biomechanical evaluation of children's bones show considerable differences in their bones' mechanical properties.

Injury in childhood

Injury can be defined as the response of tissue to kinetic energy applied to the body. The degree of injury directly parallels this kinetic energy and therefore follows basic physical laws, largely relating to the mass and, most particularly, the velocity involved. Therefore, in the assessment of an injury it is important to be aware of the circumstances in order to be able to anticipate and assess the effects of this force. The reaction of tissue to injury is manifested by inflammation, which is characterized by swelling, redness, increase in temperature, and loss of function of the injured part. The more severe the injury, the more severe is the inflammation. By definition, inflammation in the extremities can easily be observed by those in

attendance. Significant tissue damage will always be associated with a proportional degree of observable inflammation (Fig. 4).

The manner in which injuries can occur can be classified into three groups.

Type 1 injuries

Type 1 injuries occur as a result of a direct blow. This type of injury is quite common in sport, and can result from being struck by a ball, a stick, a racket, or by striking the knee directly on the playing surface. This type of injury is the easiest to prevent in that vulnerable areas (which are sports specific) can be identified and protected. Examples of protective equipment are helmets in American football and shin pads in soccer or ice hockey.

Type 2 injuries

Type 2 injuries occur as a result of an indirect blow, for example when a fall on the outstretched hand leads to an injury of the elbow

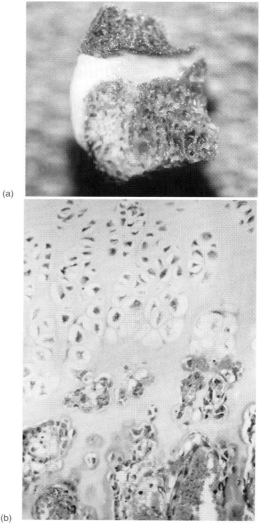

(a)

(b)

Fig. 3 (a) Actual human growth plate clearly showing the cartilage plate separating the ebony metaphysis from the epiphysis. (b) Microscopic appearance of the growth plate. Lower part of photomicrograph shows gradual conversion of cartilage to bone. This is the most common area of injury as it is weakest.

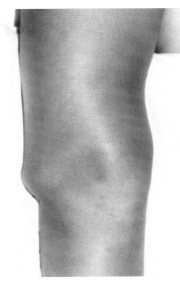

Fig. 4 Fracture dislocation of the elbow showing the easily demonstrated signs of inflammation.

or shoulder. In this case, the force is transmitted along the skeleton to a point distant from the original contact. Similarly, twisting the body around the planted foot frequently leads to knee injuries. These injuries may be prevented by altering footwear or playing surfaces. Administrative changes may also help to reduce these injuries by, for example, establishing rules preventing blocking from behind in football and checking from behind in ice hockey which have been commonly associated with injury—often severe.

Type 3 injuries

Type 3, or chronic repetitive injuries, are the common overuse injuries which are so frequently presented to health-care professionals.[2] The confusion between adults and children is most prevalent in this type of injury. Many therapeutic modalities which are effective in these types of injuries in adults may be inappropriate when used in the growing child. Again, this largely relates to the more frequent bony expression of injury resulting from chronic repetitive injury compared with soft-tissue expressions in adults. For example, patellar tendinitis, which is common in adult jumping athletes, would be more likely to express itself as Osgood–Schlatter's disease, a bony injury, in the growing athlete.

Epidemiology

Introduction

Unprecedented interest in high-performance sporting activity has developed during the second half of the twentieth century. This is the result of increased leisure time, the pervasive influences of television in our society, and, unfortunately, the political influence of competing cultures and economic units. Many national sports organizations have encouraged high-level competition with professional coaching at a very young age, creating a subclass of athletes who are streamed into highly specialized sporting activity while still very young. This has resulted in successful international competi-

tion and the achievement of national sporting goals focused on gaining international success. These programmes rely on the development of child athletes as the raw material from which to develop these young élite performers. Although these programmes have been superficially successful, there have been significant failures. Intensive training and the increased frequency of exposure has led to career-ending injuries.[3,4] Tragically, and perhaps less well known, many athletes have failed to develop into well-rounded and mature adults or have had difficulties in adjustment following the completion of a highly profiled career or the failure to achieve early international success. Cheating as a result of the credo that 'winning is everything' are further contradictions of the aims of sport in childhood.

Research into injuries in growing athletes is poorly developed. However, some general observations can be made. Clearly, the rate of injuries increases exponentially with age; the frequency of injury is low in very young children and the injuries which are incurred tend to be of a minor degree of severity.[5-8] Therefore it appears that as increasing maturity, size, and competitiveness result in increasing collision forces, the injury levels increase appropriately.[9-12] Evidence exists suggesting that the greater the frequency of participation, the greater is the rate of injury.[13]

The difficulty of assessing the epidemiology of athletic injuries is further compounded by the variability of the maturation rate. In the interests of fairness, sports administrative bodies insist upon careful categorization of participation based upon chronological age. This is frequently and rigidly enforced by checking birth certificates. However, this practice is confounded by the observation by Hyndman and Armstrong (unpublished) that in contact sports such as ice hockey, a chronological age range of 13 to 15 years may, in fact, represent a biological age of 13 to 19 years. Furthermore, high-school football players have been shown to be physically more mature than age-matched non-participants. These biological variations certainly influence selection, participation, and potential injury rates in growing children. Sporting activities requiring aerobic efficiency are also affected by biological variation. Aerobic efficiency is not related to size, and, regardless of age, immature athletes cannot generate the same efficiency as those who are physically mature.[15,16]

Therefore the epidemiology of injuries must take into account not only the paradox of physical differences between growing athletes and mature athletes but also the biological variation in the rate of this maturation process. Recognizing these paradoxes emphasizes that the whole area of understanding, treating, and preventing injuries in the child athlete is a very complex affair. While maturation screening can be used to match athletic participation to biological maturity, this methodology has not been adequately tested scientifically nor is it likely to be sociologically acceptable.[17]

The development of preventive measures and equipment have been confounded by these variables, and, with notable exceptions, many of the measures recommended have not been properly evaluated despite their well-intentioned institution. Indeed, in some instances (collision sports) they may even be a factor in causing injury as a result of misplaced confidence in the protective equipment and resulting reckless behaviour.

Essentially, the factors influencing the occurrence of injury in athletes can be divided into two groups. First there are intrinsic factors, namely those relating to the structure of the participants, and, second, extrinsic factors which relate to the nature of the activity itself and to the competitive environment.

Intrinsic factors

Much research effort has been expended in an attempt to define whether or not certain types of body habitus or joint stability are factors in the genesis of injury. Despite these efforts, no conclusive evidence has been obtained to show that there are intrinsic risk factors in the physical make-up of some athletes which makes them susceptible to injury. There is also no conclusive evidence that time-honoured preparation strategies, including preperformance stretching and warming-up, have a significant effect on the prevalence of injury.[5,18-21]

Interestingly, one area where there is increasing evidence of a direct relationship with the prevalence of injury is in the area of associated or coexisting stressful life events. These psychological factors are clearly implicated in the prevalence of injury, a fact that must be understood by coaches, trainers, physicians, and parents.[22]

Extrinsic factors

The assessment of extrinsic factors in the genesis of sports injuries has been widely documented. Injuries of type 1 (due to a direct blow) are the easiest to prevent.

Recognition of the sometimes tragic consequences of eye injuries in sports such as squash and ice hockey has led to changes in protective equipment, resulting in a substantial decrease in the frequency of injuries.[23-28] The definition of the problem, the institution of remedial action, and the resultant effect have well described by Pashby.[28-30]

Extrinsic factors involving type 2 injuries (indirect force) are, by their very nature, more difficult to prevent. Protective equipment may not have the desired effect as the forces are transmitted longitudinally through the skeleton, with their adverse effect taking place somewhere distant from the origin of the force. An example of this difficulty is the use of prophylactic knee braces in American football. What seemed to be a reasonable idea has, in fact, been shown to be ineffective; indeed, they may even have adverse effects.[31] However, significant injuries to the knee in American football may well be minimized by rule changes, such as making blocking from behind illegal. The interface between the shoe and the playing surface is also important in the genesis of injuries due to indirect forces, since too much adhesion may result in the transmission of forces indirectly to the knee rather than a fall which would, paradoxically, prevent the injury.

These changes in equipment designed to prevent type 1 injuries may enhance the potential for type 2 injuries, because the protection provided may lead to a loss of fear of injury. Consequently, high-velocity collisions can lead to type 2 injuries—such as the neck injuries associated with spearing in American football and checking from behind in ice hockey—which, tragically, may contribute to devasting injury such as paraplegia.[32,33]

Type 3 injuries (chronic repetitive injuries) in growing athletes have clearly been shown to have the potential to lead to serious injury and disability, such as that shown in the condition known as 'little leaguer's elbow'. The recognition of this has led to administrative control of the frequency of pitching, thereby minimizing the

adverse effects. Other examples where chronic repetitive activity can lead to significant complications include the use of inappropriate footwear by élite, immature distance runners, epiphyseolysis of the distal radius and potential growth arrest in gymnasts, and spondylolysis and spondylolisthesis which appear to be associated with repetitive hyperextension of the lower spine. Careful examination should be performed to ensure the identification and early recognition of these potentially serious injuries to try to minimize adverse results of sporting activity and to encourage the continual safe development of the athlete.[34-36]

A large study of sports injuries in Ireland showed that only 35 per cent of injuries in children can be related to facilities and equipment.[37] When this result is coupled to the inability to define an injury-prone habitus, the variability of injury at various developmental stages, the wide biological variation in the achievement of these developmental stages, and the increasing evidence of the importance of psychological factors in the genesis of injury, all health-care professionals, coaches, trainers, and athletes must recognize the complexity of the epidemiology of injury in the growing athlete. It should be clearly emphasized that an holistic approach to the assessment, treatment, and prevention of injury in growing athletes is essential if the desired aims of the athlete, the team, and society are to be balanced with the healthy development of a well-rounded mature adult.

Injuries to the growing athlete
Clinical application

Having reviewed the anatomy of the growing athlete and the basic mechanisms and epidemiology of injuries, we must now discuss the practical management of common problems seen in child athletes. The management of all macro injuries of type 1 (direct force) or type 2 (indirect force) is beyond the scope of this book and the reader is referred to standard paediatric fracture texts. Macro injuries which have major implications for sport will be described in detail. Particular attention will be paid to type 3 injuries (chronic repetitive stress) as these form by far the largest group presenting for management and about which there is the most controversy.

Clavicle
The clavicle is frequently injured in sports activities. In the growing athlete, fractures to the clavicle can be treated simply with a triangular bandage sling and/or the addition of a figure-of-eight bandage. There is virtually no risk of non-union, although a palpable mass of clavicle is frequently associated with the early stages of healing (Fig. 5).

The most difficult part of the management of children with clavicle fractures is when to allow them to return to sport. The risk of refracture is real, and before return is allowed the athlete should demonstrate the ability to stress the clavicle repeatedly by, for example, performing 15 to 20 unrestricted push-ups. Fractures of the distal clavicle do not have the same ominous implications as they do in adults, and can usually be simply treated using the same methods as those applied to the shaft of the clavicle. Rare cases of fracture dislocation involving the sternoclavicular joints may occur, but they are difficult to define other than with specialized techniques such as CT scans. Symptomatic treatment is usually all that is necessary (Fig. 6).

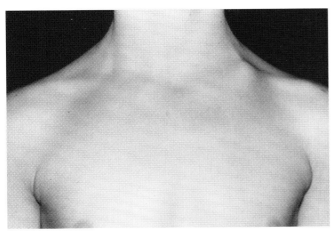

Fig. 5 Typical prominence associated with a healing clavicle in a 13-year-old hockey player.

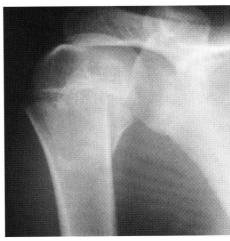

Fig. 7 Typical fracture of the proximal humerus with minimal displacement.

Shoulder

Dislocations in the shoulder region, including the acromioclavicular and glenohumeral joints, are unusual in patients with open growth plates. The different shoulder injuries sustained by these athletes are a good example of the pattern of injuries in children being distinct from injuries in adults caused by the same mechanism. Fractures of the proximal humerus are simple to treat unless grossly displaced and have very few long-term sequelae (Fig. 7).

The remodelling potential of the proximal humerus is well known, and therefore most fractures can be treated simply with a Velpeau bandage or some similar symptomatic treatment, with the expectation of a fairly early return to vigorous sporting activities (Fig. 8).

Pathological fractures of the proximal humerus secondary to a unicameral bone cyst frequently present significant concerns to attending personnel as to the suitability of the patient to participate in sports following healing of the fracture. This is a matter of judgement. There is no good evidence that the pathological fractures which can occur consequent to these injuries are associated with any long-term complications. These fractures usually heal in 2 to 3 weeks and, depending on careful informed consent, it may be appropriate to allow these young athletes to return to their sport. The complications of refracture must be balanced against the legitimate aims and wishes of the athlete. We do not hesitate to allow children with unicameral bone cysts of the humerus to participate

fully and feel that, in the vast majority, the benefits outweigh the risks. Ancillary treatment, such as the injection of hydrocortisone, may speed the healing of these benign cysts (Fig. 9), but surgical intervention is very rarely indicated unless the cyst is in the proximal femur where complications of fracture are quite common.

Elbow

It is well known that sports such as baseball which involve repetitive stressful overhand throwing can produce a non-specific painful and stiff elbow which may have important implications in the long term. This is a good example of a type 3 injury which can be prevented by limiting the activity of the athlete by legislative means in order to prevent, or minimize, the likelihood of this potentially career-ending injury (Fig. 10).

Wrist

Repetitive injuries to the wrist are analogous to repetitive injuries of the elbow (Fig. 11).

These injuries have been well documented in young gymnasts undergoing extreme training; changes can develop in the distal radial growth plate that are related to the severity and intensity of the training programmes.[36] As with the elbow injuries, they need to be identified and can be prevented by careful attention to training regimens. Periods of rapid growth may be associated with an increased vulnerability to this type of injury. This is analogous to other chronic stress-related, growth-plate disturbances such as Osgood–Schlatter's disease.

Hand

Fractures involving the small metacarpals frequently result from both sanctioned and more commonly unsanctioned pugilistic endeavours in young athletes (Fig. 12).

Many fracture texts recommend aggressive therapy for these punch fractures. However, in children, a rapid return to sports with no long-term complications is expected unless the adjacent finger is significantly rotated, in which case the rotational deformity must be corrected (Fig. 13).

Spine

The two areas of concern with regard to spinal problems in the growing athlete, in addition to macro injuries, are Scheurmann's disease and spondylolisthesis.

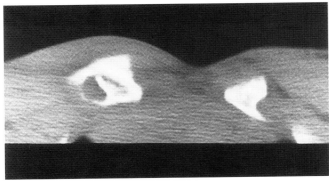

Fig. 6 Unusual fracture dislocation of the left sternoclavicular joint. Note soft-tissue swelling anteriorly. The injury healed promptly with non-operative treatment.

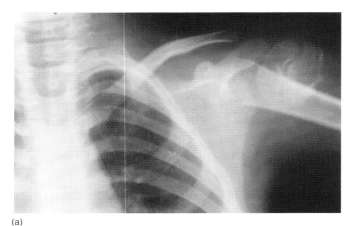

(a)

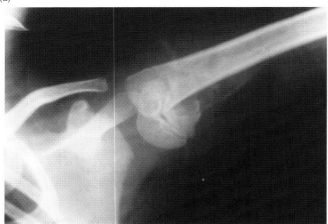

(b)

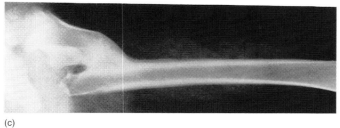

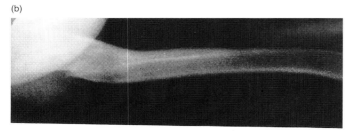

(c)

Fig. 8 A series of radiographs indicating a grossly displaced fracture of the proximal humerus treated without reduction, showing prompt healing and ultimate remodelling potential. While not the ideal management, this is a good example of remodelling seen in growing children.

Scheurmann's disease

Much confusion exists with respect to this so-called disease. Essentially, Scheurmann's disease is yet another expression of the rapid growth of the athlete, specifically the vertebral bodies. In athletes, Scheurmann's disease usually affects the lumbar spine and presents

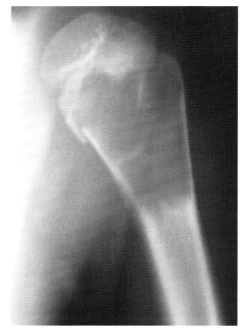

Fig. 9 Simple bone cyst of the proximal humerus showing pathological fracture.

with chronic, activity-related back pain and irregular ossification of the vertebral bodies (Fig. 14).

It is important to recognize that this is a self-limiting condition with no evidence of any long-term complications or predisposition to chronic, back-pain syndromes. Treatment is simple and symptomatic. It is not necessary to preclude participation in sport, but it may be advisable to limit it to some extent dependent upon symptoms. Weight training may aggravate the symptoms and probably should be curtailed temporarily. In some cases, an external support, such as a thoracolumbar brace, may be worn to allow continued participation. With maturation, symptoms and radiographic changes disappear.

Spondylolisthesis

Spondylolisthesis is the other major cause of mechanical back pain in children. Evidence has accumulated that spondylolisthesis is

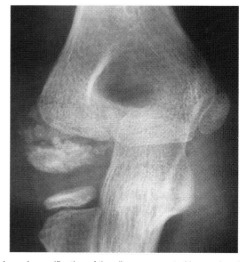

Fig. 10 Irregular ossification of the elbow aggravated by overhand throwing.

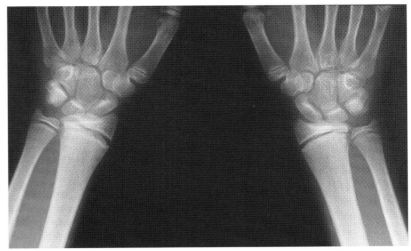

Fig. 11 Note widening of the growth plate in this painful wrist of a highly competitive gymnast.

associated with chronic, repetitive, hyperextension activities such as those performed by gymnasts. As spondylolisthesis may be progressive, it can be associated with very significant long-term spinal problems and its presence may be sufficient to curtail participation in competitive gymnastics. However, spondylolysis without spondylolisthesis does not necessarily require the athlete to discontinue gymnastics, but rather symptomatic treatment and close follow-up should be instigated (Fig. 15).

Pelvis and hip

Avulsion fractures of the pelvis

Violent muscle contractions, which occur in sports such as sprinting, can occasionally result in the avulsion of the attachment of major muscle groups from the pelvis. This is associated with acute pain and is a good example of a type 2 injury (indirect force). Symptomatic treatment with rest and a gradual return to activity is all that is required (Fig. 16).

Slipped epiphysis

Slipped epiphysis, or more correctly slipped proximal femoral physis, may present either acutely or chronically in association with athletic participation. Frequently, the symptoms may be subtle and associated with a limp and decreased performance. As the process increases, the pain experienced by the athlete may be referred to the knee. These athletes tend to be in the rapidly growing adolescent phase and are frequently overweight. Slipped epiphysis is a potentially very serious problem which requires immediate treatment and securing of the epiphysis with some form of fixation to prevent further slippage. Failure to recognize and treat this relatively common condition can result in serious arthritis and consequent permanent disability. Athletes in whom this condition is suspected should be issued with crutches immediately and referred for radiological confirmation (Fig. 17).

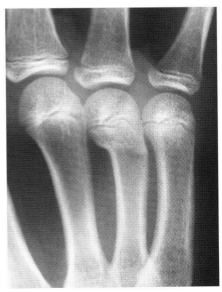

Fig. 12 Typical punch fracture in a 12-year-old.

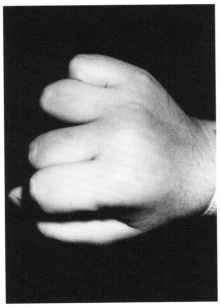

Fig. 13 Rotational malalignment secondary to malunion of a metacarpal fracture.

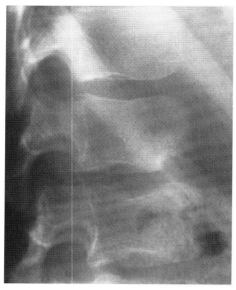

Fig. 14 Typical changes of Scheurmann's disease in a 12 year old.

Operative treatment with pin fixation is the standard treatment for this condition. Many types of pins have been used and there is no consensus favouring one system over another.

Thigh

Myositis ossificans

Myositis ossificans is a relatively common problem and almost always results from a type 1 direct blow to the thigh. The history is very characteristic: consequent to this type of injury there is persistent pain and dysfunction in the extensor apparatus of the thigh; later, radiography shows the characteristic formation of new bone

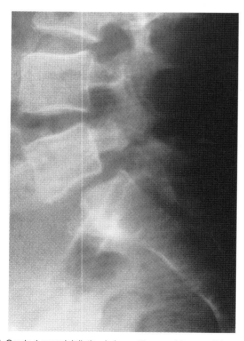

Fig. 15 Grade 1 spondylolisthesis in an 11-year-old competitive gymnast.

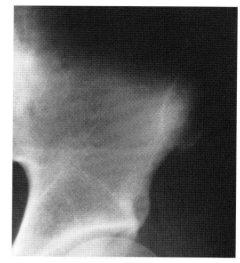

Fig. 16 Avulsion fracture of the anterosuperior iliac spine. The patient is a 15-year-old soccer player.

outside the periosteum. Thus confusion in diagnosis is usually unlikely. No long-term effects are expected (Fig. 18), but care

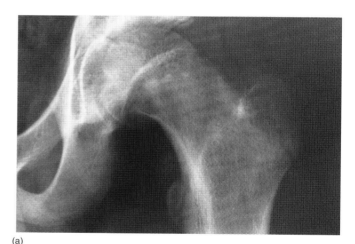

(a)

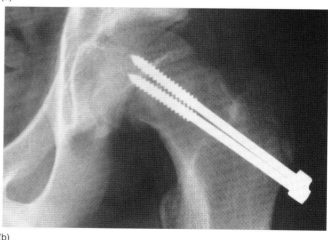

(b)

Fig. 17 (a) Slipped proximal femoral physis. (b) Following fixation with Knowles' pins.

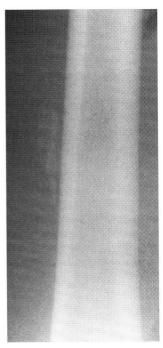

Fig. 18 Radiograph of myositis ossificans showing new bone formation within the muscle differentiated from the bone by the periosteal space.

should be taken not to attempt too aggressive rehabilitation of the muscle as this will delay the return to sport as a result of recurrent micro injury and pain.

Knee

Knee pain in athletes is perhaps the most common presentation to coaches, trainers, and physicians. The human knee is subject to tremendous mechanical stress and its particular design makes it vulnerable to injury. When the mechanical weakness inherent in the growing knee is added to this, the frequency with which problems occur in the knee joint can be readily understood. The symptoms may relate to a variety of well-defined chronic problems such as Osgood–Schlatter's disease, osteochondritis dissecans, jumper's knee, and patellofemoral instability. All these conditions can easily be diagnosed either clinically or with simple radiography.

Osgood–Schlatter's disease

Osgood–Schlatter's disease is particularly common in adolescent boys. Much has been written about this condition, often confusing and contradictory. Essentially, it can best be envisaged as a stress fracture, resulting from chronic repetitive stress due to tension developed in the extensor mechanism as it attaches to the growing tibial tubercle. Developmental age is important in that during rapid growth the bone structure of the tibial tubercle is mechanically weak and can fail. Treatment ranges from short-term immobilization to restricted activity. Some athletes may suffer pain which is severe enough to preclude competition. In such patients, it has been found that a faster return to competition is obtained with the use of plaster casts or other forms of immobilization than with treatment by other modalities[39] (Fig. 19). It is important to emphasize that the joint itself is not involved and that there are no serious long-term complications connected with this very common syndrome.

Osteochondritis dissecans

Osteochondritis dissecans presents with pain, a tendency for the knee to give way, and sometimes a limp. The diagnosis is usually established with plain radiography of the knee. In children, it is possible to correct the condition by immobilization. Although treatment by fixing these fragments with various forms of pins is performed, this form of treatment has not been adequately tested in clinical trials. In some cases, the fragment will become loose and require excision (Fig. 20).

Jumper's knee (Sinding-Larsen–Johannson disease)

Jumper's knee is another example of a chronic repetitive stress (type 3) injury at the patellar attachment to the patellar tendon. The injury is treated in a similar fashion to Osgood–Schlatter's disease. In this age group it is self-limiting and therefore treatment is symptomatic. It is important to emphasize to parents that in Osgood–Schlatter's and jumper's knee the actual joint is not involved, given the significant and justified concern they will have regarding knee injuries in general.

Patellofemoral instability

Patellofemoral instability is also relatively common in the growing athlete. It frequently presents with an acute dislocation which requires reduction (Fig. 21).

Following reduction, a radiograph should be taken to define whether or not an osteochondral fracture has occurred. Joint aspiration may be helpful for comfort and for clinical evaluation of the knee. After a short period of immobilization, rehabilitative exercises are very important to prevent recurrences of this condition. Isometric exercises in extension are very helpful in preventing chronic symptoms in those patients who present with instability but without dislocation. Persistent instability, despite adequate rehabilitation, may require soft-tissue surgical reconstruction as the growth plates preclude bony procedures, although surgical intervention is frequently unnecessary if adequate muscle rehabilitation takes place.

Tibiofemoral instability

Major ligamentous disruptions of the knee can occur in children.[40] However, an injury which would lead to an unstable knee in an adult generally results in a fracture in a child (Fig. 22). The advantage of fracture is that, when healed, the knee returns to full stability. On the other hand, in the knee particularly, growth disturbance consequent to the fracture is much more common than in other parts of the body.

Avulsion fractures of the tibial spine are, by definition, isolated, anterior cruciate ligament injuries. Because the ligament itself is detached from its insertion and can be replaced by either operative or non-operative means, the long-term complications of this type of injury are less significant than they are in an adult, where the actual ligament is disrupted. While children who suffer these injuries frequently have lax anterior cruciates, on examination, paradoxically they rarely have symptoms or limitations consequent to this instability. However, if they are symptomatic, reconstructive surgery can take place.

Anterior cruciate disruption

Clearly, children do sustain primary anterior cruciate ligament disruption (as opposed to bony avulsions). They are unusual enough that clear treatment guidelines are difficult to establish, but if there

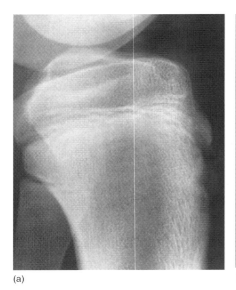
(a)

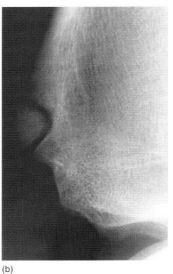
(b)

Fig. 19 (a) Early changes of Osgood–Schlatter's disease in a 13-year-old. Note fragmentation of the tibial tubercle. (b) Residual Osgood–Schlatter's disease with loose bone formation in an adult; this occasionally requires excision.

is functional instability they may require similar stabilizing treatments as adults, if sporting activity is to be maintained (that is to say, bracing and surgery may be necessary). In the young child where sufficient growth remains, the surgery may more safely be carried out by extra-articular procedures, whereas in the older child, with little growth remaining, similar intra-articular procedures to adults may be utilized successfully.

Peripatellar pain syndrome

The most problematical of all the injuries that occur in this age group are those associated with chronic knee pain without evidence of obvious clinical abnormality. Considerable experience is required to define the true pathogenesis of the pain in syndromes of this type. The development of arthroscopic examination and magnetic resonance imaging (**MRI**) has assisted tremendously in defining internal derangements of the knee, such as torn menisci, discoid menisci, and other soft-tissue abnormalities (for example, cruciate disruptions). It is in these enigmatic syndromes, where the athlete is disabled and yet there are no objective findings in any of the usual

parameters, that clinicians must be aware of the subtleties of pain interpretation and the many factors which may modify it. This is discussed more completely in the section on somatization disorders.

Stress fractures

Stress fractures occur in growing athletes in the same way as in adults. Treatment is symptomatic, with footwear and activity modifications. Persistent symptoms can easily be treated by a short period (2 weeks) of immobilization in plaster and resolution is usually rapid (Fig. 23).

Stress fractures in children may be associated with other adjacent pathologies such as benign tumours, tarsal coalition, and the presence of internal fixations. The judicious and short-term use of

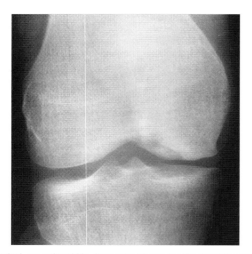

Fig. 20 Typical osteochondritis dissecans on the medial femoral condyle. Note early evidence of arthritis in this untreated patient.

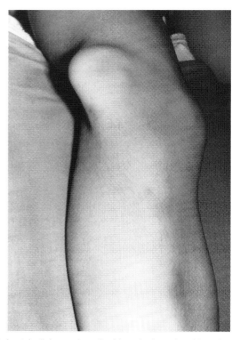

Fig. 21 Acutely dislocated patella. Note the lateral position of the patella.

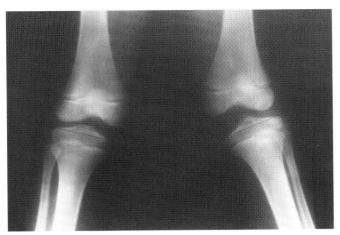

Fig. 22 Stress radiographs showing that, while unusual, ligamentous injuries can occur in growing athletes.

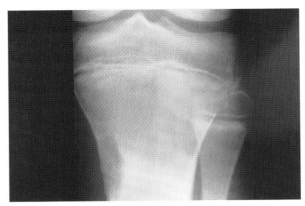

Fig. 24 Stress fracture of the proximal tibia through a non-ossifying fibroma.

plaster casts in growing athletes should not be feared (Figs 24, 25, and 26).

Osteochondroses

Osteochondroses is a regrettable term which is used to identify the similarly appearing radiographs obtained for a wide group of conditions such as Osgood–Schlatter's disease, Legge–Perthes' disease, osteochondritis dissecans, Scheurmann's disease, Frieberg's disease, and Panner's disease. Actual pathology differs, despite the similar radiographic images and therefore as it is a non-discriminating term it should probably be abandoned. It is, however, included here for the readers' clarification.

Osteochondritis dissecans

Osteochondritis dissecans can occur in the ankle joint as well as the knee. In many instances it can be treated symptomatically with either a plaster cast or, preferably, an ankle foot orthosis. Surgical removal may be necessary if the lesion is displaced (Fig. 27).

Frieberg's disease

Frieberg's disease is an unusual condition of unknown cause that usually affects the second or third metatarsal head of 13-year-old females. There is collapse of the subchondral bone and swelling and discomfort in this region (Fig. 28).

Treatment is symptomatic, and a properly designed orthosis with a metatarsal pad will usually alleviate the symptoms. Surgical treatment is necessary in very rare instances.

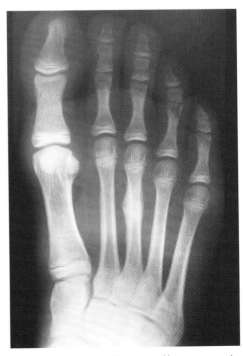

Fig. 23 Stress fracture of the third metatarsal in a cross-country runner.

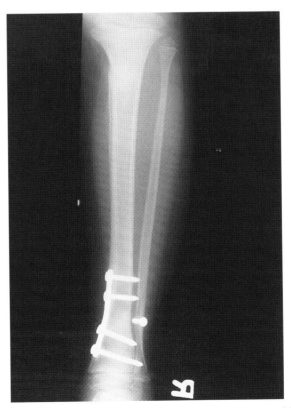

Fig. 25 Unusual open reduction of a fracture of the tibia showing stress shielding of the plate and a stress fracture of the proximal tibia. The presence of the plate affects the normal bone mechanics.

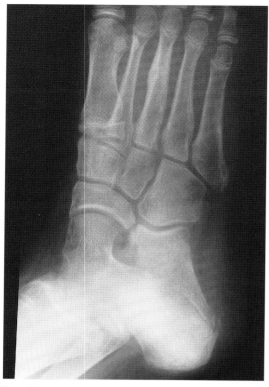

Fig. 26 Stress fracture of a metatarsal with adjacent calcaneonavicular coalition. Stiffness in the foot increases stress on adjacent bones.

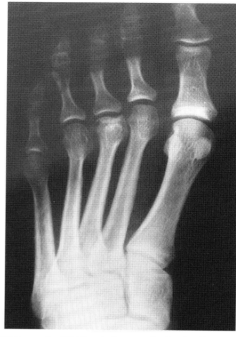

Fig. 28 Typical example of Frieberg's disease affecting the third metatarsal head.

Sever's disease

Sever's disease is similar to Osgood–Schlatter's disease, but occurs at the insertion of the Achilles tendon and is associated with rapid growth of the calcaneus. It is frequently confused with tendinitis. Normal irregular ossification is often interpreted as pathology (Fig. 29).

Treatment is symptomatic and is designed to decrease impact loading of the heel. The condition is self-limiting and there are no long-term sequelae. Most commonly it occurs in a patient who is younger than the typical patient with Osgood–Schlatter disease, as this reflects the earlier growth spurt in the foot compared with the leg.

Drugs and rehabilitation

Prescription drug therapy should be used rarely in the growing athlete. An understanding of the pathogenesis of symptoms and their

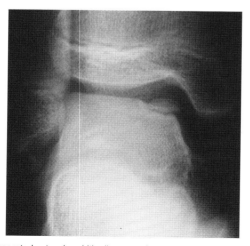

Fig. 27 Separated osteochondritis dissecans fragment. Pain and ankle instability are frequent.

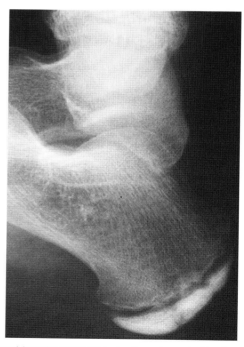

Fig. 29 Normal irregular ossification of calcaneal apophysitis. Rapid growth is associated with this appearance.

frequent bony origin should modify the enthusiasm for non-steroidal anti-inflammatory drugs and other drugs designed for the treatment of soft-tissue inflammation. There is little evidence that these drugs have any salutary effect on conditions encountered with growing athletes, and not only is their cost–benefit ratio questionable but, more importantly, their use frequently prevents a true understanding of the pathogenesis of the problem being obtained.

Perhaps the most difficult problem with the rehabilitation of growing athletes after injury is tempering their enthusiasm for an early return to their particular sport. The physician and training and coaching personnel must understand that objective evidence of sufficient healing must be demonstrated before the athlete resumes training if further or sequential injury is to be avoided. An over-enthusiastic early return is frequently associated with a sequence of nagging injuries and consequent diminished performance for a period longer than would have been the case with a more cautious return.

The objective evidence of healing is the reversal of those signs of tissue damage which indicated the presence of the injury in the first instance. Full return of range of movement following immobilization, absence of swelling, and atrophy of adjacent muscle groups are prerequisites for return to preinjury training regimes. Traditional physical therapy methods may be helpful in enhancing range of motion and strength rehabilitation. Many other modalities frequently used have not been adequately scientifically tested and are probably of little value in this age group.

Weight training is a common method for enhancing strength and athletic performance. It is often felt that this training will assist in the prevention of injury, although there is no evidence to support these claims. Injuries in the growing athlete usually occur in the bone component of the musculoskeletal system. Therefore weight training as part of an overall regime is reasonable to the limit defined by the absence of bone pain syndromes. Regimens that emphasize strengthening with less resistance are preferred to very heavy power lifting. (POSNA statement.)

Clearly, injury rates increase with increasing performance.[11] Higher, faster, and stronger do have limits, and the challenge is to recognize the limit for each athlete and the individual growth and development phase that athlete is experiencing.

Somatization disorders

Psychological factors are clearly important in achieving high-level athletic performance, and successful coaches are often known for their skill in psychological motivation. The recognition that psychological factors are also important in the genesis of injury underlines the importance of recognizing when such factors can become negative. In the extreme, extrinsic psychological stress placed on the young athlete by either parents or coaches can be a form of child abuse.

The expression of these factors has to be measured against the more obvious tissue physical injury which has been discussed previously. This area of expression of psychological stress, as manifested by somatic complaints in the absence of evidence of tissue injury, is called somatization.

Somatization disorders are syndromes of somatic complaints expressed by patients who are experiencing underlying psychological stress. They must clearly be differentiated from malingering as the patients do not appreciate the dynamics of the pathophysiology of their complaints. Most frequently the patient will complain of pain. Usually there is a definable cause for the pain, but the definable pathology cannot validate the degree of disability which is frequently associated with these conditions. This syndrome is extremely common, particularly in growing athletes whose physical maturity is almost complete. It is important to re-emphasize that these disorders are not voluntary but rather, through mechanisms which are not well understood, they express and amplify somatic complaints to the point of disability when, in fact, there is no definable objective pathological process present which would normally lead to the level of disability observed.

In some cases these disabilities are very dramatic, such as the presentation of a patient with the knee locked in full extension. Empirical evidence clearly shows that any acutely injured knee would never lock in full extension but, in order to achieve comfort, in some degree of flexion. Therefore presentation of a young athlete with the knee acutely locked in full extension is never an indication of serious intra-articular pathology, but rather a significant indication of a stressful life experience being expressed as, or somatized as, an acute musculoskeletal problem. Not all somatization disorders present in such a dramatic fashion. Surprisingly, one of the major advances in our understanding of these disorders has come with the development of the arthroscope. The ability to obtain a complete history and to perform a careful physical examination, coupled with a careful review of up-to-date radiographs and supplemented by a definition of the internal architecture of the knee joint with the arthroscope, has allowed a much greater depth of understanding of the pathogenesis of chronic pain in the knee. This presentation is a complex syndrome frequently seen in the growing athlete. The ability to objectively grade inflammation as a result of direct arthroscopic evaluation with widely disparate clinical histories has allowed the recognition that many of the painful clinical syndromes, such as chondromalacia of the patella, are, in fact, related to no definable pathology either within or adjacent to the knee. Indeed, they may frequently reflect a more global problem with respect to the interpretation of pain. All normal humans experience pain, but the interpretation of this pain varies widely.

Technetium-polyphosphate bone scanning and MRI scans have also been helpful in interpreting these syndromes, in that they are extremely sensitive to bone pathology. Thus a normal examination almost excludes substantial underlying pathology of the bone (Fig. 30). Modern diagnostic methods should therefore be able to define all known pathological causes of pain.

Many unscientific and expensive treatments have been prescribed for these ill-defined pain syndromes. Frequently, these treatments are successful in that they provide at least a transient alleviation of the symptoms. However, this is not always of benefit to the patient or athlete in that the underlying problem has not been addressed. Clearly, coaches, trainers, and health-care professionals must be aware that somatization disorders exist, and, whilst they may not reflect serious musculoskeletal pathology, they may well indicate a perverted expression of psychological stress which may result from any number of adverse life experiences. In some instances these may be of a minor nature, such as those associated with competition anxiety. However, they may reflect serious background psychopathology resulting from family separation, abusive family settings, real or perceived school failure, and conflicts in the

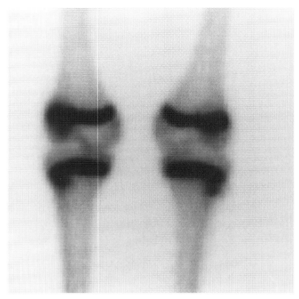

Fig. 30 Normally increased uptake of radioisotopes in growing knees clearly reflecting the concentration of metabolic activity in the growth plates.

development of the unique personality which is characteristic of mature adults.

The recent explosive revelations of the systematic sexual abuse of junior hockey players by a Canadian coach serve to underline the vulnerability of young high-performance athletes.[41] The substantial imbalance of power, coupled with the isolation of the young athlete, who in many cases was sent long distances to join an élite programme, places the athlete at risk for all sorts of abuse—in this case of the most perverse nature. This grotesque example of violation of trust serves to emphasize the complexity of the environment in which the developing athlete either succeeds or fails, and it also serves to emphasize the complexity of evaluating the symptoms which frequently accompany these stressed athletes.

There are many other less dramatic, stressful life events which influence the rate of injury, its affect on performance, and the recovery from injury, and it behoves attendant adults, particularly parents, to recognize the strong inter-relationship of the mind and body. This relationship is perhaps the most important and ill-understood component in the evaluation of athletic injury and performance. The approach to any athletic injury and, most particularly, injuries of the immature athlete must be holistic in the truest sense.

Thus the growing athlete is unique not only because he or she is growing physically and hence expresses a specific pattern of injuries unique to his or her age, but, additionally, the young athletes are developing concepts of self-worth and of their place in the world around them. They are growing people as well as growing bodies. Adults who are charged with the responsibility for encouraging the full potential of young athletes and for evaluating and preventing injury must recognize the scope of these responsibilities. The ultimate challenge is to encourage maximum performance without adversely affecting the development of the whole person and to encourage the growth of a healthy, well-rounded adult citizen who can apply the positive experiences attained in childhood athletics to the greater challenges of life. Failure to understand the dynamics of

growth and development can, and does, lead to an enhanced rate of injury and confusion of the true pathology. Mature clinicians, therapists, and coaches can best be part of the solution by having a full understanding of the potential problems and their complex inter-relationships.

Conclusions

Child athletes are different from adult athletes simply because they are growing. The difference in the bone tissue necessitated by the ability to grow creates a completely different reaction to physical stress and injury. The rate of growth in the growing athlete and the attainment of full maturity are widely disparate and the injury patterns are defined by these very disparities. Adult physicians, trainers, and coaches must exercise mature judgement in assessing the genesis of athletic dysfunction. Failure to understand the nature of the presenting complaints may lead, at best, to failure in achieving ultimate athletic performance, and at worst to a lifetime of disability caused by a potentially unnecessary injury. Perhaps even more important than physical injury is the failure to achieve the greater aim of enabling the young athlete to develop into a well-rounded and productive member of society. There is little doubt that many of these undesirable traits originate early on, and that only through a clear understanding of the differences in growing children can these effects be avoided.

References

1. Bailey DA, *et al*. The relationship of fractures of the distal radius to growth velocity in children. *Canadian Journal of Sports Sciences* 1988; **3**: 40–1.
2. Kannus P, Nittymaki S, Jarvinen M. Athletic overuse injuries in children—a 30 month prospective follow-up study at an outpatient sports clinic. *Clinical Pediatrics* 1988; **27**: 333–7.
3. American Academy of Pediatrics Committee on Accident and Poison Prevention. Skateboard injuries. *Pediatrics* 1989; **83**: 1070–1.
4. Kvist M, *et al*. Sports related injuries in children. *International Journal of Sports Medicine* 1989; **10**: 81–6.
5. Paulson JA. The epidemiology of injuries in adolescents. *Pediatric Annals* 1988; **17**: 84–6, 89–96.
6. Sutherland GW. Increased hockey injuries with age. *American Journal of Sports Medicine* 1976; **4**: 264–8.
7. Buncher CR. Statistics in sports injury research. *American Journal of Sports Medicine* 1988; **16**: 105–12.
8. Backous DD, Friedl KE, Smith NJ, Parr TJ, Capine WD Jr. Soccer injuries and their relation to physical maturity. *American Journal of Diseases of Children* 1988; **142**: 839–42.
9. deLos M, Goldie I. Incidence rate of injuries during sport activity and physical exercise in a rural Swedish community; incidence rate in 17 sports. *International Journal of Sports Medicine* 1988; **9**: 461–7.
10. Wetterhall SF, Waxweiler RJ. Injury surveillance at the 1985 Boy Scout Jamboree. *American Journal of Sports Medicine* 1988; **16**: 534–8.
11. Watson MD, DiMarino PP. Incidence of injuries in high school track and field athletes and its relation to performance ability. *American Journal of Sports Medicine* 1987; **15**: 151.
12. Chalmers DJ, Cecchi J, Langley J, Silva PA. Injuries in the 12th and 13th years of life. *Australian Pediatric Journal* 1989; **25**: 14–20.
13. McCauley E, *et al*. Injuries in women's gymnastics. The state of the art. *American Journal of Sports Medicine* 1988; **16**: 124–31.
14. Malina R, *et al*. Athletes tend to be more physically mature than non-athletes. *Pediatric Clinics of North America* **29**: 1321.

15. Storey WB. Evaluation in athletics—cardiovascular. *Pediatric Clinics of North America 19;* **29(6)**: 132.

16. Rowland TW. Developmental aspects of physiological function relating to aerobic exercise in children. *Sports Medicine* 1990; **10**: 255–66.

17. Kriepe RE, Gewanter ML. Physical maturity screening for participants in sports. *Pediatrics* 1985; **75**: 1076–80.

18. Gallagher SS, Finison K, Guyer B, Goodenough S. The incidence of injuries among 87 000 Massachusetts children and adults: results of the 1980–81 Statewide Childhood Injury Prevention Program Surveillance System. *American Journal of Public Health 19;* **74(12)**: 1343.

19. Tames, *et al*. Injuries to runners. Stretching good–no good. *American Journal of Sports Medicine* 1978; **6**: 40–50.

20. Snellock FG, Prentice WE. Warming-up, stretching for improved physical performance of sports related injuries. *Sports Medicine* 1985; **2**: 267–78.

21. Taimela S, Kujala UM, Osterman K. Intrinsic factor and athletic injuries. No conclusive evidence exists re these factors. *Sports Medicine* 1990; **9**: 205–15.

22. Kerr G, Fowler B. *Sports Medicine* 1988; **6**: 127–33.

23. Maestrello-deMoya MG, Primosch RE. Oralfacial trauma and mouth protector wear among high school varsity basketball players. *ASDC Journal of Dentistry for Children* 1989, **56**: 36–9.

24. Sane J. Comparsion of maxillofacial and dental injuries in four contact team sports: American football, bandy, basketball, and handball. *American Journal of Sports Medicine* 1988; **16**: 647–51.

25. Sim FH, Simonet WT, Melton LJ III, Lehn TA, Hockey injuries. *American Journal of Sports Medicine* 1988; **16**: 86–96.

26. DeRespinis PA, Caputo AR, Fiore PM, Wagner RS. A survey of severe eye injuries in children. *American Journal of Diseases of Children* 1988; **143**: 711–16.

27. Jones N. Eye injuries in sports—90 per cent preventable. *Sports Medicine* 1988; **7**: 163–81.

28. Pasby TJ. Eye injuries in Canadian hockey. *Canadian Medical Association Journal* 1975; **113**: 663.

29. Pasby TJ. Eye injuries in Canadian hockey. Phase II. *Canadian Medical Association Journal* 1977; **117**: 671.

30. Pasby TJ. Ocular injuries in hockey. *Canadian Medical Association Journal* 1979; **121**: 643–4.

31. Grace TG, Skipper BJ, Newberry JC, Nelson MA, Sweeter ER, Rothman ML. Prophylactic knee braces and injury to the lower extremity. *Journal of Bone and Joint Surgery* 1988; **70A**: 422–7.

32. Goldberg B, Rosenthal PP, Robertson LS, Nicholson JA. Injuries in youth football. *Pediatrics* 1988; **81**: 255–61.

33. Thompson N, Halpern B, Curl WW, Andrews JR, Hunter SC, MacLeod WD. High school football injuries evaluation. *American Journal of Sports Medicine* 1988; **16**: 97–104.

34. Sowinski, *et al*. Minimize age levels for young marathon runners. *New Studies in Athletics* 1986; **4**: 91–100.

35. Cahill BR, *et al*. Little League shoulder: lesions of the proximal humeral epiphyseal plates. *Journal of Sports Medicine and Physical Fitness* **2**: 150–4.

36. Albanese SA, *et al*. Wrist pain and distal plate closure of the radius in gymnasts. *Journal of Pediatric Orthopedics* 1989; **9**: 23–8.

37. Watson A, Sports injuries in 6799 Irish schoolchildren. *American Journal of Sports Medicine* 1984; **4**: 91–100.

38. Osgood RB. Lesions of the tibial tubercle occuring during adolescence. *Boston Medical and Surgical Journal* 1903; **148**: 114–19.

39. Ehrenborg G. The Osgood Schlatter lesion: a clinical and experimental study. *Acta Chirurgica Scandinavica* 1962; **28**: 1–26.

40. Brown DCS, Hyndman JC. Ligamentous injuries in children. *Journal of Bone and Joint Surgery* 1978; **61B**: 245.

41. Shoalts DK. There are more victims. *Toronto Globe and Mail* 1997; **9 January**: A17.

6.3 Women and sports

6.3.1 The female athlete

Constance M. Lebrun

The successful integration of female athletes into both recreational and competitive sport has not always proceeded smoothly. In addition to gender-specific physiological differences, sporting women have had to deal with sociological considerations, cultural expectations, gender equity issues and, at times, sexual harassment. Fortunately, with the advent of progressive equality legislation, both in Europe and in North America, there has been a notable trend towards increasing participation of women and girls in organized sport and physical activity. In some countries, however, there is still hesitation to wholeheartedly welcome women into the world of sport. Practitioners and paramedical personnel who care for female athletes at any level must have a special understanding of the unique sports medicine needs of this diverse population.

Females derive similar health benefits from regular exercise as do males—enhanced cardiorespiratory fitness, increased longevity, lowered blood pressure, and decreased percentage body fat. Although most research findings are based primarily on male subjects, there is mounting evidence that even moderate amounts of physical activity may confer protection against a variety of diseases, including coronary artery disease, diabetes mellitus that is not insulin dependent, and possibly some cancers. In addition, there are numerous positive spin-offs, particularly in adolescents, in terms of enhancement of confidence and self-esteem, and a reduction in risk-taking health behaviours.

Certain inherent physiological differences do exist between the sexes, but at the élite level, these variations are actually smaller than those within the population at large. The physical demands of rigorous training and competition are comparable for athletes, regardless of gender, and produce similar adaptations. As a consequence of increased opportunities, female athletes have made great strides towards 'catching up with the men'. Over the past few decades, there has been an explosion in the body of knowledge involving women and sport. This chapter will address the most important medical and orthopaedic issues for active and athletic women of all ages. Recent findings and pertinent research questions will also be discussed.

History of women in sports

The progress of women in sport has been beset with moral, social, biological, and religious road-blocks.[1-3] Permissible sporting and recreational activities have varied with the population, era, culture, climate, and geographical location. In ancient Egypt and Sparta, women were only allowed to participate in gymnastics, calisthenics, swimming, and similar competitive games, in the belief that these activities would improve their reproductive capabilities. During the Golden Age of Greece (776 BC, participation in any Olympic events was forbidden. Even the mere act of watching was punishable by being hurled off a cliff. Beauty and femininity were defined by the womanly qualities of 'chastity, modesty, obedience, and inconspicuous behaviour'.

The past two centuries have witnessed a progressive evolution in these mores. From a purely puritanical point of view, sport with its attendant opportunities for coeducation, freedom of action, revealing attire, frequent absences from home, and loosening of parental control was initially looked upon with disfavour. British literature at the turn of the century was replete with admonitions that women should not impair their ability to have children through sporting activity. The medical profession also helped to propagate such myths about the 'biological unknown'. Many limiting religious beliefs and practices, such as the traditional clothing that must be worn by Islamic women, have persisted well into the 20th century.

The 1800s

The 'true woman' of Victorian ideal was passive and frail. A physically weak, pale, and helpless body was visible evidence of material success. She and her middle-class or upper-class urban husband could afford servants, and she didn't have to work for a living. Protection of the 'female organs' was also paramount as all illness, headaches, heart conditions, etc. were somehow related to the uterus. Victorians believed that women should refrain from both physical and mental activity during menses, that they should consider themselves 'indisposed' during pregnancy and the postpartum period, and that there was a need to 'recuperate' from the physical trauma of childbirth.

Both sporting activities and clothing were severely regulated, the most notable example being the 'bathing costume'. Genteel sports such as archery, croquet, bowling, tennis, and golf were permissible forms of recreation, but often served more as social encounters than as actual physical exercise. Sport for this class of women was not meant to be strenuous, competitive, or active. Significant progress for females in sports did not begin until the late 1800s, coincident with higher education for women.

A conspicuous incongruity existed, however, between this value system and the sometimes stark reality of the era for the lower classes.[1,2] In Europe, it was primarily the women who toiled in the factories for 14 h per day, keeping the wheels of industry well oiled. In America, hardy pioneer women were forging the way west—chopping wood, hauling water, growing crops, and building and defending homesteads. For black women labouring in the fields, often as slaves, physical strength and endurance were valued commodities. Survival was a full-time pursuit, and leisure activity a luxury for which they had no time.

The early 1900s

At the turn of the century, sport for men was becoming increasingly popular, but prevailing ideologies of 'proper' female behaviour still placed women squarely on the sidelines. Paradoxically, it was still not considered contradictory for working-class women to do housework or labour outside the home. Farm women and black women were similarly 'privileged'.[4] Women who were professional physical educators in those days aligned themselves closely with the medical field in their opinions about women's inability to endure strenuous physical activity. The increase in elitism, commercialism, and violence in men's sport tended to reinforce this perception. There was a significant shortage of funding for women's sports, and limited opportunities for international competition.[4]

The history of women in the modern Olympic Games is fascinating[2] and is further detailed in Table 1. In 1920, Baron Pierre de Coubertin excluded women based on their lack of participation in the ancient games, and his firm belief that they were not athletes. When the first modern games were held in Athens in 1896, the only woman competitor was Melpomene, an unofficial runner, who completed the 40 km from Marathon to Athens in 4.5 h, about 1.5 h slower than the winner, but ahead of other male contestants. She stands as a celebrated figurehead for scores of female athletes who have literally followed in her footsteps.

In the 19th century, the customary attire for women in the United States and Europe featured long heavy skirts and pinched waists, consequently dictating a somewhat inactive lifestyle. The advent of the bicycle age encouraged the debut of more functional sporting apparel, such as bloomers with split legs and elastic bottoms. Women in the lower classes, however, continued to be restricted from sporting endeavours. Between 1900 and 1910, the suffrage movement gained momentum, with more and more women entering the employment setting. During the First World War, women went to work in the factories, where, in addition to physical labour, they received more exposure to recreational and team sports. The right to vote further boosted women to a new level of autonomy and social release.

The mid-1900s

The 1920s brought relaxed standards of dress and activity, increased independence for women, acceptance of recreational pursuits in leisure time, and the emergence of women as 'professional' sports figures. Women physical educators joined together to form the Women's Division of the National Amateur Athletic Federation. The mandate of the day was: 'a game for every girl and every girl in a game'. Prior to 1960, however, the image of women remained weak, fragile, timid, and unsuited for vigorous sport. Barriers persisted during the decades from 1920 to 1940. Colleges restricted specific athletic competition in favour of more general physical activity, and as already discussed, there was tremendous resistance to the inclusion of women in the Olympics.

The economic depression of the 1930s further discouraged the rivalry of women for 'men's tasks'. The outbreak of the Second

World War put an abrupt end to such perceptions of women's roles. Suddenly there was an acute need for female workers to fill jobs, including those demanding physical strength and endurance. Between 1940 and 1942, 4 million women entered the work force. For entertainment of the masses left at home, women were also allowed to take up certain sports. An all-women's professional baseball league was formed and lasted 12 years. In the post-war era, however, women were once again relegated to the domestic scene, while the world of men's athletics, especially professional and commercial sports, mushroomed.

The late 1900s

Numerous legislative and institutional changes in the 1970s marked the dawn of the age of awakening, or 'the Golden Age', for women in sports. In 1971, the Association for Intercollegiate Athletics for Women (AIAA) was formed. It began with 280 members, but by 1979, 859 member institutions were participating, with 27 championships in 14 different sports. The year 1972 was also a significant watershed for female athletes.[5] Title IX of the Educational Assistance Act in the United States decreed that all institutions receiving federal money were obliged to offer equal opportunities to both sexes in programming, including athletics (facilities, budgets, coaches, and uniforms). This legislation had three basic stipulations: equality of participation opportunities, scholarship dollars, and other athletic programme benefits; proportional to the enrolment and athletic involvement of women and men in that particular institution.

Participation rates for girls and women in sport increased dramatically during this time. Women were taking their rightful place in the athletic arena. In 1973, Billie Jean King beat one of the greatest male chauvinists of all time—Bobby Riggs—in three straight sets in tennis. This amazing feat helped to pave the way for other professional women tennis players. In 1974 she, along with other élite female athletes such as Donna de Verona, founded the Women's Sports Foundation. This organization advocates advancement and promotion of opportunities for girls and women in sports everywhere, and continues to expand its efforts and programmes to the present time. *WomenSports* magazine also began to highlight the achievements of female athletes. About this time, physical education started its gradual transformation from a profession into a respected academic discipline. Concurrently, research related to women active in sports was being initiated. In 1982, the Melpomene Institute for Women's Health Research was founded with the mandate of filling gaps in the existing knowledge base on women's sports-related issues.

The 1980s witnessed a slowdown in this forward momentum. There was somewhat of a backlash against the edicts of Title IX, and an ambivalence about the proper place of women in sport. In 1981, the National Collegiate Athletic Association (**NCAA**) voted to begin championships for women in the division I programmes, effectively putting the Association for Intercollegiate Athletics for Women out of business. The principles of Title IX were subsequently challenged by the NCAA. In 1984, the Supreme Court deemed athletic programmes exempt from Title IX because they did not receive direct federal funding. This ruling severely weakened the impact of Title IX for women in sport and recreation. There followed a general decline in women in coaching and admin-

Table 1 History of women in the Olympic Summer Games

Year	Females	Sports/events for women	Significant milestones
1896	0	0	
1900 Paris	11 (8.3%)	Golf, lawn tennis, yachting	Margaret Abbott—1st American woman to compete in Olympics (golf) Charlotte Cooper (GB)—1st woman to win gold (tennis)
1904 St. Louis	8 (1.3%)	Archery	
1908 London	36 (1.8%)	Archery, tennis, figure skating, gymnastics exhibition	US Olympic Committee article in *New York Times*: 'opposed to women taking part in any event in which they could not wear skirts'
1912 Stockholm	57 (2.2%)	Included swimming, diving, tennis	Women from 10 countries, not US
1916			Games suspended—World War I
1920 Antwerp	64 (2.45%)	Figure skating, tennis, swimming, diving	
*			
1924 Paris	136 (4.4%)	Fencing added	Games separated: winter and summer
1928 Amsterdam	290 (9.6%)	5 track and field events added	Several women collapse after 800-m race from heat exhaustion, IOC votes that women cannot compete in races longer than 200 m
1932 Los Angeles	127 (9.0%)	2 more track and field events added	Mildred 'Babe' Didrickson: gold in javelin and 80-m hurdles, silver in high jump due to illegal 'head-first' dive
1936 Berlin	328 (8.1%)	4 sports: athletics, swimming, fencing, gymnastics	
1940, 1944			Games suspended: World War II
1948 London	385 (10.4%)	5 sports for women, (12.7% of total events), 18 for men	Fanny Blankers-Koen of Holland (30-year-old mother of two children) wins three gold medals Alice Coachman—1st black gold medalist (high jump)
1952 Helsinki	518 (10.5%)	Individual gymnastics and equestrian events added	Women from 41 countries, Russian women dominate
1956 Melbourne	384 (11.5%)		Betty Cuthbert (Australia's Golden Girl) wins gold in 100m & 200m
1960 Rome	610 (11.4%)	800m race added back	Wilma Rudolf, dubbed the 'black gazelle', who as a child overcame partial paralysis of her left leg wins 3 gold medals
1964 Tokyo	683 (13.3%)	Volleyball added	US women dominate swimming; Ewa Klobukowska, Polish runner, fails gender test 3 years later
1968 Mexico City	781 (14.1%)		Gender testing begins: buccal smear
1972 Munich	1299 (15%)	Archery added again	Olga Korbut introduces more aerobatic style to gymnastics
1976 Montreal	1251 (20.6%)	13 sports: rowing, basketball and team handball added	Nadia Comaneci of Romania scores 7 perfect 10s. Only 65% of nations send female competitors
1980 Moscow	1088 (20.3%)	Field hockey added	Games boycotted by US, West Germany, and Japan
1984 Los Angeles	1620 (22.9%)	3000 m and marathon added, also cycling, synchronized swimming, rhythmic gymnastics	Joan Benoir wins 1st womern's Olympic marathon. Games boycotted by 17 countries
1988 Seoul	2476 (25.8%)	1000-m cycling sprints added, 10 000-m track race, heptathlon, team archery, air pistol, 50-m freestyle swimming, singles and doubles table tennis, separate yachting event (470 class)	Rosa Mota wins marathon Florence Griffith-Joyner and Jackie Joyner-Kersee dominate track & field
1992 Barcelona	3008 (28.5%)	Badminton and judo added, 23 sports open to women	34 countries had no women participants Hassiba Boulmerka of Algeria wins 1500m
1996 Atlanta	3700 (36.5%)	Beach volleyball, soccer, softball, mountain bike racing added	27 countries with no women participants Ghada Shouaa won heptathlon (1st Syrian to win gold medal)

* Women's Olympics: four sets of games held from 1922 to 1934.

istrative positions as well. With the merging of the men's and women's athletic programmes, men were more often named to head programmes, an unpredicted negative impact of Title IX legislation. Much of this backslide was secondary to structural barriers, such as unconscious discrimination in the selection process, and the lack of suitable opportunities for training for women.

Current trends are less encouraging than earlier successes. Progress has been made in terms of participation of women in traditional male sports such as hockey, football, and rugby. Marketing of sporting equipment and apparel specifically designed for women has evolved into a lucrative commercial venture. Nevertheless, there remain significant prejudices in college and university budgets, the amount of prize money at competitions, media coverage, and family and community concerns regarding girls and sports. The debate continues as to whether or not such partiality is the result of, or the cause of, the continuing inequity between male and female athletes.

Sociological considerations

'Sport socialization' is the mechanism whereby individuals are encouraged to participate in a sport or physical activity, whether at the recreational or competitive level.[6] This process is influenced by the larger social environment of family members, peers, teachers, coaches, as well as by the mass media, and the advertising industry. Sport administrators, such as athletic directors, help to shape sport and recreation programmes, including policies and practices. They must necessarily take into account various potential systemic barriers, such as sexism, racism, classism, and heterosexism. There are marked gender-related differences in the interests, values, and priorities of individuals who engage in sport. It is neither possible nor acceptable to generalize from research on the behaviour and experiences of male athletes to the female athletic population.[7]

The myth of female inferiority or the 'female deficit' paradigm lingers on, despite lack of evidence that the male model is the ideal. The words 'male' and 'female' indicate actual biological differences, while 'masculinity' and 'femininity' are more representative of culturally 'appropriate' stereotypes of behaviour. The latter terms in particular, are more relative than mutually exclusive. Other social and biological factors interact in many ways. Physical training promotes muscular development which is an indicator of physical maturation in a young man. The same level of training in a young woman may overload the reproductive axis, and slow down the development of breasts and hips. Female hormonal changes around the time of puberty lead to increased deposition of body fat. The susceptible individual may develop an unhealthy preoccupation with body size, shape, and composition.

Sport is a bastion where boys have traditionally learned about teamwork, goal-setting, the pursuit of excellence, and other achievement-oriented behaviours. These are essential skills for success in the workplace for both sexes, but women have sometimes been more ambivalent about both business and sporting achievements. In team selection situations, the strategies of some women, girls, and adolescents in particular, has been to pick their friends first, rather than the best players. For women socialized in the conventional mode, competitive sport may pose a potential threat to relationships, while for males it represents a traditional and safe mode of interpersonal contact.

Psychological models have examined attitudes towards sporting women, personality traits of female athletes, and their specific incentives for involvement. These are largely descriptive studies, and consequently scientifically undependable. There are often cultural constraints on behaviour that contribute to the problem. Successful women athletes are sometimes compelled in justification to overemphasize their feminine side, in terms of dress, make-up, colours, the importance of the dominant male figure in their life, etc. This characterization continues to be propagated today by media coverage that utilizes differential descriptive terms for elite male and female athletes. Even in sports such as intercollegiate basketball or professional tennis, journalists are more preoccupied with sportswomen's appearance and sexual attractiveness than with their athletic prowess. In Canada, this practice has induced Sport Canada to issue special guidelines for the media on non-sexist language.

Many barriers still remain for women who wish to become physically active. These include lack of time and money (double or triple workdays—paid employment, unpaid domestic duties and childcare, and/or part-time studies), threat of sexual harassment or assault, heterosexualism, and homophobia. In certain 'male-dominated' sports, women are more prone to being viewed as intruders. Feminism is not uncommonly equated with lesbianism.

It is critical for female athletes to have a 'role model' and 'positive example', including assistance for the beginner, and interaction with more qualified women as coaches and teachers. There is a need for more national conferences, journals, and textbooks on physically active women and girls. Specific exercise physiology and sport gynaecology topics are especially important to circulate in the women's health movement literature. For example, articles on menopause should discuss the benefits of regular physical activity for relief of menopausal symptoms and preservation of bone density. Women must recognize and accept the importance of self-care through sport and recreation, in order to realize the associated sense of self-worth and entitlement. The ultimate goal is not necessarily 'catching up with the men', but unhampered access to the same knowlege and facilities that men have enjoyed.

Gender equity issues and harassment in sport

Prejudices and intolerances in sport unfortunately persist as ongoing obstacles. Many sporting systems and practices still reflect and reinforce white male heterosexist superiority. Women may be discriminated against on the basis of social class, race, gender, sexual orientation, and (dis)ability. Sexist and racist partiality is particularly dominant in sport and recreation research. For example, relatively little is known about the influence of physical activity and exercise in culturally diverse populations. Women of ethnic minorities (black, Hispanic, Asian, Native American, or Muslim women) are frequently underprivileged in terms of exposure to sport, resources, and opportunities for training. System-wide affirmative action initiatives, such as leadership training programmes designed by and for minority women in coaching and administration, will help to diminish these inequalities.

Gender issues in sport

Gender relations in sport often reproduce societal patterns of domination and subordination. Witness the popularity of diminutive 'feminine' forms of physical activity, such as gymnastics. The aesthetic sports of gymnastics, figure skating, and synchronized swimming are especially vulnerable to this genre of representation. Judging is largely qualitative and based more on socially constructed concepts of feminine/heterosexual attractiveness, rather than on true athletic ability. Establishment of such artificial standards, in concert with societal pressures, the influence of the coach, preoccupation with weight, public weigh-ins, and other coercive measures may precipitate eating disorders and other maladaptive behaviours in susceptible individuals. A recent book by Joan Ryan, *Little girls in pretty boxes: the making and breaking of élite gymnasts and figure skaters,*[8] provides a fascinating but frightening exposé of this fantasy world.

The frequently macho image of men's professional sports, in combination with biased media coverage of athletes' private and professional lives, tends to relegate women to the role of 'sex object, cheerleader, onlooker and spectator, non-participants'.[5,9] Sport can be a setting for the formulation of untoward antifemale sentiments. Many rugby rituals, for example, show contempt and disrespect for women in their images of male dominance and female subordination, or the crudeness of their drinking songs. Football coaches, players, and fans may use misogynist and/or homophobic obscenities to insult opponents and 'fire-up' the home team. There appears to be a correlation between domestic violence against women and the staging of major male sporting events such as the Super Bowl.

Sexual exploitation of female athletes ranges from inappropriate media coverage to intrusive touching to outright sexual abuse. Sexual aggression is often more of a problem with male intercollegiate and professional athletes. Violence against women is further compounded by harassment or discrimination on the basis of race/ethnicity, social class, or sexuality. Many women, out of a concern for personal safety, are forced to alter their leisure needs and habits strictly as a survival strategy, such as jogging during daylight hours when the risk of sexual assault is lower.

Professional inequity

Despite growing participation and increased opportunities for women, advancement of women in decision-making and leadership roles within sport has not followed step for step. Women are still significantly underrepresented in management, coaching, and officiating, particularly at the higher levels. Sex-stereotypical beliefs tend to promulgate certain fallacies, such as the paucity of qualified female coaches; their unwillingness to recruit and travel and to apply for jobs; and the constraints of their domestic responsibilities. Other reasons cited by women for leaving the profession are poorer existing working conditions, lack of time for their friends and families, and lower financial incentives.

Even with removal of systemic barriers and the establishment of affirmative action programmes, it is not enough just to 'open the door' for women in sport. It is imperative to raise the awareness of both men and women about these subjects. Policies and procedures to combat sexual harassment are beneficial, as are broad-based educational campaigns. A critical mass of female representation in leadership and positions of power and authority within sport and recreation must be fostered. Concerns regarding gender inequity, limiting factors to sport participation (such as lack of adequate child

care facilities), and issues of sexual harassment are thus more likely to be addressed.

Positive trends

Fortunately, values are slowly shifting as the gender gap decreases. Title IX legislation had mixed effects on American intercollegiate sport. Funding, scholarships, and media coverage of women's sports increased, but paradoxically, the number of female coaches and administrators declined. The university sport system became more bureaucratic, commercial, and competitive. One rejoinder was the development of specific programmes geared for education and training of this group. In 1987, the Canadian Association for the Advancement of Women in Sport established the National Coaching School for Women to promote more females in coaching and administration. In a supportive environment, female coaches learn sport-specific coaching techniques, but also cover topics such as homophobia in sport and recreation, and sexual harassment. Other advancements involve the preparation of new courses in the field of physical education, dealing with the psychology, sociology, and history of women in sport, as well as with the exercise sciences.

The progress of sportswomen can also be tracked by their increasing level of participation in both competitive and recreational sports. In Canada, the Canadian Intercollegiate Athletic Union sanctions 10 sports for men, 7 for women. In 1994 to 1995, there were 5965 male athletes compared with 3195 females, and 44 more men's teams than women's. Swimming and volleyball were the only sports attracting more women than men. Women's soccer had the highest number of female participants of any university sport (695), and was played at 33 institutions. Possible additions to the competitive programme include women's rugby, wrestling, and ice hockey. In the United States, the National Collegiate Athletic Association data is similarly encouraging.

Institutional progress

National and international sporting and professional organizations have been instrumental in advancing the cause of female athletes. In 1982 the American College of Sports Medicine issued an opinion statement supporting full participation of women in distance events. This action was partly responsible for the inclusion of a women's marathon in the 1984 Olympic Games. In 1986, Sport Canada, a branch of the Department of Canadian Heritage, adopted a Women and Sport Policy, promoting participation and equality of women in sports.

In 1991, another notable barrier was brought to the forefront and resolved. Ann Peel, a national calibre racewalker who was also a lawyer, challenged the practice of the Athlete Assistance Program of Sport Canada regarding federal financial aid to pregnant athletes. The rules of the day allowed for full support for an injured athlete (who was possibly unable to train and whose return to health was unpredictable), while progressively cutting funding for an élite female athlete during a first or subsequent pregnancy. With substantial media coverage, this event led to implementation of the new Athlete Assistance Policy on Curtailment of Training and Competition for Health-Related Reasons. The aim was to establish a consistent approach to dealing with health-related situations, such as injury, illness, or pregnancy, where the athlete was unable to fulfil his or her normal training or competition obligations. At the same time, Sport Canada also produced a specific maternity policy.

New directions

In 1994 WomenSport International was formed. This diverse group is dedicated to bringing about positive change for women and girls in sport and physical activity at all levels of involvement. Women-Sport International is both an issues and an action oriented organization. Key activities include identifying issues of importance to women and girls in sport and physical activity, and developing networks and avenues of communication between member groups and countries for sharing information. In addition, they serve as an advocacy group promoting greater opportunities for participation in sport, and more research into specific problems. Where appropriate, they are instrumental in recommending, designing, and implementing strategies for change.

The latest advances in the field of women in sport have come from Europe. The 1994 Brighton Declaration on Women and Sport was the outcome of the First International Conference on Women and Sport ('Women, Sport and the Challenge of Change'). This meeting, organized by the British Sports Council, with support from the International Olympic Committee, brought together 280 delegates, and policy and decision makers from 82 countries for 4 days in May. This group addressed means to accelerate the process of change to redress the imbalances facing women in their participation and involvement in sport, and to help create a more equitable sporting culture worldwide. In addition to the Declaration, this group developed an International Strategy for Women in Sport, and proposed the establishment of an International Working Group on Women and Sport to encourage development and sharing of model programmes among nations and sport federations. The working policy is the right of every woman to participate and be involved in sport, regardless of race, colour, language, religion, creed, sexual orientation, age, marital status, disability, political belief or affiliation, national or social origin. To further this aim, Women and Sport Confederations were also formed from such nations as Africa, Asia, and South America.

Even the International Olympic Committee (**IOC**) has acknowledged the need to increase representation of women within sport and its technical and administrative structures. One portion of a proposal, submitted at the IOC session in July 1996 in Atlanta, states that 'National Olympic Committees must reserve to women . . . at least 10 per cent of the office in all their decision-making structures by December 31, 2000 . . . this proportion is to reach 20 per cent by December 31, 2005'. There is also the intention to amend the Olympic Charter to take into account the need to maintain equality between men and women. It remains to be seen whether these noble aspirations will be attained, but at least they are a positive step.

Physical and psychological benefits of exercise for women

Physical activity, in humans or any other population, is a complex and multidimensional behaviour that is difficult to measure accurately. It involves bodily movement, results in energy expenditure, and is correlated with physical fitness. Exercise is a defined set of movement patterns that can be more readily quantified, and physical fitness can be further characterized using a variety of standardized laboratory and field tests. Importantly, even moderate levels of physical activity and exercise will result in numerous physical and psychological health benefits for the active woman, regardless of her age or previous level of fitness.

The role of sport in society

The Brighton Declaration on Women and Sport described sport as a cultural activity, with the potential to enrich society and promote friendship between nations. Sport offers individuals opportunities for self-knowledge, self-expression, and fulfilment; personal achievement, skill acquisition, and demonstration of ability; social interaction, enjoyment, good health, and well being. Sport promotes involvement, integration, and responsibility in society and contributes to the development of the community. The positive effects on self-esteem, confidence, and control are well documented for women of all ages.

Prepubescent girls learn co-operation and teamwork by participation in games and sports with boys. School-age children who are well socialized in sport have a greater chance of remaining physically active throughout their lifetime. Physically active adolescents are less at risk of engaging in unhealthy behaviours, such as smoking, alcohol and drug abuse, or promiscuous and irresponsible sexual activity. High school girls who play sports are 80 per cent less likely to be involved in an unwanted pregnancy, and 92 per cent less likely to abuse drugs. The most active or most fit females are less likely to start smoking cigarettes. Surprisingly, the more active male adolescents are more likely to consume alcohol than their less active counterparts.[10]

Exercise in college-age women offers an outlet for the stress of university life and an opportunity for socialization and creativity, as well as mastery of new skills and competition. During pregnancy, regular physical activity can help control weight gain and low back pain, and improve mood and body control during labour and delivery. Early return to exercise postpartum facilitates attainment of prepregnancy weight and state of fitness. Perimenopausal and postmenopausal women find that many of their physical and emotional symptoms are ameliorated by exercise.[11]

Physical activity is also critical in those aged over 65 years. Older women benefit enormously from the improvement in cardiovascular fitness and balance, as well as the bone-building effects of weight-bearing exercise. With a growing elderly population, the majority of whom are women, there is an ever-increasing societal need to enhance their functional independence, to improve musculoskeletal integrity, and to prevent falls with their consequent morbidity and mortality.

Health considerations

A sedentary lifestyle is defined as either no reported physical activity, or very irregular activity that is less than three sessions per week or less than 20 min per session during the past month. Physical inactivity is the only modifiable risk factor for coronary heart disease that has increased in prevalence over the past decade. Regular activity can aid in prevention and management of coronary heart disease, hypertension, non-insulin-dependent diabetes, osteoporosis, obesity, and mental health problems such as depression and anxiety.[12] A moderate level of cardiovascular fitness has been shown to be associated with reduced all-cause mortality and all cancer mortality in physically active American, Swiss, Italian, Finnish, and Chinese women. It has also been related to lower rates of colon, breast, and certain reproductive or oestrogen-dependent cancers (ovary, uterus, breast).[13]

As little as 2 h of exercise a week on the part of a teenage girl may reduce her lifelong risk of breast cancer. Suggested mechanisms for the decrease in oestrogen-dependent cancers include: (i) maintenance of low body fat and moderation of extraglandular oestrogen; (ii) reduction in number of ovulatory cycles and subsequent diminution of gynaecological age and lifetime exposure to endogenous oestrogen; (iii) enhancement of natural immune function; and (iv) the association of other healthy lifestyle habits, such as better nutrition, regular physical examinations, etc.[14] Occupational and non-recreational physical activity appears to offer more protection than vigorous non-occupational or recreational activity.

It can be difficult to measure the role of exercise alone compared with other confounding factors. Extraneous variables are both a risk factor for the disease and associated with the variable in question, but not as a consequence of it. There is a possible synergistic effect of diet and exercise in the prevention and treatment of dyslipidaemia, hypertension, diabetes, obesity, and osteoporosis.[12] Although the majority of research has been carried out in white middle-aged males, at least a few recent studies have focused exclusively on women as subjects. There are numerous methodological problems in research of this nature, including interaction of variables, statistical difficulties with large populations, etc. The question still remains: 'Are people healthy because they exercise, or do they exercise because they are healthy?'

Promotion of physical exercise for women and girls

Common leisure-type activities reported by many women include walking, gardening, aerobics, bicycling, and running/jogging. Many other types of exercise, depending on availability, cost, and access can provide similar health benefits. In the United States, the Center for Disease Control in Atlanta (Office of Disease Prevention and Health Promotion) released *Healthy People 2000* in September of 1990. This is a document summarizing the year 2000 health objectives for the Nation, compared with a 1985 baseline epidemiological survey. One of the priority areas is 'physical activity and fitness'. Objectives are to raise the percentage of the population engaging in regular (preferably daily), light to moderate activity in addition to those participating in physical activity vigorous enough to promote enhanced cardiovascular fitness and muscular strength; while decreasing the proportion of the population engaging in no leisure-time physical activity. Overweight women (and men) are targeted and encouraged to combine a programme of sound dietary practices with regular physical activity to attain an appropriate weight. Other recommendations include an increase in the quantity and quality of daily physical education in schools, as well as the proportion of worksites offering employer-sponsored physical activity and fitness programmes. Increased community availability and accessibility of activity and fitness facilities is also recommended. It is critical to ensure that these programmes are carried out with equal consideration for both men and women.

Gender-specific physiological and physical attributes

In the days of the ancient Greeks and Romans, women were regarded more as objects of art and beauty than as potential participants in athletic activity. Little was known then about their exercise capacity or trainability. In Victorian times, there was more concern about possible detrimental effects of exercise on the reproductive system. More recently, significant inroads have been made in information related to sex-specific physical and physiological differences. Such factors must be considered when assessing sports and activity programmes for females, to serve as guidelines across both sport and gender.[15]

The effects of hormones

The response to exercise training is basically the same in men and women.[16] There may be more differences between two members of the same sex than between a male and a female athlete. The majority of the physiological changes in variables, such as the maximal aerobic capacity, occur during puberty, under the influence of the sex steroids. Until the age of 12 or 14 years there is no substantial difference between the sexes in height, weight, girth, bone width, or skinfold thickness.[16] Testosterone enhances bone formation, leading to larger heavier bones, and also promotes protein synthesis, thereby enlarging muscle mass. Oestrogen acts to broaden the pelvis, stimulate breast development, increase fat distribution on the thighs and hips, and elevate lipoprotein lipase. Its effect on bone is to accelerate the growth rate, causing closure of the epiphyses. Final bone length in women is reached 2 to 4 years after the onset of puberty.

Oestrogens have been theorized to play a role in diminishing exercise-induced muscle damage, because of their potential to stabilize muscle membrane and their antioxidant activity. The lower incidence of atherosclerosis seen in premenopausal females in comparison with males results in part from the ability of oestrogens to diminish peroxidation of low density lipoprotein (LDL). To date, evidence for such activity in muscle has come mainly from animal studies, but it is interesting to speculate on potential implications for female athletes in rigorous training and competition.[17]

Aerobic capacity

Aerobic capacity ($\dot{V}o_2$max) reflects the attainment of maximal aerobic energy transfer, and requires integration of the respiratory, cardiovascular, and neuromuscular systems. In contrast, anaerobic energy metabolism proceeds in the absence of oxygen. Prepubescent boys and girls have similar aerobic and anaerobic capacities. In fact, in the sport of swimming, winning times are similar for all strokes in this age group, and times for girls of 8 years and younger may be even faster.

Absolute $\dot{V}o_2$max, or maximal aerobic capacity, peaks between the ages of 16 and 20 years, with males reaching a value approximately 50 per cent higher than females. This is primarily due to sex differences in body composition (greater body fat in women, less muscle mass to move it) and the oxygen transport system (reduced oxygen-carrying capacity). If corrected for body weight and expressed as millilitres of oxygen per kilogram of body weight, the maximal aerobic capacity of top female athletes may be only about

16 to 20 per cent lower than their male counterparts. If the percentage of body fat is taken into account and aerobic capacity expressed in terms of lean body mass, then the difference shrinks to 9 per cent.[18] Interestingly, female black girls have been found to have lower aerobic fitness relative to body weight than white girls, and less ability to utilize oxygen at a given fat-free mass. This suggests that the fat-free mass in black girls is made up of denser bone and less actual skeletal muscle.[19]

Cardiovascular and pulmonary differences

In addition to body mass and composition, maximal aerobic capacity is affected by peak cardiac output, oxygen carrying capacity, and oxidative capacity of the skeletal muscles. Women have smaller hearts and smaller stroke volumes, therefore they also have lower cardiac outputs. They have a smaller left ventricular mass both in absolute terms and in relation to lean body mass. One compensatory adaptation noted in women is a higher heart rate at the same percentage of maximal aerobic capacity. This has practical implications in terms of utilization of the heart rate method of prescribing exercise. At lower exercise intensities such as walking and jogging, these guidelines may still be accurate, but in more strenuous activities such as aerobic dance, the heart rate may be disproportionately high. Therefore, it may be necessary to prescribe a sustained intensity level of 75 to 80 per cent of maximum heart rate, in order to achieve the desired training effect.

Mean blood pressure levels are lower in women between the ages of 12 and 54 years, but between the ages of 55 and 74, the levels are higher. Black women between the ages of 25 and 74 years have higher blood pressure than white women of the same age. Women also have a higher incidence of certain cardiac conditions such as mitral valve prolapse. Aerobic exercise has been found to exert a positive influence in the management of symptomatic women with this condition.

Mainly because of the difference in body sizes, the 'reference' woman has a smaller thoracic cage and lower lung volumes, but also less blood and tissue to oxygenate than the average male. Vital capacity (the volume of air moved through the lungs from maximal inspiration to maximal expiration) is about 10 per cent less in the female than in a male of the same size and age. Women also breathe more shallowly, using primarily the upper part of their chest, while men tend to breathe more deeply, with greater utilization of the diaphragm.

Haematological differences

Haemodynamically, women are also somewhat challenged. Men have approximately 6 per cent more red blood cells and a 10 to 15 per cent higher haemoglobin concentration and haematocrit than women. A lower haemoglobin level, lower oxygen carrying capacity, and a higher heart rate at the same percentage of maximal aerobic capacity, selectively impact the aerobic capacity of women.[15] Maximal aerobic capacity, however, is but one determinant of performance. There may be additional gender differences in arteriovenous oxygen difference—at rest, 4 to 5 ml of oxygen per 100 ml of blood for both men and women. During exercise, oxygen extraction can average 17 ml in trained athletes. During submaximal exercise the difference is higher in females, while at maximal work, females have a lower arteriovenous oxygen difference.

Running economy

Other factors, such as economy of movement or running economy and lactate threshold, also come into play, especially in distance running. Running economy is the relationship between the rate of oxygen consumption and the velocity of running at a given submaximal steady-state running speed. Men and women athletes have similar running economies when expressed in millilitres of oxygen per kilogram of body weight per minute at intensities up to and more than the marathon distance. At a common absolute running velocity, men are 6 to 7 per cent more economical than women, with a lower heart rate, blood lactate, and oxygen cost of exercise.[20] Differences in economy can explain differences in performance when data for maximal aerobic capacity are equal, as well as equal performance among individuals with different maximal aerobic capacity levels. A better predictor of running success may be the velocity at maximal aerobic capacity.

Response to training

Women are able to experience major increases (10 to 40 per cent) in maximal aerobic power and endurance capacity with aerobic training. The magnitude of change is dependent on initial level of fitness, intensity and duration of the training sessions, frequency of the training, and length of the study. The rapid improvement in performances and times by women over the last 20 years is largely a result of improved competitive opportunities and harder training regimens, including strength training. Women are also beginning participation in sport at an élite level at much younger ages than in previous eras. Whipp and Ward, in their article in Nature in 1992,[21] rocked the scientific and athletic community with their bold prediction that by the year 2025 female athletes would perform as well as their male counterparts over distances of 100 to 1500 m. If lifelong competitive possibilities for women (throughout the world) continue to expand, then records attained by women may still improve at a relatively faster rate than those set by men for some time yet.

Females may actually be better suited than males for ultraendurance-type exercise, because of their unique endocrine characteristics. For example, Paula Newby-Fraser came 11th overall in the 1989 Hawaii Ironman World Championships in a field of both men and women. A recent study demonstrated that women (matched to men at 42.2 km, marathon distance) tended to outperform their male counterparts over a longer distance of 90 km, and had a lower concentration of free fatty acids in their blood.[22] In theory anyway, the plasma concentration of free fatty acids reflects a balance between the rate of fat mobilization (similar in both sexes) and the rate of fat utilization for energy. The female subjects had a lesser aerobic capacity, but a similar running economy and endurance-training history. These findings were attributed to the women's ability to sustain a greater fraction of maximal aerobic capacity, and to their better (more efficient) utilization of fat as a substrate, a fact that has been observed previously.

Anaerobic capacity

The anaerobic system is important for success in short-term high-intensity exercise. In absolute terms, men exhibit significantly greater performance capability than women. When expressed relative to body size, composition, or size of the involved musculature, the findings are more equivocal. Fat-free mass is the best predictor of anaerobic performance. In adolescent populations, it is necessary to match subjects for Tanner stage as well as body mass or fat-free mass, especially in the lower body.[23] Testosterone has an anabolic effect on growth and development of muscle mass, while oestrogen, besides increasing adipose tissue, retards the effect on lean mass and reduces glycogenolysis. Testosterone has the additional action of tranforming type II muscle fibres to a more glycolytic profile, and increasing the level of lactate dehydrogenase. The question of whether or not true physiological or biochemical differences exist between male and female muscle tissue is still being actively researched.

There are also possible sex or gender differences in myoneural factors, such as activation of high-threshold motor units, electromechanical delay, and the rate of force development. This is postulated to be the result of more frequent and intense levels of physical activity in men, another variable that may change with women becoming generally more active. Exercise training leads to enhanced activities of the enzyme muscle phosphofructokinase (ATPase), increased maximal muscle lactate and muscle buffer capacity, as well as increases in both creatine phosphate and adenosine triphosphate (ATP) stores. A potentially confounding consideration in many of the studies is failure to adequately quantify the training status, Tanner stage, and physical activity history of the test subjects. One study of peak power output in an all-out 30-s cycle ergometer test used allometric scaling to remove the influence of disparate body dimensions, and still found that males had a superior anaerobic capacity.[24]

Strength differences between males and females

In women, muscle fibre area and total muscle cross-sectional area average 60 to 85 per cent of male values, but the relative proportion of fast-twitch (glycolytic) and slow-twitch (aerobic) fibres are equal.[15] Although females have generally only about 70 per cent of the lower body strength, sex differences are minimized if absolute strength is expressed relative to fat-free body mass. Appropriate strength training can further decrease these differences, based on ratios to body weight. Highly trained male and female athletes have similar lower body strength relative to body mass (per unit of body weight), cardiovascular endurance capacity, body composition, and muscle fibre type. However, upper body strength in women, even with training, has remained only 30 to 50 per cent that of men. Men have greater upper body muscle mass, as well as chest and shoulder girth. Adolescent boys, matched for Tanner stage with girls, possess significantly greater (30 per cent) arm and leg bone-free cross-sectional area.[23]

Weight (resistance) training in women gives similar relative gains in strength and muscle hypertrophy. It is therefore desirable to include it in a fitness programme for enhancement of athletic performance. A higher muscle mass promotes higher bone density, and a resistance training programme will slow muscle loss in elderly and dieting women. It is a myth that strength training will masculinize women. On account of the sex steroid differences, increases in strength in women are not necessarily accompanied by same amount of muscle hypertrophy as in men.

Thermoregulation

Heat tolerance varies with gender, age, size, cardiovascular fitness, and hormonal factors. Girls appear to have a larger surface area to body mass ratio, a slower onset of sweating, and a smaller sweat rate, features that may disadvantage them in conditions of extreme heat and humidity. In some studies, men have been found to have a higher sweat concentration of sodium and chloride, but a lower potassium concentration than women. Within the same maturational group, however, there are no gender differences in sweat electrolyte losses.[25] In postpubertal women, the thermogenic effects of progesterone also come into play. During pregnancy, and especially during the luteal phase of the menstrual cycle, there is an elevation in the resting core temperature of 0.3 to 0.4°C. Because of this higher starting threshold, thermoregulation may be compromised during prolonged exercise in the heat or heat exposure during the luteal phase. Women on oestrogen replacement therapy have a lower set-point temperature for initiation of sweating and vasodilation during exercise than when they are not taking such therapy. In hot climates, women gain heat faster, and because of their greater body surface area to weight ratio, have a smaller mass in which to store it. In cold environments, increased subcutaneous fat enhances insulation, but increased body surface area to weight ratio allows greater heat loss. Men and women with equal body fat percentages demonstrate no differences in metabolic rate, rectal temperature, or skin temperature.

Body composition

Body composition pertains to both the amount and the distribution of fat, as well as fat-free mass. Essential fat is the body fat stored in the bone marrow, heart, lungs, kidneys, intestines, muscles, and central nervous system, while the remainder of the fatty tissue is storage fat. Women generally have 9 to 12 per cent essential fat, compared with 3 per cent for men.[15] The 'reference' or 'idealized average' man is 10 cm taller and roughly 14 kg heavier than an average woman. Half of this weight increment is reflected in bone density, and half in a larger muscle mass. The 'reference' woman has a higher total percentage of body fat relative to males, 10 to 12 per cent derived from differential hormonal effects of androgens and oestrogens. The same volume of bone in men is 1.23 to 1.5 times heavier (denser) than female bone. Overall, women have 8 to 10 per cent more body fat than males. From 18 to 22 years old, this is usually in the range of 22 to 26 per cent, compared with 12 to 16 per cent for males. Active women have less fat than sedentary college-age women (23 to 27 per cent), and female athletes may average between 15 and 18 per cent body fat depending upon the sport.[15] Endurance athletes may have between 12 and 18 per cent body fat, and élite female runners as low as 6 to 8 per cent, while levels in volleyball and basketball players are frequently as high as 18 to 24 per cent. A higher percentage of body fat may confer an additional competitive advantage in terms of flotation in water sports such as swimming.

There are many inherent imprecisions in the current methods of measuring body composition. The error of estimations made from skinfold measurements may be as high as 14 to 28 per cent.[26] Methods include the Jackson–Pollack sum of skinfolds (five or seven sites) and the Yuhasz equation.[27] Potential sources of error have led to a critical analysis and review of these methods and equations.[28] Precise and accurate anatomical landmarks are needed, with a standard terminology for the various sites. Caliper application, pinch, and the timing of reading are all important. There is a greater likelihood of error with a thicker fat pad. The sum of skinfolds is a better tool to assess the individual athlete's adiposity, and the relative changes over time with diet and/or training.

Regional differences in fat distribution also exist between the sexes. The gynaecoidal (femoral) pattern of fat in the hips and thighs is typically seen in women, while in the androidal (abdominal) pattern, fat accumulates primarily in the abdominal area. This latter profile is more characteristic in men, but it is also seen in women after menopause. The type of fat pattern has implications for health and fitness. Androidal obesity is associated with a higher prevalence of cardiovascular disease, hypertension, blood lipid abnormalities, glucose intolerance, and insulin insensitivity. Nevertheless, the heightened lipolytic activity of the adipocytes in the abdominal region permits an easier reduction through exercise. In contrast, the increased number of normal-sized adipocytes with low lipolytic activity in gynaecoidal obesity are much more resistant. These distribution patterns are frequently expressed as the ratio of waist circumference to hip circumference, where a higher number indicates a greater risk of related diseases.[15]

Underwater weighing—the so-called 'gold standard'—still has an estimated error range of 2 to 4 per cent.[28] In young women, this may be compounded by the intrinsic shortcomings of formulae based on the assumption of a standard value for bone density. This model breaks down in certain situations. Young adult black women, who have dense bones, are well predicted by the traditional Siri formula.[26] Young adult black men, on the other hand, have denser bones, and consequently are underpredicted. In amenorrhoeic athletes who may well have osteopenia or frank osteoporosis, the calculations tend to overestimate the percentage of body fat, unless a corrective factor is used in the equations.[29] As will be discussed, there is a real danger in advocating an optimal body weight or percentage of body fat for this population of female athletes. In susceptible individuals, this has the potential to precipitate and encourage disordered eating patterns.

Furthermore, the norms for body fat gathered from testing a large, broad 'normal' population are not necessarily relevant for a select group of athletes. Women training for certain sports may have a male type of fat distribution. The norms for children and adolescents are also distinctly different. Values for a given sport should be population specific, but must also account for improved fitness, and individuality in body somatotypes. Little research exists on the relationship between changes in body fat and enhanced performance. Coaches, athletes, and sporting organizations cannot offer any satisfactory scientific evidence for an optimal percentage of body fat for their particular sport. The measured 'norms' simply reflect the average values for the élite athletes of the day, which may well be pathological. The ideal body weight for appearance, performance, and good health are not all the same.

Metabolic rate

Resting metabolic rate in women is 5 to 10 per cent lower than in men, not owing to gender, but because of a variability in metabolic activity of specific tissues. Muscle tissue is much more active than adipose tissue. As with other physiological variables, if the resting metabolic rate is expressed proportional to fat-free mass, the discrepancies between males and females disappear. As the energy cost of any exercise is directly correlated with weight, women may expend 40 per cent more calories than men for the same level of activity. Regular aerobic or endurance exercise in both sexes leads to a chronic increase or higher set-point in the resting metabolic rate. Even a single bout of exercise will increase postexercise energy expenditure in proportion to the intensity and duration of the exercise. Women or men who attempt to lose weight by dieting may experience a decrease in the resting metabolic rate, as the body attempts to adapt to a changing energy load.

Biomechanical differences

Men and women have some gender-specific biomechanical characteristics that are frequently emphasized, but which do not hold true in every case. These have been postulated to account for variations in sports performance and athletic injuries. In general, women have a wider, shallower pelvis than men, however the variation of pelvis shapes among women is greater than the difference between sexes. They also have a potentially greater Q angle (angle between the femur and tibia). Successful female and male track and field athletes, however, are found to have similar physiques (hip and shoulder widths). Many female athletes have narrower shoulders, but not necessarily a greater carrying angle at the elbow. Females are thought to have a lower centre of gravity because of a shorter relative leg length. This feature would be of benefit in sports requiring balance. However, centre of gravity is determined more by an individual's height and body type than by gender. In male and female athletes of similar heights, the actual difference in centre of gravity has been calculated to be less than 2.5 cm.

Musculoskeletal injuries in female athletes

The majority of musculoskeletal injuries are characteristic of participation in the sport rather than gender. Sport-specific biomechanics are also extremely important. Factors which have already been discussed, such as lower extremity alignment differences and less upper body strength, as well as nutritional and hormonal variations, may increase the probability of certain overuse injuries. For example, prepubertal gymnasts suffer from more upper extremity injuries, and amenorrhoeic runners are more prone to stress fractures.

Epidemiology of injuries

Much of the current knowledge of injury incidence comes from the injury surveillance database of the National Collegiate Athletic Association (NCAA), which has been in operation for more than 10 years. At present in the university system in the United States, there are only two female-only sports (field hockey, softball), and five male-only sports (water polo, baseball, American football, ice hockey, and wrestling). In comparison, in the Olympics, there are only women competing in rhythmic gymnastics and synchronized swimming; while baseball, bobsled, boxing, modern pentathlon, ski jumping, Nordic combined skiing, water polo, weight lifting, and wrestling remain male domains. Women's ice hockey will be introduced for the first time in the 1998 Nagaro Winter Olympics.

Current NCAA epidemiological data indicates that in women, the highest overall injury rate is in gymnastics, followed by soccer, basketball, field hockey, volleyball, lacrosse, and softball. Men are most frequently injured during 'spring football' (American football played in the spring) and wrestling. There is a relatively equal percentage of injuries during practice and games in soccer, lacrosse, field hockey, softball, and baseball, but interestingly, in gymnastics, 80 per cent of injuries occurred in practice. Sport differences also play a role, for example the landing manoeuvres on the balance beam in gymnastics frequently cause medial dislocation and instability of the first metatarsophalangeal joint. Long-term sequelae of these musculoskeletal problems can be significant. A 1993 follow-up study of a collegiate gymnastics team found that half of athletes had less than fully recovered from their injuries 3 years after stopping competition.[30]

Foot and ankle injuries

In terms of specific body areas, the ankle is the most commonly injured joint, particularly in basketball, volleyball, field hockey, gymnastics, and track and field events. Women's gymnastics has a relatively high rate of foot injuries, in addition to lower back problems. Women in the military services (navy or cadets) suffer from more stress fractures and other lower extremity injuries than do the males in these programmes. Just as with female collegiate distance runners and dancers, there is frequently an association with menstrual irregularity and/or disordered eating in this population. Competitive sports with excessive axial loading can cause other foot and ankle problems, such as tibiotalar impingement syndrome. Ballet dancers, owing to the demands of their activity, often incur posterior impingement of the os trigonum, as well as pain and tendinitis in the flexor hallucis longus tendon. Dancers with feet of the pes planus type may develop posterior tibial tendinitis, while those with a cavus foot may have more difficulty with Achilles tendinitis. Accessory ossicles can also create pressure points and painful areas in the foot. Specific stress fractures may be more common in certain sports. In dancers for example, a second metatarsal stress fracture can occur at the Lisfranc joint.[31] Bunions and underlying hallux valgus deformities are more prevalent in women, in part because of their preferred footwear. Management generally includes conservative measures such as orthotics and metatarsal pads, with surgical correction reserved for cosmetic purposes only.

Lower leg injuries

Both male and female athletes in jumping sports like volleyball and basketball may initially present with what looks like a 'high' ankle sprain, which on further investigation turns out to be a fibular stress fracture. More commonly, stress fractures occur anywhere along the tibia. Tibial stress fractures in the lower medial third, as well as in the proximal tibia, are reasonably benign, and heal well with conservative therapy. It is critical, however, to recognize mid-third anterior cortex fractures, with point tenderness and anterior tibial bowing. The radiographic finding of the 'dreaded black line' indicates a distraction type of stress injury, which has the potential to go on to complete fracture. Other causes of 'shin splints', or pain in the lower leg, such as chronic compartment syndrome or popliteal artery entrapment syndrome do not seem to have a selectively female preponderance.

Hip and pelvis injuries

Pain in the hip and pelvis can arise from a multitude of causes, including gynaecological, gastrointestinal, and urinary sources,[32] or it can be referred from other structures including the low back. Laboratory and radiological investigations are indicated by positive findings from a complete history and physical examination. A high index of suspicion for femoral neck stress fractures is necessary for runners who present with exercise-induced hip, groin, or thigh pain. In one study,[33] 58 per cent of these occurred in females. The 'hop' test had a sensitivity of 70 per cent in these athletes, but radiographs were only positive in 24 per cent of cases, and bone scans were required for definitive diagnosis. A fracture or partial fracture on the compression side of the bone is treated conservatively, with forms of rehabilitation that are not weight bearing, such as cycling, swimming, or running in water. An injury on the superior or tensile side, however, is much more serious, and percutaneous pinning is recommended before it goes on to fracture displacement. Nutritional counselling is important, and in amenorrhoeic athletes, oral contraceptives may be necessary to help preserve bone density.

Knee injuries

Although not universally true, the tendency for the female athlete to have a wider pelvis, increased flexibility, less well-developed musculature (especially the vastus medialis obliquus), genu valgum, and external tibial torsion cause a propensity towards anterior knee pain. Patients with patellofemoral pain syndrome typically complain of crepitus and aching in the knee, pain going up or down stairs, stiffness and retropatellar pain after sitting (the 'theatre sign'), and a subjective feeling of instability. The differential diagnosis includes inflammatory conditions (bursitis, tendinitis, synovitis), mechanical causes (patellofemoral syndrome, subluxation, dislocation, plica), and miscellaneous entities.[34] The so-called 'miserable malalignment syndrome' (Fig. 1) also involves forefoot pronation, tibial torsion, Q angle greater than 15°, increased femoral anteversion, and heel valgus. The Q angle is measured from the anterosuperior iliac spine to the central portion of the patella to the tibial tubercle. Ligamentous laxity or hypermobility syndrome is found in some women, and may also contribute to an increased incidence of patellofemoral tracking problems. During the third trimester of pregnancy, the circulating hormone relaxin may have a similar effect.

Women have a higher incidence of tears of the anterior cruciate ligament, although there is no conclusive or inclusive explanation for this phenomenon. A National Collegiate Athletic Association survey found that the anterior cruciate ligament was injured 3.5 times more often in basketball, and 2.0 times more often in soccer than in male athletes, as measured by rates per athletic exposure.[35] Females rely more on the anterior cruciate ligament for deceleration in sports with lots of starting and stopping, and less on hamstring control. They were found to have a greater risk of non-contact tears of the anterior cruciate ligament in both sports, compared with their male counterparts. Postulated causative factors include both extrinsic variables (body movement, muscular strength and co-ordination, shoe-surface interface, and skill level) and intrinsic influences (joint laxity, proprioception, limb alignment, notch dimension, ligament size). A common femoral notch shape associated with injuries of the anterior cruciate ligament is A-shaped, but H-shaped, reverse U-, or C-shaped notches may also cause a higher risk. Ratios of the

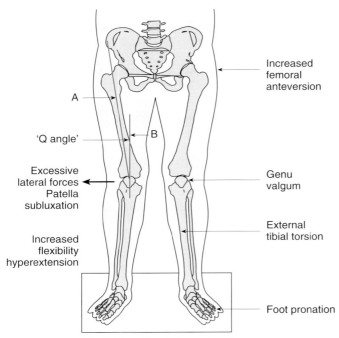

Fig. 1 Miserable malalignment syndrome.

notch-to-femoral width have been used to predict injuries of the anterior cruciate ligament and the incidence of bilaterality, but a better indicator may be the ratio of the notch width to ligament size.

Back injuries

With regards to lower back problems, scoliosis is more common in females, and there is also an association with menstrual dysfunction.[36] Persistent back pain with hyperextension in sports such as gymnastics and diving should prompt further investigations to rule out spondylolysis or stress fracture of the pars interarticularis. A nuclear medicine bone scan with SPECT (single photon emission computed tomography) is the most sensitive diagnostic tool, followed by oblique radiographs of the lumbosacral spine, or a localized CT scan. It is debatable whether or not this acquired spondylolysis progresses to spondylolisthesis at the same rate as the congenital variety. Spondylolysis and sciatica can occur simultaneously in a patient. It is therefore important to carry out a full neurovascular examination in these patients.

Upper extremity injuries

In the upper extremity, 'impingement syndrome', multidirectional instability, rotator cuff weakness, and other shoulder injuries occur secondary to increased laxity of the ligamentous structures and decreased strength. The vicious cycle of physiological instability, rotator cuff weakness, and pain leads to posterior capsular tightness and further muscle imbalance. Both male and female rowers may experience stress fractures of the ribs as a result of excessive pull of the slips of the serratus anterior muscle on the bone. In the elbow, females will sometimes have an increased valgus carrying angle and ligamentous laxity. Repetitive axial loading injuries in sports such as

gymnastics can lead to osteochondritis dissecans and loose body formation, in the same way as excessive throwing can cause 'little leaguer's elbow' in boys. Cheerleading, an activity where the women are frequently thrown up high in the air, and then caught again after a series of mid-air gyrations, has the potential for serious musculoskeletal injuries including elbow dislocations.

Distal radial epiphyseal fractures (Salter I type) and stress syndromes are not uncommon in young gymnasts. It is important to diagnose this injury early as there can be subsequent radial growth arrest and ulnar overgrowth. These young women may also experience wrist pain secondary to fractures of the navicular or scaphoid bone. Dorsal taping or splinting to block full dorsiflexion of the wrist, along with physiotherapy and relative rest, is the treatment of choice. An astute clinician and the proper investigations will help detect these problems before permanent disability occurs. Recent rule changes took effect after the 1996 Olympics, increasing the age of international competition from 14 to 16. This may alleviate some of the current overuse injuries seen in prepubescent athletes with immature skeletons and vulnerable growth plates.

Breast injuries

Both male and female athletes have a need for gender-specific care and protection for their reproductive organs. Breast disorders in women include trauma, discomfort related to sports activities, and nipple irritation caused by friction of overlying clothing. Fibrocystic disease has a similar incidence in athletes as in the general population, but the symptoms can be ameliorated somewhat by controlling the intake of xanthines in foods like caffeine or chocolate. Galactorrhoea, although less common, should be followed up by serial prolactin levels, especially if accompanied by oligomenorrhoea or amenorrhoea. Radiological investigations may uncover a pituitary microadenoma, which then mandates appropriate medical or surgical management.

Trauma to the breasts can lead to ecchymosis, haematoma formation, and occasionally fat necrosis, with induration and scarring. The nipples may be traumatized by friction, causing abrasions and bleeding. This condition is seen in male runners as well, and may be managed with the use of Vaseline, tape, or band-aids over the nipples. Thermal injury to the nipples, the so-called 'bicyclists' nipples' is sometimes also a problem. In addition to these acute and chronic conditions in the female athlete, it is important to emphasize the value of regular breast self-examination as a preventative health care measure.

It is not possible to change the size of the breast with exercise programmes or with pectoralis-specific strengthening, but it may be possible to improve the muscle tone to prevent sagging. Some requisite features of a proper sports bra are firm support of the breasts, limitation of breast motion, and a soft material that will not abrade the skin. Small-breasted women may do better with a compression-type bra, such as the Jogbra, while larger-breasted women usually require some form of encapsulation bra with circumferential support and a criss-cross or Y construction to limit motion of the breast to 2 cm in the vertical plane. Other important details include unstretchable straps, breathable material, no seams at the nipple area, no hooks or fasteners, and of course, an individualized fit. Protective chest pads or light-weight plastic cup bras are recommended for sports such as softball, hockey, and other contact sports.

Nutritional concerns

Female athletes may have several common nutritional problems, such as inadequate intake of fluids and carbohydrates, in combination with an excess relative fat intake. Low-calorie diets do not provide enough energy or adequate daily amounts of certain vitamins and minerals for the demands of the high performance athlete. Carbohydrate deficiency leads to earlier depletion of glycogen stores and increased onset of muscular fatigue. The recommended daily intake of protein is 1.1 to 1.65 g/kg of body weight, but this may need to be increased in sports where muscle bulk is required. A higher protein intake during times of intense competition and stress may help to prevent overtraining syndrome.[37]

Low calcium intake has been associated with stress fractures and osteoporosis. The recommended daily allowance for calcium in the United States is 1200 mg/day for women aged from 11 to 24 and 800 mg/day for women aged 25 years and older. Hypo-oestrogenic athletes such as amenorrhoeic runners, or postmenopausal women not on hormonal replacement therapy require 1500 mg/day. Pregnant and lactating women also have increased calcium needs. Zinc deficiency has been linked to increased injuries from microtrauma as well as changes in immune function. Iron deficiency causes anaemia and poor thermoregulation, especially during exposure to cold. Physically active women who do not eat red meat two or three times a week should take an iron supplement.

Exercise-associated anaemias

Female athletes are at higher risk of developing true anaemia than male athletes. Iron deficiency itself may occur in as many as one in four female athletes, primarily as a result of increased monthly menstrual losses combined with inadequate intake. These conditions must be differentiated from the so-called 'athletic anaemia' or 'pseudoanaemia', a physiological response to training commonly seen in endurance athletes of both sexes. Initially, exercise induces a haemoconcentration secondary to fluid loss. The body compensates by releasing renin, aldosterone, and vasopressin, which act to conserve salt and water and expand plasma volume. A new haemodynamic equilibrium is established at a lower haemoglobin level, although the absolute number of red blood cells changes little.[38] The rise in plasma volume correlates with the amount and intensity of habitual exercise, and athletes who train the hardest have the lowest haemoglobin levels. The disadvantage of a lower haemoglobin per unit of blood is counterbalanced by the positive physiological consequences. A larger blood volume causes a higher stroke volume, and consequently a greater cardiac output. The dilution of fibrinogen and other clotting factors in the blood lowers the risk of thromboembolism.

Normal values

Women generally have a lower haemoglobin concentration with 95 per cent falling into the range from 12 to 16 g/dl, compared with 14 to 18 g/dl for men. Haematocrit values are also lower in females (37 to 47 per cent) than in males (40 to 54 per cent). Each individual, however, has his or her own 'optimal' value, below which athletic performance may be compromised. It is advisable to screen for causes of anaemia in females if the haemoglobin is less than 12.5 g/dl. Adolescent athletes in particular may be further investigated by measuring serum ferritin levels.

History

Clinical manifestations of anaemia may include exercise fatigue, sensations of 'burning muscles', dyspnoea, and nausea. Pica, or a craving for ice chips, may be present in up to 50 per cent of iron-deficient patients. Important queries on history include family history of anaemia, prior episodes of anaemia, medication use (non-steroidal anti-inflammatory drugs, aspirin, iron), trauma, exercise activity, bleeding episodes (especially gastrointestinal bleeding), and menstrual history (menorrhagia). Blood donations, recent infections, pregnancies, and lactation may also deplete iron stores. Women with disordered eating patterns and dietary restrictions such as vegetarianism do not take in sufficient replacement iron. Although much more rare, intestinal parasites such as hookworms and tapeworms should be considered in the anaemic female athlete with a history of recent travel.

Physical examination and laboratory findings

Physical examination may reveal conjunctival pallor, evidence of bleeding or bruising, or enlarged lymph nodes. A rectal examination, as well as a stool test for occult blood, are part of a thorough gastrointestinal evaluation. Appropriate laboratory investigations include a reticulocyte count, red blood cell indices, and an examination of the peripheral smear. An increased reticulocyte count can occur with a haemolytic anaemia related to exercise. This presents as a postexercise low-grade haemolysis with shortened survival times of red blood cells, and is commonly seen in runners and during times of intense competition. Other findings are a low serum haptoglobin, and macrocytosis. In addition there may be high plasma haemoglobin, bilirubin, and lactate dehydrogenase, and haemoglobin and haemosiderin in the urine.

Congenital haemolytic anaemias such as sickle cell or thalassaemia syndromes, or a glucose 6-phosphate deficiency with drug-induced haemolysis, will also present with an increased reticulocyte count. It is crucial to remember that these patients may be iron depleted at the same time. A high reticulocyte count is also a normal physiological reaction to ongoing loss of red blood cell bloods from any cause, including the occult blood loss seen in up to 20 per cent of marathon runners, and urinary loss through microhaematuria. A normal reticulocyte count in the face of a normochromic normocytic anaemia suggests the 'pseudoanaemia' already described. Other red blood cell indices and serum ferritin will be normal in these cases. Macrocytic anaemias occur as a result of a lack of vitamin B_{12} or folate. A hypochromic microcytic anaemia reflects iron deficiency, and can be seen in up to 20 per cent of women and 50 per cent of pregnant women. Iron depletion without anaemia is also found in 20 to 62 per cent of high school and college-age women, and in up to 80 per cent of endurance athletes.[38]

Serum ferritin levels

The average serum ferritin level is 30 ng/ml. A value of less than 12 ng/ml correlates with no iron in the bone marrow, 12 to 20 ng/ml with minimal or no iron in the bone marrow, and greater than 20 ng/ml with sufficient iron stores in the bone marrow. A level of 1 ng/ml of plasma ferritin represents approximately 10 mg of iron stores. There can be some variation between different laboratories in ferritin measurements. Levels are also elevated in acute inflammation (usually above 50 ng/ml), and in liver disease.

Three levels of disease have been defined: iron depletion (ferritin less than 20 ng/ml); iron deficiency without anaemia (ferritin less than 12 ng/ml), but no impairment in performance; and finally, iron deficiency with florid anaemia and its repercussions on performance. Iron is also an essential element of myoglobin and cytochromes, as well as several coenzymes of the energy systems. There has been much debate about significant performance impairment with levels between 20 and 60 ng/ml. Differences have been seen in animal models, but in humans, any observed changes seem to reflect correction of a mild underlying anaemia.[39] If there is any doubt, an empirical trial of iron therapy for 2 months is warranted. An increase in haemoglobin of at least 1 g/dl intimates that iron deficiency anaemia was present.[38]

Iron requirements

The average man requires 10 mg/day of elemental iron, while menstruating women need 15 to 18 mg/day. The actual loss during menses can be as much as 35 to 60 ml of blood per cycle, or 1.2 to 2 mg of iron per day. Without sufficient replenishment, this may cause an overall drop in haemoglobin of 1 to 2 g/dl. Athletes generally have higher iron needs. Up to 0.25 to 1.0 mg/day can be lost in sweat, but an individual would have to sweat between 5 and 50 l/day in order to lose this amount.[38] Other sources of blood loss (and therefore iron loss) are haematuria, haemolysis, and gastrointestinal bleeding. Endurance runners are thought to have less iron absorption and faster iron loss from the gastrointestinal system. The average American diet contains 6 mg of iron/1000 kcal. Many female athletes with restrictive eating patterns consume less than 2000 kcal/day, and will therefore have additional iron requirements. Women who pursue modified vegetarian diets are also at increased risk because the iron that is consumed is not highly bioavailable.

Therapy

The primary therapy for iron deficiency with or without anaemia is to increase the amount of dietary iron. Haem iron such as that found in red meat has better absorption (15 to 33 per cent) than non-haem iron (2 to 20 per cent). Iron-fortified cereals and breads provide an artificial source of iron, whereas cooking acidic foods like tomato sauce in iron pans adds iron naturally to the food. Vitamin C enhances iron absorption while tannic acid (in black tea) and phytates (in green leafy vegetables) are inhibitory. Eating poultry or seafood with dried legumes will increase the absorption of iron from the vegetables.[38]

Supplementation with 30 to 60 mg elemental iron/day is recommended for any woman who does not eat meat, fish, or chicken daily.[40] Oral iron is converted from the ferric to the ferrous form in the stomach, and is then absorbed in the duodenum. Sustained release preparations do not dissolve in the stomach, and therefore are not as well absorbed in the duodenum. The athlete can maximize absorption of oral iron supplements by taking them with 200 mg vitamin C, on an empty acidic stomach, without other vitamins or minerals such as calcium or magnesium as 'competitors'. Ferrous sulphate is the cheapest form, and compliance may be enhanced by building up the dose gradually to increase tolerance.

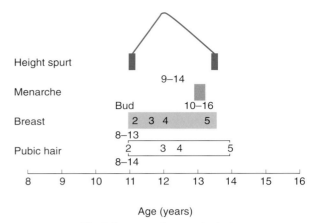

Fig. 2 Sequence of events at puberty.

Prophylactically, it may be given in doses of 325 mg three times per week. Approximately 15 per cent of administered iron is absorbed in the first 3 to 4 weeks, then absorption declines to 5 to 10 per cent, proportional to to the remaining iron deficiency. Monitoring of the haemoglobin and reticulocyte count 3 to 4 weeks after beginning therapy will help to measure the progress of therapy. Serum ferritin measurements at intervals will prevent iron overload and iatrogenic haemochromatosis. Up to 6 months of oral therapy may be necessary to replenish iron stores, and rarely is parenteral administration of iron required.

The developing female athlete

Puberty is the landmark that both figuratively and literally separates the men from the boys, but more importantly, the women from the men. Peak height velocity for girls coincides with ages 10.5 to 13 years, while for boys it occurs slightly later, at ages 12.5 to 15 years. Menarche occurs approximately 1 year after peak height velocity is achieved (Fig. 2).[41] Skeletal maturity is generally completed by the age of 18 or 19 in girls, and 21 to 22 in boys.[15] During puberty, girls may increase in height approximately 20 per cent, but after menarche, growth is limited to under 7.5 cm. The average growth spurt lasts from 24 to 36 months. This is frequently the time of life during which many athletes are first exposed to sport. Rapid growth can be associated with decreased flexibility, muscle–tendon imbalance, and increased risk of injury. Repetitive forces at the epiphyseal plate or joint surface can cause chronic problems, such as premature closure of the distal radial epiphysis in gymnasts, or osteochondritis dissecans. Tight muscle–tendon units exacerbate the traction on susceptible apophyses like the tibial tubercle (Osgood–Schlatter's disease) and calcaneus (Sever's disease).[42]

Maturation of the reproductive organs and systems follows a predetermined sequence that is better characterized by physiological stage than by chronological age (Table 2).[41] In sports, Tanner staging can be theoretically helpful in separating prepubescent and postpubescent female athletes for contact and collision sports such as field hockey, martial arts, and ice hockey. Such usage might enhance safety, because physically immature athletes with open growth plates are potentially at higher risk of injury. In practice, it may be embarrassing for young girls (and boys) to be examined in this fashion. Self-ratings of sexual maturity by comparison with a

Table 2 Tanner classification of sexual maturity stages in girls

Stage	Pubic hair	Breasts
1	None	Prepubertal; no glandular tissue
2	Sparse, long, straight, lightly pigmented on labia majora	Breast bud; small amount of glandular tissue
3	Darker, beginning to curl, extend laterally	Breast mound and areola enlarged, no contour separation
4	Coarse, curly, abundant, less than adult	Breast enlarged; areola and papilla form mound projecting from breast contour
5	Adult type and quantity, extending to medial thigh	Mature; areola part of breast contour

chart of stages has been shown to correlate well with those determined by a physician.[43]

The preparticipation physical examination in females

The preparticipation physical examination for the female athlete must consider these special matters, in addition to others. A detailed ancillary questionnaire may be administered, not only to identify current health problems, but to ascertain also other risk-taking behaviours (Table 3).[42] Specific concerns to be addressed for young girls and adolescents in particular are adequacy of nutrition (iron, calcium, calories), risk of disordered eating, menstrual disorders, psychosocial stress issues, and biomechanical factors (gynaecoid pelvis, femoral neck anteversion, genu valgum, increased Q angle). Other issues are exercise habits, safe sex, breast self-examination, regular Pap smears, smoking reduction, self-esteem building, body image, and protection from violence. The health care needs of women in their reproductive years include screening for gynaecological cancers and sexually transmitted diseases, advice on contraception, exercise and pregnancy, menopause, prevention of osteoporosis, and prevention of heart disease. Active women of all ages profit from sport-specific guidance, advice on proper equipment, and education on the health benefits of exercise. It is critical for the health care professional to understand the female athlete's needs, exercise goals, and barriers.

The menstrual cycle and the female athlete

The average age of menarche in the United States is 12.8 years, which is 1.2 to 1.3 years after peak growth velocity is attained. A menstrual cycle averages 28 days, but may range from 20 days to as long as 45 days in length. The follicular or proliferative phase lasts from menses to ovulation, and the luteal phase or secretory phase, from ovulation through to menses. The normal duration of the luteal phase is about 14 days, but shortening of the luteal phase can

occur in regularly cycling athletes, and is often the first manifestation of menstrual dysfunction.

Hormonal events

At the hormonal level, many events are occurring simultaneously. There are numerous feedback loops, both positive and negative. The hypothalamus secretes gonadotrophin-releasing hormone (**GnRH**) throughout the entire cycle. Follicle-stimulating hormone (**FSH**) and luteinizing hormone (**LH**) are subsequently secreted from the anterior pituitary gland, and stimulate accelerated growth in one or more of the ovarian follicles containing eggs. The ovary secretes oestrogen and progesterone in response to FSH and LH in another feedback loop.

During the follicular phase there is a gradual decline in FSH and LH levels, until just before ovulation, when a sudden increase in LH (6- to 10-fold) ensues together with a concurrent twofold increase in FSH. The biological action of FSH is to promote growth of the ovarian follicle(s) and the synthesis of oestrogen from androgen precursors, whereas LH stimulates androgen production from the ovary. Meanwhile, oestrogens are causing development and maturation of the endometrial surface. The sudden surge in LH results from the positive feedback of the high oestrogen levels, and precipitates ovulation, with subsequent formation of the corpus luteum. The corpus luteum secretes both oestrogen and progesterone, which stabilize the endometrium for implantation of the fertilized egg. There is also a decrease in FSH and LH secretion by the anterior pituitary at this time. Blood levels of oestrogen and progesterone drop off sharply by the end of the luteal phase, triggering desquamation of the endometrium, or menstruation. The complex interactions of the various hormones and the significant events of the menstrual cycle are illustrated in Figs 3 and 4.[44]

Premenstrual symptoms

During the luteal phase, increased levels of the female sex steroids cause symptoms such as lateral breast tenderness, fluid retention, mood swings, and carbohydrate cravings, collectively called molimina. In moderation, the presence of these hormone-mediated symptoms is good clinical evidence that the neuroendocrine system is functioning as it should. When these symptoms become excessive or troublesome, they are termed premenstrual syndrome (**PMS**). In practice it is often useful to ask a woman if she can tell if her period is coming, in order to determine whether or not ovulation is taking place. Regular or irregular menstrual bleeding may still occur even without ovulation, but there are only low baseline levels of both oestrogen and progesterone present throughout the cycle.[45]

Menstrual disturbances

The entity of 'athletic amenorrhoea' or 'exercise-associated amenorrhoea' has been described relatively recently. Amenorrhoea itself occurs in approximately 5 per cent of the general population, while it may be present in up to 20 per cent of women who exercise, and up to 50 per cent of élite athletes.[46] The discrepancies in the prevalences quoted in the literature in athletic women (5 to 62 per cent in some series, 10 to 44 per cent in others) are primarily due to the lack of a standard definition between studies, as well as differences in the populations surveyed.[47] Researchers have now agreed to a common usage of terms. In primary amenorrhoea, menstruation has

Table 3 Health history for the female athlete

Name: _____ Age: _____

Directions: Please answer the following questions to the best of your ability.

1.   How old were you when you had your first menstrual period? _____

2.   How often do you have a period? _____

3.   How long do your periods last? _____

4.   How many periods have you had in the last year? _____

5.   When was your last period? _____

6.   Do you ever have trouble with heavy bleeding? _____

7.   Do you have questions about tampon use? _____

8.   Do you ever experience cramps during your period? _____

     If so, how do you treat them? _____

9.   Are you on birth control pills or hormones? _____

10. Do you have any unusual discharge from your vagina? _____

11. When was your last pelvic examination? _____

12. Have you ever had an abnormal Pap smear? _____

13. How many urinary tract infections (bladder or kidney) have you had? _____

14. Have you ever been treated for anaemia? _____

15. How many meals do you eat each day?_____ How many snacks? _____

16. What have you eaten in the last 24 hours? _____
     _____

17. Are there certain food groups that you refuse to eat (meat, breads, etc.?) _____
     _____

18. Have you ever been on a diet? _____

19. What is your present weight? _____

20. Are you happy with his weight?_____ If not, what would you like to weigh?_____

21. Have you ever tried to loss weight by vomiting? _____

     Using laxatives?_____ Diuretics? _____

     Diet pills?_____

22. Have you ever been diagnosed as having an eating disorder?_____

23. Do you have questions about healthy ways to control your weight? _____

24. How often do you drink alcohol? _____

25. How often do you use drugs? _____

     Smoke cigarettes? _____

26. Do you wear your seat belt when in a car? _____

27. Do you wear a helmet when you bicycle? _____

28. Do you have any questions about health or personal issues? _____

29. Do you own any guns? _____

not occurred by the time the woman has reached the age of 16; secondary sexual characteristics such as breast enlargement or development of pubic hair are not present by the age of 14. In secondary amenorrhoea, menarche has been attained and normal menstruation has ensued in the past, but has now ceased for some reason. Amenorrhoea is defined as less than three periods in 1 year, or 6 months without a period. Oligomenorrhoea, or infrequent periods, is fewer than six periods in 12 months, or cycles at intervals of 39 to 90 days. Eumenorrhoeal women generally have cycle lengths of 25 to 38 days. Dysmenorrhoea refers to painful, crampy

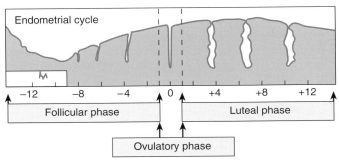

Fig. 3 The normal menstrual cycle.

menstrual periods, caused by local release of prostaglandins and contraction of the smooth muscle of the myometrium.

There is a continuum of menstrual dysfunction. Luteal phase length is affected first, decreasing to 10 days or less. The next manifestation may be euoestrogenic anovulatory cycles, where menstrual bleeding occurs at irregular intervals, without any prior warning symptoms. Finally, hypo-oestrogenic amenorrhoea results, creating a hormonal climate similar to that in the postmenopausal woman. It

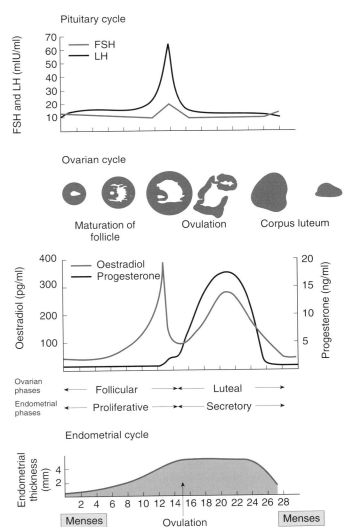

Fig. 4 Hormonal events of the menstrual cycle, phases of the ovarian and endometrical cycle and endometrial height throughout the menstrual cycle.

is difficult to detect the earliest stages, and there are no valid scientific studies that can document or predict the length of time required to progress through all three.[45,48]

Pathophysiology of athletic amenorrhoea

The most probable site of suppression of the reproductive axis is at the level of the hypothalamus or above. There are two current hypotheses regarding initiation of these hormonal changes.[49] Adrenal axis activation and catecholamine release (especially noradrenaline) during exercise inhibits the hypothalamic generation of GnRH pulses and may interact to suppress LH release. Decreases in prolactin, LH, and FSH during strenuous exercise have been found, as well as increases in catechol oestrogens and β-endorphins. Endurance training alters pulsatile release of LH owing to a central inhibitory effect.[47,50,51] It has been postulated that luteal suppression may not be the intermediate point along the progression to athletic amenorrhoea, but may represent the endpoint of successful adjustment to athletic training.[49]

Others espouse the concept of 'energy drain', where amenorrhoea is a physiological adaptation to a negative energy balance, resulting from inadequate food intake in combination with increased daily energy expenditure. Female athletes may have mean total calorie intakes that fluctuate from 5325 kJ/day (1272 kcal/day) to well over 10 000 kJ/day (2400 kcal/day). The energy demands of different sports and training regimens are also variable. Some women may fail to compensate adequately in their the diet for the additional energy cost of exercise. In situations where the intake and output of calories are discordant, the question arises whether or not compensatory reduction of resting metabolic rate occurs in response to food restriction.[52] Alternatively, the athlete may be either underreporting food or restricting energy intakes. Additionally, the 'energy drain' hypothesis may have an important modulatory effect on the hypothalamic pituitary set-point. In one study of dancers with 6 months of secondary amenorrhoea, menses recurred during periods of prolonged rest, without a change in weight or percentage body fat.[53]

It was previously thought that an absolute critical level of fat was required for initiation and maintenance of menstruation.[54,55] This theory was based on the fact that peripheral fat stores serve both as a ready source of energy, and as the site of conversion of androgens to oestrogen. Attainment of a critical weight (with a suggested minimum of 17 per cent body fat for menarche, and 22 per cent for secondary amenorrhoea) would therefore result in a change in the metabolic rate, decreasing the sensitivity of the hypothalamus to oestrogen and restoring the menstrual cycle. This hypothesis has since been disproven on a number of grounds, including analysis of the statistical methods and calculation of the regression equation. Measurements of body fatness were also based on estimates from height and weight, and not on actual measurements. Several subsequent studies have further refuted this 'critical weight' theory.[56]

Risk factors for menstrual dysfunction

Risk factors for exercise-associated amenorrhoea are complex, and include training regimen, reproductive maturity, body weight and composition, dietary practices, and emotional and psychological stress, among others.[57] It is frequently difficult to isolate a sole precipitant. There is some sport-specificity, with a higher prevalence in runners compared with athletes such as swimmers or cyclists, but there is little correlation with weekly distance, pace, or years of training. Some investigators, however, have found an inverse relationship between weekly training distance, especially during the luteal phase, and the length of the luteal phase.[58] A sudden onset of intense training may not allow sufficient time for adaptation of the reproductive axis. One prospective study, looking at luteal phase changes with training, was able to utilize strenuous exercise to cause reversible changes in the menstrual cycle, but unfortunately these data were somewhat confounded by concomitant weight loss in the subjects.[59] Other studies in this area are equivocal as to cause and effect of exercise-related menstrual disturbances, and are reviewed elsewhere.[49,50]

Non-athletes attain menarche significantly earlier than high school or college and Olympic athletes.[60] Olympic athletes begin menstruation at an average of 14.8 years. However, the physical characteristics associated with later maturation also make these women better athletes. With regards to age of menarche and age of initiation of training, there may be an inherent bias in most studies. Later menarche appears to be coincident with, or related to, some factor that selects for superior performance or permits continued participation in the sport.[61]

The pretraining menstrual pattern is the best predictor of menstrual function during training, suggesting that maturation of the hypothalamic–pituitary–ovarian axis is a critical determinant. The athletes most at risk begin training early, (prior to menarche at 12 to 16 years), have intense training programmes, consume few calories, and have the lowest body weight. Stress and poor nutrition may also play a role in decreasing hormonal secretion. The only unbiased approach to studying this issue is through randomized, prospective, cohort, experimental designs. Regardless, it is extremely likely that each athlete has her own individual threshold of energy balance, weight, fatness, physical and psychological stress, where ovulation and her ability to reproduce are compromised.

From a purely scientific point of view, there are many unanswered questions about the effects of exercise and the interaction of other variables with a woman's reproductive system. In addition to variability in the definition of amenorrhoea, the description of 'low body weight' is not universally standard. To document accurately the amount of exercise necessary to induce menstrual dysfunction, it is necessary to quantitify reliably the individual's degree of exertion and intensity of training, utilizing the parameters of heart rate and/or maximal aerobic capacity. The role of eating disorders is not clear, as many of the earliest studies looking at menstrual function specifically excluded subjects with this history. Another substantial concern with survey-type studies is the necessity of relying on a subject's memory for data about her diet, training, and menstrual history.

There are also a number of methodological problems in measuring hormonal concentrations. Both oestrogen and progesterone are bound to sex hormone-binding globulin, and only the free hormones are biologically active. Observed changes in concentration may represent a change in clearance or secretion, a failure to account for plasma volume shifts following exercise, or some other extraneous factor. The gonadotrophins, ovarian, adrenal, and thyroid hormones, as well as the endogenous opiates and neurotransmitters have complex, sometimes synergistic or antagonistic actions. There is no assurance that peripheral concentrations reflect bio-

logical activity at any target organ, or that discrete effects can be corroborated with hormonal levels. There is a need for future studies controlling for these variables; prospective, randomized, longitudinal trials where training is carefully quantified and prescribed, with concurrent measurement of basal hormonal levels.

Health consequences of menstrual dysfunction

The issues of reversibility of athletic amenorrhoea and/or any potential harmful effects have important implications for the exercising female. Evidence to date indicates that neither amenorrhoea nor luteal phase deficiency are permanent barriers to fertility, but that osteopenia (premature osteoporosis) may be a significant long-term repercussion of these conditions. Osteopenia, by definition, is a decrease in bone mass below normal, usually because of a decrease in the rate of osteoid synthesis. Osteoporosis is abnormal diminution in bone density and weight, most commonly seen in the elderly. There is weakening of the bone structure and integrity, with an increased risk of fracture. The stages of this disease are discussed in more detail later in the chapter.

The morbidity and mortality related to these particular problems, as well as to disordered eating (which may also contribute to the amenorrhoea), are elaborated on in a later section of this chapter. In addition to the risk of osteoporotic fractures at an earlier age, athletes with menstrual irregularities have an increased incidence of concurrent musculoskeletal injuries (including stress fractures).[62,63] One study of ballet dancers documented a 24 per cent prevalence of scoliosis, and delayed menarche by an average of 2 years. There was also an association between age of menarche and frequency of scoliosis.[36]

There are other significant health consequences of menstrual dysfunction. Chronic anovulation with its attendant unopposed oestrogen secretion tends to promote endometrial proliferation, potentially increasing the risk of endometrial hyperplasia and adenocarcinoma. A prolonged hypo-oestrogenic state in the premenopausal years can theoretically be a factor in increased cardiovascular disease as well, due to the loss of the protective effect of oestrogens on the cholesterol profile. It will be decades yet before the true impact of menstrual disorders in athletes is fully evident.

Premenstrual syndrome in the athletic female

PMS refers to the constellation of physical and emotional manifestations occurring in the week or two before menstruation. Approximately 40 to 90 per cent of all women have one or more PMS symptoms, and in 2 to 4 per cent, these can be severe. The most common theories are that PMS is caused by water retention, hypoglycaemia, vitamin B_6 deficiency, oestrogen excess, progesterone deficiency, or alterations in central nervous system neurotransmitters, including endorphin withdrawal.[64] Regardless of pathophysiology, PMS is now widely accepted as a legitimate diagnosis and a real entity. Emotional instability is regarded as a side-effect of the physiological phenomena.

As previously discussed, molimina is the term used for similar, but less intense, physical and emotional changes occurring before normal menstruation. Physical symptoms may include headache, backache, abdominal bloating, food cravings, constipation, fatigue, and swelling of the hands, feet, and breasts. Emotional manifestations range from tearfulness, anger, irritability, and tension to depression. Conditioning exercise can ameliorate both PMS and moliminal symptoms, by producing relaxation, decreasing food cravings, and enhancing feelings of self-control.[65] Physical activity may also relieve PMS by altering the pulsatile pattern of gonadotrophin-releasing hormone. As PMS is at least partly induced by stress, exercise may have an additional effect of enhancing feelings of well being by elevation of endorphins. A consistent pattern of physical activity (i.e. a 20 to 30 min aerobic workout at least four times a week) is needed to attain these benefits.[65]

There are relatively few well-controlled studies on other therapies for PMS in the literature. This area is difficult to study, in part because there is such a wide range of symptomatology, which may vary significantly from one menstrual cycle to another. Methodologically, it is hard to disguise exercise in a study in order to compare exercise, pills, and placebos. Use of a daily menstrual diary may be helpful for the individual athlete, to see if a predictable pattern emerges. Some clinicians advise a decrease in caloric intake,[45] while others suggest a reduction in salt consumption, and avoidance of caffeine and alcohol. In terms of medications, spironolactone, oestrogen, and bromocriptine may be effective in women with breast pain, while vitamin B_6 may help stabilize mood. Progesterone vaginal suppositories have also been advocated, and recently fluoxetine has been successfully used in doses of 20 to 60 mg/day.[66]

Management of menstrual dysfunction in the athlete

In addition to treatment of musculoskeletal injuries, it is also essential for the health care professional who deals with female athletes to screen for gynaecological problems, specifically menstrual dysfunction. The history should include the age of menarche, frequency of menstrual periods, number of periods in the last year, and the date of the last period. Further medical evaluation of the adolescent woman is recommended if she is age 14 and prepubertal, without development of secondary sex characteristics, or age 16 and premenarchal. Secondary amenorrhoea, with no periods for 3 to 6 months also warrants attention. The physician and the athlete can suspect luteal phase deficiency if menses are frequent—every 21 to 23 days. Lack of moliminal symptoms and irregular heavy bleeding suggest anovulatory cycles. Medical evaluation is necessary to rule out other causes of menstrual dysfunction, including pregnancy. It is important to include questions related to disordered eating and low nutrient intake (Table 3). Subsequent investigations are dependent upon the history and physical findings (Table 4).[44]

Further testing of the hypothalamic–pituitary–ovarian axis may include a progesterone challenge test. The administration of 10 mg of medroxyprogesterone (Provera) for 5 days should result in a withdrawal bleed within 2 to 7 days, indicating sufficient oestrogen to promote development of the endometrium. If this test is negative, it may be repeated following oestrogen priming of the endometrium with 0.625 mg of oestradiol for 16 days. Hypothyroidism is treated with synthetic thyroxine, and monitored by serial levels of thyroid-stimulating hormone.

Therapy, to some extent, will be determined by the requirements of the athlete. Symptoms of dysmenorrhoea can be successfully ameliorated with antiprostaglandin medications. There is also evidence that regular aerobic exercise is beneficial for dysmenorrhoea.[65] The mechanism of exercise-associated menstrual dysfunction itself is multifactorial. Each individual athlete may have her own 'sensitivity threshold' regarding each of the variables studied. In some cases, resumption of menses can be accomplished by gaining 1.5 to 2.5 kg in weight or with a 5 per cent decrease in training duration or intensity. A cross-sectional questionnaire-based study of 562 of 618 competitors in an ultramarathon found that an athlete's risk of menstrual dysfunction increases with the presence of more risk factors, but that no single risk factor is more important than another. The author suggests that all risk factors be considered equally, and that simply reducing the number of risk factors rather than trying to eliminate them all, offers an alternative method of managing menstrual dysfunction that may be more acceptable to both athletes and clinicians.[67]

Women who continue to be amenorrhoeic despite these non-invasive interventions should be treated with replacement hormones, either in the form of cyclic oestrogen and/or progesterone, or oral contraceptives. The oestrogen dose required is similar to that for postmenopausal women at 0.625 mg/day from days 1 to 25, with the addition of medroxyprogesterone at 10 mg/day from days 16 to 25. In women with anovulatory cycles and adequate levels of oestrogen, cyclic progesterone for 10 days out of the month is recommended to induce regular withdrawal bleeding.[68] Such a regimen is thought by some to prevent endometrial cancer and significantly increase bone density.[69,70] Measurement of bone density may be appropriate to document risk of osteoporosis, and monitor the effects of therapy.

If the athlete wishes to become pregnant, then stimulation of ovulation with clomiphene may be necessary. Oral contraceptives can be prescribed for treatment of menstrual dysfunction, as well as for purposes of birth control. There are no firm guidelines regarding therapeutic use of these medications for maintenance of bone density in amenorrhoeic or oligomenorrhoeal women. In many studies on bone density, the authors have systematically excluded subjects with a history of oral contraceptive use. The research findings to date will be reviewed in a later section of this chapter. Although hormone replacement therapy in the older woman has been shown to be protective for bone, together with adequate calcium intake and regular weight-bearing exercise, there is still some controversy regarding the relative roles of oestrogen and progesterone in bone metabolism.

Contraception in the athletic female

Sexually active women must be made aware of the need for contraception, even if they are not menstruating on a regular basis. Ovulation can resume before menses, and it is not unusual for athletic women to ovulate some months and not others. Unprotected intercourse may result in unwanted pregnancy. The morning-after pill (Ovral two tablets initially and two after 12 h), administered within 72 h of unprotected intercourse will prevent pregnancy in more that 95 per cent of cases.[71] The intrauterine device, or IUD, is less popular as a mode of contraception in athletes because of the increase in menstrual cramping and blood loss, consequently leading to a

Table 4 Evaluation of amenorrhoea

History

Gynaecological history (age of menarche, development of secondary sexual characteristics, length and timing of menstrual cycles, presence of moliminal symptoms, sexual history, contraception, pregnancies)

Family history—late menarche, menstrual disorders

Physical activity—frequency, duration, intensity, type, age of onset, any recent changes

Weight—lowest, highest, recent changes (6–12 months prior to onset of amenorrhoea)

Nutritional history—vegetarianism, potential eating disorders, check for adequacy of calcium and iron intake

Social history—conflicts and support systems at home, at work, in social environment, sources of self-esteem, coping skills and methods, history of depressive symptoms, physical or sexual abuse

Medications—including past history of oral contraceptives

Galactorrhoea, headaches, visual changes, altered sense of smell

Symptoms of oestrogen deficiency—vasomotor symptoms, vaginal atrophy, dyspareunia

Symptoms of androgen excess—hirsutism, oily skin, acne

Symptoms of decreased thyroid function—cold intolerance, constipation, dry hair and skin

Physical examination

General physical examination—height, weight, body mass index, body composition

Stigmas of chromosomal abnormalities, such as Turner's syndrome—short stature, webbed neck, increased cubital angle

Fundi (papilloedema), visual fields by confrontation

Thyroid—enlargement, nodules

Breasts—galactorrhoea

Tanner staging—breast development, pubic and axillary hair growth

Pelvic examination—presence of normal sexual organs, polycystic ovaries, clitoromegaly, vaginal dryness/atrophy (oestrogen deficiency)

Hirsutism—also male pattern alopecia

Acne (androgen excess), dry hair and skin (thyroid deficiency)

Investigations

Pregnancy test (βHCG—urine or serum test)

Thyroid function studies (T_4, thyroid-stimulating hormone)

Prolactin (serial a.m. values)—To rule out microadenoma (if elevated: CT scan or MRI of sella)

Gonadotrophins—Follicle-stimulating hormone (FSH), luteinizing hormone

Karyotype—in women under 30 with amenorrhoea and high FSH, or absent uterus, or stigmas of chromosomal abnormalities

Testosterone and dehydroepiandrosterone sulphate (DHEAS)—if signs of androgen excess

Oestradiol (check for hypo-oestrogenic state) and/or progesterone (document luteal phase)

greater risk of iron deficiency anaemia. There is also a higher incidence of infection, and tubal pregnancies may still occur.

Barrier methods, such as condoms, the diaphragm or the cervical cap demand consistency of usage in order to be most effective. The vaginal sponge has recently been removed from the market due to complications related to infection and breakdown of the material. The diaphragm and vaginal sponge, in particular, may contribute to the development of urinary tract infections. Pregnant women are also more at risk of bladder infections. Proper perineal hygiene, and regular emptying of the bladder, especially after intercourse, will help prevent this. All sexually active women should be counselled on the risks of sexually transmitted diseases including acquired immunodeficiency syndrome (AIDS) and hepatitis, and should be encouraged to practice 'safe sex'. The use of condoms should be promoted for protection against disease, in addition to their role in birth control.

Oral contraceptives

Oral contraceptives are frequently utilized to regulate the menstrual cycles, as well as for contraception. Current recommendations are to use a low-dose combination pill, with 30 to 35 µg of ethinyl oestradiol, and 0.4 to 1.0 mg of a progestogen. If necessary, menstruation can be delayed around important events for up to 10 days by continuing on with either a monophasic pill, or the highest concentration of a triphasic pill. As there is some risk of breakthrough bleeding with this technique, another approach is to shorten the cycles progressively in the months leading up the the critical time, so that the pills can be discontinued and menstrual bleeding will occur in advance of the competition. Most of the synthetic hormones contained in the oral contraceptives will also have cleared from the system by then.

Side-effects of oral contraceptives

Many female athletes are still resistant to the use of oral contraceptives. There is a fear of unacceptable side-effects, such as weight gain and fluid retention; a desire 'not to put anything artificial into their bodies'; and concerns about possible adverse effects on athletic performance. Other complications related to birth control pills include breakthrough bleeding, alteration in carbohydrate metabolism and lipid profile, as well as changes in haemostatic mechanisms. To improve compliance, it is often helpful to point out some of the beneficial effects of the pill, such as control of the menstrual cycle; decrease in dysmenorrhoea, blood loss, and the risk of anaemia; lower incidence of benign breast disease, polycystic ovarian disease, sexually transmitted diseases, ectopic pregnancies, and for some reason, rheumatoid arthritis. The most important benefit for the woman with chronic anovulation is the decrease in endometrial hyperplasia, and the possible protection of bone density.[72]

The older, higher dosage formulations were more likely to have adverse effects, but the incidence of these is significantly reduced with the current medications. Modern oral contraceptives come in a variety of preparations, including triphasic, biphasic, low oestrogen (20 to 35 µg of ethinyl oestradiol), and progesterone-only mini-pills. There are also long-acting, injectable, progesterone-only preparations that can be injected (Depo-Provera) once every 3 months. A subdermal implant (depo-medroxyprogesterone or Norplant) is also available in some countries. The newer third-generation progesterones, norgestimate, gestodene, and desogestrel have significantly less impact on cardiovascular risk factors such as lipid levels.

Oral contraceptives and the adolescent

In the adolescent population, there remain some important unanswered questions. There is a potential fear that administration of oral contraceptives might cause premature epiphyseal closure and loss of potential height. Arguments against this possibility include the fact that most women only grow about a centimetre after menarche. Theoretically the oestrogen milieu of pregnancy could also increase the rate of closure of the growth plates. Some physicians and scientists believe that oral contraceptives given to young adolescents might have permanent adverse effects on the hypothalamic–pituitary–ovarian axis. Most researchers, however, believe that these are independent and idiopathic effects. The American Academy of Pediatrics has recommended that amenorrhoeic women over the age of 16, or 3 years postpuberty, can and should be treated with oral contraceptives.[73] Another confusing area regarding contraception is whether usage of oral contraceptives decreases condom use. Finally, there is the question of how clinicians can improve compliance with oral contraceptives in this population.

Oral contraceptive use in older women

Perimenopausal women without any contraindications such as smoking or cardiovascular disease may now continue to use oral contraceptives indefinitely up until menopause. They increase control of erratic ovarian function, stabilize some of the vasomotor symptoms, and prevent decreased bone mass.[74] There is a concomitant diminution in menorrhagia, dysmenorrhoea, and PMS, as well as a reduction in gynaecological surgical procedures with their attendant morbidity and mortality. These properties are all advantageous to women in this age group who wish to either become or remain physically active.

Other gynaecological concerns

Stress incontinence and other pelvic floor problems are frequent sequelae from the perineal trauma of childbirth. Women may be embarrassed to bring up such topics, but they can be seriously inhibited from exercising because of these disorders. There are a number of helpful different treatments, ranging from Kegel exercises that the woman can perform herself at home, to sophisticated biofeedback machines to retrain the pelvic floor muscles. Uterine prolapse in the older exercising woman can be managed initially with the use of a pessary, but may eventually require surgical correction.

Menstrual cycle phase and oral contraceptives: effects on athletic performance

Female athletes are unique in many aspects, not the least of which is their hormonal make-up. From puberty through adolescence, the reproductive years, and postmenopausal years, the female athlete must train and compete against a background kaleidoscope of ever-shifting hormones. The female sex steroids vary considerably, whether during different phases of the menstrual cycle, or during administration of oral contraceptives, or during hormonal replacement therapy. Both oestrogens and progestogens have individual, interactive, and frequently opposing physiological actions of conceivable significance for the exercising female.

Actions of oestrogen

Oestradiol and its congeners have a number of metabolic effects: increased glycogen storage and uptake in liver and muscle, glycogen-sparing effect at rest, and inhibition of gluconeogenesis and glycogenolysis.[75] Oestrogen also spares glycogen through shifting metabolism more towards free fatty acids for fuel, through increased lipid synthesis, and enhanced lipolysis in muscle and adipose tissue. It therefore promotes a greater reliance on fat for energy at the same relative exercise intensity, as well as increasing actual lipid availability. In terms of fluid homeostasis, oestrogen has a fluid-retaining effect, possibly through an effect on the kidneys, or an alteration in the synthesis or release of antidiuretic hormone. Its actions in bone homeostasis have already been discussed. Beneficial actions on the cardiovascular system include relaxation of vascular smooth muscle and favourable alterations in the cholesterol profile, and are covered in more detail later. Oestrogen has also been noted to have a positive effect on cognitive function and memory.[76] It appears to influence the biochemistry of the brain by altering concentrations and availability of neurotransmitter amines, including serotonin.

Actions of progesterone

Progesterone enhances glycogen storage and uptake, both in animals and in humans. It affects several aspects of respiratory function: minute ventilation, maximal exercise response, respiratory drive, and respiratory muscle endurance.[77,78] It has recently been found to affect diffusing capacity of carbon monoxide, especially during menses when both oestrogen and progesterone are low.[79] Many of these respiratory effects are reproducible in male subjects with administration of medroxyprogesterone acetate.

Progesterone has been implicated in the hyperventilation seen during pregnancy and the luteal phase of the cycle, although it has not been possible to correlate actual progesterone levels directly with the alteration in ventilation or ventilatory responsiveness. Endurance athletes are known to have blunted ventilatory responses in reaction to hypoxia and hypercapnia as an adaptive phenomenon to rigorous training. A less sensitive respiratory drive allows them to desaturate at very intense levels of exercise, without experiencing limiting dyspnoea. During the luteal phase of the menstrual cycle, as well as with administration of medroxyprogesterone acetate to male subjects, ventilatory drives are enhanced by the higher levels of progesterone. This has a potential maladaptive effect for athletic performance, although significant limitation has been demonstrated in non-athletes only, suggesting that there is some element of training and acclimatizion to this small effect.

The thermogenic effect of progesterone is the cause of the elevated basal body temperature during pregnancy and during the luteal phase of the cycle. In the luteal phase, there are also increased aldosterone levels, both at rest and during exercise. The higher progesterone levels during this phase act at the level of the kidney to block the action of aldosterone, resulting in a loss of sodium and water. This in turn stimulates the renin/angiotensin system to increase secretion of aldosterone, and at the same time promotes an increase in antidiuretic hormone. This mechanism is partially responsible for the fluid retention during the luteal phase.

Hormonal changes during the reproductive years

Over the course of a normal menstrual cycle, there are several different hormonal scenarios. During the follicular phase, concentrations of both hormones are low. At ovulation, oestradiol levels peak, but progesterone remains low. During the luteal phase, both hormones are high, with concentrations dropping off just before menstruation. Menstruation itself is complicated by the actions of prostaglandins. In women with shortened luteal phases and/or anovulation, the patterns of hormonal shifting are different again. Pregnancy promotes extreme changes in hormone levels that continue through the puerperium. Menopause has its own unique considerations as a result of oestrogen deficiency. The addition of exogenous hormones for therapeutic reasons is difficult to compare with the effects of physiological levels of endogenous hormones.

Effects of hormones on performance

There are many influences in an athlete's training and competitive schedule that can affect performance. Disruption of circadian rhythms, such as by crossing time zones, is more likely to have a significant impact through alteration of the sleep–wake cycle and other endogenous hormonal variations than through changes in the timing of the menstrual cycle. In terms of the menstrual cycle itself, about one-third of all athletes believe that menstruation affects performance in an adverse manner. Nevertheless, gold medals have been won and world records set at all phases of the cycle.[78]

The first studies in this area were either anecdotal reports or retrospective surveys, and therefore unreliable in a pure scientific sense because of their very nature. Early work attempting to document measurable changes in performance (with a variety of physiological tests at either submaximal or maximal workloads) was carried out with inconsistent classification of menstrual cycle phases. Basal body temperature curves, further enhanced by computerized interpretations, have been used effectively to establish the phase of the cycle.[80] Recently, the use of kits to test for luteinizing hormone in the urine have made prediction of ovulation even more reliable.[81] Nevertheless, the only acceptable criterion for documentation of menstrual cycle phase is accurate measurement of serum hormonal levels. It is important to measure these in a resting state, as concentrations of both oestrogen and progesterone are known to increase with exercise.

Early investigations did not generally substantiate any dramatic effects of menstrual cycle phase on performance, although subjectively, if there was a decrement, it was generally during the luteal phase and the first few days of menstruation. Some women are more bothered by dysmenorrhoea during their period, while others find the premenstrual symptoms in the week or two before menstruation to be the cause. It is important to point out in reviewing these studies that for many recreational athletes, any alterations in performance have minimal impact, but for an élite or professional athlete, the difference between first and second place is often measured in tenths of a second. This difference may not be statistically significant in the true sense of the word, but it is definitely critical to the success of that particular athlete.

Cardiovascular variables, such as heart rate, stroke volume, plasma volume, blood pressure, and haemoglobin concentration are affected primarily by the fluid balance shifts that take place in response to hormonal alterations. The impact of such changes on performance appears to be minimal, although they are probably mitigated by compensations in other systems. There have also been suggestions that the maximal aerobic capacity is slightly lower during the luteal phase,[82] but the implications of this finding are not clear, especially as maximal aerobic capacity is not the best determinant of performance. Running economy may also be affected.

Basal metabolic rate is elevated in the postovulatory or luteal phase compared with preovulatory or follicular phases, and is lower just before ovulation. Increases in 24-h energy expenditure during the luteal phase have also been documented under controlled sedentary conditions. Spontaneous energy intakes of women vary according to phase of the menstrual cycle, higher during the luteal phase than during the follicular phase.

Energy metabolism

Theoretically, metabolism should be most efficient during the mid-luteal phase. High concentrations of both oestrogen and progesterone promote glycogen storage and sparing during exercise, which should be advantageous for prolonged endurance exercise. Higher muscle glycogen levels and enhanced performance with lower blood lactate levels during the luteal phase have been documented by some researchers, but many others have not found the same difference (for reviews, see references 77, 78 and 83). Results are also affected by modification of the pre-exercise nutritional status of the athlete, and initial muscle glycogen levels. Changes in blood glucose levels during exercise in different phases of the cycle are similarly affected, and are also impacted upon by the complex reactions of other hormones such as insulin, cortisol, growth hormone, and plasma catecholamines. Studies of substrate turnover and hormonal metabolic clearance rates would help clarify the processes that are happening at these times.

Thermoregulation

The higher progesterone levels in the luteal phase result in an elevation of core body temperature by about 0.3°C. This may disadvantage women for prolonged exercise in an environment with a high ambient temperature. Indeed, some studies have shown an elevated heart rate, higher aerobic capacity, and increased rating of perceived exertion in strenous exercise during this phase. Because of a higher muscle temperature, some have postulated a decrement in strength during the luteal phase, but this has not been substantiated. The more likely determinants of strength are genetic predisposition, nutritional status, and patterns of training.

Oral contraceptives

Most oral contraceptives contain a combination of an oestrogen and a progestogen. There is no doubt that these medications diminish PMS symptoms, monthly dysmenorrhoea, and blood loss, and regulate the cycle in a predictable fashion. These may be the mechanisms for the reduction in musculoskeletal injuries in women on oral contraceptives seen in some studies. The consequences for various forms of athletic performance are less clear. Investigators are not in agreement on either quantitative or directional effects of these medications on a variety of physiological parameters. This field is complicated further by the diversity in the strength and preparation of the oestrogen and progesterone components used.

Early studies with much higher dosage pills did demonstrate a small decremental effect on the maximal aerobic capacity, but more recent studies have shown this impact to be lessened with lower dosages. It is likely that as the troublesome side-effects of the pill are diminished by newer and better preparations, so too are any significant decrements in athletic performance. The positive health benefits of oral contraceptives probably far outweigh any adverse effects, particularly in terms of prevention of iron deficiency anaemia by decreasing excessive menstrual bleeding, and protection of bone density in amenorrhoeic athletes. However, there may be marked individual effects in some women.

The androgenic component of the pills has been postulated to have a potentially favourable influence on strength, but this has now been largely discounted. In 1987, the International Olympic Committee placed norethindrone on the list of banned drugs as a performance-enhancing agent, on the premise that the metabolic by-products could either give an anabolic steroid effect or mask other anabolic steroids from detection. This ruling was successfully challenged by physicians and scientists. There was a recent furore at the 1994 World Masters' Games in Australia, where some competitors were taking hormonal replacement therapy containing small doses of testosterone in addition to the oestrogen. Basically, any substance that is perceived to give even a small competitive advantage is suspect in high-performance sport and international competition.

Cardiovascular and ventilatory alterations due to oral contraceptives have not been shown to be significant in terms of performance. Effects on blood pressure, triglycerides, and lipids are minimized by lower doses and by the newer progestogens. Regular conditioning exercise also ameliorates any of these observed changes. The impact on blood glucose is a bit more complicated. Glucose production is primarily determined by insulin, although other homones such as thyroxine, cortisol, the catecholamines, and growth hormone have a counter-regulatory effect. Progesterone acts to reduce insulin binding secondary to a decrease in insulin receptor concentration, similar to its mode of action during the luteal phase of the cycle. Growth hormone levels can be increased by large doses of oestrogen, and decreased by progestogens. Apart from the adverse effects on glucose tolerance in some genetically susceptible individuals, there does not seem to be any significant impact on athletic performance. Energy metabolism is another area with confusing results. Similar to during the luteal phase of the cycle, the glycogen-sparing effect and enhancement of lipolysis secondary to the oestrogen and progesterone component of birth control pills may actually confer a metabolic advantage, especially in relation to high-intensity exercise of prolonged duration.

Conclusions

In conclusion, there may be subtle physiological variations in vascular volume dynamics, substrate metabolism, ventilation, and thermoregulation in response to the endogenous shifts in oestrogen and progesterone during the different phases of the cycle. Women taking oral contraceptives, or hormonal replacement therapy, may also experience fluctuations in some of these variables, depending upon the formulation used, and the relative concentrations of oestrogen and progestogens. In the élite female athlete, there may be small effects on performance, but the majority of women exercising at a less competitive or recreational level will not be affected.

The large interindividual variation in response to the biological effects of both the endogenous hormonal shifts of the normal menstrual cycle and exogenous female hormones in oral contraceptives mandates an individualized approach to the female athletic patient who comes in with such questions. Current oral contraceptives contain 30 to 50 per cent less hormone than earlier formulations, and have a corresponding decrease in other nuisance side-effects. Their usage is now being promoted well into the perimenopausal years in women who do not have any other significant risk factors, for protection of bone density. There is no current evidence that would mitigate against this.

More prospective controlled trials using serum concentrations of oestrogen and progesterone are necessary to give definitive answers in this area. Given the variation in pill formulations and the newer preparations, a tremendous amount of research has yet to be done in terms of oral contraceptives and athletic performance. Future investigations should focus on the potential mechanisms of any observed effects. Follow-up testing after discontinuation of the medication is also needed to investigate further the reversibility, and time-frame for any performance changes. It is also extremely important that investigators carrying out other unrelated studies on female athletes standardize both the phase of the cycle, and the use or non-use of oral contraceptives, in order to avoid potentially confounding results due to the variation in female sex steroids.

Disordered eating patterns in the female athlete

Athletes display a heightened body awareness which, in combination with pressure to meet body weight expectations for their sport, can lead potentially to disordered eating patterns. There is also a relationship between compulsive athleticism and eating disorders.[84] Between 90 and 95 per cent of all eating disorders are found in females. Prevention and detection are extremely important because of the natural history of this affliction. The prognosis for full-blown eating disorders is not well established, but is not overly optimistic. It is thought that approximately 40 per cent of patients will recover, 30 per cent will recover but have relapses, and 30 per cent will be chronically affected. Between 10 per cent and 18 per cent may actually die of their disease, as a result of suicide, cardiovascular collapse or arrest, sepsis, or gastric or intestinal perforation.[85,86] Importantly, there is a spectrum of 'disordered eating' ranging from abnormal eating behaviour or poor nutritional habits at one end, to the frank eating disorders of anorexia and bulimia. All afflicted women are at risk of serious metabolic, endocrine, skeletal, and psychiatric problems.

There are many similarities in psychopathology between amenorrhoeic athletes and patients with frank anorexia nervosa or bulimia. These are: ritualized dietary habits, compulsive behaviour, low food intake, heightened energy expenditure, and amenorrhoea.[84] There are similarities in the reproductive and stress hormones as well.[62] Amenorrhoea begins early in the course of anorexia nervosa and, in 25 to 35 per cent of women, can occur before any actual weight loss. Studies in athletes reveal a higher incidence of eating disorders than in the general population, especially when looked for in conjunction with menstrual dysfunction. Major affective dis-

orders have also been documented in amenorrhoeic runners. A study of dancers compared with non-dancers, both with eating disorders, has shown increased substance abuse (amphetamines, barbiturates, tranquilizers, hallucinogens, and cocaine) and emotional distress in non-dancers.[87] This was thought to be due to the fact that disordered eating is normative in the world of dance because of the professional pressure to be thin, and therefore did not create as much psychological distress. The end points of this restricted pattern of eating are still the same, however, in terms of weight loss and amenorrhoea.

Definitions

Under the new DSM-IV classification system (Table 5,[88]) only 1 per cent of the general population meet the strict psychiatric criteria for anorexia nervosa, while 3 per cent fit the definition of bulimia nervosa. The true incidence in athletes is probably not known, as much of the work to date has been carried out using the previous definitions. The old DSM-IIIR classification of anorexia (15 per cent below normal weight for age and height) probably underrepresented the extent of the problem in athletic women. In addition to the usual denial mechanisms, athletes have a higher muscle mass from training and may not look as emaciated, thereby making detection more difficult. There are also known difficulties with the questionnaires in common usage—the standard eating disorder questionnaire (Eating Attitudes Test),[89] the Eating Disorder Inventory (EDI), and the EDI-2[89,90]—including the possibility of response distortion.[91] Nevertheless, high scores on some scales, such as the Drive for Thinness (DFT) scale are useful in screening for potential problems.

Health care professionals must be vigilant and sensitive to early warning signals of both anorexia and bulimia such as weight loss, excessive preoccupation with food and weight, unexplained changes in personality (depression, anxiety, or self-criticism), the wearing of baggy or layered clothing, and excessive exercise outside of normal practice hours. The binge–purge cycle begins with a 'diet', which then creates physiological hunger, followed by a binge, frequently involving 'forbidden' or pleasure-type foods. Some athletes may consume as many as 4000 to 5000 kcal at a sitting, giving immediate psychological relief. The resultant depression and guilt reaction subsequently provoke the purging behaviour (vomiting, laxative use, diuretics) and/or excessive exercise in compensation.

Risk factors

The more élite the level of competition and the higher the stakes (i.e. college scholarship or a gold medal), the more the athlete is willing to risk in order to win. Sports at risk include the appearance sports (gymnastics, figure skating, ballet), endurance sports (track and field, cross-country skiing), and sports with weight classifications (rowing, martial arts). In this latter group, disordered eating patterns are frequently seen in male athletes as well. Importantly, no sport is exempt from the possibility that its athletes may develop disordered eating.

Contributing factors (especially in Western society) include sociocultural norms and media-driven expectations. Thinness is equated with control, success, goodness, power, and beauty. There are thought to be biological factors as well: hormonal (10 to 1; female to male incidence); and imbalances in the neurotransmitters

Table 5 DSM-IV diagnostic criteria for eating disorders

307.1   Anorexia nervosa

A.   Refusal to maintain body weight at or above a minimally normal weight for age and height (e.g. weight loss leading to maintenance of body weight at less than 85% of that expected; or failure to make expected weight gain during period of growth, leading to body weight of less than 85% of that expected).

B.   Intense fear of gaining weight or becoming fat, even though underweight.

C.   Disturbance in the way in which one's body weight or shape is experienced, undue influence of body weight or shape on self-evaluation, or denial of the seriousness of the current low body weight.

D.   In postmenarchal females, amenorrhoea, i.e. the absence of at least three consecutive menstrual cycles. (A woman is considered to have amenorrhoea if her periods occur only following hormone, e.g. oestrogen, administration.)

Specify type:

Restricting type: during the current episode of anorexia nervosa, the person has not regularly engaged in binge-eating or purging behaviour (i.e. self-induced vomiting or the misuse of laxatives, diuretics, or enemas).

Binge-eating/purging type: during the current episode of anorexia nervosa, the person has regularly engaged in binge-eating or purging behaviour (i.e. self-induced vomiting or the misuse of laxatives, diuretics, or enemas).

307.51   Bulimia nervosa

A.   Recurrent episodes of binge eating. An episode of binge eating is characterized by both of the following:

(1)   Eating, in a discrete period of time (e.g. within any 2-h period), an amount of food that is definitely larger than most people would eat during a similar period of time and under similar circumstances.

(2)   A sense of lack of control over eating during the episode (e.g. a feeling that one cannot stop eating or control what or how much one is eating).

B.   Recurrent inappropriate compensatory behaviour in order to prevent weight gain, such as self-induced vomiting; misuse of laxatives, diuretics, enemas, or other medication; fasting; or excessive exercise.

C.   The binge eating and inappropriate compensatory behaviours both occur, on average, at least twice a week for 3 months.

D.   Self-evaluation is unduly influenced by body shape and weight.

E.   The disturbance does not occur exclusively during episodes of anorexia nervosa.

Specify type:

Purging type: during the current episode of bulimia nervosa, the person has regularly engaged in self-induced vomiting or the misuse of laxatives, diuretics, or enemas.

Non-purging type: during the current episode of bulimia nervosa, the person has used other inappropriate compensatory behaviours, such as fasting or excessive exercise, but has not regularly engaged in self-induced vomiting or the misuse of laxatives, diuretics, or enemas.

307.50   Eating disorder not otherwise specified

This category is for disorders of eating that do not meet the criteria for any specific eating disorder. Examples include:

1.   For females all of the criteria for anorexia nervosa are met except that the individual has regular menses.

2.   All of the criteria for anorexia nervosa are met except that, despite significant weight loss, the individual's current weight is in the normal range.

3.   All of the criteria for anorexia nervosa are met except that, the binge eating and inappropriate compensatory mechanism occur at a frequency of less than twice a week or for a duration of less than 3 months.

4.   The regular use of inappropriate compensatory behaviour by an individual of normal body weight after eating a small amount of food (e.g. self-induced vomiting after the consumption of two cookies).

5.   Repeatedly chewing and spitting out, but not swallowing, large amounts of food.

6.   Binge-eating disorder: recurrent episodes of binge eating in the absence of the regular use of inappropriate compensatory behaviours characteristic of bulimia nervosa (see Appendix B in DSM-IV for suggested research criteria).

serotonin and noradrenaline, and possibly melatonin. Athletic participation by itself does not cause this bizarre behaviour, rather it can precipitate it. Susceptible individuals frequently come from a family with extreme difficulty in resolving conflict. It is also necessary to explore the possibility of a history of sexual or physical abuse.

These women have not developed good coping skills for stress, and consequently suffer from a lack of assertiveness and low self-esteem. Their sense of self-worth tends to be derived from external feedback, especially in the domains of appearance or performance. They gain an illusion of control by manipulating their weight or food intake. They generally lack any identity outside of their sport, and have few other support systems. This is especially important at times of injury or pending retirement from an athletic career. Their obsessive–compulsive nature helps maintain the restrictive eating behaviours and the overexercising pattern.

Some of the triggers associated with the onset of eating disorders in athletic women have been characterized and include: prolonged periods of dieting, frequent weight fluctuations, sudden increases in training volume, and traumatic events such as an injury or the loss of a coach.[92] Either blatant or inadvertent comments from others, such as coaches, parents, or peers may precipitate a preoccupation with body weight, size, and composition. Compared with sedentary controls, athletes with eating disorders begin their sport-specific training and dieting at an earlier age. Many feel that puberty occurred too early for optimal achievement in their sport. In terms of athletic performance, there is often an initial 'honeymoon period' where it is improved, and the athlete receives positive feedback from everyone concerned, and so continues her maladaptive behaviour. Eventually, however, both the health and the performance of the athlete will suffer.

Signs and symptoms

Screening for these disorders during the preparticipation examination should be implemented. Specific health questions in the questionnaire and a brief nutritional screen (24-h recall) will serve to identify athletes at risk. The history and physical examination should be complete, and directed towards common signs and symptoms of restricted food/energy intake. These include obsession with weight and food intake, unexplained fatigue, sensation of bloating after eating (probably due to decreased gastric motility), amenorrhoea or other menstrual irregularities, fat and muscle loss, dry hair and skin, brittle nails, cold purplish hands and feet, decreased body temperature or cold intolerance, light-headedness, and decreased ability to concentrate. Suspicious symptoms suggesting purging are swollen parotid glands, chest pain, sore throat, abdominal pain, face and extremity oedema (rebound fluid retention or secondary aldosteronism), diarrhoea, and/or constipation. A heart rate of less than 50 beats/min is suggestive of an eating disorder until proven otherwise. The differential diagnosis for these findings should encompass metabolic disease, malignancy, inflammatory bowel disease, infection, and achalasia.[85,86]

Patients may present to their dentist first with erosion of the dental enamel at the back of the teeth from regurgitation of acidic stomach contents. Oesophagitis and Mallory–Weiss tears of the oesophagus can occur from excessive retching. Occasionally callouses on the back of the hand (Russell's sign) from inducing the gag reflex are seen, but the majority of women train themselves to vomit spontaneously. 'Chipmunk cheeks' are due to swollen parotid glands. Other physical signs in addition to a low body weight are decreased subcutaneous fat and muscle, hypothermia, bradycardia, lanugo hair (fine raised white hair, particularly on the chest and trunk), orthostatic blood pressure changes (due to dehydration), and cold, discoloured hands and feet. Bulimic patients may be of normal weight for their size.

Laboratory findings

Blood tests frequently reveal non-specific changes: leucopenia, anaemia, thrombocytopenia, and elevation of blood urea nitrogen, serum carotene, serum cholesterol, and transaminases. Hyponatraemia can be seen in women who are overloading with fluid, while excessive vomiting may cause hypokalaemia, and hyperchloraemic metabolic alkalosis. Laxative abuse may lead to metabolic acidosis. Gonadotrophins (follicle-stimulating hormone and luteinizing hormone) and some thyroid hormones (T_4 and thyroid-stimulating hormone) are usually normal. Concentrations of T_3 are low as a result of decreased peripheral conversion of T_4 to T_3 secondary to malnutrition. Urinalysis often reveals pyuria, haematuria, proteinuria, and elevated urine pH. An electrocardiogram (**ECG**) is indicated if the pulse is less than 50 or there is any electrolyte abnormality, particulary in the athlete with purging behaviour. Athletes will frequently notice decreased aerobic capacity and maximal heart rate. Common ECG abnormalities are bradycardia (60 beats/min or below), low voltage, low inverted T-waves, and prolonged QT interval. Amenorrhoeic women may require bone densitometry, both to establish a baseline and to monitor effects of treatment.

Treatment

Management of an athlete with disordered eating is facilitated by involving a multidisciplinary team. The team physician, coach, athlete, parents, nutritionist, psychologist, exercise physiologist or strength coach, and school administrator all have an important role to play, and should ideally be organized as an easily accessible and cohesive network. Confrontation of the athlete with evidence of her pattern of behaviour can be difficult, and requires a sensitive, caring approach, demonstrating concern about her well being. It is frequently useful to begin by discussing the concepts of energy deficit and energy expenditure. Too rapid a change in body composition will result in the loss of lean muscle mass as well as fat. Another successful strategy may be to focus on the performance aspects of proper nutritional habits and appropriate levels of training. It is usually possible to link exacerbations of the eating patterns with stress. It is important to discuss the unreality of societal expectations with their overemphasis on body size and composition.

The physician may limit sport participation if there is an electrolyte or ECG abnormality present. Investigations of the amenorrhoeic athlete have already been discussed, and hormone replacement is encouraged for patients intractable to other methods of medical management. Nutritional counselling from a suitably qualified professional can be directed towards appropriate body composition. It should emphasize lean body mass, calorie needs, healthy weight range, education, scheduling of meals and snacks, and guidelines on healthy food choices. With guidance from the exercise physiologist and/or strength trainer, strength and fitness can be maintained while the athlete attempts to alter her eating behaviour towards a healthier pattern. Psychological evaluation takes account of other stress factors (school, family, social), and promotes development of healthy coping behaviours, self-esteem, and assertiveness skills. Admission to hospital of the anorexic or bulimic individual is suggested for weight loss below 30 per cent of normal,

Table 6 Risk factors for osteoporosis
Female gender
Advanced age
Menopause (surgical or natural)
White or Oriental woman
Diet low in calcium
Smoking
Alcoholism
Immobilization
Amenorrhoea/hypo-oestrogenic states
Anorexia nervosa
Prolonged corticosteroid use

the presence of cardiac compromise, hypotension, dehydration, or significant electrolyte abnormalities, or the failure of outpatient treatment after 3 months of therapy.

Bone health in the female athlete

Osteoporosis is a major public health burden that is unfortunately escalating with the current increased longevity for men and women alike. Thirty-three per cent of women older than 65 will sustain one or more vertebral fractures during their remaining life, and the same proportion of women older than 85 will sustain a hip fracture In the United States alone, there are 1.5 million hip fractures per year, generating significant health care costs. The choice for older females unfortunately seems to lie between 'living longer or dying longer'. For many women, a hip fracture signals not only pain and disability, but a major loss of independence. It is frequently 'the beginning of the end'.

Bone pathophysiology

The peripheral or appendicular skeleton is 80 per cent comprised of cortical, or compact bone. Cortical bone is primarily found in the shafts of long bones. The axial skeleton, which accounts for the remainder of skeletal mass, is approximately 70 per cent trabecular or cancellous bone. As such, it is more subject to incomplete modelling and more prone to fracture. Factors determining peak bone mass include age, race, sex, cigarette use, nutritional and hormonal status, alcohol intake, muscular strength, and body composition (Table 6). Key substances active in bone metabolism are: parathyroid hormone; growth hormone; vitamin D_3; thyroid, gonadal, and adrenal hormones.[93] The strongest positive correlations with axial bone mineral density are weight, oestrogen exposure, physical activity, and calcium intake, while a family history of osteoporosis is associated with a lower bone mineral density.[94]

More than 90 per cent of peak skeletal mass is present by 18 years of age, with bone density increases of 6 to 8 per cent per year during growth,[95] and peak bone aquisition in the lumbar spine and femoral neck occurring in females between the ages of 11 and 14. As up to 48 per cent of skeletal mass and 15 per cent of adult height is attained during the adolescent years, athletes in this age group have a 'window of opportunity' to build up their bone banks. Losing bone mass when bone should be becoming denser may permanently compromise maximal bone mineral density, and offer less

protection against fractures of the vertebrae, hip, and wrist in the postmenopausal years.

Peak bone mass is generally achieved by the third decade of life. A small gain can occur during the thirties, even though the estimated age when mineral acquisition ceases is between 28.3 and 29.5 years. Physical activity and dietary calcium exert a positive effect, while the use of oral contraceptives may have a further independent positive effect.[76] Milk consumption and calcium supplementation during the critical years result in a higher bone density at maturity.[96,97] After this time a biphasic pattern of loss is seen. Beginning at approximately age 40, there is a protracted slow phase, with a transient accelerated phase after menopause. Trabecular bone loss begins a decade sooner than cortical bone loss. Cortical bone is somewhat protected by athletic activity, but trabecular bone, which comprises up to 42 per cent of the lumbar vertebrae is not. Trabecular bone also seems to be more sensitive to changes in hormonal concentration.

During the course of the average lifetime, women lose 50 per cent of cancellous bone and 30 per cent of cortical bone; while men lose about 30 per cent and 20 per cent respectively. Bone loss averages 3 per cent per decade for women. The higher rate of bone loss in women is related to the difference in lifetime bone metabolism, including a lower dietary intake of calcium, participation in weight-reducing diets, the drains of pregnancy and lactation on calcium reserves, and finally bone mineral loss associated with cessation of ovarian function at menopause. There is also regional variablity in the pattern of bone mineral decrease in the lumbar spine, femoral neck, and femoral shaft. It is therefore essential to maximize the adult bone mass, so that these women do not enter into the postmenopausal years at an already disadvantaged starting point.

Measurement of bone mineral density

Bone mineral density can be measured by utilizing a variety of methods: radiographic testing, single-photon absorptiometry, dual-photon absorptiometry, quantitative computed tomography, and dual-energy X-ray absorptiometry (**DEXA**).[98] DEXA is the current 'gold standard'. The enhanced precision (0.5 to 2.0 per cent) and accuracy (3 to 5 per cent) allow for site-specific measurement as well as evaluation of the entire skeleton. In a relatively short time period, and with a small dose of radiation, cortical and trabecular bone can be assessed, in addition to regional and total body composition.

Recently, the World Health Organization has clarified the classification of bone density values as follows:[99,100]

Normal: patients with a bone mineral density within one standard deviation of their predicted mean peak bone mass.

Osteopenia: patients with a bone mineral density between 1.0 and 2.5 standard deviations below their predicted mean peak bone mass.

Osteoporosis: patients with a bone mineral density lower than 2.5 standard deviations below their predicted mean peak bone mass.

Severe osteoporosis: those patients having a bone mineral density greater than 2.5 standard deviations below their predicted mean bone mass, plus one or more fragility fractures.

A woman is at serious risk for fracture when the bone mass in any given area is reduced by 20 to 30 per cent of normal for women at peak bone mass. In women over the age of 65, each decrease of one standard deviation in bone density increases the age-adjusted risk for hip fracture by 2.6.[94]

Effects of exercise on bone density

There is a small, but significant, protective influence of regular exercise on bone mass. Physical activity under the influence of gravitational force is an important influence on bone mass and architecture, but the frequency, duration, and magnitude of skeletal loading must be taken into account. Active load type exercises (such as swimming) are less effective than impact load activities (using at least three times body weight).[101] Mechanical stress stimulates bone remodelling, but the magnitude of the response is influenced by the hormonal and nutritional milieu. Weight-bearing activity such as walking, running, and dancing are best, but the effect may be limited to specific bones that are mechanically loaded. High impact activity or weight training may therefore be even more consequential in premenopausal women, and the duration of involvement may be significant as well.[102] Increased aerobic power is also associated with greater bone mass. There are independent effects of muscle strength, physical fitness, and body mass on bone density, and age itself mediates its effects through associated changes in these factors. Muscle mass is more closely associated with bone mass in men, while in women, correlations are greater with fat than with muscle.[103] Therefore, increased body fatness may be somewhat beneficial to older women not taking oestrogen, in that there is increased peripheral conversion of androgens to oestrogen in fatty tissue.

Professional tennis players (male and female) have been noted to have an increase in the density of bone substance and bone diameter as well as in actual length in their dominant stroke arm.[104] This is a biopositive adaptation, resulting from a combination of mechanical strain and hyperaemia from exercising the limb, with a net stimulatory effect on the epiphyseal plate. The age at which physical activity begins can also affect bone mineral content.[105] A Finnish study[106] of 105 national squash and tennis players and 50 controls found a substantial difference in bone mineral density between the dominant and the non-dominant arm. The bone mineral density of the humerus was two to four times greater in players whose careers began before menarche, than 15 years after.

Appropriate mechanical loading is therefore essential during the critical period of rapid skeletal growth. High school athletic participation is a significant predictor of the bone mineral density of the femoral neck, and possibly the bone mineral density of the total body and spine[107] Remodelling of trabecular bone is thought to occur within 16 to 18 weeks, but the time required for an actual increase in bone mineral density is not known.[93,108] One group measured a small increase in lumbar bone mineral density in 11 gymnasts after 27 weeks of training.[109] To a certain extent, regular weight-bearing exercise can offset the negative effects of amenorrhoea and low hormonal state. A group of 26 college-age gymnasts had significantly higher bone mineral density than age-matched controls, despite insufficient dietary calcium, and a higher propensity to have interruption of their menstrual cycles.[110]

Exercise and high dietary calcium may preferentially alter bone density at different skeletal sites. In one study, women who exercised maintained trabecular bone mineral density, calcium intake affected the bone mineral density of the femur, but there was no effect of either on bone mineral density of the distal radius.[111] Fat-free weight (including muscle) is significantly correlated with bone mineral content in the non-dominant radius, femurs, and lumbar vertebrae.[112] Interestingly, black women have 16.7 per cent more total body calcium than age-matched white women. There is minimal documentation in the literature of bone density in other ethnic groups, but it is well known that women of Asian or Caucasian descent have a higher risk of osteoporosis.

The current thinking is that exercise training either increases bone mineral density or retards bone loss. This is important for women of all ages and races, especially during the postmenopausal years. There is still a need for rigorous testing of this hypothesis. In a critical review of the literature, Marcus *et al.*[113] examined the scientific evidence for the relationship between exercise and bone density. In many studies, emphasis was placed on aerobic training and flexibility rather than skeletal loading, and' bone density was measured in limbs that were not loaded. Other potential sources of confusion were insufficient training duration and a lack of randomization. Studies correlating bone mineral density with activity level should also control for oral contraceptive use, hormonal conditions, and menopausal status.

Effects of hormones on bone density

Spine mineral deficits reflect not only bone loss, but also inadequate acquisition during adolescence and early adulthood. Even prolonged weight-bearing exercise may not maintain bone mineral density in the face of insufficient hormonal production. Low bone mass has been associated with late age of menarche, and/or subsequent amenorrhoea, cumulative duration of oligomenorrhoea, and initiation of exercise training in proximity to menarche. Low bone mineral density has been documented in the appendicular weight-bearing bones of amenorrhoeic athletes, as well as in the spine.[114]

The actions of the reproductive hormones in bone metabolism are complementary. Oestrogen affects primarily bone mineralization, and acts peripherally to prevent bone resorption and decrease bone remodelling. Oestrogen receptors are present in the osteoblasts. Oestrogen stimulates secretion of calcitonin and antagonizes the peripheral action of parathyroid hormone. Low oestrogen levels thus lead to increased calcium resorption from bone, as well as decreased calcium absorption from the intestine and decreased calcium reabsorption from the kidney (secondary to decreased conversion of vitamin D to 1,25-dihydroxy vitamin D). Progesterone may impact trabecular bone density by promoting bone formation and accelerating bone remodelling.[68,70] It may also act to inhibit bone resorption. Chronic exercise training decreases serum concentrations of both oestrogen and progesterone.[115]

Other hormones play an ancillary role in the homeostasis of bone. Inadequate levels of parathyroid hormone as well as increased amounts of corticotrophin have been shown to accelerate bone loss. Cortisol and β-endorphins, which are elevated with exercise, exert a negative feedback effect at the hypothalamus and pituitary in terms of secretion of gonadotrophins. Fasting or reduced calorie intake increases the serum sex hormone-binding globulin, which reduces the level of biologically active oestrogen, progesterone, and testosterone. An increase in sex hormone-binding globulin also occurs in athletes on a high fibre diet and a low meat and protein diet, i.e. vegetarians.

Amenorrhoeic individuals who exercise do have higher vertebral bone densities than sedentary amenorrhoeic women, but the hypogonadal state in these athletes is still associated with lower bone mineral densities. Amenorrhoeic women have lower lumbar and femoral bone mineral densities than controls, and a greater number of stress fractures. Drinkwater[61] documented lumbar bone mineral density to be 14 per cent lower in amenorrhoeic women, despite running a greater total distance per week than regularly menstruating athletes (67.1 compared with 40.0 km). Cann[116] found spinal (trabecular) bone mass to be reduced by 20 to 30 per cent and peripheral mineral values by 5 to 10 per cent in amenorrhoeic groups. Other compounding factors, in addition to late menarche and oligo/amenorrhoea, are a low percentage of body fat, non-use of contraceptives, and low dietary calcium.

Anovulatory menstrual cycles and low progesterone levels are also related to trabecular bone loss in 'normally' menstruating women. Early menstrual dysfunction, such as shortened luteal phase or anovulatory cycles, is extremely difficult to detect clinically but can have a cumulative effect on bone density.[117] This is an important area for more research, as bone mineral density has been shown to be proportional to the total number of normal menses.[118] Prior menstrual history is the best predictor of trabecular bone density. These effects, however, seem to be limited to the vertebrae, whereas postmenopausal osteoporosis affects the radius and the vertebrae. In theory, women who are active physically should have a higher bone density, so the true effect of amenorrhoea may be underestimated. Many women who experience amenorrhoea also exercise compulsively and overtrain. They may ignore signs of impending injury, leading to an increased incidence of musculoskeletal injuries and stress fractures, despite 'normal' bone density.

Treatment of osteoporosis

Treatment of established osteoporosis is controversial. Bone loss as a result of amenorrhoea appears to be at least partially irreversible. When amenorrhoeic athletes regain normal menses (either through reduced training or an injury preventing training), there is a 6.3 per cent increase in bone mineral density compared with a 3.4 per cent decrease in women who remain amenorrhoeic. Both values are still lower than age-matched eumenorrhoeal controls.[119] No long-term study to date has shown that amenorrhoeic individuals can fully regain lost bone mineral density, despite returning to a normal reproductive status. The risk is especially critical for the adolescent or young adult athlete, in whom attainment of peak bone mass is essential.

Oestrogen/progesterone replacement therapy can maintain bone mass and decrease the fracture rate in postmenopausal women. There appears to be a critical dose necessary for this effect. In one study,[120] low dose (0.3 mg/day of oestradiol) therapy prevented radial bone mass loss, but a moderate dose (0.625 mg oestradiol) was required to increase lumbar spine bone mass as well.[120] Calcium supplementation and regular weight-bearing exercise will augment these results, but are not effective therapies in the absence of the hormones. Menstruating female athletes require at least 1000 mg/day of calcium, while the recommendation for non-menstruating and postmenopausal women is 1500 mg/day. Athletes consuming less than 2000 kcal/day will usually require supplementation. A single regular-strength Tums® (indigestion) tablet con-

tains 200 mg of elemental calcium, the same as 250 ml of milk, or 125 g of cheese.

Even normal daily walking is associated with greater bone mineral density of the lumbar spine and femoral neck. Short-term weight-bearing exercise training increased bone mineral content in postmenopausal women (55 to 70 years) by 5.2 per cent over 9 months compared with -1.4 per cent in controls; after 22 months, bone mineral density increased by 6.1 per cent. Unfortunately, these impressive results are lost after training ceases. After 13 months of decreased activity, the bone mineral density in the exercising group was only 1.1 per cent above baseline. The Lanyon hypothesis states that bone mass will increase to meet the demand from mechanical loading, but only for as long as the stimulus is continued.[121] In other words, women of any age have to maintain adequate activity for bone adaptations as a result of training to persist. Non-loading exercises are generally ineffective in preventing vertebral bone loss in postmenopausal women. Muscular forces as well as gravitational forces lead to bone hypertrophy in healthy postmenopausal women. Inclusion of both aerobic and strength-training activity in an exercise programme will therefore help to maintain bone density, as well as improving balance.[122]

Management of the young athlete with decreased bone density

Dilemmas arise in the management of the young amenorrhoeic or premenarchal athlete. Optimal therapy is not yet well established on the basis of research findings. A survey of current clinical practice amongst a group of primary care sports medicine physicians[123] indicated that the majority would favour hormonal replacement for the individual resistant to other treatments. They were divided between oestrogen and progesterone combinations in various dosages, or the usage of oral contraceptives. Few, if any, would administer either therapy to women under the age of 16, and many were concerned about suppression of the hypothalamic–pituitary–ovarian axis, even in older athletes. There is also support for the administration of progesterone alone, for preservation of bone density in anovulatory athletes.[68]

Oral contraceptives may have a role in prevention and treatment of premature osteopenia or osteoporosis in both anorexic and amenorrhoeic individuals. In eumenorrhoeal premenopausal women, oral contraceptives either slightly elevate or have no effect on bone mineral density. A recent review[124] suggests that the use of oral contraceptives in women aged 30 to 40 years may stabilize or even increase bone mass, in a dose-related fashion. The recommended regimen is 20 to 35 μg of ethinyl oestradiol, in combination with norethindrone, a progestogen that is known to have a positive effect on bone mass. There is also probably an interaction between the amount and type of exercise, menstrual function, and attainable benefit from hormone replacement therapy. The administration of oral contraceptives may slow bone loss, but the question remains of whether they can increase it to normal.

New therapies for osteoporosis

Newer medications such as etidronate, alendronate, and calcitonin are being investigated in the postmenopausal woman, but little information exists on the indications, dosage, or length of therapy for the younger athlete. Bisphosphonates are a new class of drugs characterized by a phosphorus–carbon–phosphorus bonding. As they are analogues of pyrophosphates, they bind strongly to hydroxyapatite crystals and function to inhibit bone resorption. Their effect on bone deposition is not clearly known. Etidronate has been approved for use in the older patient in many European countries and in Australia. Alendronate (Fosamax) is now available in Canada. Other bisphosphonates on the horizon include clodronate, tiludronate, and risedronate. Years of study will be required in order to document their long-term actions as well as side-effects, especially in the premenopausal young adult population.

Calcitonin is a long-chain peptide hormone which is produced in the parafollicular cells of the thyroid gland. It functions to inhibits bone resorption by a direct action on the activity of the osteoclasts. Calcitonin therefore stabilizes bone mass in both the axial and appendicular skeleton. It also has an analgesic effect, and is commonly used in symptomatic Paget's disease, or during the first several months after an osteoporotic fracture. Development of a suitable route of administration has proceeded slowly. Calcitonin is degraded by gastric juices if given by mouth, while injected calcitonin causes transient side-effects lasting from 30 min to a couple of hours in about 50 per cent of treated patients. These may consist of vasomotor symptoms, hot flushes or reddening of the face and hands, dizziness, or gastrointestinal symptoms like nausea and vomiting. Nasal spray calcitonin shows some promise as a therapeutic modality. A dosage of 200 IU/day increases bone density in young amenorrhoeic athletes, compared with placebo, without any significant side-effects. There does not seem to be any change in bone density in postmenopausal women. Outcomes research, and more double-blind, placebo-controlled trials are necessary to relate immediate side-effects relative to the risk for long-term disability (i.e. hip fracture).

The 'female athlete triad'— disordered eating, amenorrhoea, and osteoporosis

Regular physical activity provides numerous positive health benefits for men and women of all ages. Nevertheless, sports physicians and scientists are becoming increasingly concerned about a 'triad' of problems occurring in susceptible athletes, primarily young females, in association with pursuit of their sporting dreams. This phenomenon has only recently been described in the literature, but had been silently observed by coaches, parents, team physicians, and athletes for some time. The three conditions are disordered eating, amenorrhoea (or absence of menses), and premature osteoporosis. Although they are discrete medical entities, there is enormous potential for these problems to be interrelated in the same sport, as well as in the same individual.[85,125]

A preoccupation with excessive thinness can precipitate a range of poor nutritional behaviours including the frank eating disorders of anorexia nervosa and bulimia nervosa. Food restriction, binging or purging, laxative or diuretic abuse, and even excessive exercise are used as methods to lose weight, ostensibly to improve performance. Pressure to 'be thin to win' can come from the athlete, the coach, and/or the parents, and is often reinforced by cultural, societal, and sport-specific expectations. The subsequent imbalance between nutrient intake and energy expenditure can induce amenorrhoea (or other menstrual abnormalities). Loss of the protective effect of the female hormones on calcium metabolism then leads to premature loss of bone mass or osteoporosis, which has been shown to be at least partially irreversible, even with the resumption of normal menstrual cycles.

Current diagnostic criteria, the medical consequences, and the prevalence of each of the triad disorders in the athletic population have been presented separately. This section will focus on significant warning signs, treatment, intervention, and preventative strategies. Substantial work has been done in this area by the Women's Task Force of the American College of Sports Medicine. In June of 1992, a panel of experts was convened in Washington, DC, to discuss the triad. In the setting of a comprehensive conference format, participants addressed the subjects of prevention, screening, risk profiles, diagnostic parameters, training dynamics, treatment, educational gaps, and research needs.[125,126] The young female athlete, at risk because of the 'pressure to excel' and the 'win at any cost' type of mentality is driven to achieve or maintain an 'ideal' body weight and/or an 'optimal' level of body fat. Adolescence in particular, is a sensitive period, a 'window of vulnerability' for development of these problems.

The assumption that continued weight loss ensures continued improvement in athletic performance is dangerous and should be discouraged. There is only a mild to moderate negative association between body fat content and performance ($r = -0.40$ to -0.68), and the percentage of body fat accounts for only 16 to 46 per cent of the variation in performance. The fallacy that every sport has an 'ideal percentage of body fat' is also not based on sound scientific principles. Instead, there is a need to take into consideration individual variation in body type and composition.[28] With dieting, muscle mass as well as fat is lost. Other side-effects of poor nutrition include fatigue, anaemia, electrolyte abnormalities, and depression. These will all eventually lead to a decrement in performance.

Prevention of the triad disorders starts with awareness and sensitivity to the pertinent issues. Athletic females with any one component of the triad should be questioned regarding the other entities. The preparticipation physical examination offers the ideal opportunity for the team physician to screen for these problems. It is important to de-emphasize low body fat, and to educate athletes thoroughly on nutrition and training principles, the development and maintenance of normal menstrual cycles, and the prevention of osteoporosis. A co-ordinated team approach, using the coach, athlete, parent, physician, nutritionist, etc., works best. School administrators and athletic directors have a responsibility to discourage coaching practices that rely on potentially harmful training techniques, or encourage inadequate nutrition, weight loss, and disordered eating. National governing bodies of sport and the International Olympic Association should also focus less on the leanness of the athlete in certain aesthetic sports, and more on her athletic performance.

At this inaugural conference on the triad, specific strategies were outlined in the areas of prevention, research needs, health consequences, medical care, education, and agency/administration responsibilities. The role of social isolation, specific psychological profiles of the athlete at risk, and the potential for sport–athlete mismatch were also deliberated. It was concluded that women must realize the full physiological, social, and psychological benefits of sports and exercise, and should be encouraged to strive for excellence, but not at the cost of their long-term health. Priorities of the conference included the preparation of suitable educational materials for athletes, parents, coaches, trainers, and administrators, as well as identification of physicians and scientists able to address lay and professional audiences on the issues. It was deemed critical to develop guidelines for team and primary care physicians to follow for preparticipation examinations of female athletes, and for prevention, identification, and treatment of these disorders. It was also decided to work with the appropriate medical specialty groups to address these same issues. Another initiative was the preparation of a position paper endorsed by the American College of Sports Medicine establishing a standard of conduct for those responsible for coaching and/or training of female athletes. A research agenda in the areas of surveillance, body composition, weight management, disordered eating, menstrual dysfunction, and osteoporosis was also outlined.[126]

To date, a slide series entitled 'The female athlete triad', of 80 slides plus an associated text has been developed for physicians to be able to present in their communities. More than 200 copies of this presentation have been distributed through the office of the American College of Sports Medicine (ACSM). The set has been translated into French by the Canadian Academy of Sport Medicine (CASM). Other educational materials are currently under production, including a guide for coaches and a videotape on the triad. A position stand on osteoporosis and exercise has been published by the ACSM in their journal *Medicine and Science in Sports and Exercise*,[127] and one specifically addressing the triad has recently been approved.[128] Numerous television and radio presentations, and newspaper and magazine articles have also helped to publicize the issues to the general population.

Slowly but surely, sporting organizations are expressing interest. Following the death of gymnast Kristy Henrich from bulimia in 1994, the United States Gymnastics Federation has instituted some preventative measures. Recent books have critically exposed some of the pathological coaching behaviours and training regimes in sports such as figure skating and gymnastics.[8] Some rule changes that have come into effect following the 1996 Olympics include raising the age of competition in gymnastics to 16. WomenSport International, with the aid of the International Olympic Association, held a conference on the Female Athlete Triad in September 1995. Out of this, a joint task force has been appointed to oversee further exploration of the problem, and potential solutions. In other sports, efforts have also been made to protect the young female player at risk. The Women's Tennis Council's Age Eligibility Commission was formed to review the age eligibility rule, and determined that girls of 14 and 15 are not yet ready to handle the physical and psychological demands of the professional tennis circuit. Measures such as these may decrease the incidence of the triad disorders, by discouraging extreme levels of competition at too young an age.[129]

Exercise and the postmenopausal woman

The term 'menopause' refers to the last spontaneous menstrual period that occurs as a result of the loss of ovarian function, while the 'climacteric' is the span of the entire transition from the reproductive to the postreproductive interval of a woman's life. The mean age of menopause is 51 years. Over 90 per cent of women live past this age, with an average life expectancy of 28 years beyond this critical event. Exercise during the menopausal and postmenopausal years can improve the quality of life, cardiovascular fitness, decrease body fat, lower blood pressure, reduce the risk of coronary artery disease, and prevent osteoporosis. Evidence is accumulating that hormonal changes do not contribute to cardiorespiratory decline, and that menopause has no effect on maximal aerobic capacity. Rather, it is the effect of ageing combined with a decrease in physical activity. Possible reasons include a change in body composition (gain in body fat; decrease in fat-free mass, specifically muscle), decreased physical activity, decreased cardiac contractility (affecting the maximal heart rate, stroke volume, and cardiac output), and a change in pulmonary function (decrease in maximum ventilation).[18] Older masters athletes have cardiorespiratory fitness values equivalent to or higher than moderately active and sedentary women 20 to 30 years younger.[130]

Many older women have not had the opportunity in their youth to be as active as they can be today. At present, with increased leisure time, retirement, increased opportunities, and access to facilities, many postmenopausal women are turning to physical activity for the first time. It behooves the family physician or sports medicine specialist to encourage such participation, and to know of the specific advantages and risks of exercise in this age group. Even septuagenarian women can benefit from a long-duration combined aerobic and resistance exercise programme to increase their maximal aerobic capacity and thigh muscle strength, speed, and force development.[131] This information is important, as strength is a probable risk factor in falls in the elderly. At all ages, women are weaker than men, and the incidence of falls and hip fractures in women is two to three times that in men. Quadriceps strength, in particular, is required for normal day-to-day activities such as walking and stair climbing.

The constellation of changes accompanying the menopause include vasomotor instability (hot flushes), fatigue, sweating, headache, insomnia (decrease in rapid eye movement sleep), nervousness, irritability, myalgias, arthralgias, palpitations, and dizziness, plus weight gain from decrease in activity. Exercise is helpful in ameliorating these symptoms.[11] Underlying mechanisms include haemodynamic changes, sympathetic nervous system activity, baroreceptor function changes, and release of endogenous opiates (endorphins). Hot flushes may be managed satisfactorily with progesterone (20 mg of medroxyprogesterone acetate/day) or with clonidine (0.1 to 0.4 mg/day). Norethindrone in dosages of 5 mg twice daily may also prevent postmenopausal bone loss.

Before starting an exercise programme, any women over 50 with two or more coronary risk factors and/or symptoms or signs suggesting cardiopulmonary or metabolic disease should have a complete history taken and physical examination, including a cardiac stress test. There is a need to start slowly and progress gradually. Specific guidelines are important and will help reduce the risk of drop-out and overuse-type injuries. Current recommendations are: participation in some type of continuous aerobic activity utilizing large muscle groups, for a minimum of 20 min/day, 3 days/week, at an intensity of 70 to 85 per cent of maximal heart rate. Patients should be encouraged to 'do what they want to do', not what the physician wants them to do.

Physically, the postmenopausal woman who undertakes an exercise programme may be prone to specific inconveniences that should be addressed by the supervising physician. Age and hormone-related changes in the lower urinary tract may cause stress incontinence and atrophic cystitis or urethritis with urinary frequency. Muscles and ligaments supporting the pelvic contents may atrophy and weaken, increasing the tendency for uterine prolapse. Loss of breast tissue and decreasing tissue elasticity may result in breasts becoming more pendulous. However, there is really no evidence that high-impact strenuous exercise such as running or jumping can cause uterine, rectal, or urinary bladder prolapse. Kegel exercises are recommended to retrain weak pelvic diaphragmatic muscles—25 Kegel exercises twice daily, holding each contraction for 8 to 10 s. Postmenopausal women also need adequate breast support during running or jumping activities.

Hormone replacement therapy

Hormone replacement therapy is the cornerstone of therapy in relation to preservation of bone density. There are other salient health concerns related to the menopausal years. Oestrogen deficiency causes immediate and delayed effects on the reproductive system, such as changes in the epithelial cells, thinning of the vaginal lining, and shrinking of the vaginal vault in both length and width. Dryness and an elevation of the pH to over 5.0 increase the risks of bacterial infection, and are associated with itchiness, burning, and painful intercourse. Hormonal replacement therapy can ameliorate many of these symptoms. Where systemically administered oestrogens are contraindicated (such as in the woman with a history of breast or uterine cancer), oestrogen cream may offer some relief for these problems.

The principal natural oestrogen produced by the ovary is 17-β-oestradiol. Circulating levels are generally between 40 to 400 pg/dl prior to menopause, and drop afterwards to less than 30 pg/dl. Oestrone is derived from the metabolism of 17-β-oestradiol, and the aromatization of androstendione in adipose tissue. Replacement oestrogen comes in a variety of preparations. Parenterally, it can be administered as oestradiol esters in oil, for sustained release. Oral forms include oral micronized oestradiol, oestrone, and quinoestrol, an oral steroidal oestrogen that is stored in adipose tissue and gradually released into the circulation. For topical application, there are vaginal creams containing conjugated equine oestrogens, oestropipate, dienoestrol, or 17-β-oestradiol. Some women are taking large amounts of wild yams, which contain a high concentration of natural oestrogen.

Therapeutic regimens usually include some form of oestrogen for days 1 to 25 of the cycle, and concomitant progesterone therapy to protect the endometrium from the effects of continuous oestrogen. This frequently necessitates induction of withdrawal bleeding at intervals, a side-effect that is not always appreciated by the woman, especially an athletically active woman, who thought that she was finally finished with this monthly problem. Progesterone is usually given in dosages of 5 to 10 mg from days 13 or 16 to day 25, although more recent programmes have tried continuous medroxyprogesterone acetate at 2.5 mg/day. Long-term unopposed oestrogen therapy is also thought to increase the risk of breast cancer,[132] although a recent review of the epidemiological data has suggested that this may be the result of either prevalence or surveillance bias.[133]

Oestrogen alone or in combination with progesterone retards postmenopausal bone loss. It is most expedient if prescribed in the early postmenopausal years. The minimal effective doses to protect both the appendicular and the axial spine are 0.625 mg/day of conjugated equine oestrogens, or 0.05 mg of transdermal oestrogen. Bone resorption is diminished when circulating levels of oestradiol reach a value of 60 pg/ml, similar to the last days of the follicular phase. Physical exercise in addition to oestrogen treatment does not result in further increases in bone mineral density, but timing and duration of oestrogen therapy are important. At least 7 years of oestrogen therapy appear necessary for maximal benefit, but this may still not be enough to protect women of 75 years and older from fracture.

There is also a higher incidence of coronary artery disease in women not receiving hormone replacement therapy.[134] At least one of the protective effects of oestrogens is owing to increased levels of high-density lipoprotein (**HDL**) cholesterol, and lowered LDL cholesterol.[135,136] The addition of various forms of progesterone to the therapeutic regime does not seem to alter this effect significantly.[137] This area is difficult to study because of numerous confounding factors including hereditary predisposition to coronary artery disease, obesity, hypertension, diabetes mellitus, smoking, hyperlipidaemia, inactivity, and stress. Exercise by itself also elevates HDL levels.

Cardiovascular disorders in women

Cardiovascular disease is the leading cause of death in women, ahead of cancer and other diseases, with one in nine women between the ages of 45 and 64 having clinical evidence of coronary artery disease, and one in three women over the age of 65. The lifetime risk of coronary artery disease is 31 per cent, compared with 2.8 per cent for hip fracture, 2.8 per cent for breast cancer, and 0.7 per cent for endometrial carcinoma.[138] In general, the onset of coronary heart disease is later in women than in men—10 years for any clinical manifestation, and 20 years for myocardial infarction. Unfortunately, women who do sustain myocardial infarctions have a substantial increase in morbidity and mortality, as well as increased mortality after coronary artery bypass grafts, and lesser success with coronary angioplasty. Female gender is the most powerful predictor of adverse outcome from coronary artery bypass grafts.[134,136,138]

Approximately 40 per cent of all coronary events in women are fatal, and 67 per cent of all sudden deaths in women involve those not previously known to have coronary artery disease. It is not known if the excess mortality for women reflects a true gender effect, or other factors, such as older age, greater number of concomitant diseases, differences in access to medical care or hospital facilities, or potential non-compliance or suboptimal use of medical therapies.[138] As the first presentation of coronary artery disease is frequently a heart attack and/or sudden death, it is essential to detect this disease sooner in women. Cigarette smoking triples the risk of a myocardial infarction, and women who smoke undergo menopause at an earlier age, thereby spending more years in the postmenopausal state. Former smokers will regress to a comparable rate of myocardial infarction and fatal coronary disease as women who never smoked.

Protective effects of female sex steroids on coronary artery disease

Coronary risk factors unique to women are oral contraceptive use, hysterectomy with oophorectomy, menopause, and oestrogen replacement therapy. The female sex steroids, oestrogen and progesterone, have complex protective and interactive actions on various parameters. Once the level of these hormones drop after menopause, a woman's risk for cardiovascular disease increases dramatically. The duration of oestrogen deprivation is also a factor, and women with premature menopause or early surgical menopause have a much greater incidence of disease. Oestogen replacement therapy is known to decrease coronary heart disease and stroke by 40 to 60 per cent, and this lower incidence persists into the eighth decade of life.[136] Patients with established cardiovascular disease benefit most from oestrogen replacement therapy. In addition to improvements in lipoprotein metabolism and coronary risk, oestrogen replacement therapy has favourable effects on blood pressure, clotting factors, diabetes, and osteoporosis. Women on long-term postmenopausal oestrogen replacement therapy have a statistically significant reduction in all-cause mortality, largely due to its effect on coronary artery disease. Overall, the cancer mortality in this group is similar to non-users, although users had a higher risk of death from breast cancer, and a lower risk from lung cancer.[139]

Oestrogen increases the high-density lipoprotein (**HDL**) component of cholesterol by 13 to 16 per cent through the degradation of hepatic lipase, and decreases low-density lipoprotein (**LDL**). Progesterone modifies these values in the opposite direction. Levonorgestrel has a larger effect than medroxyprogesterone acetate, but micronized progesterone does not alter lipids at all. LDL cholesterol is atherogenic, while HDL plays a role in removing excess cholesterol and transporting it back to the liver where it is degraded and reformed into other lipoproteins.

The effects of oestrogen on HDL/LDL ratios only explain approximately 30 to 50 per cent of the cardioprotective influence of this hormone. At least as important is its action on vascular reactivity and permeability. Oestrogen acts to increase hepatic angiotensinogen release. It elevates local production of prostacyclin, which acts as a vasodilator, and inhibits platelet aggregation. In addition, there is thought to be decreased lipid uptake into the vascular wall as a consequence of the membrane-stabilizing effects of oestrogen. Oestrogen acts via endothelial-derived relaxation factor and receptors in the vessel walls to produce coronary vasodilatation. Progesterone receptors are also present in the vessel wall, but there is less available information on the impact of combined oestrogen/progesterone regimens.[135]

The combination of hormones in oral contraceptives have implications for cardiovascular and metabolic disease as well. A small elevation in blood pressure is sometimes seen in individual patients, but this can easily be detected on follow-up vists, and the medication changed or discontinued. More often, there is a vasodilatation effect. Thromboembolism remains a small risk with the higher dosage formulations, particularly in women over the age of 35 who smoke, but this is minimized if the ethinyl oestradiol concentration is less than 35 µg. In terms of glucose metabolism, oestrogen increases pancreatic insulin secretion and improves insulin sensitivity. Depending on the androgenicity of the steroid used, the progestin component increases pancreatic insulin secretion, but may also increase insulin resistance.[135]

Similarly to oestrogen replacement therapy, the oestrogen in the pill acts to increase HDL cholesterol and decrease LDL cholesterol, with a small increase in triglycerides. Like physiological oestrogen, it also inhibits the uptake of cholesterol into the vessel walls. Progesterone counteracts the effect of oestrogen, and causes a decrease in HDL cholesterol, with the androgenicity of the progesterone determining its ultimate impact on the lipid profile. The newer progestogens (desogestrel, gestodene, and norgestimate) have neutral or even favourable consequences for key lipid and lipoprotein levels. The most recent formulations are thought to be safe even into the perimenopausal years. Recent work suggests that there may even be a protective effect on coronary artery disease.[72]

Prevention of heart disease in women

Primary prevention of heart disease includes emphasis on exercise for coronary protection for women. The epidemiological studies on the interaction of physical activity and coronary heart disease meet all the classic criteria for determining causality—consistency, strong exposure–response gradient, repeatability, specificity, assessment of exposure before endpoints, and control of confounding variables.[12] Exercising women with comparable cholesterol levels to sedentary counterparts generally have better outcomes. In the 1950s to 1970s, many women were homemakers and gained physical activity through housework or childcare. Today's woman has a multitude of choices in terms of exercise for her leisure time.

Regular physical exercise facilitates weight reduction or maintenance, improves lipid profile and insulin sensitivity, and decreases blood pressure. Long-term regular physical exercise of moderate intensity lowers blood pressure by an average of 10 mmHg, independent of weight loss, due to a reduction of sympathetic outflow activity. The acute action of dynamic aerobic exercise, such as walking, swimming, cycling, or stair climbing, is to increase the systolic and lower the diastolic pressure. Isometric exercise as in resistance training, weight training, and calisthenics, increases both systolic and diastolic blood pressure, and should not be prescribed in isolation. Other risk reductions, especially important for the diabetic population, include smoking cessation, and weight reduction. This in turn decreases hypertension, glucose intolerance, and hyperlipidaemia.

Summary

A decade ago, influential scientists were posing numerous questions relating to the female athlete. Today, some of these have been answered, but many more questions have arisen in their place. The inclusion of a chapter on the female athlete in a textbook such as this, surely represents a step forward in terms of our understanding of the unique characteristics of women in sports. Hopefully, some of the topics that have been discussed will pique the interest of a student or future researcher perusing these pages to carry on with the work done to date in this area. The number of potential investigations is limited only by the imagination.

Are there inherent biological factors that restrict the ability of women to transport and utilize oxygen, or do the observed variations represent some feature amenable to training? What are the most appropriate methods to match male and female subjects on the fitness factor? What cardiorespiratory, thermoregulatory, and metabolic alterations result from the myriad of hormonal shifts that the exercising female encounters throughout her reproductive life? Does the human body, with all its intricacies and duplication of systems, somehow compensate in some areas for adverse effects in others? Is athletic amenorrhoea a manifestation of a successful adaptation to training? Like the horse losing all but its middle toe to run on—is it nature's way of trying to even out physiological imbalances that may negatively impact on performance? Perhaps even the effect on bone density is an accommodative phenomenon, in that a lighter frame is easier to move through space! How can the female athlete ensure realization of the multitude of health benefits of regular exercise participation, without incurring either acute or chronic musculoskeletal injuries, or medical problems such as disordered eating, amenorrhoea, or premature osteoporosis?

In the past, there have been finite opportunities for women as leaders, executives, high performance coaches, senior decision-makers in sport, and researchers; as well as limited participation in sport by women at the school, university, and élite level. Overall there are still less Olympic sports for women, fewer resources for women's sport, a lack of female role models in sport and administration, and stratification of sport based on sex. Nevertheless, tremendous advances have been made, especially in the last few decades, towards a more balanced sporting culture. In the future, it is hoped that women at all levels will have equal access to the sport system, whether as a participant, coach, official, administrator, physician, therapist, or scientist. Sex-integrated sport, leadership development, and expanded opportunities for high-performance competition will continue to benefit the more competitive female athlete. In the final analysis, however, increased resource allocation to research issues, educational initiatives, and promotion for women in sports, will impart long-term gains for all active women in the population.

References

1. Lutter JM. History of women in sports: societal issues. *Clinics in Sports Medicine* 1994;**13(2)**: 263–79.
2. Jaffe R. History of women in sports. In: Agostini R, ed. *Medical and orthopedic issues of active and athletic women*. Philadelphia: Hanley & Belfus, 1994: 1–5.
3. Lutter JM. Sociologic considerations on women and sports. In: Agostini R, ed. *Medical and orthopedic issues of active and athletic women*. Philadelphia: Hanley & Belfus, 1994: 6–12.
4. Birrell SJ. Discourses on the gender/sport relationship. *Exercise and Sport Sciences Reviews* 1988; **16**: 459–502.
5. Lopiano DA. Equity in women's sports: a health and fairness perspective. *Clinics in Sports Medicine* 1994; **13**: 281–96.
6. Barnett NP, Wright P. Psychological considerations for women in sports. *Clinics in Sports Medicine* 1994; **13**: 297–313.
7. Lenskyj, HJ, Sport Information Resource Centre, Sport Canada, Canadian Heritage, eds. *Women, sport and physical activity: selected research themes. Summary of selected research themes, and bibliography*. Gloucester, Ontario: Minister of Supply and Services Canada., 1994: 5
8. Ryan J. *Little girls in pretty boxes: the making and breaking of elite gymnasts and figure skaters*. New York: Doubleday, 1995.
9. Lopiano DA. Gender equity in sports. In: Agostini R, ed. *Medical and orthopedic issues of active and athletic women*. Philadelphia: Hanley & Belfus, 1994: 13–22.
10. Aaron DJ, Dearwater SR, Anderson R, Olsen T, Kriska AM, Laporte RE. Physical activity and the initiation of high-risk health behaviors in adolescents. *Medicine and Science in Sports and Exercise* 1995; **27**: 1639–45.
11. Hargarten KM. Menopause: how exercise mitigates symptoms. *The Physician and Sports Medicine* 1994; **22**: 49–67.
12. Blair SN, *et al*. Physical activity, nutrition, and chronic disease. *Medicine and Science in Sports and Exercise* 1996; **28**: 335–49.
13. Bernstein L, Henderson B, Hanisch R, Sullivan-Halley J, Ross R. Physical exercise and breast cancer in young women. *Journal of the National Cancer Institute* 1994; **86**: 1403–8.
14. Kramer MM, Wells CL. Does physical activity reduce risk of estrogen-dependent cancer in women? *Medicine and Science in Sports and Exercise* 1996; **28**: 322–34.
15. Sanborn CF, Jankowski CM. Physiological considerations for women in sport. *Clinics in Sports Medicine 1994*; **13**: 315–27.
16. Wilmore JH, Costill DL, eds. Gender Issues and the Female Athlete. In: *Physiology of sport and exercise*. Champaign, Ilinois: Human Kinetics, 1994: 442–66.
17. Tiidus PM. Can estrogens diminish exercise induced muscle damage? *Canadian Journal of Applied Physiology* 1995; **20**: 26–38.
18. O'Toole ML. Exercise and physical activity. In: Douglas PS, ed. *Cardiovascular health and disease in women*. Philadelphia: W.B. Saunders, 1993: 253–67.
19. Pivarnik JM, Bray MS, Hergenroeder AC, Hill RB, Wong WW. Ethnicity affects aerobic fitness in US adolescent girls. *Medicine and Science in Sports and Exercise* 1995; **27**: 1635–8.
20. Daniels J, Daniels N. Running economy of elite male and elite female runners. *Medicine and Science in Sports and Exercise* 1992; **24**: 483–9.
21. Whipp B, Ward S. Are women catching the men? *Nature* 1992; **355**: 25.
22. Speechly DP, Taylor SR, Rogers GG. Differences in ultra-endurance exercise in performance-matched male and female runners. *Medicine and Science in Sports and Exercise* 1996; **28**: 359–65.
23. Nindl BC, Mahar MT, Harman EA, Patton JF. Lower and upper body anaerobic performance in male and female adolescent athletes. *Medicine and Science in Sports and Exercise* 1995; **27**: 235–41.
24. Batterham AM, Birch KM. Allometry of anaerobic performance: a gender comparison. *Canadian Journal of Applied Physiology* 1996; **21**: 48–62.
25. Meyer F, Bar-Or O, MacDougall D, Heigenhauser GJF. Sweat electrolyte loss during exercise in the heat: effects of gender and maturation. *Medicine and Science in Sports and Exercise* 1992; **24**: 776–81.
26. Lohman TG. *Advances in body composition assessment*. Champaign, Illinois: Human Kinetics, 1992.
27. Jackson AS, Pollock ML, Ward A. Generalized equations for predicting body density of women. *Medicine and Science in Sports and Exercise* 1980; **12**: 175–82.
28. Barr SI, McCargar LJ, Crawford SM. Practical use of body composition analysis in sport. *Sports Medicine* 1994; **17**: 277–82.
29. Cote KD, Adams WC. Effect of bone density on body composition estimates in young adult black and white women. *Medicine and Science in Sports and Exercise* 1993; **25**: 290–6.
30. Wadley GH, Albright JP. Women's intercollegiate gymnastics: injury patterns and 'permanent' medical disability. *American Journal of Sports Medicine* 1993; **21**: 314–20.
31. Kadel NJ, Teitz CC, Kronmal RA. Stress fractures in ballet dancers. *American Journal of Sports Medicine* 1992; **20**: 445–9.
32. Short JW, Pedowitz RA, Strong JA, Speer KP. The evaluation of pelvic injury in the female athlete. *Sports Medicine* 1995; **20**: 422–8.

33. Clement DB, *et al.* Exercise-induced stress injuries to the femur. *International Journal of Sports Medicine* 1993; **14**: 347–52.

34. Reid DC. The myth, mystic and frustration of anterior knee pain. *Clincal Journal of Sport Medicine* 1993; **3**: 139–43.

35. Arendt E, Dick R. Knee injury patterns among men and women in collegiate basketball and soccer: NCAA data and review of literature. *American Journal of Sports Medicine* 1995; **23**: 694–701.

36. Warren MP, *et al.* Scoliosis and fractures in young ballet dancers: relation to delayed menarche and secondary amenorrhea. *New England Journal of Medicine* 1986; **314**: 1348–53.

37. Adlercreutz H. Effect of diet and exercise on hormones: implications for monitoring training in women. *Clinical Journal of Sport Medicine* 1991; **1**: 149–53.

38. Eichner ER. Sports anemia, iron supplements, and blood doping. *Medicine and Science in Sports and Exercise* 1992; **24**: S315–18.

39. LaManca JJ, Haymes EM. Effects of iron repletion on Vo_2max, endurance and blood lactate in women. *Medicine and Science in Sports and Exercise* 1993; **25**: 1386–92.

40. Shangold MM, Mirkin G, eds.*Women and exercise: physiology and sports medicine.* 2nd edn. Philadelphia: F.A.Davis, 1994.

41. Tanner JM. *Growth at adolescence.* 2nd edn. Oxford: Blackwell Scientific Publications, 1962.

42. Johnson MJ. Preseason sports examination for women. In: Agostini R, ed. *Medical and orthopedic issues of active and athletic women.* Philadelphia: Hanley & Belfus, 1994: 35–49.

43. Duke PM, *et al.* Adolescent's self-assessment of sexual maturation. *Pediatrics* 1980; **66**: 918–20.

44. Lebrun CM. The female athlete: exercise, osteoporosis and birth control. In: Mellion MB, ed. *Sports medicine secrets.* Philadelphia: Hanley & Belfus, 1994: 36–42.

45. Prior JC, Vigna YM, McKay DW. Reproduction for the athletic woman: new understandings of physiology and management. *Sports Medicine* 1992; **14**: 190–9.

46. Highet R. Athletic amenorrhea: an update on aetiology, complications and management. *Sports Medicine* 1989; **7**: 82–108.

47. Loucks AB, Horvath SM. Athletic amenorrhea: a review. *Medicine and Science in Sports and Exercise* 1985; **17**: 56–72.

48. Prior JC, Vigna YM. Ovulation disturbances and exercise training. *Clinical Obstetrics and Gynecology* 1991; **34**: 180–90.

49. Loucks AB, *et al.* The reproductive system and exercise in women. *Medicine and Science in Sports and Exercise* 1992; **24**: S288–93.

50. Loucks AB. Effects of exercise training on the menstrual cycle: existence and mechanisms. *Medicine and Science in Sports and Exercise* 1990; **22**: 275–80.

51. Keizer HA, Rogol AD. Physical exercise and menstrual cycle alterations: what are the mechanisms? *Sports Medicine* 1990; **10**: 218–35.

52. Wilmore JH, *et al.* Is there energy conservation in amenorrheic compared with eumenorrheic distance runners? *Journal of Applied Physiology* 1992; **72**: 15–72.

53. Warren MP. The effect of exercise on prepubertal progression and reproductive function in girls. *Journal of Clinical Endocrinology and Metabolism* 1980; **51**: 1150–7.

54. Frisch RE, *et al.* Delayed menarche and amenorrhea of college athletes in relation to age at onset of training. *Journal of the American Medical Association* 1981; **246**: 1559–63.

55. Frisch RE, McArthur JW. Menstrual cycles: fatness as a determinant of minimum weight for height necessary for their maintenance or onset. *Science* 1974; **185**: 949–51.

56. Sanborn CF, Albreght BH, Wagner WW. Athletic amenorrhea: lack of association with body fat. *Medicine and Science in Sports and Exercise* 1987; **19**: 207–12.

57. Fruth SJ, Worrell TW. Factors associated with menstrual irregularities and decreased bone mineral density in female athletes. *Journal of the Orthopedic Society of Physical Therapy* 1995; **22**: 26–38.

58. Shangold MM, Levine HS. The effect of marathon training upon menstrual function. *American Journal of Obstetrics and Gynecology* 1982; **143**: 862–9.

59. Bullen BA, Skrinar GS, Beitins IZ, Von Mering G, Turnbull BA, McArthur JW. Induction of menstrual disorders by strenuous exercise in untrained women. *New England Journal of Medicine* 1985; **312**: 1349–53.

60. Malina RM. Menarche in athletes: a synthesis and hypothesis. *Annals of Human Biology* 1983; **10**: 1–24.

61. Stager JM, Wigglesworth JK, Hatler LK. Interpreting the relationship between age of menarche and prepubertal training. *Medicine and Science in Sports and Exercise* 1990; **22**: 54–8.

62. De Souza MJ, Metzger DA. Reproductive dysfunction in amenorrheic athletes and anorexic patients: a review. *Medicine and Science in Sports and Exercise* 1991; **23**: 995–1007.

63. Rigotti NA, Neer RM, Skates SJ, Herzog DB, Nussbaum SR. The clinical course of osteoporosis in anorexia nervosa: a longitudinal study of cortical bone mass. *Journal of the American Medical Association* 1991; **265**: 1133–8.

64. Cowart VS. Can exercise help women with PMS? *The Physician and Sports Medicine* 1989; **17**: 169–78.

65. Prior JC, Vigna YM, Sciarretta D, Alojado N, Schultzer M. Conditioning exercise decreases premenstrual symptoms: a prospective, controlled 6-month trial. *Fertility and Sterility* 1987; **47**: 402–8.

66. Steiner M, *et al.* Fluoxetine in the treatment of premenstrual dysphoria. *New England Journal of Medicine* 1995; **332**: 1529–34.

67. Myburgh KH, Watkin VA, Noakes TD. Are risk factors for menstrual dysfunction cumulative? *The Physician and Sports Medicine* 1992; **20**: 114–25.

68. Prior JC, Vigna YM, Barr SI, Rexworthy C, Lentle BC. Cyclic medroxyprogesterone treatment increases bone density: a controlled trial in active women with menstrual cycle disturbances. *American Journal of Medicine* 1994; **96**: 521–30.

69. Prior JC, Vigna YM, Alojado N. Progesterone and the prevention of osteoporosis. *Canadian Journal of Obstetrics, Gynecology and Women's Health Care* 1991; **3**: 178–84.

70. Prior JC. Progesterone as a bone-trophic hormone. *Endocrine Reviews* 1990; **11**: 386–98.

71. Grou F, Rodrigues I. The morning-after pill—how long after? *American Journal of Obstetrics and Gynecology* 1994; **171**: 1529–34.

72. Burkman RT. Noncontraceptive effects of hormonal contraceptives: bone mass, sexually transmitted disease and pelvic inflammatory disease, cardiovascular disease, menstrual function and future fertility. *American Journal of Obstetrics and Gynecology* 1994; **170**: 1569–75.

73. Committee on Sports Medicine of the American Academy of Pediatrics. Amenorrhea in adolescent athletes. *Pediatrics* 1989; **84**: 394–5.

74. Gambacciani M, Spinetti A, Taponeco F, Cappagli B, Piaggesi L, Fioretti P. Longitudinal evaluation of perimenopausal vertebral bone loss: effects of a low-dose oral contraceptive preparation on bone mineral density and metabolism. *Obstetrics and Gynecology* 1994; **83**: 392–6.

75. Bunt JC. Metabolic actions of estradiol: significance for acute and chronic exercise responses. *Medicine and Science in Sports and Exercise* 1990; **22**: 286–90.

76. Kampen DL, Sherwin BB. Estrogen use and verbal memory in healthy menopausal women. *Obstetrics and Gynecology* 1994; **83**: 979–83.

77. Lebrun CM. The effect of the phase of the menstrual cycle and the birth control pill on athletic performance. *Clinics in Sports Medicine* 1994; **13**: 419–41.

78. Lebrun CM. Effect of the different phases of the menstrual cycle and oral contraceptives on athletic performance. *Sports Medicine* 1993; **16**: 400–30.

79. Sansores RH, Abboud RT, Kennell C, Haynes N. The effect of menstruation on the pulmonary carbon monoxide diffusing capacity. *American Journal of Respirology and Critical Care Medicine* 1995; **152**: 381–4.

80. Prior JC, Vigna YM, Schultzer M, Hall JE, Bonen A. Determination of luteal phase length by quantitative basal temperature methods: validation against the midcycle LH peak. *Clinical and Investigative Medicine* 1990; **13**: 123–31.

81. Miller PB, Soules MR. The usefulness of a urinary LH kit for ovulation prediction during menstrual cycles of normal women. *Obstetrics and Gynecology* 1996; **87**: 13–17.

82. Lebrun CM. Effects of menstrual cycle phase on athletic performance. *Medicine and Science in Sports and Exercise* 1995; **27**: 437–44.

83. Lebrun CM. Effects of the menstrual cycle and birth control pill on athletic performance. In: Agostini R, ed. *Medical and orthopedic issues of active and athletic women.* Philadelphia: Hanley & Belfus, 1994: 78–91.

84. Yates A, Shisslak C, Crago M, Allender J. Overcommitment to sport: is there a relationship to the eating disorders? *Clinical Journal of Sport Medicine* 1994; **4**: 39–46.

85. Putukian M. Female athlete triad. *Sports Medicine and Arthroscopy Review* 1995; **3**: 295–307.

86. Sundgot-Borgen J. Eating disorders in female athletes. *Sports Medicine* 1994; **17**: 176–88.

87. Holderness CC, Brooks-Gunn J, Warren MP. Eating disorders and substance use: a dancing versus a nondancing population. *Medicine and Science in Sports and Exercise* 1994; **26**: 297–302.

88. American Psychiatric Association, ed. *American Psychiatric Association diagnostic and statistical manual.* 4th edn. Washington, DC: American Psychiatric Association, 1994.

89. Garner DM, Olmsted MP, Polivy J. Development and validation of a multidimensional eating disorder inventory for anorexia and bulimia. *International Journal of Eating Disorders* 1983; **2**: 15–34.

90. Garner DM, Garfinkel PE. The eating attitudes test: an index of the symptoms of anorexia nervosa. *Psychological Medicine* 1979; **9**: 273–9.

91. O'Connor PJ, Lewis RD, Kirchner EM. Eating disorder symptoms in female college gymnasts. *Medicine and Science in Sports and Exercise* 1995; **27**: 550–5.

92. Sundgot-Borgen J. Risk and trigger factors for the development of eating disorders in female elite athletes. *Medicine and Science in Sports and Exercise* 1994; **26**: 414–19.

93. Snow-Harter C. Bone health and prevention of osteoporosis in active and athletic women. *Clinics in Sports Medicine* 1994; **13**: 389–404.

94. Orwoll ES, Bauer DC, Vogt TM, Fox KM. Axial bone mass in older women. *Annals of Internal Medicine* 1996; **124**: 187–96.

95. Bonjour J, Theinz G, Buchs B, Slossman D, Rizzoli R. Critical years and stages of puberty for spinal and femoral bone mass accumulation during adolescence. *Journal of Clinical and Endocrinological Metabolism* 1991; **73**: 1330–3.

96. Johnston CC, Jr. *et al.* Calcium supplementation and increases in bone mineral density in children. *New England Journal of Medicine* 1992; **327**: 82–7.

97. Lloyd T, *et al.* Calcium supplementation and bone mineral density in adolescent girls. *Journal of the American Medical Association* 1993; **270**: 841–4.

98. Notelovitz M. Osteoporosis: screening, prevention and management. *Fertility and Sterility* 1993; **59**: 707–25.

99. Kanis JA. *Osteoporosis.* Oxford: Blackwell Science, 1994.

100. WHO. Assessment of osteoporotic fracture risk and its role in screeing for postmenopausal osteoporosis. Geneva: *WHO Technical Report Series*, 1994; No. 843.

101. Grimston SK, Willows ND, Hanley DA. Mechanical loading regime and its relationship to bone mineral density in children. *Medicine and Science in Sports and Exercise* 1993; **25**: 1203–10.

102. Alekel L, *et al.* Contributions of exercise, body composition, and age to bone mineral density in premenopausal women. *Medicine and Science in Sports and Exercise* 1995; **27**: 1477–85.

103. Baumgartner RN, Stauber PM, Koehler KM, Romero L, Garry PJ. Associations of fat and muscle masses with bone mineral in elderly men and women. *American Journal of Clinical Nutrition* 1996; **63**: 365–72.

104. Krahl H, Michaelis U, Pieper H, Quack G, Montag M. Stimulation of bone growth through sports: a radiological investigation of the upper extremities in professional tennis players. *American Journal of Sports Medicine* 1994; **22**: 751–7.

105. Slemenda CW, Miller JZ, Hui SL, Reister TK, Johnston CC, Jr. Role of physical activity in the development of skeletal mass in children. *Journal of Bone and Mineral Research* 1991; **6**: 1227–33.

106. Buchanan J, Myers C, Lloyd T, Leuenberger P, Demers L. Determinants of peak trabecular bone density in women: the role of androgens, estrogen and exercise. *Journal of Bone and Mineral Research* 1988; **3**: 673–80.

107. Teegarden D, *et al.* Previous physical activity relates to bone mineral measures in young women. *Medicine and Science in Sports and Exercise* 1996; **28**: 105–13.

108. Snow-Harter C, Marcus R. Exercise, bone mineral density and osteoporosis. *Exercise and Sport Sciences Reviews* 1991; **19**: 351–89.

109. Nichols DL, Sanborn CF, Bonnick SL, Ben-Ezra V, Gench B, DiMarco NM. The effects of gymnastics training on bone mineral density. *Medicine and Science in Sports and Exercise* 1994; **26**: 1220–5.

110. Kirchner EM, Lewis RD, O'Connor PJ. Bone mineral density and dietary intake of female college gymnasts. *Medicine and Science in Sports and Exercise* 1995; **27**: 543–9.

111. Dalsky GP. Effect of exercise on bone: permissive influence of estrogen and calcium. *Medicine and Science in Sports and Exercise* 1990; **22**: 281–5.

112. Heinrich CH, Going SB, Pamenter RW, Perry CD, Boyden TW, Lohman TG. Bone mineral content of cyclically menstruating female resistance and endurance trained athletes. *Medicine and Science in Sports and Exercise* 1990; **22**: 558–63.

113. Marcus R, Drinkwater BL, Dalsky GP, Dufek J, Slemenda CW, Snow-Harter C. Osteoporosis and exercise in women. *Medicine and Science in Sports and Exercise* 1992; **24**(Suppl.): S301–7.

114. Myburgh KH, Bachrach LK, Lewis B, Kent K, Marcus R. Low bone mineral density at axial and appendicular sites in amenorrheic athletes. *Medicine and Science in Sports and Exercise* 1993; **25**: 1197–202.

115. Montagnani CF, Arena B, Maffuli N. Estradiol and progesterone during exercise in healthy untrained women. *Medicine and Science in Sports and Exercise* 1992; **24**: 764–8.

116. Cann CE, Martin MC, Genant HK, Jaffe RB. Decreased spinal mineral content in amenorrheic women. *Journal of the American Medical Association* 1984; **251**: 626–9.

117. Prior JC, Vigna YM, Schechter MT, Burgess AE. Spinal bone loss and ovulatory disturbances. *New England Journal of Medicine* 1990; **323**: 1221–7.

118. Drinkwater BL, Bruemner B. Menstrual history as a determinant

of current bone density in young athletes. *Journal of the American Medical Association* 1990; **263**: 545–8.

119. Drinkwater BL, Nilson K, Ott S, Chesnut III CH. Bone mineral density after resumption of menses in amenorrheic athletes. *Journal of the American Medical Association* 1986; **256**: 380–2.

120. Beaumont LF, Blake JM, Webber CE. Bone mass, serum lipids, and lipoproteins during three years of opposed estrogen replacement. *Journal of the Society of Obstetricians and Gynecologists of Canada* 1996; **18**: 353–9.

121. Lanyon LE. Bone loading, exercise, and the control of bone mass: the physiological basis for the prevention of osteoporosis. *Bone* 1989; **6**: 19–21.

122. Nelson M, *et al.* High-intensity strength training to reduce risk factors for osteoporotic fractures. *Journal of the American Medical Association* 1994; **272**: 1909–14.

123. Haberland CA, Seddick D, Marcus R, Bachrach LK. A physician survey of therapy for exercise-associated amenorrhea: a brief report. *Clinical Journal of Sport Medicine* 1995; **5**: 246–50.

124. DeCherney A. Bone-sparing properties of oral contraceptives. *American Journal of Obstetrics and Gynecology* 1996; **174**: 15–20.

125. Lebrun CM. The female athlete triad: disordered eating, amenorrhea, and osteoporosis. *Orthopaedics International* 1994; **2**: 519–26.

126. Yeager KK, Agostini R, Nattiv A, Drinkwater B. The female athlete triad: disordered eating, amenorrhea and osteoporosis. *Medicine and Science in Sports and Exercise* 1993; **25**: 775–7.

127. American College of Sport Medicine. Position stand on osteoporosis and exercise. *Medicine and Science in Sport and Exercise* 1995; **27**: i–vii.

128. American College of Sport Medicine. Position stand on the female athlete triad. *Medicine and Science in Sport and Exercise* 1997; **29**: i–ix.

129. Skolnick AA. Health pros want new rules for girl athletes. *Journal of the American Medical Association* 1996; **275**: 22–4.

130. Wells CL, Boorman MA, Riggs DM. Effect of age and menopausal status on cardiorespiratory fitness in masters women runners. *Medicine and Science in Sports and Exercise* 1992; **24**: 1147–54.

131. Cress ME, *et al.* Effect of training on $\dot{V}o_2$max, thigh strength, and muscle morphology in septuagenarian women. *Medicine and Science in Sports and Exercise* 1991; **23**: 752–8.

132. Colditz GA, *et al.* The use of estrogens and progestins and the risk of breast cancer in postmenopausal women. *New England Journal of Medicine* 1995; **332**: 1559–93.

133. Speroff L. Postmenopausal hormone therapy and breast cancer. *Obstetrics and Gynecology* 1996; **87** (Suppl.): 44S–54S.

134. Douglas PS, *et al.* Exercise and atherosclerotic heart disease in women. *Medicine and Science in Sports and Exercise* 1992; **24**(Suppl.): S266–76.

135. Wild RA. Estrogen: effects on the cardiovascular tree. *Obstetrics and Gynecology* 1996; **87**(Suppl.): 27S–35S.

136. Sullivan JM, Fowlkes LP. The clinical aspects of estrogen and the cardiovascular system. *Obstetrics and Gynecology* 1996; **87**(Suppl.): 36S–43S.

137. Paganini-Hill A, Dworsky R, Krauss RM. Hormone replacement therapy, hormone levels, and lipoprotein cholesterol concentrations in elderly women. *American Journal of Obstetrics and Gynecology* 1996; **174**: 897–902.

138. Wenger NK. Preventive coronary interventions for women. *Medicine and Science in Sports and Exercise* 1996; **28**: 3–6.

139. Ettinger B, Friedman GD, Bush T, Quesenberry CP. Reduced mortality associated with long-term postmenopausal estrogen therapy. *Obstetrics and Gynecology* 1996; **87**: 6–12.

6.3.2 Exercise and pregnancy— What do I tell my pregnant patient?

Michelle F. Mottola

Traditional medical advice has been for pregnant women to rest during pregnancy.[1] However, that outdated medical advice does not address the increasing participation of women in sports and recreational activities, as well as women who work throughout pregnancy in strenuous and non-traditional occupations (such as the police work, fire fighting, military service, etc.). Because pregnancy is such a unique process in which almost all of the control systems of the body are modified in order to maintain maternal and fetal homeostasis, the addition of exercise may represent a significant challenge to maternal and fetal well being, especially at the higher intensities of physical work. Several potential risks have been identified in the literature and each appears to have a dose–response relationship to the intensity of maternal exercise, in that, as the intensity of maternal exercise increases, the risk of the hypothetical effects also is augmented. Wolfe *et al.*[1,2] and Clapp[3] provide excellent reviews on the effects of maternal exercise on maternal and fetal well being.

Figure 1 shows a flow chart of three major hypothetical risks that may occur to fetal growth and development during maternal exercise. Three different mechanisms are proposed.[1,2] The first (Fig. 1, middle panel) occurs as a result of increased catecholamine release which causes a redistribution of maternal blood flow from the gut and uterus to the working muscles of the mother.[4] This blood flow redistribution appears to be a dose–response relationship. As the intensity and duration of maternal exercise increases, the amount of blood shunted from the uteroplacental area to the working muscles of the mother is also augmented.[5] Maternal training does not seem to alter this phenomenon because Jones *et al.*[6] showed that, in rats, chronic maternal exercise did not change the amount of blood shunted from the gut to the working muscles of the mother compared with sedentary animals performing acute maternal exercise.

Oxygen delivery to the uteroplacental area is directly proportional to uterine blood flow.[7] A hydraulic occluder was placed on the uterine vasculature of pregnant sheep. Quantitative assessments of acute placental blood flow and fetal responses showed that the changes in fetal Po_2 and oxygen content were directly related to the magnitude of vascular occlusion. Fetal β-endorphin (a marker for fetal distress) was not released until uteroplacental blood flow was reduced by 65 per cent.[8] The relationship of this to maternal exercise intensity must be verified but it appears to be approximately 80 per cent $\dot{V}o_2$max in the exercising pregnant sheep.[9] With a reduced uteroplacental blood flow, there may be a reduction in fetal oxygenation and decreased placental oxygen diffusion capacity, which may lead to altered growth and development.[1] Many studies have shown that women who exercise at higher intensities and after 28-weeks gestation[10] give birth to smaller babies.[10,11]

The second hypothetical effect (Fig. 1, left) results from an increase in maternal blood glucose utilization as a metabolic fuel by the working muscles of the mother. With strenuous maternal exercise this may lead to maternal hypoglycaemia, which would decrease fetal glucose availability. Since the fetus utilizes maternal blood glucose as a major energy source for growth and development, regular exposure to reduced maternal blood glucose values may lead to fetal malnutrition, intrauterine growth restriction, and reduced birth weight.[12]

Finally, an increase in maternal body core temperature (Fig. 1, right) may occur with maternal exercise. As the intensity and duration of exercise increases, maternal body core temperature augments accordingly. At rest, fetal body core temperature is normally about 0.6°C higher than maternal because of augmented fetal metabolic rate as a result of growth and development.[13] This maintains the normal heat gradient and ensures that heat dissipation is from higher to lower, that is, fetal to maternal heat dissipation. As maternal body temperature increases, a latent response occurs in fetal body core temperature, such that maternal body core temperature is higher than fetal. This reverses the normal temperature gradient between fetus and mother, so that the fetus now receives heat from the mother.[13] This may increase fetal body temperature and may alter fetal development especially in the first trimester.[14]

As no threshold in intensity and duration of maternal exercise above which problems occur has been determined, it is important that medical screening take place to ensure a healthy pregnancy before maternal exercise. The literature suggests that the higher the intensity and duration of maternal exercise, the greater the risk of these potential effects occurring. Guidelines promoting exercise intensities of 60 to 70 per cent of $\dot{V}o_2$max are within accepted levels for healthy pregnancies.

Medical prescreening

An important medical screening tool that physicians can use to monitor patients regarding exercise during pregnancy is the *Par-med-X for pregnancy*. This document was developed by Dr Larry Wolfe from Queen's University and Dr Michelle Mottola from the University of Western Ontario. The Canadian Society for Exercise Physiologists (**CSEP**) now holds the copyright for this document which is also endorsed by Health Canada. It includes a prescreening questionnaire to identify contraindications to exercise during pregnancy, a list of safety considerations, and aerobic and muscle conditioning guidelines. (This document can be ordered from: the CSEP Office Suite 202 – 185 Somerset St West, Ottawa, Ontario, Canada K2P 0J2; telephone: 613 234 3755, fax: 613 234 3565.) In addition, the Canadian Academy of Sports Medicine (CASM) is

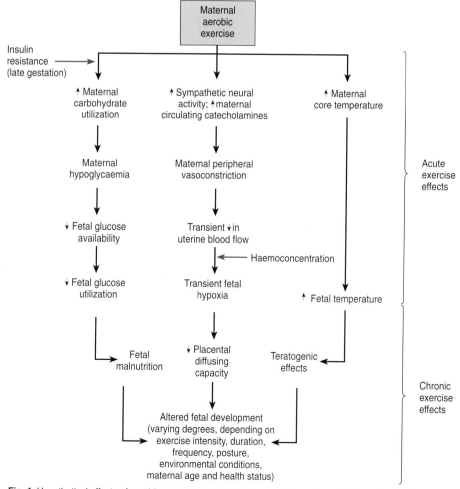

Fig. 1 Hypothetical effects of aerobic exercise on fetal development (reproduced with permission from ref. 2).

Table 1 Contraindications for exercise during pregnancy	
Absolute contraindications	**Relative contraindications**
Permanent or temporary restriction until control is treated, stable, and/or past acute phase. Please circle any that pertain to your patient:	Risks may exceed benefits of fitness conditioning. Decision to exercise or not should be made with qualified medical advice. Please circle any that pertain to your patient:
1. Clinically significant valvular or ischaemic heart disease	1. History in previous pregnancies of premature labour, intrauterine growth restriction
2. Type I diabetes mellitus, peripheral vascular disease, thyroid disease, uncontrolled hypertension, or other systemic disorders (hepatitis, mononucleosis, etc.)	2. Anaemia or iron deficiency (haemoglobin < 10 g/dl)
3. An incompetent cervix (multigravid patients)	3. Clinically significant pulmonary disease (e.g. chronic obstructive pulmonary disease)
4. A history of two or more spontaneous abortions	4. Mild valvular or ischaemic heart disease, significant cardiac arrhythmia
5. Bleeding or placenta previa	5. Very low physical fitness prior to pregnancy
6. Ruptured membranes or premature labour	6. A prescription of drugs which can alter cardiac output or blood flow distribution
7. Toxaemia or pre-eclampsia (current pregnancy)	7. Obesity and/or 'type II' diabetes prior to pregnancy
8. Evidence of fetal growth restriction (current pregnancy)	
9. Very low percentage of body fatness, eating disorders (i.e. anorexia)	
10. A multiple pregnancy	

Modified from source: *Par-med-X for Pregnancy*, 1996. Reprinted by permission from the Canadian Society for Exercise Physiology.

publishing a position paper on exercise during pregnancy in the autumn of 1997 and will include the *Par-med-X for pregnancy* document.

Contraindications for exercise and safety considerations

Table 1 shows contraindications for exercise during pregnancy, Table 2 shows reasons to discontinue exercise and consult a physician and Table 3 indicates safety considerations for maternal exercise. No supine exercise past 4 months of pregnancy has been suggested by the American College of Obstetricians and Gynecologists,[15] because of possible blocking of the inferior vena cava and/or the abdominal aorta while exercising in the supine position. The symptoms associated with the blocking of the inferior vena cava are light-headedness and dizziness; while there are no symptoms for blocking of the abdominal aorta, which may decrease blood flow to the uteroplacental area. The cautionary note at the bottom of Table 3 suggests monitoring of the temperature of heated pools. This is based on an animal study[16] which found an increase in teratogenic problems in animals exercised (swim-trained) in warm water (37.4°C).

Table 2 Reasons to discontinue exercise and consult a physician	
♦ Bloody discharge from the vagina	♦ Excessive fatigue, palpitations, or chest pain
♦ Persistent contractions	♦ Unexplained abdominal pain
♦ Absence of fetal movement (after initial detection)	♦ Sudden swelling of ankles, face, or hands
♦ Persistent headaches and/or visual disturbances, unexplained dizziness, or fainting	♦ Any 'gush' of fluid from the vagina (premature membrane rupture)
♦ Elevation of pulse rate or blood pressure persisting after exercise	♦ Swelling, pain, and redness in the calf of one leg
♦ Insufficient weight gain (< 1 kg/month during the last two trimesters)	

Modified from source: *Par-med-X for Pregnancy*, 1996. Reprinted by permission from the Canadian Society for Exercise Physiology.

Table 3 Safety considerations	
♦ Avoid prolonged or strenuous exertion during the first trimester	♦ Avoid exercise while lying on your back past 4th month of pregnancy
♦ Avoid isometric exercise or straining while holding your breath	♦ Avoid activities that involve physical contact or danger of falling
♦ Maintain adequate nutrition and hydration—drink fluids before and after exercise	♦ Periodic rest periods may help to minimize possible hypoxic or temperature stress to the fetus
♦ Avoid exercising in warm/humid environments	♦ Know reasons to stop exercise and consult your physician immediately if they occur

Caution—It is important to monitor the temperature of heated pools. Maternal body temperature during exercise may be increased *more* by exercising in a warm environment.
Modified from source: *Par-med-X for Pregnancy*, 1996. Reprinted by permission from the Canadian Society for Exercise Physiology.

FREQUENCY	INTENSITY	TIME	TYPE
Begin at three times per week and progress to four or five times per week.	Exercise within an appropriate RPE range and/or target heart rate zone.	Attempt 15 minutes even if it means reducing the intensity. Rest intervals may be helpful.	Non-weight bearing endurance exercise using large muscle groups (e.g. stationary cycling, swimming, aquatic exercise) or walking or low impact aerobics.

PRESCRIPTION/MONITORING OF INTENSITY

The best way to prescribe and monitor exercise is by combining the heart rate and rating of perceived exertion (RPE) methods:

TARGET HEART RATE ZONE

The heart rate zones shown below are appropriate for most pregnant women. Exercise at the lower end of the HR range at the beginning of a new exercise programme and in late pregnancy.

AGE	HEART RATE
< 20	140–155
20–29	135–150
30–39	130–145
≥ 40	125–140

PERCEPTION OF EXERTION

Check the accuracy of your heart rate target zone by comparing it to Borg's RPE scale. A range of about 12 to 14 ('somewhat hard') is appropriate for most pregnant women.

6	
7	Very, very light
8	
9	Very light
10	
11	Fairly light
12	
13	Somewhat hard
14	
15	Hard
16	
17	Very hard
18	
19	Very, very hard
20	

'TALK TEST' A final check to avoid over-exertion is to use the talk test. The exercise intensity is excessive if you cannot carry on a verbal conversation while exercising.

RATE OF PROGRESSION The best time to progress is during the second trimester since the risks and discomforts of exercise are the lowest at this time. It is not advisable to begin a new exercise programme or increase the amount of exercise prior to the 12th week or after the 28th week. Aerobic exercise at target HR should gradually and progressively be increased during the second trimester from a minimum of 15 minutes per session to a maximum of approximately 30 minutes per session.

WARM-UP/COOL-DOWN Aerobic activity should be preceded by a brief, 10–15 minute warm-up and followed by a short 10–15 minute cool-down. Low intensity, stretching, and relaxation exercises should be included in the warm-up/cool-down.

Fig. 2 Aerobic physical activity prescriptions for pregnancy. Source: *Par-med-X for pregnancy*, 1996. Reprinted by permission from the Canadian Society for Exercise Physiology.

Exercises for sedentary women and athletes

Healthy sedentary pregnant women who wish to start an exercise programme should be treated differently than the recreational athlete or the well-conditioned pregnant athlete. The following guidelines are suggested for each of these population groups for aerobic exercise and muscular conditioning exercise.

Sedentary women—aerobic exercise guidelines

Previous medical advice was that sedentary pregnant women should not start an exercise programme during pregnancy. However, recent scientific literature and guidelines suggest that if no contraindications to exercise exist and the pregnancy is healthy, women may start an exercise programme in the second trimester.[17] Exercise should not be started in the first trimester because of the potential heat risk and the increased risk of miscarriage. Many women do not feel well in the first trimester and may be discouraged from exercise if the exercise is started at that time. The best time to start an exercise programme is in the second trimester, around 16 weeks.

The frequency of exercise should be approximately 3 times per week, increasing until a maximum of four to five times per week. Intensity of exercise should be monitored by heart rate (pulse rate), which should be targeted within specific target heart rate zones based on age (Fig. 2). These target heart rate zones are approximately 60 to 70 per cent of peak oxygen consumption based on age.

Table 4 Example of gradual increase in aerobic exercise quantity during the second trimester for a previously sedentary woman

Week of gestation	Duration (min/session)	Frequency (sessions/week)
Do not begin a new exercise programme or increase habitual quantity and quality prior to the 15th week.		
16	15	3
17	17	3
18	19	3
19	21	3
20	23	4
21	25	3
22	26	4
23	27	3
24	28	4
25	29	3
26	30	4
27	30	3
28	30	4
Do not increase exercise duration or frequency after the 28th week of gestation. If necessary, reduce exercise quantity and quality to avoid chronic fatigue in late gestation.		

Adapted from Wolfe LA. Pregnancy. In: Skinner JS, ed. *Exercise testing and exercise prescription for special cases: theoretical basis and clinical application*, 2nd edn. Philadelphia: Lea & Febiger, 1993, with permission.

A sedentary woman should begin at the lower end of the target heart rate zone.[17] Coupled with target heart rate zones should be the rating of perceived exertion scale.[18] Out of a scale of 20, pregnant women should be exercising at an intensity of between 12 and 14 (somewhat hard); on the 10-point scale, between 3 and 4.[19] In addition, one final check of intensity is the 'talk test'. If the pregnant woman cannot carry on a conversation while exercising, without being out of breath, she should reduce the intensity.

The duration of exercise should be approximately 15 min per session at the target heart rate, increasing by 2 min every week until a maximum of 30 min per session at the target heart rate is achieved. Intensity or duration of exercise should not be increased past the 28th week of gestation[19] because of fatigue. Table 4 shows an example of frequency and duration increases for healthy pregnant women who were previously sedentary.

Each exercise session should start with 5 to 15 min of warm-up and end with 5 to 15 min of cool-down exercises at a lower intensity. The types of aerobic exercises recommended are walking, low impact aerobics, and exercise where body weight is supported, such as cycling and swimming. McMurray *et al.*[20] suggested that 40 min of walking or aerobic dance (heart rate averaged 135 ± 5 beats/min) did not adversely affect the mother metabolically in pregnant untrained women of 22 to 28 weeks gestation. All pregnant women should know the safety signs and consult a physician should any contraindications occur (Table 2).

Precautions for muscular conditioning exercise

The precautions listed in Table 5 for muscular conditioning exercise suggest modifications during pregnancy. Joint laxity may occur during pregnancy. Schauberger *et al.*[21] suggested that joint laxity was found in five of the seven peripheral joints studied over the course of pregnancy and postpartum, but there was no correlation with serum relaxin levels. Joint laxity was not influenced by parity, maternal age, or prepregnancy exercise levels.[21]

If diastasis recti develops during pregnancy, abdominal exercise is not recommended. Tearing of the linea alba occurs with this condition, which gives the bulging or rippling along the midline. Continuing to strengthen the rectus muscles through abdominal exercises may worsen this condition as the pregnant abdomen continues to protrude, because tearing will occur at the weakest point which is the connective tissue (linea alba).

Posture is important and a 'neutral' pelvic alignment is suggested rather than the pelvic tilt position. The use of the pelvic tilt is controversial because this position may decrease the normal lordotic curvature in the spine and place undue stress on the vertebral ligaments in the lumbar region.

Weight lifting is another area that sparks controversy. Weight lifting that occurs while lying on the back should be modified to either a sitting, standing, or side-lying position if possible. The use of a resistive tool such as low-weight free weights or a dynaband are recommended. Low resistance weight and high repetitions are also recommended for free weights and weight machines. Table 6 gives examples of muscular conditioning exercises.

Recreational athletes—aerobic exercise guidelines

Women who have been exercising prior to pregnancy at a mild to moderate intensity have been advised by the medical profession to continue exercise during pregnancy. However, it is necessary to determine frequency, intensity, duration, and type of exercise, before advising pregnant women to continue. In addition, medical prescreening must occur to rule out contraindications. The aerobic guidelines presented for sedentary women are also suggested for the recreational athlete. They may be able to exercise at the higher end of the target heart rate zone based on age, for the maximum of 30 min for four to five times per week. The type of exercise suggested is similar to that for sedentary women. However, if a woman has been jogging before pregnancy, she may continue within the aerobic exercise guidelines, unless she develops joint problems or is uncomfortable with this mode of exercise. Switching to stair climbing (with no jarring movements) or to exercises that support body weight would be recommended. The muscle conditioning precautions for the recreational athlete are the same as above for the sedentary woman.

Athletes and strenuous exercise

Pregnancy is not the time for engaging in athletic competition or strenuous activity that would place the mother at risk for bodily injury. There are also no known benefits to the fetus of maternal

Table 5 Precautions for muscular conditioning during pregnancy

Variable	Effects of pregnancy	Exercise modifications
Body position	In the supine position (lying on the back), the enlarged uterus may decrease the flow of blood returning from the lower half of the body as it presses on a major vein (inferior vena cava)	Past 4 months of gestation, exercises normally done in the supine position should be altered; such exercises should be done side-lying or standing
Joint laxity	Ligaments become relaxed due to increasing hormone levels	Avoid rapid changes in direction and bouncing during exercise
	Joints may be prone to injury	Stretching should be performed with controlled movements
Abdominal muscles	Presence of a rippling (bulging) of connective tissue along the midline of the pregnant abdomen (diastasis recti) may be seen during abdominal exercise	Abdominal exercises are not recommended if diastasis recti develops
Posture	Increasing weight of enlarged breasts and uterus may cause a forward shift in the centre of gravity and may increase the arch in the lower back; this may also cause shoulders to slump forward	Emphasis on correct posture
Body temperature	Increases in maternal body temperature causes increases in fetal temperature	Emphasis on drinking water every 15–20 min throughout exercise
	Prolonged increases in maternal body temperature, especially during the first trimester, may cause abnormal fetal development	Heart rate should not go beyond limits listed for aerobic exercise
		Core body temperature should not go above 38°C
Weight-lifting precautions	Emphasis must be placed on continuous breathing throughout exercise	
	Exhale on exertion, inhale on relaxation	
	Valsalva manoeuvre (holding breath while working against a resistance) causes an increase in blood pressure and therefore should be avoided	
	Avoid exercise in supine position past 4 months gestation	

Modified from source: *par-med-X for Pregnancy*, 1996. Reprinted by permission from the Canadian Society for Exercise Physiology.

exercise past 80 per cent of $\dot{V}O_2$max. In fact, as previously suggested, the animal literature indicates that at this high intensity the fetus may be in distress and uteroplacental blood flow may be reduced by 65 per cent.[8] The physician must ask the athlete why she wants to pursue such high-intensity training while pregnant. In this situation the risks to the fetus far outweigh any maternal benefits and reduction in intensity and duration would be highly recommended. If the physician or exercise professional has access to

Table 6 Prescription for muscular conditioning during pregnancy

It is important to condition all major muscle groups during both prenatal and postnatal periods

Warm-ups

Range of motion: neck, shoulder girdle, back, arms, hips, knees, ankles, etc.	Static stretches: all major muscle groups (Do not overstretch)

Muscular strength and endurance

Upper back: shoulder blade pinch	Lower back: modified standing, opposite leg and arm lifts	Abdominal: curls-ups, head raises in side-lying or standing position
Pelvic floor: Kegel exercises	Shoulders/arms: shoulder rotations, modified push-ups against a wall	Buttocks/legs/feet: buttocks squeeze, standing leg lifts, heel raises

Modified from source: *par-med-X for Pregnancy*, 1996. Reprinted by permission from the Canadian Society for Exercise Physiology.

equipment that can assess cardiorespiratory responses to a peak exercise test in combination with blood lactate levels, it would be advisable to determine the anaerobic threshold. Exercise can then be prescribed for the individual pregnant athlete below her level of anaerobic threshold. For an athlete who is highly motivated, this may be a safe way to prescribe exercise outside the guidelines suggested above for aerobic actvity. The muscle conditioning precautions for the well-conditioned athlete are the same as above for the sedentary woman.

The literature describing the effects of strenuous exercise on mother and fetus is limited. Most of the studies presented are case studies of women athletes and are retroactive reports, not randomly designed trials. A recent study assessed the effects of a vigorous exercise programme continued into late pregnancy on birth weight. The results suggested that women who exercised vigorously, for more than four sessions per week past 25 weeks gestation, gave birth to babies weighing 315 g lower than controls.[22]

Occupation and physical activity

The *Par-med-X for pregnancy* document has a question about activity performed in the pregnant woman's job, whether it be homemaker, or nurse working 12-h shifts and lifting patients. Determining the activity level of the pregnant woman as she performs everyday activities is important and must be considered when prescribing an exercise programme. If the pregnant woman is engaging in high-intensity physical activities in her occupation, it is important to prescribe an exercise programme to complement the activities performed in everyday life. This will prevent unnecessary fatigue, overuse injuries, and decrease the potential risk to the fetus.

The effects of occupation on pregnancy outcome is reviewed in Wolfe *et al.*[1] Additional recent studies suggest that occupational physical activity may play an important role in pregnancy outcome. Military women in active duty who gained less than 11.5 kg during pregnancy developed preterm labour more often.[23] The risk of preterm labour was also increased in women who worked regularly in the evening or at night and had occupations with long hours of standing; work continued through late gestation also increased the risk of delivering a preterm infant.[24]

In a national survey of United States nurses, factors significantly associated with preterm birth included number of hours worked per week, per shift, and while standing. Other factors were noise level, physical exertion, and occupational fatigue.[25] In addition, Spinillo *et al.*[26] associated moderate to high physical activity in the work place with a twofold increase in the risk of severe pre-eclampsia, compared with mild activity at work. In a review article on physical work and pregnancy outcome, Alborg[27] concluded that the epidemiological evidence suggests that occupations including prolonged standing and/or walking continued into late gestation, as well as work encompassing several strenuous factors in combination, appear to increase the risk of preterm delivery. Alborg[27] recommends that working pregnant women avoid extremely heavy physical exertion (close to maximum) in early pregnancy and late gestation. Occupational heavy lifting and the impact on spontaneous abortion is inconclusive and requires further study. Thus, before exercise can be prescribed for pregnant women in the work force, it is important to determine how physically active they are in their current occupation so that overexertion and undue fatigue are avoided.

Postpartum exercise

Many pregnant women are concerned about when they can safely return to exercise after the baby is born. The period of time before exercise can be restarted depends upon the number of complications during labour and delivery. If labour and delivery are uncomplicated, a postpartum woman can return to aerobic exercise usually once vaginal bleeding from delivery has stopped, and/or her postpartum check-up is normal. It is recommended that she begin her exercise programme at the lower intensity heart rate range (Fig. 2) and follow the same guidelines as if she were pregnant. Avoiding unnecessary fatigue is an important consideration for any new mother, and starting off with walking while pushing a baby carriage is an excellent way to regain activity. If the postpartum woman has had a caesarean section, or complications during labour and delivery, it is recommended to wait at least 10 weeks or until labour and delivery complications have healed or returned to normal.

Muscular conditioning exercises are also recommended for the postpartum woman, and return to these exercises is suggested after the first postpartum check-up and vaginal bleeding due to delivery has stopped. Kegel exercises are important to continue and can be started again as soon as the postpartum woman feels well enough to start them. Theses exercises may help to strengthen weakened pelvic floor muscles from delivery and may help postpartum incontinence. Abdominal exercises can be started as well and may be performed in the supine position. Women who have experienced diastasis recti during pregnancy are advised to proceed with caution and start abdominal exercise slowly, gradually building up the number of repetitions.

Lactating women have been shown to have a reduced level of noradrenaline, indicating that neurohormonal systems are restrained.[28] This may explain why exercise has little adverse effect on milk quality, quantity, or on infant weight gain.[29]

Infants detect sweet and sour tastes.[30] The literature has suggested that infants may refuse to nurse, or be restless, during a feeding postexercise because of an increase in the lactic acid content of the milk, which may produce a sour taste.[30] Maximal exercise has been shown to increase the amount of lactic acid in breast milk postexercise, which leads to decreased acceptance of this milk.[30] However, aerobic exercise at 60 to 70 per cent of $\dot{V}o_2$max, performed four or five times per week beginning 6 to 8 weeks postpartum, had no adverse effect on lactation.[29] It would seem that mild to moderate exercise is well tolerated postpartum, but strenuous (near maximum) aerobic activity should be avoided until lactation is terminated.

References

1. Wolfe LA, Brenner IKM, Mottola MF. Maternal exercise, fetal well-being and pregnancy outcome. *Exercise and Sports Sciences Reviews*, 1994; **22**: 145–94.
2. Wolfe LA, Ohtake PJ, Mottola MF, McGrath MJ. Physiological interactions between pregnancy and aerobic exercise. *Exercise and Sport Sciences Reviews* 1989; **17**: 295–351.
3. Clapp JF. Exercise during pregnancy. In: Bar-Or O, Lamb D, Clarkson PM, eds. *Exercise and the Female—A Lifespan Approach. Perspectives In Exercise Science and Sports Medicine*, Vol. 9. Carmel, IN: Cooper Publishing Group, 1996; 413–51.

4. Lotgering F, Gilbert R, Longo L. Exercise responses in pregnant sheep: oxygen consumption, uteroplacental blood flow and blood volume. *Journal of Applied Physiology* 1983; **55**: 834–41.

5. Jones MT, Rawson RE, Robertshaw D. Determination of maximal oxygen consumption in exercising pregnant sheep. *Journal of Applied Physiology* 1992; **73**: 234–9.

6. Jones MT, Norton KI, Dengel DR, Armstrong RB. Effects of training on reproductive tissue blood flow in exercising pregnant rats. *Journal of Applied Physiology* 1990; **69**: 2097–103.

7. Mostello D, Chalk C, Khoury J, Mack CE, Siddiqi TA, Clark KE. Chronic anemia in pregnant ewes: maternal and fetal effects. *American Journal of Physiology* 1991; **261**: R1075–83.

8. Skillman CA, Clark KE. Fetal β-endorphin levels in response to reductions in uterine blood flow. *Biology of the Neonate* 1987; **51**: 217–23.

9. Jones MT, Rawson RE, Riplog S, Robertshaw D. Oxygen consumption and uterine blood flow in exercising pregnant sheep. *Medicine and Science in Sports and Exercise* 1991; **23**(Suppl.): S169.

10. Clapp JF, Dickstein S. Endurance exercise and pregnancy outcome. *Medicine and Science in Sports and Exercise* 1984; **16**: 556–62.

11. Clapp J, Capeless E. Neonatal morphometrics after endurance exercise during pregnancy. *American Journal of Obstetrics and Gynecology* 1990; **163**: 1805–11.

12. Clapp JF, Wesley M., Sleamaker R. Thermoregulatory and metabolic responses to jogging prior to and during pregnancy. *Medicine and Science in Sports and Exercise* 1987; **19**: 124–30.

13. Lotgering F, Gilbert R, Longo L. Exercise responses in pregnant sheep: blood gases, temperature and fetal cardiovascular system. *Journal of Applied Physiology* 1983; **55**: 842–50.

14. Bell AW Consequences of severe heat stress for fetal development. In: Hales JRS, Richards D, eds. *Transactions of the Menzies Foundation*. Melbourne: Menzies Foundation, 1987: 149–59.

15. American College of Obstetricians and Gynecologists. Exercise during pregnancy and the postpartum period. *ACOG Technical Bulletin* 1994; **189**(Feb.): 2–7.

16. Mottola MF, Fitzgerald HM, Wilson NC, Taylor AW. Effect of water temperature on exercise-induced maternal hyperthermia on fetal development in rats. *International Journal of Sports Medicine* 1993; **14**: 248–51.

17. Mottola MF, Wolfe LA. Active living and pregnancy. In: Quinney HA, Gauvin L, Wall AE, eds. *Toward active living. Proceedings of the International Conference on Physical Activity, Fitness and Health*. Champaign, IL.: Human Kinetics Publishers, 1994: 131–40.

18. Borg G. A category scale with ratio properties for intermodal and interindividual comparison. In: Geissler H-G, Petzold P, eds. *Psychophysical judgement and the process of perception*. Berlin: VEB Deutscher Verlag du Wissenschaften, 1962.

19. Wolfe LA, Mottola MF. Aerobic exercise in pregnancy: an update. *Canadian Journal of Applied Physiology* 1993; **18**: 119–47.

20. McMurray RG, Hackney AC, Guion WK, Katz VL. Metabolic and hormonal responses to low-impact aerobic dance during pregnancy. *Medicine and Science in Sports and Exercise* 1996; **28**: 41–6.

21. Schauberger CW, Rooney BL, Goldsmith L, Shenton D, Silva PD, Schaper A. Peripheral joint laxity increases in pregnancy but does not correlate with serum relaxin levels. *American Journal of Obstetrics and Gynecology* 1996; **174**: 667–71.

22. Bell RJ, Palma SM, Lumley JM. The effect of vigorous exercise during pregnancy on birth-weight. *Australian and New Zealand Journal of Obstetrics and Gynaecology* 1995; **35**: 46–51.

23. Magann EF, Winchester MI, Carter DP, Martin JN, Nolan TE, Morrison JC. Military pregnancies and adverse perinatal outcome. *International Journal of Gynaecology and Obstetrics* 1996; **52**: 19–24.

24. Fortier I, Marcoux S, Brisson J. Maternal work during pregnancy and the risks of delivering a small-for-gestational-age or preterm infant. *Scandinavian Journal of Work Environment and Health* 1995; **21**: 412–18.

25. Luke B, *et al*. The association between occupational factors and preterm birth—a United States nurses study. *American Journal of Obstetrics and Gynecology* 1995; **173**: 849–62.

26. Spinillo A, Capuzzo E, Colonna L, Piazzi G, Nicola S, Baltaro F. The effect of work activity in pregnancy on the risk of severe pre-eclampsia. *Australian and New Zealand Journal of Obstetrics and Gynaecology* 1995; **35**: 380–5.

27. Ahlborg G. Physical work load and pregnancy outcome. *Journal of Occupational and Environmental Medicine* 1995; **37**: 941–4.

28. Altemus M, Deuster PA, Galliven E, Carter CS, Gold PW. Suppression of hypothalamic–pituitary–adrenal axis responses to stress in lactating women. *Journal of Clinical Endocrinology and Metabolism* 1995; **80**: 2954–9.

29. Dewey KG, Lovelady CA, Nommsen-Rivers LA, McCrory MA, Lonnerdal B. A randomized study of the effects of aerobic exercise by lactating women on breast-milk volume and composition. *New England Journal of Medicine* 1994; **330**: 449–53.

30. Wallace JP, Inbar G, Ernsthausen K. Infant acceptance of post-exercise breast milk. *Pediatrics* 1992; **89**: 1245–7.

6.4 The ageing athlete

Darrell Menard

'Age is not a barrier to performance, only an inconvenience.'[3]

Introduction

It is estimated that there are more than 30 million North Americans over the age of 65 and that this number is increasing on a daily basis.[1] Both the absolute and the relative number of older individuals is increasing so rapidly that by the year 2030 more than 20 per cent of the population will be over 65 years of age—a number in excess of 60 million people![2] In addition, the most rapidly growing segment of our society is the over-85 age group.[3] To confirm that our society is ageing, one only has to realize that over 50 per cent of the people who have ever been older than 65 are alive today.[4] This enormous segment of humanity has begun to challenge the paradigm that people should grow old gracefully and is no longer content with the prospect of retiring to rocking chairs and living a life of leisure. Instead, many of them are turning to sports in search of fun, fitness, self-fulfilment, and new challenges. Some go so far as to complete the Ironman triathlon, run marathons, climb mountains, win Olympic medals, swim the English Channel, or cycle across North America. Nearly 40 years after Roger Bannister became the first person to run a sub-4 minute mile, Eamonn Coghlan accomplished the same feat at the age of 40 on an indoor track. At one time, including a masters age group event at a sports competition was a concession reluctantly made by the event director. Things have evolved to the point where masters categories are now considered a routine feature at most competitions and the number of senior participants frequently rivals that of the young. Globally, we now find events organized exclusively for older athletes.

The World Senior Games was first held in 1970 with 200 competitors taking part. Twenty-five years later, Buffalo, New York, hosted the 11th World Veterans Athletics Championships in which 5335 masters athletes from 79 nations gathered to test their athletic abilities and celebrate the joy of sports. This event was rated the second largest track and field event in history, second only to the 10th World Veterans Athletics Championships held in Miyazaki, Japan. Participants were between 35 and 93 years of age, and at the end of this 11-day sports extravaganza 58 new, age-class world records had been established. In the articles written about these games, it was remarkable how often the authors referred to the competitors as possessing child-like enthusiasm despite their obvious ages. Many of the athletes came to test themselves and were not preoccupied with the 'win at all costs' philosophy that is corrupting our younger generation of athletes. This does not imply that ageing athletes do not take their sports participation seriously. On the contrary, watching them perform would convince anyone of their intensity and determination. What they do possess is a realistic perspective on their efforts. The masters athletic movement offers its participants more than the obvious fitness and social advantages. It also offers them one of the elixirs of life—fun and something to look forward to as they age. In addition, they have a chance to interact with athletes many years their junior, an opportunity which is mutually beneficial.

Masters athletes have become the focus of considerable media interest in the last 20 years. The general public is genuinely captivated by the life stories and achievements of many older competitors. This is possibly because these individuals serve as role models, reminding us all of what can be accomplished if we refuse to accept physical limits and perform to our capabilities. Some people may feel a little younger and more worthwhile when they see a senior competitor outperform opponents 20, 30, or 40 years their junior. Some people may even be inspired to question if they really are 'over the hill'. The success of ageing athletes reminds all of us that great things are possible with a little effort, dedication, and self-confidence.

Consider, for example, the story of Priscilla Welch. Although she was 30 pounds (13.6 kg) overweight, a heavy smoker, and never before active, she took up jogging at the age of 34. She did not remain a jogger for long, and at the age of 39 was selected for the 1984 British Olympic Team. She finished sixth in the marathon at the Los Angeles Olympics, establishing a British national record. Her marathon personal best of 2 h 26 min 51 s was run at the age of 42. Even into her mid-40s she remained one of the finest distance runners in the world and believes that age had a minor influence on her performances. Individuals like this provide important role models for our older citizens. Publicizing their achievements demonstrates that much can be accomplished beyond the age of 40.

The scientific community has also taken an interest in the ageing process and how it affects athletic performance. This is reflected in the increasing volume of literature that is being written on the subject. Sports magazines, scientific journals, and reference texts frequently include discussions of the ageing athlete, a fact which attests to the increasing importance of this growing group of competitors. There is a National Institute on Aging in the United States, and this organization actively encourages research and symposia on the ageing process. Unfortunately, until recently, much of the research and literature in this field was focused on the benefits of exercise in terms of promoting cardiovascular health and longevity. Very little was focused specifically on the ageing athlete. This has left many important questions unanswered, offering the scientific community an almost limitless opportunity for meaningful research. This chapter is dedicated to addressing a number of these questions in the hope of providing a more thorough understanding of this unique entity in the world of sports—the ageing athlete.

Ageing

Considerable research has been directed towards understanding the ageing process and the many changes it produces in the human body. One of the most surprising consequences of recent research is that almost everything we once believed about the ageing process is now being challenged. Many of the changes that were once attributed to the ageing process are now known to be the results of disease processes, environmental influences, and physical inactivity. Earlier researchers often failed to control for these variables, and as a result many of their conclusions were incorrect. As more masters athletes push the 'envelope of ageing' to its limits and more research is performed, it is almost certain that many of the changes currently attributed to the ageing process will be found to be the result of other factors.

Before the structural and functional changes associated with the ageing process can be appreciated adequately, it is necessary to understand the concept of ageing. Contrary to popular belief, ageing is not a metamorphosis that suddenly occurs upon reaching some significant milestone in life, such as the age of 40. Rather, it is an inevitable and continuous process that begins at conception and continues through infancy, childhood, adolescence, maturation, and old age. It cannot be avoided, reversed, or even postponed. Research shows that, with certain lifestyle changes, the best that can be hoped for is a reduction in the rate at which the process occurs.

There are almost as many definitions of ageing as there are authors who write on the subject. Most of them state something to the effect that ageing involves an impairment of an organism's ability to respond appropriately to environmental stresses. After careful consideration, however, many of these definitions fall considerably short of being complete. In fact, what many of them do is simply state the net result of ageing. Strehler recognized this fact and offers one of the simplest and yet most complete descriptions of the ageing process. He states that the ageing process has four basic properties: 'Ageing is universal, decremental, progressive and intrinsic'.[5] In other words, everyone ages; structural and functional losses occur and relentlessly progress with the passage of time, and the ageing phenomenon is innate to our genetic make-up, not a pathological process. Any change in an older person that fails to meet these criteria cannot be attributed to the ageing process. The net result of ageing is a gradual eroding of the functional reserves of all our organ systems such that it is progressively more difficult to compensate for environmental stresses, metabolic disturbances, disease processes, and anything else that can disrupt homeostasis. Several investigators have shown that there is a linear decline in the functional reserves of most body systems after the third decade of life.[6,7] These decrements remain obscure until the individual is placed under a sufficient volume of physiological stress. At this point, the individual's ability to respond will be less effective than it was when he or she was younger. Ageing is an extremely complex process that involves

changes at the molecular and cellular levels, and the exact mechanism by which it occurs is still uncertain.

Ageing theories

The concept of ageing and why it occurs has probably been a subject of curiosity to mankind since time began. The gifted intellectual Leonardo da Vinci was one of the first people to take a scientific interest in the investigation of ageing. He conducted an experiment where he dissected the bodies of 30 older adults in an effort to discern what anatomical changes accompany the ageing process. On completion of his study, he concluded that ageing was due to thickening of the blood vessels.[8] Since then, many scientists have unsuccessfully attempted to unravel the mystery behind why organisms age. With the recent explosion of knowledge in the fields of genetics, nuclear medicine, biochemistry, immunology, and molecular biology, tools and investigational techniques are being developed that could help to explain the ageing process. Techniques that may prove important include recombinant DNA, cell fusion, and cell hybridization. Until a definitive explanation can be provided, we shall have to content ourselves with a number of hypotheses.

As a general rule, if something is poorly understood there will be numerous theories attempting to provide all the answers, and the ageing process is no exception. While many ageing theories have been proposed, none adequately explains what has been observed experimentally. It is possible that a process as complex as this may be governed by multiple mechanisms. The following is a brief review of some of the more popular theories which attempt to explain the mechanism of ageing.

1. The free-radical theory
Free radicals are atoms or molecules that contain an unpaired electron and so are highly reactive. Within a cell, free radicals will randomly react with other structures and damage them. Free-radical damage in connective tissues can induce the cross-linkage of macromolecules such as collagen. This can render these tissues increasingly brittle. Free radicals can also inactivate enzymes, break DNA molecules, peroxidize lipids, and injure cellular membranes. In order to combat free-radical damage, the cell is equipped with a number of defence mechanisms, including antioxidants and DNA repair enzymes. Over time, however, continual bombardment of the cellular components by free radicals will render the cell progressively less able to function under stress. In addition to damaging cellular structures, these reactions are costly in terms of the energy and materials that are required to effect repairs. The net result of these cellular injuries is a reduced ability to function efficiently and replicate genetic material reliably. Since this effect is occurring throughout the body, there is a global reduction in its ability to cope with physical stresses.

2. The ageing-programme theory
This theory contends that the ageing process is actually programmed into each organism's genetic make-up. Our chromosomes may contain 'ageing' or 'senescence' genes which function as biological chronometers setting the unique pace at which each of us ages. In support of this, researchers have observed that members of various species exhibit a relatively constant lifespan, which suggests some genetic control over longevity. The strongest evidence supporting this theory was provided when Hayflick and Moorhead[9]

demonstrated that human embryonic fibroblasts grown in culture lived a finite period of 50 ± 10 replications. They also found that the cells taken from older donors were capable of fewer replications before dying. Their findings have been reproduced by other investigators.[10] In diseases such as diabetes, progeria, and Down's syndrome, premature ageing occurs at the cellular level. Perhaps understanding the genetics behind these conditions will help us better understand the ageing mechanism.

3. *The neuroendocrine theory*

The central premise of this theory is that because the neuroendocrine system is essential to nearly all of an organism's functions, any alterations in the controls exerted by this system will have far-reaching effects at the molecular, cellular, and organ levels. The functioning of this system does decline with age, which could explain the drop in physiological efficiency noted during the ageing process. While this theory can potentially explain the wide range of changes that occur with ageing, it fails to address how cells which have been isolated from the influence of the neuroendocrine system and grown in culture can still experience typical age-related alterations.[10]

4. *The altered-protein theory*

Proponents of this theory conjecture that, as we age, altered protein formation occurs. Since proteins play a central role in the structure and function of all organisms, it seems reasonable that alterations in normal protein synthesis will have widespread ramifications in terms of cellular function. Consider, for example, enzymes which are specialized proteins responsible for effecting a multitude of bodily reactions. Alterations in their structure will greatly interfere with the normal physiological operation of the cell. It is possible that intrinsic or extrinsic factors which cause DNA damage lead to errors in the synthesis of various proteins, including enzymes. Defective cellular products are not as efficient and so will handicap the cell's ability to adapt to various stresses.

5. *The waste-product accumulation theory*

This theory contends that with ageing there is a progressive accumulation of ineffective biological materials within each cell and that this ultimately impedes the cell's optimal functioning. One such compound is lipofuscin, which is a byproduct of free-radical damage. The volume of this material increases in ageing cells and can account for 7 per cent of the total intracellular volume of biological materials by the age of 90.[10] To date, there is no evidence that lipofuscin has any deleterious effect on cellular function. However, as part of this process cells may accumulate a number of materials which are noxious. The build-up of these harmful substances could inflict progressively greater amounts of damage on the cell, rendering it less efficient.

6. *The cross-linkage theory*

In this theory, it is believed that the formation of inter- and intramolecular cross-linkages is enhanced with ageing, leaving macromolecules increasingly resistant to normal degradation and turnover. Cross-linkages affect many types of macromolecules including collagen, elastin, and other connective tissue elements. As a result of this process, tissues are rendered increasingly brittle and membranes more difficult to cross. Cross-linkages also occur in molecules that are essential for cellular replication, such as DNA and RNA. It is possible that linkage of these molecules interferes

with or prevents the transcription of genetically encoded information and so drastically interferes with normal cellular functioning. Further study is required in this area.

7. *The immunological theory*

Walford proposed that age alters immunoregulatory genes such that organisms lose their ability to discriminate between self and non-self.[11] The net result of this change is an increase in the incidence of autoimmune reactions. Consequently, there is a reduction in the efficiency with which the various target organs function and the individual becomes increasingly susceptible to diseases, infections, and neoplasms. Further research is required to determine whether this theory can explain the diversity of changes seen in ageing.

The above theories represent the most popular attempts at explaining the mechanisms by which ageing occurs. Other possible explanations include DNA methylation, protein racemization, non-enzymatic glycosylation, dysdifferentiation, codon restriction, loss of ribosomal RNA genes, genetic mutation, and errors in transcriptional and translational processes.

While the above theories do not provide a definitive explanation on how and why we age, they do serve to illustrate how complex the ageing process may be. Ageing is not pathological but rather an inevitable event in which numerous factors play a role. Everyone ages in a unique pattern and it is impossible to predict the course that any individual will follow. Regardless of the individual pattern, the structural and physiological changes associated with ageing have important implications for athletic performance. The very nature of the ageing process dictates that the ageing athlete differs biologically from the younger competitor.

Inactivity

An inactive lifestyle is a far greater threat to one's continued health than the ageing process. This is disconcerting because in our highly automated society inactivity is almost a cultural objective. Why take the stairs when you can use the escalator? Why push a lawnmower when you can drive it? Why rake leaves when you can blow them away with a machine? Why walk to the corner store when you can drive? There is a time and a place for every labour-saving innovation, and individually they do not significantly alter our daily physical activity. However, collectively, these devices greatly reduce the physical activity required of the average person. Labour-saving devices were originally intended to improve efficiency and provide people with time to pursue more pleasurable pastimes. Instead of dedicating some of this free time to active living, many people elect to pursue largely sedentary interests and assume the accompanying health risks. Data from the Framingham study, and other investigations, so clearly indicates the relationship between health and physical activity, that inactivity is now considered an independent, health-risk factor.[7] Inactivity and its associated health problems are so endemic to our culture that people have begun to use the term 'hypokinetic diseases'. Conditions such as osteoporosis, atherosclerosis, obesity, hypertension, hyperlipidaemias, depression, inflexibility, and chronic fatigue are often closely associated with a sedentary lifestyle.

In addition, it is distressing that the majority of our society continues to accept inactivity as a natural consequence of ageing. So much so, that the older adult who remains physically active is often thought to be eccentric. This misconception is so firmly entrenched in our culture that many people feel ageing exercisers are gambling with their lives when, in fact, the opposite is true. It is not uncommon for an older person to be told that participating in regular exercise is unnatural. Nothing could be further from the truth. Maintaining a physically active lifestyle throughout one's life is one of the secrets to remaining healthy and productive. Staying physically active may be viewed as an option for the young, but it is essential for the maintenance of an ageing individual's health. Failing to remain active permits an excessive rate of structural and physiological loss that will threaten a person's ability to remain independent in later years. Regular exercise is one way in which the elderly can continue to live and enjoy life rather than being limited to simply existing.

Many of the changes attributed to the ageing process are actually the direct result of a sedentary lifestyle. It is estimated that inactivity accounts for more than 50 per cent of the structural and physiological decrements that can be demonstrated in a sedentary adult.[6,12] This relationship was not well recognized until a few years ago, and consequently much of the ageing research performed prior to this was biased by this 'inactivity factor'. An excellent illustration of the relative roles of ageing and inactivity in the deterioration of physiological function is provided by Kasch *et al.*[1] in a study on the effect of exercise and inactivity on the aerobic power of older men. The study consisted of two sets of 15 men and took place over a period of 23 years. One group participated in an aerobically oriented fitness programme, while the other group did no regular exercise during the study period. At the conclusion of the study the two groups were tested and the results are shown below.[1]

1. The exercisers reduced their bodyweight by an average of 3.4 kg while the non-exercisers gained an average of 3.2 kg.

2. The exercisers had an average of 15.9 per cent body fat while the non-exercisers averaged 25.7 per cent.

3. The exercisers had an average resting pulse rate 10 beats/minute lower than that of the non-exercisers.

4. Blood pressures were noted to be higher in the non-exercisers, with 9 of the 15 being clinically hypertensive at the conclusion of the study.

5. The maximum oxygen uptake ($\dot{V}O_2$max) of the exercisers decreased by an average of 13 per cent, while the non-exercisers showed an average decline of 41 per cent.

6. The maximum attainable heart rate of the exercisers was an average of 20 beats/min higher than that of the non-exercisers.

Despite the small number of subjects involved in this study, the results strongly suggest that inactivity makes a large contribution to the physical changes that we see in many ageing individuals. The $\dot{V}O_2$max results are particularly striking because they suggest that only 32 per cent of the loss seen in the non-exercisers could be attributed to ageing, with the remaining 68 per cent of the loss resulting from disuse. This suggests that the effect of disuse on the structural and physiological decrement may be even greater than originally estimated. Dr Cooper has conducted extensive physiological evaluations of numerous world-class athletes. Based on his findings, he concludes that, 'Most of the decline that comes with age isn't inevitable at all. It's caused by disuse.'[13]

One question that needs to be addressed is: 'Why do these disuse changes occur in the first place?' The answer lies in the fact that one of the basic rules governing the economical operation of the body is the 'use it or lose it' principle. Management of the entire body is controlled by this unavoidable biological law. In practical terms, this law states that if a particular tissue is not being used then why waste energy and materials maintaining it. This is inefficient and as such is bad biological business. Anyone who has worn a cast can attest to the enthusiasm with which the body adheres to this principle. After only 6 weeks' immobilization the injured limb usually emerges with marked atrophy and a significantly reduced range of motion. The body appears to make no distinction between inactivity and immobilization. In both cases, a given body part is not being used and therefore some of its components could be better utilized elsewhere, or eliminated. In our current economic climate, many corporations are employing the same principle in order to remain competitive.

Structural and physiological changes

A number of well-documented structural and physiological changes occur in the ageing body. These changes are probably initiated at the cellular level and are quantitative, qualitative, and regulatory in nature. The net result is a reduction in the ageing individual's functional reserves such that he or she is less able to handle physiological stresses. It should also be noted that age-related changes have been identified in virtually every organ system, and individually these changes can have significant implications. A good example of this would be changes in the neuroendocrine system which impacts on virtually every cell in the body. However, since the effective operation of the body depends on a collection of highly complex and integrated activities, no change in one component should be considered in isolation from changes in the others. Thus, even if researchers are able to identify the specific changes that occur as a result of ageing, interpreting their significance will be very complicated. When reviewing the changes associated with ageing, it is important to recognize that ageing is not a disease and that there are no specific symptoms or sensations permitting an individual to suddenly identify that he or she is ageing. All the alterations occur so subtly that the individual fails to recognize them. It is only when the person is subjected to evaluation with sophisticated equipment or to the maximal demands of an athletic event that functional losses become undeniable. It also important to note that people appear to age at different rates. In other words, two individuals with the same chronological age may be biologically many years apart.

Cardiovascular changes

Age-related alterations in the cardiovascular system have been the focus of attention for many years. This is undoubtedly because cardiovascular disease is a major cause of morbidity and mortality. There is considerable contradictory information in this area because it is often difficult to distinguish between changes due to ageing, inactivity, disease processes, or a combination of these factors. Physiologists consider that $\dot{V}O_2$max is the single most reliable indicator of cardiovascular fitness. Evidence indicates that beyond 35 years of age there is an inevitable decline in $\dot{V}O_2$max such that by the age of 60 it is often 80 per cent of what it was at the age of 20.[14-16] This represents a rate of decline of 0.5 to 1.0 per cent annually and has important implications in events requiring maximum aerobic effort. The $\dot{V}O_2$max of deconditioned or sedentary individuals may decrease at a rate in excess of 1 per cent annually. The more active an individual is, the slower the rate at which his or her $\dot{V}O_2$max will decline. For élite masters athletes the annual rate of decline may be less than 0.1 per cent, a tenth of the rate of loss seen in inactive people.[7,17] One of the critical factors in minimizing this loss of $\dot{V}O_2$max appears to be the maintenance of a high-intensity, training programme.[17]

Several investigators contend that this reduction in $\dot{V}O_2$max is due to the linear decline in maximum attainable heart rate (**MAHR**) that occurs with age.[18] The MAHR can be roughly estimated using the formula:

$$MAHR = 220 - \text{years of age} \pm 10.$$

While the reduction in MAHR is undoubtedly a factor in the age-related decline in $\dot{V}O_2$max it is unlikely to be the only factor. $\dot{V}O_2$max is a complex value that depends on a number of physiological variables including cardiovascular, pulmonary, and muscle function, as well as aerobic fitness. Since ageing is associated with diminished capacity in all these areas, it seems more reasonable to assume that the cause of the age-related decline in $\dot{V}O_2$max is multifactorial. Research has clearly demonstrated that with proper training older exercisers are capable of making significant increases in their aerobic power.[19] Green and Crouse[20] conducted a meta-analysis and found that 30 min of aerobically demanding exercise three times a week was sufficient to produce improvements in $\dot{V}O_2$max and that it did not matter what the aerobic activity was.

Cardiac output is a measure of how much blood the heart can pump in a given period of time. Mathematically, it is calculated as the product of stroke volume and heart rate. Research suggests that as we age stroke volume and heart rate are reduced at high workloads and so cardiac output must also decline.[18,21,22] This reduction in cardiac output will profoundly affect an athlete's aerobic work capacity because it reduces the amount of oxygen-rich blood that can be delivered to the working tissues. It should be noted that while MAHR does not improve with regular exercise, stroke volume can be improved through changes in preload and afterload.[23] With ageing, the heart returns to resting rates more slowly following maximal and submaximal efforts. This has important implications for ageing competitors who incorporate interval-type training into their programmes. In general, masters athletes will require longer recovery times between intervals than will younger athletes of a similar fitness status. To ensure that adequate recovery periods are taken between intervals, all athletes should be taught to monitor their heart rate.

Excluding disease processes, the functional changes noted above seem to occur with only minor structural alterations to the heart itself. The interstitial volume of collagen, reticulin, and elastin fibres increases, resulting in a condition known as fibrosis. While these increases are generally small, they do render the myocardium less compliant. This may be functionally insignificant at rest, but when the cardiovascular system is operating maximally it could limit ventricular filling and so reduce cardiac output. In support of this, several authors have noted an age-related decline in cardiac ejection fraction at high workloads only.[24] Ageing myocardium accumulates lipofuscin, the significance of which is uncertain. Amyloid is another protein which is found in the hearts of most people over 90 years of age, but seldom in those under 60.[25] This change is also

of uncertain significance. The cardiac conduction system is also influenced by the ageing process. In general, collagen, elastin, reticulin, and fatty tissues infiltrate the conducting tissues. This fibrotic process occurs in conjunction with a loss of the specialized conducting tissues. For instance, between the ages of 20 and 75, up to 90 per cent of the pacemaker cells located in the sinoatrial node may disappear.[25] While the significance of these changes is unknown, they may contribute to the age-related decline in maximum heart rate. Controversy exists as to whether the contractile properties of the myocardium decrease with age.[18,25,26] In addition to the changes discussed above, the following have also been observed.

1. Myocardial responsiveness to catecholamine stimulation is reduced.[18,22,25]

2. The collagen fibres of the pericardium straighten, rendering the pericardium thicker and less compliant.[25]

3. The valvular structures experience collagen deposition and degeneration, lipid accumulation, and calcium deposition. These changes serve to stiffen these tissues, but their effect on performance is unknown.[25]

4. The circumference of all four cardiac valves increases.[25]

5. The ageing heart may undergo geometric alterations: it may shorten, ventricular septal thickness increases, the left atrium dilates, and the volume of the left ventricle is diminished.[25]

6. There are reduced tissue levels of noradrenaline, acetylcholine, and adenyl cyclase.[18]

It is difficult to be certain whether these changes are the direct result of the ageing process, disease, inactivity, or a combination of factors. It is also difficult to determine how much, if any, impact they have on performance. However, when considering the issue of maximum performance, even minor alterations may have significant implications. On the whole, the observed cardiac changes serve to reduce myocardial compliance, reduce the maximum attainable heart rate, decrease cardiac output, and lower $\dot{V}O_2$max. A direct consequence of this is that the ageing heart must work harder to meet the metabolic demands of the body at any given workload. This loss of cardiovascular efficiency is a major factor in the progressive decline in aerobic performance noted with increasing age and is clearly evident in the marathon records for various ages (Fig. 1).

Research by Zauber and Zauber[27] strongly suggests that the haematological values of healthy subjects over the age of 85 are the same as those of young adults. This includes values for blood volume, red blood cell count, haemoglobin, haematocrit, serum iron, erythrocyte sedimentation rate, and white blood cell count. Zauber and Zauber[27] also found no significant reduction in the haematological response to stress with ageing. This indicates that the ageing competitor will probably be able to elevate his or her haemoglobin levels in response to regular, aerobically demanding exercise.

The vascular system is by no means exempt from the relentless alterations of the ageing process. In fact, this is one area where considerable change is often noted. However, care must be taken to differentiate age-related modifications from those caused by pathological processes such as atherosclerosis. While atherosclerosis is a disease process, its universality has led some authors to question

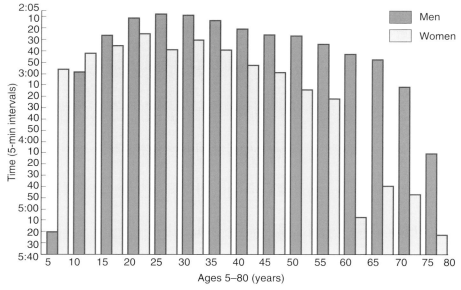

Fig. 1 Marathon records by age—United States records taken at ages 5 to 80 in 5-year intervals, and correct to 1 January 1983.

whether it should be considered as a normal part of ageing. While this distinction may be academic, the reality is that virtually every ageing adult, regardless of his or her lifetime activity pattern, will have some degree of atherosclerotic change in his or her vascular system. The extent of this disease in asymptomatic individuals varies enormously. An insidious process, atherosclerosis narrows the lumens of blood vessels, leaving them less able to supply blood to a given area. At the same time, it also reduces vessel-wall extensibility. These changes begin well before the age of 40 and have been noted during autopsies of teenagers. Independent of this disease process, the vasculature experiences enhanced collagen deposition. This collagen becomes progressively more rigid as its cross-linkages mature and undergo stabilization. Calcium is also deposited into the elastin fibres found in vessel walls, a phenomenon referred to as elastocalcinosis. The end result of these changes are vessels which are narrower and offer greater resistance to blood flow. In terms of maintaining adequate circulation, greater kinetic energy will be required to overcome vascular resistance, and therefore cardiac workload is noticeably increased with no corresponding increase in cardiac output.

Injection studies, where the blood supply to various organs and tissues are injected with media, have also shown that ageing is associated with a concomitant decline in the microvascular supply to muscle, major organs, and peripheral tissues.[15] This has a number of important implications. First, it is a major factor in limiting the body's functional organ reserves, making it increasingly difficult to maintain homeostasis when stressed. Second, it reduces the volume of blood that can be delivered to the working tissues. Without a continuous supply of oxygen and substrates, these tissues would be unable to function at an intense level for very long. This blood flow is also essential for removing many of the waste products generated in the working tissues, which if allowed to accumulate would seriously hinder performance. In addition, these changes reduce the body's ability to respond to an injury and so may alter the rate of recovery.

Connective tissue changes

Connective tissues function to provide support and structure to the various components of our body. Since connective tissues are major constituents of most body tissues, they make a major contribution to their mechanical properties. In fact, the different mechanical properties of numerous tissues are largely dictated by their unique combination of connective tissues. This is an economical design because by using the same basic ingredients and arranging them in unique combinations the body is able to adapt and meet its various structural and support requirements. Employing this amazing versatility, the connective tissues can satisfy the enormously different physical requirements of structures as dissimilar as the cornea and the medial meniscus.

Connective tissues such as fasciae, tendons, and ligaments were once thought to be entirely inert structures. After synthesis they were believed to reside passively in the body, performing their structural and support roles. We now know that these tissues are highly dynamic in nature. They are constantly undergoing modifications in an effort to adapt to the stresses to which they are subjected. As a rule, physical activity serves to stimulate connective tissue hypertrophy while inactivity promotes atrophic changes. This is yet another example of the 'use it or lose it' principle that is such an innate part of our physical well being.

It is obvious from the above that not all connective tissues are the same. Their compliance and tensile strength are determined by their unique combination of proteins such as elastin, connectin, collagen, and proteoglycans. These basic macromolecules are arranged in a variety of combinations to create the framework for most of the body's tissues. Collagen accounts for approximately 30 per cent of our total body protein, making it by far the most abundant connective tissue element. It is a major component of basement membranes, intervertebral discs, blood vessels, teeth, bone, cartilage, tendon, skin, and ligaments. It is also present in nearly all organs where it serves to hold cells together in discrete units. In all, five major types of collagen are recognized. Each differs in its amino-acid composition and sequencing, as well as the type and extent of cross-linkage bonding.[28,29] Their individual molecular designs provide each type of collagen with unique properties of compliance and tensile strength. The degree of either of these properties is determined by the amount of cross-linkage bonding present. The greater the amount of tissue rigidity required, the greater the cross-linkage bonding. Thus the collagen found in bone is far more heavily cross-linked than that found in tendons. These cross-linkages occur both inter- and intramolecularly and provide collagen with a greater tensile strength than steel. It is estimated that a load of 10 to 40 kg is required to rupture a collagen fibre 1 mm in diameter.[30,31]

Many of the age-related alterations that occur in collagen are focused on the cross-linkages. As collagen ages, its molecular stability increases and so the tissue in which it resides becomes less compliant. The physical evidence supporting this change is that ageing collagen is increasingly less soluble and thermally more stable.[32] This enhanced stability was initially attributed to an increase in the number of cross-linkages present in the collagen molecule. It has since been shown that shortly after being synthesized a collagen fibre processes all the cross-linkages it will ever have. It is believed that during maturation cross-linkages that were once reducible undergo stabilization, leaving the collagen fibre progressively less compliant.[18,29] It should also be noted that protein cross-linkage also occurs via free-radical damage and non-enzymatic glycosylation processes.[33] Ageing also reduces the volume of ground substance surrounding collagen fibres such that the gel–fibre ratio is decreased. A high gel–fibre ratio helps to keep the collagen fibres separated, while a low ratio may allow for increased intermolecular bonding between collagen fibres and other molecules.

The rate at which collagen loses its compliance can be influenced by several factors, such as physical activity and hormonal changes. Exercise seems to enhance the rate of collagen turnover. In this way, exercise shortens the lifespan of collagen molecules and retards the process of maturational stabilization. This suggests that exercise will help maintain the youthfulness of these tissues. Hormones such as insulin, thyroxine, and corticosteroids have also been implicated in the ageing of collagen. Hamlin *et al.*[34] found that collagen isolated from the tissues of a 40-year-old, diabetic patient resembled those found in healthy individuals over 100 years old. Excessive, non-enzymatic glycosylation occurs in the diabetic state and may be the mechanism by which the collagen of a diabetic person ages so rapidly. Since hormonal changes accompany the normal ageing process, it is reasonable to postulate that these changes may influence the collagen structure of the senior athlete.

Elastin is found in most connective tissues. It is the major component of the elastic fibres found in large quantities in the skin, vasculature, and ligaments. These unique fibres possess physical properties which allow them to stretch several times their length and then return to their original size once the traction forces are withdrawn. Elastin molecules undergo age-related changes similar to those seen in collagen. More specifically, their cross-linkages undergo maturational stabilization. They also experience an increase in their polar amino-acid composition.[35] Microscopic examination shows that ageing elastic tissues lose their regularity and that their lamellae are visibly ragged and slender. The net result of all these changes is that ageing elastin fibres become increasingly brittle and more easily subject to fracture.[29] This has significant

implications for ageing athletes who depend on their vascular and ligamentous tissues during all athletic performances.

Ageing connective tissues also experience a reduction in their water content. The consequences of this change include a reduction in shock-absorbing capacity and a loss of tissue compliance. Both of these losses will substantially alter the ageing body's ability to effectively absorb and neutralize the forces generated during physical activity. Considered in their totality, all the age-related alterations in connective tissue are important because they significantly alter the mechanical properties of many tissues and render the ageing competitor increasingly vulnerable to injury.

Skin changes

Skin is not an organ in the classic sense, but it is often referred to as a functional organ because of the number of critical functions that it plays. This is especially evident when a person experiences extensive burns and requires extraordinary medical efforts to ensure survival. Skin functions as a protective barrier against trauma, an energy storage site, a boundary against infection, a barrier against environmental insults such as ultraviolet light and rain, and as an important component of our thermoregulatory system. With so many roles to play, any age-related skin change could have far-reaching implications.

Skin ages as a result of intrinsic structural and functional changes in combination with extrinsic influences such as ultraviolet light, wind, and thermal stresses. While these extrinsic factors are not innate to the ageing process, they are mentioned because of the universality with which people are exposed to them. The very nature of most sporting activities exposes ageing competitors to more sun, wind, and cold than the average inactive person.

Wrinkling is an obvious superficial feature that we all identify as a sign of ageing. However, most age-related changes occur below the skin surface and have direct applications to the ageing athlete. One of the most evident morphological changes is the thinning of the epidermal, dermal, and subcutaneous skin layers.[36] This thinning substantially compromises the skin's insulatory ability, leaving the person more vulnerable to cold injury. It also reduces the trauma cushion that skin provides for the underlying tissues, and body contact of insufficient magnitude to cause a contusion in a younger person might cause one in an older competitor. Ageing skin also has fewer elastin fibres and increasing maturational stabilization of its collagen fibres. These changes alter the viscoelastic properties of ageing skin such that it is less able to respond to deforming forces. Thus the ageing process leaves skin increasingly fragile and so more susceptible to damage from even mild trauma. Bumps, scratches, shearing forces, and wear and tear are unavoidable facts of life for every athlete. When exposed to these forms of mechanical trauma, ageing skin can tear at intensities that would leave younger skin unaffected. This should be kept in mind, particularly when applying adhesive tape to the skin of an ageing athlete. All adhesive tape should be removed very carefully to avoid tearing the underlying skin, as its adhesive properties may exceed the skin's mechanical strength.

The interdigitations, or rete pegs, between the epidermis and the underlying dermis (Fig. 2) ensure that these two skin layers adhere to each other. With ageing, these interdigitations diminish, making it easier to separate the epidermis from the dermis, a phenomenon

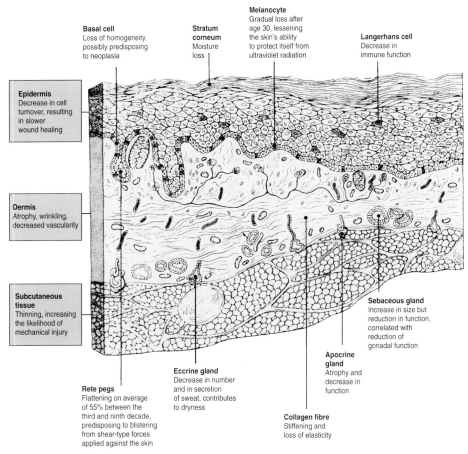

Basal cell
Loss of homogeneity, possibly predisposing to neoplasia

Stratum corneum
Moisture loss

Melanocyte
Gradual loss after age 30, lessening the skin's ability to protect itself from ultraviolet radiation

Langerhans cell
Decrease in immune function

Epidermis
Decrease in cell turnover, resulting in slower wound healing

Dermis
Atrophy, wrinkling, decreased vascularity

Subcutaneous tissue
Thinning, increasing the likelihood of mechanical injury

Sebaceous gland
Increase in size but reduction in function, correlated with reduction of gonadal function

Apocrine gland
Atrophy and decrease in function

Rete pegs
Flattening on average of 55% between the third and ninth decade, predisposing to blistering from shear-type forces applied against the skin

Eccrine gland
Decrease in number and in secretion of sweat, contributes to dryness

Collagen fibre
Stiffening and loss of elasticity

Fig. 2 Anatomy of skin and the ageing process. (Reproduced from Femtu NA, *et al.* Common problems of aging skin. *Patient Care* 1990: 33, with permission.)

that occurs when blisters form. This increased tendency to blister will hamper performance in sports where friction forces are a major factor. Once formed, an older competitor's blisters will heal more slowly and are more likely to become infected. With ageing, the capillary density in the peripheral tissues is diminished and the remaining vasculature is thinner and more fragile. These changes increase the ageing competitor's tendency to bruise following trauma. Some loss of sensory acuity may occur in ageing peripheral tissues, which means that ageing athletes can experience greater injury to their cutaneous tissues before becoming aware of it. The number of immunocompetent cells present in the skin is also reduced during ageing. There is diminished T-cell function and Langerhans cells die off, rendering the older individual more vulnerable to skin infections and neoplasms. Fingernails and toenails are extensions of the skin and are also altered with age. Ageing nails are thinner and so more prone to injury. Since ageing nails grow more slowly, the recovery from such an injury is often delayed.

Ageing skin is also less able to protect the body from the damaging effects of ultraviolet light. After the age of 30, an individual loses approximately 2 per cent of his or her melanocytes annually.[36] Melanocytes are specialized skin cells that produce the pigment melanin when exposed to ultraviolet radiation. The resultant 'sun tan' is a protective mechanism designed to shield the body from further ultraviolet injury. The age-related reduction in the melano-

cyte population leaves a person increasingly susceptible to sun damage. To make matters worse, ageing skin displays a reduced inflammatory response to injury. Sunburn is a typical example of such a response. Thus the ageing person will tolerate longer exposures to the sun before becoming sunburned. People frequently misinterpret this change as indicating they have developed greater sun tolerance, when in reality, they are still experiencing ultraviolet-induced damage. Thus older skin is at increased risk of injury, not only because it has a reduced defence capacity but also because its early warning systems do not work as well. This is of concern for two reasons. First, athletes tend to spend more time in the sun than non-athletes. Second, the cumulative effect of sun damage is important. The older people become, the greater the volume of damage that accumulates and the greater the risk of developing skin cancers. Ageing athletes can reduce their risk of skin injury in several ways.

1. Wear a hat or cap when out in the sun, particularly for prolonged activities such as 18 holes of golf or a triathlon.

2. Wear light-coloured clothing to reflect as much of the sun's rays as possible.

3. Exercise during periods of the day when the sun is the least intense, i.e. before 10 a.m. and after 4 p.m.

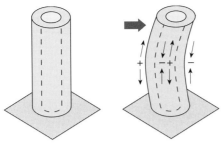

Fig. 3 The response of bone to compressive and tensile forces. (The large arrow represents a force applied to the bone.) The concave surfaces of the bone cylinder carry a negative charge, and the convex surfaces carry a positive charge. These charges affect the loss and gain of bone tissue. (Redrawn from ref. 41, with permission.)

4. Use a sunscreen with a minimum sun-protective factor (**SPF**) of 15 that protects against both UVA and UVB rays.

5. Have skin lesions that are slow to heal or moles that develop changes, examined by a physician.

Skeletal changes

Some of the best understood age-related alterations occur in the skeletal system. Bony tissue is a complex matrix of organic and inorganic materials. This combination yields a product that is lightweight and yet capable of withstanding a lifetime of mechanical stress. Bones are dynamic tissues and will undergo structural adaptations in direct response to the physical demands placed upon them. This quality was recognized over 100 years ago when Wolff's law of anatomy was first proposed. This law basically states that: 'The robustness of bone is in direct proportion to the physical forces applied to it'.[37] Bones become mechanically stronger when regularly stressed and weaker when left unchallenged. This hypertrophic response will only occur in the specific areas of the skeleton that are experiencing the extra forces. The best example of this is the unilateral bony enlargement that occurs in the dominant arms of baseball pitchers and tennis players. This is undoubtedly a protective response aimed at preparing the dominant arm to cope with the stresses to which it is being subjected. Bassett and Becker[38] suggest that the mechanism for the local control of bony growth is electrical. They believe that osseous tissues function like piezoelectric crystals that convert mechanical stresses into electrical energy. When a bone is mechanically stressed, the segment that undergoes compressive forces produces a negative electric charge while the segment under tension becomes positive. It is this distribution of charges that controls the level of cellular activity in bone and permits them to respond and adapt to the specific stresses that they encounter (Fig. 3). Any condition that compromises a bone's architecture or its adaptability will reduce its resilience to mechanical stresses and leave it vulnerable to structural breakdown. These breakdowns can occur gradually, as seen in overuse-induced stress fractures, or instantly, as in traumatic fractures.

Without a doubt, the greatest threat to the skeletal integrity of the ageing adult is osteoporosis. Osteoporosis is an idiopathic condition in which the rate of bone resorption exceeds the rate of bone formation. This imbalance leads to a progressive loss of bone mass and is a major concern because bone strength is directly related to the volume of bone mass. It is an insidious condition that affects over 25 million North Americans, and often the first indication of its existence is when a fracture occurs following a relatively minor trauma. These initial fractures often involve the hip or vertebral body, and are associated with a high rate of morbidity and mortality. Until recently, it was believed that the rate of bone loss in osteoporosis was gender specific, with women experiencing losses two to three times more rapidly than men. It now appears that there are two different types of osteoporosis. Type I osteoporosis affects women only and occurs with the loss of oestrogen production that accompanies the menopause. This process involves an annual reduction in bone mass of approximately 0.6 per cent.[39] Type II osteoporosis affects both sexes and occurs as a direct result of the ageing process. It is believed that this loss is the result of an age-related decline in osteoblast activity and accounts for an annual reduction in bone mass of approximately 0.3 per cent.[39] Clearly, the rate of bone-mass depletion experienced by the average woman exceeds that of the average man. The injustice does not end here. Often, men do not appear to experience bone-mass losses until the age of 50, often with no sequelae until the eighth decade of life. Women, however, frequently begin losing bone mass in their early thirties. The combination of an earlier onset and higher rate of loss, means that by the time many women have reached their seventies they have lost more than 30 per cent of their total bone mass and are considerably more vulnerable to fracture than they were at age 20.[40–42] The sedentary lifestyle so commonly associated with advancing age is also a major factor in the loss of bone mass. In studies involving individuals who have been immobilized for various reasons (astronauts, quadriplegics, and people with casts) dramatic bone-mass depletion has been observed over relatively short periods. Clearly, age-related bone loss is a serious threat to every ageing individual, including ageing athletes.

The aetiology of osteoporosis appears to be multifactorial. Reductions in skeletal blood flow, insufficient calcium intake, decreased gastrointestinal calcium absorption, hormonal factors such as reduced oestrogen, physical inactivity, and genetics have all been implicated in this process. As far as ageing athletes are concerned, several critical concepts should be kept in mind.

1. Since the age-related loss of bone mass is a universal process, it must be assumed that every ageing athlete is to some extent osteoporotic.

2. With all the variables involved in this process, no two individuals of the same age will have experienced the same volume of losses.

3. Almost without exception, ageing female athletes will have greater bone-mass losses than men of the same age.

4. There are no obvious symptoms indicating that an individual is seriously osteoporotic. Often the first indication of a problem is when the competitor experiences a fracture following minimal trauma.

5. Loss of bony mechanical strength is a significant threat to people who have lived largely sedentary lives and begin exercising after the age of 50. It is critical that they control their initial enthusiasm and 'start slowly and progress gradually'. This strategy will allow their skeletal systems sufficient time to adapt and so reduce the incidence of stress fractures.

6. Ageing bone does not appear to lose its ability to respond to mechanical stresses. Individuals in their eighties have experienced bone-mass improvements in response to activities involving muscular traction and gravitational forces.[43] These changes include increases in such things as thickness, strength, calcium concentration, nitrogen concentration, and hydroxyproline and DNA content. Thus it appears that regular physical activity not only slows down the rate of bony demineralization but, to some extent, may even reverse it. Given this potential, exercise offers the ageing individual a greater opportunity to maintain skeletal integrity than any pharmaceutical agent.

Respiratory changes

While a functioning respiratory system is a requisite for life, an efficient respiratory system is essential for athletic success. Unfortunately, with the passage of time, the respiratory system falls prey to the deleterious influence of a number of factors, including previous pulmonary illnesses, environmental pollutants, tobacco smoke, a sedentary lifestyle, and the ageing process. No one is certain how much each of these factors contributes to the respiratory alterations that accompany ageing. However, studies have attempted to control for the above variables and concluded that there is a progressive deterioration in respiratory function that is directly attributable to the ageing process.[44] Many of these changes manifest themselves as an increased sense of respiratory effort during physical exertion. Consequently, ageing athletes tend to experience breathlessness at lighter workloads than when they were younger.

A number of architectural alterations occur in ageing pulmonary tissues. For example, there is a progressive degradation of the collagen and elastin fibre content of the pulmonary parenchyma.[29,40,45] In its most advanced state this deterioration is referred to as senile emphysema. The rate at which this degradation occurs is increased considerably in individuals whose lungs are repeatedly insulted by tobacco smoke and the multitude of environmental pollutants present in the atmosphere. While this is not truly an age-dependent phenomenon, it is included here because these noxious agents have a cumulative effect on everyone living in an industrialized society.

This damage to the pulmonary tissues significantly compromises the structural integrity of the lung and reduces its capacity for elastic recoil. The lung depends on elastic recoil to aid expiration. Since recoil requires no energy, it reduces the active workload associated with breathing. As progressively greater amounts of elastic recoil are lost, the work associated with breathing increases. This loss of structural support for the pulmonary tissues will also permit airway closure at higher lung volumes and so increase the older adult's residual lung volumes. While this is occurring, there is a generalized increase in the rigidity of many of the chest-wall structures. The intercostal musculature becomes less compliant, the costovertebral joints stiffen, and the costochondral cartilages become less elastic. Consequently, greater physical effort is needed to overcome chest-wall resistance during inspiration. Thus ageing is clearly associated with an increased workload during both inspiration and expiration. deVries[47] believes that this could account for as much as a 20 per cent increase in respiratory effort. These changes will obviously hinder the performance of older athletes who compete in aerobically demanding activities.

Ageing respiratory musculature experiences both a loss of strength and a progressive increase in its connective tissue content. These weaker and stiffer muscles are less able to generate the inspiratory pressures needed to ventilate the lower lung segments where blood perfusion is the greatest. This leads to ventilation–perfusion mismatches whereby blood is delivered to lung tissues that are not being inflated with oxygen-rich air. Consequently, respiratory gas exchange is less efficient. With ageing there is a reduction in the small vessel density of the lung parenchyma. Collagen deposition may also occur at the level of the alveolar capillary basement membrane. If this occurs, it will increase the diffusion barrier over which O_2 and CO_2 must be exchanged during respiration.

The above changes in the respiratory system manifest themselves in a number of specific functional decrements.

1. Inspiratory capacity is reduced.
2. Forced expiratory volume in 1 second (FEV_1) (a measure of the volume of air that can be forcibly exhaled in 1 s) is reduced.
3. Residual lung volume is increased.
4. Total lung capacity is reduced.
5. Tidal volume (the volume of air exchanged with each normal respiration) is reduced, which means that the older person must breathe more frequently in order to maintain an adequate volume of oxygen exchange.
6. Vital capacity is reduced (vital capacity may decline by as much as 25 ml annually beyond the age of 20[6,45]).
7. Inspiratory airflow is reduced.

The importance of many of the specific changes that occur in the ageing respiratory system is uncertain. Collectively, however, these changes gradually reduce the respiratory system's functional reserve. This reserve is normally large enough to ensure that there are no apparent functional changes while the individual is at rest. However, when ageing exercisers begin an aerobically demanding activity, such as cross-country skiing, they will experience respiratory distress at a lower physiological workload than they would have in their twenties or thirties. Basically, the ageing competitor's respiratory system is less efficient and progressively less able to deliver oxygen to the body's working tissues. This is one of the major reasons for the age-related deterioration in performance seen in events demanding maximum aerobic efforts. A comparison of the winning times in the men's marathon at the 1995 World Veterans Athletics Championships for the age group 40 to 44 (2 h 30 min 29 s) and 80 to 84 (4 h 38 min 43 s) serves to illustrate just how significant these changes are. It must be clearly understood that the rate at which many of these respiratory changes occur is considerably increased in the sedentary individual. Regular exercise substantially reduces the extent of these losses, with the most significant contribution being the strengthening of the respiratory musculature.

Skeletal muscle changes

Skeletal muscle is a vital element in athletic performance, regardless of the age of the competitor or the event. There has been considerable research in this area and a great deal is known about the ultrastructure of muscle fibres and how they function during muscular contraction. Unfortunately, our understanding of the age-related changes in muscle tissue has been confused by the failure of many researchers to control for the deleterious influence of inactivity. In fact, many of the muscle changes attributed to the ageing process occur in younger individuals who are immobilized for even brief periods. It appears that the ageing process is accompanied by a number of alterations in muscle tissue and that a sedentary lifestyle enhances the rate at which they occur.

Ageing is accompanied by a loss of muscle tissue such that by 60 to 70 years of age, muscle mass has decreased by 25 to 30 per cent.[46] Superficially, this loss may not be apparent because many muscle fibres are replaced by fat or connective tissues and so muscle girth is maintained. At the cellular level there is a loss of muscle fibres and those that do remain undergo atrophic change.[47] It should be noted that the elements remaining show no apparent alterations in contractile protein.[48] Larsson et al.[49] have shown a selective loss of the type II (fast-twitch) fibre population, with the type I (slow-twitch) fibre population remaining fairly stable. As a result of this shift, there is a relative increase in the type I fibre population. This change is probably unrelated to the ageing process and more likely due to a combination of motor-unit remodelling and the differential use made of these fibre types during ageing. Type I fibres are recruited extensively for the postural and lower intensity activities that dominate the lives of most elderly people, whereas type II fibres are employed in more explosive activities such as sprinting and are utilized less frequently as people age. As motor-unit remodelling occurs, the regularly used type I fibre population will maintain its innervations, while the less utilized type II fibre population experiences denervation atrophy.[46] Thus, with advancing age, less muscle is available for use and what remains available is increasingly dominated by the type I fibre population. Research has shown that regular use of the fast-twitch fibre population will help prevent its relative loss.[48,50] Hormonal changes may also play a role in the age-related loss of muscle mass. The anabolic properties of testosterone and growth hormone make them important factors in the maintenance of muscle mass. Both these hormones are produced in diminishing quantities as people age.[51]

Muscle remains biochemically stable during ageing. The levels of both the aerobic and anaerobic muscle enzymes are consistent with those of younger individuals in terms of their activity per unit of muscle weight.[48] In other words, while older athletes have less muscle tissue available, the muscle they do have retains its normal enzyme levels. This suggests that with appropriate training, ageing muscles should have considerable potential for improvement in the areas of strength and endurance—something which experience and research have proven to be true.

The capillary-to-fibre ratio refers to the number of capillaries that make contact with a given muscle fibre. This is an important concept because it determines the maximum distance over which oxygen and nutrients must diffuse before reaching each working muscle fibre. The larger this ratio, the greater the volume of oxygen that can be delivered to working tissues and the greater is the capacity for aerobic work. Plyley[52] has reported a very small decrease in the capillary-to-fibre ratio in older sedentary men compared with younger sedentary men. However, he did not compare younger and older athletes. According to Plyley, ageing individuals can respond to the stimulus of regular exercise by increasing their capillary density. Based on this, there is no reason to suspect that ageing is responsible for a significant change in capillary-to-fibre ratios. However, it is possible that the increase in the non-muscle tissue within muscle will serve to increase the distance over which gas exchange must occur and that this can contribute to the $\dot{V}O_2$max reductions noted with ageing.[53]

A motor unit consists of a motor nerve and all the muscle fibres that it innervates. With ageing, there are fewer available muscle fibres in each motor unit and possibly fewer motor units.[26] Because of these changes, less contractile tissue can be utilized when a motor unit is recruited. While the bottom line here is a progressive loss of strength, these losses are not as dramatic as might be anticipated. Meltzer studied the performances of American Olympic-style weightlifters and found their performances declined, on average, 1.0 to 1.5 per cent annually beyond the age of 30.[54] This rate remained relatively constant until the age 70 when it increased significantly. Grassi found similar results studying the vertical-jump performances of masters track and field athletes competing in power-oriented events.[54] Studies show that, with training, older adults can experience significant improvements in their strength. It appears that the mechanism by which ageing athletes achieve strength-gains differs from that of younger competitors. Young athletes realize strength-increases primarily through muscular hypertrophy, whereas older athletes appear to increase their strength mainly through improved motor-unit recruitment. Thus young athletes improve by developing more contractile elements, while ageing athletes must learn to use what muscle they have more efficiently.[26] These observations were made on the basis of studies of relatively short duration. Long-term investigations are required to determine whether ageing athletes are capable of muscular hypertrophy.

The contractile speed of muscle decreases with age, and this may, in part, result from a delay in nerve impulse transmission at the motor end-plate. This has enormous implications for athletic performance. Power is the ability to do work over time. In an explosive event such as the javelin, the most successful competitors can apply the greatest amount of force to the javelin over the maximum velocity of muscle contraction. Damon[55] has shown that the maximum velocity of muscle contraction possible against any given mass decreases with age. These detriments exist for isometric, concentric, and eccentric muscle contractions. In other words, ageing javelin throwers will be unable to accelerate the javelin as rapidly as they once could, and so their performance will suffer. This may serve to explain why it has been the power events in which ageing athletes have traditionally fared the poorest in comparison with their younger opponents.

Some of the other muscle structural changes that have been attributed to the ageing process are described below.

1. Grouping of fibre types has been observed on muscle biopsy, supporting the possibility that neurogenic changes occur as muscle ages.[56]

2. Alnaqeeb et al.[32] have shown that there is an increase in the collagen content of ageing muscle. Since collagen is a relatively non-compliant substance, the musculature of ageing athletes becomes progressively stiffer. This will hamper performance and increase the potential for injury.

3. Ultrastructural alterations have been reported by Sato *et al.*[57], but their athletic significance is unknown. Type I fibres show Z-band streaming and the formation of nemalin-like structures. Type II fibres exhibit fragmentation, increased lipofuscin, and loss of Z-materials.

4. Lipofuscin granules develop, but the significance of this is unknown.[33]

5. Mitochondria are one of the principal intracellular organelles responsible for energy production. Studies have shown no change in their density within ageing muscle, but it is uncertain whether or not their volume decreases.[58]

To reiterate, many of the structural alterations attributed to ageing muscle have also been noted in the musculature of immobilized younger individuals. How much of the changes are truly the result of ageing or disuse is difficult to say. It should be noted that in studying ageing muscle tissue, Klitgaard *et al.*[59] found that the muscle biopsies of older men who had done resistance training for most of their lives resembled those of 20-year-olds, while the biopsies of the sedentary older men participating in the study showed the changes that have typically been labelled as age-related. The net result of the observed age-related changes is a loss of strength, endurance, mass, compliance, and speed of contraction. These losses translate into a significant deterioration in physical performance potential. The good news is that ageing muscle tissue appears to retain its ability to respond to training stimuli such that structural and functional improvements can be achieved at any age.[26]

Nervous system changes

The nervous system is a complex collection of several billion cells that function as the body's internal communication network. Even more impressive are the innumerable synaptic connections that permit the nervous system to communicate with every cell in the body. Any process that affects the operation of this system will have far-reaching effects on the functioning of the entire body. Research shows that structural and functional changes occur in the ageing nervous system. The structural changes include the following:

(1) a reduced rate of cerebrospinal fluid production and turnover;[60]

(2) increased size of the brain's ventricles;[61]

(3) decreased brain weight by as much as 20 per cent between the ages of 45 and 85, most of which is attributed to a loss of extracellular fluid rather than neurones;[61] and

(4) loss of 50 000 to 100 000 neurones daily from the cerebral cortex, spinal cord, and peripheral nerves.[61]

The impact of these alterations on the operation of the nervous system is uncertain.

The senses are also affected by the ageing process. Age-related hearing loss is referred to as presbycusis and is extremely common. To compound matters, our ears are continually bombarded by numerous sources of sound pollution. These two processes combine to produce a hearing decrement in virtually every older individual. Hearing loss is particularly relevant to athletic performance because many of the cues that athletes rely upon are auditory in nature. Opponents' breathing patterns, team-mates calling for a pass, the

dribble of a basketball, or the cheer of the crowd are all important to athletic success.

Normal age-related changes in vision are known as presbyopia and result in decreased visual acuity and accommodation. As we age the crystalline lens of the eye becomes increasingly brittle and so will not change shape as readily to permit accommodation. Good vision is a prerequisite to success in most sports because athletes rely heavily upon visual cues to influence their actions and reactions. Fortunately for ageing competitors with visual or auditory deficits, the technology exists to help them overcome all but the very worst of losses.

One of the most valued athletic abilities is reaction time, and this clearly slows with advancing age.[47] This slowing is the result of several changes within the ageing neuromuscular system:

(1) a reduced rate of muscular contraction;

(2) a decrease in the rate of nerve impulse propagation;

(3) a reduction in the rate of perceptual processing;

(4) a decrease in the conduction rate of sensory nerves; and

(5) an increase in the central processing time for sensory stimulation.

In other words, every element in the reflex loop is hindered, to some extent, by the ageing process. It appears that the increase in the time required for central processing is the major contributor to the overall slow-down. Research also shows that when a choice of possible reaction-timed responses exists, the older person's reaction time slows much more than that of a younger person. This is the result of an even further increase in the central processing required for a response to occur. Thus the ability to make split-second decisions and react is significantly impaired with increasing age, particularly if it involves a novel situation. This has major implications for the older athlete performing in the read-and-react situations so commonly encountered in sports like hockey, soccer, football, squash, basketball, and volleyball. It should be noted that the reaction times of older athletes have been shown to be shorter than those of younger sedentary individuals, but not shorter than those of younger athletes.[62] This strongly suggests that reaction time, like so many other physical abilities, also deteriorates with disuse.

There appear to be differences in the way that ageing athletes cope with the attentional or focusing stresses demanded of them, particularly in highly stressful competitive situations. Molander and Backman[50] conducted a study in which older and younger athletes were monitored during the performance of a precision sporting activity. Although both groups reported an increase in their state of arousal during the competitive phase, the older athletes differed in two notable ways:

1. During the competitive phase of the activity their heart rates did not decrease as much as the younger subjects.

2. Their motor performance deteriorated from the training to the competitive situation, while that of the young group remained unchanged or improved.

Molander and Backman conjecture that this deterioration in performance may reflect an age-related change in attentional functioning (focusing skills). It seems that older athletes are less efficient at focusing their attention on a specific task during a stressful situation. They also postulate that the deteriorating motor skills of the ageing athlete require the commitment of greater amounts of mental energy towards rehearsing and attempting to retrieve the required neural patterns, leaving them less mental energy to commit to dealing with external variables such as the crowd. Regardless of the actual mechanism, these losses are important because they suggest that even the most highly skilled ageing athlete will probably experience performance deficits while competing in highly stressful situations. These deficits will probably increase substantially as the athlete's skill decreases because he or she must concentrate more to properly perform technical skills rather than dealing with the event in its entirety. This can be very frustrating for older athletes, particularly if they find that their training performances are superior to their competitive efforts. They may begin to consider themselves 'chokes' who can no longer handle the pressure of competition. If these individuals become frustrated, their performance will deteriorate even further and a vicious circle of decaying performance will be established. A reasonable coaching approach to this situation would be to make the athlete aware that this phenomenon is a normal consequence of ageing. While this does not change the situation, it may serve to reduce the athlete's frustration level and improve their performance. Coaches might also try structuring training sessions to regularly expose their older athletes to stressful situations, providing them with the opportunity to learn to cope better with distractions and pressures.

Crystallized intelligence refers to the knowledge that individuals accumulate through their lifetime experience. This form of knowledge is maintained into old age and may even improve with the passage of time.[63] Fluid intelligence refers to a person's ability to solve new and complex problems, particularly those requiring abstract thought. This form of intelligence declines with age, lending support to the old adage that 'you can't teach an old dog new tricks', or at least not easily. This change is very relevant to coaching and competitive situations. On one side, the coach will generally find it more difficult to teach new skills and tactics to an older competitor. On the other side, the ageing athlete will have greater difficulty coping with novel competitive situations. Both these changes will handicap the older competitor's performance, particularly in complex sporting activities.

Sleep architecture is altered with age, such that total sleep remains relatively unchanged but sleep efficiency decreases.[64] In other words, more time must be spent in bed to attain the same volume of sleep. Older individuals often find remaining asleep more difficult than falling asleep, they wake more often, and, once awakened, they remain awake longer than younger individuals. Their sleep pattern also becomes more fragmented. This may occur because of a gradual loss of deep delta sleep, a change which provides them with a lighter quality of sleep. The sleep requirement for an individual does not appear to change with increasing age[55] and rapid eye movement (**REM**) sleep remains constant throughout life. These changes in sleep patterns are relevant because they can interfere with an ageing athlete's ability to recover from training and competitive efforts.

In summary, the nervous system undergoes many age-related changes. In addition, there appears to be considerable evidence suggesting that the 'use it or lose it' principle governs the functions of neurones as much as it does muscle fibres. Neurophysiologists have demonstrated that regular stimulation delays the involution of neurones, and that hypertrophy may occur with sufficient stimulation.[47] Decreases in fluid intelligence, selective and divided attention, the senses, and reaction time all affect athletic performance. These changes occur very subtly and may not be clinically apparent in a sedentary person until he or she is over 65. However, they will be evident in the athletic arena at a much earlier age because in this environment microadvantages often separate the winners from the losers.

Tendon and ligament changes

Ligaments and tendons are important structures because they play essential roles in the day-to-day operation of the musculoskeletal system. By definition, tendons are bands of connective tissue that anchor muscles to bones. In doing so, they function as energy-transmission mechanisms. Ligaments are connective tissue bands that attach one bone to another. As connective tissue structures, both consist primarily of collagen and will experience all of collagen's age-related alterations. Ageing tendons and ligaments become progressively less compliant and increasingly more vulnerable to injury. Once injured, ageing tendons and ligaments are relatively unforgiving. Severely traumatized ligaments will never return to their original length, their stress–strain characteristics will be permanently disrupted, and microscopic examination will reveal evidence of collagen fibre failure.[65] Ageing also appears to be associated with a reduction in the glycosaminoglycans concentration found in tendons.[66] The significance of this change is uncertain.

Ligaments and tendons are by no means exempt from the deleterious effects of an inactive lifestyle. Research has identified a number of alterations which include:

(1) a reduced rate of collagen turnover so that there is a greater opportunity for cross-linkage stabilization to occur, thus rendering these structures increasingly brittle;

(2) bony resorption at the site of tendon/ligament insertion so that less tension is required to produce a complete disruption or avulsion fracture;

(3) a decreased number of cellular elements;

(4) diminished collagen fibre thickness;

(5) reduced tissue capillarization;

(6) decreased glycosaminoglycans concentration; and

(7) lower tissue water content.

All these changes considerably hinder the ability of tendons and ligaments to withstand the stresses applied to them during periods of physical exertion, therefore leaving them at increased risk of injury. However, these changes have all been shown to regress when tendons and ligaments are regularly exposed to the stresses and strains of physical activity. Viidik[29] has developed several animal models which illustrate that training increases the tensile stress tolerance of both ligaments and tendons. The ageing exerciser will develop stronger, thicker, and more supple tendons and ligaments. In this state, these structures are able to tolerate considerably more wear and tear before tissue breakdown occurs. This is important for all athletes, but particularly for ageing athletes involved in sports requiring a high volume of repetitive movements such as swimming and running.

Flexibility changes

Flexibility can be thought of as the range of motion possible for any joint (for example, the hip) or set of joints (for example, the spinal column). In any individual, flexibility varies considerably depending upon the joint. The athlete's specific flexibility needs are dictated by the athletic event in which he or she participates. For instance, superior hip flexibility is important for a hurdler, but of little value to an archer. The movement possible about any joint is determined by a number of factors including the following:

1. Bony structures—the olecranon in the elbow is a classic example of a bony structure that restricts joint movement.

2. Muscle and fascia—inflexible muscle tissue will limit joint movement.

3. Ligaments, tendons, and joint capsules—non-compliant connective tissues also restrict joint movements.

Any changes in the body which promote the above alterations will limit flexibility. The consequences of reduced flexibility for an athlete are numerous and potentially costly. For example, consider the effects of limited shoulder range of motion on a tennis player's ability to serve. Athletes who cannot assume certain positions will be less effective. The high jumper with limited back extension will have trouble performing the 'Flop' technique. Inflexible people encounter greater resistance to work and so expend more energy to accomplish a given task. The final consideration is that injury rates increase as flexibility decreases. Non-compliant tissues appear to be more easily damaged.

There is a paucity of well-controlled research addressing whether flexibility changes with age and quantifying those changes in specific joints. Controversy exists over whether flexibility is altered by the ageing process at all, or whether inactivity is responsible for all the losses that have been observed. While some studies report increased passive resistance to movement, others do not.[2] It seems reasonable that if muscle, fascia, ligaments, tendons, and joint capsules become less compliant with age, flexibility must also diminish. This is consistent with the frequently noted observation that flexibility declines steadily after childhood. While there is undoubtedly an innate component to the flexibility losses noted with age, it appears that inactivity is the dominant factor in the average person. Generally, the less active people are, the more rapidly their flexibility will deteriorate. While the age-induced losses are permanent, the inactivity-induced losses are not. Studies in which older individuals were given range-of-motion exercises demonstrated significant improvements in flexibility within relatively short periods of time.[26] The greatest gains were observed in those individuals who had lived the least active lives. It should be noted that studies have shown that increasing the temperature of a joint will enhance tissue compliance and so improve flexibility.[2] This supports the importance of a warm-up, particularly for the ageing athlete whose tissues are usually less compliant. Failing to warm up adequately is a mistake that a younger athlete may get away with, but for the ageing athlete this error often proves costly in terms of unnecessary time lost to injury.

Cartilaginous changes

Articular cartilage is an ingenious combination of collagen fibres embedded in a matrix of ground substance rich in chondroitin sulphates and mucoproteins. This blend provides it with the physical properties of a gel which is anchored to the underlying bony tissues and permits joints to function as lubricated bearings during movement. It also provides articular cartilage with mechanical properties ideally suited to shock absorption.

Articular cartilage differs from most body tissues in that it lacks a direct blood supply and so depends entirely on imbibition and diffusion processes to meet its nutritional needs. Both these processes are facilitated by the mechanical loading and unloading of the joint surface. When exposed to regular mechanical stimulation, articular cartilage will respond by thickening in much the same way as bone does. Hall's research[67] supports the contention that articular cartilage will remain healthy if regularly subjected to compressive and decompressive forces. His work also illustrates that, deprived of such stimulation, cartilage will atrophy and become more vulnerable to injury. Regardless of age, cartilage is fatiguable and will fail structurally when exposed to excessive mechanical stress. This overuse causes fractures of collagen fibres, reduces the volume of proteoglycans on the cartilaginous surface, and damages chondrocytes. The cartilaginous damage associated with overuse will be even greater if some degree of joint malalignment exists for congenital or traumatic reasons. For instance, a torn medial meniscus substantially alters the mechanics within the knee joint such that whenever the knee is extended, the femur is forced into the tibial plateau. This high-contact force causes excessive wear and tear of the underlying articular cartilage and promotes the development of early degenerative changes. Following a complete menisectomy, the contact pressure on the menisectomized side of the joint is increased and once again the articular cartilage is subjected to excessive wear and tear. The partial menisectomies that are performed today attempt to preserve as much of the viable meniscus as possible in an effort to minimize the disruption of normal knee-joint mechanics.

Research demonstrates that articular cartilage experiences a number of age-related alterations. The most important of which is the loss of tissue compliance that occurs as a result of the cross-linkage stabilization of collagen molecules. This stabilization renders cartilage increasingly brittle and less able to cope with repetitive stresses. Articular cartilage in this state is increasingly vulnerable to the structural failure that can occur with overuse injuries. Ageing cartilage also contains less water and has increased concentrations of keratosulphate and chondroitin sulphate. All these changes reduce the compliance of articular cartilage, rendering it less able to perform its critical role of shock absorption. While the ageing process does produce cartilaginous changes, inactivity makes the greatest contribution to cartilaginous deterioration.

Psychosocial factors

Psychosocial issues play a major role in the performance of all athletes, but are particularly relevant to the success and failure of the ageing athlete. It is critical that health-care professionals, coaches, and trainers recognize that the ageing sports enthusiast lives, works, trains, and competes in a psychosocial environment very different from that of his or her younger opponents. Compare, for example, the pressures on a 46-year-old, single mother with three children who works full time and is training for a triathlon, with those of the average 20-year-old collegiate basketball player. Ageing competitors almost always have more financial, professional, social, and family obligations than their younger rivals. This translates into more distractions, disruptions, preoccupations, concerns, commitments, time compression, and fatigue. None of these stressors is compatible with optimal training or competing. Pressured athletes often train inconsistently. They frequently miss workouts and when they do train they often hurry their warm-ups, ruminate during their workouts, and then cut their cool-downs short. This puts them at increased risk of becoming injured. In addition, harried athletes often fail to experience the pleasure and relaxation commonly derived from a good workout. Despite the potential for this problem, many ageing athletes actually look to their training as a form of stress management which helps them cope with the demands of the rest of their life. This section will review a number of psychosocial factors which are apparent in the masters sporting environment, in the hope that this insight will better prepare the reader to understand ageing athletes and their problems.

Active living not only provides ageing citizens with many structural and physiological benefits, it also offers them a number of psychosocial rewards. Studies have shown that élite and recreational runners, regardless of their weekly mileage, score lower on measures of tension, fatigue, depression, confusion, and anger, and higher on items that estimate vigour (Fig. 4).[68] These benefits occur regardless of the runner's age. One of the unpleasant realities of ageing is that it leaves many individuals alone in the world. In the United States, one in seven males and one in three females live alone.[69] This is very disconcerting for many individuals and provides significant motivation for participation in team sports. A sense of belonging with other human beings is an essential feeling for most people. Kavanagh and Shephard[70] conducted studies on the participants at the 1985 World Veterans Athletics Championships and found that the top three reasons for participating in the games were as follows:

(1) to belong to a group, 92.8 per cent;

(2) to enhance mood, 90 per cent; and

(3) fitness, 54 per cent.

These are radically different from the top three responses that would have been given if the athletes interviewed had been young Olympic hopefuls. It appears from the responses that the ageing competitor is generally more concerned with the psychosocial benefits of sports involvement than the physical benefits. Sports participation offers older people the opportunity to get out of the house, meet people, have fun, and keep in touch with athletes many years their junior. Regular exercise often leads to improvements in physical appearance and, in some instances, athletic success. Both of these serve to enhance an individual's feeling of self-confidence and worth. In a culture which extols the virtues of remaining eternally youthful, maintaining a positive self-image can be very difficult as we age. This is where participating in sports and fitness programmes can be particularly beneficial to the ageing individual.

Why is it uncommon for world-class athletes to carry on to become world-class masters athletes? Why are there not more athletes like Gordie Howe, Nolan Ryan, Precious McKenzie, Joyce Smith, and Arnold Palmer competing into their forties and fifties?

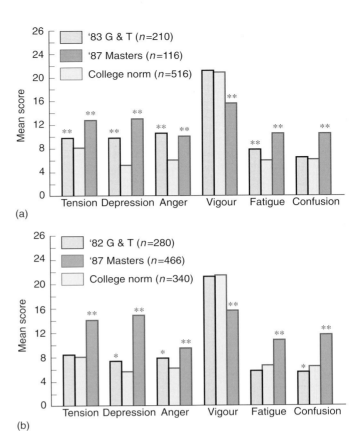

(a)

(b)

Fig. 4 Comparison of group means on the Profile of Mood States. (a) Male athletes $**p < 0.001$, two-tailed t tests comparing this group's mean scores with masters' mean scores. (b) Female athletes $*p < 0.05$, $**p < 0.001$, two-tailed t tests comparing this group's mean scores with the masters' group mean scores. (Reproduced from ref. 88, with permission.)

The physiological and structural changes that occur with ageing are not sufficient to explain the large drop-out of high-level competitors before the age of 40. The answer lies in a loss of motivation. Many of these individuals devoted their younger years to endless hours of training and competing in an effort to become and remain a world-class athlete. During this time, important issues such as education, marriage, family, business, recreation, and socializing are often forced into second place. They are often able to justify putting the rest of their life on hold by promising themselves that things will be different after they achieve their athletic goals. Once these goals are reached there is often considerable pressure and little incentive to resist retiring from sports and living a normal life. As one athlete put it: 'My motto used to be that I wouldn't let my job interfere with my running. Now I do not let my running interfere with my job. My family also takes precedence over my running'.[71] In this particular case, sport has gone from first to third place on this person's priority list. This change in status greatly affects the quality and quantity of training that a person will consistently perform. This attitude differs significantly from that of individuals who begin their athletic careers later in life. In many cases, these people gave up sports during their youth, while they attended to the other distractions of life. Once they are educated, become secure in their jobs, and their children have grown up, they find themselves looking for a new challenge—and sports provides the answer.

Numerous terms have been used to describe the loss of internal drive which often affects the ageing athlete's ability to perform. Burnout, lack of motivation, losing the competitive edge, lacking the killer instinct, and just not having 'it' any more are but a few of the excuses frequently made for declining athletic performance. These individuals often retain their desire to achieve but lose their drive. This phenomenon is not unique to the sporting world; it is a well-documented fate for many young business executives who spend years working day and night and eventually can no longer handle the load. Russell and Branch[72] summarized this process nicely: 'Rarely will you see an athlete who hasn't put on 10–15 pounds over a full career but even rarer are the ones who don't put on the same amount of mental fat. That's the biggest killer of ageing champions because it works on your concentration and mental toughness, which are the margins of victory; it prevents you from using your mind to compensate for your diminishing physical skills'. 'Mental fat' or lack of motivation has forced the retirement of many ageing athletes long before their bodies failed them.

Several authors have studied the psychological reactions of people who suffer significant losses.[73] While the terms used may vary, the results consistently point to a typical grief reaction containing three basic phases: (1) denial; (2) anger; and (3) acceptance. While these grief reactions were first described in individuals who were told they were dying, they are no less applicable to athletes facing the reality that they are no longer capable of improving their performance. Every athlete eventually slows down, and some will slow down faster than others. When this point is finally reached, athletic improvement is no longer possible. This can be extremely frustrating because improvement is often the athlete's *raison d'etre*, and when this possibility no longer exists many lose interest in competing. Such a realization can be a major psychological crisis for athletes who have overvalued their athletic involvement. It is easy to believe that athletes can undergo grief-like reactions when experiencing a loss of this magnitude. One only has to watch their emotional reactions when they announce that they are retiring to realize the pain they are experiencing. These reactions can occur in any athlete who faces the reality of no future improvement, regardless of his or her age. Consider, for example, how an 18-year-old National Hockey League draft-pick feels when he experiences a career-ending knee injury. People who have competed for decades will often experience this reaction in their late thirties and early forties when they realize that they are struggling to stay competitive rather than improving.

Individuals who do not begin competing until they are older undergo an entirely different process. They often enjoy several years where they physiologically adapt to their sport and their performances continue to improve. These people often describe themselves as feeling nearly immortal because while everyone around them is physically deteriorating, they are actually achieving personal bests. It is not difficult to imagine that when these individuals reach the point beyond which athletic improvement is no longer physically possible, they often undergo an intense grief reaction.

The initial response of grieving older athletes is to deny that they have reached their physiological peak. They do not accept that their inability to establish personal best performances is the result of biological changes associated with the ageing process. Instead, they typically attribute their faltering performances to a variety of factors including inferior training, a bad season, not enough miles run,

insufficient weight training, not enough competitions, too little speed work, preoccupation with the family, work-related problems, illness, etc. They believe all that is needed to regain their form is to train harder, longer, faster, further, and more frequently. When athletes adopt this approach, they usually overtrain, their performances worsen, and their chances of becoming injured increase dramatically. Eventually, the athlete ends up in the second phase of grieving, which is anger. Unable to accept that they can no longer perform at a given level, these athletes feel that they are the victims of a great injustice. They are angry because the skills that they have worked so hard to develop are slowly slipping through their fingers and, despite their best efforts, there is absolutely nothing that they can do about it. No amount of training, dieting, self-sacrifice, or dedication can restore their former athletic ability. They may also be angry because others around them continue to improve while they cannot. They have lost control of the situation and begin to ask: 'Why is this happening to me? I have done nothing to deserve this punishment.' It is in this state of mind that the grieving athlete is at the greatest risk of abandoning sport entirely. 'Why bother if you can't perform at your best? I don't want to be remembered as a has-been. I should retire quietly before someone asks me to...' are commonly heard expressions from individuals in the anger phase. It is at this critical point that the ageing competitor would benefit most from contact with someone who has survived the grieving process and is still actively enjoying sports. This role model can help the athlete make a successful transition into the acceptance phase of the grieving process. Unfortunately for the ageing athlete, such people are few and far between.

During the acceptance phase, the ageing athlete comes to accept that the ageing process affects everyone and that nothing can be done to change his or her situation. The maturation required here often permits the individual to focus on new challenges and accept that the quality of his or her future performances must be considered in the light of physiological limits. Basically, a new set of realistic performance expectations is developed. These athletes are often the happiest because they have come to realize the greatest satisfaction that an athlete can derive from a competition is to give his or her best effort, regardless of winning. While the above sounds theoretical, it is in fact a very normal occurrence that has been repeating itself since people first began competing. Anyone who coaches, trains, manages, or treats older competitors must be aware of this process. With some understanding and guidance many individuals will survive this phase and continue to enjoy rewarding sporting lives.

The ageing process offers the athlete two major competitive advantages: maturity and experience. The knowledge acquired through a lifetime of experience is a treasure that every coach values and would love to be able to instil automatically into his or her novices. Unfortunately for coaches, experience cannot be acquired from a pill, injection, ointment, textbook, or a well-delivered 'pep talk'. It can only come from successes and failures experienced during years of training and competing. This is where ageing competitors often make major contributions in team sports. They are reservoirs of knowledge, to whom younger players can turn for instruction and inspiration. The younger players often have the raw physical talent but lack the refined physical skills, maturity, and the gamesmanship required to be successful in a given sport. Skills like bluffing, surprise, anticipation, patience, concentration, focusing, taking advantage of an opponent's lapses, and making opponents play your game all take time to develop. In this regard, older athletes often function as teachers and stabilizing influences on a team. From experience they know what must be done in order to be victorious in specific game situations. Experienced competitors often possess an advanced level of self-understanding. As individuals they understand their body responses, when they need to work hard, when they need to rest, and the price that must be paid to be successful. This intimate knowledge goes a long way towards negating the physical advantages of youth. Sheehan[74] summarized the value of experience when he stated:

In the September of my life I am all that the past has taught me. I know things that were a mystery before. Every year has become an asset, every experience a treasure. I am no longer a rookie, no longer a neophyte and I no longer look to veterans for guidance—I am a veteran, a master at my own game.

With the growing popularity of masters sports has come an increasing volume of media coverage and the greater possibility of monetary rewards. It is now possible for a successful ageing athlete to become both rich and famous. The lure of these desirable elements is providing considerable motivation for many older competitors to continue competing or to come out of retirement. The Senior Golf Tour and the American Road Running Circuit both provide opportunities for masters athletes to achieve fame and fortune. The Senior Golf Tour annually offers several million dollars in prize money, and some golfers are earning more than they did on the Open PGA Tour. For example, Al Geiberger joined the tour at the age of 50 and in his first year earned more than in any of his previous 28 years on the PGA Tour. The American Road Running Circuit provides us with possibly the best example of the fame that can be attained by an ageing competitor. John Campbell had retired from running on three occasions and, before becoming a masters competitor, could best be described as a relatively obscure distance runner from New Zealand. Since turning 40, however, this determined competitor has earned the status of a running superstar. His 2 h 11 min 4 s marathon is the fastest ever run by a masters athlete and rates a world-class performance at any age. In 1990 he was undefeated in 20 races and established age-class, world records at six different distances. One of the secrets of his success was an arduous training schedule in which he ran 140 miles a week. While the availability of money and recognition will help the masters sporting movement grow at the élite level, they will also increase the possibility that the problems corrupting the younger athletic world will diffuse into masters sports. While the numbers are smaller, problems such as overtraining, blood doping, steroids, and the use of other ergogenic aids is almost certainly occurring in masters sports.

A review of the literature concerning ageing athletes reveals that an individual's attitude towards ageing is of paramount importance in determining how well he or she copes. If the person views ageing as an inevitable tragedy in which all the virtues of youth are lost, then he or she will probably handle the ageing process poorly. We live in a world which cherishes the attributes of youth, and billions of dollars a year are spent convincing people that they should use various products to maintain a youthful image. This negative attitude towards growing older has convinced many people that ageing is something to dread. This attitude is by no means new. Shakespeare sums up our society's attitude towards ageing in his poem

The Passionate Pilgrim[75] 'Age, I do abhor thee, youth, I do adore thee'. Berman *et al.*[61] state that, as a result of this pervading attitude, a significant number of older adults suffer from the 'brainwashed elderly syndrome'. In this mental set, people believe that ageing is associated with wrinkles, retirement, rocking chairs, inactivity, unattractiveness, diminished mental capacity, and lack of worth. These people are also convinced nothing can be done to avoid this fate and they frequently live a self-fulfilling prophecy. Tragically, this conditioned thinking is so powerfully ingrained in our culture that people are frequently convinced that they are decrepit by the age of 30. The biographies of successful older athletes provides a striking contrast to this self-deprecating attitude. These people are remarkably consistent in their positive mental outlook. They are not focused on all the things that ageing is taking away from them but rather strive to enjoy the many things it provides. They generally think younger, act younger, dress younger, and partake of activities commonly identified with the younger generation. There appears to be more to growing old successfully than maintaining good physiology; it would also appear that maintaining a positive attitude is a necessary prerequisite.

Ageing and altitude

Since people are retiring earlier and the opportunity for travel is increasing, larger numbers of ageing individuals will be participating in high-altitude recreation and sport. This includes such things as hiking excursions in mountainous regions, mountain climbing, and competitive events held at higher altitudes. While mountain climbing is undeniably one of the most physically demanding athletic events, this has not prevented ageing athletes from achieving some impressive feats. One of the most impressive accomplishments was by Ramon Blanco of Spain, who, at the age of 60, became the oldest person to conquer Mount Everest, a gruelling climb of 8848 m.

Surprisingly little research has been undertaken on ageing and altitude tolerance. The investigations that have been performed suggest that increasing age offers mixed blessings in terms of coping with the stresses of altitude. On the positive side, researchers have found that ageing is associated with a decreased incidence and severity of acute mountain sickness.[76] This benefit appears to be unrelated to the rate of ascent, disproving the commonly held belief that the young are more susceptible to altitude illness because they climb faster than their older colleagues. Acute mountain sickness is a condition commonly experienced by individuals who ascend to altitudes in excess of 3000 m. The afflicted person experiences symptoms of headache, anorexia, nausea, vomiting, weakness, and insomnia within 6 to 96 h of arriving at altitude. This condition is usually self-limiting; however, some individuals go on to develop high-altitude pulmonary oedema or high-altitude cerebral oedema, both potentially life-threatening conditions. The mechanism by which increasing age protects against altitude-related illnesses is uncertain.

On the negative side, altitude will compound the oxygen-delivery problems of the ageing athlete. Ageing is associated with a reduction in an individual's arterial partial pressure of oxygen.[76] Basically, older competitors are unable to deliver the same volume of oxygen to their working muscles as younger people in the same state of health. To complicate matters, as altitude increases the partial pressure of oxygen in the atmosphere decreases, and so less oxygen is available for the cardiorespiratory system to capture and deliver to the working tissues. This double disadvantage serves to handicap, or at least greatly challenge, the ageing athlete who is exercising at altitude. To put into perspective how much of a disadvantage age-related changes are to physical performance at altitude, research indicates that the ability to tolerate the physiological demands of altitude depends more on people's general health and fitness than on their age.[76]

Thermal stress

Thermoregulation is an essential body function, and can be defined as the ability to maintain a normal body temperature by balancing heat-dissipating and heat-generating mechanisms. This is necessary because the body is designed such that cellular structures, enzymes, and chemical reactions function optimally within a narrow band of temperatures. In humans, the optimal physiological operating temperature is approximately 37 °C. When thermoregulatory mechanisms fail to hold the body at this temperature, optimal physiological function is impossible and athletic performance deteriorates. Independent of age, this functional deterioration will be greatly facilitated if the athlete starts the workout or competition underhydrated, ill, hung-over, tired, unacclimatized, or in poor physical condition. Thermoregulatory failure leaves the individual vulnerable to thermal injuries such as heat cramps, heat exhaustion, heat stroke, frostbite, or hypothermia. A wide variety of athletic events are held in environments where the ambient temperatures range from –30 °C to +40 °C. At the extremes of this temperature range, the risk of thermal stress-related problems is high. With more ageing athletes participating in these events, it behoves us to determine whether the ability to tolerate thermal stresses is altered with age.

Ageing has traditionally been associated with reduced heat tolerance. It has been observed that during heatwaves older individuals are more susceptible to thermal injuries and related fatalities than younger people.[77] However, this trend does not indicate whether the reduction in tolerance is the result of the ageing process or other variables such as illness or poor physical fitness. Relatively little research has been done in this area, and of the studies that have been performed many were poorly designed in that they failed to control for important variables such as cardiovascular fitness, state of acclimatization, disease processes, and body composition. These variables significantly influence an individual's ability to tolerate heat stress. A review of the well-controlled investigations suggests that the ageing process is responsible for some reduction in heat tolerance, but that this loss is not as significant as the losses attributable to poor physical fitness, disease processes, and lack of acclimatization.[77] The exact mechanism by which this age-related decline occurs is uncertain, but it seems reasonable to assume that, since thermoregulation is a complex process, the cause is multifactorial.

Researchers have pointed to changes in the ability of the ageing athlete to dissipate heat through perspiration. Apparently, sweat responses to exercise are both delayed and diminished with ageing.[78] Both of these changes hinder the athlete's ability to dissipate body heat. However, it has been shown that, with physical training, sweat glands will respond to exercise earlier and show no decline in their capacity for sweat production.[77] Kenny and Anderson[79] have demonstrated that ageing athletes competing in hot and humid environ-

ments sweat the same volumes as younger competitors. However, when the environment is hot and dry, ageing competitors produce substantially less sweat than their younger opponents. This difference could be the result of an inability to handle the volume of sweating required because of the relatively underhydrated state of the average older person. Goldman[15] reported that total body water decreases from 62 per cent of total bodyweight at age 25 to 53 per cent at age 75. Berman et al.[18] put it another way, stating that the average 35-year-old weighing 70 kg has as much as 7 to 8 litres more body water than a 75-year-old of the same weight. This has considerable relevance to athletic performance, particularly since ageing is also associated with a reduced sensation of thirst. Thus ageing athletes competing in hot, dry environments may become significantly dehydrated before the sensation of thirst motivates them to drink. Experience from the 1989 World Veterans Athletics Championships supports this, in that the competitors were reported to be less aware of when they were overheating and in need of fluids.[80]

In view of the serious consequences of heat injuries and the ageing athlete's unique physiology, a number of important recommendations can be made for older individuals training and competing in hot environments.

1. Athletes should hydrate well before, during and after their event.

2. During the competition, athletes should begin taking in replacement fluids long before they feel thirsty. If they wait until thirst develops, they will already be in trouble and unable to compensate enough to correct their fluid depletion.

3. Ideally, competitions and training sessions should be held during the coolest time of the day.

4. Fluid intake should never be restricted during hot weather practices.

5. Athletes should remain in the shade as much as possible and wear light-coloured clothing.

6. Whenever possible, athletes should wear a hat to protect their head from the sun.

7. Participants should realistically assess their fitness level and understand that the less fit they are the lower their heat tolerance will be.

8. Competitors should be familiar with the early symptoms of heat stress, such as muscle cramps, dizziness, cool skin, dry skin, elevated pulse, nausea, excessive thirst, weakness, and fatigue.

9. Athletes should monitor their bodyweight closely, as rapid losses indicate they are not drinking enough to replace their losses.

10. Athletes should closely monitor the colour of their urine. Urine which becomes dark yellow, is concentrated and indicates the athlete needs to increase his or her fluid intake.

Very little research has addressed the issue of age-related alterations in cold tolerance. However, some facts are available for consideration. The ageing competitor is at increased risk of experiencing localized cold injuries such as frostbite for several reasons. First, although it is not specifically an age-related change, atherosclerosis reduces the volume of warm blood that can be delivered to cooling peripheral tissues. It has also been suggested that as individuals age, their perception of cold may be diminished.[18] Finally, with increasing age there is a gradual reduction in subcutaneous adipose tissue which functions as a layer of insulation for the body. These changes render the ageing competitor's peripheral tissues more vulnerable to cold injury. Since ageing is associated with a reduction in our ability to handle physiological stresses, it would be reasonable to assume that ageing may be associated with diminished physical performance in cold environments. More research is required before many of the questions in this area can be answered.

Injuries

Ageing not only renders masters athletes physiologically, structurally, and psychosocially different from younger athletes, but it also leaves them increasingly vulnerable to injury. Stiffer tendons, muscles, joint capsules, brittle ligaments, a reduced rate of tissue repair, decreased joint flexibility, and loss of bone mass all contribute to this vulnerability. As athletes age, they are often able to maintain specific performance levels only by working closer to their physiological maximum. Working at this intensity places any athlete at an increased risk of injury. To make matters worse, injured ageing athletes also appear to be at greater risk of developing complications such as infections. This may be the result of the ageing person's altered physiological ability to respond to the stress of injury. In view of the above, it is not surprising that the injury pattern experienced by masters competitors differs significantly from that of their younger opponents. In this section, we will not consider specific injuries but rather focus on how the ageing athlete's injuries differ from those seen in younger adults.

Masters competitors are potentially the victims of two distinct types of injury: those resulting from their current training and competing, and those that occurred in their youth and return later to haunt them. Either type of injury can be sufficient to cause considerable discomfort, hamper proper training, and ultimately force a premature retirement from sports. Consider, for example, a high-school athlete who experiences a major joint injury such as an anterior cruciate ligament disruption. Even with the finest treatment, the damaged knee's structural integrity will remain permanently compromised. Once healed, these major joint injuries often remain quiescent until middle age, when the individual begins to notice that his or her joint can no longer tolerate repetitive stresses such as those placed on the knee in running sports. The frustrating reality for many ageing competitors is that the major injuries of their youth often dictate what athletic activities they can tolerate in their later years.

Clinical experience suggests that younger athletes suffer from a much higher incidence of traumatic musculoskeletal injury than their older colleagues. This occurs despite the younger athlete's connective tissues being generally more supple. Since the injuries that athletes experience are largely dictated by the sports in which they compete, it is not surprising to find that younger athletes tend to participate in sports with a greater potential for body contact and trauma. Additionally, their relative lack of competitive experience and their tendency to participate with more reckless intensity puts them at greater risk of experiencing traumatic injuries. Masters ath-

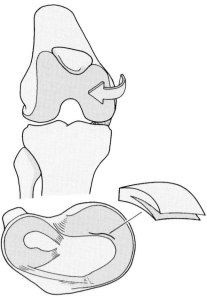

Fig. 5 Degenerative horizontal cleavage tear. (Reproduced from Sutton JR, Brook RM. *Sports medicine for the mature athlete.* Philadelphia: Benchmark Press, 1986; 283, with permission.)

letes are by no means immune to traumatic injuries such as internal joint derangements; however, these types of injury are uncommon and when they occur the individual may not present with a classic history. This is one reason why health-care professionals often overlook the diagnosis of significant joint injuries in ageing athletes and mistakenly attribute their signs and symptoms to degenerative processes. This can lead to treatment delays and cause major disruptions to training schedules. Rotator-cuff tears are an excellent example. The ageing athlete's rotator cuff is increasingly brittle and almost certainly weakened from repetitive microtrauma. It is often torn when the ageing individual's arm is forced into abduction, as occurs when skiers attempt to break their fall using an outstretched arm. These injuries are frequently incorrectly diagnosed as muscle strains, sprains, contusions, or tendinitis.

The musculoskeletal system is designed to be used, and its components require regular mechanical loading and unloading to remain healthy. Deprived of this stimulation they experience atrophic change. These tissues have their limitations and if overused they will break down faster then they can be repaired. This process of overuse and the degenerative tissue changes it induces is an enormous threat to the ageing competitor. Postural malalignments serve to exacerbate this threat by overloading various components of the musculoskeletal system. For example, runners with genu varus (bowed legs) repeatedly subject the medial compartments of their knees to excessive mechanical stresses. This repetitive overloading of the medial compartment will considerably shorten its lifespan. Eventually, the medial meniscus will break down (as shown in Fig. 5) and osteoarthritic degeneration develops. Research by DeHaven and Littner[81] indicates that the incidence of inflammatory problems increases with ageing, until by the age of 70 the top five athletically associated maladies are inflammatory in nature. Anyone working with masters athletes should beware of the 'evil itises'— arthritis, tenosynovitis, fasciitis, bursitis, capsulitis, and tendinitis. These injuries commonly begin as small nagging problems. If they are identified at this stage and treated effectively, they usually resolve with no sequelae. If they are ignored or inadequately treated, these small problems can progress to become major injuries and the athlete may be sidelined indefinitely.

The most effective strategy for dealing with athletic injuries is to prevent their occurrence in the first place. This is an especially important consideration for ageing competitors because their injury recovery rate is slower. Many of the structural changes associated with ageing leave tissues with reduced compliance and a diminished blood supply. In view of these changes, it is important for ageing athletes to perform an adequate warm-up before every workout or competition to increase the blood supply and temperature of their working tissues. Both these adjustments prime the tissues for work, enhance their viscoelastic properties, and so prepare them for use. Compliant muscles and tendons are far more difficult to injure. The value of having compliant tissues reinforces the importance of including some flexibility training in every ageing athlete's programme. The time invested in stretching will yield large dividends in terms of time saved through injury prevention.

Healing and ageing

Research indicates that ageing has a detrimental effect on the healing process. The body's normal response to injury is described as occurring in three phases:

(1)   the inflammatory phase;

(2)   the proliferative phase; and

(3)   the remodelling phase.

All three phases are adversely affected by the ageing process. With ageing there is dampening of the inflammatory phase. There is also a delay in the cellular migration, proliferation, and maturation that occur during the proliferative phase. In the remodelling phase, collagen is laid down less rapidly, in smaller volumes, and with altered binding patterns.[4] The net result of these changes is that, as we age, the events associated with the healing process begin later, proceed more slowly, and do not achieve the same level. Studies involving rats have shown that following a muscle contusion the proliferation of muscle fibres, fibroblasts, and blood vessels occurs more rapidly in the young.[4] Some researchers have suggested that the age-related delays in the healing process occur because of increases in the time that it takes to prime the system for the regenerative process.[4] Regardless of the aetiology, the bottom line is that, when injured, the older athlete's body still effects a quality repair but it takes longer than it used to. Al Oerter, the great discus champion, noticed this in his training, in that the injuries he developed in his forties and fifties seemed to require a longer time to heal. Just as there are large variations in the rate at which individuals age, there are also wide variations in the rate at which they recover from injury. To complicate matters, the rate of healing is also influenced by tissue changes induced by disease processes, disuse, environmental insults, and the presence of other body stressors. Any process that reduces tissue capillary density will reduce the rate at which oxygen and repair substrates can be delivered to an injury site. Despite the above, bony tissues appear to be unique, in that once skeletal maturity is achieved in late adolescence, there appears to be no age-related decline in the rate of fracture healing.[82]

Treatment considerations

The basic treatments for most athletic injuries are well described, and since they do not vary with the age of the competitor will not be the subject of this discussion. Instead, this section will focus on a number of treatment issues that are unique to the ageing athlete.

First, beware of Ageism! Ageism is a bias towards individuals on the basis of their age and can influence the way many ageing competitors are treated by the medical system. It is ageism that prompts some health-care professionals to discard an older competitor's complaints of discomfort with the all too common phrase: 'What do you expect for someone your age?' This approach is unacceptable as there is no scientific evidence suggesting that healthy older individuals cannot participate in a wide variety of sporting events without experiencing pain. Pain is not a normal part of the ageing process, and when it occurs it usually indicates that something is wrong. Many older people will not complain of pain because they fear treatment or do not want to 'give in'. This is particularly true of ageing competitors who often view injuries as a threat to their continued participation. Health-care professionals are obliged to take athletes' complaints of injury seriously, regardless of their age. They all deserve a comprehensive evaluation, and the decision to refer for specialist consultation should always be based on the individual's symptoms and not his or her age.

It is important to recognize that dedicated masters athletes will react to injury in the same way as most athletes and so will be reluctant to simply discontinue their training and competitive schedules. Their athletic involvement has become a highly valued component of their self-image and this is seriously threatened when an injury restricts their active participation. Before health-care professionals can effectively manage these individuals they must recognize the existence of this 'athletic mind set'. To pronounce to the athlete, 'The solution is simple: if it bothers you to weight lift then stop weight lifting' is both inappropriate and insensitive. This approach does little to dissuade many athletes from participating in their sport, and, in fact, challenges some individuals to attack their event with even greater fervour in an effort to prove the medical world wrong.

As an alternative, health-care professionals should take the time to explain the problem carefully, indicating that continuing an unrestricted training programme could not only cause more extensive damage but might permanently interfere with the athlete's ability to compete and improve in their particular sport. The objective is to convince them that by accepting a short-term loss they will ultimately enjoy a long-term gain. The extent of this short-term loss can be minimized by proposing alternative athletic activities that permit competitors to maintain or even improve their fitness skills without hampering their recovery. The more sport specific these activities are, the greater their potential benefit. A good example of this would be water running sessions for a marathoner with a metatarsal stress fracture. Technique modification is another avenue that can be pursued. For example, a tennis player with chronic supraspinatous tendinitis may find switching from an overhead to a side-arm serve will allow them to continue playing with minimal discomfort. Although these adjustments do not resolve the injury, the athletes are happy because they can continue to participate without further exacerbation of their problem. If necessary, bracing can be used to provide support to areas where the normal musculoskeletal structures have been compromised. Only as a last resort should a complete change of activity be recommended.

It should be remembered that injuries of little significance to sedentary people may cause considerable problems for élite athletes regardless of their age. An injury that could normally be satisfactorily treated with a conservative approach may require definitive correction in ageing athletes because it hinders their ability to perform at a desired level of competence. Left untreated, these individuals will often experience the same depressive symptoms seen in younger competitors under the same circumstances. To dismiss this reaction as immature, exaggerated, or hypochondriacal is irresponsible. One must be aware that ageing athletes often take their sporting involvement very seriously and deserve at least the same level of concern from the health-care profession.

As noted earlier, inactivity poses a considerable threat to the structural integrity of the ageing individual because it clearly accelerates the rate at which many decremental processes occur. Understanding this concept is important to the effective management of the injured ageing athlete. Immobilization is frequently needed for injuries such as fractures and severe ligamentous sprains. While in many instances immobilization cannot be avoided, it should be used only when necessary and for as brief a period as possible. The treatment of shoulder dislocations provides an excellent example. The standard protocol for younger individuals who experience a glenohumeral dislocation, involves 6 weeks in a sling, immobilized in adduction and internal rotation. The objective is to maximize future stability by facilitating as snug a repair of the joint capsule as possible. When the same injury occurs in someone older, the objective is to maximize joint range of motion through early mobilization. To this end, Valaschini and MacIntyre give their older patients with shoulder dislocations a sling for comfort only, starting them on range-of-motion and strengthening exercises within 3 days of the injury.[83] Not only does immobilization threaten the ageing competitor with all the changes associated with inactivity, it is also a major source of frustration. Knortz[58] has pointed out that immobilized geriatric patients are at a dual disadvantage in terms of muscle fibre alterations. Not only do they continue to experience the selective fast-twitch fibre atrophy that occurs with ageing, but they also experience slow-twitch fibre atrophy in response to their immobility. This supports the need for early and aggressive physiotherapy to ensure that joint range of motion is maintained, muscular strength is preserved, and bone-mass loss is minimized.

A regular exercise programme is one way in which individuals can reduce their risk of developing problems such as coronary artery disease, but it is by no means an absolute guarantee that these problems will never occur. The adage: 'We all must die of something' is as true today as it was 5000 years ago. Health-care professionals must keep this in mind when dealing with ageing athletes. These people can present for the first time with the signs and symptoms of a significant underlying illness, and their involvement in sport can confuse the issue. For example, shortness of breath on exertion is a classic feature of advanced coronary artery disease. It is also commonly experienced by athletes participating in aerobically demanding sports. Shortness of breath in elderly athletes should never be superficially dismissed as indicating that they are unfit, particularly if it has never occurred before and is hindering their ability to train. These individuals merit a thorough examination to establish whether there is a pathological explanation for their respiratory problem such as coronary artery disease, anaemia, exercise-induced asthma, etc. This concern extends to a number of symptoms including unexplained weight loss, chronic fatigue, dramatic decline in physical performance, loss of motivation, and persistent pain. While all these symptoms can be attributed to the stress of training, in the ageing individual, they have a higher probability of indicating the presence of disease and so merit more than a superficial review.

Rehabilitating an injured athlete is perhaps the most important aspect of treatment. It often determines how quickly the athlete can return to competition, and, in some cases, determines if they will return at all. The aim of rehabilitation is to restore normal function in the shortest possible time. This is critically important to ageing athletes because the longer that they are unable to train properly, the harder they must work to regain their level of performance. Rehabilitative efforts should be initiated as soon as possible following an injury and the entire range of available treatment modalities should be considered. As noted earlier, ageing athletes heal slower and rehabilitation programmes must be adjusted accordingly. As a general guideline, when estimating the rehabilitation time required for an older athlete, twice as much time should be allowed for someone aged 60 as for someone aged 20. Athletes who are 75 or older will probably require three times the standard time.[80] These estimates apply to almost all injuries and can be a source of frustration to the athlete and therapist if neither is aware of them from the start.

Medication considerations

The use of medication is a concern for athletes of all ages. However, it is a particularly important topic for the ageing athlete. The entire pharmacotherapy process is significantly influenced by age, disuse, disease, and environmentally related alterations to a person's structure and physiological function. Generally speaking, in our society, the older people become, the more medication they regularly consume. Combine this fact with the anatomical, physiological, and pathological changes that occur in older individuals and it is not surprising to see an increase in the incidence of adverse drug reactions. The following are a number of the pharmacokinetic changes associated with the ageing process.

1. Reduced absorption—this occurs as a result of decreased gastric acid production, increased stomach-emptying time, reduced intestinal absorptive surface area, and decreased intestinal mucosal blood flow.[24] In theory, these changes can substantially reduce the rate at which many drugs are absorbed, but in practice the healthy older person appears to experience only minor reductions.

2. Altered distribution—with ageing there is usually a reduction in total body water, an increase in body fat, and a loss of lean body mass.[24] Water-soluble medications will therefore be distributed over a smaller volume and will have a greater effect per dose. Fat-soluble medications, however, will be dispersed over a larger body volume and so have a diminished effect per dose.

3. Plasma binding proteins—these bind to medications and assist in their distribution throughout the body. The concentration of these proteins remains unchanged in many

older adults and when reductions do occur, they are usually minor.[24]

4. Reduced renal clearance—ageing is associated with a loss of renal tissue and a reduced glomerular filtration rate.[24] As a result, drugs that require renal clearance are handled more slowly. This is particularly true of many antibiotics.

5. Reduced hepatic clearance—with ageing there is a loss of hepatocytes and a reduction in the volume of blood flow they receive.[24] Thus drugs that require hepatic metabolism will be handled more slowly.

6. Reduced cell receptors—the number of drug receptors on various cells may decrease with ageing.[24] This reduces the amount of drug that can enter these cells and so reduces the effectiveness of the medication.

The above changes combine to significantly influence how an older individual responds to certain medications. Since the body relies primarily on hepatic metabolism and renal excretion to eliminate drugs, these functional alterations will serve to increase the half-life of many medications in ageing individuals.

Inflammatory conditions are the most common problems affecting ageing athletes and non-steroidal anti-inflammatory drugs (NSAIDs) are commonly used in their treatment. These agents include ibuprofen, acetylsalicylic acid, naproxen, indomethacin, and several others. Although these medications are frequently prescribed, they should be used with caution for several reasons. First, NSAID-induced gastrointestinal complications (for example, gastric ulceration) occur more frequently in older people, particularly women or individuals with a history of peptic ulcer disease.[84] This is partially due to an age-related reduction in gastric vascularization that compromises gastric mucosal protective mechanisms. These protective mechanisms are also compromised by an NSAID-induced reduction in prostaglandin synthesis. With less gastric mucosal protection, the stomach is at increased risk of injury. Second, ageing is associated with an increased incidence of adverse reactions to NSAIDs. Third, the anti-inflammatory and analgesic effect of NSAIDs may reduce or eliminate the sensation of pain—nature's warning signal that it is time to stop. Without these reminders, people often continue to be active and may exacerbate their injuries. This is particularly true when the individual is suffering from a degenerative joint problem such as osteoarthritis. A safer approach in these cases is to prescribe a very light dose or none at all prior to exercise and then a full dose after the workout to limit the pain and inflammation.

The following are some general principles for prescribing medications to ageing athletes.

1. Use as few medications as possible.

2. Use as low a dose as possible.

3. Medication responses may be less dramatic than in the young.

4. Beware of side-effects and possible drug interactions.

5. If a medication is not accomplishing what is required, discontinue it and try another.

Training principles

Volumes have been written on the principles of safe and effective training. It is beyond the scope of this chapter to discuss all these principles, but it is worthwhile highlighting a number of issues of particular importance in the training of ageing athletes.

Just as ageing athletes experience decrements in their organs' functional reserves, their ability to compensate for training errors is also reduced. The ageing competitor cannot expect to make the same training mistakes as many younger athletes and survive uninjured. Competing too frequently, training too long and intensely, failing to rest and permit recovery, ignoring flexibility work, training inconsistently, and avoiding strength training are common training errors. These errors often leave younger athletes performing suboptimally or at the very worst with minor injuries. Conversely, masters competitors may pay a much heavier price for making the same mistakes. Frequently, their performances will deteriorate considerably and their chances of developing a serious injury are much greater. Frank Shorter, the 1972 Olympic marathon champion, discovered this when he entered masters competition. He stated:[85]

You can't train the same way you did when you were 23. It just isn't going to work. All you do when you're 23 is go out the door, turn left, turn right and go as hard as you can till you start to break down. Then you take a day or two of easy running till you heal up. But that's not what happens when you get to be a master.

Until his retirement at the age of 46, Nolan Ryan was one of baseball's finest pitchers and the all-time leader in strike-outs. He attributed his competitive longevity to his commitment to a year-round training programme. His programme emphasized a combination of weight-training, running, stretching, and regularly scheduled rest days. He consistently performed this programme regardless of how his pitching game was going. Ageing athletes are undeniably unique and must be mature enough to recognize and accept this fact if they intend to enjoy the many fruits of competitive effort.

If there was a set of commandments governing the rules for training older athletes, the first commandment would be: 'Thou shalt start low and progress slowly'. This is a critical concept that applies to the development of all athletes, regardless of their age, sport, or level of expertise, but it is particularly important for the older competitor. All body tissues are capable of adapting to the various training stresses to which they are subjected. However, two points should be remembered. First, athletes will adapt to the stresses of training at their own unique rate. Since older athletes have a greater potential for structural and functional diversity, the variation in their rate of adaptation will be greater than that seen in younger competitors. Second, there are considerable differences in the rate at which different body tissues adapt to the stresses of exercise. For instance, the cardiovascular and respiratory systems respond much faster to training stimuli than the musculoskeletal system. This rapid cardiorespiratory adaption leaves athletes feeling capable of greater volumes of exercise, long before their muscles, tendons, and bony tissues have had sufficient time to adapt. In practical terms this means the 'motor' is ready to train long before the 'chassis' can handle the strain. This difference in the rates of adaptive response leaves the ageing athlete vulnerable to injury during this time.

People who have been sedentary for prolonged periods must be especially careful not to overdo it in the early part of their programme. Unfortunately, many people ignore this advice and end up injured long before they have had a chance to enjoy the many benefits regular exercise has to offer. To illustrate a safe approach to becoming active, let us consider a 45-year-old woman who has been inactive for 20 years, decides she would like to start running to get back in shape and comes to your office for some sound advice. After congratulating her on the decision to become active, I would spend some time convincing her of the importance of gradually introducing her body to the stresses of exercise. In particular, I would explain to her that time and her inactive lifestyle have altered her body and left it more vulnerable to injury. I would strongly encourage her to start out with a walking programme which gradually has her doing longer distances and faster cadences. Once she becomes comfortable with this, begin to introduce brief periods of running in a pattern such as walk for 5 min, jog for 2 min, walk for 5 min, etc. Each week she can increase the distances and the relative amount she is running until several months later she is safely running the entire workout. This is a cautious approach, but it makes good physiological sense. By adhering to the principle of starting low and progressing slowly, an athlete can often avoid unnecessary injuries and enjoy a more rewarding sporting life. Athletes who ignore this principle may enjoy a rapid initial improvement but often find their further progress hindered by injuries. As a general rule, the older and less fit the individual, the lower they should start out and the more slowly they should progress.

One of the questions addressed in the literature is how responsive are older athletes to training stimuli. Do they respond in the same way and to the same extent as their younger opponents? There are a number of studies demonstrating that, regardless of age, older individuals who begin training are capable of making noteworthy physiological improvements.[43,86] These improvements include the following:

(1) reduced resting heart rate;

(2) improved $\dot{V}O_2$max;

(3) increased vital capacity;

(4) decreased percentage body fat;

(5) improved work capacity;

(6) reduced blood pressure;

(7) increased strength;

(8) increased endurance; and

(9) increased flexibility.

These improvements even occur in individuals with clinically evident cardiovascular disease, although to a lesser extent than in disease-free individuals.[43] It has long been recognized that participating in aerobic activities such as cycling, cross-country skiing, walking, swimming, in-line skating, and running can provide substantial physiological benefits regardless of the participant's age. However, strength training was an area of uncertainty in this regard. Studies of strength training in older subjects have demonstrated that older athletes are capable of strength improvements at a rate equal to or faster than some younger athletes (Fig. 6).[49,51,87] This is

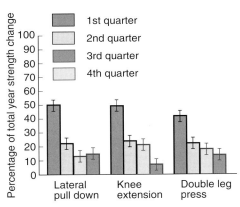

Fig. 6 Percentage of total strength change for the strength-training group over the year, divided into quarters in the lateral pull-down, knee extension, and double leg press.

encouraging because the ability to make strength improvements is an important factor in many athletic activities. The benefits are obvious for events such as shot-put, discus, and power lifting, but are also important in curling, swimming, mountain climbing, and soccer. The need for strength training is perhaps more imperative for ageing athletes than for the young. As noted earlier, ageing skeletal muscle changes so that the fast-twitch fibre population diminishes in diameter and number. The rate of this loss is accelerated by an inactive lifestyle.

Ageing does not appear to affect the frequency with which resistance training can be performed. As a basic guideline, older athletes can complete three resistance training sessions/week for each muscle group. These sessions should be performed on alternate days to permit adequate time for tissue repair and adaptation. If the older athlete finds this schedule to be too demanding they should increase the rest period between sessions. The research of Morganti *et al.* on older women suggests that resistance workouts should consist of three sets of 8 to 10 repetitions, with the person working at 80 per cent of their one repetition maximum.[87] From the standpoint of strength gain, it does not appear to matter what type of equipment is used (free weights, resistance machines, etc.) What is important is that the resistance can be progressively increased as the person gets stronger. Training programmes that regularly utilize the fast-twitch muscle fibre population will minimize the rate at which these losses occur. This is an aspect of training that many athletes neglect, and it often proves to be the deciding factor between victory and defeat. This holds true regardless of the age of the competitor. Maintaining muscle strength is also an important factor in injury prevention. Muscle functions as an important shock absorber, particularly in sports which involve running activities. Weak muscles are less able to absorb mechanical stresses and so greater volumes of these stresses are transmitted to other components of the musculoskeletal system such as cartilage and bony tissues. Under this increased load these tissue will experience premature wear and tear.

One of the most frequently employed training guides is monitoring the response of the athlete's heart rate to exercise. Athletes can easily be taught to take their pulse before, during, and after workouts, or they can rely on one of the numerous heart-rate monitors that are commercially available. A person's maximum heart rate can be estimated using the formula MAHR = 220 – age in years (plus or minus 10). For example, a 40-year-old can expect to have a maximum heart rate in the range of 170 to 190 beats/min. Using this number, it is possible to estimate the heart rate that a person should maintain during workouts of various intensity. For example, during long swims aimed at improving aerobic capacity a heart rate of 70 to 80 per cent of the estimated maximum attainable heart rate should be maintained. It is important to remember that this formula is only an approximation, and that there are many individuals for whom it will not provide a reasonable estimate. In people over 60 years of age, maximum heart rates can range from over 200 to as low as 105 beats/min.[26] This is an enormous variation. Thus target heart rates based on age alone will often under- or overestimate an individual's ideal exercise intensity, neither of which is desirable. In addition, individuals on beta-blockers have their maximum attainable heart rate pharmacologically suppressed. These people are often frustrated because they cannot exercise hard enough to attain heart rates in the target zone. This is both discouraging and potentially dangerous. A safer operating guide is to advise participants to exercise initially at an intensity that permits them to carry on a reasonable conversation. Once a reasonable level of fitness has been achieved, they can then begin to test the parameters of their cardiac response to exercise and so discover their limits.

'No pain, no gain' is a commonly quoted training philosophy. While this motto is intended to remind us that it takes sacrifice and dedication to improve, some people interpret it literally. The latter approach is dangerous as it encourages people to ignore pain, one of the body's important warning signals. Encouraging individuals to train to the point of pain is inappropriate, especially when dealing with adults who have just abandoned their sedentary lifestyle in pursuit of the benefits of active living. Many of these people have never been in good physical condition and every exposure they have ever had to exercise has been painful. Many of them believe that everyone who exercises experiences pain and they cannot comprehend why anyone would voluntarily do this on a regular basis. This is one reason why many people who become involved in fitness programmes give up before they are fit enough to realize how enjoyable it can be. Physical educators and health-care professionals must encourage older adults to begin training at a level they enjoy and will want to come back to. If this approach is taken, more older adults will become enthusiastic about fitness and perhaps the news will spread that exercise does not have to be a 'near death' experience.

One strategy that more and more athletes are employing to avoid injury is cross-training. The basic principle here is to vary the types of stresses applied to the body as well as the parts of the body they are applied to. To this end, athletes combine a variety of activities including such things as swimming, running, walking, cycling, aerobics, stair-climbing, rowing, cross-country skiing, and in-line skating. Cross-training offers the athlete a number of advantages including a reduction in injury rate, increased variety, and the ability to train intensely more frequently. This approach to training makes sense at every age, but it makes particular sense for ageing athletes who need increasingly longer recovery periods between intense workouts in order to avoid becoming injured. This ever-increasing need to recover means that the ageing competitor is able to train intensely less often and this will adversely affect performance. By incorporating cross-training into their programmes ath-

letes can continue to train relatively intensely at one activity while recovering from another. The 1972 Olympic Marathon Gold Medallist, Frank Shorter, is now a masters athlete and his training programme consists of a balance between running and cycling. Prior to this change in approach, he found himself plagued by an ever-increasing number of injuries. With the incorporation of regular cycling sessions into his schedule, he has had no major injury problems and his running performances have not suffered appreciably. Cross-training also encourages the development of muscle balance and flexibility—two important elements in the prevention of injury. The psychological benefits of varying your training cannot be over-emphasized. Athletes who are mentally fresh approach their training with enthusiasm and are less likely to experience overtraining syndrome. Ageing competitors who wish to extend their competitive careers would be wise to regularly employ cross-training in their programmes and they will find the need for this variety will increase the older they get.

Rest is a critical component of every athlete's training programme. The very nature of a training programme involves subjecting the body to stresses sufficient to cause tissue breakdown. The athlete must then ease off to allow the body sufficient time to replace, repair, reinforce, and recover. The body undergoes its adaptive responses during the recovery phase. Athletes who fail to incorporate rest and recovery into their programme often experience tissue breakdown at a rate faster than tissue repairs can be effected. With this imbalance, it will not be long before injuries occur and the athlete is forced to rest. The recovery needs of each athlete are extremely variable. Some individuals can only work intensely twice a week and require easier sessions on the other 5 days. Others can work hard for 6 days, take a day off, and then start again. Despite this wide variation in rest requirements, one thing is certain: the capacity to recover from intense workouts is significantly reduced with ageing. Athletes who were training hard on alternate days in their thirties often find that they can only work hard every fourth or fifth day in their forties. The reason for this change is uncertain, but it could be conjectured that the body's ability to initiate the protein synthesis needed for cellular repair may slow with increasing age. Regardless of the mechanism, anyone coaching ageing athletes must recognize that they cannot be placed on the same training schedule as younger athletes. If they are, it is probable that insufficient recovery time will be provided and the athletes will soon be injured or overtrained.

The final comment on training focuses on the need for a pre-programme medical evaluation. It is recommended that all older individuals who have never been active or who are returning to an active lifestyle be given a thorough medical assessment. Many of these individuals will have disease processes and orthopaedic problems that should be addressed before they begin a vigorous training programme. An evaluation of this type should include the following:

(1) an assessment of risk factors for cardiovascular disease, respiratory problems, and diabetes;

(2) a general medical examination with attention focused on the cardiovascular, respiratory, and musculoskeletal systems;

(3) a general assessment of strength and flexibility;

(4) an electrocardiogram; and

(5) a stress test if anything in the history or physical examination suggests potential cardiovascular compromise.

This evaluation also affords the assessor the opportunity to reinforce some of the basic training principles with the individual. It is hoped that this screening process will identify individuals with problems before they injure themselves. It is also hoped that those who are given clean bills of health will feel more confident as they embark on the road to fitness.

Conclusions

In this chapter we have addressed the phenomenon of ageing and how it potentially influences the athletic performance of the older competitor. After careful consideration, it is clear that the ageing athlete is a unique entity in the world of sport. The masters athletic movement is growing rapidly, and it will continue to grow as our population continues to age. Some élite masters are capable of world-class performances and several have won medals in international competition. We have seen that ageing is a universal, intrinsic, progressive, and deleterious process. Notwithstanding this, the specific mechanism by which ageing occurs remains uncertain. A well-defined collection of structural and physiological changes occur with ageing, and many of these alterations are associated with declining athletic performance. In addition, ageing athletes live in a psychosocial environment very different from their younger opponents. In this environment, issues such as loss of motivation can prove to be more debilitating than all the physical alterations combined in producing a deterioration in athletic performance. The ageing competitor appears to be less able to handle the stresses associated with performing in the heat, the cold, or at altitude, but the age-related changes that are involved here are not nearly as important as the effects of diminished cardiovascular fitness, disease processes, and lack of acclimatization. All these changes influence injury patterns, healing rates, and treatment approaches. The reader is reminded that much of the research in this area has been biased by poorly designed studies that failed to control for confounding variables such as disease processes, environmental influences, medications, lifestyle habits, and inactivity. Of these, the influence of inactivity is probably the most underestimated and potentially the most easily corrected.

The structural and physiological changes associated with an inactive lifestyle may be the greatest health threat facing our ageing population. Aristotle recognized this fact several thousand years ago when he wrote that 'life is motion'. In the ensuing years science has produced no evidence to dispute this basic truth. More recently, Shephard, a leader in the field of exercise physiology, has stated that:[70] 'Physical activity has more potential for promoting healthy ageing than anything else science or medicine has to offer today'. There can be no denying that the body was designed such that its structure and function are improved with regular use and that, deprived of this stimulus, it will undergo many degenerative changes. Active living is a prescription for life, and it is one of those miracle medicines that does everything we ask of it with very few side-effects. It is truly a fountain of youth that is available to us all. In sharing his secret of successful ageing, Sheehan[74] offers this inspiring advice.

The best way to play the aging game is to concede nothing. Never make it easy for yourself. Should your body suggest it is too old for this effort, say 'Nonsense!'

Should your mind decide it is too late to learn new tricks, say 'Balderdash!' Should your soul say it needs a respite from duty and obligation, say 'Rubbish'.

If we follow this advice it may be possible to live up to the motto of the American Health Foundation which states: 'The art of living consists of dying young, but as late as possible'.

References

1. Kasch FW, Boyer, JL, Van Camp SP, Verity LS, Wallace JP. The effect of physical activity and inactivity on aerobic power in older men (a longitudinal study). *Physician and Sportsmedicine* 1990; **18**: 73–83.
2. Chesworth BM, Vandervoort AA. Age and passive ankle stiffness in healthy women. *Physical Therapy* 1989; **69**: 217–24.
3. Gorman KM, Posner JD. Benefits of exercise in old age. *Clinics in Geriatric Medicine* 1988; **4**: 181–92.
4. Eaglestein WH. Wound healing and ageing. *Clinics in Geriatric Medicine* 1989; **5**: 183–8.
5. Strehler BL. *Time, cells and ageing.* New York: Academic Press, 1962.
6. Siegel AJ, Warhol MJ, Lang E. Muscle injury and repair in ultra long distance runners. In: Sutton JR, Brock RM, eds. *Sports medicine for the mature athlete.* Indianapolis: Benchmark Press, 1986: 35–43.
7. Stauss RH. *Sports medicine.* Philadelphia: WB Saunders, 1984.
8. Belt E. Leonardo da Vinci's studies of the ageing process. *Geriatrics* 1952; **7**: 205–10.
9. Hayflick L, Moorhead PS. The serial cultivation of human diploid cell strains. *Experimental Cell Research* 1961; **25**: 585–621.
10. Makinodan T. Biology of ageing. In: Meakins JL, McClaran JC, eds. *Surgical care of the elderly.* Chicago: Year Book Medical Publishers, 1988.
11. Walford RL. *The immunologic theory of ageing.* Copenhagen: Munksgaard, 1969.
12. McArdle WD, Katch FI, Katch VL. *Exercise physiology—energy, nutrition and human performance.* 2nd edn. Philadelphia: Lea and Febiger, 1986.
13. Fixx JF. The test of time. *Runner* 1984; **May**: 58–62.
14. Astrand PO. Exercise physiology of the mature athlete. In: Sutton JR, Brock RM, eds. *Sports medicine for the mature athlete.* Indianapolis: Benchmark Press, 1986: 3–16.
15. Goldman R. Speculations on vascular changes with age. *Journal of the American Geriatric Society* 1970; **18**: 765–9.
16. Schuman JE. Some changes of ageing. *Journal of Otolaryngology* 1986; **15**: 211–13.
17. Jackson AS, Beard EF, Wier LT, Ross RM, Stuteville, Blair SN. Changes in aerobic power of men, ages 25–70 yr. *Medicine and Science in Sports and Exercise* 1995; **27**: 113–20.
18. Berman R, Haxby JV, Pomerantz RS. Physiology of ageing. Part 1: Normal changes. *Patient Care* 1988; **22**: 20–36.
19. Babcock MA, Paterson DH, Cunningham DA. Effects of aerobic endurance training on gas exchange kinetics in older men. *Medicine and Science in Sports and Exercise* 1994; **25**: 447–52.
20. Green JS, Crouse SF. The effect of endurance training on functional capacity in the elderly: a meta-analysis. *Medicine and Science in Sports and Exercise* 1995; **27**: 920–6.
21. Bortz WM II. Disuse and ageing. *Journal of the American Medical Association* 1982; **248**: 1203–8.
22. Sheppard JG, Pacelli LC. Why your patients shouldn't take ageing sitting down. *Physician and Sportsmedicine* 1990; **18**: 83–91.
23. Tate CA, Hyek MF, Taffet GE. Mechanisms for the responses of cardiac muscle to physical activity in old age. *Medicine and Science in Sports and Exercise* 1994; **26**: 561–7.

24. McClaren JC. Clinical profile of the elderly. In: Meakins JL, McClaran JC, eds. *Surgical care of the elderly.* Chicago: Year Book Medical Publishers, 1988.

25. Kitzman DW, Edward WD. Age-related changes in the anatomy of the normal human heart. *Journal of Gerontology* 1990; **45**: M33–9.

26. Brooks GA, Fahey TD. *Exercise physiology, human bioenergetics and its applications.* New York: Macmillan, 1985.

27. Zauber NP, Zauber AG. Hematologic data of healthy very old people. *Journal of the American Medical Association* 1987; **257**: 2181–4.

28. Torp S, Baer E, Friedman B. Effects of age and mechanical deformation on the ultra structure of tendon. *Proceedings of 1974 Colston Conference on Structure of Fibrous Biopolymers.* London: Butterworths, 1975: 223–50.

29. Viidik A. Connective tissues—possible implications of the temporal changes of the ageing process. *Mechanisms of Ageing and Development* 1979; **9**: 267–85.

30. Stryer L. *Biochemistry.* 2nd edn. San Francisco: WH Freeman, 1981.

31. Turek SL. *Orthopedics—principles and their application.* 4th edn. Philadelphia: JB Lippincott, 1984.

32. Alnaqeeb MA, Al Zrid NS, Goldspink E. Connective tissue changes and physical properties of developing and ageing skeletal muscle. *Journal of Anatomy* 1984; **139**: 677–89.

33. Balin AK, Allen RG. Molecular basis of biologic ageing. *Clinics in Geriatric Medicine* 1989; **5**: 1–18.

34. Hamlin CR, Kohn RR, Luschin JH. Apparent accelerated ageing of human collagen fibers. *Diabetes* 1975; **24**: 902.

35. Nejjar I, Pieraggi MT, Thiers JC, Bouissou H. Age-related changes in the elastic tissue of the human thoracic aorta. *Atherosclerosis* 1990; **80**: 199–208.

36. Fenske NA, Lober CW. Skin changes of ageing: pathological implications. *Geriatrics* 1990; **45**: 27–32.

37. Wolff J. *Das Gesetz der Transformation der Knochen.* Berlin: A Hirschwald, 1892.

38. Bassett CA, Becker RO. Generation of electric potentials by bone in response to mechanical stress. *Science* 1962; **137**: 1063–4.

39. Stillman RJ, Lohman TG, Slaughter MH, Massey BH. Physical activity and bone mineral content in women aged 30 to 85 years. *Medicine and Science in Sports and Exercise* 1986; **18**: 576–80.

40. Beyer R, Huang JC, Wilshire EB. The effect of endurance exercise on bone dimensions, collagen and calcium in the ageing male rat. *Experimental Gerontology* 1985; **20**: 315–23.

41. Smith EL. Exercise for the prevention of osteoporosis: a review. *Physician and Sportsmedicine* 1982; **10**: 72–9.

42. Twomey L, Taylor J. Age changes in lumbar intervertrebral discs. *Acta Orthopaedica Scandinavica* 1985; **56**: 496–9.

43. Sager K. Senior fitness—for the health of it. *Physician and Sportsmedicine* 1983; **11**: 31–6.

44. Knudson RJ, Clark DF, Kennedy TC, Knudson DE. Effect of ageing alone on mechanical properties of the normal adult human lung. *Journal of Applied Physiology* 1977; **43**: 1054–62.

45. Jones PL, Millman A. Wound healing and the aged patient. *Nursing Clinics of North America* 1990; **25**: 263–77.

46. Brooks SV, Faulkner JA. Skeletal muscle weakness in old age: underlying mechanisms. *Medicine and Science in Sports and Exercise* 1994; **26**: 432–9.

47. deVries HA. *Physiology of exercise for physical education and athletics.* 4th edn. Dubuque, Iowa: WC Brown, 1986.

48. Wiswell RA, Jaque SV, Hamilton-Wessler M. Exercise and muscle strength. In: Morley JE, Glick Z, Rubenstein LZ, eds. *Geriatric nutrition.* New York: Raven Press, 1990: 447–56.

49. Larsson L, Sjodin B, Karlsson J. Histochemical and biochemical changes in human skeletal muscle with age in sedentary males, age 22–65 years. *Acta Physiologica Scandinavica* 1978; **103**: 31–9.

50. Molander B, Backman L. Age differences in heart rate patterns during concentration in a precision sport: implications for attentional functioning. *Journal of Gerontology* 1989; **44**: P80–7.

51. Munnings F. Strength training—not only for the young. *Physician and Sportsmedicine* 1993; **21**: 133–40.

52. Plyley MJ. Fine-tuning muscle capillary supply for maximum exercise performance. *Cardiology* 1990; **6**: 25–34.

53. Babcock MA, Paterson DH, Cunningham DA, Dickinson JR. Exercise on-transient gas exchange kinetics are slowed as a function of age. *Medicine and Science in Sports and Exercise* 1994; **26**: 440–6.

54. Meltzer DE. Age dependence of olympic weightlifting ability. *Medicine and Science in Sports and Exercise* 1994; **26**: 1053–67.

55. Damon EL. An experimental investigation of the relationship of age to various parameters of muscle strength. Doctoral dissertation, University of Southern California, 1971.

56. Green HJ. Characteristics of ageing human skeletal muscles. In: Sutton JR, Brock RM, eds. *Sports medicine for the mature athlete.* Indianapolis: Benchmark Press, 1986: 17–26.

57. Sato T, Akatsuh H, Kito K, Tokoro Y, Tauchi H, Kato K. Age changes of myofibrils of human minor pectoral muscle. *Mechanisms of Ageing and Development* 1986; **34**: 297–304.

58. Knortz KA. Muscle physiology applied to geriatric rehabilitation. *Topics in Geriatric Rehabilitation* 1987; **2**: 1–12.

59. Klitgaard H, Mantoni M, Schiaffino S, *et al.* Function, morphology and protein expression of ageing skeletal muscle: a cross-sectional study of elderly men with different training backgrounds. *Acta Physiologica Scandinavica* 1990; **140**: 41–54.

60. May C, Kaye JA, Atack JR, Schapiro MB, Friedland RP, Rapoport SI. Cerebrospinal fluid production is reduced in healthy ageing. *Neurology* 1990; **40**: 50–2.

61. Berman R, Haxby JV, Pomerantz RS. Physiology of ageing. Part 2: Clinical implications. *Patient Care* 1988; **22**: 39–66.

62. Spirduso WW, Clifford P. Replication of age and physical activity effects on reaction and movement time. *Journal of Gerontology* 1978; **33**: 26.

63. Hofland B, Willis S, Baltes P. Fluid intelligence performance in the elderly: intra-individual variability and conditions of assessment. *Journal of Educational Psychology* 1981; **73**: 573–86.

64. Dinner DS, Erman MK, Roth T. Help for geriatric sleep problems. *Patient Care* 1990; **2**: 24–31.

65. Booth FW, Gould EW. Effects of training and desire on connective tissue. *Exercise and Sports Science Review* 1975; **3**: 83–112.

66. Vailas AC, Perrini VA, Pedrini-Mille A, Holloszy JO. Patellar tendon matrix changes associated with ageing and voluntary exercise. *Journal of Applied Psychology* 1985; **58**: 1572–6.

67. Hall MD. Cartilage changes after experimental relief of contact in the knee joint of the mature rat. *Clinical Orthopedics* 1969; **64**: 64–76.

68. Ungerleider S, Porter K, Golding J, Foster J. Mental advantages for masters. *Running Times* 1989; July: 18–20.

69. Edelstein JE. Foot care for the ageing. *Physical Therapy* 1988; **68**: 1882–6.

70. Kavanagh T, Shephard RJ. Can regular sports participation slow the ageing process? Data on masters athletes. *Physician and Sportsmedicine* 1990; **18**: 94–104.

71. Tymn M. Carl Hatfield: never beaten by a McCoy. *National Masters News* 1988; May: 18.

72. Russell B, Branch T. *Second wind.* New York: Ballantine, 1980.

73. Kubler-Ross E. *On death and dying.* New York: Macmillan, 1969.

74. Sheehan G. *Personal best.* Emmaus, PA: Rodale Press, 1989.

75. *The Works of Shakespeare.* Shakespeare Head Press Edition, Oxford University Press, 1938: 1249.

76. Balcomb AC, Sutton JR. Advanced age and altitude illness. In: Sutton JR, Brook RM, eds. *Sports medicine for the mature athlete.* Indianapolis: Benchmark Press, 1986: 213–24.

77. Kenny MJ, Gisolfi CV. Thermal regulation: effects of exercise and age. In: Sutton JR, Brock RM, eds. *Sports medicine for the mature athlete*. Indianapolis: Benchmark Press, 1986: 133–41.

78. Astrand PO, Rodahl K. *Textbook of work physiology*. Singapore: McGraw Hill, 1986.

79. Kenny WL, Anderson RK. Responses of older and younger women to exercise in dry and humid heat without fluid replacement. *Medicine and Science in Sports and Exercise* 1988; **20**: 155–60.

80. Brown M. Special considerations during rehabilitation of the aged athlete. *Clinics in Sports Medicine* 1989; **8**: 893–901.

81. DeHaven KE, Littner DM. Athletic injuries: comparison by age, sport and gender. *American Journal of Sports Medicine* 1986; **14**: 218–24.

82. McRae R. *Practical fracture treatment*. New York: Churchill Livingstone, 1981.

83. Valaschini G, Macintyre J. Immediate reduction of shoulder dislocation. *Physician and Sportsmedicine* 1995; **23**: 61–5.

84. Huang SHK. Preventing NSAID-induced gastropathy before it becomes a pain in the gut. *Canadian Journal of Geriatrics* 1989; **5**: 29–34.

85. Tymn M. Frank Shorter is looking ahead. *National Masters News* 1987; May: 6.

86. Thomas SG, Cunningham DA, Rechnitzer PA, Donner AP, Howard JH. Determinants of the training response in elderly men. *Medicine and Science in Sports and Exercise* 1985; **17**: 667–72.

87. Morganti CM, Nelson ME, Fiatarone MA, *et al*. Strength improvements with 1 yr of progressive resistance training in older women. *Medicine and Science in Sports and Exercise* 1995; **27**: 906–12.

88. Ungerleider S. Mood profiles of masters track and field athletes. *Perceptual and Motor Skills* 1989; **68**: 607–17.

6.5 Athletes with a disability

Darren W. Booth and Basil J. Grogono

A challenge for sports medicine

Introduction

The ability of the human spirit to overcome every conceivable barrier is nowhere more evident than in the explosion of athletic activites performed by men, women, and children who are disadvantaged by physical or mental disability. It is ability rather than disability that should be universally recognized.

During the past decade, with advances in rehabilitation, coaching techniques, and concomitant technological improvements in sports equipment, disabled athletes can compete effectively in an incredibly wide variety of sports. Improvements in wheelchair design allow wheelchair athletes to race with unheralded speed in sprint races and outpace the able-bodied in marathon races. New prostheses bring enhanced performance for the amputee. Specialized adaptations permit the enthusiast to participate in sailing and ocean racing, paragliding and microlight flying (Fig. 1), scuba diving, winter sports, etc.

Furthermore, there has been an awakening of the medical and scientific communities, allied professionals, and the general public to the full potential of the disabled athlete. Not every disabled person aspires to become an international star. It requires tremendous dedication and prolonged effort to reach the standards of the Para-

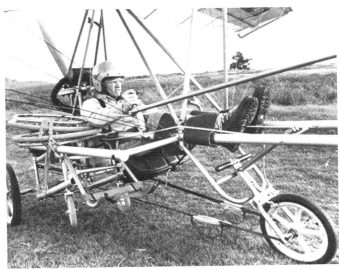

Fig. 1 Disabled people can fly a microlight aircraft.

lympics. Yet élite athletes are a role model, and success in sport has been recorded as improving morale and adjustment for many individuals.

Thus potential athletes can be divided into:

(1) recreational

(2) competitive

(3) élite with national and global ambitions.

It is the élite athlete who gains recognition and for whom vast funds are raised. However, with ingenuity and imagination, relatively simple facilities and devices can initiate local competition and team events. It is from simple beginnings that the whole 'sports for the disabled' movement began.

Historical perspective: evolution of sports for disabled people

The origin of competitive sport for disabled people is directly related to the rehabilitation of Second World War veterans with spinal cord injuries, although there are earlier examples of outstanding disabled athletes and sports organizations for the disabled.[1] However, it was the renewed interest in sport as therapy after the war in the United Kingdom and the United States that opened the way for the present widespread adoption of sport for the disabled.

The young and enthusiastic Dr Ludwig Guttman, Director of the Spinal Injury Centre at the Stoke Mandeville Hospital in England, instituted wheelchair basketball, archery, bowling, and fencing in his rehabilitation programme during the Second World War. In 1948, he organized the first international sporting event with an archery competition between the resident paraplegics and similarly disabled Dutch athletes. Concurrent developments in the United States[2] involved the beginnings of wheelchair basketball competitions between the Veterans' Administration Hospitals. A prominent figure in this movement was Professor Timothy Nugent of the University of Illinois. He was responsible for organizing the first National Wheelchair Basketball Tournament in Illinois in 1949. It is interesting to note that, whereas wheelchair sports were confined to spinal cord victims in Stoke Mandeville, amputees were allowed to participate in the United States.

The Stoke Mandeville Games grew in success to include an ever-increasing number of countries, and in 1956 the Games were formally recognized by the International Olympic Committee with the presentation of the Fearnley Cup, a symbol of the aim of the

Olympic movement. Similar developments in the United States led to the first National Wheelchair Games in New York, where competitions included basketball, track and field events, swimming, table tennis, and archery.

The birth of key organizations

The National Wheelchair Athletic Association (**NWAA**) in the United States was formed in 1958, and the International Stoke Mandeville Games Committee (**ISMGC**) was created in 1960. They combined in their early phases of development and became officially affiliated, thus the Games took another giant step forward in their remarkable international progress. In this same year, a deliberate attempt was made to connect the Olympics and the 'Paralympics' when the first Paralympics were held in Rome, Italy.

International Sports Organization for the Disabled (ISOD)

The Paralympics held in Japan in 1964 provided the impetus to the inauguration of this organization.

International Coordinating Committee (ICC) for World Sport

The 'Paralympics' were established under the control of this one body in 1982 after agreement by the International Olympic Committee (**IOC**). The 1984 games in New York and Stoke Mandeville were the first to benefit.

International Paralympic Committee (IPC)

This committee has now replaced the IOC and was responsible for awarding the X Paralympics to Atlanta in 1996. Over 3310 athletes from 104 nations attended this milestone in the history of sports for the disabled.

Committee International de Sports des Sourds (CISS) (International Committee of Sports for the Deaf)[3]

Sports for the deaf were inaugurated in Paris as long ago as 1924 when seven nations competed in athletics, cycling, football, shooting, and swimming events.[4]

The CISS was founded in 1926. Since then, the 'Silent Games' have been held every four years. An agreement was reached in 1990 between the IPC and the CISS at an extraordinary meeting held in Germany, when:

1. The CISS was recognized as the supreme authority for the deaf.

2. The World Games for the Deaf (summer and winter) were given the same status as the Paralympics.

3. Funding for sports for the disabled was to be shared with the CISS on a proportional basis.

The most recent World Games for the Deaf were held between 13 and 16 July 1997, in Copenhagen.

CISS is no longer affiliated with the International Paralympic Committee (IPC). It is recognized by the International Olympic Committee (IOC).

In his book 'Deaf Sports' David Stewart explain: 'Sports for the Deaf' is a vehicle for understanding the dynamics of being deaf.[5] It serves as a catalyst for socialization, provides access to support sys-

Date	Place		Number of countries	Number of athletes
1949	Seefeld	Austria	5	33
1953	Oslo	Norway	6	43
1955	Oberammegau	Germany	8	57
1959	Montana-Vermala	Switzerland	8	56
1963	Are	Sweden	8	53
1967	Berchesagarten	Germany	12	86
1971	Adelboden	Switzerland	13	92
1975	Lake Placid	USA	15	268
1979	Meribel	France	14	94
1983	Madonna di Campiglio	Italy	16	143
1991	Banff	Canada	16	
1995	Yllas	Finland	19	267
1999	Davos	Switzerland	—	—

Table 1 CISS Winter World Games

tems, and plays an important part in the education of children and adults. The World Games for the Deaf bringing together the Deaf community are held every fourth year. There are winter and summer games. Tables 1 and 2 document the success of these wonderful events.

A world of silence and signs

Contestants in these games are not allowed to wear hearing aids while competing and must have at least 55 dB hearing loss in the best ear. Further information is available on the Internet.

The Paralympics and other international competitions (Table 3)

Whilst international competitions were subsequently held at Stoke Mandeville every 3 years, the Paraplegic Olympic Games (Paralympics) became established every 4 years. In 1960, the first Paraplegic Games were held just a few weeks after the Rome Olympics. A total of 400 wheelchair athletes from 23 countries participated. They lived in the Olympic village and competed in the Olympic stadium. Sir Ludwig Guttman was saluted by His Grace Pope Paul who compared him with the founder of the Olympic Movement declaring: 'You are the 'de Coubertin' of the paralysed!'

In 1964, the II Paralympics were held in Tokyo and were supported by the Japanese royal family. These Games were meticulously planned, and there was an independent Paralympic village for the first time. The Paralympic flag, anthem, and poster heralded another step forward and served as an impetus for the formation of the International Organization for Sports for the Disabled (**ISOD**).

The Paralympics were hosted by Tel Aviv in 1968 and by Heidelberg in 1972. On this latter occasion there were over 1000 competitors from 44 countries who were housed in a splendid university which is specially adapted for wheelchair students. Demonstration sports, involving amputee and blind athletes of the German disabled sports movement, conveyed their need for international competition.

The first true Olympic Games for the disabled took place at the

Table 2 CIIS World Summer Games for the Deaf

	Date	Place		Number of nations	Number of athletes
1.	1924	Paris	France	9	133
2.	1928	Amsterdam	Holland	10	210
3.	1931	Nuremburg	Germany	14	316
4.	1935	London	United Kingdom	12	283
5.	1939	Stockholm	Sweden	13	264
6.	1949	Copenhagen	Denmark	14	393
7.	1953	Brussels	Belgium	16	524
8.	1957	Milan	Italy	25	626
9.	1961	Helsinki	Finland	24	595
10.	1965	Washington	USA	27	697
11.	1969	Belgrade	Yugoslavia	33	1183
12.	1973	Malmö	Sweden	32	1061
13.	1977	Bucharest	Romania	32	1118
14.	1981	Cologne	Germany	32	1213
15.	1985	Los Angeles	USA	29	1053
16.	1989	Christchurch	New Zealand	30	959
17.	1993	Sofia	Bulgaria	51	1706
18.	1997	Copenhagen	Denmark	70	2098
19.	2001	Rome	Italy	—	—

Toronto Olympiad in 1976.[6] These Games saw the participation of 1560 paralysed, amputee, and blind athletes from 40 countries in a truly international sporting event. It was held under the chairmanship of Robert Jackson, but was complicated by the withdrawal of athletes from eight countries because of the inclusion of a team from South Africa. In 1980, the Olympiad was held in Arnhem, Holland, and marked the inclusion of athletes with cerebral palsy for the first time.

The 1988 Games in Seoul and then the 1992 Games in Barcelona were heralded to be the most ambitious and successful Paralympic Games. Each attracted record numbers of athletes, participating nations, and media coverage. Barcelona was remarkable because of the sell-out crowds with a total of over a million spectators! As already mentioned, the X Paralympics held in Atlanta in 1996 saw the participation of 3350 athletes from 120 nations.

Pan American Games: the aim to foster sport in other countries

Winnipeg, Manitoba, held the first Pan American Games in 1967[7] which proved to be a great impetus for Canada and many other countries; Mexico, Argentina, Brazil, Peru, Jamaica, Tobago, and Trinidad all participated although they had very few resources.

World Games for the Deaf

Mention has already been made of these Games.

Sports for the disabled

Examples of year-round sports

Basketball (wheelchair)[8]

Wheelchair basketball involves two teams of five players and is a highly competitive and exciting game which has become a world-class sport. In 1993 the International Wheelchair Basketball Federation (IWBF) became an independent sports federation with 50 member nations. It aims to organize and develop wheelchair competitions to the highest level and increase the number of countries involved. It provides training for referees and classifiers, and sets the rules. Players are awarded 1 to 4.5 points according to degree of functional disability. No team can field a team with more than 14

Table 3 Growth in the Paralympic Games from 1960 to 1996

Paralympic Games			Athletes and support staff	Countries taking part
1960	I	Rome, Italy	400	23
1964	II	Tokyo, Japan	390	22
1968	III	Tel Aviv	1000	29
1972	IV	Heidelberg, Germany	1400	44
1976	V	Toronto, Canada	2700	42
1980	VI	Arnhem, Holland	2500	42
1984	VII	New York, USA	1700	41
	VII	Stoke Mandeville, UK	2300	45
1988	VIII	Seoul, Korea	4200	62
1992	IX	Barcelona, Spain	4158	83
1996	X	Atlanta, USA	3500 (1000 coaches and support staff, 8000 volunteers)	120

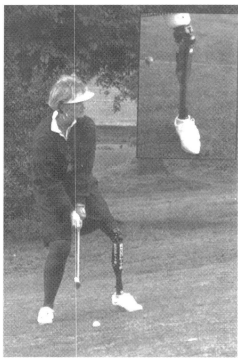

Fig. 2 Golfing (inset shows a close-up view of the prosthesis).

points. The Gold Cup for men is held every 4 years. The Gold Cup for women was held at St Etienne, France in 1990.

Boccia

This is a precision game, similar to lawn bowls, played by athletes with cerebral palsy. Boccia is very popular as it is one of the very few activities that allows those with severe disabilities to compete against each other. There are team and individual events. The athlete attempts to bowl a special leather ball as close as possible to a 'jack' by throwing or rolling it down a narrow playing field (a tube can be used to launch and direct the ball). The game requires the co-operation of the coach who is allowed to help but not direct the direction and distance traversed by the Boccia ball.

Cycling

For competition purposes, three categories are designated: cyclists with cerebral palsy; visually impaired and blind; and amputees with other athletes. It is remarkable how well many competitors with cerebral palsy can perform. They may use tricycles. Blind cyclists ride tandem with a sighted rider in front. Amputees can adapt their cycles to their needs. Timed trials and road racing events are popular.

Golf

Both amputees and the blind can participate in this sport. The amputees have a variety of different devices to assist them (Fig. 2). There is also a specially adapted cart with a swivel seat for those who want to play 'sit-golf'.

Goalball

This sport is played by all classes of visually impaired athletes and is played between two teams of three competitors. The ball contains a bell to guide the players, and the goalmouth is wide. The 'centre' of one team hurls the ball along the floor towards their opponents' goal. The defenders orient themselves to the ball's trajectory by listening to the bell. The object is to use the body to block the ball from entering the net (Fig. 3). This a very strenuous and exciting game for spectators and participants alike, and is played in silence. The referee is careful to check that all players are completely blindfolded.

Riding for the disabled

Horseback riding can be very beneficial for children, adolescents, and adults with cerebral palsy and other disabilities. Many riders who have difficulty in walking seem to gain confidence and improve their co-ordination when they entrust their talents to their steed. Expert instruction is available in many parts of the world and competitions include dressage and even some jumping.

Personal ponies is an example of a unique organization which promotes this sport. It is dedicated to providing Shetland ponies for disabled children in the United States, details of which can be found on the Internet.

Rugby (wheelchair)

Quadraplegics play this game using a volleyball. Players dribble and pass the ball and score by making a goal. It is a vigorous game also known as 'murder'.

Swimming

This is one of the longest standing and most popular sports in which all 'disabled' people can take part and compete. At the competitive level, the classification process has been very carefully designed to ensure that fellow athletes have a similar level of functional impairment. Athletes are divided into two groups: blind or visually impaired; and others. Details of this Functional Classification System can be found in the medical classification guide (IPC Assembly Executive Committee for Swimming; see also Table 4 and below).

Tennis (wheelchair)

A good game of wheelchair tennis is just as enthralling as watching Wimbledon and wonderful for the players who have conquered the art of combining strokes, wheelchair manipulation, and strategy.

The rules are the same as standard tennis except that the ball is allowed to bounce twice. Wheelchairs are designed to be instantly manoeuvrable, and racquets are light but strong. Quadriplegics can

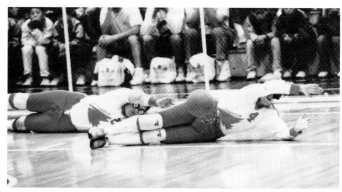

Fig. 3 Goalball played by visually impaired athletes.

Table 4 Functional Classification System (FCS)—Categories and classes

Visually Impaired

ATHLETICS

T10	No light perception; unable to recognize hand shapes
T11	2/60 and/or visual field of less than
F11	five degrees*
T12	2/60–6/60 and visual field of more
F12	than five degrees and less than twenty degrees*

Amputee

T42	Single above-the-knee; combined lower and upper limb amputations; minimum disability
T43	Double below-the-knee; combined lower and upper limb amputations; normal function in throwing arm
T44	Single below-the-knee; combined lower and upper limb amputations; moderate reduced function in one or both limbs
T45	Double above-the-elbow; double below-the-knee
T46	Single above-the-elbow; single below-the-elbow; upper limb function in throwing arm
F40	Double above-the-knee; combined lower and upper limb amputations; severe problems when walking
F41	Standing athletes with no more than seventy points in the lower limbs**
F42	Single above-the-knee; combined lower and upper limb amputation; normal function in throwing arm
F43	Double below-the-knee; combined lower and upper limb amputations; normal function in throwing arm
F44	Single below-the-knee; combined lower and upper limb amputations; normal function in throwing arm
F45	Double above-the-elbow; double below-the-elbow
F46	Single above-the-elbow; single below-the-elbow; upper limb function in throwing arm

Cerebral Palsy

T30	Severe to moderate involvement; uses one or two arms to push wheelchair; control is poor; affects both arms and legs
T31	Severe to moderate involvement; foot propelled wheelchair push; affects both arms and legs
T32	Limited control of movements; some throwing motion
T32 F32	Full upper strength in upper extremity; propels wheelchair independently; affects both arms and legs; or same side arm and leg
T33 F33	Good functional strength with minimal limitation or control problems in upper limbs and trunk; affects lower legs
T34 F34	May use assistive devices; slight loss of balance; affects lower legs or both legs and one arm
T35 F35	Walks or runs without assistive devices; balance and fine motor control problems
T36 F36	Good functional ability in dominant side of body; affects arm and leg on same side of body
T37 F37	Minimal involvement; could be present in lower legs, arm and leg on same side of body, one leg, or demonstrate problems with balance

Wheelchair

T50	Uses palms to push wheelchair; may have shoulder weakness
T51	Pushing power comes from elbow extension
T52	Normal upper limb function; no active trunk
T53	Backwards movement of trunk; uses trunk to steer; double above-the-knee amputations
F50	No grip with non-throwing arm; may have shoulder weakness
F51	Difficulty gripping with non-throwing arm
F52	Nearly normal grip with non-throwing arm
F53	No sitting balance
F54	Fair to good sitting balance
F55	Good balance and movements backwards and forwards; good trunk rotation
F56	Good movements backwards and forwards; usually to one side (side to side movements)
F57	Standard muscle chart of all limbs must not exceed seventy points**

Functional
(Swimming)

S1	Unable to catch water; restricted range of motion; no trunk control; leg drag; assisted water start
S2	Unable to catch water; restricted range of motion; no trunk control; slight leg propulsion; unassisted water start
S3	Wrist control limited; limited arm propulsion; minimal trunk control; hips below water; water start
S4	Wrist control; arms not full fluent; minimal trunk control; hips below water; better body position
S5	Full propulsion in catch phrase; limited arm movement; trunk function; leg propulsion; sit or stand starts
S6	Catch phrase present; arm movement efficient; trunk control; leg propulsion; push start, sit or stand
S7	Good hands; good arms; good trunk; hips level; stand or sit dive start
S8	Hand propulsion; arm cycle good; trunk good; hips and legs level; use of start blocks
S9	Full hand propulsion; full arm propulsion; full trunk control; propulsive kick; dive start from blocks
S10	Full hand and arm propulsion; full trunk control; strong leg kick; dive start and propulsion in turns

Visually Impaired

CYCLING, GOALBALL, JUDO & SWIMMING

B1	No light perception, unable to recognize hand shapes
B2	Visual acuity of 2/60 with less than 5 degrees field of vision
B3	Visual acuity of 2/60-6/60 and field of vision from 5–20 degrees

*   Normal field of vision is approximately 120–180 degrees
**   The extent of the disability is represented by an evaluation which tests function and strength of the muscle groups. Function and muscle strength are represented by point values for each class (i.e. less than 70 points equals an F 41 or F57 athlete)
From the Xth Paralympic Games Official Commemorative Program. Disability Today Publicity Group Inc., 1996: 79.

play this game but have to choose their own method of fixing their racquet to their wrist. They can use powered chairs. The International Wheelchair Tennis Federation promotes this sport in which more than 70 nations now participate.

Volleyball

Volleyball has been adapted for disabled athletes, largely as a result of the enthusiasm of the Dutch, and can be played by both males and females. *Sitting volleyball* is a Paralympic sport and has become one of the main team sports. It is exciting and crowd-pleasing.

Standing volleyball

A classification system has now been established to allow amputees and other people with other disabilities to compete. Above-knee amputees are now using specially designed prostheses (partly made of carbon fibre) which provide cushioning, a light foot, and a four-bar linkage.

The World Organization for Volleyball for the disabled represents countries in Europe, Asia, Africa, and North and South America. This is, indeed, a worldwide sport!

Yachting

Athletes with all types of disabilities can sail. The yachts are designed with special controls and usually have a deep keel to ensure that the yacht does not capsize.

Winter sports for the disabled athlete[9,10]

Disabled persons have often been overprotected from participating in the joys and perils of winter sports. On snow-covered mountains and frozen lakes all over the globe there are wonderful opportunities to engage in stimulating outdoor activities each winter. Fortunately, great advances have been made in the design of equipment to help disabled athletes participate and train to become avid competitors in a variety of winter sports. This chapter, however, will concentrate on skiing.

After the Second World War and the Vietnam War, pioneer amputee skiers devised ingenious adaptations of standard ski equipment.[9] Peppi Zwicknagle, an Austrian skier who lost both his legs in an explosion caused by a hand grenade, became a ski instructor in 1947 and taught on the famous ski slopes of Kitzbuhel. Over 100 disabled skiers took part in a race in Austria in 1947.[11] In the United States, this development was greatly helped by Olympic Gold Medal champion Gretchen Fraser and veteran Jim Withers,[3] who taught many injured American soldiers to ski as part of their rehabilitation process. Paul Leimkuehler[3] of Cleveland devised the three-track system, which uses one ski and two outriggers, as standard equipment for the amputee skier.

The National Handicapped Sports[3] now has 61 Chapters and 30 000 members with a wide variety of disabilities, witnessing the tremendous expansion that has taken place in the United States. Similar growth in winter sports has taken place around the world where sufficient funds and facilities exist.

Amputees
Children

Programmes devised in Denver allow children with amputations to ski with or without their prostheses. Most young children choose three-track skiing (see below) without their prostheses. Those who learn to ski around the ages of 16 or 17 prefer to use their prostheses, as they are more conscious of their overall appearance.[12] Above-knee amputees usually ski without their protheses.[13]

Upper limb amputee

These skiers have difficulty in balance and rely on their lower limbs for control. Above-elbow amputees are not allowed to use their prostheses, but below-elbow amputees can attach them to the ski pole.

Precautions
- Keep the stump warm at all times and use a double wool sock.

- Patellar-bearing prostheses may need an extra insert.

- Canting. The application of an insert to alter slightly the line of weight-bearing on the sound ski may be required in three-track skiers (see below).

Blind skiers

Totally blind athletes can become proficient skiers. They gain much pleasure from the sport and many have become experts and champions. Blind skiers are accompanied by a guide or instructor. An organization named Blind Outdoor Pleasure Development (**BOPD**)[14] based in Aspen, Colorado, provides free instruction. The basic method used is the two-track system where the instructor communicates by voice or touch. 'A ski bra' (see below) may be used to augment this system in its initial stages. Orange jackets or bibs are often worn by blind skiers, their guides, and teachers.

Adaptive skiing
Three-track skiing

Three-track skiing is designed for those people who have one sound lower limb and two functional arms. This includes athletes with a single lower limb amputation, polio affecting principally one limb, and active people with hemiplegia. The skier uses one standard ski and two outriggers for balance. If he or she has a flail limb it is held in place beside the strong limb.

The outrigger has been modified so that it can be used as a crutch when needed. An ingenious invention by Ed Paul comprises a 'ski flip'. The outriggers are used in the usual way when skiing, but they can be moved and locked in an upward position to help in standing or getting on to a ski lift.[13]

Four-track skiing

Here, skiers equalize their weight distribution and assist their balance by sharing the load on four surfaces—two skis and two outriggers. Canting is required to overcome abnormalities of muscle imbalance and spasticity. The method is suitable for those with cerebral palsy, myelodysplasia, or musculodystrophy.

'Ski-bra' aids[12]

A hook is attached to one ski which fits into an eyelet on the other, this keeps the ski tips 7.5 to 10 cm apart and prevents the skis from crossing. An elastic 'bungie cord' allows the more advanced skier greater freedom to engage in more enterprising runs. Essential garments are high-quality, well-fitting boots, and modified ski length.

Sit-ski (Fig. 4(a))

The need to use a wheelchair does not curtail the enterprising athlete from enjoying downhill skiing. There are hazards, but deter-

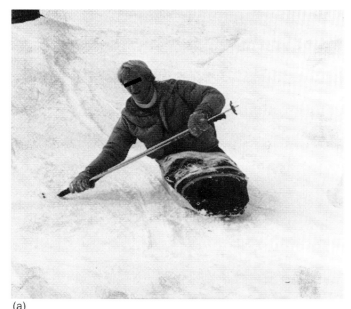

(a)

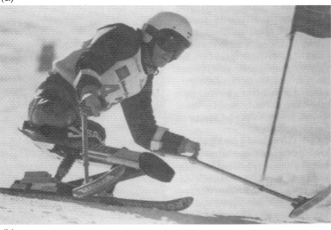

(b)

Fig. 4 (a) Sit skier (from *Sports and Spokes*, 1984; **9**:36, with permission). (b) Monoskiing.

mination, training, and skill enable the avid and irrepressible to zoom along in the snow despite severe disability. Even quadriplegics have been known to 'sit ski'. This was invented by Peter Axelson[15] (a paraplegic T10 and keen skier). The device is somewhat like a dish-sled which allows the skier some control of its gyrations. It functions like a ski boot and binding and holds the participant tightly. Cushions, pads, and foam protect the user from injury, and from cold. Special instruction is necessary and the instructor may use a tether to help his student to stop or change direction.

The reported injury rate[16] is 16 per 1000 ski-hours compared with 2 per 1000 ski-hours for other disabled skiers. Goggles and helmets are mandatory to guard against flying debris.

Monoskiing (Fig. 4(b))
This is one stage up on sit-skiing. It consists of a chassis similar to the above device but it is mounted on a single ski. Short adjustable outriggers are used to control balance and turning. It's best if the individual has some previous skiing experience before engaging in

this sport. Monoskiing is mostly used by paraplegics; those with lesions above T10 up to T4 have to use seat belts and straps to support the upper body.

Classification of athletes and selection of appropriate sport

Disabled athletes may have impaired physical, sensory, or cognitive function. The process of ensuring a fair level of competition for each individual has been difficult, highly contentious, and much debated.

Sir Ludwig Guttman[17] based his classification system of disabled athletes on the level of spinal cord lesion. He personally supervised some of the examinations which were carried out by physiotherapists and doctors in the presence of coaches. Later, with the inclusion of amputees, the blind, and people with cerebral palsy, a functional system had to be devised. The responsiblity therefore passed from the hands of a medical team alone to include athletes, trainers, and classification specialists.

The following system was used for the 1996 X Paralympic Games held in Atlanta. Athletes competed in 17 events, and two demonstration events (wheelchair rugby and yachting) were held.

Functional Classification System (FCS)[18]
Categories
1. *Visually impaired*—causes include diabetes, retinitis pigmentosa, tumours, and viral and congenital factors.

2. *Cerebral palsy*—this can be congenital or acquired early in life. The group also includes cerebral trauma and cerebrovascular accident, as well as quadriplegia or tetraplegia and diplegia—with spasticity, ataxia and/or athetosis.

3. *Amputees*—either congenital or amputation resulting from a vascular disease, trauma, infection, or tumour. The amputation can be above or below the elbow, above or below the knee—with prosthesis or with orthosis.

4. *Wheelchair athletes*—spinal cord injury or disease which has led to the loss of spinal cord nerve function. This can be caused either by congenital factors or as a result of trauma, infection, or a tumour.

5. *Les autres*—this category takes in those people with osteogenesis imperfecta, a congenital limb deficiency, muscular dystrophy, dwarfism, and arthrogryposis. These athletes compete in the cerebral palsy, amputee, or wheelchair category according to the particular assessment of disability assigned to the individual.

6. *Intellectual disability*—this group does not compete in the Paralympics and is not considered here. However, people with this disability are likely to be included in the future.

Classes
The categories described above are subdivided into classes. Each athlete is assigned to a particular class based on the results of both a medical examination and a technical assessment of ability.

Medical classification

This is conducted by a team of sports professionals to evaluate basic levels of functional ability, muscle power, balance, co-ordination, gross and fine activities, and range of motion; each level is allotted points.

Technical classification

Here, the athlete is viewed participating in their chosen sport which, coupled with the results obtained from the medical test, allows the examiner to reconsider the previous judgement. This is particularly important in swimming where classes are further sub-divided according to the athlete's ability to perform certain functions, for example S1–10 (freestyle), SB 2–10 (breaststroke), and SM 4–10 (medley). All classes are identified by a letter (for example, T, track; F, field) followed by a number. Generally, this number represents the extent of the athlete's disability, the higher the number the higher the functional ability.

Table 4 gives the outline of the Functional Classification System, but it is important to note that the classification is sport-specific.

Functional classification. Is it fair? Does it work?

1. The system is now applied to all sports, for instance track and field events, swimming, table tennis, and shooting. Special provision is made for new sports such as wheelchair tennis.

2. It also allows athletes with widely differing disabilities to compete against each other.

3. It is impossible to be completely fair to all athletes and at all times; some will tire after stress, others show different physiological responses to exercise.

4. The athlete must co-operate with the testing process and not attempt to cheat. His or her performance is checked throughout the contest and an analysis made to see if the result is within the expected range.

Selection of the appropriate sport (Table 5)

The deaf athlete The deaf athlete's hearing impairment is often the result of a sensory neural deficit caused by damage to the cochlea.[20] If there has been damage to the semicircular canals or vestibular apparatus then equilibrium deficits, with a concomitant loss of balance and co-ordination, may compound the athlete's disability. However, the greatest limitation for deaf athletes is generally their inability to communicate with other individuals. This inability can be overcome by using sign language and other methods of visual cueing. Deaf athletes can also compensate for hearing loss by maximizing their visual abilities through powers of observation and peripheral vision. Acquisition of these skill enables most deaf persons to participate in almost any athletic activity.

The visually impaired athlete: 'blind athlete'

These athletes have partial or complete loss of sight. Eligibility for athletic competition is granted only to those who have less than 10 per cent useful vision, the legal limit for blindness. Classification is carried out by an ophthalmologist (accredited by the International Blind Sports Association[21]) familiar with the system, and involves testing the individual's better eye while he or she is wearing contact or corrective lenses.

Visually impaired athletes compete in a wide variety of sports including baseball, bowling, cycling, goalball, judo, marathon

Table 5 Paralympic sports key	
Archery	**Judo**
Amputee and wheelchair	Blind and visually impaired Seven categories
Athletics	**Power lifting**
All classes Track, throwing, jumping, pentathlon, marathon	Open class Ten categories according to weight
Basketball	**Rugby (wheelchair)**[a]
Paraplegics, amputees, CP Classified according to points	
Boccia	**Shooting**
CP	Amputees, blind, visually impaired versus others
Three classes	Ten functional categories
Bowls (lawn)	**Swimming**
Amputees, wheelchair, blind, visually impaired	All athletes: blind and visually impaired versus others Ten functional categories
Cycling	**Table tennis**
Cp, visually impaired Tricycles (CP), tandem cycling (visually impaired)	All except blind Ten functional classes
Equestrian	**Tennis**
All disabilities Dressage (some jumping)	Mobility related
Fencing	**Volleyball**
Foil, sabre, épée	Standing and sitting
Football (soccer) (seven-a-side)	**Yachting**[a]
CP, ambulatory	
Goalball	
Blind and visually impaired Three players per side	

[a] Demonstration sports in the 1996 Paralympics

racing, cross-country and downhill skiing, swimming, track and field events, and wrestling. Individual events for visually impaired are the same as those for more normally sighted individuals, but with some special modifications.

1. In track races, B1 runners are accompanied by a sighted athlete acting as a guide.

2. In the 100-metre race, the blind athlete runs freely from the starting position to his coach who calls instructions from beyond the finish line.

3. In cycling, the visually impaired rider rides tandem behind the sighted guide.

Visually impaired athletes have achieved many records, and in many events they rival the performance of normally sighted individuals.

The cerebral-palsied athlete

Athletes with cerebral palsy have a centrally mediated, non-progressive neurological disorder which results in varying degrees of motor dysfunction. The variable nature and extent of the disorder is reflected in the traditional classification system established by the Cerebral Palsy Sports and Recreation Association.[22]

Functional classification allows players to compete in several sports against amputees and other disabled athletes who have similar functional capability. It is applied to shooting, swimming, table tennis, and track and field participants. Muscle spasticity, spinal stability, and the use of supportive strapping and functional aids are all taken into consideration. Participants may be ambulatory or compete in a wheelchair depending on the extent of their motor dysfunction.

Track and field and swimming are popular sports for these athletes. They also compete in cycling, powerlifting, and shooting events; the sport is virtually the same as for the able-bodied, but with some modifications. (For instance, a cyclist can use a tricycle if more severely affected.) Boccia[23] is a wonderful sport for those with cerebral palsy, even when severely handicapped.

Athletes with cerebral palsy have achieved some remarkable standards of performance in many events.

The amputee athlete

Amputee athletes have a partial or complete loss of one or more limbs. The traditional ISOD classification system for amputee athletes contained nine different classes, but it has largely been replaced by the Functional Classification System described above.

Minimum loss allowed

Loss of one or both upper extremities can be either above or below the elbow, lower extremity loss refers to above or below the knee. Minimum disability requirements for track and field athletes stipulate that the upper extremity loss must be above the wrist and the lower extremity through or above the ankle joint.

Track and field and swimming events are the most popular for this group. The rules for individual events are the same as for able-bodied competition. Amputee athletes may use a prosthesis, but no other assistive device is allowed.[24] Prosthesis use is optional, but is not permitted in the high jump (Fig. 5).

Double amputees compete in a wheelchair in, for example, basketball.

New horizons for some!

Sports participation by amputee athletes has expanded greatly in recent years thanks to an increasing awareness of their athletic ability and the amazing improvement of prosthetic design. However, many older people with vascular disease are not eligible and, in many countries, there are insufficient facilities and funds for the millions of amputees resulting from personnel mines. Athletes now compete in basketball, cycling, shooting, powerlifting, and swimming. Recent world records were achieved at Atlanta.[25]

The wheelchair athlete

These sportsmen and women were the originators of 'wheelchair sports', and have attracted much scientific and public attention.

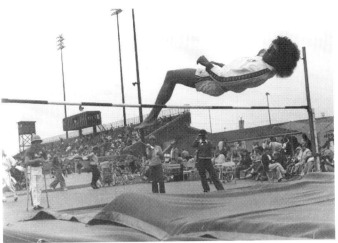

Fig. 5 High jump. Historic jump. Harry Boldt clears 1.86 m in 1976 Olympiad. (Photograph by Basil J. Grogono.)

They were the first to participate in international competition for the disabled, and today comprise one of the largest groups of physically disabled athletes. Athletes with other disabilities (double AK, amputation) may also compete in this class.

The traditional ISMGF system, with three classes for quadriplegics and five for paraplegics, has largely been replaced by the FCS based on quality and quantity of muscle function as well as the ability to perform specific movement patterns required for a given sport. It is applied to shooting, swimming, table tennis, and track and field participants and takes into consideration muscle spasticity, spinal stability, the use of supportive strapping, as well as functional aids.

Track and field and swimming events are very popular and spectacular. The new design of racing wheelchairs enable these athletes to compete at speed, outpacing runners particularly in long-distance events. Track and field participants compete in wheelchairs, with the exception of athletes who are able to throw from a standing position. Other competitive sports include basketball, fencing, marathon racing, shooting, snooker, table tennis, and powerlifting.

Les autres[19]

This title is applied to those athletes who do not fit into any of the previously designated groups. It comprises a wide variety of congenital and acquired conditions, including dwarfism, osteogenesis imperfecta, muscular dystrophy, and arthrogryposis. Functional classification allows these athletes to compete fairly against athletes in other categories.

Vista 1993[26]

This was a milestone in the development of sports for the disabled athlete. Under the chairmanship of Dr Robert Stedward, 163 internationally renowned authorities congregated in Jasper, Alberta, Canada, to discuss their views. Topics included sports performance as it applies to exercise physiology, sports medicine, advances in training techniques, technical developments, classification, integration, ethics, and organization and administration. The entire conference is compiled into *Vista 1993*, a veritable bible for those interested in athletic activities for the disabled. One of the consequences of this historic meeting was the formation of the Sport Science Committee of the International Paralympic Committee.

Exercise physiology and fitness[27]

Assessment of disabled athletes may require special adaptation of the standard techniques in order to accommodate the individual's disability. Amongst the determinants used are: body composition (mass/height ratio); muscle strength; cardiorespiratory function (maximal oxygen uptake); electrocardiogram. Arm-crank ergometers and wheelchair ergometers have been used to assess lower limb amputees and the spinal cord injured.

A number of interesting findings have been reported, including:

1. *Response to vigorous exercise*—cardiac performance is impaired by muscle weakness or a slow response caused by an alteration in the sympathetic nerve supply and an alteration in peripheral resistance.[27]

2. *Ventricular preloading*—caused by blood pooling in the paralysed extremities.

3. *Chronotropic and inotropic response*—the normal brisk increase in heart rate at the onset of exercise may be absent, due to interference with the sympathetic nerve supply (T2–T4) in paraplegic atheletes.

This is compensated for by an increase in stroke volume, but it may be difficult to sustain because of poor venous return. At this stage there is a danger of premature ventricular contractions, ST depression, and, in some cases, cardiac arrest.[28,29]

4. *Ventricular after-loading*—during ambulation, the maximum, voluntary intramuscular force of muscles concerned with arm movements interferes with their vascular supply. The after-loading of the heart is increased, blood pressure is increased, and stroke volume is restricted. It should be noted that this phenomenon occurs mainly in inactive people and is corrected in the well-trained, fit athlete who has developed powerful arm muscles.

5. *Respiratory abnormalities*—respiratory minute volume is often diminished in a disabled athlete due to the accumulation of anaerobic by-products in the active muscles.[30] This heavy ventilatory demand is an added embarrassment if the shoulder muscles are already committed to the demands of wheelchair propulsion. Partial or complete paralysis may also interfere with respiratory function.

6. *Thermoregulation: too cold or too hot*—the sympathetic nervous system plays a major role in thermoregulation,[31,32] inducing thermogenic breakdown of fat, vasoconstriction in the cold, and vasodilatation in the heat.[31,33]

Thus trainers and athletes must be aware of the dangers of heatstroke and collapse in hot humid conditions. In the cold, on the other hand, downhill skiers may suffer excessive heat loss. Undue sensitivity to catecholamines may give rise to massive cold-induced hypertension if chilling is prolonged.[34] (See also below.)

The role of sports medicine[35]

Sports for the disabled originated as part of the rehabilitation process, but both sports and competitions have become more sophisticated in recent years. The medical profession has played a role in this process; however, athletes, coaches, and sports scientists have all enabled marked improvements to be made in competitors' performances. For instance, the world record time for the 1500 metres dropped by 1 min between the 1980 and 1992 Paralympic Games.

Curtis[35] has drawn attention to the need for sports medicine specialists, athletes, and coaches to co-ordinate their efforts. Many athletes manage their own injuries without reference to medical evaluation. A sports medicine team comprising physical therapists, trainers, physicians, nutritionists, prosthetists, exercise physiologists, and biomechanists can contribute to the improvement and understanding of the needs of the disabled athlete in the same way as they have for the able-bodied.

Problems encountered by disabled athletes

(1) *Disability-related*—but occurring in competitive and/or non-competitive sports, for example urinary infection and problems of thermoregulation in a paraplegic athlete;

(2) *Disability-related, aggravated by competition*—for example pressure sores on the buttocks of a wheelchair competitor;

(3) *Not disability-related, but competition-related*—shoulder impingement syndrome in a blind, discus thrower;

(4) *Incidental*—for example allergy to a bee sting in an amputee.

Analysis and identification of these problems is now considered to be a task of the sports medicine specialist, whereas they were previously dealt with by the attending team doctor.

Urinary-tract infections

Neurological control of the urinary tract is usually deranged after spinal cord injury. Infection of the bladder, urethra, and kidneys are common complications for the paraplegic. Renal disease is the main cause of death in these people. The use of intermittent catheterization instituted by Sir Ludwig Guttman[36] decreased the frequency of these complications and gave athletes a greater sense of responsibility for good urinary-tract care. None the less, it is wise to have catheterization facilities and staff familiar with paraplegic care available at national and international meetings.

Temperature-regulation[31,32]

The loss of the autonomic nervous-system influence reduces the vasomotor and sudomotor response of insensitive skin in athletes with spinal cord injuries. The loss of sensory afferent impulses below the level of the lesion may limit the hypothalamic response to exercise and temperature. In addition, the loss of the extremity muscle pump reduces the venous return to the heart and further compromises the thermoregulatory responses. High paraplegics and quadriplegics are the most affected, particularly when exercising under extremes of temperature. Body core-temperature levels in these individuals tend to be higher than normal in the heat and cooler in the cold.

Hyperthermia[32] Regional loss of circulatory and sweating responses have been described in persons with spinal cord lesions. Some limited sweating may occur over insensitive areas, but it is not always synchronous with sweating over the normally innervated area. Core body temperature is therefore dependent on evaporative heat loss from the head, neck, arms, and dry-heat exchange from the rest of the body.[37] The athlete can help to prevent hyperthermia by:

(1) wearing minimal clothing;

(2) keeping cool with damp cloths and towels or using a water spray;

(3) staying in the shade when not competing;

(4) forcing fluids during training and competition.

Hypothermia[31] This may occur in cold, damp, and/or windy conditions. It may also arise after the athlete has competed but has to sit and wait in a wheelchair. The skin remains vasodilated and damp with sweat and other moisture. Unfortunately, the normal shivering mechanism is minimal and ineffective in these athletes. Hypothermia can be guarded against by:

(1) wrapping up well and wearing additional warm and waterproof clothes;

(2) taking a warm shower or bath after a competition;

(3) changing into dry clothing;

(4) drinking water or other replacement fluids.

Pressure sores

Pressure sore are the most common and costly complication of spinal cord injury.[38] They result from unduly prolonged pressure on an insensitive area, such as the buttocks and sacrum. The normal hydrostatic pressure of capillaries average 25 mmHg, but collapse and thrombosis of these capillaries takes place if this pressure is exceeded for more than 2 h.

Whilst wheelchair athletes, on the whole, are less prone to developing pressure sores than their non-competitive colleagues, they are not totally immune. It has been shown that wheelchair athletes who sit with their knees higher than their buttocks subject their skin to high pressures. Athletes participating in sports where large, shearing forces are incurred on the skin of the sacrum, buttocks, and hips are also candidates for this avoidable problem. Wheelchair users need to shift their position intermittently and lift the buttocks off the chair at regular intervals. The wheelchair seat should be well padded and customized to fit the individual. All seat cushions should be fitted by an expert and checked that they conform to the regulations of the particular sport.

The risk of pressure sores is increased if the athlete's skin is damp from sweat and other moisture. It cannot be emphasized how important it is for all paraplegic and quadriplegic athletes to check their skin for evidence of undue pressure and incipient pressure sores. The price of freedom from pressure sores is eternal vigilance!

Shoulder and other injuries

These are discussed below.

Injuries to the disabled athlete[39]

Many of the injuries and derangements sustained by athletes are familiar to modern orthopaedic surgeons. Dramatic improvements in the understanding, diagnosis, and management of, for example, shoulder injuries have been made in the past decade. Retrospective studies have been carried out by a number of authors on the inci-

dence, location, and prevalence of injuries sustained by wheelchair athletes. A consistent pattern has emerged.

1. Muscle soreness is a common problem, particularly in the shoulder girdle muscles, and appears to be related to the type and frequency of games played.[40]

2. The hand is the most common site of injury[41,42]. Acute sprains of the small joints occur when the fingers get caught between the spokes and rim or between wheelchairs, for instance in basketball. Cuts, abrasions, and blisters are common injuries caused by repetitive or sudden contact with wheels or tyres. The hypothenar eminence is particularly vulnerable if calluses are not developed. Protective taping, the use of padded rims, and protective gloves are essential tools to combat these frequent injuries.

3. Clinical and electrophysiological tests on the hands and wrists of wheelchair athletes demonstrated that the most common site for nerve entrapment was the median nerve in the proximal part of the carpal tunnel, corresponding to the interface between the hand and wheel rim during wheelchair propulsion. The ulnar nerve was also sometimes subject to compression in Guyon's canal in the wrist.[43]

> Rest from the aggravating activity, exercises to strengthen the wrist extensors, and flexor-splinting the wrists may be required if symptoms persist. Although a recent report found that protective padded gloves did not relieve the carpal tunnel syndrome, it is worthwhile splinting the wrist and using padded rims and gloves to prevent injury. There are no reports on the use of surgical decompression of the median nerve in this population of athletes.

> Recently, a team at Cornell University tested ways of reducing the incidence of carpal-tunnel syndrome in computer users.[44] They found that using a tilt-down keyboard, in which the wrist is held in a neutral position for most the time, reduces the mean pressure in the carpal tunnel and hence the incidence of this common malady. It would seem logical to study the ways that wheelchair athletes could likewise alter the position of their wrists when propelling their chairs.

4. The shoulder is the basic engine that drives the upper extremities in wheelchair athletes.[45] Very high loads are demanded of it, and it is not surprising that it is frequently subject to impingement syndromes, rotator cuff tendinitis, and other derangements. Perfect moment of the shoulder depends on the synchronous action of the adductor and rotator muscles whilst the abductors (deltoid and supraspinatus) elevate the arm. A recent investigation found that wheelchair athletes presenting with shoulder pain and impingement syndrome had a relative weakness of the adductors.[46] If a shoulder impingement is suspected, a vigorous exercise programme to increase the power of the internal and external rotators and adductors should be instituted together with exercises to improve the strength of the scapular retraction muscles. Stiffness of the shoulder should also be treated by appropriate stretching exercises. Overuse injuries can be prevented by adequate preparation with strength and endurance exercises and an efficient wheelchair, which minimizes abduction and rotational movements of the shoulder.[47]

Curtis and Dillon[48] reported on 128 wheelchair athletes (101 men and 27 women), 72 per cent of whom sustained one or more injuries (291 injuries in all). Thirty-two different sports were

Table 6 Injuries sustained by élite wheelchair athletes during a 1-year period[42]

Type of injury	n	Percentage
Strain	24	48
Abrasion	11	22
Contusion	5	10
Blisters	3	6
Fracture	3	6
Sprain	2	4
Laceration	1	2
Illness	1	2

involved. The highest risk sports were track, basketball, and road racing: archery, table tennis, and slalom were rarely associated with injury. Ferrara and Davis[42] studied the frequency and type of injuries sustained by 19 competitive élite wheelchair athletes over a 1-year period (Table 6). They also found that the majority of the injuries were sustained during track, basketball, and road racing. Direct impact with the floor or another chair was the most common cause of injury. All authors emphasize the importance of a comprehensive vigorous team approach to prevent these injuries.

Martinez[49] and McCormick *et al.*[50] reported a similar distribution of upper extremity injuries in wheelchair athletes participating in basketball, field events, and road racing. A more specific retrospective study of élite wheelchair athletes revealed 50 injuries in 19 athletes, 65 per cent of which were acute and usually due to collisions or falls from a chair either during the competition (48 per cent) or during practice (62 per cent).

Long-distance trail[51]

An unusual, testing week-long distance race took place in Holland in which 40 wheelchair athletes participated, 20 per cent of whom sustained injures. Of these, half were acute injuries (wheelchair collisions) and half due to overuse. Most injuries were to the shoulders, elbow, and hands. Blisters of the hands were common. Problems of pressure sores and temperature regulation reinforced the need for medical teams to be in attendance during such long-distance events. Injuries are common in all wheelchair sports. In a cross-disability study, Ferrara *et al.*[47] found that 32 per cent of all athletes questioned recalled at least one injury during practice, training, or competition. Likewise, Burnham found that 182 injuries had occurred in 116 wheelchair basketball players.[39] Of the athletes reported, 82 per cent sustained at least one injury during a single season.

Paralympics[50,52]

These Games, as with other major competitions, provide a great opportunity to study the incidence of injuries in athletes.

Athletes with Disability Register (ADIR)— prospective study[53]

This is a sports-injury surveillance model with specific modifications for the disabled athlete. It is sponsored by the United States Olympic Foundation through the USA Cerebral Palsy Association.

Each athlete records and reports data directly to the ADIR. As injury patterns emerge, adjustments can be made to training techniques, rules, or equipment. New avenues of research can be instituted and new ideas tested. However, uniform definitions are important for practice-reportable injury, for instance does the phrase 'full return to sport' mean the same to different people?

Over 300 athletes from the National Handicapped Sports (**NHS**) association, the National Wheelchair Basketball Association (**NWBA**), the United States Association for Blind Athletes (**USABA**), and the USA Cerebral Palsy Association (**USACPA**) participated in this prospective study (Table 7).

Conclusions This prospective study is a model for the future. Not only does the ADIR database provide a great stimulus to the understanding of the pattern of injuries sustained by disabled athletes, but it also highlights the current trends in training and provides a basis for future developments.

Training

Appropriately graded training can lead to substantial improvements in both muscle function and cardiovascular function.[54-56]

Muscle function

The training programme for a disabled athlete follows the standard principles of that for an able-bodied athlete. Hypertrophy of the arm muscles can be quite remarkable, especially in wheelchair athletes; in some cases, the cross-sectional area of a simple upper extremity muscle fibre has averaged three times more than that seen in a typical athlete.[57]

Obviously, gains in explosive power and in strength endurance are of advantage in sprint and long-distance races, respectively. However, any improvement in muscle strength for everyday living can also be appreciated. Often, an inactive person with a visual impairment may have difficulty in mounting kerbs and ramps, whereas the fit athlete sails up these with ease.

Cardiovascular

Rigorous training leads to a marked gain in maximal oxygen consumption compared with the inactive disabled person.[54,55] Not only does it lead to a greater functional capacity overall, but it also gives a general sense of well being and an improvement in mood; an increase in the thickness of the left ventricular wall is regarded as beneficial. Wheelchair athletes exhibit a substantial increase in the size of the upper body blood vessels but have smaller lower body vessels when compared with controls. Zeppilli *et al.* found that long-distance wheelchair athletes had larger abdominal aortae and vena cavae than their wheelchair baseball colleagues.[58]

Training guidelines

1. *Upper body flexibility and strength*—stretching and resistance exercises prepare the athletes for competition and help prevent injury to muscles, tendons, and ligaments.[48,59] Particular attention should be paid to improving and maintaining muscle flexibility of the trunk and upper extremities. Stretching programmes for the trunk, shoulders, elbows, and wrists should be part of both the warm-up and cool-down processes. Individual exercises are performed whilst athletes are in their wheelchairs.

Resistance exercises are designed to increase the strength, power, and endurance of the trunk and upper extremities.[60,61] Weight training will provide a good-quality workout and requires a min-

Table 7 ADIR—prospective study[a,b] of 300 athletes[53]

Risk of injury			
(per 1000 athlete exposures)	9.45 for disabled sportspersons (participating in trial)		
	12.15 for football palyers		
	14–17 for ice hockey		

Injury	Time lost	Able-bodied (%)	Disabled (%)
Minor	less than 7 days	70	52
Moderate	8–21 days	20	27
Severe	22 or more	10	21

Mean days lost	2 Years	1990–1992	
National Wheelchair Association	15.1		
National Handicapped Sports	26.8		
National Wheelchair Basketball Association	8.8		
United States Association for Blind Athletes	7.17		
United Cerebral Palsy Association	10.65		
Musculoskeletal-related injuries	75 (59%) (upper extremity, 36 (48%)#)	300	
Disability-related occurrences	52 (41%)		

[a] Disabled Sport Organizations of USA Olympic Committee.
[b] Individual athletes' records reported to trained instructor and entered into database.

imum of modification to existing equipment. Another person (a 'spotter') should be present to ensure safety when using free weights and to provide assistance, when required, with the secure fitting of straps, belts, etc.

2. Special considerations

- Athletes with high spinal injuries may tire easily and require longer rest periods.

- Measurement of the heart-rate responses to exercise may not be an accurate indicator of training progress.

- Careful records should be kept of training times, number of repetitions during training sessions, etc.

- Additional factors include the need to be alert to dizziness, ataxia, depression, and the potential side-effects of medication, as well as the management of spasticity.

Conclusion

The advantages of expert training for the athlete are manifest, but demand great dedication, skill, and enthusiasm of all concerned.

Technical developments

The wheelchair
Biomechanics

Wheelchair locomotion is an inefficient means of transportation, even when employed by experienced athletes. The mechanical efficiency of wheelchair locomotion is, at best, compared with the minimum of 20 per cent for walking or cycling at similar speeds. Mechanical efficiency depends on numerous intrinsic factors including: wheelchair mass and design; the athlete's mass, propulsion technique; and physiological efficiency. Extrinsic factors, such as the nature and grade of the ground surface, must also be considered.

The physiological inefficiency of wheelchair locomotion is largely the result of the dependence on the upper extremities to provide the necessary propulsion force. Upper extremity muscles generally require more energy and tire more quickly than do lower limb muscles. This leads to more costly energy requirements and the working muscles are more susceptible to injury.

Sport-wheelchair design

An excellent analysis of the factors involved in the design of wheel-chairs is given by Higgs.[62] Matching the disabled athlete's body to the demands of a particular sport has parallelled that of the able-bodied.

Sportsmen and women with large muscle mass are attracted to throwing events, such as the javelin and discus, in which disabled athletes compete from a static chair; sprinters and marathon runners require light but sturdy wheelchairs; tennis players require instant manoeuvrability and basketball players likewise need to twist, turn, and stop like acrobats.

Thus specialization of equipment and techniques has evolved. There are now a wide variety of wheelchairs available commercially, each designed for specific sports such as basketball, tennis, and racing.

Propulsion A six-phase cycle is now proposed, divided into:

(1) acceleration

(2) impact

(3) drive phase

(4) rotation production phase

(5) disengagement phases

(6) the back swing.

At low velocities it is possible to apply large amounts of force for long periods—the hand rim is 'grabbed' and pushed. As velocity increases it becomes more difficult to catch up with the hand rim, most of the energy being deployed in the kinetic energy required to move the limbs. A maximum speed is attained when all the energy is used to accelerate the limbs, which is then available for transfer to the hand rim.

Retarding forces Rolling resistance is of chief importance at low speeds and is dependent on the size and camber of the wheels, as well as the interphase between the tyres and the surface on which the wheelchair is running. On a compliant surface, using higher tyre pressures, tyres tend to cut into the track surface. On a hard surface there is less deformation of the tyre wall and thus less energy loss. Higgs has found that the lowest rolling resistance for compliant surfaces, such as at Stoke Mandeville, results with a tyre 28 mm wide, a pressure of 5 to 6 bar (75 to 90 p.s.i.) and a camber of 12 to 15 degrees.[41]

Aerodynamic resistance is of most importance at high speeds. The aerodynamic flow is quite complicated. At low speeds, such as a quadriplegic may achieve, the air around the wheelchair and athlete clings to the surface and streamlining is not of importance; in fact, a rough surface may produce a reduction in drag. However, at faster speeds, as in sprinting, streamlining may reduce the drag.

Conclusions

Improvements in wheelchair design should include: a custom ergo-nomic design to fit the athlete's body shape; refinement of the seat to allow optimum transfer of energy from the body of the wheel-chair; increased rigidity of the wheels; reduced aerodynamic drag; improved steering through weight shifting of the competitor; reduced rolling resistance by matching the tyre width to specific demands of the track surface.

One shape fits all and hoorah for the superspeedster!

One of Higgs' suggestions is to allow athletes to compete in two classes: one in which there are the same, strict wheelchair specifications for all, and another 'open' class for the most technologically advanced wheelchairs allowed.

Developments in prosthetic and orthotic design[63,64]

While many amputee sports (for example swimming or jumping) are performed without prostheses, an increasing number of activities are enjoyed with greater efficiency and pleasure because of the revolution in design and manufacture of prostheses and special orthoses for the upper or lower limb. These new systems have proved highly successful in many competitive sports. New materials such as carbon fibre and titanium allow fabrication of lighter and stronger devices compared with those made from traditional materials.

Different sports require different designs for prostheses. A runner with an above knee amputation needs his or her prosthesis to provide quick extension of the knee as well as a smooth controlled flexion. This requirement is supplied by a hydraulic control of flexion and energy saving 'bounce back' at terminal impact. A golfer, however, requires controlled torsional movement of the knees as the trunk pivots in the natural swing. The knee must be stabilized in in the partially flexed position while the ball is struck but the distal knee needs to extend at the completion of the swing. An 'intelligent' prosthesis has recently been developed using a microprocessor which controls the knee automatically in swing phase whatever the demands of the terrain.

Similarly the design of ankle and foot devices should suit the sport for which they are used. For example, in scuba diving, skiing, or rowing a special design will allow the angle of the ankle to be altered easily.

A variety of prostheses and orthoses is now available for the upper limb also. Myoelectric prostheses have been perfected for both children and adults although simpler devices are more suitable for the aspiring amputee athlete.

Doping and 'boosting'[52]

In the early days of wheelchair games the athletes, the coaches, and their supporters were so delighted to be competing in any event that little attention was paid to the medication which the athlete might be taking. A number of athletes competing in the First National Games held in Canada were not fit for competition because of acute urinary infections or pressure sores. Several athletes were taking medication for complications of their spinal cord injury. All this has changed. The competitors are fit, well-trained individuals who have to undergo drug testing to the same standards as able-bodied athletes.

Banned substances[65] (Tables 8, 9)

A full investigation for the use of banned substances by medal winners was conducted at the Paralympics in Barcelona in 1992 and Atlanta in 1996. The IPC policy is that these substances are the same as those in the IOC list.

Table 8 Protocols for collecting specimens for drug-testing from disabled athletes

1. Condom drainage	Leg bag sample not used	Condom disconnected and a fresh bladder sample taken
2. Self-catheterization	Premitted to use own catheter	Empty bladder and take the next sample
3. Blind athletes	Cannot assert they have seen testing!	Their representative legally permitted to sign document on their behalf
4. Mentally disabled	Must be accompanied by team representative.	

Doping 'a la carte'

Blood doping has been tried by some athletes participating in able-bodied sports, but it is definitely banned in all competitions. The method consists of drawing off blood from the athlete some time before the competition, storing it, and replacing it just prior to the event. The increased oxygen-carrying capacity gained by this illegal procedure would benefit the long-distance racer. The procedure can be hazardous; one athlete developed septic shock during the Olympic Games at Alberville.

Athletes and therapeutic medication

The rules on this thorny problem are still under discussion, and, at present, are subject to those laid down by each hosting authority.

Boosting[66]

Intentional induction of autonomic dysreflexia in quadriplegic athletes

Autonomic dysreflexia is a unique phenomenon affecting individuals with spinal cord injuries above the splanchnic sympathetic outflow (T6), for example quadriplegics and paraplegics C2 down to T6. It is triggered by a nociceptive stimulus distal to the level of injury. These impulses ascend the spinal cord giving connections to the sympathetic cell bodies, which results in a massive sympathetic

Table 9 List of substances banned by the IOC and IPC

Androgenic steroids

Stimulants

Narcotics/analgesics

— heroin, morphine, cocaine

— codeine is allowed under special circumstances

Diuretics unless specially prescribed

Peptide hormones and analogues (salbutamol and chorbutamol)

Human growth hormone

Erythropoietin

discharge. This is further exaggerated by the lack of supraspinal inhibitory control and the formation of abnormal synaptic connections.[66] Autonomic dysreflexia is manifested by:

- peripheral vasoconstriction;

- gooseflesh shivering and pallor distal to the level of injury;

- hypertension leading to stimulation of the aortic and carotid baroreceptors and activation of the parasympathetic nervous system resulting in nasal stuffiness and bradycardia.

Vasodilatory impulses from the medullary vasomotor centre in the thoracic cord are unable to respond so that vasoconstriction persists.

Boosting to win Hitherto, this autonomic dysreflexia was regarded as a major emergency in spinal cord medicine because of the danger of producing uncontrolled hypertension, cerebral haemorrhage, blindness, aphasia, cardiac dysrhythmia, and possibly death. Impaired sweating may also lead to hyperthermia. Recently, quadriplegics have been triggering this phenomenon to gain advantage in their sports. Methods used to produce this enhanced state include bladder overdistension, tight leg straps, and sitting on sharp objects.

Experimental boosting

The effects of 'boosting' and the mechanism of its induction were investigated by Burnham et al.[66] in eight quadriplegic athletes with lesions between C6 and C8. They performed a simulated wheelchair 7.5-km race in the laboratory in the 'unboosted' and 'boosted' states. Results obtained showed that quadriplegic athletes enhanced their performance. 'Boosting', however, is potentially very dangerous and could give rise to severe hypertension. Serge Raymond,[67] a tetraplegic (quadriplegic) himself, emphasizes that the use of reflex dysreflexia amongst athletes has enabled these competitors to significantly improve their performance in marathon racing during the past 10 years. Boosting remains an ethical, medical, and regulatory dilemma.

This social problem shows the difficult dilemma which authorities face in deciding how to deal with a physiological reflex response. Reflex dysreflexia is a practice which is almost impossible to regulate and cannot be considered as doping per se, despite the incipient dangers as well as the unfairness to those who cannot or do not practise it.

Integration: its pros and cons[68-70]

Sports for the disabled are now well established. Athletes with many different disabilities, including cerebral palsy, visual impairment, neurological diseases, and spinal injuries, now have a world-recognized system in which they can compete with fairness against any other competitor with a similar functional capacity. The élite athletes amongst this group compete in the Paralympics and therefore feel they should have Olympic status for any medals won. The question arises as to whether sports for the disabled should remain separate or be fully or partially integrated into events for the able-bodied. There are several aspects to this dispute.

1. No disability is barred. In the original Stoke Mandeville Games only those with spinal injuries were eligible. Since 1985 all those who have more than a minimum disability can

compete in international sports events whatever the cause of their disability.

2. The Functional Classification System provides a fair assessment of each athlete.

3. Olympic-status exhibition events of specific disabled sports have been presented at the past two Olympic Games. There is a strong movement to include at least some Paralympic sports into the traditional Olympic Games themselves.

4. Some disabled people can compete against an able-bodied person, in some sports such as rifle-shooting or archery, without any handicap.

5. There is a movement to join the different sports organizations and clubs under one roof. Whilst this might improve efficiency it would destroy the personal nature of the parent club.

Conclusions and outlook for the future

We live in a world of change. The past decade has seen a dramatic expansion and increased sophistication of sports for the disabled. Current research into the mechanism and management of spinal cord injuries is at last beginning to bear fruit, but it is unlikely that any rapid procedure or regimen will be available to alter the inevitable permanence of complete spinal cord injuries for some years.

Sporting activities, for both the amateur and professional athlete, offer a tremendous source of pleasure and motivation for the millions of disabled all over the world. It is hoped that this chapter will stimulate potential athletes, amateur athletes, and medal winners, together with trainers and sports professionals, to share their knowledge and enthusiasm.

In 1996, 3500 Paralympic athletes demonstrated the 'Triumph of the Human Spirit' in Atlanta. Now it's up to all of us to apply our enthusiasm, ideas, and knowledge to this wonderful world of Sport!

References

1. Guttman I. The development of sport for the disabled—historical background. In: Guttman I. ed. *Textbook of sport for the disabled*. Aylesbury: HM Publishers, 1976: 14–20.
2. Labanowich S. The physically disabled in sports, tracing the influence of two tracks of a common movement. *Sports and Spokes* 1987; **12**: 33–44.
3. McConkey J. The concise authorised history of the National Handicapped Sports and Recreation Association. *Handicapped Sports Rep*. 7: 22–6.
4. Dresse A. CIIS *History of the International Committee of Sports for the Deaf*. CIIS Bulletin 1993; **July**: A1/1–7.
5. Stewart D. *Deaf Sport. The impact of Sports within the Deaf Community*. Washington, 1991.
6. Jackson RW, Fredrickson A. Sports for the physically disabled: the 1976 Olympiad (Toronto). *American Journal of Sports Medicine* 1979; 7: 293–6.
7. Grogono BJS. The first Pan Am Wheelchair Games, Winnipeg, Manitoba, 1967. *Manitoba Medical Review* 1968; **June/July** (Suppl.).
8. Wheelchair Basketball Federation. *Wheelchair basketball to the year 2000*. Wheelchair Basketball Federation, 1 Meadow Close, Shavington, Crewe, Cheshire, CW2 5BE, UK
9. Laskowski ER. Snow skiing for the disabled. *Mayo Clinic Proceedings* 1991; **96**: 160–72.
10. Kray MH, Messner DG. Skiing for the physically handicapped. *Clinical Sport Medicine* 1982; **1**: 3219–332.
11. Lessard B. The history and development of three-track skiing. In: Stieler WE, ed. *Kick the handicap learn to ski! A handbook of information for the physically handicapped*, 2nd edn. Marlette, Michigan: Adapted Sports Association 1977: 105–11.
12. Ryan AJ, Jackson RW, McCann BC, Messner DG, Beavor DP. Sport and recreation for the handicapped. *Physician and Sportsmedicine* 1978; **6**: 44–48, 51–5, 58–61.
13. Kegel B. *Sports for the leg amputee*. Redmond, Washington: Medical Publishing Company.
14. Blind Outdoor Leisure Development (Informational brochure). Aspen, Colorado: BOLD Inc., 1981.
15. Axelson P. Sit-skiing. Part 1. *Sports and Spokes* 1984; **10**: 28–31.
16. McCormick DP. Skiing injures in sit-skiers. *Sports and Spokes* 1985; **11**: 20–1.
17. *ISMGF guide for doctors*. Aylesbury: Stoke Mandeville Games Federation, 1982.
18. Xth Paralympic Games. *The official commemorative program*. Disability Today Publishing Group Inc., 1996: 78–9.
19. Xth Paralympic Games. *The official commemorative program*. Disability Today Publishing Group Inc., 1996: 79.
20. Shapira W. Competing in a silent world of sports. *Physician and Sportsmedicine* 1975; **3**: 99–105.
21. *International Blind Sports Association handbook*. Madrid: International Blind Sports Association, October 1989.
22. *General and functional classification guide*. IX Paralympic Games, Barcelona 1992.
23. Oglesby SE. *Boccia the game for all. An introductory guide*. International Boccia Federation, Georgia State University, Atlanta, Georgia, USA.
24. Kegal B. Physical fitness, sports and recreation for those with lower limb amputation or impairment. *Journal of Rehabilitation and Development*.1985; **Clin. Suppl**. 1: 1–125.
25. Atlanta records from the Xth Paralympics. www.paralympic.org./history.htm
26. Steadward D, Nelson ER, Wheeler DW, eds. *Vista 93: the outlook*. University of Alberta, Canada: Priority Printing, 1993.
27. Shepherd RJ. Exercise physiology in athletes with disabilities. In: Steadward D, Nelson ER, Wheeler DW, eds. *Vista 1993: the outlook*. University of Alberta, Canada: Priority Printing, 1993: 20–35.
28. Blocker SN, Merrill JM, Krebs MA, Cardus DP, Osterman HJ. An electrical review of patients with spinal cord injury. *American Corrective Therapy Journal* 1983; **37**: 101–4.
29. van Alste JA, la Haye MW, de Vries J, Boom HBK. Exercise electrocardiography using rowing ergometer for leg amputees. *International Journal of Rehabilitation Medicine* 1985; 7: 1–5.
30. Hjeltnes N. Oxygen uptake and cardiac output in paraplegics with low level spinal lesions. *Scandinavian Journal of Rehabilitation* 1977; **9**: 107–9.
31. Sanka MN, Lazka WA, Pandolf KB. Temperature regulation during upper body exercise in able-bodied and spinal injured. *Medicine and Science in Sports and Exercise* 1989; **21**: 431–40.
32. McCann BC. Thermoregulation in spinal injury: the challenge of the Atlanta Olympics. *Spinal Cord* 1996; **34**: 433–6.
33. Shephard RJ. *Physiology and biochemistry of exercise*. New York: Praeger, 1982.
34. Mathias CJ, Hillier K, Fraenkel HL, Spalding, JMK. Plasma prostaglandin E during neurogenic hypertension in tetraplegic man. *Clinical Science and Molecular Medicine* 1975; **49**: 625–8.
35. Curtis KA. The role of sports medicine team members in sports for persons with disabilities. In: Steadward D, Nelson ER,

Wheeler DW, eds. *Vista 93: the outlook*. University of Alberta, Canada: Priority Printers, 1993: 196–203.

36. Guttman Sir LG. The non-touch technique of intermittent catheterization. In: *Spinal cord injuries*. Oxford: Blackwell Scientific, 1973: 345–57.

37. Cooper DM, Watt RC, Altercu V. *Guide to wound care*. Chicago: Hollister, 1983: 59–60.

38. Guttman Sir LG. Pressure sores. In: *Spinal cord injuries*. Oxford: Blackwell Scientific, 1973: 485–512.

39. Burnham RS. Injuries in athletes using wheel chairs. In: Steadward D, Nelson ER, Wheeler DW, eds. *Vista 93: the outlook*. University of Alberta, Canada: Priority Printing, 1993: 216–20.

40. Hoeberigs JH, Debets-Egen HBL, Verstappen FTJ. Muscle soreness in wheelchair basketballers. *International Journal of Sports Medicine* 1984; Suppl.: 177–9.

41. Botwin Madorsky JG, Curtis KA. Wheelchair sports medicine. *American Journal of Sports Medicine* 1984; **12**: 128–32.

42. Ferrara MS, Davis RW. Injuries to elite wheelchair athletes. *Paraplegia* 1990; **28**: 334–41.

43. Aljure JS, Eltoria I, Bradley WE, Lin JF, Johnson B. Carpal tunnel syndrome in paraplegic patients. *Paraplegia* 1985; **23**: 182–6.56.

44. Editorial. Research finds solution to carpal tunnel syndrome for computer users. In: *Revue Canadienne d'information medicale* 1995; March/April: 46.

45. Hawkins RJ, Kennedy JC. Impingement syndromes in athletes. *American Journal of Sports Medicine* 1980; **8**: 151–8.

46. Burnham RS, May L, Nelson E, Steadwood RD, Reid DC. Shoulder pain in wheelchair athletes—the role of muscle imbalance. *American Journal of Sports Medicine* 1993; **21**: 238–42.

47. Ferrara MS, Buckely WE, McCann BC, Limbird TJ, Powell JW, Robl R. The injury experience of the competitive athlete with a disability: prevention implications. *Medicine and Science in Sports and Exercise* 1992; **24**: 184–8.

48. Curtis KA, Dillon DA. Survey of wheelchair injuries: common patterns and prevention. *Paraplegia* 1985; **23**: 170–5.

49. Martinez SF. Medical concerns among wheelchair users. *Physician and Sportsmedicine* 63–8.

50. McCormack DAR, Reid DC, Steadward RD, Syrotuik DG. Injury profiles in wheelchair athletes: results of a retrospective study. *Clinical Journal of Sport Medicine* 1991; **1**: 35–40.

51. Hoeberigs SF, Debets-Egen HBL, Debets PML. Sports medical experiences from the International Flower Marathon for disabled wheelers. *American Journal of Sport Medicine* 1990; **18**: 418–21.

52. Schaffer RS, Proffer DS. Sports medicine for wheel chair athletes. *American Family Physician* 1989; **39**: 239–45.

53. Ferrara M, Buckely WE. Athletes with disabilities injury register. In: Steadward D, Nelson ER, Wheeler DW, eds. *Vista 93: the outlook*. University of Alberta, Canada: Priority Printing, 1993: 205–14.

54. Davis GM, Shepard RJ. Cardiorespiratory fitness in highly active versus less active paraplegics. *Medicine and Science in Sports and Exercise* 1988; **20**: 463–8.

55. Davis GM, Shepard RJ. Strength training for wheelchair users. *British Journal of Sports Medicine* 1990; **24**: 25–30.

56. Davis GM, Plyley MJ, Shepard RJ. Gains in cardiorespiratory fitness with arm crank training in spinally disabled men. *Canadian Journal of Sport Science* 1991; **16**: 64–72.

57. Taylor A. Physical activity for the disabled. In: *Report of the research priority development conference*. Ottawa: Fitness and Amateur Sport, 1981: 15–21.

58. Zeppilli P, Vanicelli R, Santini C, *et al*. The echographic size of conductance vessels in athletes and sedentary people. *International Journal of Sports Medicine* 1995; **Jan. 16** (1): 38–44.

59. Walsh CM, Hoy DJ, Holland IJ. *Get fit flexibility exercises for the wheel chair user* Edmonton Research and Training Centre for the Physically Disabled, University of Alberta, Canada, 1982.

60. Walsh CM, Steadward RD. *Get fit. Muscular exercises for the wheel chair user*. Edmonton Research and Training Centre for the Physically Disabled, University of Alberta, Canada, 1984.

61. Skuldt A. Exercise limitations of quadriplegics. *Sports and Spokes* 1984; **10**: 19–20.

62. Higgs C. Sport performance: technical developments. In: Steadward D, Nelson ER, Wheeler DW, eds. *Vista 1993: the outlook*. University of Alberta, Canada: Priority Printing, 1993: 168–83.

63. Chadderton C. What's new in prosthetics? *Camps Newsletter* 1993; **November**: 1–24.

64. Tiessen J. Orthotics and and Prosthetics. Fit and Fashion join a tradition of function. *Disability Today* 1966; **5** (Winter): 23–5.

65. Riding M. *The doping issue. Vista 1993: the outlook*. University of Alberta, Canada: Priority Printing, 1993; 396–9.

66. Burnham R, Wheeler G, Bhambhani Y, Belanger M, Erickson P, Steadwood R. Intentional induction of dysreflexia among quadriplegic athletes: enhancement, efficacy, safety, and mechanism. In: Steadward D, Nelson ER, Wheeler DW, eds. *Vista 93: the outlook*. University of Alberta, Canada: Priority Printing, 1993: 224–38.

67. Raymond S. 'Boosting'. In: Steadward D, Nelson ER, Wheeler DW, eds. *Vista 93: the outlook*. University of Alberta, Canada: Priority Printing, 1993: 242–7.

68. Dendy E. Integration issues in sport for people with disabilities. An overview. In: Steadward D, Nelson ER, Wheeler DW, eds. *Vista 93: the outlook*. University of Alberta, Canada: Priority Printing, 1993: 359–65.

69. Lindstrom H. Integration of persons with disabilities: an overview. In: Steadward D, Nelson ER, Wheeler DW, eds. *Vista 93: the outlook*. University of Alberta, Canada: Priority Printing, 1993: 333–43.

70. Labnowich S. Integration: anomalies and realities. In: Steadward D, Nelson ER, Wheeler DW, eds. *Vista 93: the outlook*. University of Alberta, Canada: Priority Printing, 1993: 345–50.

Further reading

Official commemorative programmes, especially to the:

X Paralympic Games Official Commemorative Program, Atlanta. Disability Today Publishing Inc., 1996

IX Paralympic Games, Barcelona

1998 VIII Paralympic Games, Seoul. *Sports and Spokes* 1989; **14** (5): 5–29.

1976 V Paralympic Games, Toronto. Bell Canada (Organizing Committee for the Physically Disabled Toronto).

7

Special considerations in sports injuries

7.1 Introduction

William D. Stanish

Over the years it has become obvious that there are areas of special concern that particularly apply to sports medicine. On one hand there is the management of sports injuries and on the other there is a requirement for understanding the principles of sport fitness/health. Fundamental to the practice of sports medicine is the understanding and comprehension of emergencies of the musculoskeletal system, maxillofacial injuries, pulmonary and abdominal insults, and trauma to the spine and head.

Historically, fractures about the face were misunderstood and under appreciated, frequently resulting in considerable residuum. A malunited fracture of the mandible, for example, would commonly result in malocclusion of the bite, triggering degeneration of the temporomandibular joint with considerable discomfort and dismay. Diplopia can occur if and when the zygomatic arch is fractured and not anatomically realigned. Contemporary oral medicine/surgery emphasizes the importance of intricate appraisal and definitive management of facial injuries. Appreciation of the importance of the soft tissue insult—as well as the bony injury—is fundamental. There has been considerable attention directed towards preventative measures, not the least of which are protective mouth guards. Widespread in their application, form-fitting mouth protectors have been fundamental in decreasing injuries to the teeth, jaw, and cerebrum. The ability of the semirigid mouth orthotic to decrease the effects of impact from sport has been well documented. Facial trauma resulting from injuries in ice hockey have been reduced dramatically by the rigid implementation of the use of protective face guards and masks.

Injuries to the eyes and teeth are seen far less frequently since the introduction (as a consequence of rule changes) of face masks. However, if an injury does occur, an orderly physical examination, combined with systemic radiographic analysis, still affords the best means of achieving a successful clinical outcome.

Head and spine trauma, occurring during athletics, can have devastating morbidity. Protective head gear, once felt to be the most important method for guarding against injury, has been de-emphasized with more emphasis being placed on stringent application of regulations. This is particularly true in such contact sports as American football, amateur boxing, and ice hockey, for example, in many jurisdictions it is now mandatory to use properly designed head protectors in bicycling. Nevertheless, major research thrusts have been directed towards more appropriate protective head appliances which are designed to decrease the concussion to the cerebrum and protect the soft tissues of the head . The incidence of sport-related head and spine trauma has been reduced, principally as a result of changes in rules and regulations. For example, American football was notorious for teaching techniques which emphasized the use of the head/helmet as a battering ram. Rules have been introduced which outlaw this technique—spearing—with consequent reduction of trauma to the head and neck. However, even with proper coaching, ideal equipment, and appropriate technique, injuries to the head and neck do occur, particularly in sports which involve collision.

When an injury does occur correct first aid must be initiated. On-field medical analysis of the injured athlete is very important. An improper technique for transporting the athlete with a neck injury, for instance, can add considerably to his or her long-term morbidity. An unrecognized unstable fracture of the cervical spine could result in complete quadriplegia if not handled correctly and appropriate techniques for analysing the athlete and splinting the spine with proper airway control are a fundamental requirement.

Somewhat less obvious, but equally concerning, are athletic injuries to the chest and abdomen. A blunt trauma to the thorax and kidney region is commonly underestimated in terms of severity. Deceleration injuries are also poorly appreciated in terms of the damage that they may afford. Particularly troublesome, in terms of diagnosis and management, are visceral injuries in the adolescent athlete. The younger individual/athlete has enormous physiological reserve, and a ruptured spleen as a consequence of blunt trauma in sport may remain indolent for hours until haemorrhagic shock occurs—suddenly and dramatically.

The skilled and well-trained sport medicine practitioner must be prepared to manage The Fallen Athlete. The fundamentals of first aid transcend all subspecialities of medicine and must be closely followed when functioning as a team physician. Constant vigilance must be maintained with respect to subtle pathology, whether to the brain, spine, abdomen or chest, that may manifest itself minutes or even hours later. These special problems in sports medicine are evaluated in the following Section.

7.2 Emergencies of the musculoskeletal system in sport: 'the fallen athlete' (Rodin)

Robert M. Brock

Introduction

The subtitle 'the fallen athlete' refers to the sculpture of the same name by Rodin. I was at the 1989 world figure skating championships in Paris as an attending sports medicine physician. At the Rodin museum, I was moved by the amazing sensitivity of this sculptor in depicting the pain, strain, and anxiety experienced by the injured athlete. The figure is real. The reality of sport is that it encompasses the hope and dreams of mankind. When sudden injury occurs, the sports medicine physician will most certainly have a 'fallen athlete'.

Fortunately, the incidence of true emergency situations is low. In my view, crisis situations only constitute an emergency if immediate intervention can alter the clinical outcome. The *Oxford dictionary of current English* defines an emergency as a '. . . sudden state of danger, requiring immediate action'.[1] This is the criterion for inclusion of topics in this chapter. Practical remarks will focus on the early recognition, on-the-field clinical assessment, and transport. Following injury, athletes, coaches, and parents are anxious to know when sport can be resumed. Some of the athletes will be able to return to the same sport after appropriate management. Unfortunately, others will only be able to return to alternative sports with permanent limitations.

Philosophy: approach to the acutely injured athlete

It is common to be distracted by the gross deformity of a fracture, but it must be remembered that the trauma causing the limb injury may have injured the airway or caused life-threatening head, chest, or abdominal injuries. Multiple injuries are expected in the motor-cycle racer. However, these risks are no less prevalent in the down-hill skier who is travelling at 100 km/h, constantly on the edge of a sudden catastrophe. In orthopaedic medicine, we become so focused on the problems of the extremities that we can forget that there is a human body attached to that injured limb.

Emergencies of the musculoskeletal system are often seen in conjunction with emergencies of other systems. In dealing with an injured athlete at the scene of the accident, listen to the athlete and identify the primary area of concern while assessing the 'A, B, Cs' (airway, sites of bleeding, and circulation). The history of the mechanism of injury, and the degree and direction of forces are of great importance in determining the severity and the nature of the injury. Often, information from team mates or officials will be helpful. Advance knowledge of any pre-existing conditions of the athlete is helpful.

On the field, after you have gleaned the medical history and performed the 'A, B, Cs', a limited examination of the injured limb is essential. Look for gross deformity and feel for crepitus suggesting fractures. Note the gross function of the joint, including the range of motion and neuromuscular performance. Examine the pulses and capillary perfusion. Are there any associated injuries to the same or to other limbs? Decisions about the form of splinting needed and the mode of transport are made only after adequate assessment.

It is fundamental to focus on the athlete's needs, not the needs of others. Amid the confusion of acute emergencies, several groups have their own priorities. Unfortunately in many sporting activities the media influence the timing of the events. Some become very upset if there is a pause in the action. The primary concern of the sports physician should be to ensure that proper medical attention is given to the fallen athlete.

Preparation for sports medical coverage

Preparation for a potential medical disaster is necessary both before and during the event. The incidence of critical injuries is low, thus when a crisis does occur, mass confusion often follows. Be prepared! In fact, this may be the most important way of dealing with an emergency.

Before the sports event

One of the simplest parts of any disaster plan is often underestimated in its importance. It is the list of all the emergency telephone numbers. Before the event, local hospitals and physicians should be notified about the potential of serious injuries presenting to their institutions. Emergency transport systems differ in their responsiveness and must be forewarned. All this must be arranged in advance of the competition.

Another important aspect is the disaster plan that covers a sudden and unexpected emergency. Every disaster plan has problems when put into action. It must be written and rehearsed. At one event all the emergency supplies had been gathered in one place. These supplies included oxygen, a fracture board, and the available telephone to make the necessary calls. When an emergency arose, no one could find the key to the room to get at the supplies. Simple tasks can be easily overlooked if the plan is just written or, worse still, just talked about and not actually rehearsed. Often at a major event there are many volunteers who have medical skills and great interest, but have little experience at an actual sports event. Taking a skater off a busy practice rink is different from taking the injured diver from a pool. The injury might be the same but the practical implementations of the disaster plan are very different.

Similarly, when travelling with a team outside your own health care system (country), it is very important that before the event the sports physicians should familiarize themselves with the local arrangements. We have been at world competitions where the attending doctor was not a practising clinician. Being forewarned is an enormous advantage in being prepared.

Lack of communication between the medical team and the organizing committee of the event can be a problem. As with many volunteer situations the expectations of the sports organization and the medical volunteers are usually different. Before the event it is crucial to have all the concerns expressed. Issues such as expected times of coverage and budget for supplies are very real. At the outset these issues must be resolved with frequent and clear communication.

At the sports event

Being prepared for a competition means having the proper coverage. This includes personnel as well as equipment and communication systems.

Personnel

Sports medicine is a recognized medical specialty. In Canada there are many individuals who have gone through an accreditation process[2] and are interested in covering competitions. These people should form the core of your medical staff. Emergency room physicians often have an interest and are adroit in the early management of acute injuries. They are, therefore, excellent sources of physician coverage. Sport physiotherapists and athletic trainers are invaluable. Some authorities have personnel who are specialists in evacuation of injured people. These people can often contribute to the team. Remember, medical care, especially sports medicine care, is really a team approach.

Equipment

Each event has its own special needs. The equipment for aquatic championships is different from that for a skiing event or a marathon. Types and rates of sport-specific injuries will help determine what personnel and equipment should be on site. Emergency resuscitation equipment, splints, and emergency transportation must be provided. Minor trauma equipment may be helpful (laceration sets, splints). In stressful athletic challenges such as marathons, hyperthermia and hypothermia are potential problems. Specific therapeutic modalities for temperature extremes should be available at the site of competition.

Communications

Communication is very important in any crisis situation and should be in place prior to the event (and tested). Excellent communications systems are a cornerstone of any disaster plan.

Many events have a site that is extended over a large geographical area. Examples include road cycling and downhill skiing. It may be important to ensure that an injury sustained on any part of the course is readily identified and reached. Internal communications by walkie-talkies may be necessary. Knowledge beforehand of the placement of available emergency telephones and telephone numbers is critical. This alone could save a life.

When a patient is taken from the site of an event to a medical facility, written documentation must be sent along with the patient. Information on the general state of the patient and the status of the neurovascular structures are of vital importance. Vital signs taken on arrival at the institution have much more meaning when they can be compared with the situation at the time of injury. If the athlete has sustained a significant injury at an event, which requires treatment, it is important to send with him a written report of that treatment for his own doctor.[3]

The essential element of management of emergencies of the musculoskeletal system is to be prepared to deal with a crisis when it arises, as it always does, unexpectedly. One needs to recognize the inherent risks in each sport. When approaching the acutely injured athlete, we need to use the clinical skills basic to all of medicine. Taking a good history and doing the appropriate physical examination takes practise which is enhanced by experience. Acute treatment and communication are skills to be practised.

In this chapter, acute injuries of shoulder, elbow, and knee will be discussed. In addition, the acute compartment syndrome is an additional preventable cause of tragic outcomes in sport injures. Frostbite is another preventable emergency condition which is usually seen in weekend athletes who are not as well trained or equipped as the élite athletes. A few words will be added about the immediate handling of frost-bite as well as the rare amputation necessitated by sports trauma.

An attempt to be as practical as possible with each crisis situation is the approach. As with most situations in medicine, the approach to the problems is as important as achieving the actual diagnosis. (This is just like some judges of athletic performance who feel that style is more important than technique!) Each section will stress the setting, 'on-the-field' clinical assessment, sideline management transportation, and prognosis.

Most emergencies start suddenly with a shout of 'player down'. Frantic officials, glaring lights, concerned coaches, distraught parents, and scrambling confusion, follows. As a sports medicine practitioner, you need to analyse the crisis objectively with clinical clarity and bring order to the management of the musculoskeletal emergency.

Acute injuries to the shoulder

The setting

Acute injuries to the shoulder are the second most common musculoskeletal complaint in both emergency departments and sports injury clinics. Acute shoulder injuries in contact sports are especially common. The patient has had contact either with another player or the playing surface. The actual mechanism may not have been witnessed by persons on the sideline. At the time of injury the setting usually includes a fall on an outstretched arm or collision with another player, or is the result of a 'pile-up' in either football or hockey. Each sport has its own shoulder risk. A volleyball player may be 'digging' for a volley, a figure skater missing a landing from a triple axle jump, a hockey player receiving a check into the boards, or the football player crunched during a tackle.

On-the-field clinical assessment

In all subsequent discussion, we shall assume that the injured athlete has only one injury at a time. Never forget that in a real situation multiple areas of injury often occur. The other areas of the patient may take precedence over the musculoskeletal areas (airway, bleeding, etc.).

The medical team usually has to deal with a player lying on the playing surface. Initial inability to move their arm and a great deal of pain are the common symptoms. Glenohumeral dislocation is the commonest problem seen in the 15- to 30-year-old age group. In younger patients a fracture of the proximal humerus or fractured clavicle are the usual problems. In my experience, glenohumeral dislocation for the first time is less common in the younger age groups.

Patients may complain of pain in the shoulder area. At the outset, one must ask about a presence of neck pain or dysfunction in the other extremities. Patients may complain of pain over to the sternoclavicular area or down their arm. Questions about the distribution of the pain and the character of the pain are important. The ability to function is equally important. The advantage of initial assessment includes the ability to note significant defects of neurological function, particularly the axillary nerve, secondary to an acute shoulder injury. Many of these are transient after initial injury and may only last from seconds to minutes; very few persist for a long period of time. Patients may relate that they are unable to move their arm, either in external rotation or abduction; they may complain of numbness compatible with a 'dead arm' syndrome.

Often in the heat of the moment the details of the mechanism of injury are difficult to ascertain. Distinguishing between various mechanisms such as a fall on the shoulder itself or a fall on the outstretched arm is very helpful in deciding the actual diagnosis. In the individual athletic sports such as boxing, the actual mechanism is apparent. In multiple person collisions, as seen in team sports, the actual mechanism is sometimes more difficult to identify. Information on a previous history of injury can be helpful.

While at the scene of injury, inspection of the injury is fundamental. One looks for deformity. Squaring of the shoulder with the associated anterior bulge or fullness is associated with anterior dislocation of the glenohumeral joint. Sometimes athletic clothing prevents a visual appraisal of the shoulder until the competitor is removed to the sidelines. One may see obvious deformity of the clavicle, or the patient may be short of breath with marked pain over the medial aspect of the clavicle.

Crepitus is not usually felt in a simple shoulder dislocation, but is obviously felt in fractures of the humerus and clavicle.

It is reasonable to do a quick assessment for gross function of the neurological status on the field, looking for paraesthesia and gross weakness. In the event of any kind of brachial plexus injury the neurological deficit may not follow a specific pattern but in fact may be patchy in its presentation.

It is unlikely to find an open wound in an acute shoulder injury, although the rare clavicular fracture may either tent the skin or be associated with a skin abrasion and should often be considered an open wound.

Differential diagnosis of acute injuries of the shoulder

- glenohumeral dislocation
- acromioclavicular dislocation
- fractured clavicle
- fractured proximal humerus
- brachial plexus injury
- sternoclavicular dislocation

Based on the history and physical findings it is usually possible to determine whether this is a straightforward dislocation or a fracture dislocation of the proximal humerus. Radiography is essential. Most fractures of the clavicle are easily discernible. Shoulder tip pain with or without deformity represents acromioclavicular pathology. The brachial plexus injury may not have any obvious deformity at the time of first assessment. Patchy numbness with weakness of the shoulder, sometimes associated with a lot of pain, may be seen with nerve injuries. Often the shoulder has been dislocated but has reduced spontaneously.

Transportation

The patient is usually able to walk from the playing field. Given that the shoulder is the only area of injury, it is reasonable to remove the athlete from the playing field after splinting their forearm with the opposite hand or having another person splint the forearm, steadying it to decrease the motion at the shoulder area. Applying a sling and swathe will add comfort. In the case of the multiply injured athlete, splinting is mandatory before transport from the playing area.

Treatment

Sideline management

At the sidelines one must re-evaluate more thoroughly the history and physical findings. A more comprehensive physical examination can be obtained. A complete neurovascular examination is conducted with better exposure of the injured area. After this examination better splinting can be applied.

A diagnosis of anterior dislocation is often made. When certain of the diagnosis of a glenohumeral dislocation, particularly in the recurrent dislocator, it is often very easy to reduce the shoulder gently with the following technique. The patient should be removed to a quiet area and made comfortable in a supine position, then firm but gentle traction is applied. When the shoulder is reduced promptly and gently, less soft tissue damage and subsequent swelling will occur. Rehabilitation will be swifter. This is certainly true if there is neurovascular compromise. The earlier the reduction, the less damage to the vital structures. If, on the other hand, the diagnosis is uncertain or fracture is suspected (or any significant resistance is met in attempted reduction), then the patient should be transported to a facility for more definitive diagnosis and treatment. It is important to note the neurovascular status of the patient at the time of injury (even if normal) and to follow this until more definitive care can be arranged. Once reduced, a modified Velpeau shoulder dressing and ice pack will keep the athlete comfortable until further care is rendered.

When the diagnosis is a fracture of the clavicle, then this can be managed by an ice pack and sling until radiography is performed. If the wound is compounded, urgent surgical treatment is indicated.

Dislocation of the acromioclavicular joint, with or without fracture of the distal clavicle, can be treated as a fractured clavicle. If the neurovascular status is normal, there is no need to evacuate the patient immediately.

The most serious of all these shoulder injuries, posterior sternoclavicular dislocation, is fortunately rare. When present it is potentially deadly. This dislocation occurs secondary to direct force at the medial end of the clavicle. The acute symptoms are pain, and possibly respiratory distress. This requires immediate reduction with longitudinal traction, moderate abduction, and extension of the shoulder. Sometimes it is necessary to use a towel clip to reach the medial end of the clavicle and pull it anterior. If the situation is still unstable after reduction, lie the patient with rolled towels or sand bags between the scapulas. The shoulder should be extended and abducted. A 25 per cent (16/60) rate of serious complications of the trachea, oesophagus, or great vessels has been reported.

Anterior dislocation of the sternoclavicular joint is the more common injury. This position is noted by the pain and prominence of the sternoclavicular joint. Sometimes there is very little deformity, minimal pain, and full range of motion and function. Unless a major deficit was initially present, return to the present game may be allowed with caution.

Definitive management

More definitive treatment of the dislocated shoulder is indicated if reduction is not accomplished at the sidelines. Appropriate analgesia or anaesthesia is needed to allow a successful reduction. Arguments exist as to the necessity of immobilization of the first-time dislocation. Some feel that a first-time dislocation is best managed with 6 weeks of rest, immobilized in a sling in adduction and internal rotation. Others suggest that the best treatment for even the initial dislocation is early movement. Patients suffering recurrent dislocations need early rehabilitation, with consideration for surgical repair when recurrence is a functional handicap. If the athlete with a first-time dislocation is over 30 to 35 years old there is little to be gained by 6 weeks of immobilization as the recurrence rate is relatively low.[4]

In the patient with recurrent dislocations it can be argued that radiological evaluation is not necessary, especially if reduction was obtained very easily and quickly. However in all other situations, radiographs should be taken to look for evidence of fracture and associated pathology.

Fractures of the clavicle may need a clavicle strap or a simple sling depending on the nature of the fracture. Non-unions are rare. Open reductions are done only in exceptional circumstances, for example vascular injury.

Most centres do not generally perform open reductions on acromioclavicular separations (R.J. Hawkins, personal communication). The exceptions are in the types that are caught in the trapezius (Rockwood type IV and V) or with the extremely rare type VI, when the distal clavicle is below the coracoid.[5]

After injury, the player would not return to play, especially if there is any suspicion of a fracture or neurological deficit. This holds true even in the situation of recurrent dislocations if there is any suspicion of neurological deficit or fracture.

A patient with recurrent shoulder dislocations will be able to return to their sport within 10 to 14 days. Aggressive physiotherapy is used in the first few days, progressing to graduated functional utilization for both activities of daily living and sport. In our clinic, a first-time anterior dislocation is immobilized for 4 to 6 weeks in internal rotation and adduction. Recently, we are mobilizing these patients more often at 10–14 days with early rehabilitation. A great deal of discussion exists about the length of time of immobilization in the first-time dislocation. In theory the damage is already done, especially to the anterior glenoid labrum. Hence many surgeons do not immobilize the shoulder for any prolonged length of time. In either case, during that period of time, isometric exercises can be done in the sling. Following release from immobilization, range of motion and progressive exercise can occur.

Fractured clavicles heal in the skeletally mature athlete in about 6 weeks. The amount of exercise of the shoulder permitted during this period depends upon the amount of displacement and the amount of pain the patient is experiencing. Although non-union of the clavicle is frequently feared, in actual practice it is not very common. Early range of motion of the shoulder does not inhibit fracture healing. Muscle strengthening exercises that are not causing any pain, and hence little motion at the fracture site, are to be encouraged. The clavicles of children that are non-skeletally mature heal very rapidly. Return to sport is based on clinical and radiological evidence of healing. It is my view that most athletes should not go back until the clavicle is clinically solid and the appropriate muscles rehabilitated. This may take as long as 12 weeks for optimum fracture healing and rehabilitation of muscle strength.

Much has been written about the dislocating shoulder. In our practice we rehabilitate this injury very quickly, allowing a few days of rest for the initial discomfort to settle. This is followed by progressive exercises, especially of the external rotators. We find that the defect in external rotator strength is usually the greatest and needs rehabilitation the most. We have seen a number of 'failed' shoulder separations when treated conservatively. When a regime of infraspinatus strengthening has been undertaken, non-operative care has been successful.

Prognosis

As with all injuries the prognosis depends upon both the pathology and the sport requirements. Overall, when patients have reached approximately 85 per cent function and strength of the non-injured shoulder, they can return to full activity.

When patients have an injured shoulder it does not preclude the maintenance of their cardiovascular fitness. If patients ignore their cardiovascular fitness there will be a prolonged delay in returning to sport. Upper extremity injuries allow continuance of lower extremity workouts. Bicycle riding and running must continue for the maintenance of cardiovascular fitness. Weight lifting of the non-injured limbs is also important. The athletic population is distinguished from other patient populations by asking 'What can I do?' rather than 'What shouldn't I do'!

Elbow injuries

The setting

Falls from heights as in gymnastic dismounts, especially the non-intentional dismounts, often cause significant injuries to elbows. Wrestlers, high-jumpers, and pole-vaulters also present with serious elbow injuries.

On-the-field clinical assessment

After an acute elbow injury, pain is usually in the local area but may not be well localized to one aspect of the elbow. Injuries involving fractures to the radial head or olecranon often are well localized to that anatomical area; however, subluxations, dislocations, and supracondylar fractures may have pain and swelling not well localized to the area of injury.

Many elbow injuries appear in the locked position, that is to say there is great reluctance for the patient to move the elbow. A history of a previous injury is usually non-contributory in terms of elbow injuries as recurrent dislocations are very unusual. The mechanism of injury is very important in that fracture of the olecranon usually occurs with direct trauma and most of the other injuries occur with indirect trauma, for example landing on the outstretched hand. Numbness, tingling, or lack of power are common complaints at the time of initial injury to the elbow. This can result from specific neurological deficit or more likely the trauma of the injury. Seven per cent of supracondylar injuries have some degree of neurological defect.[6]

On examination, deformity is often present at the elbow. At 90 degrees of flexion, the lateral epicondyle, the medial epicondyle, and the tip of the olecranon form an anatomical equilateral triangle. In dislocations this relationship is altered. In the common types of transverse supracondylar fracture this relationship is often maintained. Radial head fractures can occur either alone or in combination with a dislocation. When they occur alone, usually pain is localized to the radial head and is worse with supination or pronation of the forearm. In the presence of an olecranon or supracondylar humeral fracture, crepitus can sometimes be felt. Palpable defects are felt in a fractured olecranon or if there is an acute triceps tear (as occurs in the older population). The gross function is usually poor after a significant elbow injury because of spasm, let alone anatomical derangement. Open wounds are more common because of the proximity of the olecranon to the subcutaneous tissue in the skin. Even small abrasions over an acute fracture area must be considered as an open fracture until proven otherwise.

Differential diagnosis of injuries about the elbow

- epicondyle fractures
- radial head fractures
- olecranon fractures
- supracondylar fractures of the humerus
- elbow dislocations
- radial head dislocations
- elbow joint intra-articular fractures

- other osteochondral injuries (e.g. Pannier's disease)

Based on the history and physical examination, a single bone fracture (i.e. radial head or olecranon) can be diagnosed. This is confirmed by radiography, which also can be used to ascertain the more serious dislocation. Often an osteochondral fracture is in combination with a dislocation. This too will be confirmed by radiological investigation.

Transportation

When there is a suspected fracture and/or dislocation, a decision must be made as to the method of transporting the patient. Splinting before removing from the playing field is advised. One must be cautious because neurovascular complications with elbow injuries are frequent. The ulnar nerve often has a transient defect to some degree.[6] In supracondylar fractures one must always be concerned about the vascular supply, even if the vessel is not acutely torn.[7,8] On-field notation of the presence (or absence) of pulses as well as gross function of the nerves is important for subsequent evaluation.

After the serious injury is splinted, some athletes will be able to walk. However if this is not possible, a stretcher must be used.

Treatment

Sideline treatment

The elbow may have fairly normal alignment. Localized pain over a specific anatomical area may indicate a specific fracture. Radial head fractures present with local pain and decreased pronation/supination. Fractures of the olecranon have local pain and decreased flexion/extension.

The skeletally immature patient may rapidly develop a huge elbow. This is painful, swollen, and purple-blue in colour and will have a fracture even if it cannot be seen on radiography. Therefore, if injured players develop early swelling but have good range of motion and minor pain, do not permit them to return to action until an additional radiological examination is performed.

At the sideline, neurovascular monitoring must continue. If there is gross deformity and the anatomical triangle is not intact, posterior dislocation is to be suspected. One might consider an immediate reduction. Remove the athlete to a quiet place and attempt a reduction. Often, early gentle reductions are very easy. Pain, swelling, and complications are lessened by this early reduction. Gentle longitudinal traction is applied to the forearm, while forward flexing the elbow. If any significant force is necessary or there is crepitus it is better to move the patient to a facility where an orthopaedic consultation can occur. Appropriate splinting and monitoring of the neurovascular status must be continued. This may be forgotten if a 'sideline reduction' was easily attained. In all significant elbow trauma, radiological evaluation must be carried out to look for evidence of fracture and adequacy of reduction. Return to sport must not occur until the radiographs have been assessed. A displaced fracture or a loose body can prevent congruent reductions. Unstable reductions require open surgery with internal fixation in some cases.

Gross deformity of the elbow may have an intact anatomical triangle. Here the deformity usually represents a displaced supracondylar fracture of the humerus. In the emergency situation the pulse may be absent. If this is the case, gross overall alignment should be regained gently with traction and a little flexion. One would expect that the pulse will return. If on the other hand, in an attempt to restore gross alignment the pulse disappears as one flexes the elbow, then the reduction should be positioned until the pulse is restored. Needless to say, in clinical evaluation, as important as the presence or absence of pulses is the adequacy of capillary circulation. A patient with inadequate capillary circulation regardless of pulses is in a true emergency situation and should be treated appropriately with immediate evacuation from the playing field to a facility for definitive care. Fortunately, these vascular emergencies are rare.[9] Constant vigilance will decrease the potential complications of inadequate circulation of a limb.

Definitive treatment

Displaced fractures and dislocations about the elbow need the appropriate reduction. Congruency of the elbow joint must be obtained without loose fragments in the joint.

Only anatomical reductions can be accepted in supracondylar fractures. Treatment often requires operative intervention either with closed reduction and fluoroscopic pinning or actual open reduction and internal fixation.

Prognosis

Once again, the prognosis for return to sport is injury dependent. Patients with stable injuries can be started on early range of motion exercises as the amount of pain dictates. This should include, of course, active range of motion, without passive stretching already damaged muscles. As pain subsides and range of motion increases the patient can return to sport. In terms of gymnastics, an excellent range of painless motion is necessary before the return to sport can be contemplated. This may take 3 to 6 weeks or longer if the injury is significant.

Patients with elbow dislocations can be started on early, protected range of motion exercises without compromising the final result.

Displaced fractures need 3 weeks immobilization after open reduction. Active, not passive, range of motion exercises follow. Progressive strengthening and functional rehabilitation completes the treatment. Return to normal function may never occur, but we have seen a number of determined elite gymnasts return to their same high level of competition following displaced supracondylar fractures. This rehabilitation may take 3 to 6 months.

Undisplaced fractures of the radial head need early mobilization and return to full sport function is usually within 6 weeks. These people may never regain full range of motion, but lack usually only a few degrees in extension or flexion. In radial head fractures, pronation and supination is often reduced slightly. This may not inhibit athletic performance. In throwing sports, any decrease in range of motion may prove significant. In some artistic sports, such as artistic gymnastics, figure skating, and synchronized swimming, the lack of 10 to 20 degrees of extension may cost the athlete marks for artistic impression. Similarly a patient with a fractured olecranon, once stabilized by open reduction, can start on early, active range of motion exercises. Clinical and radiological healing will allow a return to sport 6 to 12 weeks after injury.

It is fundamental to rehabilitate the entire athlete. Cardiovascular training can continue without interruption. Other joints and their muscle groups need functional exercises as much as the injured parts. Continue the exercise of all non-involved limbs and joints throughout the post-injury period so that when the elbow injury is healed the athlete as a whole will be ready to return to competition.

Knee emergencies

The setting

Emergency knee problems are more common than hip or ankle injuries. Contact sports (football, hockey, rugby) and high velocity sports (motor sports, downhill skiing) can cause major knee injuries which can cause permanent limb dysfunction. This type of injury also occurs in jumping sports (long jump, gymnastics).

On-the-field clinical assessment

The contact sport collision, the gymnast falling from an apparatus (such as the high bar), or a long jumper who missed a landing are all examples of situations in which to expect serious injuries to the knee. In each example, the foot is planted and the upper thigh keeps moving as a result of either a direct collision or of the body's own momentum. Violent force is necessary to dislocate a knee. Kennedy (1963)[10] demonstrated with cadaver studies that the force necessary to dislocate knees and rupture cruciate ligaments could cause complete rupture of the popliteal artery above the trifurcation. Other severe associated injuries can occur. Supracondylar fractures of the femur are not uncommon. In the skeletally immature athlete, the distal femoral or proximal tibial epiphyseal plate is weaker than either the bone in the supracondylar area or the ligamentous structures about the knee.[11,12] In these cases separation of the epiphyseal growth plate can occur before diaphyseal fracture or ligamentous disruption. All these situations are true emergencies.

The fallen athlete who complains about severe pain diffusely around the knee can have a gross deformity. However, a knee dislocation can spontaneously reduce before medical attention arrives. In fact, most complex knee ligament disruptions were knee dislocations that spontaneously reduced at the time of injury. A history of previous injury will sometimes be recorded if there has been a previous anterior cruciate injury. However, recurrent tibial–femoral dislocations are not a problem. If the patient gives the story that they have had 'this problem before' one should consider recurrent patellar dislocations or anterior cruciate injury.

Deformity is usually present if either the knee dislocation is not reduced or if there is a fracture. Sometimes to the unfamiliar eye the deformity is relatively subtle, especially if immediate swelling has occurred.

Crepitus is felt as a fracture is aligned. Functional assessment at the scene reveals gross abnormality. The range of motion will be poor. Approximately half of the dislocations are anterior, and the major vessel area is at greatest risk in this type of dislocation.[13] Neurovascular function must be assessed thoroughly; 20 to 35 per cent of patients have vascular impairment.[5] Pulses may or may not be present. Capillary function is very important in assessing vascular adequacy. However, neither intact capillary perfusion nor presence of pulses guarantees that there is vascular continuity. Neurological complications, such as drop foot and paraesthesia, may be noted in 25 to 35 per cent.[5] Posterolateral dislocations stretch the peroneal nerve over the lateral femoral condyle.[5] Observe carefully for popliteal swelling as a sign of popliteal artery injury. Remember that the dislocated patella can cause deformity. If the assault to the knee is small, careful examination makes patellar dislocation obvious. The knee will be flexed, the medial femoral condyle will be prominent, and the laterally displaced patella may be observed and palpated.

Puncture wounds from displaced femoral fractures are occasionally present. Remember that even the smallest of puncture wounds represents a compound fracture.

Differential diagnosis of acute injuries about the knee

- knee dislocation

- displaced fracture of distal femoral epiphysis

- displaced fracture of proximal tibial epiphysis

- supracondylar femoral fracture

The exact diagnosis may be difficult at the scene. On-the-field assessment will usually indicate the occurrence of a very significant lesion. Differentiating between dislocation and a displaced fracture can sometimes be done by determining the point of maximum deformity.

Transportation

Many complications can result from the initial knee injury. Initial treatment can also result in further problems. Further compounding of the wound or damage to the neurovascular structures can occur. Traction to realign either a dislocation or a displaced fracture is appropriate. This is especially true if the dislocation is associated with arterial compromise. If a pulse is initially present but disappears after traction, remove the traction and allow some deformity until the pulse returns. On-field alignments should be carried out gently and easily. If marked resistance is met or great force is needed then it is better to leave the deformity as it lies. Some posterolateral dislocations are not reducible by closed means. Forcing these can result in further damage to the popliteal nerve. Medial capsular enfolding can prevent reductions.[14]

Splinting should be done with proper long leg splints. Splints appear in many types, but it is important that the type is familiar to the physician applying it. Important features of a splint include lightness, ease of position, and non-constriction. There are many commercial types available. Commonly used in North America are air splints and cardboard materials. The latter is easily shaped into the appropriate size. If a prefabricated splint is not available, splinting to the good leg with cloth ties is an option. If air splints are not used with the appropriate inflation pressures, severe constriction of the limb can occur. In addition, pressure blisters are seen more commonly under splints which are too tight. Immediate transport to a definitive facility via fracture board or a stretcher is mandatory. Document the neurovascular status and send support staff with the patient to the hospital with this written information. Competition officials should not be allowed to influence medical decisions. It is fundamental to take the time to stabilize the injury properly, although there will be many pressures to resume competition to satisfy the media, sponsors, etc.

Treatment

Sideline management

On the sideline the application of ice is appropriate. Proper splinting should be well padded and not too rigid. This allows for the massive swelling that will develop. Continue to monitor the neurovascular status. Patient evacuation to the appropriate facility is a matter of urgency as when there is vascular compromise, the complications increase exponentially with time.

As suggested above, many of these serious injuries are disabling enough to require splinting on the field. However, one is often surprised by the athlete who is brought to your attention after being helped to the sidelines with a knee injury without deformity. A knee injury that is examined on the sidelines may have a fracture or a multiple ligament disruption. Occasionally, knees will be examined that have damage to both cruciates with or without a collateral ligament injury. These knees were probably dislocated at the time of impact. The danger of vascular complications in the case of multiple ligament disruption is identical to the knee found displaced at the scene. Therefore, if the knee demonstrates a severe degree of laxity, assume this was a dislocation of the tibial–femoral joint. Treat this as you would any other potentially emergency injury.

Definitive management

Motorcycle racers and downhill skiers often have major injuries to more than one system. Catastrophic knee injuries may be associated with other major injuries of the chest and head. Obviously, these other areas take priority in treatment. However, while other injuries are being assessed or treated, fractures and dislocations should be stabilized.[15] Continual monitoring of the vascular supply and the potential for compartment syndromes should not be forgotten.

Not all vascular injuries are initially obvious. Welling *et al.*[16] described 14 cases of dislocated knee of which seven had palpable pulses. Constant vigilance must be undertaken and vascular complications should be dealt with promptly. Arterial perfusion must be restored within 6 h. This time window will allow salvage of most function.[13,17] Fracture stabilization after vascular repair is the current preferred course of action.[5] Compartment decompression by fasciotomy is crucial if vascular injury has occurred.[18] Intraoperative, intra-arterial bolus injection of contrast appears to be as good as a formal angiogram in these injuries, especially as the time taken to arrange a formal angiogram can be excessive. Today, the most common method of intervention is to identify the area of lesion in the operating room with an intraoperative arteriogram, but this approach will vary between institutions. This is followed by a medial approach. Lesions are dealt with by a reverse saphenous graft. Some method of knee stabilization should then be used to protect the graft.[8] The patient is at risk of developing a compartment syndrome up to at least 72 h, either post-injury or postoperatively. Most surgeons will do a fasciotomy at the time of initial vascular repair.

Epiphyseal displacements can sometimes be stabilized by closed reduction with or without pin fixation. Fractures about the knee are treated by open reduction and internal fixation.[11,12]

Neurological defects can be present. Most nerve lesions are neurapraxias or lesions in continuity. Unfortunately, the common peroneal nerve is easily damaged. Nizt *et al.*[19] showed with grade III ankle sprains that only a 6 per cent change in the length (elongation) adversely affected nerve function. Some neurosurgeons will elect to explore these nerves, usually on a delayed basis, but this decision may be modified by the electromyographs and clinical picture.

Fractures into and about the knee are treated by open reductions with internal fixation. Different methods of fixation are used depending on the character of the fracture. If the fracture is in the diaphysis, a locked intramedullary rod is used. If the fracture is intercondylar or truly supracondylar, a blade plate is fixed to the lateral cortex of the femur. Occasionally, a cast brace may be used if the fracture is not stable. The goal is to mobilize the knee as early as possible. If feasible, early partial weight bearing is preferable to none.

The definitive care of knee dislocations is controversial. Difference of opinion exists on primary compared with delayed ligament repair.[20] Some orthopaedic surgeons prefer to repair the ligaments after 2 weeks when collateral circulation is established.[5] Others will cast the injuries in 30 degrees of flexion for 6 weeks.[21] A delayed repair for functional defects can then be performed as necessary.

Prognosis

Patients with epiphyseal fractures have a better prognosis than those with multiple ligament disruption. Epiphyseal injuries are usually in younger athletes and long-term complications of growth are possible.[11] However, with a well-reduced femoral epiphysis, angular problems usually do not occur. The femoral epiphysis usually closes after this injury, but the tibial side does not recover so easily. Even with a perfect reduction, abnormal growth can occur secondary to the altered blood flow in this area (either increased or decreased). As the patients with tibial epiphyseal injury are younger, closure is further off, and there is a longer time for abnormal growth to occur. For example, sometimes the resultant increased blood supply to the proximal metaphysis will stimulate increased growth through the epiphyseal plate.

If the reduction of the fracture is stable, range of motion exercises and muscle strengthening can be commenced immediately postoperatively. In the adult, fractures will need at least 12 weeks to become solid enough to afford full unrestricted weight bearing. Water exercises and cycling may be started before this time. Both are necessary to maintain cardiovascular fitness. Cycling and swimming will help regain hip, knee, and ankle range of motion. Return to sport is possible for most fractures. If an internal fixation device is used, this should possibly be removed before full sport participation. The whole process may take as long as 18 months to 2 years depending on the fracture.

Complex ligamentous injuries have poor prognoses in terms of regaining full function. This seems to be true regardless of treatment. Stiffness of range of motion or instability from residual ligament pathology is common. However, if there are no complications (artery or nerve), return to some sport is a reasonable goal. In our practice we advocate extensive use of bracing. Some sports (e.g. rugby) and some patients will not tolerate bracing. However, we recommend bracing for 2 years post-injury.

The prognosis is poor if there is a vascular injury associated with these knee injuries. Kennedy, in 1963,[10] wrote that there was a 50 per cent amputation rate with knee dislocations. More recently, with earlier recognition, improved imaging, and more skilled vascular surgeons, this rate should be much lower. Savage (1980)[8] saw an 85 per cent salvage rate of knee dislocation with arterial compromise.[8,10] Open knee dislocations have a very poor prognosis.[22]

It is also of note that the compound fractures associated with major vascular injuries may need amputation. O'Brien suggests that amputation may be better than multiple procedures on the major compound injury that is limb threatening.[23,24]

Although nerve injuries are usually lesions without gross disruption, mostly neurapraxia and axonotmesis, the peroneal nerve problems are slow to recover. Many need surgical exploration to look for intraneural neuromas; however, this issue is controversial.

Sport is one of the main sources of catastrophic knee injuries. Armed with suspicion, early recognition is usually possible. The hidden injury may be the multiple ligament disruption that was dislocated at the time of injury but reduced by the time of the medical examination. If early aggressive treatment is instituted, return to sport may be possible. However, with any complications present, full return to the demands of sport is unlikely.

Compartment syndrome

The setting

The end results of compartment syndromes were first identified by Volkmann in 1881.[25] He described the paralyses and contractures that occurred in the upper extremity when bandages were bound too tight. He stated: 'The paralysis depends on the fact that the primary muscle groups die when deprived of oxygen for too long. . .'.[25] In 1909, Thomas[26] reviewed the world literature noting only a few cases of leg compartment syndromes. Since that time ischaemic contracture has been identified with constricting bandages and casts. Other causes,[5,27] which include primary vascular compromise, toxins, burns, and many others, have also been recognized. However, in the realm of sports medicine, closed injury by direct blunt trauma is the cause of acute compartment syndromes.

Compartment syndrome is defined as a condition in which the circulation and function of tissues within a closed space are compromised by an increased pressure within that space. This usually involves the calf or the forearm. Foot and thigh compartment syndromes have also been described.[28,29]

Relatively minor trauma or trauma without fracture can be the precipitating event. Contusions in contact sports, such as soccer,[30] or ruptured muscles in racket sports are examples of sports situations causing acute compartment syndromes.[31]

On-the-field clinical assessment

The initial injury can be a fractured tibia, radius, or distal humerus. The tissue perfusion can be interrupted directly or secondarily as the result of pressure from constrictive dressings. However, the initial injury may not be that severe. The kicked shin or contused calf are examples of presenting injuries in our emergency department. There may be involvement of a number of upper extremity injuries, but supracondylar fractures, forearm fractures, contusions, or crush injuries are the most common. The descriptions that are given below also apply to the upper extremity injuries.[32]

One tennis player was accelerating towards the net and tore the mid-portion of the gastrocnemius. Massive swelling in the closed superficial posterior compartment resulted in a compartment syndrome.

At the scene of the sporting event, complaints may be minimal.

Over the following hours, the bleeding into the fascial space continues to raise the intracompartmental tension to critical levels. The player may wake up in the middle of the night in agony. After the game, the hot shower adds to the swelling. The bus ride home may be accompanied by increasing pain. The signal of rising intracompartmental pressure is pain, which is out of proportion to the injury. Even a fracture, once splinted, usually does not cause a great deal of pain. If the normal doses of analgesia are not controlling the pain, consider the possiblity of compartment syndrome until proven otherwise. It can take up to 72 h after the injury for a compartment syndrome to manifest itself. Complaints of numbness, tingling, coldness, and paralysis are all late symptoms.

The pathophysiology has been well described. Compartments are bounded by bone and dense unforgiving fascia. Pressure will increase as the bleeding continues. When the venule pressure is exceeded by the intracompartmental pressure, the venules collapse causing further increase in interstitial and compartment pressure. Next the arterioles close and cause muscle ischaemia, releasing histamine-like substances. These substances increase capillary permeability, further increasing the compartment pressure.

The primary ischaemia is from the arteriole level. Therefore, the major clinical findings of pallor, absence of pulse, paraesthesiae, and paralysis are late signs. The first sign is the pain associated with passive stretch of the muscles in the affected compartment. This will occur long before the pressure is high enough to cause permanent damage to the enclosed structures. Sometimes this early stretch pain is associated with a cyanotic tinge to the extremity. Normal pulse and nerve function is found in the early salvageable stages. Palpation of a compartment for tenseness is very subjective and not reliable. Accurate measurements of pressures are easily obtained. Manometric evaluation of the pressures should be made if there is any question of the diagnosis.

Differential diagnosis of compartment syndrome

- compartment syndrome
- major arterial injury
- isolated partial nerve injury
- ruptured muscle
- undiagnosed fracture

Acute compartment syndrome can be an isolated event or occur secondary to a major arterial injury. If blood supply is not restored with an arterial repair within 6 h, the muscles undergo further swelling. This further compromises the compartment blood supply by increasing the pressure, and a vicious cycle is established. Occasionally, athletes will have an isolated contusion or stretch of the peroneal nerve causing severe pain and neural dysfunction. This may be confused with a primary compartment problem. An isolated partial rupture of muscles (e.g. medial head of gastrocnemius) is commonly seen. This usually causes pain but is relatively easily managed with rest, ice, compression, and elevation. Low velocity trauma, enough to cause a fracture but not enough to cause disruption of the compartment sheath or interosseous membrane, will predispose to a compartment syndrome. This is because in a displaced fracture the compartments are torn and disrupted enough to self-decompress.

Transportation

As stated above, this diagnosis is more likely to present after the competition. However, it is one of the few true emergencies in sports medicine. When the diagnosis is seriously suspected it must be treated aggressively. If there has been a circumferential cast or dressing applied for a fracture or wound, then while the patient is being transferred to the hospital, the cast or bandages should be split and possibly removed. Skin must be seen from one end of the cast to the other.

The position of the leg during transportation is also important. If there is vascular impairment the limb probably should be kept at a neutral level with respect to the heart. There is a relative decrease in arterial flow to a limb associated with elevation. Dependency increases venous congestion, which would compound the problems in compartment syndromes. Hence a neutral position of the limb is desired.

Treatment

Sideline management
At the sideline, preventive measures are possible. Early elevation of an injured extremity will decrease the likelihood of venous congestion. Early application of ice and compression of a contusion to stop bleeding will also decrease the risk of an expanding compartment. Splints which are not circumferential are also helpful.

Definitive management
Usually, the diagnosis can be made clinically. When present, pain out of proportion to the injury and pain with passive stretch of muscles in the tight compartment are the classic findings. Sometimes there is doubt about the clinical findings. There are several methods to measure compartment pressures directly. Whitesides (1975),[33] Murbarak and Owen (1978),[34] and Rorabeck (1981), have described methods of compartment pressure measurement in static fashion. Occasionally, a patient may be obtunded from a head injury or be in a period of cardiovascular shock. In these situations a dynamic method of an indwelling wick catheter to monitor the pressures is indicated.

Normal resting compartmental pressure is 4 mmHg. In the emergency situation a compartment pressure of over 30 mmHg demands fascial decompression. When the patient is in shock, if the compartment pressure is measured within 10 to 30 points of the diastolic, then this patient should have a fasciotomy.

With normal exercise the readings can reach 50 to 60 mmHg, but it falls quickly with the cessation of activity. In the presence of chronic compartment syndromes the pressures elevate to between 75 and 100 mmHg and their resting pressures are between 15 and 30 mmHg.[34] Styf showed some increase in pressures in patients using custom knee braces.[35] Some predisposition to compartment syndrome may be found in the anatomy of the compartment fascia.[36,37]

Some work suggests that there is a place for magnetic resonance imaging in the evaluation of chronic compartment syndromes (Vellet, personal communication).

It has been shown experimentally that when a cast is split the compartment pressures are reduced by 30 per cent.[38] When a cast, soft roll, and dressing were bivalved so that there was no circumferential constricting elements from one end to the other, up to 85 per cent reduction in compartment pressures occurred.

It is a surgical emergency when the diagnosis is made either clinically or by objective measurement. The definitive treatment is fasciotomy. In the calf there are four compartments (five if you count the posterior tibial muscle to be in a separate compartment).[18,31] If the diagnosis is made objectively and only one or two compartments are involved, it may be reasonable to release only those compartments. Despite local measurements of only one compartment involved, Rorabeck feels that if the pressure is over 30 mmHg, then all four compartments should be decompressed.[18] In many situations it is necessary to decompress all four compartments. Double incision fasciotomy is advocated by some authors.[18,34] Kelly and Whitesides, in 1967,[39] approached the four compartments by excising the fibula. In our centre we use the two incision method. After 5 to 7 days, delayed primary closure with or without skin grafting is performed.

Prognosis

Delay in making the diagnosis or treatment can be catastrophic to the athlete. Research has shown that even 2 h will produce early muscle changes.[40] Classic Volkmann's ischaemic contractures follow 12 h of ischaemia. In practice this has been shown to be accurate. Rorabeck had excellent results in patients who were treated less than 12 h after injury.[18]

The prognosis for return to sport depends somewhat on the cause of the syndrome. In cases of muscle rupture the prognosis is not as good for return to a high level of competition. Irreversible changes to some of the muscle can occur after 6 h. The percentage of defect influences the amount of restoration of function.

The muscle rehabilitation necessary after fasciotomy is prolonged. The limb may have some chronic swelling as a result of chronic venous insufficiency. Muscle often prolapses if unconstrained by fascia. This may influence the ultimate power that can be generated.

Our definition of an emergency is a situation in which immediate intervention will produce a difference in outcome. Compartment syndrome is a good example. A delayed diagnosis and treatment is devastating to the athlete. If the diagnosis is made early and treatment is carried out within 6 h, it is reasonable to expect full return to function and sport.

Frost-bite

The setting

The setting for frost-bite is present in some part of Canada for 12 months a year. Our national ski team can train all year long on glaciers in the Canadian Rocky Mountains. For most winter sport enthusiasts it is possible to downhill, cross-country ski, or hike for 6 months of the year. The settings for cold injuries are plentiful.

There are several types of cold injuries. The individual can develop hypothermia or localized parts can develop frost-bite. In hypothermia, the core body temperature drops. In frost-bite, the core temperature may be normal while the temperature in the peripheral tissues drops, which causes local freezing of tissues.

The end result of frost-bite is destruction and death of tissue. The body attempts to preserve core temperature by decreasing blood flow to parts exposed to cold. Vasoconstriction, mediated by the sympathetic nervous system, is the mechanism by which this is carried out. Unfortunately, some patients are predisposed to problems. Smoking (or any use of tobacco), age extremes (either very young or very old), fatigue, poor nutrition, or the influence of alcohol can all predispose people to frost-bite.[41]

Destruction due to frost-bite is the end result of a sequence of events. The first pathological change is the formation of actual ice crystals in the cells. This mechanically distorts the cell and adversely affects its functions. Local vascular stasis occurs, followed by clotting and distal presentation of local hypoxia, ischaemia, and acidosis. Rewarming will cause a rebound vasodilatation and some capillary breakdown. Oedema and further tissue damage will follow. However, if the exposure continues, deeper tissues become involved. If a large vessel is frozen, a mummification process accompanied by gangrene will follow.[42]

Obviously the skier is at risk. Not so obvious are the speed skaters who have to train outdoors. The footballer, who plays outdoors in November in the middle of a snow storm, is at risk. Even the hunter who hikes over the varied terrain in the autumn and spring is at risk. Wet marshland and fields predispose to wet, cold feet. This is a perfect set-up for chilblains (trench foot).

The weekend athlete at risk is the one inexperienced in outdoor winter athletic activities. This may be the first-time skier who wears stylish clothing that is thinly insulated and tight. With their inexperience, it is common to wear ski boots that are badly designed and too tight. Similarly, gloves that are too constricting may not allow for enough movement for the fingers.

Experienced athletes get into trouble by neglect. For example, their favourite pair of cross-country ski boots may be comfortable, but they probably have worn through the insulation in areas of the toe and heel.

The environmental temperature does not need to be frigid. Repetitive exposure to water around 0°C is enough to cause trench foot. Skin will freeze if the tissue is at −2°C. Adding a wind chill to temperatures of 5 to 10°C can drop the actual temperatures to levels capable of freezing tissues.

Another measurement of the athletes at risk is even more sophisticated. The Glacier Patrol 100 km ski race over the high terrain of Switzerland gave rise to the Arolla Index. This collates the time of exposure, wind-chill factors, and measured temperature into one index.[43]

'On-the-field' clinical assessment

Commonly, the first effects of local cold go unnoticed by the affected individual. Frost-nip is the first step in local cold injury. Reversible ice crystals form on the skin surface. The frosted appearance and numb feelings are reversible if warming procedures are carried out. If not, then the process continues and freezes deeper tissues. Slight initial swelling and redness may precede the skin prickling sensations. As the process continues the skin becomes yellow and waxy. When the cold stimulus is unchecked the subcutaneous tissue will freeze and the skin will feel solid. At first there are blisters that represent superficial freezing. If capillaries are involved and they rupture, then the blisters become haemorrhagic. This represents a deeper level of involvement. If on initial assessment there is dry gangrene, larger vessels than capillaries have been compromised. In this case a degree of tissue destruction is complete.

Trench or immersion foot is found in the patient with repetitive exposure of bare skin to wet and cold around 0°C. The skin is red in the early stages. A mottled grey-blue or white occurs after extended exposures. The skin is sensitive and easily 'burns' with any temperature change. With rewarming, the foot becomes swollen and oedematous, and the skin becomes red and reactive to minimal stimuli.

Transportation

The patient with frost-bite is a true emergency. If the frozen part is in the foot and any thawing occurs, transport of the the patient will require a stretcher. A thawed area of tissue that has been frost-bitten is defenceless against mechanical forces. The trauma of simple weight bearing will increase the local tissue destruction at an alarming rate. Frost-nip can be rewarmed at the site and no evacuation is necessary. Patients with trench foot need protection from repeated exposure to the cold and wet.

Treatment

Sideline management

Prevention is the best treatment in any sports injury. Cold injury is a good example of an injury that can be prevented. Unfortunately, a key element to prevention is common sense. Preventative lubrication of chronically dehydrated skin is useful in decreasing the effects of dryness and flaking incurred with frost-nip. The wearing of adequate insulation in the form of dry, properly fitting (especially not tight) clothing is a major step in prevention. It is vital to keep moving the fingers and toes. If they become numb, take action to move them (e.g. remove boot). Use the buddy system: ski and hike with a companion that can help check your face, ears, and nose for early blanching or frosting. Remove yourself out of the wind if cold injury is suspected. This will increase the relative temperature in the tissues. Ski in areas that are protected by trees. Come down from higher altitudes until the area is rewarmed thoroughly. Alcohol stimulates heat loss but does not give significant peripheral dilatation in the presence of cold-induced vasoconstriction. Therefore, alcohol only compounds the problem. Similarly, smoking is absolutely contraindicated.

Frost-nip needs early rewarming. This is easily achieved by blowing warm exhaled air across the affected area. The armpit or the groin are two areas that can be used to rewarm a cold hand or foot. Continued monitoring by a companion is important.

Trench foot should be kept dry. Great care must be taken in skin management because the skin may be friable. Dry, padded dressing should be used for any blisters or skin breaks as the potential for superficial infection is present.

Frost-bite is a true emergency. Even worse than a frozen limb is the limb that is frozen, thawed, and refrozen. The practical point is that if the frost-bite occurs in a situation where there is the possibility of refreezing after thawing, leave the part frozen until definitive treatment can be carried out. The frozen limb can bear some weight if necessary. However, as soon as it is thawed meticulous care of tissues is necessary. The thawed foot will swell rapidly and be unlikely to fit into the original boot. The mountain climber, cross-country trekker, or the patient with a previously frozen extremity can become a great liability to the whole group.

Definitive management

The patient with frost-bite may well have central hypothermia as well as local frost-bite. Confusion, a slow mental state, and weakness that is associated with hypothermia must be noted and treated. The patient should be rewarmed as rapidly as possible. However, during this phase, ventricular fibrillation is a possibility so that one should be prepared to deal with this potential complication. Rewarming of the extremity needs to be done by immersion in warm water. The water needs to be clean (preferably sterile). The temperature should be kept at 40 to 42°C for 15 to 30 min. The water container should be large enough to include all of the frozen part at one time. Warm water will need to be added as the frozen extremity cools the first water. Do not warm the affected part against a fireplace as it will thaw unevenly. Initial blood flow into the area will make the part 'burn'. The nerves will be sensitive and capillary fragility will increase oedema into the area. Intact blisters should be left, but broken blisters should be debrided and the wounds dressed with sterile dressing. Tetanus prophylaxis should be administered.

Various agents have been investigated for enhancing revascularization. Heparin, intra-arterial reserpine, chemical and operative sympathectomy, and dextran of low molecular weight have all been tested without consistent results.

The damage has been done by the initial intracellular freezing. The cell wall membranes rupture releasing their contents. Extracellular fluid becomes hyperosmotic and clotting follows. With rewarming there is increased vascularity. Local haemorrhage and oedema causes further anoxia and cellular damage. If the freezing is in the calf or tibial area, rewarming can trigger a compartment syndrome.

If gangrene is present initially, it is usually dry gangrene that is not infected. These wounds should also be dressed and monitored as the rewarming may demarcate the area of gangrene at a different level than initially anticipated. Live tissue may be present under the layers of necrotic skin. Most authors suggest leaving amputation for weeks or months as long as secondary infection does not intervene.

If long-term pain is a problem, sometimes sympathectomy is of benefit. Pain control by non-surgical techniques should be considered (transcutaneous electrical nerve stimulation, or acupuncture).

Prognosis

Frost-nip, by definition, is reversible freezing of very superficial layers of skin. Hence treated early and adequately, full return to function is anticipated. Obviously, this is the form of frost-bite most commonly seen in the recreational skier.

Flaking and redness of the affected areas of skin often follow trench foot rewarming. Patients who have experienced trench/immersion foot have a sensitive extremity for a lengthly period. It may be prone to future cold injury. Increased vascular changes to the skin are common. Chronic hypersensitivity is a common sequelae.

Frost-bite causes permanent damage; the extent of damage depends on the amount and depth of tissue initially involved and the duration of freezing. The response to rewarming is also extremely important. Large amounts of oedema and the presence of a compartment syndrome are associated with a poor prognosis. If secondary infection occurs, the outcome depends on the organism and the extent of the infection.

When frost-bite occurs in growing bones it affects the epiphyseal plates. Characteristically, the growth plates fuse giving rise to deformities of the digits.

Frost-bite is like many sports medicine injuries. The presentation can be incidental or an emergency. If the clinical diagnosis is ignored by the athlete or the injury is misdiagnosed or mismanaged by the doctor, the results can be devastating. Fortunately, like many sports medicine injuries, it is uncommon and usually prevented by common sense.

Summary

Fortunately, major emergencies are rare; experience has taught that more than half of the battle is to be prepared for disaster.

The patient with a major limb injury may well have airway or cardiovascular troubles and these take precedence over the injured limb. Arterial injury, neurological defects, and compound fractures are the most common emergency limb injuries in sport. Appropriate clinical examination is the second step in their management. (Being prepared is the first step.) The extent and methods of rehabilitation vary with the injury, the athlete, and the sport. Prognosis varies with each specific injury.

The management must include rehabilitation of the whole individual in order to achieve the optimum outcome.

References

1. Allen RE (ed.). *The Oxford dictionary of current English*. Oxford University Press, 1985: 239.
2. Pipe A. Canadian Academy of Sport Medicine: Accreditation committee. Examination
3. Fallat ME. Transport of the injured child. *Seminars in Pediatric Surgery* 1995; **4**(2): 88–92.
4. Simonet WT, Cofield RH. Prognosis in anterior shoulder dislocation. *American Journal of Sports Medicine* 1984; **12**: 19–24.
5. Rockwood CA, Green DP. *Fractures in adults*. Vol 2. Philadelphia: Lippincott, 1984: 870–1.
6. Pritchard DJ, Linscheid RL, Svien HJ. Intra-articular median nerve entrapment with dislocation of the elbow. *Clinical Orthopaedics and Related Research* 1973; **90**: 100–3.
7. Axe MJ. Limb threating injuries in sport. *Clinics in Sport Medicine* 1989; **8**: 101–9.
8. Savage R. Popliteal artery injury associated with knee dislocation: improved outlook? *American Surgeon* 1980; **46**: 627–32.
9. Hurley JA. Complicated elbow fractures. *Clinics in Sports Medicine* 1990; **9**: 39–57.
10. Kennedy JC. Complete dislocation of the knee joint. *Journal of Bone and Joint Surgery* 1963; **45A**: 889–91.
11. Burkhart SS, Peterson HA. Fractures of the proximal tibial epiphysis. *Journal of Bone and Joint Surgery* 1979; **61A**: 996–1002.
12. Shelton WK, Conale CF. Fractures of the proximal tibia epiphyseal cartilage. *Journal of Bone and Joint Surgery* 1979; **61A**: 167.
13. Green NE, Allen BL. Vascular injuries associated with dislocation of the knee. *Journal of Bone and Joint Surgery* 1977; **59A**: 236–9.
14. Sisto DJ, Warren RF. Complete knee dislocation. *Clinical Orthopaedics and Related Research* 1985; **198**: 94–101.
15. Ryan AJ, Allman Jr. FL. *Sports medicine*. 2nd edn. San Diego: Academic Press, 1989.
16. Welling RE, Kakkasseril J, Cranley JJ. Complete dislocations of the knee with popliteal vascular injury. *Journal of Trauma* 1981; **21**: 450–3.
17. Cohen SL, Taylor WC. Vascular problems of the lower extremity in athletes. *Clinics in Sport Medicine* 1990; **9**: 449–70.
18. Rorabeck CH. The treatment of compartment syndromes of the leg. *Journal of Bone and Joint Surgery* 1984; **66B**: 93–7.
19. Nitz AJ, Dobner JJ, Kersey D. Nerve injury and grade 2 and 3 ankle sprains. *American Journal of Sports Medicine* 1985; **13**: 177–82.
20. Meyers MH, Moore TM, Harvey JP Jr. Traumatic dislocation of the knee joint. *Journal of Bone and Joint Surgery* 1975; **57A**: 430–3.
21. Taylor AR, Arden GP, Rainey HA. Traumatic dislocation of the knee. A report of forty-three cases with special reference to conservative treatment. *Journal of Bone and Joint Surgery (British Volume)* 1972; **54**: 96–102.
22. Wright DC, Covey DC, Born CT, Sadasivan KK. Open dislocation of the knee. *Journal of Orthopaedic Trauma* 1995; **9**(2): 135–40.
23. O'Brien PJ. Management of the comprimised lower extremity. *Canadian Journal of Surgery* 1995; **38**(3): 218–20.
24. Clarke P, Mollan RAB. The criteria for amputation in severe lower limb injury. *Injury* 1994; **25**(3): 139–43.
25. Volkmann R. Die ischaemischem muskellamungen und kontrakturen. *Chirurgie* 1881; **8**: 801
26. Thomas JJ. Nerve involvement in the ischemic paralysis and contracture of Volkmann. *Annals of Surgery* 1909; **49**: 330–70.
27. Matsen FA. Compartment syndrome: a unified concept. *Clinical Orthopaedics* 1975; **113**: 8–14.
28. Gardner AMN, *et al.* Reduction of post-traumatic swelling and compartment pressure by impulse compression of the foot. *Journal of Bone and Joint Surgery* 1990; **72B**: 810–15.
29. Myerson MS. Experimental decompression of the fascial compartments of the foot: the basis for fasciotomy in acute compartment syndromes. *Foot and Ankle* 1988; **8**: 308–14.
30. Leach RE, Corbett M. Anterior tibial compartment syndrome in soccer players. *American Journal of Sports Medicine* 1979; **7**: 258–9.
31. Davies JAK. Peroneal compartment syndrome secondary to rupture of peroneus longus: case report. *Journal of Bone and Joint Surgery* 1979; **61A**: 783–4.
32. Weinstein SM, Herring SA. Nerve problems and compartment syndromes in the hand, wrist and forearm. *Clinics in Sports Medicine* 1992; **11**(1): 161–88.
33. Whitesides TE, Haney TC, Morimoto K, Harada H. Tissue pressure measurements as a determinator of the need of fasciotomy. *Clinical Orthopaedics and Related Research* 1975; **113**: 43–51.
34. Mubarak SL, Owen CA. Double-incision fasciotomy of the leg for decompression in compartment syndromes. *Journal of Bone and Joint Surgery* 1977; **59A**: 184–7.
35. Styf JR, Nakhostine M, Gershuni DH. Functional knee braces increase intramuscular pressures in the anterior compartment of the leg. *American Journal of Sports Medicine* 1992; **20**(1): 46–9.
36. Hurschler C, Vanderby R Jr, Martinez DA, Vailas AC, Turnipseed WD. Mechanical and biochemical analyses of tibial compartment fascia in chronic compartment syndrome. *Annals of Biomedical Engineering* 1994; **22**(3): 272–9.
37. Turnipseed WD, Hurschler C, Vanderby R Jr. The effects of elevated compartment pressure on tibial arteriovenous flow and relationship of mechanical and biochemical characteristics of fascia to genesis of chronic anterior compartment syndrome. *Journal of Vascular Surgery* 1995; **21**(5): 810–16.
38. Garfin SR, Murarak SJ, Evans KL, Hargens AR, Akeson WH. Quantification of intracompartmental pressure and volume under

plaster casts. *Journal of Bone and Joint Surgery* 1981; **63A**: 449–53.

39. Kelly RP, Whitesides TE, Jr. Transfibular route for fasciotomy of the leg. In Proceedings of the American Academy of Orthopedic Surgeons. *Journal of Bone and Joint Surgery* 1967; **49A**: 1022–3.

40. Jepson PN. Ischemic contracture, experimental study. *Annals of Surgery* 1926; **84**: 785–95.

41. Valnicek SM, Chasmar LR, Clapson JB. Frostbite in the prairies: a 12 year review. *Plastic and Reconstructive Surgery* 1993; **92(4)**: 633–41.

42. Fritz RL, Perrin DH. Cold exposure injuries: prevention and treatment. *Clinics in Sports Medicine* 1989; **8**: 111–27.

43. Reymond M, Rigo M. The 'Arolla' index: a study of 88 cases of frostbite during a high mountain competition. *Journal de Chirurgie* (Paris) 1988; **125**: 239–44.

Suggested reading

Allman Jr. FL, Ryan AJ. The immediate management of sports injuries. In: Ryan AJ, Allman Jr. FL. *Sports medicine*, 2nd edn. San Diego: Academic Press, 1989: 281–318.

Bracker MD. Environmental and thermal injury. *Clinics in Sports Medicine* 1992; **11**: 419–26

Ernst CB, Kaufer H. Fibulectomy-fasciotomy: an import adjunct in the management of lower extremity arterial trauma. *Journal of Trauma* 1971; **11**: 365–80.

7.3 Maxillofacial injuries in sport

G.F. Goubran

Introduction

As contact and non-contact sports have become more competitive in recent years and as there is strong encouragement to participate in them from an early age, sporting injuries to the maxillofacial region and dental structures have become more common. In a recent Australian study, one-third of dental trauma was due to participation in sport.

Maxillofacial injuries due to sporting involvement may include fractures of the facial skeleton, intra- and extraoral lacerations, and dental injuries (the latter are the most common). The use of professionally fitted (custom-made) mouthguards may prevent such injuries. It is particularly important for teenagers receiving orthodontic treatment with fixed brackets (so-called 'railway tracks') to wear custom-made mouthguards during sports activities to protect soft tissues, lips for example, from lacerations and injuries which could be caused by rubbing against the orthodontic appliance.

Custom-made mouthguards are far superior in reducing maxillofacial injuries compared with the off-the-shelf types available.

The wearing of appropriate sports helmets (as worn by cricketers, American footballers, ice-hockey players, etc.) in contact and non-contact sports has made a great contribution to safety.

A resilient, plastic mouthguard acts by absorbing some of the force of a blow to the mouth at the impact site and then distributing the remaining energy throughout the mouthguard, namely to a much greater surface area than that of the actual impact. Of course, if the contact is of sufficient severity, this device will be inadequate for dealing with the forces in question and injury will not be prevented. On such occasions, the mouthguard can then only help to reduce the magnitude of injury.

In general, however, the custom-made mouthguard fitted to the upper jaw protects the upper anterior teeth during impact and helps to avoid their avulsion. It also guards against intraoral lacerations by separating the upper teeth from the soft tissues of the tongue, lips, and cheeks. The upper and lower opposing teeth are also protected from impact produced when the mandible is involuntarily and forcibly closed. The likelihood of a fractured mandible following impact from below is thus reduced.

Perhaps of greater importance, it reduces the force of mandibular impact transmitted through the mandibular joints to the skull (the very thin glenoid fossa) and brain, thus lessening the risk of concussion and other more serious head injuries.

A bimaxillary mouthguard obviously increases protection of the intraoral soft tissues and protects the maxillary and mandibular teeth. This mechanism also stabilizes the mandible to the maxilla and the rest of the skull, reducing the risk of its fracture—a property that has been confirmed experimentally. The bimaxillary mouthguard may be of special value in the boxing ring where many punches may be aimed at the mandible (uppercuts) with the intention of causing a knockout.

However, because of its bulk it causes an increase in resistance to oral airflow and thus difficulty in breathing. Custom-made mouthguards fitted to the upper jaw alone have the least detrimental effect on oral airflow and most closely approximate with not wearing a guard.

As well as benefiting physically from wearing a custom-made mouthguard and a sports helmet, sports participants may experience a significant improvement in their self-confidence and performance.

Fractures of the facial skeleton

Maxillofacial injuries in sport can result from either direct contact with an opponent or equipment (cricket ball, hockey stick, etc.) The degree of trauma can vary from a simple crack fracture, requiring no treatment (causing minimum inconvenience), to major disintegration of the facial skeleton, with involvement of overlying soft tissues and adjacent structures (for example, the eyes, sinuses, tongue, and teeth). Such injuries are relatively easy to recognize by the obvious bony deformity seen immediately after the impact, before overlying tissue becomes oedematous and swollen. Fractures should always be suspected if teeth fail to occlude normally.

For convenience the facial skeleton is divided into three parts:

(1) the lower third—the lower jaw (mandible);

(2) the middle third—the area between the superior orbital margin above and the occlusal plane below (in the case of an edentulous patient the maxillary alveolus);

(3) the upper third—the area above the superior orbital margin.

Since surgical treatment of these injuries is a highly specialized subject, in this chapter we shall concentrate only on the recognition and diagnosis of maxillofacial trauma.

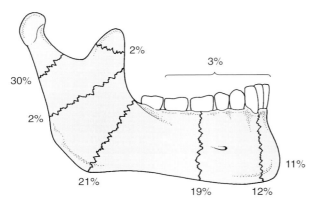

Fig. 1 Percentage of fractures at the 'mandibular site'.

Fractures of the lower third (fractured mandible)

The second most common cause of mandibular fractures is sports injury (assault being the most common). Fractures of the mandible can occur in either the ramus or the body of the mandible (Fig. 1). Fractures of the ramus are usually closed injuries, while those of the body are often compound. Fractures of these two main areas differ in their clinical presentation and thus present different management problems.

Fractures in the area of the ramus include fractures of the condylar region, coronoid process, and ramus. Fractures of the body of the mandible include the angle, midbody (molar and premolar area), midline, lateral to the midline in the incisor area, and dentoalveolar fractures. These fractures can occur singly or in any combination; the most common is a bilateral fracture involving the condylar neck on one side and the opposite angle.

Fractures of the ramus area
Condylar region fracture
The condylar region is the most common site of mandibular fracture and, unfortunately, the most frequently undiagnosed. The importance of diagnosing fractures of the mandibular condyles cannot be overemphasized, particularly in children. If they are undetected and mismanaged, they may lead to gross asymmetrical growth or ankylosis of the joint (Fig. 2).

The fractured condyle can be unilateral or bilateral and intracapsular or extracapsular. Most are extracapsular fractures of the condylar neck which may or may not be dislocated. There is pain and swelling over the fractured temporomandibular joint (Plate 2). It is tender to palpate and invariably the mandibular midline is deviated towards the fractured side. Movements are limited, particularly lateral excursion away from the injured side (Fig. 3). Anterior open bite and gagging of the occlusion on the posterior molars are indications of bilateral condylar fractures (Plate 3).

Coronoid process fracture
Fractures of the coronoid process are very rare and cannot be diagnosed on clinical examination alone. Apart from pain and limitation of mandibular movement, there is intraoral tenderness and ecchymosis over the coronoid process region.

Ramus fracture
Ramus fractures are also rare. Apart from swelling and discomfort, there is little else to see as the fractured segment is sandwiched between the masseter and the pterygoid muscles.

Fractures of the body of the mandible
Fracture of the angle
Fracture of the angle is the second most common mandibular fracture, and often occurs through an unerupted lower-third molar. The displacement is caused by the pull of the masseter and/or medial pterygoid muscles, depending on the direction of the fracture line through the bone (Fig. 4).

Midbody fracture (molar and premolar area)
Unilateral fractures can present with very little displacement as the muscles on either side of the fractured site tend to counteract each other.

Midline fracture (symphyseal)
Midline fractures can present with little displacement as the fracture line passes between the genial tubercles The pull of the genioglossus and geniohyoid muscles tends to impact the bone ends together. Although it is difficult to demonstrate such a fracture radiologically, it should be suspected in all cases where patients have sustained trauma to the point of the chin and particularly where bilateral condylar fractures are present.

Fracture lateral to the midline (parasymphyseal)
Unlike midline fractures, parasymphyseal fractures present with considerable displacement, as the muscles attached to the genial tubercles tend to displace the fractured fragment lingually (Plate 4).

The diagnosis of mandibular fractures is usually obvious as there is pain and discomfort accompanied by swelling and ecchymosis. Fractures of the body of the mandible are often compound in the mouth, and, in cases of severe facial lacerations, can be compound to the face. Invariably there is evidence of haemorrhage at the fracture site in compound fractures. Unlike the middle third, the presence of the powerful muscles of mastication inserted into the mandible produces gross displacement of the fractured fragments unrelated to the direction of the traumatic force. In fractures of the body of the mandible, abnormal movement across the fracture site can be elicited on gentle pressure. Derangement of occlusion and limitation of mandibular movement caused by pain and trismus are present. Blood-stained saliva and sublingual ecchymosis are indicative of mandibular fracture. If the inferior dental branch of the mandibular nerve is involved in the fracture, there will be paresthesia or anaesthesia to the lip. However, the precise physical signs and symptoms of mandibular fractures vary according to the site of the fracture.

Dentoalveolar fracture
In dentoalveolar fractures the teeth are avulsed, subluxed, or fractured with or without an associated fracture of the supportive alveolar bone and without a demonstrable fracture of the body of the mandible. The diagnosis of such a fracture is usually obvious because of the derangement of the occlusion, pain, and discomfort. The fractured segment is usually loose (Plate 5).

Examination of the mandible
Both sides of the lower border of the mandible are palpated from behind the patient using the fingers of both hands, starting from the

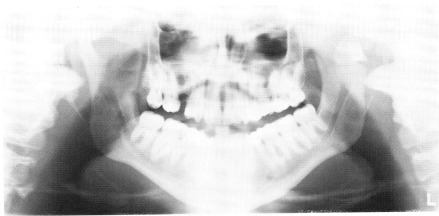

Fig. 2 Orthopantomogram showing a fracture dislocation of the left mandibular condyle.

midline and working backwards. Step deformities, particularly at the region of the angle, should be noted.

Swelling of the temporomandibular joint is observed by standing in front of the patient. Gentle palpation of the joints will reveal any tenderness. The absence or presence of movement of the condylar heads is detected by placing the little fingers in both external auditory meatus with the pulp of the finger facing forward. The patient is then asked to move the mandible in all directions. Pain, discomfort, and restricted movement are present in the region of the affected condyle. Attempting to move the jaw will worsen the pain. Intraorally, the presence of ecchymosis sublingually following trauma is pathognomonic of a mandibular fracture (Plate 6). On suspected fracture sites, particularly the symphyseal and parasymphyseal regions, the thumb and forefinger of each hand are placed on each side of the suspected fracture site and gentle pressure is used to elicit any mobility across the fracture line.

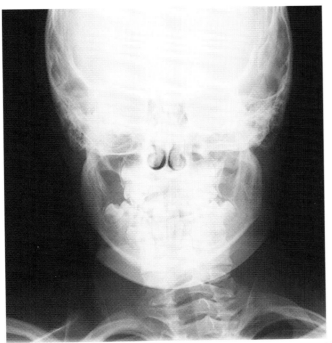

Fig. 3 Posteroanterior view showing a bilateral condylar fracture in a 10-year-old with mixed dentition.

Radiological investigation

Views at right angles to each other are needed to diagnose a fractured mandible.

Lateral oblique (right and left) The lateral oblique is centred over the angle of the mandible. As well as showing the fractured body of the mandible it may reveal fractures of the condyle (Fig. 5).

Posteroanterior The posteroanterior view will demonstrate fractures of the body and angle, together with any displacement of the fractured fragments (Fig. 6). Undisplaced fractures of the midline or lateral to the midline are not easily demonstrated on this view. The condylar head is obscured by the superimposition of the mastoid process.

Intraoral radiographs Intraoral radiographs are required to demonstrate the condition of the teeth in the fracture line. Occlusal films are invaluable for demonstrating midline or lateral to midline fractures (Fig. 7).

Orthopantomogram The orthopantomogram is invaluable in detecting fractures anywhere in the mandible. It demonstrates injuries in the condylar region unseen on other radiographic standard views, particularly those of the condyles. Unfortunately, this view cannot be obtained on bedridden or unconscious patients. A right angle view to the orthopantomogram must be obtained to supplement it (Fig. 8).

Reverse Town's views Fractures of the condylar neck are best seen on this view.

Temporomandibular joint views These are used to demonstrate condylar dislocations. If taken with the mouth closed and then open, they will demonstrate the functioning of the joint.

Tomography Tomography is the only helpful radiological view which demonstrates intracapsular fracture of the temporomandibular joint.

Fractures of the middle third

Fractures of the middle third are less common than fractures of the mandible. The middle third extends backwards to the frontal bone above and the body of the sphenoid below. It is made up of a number of bones:

(1) two maxillae;

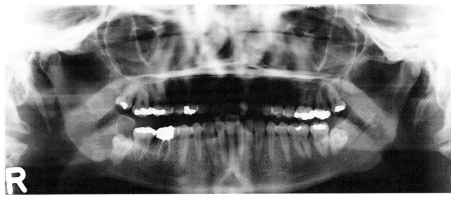

Fig. 4 Orthopantomogram showing a fracture of the right mandibular angle through an unerupted right wisdom tooth following a rugby tackle.

(2) two palatine bones;

(3) two inferior conchae;

(4) the vomer;

(5) the ethmoid and its attached superior and middle conchae;

(6) two nasal bones;

(7) two lacrimal bones;

(8) two zygomatic bones;

(9) two zygomatic processes of the temporal bones;

(10) the pterygoid plates of the sphenoid.

The majority are wafer-thin fragile bones and thus comminute

easily. They also articulate with one another in a complex manner that makes it impossible to fracture one bone on its own without disrupting its neighbours (Plate 7).

Fractures of the middle third are usually closed fractures and therefore are difficult to visualize. In severe facial fractures the facial bones can disintegrate into tens of fragments.

Classification of middle-third fractures

The middle third can be further divided into the right and left lateral block (zygomaticomaxillary) and the central block (nasomaxillary) (Fig. 9).

Fractures of the lateral middle third (zygomatic complex fracture)

The zygomatic bone (malar bone, cheek bone) usually fractures in the proximity of the zygomaticomaxillary, zygomaticotemporal, and zygomaticofrontal sutures involving the related parts of the maxillary, temporal, and frontal bones. Therefore the term 'zygomatic complex fracture' is more appropriate than zygomatic bone fracture. The zygoma, as an entity, is unlikely to fracture by itself except in severe trauma.

The zygomatic bone is usually driven inwards into the maxillary

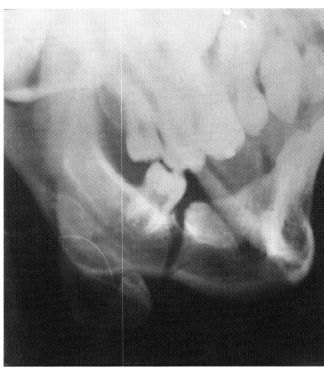

Fig. 5 A lateral oblique radiograph showing a fracture between an unerupted first and second molar.

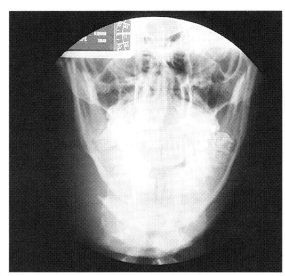

Fig. 6 Posteroanterior film showing a marked displacement of the distal fragment in a fractured mandible.

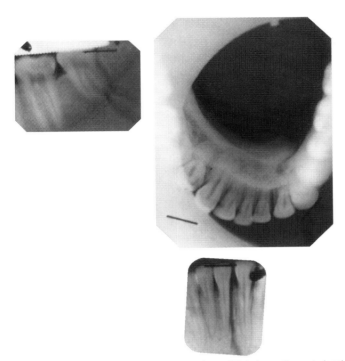

Fig. 7 Intraoral radiographs showing a fractured mandible between the central and lateral incisors as well as the third molar region.

sinus. The depression varies in degree according to the fracturing force. Fractures vary from minimally displaced to severe displacement, giving rise to an unsightly flattening of the cheek prominence, best seen by standing behind and above the patient, immediately after trauma, before it is masked by oedema and swelling (Plate 8). There is usually epistaxis on the fractured side as the maxillary sinus fills with blood (Fig. 10).

Circumorbital ecchymosis develops within a short time of injury. Unlike a black eye, which is patchy, circumorbital ecchymosis is a generalized swelling around the eye with a uniform intensity limited by the orbicularis oculi (Plate 9).

In the zygomatic complex fracture, the subconjunctival ecchymosis (bloodshot eye) occupies the outer quadrant of the eye with no limit to its extension posteriorly (Plate 10). This is demonstrated by asking the patient to look upwards and inwards. Unlike bruising elsewhere in the body, subconjunctival ecchymosis stays bright red in colour until it disappears (4 to 6 weeks) because atmospheric oxygen can pass from the air through the thin conjunctiva to oxygenate the haemoglobin.

If the fracture involves the nearby infraorbital nerve, the patient invariably complains of paresthesia or anaesthesia of the area supplied by this nerve (lower eyelid, lateral side of the nose, the cheek, and the related half of the upper lip). The inward displacement of the zygomatic bone may impinge on the mandibular coronoid process, thus interfering with the lateral movement of the lower jaw.

Temporary diplopia for 1 or 2 days is a common symptom in the early stages of zygomatic fractures and is caused by oedema and effusion in and around the eye. Involvement of the extraocular muscles or their nerve supply in the fracture site results in diplopia. If a fracture occurs in the vicinity of the frontozygomatic suture above the Whitnall's tubercle, the globe of the eye is displaced with

the fractured zygomatic bone (**Plate 11**). Severe fracture of the zygomatic complex involving the floor of the orbit can result in herniation of the orbital fat and contents in the maxillary antrum, giving rise to enophthalmos.

'Blow-out' fracture

A 'blow-out' fracture is a fracture of the orbital floor without the fracture of the orbital rim. It is caused by a sudden rise in intraorbital pressure, such as might occur when a ball or a fist hits the rim of the orbit and forces back the orbital contents without rupturing the globe of the eye. As a result, the very thin orbital floor (approximately 0.5 mm thick) is easily disrupted and its contents are displaced into the maxillary sinus (Figs 11, 12). If excess orbital fat herniates into the maxillary sinus, enophthalmos occurs. Occasionally, extraocular muscles (inferior rectus and inferior oblique) become incarcerated in the fracture line, thus limiting ocular movement, particularly in upward gaze, and giving rise to diplopia. Lacerations and abrasions of the lids as well as circumorbital and subconjunctival ecchymosis can also occur. The presence of blood in the related antrum can give rise to unilateral epistaxis.

About 20 per cent of blow-out fractures occur through the thin orbital plate of the ethmoids. Entrapment of the medial rectus is extremely rare.

Fracture of the zygomatic arch

It is not uncommon for a fracture of the zygomatic arch to occur without any other facial bone fracture. Invariably there is a circular depression (dimple) overlying the fractured zygomatic arch (**Plate 12**). The displaced fracture arch impinges on the coronoid process of the mandible, limiting the lateral mandibular excursion towards the side of the fracture (Figs 13, 14). If the fractured zygomatic arch is part of a more extensive zygomatic complex fracture or facial fracture, the above sign is replaced with the more gross physical signs of facial fractures.

Fractures of the central block

Dentoalveolar fractures

Dentoalveolar fractures present as a marked derangement of occlusion without a demonstrable fracture of the maxilla. The fractured segment is usually loose (**Plate 13**).

If a tooth is knocked out and found clean, then every attempt should be made to push it back into its socket, making sure that its correct position is restored. This is usually painless if it is done immediately following the accident. If the tooth is found dirty (that is to say, soiled), it should be rinsed in cold water or milk before gently pushing it back in place. The tooth is kept in place by gentle pressure, such as biting on a clean handkerchief, before the patient is sent to see his/her dentist as soon as possible.

If the tooth cannot be pushed back into its socket then it should be placed in a small container of milk and both the patient and tooth transfered to the nearest dentist immediately. Avulsed teeth should never be allowed to become dry or washed in disinfectant.

If a tooth is knocked out and cannot be found, then it is mandatory to obtain a chest radiograph to exclude the possibility that it has been accidentally inhaled (Fig. 15).

Le Fort type fractures

Le Fort types of fractures were first described in 1900 by Rene Le Fort in Paris, following experiments on cadavers. Since then, the

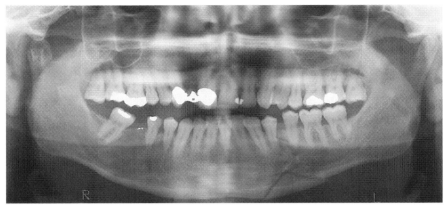

Fig. 8 Orthopantomogram showing a bilateral mandibular fracture (R condyle and L body).

pattern of these fractures has repeatedly been confirmed both clin-ically and radiologically (**Plate 14**). In all the Le Fort type fractures the backward displacement of the tooth-bearing portions leads to positioning of the upper teeth behind the lower incisors gagging on the back molars.

Le Fort type 1 (Guerin or low transverse fracture) Plate 14(a)

This is a horizontal fracture of the tooth-bearing segment of the maxilla. The line of fracture starts from the lower anterolateral edge of the nasal cavity and runs across the canine fossa to the pterygoid maxillary fissure below the zygomatic but-tress, involving the lower third of the pterygoid plates. The fracture line crosses medially above the floor of the nose to meet the lateral fracture line behind the maxillary tuberosity. Apart from the mobil-ity and downward displacement of the tooth-bearing alveolus and palate, there are none of the physical signs usually associated with Le Fort type 2 and type 3 fractures. Occasionally, the fractured seg-ment is not mobile and only a derangement of the occlusion is observed. This usually takes the form of a deviated maxillary mid-line.

Le Fort type 2 (pyramidal fracture) Plate 14(b)

Le Fort type 2 fractures separate the whole of the central block of the middle third of the face from its cranial support. The line of fracture com-mences in the inferior half of the nasal bones down on both sides across the frontal process of the maxillae, it then crosses the lacrimal bones above the nasolacrimal duct, downwards and forwards lat-erally crossing the inferior orbital margin in the region of the zygo-maticomaxillary suture by the intraorbital foramen, often involving the nerve. It then crosses the anterior wall of the maxillary antrum beneath the zygomatic buttress crossing the pterygoid–maxillary fissure and involving the pterygoid plates.

Le Fort type 3 (high transverse fracture) Plate 14(c)

This fracture separates the entire bony facial structure from the base of the skull, and occurs when a blow of great severity crashes the face backwards, involving the zygomatic bone and the nasoeth-moidal buttress. The fracture line passes through the nasofrontal suture separating the nasal bones and the frontal processes of the maxilla from the frontal bones. It then extends across the superior half of the lacrimal bone into the orbital plate of the ethmoid and continues backwards to the optic foramen. The strong ring of com-pact bone around the optic foramen deflects the line downwards to the posterior part of the inferior orbital fissure where the fracture

line bifurcates. One limb continues backwards over the upper part of the maxilla in the sphenopalatine fossa to reach the upper limit of the pterygomaxillary fissure to the pterygoid plates, causing them to fracture from the spheroid bone. The other limb of the bifurcation follows another line of weakness from the anterior part of the infer-ior orbital fissure to the lateral wall of the orbit, crossing the fronto-zygomatic suture to meet the outer line of fracture on the infratemporal surface of the greater wing of the spheroid. The sep-aration from the bone of the skull is completed by fracturing both zygomatic arches and the nasal septum, which is usually commin-uted in such fractures.

On superficial examination, Le Fort fractures type 2 and 3 appear very similar. These two fractures can only be differentiated clinically after careful examination and palpation of the zygomatic bone, which is not fractured in Le Fort type 2. This should be con-firmed by radiological investigations.

Displacement of the fractured middle third of the face is inde-pendent of the muscles of facial expression, but is determined by the degree of violence and the direction of the blow. Within a few hours of injury, patients with severe middle-third fractures assume a very characteristic appearance with three basic clinical signs.

1. *Bilateral circumorbital and subconjunctival ecchymosis*: this develops rapidly and becomes very pronounced, reaching its peak in 48 h.

2. *Balloon face*: the enriched blood supply to the face in the absence of deep cervical fascia causes the facial oedema to be gross, giving rise to characteristic ballooning of the face.

3. *Lengthening of the face*: the frontal bone and the body of the spheroid bone form an inclined plane which lies at an angle of about 45 degrees to the occlusal plane. In Le Fort fractures the facial skeleton is driven down this inclined plane. As a result of the displacement, the face is pushed in ('dished face'), which is more obvious when the oedema has subsided. The posterior teeth of the maxilla push open the mandible by premature occlusion on the mandibular teeth, causing lengthening of the face (Plate 15).

On examination, patients may complain of being unable to open their mouths, but in point of fact the mouth is already wide open with bilateral gagging of the molar teeth (Fig. 16). Closure can be achieved by elevating the displaced upper jaw forwards and upwards.

The mobility of the central block is confirmed by grasping the upper incisor teeth and/or the anterior part of the maxilla between the index finger and the thumb of one hand and moving it gently to and fro against the middle finger and the thumb of the other hand which is placed firmly on the frontonasal region.

Damage to the infraorbital nerve may lead to paraesthesia of the

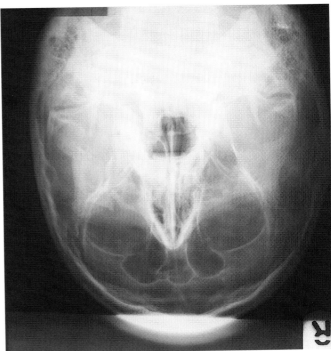

Fig. 10 Occipitomental radiograph showing a fracture of the left zygomatic complex.

cheek, the lateral wall of the nose, the lower eyelid, and the related half of the upper lip. Depending on whether there is neuropraxia or neurotmesis, recovery may take up to 18 months. Comminution of the ethmoid bone may lead to dural tear and cerebrospinal fluid rhinorrhoea (Plate 16).

Herniation of the orbital contents through a comminuted orbital floor can result in enophthalmos. Should the inferior rectus and oblique muscles become entrapped in the comminuted orbital floor, mechanical interference will prevent upward and outward rotation of the eye and cause vertical diplopia. Alteration in the level of the globe of the eye will occur if the fracture passes above the origin or the insertion of the suspensory ligament which passes from the lacrimal bone medially to Whitnall's tubercle situated laterally just below the frontozygomatic suture. As the globe of the eye drops the upper eye lid follows it downwards, giving rise to the physical sign known as 'hooding of the eye'.

A depressed fracture of the zygomatic complex in Le Fort type 3 fractures may impinge on the coronoid process of the mandible and prevent its lateral excursion towards the fractured side.

Nares are invariably blocked with fresh blood and/or dried blood, making breathing through the nose difficult.

Occasionally in severe Le Fort type 2 and 3 fractures with complex nasal injuries, the nasolacrimal duct is involved resulting in epiphora. A severe cleaving blow directed up the centre of the upper jaw can result in a split palate (Plate 17).

Nasal complex fractures

It is uncommon to fracture the nasal bones alone without fracturing the nasal process of the maxilla with disruption and comminution of the nasal septum—hence the expression 'nasal complex'.

A severe nasal complex fracture can involve the cribriform plates, resulting in dural tear and cerebrospinal fluid rhinorrhoea.

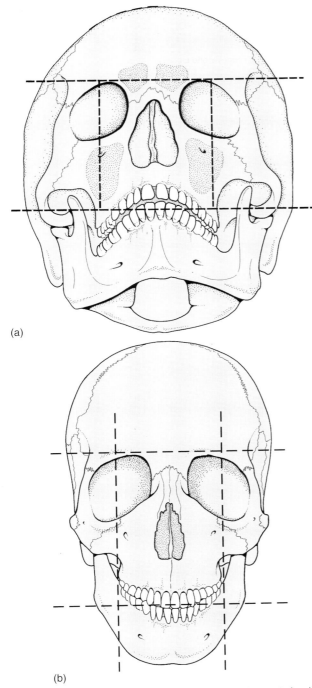

(a)

(b)

Fig. 9 Subdivision of the middle third of the facial skeleton into central and lateral blocks.

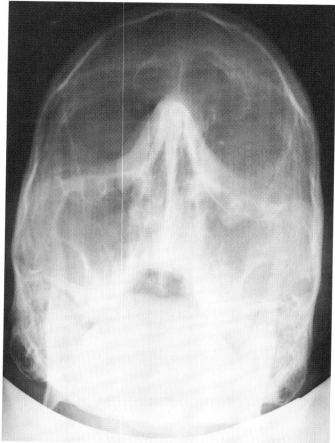

Fig. 11 Occipitomental view showing 'pearl drop' in a 'blow-out' fracture.

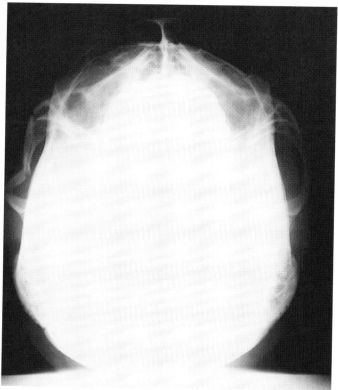

Fig. 13 Submentovertex radiograph showing fracture of the right zygomatic arch of an international soccer goalkeeper after collision with another player.

The displacement of the fractured nasal complex will depend on the direction of the fracturing force. If the fracturing force is applied directly to the bridge of the nose, the nasal complex is pushed in and the maxilla is forced out. If the fracturing force is applied laterally, the nasal complex is displaced to one side (Plate 18). Obvious deformity of the nose makes the diagnosis of such a fracture easy. However, oedema and bruising can mask the deformity. The skin

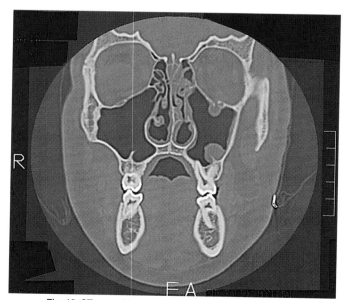

Fig. 12 CT scan of the same patient showing the 'pearl drop'.

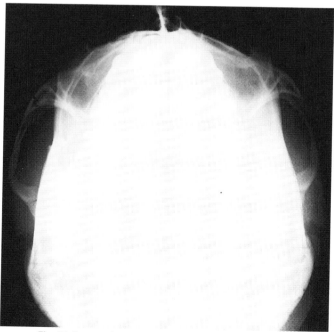

Fig. 14 Same patient as Fig. 13 after reduction of the fracture.

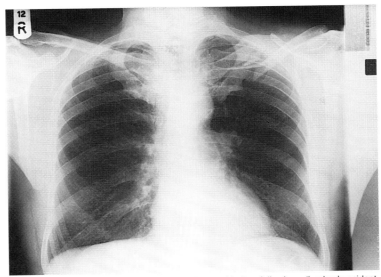

Fig. 15 Chest radiograph showing an inhaled central incisor following a 'hockey' accident.

covering the bridge of the nose is very thin and often splits. Occasionally, fragments of the nasal bones are seen through the split skin. Epistaxis occurs from both nostrils. Bilateral circumorbital and subconjunctival ecchymosis are confined to the medial half of the eye.

Rhinorrhoea

If the fracture of the perpendicular and cribriform plate of the ethmoid bone is associated with dural tears, cerebrospinal fluid will escape through the nostrils. This is difficult to recognize in recently injured patients because of the presence of epistaxis, blood clot(s), and dried blood in the nasal cavities and nares. The discharge of clear serum following the organization of the blood clot or if the patient has been suffering from acute coryza before injury can lead to confusion in diagnosis. However, if there is any doubt about the origin of the secretion from the nostrils following a middle-third

injury it should be considered as cerebrospinal fluid rhinorrhoea and treated accordingly.

Occasionally, and if the nostrils are blocked, leaking cerebrospinal fluid escapes down the throat to the posterior third of the tongue. In this case, a conscious patient may complain of a salty taste. Appropriate antibiotic therapy, which can cross the blood–brain barrier in therapeutically effective concentrations, should be administered either orally or parenterally to safeguard against meningitis. This therapy should be continued for at least 2 days after the cerebrospinal fluid leakage has ceased.

Naso-orbital deformity (telecanthus)

Severe displacement of the frontal process of the maxilla, which carries with it the insertion of the medial canthal ligament, produces telecanthus by widening of the nasal bridge.

Radiological investigations

Four radiographs are needed to diagnose middle-third fractures (Fig. 17).

10-Degree occipitomental projection

This view gives an indication of the amount of downward displacement of the facial bones. In this view the X-ray tube is angled to the feet. Therefore the central ray emerges through the infraorbital margin, displacing the petrous temporal bone downwards and clearing the alveolar segment of the maxilla.

30-Degree occipitomental projection

This view shows the associated backward displacement of the facial bones. In effect, the 10- and 30-degree occipitomental views act on the same principle applied to the radiography of long bones, namely they are taken at right angles to one another.

True lateral skull

In general, this is the most useful of the four views. Fortunately, it is a view which can be accommodated by an unconscious, ill, or uncooperative patient.

Nevertheless, complete and careful radiological diagnosis of the facial fractures can only be determined after careful examination of all four projections.

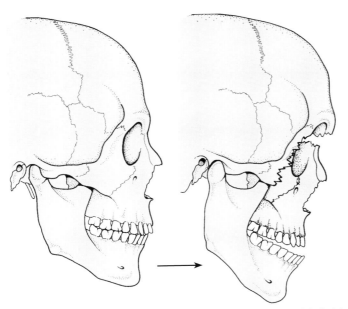

Fig. 16 The downward and backward displacement of the middle third of the facial skeleton forces the lower jaw to gag open.

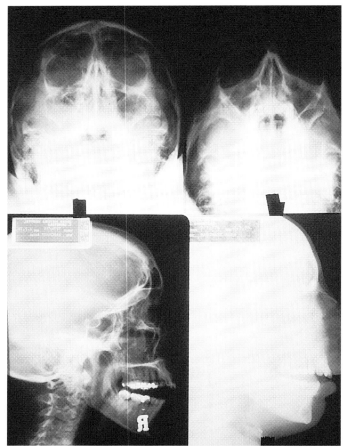

Fig. 17 The four standard radiographs for the diagnosis of facial fractures.

depends on a knowledge of the fracture patterns that may occur. An overall assessment of the four projections from a distance is important before a closer study is made of the finer aspects of the facial bones, since a discrepancy between the size and shape of the orbits, antral, etc., or an open anterior bite from a displacement of either jaw will be immediately noticeable from a distance.

The occipitomental projections are viewed first, and their interpretation should be based on the five curvilinear lines (Campbell lines) (Fig. 19). The first line curves from one frontozygomatic suture on one side along the supraorbital ridges to the opposite side. The second line follows the curve of one zygomatic arch and the infraorbital margin of one side across the nasal bones to the zygomatic complex of the other side. The third line curves through the condylar neck, the coronoid process, and the lateral and medial walls of the antrum to the opposite side. The fourth line follows the line of occlusion from one side to the other, and the fifth line follows the lower border of the lower jaw from one angle to the opposite.

Facial fractures will show on radiographs as a disturbance of the continuity along one or more of the Campbell lines.

In addition to the standard projections, it is often useful to rely on additional views.

1. *Orbital tomography*: to confirm 'blow-out' fractures.

2. *Submentovertical*: an extremely useful view to confirm zygomatic arch fractures.

3. Intraoral radiographs:

   (a) periapical film to show the condition of teeth in the line of fracture;

   (b) occlusal film to investigate a fractured palate.

Computed tomography and MRI

CT scans and MRI are able to show considerable detail of the soft tissue relating to bone and air spaces in a remarkable anatomical display which is unmatched by any other non-invasive technique.

The true lateral projection can show a fracture of the inner and/or outer plate of the frontal sinus in conjunction with a fracture of the nasal bones. Severe injuries in this region might also show a fracture of the orbital roof and cribriform plates and fractures of the anterior cranial fossa. The true lateral view also shows widening of the frontozygomatic suture in high transverse facial fractures (Le Fort type 3) and backward and downward displacement of the central block in Le Fort types 1, 2, and 3.

Whenever the central block or the zygomatic bone is fractured, the posterior walls of the antral cavity are disrupted. Disruption of the dense line of the floor of the nose is an indication of fracture of the hard palate.

The presence of the low transverse fracture (Le Fort type I) can be checked at the anterior nasal aperture. If the lateral view is projected in the supine position, fluid levels in the antral cavity can be seen as well as disruption of the pterygoid plates.

Soft-tissue lateral projection

From this lateral view, fractures of the nasal bones and spine are clearly visible. Foreign bodies (for example, broken teeth, road grit, etc.) in the soft tissues of the face, particularly the lips, can also be seen (Fig. 18).

System of interpretation

Except for a fractured zygomatic arch, complete fracture lines are not seen in facial trauma. Radiological diagnosis of facial trauma

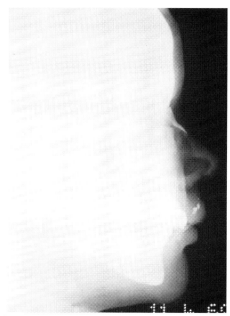

Fig. 18 Soft-tissue lateral projection showing a part of a tooth in the upper lip.

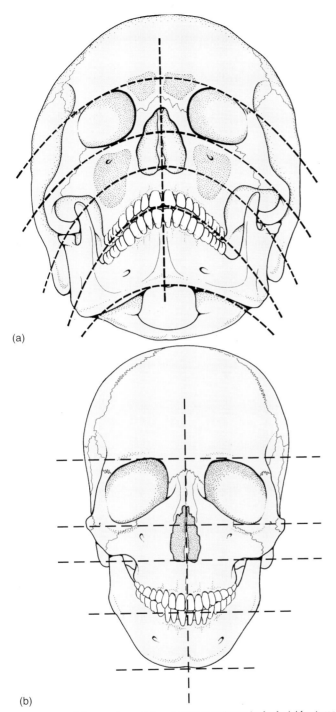

(a)

(b)

Fig. 19 Campbell lines system of interpretation of radiographs for facial fractures.

Therefore their use in maxillofacial injury, particularly in extensive fractures in the region of the midface and orbits, is invaluable.

Management of facial fractures

Facial fractures are never a life-threatening injury unless they interfere with the patency of the airway or are bleeding profusely. The immediate treatment should be directed to the patient's general medical welfare with a thorough physical examination.

Priorities in treatment

Urgent treatment

Airway

Injuries to the middle third of the face can be a source of upper-airway embarrassment, particularly if the middle third is impacted backwards and downwards, and the soft palate is in contact with the posterior third of the tongue and/or the posterior pharyngeal wall. In such cases, two fingers are inserted behind the soft palate into the posterior nasal apertures and the whole of the middle third is forcibly pulled forwards and upwards. The oral cavity should be examined for dentures (broken or whole) together with avulsed loose or broken teeth. It is important to clear the oral cavity of blood and other foreign bodies.

Constant supervision is necessary to confirm that the nasopharyngeal airway is patent. This is done by frequent aspiration. Occasionally, it is necessary to pass an endotracheal tube to secure the patient's airway. The assurance of the airway by intubation is directly related to its patency. Thus regular suction of the lower third of the tube and beyond is of vital importance to secure patency of the lumen against occlusion by blood clots and mucosa. Conscious patients should be nursed in a sitting position with the head forward, provided that there is no medical contraindication to this position, to allow any secretion to dribble out of the mouth. Unconscious patients are better nursed on their side so that blood and saliva can drain from the mouth.

The indications for tracheostomy are fewer since the introduction of soft, flexible plastic tubes which cause less irritation to the trachea and which can be left *in situ* for days. However, tracheostomy should be considered if the middle third of the facial skeleton is impacted and cannot be reduced forward manually or in cases of uncontrollable postnatal haemorrhage or severe oedema of the glottis.

Bleeding

Severe bleeding is often internal. Therefore exploration may be urgently required. However, persistence of profuse nasal or oropharyngeal bleeding may be a sign of damage to one of the large vessels associated with fractures of the base of the skull or to the anterior and posterior ethmoid vessels. The insertion of a postnasal pack containing a haemostatic agent or Surgitek (Reuter Epitek) is very effective in these cases. The advantage of the latter is that drainage as well as aspiration is possible (Plate 19).

Intracranial bleeding

Close monitoring of patients using, for example, The Glasgow Coma Scale is important to detect any deterioration in cerebral function. CT or MRI scanning may also confirm intracranial bleeding. Extradural bleeding requires urgent decompression.

Treatment needed promptly

This category includes serious injuries which need prompt attention, perhaps by multidisciplinary specialties. Examples are open fractures, chest injuries such as a pneumothorax and/or abdominal trauma, and extensive muscle wounds.

Non-urgent treatment

Maxillofacial injuries come under this category. However, it must be emphasized that fractures of the facial skeleton must be diagnosed and treated as soon as the patient's condition permits. If untreated for 3 weeks they are virtually uncorrectable. At best, cosmetic man-oeuvres to camouflage the initial injury can be utilized. Further-more, there may well be a functional disability in biting or vision (diplopia) or difficulty in breathing or lacrimation (epiphora).

Fractures of the upper third

Fractures and clinical manifestations of the upper third are beyond the scope of this chapter. However, depressed and compound fractures of the frontal bone are serious injuries which require special management and treatment.

Further reading

Le Forte R. Étude experimentale sur les fractures de la machoine super-ieure. *Revue de Chirurgie* 1900–1; **23**: 208.

Chapman PJ. The prevelance of the orofacial injuries and the use of mouthguards in rugby union. *Australian Dental Journal* 1985; **30**: 346.

Chapman PJ. Mouthguards and the role of sporting team dentists. *Australian Dental Journal* 1989; **34**: 36–43.

McGregor JC. Soft tissue facial injuries in sport (excluding the eye). *Journal of the Royal College of Surgeons of Edinburgh* 1994 (April); **39**: 76–82.

McGregor JC. Is sport good for us? A personal view on sporting injuries and how to manage them. *Journal of the Royal College of Surgeons of Edinburgh* 1995 (December); **40**: 359–62.

Kujala UO, Taimela S, Antti-Poika I, Orava A, Tuominen R, Myllynen P. Acute injuries in soccer, ice hockey, volleyball, basketball, judo and karate: analysis of National Registry data. *British Medical Journal* 1995; **311**: 1465.

7.4 Cardiopulmonary and abdominal emergencies in sports medicine

Michael F. Murphy

Introduction

The ill or injured athlete is no stranger to emergency departments. Competitive and recreational athletes comprise a substantial proportion of an emergency department's annual census. The vast majority of these are recreational athletes with a minor orthopaedic injury that prevents participation for a brief period to allow recovery. Less commonly, the condition poses a permanent threat to future athletic participation. It is exceedingly uncommon for such conditions to constitute a true emergency threatening the life or limb of the athlete, which is the focus of this chapter.

There is a necessity to undertake a complete evaluation. Health care providers involved in the care of the athlete must have an appreciation of the settings, patterns, and specific injuries likely to be encountered in each sport in order to focus the evaluation and management of the injured athlete. The limitations of the setting in which the provider is operating may impose restrictions on that provider's ability to investigate and intervene, though in many cases careful planning has the potential to mitigate this limitation. This is a particular concern of sports medicine providers involved in planning sports venues.

Scope of the problem

The incidence of cardiopulmonary and abdominal emergencies in sports medicine is related to the underlying health of the athlete, the inherent risks of the activity, and the intensity of the exertion.

Jokl, in his exhaustive review 'Sudden death of athletes', presents the historical perspective.[1] The general impression that exercise had the potential to produce primary cardiac pathology and death persisted into this century. It is now known that the majority of cases of sudden cardiac death and myocardial infarction occur in individuals with underlying cardiac disease, such as hypertrophic cardiomyopathy, rheumatic heart disease, and ischaemic heart disease. The roles of performance- enhancing medications and blunt trauma to the chest in causing sudden death of the athlete are becoming clarified. Diabetes mellitus, asthma, sickle cell anaemia, and infectious mononucleosis are known to predispose the athlete to acute emergencies.

Many sporting endeavours exposing the participant to high energy impact are inherently risky. Motorized vehicular events, augmented speed sports (skiing, snowboarding, sledding, cycling, skating, etc.), and activities such as hang-gliding and skydiving have the capacity to expose participants to substantial risk of injury. Contact sports are associated with a limited though real incidence of substantial cardiothoracic and abdominal morbidity, even in sports where impact potential is low such as baseball, soccer, and basketball.[2]

The risk of acute illness and injury in spectators may also be a concern of the sports medicine provider from both a planning and management perspective. Spirited partisan enthusiasm has been known to produce substantial injuries and care of these victims may be the responsibility of the sports medicine provider.

One would expect the intensity of exertion and zeal to stand alone as contributors to the risk of significant illness or injury. This variable fails scrutiny in comparing elite, competitive athletes with recreational athletes. The competitive athlete is an individual who participates in an organized team or individual sport in which regular competition is a component, a high priority is placed on excellence and achievement, and vigorous systematic training is required.[3] The recreational athlete is more focused on personal well being and enjoyment. The presence and severity of underlying disease and the inherent risks of the activity remain the substantive independent risk factors.

Overview of evaluation and management

The sophistication of the evaluation and management of the acutely ill or injured athlete is dependent upon three factors: (i) the training and skills of the provider, (ii) the equipment and supplies available, and (iii) the degree to which support services and personnel are available, i.e. the venue of the evaluation.

Field

The field delivery of medical care is usually categorized as first aid, basic life support, or advanced life support, though the distinctions may be blurred as one moves from one level of sophistication to the next. The first aid provider delivers just that—first aid. The provider has a basic knowledge of anatomy, physiology, and pathophysiology, and has some familiarity with medical terminology. The emphasis is on splinting, bandaging, haemorrhage control, the prevention of further injury, and preparation for transport. Some first aiders are capable of performing cardiopulmonary resuscitation. These individuals constitute the backbone of field medical support units for mass gatherings such as sporting events. Typically, they are committed volunteers who see their role as purely supportive of a more definitive system of medical care delivery.

Basic life support is the minimum level of qualification for ambulance personnel in much of the developed world. These health care providers ordinarily have been trained in basic and advanced first aid, supplemented with some anatomy, physiology, and pathophysiology. They are minimally literate in medical terminology, though to a utilitarian degree. Principles of safe extrication, splinting, haemorrhage control, and transport are well developed. Basic life support providers reliably monitor vital signs and perform cardiopulmonary resuscitation as necessary. They should be able to identify an athlete with a potentially life- or limb-threatening condition, which distinguishes them from the first aider. It is this ability that allows the basic life support provider some latitude in determining how quickly the victim must be moved to more definitive levels of care. The basic life support provider does not perform tasks normally carried out by a physician, such as endotracheal intubation, defibrillation, and intravenous therapy.

Advanced life support personnel deliver sophisticated care and may, in some systems, be physicians. These individuals have a firm grasp of anatomy, physiology, pathophysiology, relevant pharmacology, and medical terminology. What sets them apart is their ability to perform life-saving skills ('medical acts') that have traditionally been the domain of physicians. These skills generally fall into three categories: (i) advanced airway management (endotracheal intubation), (ii) direct current cardioversion and defibrillation, and (iii) intravenous drug and fluid therapy. Thus, they have the ability to deliver substantial supportive, and in some cases definitive, therapy.

The skills of the provider will generally determine the equipment and supply needs. In most cases the providers will carry the necessary equipment with them. The sports medicine health care provider must ensure that the personnel, equipment, and supplies available at the scene match the potential case mix.

Principles of field management

The field management of sports-related injuries generally focuses on the prevention of further injury and the comfort of the athlete. The care provided in this setting is not medically sophisticated and there is no particular necessity for speed. Cardiopulmonary and abdominal emergencies distinguish themselves owing to their potential for a lethal outcome.

At the first aid/basic life support level, medical care is not complex and the emphasis is on basic care and rapid transport to definitive therapy. However, as advanced life support providers and physicians become involved, the potential exists to deliver very complex care in the field. Consequently, delivery of the athlete to a health care facility may be delayed. Thus 'complexity of care' and 'speed' become competing priorities. The resolution of this dilemma rests in understanding the distinction between supportive and definitive care. Advanced life support providers deliver definitive care for many 'medical' emergencies such as cardiac arrest, acute respiratory failure, and hypoglycaemia. Time spent at the scene is justified to deliver such care and achieve an optimum outcome. However, the definitive care of the trauma victim occurs in a hospital, and often in an operating theatre. For this reason, only essential supportive care such as cervical spine immobilization and definitive airway management should precede expeditious transport of the athlete with cardiothoracic or abdominal trauma to an appropriate emergency facility.

Emergency department

The principles of management of the athlete with a cardiopulmonary or abdominal emergency are no different from those for any other patient. Knowledge of the patterns of illness or injury associated with various athletic endeavours are essential in planning a diagnostic and therapeutic course. As in the field, it is important to understand the distinction between supportive and definitive care. This is particularly true of the injured athlete where resuscitation and diagnosis occur simultaneously, while emergency physicians and surgeons determine the most appropriate course of action.

Medical emergencies

Pulmonary emergencies

Exercise-induced asthma (exercise-induced bronchospasm), pulmonary embolism (thromboembolism and air embolism), and spontaneous pneumothorax constitute the most common life-threatening emergencies in this category

Exercise-induced asthma is discussed in detail elsewhere in the text (see Chapter 3.2). However, it constitutes an important life-threatening entity and should be mentioned here. Asthma is defined as the presence of intermittent wheezing, chest tightness, and cough, together with bronchial hyperresponsiveness.[4] Pathologically, most people with asthma have infiltrates of immunocompetent cells, particularly eosinophils, neutrophils, lymphocytes, and mast cells in the bronchial mucosa, and inflammation is a prominent feature of the disease. Certain triggers cause the release of preformed substances from these inflammatory cells leading to bronchospasm. In the case of exercise-induced asthma, it is believed that exercise, hyperventilation, and dry air cause mucosal drying and cooling leading to changes in osmolarity and release of mediators. Topical and systemic steroids, sodium chromoglycate, and β_2-agonists are useful in the mitigation of exercise-induced asthma.

Despite advances in our understanding of the disease and its management, the death rate from asthma continues to remain at disturbingly high levels. Fatal or near fatal asthma has been associated with profound emotional upsets, thermal inversions, the use of β-blockers, and the ingestion of acetylsalicylic acid or non-steroidal anti-inflammatory drugs in sensitive patients. Thus far, exercise alone has not been implicated.[5] The vast majority of deaths are preventable and result form a failure of the physician, the patient, or both to recognize the seriousness of the episode.[6]

Standard management of an athlete with exercise-induced asthma should include inhaled steroids, sodium chromoglycate, and β_2-agonists as prophylaxis, as indicated. The mainstay of therapy for an acute attack is inhaled β_2-agonists. Failure of a moderate to severe attack to respond promptly to such measures should motivate urgent referral to an emergency department.

Pulmonary thromboembolism in otherwise healthy individuals is not common. It is decidedly rare in young and vigorous athletes.

However, the syndrome of pulmonary thromboembolism as a complication of 'effort thrombosis' of the upper or lower extremity is well described in athletes.[7] The death rate from untreated pulmonary thromboembolism is in the range of 20 to 30 per cent. If diagnosed and treated appropriately, the mortality is less than 10 per cent. The diagnosis of pulmonary thromboembolism is frequently elusive, in large part because of the vagaries of its presentation. Pleuritic chest pain, dyspnoea, cough, haemoptysis, or syncope may be present. Tachypnoea and tachycardia are often, but not invariably, present. Hypoxaemia is usually present on arterial blood gas measurement. However, the key to the diagnosis of pulmonary thromboembolism is vigilance and a high index of suspicion, particularly in an athlete with acute or subacute pulmonary symptoms.

Air embolism, in the context of sports medicine, is isolated to recreational scuba diving. The cause of air embolism in scuba divers has been attributed to barotrauma from overdistension of the alveoli and pulmonary venous vasculature, with subsequent air embolization induced by the negative intrathoracic pressures which occur during inspiration after surfacing.[8] Predisposing factors include uncontrolled ascent, breath-holding on ascent, lung cysts or blebs, or obstructive pulmonary disease. Once air has entered the pulmonary venous system, cardiac and distal arterial air embolization becomes a possibility. The usual presentations include focal neurological deficits, seizures, coma, and cardiac arrest at or near the time of surfacing. Definitive therapy is recompression in a hyperbaric oxygen chamber. However, in the interim the diver should be given 100 per cent oxygen and maintained head down in the left lateral position unless cardiopulmonary resuscitation is underway. This position is believed to trap the air in the apex of the left ventricle and prevent the buoyant bubbles from travelling to the brain.

A spontaneous pneumothorax, heralded by the relatively sudden onset of pleuritic chest pain and dyspnoea but not associated with trauma, is uncomfortable but usually no cause for alarm. However, if the collection of air comes under tension as additional air is forced out of the parenchymal defect into the pleural space during expiration, mediastinal shift and impedance to venous return produce a life-threatening situation. The picture is one of air hunger, shock, distended neck veins, and decreased air entry on the affected side. Tracheal deviation away from the affected side is an inconsistent sign. The immediate management is by needle thoracostomy in the second intercostal space in the mid-clavicular line. Patients with small, asymptomatic, spontaneous pneumothoraces may be followed as outpatients, provided that compliance with postdischarge instructions can be assured. Alternatively, patients may be fitted with small calibre chest tubes attached to one-way flutter valves (Heimlich valve[R]) and managed as outpatients. Patients with large or persistent pneumothoraces, or significant symptoms, require tube thoracostomy and hospital admission.

Cardiovascular emergencies

Sudden collapse and death in the athlete is a rare event, but when it does occur the predominant causes are cardiac in nature. More rarely, it is related to an intracranial catastrophe or a disorder of temperature regulation.[1] The definition of sudden death is not straightforward. The World Health Organization defines sudden death as that occurring within 24 h of the onset of illness or injury.[9]

The American Heart Association has adopted a modified definition that accounts for the majority of deaths due to cardiac disease excluding vascular causes.[10] 'Arrhythmic death' is the abrupt loss of consciousness and disappearance of pulse without prior collapse of the circulation. 'Death due to myocardial failure' is the gradual circulatory failure and collapse of the circulation before disappearance of the pulse. Time frames are not defined, nor do they appear to be relevant. For the most part, athletes who die suddenly have underlying cardiovascular disease with myocardial ischaemia as the proximate event manifesting itself as a malignant ventricular arrhythmia with collapse.[11] These cardiac arrest rhythms are ventricular fibrillation, pulseless ventricular tachycardia, ventricular asystole, and electromechanical dissociation. Cardiac arrest occurs during or immediately after exertion, and is often unheralded by premonitory symptoms. Athletes who die suddenly at less than 35 years of age usually have some form of congenital heart disease. Acquired disorders predominate in those aged over 35.

Sudden death at less than 35 years of age

These athletes are predominantly male, 1 to 18 years of age, and involved in interscholastic sports.[3] The underlying cardiac disorders include hypertrophic cardiomyopathy, idiopathic concentric left ventricular hypertrophy, and congenital anomalies of the coronary arteries. Mitral valve prolapse, myocarditis, aortic valvular stenosis, sarcoidosis, cardiac conduction system abnormalities, coronary artery disease, and aortic rupture due to 'cystic medial necrosis' (e.g. Marfan's syndrome) are rare causes of sudden death in the young athlete and are mentioned only for completeness.

In most cases hypertrophic cardiomyopathy, also known as asymmetric septal hypertrophy or idiopathic hypertrophic subaortic stenosis, is a genetically transmitted disorder following an autosomal dominant pattern with a high degree of penetrance. Pathologically, the left ventricle is markedly hypertrophied, particularly in the ventricular septum. Increased numbers of abnormal intramural coronary arteries with thickened walls and narrowed lumens are present.[3] Functionally, obstruction to left-ventricular ejection may occur and is potentiated by a reduction in left-ventricular end-diastolic volume or increased myocardial contractility (e.g. exercise). Dyspnoea, angina, presyncope, and syncope are the most common presenting symptoms, when they exist. Unfortunately, sudden death is a frequent presentation of this disorder in the athlete. The probable sequence of events is obstruction to ejection, leading to ischaemia and a malignant ventricular arrhythmia. Sudden death in a young athlete should prompt echocardiographic evaluation of first-degree relatives at a minimum.

Some investigators have found severe concentric left-ventricular hypertrophy in young athletes who die suddenly.[3] It is not characterized by genetic transmission or asymmetric left ventricular hypertrophy and may be related to severe systemic hypertension in the athlete.

Congenital abnormalities of the coronary arteries have been incriminated as the cause of sudden death in young athletes. Abnormal origin of the vessel or functional obstruction of flow are believed to lead to myocardial ischaemia and cardiac arrest.

Idiopathic mitral valve prolapse is a very common cardiac valvular disorder with a prevalence of about 5 per cent in the general population. Most (66 per cent) are female and the vast majority are asymptomatic. Although exceedingly rare, the most feared complication of mitral valve prolapse is sudden death. Available data would suggest that it is reasonable to limit athletic endeavours in patients with mitral valve prolapse with a history of syncope, disabling chest pain, complex ventricular arrhythmias (particularly if induced or worsened by exercise), significant mitral regurgitation, prolonged QT interval on the ECG, Marfan's syndrome, or a family history of sudden death.[12] The American Heart Association and the American College of Cardiology have published recommendations regarding recreational and occupational activity levels for young patients with heart disease to aid physicians in counselling.[13,]

Sudden death at more than 35 years of age

Increasing numbers of competitive recreational athletes are aged over 35. As is the case with younger athletes, these athletes may have underlying cardiovascular disease. However, the condition is more often 'known' and 'acquired' in this population, than 'occult' and 'congenital' as is the case with younger athletes. Up to 50 per cent of sudden deaths in this age group, during or immediately after physical activity and occur in persons with known or symptomatic cardiovascular disease.[15] The vast majority of deaths are due to coronary artery disease with severe atherosclerotic narrowing of one or more coronary arteries.

Substance abuse

Perhaps the most disturbing contribution to the incidence of sudden death among athletes is the growing usage of performance-enhancing medications by athletes. Predictably, the most dangerous medications are those 'stimulants' which appear to improve performance and stamina, with cocaine achieving notoriety. All stimulant-type medications, including amphetamines, phenylpropanolamines, ephedrine and its derivatives, and cocaine have the potential to cause large increases in heart rate and blood pressure with lethal outcomes. It is clear that a lethal outcome is not necessarily related to dose, route of administration, or the presence of underlying cardiovascular disease, although a correlation exists.

Traumatic emergencies

Much of the focus of sports medicine is on the care of the injured athlete. By far the most common injuries are those to the musculoskeletal system, particularly the extremities. However, the most lethal are those to the central nervous system (including spinal cord), the chest, and the abdomen. Although serious cardiopulmonary and abdominal trauma can occur in all sports, the risk of serious injury is directly proportional to the potential for high energy impact and its amount. Motorized vehicular events, augmented speed sports, and contact sports are most commonly implicated.

Death from trauma has a trimodal distribution.[16] The first peak is within seconds to minutes and is associated with such severe injury that salvage is only rarely possible even in the most sophisticated systems of emergency medical services. The second peak occurs from minutes to hours after the injury and may be significantly blunted by applying the fundamental principles of trauma care. The third peak occurs from days to weeks after the initial injury and is usually related to sepsis and multiorgan failure.[16]

Even in the emergency department of a high-volume trauma centre, injuries that are immediately life threatening are not common. The keys to the detection of life-threatening injuries and optimum outcome are index of suspicion, the recognition of important but sometimes subtle symptoms and signs, and the ability to access definitive care in a timely fashion. A prioritized approach that is rapid and comprehensive, emphasizing simultaneous evaluation and management of the injured athlete, is essential. Initially, the life threats, the settings where they are likely to occur, and their presentation will be analysed. Later, an organized and consistent approach to the injured athlete will be presented.

Cardiopulmonary trauma

Although blunt or penetrating trauma to the airway and chest would be expected to be hazards of virtually any athletic endeavour, there is scant literature on the topic. What is available relates only to blunt trauma and, in particular, blunt trauma to the heart owing to its lethal nature. The American College of Surgeons in their Advanced Trauma Life Support Course categorized airway and chest injuries into 'immediately' and 'potentially' life-threatening categories.[16]

The immediate life threats are those that produce acute cardiopulmonary failure leading to cellular hypoxia and death, and include airway obstruction, tension pneumothorax, open pneumothorax, massive haemothorax, flail chest, and cardiac tamponade. Potentially life-threatening injuries include cardiac concussion (commotio cordis), myocardial contusion, pulmonary contusion, aortic disruption, traumatic diaphragmatic hernia, tracheobronchial disruption, and oesophageal disruption.

Airway obstruction

Airway obstruction is the major life-threatening consideration in any patient presenting with neck or maxillofacial trauma. Since gunshot and stab wounds are decidedly uncommon in the athlete, the mechanism of injury will virtually always be blunt trauma. Motorized vehicular sports may produce dramatic maxillofacial or neck injuries in the setting of multiple trauma, with the potential to overlook subtle but important laryngeal signs. Projectiles such as hockey pucks, lacrosse balls, and baseballs have produced potentially life-threatening blunt laryngeal trauma. Any contact or racket sport possesses the potential to inflict serious neck injury. Regardless of how benign these injuries may appear, the potential for rapid deterioration to total airway obstruction and death must be appreciated. The threat to airway integrity with oral and maxillofacial injuries is usually evident, and is secondary to the pooling of blood and saliva in the hypopharynx, massive oedema, or foreign bodies such as teeth or dentures. Blunt neck trauma may be much more insidious. The classic presentation of impending upper airway obstruction has the patient seated, leaning forward, drooling saliva, and stridorous. It is important to realize that the athlete who is simply 'a little hoarse' after blunt neck trauma may also rapidly deteriorate. This hoarseness may be a subtle sign of serious laryngeal injury or oedema. These athletes must be expeditiously transported to a facility where a full assessment of airway integrity, including radiography and laryngoscopy, can be performed. In the unlikely event that the sports medicine caregiver is faced with a penetrating neck injury, it is axiomatic that the wound should not be probed with fingers or instruments, in case a situation that is not life threatening is manufactured into one that is. Formal evaluation in a setting where definitive care can be rendered is imperative in such situations.

Tension pneumothorax

Tension pneumothorax is an uncommon clinical condition most often encountered in the setting of a patient who is being manually or mechanically ventilated, particularly if high pressures are required to achieve adequate ventilation. Blunt chest trauma is ordinarily the aetiology in the context of sports medicine. Athletes with a past history of pneumothorax or those with underlying obstructive pulmonary disorders, such as asthma, may be at increased risk, particularly following a blow to the chest. Sports that create a setting for multiple trauma (motorized vehicular events and augmented speed sports) are also implicated. The condition develops when the visceral pleura is disrupted, allowing air to escape into the pleural space. If this air leak acts as a one-way valve with additional air entering the pleural space with each expiration (but unable to escape from the pleural space), the pressure in the pleural cavity eventually rises and compresses mediastinal structures and the opposite lung. Mediastinal compression leads to inadequate cardiac filling and shock. The loss of lung volume in the ipsilateral lung and the compression of the opposite lung lead to acute respiratory failure with hypoxaemia and hypercapnia. Tension pneumothorax is a clinical, not a radiological, diagnosis and immediate decompression is mandated.[16] The classic clinical findings include marked respiratory distress, decreased breath sounds on the affected side, tracheal deviation to the opposite side, distended neck veins, and shock. The patient who is alert with a single system injury is easily identifiable and likely to fit this mould. In the author's experience, the classic presentation is more difficult to appreciate in the setting of multiple trauma when it is necessary to work through the diagnostic possibilities for the patient with moderate to severe respiratory distress, shock, and distended neck veins (or a central venous pressure that is normal or elevated if such a line is in place). In the setting of blunt chest trauma these possibilities include tension pneumothorax, cardiac tamponade, and myocardial contusion. The diagnosis is made when the chest is vented and produces a gush of air, and the vital signs improve. Definitive therapy is tube thoracostomy with a chest tube (36 french or larger).

Open pneumothorax

Open pneumothorax is caused by a penetrating or avulsing type of injury, and has not been mentioned in the sports medicine literature to date. The priorities include consideration of additional injuries, particularly to lung, heart, and vascular structures, and the management of the pleural space. Particular hazards relate to the development of a tension pneumothorax, blood loss, or a 'sucking chest wound'. A sucking chest wound is typified by air preferentially entering the pleural cavity through the chest wall defect rather than entering the lung via the trachea during inspiration. Management involves covering the wound with an occlusive dressing. A one-way valve that allows the escape of pleural space air can be fashioned by leaving one side of an occlusive dressing unsecured. A tension pneumothorax can thus be avoided. Definitive management will range from tube thoracostomy and routine wound care to formal surgical closure, depending on the characteristics and behaviour of the wound.

Massive haemothorax is defined as the loss of more than 1500 ml

of blood into the pleural space. The disorder is exceeding uncommon, and in civilian emergency practice is almost always the result of penetrating chest trauma. Its presentation in sports medicine is in the athlete with severe blunt chest trauma. The rate and volume of blood loss are variable and depend upon the size of the injured vessel and the pressure within it. Tube thoracostomy and volume resuscitation constitute definitive therapy unless ongoing blood loss exceeds 200 ml/h, at which time thoracotomy may be indicated.

Flail chest

Flail chest should be considered not just as a chest-wall disorder secondary to multiple contiguous rib fractures, but as a syndrome of segmental chest-wall instability combined with visceral thoracic injury of varying severity. The syndrome should be considered in any athlete sustaining significant blunt trauma. Flail chest is produced by a blunt force sufficient to fracture three or more adjacent ribs, each at two points. The flail segment may be on either side of the thorax or may be central if it involves the sternum. If the disorder is unilateral, the lung is often injured, leading to hypoxia of varying degrees depending on the severity of the pulmonary contusion underlying the flail segment. Paradoxical motion of the unstable chest-wall segment with inspiration and expiration contributes to this hypoxia. The flail segment is often not visualized acutely because of the time course of compliance changes related to the lung injury. Chest wall palpation, radiographic findings, and hypoxia on arterial blood gas determination, point to the correct diagnosis. Supplemental oxygen is the initial step in management, and may culminate in endotracheal intubation and mechanical ventilation if respiratory failure progresses. The patient with a central flail segment may have sustained significant trauma to the underlying mediastinal structures at the time of the injury, most commonly myocardial contusion which will be discussed in more detail below.

Cardiac tamponade

Cardiac tamponade most commonly results from penetrating trauma and must be exceedingly rare in recreational or competitive athletics, although the scenario can be imagined. The pericardial sac is a rigid fibrous structure that encases the heart. The introduction of even small amounts of blood, other fluids, or air into this sac compresses the heart and limits its ability to fill with blood. The result is a reduction of cardiac output and, potentially, shock. The classic presentation is known as Beck's triad and consists of hypotension, elevated venous pressure, and muffled heart sounds. The key to diagnosis is index of suspicion. Initial resuscitation consists of intravenous fluids. Pericardiocentesis is indicated if these measures fail to produce haemodynamic stability. The author uses a large (e.g. 16 gauge) intravenous catheter over needle arrangement and leaves the plastic cannula in the pericardial space to provide continuous drainage.

In the setting of trauma, the patient who presents with shock and a normal or elevated venous pressure is suffering from one of three disorders: tension pneumothorax, cardiac tamponade, or myocardial contusion. If deterioration is rapid, in addition to providing supplemental oxygen and intravenous fluids, the clinician should initially needle both sides of the chest to detect and manage a tension pneumothorax. If this manoeuvre fails to produce a diagnosis, the next step is to attempt a periocardiocentesis.

Cardiac contusion

Potentially life-threatening disorders include myocardial contusion, pulmonary contusion, aortic disruption, traumatic diaphragmatic hernia, tracheobronchial disruption, and oesophageal disruption. Presentation is usually insidious rather than dramatic, although if overlooked these disorders produce an increase in mortality. With the exception of myocardial contusion, none are specifically mentioned in the sports medicine literature. However, the potential exists for any of these disorders to occur in the traumatized athlete and thus they deserve mention.

The ability of blunt, seemingly innocuous cardiac trauma to result in dysrhythmias and dysfunction must be appreciated. Sudden death has been reported in young athletes who have received blows to the chest. Some chest injuries, such as those resulting from a ball (thrown or hit), a lacrosse ball or hockey puck, or a punch during a boxing match, are seemingly trivial in degree.[17,18] Other reported causes include falling with considerable force on an object such as a football and delivering a blow to the chest.[19] Blunt myocardial injury can be divided into three entities: cardiac concussion (commotio cordis), myocardial contusion, and cardiac rupture.

Cardiac concussion is not associated with morphological evidence of injury, and cardiac enzymes are not elevated on serum testing. While the precise mechanism of cardiac arrest in commotio cordis has not been determined, it is likely that lethal arrhythmias such as ventricular fibrillation result from the blow to the chest. Myocardial contusions, however, while difficult to diagnose, are associated with morphological cell damage. Cardiac enzymes may be elevated, the ECG may be abnormal (sinus tachycardia, non-specific ST-segment and T-wave changes, and disturbances of conduction and rhythm), and echocardiography typically demonstrates segmental wall motion abnormalities. Lethal cardiac arrhythmias may result. Large contusions with significant cardiac dysfunction may lead to shock and must be differentiated from other causes of non-hypovolaemic shock in the setting of trauma, such as tension pneumothorax and cardiac tamponade.

Cardiac rupture in the setting of blunt trauma is a uniformly lethal condition. However, penetrating cardiac injury may be potentially survivable, but only in the most efficient emergency medical service delivery systems.

Pulmonary contusion

A pulmonary contusion is characterized by intrapulmonary haemorrhage and oedema. Gas exchange is compromised, and the damaged area of lung becomes stiff and non-compliant. Hypoxaemia and hypercapnia result. It may take some time for these changes to develop fully, necessitating a high index of suspicion and ongoing monitoring of the injured athlete. In fact, initial arterial blood gases and chest radiography may be normal. The association of pulmonary contusion with flail chest is described above.

Ninety per cent of those who sustain a traumatic aortic injury die at the scene of the accident. The mechanism of injury is rapid deceleration, such as a skier hitting a tree or falls from height as may occur in many sports. Of those who survive to reach hospital, 50 per cent will die if the injury is unrecognized or unrepaired.[16] Aortic rupture most commonly occurs where the ligamentum arteriosum attaches to the distal arch. Less commonly, it occurs at the aortic root or where the aorta pierces the diaphragm. The diagnosis rests on a high index of suspicion combined with radiological findings.

Symptoms and signs are non-specific and vague. Chest or back pain, dyspnoea, hoarseness, and dysphagia may be present. A difference in blood pressure between arms, or between the arms and the legs, as well as a systolic murmur or bruit may be noted. A supine anteroposterior chest radiograph taken as a matter of routine in all cases of significant trauma may reveal any of the following: superior mediastinal width exceeding 8 cm, distortion or blurring of the aortic outline, presence of a left pleural cap, elevation of the right and depression of the left mainstem bronchi, fractures of the first or second ribs, obliteration of the clear space between the pulmonary artery and the aorta, or deviation of a nasogastric tube to the right.[20] The gold standard for diagnosis remains aortography, and it should be performed if rupture is suspected. Computed tomography (**CT**), although useful for screening, is not definitive and may lull the physician into a false sense of security. Definitive therapy is surgical.

Trauma to the diaphragm, tracheobronchial tree, and oesophagus must be exceedingly rare in athletes. Even if they occur, their times frames and modes of presentation make their diagnosis and management a matter of concern for emergency physicians and surgeons rather than sports medicine personnel.

Abdominal trauma

Much more has been published in relation to abdominal trauma in the athlete than on cardiopulmonary trauma. It has been reported that 10 per cent of abdominal injuries are sports related.[21] Motorized vehicular events, augmented speed sports, and team contact sports have produced the majority of these injuries. As with cardiopulmonary injuries, penetrating trauma is rare and the vast majority of cases are the result of blunt trauma.[22] Solid and hollow abdominal and pelvic viscera, major vessels, and retroperitoneal structures have sustained substantial injuries in athletic endeavours.[23] Sledging, competitive and recreational skiing, and contact sports such as North American football and rugby predominate in the literature as settings for this type of trauma.[24-33]

The evaluation and management of an athlete with abdominal trauma is particularly challenging. Even in the face of life-threatening intra-abdominal injury, symptoms and signs may be absent or subtle. Up to 20 per cent of patients with blood in the peritoneal cavity will have a benign abdominal examination when first examined in the emergency department. Such patients often have a head injury or other painful injury that overshadows or masks the abdominal findings. The importance of a high index of suspicion in patients with abdominal trauma cannot be overemphasized. The aim of the initial assessment of patients with serious abdominal trauma is to determine that an intra-abdominal injury exists and that operative intervention is required, not to diagnose the injury acurately to a specific organ.[16] Once it is determined that immediate surgery is not required, more time-consuming and specific diagnostic manoeuvres can be undertaken to pin-point specific organ injuries.

Blunt and penetrating trauma produce much different patterns of injury. Penetrating trauma tends to be rather easier to identify in that there is outward evidence of abdominal injury, i.e. the entry or exit wound. In general terms, the injury tends to be limited to the abdominal cavity, although this is not always the case, and the organs injured tend to lie in the path of the penetrating object. Any gunshot wound violating the peritoneum, and the vast majority do, requires operative exploration because of the frequency of significant intra-abdominal injury. Peritoneal violation is more difficult to document in stab wounds unless the patient exhibits signs of peritoneal irritation or blood loss with haemodynamic instability, and operation is indicated. In most cases this is not present and the wound is explored under local anaesthesia. If the wound track is clearly entirely extraperitoneal, no further evaluation is necessary. However, if the exploration is equivocal or demonstrates peritoneal violation, a diagnostic peritoneal lavage is indicated. Some centres utilize CT scanning or ultrasound instead of peritoneal lavage at this stage, particularly in children.[34,35] The probability of organ injury can often be determined by these procedures and a decision made as to the necessity for an operation.

While penetrating trauma does not discriminate between hollow and solid viscera, blunt trauma has a decided predilection to affect solid organs such as the spleen, liver, kidney, and pancreas.[35] Direct blows coupled with shear forces related to sudden deceleration are the probable mechanisms. Hollow viscus injury is believed to occur when a sudden increase in intraluminal pressure leads to rupture. Ruptures of the large and small bowel, the gall bladder, and the urinary bladder due to sports-related trauma have all been reported.[28,35,36,37]

The appropriate evaluation and management of abdominal trauma depends on a clear understanding of the anatomy involved and the patterns of injury as discussed above. The abdomen has several distinct regions: the peritoneal cavity, the retroperitoneum, and the pelvis. The peritoneal cavity is divided into intrathoracic and abdominal compartments. At the limit of expiration the intrathoracic abdomen extends from the fourth intercostal space to the inferior costal margin. Thus the rib cage affords an element of protection for the liver, spleen, stomach, and transverse colon if blunt force is applied. However, it is important to recognize that penetrating chest trauma below the fourth intercostal space (nipple level anteriorly, inferior tip of scapula posteriorly) may violate the diaphragm and produce intra-abdominal injury. These diaphragmatic injuries heal poorly and produce an opportunity for internal herniation of the gut into the chest. Subsequent strangulation of the herniated gut is not infrequently fatal, emphasizing the importance of diagnosing and repairing such injuries at the time that they present. CT scanning and diagnostic peritoneal lavage are manoeuvres employed to establish the diagnosis; the latter is more sensitive in the author's experience. The retroperitoneum contains the great vessels, the pancreas, the kidneys and ureters, and portions of the duodenum and colon. The pelvis houses the rectum, the urinary bladder, the major pelvic vessels and, in the female, the internal genitalia.

Approach to an athlete with an actual or potential life threat

The evaluation and resuscitation of the critically ill or injured athlete is strongly dependent on the ability of the provider to undertake both tasks simultaneously. The ultimate outcome will rely on the ability to undertake a rapid and prioritized assessment, intervene as appropriate, and make key decisions as necessary. The knowledge base and skills of the provider, the equipment and supplies available, the presence of qualified help, and the setting of the resuscitation are powerful determinants of the outcome. Preplanning has the effect of favourably influencing some or all of these. The standardized approach developed by the American Heart Association for Advanced Cardiac Life Support (ACLS) and the Committee on Trauma of the American College of Surgeons for Advanced Trauma Life Support (ATLS) provides an excellent preparation for such providers.[10,16] The principle of simultaneous prioritized evaluation and treatment are equally applicable to trauma and non-trauma situations.

The initial phase of the evaluation which addresses the immediate priorities of airway, breathing, and circulation (**ABCs**) is known as the primary survey and is common to both types of emergencies. Trauma and non-trauma strategies tend to diverge at this point. Life-threatening non-perfusing cardiac arrest rhythms make up the majority of the non-trauma emergencies and lend themselves well to early definitive electrical and pharmacological interventions. Successful resuscitation is followed by post-resuscitation management.

For the traumatized athlete the primary survey identifies the immediate life threats, dictates definitive airway management, and initiates haemodynamic support as needed. The primary survey then blends imperceptibly into the resuscitation phase where the issues of haemorrhage control, shock management, and respiratory support continue to be addressed. The secondary survey, or head-to-toe evaluation, is then undertaken to determine potential threats to life or limb and subsequent investigative and therapeutic initiatives. This final phase addresses the indications for, and urgency of, operative and non-operative care, as well as stabilization of the patient in preparation for transfer to a facility able to provide more sophisticated care if required.

Primary survey

The primary survey is a rapid evaluation designed to detect and attempt to reverse immediate life threats. The ABCs are the focus, and at each step of the evaluation the provider employs the 'look, listen, and feel' format. Life-saving interventions are performed as the need is determined. On approaching the ill or injured athlete the provider immediately surveys the scene for hazards, and if safe proceeds to the victim's head. While ascertaining the circumstances of the event, the provider observes the victim and gently places a hand on either side of the head to maintain cervical spine alignment and provide reassurance. Depending on the setting and expertise of available personnel, two large-bore intravenous infusions should be initiated, 100 per cent oxygen applied, and the patient placed on a monitor and undressed. While listening to available history, verbalization by the patient is noted and if not spontaneous, solicited. If the patient is able to speak, airway and breathing are sufficient to render immediate intervention unnecessary. If the patient does not speak, the chest is observed for respiratory effort and a hand is placed near the mouth and nose to feel for air movement. One listens for a stridorous or obstructive quality to the breathing. A decision is then made as to the adequacy of the airway.

Management of the airway is coupled with a consideration of the likelihood of cervical spine instability because airway manoeuvres may also cause cervical spine movement. In most cases the decision as to whether precautions are necessary is clearly evident. However, when in doubt one should err on the side of caution and maintain cervical spine immobility. The cervical spine moves in six directions: flexion and extension, right and left lateral flexion, and right and left rotation. A variety of immobilizing devices are commercially available but offer little advantage over simply taping the forehead to either side of the backboard or stretcher, and in the case of the non-cooperative patient, having an attendant apply manual immobilization.

An inadequate airway requires immediate intervention. Ideally, such intervention would follow an adequate cross-table lateral radiograph of the cervical spine, although this is not always possible. The airway may just require simple opening manoeuvres such as a head tilt or jaw thrust, coupled with upper airway suctioning. In the patient with a potential cervical spine injury the jaw thrust manoeuvre is modified. With a hand stabilizing each side of the head, the index fingers of both hands elevate the angles of the mandible while cervical spine alignment is maintained. Simple airway manoeuvres may be augmented or replaced by the use of nasopharyngeal or oropharyngeal airways. The former are much better tolerated by patients with active airway protective reflexes such as an intact gag reflex.

Failure to secure an adequate airway or demonstrate effective breathing leads to the institution of manual ventilation and preparation for endotracheal intubation. Manual ventilation may be in the form of mouth to mouth, mouth to mask, or bag and mask. The route of endotracheal intubation will depend on patient condition and operator skill. When cervical spine stability is not a concern, traditional direct laryngoscopy and orotracheal intubation is the norm. If cervical spine integrity is in question, 'in line' stabilization (not traction) of the head–neck unit with orotracheal intubation is performed. Blind nasal intubation may be attempted unless significant mid-facial trauma provides the potential for the tube to be passes intracranially. In this case cricothyroidostomy or percutaneous transtracheal jet ventilation should be considered. Orotracheal intubation aided by a light wand is a superior technique that produces little spine movement and may be an acceptable alternative in skilled hands.

No discussion of endotracheal intubation is complete without reference to the principles of 'rapid sequence intubation'. The aims of this technique are rapid airway control, maintenance of oxygenation, airway protection, and attenuation of adverse cardiovascular and intracranial pressure responses to intubation. The complete algorithm can be seen in Table 1. The skill set and knowledge base of the operator and the clinical scenario affect the application of the components of the algorithm. For some patients the entire sequence is appropriate, while for others none of it may be (e.g. cardiopulmonary arrest).

Once airway patency has been established or ensured, adequacy of breathing must be evaluated following the 'look, listen, and feel' approach. If the patient is apnoeic, manual ventilation must be instituted as described above. Three traumatic conditions should be considered at this point: tension pneumothorax, open pneumothorax, and flail chest.

Circulation is evaluated by assessing the level of consciousness, skin colour, the presence and quality of the pulse, and blood pressure. In the absence of vital signs, cardiopulmonary resuscitation is initiated unless blunt trauma is the proximate event. In such cases, the success rate of even maximal resuscitation is so dismal that

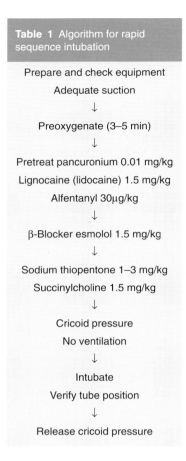

Table 1 Algorithm for rapid sequence intubation

Prepare and check equipment
Adequate suction
↓
Preoxygenate (3–5 min)
↓
Pretreat pancuronium 0.01 mg/kg
Lignocaine (lidocaine) 1.5 mg/kg
Alfentanyl 30μg/kg
↓
β-Blocker esmolol 1.5 mg/kg
↓
Sodium thiopentone 1–3 mg/kg
Succinylcholine 1.5 mg/kg
↓
Cricoid pressure
No ventilation
↓
Intubate
Verify tube position
↓
Release cricoid pressure

measures short of immediate thoracotomy, open-chest cardiac massage, and thoracic aortic cross-clamping are futile.

External haemorrhage should be controlled and obvious fractures splinted during the primary survey. It is important at this juncture to recall the principles of field management mentioned earlier as they apply to the athlete with chest or abdominal trauma. In the field, only essential supportive care such as cervical spine immobilization and definitive airway management should precede expeditious transport to a centre that is capable or providing definitive care.

Advanced cardiac life support

The primary survey in an athlete who suddenly collapses in cardiopulmonary arrest is neither complex nor difficult. It is usually clear that the situation is non-traumatic and primarily neurological or cardiac in nature. Once it is recognized that the athlete is not breathing and has no pulse, cardiopulmonary resuscitation is initiated and help summoned. Ideally, a direct current defibrillator and medications needed for resuscitation will be available at the scene of the event or arrive with first responders (e.g. fire and police) or ambulance personnel.

There are four common cardiac arrest rhythms: ventricular fibrillation, pulseless ventricular tachycardia, asystole, and pulseless electrical activity (formerly electromechanical dissociation). The factors that most affect the chances for successful resuscitation are, in order of importance: rapid defibrillation for ventricular fibrillation or pulseless ventricular tachycardia, early onset and continued

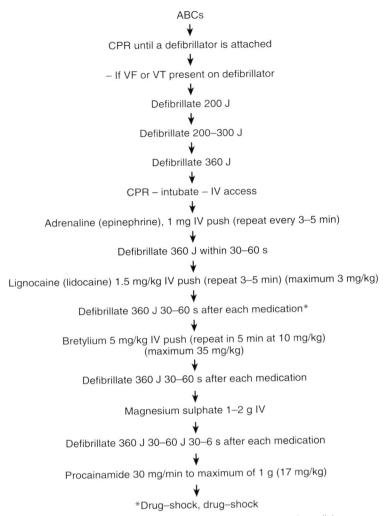

ABCs

CPR until a defibrillator is attached

– If VF or VT present on defibrillator

Defibrillate 200 J

Defibrillate 200–300 J

Defibrillate 360 J

CPR – intubate – IV access

Adrenaline (epinephrine), 1 mg IV push (repeat every 3–5 min)

Defibrillate 360 J within 30–60 s

Lignocaine (lidocaine) 1.5 mg/kg IV push (repeat 3–5 min) (maximum 3 mg/kg)

Defibrillate 360 J 30–60 s after each medication*

Bretylium 5 mg/kg IV push (repeat in 5 min at 10 mg/kg)
(maximum 35 mg/kg)

Defibrillate 360 J 30–60 s after each medication

Magnesium sulphate 1–2 g IV

Defibrillate 360 J 30–60 J 30–6 s after each medication

Procainamide 30 mg/min to maximum of 1 g (17 mg/kg)

*Drug–shock, drug–shock

Fig. 1 Ventricular fibrillation (and pulseless ventricular tachycardia)

effective cardiopulmonary resuscitation, early definitive airway management with endotracheal intubation and 100 per cent oxygen, and adrenaline in adequate dosage to maintain coronary and cerebral blood flow.[10] Figures 1, 2, and 3, which are adapted from the American Heart Association Textbook of Advanced Cardiac Life Support,[10] show the algorithms for the management of the cardiac arrest rhythms. The algorithm for the management of sustained ventricular tachycardia with a pulse is included for completeness (Fig. 4).

The aetiology of the arrest in an athlete is usually related to the presence of underlying heart disease, as discussed earlier. However, aggravating or initiating factors such as dehydration or hypovolaemia, electrolyte abnormalities, acidosis, hypoxaemia, tension pneumothorax, or cardiac tamponade may be present and correctable.[10]

Resuscitation phase

This term applies specifically to the period of time following the primary survey of a traumatized athlete. Interventions initiated during the primary survey are continued during this phase. The spe-

cific actions that occur at this time relate to the management of shock and obtaining essential radiographs.

Shock is initially managed with warmed crystalloid solutions such as Ringer's lactate or normal saline, ideally delivered under pressure to the unstable patient. Hypotonic solutions are not used for resuscitation. These fluids are continued to a limit of 40 ml/kg or about 3 litres in the average adult at which point ongoing shock management involves the use of blood products.

At this time a severely traumatized athlete may have a nasogastric tube inserted to decompress the stomach, if not contraindicated by a mid-face fracture. A urinary catheter may also be inserted unless contraindicated. The patient in shock should also be considered for central venous pressure line insertion and measurement, particularly if there has been blunt trauma to the chest and cardiac tamponade and myocardial contusion are diagnostic possibilities.

Three plain film radiographs are indicated at this time in all blunt trauma cases: a cross-table lateral cervical spine, an anteroposterior chest, and an anteroposterior pelvis film. These are obtained in the resuscitation suite using fixed or portable apparatus. Additional films may be of interest in an athlete sustaining a gunshot

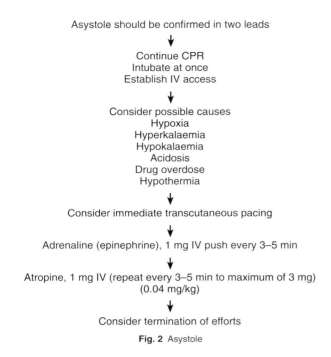

Fig. 2 Asystole

wound to the trunk or head in order to determine the trajectory of the missile and potential organs injured.

Secondary survey

The secondary survey does not begin until immediate life threats have been addressed, resuscitation initiated, and the need for immediate operation dispelled. This evaluation is a head-to-toe survey employing the 'look, listen, and feel' format to determine the extent of injury and the need for definitive care.

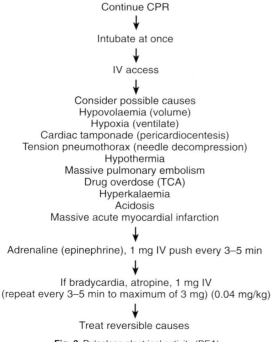

Fig. 3 Pulseless electrical activity (PEA)

Evaluation of the head and neck documents pupil size, reaction, and equality, the presence or absence of blood behind the tympanic membranes, symmetry of neurological function and a Glasgow coma scale score (Table 2). Airway patency is re-evaluated and cervical spine status confirmed radiologically.

The chest is inspected for symmetry of motion, the presence of segmental paradoxical motion, and adequacy of ventilation. Palpation and auscultation confirm bony integrity and symmetry, detect tenderness, and assess equality and adequacy of air entry. Pulse oximetry and arterial blood gases are indicated to confirm adequate oxygenation and ventilation. The chest radiograph should be carefully studied.

The spleen and liver are the most frequently injured intraperitoneal organs. The fragile nature of the spleen makes it particularly susceptible to damage from blunt trauma sustained in all types of sporting events, but particularly contact sports and augmented speed sports such as skiing and cycling. The increased susceptibility of the spleen to rupture in athletes contracting infectious mononucleosis is a matter of some concern. However, a review of the literature suggests that the following recommendations are reasonable: in the absence of marked symptomatic splenomegaly, mild activity may be resumed after the 21st day of illness; non-contact sports may be resumed 1 month after the onset of symptoms; resumption of strenuous contact sports may also begin after 1 month provided that the spleen is neither palpable nor enlarged by abdominal ultrasound examination.[38,39]

The abdominal examination may be difficult and misleading. The aim is to determine whether surgical intervention is required. Close observation and frequent re-evaluation are important principles in the ongoing management of abdominal trauma. An athlete with an altered sensorium is a particular dilemma. Inspection, palpation, auscultation, and rectal examination are integral aspects of the examination. Positive findings are useful and may dictate management. Negative findings are suspect and demand re-evaluation. Rectal examination is of particular importance and should address specific issues: the quality of rectal sphincter tone, the presence or absence of blood, and, in the male, prostate position. Diagnostic peritoneal lavage is a useful adjunct in the evaluation of abdominal trauma and in determining the need for laparotomy. However, it is an operative procedure that significantly alters subsequent abdominal examination. Therefore it should be performed by, or on the direction of, the surgeon who will act on its results.

Physical examination of the pelvis consist of three manoeuvres: compressing the iliac wings, distracting the iliac wings, and applying pressure to the symphysis pubis in an anteroposterior direction. Radiography of the pelvis is essential in ruling out a pelvic fracture.

Injuries to the kidney are relatively common in athletes sustaining blunt trauma to the trunk, particularly the flanks. The hallmark of trauma to the urinary system is haematuria. Dipsticks used to detect blood in the urine actually react to haemoglobin released into the urine by lysed red cells. The reaction is not specific for haemoglobin, as it also gives a positive response to myoglobin. For this reason it is essential to confirm the presence of red cells in a dipstick-positive urine by microscopy. The severity of genitourinary trauma does not correlate with the amount of blood in the urine; thus an intravenous pyelogram, renal scan, or renal flow Doppler ultrasound and a cystogram must be obtained if haematuria is pres-

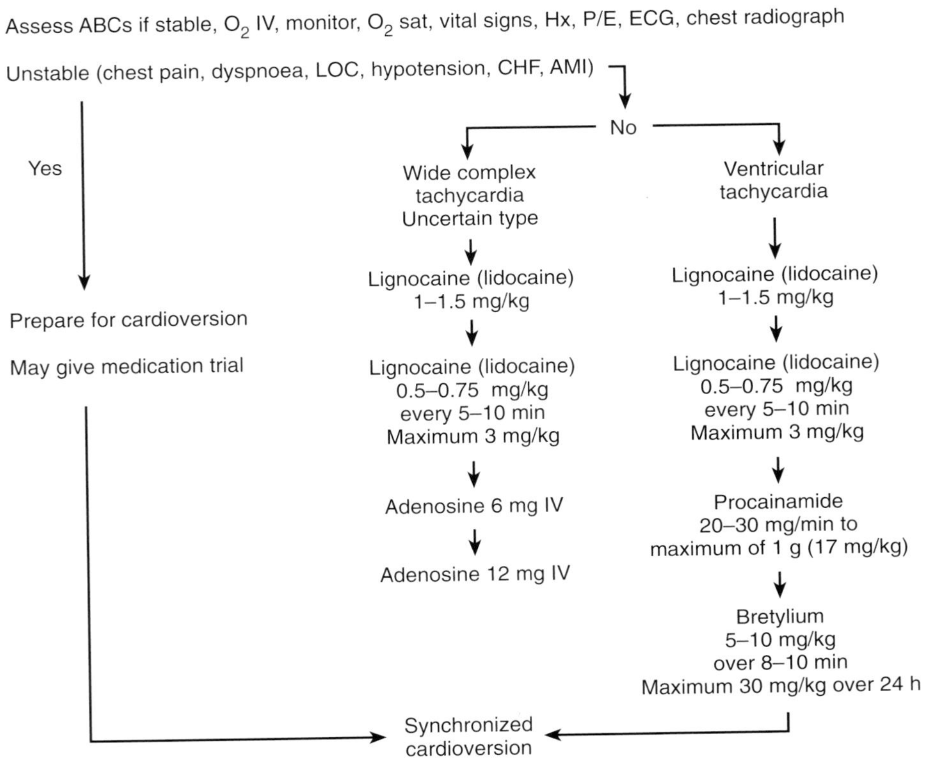

Assess ABCs if stable, O$_2$ IV, monitor, O$_2$ sat, vital signs, Hx, P/E, ECG, chest radiograph

Unstable (chest pain, dyspnoea, LOC, hypotension, CHF, AMI)

No

Yes

Wide complex tachycardia Uncertain type

Ventricular tachycardia

Prepare for cardioversion

May give medication trial

Lignocaine (lidocaine) 1–1.5 mg/kg

Lignocaine (lidocaine) 1–1.5 mg/kg

Lignocaine (lidocaine) 0.5–0.75 mg/kg every 5–10 min Maximum 3 mg/kg

Lignocaine (lidocaine) 0.5–0.75 mg/kg every 5–10 min Maximum 3 mg/kg

Adenosine 6 mg IV

Procainamide 20–30 mg/min to maximum of 1 g (17 mg/kg)

Adenosine 12 mg IV

Bretylium 5–10 mg/kg over 8–10 min Maximum 30 mg/kg over 24 h

Synchronized cardioversion

Fig. 4 Wide complex tachycardia

ent in an athlete who presents with trauma. The issue is clouded by the fact that occult haematuria is commonly detected in athletes after many types of sporting events (e.g. boxing, basketball, football, long-distance running). Of course, the difference is that those who present for evaluation have sustained an injury that is perceived as being out of the ordinary and a full examination is thus indicated.

Fortunately, the majority of patients have renal contusions or minor parenchymal injuries which produce microscopic haematuria, and can be managed as outpatients. A most devastating injury which requires expeditious diagnosis and operative intervention to salvage the kidney is a renal pedicle injury. This injury may reduce or eliminate blood flow to the kidney, leading to organ necrosis if not reversed within 4 to 6 h.

The usual means of obtaining a urine specimen from a trauma victim is via a urethral catheter. Injury to the female urethra is uncommon even in perineal trauma, and the most frequently encountered impediment to bladder catheterization is an inability to gain access to the urethral meatus because of fracture of the pelvis, hip, or femur. The male urethral meatus is not usually very difficult to find, but careful consideration is necessary before inserting a urethral catheter into a traumatized male. Blood at the meatus or a high-riding prostate on rectal examination mandate a urethrogram prior to the procedure. If radiography shows a pelvic fracture, the prostate is normal, and there is no blood at the meatus, a careful attempt at catheterization can be made. If resistance is encountered, the attempt should be abandoned and a urethrogram obtained.

Traumatic pancreatitis has been associated with bicycle handle-bar injuries in children, contact sports such as karate and American football, and non-contact sports including soccer and skiing.[30,40–42] The diagnosis may be overlooked on initial examination as symptoms and signs may be gradual in onset. An index of suspicion for pancreatic injury in cases of blunt upper abdominal trauma produces an earlier diagnosis. Typical symptoms and signs of abdominal pain and tenderness combined with elevated serum amylase establish the diagnosis. Associated injuries such as duodenal haematoma and rupture must be considered. Surgical consultation is

Table 2	Glasgow Coma Scale	
	Reaction	**Score**
Eye opening	Spontaneous	4
	To voice	3
	To pain	2
	None	1
Verbal response	Oriented	5
	Confused	4
	Inappropriate words	3
	Incomprehensible sounds	2
	None	1
Motor response	Obeys command	6
	Localizes pain	5
	Withdraw (pain)	4
	Flexion (pain)	3
	Extension (pain)	2
	None	1

essential for all patients with traumatic pancreatitis owing to the incidence of surgically correctible pancreatic lesions and the development of serious complications such as haemorrhage, pseudocyst formation, and pancreatic abscesses.

The evaluation of the extremities includes the palpation of all bones and joints, with particular attention being paid to the elbows and knees for occult dislocation and relocation. A particular concern in these cases is the integrity of vascular and neurological structures in proximity to the joint. All peripheral pulses are palpated and major peripheral nerves evaluated where possible.

Definitive care

Following the secondary survey an inventory of injuries sustained by the athlete can be compiled and prioritized for management. Fracture stabilization and operative interventions that are required are undertaken in this phase. In addition, stabilization of the patient in preparation for transfer to a more appropriate facility is completed.

Post-resuscitation care

In the immediate post-resuscitation period attention must be focused on several priorities. Oxygenation and ventilation must be maintained effectively by the athlete as long as he or she is able to do so unassisted. Ongoing failure of the victim to recover consciousness and spontaneous respiration despite an adequately perfusing rhythm should alert the provider to the possibility of an intracranial catastrophe or anoxic brain injury. Basic manoeuvres to manage intracranial hypertension should be initiated, including hyperventilation to a $PaCO_2$ of 30–34 mmHg, 15 degrees of head-up tilt, and the maintenance of oxygenation. Hypotension is not uncommon immediately after a rhythm is re-established, and often recovers with time, intravenous fluids, or pressors as required. Hypertension may exist, particularly if resuscitation is prompt and adrenaline was used. This usually settles quickly without specific therapy. Antiarrhythmic agents utilized during the resuscitation are continued as infusions. Whether or not they should be instituted as a prophylactic measure is controversial, but is not the habit of the author.

Malignant dysrhythmias such as ventricular tachycardia with a pulse, multiform premature ventricular contractions (PVCs), and R-on-T PVCs are treated as they arise with the appropriate antiarrhythmic agents.

Summary

Cardiopulmonary and abdominal emergencies of sufficient magnitude to constitute a threat to the life of the athlete are not common. However, the fact that they exist demands that those who care for these athletes have an appreciation of the disorders that may present, the settings in which they occur, and the management required. When the sports medicine health care provider is armed with this knowledge, his or her ability to serve the athletic community is greatly enhanced as is the safety of the individual athlete.

References

1. Jokl E. *Sudden death of athletes*. Springfield: Charles C. Thomas, 1985.
2. Mustalish AC, Quash ET. Sports injuries to the chest and abdo-
men. In: Scott NW, Nisonson B, Nicholas JA, eds. *Principles of sports medicine*. Baltimore: Williams & Wilkins, 1984.
3. Maron BJ, Epstein SE, Roberts WC. Causes of sudden death in competitive athletes. *Journal of the American College of Cardiology* 1986; **7**: 204–14.
4. Woolcock AJ. Asthma. In: Murray J, Nadel JA, eds. *Textbook of respiratory medicine*. Philadelphia: WB Saunders, 1988.
5. Benatar SR. Fatal asthma. *New England Journal of Medicine* 1991; **314**: 423–9.
6. McFadden ER. Fatal and near fatal asthma. Editorial. *New England Journal of Medicine* 1991; **324**: 409–11.
7. Johnson PR, Krafcik J, Green JW. Massive pulmonary embolism in a varsity athlete. *Physician and Sports Medicine* 1984; **12**: 61–3.
8. Cales RH, Humphreys N, Pilmanis HA, Heilig R. Cardiac arrest from gas embolism in scuba diving. *Annals of Emergency Medicine* 1981; **10**: 589–92.
9. World Health Organization. *Manual of the international statistical classification of diseases, injuries and causes of death: based on the recommendations of the 9th Revision Congress, 1975, and adopted by the 29th World Health Assembly*. 1975 Revision. Geneva: World Health Organization, 1977: 40.
10. Lundberg GA, ed. Guidelines for cardiopulmonary resuscitation and emergency cardiac care. Recommendations of the 1992 National Conference; American Heart Association. *Journal of the American Medical Association*, 1992; **268**: 2171–302.
11. Cobb LA, Weaver D. Exercise: a risk for sudden death in patients with coronary heart disease. *Journal of the American College of Cardiology* 1986; **7**: 215–19.
12. Jeresaty RM. Mitral valve prolapse: definition and implications in athletes. *Journal of the American College of Cardiology* 1986; **7**: 231–6.
13. American Heart Association. Recreational and occupational recommendations for young patients with heart disease. A statement for physicians by the Committee on Congenital Heart Defects of the Council on Cardiovascular Disease in the Young. *Circulation* 1986; **74**: 1195A–8A.
14. Maron BJ, Mitchell JH. Revised eligibility recommendations for competitive athletes with cardiovascular abnormalities. *Journal of the American College of Cardiology* 1994; **24**: 848–50.
15. Northcote RJ, Flannigan C, Ballantyne D. Sudden death and vigorous exercise—a study of 60 deaths associated with squash. *British Heart Journal* 1986; **55**: 98–203.
16. *Advanced trauma life support student manual*. Chicago: American College of Surgeons, 1989.
17. Green ED, Simson LR, Kellerman HH, Horowitz RN, Sturner WQ. Cardiac concussion following a softball blow to the chest. *Annals of Emergency Medicine* 1980; **9**: 155–7.
18. Maron BJ, *et al*. Blunt impact to the chest leading to sudden death from cardiac arrest during sporting activities. *New England Journal of Medicine* 1995; **333**: 337–42.
19. Finn WF, Byrum JE. Fatal traumatic heart block as a result of apparently minor trauma. *Annals of Emergency Medicine* 1988; **17**: 59–62.
20. Rosen P, Murphy MF. Thoracic vascular pathologies. *Emergency Medicine Clinics of North America* 1983; **1**: 417–30.
21. Bergqvist D, Hedelin H, Karrlson G. Abdominal trauma during 30 years: analysis of a large case series. *Injury* 1981; **13**: 93–9.
22. Higgins JR, Halpin DM, Kapff PD. Penetrating injury on an artificial ski slope. *Injury* 1987; **18**: 342–43.
23. Diamond DL. Sports related abdominal trauma. *Clinics in Sports Medicine* 1989; **8**: 91–9.
24. Scharplatz D, Thurleman K, Enderlin F. Thoracoabdominal trauma in ski accidents. *Injury* 1978; **10**: 86–91.
25. Matter P, Ziegler WJ, Holzach P. Skiing accidents in the past 15 years. *Journal of Sports Science* 1987; **5**: 319–26.

26. Wright JR, Hixson EG, Rand JJ. Injury patterns in Nordic ski jumpers. A retrospective analysis of injuries occurring at the Intervale Ski Jump Complex from 1980 to 1985. *American Journal of Sports Medicine* 1986; **14**: 393–7.

27. Hedges JR, Greenberg MI. Sledding injuries. *Annals of Emergency Medicine* 1980; **9**: 131–3.

28. Griffith CD, Saunders JH. Cholecystoduodenocolic fistula following abdominal trauma. *British Journal of Surgery* 1982; **69**: 99–100.

29. Pliskin M, D'Angelo M. Atypical downhill skiing injuries. *Journal of Trauma* 1988; **28**: 520–2.

30. Bergqvist D, *et al.* Abdominal injury from sporting activities. *British Journal of Sports Medicine* 1982; **16**: 76–9.

31. Prall JA, Winston KR, Brennan R. Severe snowboarding injuries. *Injury* 1995; **26**: 539–42.

32. Kim PC, *et al.* Tobogganing injuries in children. *Journal of Pediatric Surgery* 1995; **30**: 1135–7.

33. Tan DT, Kim HS, Richmond D. Gastric mucosal lacerations from blunt trauma to the abdomen. *American Journal of Gastroenterology* 1975; **63**: 246–8.

34. Kane NM, *et al.* Pediatric abdominal trauma: evaluation by computed tomography. *Pediatrics* 1988; **82**: 11–5.

35. Foley LC, Teele RL. Ultrasound of epigastric injuries after blunt trauma. *American Journal of Roentgenology* 1979; **132**: 593–8.

36. Kenney P. Abdominal pain in athletes. *Clinics in Sports Medicine* 1987; **6**: 885–904.

37. Grossman JA, *et al.* Equestrian injuries. Results of a prospective study. *Journal of the American Medical Association* 1978; **240**: 1881–2.

38. Maki DG, Reich RM. Infectious mononucleosis in the athlete: prognosis, complications and management. *American Journal of Sports Medicine* 1982; **10**: 162–73.

39. Haines JD. When to resume sports after infectious mononucleosis. How soon is safe. *Postgraduate Medicine* 1987; **81**: 331–3.

40. Mclatchie GR, Davies JE, Culley JH. Injuries in karate—a case for medical control. *Journal of Trauma* 1980; **20**: 956–8.

41. Mclatchie GR. Karate and karate injuries. *British Journal of Sports Medicine* 1981; **15**: 84–6.

42. McLatchie GR. Analysis of karate injuries sustained in 295 contests. *Injury* 1976; **8**: 132–4.

7.5 Spine injuries

David C. Reid and Chris Osinga

Spine trauma, even without neurological injury, presents a challenging clinical situation, and when associated with paralysis is one of the more serious medical problems. The paradox of these injuries occurring in association with sports and recreation lends even more tragic overtones. Spine fractures are encompassed within the classification of catastrophic injury.

The term catastrophic injury is defined as any injury incurred during participation in sport in which there is a permanent severe functional neurological disability (non-fatal) or a transient but not permanent functional neurological disability (serious).[1] An example of a serious catastrophic injury would be a fractured vertebra with no paralysis, while a similar injury with associated partial or complete quadriplegia would be a non-fatal catastrophic injury. Fatalities are the final group of catastrophic injuries and are subdivided into those resulting directly from participation in the skills of sport, or indirect fatality which is caused by a systemic failure as a result of exertion while participating in a sport. In a review of 1081 spine fractures, 134 (12 per cent) had sporting or recreational causes[2] (Table 1). Sports and recreation was the fourth most common cause of sustaining a spine fracture and second only to motor vehicle acci-

dents in producing paralysis (Fig. 1). In many areas, these catastrophic injuries are decreasing in numbers and severity, while in some sports there is considerable concern about the possibility of rising statistics.[1,3-6]

Spine fracture in selected sport
Diving and swimming

World-wide, diving is the sport with the highest frequency of catastrophic injury, accounting for about 25 per cent of the fractures in our series; an alarming 71 per cent of these were associated with neurological deficiencies.[2,5,7] Thus diving injuries account for about 45 per cent of the spine trauma in sports and recreation or about 9.2 per cent of overall spinal cord injuries from all causes. While to some degree the figure correlates with hours of sunshine, private pools, and the prevalence of water sports on lakes and rivers, most series still feature an incidence of diving accidents (Table 2).

The profile of an average diving injury is a cervical fracture, usually between C4 and C6 with an associated complete motor and sensory lesion with a very poor prognosis for functional useful

Table 1 Spine fractures and neurological deficits related to sport

Sport/recreation	Absolute frequency	Percentage	Percentage with neurolocial deficit for particular sport	
			Absolute frequency	Percentage
Diving	34	25	24	71
Snowmobile	16	12	7	44
Equestrian	16	12	4	25
Parachute/skydiving*	14	10	3	21
All-terrain vehicles‡	12	9	4	33
Toboggan	11	8	1	10
Bicycle	4	4	1	25
Rugby	4	4	1	25
Ice hockey	3	2	1	33
Downhill skiing	3	2	1	33
Surfing	3	2	1	33
Football	2	1	0	0
Mountaineering	2	1	1	50
Other†	10	8	4	40
Total	134	100	53	

* Includes hang-gliding and ultralite plane.
‡ Includes motocross racing, dirtbike and all-terrain (3-wheel) vehicles each with 4 cases.
† Includes only 1 case of trampoline injury.

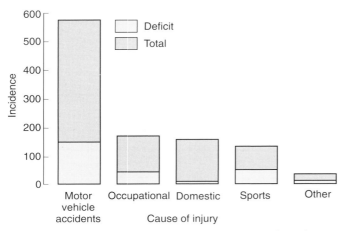

Fig. 1 Sports and recreation are the fourth most common cause of spine fracture, and the second most frequent cause of sustaining associated paralysis.

recovery (Fig. 2). It is this last fact that makes it such a disastrous statistic. Diving off a beach or a pier or into a private pool and striking the bottom is the most common mechanism, invariably secondary to water which is too shallow.

In the recreational setting, alcohol abuse often contributes to poor judgement. In 1994, Kluger *et al.* reported 74 per cent of patients in their series had a measurable blood ethanol level.[9] From this perspective, it is obvious that most of these injuries are preventable and public education programmes will play an important role. A group of neurosurgeons have embarked upon a very aggressive education campaign aimed mainly at teenagers using the slogan 'feet first—first time' and they claim to have reduced the incidence of spinal cord injuries by about 40 per cent. Similar slogans have been adopted in various parts of the world in attempts to reduce this unnecessary statistic.

In a report by Mueller and Cantu,[1] swimming accounts for a second significant number of catastrophic injuries which involved swimmers practising racing starts in the shallow end of the pool. With the current use of a deeper dive for the racing start, it is imperative that, in both practice and competition, racing starts are carried out in the deep end of the pool only. Most pools with a diving tank are of sufficient depth to allow the diver to avoid col-

lision with the bottom. Nevertheless, poor technique from a high dive may result in contact even in adequately designed areas. The water does not slow the diver's speed significantly until at least a depth of 1.5 m (5 feet) has been reached. The force of impact with the water spreads the unskilled diver's arms apart and the head may contact the bottom. Many drownings are due to quadriplegia secondary to the burst on impact. Once again, emphasis on technique is the key to reducing risk.

Bodysurfers are a distinct group of swimmers at risk. Cervical spine injuries have recently been reported in ocean-surfers. When diving into tumbling waves, the body is exposed to powerful forces which may produce an uncontrolled collision of the head with the ocean bottom. Cheng *et al.* reported a series of predominantly older men, especially those with previously narrowed spinal canals, who sustained cervical spine injuries and cord damage.[10] Scher reported on three patients, who were older and had evidence of osteoarthrosis, who experienced central cord syndrome secondary to bodysurfing accidents.[10] Education of the public against this risk would be the cornerstone of prevention.

Rugby football

Rugby spine trauma parallels the popularity of the sport in different countries. Thus in British Columbia, Sovio *et al.*[12] reviewed 390 spine fractures and found only nine due to rugby. However, figures reported in the United Kingdom, New Zealand, and Australia are sufficiently high to raise considerable concern.[13-19] Frequently, these injuries are severe enough to cause either death or complete quadriplegia. There is a suggestion that the incidence is increasing. The vulnerable age for a rugby player is between 15 and 21, and the injuries are often related to aggressive and dangerous play, particularly in the scrums. Hyperextension of the neck can occur with charging in when the scrum is engaged or flexion compression injuries may occur with collapse of the scrum.[20] For this reason new rules have been introduced to 'de-power' the scrums, such as the 'crouch, touch and engage' method, as well as attempts to control rucks and mauls. These rules are gradually being adopted for international competition. The rule changes include keeping the head

Site	Reference	Total cases (all causes)	Percentage due to	
			Sport	Diving
United States	6	318	5.0	2.2
Norway	9	725	8.2	4.4
England	10	619	6.9	5.3
Austria	11	112	10.7	8.0
Australia-(Victoria)	12	325	12.6	8.3
Alberta	13	262	21.0	9.2
Ontario	7	358	15.4	10.6
Australia (Brisbane)	14	207	17.9	14.0

Table 2 Diving as a cause of traumatic spinal cord injury*

* Taken for other sports from Tator and Palm[7] and Kurtzke.[8]

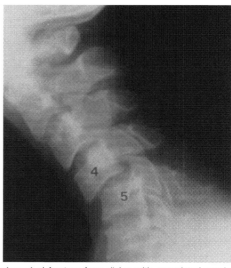

Fig. 2 Typical cervical fracture from diving with associated paralysis and poor prognosis for recovery.

and shoulders above the level of the hips, no charging, and penalties for collapsing, popping, or wheeling the scrum. The importance of these rule changes cannot be overemphasized since rugby is probably a major cause of sport-related spine trauma worldwide.[13,18] In the club system, when a substitute is required for a regular member of the scrum, care should be taken to ensure that the individual has sufficient experience and neck musculature, and is relatively strength-matched, if unnecessary risk is to be avoided. Relatively older and more experienced players are better able to maintain the integrity of the scrum. Further, players who are unfamiliar with playing with each other are more likely to unsettle the scrum and lead to dangerous scrum collapses.[20] Furthermore, there are now safer techniques that can be used in 'locking' the scrum, so that there is less chance of injury during inadvertent collapse.

American football

Football has always been associated with a large number of injuries and this is reflected in the catastrophic injury data.[21-29] In 1931, the American Football Coaches Association (**AFCA**) initiated the first annual survey of football fatalities, and in 1977 the National Collegiate Athletic Association (**NCAA**) initiated a national survey of catastrophic football injuries.[1,29] As a result of these projects, important contributions to the safety of the sport have been made. The most noticeable of these were the 1976 rule changes concerning tackling and blocking with the head.[1] They also established safety standards for football helmets and suggested improvements in medical care and coaching techniques.[30] In more current series, the low frequency of football-related catastrophic injuries is encouraging. This is particularly interesting in view of the high frequencies reported in many of the older sources.

The mechanism of injury is usually axial loading with the cervical spine slightly flexed (Fig. 3).[31] This aligns the spine in such a way that a burst type injury is frequently the result of a massive impact. In the past, the fulcrum supplied by a single-bar face-mask (Schneider's hyperflexion injury), as well as the guillotine mechanism of hyperextension with the posterior ridge of the football helmet forming a fulcrum in the upper cervical area have gradually been eliminated by changes in equipment manufacturing and fitting.[24] The number of permanent quadriplegics in our study decreased from 34 in 1976 to 5 in 1984, supporting Murphy's contention[5] that preventive programmes involving rule and equipment changes are effective.

As well as the potential efficacy of preventive programmes involving rules and equipment changes, the importance of cervical muscle strength has been repeatedly emphasized and incorporated more frequently into preseason training and as ongoing conditioning throughout the season. These rule changes and careful training in tackling techniques are particularly important in the younger age group. While neck rolls may protect against cervical plexus root and cord traction injuries to some degree, they offer very little protection against cord damage secondary to fracture and fracture dislocation.

A recent report[32] on late progressive instability of the cervical spine in a high jumper illustrates the potential for an insidious onset of neurological signs, and we should be aware of this with football.[32] Sports which involve repetitive flexion stresses to the cervical spine can cause this problem. Complaints of intermittent peripheral par-

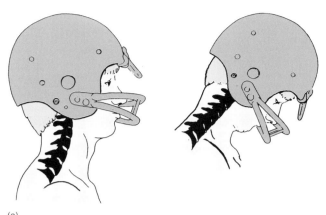

(a)

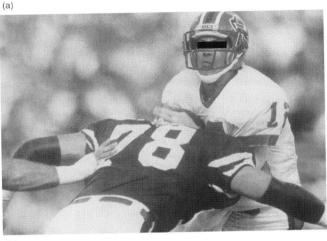

(b)

Fig. 3 (a) The neutral position of the cervical spine is characterized by lordosis. With slight forward flexion the cervical vertebrae are reduced to a vertical column. (b) In tackles during which the head is the first point of contact (spearing), the cervical spine is at risk.

aesthesia, neck pain, and central neurological signs, and the presence of slight anterior subluxation, wedging, or subtle kyphotic angulation at one level should alert the physician to this diagnosis.

Gymnastics and trampolining

Most fatal injuries in gymnastics are the result of head trauma, with males sustaining injury on the high bar, or parallel bars in particular, and females injured whilst performing on the uneven bars.[1,33] Occasionally, spinal injury is the result of a mistimed vault. The use of trampolines, either in association with gymnastics and diving training or as a recreational pursuit, has also resulted in an ever-increasing number of spine injuries, and the high risks with this equipment have been discussed.[22,33,34] A virtual ban on trampolines in the high-school system and better awareness of spotting techniques and safety rules have led to a decreased incidence. However, inasmuch as trampolines are often used in practising very difficult moves in gymnastics and diving, it is important that an ongoing appreciation of the safety precautions must be present. Furthermore, care to ensure adequate supervision, particularly in the younger age groups, and the presence of experienced or well-trained spotters and catchers during practice sessions will eliminate many injuries.

Skydiving

Skydiving accounted for 10 per cent of the injuries in our series and these were all thoracolumbar fractures. Parachuters usually land feet first with the legs together as they absorb the shock with the parachute landing fall. This involves slight flexion of the hips and spine, sudden rotation to the side, and a roll onto the ground. Thus the injury mechanism, theoretically, usually involves flexion and rotation producing either a wedge compression or burst type fracture.[35] Many of the injuries involve a combination of minor equipment malfunction and inexperience. Inasmuch as many programmes require very little training before the first jump is allowed, it is surprising that this figure is as low as the data suggest.

Pole vault

Because of the number of injuries in high-school pole vaulting, the National Federation of State High School Associations passed a rule that, beginning with the 1987 season, all individual units in the pole vault landing area must include a common cover or pad extending over all sections of the pit.[1] This has had the effect of dramatically reducing the number of catastrophic injuries in this sport, and is a special reminder that physicians and therapists in attendance at meetings have a duty to ensure and check the safety of equipment. This, in turn, requires a detailed knowledge of the sport.

Winter sports

Many sports have their main season during the winter months, but the traditional winter sports are those activities requiring ice or snow as a playing surface.[36] Because of the physical characteristics of this frozen water, most winter sports (with notable exceptions) have evolved into high-speed events. Velocity in sports such as skiing, the hard ice surface and the physical contact of hockey, the speed and height of landing in ski-jumping, and the bullet-like, but relatively exposed, projectile in bob-sleigh would lead one to suspect that there would be an unacceptably high incidence of spine trauma. Nevertheless, considering the large number of participants in these pastimes, the relative incidence of spine fracture is low. However, the increasing popularity of the snowmobile as a recreational vehicle has added an alarming dimension to the previously unremarkable statistic.[36,37]

Ice hockey

There has been concern that the incidence of spine fractures in ice hockey is increasing.[38] In 1991 Tator et al.[39] reported on national surveys of Canadian hockey conducted in 1982, 1984, and 1986. Major injuries to the spine were rare in the 1960s and 1970s, but between 1982 and 1986 they occurred at a rate of approximately 15 per year.[39] Indeed, on a *per capita* basis, ice hockey now causes between two and three times as many cases of quadriplegia annually in Canada as does football in the United States.[39-42] There has been much speculation on the reasons for this apparent sudden surge in hockey-related spine trauma, including larger, stronger players, changes in the attitude of coaches and referees, and improved helmets and face-masks leading to a false sense of security. There is a strong concern that full face masks have prompted rough and violent hockey play.[43,44] Although the hockey helmet protects the skull,

Table 3 Factors related to spine injury with skiing
Landing poorly from a jump
Losing control; skiing too fast
Collision with trees, lift-posts, or rocks
Collision with hidden skiers over the crest of a hill
Collision where side-runs join main runs
Collision due to overcrowding of slopes
Novice skiers crossing the slopes in path of fast skiers
Alcohol use
Wearing earphones and being unaware of auditory clues
Poorly groomed slopes; inadequate snow
Inadequately taught or poorly practised ski etiquette

it does not appreciably alter the dynamics of the neck.[45] Inevitably, the mechanism of injury is an axial loading or flexion injury as the individual collides with the boards. Tator et al. found that 73 per cent of injuries occurred in organized games, and that a push or check leading to the head colliding with the boards was the most common mechanism.[39] A new rule has now been implemented in ice hockey forbidding checking from behind into the boards as well as greater enforcement of boarding, cross-checking, and other stick penalties. There also has been a very serious effort to educate people involved in hockey—players, coaches, and referees—about the seriousness of the problem.[46] As with so many hockey injuries, abiding by and enforcing existing rules would make a major impact on the statistics. Further, players can be taught defensive tactics for avoiding spinal injuries and encouraged to perform exercises to strengthen the neck muscles.[39]

Alpine skiing

Spine fractures comprise a small but devastating percentage of skiing injuries. The incidence in alpine (downhill) skiing has ranged from zero to 5.2 per cent in the reported series.[47-50] The number appears to be increasing slowly over the 7 years of our study. In 1992, Myles et al. found that the highest number of injuries occurred in the years with the greatest number of skier days.[51] The most common mechanisms of injury include attempting a jump and landing poorly, and losing control and hitting a tree. (Table 3). The other contributing factors are: (1) collision with stationary or slower skiers who were just over the edge of a slope and therefore invisible until the last minute; (2) novice skiers crossing the slopes in the paths of fast skiers on the main run; (3) overcrowding of the slopes, particularly at the junction of two runs, with fast skiers coming into the same flow pattern as the slow skiers; and (4) collision with the lift supports, rocks, and grooming or snow-making equipment.

These aetiological factors are basically of two varieties. The first is essentially related to poor judgement and this in turn is linked to youth, alcohol, and in many cases poor teaching, lack of awareness of others, poor ski etiquette, or pure selfishness. The second factor is the ski slope design, with too many runs converging and overcrowding of some parts of the slope. Added to this is inadequate policing of the activities of skiers when dangerous mini-jumps have been made or when obvious and inappropriate behaviour has developed on crowded slopes.

The same factors that generate spine injuries also lead to head injury and death. Morrow reported on 22 fatalities among alpine

Table 4 Associated injuries with spine fractures

Degree and site of injury	Snowmobiles	Toboggan	Alpine skiing	Ice hockey	All winter sports
None present	10	7	5	5	27(56%)
Associated injuries	10	4	6	1	21(44%)
Another vertebra	—	2	1	—	3
Thoractic trauma	4	2	2	—	6
Head injury	2	2	—	1	5
Long bone fracture	5	1	2	—	8
Abdominal trauma	3	—	1	—	4
Pelvic trauma	2	—	—	—	2
Facial injury	1	—	1	—	2
Brachial plexus	1	—	1	—	1
Urinary tract	—	—	1	—	1
Knee ligaments	—	—	1	—	1
Total injuries	17	5	10	1	33
Multiple trauma	6	1	3	0	10(21%)

Adapted from ref. 36.

skiers in Vermont from 1979–80 to the 1987–8 ski seasons.[52] However, alpine skiing fatalities do not usually occur in the typical recreational skier but in the highly skilled young adult, capable of skiing at very high speeds. There is an estimated rate of one death per 1.6 million skier days. In addition to the factors cited, Shealy[53] noted that these accidents also resulted from falls on slopes that were rated above the skier's abilities and crashes while racing informally with other skiers, as well as while making practice runs prior to competition. The cause of death is mainly from blunt trauma to the head (82 per cent) and occasionally to the chest and abdomen.

While cervical spine fractures occur frequently, burst fractures of L1, signifying actual loading with or without a flexion component, predominate in most series. When cervical fractures do occur they are usually midcervical.[2,54] They are often associated with head injuries and normally with direct impact to the face or forehead. The skier's position at high speed is usually with the head forward and the shoulders raised, and it is suggested that a helmet with an extended posterior rim design may afford some protection against cervical spine injuries.[55,56]

In our series, the average age was 20.2 years with the youngest being 13 years. This series includes several teenagers but no one over the age of 26 years.[34] Ellison[55] and Margreiter et al.[57] reported 1.8 per cent and 4.7 per cent, respectively, in their series of skiing injuries involving the spine in children and teenagers. Injuries to the spine in young individuals require considerable energy input, but are frequently less severe with a relatively less prolonged morbidity.[58]

Associated injuries are present in about 60 per cent of individuals sustaining a spine fracture, with approximately one-third having a neurological deficit (Table 4). Long bone fractures, thoracic injuries, abdominal injuries, and ligament damage to the knee are frequent concomitant injuries, and point to the need for careful evaluation before moving the injured individual as well as skilled management of the transport down off the ski slopes.[56] There does not appear to be a specific relationship to the time of day or, with the exception of head injuries, to the type of helmet and equipment used. In western Canada a higher incidence of injuries was linked to

areas in 'chinook zones', which is hypothesized to produce more icy conditions through frequent temperature changes.[51]

One of the most important factors for ski patrollers is to understand that, first, spine fracture does not have to be associated with paralysis. Hence, careful assessment is always necessary before moving an individual. Second, spine fractures are often accompanied by at least one other major injury.[58–61] These associated injuries are frequently more obvious. A rapid but diligent assessment of the entire skier is necessary in these cases. Otherwise, dramatic peripheral injuries may lead to overlooking the spine fracture with its potentially disastrous result. Ski patrollers must be trained carefully in the difficult task of transporting the skier with spine fractures and associated multiple trauma.

Freestyle skiing

The acrobatic nature of freestyle skiing and the temptation for unskilled individuals to mimic the dramatic manoeuvres seen in the professional results in the greatest number of spine injuries in freestyle skiing. As the sport gains in popularity, we can expect the incidence of injuries to rise. Thoracolumbar fractures alone account for 8 per cent of all time-lost injuries in some series. This high figure, cited by Dowling,[62] was obtained without the inclusion of inverted aerials (flips). These aerials have caused a number of serious spine fractures and have been banned by the United States Skiing Association. Inverted aerials are still included in World Cup competitions held in Canada and European countries. This event in freestyle skiing is controversial, and careful statistics of injuries, related to the number of exposures, should be monitored. The risk from freestyle skiing may be reduced to some extent by good training programmes that include adequate dry land gymnastic skills and carefully supervised competition with attention to weather conditions, visibility, and snow conditions in the take-off and landing areas.

Ski jumping

Cross-country and alpine skiing are enjoyed by millions of people for recreational purposes. In contrast, ski jumping is almost exclusively a competitive sport with a limited number of performers.[62] These jumpers may perform on average about 400 jumps per year.

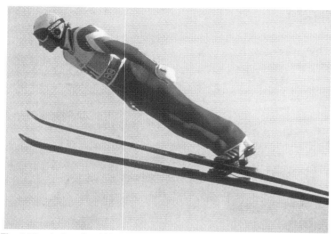

Fig. 4 The design of a ski jump allows landing with minimal impact by maximizing the transition area. This, together with airfoil techniques, has made ski jumping safer.

Special facilities are required for nordic ski jumping (Fig. 4). A skier begins at the top of the in-run, which is a ramp supported by scaffolding or conformed ground. On the in-run, the jumper crouches to minimize wind resistance and hence maximize take-off speed. At the end of the in-run the skier must time the jump perfectly and, almost simultaneously, press the body forward over the skis to make an airfoil and generate lift. This leaning position is maintained for as long as possible (Fig. 4). Towards the end of the flight, the hips are pressed forward, the shoulders are raised, and the trunk is extended into a position perpendicular to the slope of the hill. With a crouched movement, one foot is brought slightly ahead of the other as the ski touches the landing hill. The run is completed by skiing through the transition curve and into the long, flat out-run. This allows deceleration. Two jumps are completed, and points are awarded for style and distance.

To the casual observer the ski jump would appear to be a natural setting for catastrophic injuries. However, because of the skill level of the ski jumper, proper hill maintenance, and good judgement on the part of the officials, spine fracture is rare.[63-68] Indeed, in the 1980 Lake Placid Winter Olympics, over 5000 jumps were made with only two injuries—a mild concussion and a fractured clavicle. At the Intervale ski jump complex, the largest ski jumping complex in North America a 5-year record of ski jumping injuries does not include a cervical spine fracture or dislocation in its statistics. Nevertheless, in sports where take-off speeds of 50 to 56 miles/hour are achieved on 70-m hills and 45 to 55 miles/hour on the 50 to 60-m hills, followed by up to 70 to 90 m in the air, there is always the potential for catastrophic injuries.[67-73]

In Wester's study[65] of a series of ski jumping injuries in Norway, the risk of being seriously injured was approximately 5 per cent in a 5-year period (1977 to 1981) and was higher in the age group 15 to 17 years. The first jump of the day is particularly dangerous, but most of the serious injuries occur in jumps where the jumper has previously experimented. It is possible that the jumper meets unexpected snow conditions on a jump that is felt to be familiar. Other possibilities include the need for a couple of jumps to 'remember' or 'get the feeling of' a particular jump. When spine fractures do occur, they are usually middle to low cervical and are associated with

concussion and paralysis. Only six fatalities occurred during a 50-year period in the USA; four of these were associated with cervical spine injuries, and at least three were in the C1 to C2 area. The overall fatality rate for nordic jumping is estimated at about 12 per 100 000 participants annually, which is within the range for other 'risky' outdoor sports.[69]

Injuries are not common in the age group 12 and under. These youngsters compete on relatively small jumps, with lengths up to 30 to 35 m, which are naturally associated with correspondingly lower speeds. With flexibility of the young spine structures and light body weights, the resultant kinetic energy is low. Ages 15 to 17 seem to present the greatest risk, with poor judgement and attempts at longer jumps than those for which they are physically or technically qualified being the main contributing factor. The need for careful observations and control by coaches, and progression only once sufficient skill has been obtained, are obvious factors in reducing injuries. Despite the fact that many skiers blame personal faults such as rotation of the take-off, too early take-off, and asymmetric ski placement as the main causes of injury, it is frequently poor judgement regarding their own ability that results in problems for the skier. Lack of practice may account for early season problems. Changing snow conditions are more prevalent at both ends of the season. The quality of the in-run, the development of ruts, and the uniformity of packing can all alter the velocity and balance during the critical moments prior to take-off. At the end of the season, or after a heavy snowfall, the landing area can develop gnarls or irregularities, or the snow can allow the skis to sink upon impact with the ground, all of which may disturb balance or cause deceleration. Only careful inspection and grooming of the run will overcome these difficulties.

Increasing confidence and efforts to achieve or surpass personal-best distances may influence the rise of injuries towards the end of the season. This factor, along with the fact that over 50 per cent of severe injuries occur on the first jump, indicates the need for jumpers to examine all aspects of the jump thoroughly, including the in-run and landing areas, before committing themselves to attempting the course. Equipment is another key factor and there has been a remarkable improvement in this area. Skis, bindings, clothing, and above all good head protection have added a dimension of protection that unfortunately can sometimes lead to recklessness. Previous experiments with high heel blocks allowing early retainment of the floating position seems to increase the incidence of dangerous falls during take-off, particularly when small decelerations are encountered on the in-run. Apart from the skier's equipment, the construction of rails, shields, and fences in all areas of the jump should make it impossible for skis or body parts to become stuck in the case of a fall.[66]

One of the most significant factors in reducing ski jumping injuries is the improvement in technique. The older, less aerodynamic-efficient ski jumping techniques, requiring that the jumper be projected high into the air and then free fall while flying horizontally, has been replaced with a modern jump in which the idea is to mimic an airfoil and generate lift. Therefore, it is possible to fly further without needing so much altitude. The vertical component of the flight curve relative to the horizontal component has been decreased. This, in turn, has allowed the jumping hill to be redesigned. The modern ski jumping hill is not so steep and as a

Table 5 Sport and recreational acquired spine fractures related to age

Sport	Mean	SD	Range
Diving	22.00	5.85	12–39
Equestrian	35.81	11.69	17–52
Snowmobile	26.93	7.71	12–39
Parachute/skydiving	26.00	5.72	19–41
All-terrain vehicle	27.33	9.35	16–46
Toboggan	20.82	9.29	8–35
Bicycle	42.00	26.91	12–64
Rugby	26.75	2.50	24–30
Downhill skiing	18.33	6.81	13–26
Ice hockey	19.33	4.51	15–24
Surfing	40.00	17.06	26–59
Mountaineering	24.00	5.66	20–28
Football	17.00	1.41	16–18
Soccer	24.00*		
Water skiing	28.00*		
Frisbee	27.00*		
Dancing	14.00*		
Badminton	72.00*		
Caber throw	50.00*		
Trampoline	5.00*		
Wrestling	20.00*		
Rope swing	21.00*		

* One subject only.
Adapted from ref. 2.

result the transition area is flatter and longer. This has increased the margin of safety since the landing hill more closely resembles the flight curve of a broader range of jumps, including the very long and the very short attempts.

Off-road vehicles

Off-road motor vehicles made their appearance in the late 1960s and early 1970s and have gained rapidly in both popularity and as a cause of spine fracture.[36,71,74] The predominant reason for this increase is the all-terrain vehicle. They form up to 10 per cent of sport- and recreational-induced spine fractures, and in some publications 35 per cent of these have associated neurological injury. However, there are also over 2 million snowmobiles in use in the United States and a larger *per capita* number in Canada.[64] Typically, the snowmobiler is injured while driving at night (52 per cent), driving under the influence of alcohol (53 per cent), and driving in unfamiliar terrain.[70–72] In 1973 Wenzel and Peters[71] reported that 11 per cent of the injuries occurred in children aged 10 or less (Table 5). The incorrect image of the snowmobile as a safe piece of equipment and easy to drive leads many parents to view it almost as a toy.[71–81] Ultimately, the key to reducing the number of snowmobile injuries and fatalities may be setting an age limit and educating drivers.[72–77,82] Going off embankments, tipping on steep terrain, colliding with another snowmobiler, hitting an object (frequently a tree), or becoming airborne are the most common mechanisms of sustaining spine fractures. Occasionally, the machine may roll on to the driver. Because of the cold weather conditions, compliance with wearing protective headgear is good, but frequently the impact is so great that these do not eliminate spine injury, head injury, or even fatalities.

Throughout North America, there is a general paucity of legislation relating to the use of off-road motor vehicles. Legislation, better equipment, and public education has made snowmobiling a safer sport over the last few years.[83–87] The following recommendations may further improve this record:

(1) a review of snowmobile legislation to ensure the requirement for safety and training programmes for all drivers;

(2) stricter enforcement and regulations of snowmobilers on public highways;

(3) the development of designated areas and trails for snowmobiles;

(4) improved safety designs of equipment, including helmets, as well as education for the snowmobiler.

Tobogganing

As would be anticipated, tobogganing injuries frequently involve very young individuals and approximately one-third of the spine fractures in our series occurred in children under the age of 15 years. Poor judgement features highly in the mechanism of injury which frequently involves collision with a post, fence, or tree.[2] Properly cleared and designated areas are the single most important factor in reducing injury.

Transient quadriplegia

In 1986, Torg *et al.*[88] reported 32 cases of athletes who had experienced transient quadriplegia. The quadriplegia lasted for as little as 1 min to as long as 48 hours. and in all cases resolved completely. Magnetic resonance imaging (**MRI**) was performed for only one patient and this did not reveal intrinsic cord abnormalities. Of the 32 athletes, 4 showed evidence of ligament instability, 6 had acute or chronic intervertebral disc disease, and 5 had congenital cervical anomalies. A total of 17 of the 32 athletes were identified as having relative cervical spine canal stenosis. The mechanism of injury was postulated to be a neuropraxia of the cervical cord secondary to developmental narrowing of the spinal canal (also known as relative spinal stenosis). A pincer mechanism is proposed as follows:

1. The distance between the posteroinferior margin of the superior vertebral body and the anterosuperior aspect of the spinolaminar line of the subjacent vertebra decreases with hyperextension and compresses the cord.

2. In hyperflexion the lamina of the superior vertebrae and the posterosuperior margin of the vertebral body approximate as pincers.[89,90]

In 1991 Scher reported on nine cases occurring in South African rugby players. Of these, five players had radiographic spinal stenosis, two had pre-existing intervertebral disease, one had congenital fusion of posterior elements of C2 to C3, and two patients had no plain film abnormality.[91]

Torg *et al.*'s criterion for relative spinal stenosis was that the ratios of spinal canal to vertebral midbody in these individuals were less than 0.80 (Fig. 5).[92] This is compared with a ratio of 0.98 or more in a control group of athletes. Ladd and Scranton, Cantu, and

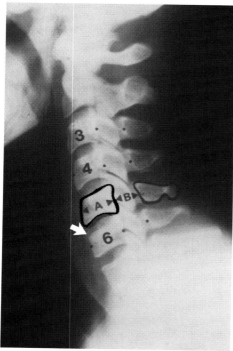

Fig. 5 Relative spinal stenosis as indicated by the ratio of the spinal canal to the width of the vertebral body. A value of less than 0.8 is considered to be abnormal.

Walsh[44,93–95] have gone so far as to suggest that any individual with identifiable relative spinal stenosis of the cervical spine should be advised to discontinue participation in contact sports. However, a more recent study by Odor *et al.* who reviewed the Torg ratio in 224 football players noted that approximately 33 per cent of them had a ratio of less than 0.8 at one or more levels of the cervical spine.[96] In 1996, Torg *et al.*[90] compared a cohort of 45 patients having had an episode of transient quadriplegia to cohorts of asymptomatic players as well as 77 former football players who were permanently quadriplegic secondary to injury. In the symptomatic group the sensitivity of a ratio less than 0.8 was 93 per cent. However, the specificity in the asymptotic college player was only 59 per cent, and in asymptotic professional players only 58 per cent. The cohort with spinal paralysis had a significantly larger mean ratio than the three cohorts aforementioned. The positive predictive value of relative spinal stenosis as defined by a ratio of less than 0.8 was only 0.2 per cent. Further, none of the 45 symptomatic players had had a catastrophic spinal injury at follow-up. In retrospect, none of the quadriplegic group could recall having experienced transient quadriplegia prior to injury. Developmental cervical stenosis in a stable cervical spine does not seem to predispose to catastrophic neurological injury.[90,97]

It is possible that the large size of the cervical vertebral body of these heavily developed individuals gives apparent narrowing of the canal and decreased Torg ratio when indeed the canal width is more than adequate. In any event, in view of the fact that a large number of asymptomatic football players have a ratio less than 0.80 and the test's low positive predictive value, the utility as a predictor of an athlete suffering transient or permanent neurological sequelae is not shown.

In 1991 Bailes *et al.*[98] pointed out that vigilance is required in both clinical and radiological assessment to ensure that such injuries are truly transient. They feel, in the absence of a neurological deficit or radiological evidence of injury and no congenital spine anomaly, that return to contact sports is possible. Torg[97] recommends that continued participation in contact activities be restricted in the following patient populations, those with:

(1) documented ligamentous laxity;

(2) intervertebral disc disease associated with cord compression or significant degenerative changes;

(3) MRI evidence of cord defect or swelling;

(4) symptoms or neurological findings lasting more than 36 h; and

(5) more than one occurrence.

All cases deserve individual consideration, and any decision for return to play or advice regarding vulnerability to further injury should include factors other than the simple plain radiographs.

Burners and stingers (traumatic radiculopathy)

In 1983, a survey of over 3000 secondary school and varsity football teams found that 25 per cent of the players had a history of neck injury.[99] Most reported neck pain, numbness, tingling, burning, or weakness in one upper limb. Usually, this was related to tackling using the head as the first point of contact, or in collision with forced side-flexion of the neck and depression of the shoulder of the contralateral side (Fig. 6).[100,101] These episodes were clumped together under the heading of burners and stingers.[102] They have often tended to be regarded as benign and are treated with an uncharacteristic lack of respect compared with that given to most neurological traumas.

The symptoms range from a brief 'knife-like' shooting pain confined to the shoulder to transient numbness and paralysis of the whole arm. For the most part the symptoms clear up quickly, although with careful testing it can be seen that there is frequently detectable pathology lasting over 48 h and electrophysiological changes which may persist for several months (Table 6). At various times the pathophysiology of the lesion has been located in the spinal cord, the nerve root, the brachial plexus, or the peripheral nerve level. It is common for the athlete to admit to sustaining burners as frequently as one per game for an entire season without ever having received a detailed neurological assessment or any specific therapy.

The management and advice varies from uninterrupted continuation of play to complete cessation of sport. Typically, however, there is a brief assessment on the field followed by a return to play. The athlete may receive bolstering of the cervical spine or shoulder and instruction on improving tackling techniques. Rarely is there rigid immobilization until fracture or dislocation has been ruled out. In our series a significant number of the athletes tested had persistent neurological signs and symptoms 3 weeks after their latest burner episode.

The C5 to C6 area is most commonly affected with both radiographical abnormalities and electrophysiological changes. The lesions are in the upper trunk in over half the cases, and nerve root lesions and peripheral nerve involvement are equal in frequency.[103-106] Thus the locations and severity of the neurological injury following a forced cervical compression or flexion injury is variable, and the diagnosis of burner or stinger does not imply a specific nerve injury or prognosis. Individuals sustaining recurrent burners should have a thorough investigation, the findings should be reviewed, and the athlete should be advised regarding the potential risks to the neural system.

Table 6 Duration of symptoms from burners		
Symptoms	**Duration**	**Frequency (%)**
Initial dysthetic pain	≤ 1 min	57
	5 min or more	35
	Unknown	18
Continued subjective weakness	None	34
	8 h	12
	24 h	12
	≥ 2–3 weeks	42

In any event, when such an episode occurs, the person responsible for medical care should make sure that the athlete is removed from play and properly assessed and not allowed to return until a definitive diagnosis is made.

Naturally, the major concern is to separate mild transient injuries from those which may lead to permanent paralysis if inadequately managed. The following points are helpful.

1. When in doubt do not make the final decision on the field or sidelines where things are often hectic. The subtle pressures from athlete and coach are significant and there is a tendency to be hurried. Take the player to the dressing room and carefully reassess. Do this immediately and not at the end of the game.

2. Adequately undress the player in order to palpate and inspect the area; this often requires careful removal of equipment.

3. Where there is concern that the symptoms do not fit the classic pattern or are more than transient, send the player for radiography.

4. If there appear to be any residual symptoms, make a decision which errs on the side of safety.[107-109]

The following points should arouse suspicion of a more severe injury. Significant tenderness over the trapezius and sternomastoid, particularly if associated with a restricted range of functional motion, should be noted. Any obvious midline deformity to palpation, specifically a step or a gap between the spinous processes, should be taken as evidence of spinal instability, and appropriate splinting and precautions taken. Even extreme tenderness in the midline, over the ligament nuchae and the spinous processes, is uncharacteristic of the usual burner and stinger and must be treated with caution. Weakness, paralysis, and paraesthesia in more than one extremity should be assumed to be spinal cord damage until proved otherwise.

During preseason medicals, those individuals with a history of multiple burners and stingers, or those who are in vulnerable positions such as linebackers or fullbacks, must have a very careful neurological examination and appropriate radiography. These individuals require a special neck-strengthening programme and their contact time in practice should be minimized. The emphasis should be on teaching correct techniques of blocking and tackling which minimize the use of the head as a major weapon. Occasionally neck

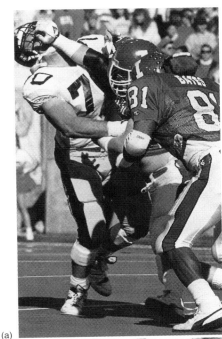

(a)

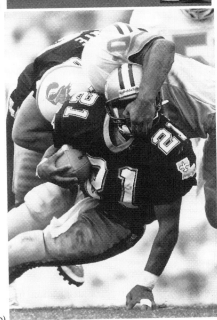

(b)

Fig. 6 While direct compressive loading of the cervical spine may be a common cause of the 'burner' syndrome, (a) forced extension with shoulder depression and (b) rotary torques may also generate symptoms in the susceptible individual.

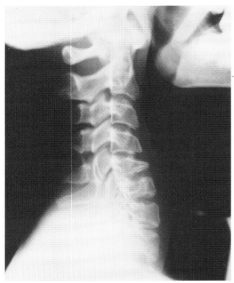

Fig. 7 Old trauma to C5 has resulted in deformity. Careful flexion and extension films will reveal any associated instability.

rolls and cervical collars seem to reduce the frequency of episodes.[110] Nevertheless in those injury-prone individuals who continue to have problems, wherever possible a change in position should be contemplated which may have the effect of placing them at less risk.

Torg et al.[31] have estimated that the compressive load limits for the cervical vertebral bodies are between 750 and 1000 pounds (1.65 to 2.2×10^3 kg). If this load has reached a maximal compressive mode, with the head slightly flexed, a compression fracture of the vertebral body may occur. Extending the neck to keep the face up may create uneven forces, and tackling with the head laterally flexed may also leave the cervical spine in a vulnerable position. Thus it is not always possible to protect the neck. The main points of emphasis should be anticipating contraction of the large neck muscles, hunching the shoulders, and using the arms for the initial contact in blocking and tackling.

Where the radiographs show changes in the shape of the vertebral body, which may be related to old or new trauma, flexion and extension films may help to reveal minor instabilities (Fig. 7).

Where the symptom complex suggests a more proximal pathology than the traditional midcervical area, careful views of the C1 to C2 area are required. Individuals with degenerative spondylosis need to be considered on an individual basis. There is an increased incidence of facet joint change, joint space narrowing, and osteophyte formation in many individuals who have spent a large number of years playing football, wrestling, or soccer. While there is no direct relationship between radiographic changes and symptomatology, significant degenerative changes combined with chronic nerve root irritation can ultimately affect their activities of daily living. Thus athletes should be alerted to this possibility so that they can decide whether or not to continue their sport should there be a definite risk of the development of significant symptomatic degenerative changes. Individuals with degenerative spondylosis need to be counselled on an individual basis. Similarly, any congenital abnormality must be considered on an individual basis (Fig. 8).

Essentially, the common, symptom complex known as 'burners or stingers' should never be taken lightly, and no player should be returned to the field of contact until a careful neurological examination has been carried out.

Principles of moving a spine injury athlete

It is incumbent upon the senior medical person attending any contact sporting event which carries a risk of spinal injury to ensure that a protocol has been set up for handling significant emergencies. The location of the nearest telephone, hospital, and access for stretcher or ambulance must be established. Furthermore, the field of play must be examined for hazards and safety. Should a potentially catastrophic injury to the spine occur, the playing surface will dictate potential difficulties with transferring the athlete safely.[3] Rescuing somebody from the water or a jumping pit presents a very different challenge to that of moving an ice hockey player on an ice surface, moving someone from the ski slopes, or dealing with the cumbersome helmet and shoulder pads of football players. Only familiarization, training, and rehearsal will equip the medical personnel sufficiently to handle the situations smoothly and efficiently.

The unconscious patient with a potential neck injury presents a further challenge. All unconscious athletes must be assumed to have a cervical spine injury and be handled accordingly (Fig. 9). Further, any patient sustaining an injury above the clavicle or any patient injured at high speed should arouse suspicion of an associated spine or spinal cord injury.[111] The initial screen of the individual establishes the adequacy of the airway and then spinal tenderness, the athlete's ability to move all limbs, and the presence or absence of sensation are carefully sought. The most experienced person pres-

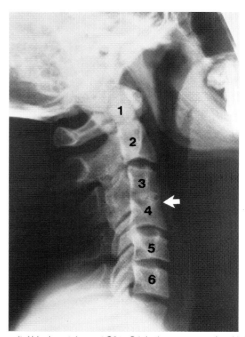

Fig. 8 Congenital block vertebrae at C3 to C4. In the presence of multiple episodes of 'burners' this may be a contraindication to continued participation.

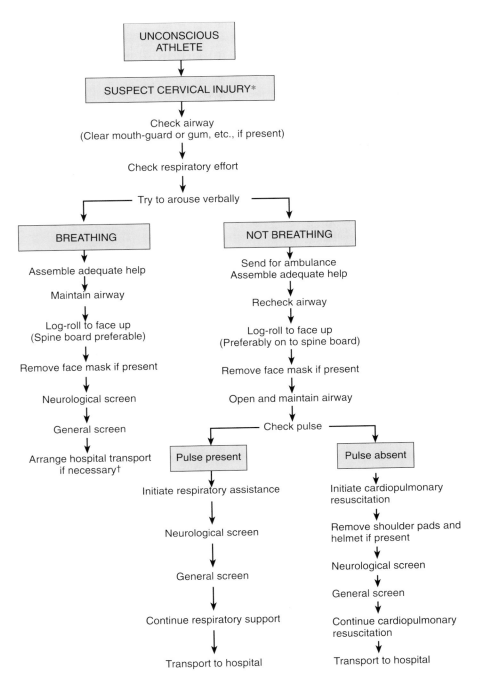

Fig. 9 Decision matrix for on-site management of the unconscious athlete. *Any significant suspicion of a cervical injury should prompt all spinal precautions and arrangements for transport to medical facility. †Other than very transient loss of consciousness or grade I to II concussions, full assessment at hospital is advisable.

ent should take command. Any evidence of head and neck problems requires immediate stabilization of the cervical spine while a more detailed secondary screen is carried out to assess the extent of the injury. If necessary, turning is organized along with transfer to a spine board or stretcher. It is recommended that four people be involved in applying a spine board using the modified log-roll technique:[111]

(1) one to maintain manual, in-line immobilization of the head and neck;

(2) one for the torso;

(3) one for the pelvis and legs; and

(4) one to direct the procedure and position the spine board.

It should be remembered that high-speed motor sports and skiing produce combined injuries to the viscera and appendicular skeleton as well as the cervical spine. Thus it is important not to be distracted completely from the assessment of the total athlete when a cervical spine injury has been identified and, conversely, a seriously deformed fractured limb should not divert suspicion away from the cervical spine until an injury to this area has been specifically ruled out.

Finally, it should be pointed out that significant disruption of the vertebral column can occur without associated paralysis and often the clinical signs of local tenderness may be the only clue to an underlying unstable spine.

Summary

In this chapter we have emphasized the high incidence of potentially serious and catastrophic injuries sustained in sport. Several points have emerged, including the fact that spine trauma need not necessarily be associated with paralysis and thus may be overlooked unless a diligent and careful examination is made. Second, the events leading up to a spine injury in high-velocity sports such as skiing may be associated with many other problems. Thus in the excitement of managing a peripheral injury, there may be a tendency to miss the cervical or lumbar spine problem.

Most individuals do not encounter spine injuries on a frequent basis and, therefore on the occasion that it occurs when they are in charge of supervising a sport, they are often caught unprepared. Rescue and immobilization procedures on ice, gymnastic mats, ski slopes, and football fields should be practised on a regular basis to ensure familiarity with the problems and nuances of these different environments. It is a sad fact that many of the injuries that occur in sports and recreation are eminently preventable if elementary precautions are taken. Nowhere is this more true than in the frequent injuries associated with diving or those incurred on recreational all-terrain vehicles.

Finally, this chapter should serve as a reminder for anybody in charge of a sports facility to ensure and check that adequate triage procedures are in place before any game or competition commences, so that, in the event of a serious injury, expeditious and safe transport can be arranged.

References

1. Mueller FO, Cantu RD. Catastrophic injuries and fatalities in high school and college sports. Fall 1982–Spring 1988. *Medical Science in Sports and Exercise* 1990; **22**: 737.
2. Reid DC, Saboe L. Spinal trauma in sports and recreation. *Journal of Clinical Sports Medicine* 1991; **1**: 75.
3. Reid DC. *Sports injury, assessment and rehabilitation.* New York: Churchill Livingstone, 1991.
4. Tator CH, Edmonds VE. Sports and recreation are a rising cause of spinal cord injury. *Physician and Sportsmedicine* 1986; **14**: 157.
5. Murphy P. Still too many neck injuries. *Physician and Sportsmedicine* 1985; **13**: 29.
6. Key AG, Retief PJM. Spinal cord injuries: An analysis of 300 new lesions. *Paraplegia* 1970; **7**: 243.
7. Tator CH, Palm J. Spinal injuries in diving. Incidence high and rising. *Ontario Medical Review* 1981; **48**: 628.
8. Kurtzke JF. Epidemiology of spinal cord injury. *Experimental Neurology* 1975; **88**: 163.
9. Kluger Y, Jarosz D, Paul DB, Townsend RN, Diamond DL. Diving injuries: a preventable catastrophe. *Journal of Trauma* 1994; **36**: 349–51.
10. Cheng CL, Wolf AL, Mirvis S, Robinson WL. Bodysurfing accidents resulting in cervical spinal injuries. *Spine* 1992; **17**: 257–60.
11. Scher AT. Bodysurfing injuries of the spinal cord. *South African Medical Journal* 1995; **85**: 1022–4.
12. Sovio OM, Van Peteghan PK, Schweigel JF. Cervical spine injuries in rugby players. *Canadian Medical Association* 1984; **130**: 36.
13. Burry HC, Gowland H. Cervical injury in rugby football—a New Zealand survey. *British Journal of Sports Medicine* 1981; **15**: 56.
14. Carvell JE, Fuller DJ, Duthie RB, Cockin J. Rugby football injuries to the cervical spine. *British Medical Journal* 1983; **286**: 49.
15. Kewalramani LS, Drauss JF. Cervical spine injuries resulting from collision sports. *Paraplegia* 1981; **19**: 303.
16. McCoy GF, Piggot J, Macafee AL, Adair IV. Injuries of the cervical spine in schoolboy rugby football. *Journal of Bone and Joint Surgery* 1984; **66B**: 500.
17. O'Carroll PF, Sheehan JM, Gregg TM. Cervical spine injuries in rugby football. *Irish Medical Journal* 1981; **74**: 377.
18. Scher AT. Rugby injuries to the cervical spinal cord. *South African Medical Journal* 1980; **57**: 37.
19. Silver JR. Injuries to the spine sustained in rugby. *British Medical Journal* 1984; **288**: 37.
20. Milburn PD. Biomechanics of rugby union scrummaging, technical and safety issues. *Sports Medicine* 1993; **16**: 168–79.
21. Albright JP, McAuley E, Martin RK. Head and neck injuries in college football: an eight year analysis. *American Journal of Sports Medicine* 1985; **13**: 147.
22. Alley R H Jr. Head and neck injuries in high school football. *Journal of the American Medical Association* 1964; **188**: 418.
23. Clarke KS. An epidemiologic view. In: Torg JS, ed. *Athlete injuries to the head, neck and face.* Philadelphia: Lea and Febiger, 1982: 15–25.
24. Schneider RC, ed. *Head and neck injuries. Football: mechanisms, treatment and prevention.* Baltimore: Williams and Wilkins, 1973: 77–125.
25. Funk FJ, Wells RE. Injuries of the cervical spine in football. *Clinical Orthopaedics and Related Research* 1975; **109**: 50.
26. Nine KM, Veqsgo JJ, Sennett B, Torg JS. Prevention of cervical spine injuries in football. A model for other sports. *Physician and Sportsmedicine* 1991; **19**: 54–64.
27. Schneider RC. Serious and fatal neurosurgical football injuries. *Clinical Neurosurgery* 1964; **12**: 226.
28. Schneider RC, Reifel E, Crisler HO, Oosterbaan BG. Serious and fatal football injuries involving the head and spinal cord. *Journal of the American Medical Association* 1961; **177**: 362.
29. Torg JS, Vegso JJ, Sennett B, Das M. The National Football Head and Neck Injury Registry 1971–1984. *Journal of the American Medical Association* 1985; **254**: 3439–3.
30. Clarke KS, Powell JW. Football helmets and neurotrauma, an epidemiological overview of three seasons. *Medicine and Science in Sports and Exercise* 1979; **11**: 138.
31. Torg JS, Vegso JJ, O'Neill MJ, Sennett B. The epidemiologic, pathologic, biomechanical and cinematographic analysis of football induced cervical spine trauma. *American Journal of Spine Medicine* 1990; **18**: 50–7.
32. Paley D, Gillespie R. Chronic repetitive unrecognized flexion injury of the cervical spine (high jumpers' neck). *American Journal of Sports Medicine* 1986; **14**: 92.
33. Hodgson VR. Reducing serious injury in sports. *Interschool Athletic Administration* 1980; **7**: 11.
34. Saboe LA, Reid DC, Davis L, Warren S, Grace MG. Spine trauma and associated injuries. *Journal of Trauma* 1991; **31**: 43–8.
35. Rodrigo J, Boyd R. Lumbar spine injuries in military parachute jumpers. *Physicians and Sportsmedicine* 1979; **7**: 9.
36. Reid DC, Saboe L. Spine fractures in winter sports. *Sports Medicine* 1989; **7**: 393.
37. Allan DG, Reid DC, Saboe LA. Off-road recreational motor vehicle accidents: hospitalization and deaths. *Canadian Journal of Surgery* 1988; **31**: 233.

38. Feriencik K. Trends in ice hockey injuries: 1965 to 1977. *Physician and Sportsmedicine* 1979; **7**: 81.

39. Tator CH, Edmonds VE, Lapczak L, Tator IB. Spinal injuries in ice hockey players, 1966–1987. *Canadian Journal of Surgery* 1991; **34**: 63–9.

40. Tator CH, Ekong CE, Rowed DW, Schwartz ML, Edmonds VE, Cooper PW. Spinal injuries due to hockey. *Canadian Journal of Neurological Science* 1984; **11**: 34–41.

41. Reid DC, Saboe SA. Spine injuries resulting from winter sports. In: Torg JS, ed. *Athletic injuries to the head, neck and face.* 2nd edn. Chicago: Mosby Year Book, 1991.

42. Tator CH, Edmonds VE. National survey of spinal injuries in hockey players. *Canadian Medical Association Journal* 1984; **30**: 875.

43. Reynen PD, Clancy WG Jr. Cervical spine injury, hockey helmets, and face masks. *American Journal of Sports Medicine* 1994; **22**: 167–70.

44. Walsh S. A proposal for the use of the half face, clear plastic visor for national collegiate athletic association hockey. In: Castaldi CR, Hoerner EF, eds. *Safety in ice hockey.* Philadelphia: American Society for Testing & Materials, 1989: 55–7.

45. Bishop PJ, Norman RW, Wells R, Raney D, Skleryk B. Changes in the centre of mass and movement of inertia of a headform induced by a hockey helmet and face shield. *Canadian Journal of Applied Sports Science* 1983; **8**: 19.

46. Hayes D. Reducing risks in hockey. Analysis of equipment and injuries. *Physician and Sports Medicine* 1978; **6**: 67.

47. Frymoyer JW, Pope MH, Kristiansen T. Skiing and spinal trauma. *Clinics in Sports Medicine* 1982; **1**: 309.

48. Davis MW, Litman T, Drill FE, Mueller JK. Ski injuries. *Journal of Trauma* 1977; **17**: 802.

49. Gutman J, Weisbuch J, Wolf M. Ski injuries in 1972–73: a report analysis of a major health program. *Journal of the American Medical Association* 1974; **230**: 1423.

50. Howarth B. Skiing injuries. *Clinical Orthopaedics and Related Research* 1965; **43**: 171.

51. Myles ST, Mohtadi NG, Schnittker J. Injuries to the nervous system and spine in downhill skiing. *Canadian Journal of Surgery* 1992; **35**: 643–8.

52. Morrow PL. Downhill ski fatalities: The Vermont experience. Presented at the National Association of Medical Examiners Annual Meeting, Boston, 5 November 1988.

53. Shealy JE. How dangerous is skiing and who's at risk? *Ski Patrol Magazine* 1985; **2**: 21.

54. Oh S. Cervical injury from skiing. *International Journal of Sports Medicine* 1984; **5**: 268.

55. Ellison AE. Skiing injuries. *Clinical Symposium* 2977; **29**: 1.

56. Clancy WG, McConkey JP. Nordic and alpine skiing. In: Schneider RCS, Kennedy JCK, Plant MLP, eds. *Sports injuries— mechanisms, prevention and treatment.* Baltimore: Williams and Wilkins, 1985.

57. Margreiter R, Raas E, Luger LJ. The risk of injury in experienced alpine skiers. *Orthopedic Clinics of North America* 1976; **7**: 51.

58. Garrick JG, Requa RK. Injury patterns in children and adolescent skiers. *American Journal of Sports Medicine* 1979; **7**: 245.

59. Henderson RL, Reid DC, Saboe LA. Multiple contiguous spine fractures. *Spine* 1991; **16**: 128–31.

60. Keen JS. Thoracolumbar fractures in winter sports. *Clinical Orthopaedics and Related Research* 1987; **216**: 39.

61. Harris JB. Neurological injuries in winter sports. *Physician and Sportsmedicine* 1983; **11**: 111.

62. Dowling PA. Prospective study of injuries in United States Ski Association freestyle skiing, 1976–77 to 1979–80. *American Journal of Sports Medicine* 1982; **10**: 268.

63. Reif AE. Risks and gains. In: Vinger PF, Hoerner EF, eds. *Sports injuries: the unthwarted epidemic.* 2nd edn. Littleton, MA: PSG, 1986.

64. Rich P. Canada leads field in sports-related spinal injuries. *Medical Post* 1985; Sept. 3: 50.

65. Wester K. Serious ski-jumping injuries in Norway. *American Journal of Sports Medicine* 1985; **13**: 124.

66. Wright JR, Hixson EG, Rand JJ. Injury patterns in nordic ski-jumpers. A retrospective analysis of injuries occurring at the Intervale Ski Jump Complex from 1980–1985. *American Journal of Sports Medicine* 1986; **14**: 393.

67. Wester K. Improved safety in ski-jumping. *American Journal of Sports Medicine* 1988; **16**: 499.

68. Eriksson E. Ski injuries in Sweden: a one year survey. *Orthopedic Clinics of North America* 1976; **7**: 3.

69. Wright JR, Hixson EG, Rand JJ. Injury patterns in nordic ski jumpers. *American Journal of Sports Medicine* 1986; **14**: 292.

70. Write JR. Nordic ski-jumping fatalities in the United States: a 50 year summary. *Journal of Trauma* 1988; **28**: 848.

71. Wenzel FJ, Peters RA. A ten-year survey of snowmobile accidents, injuries and fatalities in Wisconsin. *Physicians and Sportsmedicine* 1986; **14**: 140.

72. Kritter AE, Carnesale PG, Prusinski D. Snowmobile: Fund and/ or folly. *Wisconsin Medical Journal* 1972; **71**: 230.

73. Trager GW, Grayman G. Accidents and all-terraine vehicles (C). *Journal of American Medical Association* 1986; **225**: 2160.

74. Reid DC, Saboe LA, Allan DG. Spine trauma associated with off-road vehicles. *Physician and Sportsmedicine* 1987; **16**: 143.

75. Hamidy CR, Dhir A, Cameron B, Jones H, Fitzerald GWN. Snowmobile injuries in Northern Newfoundland and Labrador. An 18 year review. *Journal of Trauma* 1988; **28**: 1232.

76. Haynes CD, Stroud SD, Thompson CE. The three wheeler (adult tricycle): An unstable, dangerous machine. *Journal of Trauma* 1986; **26**: 643.

77. Chism SE, Soule AB. Snowmobile injuries: hazards from a popular new winter sport. *Journal of the American Medical Association* 1969; **209**: 1672.

78. Wiley JJ. The dangers of off-road vehicles to young drivers. *Canadian Medical Association Journal* 1986; **135**: 1345.

79. Dominici RH, Drake EH. Speed on snow: The motorized sled. *American Journal of Surgery* 1970; **119**: 483.

80. Damschroder AD, Kleinstiver BS. Homo snomoblilius. *American Journal of Sports Medicine* 1976; **4**: 249.

81. Percy EC. The snowmobile. Friend or foe? *Journal of Trauma* 1972; **12**: 444.

82. Stevens WS, Rodgers BM, Newman BM. Pediatric trauma associated with all-terrain vehicles. *Journal of Pediatrics* 1986; **109**: 25.

83. Speca JM, Cowell HR. Minibike and motorcycle accidents in adolescents. A new epidemic. *Journal of the American Medical Association* 1975; **232**: 55.

84. Golladay ES, Slezak JW, Mollitt DL, Siebert RW. The three wheeler—a menace to the preadolescent child. *Journal of Trauma* 1985; **25**: 232.

85. Westman JA, Morrow G III. Moped injuries in children. *Pediatrics* 1984; **74**: 820.

86. Wiley JJ, McIntyre WM, Mercier P. Injuries associated with off-road vehicles among children. *Canadian Medical Association Journal* 1986; **135**: 136.

87. Withington RL, Hall LN. Snowmobile accidents: a review of injuries sustained in the use of snowmobiles in northern New England during the 1968–69 season. *Journal of Trauma* 1970; **10**: 760.

88. Torg JS, Quedenfeld TC, Burstein A, Spealman A, Nichols C III. National Football Head and Neck Registry: Report on cervical quadriplegia. 1971 to 1975. *American Journal Sports Medicine* 197; **7**: 127.

89. Penning L. Some aspects of plain radiograph of the cervical spine in chronic myelopathy. *Neurology* 1962; **12**: 513–19.

90. Torg JS, Naranja RJ, Palov H, *et al.* The relationship of developmental narrowing of the cervical spinal canal to reversible and irreversible injury of the cervical spinal cord in football players. *Journal of Bone and Joint Surgery* 1996; **78A**: 1308–14.

91. Scher AT. Spinal cord concussion in rugby players. *American Journal of Sports Medicine* 1991; **19**: 485–8.

92. Torg JS, *et al.* Neurapraxia of the cervical spinal cord with transient quadriplegia. *Journal of Bone and Joint Surgery* 1986; **68A**: 1354–70.

93. Ladd AL, Scranton PE. Congenital cervical spinal stenosis presenting as transient quadriplegia in athletes. Report of two cases. *Journal of Bone Joint Surgery* 1986; **68A**: 1371–4.

94. Ladd AL, Scanton PE. Congenital cervical stenosis presenting as transient quadriplegia in athletes. *Journal of Bone Joint Surgery* 1986; **68A**: 1731.

95. Cantu RC. Head and spine injuries in youth sports. *Clinics in Sports Medicine* 1995; **14**: 517–32.

96. Odor JM, Watkins RG, Dillin WH, Dennis S, Saberi M. Incidence of cervical spinal stenosis in professional and rookie football players. *American Journal of Sports Medicine* 1990; **18**: 507–9.

97. Torg JS. Cervical spinal stenosis with cord neurapraxia and transient quadriplegia. *Sports Medicine* 1995; **20**: 429–34,

98. Bailes JE, Hadley MN, Quigley MR, *et al.* Management of athletic injuries of the cervical spine and spinal cord. *Neurosurgery* 1991; **29**: 491–7.

99. Gerberich SG, *et al.* Spinal trauma and symptoms in high school football players. *Physician and Sportsmedicine* 1983; **11**: 122.

100. Bergfeld JA, Hershman EB, Wilbourn AJ. Brachial injuries in athletes. *Orthopaedic Transactions* 1988; **12**: 743–4.

101. Chrisman OD, *et al.* Lateral-flexion neck injuries in athletic competition. *Journal of the American Medical Association* 1965; **192**: 117–19.

102. Poindexter DP, Johnson EW. Football shoulder and neck injury. A study of the 'Stinger'. *Archives of Physical Medicine and Rehabilitation* 1984; **65**: 601–2.

103. Robertson WC Jr, Eichman PL, Clancy WG. Upper trunk, brachial plexopathy in football players. *Journal of the American Medical Association* 1976; **241**: 1480–2.

104. DiBenedetto M, Markey K. Electrodiagnostic localization of traumatic upper trunk brachial plexopathy. *Archives of Physical Medicine and Rehabilitation* 1984; **65**: 15–17.

105. DiBenedetto M, Chardhry U, Markey K. Proximal nerve conduction. Brachial plexus. *Muscle and Nerve* 1982; **5**: 564.

106. Hu R, Burnham R, Reid DC, Grace M, Saboe L. Burners in contact sports. *Clinical Journal of Sports Medicine* 1991; **1**: 236–42.

107. Masoon JC, Kevin T, Rehhopf P. System for preventing acute neck injury. *Physician and Sportsmedicine* 1977; **5**: 76.

108. Feldick HG, Albright JP. Football survey reveals 'missed' neck injuries. *Physician and Sportsmedicine* 1976; **4**: 77.

109. Reid DC, Henderson R, Saboe L, Miller JDR. Etiology and clinical course of missed spine fractures. *Journal of Trauma* 1987; **27**: 980–6.

110. Gibbs R. A protective collar for cervical radiculopathy. *Physician and Sportsmedicine* 1984; **12**: 139.

111. (ATLS) *Advanced Trauma Life Support Course for Physicians, Student Manual.* Committee on Trauma, American College of Surgeons, 1993: 214–15.

7.6 Head injuries in athletics

Michael L. Schwartz and Charles H. Tator

Introduction

In industrial societies today there is a greater democratization of athletic activity than ever before. With a shorter work-week and increased leisure time and the perception by the public that physical activity need not cease when formal education finishes, older people are remaining active or resuming sporting activities. Furthermore, through television, there is a greater emphasis on high-performance competition that influences the behaviour of athletic participants of all ages and predisposes to more serious injuries.

Epidemiology

Athletic activities, needless to say, vary from one part of the world to another and are influenced by climate, geography, and culture. Reviews of catastrophic sporting injuries in the province of Ontario, Canada conducted by one of us (CHT) in 1986, 1989, and 1992[1,2] found that head injuries comprised 20 per cent. The proportion of head injuries remained nearly constant across all three reviews and accounted for 21.3 per cent of the total (Fig. 1). The head injuries resulted from a range of activities illustrated in Fig. 2. Motor sports proved most dangerous, accounting for 115 of the 413 head injuries, with snowmobiling (68) and the use of off-road all-terrain vehicles (28) making up 83.4 per cent of the 115 injuries. Pedal bicycling accounted for 102 injuries. Winter sports, including alpine skiing

(19) and hockey (16), accounted for 62 injuries, water sports for a total of 33 injuries, and a miscellaneous group accounted for 101 additional head injuries (Fig. 3). This report,[1] produced by surveying Ontario neurosurgeons, orthopaedic surgeons, emergency physicians, coroners, and other health-care professionals who might be expected to see catastrophic injuries, is by no means complete. Nevertheless, the identification in the 1986 review that the use of all-terrain vehicles (**ATV**), especially those with three wheels, was a particularly dangerous activity led to the withdrawal of three-wheel ATVs from the Ontario, Canada market.

This study surveyed the use of alcohol among those suffering catastrophic injuries. In cases with specific information (1130 of 1594), there was definite evidence of alcohol consumption in 14.6 per cent of 775 survivors and in 45.9 per cent of 355 fatalities.[1]

The recognition of trends in the incidence of injury from particular activities may permit the evaluation of preventive measures. Diving injuries which accounted for 3 per cent of all head injuries in 1986 now comprise fewer than 1 per cent of the total. This improvement may be due, in part, to 'Water smart', a specific prevention programme begun in Ontario during 1989 by a coalition of partners

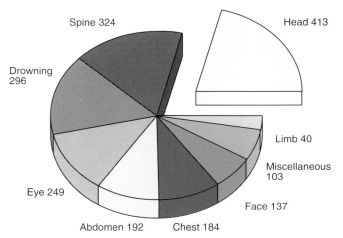

Fig. 1 Reviews of catastrophic sporting injuries in the Province of Ontario, Canada were conducted in 1986, 1989, and 1992. Head injuries accounted for 21.3 per cent of the total and remained a constant proportion of catastrophic sporting injuries in each epoch.

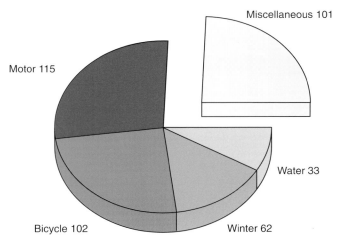

Fig. 2 Head injuries occurred in participants in a variety of activities with motor sport, bicycling, and a miscellaneous category accounting for 77 per cent of 413 head injuries. Diving injuries, which accounted for 3 per cent of all head injuries in 1986, now comprise fewer than 1 per cent of the total and are included under water-sport injuries. Hockey injuries, which accounted for 6 per cent of all head injuries in 1986, now comprise only 2 per cent of the total and are included under winter-sport injuries.

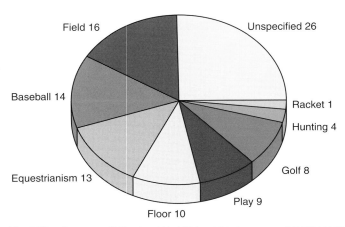

Fig. 3 Miscellaneous activities in which 101 head injuries occurred. Field sports include American football and rugby.

led by the Royal Life Saving Society of Canada, Ontario Branch. Similarly, the reduction in head injuries resulting from ice hockey, which accounted for 6 per cent of all head injuries in 1986, to 2 per cent of the current total may, in part, be attributed to prevention programmes that include rule changes disallowing checking or pushing from behind, dissemination of a video tape entitled 'Smart hockey' detailing the mechanism of catastrophic injuries, and the encouragement of helmet use by players at all levels of expertise, including professional players. It is desirable that individuals who have an interest or supervisory role in athletics survey the patterns of injury where they live and work so that dangerous activities may be identified, safe practices promoted, and the efficacy of prevention programmes evaluated.

Role of the physician

Because head injuries, even apparently minor ones, may be so devastating and irrevocable,[3,4] the physician's role must include the advocacy of safe practices which enhance prevention and mitigation of brain injuries. Physicians involved in athletics must also understand the pathophysiological mechanisms of brain injury and be familiar with the principles and practice of early treatment.

Pathophysiology

The vast majority of sporting head injuries are blunt injuries, caused by falls or collisions. In general, if the head is buttressed and acceleration of the cranium and its contents is prevented, there is no significant injury to the brain unless there is mechanical failure of the cranium, that is, a depressed skull fracture. In such a case, there may be a focal injury to the brain underlying the depressed fragment.

In the majority of head injuries that occur in athletics there is violent acceleration (or deceleration) imparted to the head. Even though it is encased within the rigid, bony shell of the cranium and floats in the watery medium of the cerebrospinal fluid, the human brain has evolved by increasing in size and complexity, to the point where it is vulnerable to injury when the head is subjected to violent acceleration or deceleration. Diffuse damage may occur, even without violation of any of the coverings of the brain. The brain parenchyma is composed of a delicate network of interconnecting axons. Because of the high metabolic requirements of neurones,

there is a rich, but very delicate, vascular network of fine capillaries that conduct oxygen and glucose to them. There is no fibrous or tough internal structure to the brain. As a result, when a person suffers a blow to the head or falls and strikes his head on the ground, the brain is literally torn to pieces by the internal shearing forces that are generated on impact.[5]

Figure 4 shows the computed tomographic (**CT**) scan of a somewhat unusual case where a hockey player, properly equipped with a helmet, fell and struck his head on the ice. One can see the white, irregular haemorrhages that resulted from tearing of blood vessels within the brain parenchyma. As these lesions are located subjacent to the cerebral cortex subserving leg function, the boy's legs were stiff and spastic but his arms (the relevant cortex is shown in the CT slice on the right) were unaffected. Because of the disparity between arm and leg function it was thought at first that the athlete had suffered a spinal cord injury.

The damage caused by deceleration injury may be widespread, but the shape of the cranial cavity tends, in addition, to focus the shearing forces in the frontal and temporal lobes as indicated in Fig. 5. Figure 6 shows the CT scan of a person who has suffered an injury that is predicted by the model illustrated in Fig. 5. The left-hand CT slice passes through the inferior portion of the frontal lobes where fresh haematomas (white) are surrounded by (dark) oedema. The middle slice, passing through the temporal lobes, shows bruising anteriorly at the poles. The right-hand slice at the level of the midbrain where the ambient cerebrospinal fluid cisterns can no longer be clearly seen surrounding the brainstem, indicates raised intracranial pressure.

The focusing effect of skull shape on the shearing forces may also produce damage on the side of the head opposite to where the blow was struck, a so-called 'contrecoup' injury. Figure 7 illustrates a subgaleal haematoma, on the observer's left, over the patient's right parieto-occipital region. A traumatic intracerebral haematoma is visible in the contralateral temporal lobe.

Biomechanical studies show that punches and kicks to the head may exceed a force of 100 G.[6] From impact tests on head forms containing accelerometers used in helmet design, it has been determined that the peak force on impact in an unrestrained fall from standing height when the head strikes a hard flat surface may exceed 300 G. In fact, the Canadian Standards Association (**CSA**) standard for cycling helmets requires only that in a fall from a height of approximately 1.5 m (80 joule impact) the force of acceleration be mitigated to 250 G.[7] This corresponds to the force to which the head of an unrestrained passenger might strike the dashboard in an automobile collision at low speed. In short, very severe forces may be applied to the brain as a result of blows to the head and falls in which the head strikes the ground.

In evaluating patients with head injuries there are two aspects to consider. The first is the focal injury, that is to say the damage done to a specific part of the brain that subserves a particular function. For example, an injury to the posterior part of the left frontal lobe results in impaired control or even paralysis of the right side of the body, and in most people, produces a deficit in the production of speech. An injury to the occipital lobe may cause haemianopia and so on. If a focal injury is caused without acceleration of the whole brain, there may be no loss of consciousness. The second aspect to consider is the amount of diffuse brain damage caused by acceleration. In the case of focal or diffuse brain damage, there is some loss

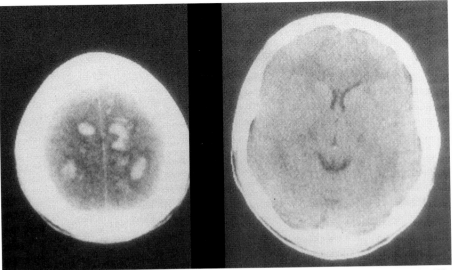

Fig. 4 On the left, the white irregular regions within the brain parenchyma represent blood that has extravasated from vessels within the brain parenchyma torn by shearing forces generated on impact when this hockey player's head struck the ice. These lesions are subjacent to the cerebral cortex subserving leg function. As a result, his legs were stiff and spastic but his arms were unaffected. The CT scan slice on the right in represents a cross-section through the portion of the motor strip subserving arm function where there has been no significant injury.

of function caused by brief mechanical distortion that make neurones refractory to stimulation. This is, indeed, reversible. More severe shearing forces result in the tearing of axons and the death of neurones. The initial effect is coma and/or amnesia. The lasting effect of diffuse axonal injury, particularly to the frontal lobes, is a lack of resilience in adapting to novel situations with slow and erratic performance.[8] Focal and diffuse injury often coexist and may result in persisting deficits that range from subtle personality changes through obvious deficits of intellect and memory, or even persistent coma.

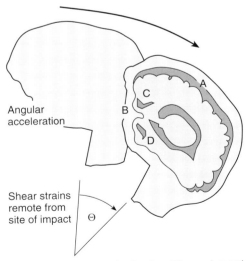

Fig. 5 When angular acceleration or deceleration of the cranium and its contents occurs, the brain rotates within the cranial cavity. Bridging (A) veins from the surface of the brain to the major venous sinuses may be stretched and torn with the release of blood into the potential subdural space. The sphenoid wing (B) impedes rotation and focuses shear strains within the frontal lobe (C) and the temporal lobe (D). The traumatic intracerebral haematomas that occur within the substance of the brain, remote from the site of impact, are called 'contrecoup' lesions.

A 'second injury'[9,10] may result from hypoxia caused by inadequate ventilation immediately after impact, or from ischaemia resulting from cerebral oedema and raised intracranial pressure. If intracranial blood vessels are torn, then an expanding intracranial haematoma may compress and distort the brain producing focal damage at the site of the haematoma or more diffuse damage by intracranial hypertension.

Temporal skull fractures may tear the middle meningeal artery with release of blood outside the dura, an epidural haematoma. Figure 8 shows a right epidural haematoma (on the observer's left). The blood clot, which appears lentiform or lens-shaped on cross-section, has that shape because it is bounded laterally by the inner table of the skull and medially by the dura. Despite the limiting effect of the dura, the brain is compressed and distorted. The lateral ventricles, seen in cross-section, which should straddle the midline, are compressed and displaced towards the patient's left.

Rupture of bridging veins from the surface of the brain to dural sinuses may release blood beneath the dura over the surface of the brain, that is, a subdural haematoma. An immense, right acute subdural haematoma is illustrated in Fig. 9. There is a dramatic shift of the ventricles toward the patient's left.

Shearing forces that tear significant blood vessels within the substance of the brain may produce traumatic intracerebral haematomas as illustrated in Figs 6 and 7. Any of the above processes may produce both focal and diffuse effects. Increasing distortion and rising intracranial pressure generally result in an increasing neurological deficit and a declining level of consciousness, which should prompt a neurosurgical consultation and possibly a CT scan.

Distortion of the oculomotor (3rd cranial) nerve by transtentorial herniation of the temporal lobe causes pupillary dilatation and is an ominous sign requiring immediate neurosurgical attention.

Once intracranial pressure has been relieved, resolution of cerebral oedema and recovery may begin. Recovery is thought to occur by axons of surviving neurones sprouting to form new connections,

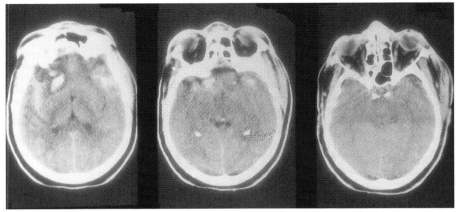

Fig. 6 The left-hand CT slice passes through the inferior portion of the frontal lobes where fresh haematomas (white) are surrounded by (dark) oedema. The middle slice, passing through the temporal lobes, shows bruising anteriorly at the poles. The right-hand slice at the level of the midbrain where the ambient cerebrospinal fluid cisterns can no longer be clearly seen surrounding the brainstem, indicates raised intracranial pressure.

that is 'rewiring' of the brain, or by an increase in the role of surviving neurones which subserve new functions formerly carried out by the neurones that have been lost.[11] Recovery from a brain injury continues for many months, although, in general, the greatest improvement occurs within the first weeks after injury. Even in the face of a relatively good recovery, effective return to preinjury activities may be hampered by the psychological effects of diffuse brain injury.[12]

Initial evaluation

It is the task of the physician who begins resuscitating a patient with a head injury to determine the likelihood of there being a condition requiring treatment, such as a traumatic intracranial haematoma. The first step is to obtain a history of the mechanism of injury. A

rugby player who has been stunned by a blow to the head and is dazed only momentarily is less likely to have suffered a severe injury than a cyclist who has come off his bike at 50 km per hour. If the patient was initially conscious and is sinking into coma, or if he initially moved all his limbs and has now become hemiplegic, it is likely that there is an expanding intracranial haematoma which is progressively distorting the brain and raising the intracranial pressure. Such a patient must be transferred immediately to a neurosurgical unit for assessment.

The Glasgow Coma Score[13,14] (**GCS**) is useful in deciding whether a patient is improving, staying the same, or deteriorating. In effect, it is an operational definition of consciousness that has the observer repeat, at intervals, a series of easy, stereotyped observations. By assessing and reporting whether a patient opens his eyes to

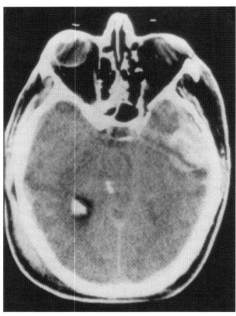

Fig. 7 A subgaleal haematoma can be seen, on the observer's left, over the patient's right parieto-occipital region. A traumatic intracerebral haematoma, a so-called 'contrecoup' injury, is visible in the contralateral temporal lobe.

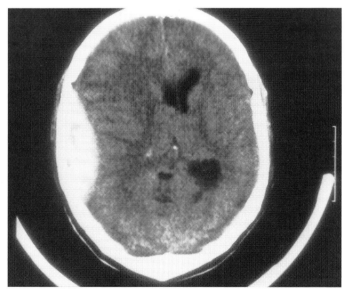

Fig. 8 A right epidural haematoma can be seen on the observer's left. The blood clot, which appears lentiform or lens-shaped on cross-section, has that shape because it is bounded laterally by the inner table of the skull and medially by the dura. Despite the limiting effect of the dura, the brain is compressed and distorted. The lateral ventricles, seen in cross-section, which should straddle the midline, are compressed and displaced toward the patient's left.

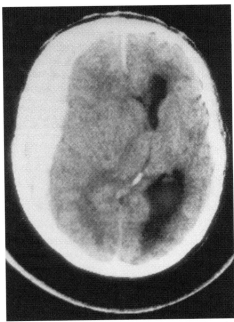

Fig. 9 An immense, right acute subdural haematoma. There is a dramatic shift of the ventricles toward the patient's left.

certain stimuli, answers questions appropriately, or moves his limbs in a certain way, the observer can base therapeutic decisions on the patient's improvement or decline. A 15-point scale has been developed.

If the patient's eyes are spontaneously open, a full score of 4 is assigned by the observer. If the eyes are closed during the period of observation but the patient responds to voice (not necessarily an instruction to open the eyes) by opening them, a score of 3 is given. If a painful stimulus is required for eye-opening, then 2 is given. No eye-opening receives a score of 1.

The best motor response (on the good side if the patient is hemiparetic) is assigned a score of 6 on compliance with a simple verbal instruction. Localization of a painful stimulus, such as reaching up to attempt to remove the examiner's hand pressing on the superior margin of the orbit, receives a score of 5. Withdrawal of the hand from nailbed compression is scored as 4 and spastic flexion of the elbow, a stereotyped, reflex response is scored as 3. Spastic extensor posturing receives 2 and no motor response is scored 1.

If in conversation, the patient is oriented to person, place, and time, a score of 5 is given. A score of 4 is assigned to the patient who converses but is disoriented. A score of 3 is given for single words (often expletives) and a score of 2 for incomprehensible sounds. A score of 1 indicates no verbal response. As may be readily appreciated, the verbal portion of the Glasgow Coma Score may be at variance to the eye and motor scores if an apparently conscious patient is very young, lacks facility in the examiner's language, or is aphasic.

The sum of the eye (**E**), motor (**M**), and verbal (**V**) scores may be computed, or the three may be evaluated and graphed separately hour by hour or more frequently as required. Practical advice on the use of the scale is documented in many sources.[15] A deteriorating GCS is an indication for prompt transfer of an athlete under observation to a medical facility.

First aid

In the management of any head injury, certain priorities govern treatment.[15] Of prime importance is maintenance of the airway, ensuring that there is adequate ventilation and making certain that the blood pressure is adequate. In the formal setting of an organized athletic competition the physician providing medical coverage should have a prearranged emergency plan that includes personnel, procedures, and equipment appropriate to the sport, the level of competition, and the weather.[16] Communication with local emergency services is essential. The availability of support personnel with additional equipment will determine the extent of treatment that can be provided by the sideline physician. The sideline physician's training should be commensurate with the level of responsibility expected.

As for equipment for the management of head injuries, a sphygmomanometer is recommended. A mask that can be tightly applied to the face and a bag to provide positive-pressure ventilation should be available. Whether endotracheal intubation and the capacity to maintain an intravenous line will be options in field-side management should be determined in advance. In the vast majority of cases, blood loss will not be an issue, and the person rendering first aid will deal only with airway and ventilation.

Since a blow sufficiently severe to render a person unconscious is also strong enough to cause a cervical spine fracture, one should assume that any unconscious person also has a broken neck. During resuscitation and transport of the fallen athlete, distortion of the neck should be avoided and removal of helmets and other protective equipment (but see below) should be done with gentle in-line manual traction to maintain cervical alignment. If physicians are responsible for the care of American football players, they should familiarize themselves with the design and disassembly of helmets and face masks in use by the teams they serve. Specific equipment such as screwdrivers, electricians' wire cutters, and bolt cutters should be kept available.[17] The hazards of helmet removal must be understood.[18] Several people are required to safely remove the helmet of an unconscious athlete.[19] One individual maintains in-line traction on the neck, a second removes the chinstrap, mouthpiece, face mask, etc. and cuts away all equipment impairing the airway access. Another person slides a hand under the occiput to support the head and neck in a neutral position while the helmet is spread at the earholes and gently withdrawn. With airway and ventilation assured, unconscious competitors should be transferred forthwith to the emergency department of a hospital with a neurosurgical service.

Evaluation of severity

In virtually every significant diffuse brain injury there is a period of amnesia that surrounds the impact that caused it.[20,21] As we record new memories, they are initially somewhat volatile. With a significant blow to the head, the last memories prior to impact are lost. This backward loss of memory is called retrograde amnesia (**RGA**). The retrograde amnesia may initially be of long duration but tends to shrink with the passage of time. It is generally considered to be less reliable an indicator of the severity of injury than the memory gap that follows the injury, the period of post-traumatic amnesia (**PTA**). Even though a head-injury patient may superficially appear to be normal, if one questions the subject, say 3 months after injury,

Table 1	Severity of concussion	
Grade	LOC	PTA
1—Mild	No	< 30 min
2—Moderate	< 5 min	> 30 min
3—Severe	> 5 min	> 24 h

From ref. 25. LOC, loss of consciousness; PTA, post-traumatic amnesia.

one may discover that the patient has no recall of a period of several days or even several weeks. In the mildest cases, there may be no loss of consciousness but there may be a period of amnesia.

The duration of PTA is thought to depend on, or is taken as an indication of, the severity of brain injury. In clinical practice it is usually determined in retrospect. A 'real time' measure of emergence from PTA has recently been described[22,23] and compared to the standard instrument for the determination of the duration of post-traumatic amnesia, the Galveston Orientation and Amnesia Test (**GOAT**).[24] Injured athletes may be asked to recall three simple words as a test of their ability to record new memories. Each word should be looked at for 10 s and read aloud. Immediate and 24-h recall should then be tested. Failure to recall all three words perfectly means that PTA persists and further exposure to risk, that is, return to play, should be deferred. The three-word test may be repeated until the words are recalled correctly.

Concussion may be classified as mild, moderate, or severe, as indicated in Table 1.[25] In the mild category, there is only a brief memory gap without loss of consciousness. In severe concussion there is coma and PTA. In the past, it was believed that a brief loss of consciousness was the result of a physiological disruption of brain function only, and that 'concussion' was a completely reversible condition. We now know that recovery after a concussion is not complete, but rather there is death of some neurones and a cumulative effect if concussion is repeated.[26,27]

Since 1975, neuropsychological tests which evaluate the subject's ability to rapidly process information have been available.[28] These tests, applied to athletes who have suffered repeated concussions, indicate that the effect of repeated injury is cumulative and that recovery occurs more slowly and less completely with each successive injury. It has been well known for a long time that injury severity correlates well with the length of a boxing career and the number of bouts fought.[29] Figure 10 shows the severe cerebral atrophy and cavum septum pellucidum that may result from repeated blows to the head.

Return to play guidelines

Any confusion, loss of consciousness, or focal neurological deficit in a player is sufficient cause for withdrawal from the game. A series of guidelines for return to play after concussion is shown in Table 2. The guidelines are predicated on the observations that the effect of repeated concussion is cumulative and that, infrequently, a minor blow to the head shortly after a significant head injury may be catastrophic.[30,31] It is known from animal experimentation that following a brain injury, autoregulation (that is to say, the maintenance of constant cerebral blood flow through a range of systemic arterial

pressures) is lost.[32] It is thought that impaired autoregulation may predispose to fulminant cerebral oedema following a concussion. The recovery of autoregulation after a cerebral insult may take several weeks.[33] We propose that 6 weeks is likely to be sufficient time for the restitution of normal cerebral vascular reactivity. Should second-impact syndrome be suspected, rapid intubation, hyperventilation, and an intravenous osmotic diuretic are recommended.[34]

After a mild concussion, a player may return to play if he is well for 1 week. Persistent headache, difficulty concentrating, memory impairment, or neurological deficit after 1week not only precludes return to play but is an indication for a complete neurological examination and possibly a CT scan. A second mild concussion warrants a longer recess from competition, and a third concussion, longer still. For moderate concussions, a recess of 2 weeks is recommended after the first injury, 6 weeks after the second, and suspension for the season after the third. For severe concussions, a suspension of 6 weeks is recommended to allow for the restoration of autoregulation. A second severe concussion, at minimum, requires suspension of play for the duration of the season and should lead to consideration of abandoning the sport altogether. A third severe concussion precludes further play for the individual in all contact sports. It should be recognized that certain individuals are at greater risk than their companions in the performance of particular athletic activities. Those who suffer repeated injuries should be directed to other less dangerous sports.

Advocacy

Many sports can be made safer by rule changes, improved equipment, or the recognition by coaches that certain practices are dangerous. For example, North American football players used to be directed to tackle by striking the numbers on the opposing player's jersey with their helmets. While often effective in stopping the oncoming runner, the practice, called spearing, sometimes resulted in a broken neck for the tackler. As a result of coaching and rule changes, the incidence of such injuries in North American football has declined.[35] It is important that coaches be reminded and that rules are enforced if the benefits to players are to be maintained.[36]

Some activities, by their very nature, are unacceptably hazardous

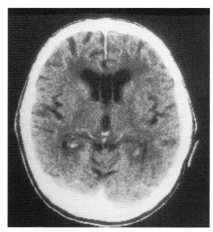

Fig. 10 There is severe cerebral atrophy and a cavum septum pellucidum, findings that may result from repeated blows to the head. Such changes may be correlated with the length of a boxing career and the number of bouts fought.

Table 2 Return to play after concussion

	First concussion	Second concussion	Third concussion
Grade 1 (mild)	Play if OK for 1 week	Play if OK for 2 weeks	Off 6 weeks, then play if OK for 1 week
Grade 2 (moderate)	Play if OK for 2 weeks	Off 6 weeks, then play if OK for 1 week	Off for the season, play next year if OK
Grade 3 (severe)	Off 6 weeks, then play if OK for 1 week	Off for the season, play next year if OK	Desist from contact sports

Modified from ref. 25.

and should be discontinued. With the knowledge that repeated head blows are cumulative in their effect, one cannot condone boxing as a civilized sporting activity. Proponents and opponents of boxing tend to focus on the infrequent catastrophic ring injuries, but, in fact, the repeated head blows suffered by thousands of participants (in the belief that they are getting healthy exercise and building character) are of much greater concern.[37] Since the object in a boxing match is to knock out one's opponent, that is to inflict permanent brain damage, the activity must be repugnant to all responsible physicians. In preventing injury, the ringside physician is about as effective as the priest at a judicial hanging.

Bicycling, which has always been a popular sport in Europe, is now being practised by an increasing number of people in North America. It is estimated that 85 million people in the United States ride bicycles and that bicycling injuries accounted for an estimated 574 000 emergency-room visits and 1300 deaths in the United States during 1985.[38] The most common cause of death and serious disability in those bicycle accidents was head injury. The use of bicycle helmets significantly reduces the severity of head injuries among cyclists,[38] but many people, especially children, are reluctant to wear them. Although children attending a summer day-camp were educated about helmets and were compliant during camp, they ceased wearing them as soon as camp was over.[39] A British study compared injury patterns in cyclist wearers and non-wearers of helmets attending an emergency department. Wearing a helmet decreased the odds of suffering a head injury by a factor of 3.25.[40] In Queensland, Australia, where wearing bicycle helmets became compulsory in 1991, the incidence of bicycle-related head injuries in children dropped from 47 per 100 000 population to 18 per 100 000.[40,41]

The modification of public opinion and practice in bicycling is beginning to produce benefit, but attitudes regarding the use of helmets for Western-style equestrianism lag behind. Only 2 out of 155 patients involved in horseback riding injuries were wearing helmets, although head injury occurred in 92 per cent of the injured riders and accounted for 11 deaths.[42] Acceptance of helmets by English-style riders are somewhat better.[43]

Helmets produce their effect as the liner is crushed on impact. Deceleration of the head is spread over the time and distance that the liner is crushed, and hence the peak acceleration of the skull and its contents is reduced. Helmets containing head forms equipped with accelerometers are tested by dropping them on hard surfaces or anvils.[44] In this way, the effect upon deceleration of design and material changes can be evaluated. The crushable material is chosen to be appropriate for the particular impact against which it is

intended to protect. Motorcycle helmets, for example, have much stiffer linings than those intended for bicycling because they must cushion against impact at higher speeds. At the high-speed impacts expected in motorized vehicle collisions the wearer's head would completely crush the helmet's polystyrene foam (Styrofoam) liner and 'bottom out' against the hard outer shell resulting in an abrupt deceleration and worse brain injury. Bicycle helmets are intended to mitigate the impact when a cyclist falls off the bicycle and strikes the ground. If, in a collision, the cyclist is swept up on the front of the car and accelerated to the speed of the car, the helmet will provide insufficient protection on impact with the ground. All helmets are a compromise in that sufficient padding to render a blow completely harmless would be too bulky and heavy to be worn.

The most effective helmets currently available have certain features. An external hard plastic shell is necessary to diffuse, over a wider area, the impact of striking or being struck by a relatively small object. Penetration of a relatively sharp object may also be prevented by a hard but not a 'soft shell' of netting or cloth. As the crushable liner has been designed to be appropriate to the expected deceleration forces that are most likely to occur on impact during a particular activity, a helmet intended for one activity should not be used for another purpose. Once crushed, the liner no longer cushions adequately and the helmet should not be reused. As a rule, one should choose a helmet certified for a particular sport by a responsible agency in one's own country, for example the Canadian Standards Association (**CSA**), the American National Standards Institute, Inc. (**ANSI**), the Snell Memorial Foundation, Inc., and so on. These agencies also specify testing procedures for the chin strap and harness. Approval means that the helmet is less likely to slip or fly off at the moment of impact.

After the safety criteria have been met, then style and comfort are also factors to consider. Look for adequate ventilation, unobstructed vision, and attractive colour. If the user looks and feels good, the helmet is more likely to be worn.

Helmets do not attenuate the forces applied to the cervical spine sufficiently to prevent neck injuries. After the introduction of helmets to ice hockey there was an increase in the number of cervical spine fractures because players felt invulnerable. Physicians should caution against unreasonable expectations for protective equipment.

Recreational athletic activity is fun and healthy for almost all participants. High-level competition adds increased enjoyment for those athletes who are sufficiently trained and skilful. Head injuries, even apparently mild ones, are so devastating that they must be avoided at all costs. Responsible physicians must promote only those recreational activities where the risk of head injury does not out-weigh the benefits of participation.

References

1. Tator CH. *Report of the Ontario Sport Medicine Advisory Board*, Vol. II. Province of Ontario: Ministry of Tourism and Recreation, 1987.

2. Tator CH, Edmonds V, Lapczak L. Analysis of 1594 cases of catastrophic injuries in sports and recreation with a view to injury prevention. *The Canadian Journal of Neurological Sciences* 1996; **23** (Suppl. 1): S31.

3. Benton AL. Historical notes on the postconcussion syndrome. In: Levin HS, Eisenberg HM, Benton AL, eds. *Mild head injury.* New York: Oxford University Press, 1989: 3–7.

4. Dacey RG Jr. Complications after apparently mild head injury and strategies of neurosurgical management. In: Levin HS, Eisenberg HM, Benton AL, eds. *Mild head injury.* New York: Oxford University Press, 1989: 83–101.

5. Strich SJ. Cerebral trauma. In: Blackwood W, Corsellis JAN, eds. *Greenfield's neuropathology.* Chicago: Year Book Medical Publishers, Inc., 1976: 327–60.

6. Schwartz ML, Hudson AR, Fernie GR, Hayashi K, Coleclough AA. Biomechanical study of full-contact karate contrasted with boxing. *Journal of Neurosurgery* 1986; **64**: 248–52.

7. Canadian Standards Association. *Cycling helmets.* Toronto, Ontario: Publication No. CAN/CSA-D113.2-M89, September 1989.

8. Stuss DT, Ely P, Hugenholtz H, Richard MT, LaRochelle S, Poirer CA, Bell I. Subtle neuropsychological deficits in patients with good recovery after closed head injury. *Neurosurgery* 1985; 41–7.

9. Jennett B, Teasdale G. Dynamic pathology. In: Jennett B, Teasdale G, eds. *Management of head injuries.* Philadelphia: FA Davis Co., 1981: 45–75.

10. Alexander MP. The role of neurobehavioral syndromes in the rehabilitation and outcome of closed head injury. In: Levin HS, Grafman J, Eisenberg HM, eds. *Neurobehavioral recovery from head injury.* New York, Oxford: Oxford University Press, 1987: 191–205.

11. Devor M. Plasticity in the adult nervous system. In: Illis LS, Sedgwick EM, Glanville HJ, eds. *Rehabilitation of the neurological patient.* Oxford: Blackwell Scientific Publications, 1982: 44–84.

12. Prigatano GP. Psychiatric aspects of head injury: Problem areas and suggested guidelines for research. In: Levin HS, Grafman J, Eisenberg HM, eds. *Neurobehavioral recovery from head injury.* New York, Oxford: Oxford University Press, 1987: 215–31.

13. Teasdale G, Jennett B. Assessment of coma and impaired consciousness: A practical scale. *Lancet* 1974; **2**: 81–4.

14. Jennett B, Teasdale G. Assessment of impaired consciousness. In: Jennett B, Teasdale G, eds. *Management of head injuries.* Philadelphia: FA Davis Co., 1981: 77–93.

15. Committee on Trauma. *Advanced trauma life support instructor manual.* Chicago: American College of Surgeons, 1994.

16. Rubin A. Emergency equipment: What to keep on the sidelines. The *Physician and Sportsmedicine* 1993; **21**: 47–54.

17. Putman LA. Alternative methods for football helmet face mask removal. *Journal of Athletic Training* 1992; **27**: 170–2.

18. Segan RD, Cassidy C, Bentkowski J. A discussion of the issue of football helmet removal in suspected cervical spine injuries. *Journal of Athletic Training* 1993; **28**: 294–305.

19. Feld F. Management of the critically injured football player. *Journal of Athletic Training* 1993; **28**: 206–12.

20. Corkin SH, Hurt RW, Twitchell TE, Franklin LC, Yin RK. Consequences of nonpenetrating and penetrating head injury: Retrograde amnesia posttraumatic amnesia, and lasting effects on cognition. In: Levin HS, Grafman J, Eisenberg HM, eds. *Neurobehavioral recovery from head injury.* New York, Oxford: Oxford University Press, 1987: 318–29.

21. Crovitz HF. Techniques to investigate posttraumatic and retrograde amnesia after head injury. In: Levin HS, Grafman J, Eisenberg HM, eds. *Neurobehavioral recovery from head injury.* New York, Oxford: Oxford University Press, 1987: 330–40.

22. Schwartz ML, Stuss DT, Carruth F, *et al.* The course of posttraumatic amnesia. *Canadian Journal of Neurological Sciences* 1995, **22** (Suppl. 1): S20.

23. Schwartz ML, Stuss DT, Carruth F, *et al.* The course of posttraumatic amnesia: three little words. *Canadian Journal of Neuroscience* 1996 (In press.)

24. Levin HS, O'Donnell VM, Grossman RG. Galveston Orientation and Amnesia Test: A practical scale to assess cognition after head injury. *Journal of Nervous and Mental Diseases* 1979; **167**: 675–84.

25. Cantu RC. Guidelines for return to contact sports after a cerebral concussion. *The Physician and Sportsmedicine* 1986; **14**: 75–83.

26. Gronwall D, Wrightson P. Cumulative effect of concussion. *Lancet*, November 1975; **ii**: 995–7.

27. Gronwall D. Cumulative and persisting effects of concussion on attention and cognition. In: Levin HS, Eisenberg HM, Benton AL, eds. *Mild head injury.* New York: Oxford University Press, 1989: 153–62.

28. Gronwall D, Wrightson P. Memory and information processing capacity after closed head injury. *Journal of Neurology, Neurosurgery and Psychiatry* 1981; **44**: 889–95.

29. Corsellis JAN, Bruton CJ, Freeman-Browne D. The aftermath of boxing. *Psychological Medicine* 1973; **3**: 270–303.

30. Saunders RL, Harbaugh RE. The second impact in catastrophic contact-sports head trauma. *Journal of the American Medical Association* 1984; **252**: 538–9.

31. Kelley JP, Nichols JS, Filley CM, Lillehei KO, Rubinstein D, Kleinschmidt-DeMasters BK. Concussion in sports: Guidelines for the prevention of catastrophic outcome. *Journal of the American Medical Association* 1991; **266**: 2867–9.

32. Lewelt W, Jenkins LW, Miller JD. Autoregulation of cerebral blood flow after experimental fluid percussion injury of the brain. *Journal of Neurosurgery* 1980; **53**: 500–11.

33. Paulson OB, Lassen NA, Skinhøj E. Regional cerebral blood flow in apoplexy without arterial occlusion. *Neurology* 1970; **20**: 125–38.

34. Cantu RC. Second impact syndrome: Immediate management. *The Physician and Sportsmedicine* 1992; **20**: 55,58,66.

35. Schneider RC, Peterson TR, Anderson RE. Football. In: Schneider RC, Kennedy JC, Plant ML, eds. *Sports injuries.* Baltimore, MD: Williams and Wilkins, 1985: 1–63.

36. Heck JF. The incidence of spearing by high school football ball carriers and their tacklers. *Journal of Athletic Training* 1992; **27**: 120–4.

37. Barth JT, Alves WM, Ryan TV, *et al.* Mild head injury in sports: Neuropsychological sequelae and recovery of function. In: Levin HS, Eisenberg HM, Benton AL, eds. *Mild head injury.* New York: Oxford University Press, 1989: 257–75.

38. Thompson RS, Rivara FP, Thompson DC. A case-control study of the effectiveness of bicycle safety helmets. *New England Journal of Medicine* 1989; **320**: 1361–7.

39. Winn GL, Jones DF, Bonk CJ. Taking it to the streets: Helmet use and bicycle safety as components of inner-city youth development. *Clinical Pediatrics* 1992; **31**: 672–7.

40. Maimaris C, Summers CL, Browning C, Palmer CR. Injury patterns in cyclists attending an accident and emergency department: A comparison of helmet wearers and non-wearers. *British Medical Journal* 1994; **308**: 1537–40.

41. Pitt WR, Thomas S, Nixon J, Clark R, Battistutta D, Acton C.

Trends in head injuries among child bicyclists. *British Medical Journal* 1994; **308**: 177–8.

42. Hamilton MG, Tranmer BI. Nervous system injuries in horse-back-riding accidents. *Journal of Trauma* 1993; **34**: 227–32.

43. Nelson DE, Rivara FP, Condie C. Helmets and horseback riders. *American Journal of Preventive Medicine* 1994; **10**: 15–19.

44. Bishop PJ, Briard BD. Impact performance of bicycle helmets. *Canadian Journal of Applied Sports Science* 1984; **9**: 94–101.

7.7 Injuries to the wrist and carpus

Gary R. McGillivary

Introduction

The wrist is very prone to injury in all walks of life, and athletic endeavours are no exception to this. In collision sports, the wrist is frequently injured because we naturally defend ourselves by raising our arms and hands. In non-collision sports, falls are very common and most of them occur with an outstretched hand in a dorsiflexed position with the wrist bearing the brunt of the force. In sports in which clubs, bats, or sticks are used, both direct and indirect blows to the wrist may be incurred. In indirect blows, the force is transmitted through the club to the wrist. Given the frequency with which this area is injured, it is essential that anyone treating athletes becomes familiar with the large variety of injuries that may occur.[1] Many of the injuries are rather unusual, and exact diagnosis and treatment may only be obtainable from someone seeing large numbers of patients with such injuries. None the less, it is important for those involved in the primary care of athletes to have an appropriate level of awareness and concern about the types of pathology that may be present.

As entire textbooks have been written about wrist injuries, we shall highlight only the diagnosis and treatment possibilities in this chapter. For an in-depth review of any given injury, the reader is referred to the large number of textbooks and treatises available on the various subjects (see Further Reading and refs 2 and 4).

Anatomy

The bony and ligamentous anatomy of the wrist is very complex and in many ways is still not completely understood. Controversy surrounds the exact description of the various ligamentous structures and the functional anatomy of the write.[2-4] For the most part, however, the details of these controversies will not affect the day-to-day treatment of athletes, at least at this point, and therefore will not be dealt with in detail.

In teaching health professionals, physicians, residents, and other orthopaedic surgeons about the wrist and its anatomy, the single most important anatomical fact to be addressed is that it is not a single joint. Thus we refer to the wrist area and not to the wrist joint.

The wrist is a complicated arrangement of the radius and ulna articulating with one another at the distal radio-ulnar joint and in turn articulating with the scaphoid, lunate, and triquetrum at the radiocarpal joint. The radiocarpal joint itself also has specific joints each with their own problems and pathology, such as the radio-scaphoid joint, the radiolunate joint, the ulnolunate joint, and the ulnotriquetral articulation. In addition, the scaphoid, lunate, and triquetrum all articulate with each other. The pisiform bone resides as a sesamoid in the flexor carpi ulnaris tendon and articulates with the triquetrum at the pisotriquetral joint. Moving distally, one encounters the so-called midcarpal joint, which again is a series of articulations comprised of the scaphotrapeziotrapezoid joint and the scaphocapitate and capitolunate joints, and finally the four-quadrant area of the wrist where the capitate, lunate, triquetrum, and hamate all meet.

This network of bones and joints is supported by a complicated series of ligamentous structures. The most vital ligaments are the stout palmar-sided wrist ligaments. The exact course and appropriate nomenclature for each of these ligaments is still controversial, but there is no controversy surrounding the fact that these ligaments are critical in maintaining the normal relationships between carpal bones and therefore maintaining normal wrist kinematics.

In addition to the palmar ligaments, there are significant interosseus ligaments between the scaphoid and the lunate and between the lunate and the triquetrum (Fig. 1). These run in a sheet-like fashion from the dorsal to volar side between the carpal bones discussed above. The mid-portion of these ligaments is less stout and

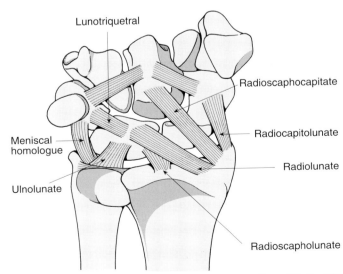

Fig. 1 A schematic of volar wrist ligaments (redrawn from Green DP. *Operative hand surgery*, New York: Churchill Livingstone, 1985: 14, with permission).

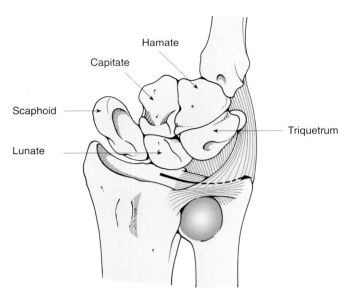

Fig. 2 A diagrammatic representation of the structures comprising the triangular fibrocartilage complex (redrawn from Green DP. *Operative hand surgery*. New York: Churchill Livingstone, 1988: 946, with permission).

more of an interosseus membrane than a ligament. The dorsal ligaments are less well defined and of much less clinical importance than the volar and interosseus ligaments.

Arising from the ulnar surface of the radius and extending distal to the distal ulna and blending with the ulnar and volar wrist ligaments is the triangular fibrocartilage complex (Fig. 2). This structure is comprised of a number of different components and serves a number of vital functions in this area, ranging from acting as a shock absorber on the ulnar side of the carpus to aiding in the stabilization of the carpus and the distal radio-ulnar joint.[5] This structure may become involved in a number of pathological processes, both degenerative and acute injuries alike.

In summary, the anatomy of the wrist is very complex and intricate. Multiple articulations are present, all of which must be considered individually when discussing any significant wrist pathology, and the ligamentous structures in the wrist are significant structures which contribute in an important fashion to normal wrist kinematics and therefore to wrist function. The importance of envisaging the wrist not as a joint but as a series of small joints cannot be overemphasized.

History and physical examination

As in all patient encounters, the initial history and physical examination are the most important part of arriving at a diagnosis and embarking on a plan of treatment in dealing with an athlete with an acutely injured or chronically painful wrist.

The history should include whether there has been a significant injury recently or remotely and the exact nature of this injury, if possible. Details of the amount of force involved and, if possible, the position of the hand and wrist and upper extremity at the time of the injury should be obtained. In addition to this information, it is critical to enquire as to the exact nature and location of the pain; it is not enough simply to ascertain that it is the wrist that is sore, it should also be ascertained whether it is the dorsal radial or the volar radial aspect of the wrist. The patient should simply be asked to

indicate the area from which the pain appears to be emanating. In this way information is obtained as to where the patient locates the source of the pain. In addition to this, in many patients who have complaints of chronic pain rather than an acute injury, the magnitude of the pain and the amount of disability it produces are important pieces of information. It is important to decide whether the patient is having pain that can be described as a nuisance, or whether the pain is disabling the individual and has prevented him or her from performing normal activities.

Of course, inquiries must also be made about the presence or absence of neurological symptoms, vascular symptoms, symptoms elsewhere in the extremity, and general functions as would be done in any initial encounter with a patient.

Physical examination of the wrist should be careful, methodical, and very precise, as, unlike most other areas of the body, we are dealing with a very large number of structures confined in a very small space. Precise examination is of the utmost importance.

The first component of the examination is inspection. On initially examining the wrist one should look carefully for any signs of deformity and any areas of localized discoloration or swelling, and note how the patient uses the hand and wrist and entire upper extremity as he or she carries on normal activities throughout the interview. Valuable information can be gained in this fashion. Noting the exact location and the exact nature of any deformities or swellings is of critical importance.

The next step in the physical examination should be careful assessment of the neurological and vascular status of the hand involved. This includes not only checking pulses and capillary refill but examining the extremity to determine whether it is warmer or colder than the opposite extremity, again noting any discoloration present. The neurological examination should check specific muscle function, in particular the thenar musculature innervated by the median nerve and the ulnar innervated musculature. Two-point discrimination in all digits is quickly and easily assessed and is a reasonably sensitive method for assessing sensation in the hand.

A careful assessment of both an active and a passive range of motion of the wrist should be performed and it should always be compared with the opposite wrist, noting in the history whether there had been any problems with the opposite extremity. Specifically, all planes of motion in the wrist should be checked, including dorsiflexion, palmar flexion, radial deviation, and ulnar deviation, pronation and supination. A note should be made of whether any discomfort is present with any of these motions and whether it is limited to the extremes of movement.

When palpating the wrist, one should begin well away from the area where the patient claims to have the most discomfort. All the specific areas of the wrist should be carefully examined with pinpoint thumb pressure and the source from which the pain seems to emanate should be noted as exactly as possible. If this is done quickly or in a cursory fashion, not much information will be gained. If this technique is practised and is applied carefully and precisely, a great deal of information can be gained about the specific and exact location of pathology from this part of the examination. Specific areas that should be carefully examined are the distal radio-ulnar joint; the distal ulna; the region just distal to the distal ulna, where the triangular fibrocartilage complex lies; the distal radius itself; the radioscaphoid area; the scapholunate area; the radiolunate

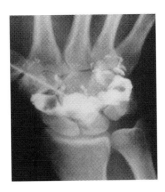
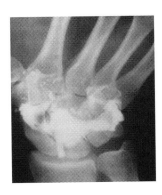
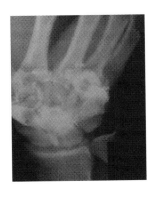

Fig. 3 A typical wrist arthrogram.

area; and the lunotriquetral area. In addition to this, the pisiform bone should be grasped and compressed against the triquetrum and moved in a radial and ulnar direction to see whether there is any pain or tenderness in the pisitriquetral joint. This pinpoint examination can be carried out dorsally, radially, ulnarly, and volarly.

There are a number of special tests that can be carried out on physical examination of the wrist which should also be carefully checked, particularly in patients presenting with a history of a recent or removed injury. The first of these is the triquetral ballotment test. This is a specific test for lunotriquetral ligament integrity and whether or not there is lunotriquetral instability. To perform this test the lunate and carpus of the involved wrist are stabilized with the thumb and index finger of one hand. The triquetrum and pisiform can easily be grasped and moved in a dorsal and volar direction with the thumb and index finger of the other hand. Some practice is required to perform this test properly and to learn to assess it, but with experience one can determine whether the amount of motion present is excessive and also whether there is any crepitation associated with this manoeuvre and whether it produces pain. A great deal of information can be obtained in this fashion.

The next specific test is known as the Watson manoeuvre. This test (first described by Dr Kirk Watson) is a specific test for scapholunate ligamentous disruption, or scaphoid instability. The manoeuvre is performed by having the patient supinate the forearm; the affected wrist is then moved into ulnar deviation and pressure is applied to the volar aspect of the scaphoid (the scaphoid tubercle), with one thumb. With pressure applied in this manner, the wrist is then forcibly moved from ulnar deviation into radial deviation. In changing from ulnar to radial deviation the normal scaphoid tubercle will move in a volar direction as the scaphoid palmar flexes to avoid impinging upon the radial styloid as the wrist moves into radial deviation. If a scapholunate dissociation is present or if the scaphoid is unstable, pressure on the volar aspect of the scaphoid with the thumb will prevent this normal palmar flexion of the scaphoid and an audible 'clunk' will be produced and/or the patient will experience pain.

The final special test is for midcarpal instability, which is very uncommon. The examiner grasps the patient's distal forearm with one hand, and with the other takes the patient's hand. The patient is asked to relax. Once the patient has relaxed, pressure is applied to the distal hand in a volar direction. If there is any associated midcarpal instability, there will be an obvious 'clunk' with a zigzag deformity produced in the wrist. This is a rather dramatic physical finding when present.

Radiographic and ancillary investigations

Following a careful history and physical examination, one has a large amount of information available with which to approach the diagnosis and treatment of a patient with an injured or painful wrist. Further information can now be gained using radiographic and other investigations as seem to be indicated.

Simple anteroposterior and lateral radiographs of the involved wrist are very useful. Review of these radiographs will allow not only the diagnosis of some of the more obvious and dramatic wrist injuries, but also may reveal very subtle abnormalities or signs which may offer clues as to the exact diagnosis in many patients with subtle or rare injuries. These radiographs can only be interpreted after appropriate teaching and experience.

Following physical and radiographic examination a significant number of individuals will require further investigation to determine their diagnosis. A large number of ancillary investigations are possible and not all of these are useful in any one individual. Therefore the investigation should probably proceed on an individual basis.

Technetium pyrophosphate scanning has become increasingly useful to help localize wrist pathology in some patients and has also been used as a screening device in chronic wrist pain. Cineradiography, CT, magnetic resonance imaging (**MRI**), and cine-MRI are all possible methods which can be used in the investigation of individual patients, but the indications for these modalities are somewhat limited.

Wrist arthrography has been used extensively to investigate wrist pathology, particularly for injuries to various ligamentous structures such as the lunotriquetral ligaments, the scapholunate ligaments, and the triangular fibrocartilage complex (Fig. 3). In recent years techniques have been improved and the information gained has been more beneficial. However, because of the advent of wrist arthroscopy, the present author has not used wrist arthrography to any great extent. Arthroscopy of the wrist has become increasingly popular over the past few years as a means of not only arriving at specific diagnoses but also carrying out arthroscopic surgery to treat certain kinds of pathology.

A number of studies[6,7] have shown that wrist arthroscopy provides more specific and better information than wrist arthrography. The radiocarpal joint, including the volar wrist ligaments and interosseus ligaments as well as the triangular fibrocartilage complex, can all be directly assessed through a variety of portals. In addition, the midcarpal joint can also be carefully examined directly using the arthroscope. This has led to a better understanding of the various kinds of pathology affecting the wrist, particularly ligamentous injuries and injuries to the triangular fibrocartilage complex.

Fractures

Fractures about the wrist are extremely common and athletes are no exception to this. Falls on the outstretched dorsiflexed hand are the most common source of these injuries, but some are produced by indirect trauma. Detailed accounts of the treatment of many of these injuries are given in standard orthopaedic textbooks and no attempt will be made here to supplant these.

Distal radial fractures

Fractures of the distal radius are the most common fracture occurring in the upper extremity. The diagnosis of these injuries is generally straightforward, with the patient presenting after a fall on the outstretched hand. The patient will describe an immediate onset of pain, swelling, and frequently deformity.

Physical examination will reveal marked swelling and often a significant deformity through the region of the wrist. The neurological and vascular status of the hand should be very carefully examined as some of these injuries will be associated with significant soft tissue injury, including injuries to the nerve and blood vessels crossing the region of the injury. Radiography confirms the diagnosis and reveals the degree of angulation, displacement, and comminution present at the fracture site. All this information should be carefully and specifically noted. Particular attention should be paid to whether the fracture extends into any of the joints, and specifically whether it is a radioscaphoid joint or, more importantly, the lunate fossa of the radius. In addition, one must remember to assess whether the fracture is intra-articular at the distal radio-ulnar joint. Frequently, the fact that these fractures are intra-articular is not noted.

Traditional treatment has been closed reduction and cast immobilization. More recently, however, clinical reviews of fractures treated in this fashion have shown a high incidence of unsatisfactory results; specifically, in one series only approximately 5 per cent of all patients sustaining a fracture of the distal radius had what could be considered an excellent outcome.[8] Studies have generally shown poor results in these fractures, particularly in young active patients. This has led to a more aggressive approach to the treatment of 'simple' fractures, particularly in young people.

When an athlete presents with such an injury the aim is obviously to restore function to as normal a state as possible as quickly as possible. Most studies support the fact that the best way of achieving this aim is to restore anatomy as closely as possible to normal, to attain early union, and, if possible, to begin early motion.

A number of classification systems have been developed for fractures of the distal radius and a large number of eponyms are associated with them. The present author prefers to avoid the use of eponyms when dealing with fractures of the distal radius, because they imply a certain amount of familiarity and disdain toward some very complex fractures. More often than not, one will hear phrases such as 'It's just a Colles' fracture' to describe what can be a potential career-ending injury for a young athlete. After the initial history, the physical examination, and a careful review of the radiographs have been completed, a plan should be formulated as to how best to manage the individual fracture. Consideration is given to such factors as fracture stability, comminution, and whether the fracture is intra-articular.

As in all fractures, the initial aim is to obtain an acceptable reduction. In a young adult this would include restoring the length of the radius to normal and correcting to neutral the angulation of its distal articular surface as viewed on a lateral radiograph, that is, ensuring that the distal articular face is perpendicular to the long axis of the radius. Normally, the distal articular surface of the radius tilts 10 to 14° in a palmar direction (Fig. 4). Correction to neutral is not an arbitrary requirement. Long-term follow-up of fractures of the distal radius with dorsal angulation, that is, angulation of the distal articular surface beyond neutral, reveals that these patients develop further problems with the carpus. The dorsal tilt of the distal radial surface leads to a dorsal tilt of the lunate and subsequently to palmar flexion of the capitate so that the hand is lined up with the radius. This produces the so-called zigzag collapse deformity of the capitate, lunate, and distal radius. This collapse deformity can subsequently lead to pain, ligamentous instability, and occasionally degenerative change in the carpus. If there is an intra-articular component to the fracture it has been shown that a step deformity of greater than 1 to 2 mm is unacceptable as this will lead to accelerated degenerative change.[9] The most critical joints to restore anatomically are the radiolunate joint, or the lunate fossa of the distal radius, and the distal radio–ulnar joint as reconstructive procedures for pain and arthrosis are often based around these two joints.

A closed reduction of the fracture is attainable and this reduction must be maintained. As stated earlier, it is generally believed that the results of cast immobilization in young patients, except for the most minor fractures, are unacceptable as the fractures lose their excellent reduction with simple cast immobilization (Fig. 5). Therefore the majority of these patients should be treated with an external fixation device to maintain the reduction in an acceptable position. If a reduction cannot be attained or maintained in this fashion, then formal open reduction with internal fixation may be required[10] (Fig. 6).

Complications of these fractures are frequent. Neurological injury, particularly median nerve dysfunction, occurs, although fortunately, vascular injury and compartment syndrome are both unusual. The more common complications include restriction of motion, arthrosis from non-congruent articular surfaces or as a result of excessive residual dorsal angulation, and ulnar-sided wrist pain and impingement due to lack of restoration of adequate radial length.

In summary, cavalier treatment of these fractures may lead to significant hand and wrist dysfunction, particularly in the young athlete. An aggressive approach seems indicated from the outset.

Scaphoid fractures

Scaphoid fractures occur very frequently. Again, these mainly occur as a result of a fall on the outstretched hand.

The initial presentation of a fractured scaphoid may be relatively minor symptoms of slight wrist discomfort on the radial aspect of the wrist with little or no swelling; the only physical finding may be slight discomfort over the volar tubercle of the scaphoid or in the region known as the anatomical snuff-box. If the initial radiograph

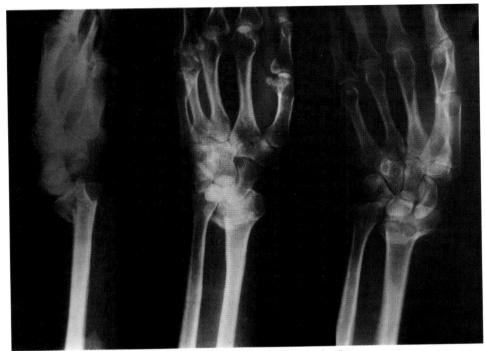

Fig. 4 An extra-articular fracture of the distal radius.

of the wrist reveals a fracture, then the diagnosis is fairly straight-forward. However, if the initial radiographs are normal, the situation may be more complicated. A patient with the above symptoms and physical findings and a normal radiograph is best treated by immobilization for 2 weeks followed by repeat radiographs in an effort to identify the fracture. If the patient remains symptomatic and the radiographs are still normal, a bone scan may be beneficial.

The aim of treating a scaphoid fracture is to attain anatomical union (Fig. 7).[11] The best treatment depends on a number of factors, such as the location of the fracture within the scaphoid and whether it is displaced or undisplaced. Displacement is far more important than location.

According to standard dogma 99 per cent of undisplaced scaph-

oid fractures will unite if treated appropriately from the time of injury. Appropriate treatment is said to consist of cast immobilization from the time of initial presentation until fracture union has occurred. The type of immobilization has varied over the years from a below-elbow thumb spica with the interphalangeal joint of the thumb free, to above-elbow casting to include immobilization of the interphalangeal joint of the thumb as well as the index and long fingers. More recent data suggest that the use of an above-elbow cast to include immobilization of the interphalangeal joint of the thumb for 3 weeks and subsequently a below-elbow version of the same spica would be adequate treatment.

The total time of immobilization required to gain union is extremely variable. It may be as short as 6 weeks or as long as a year,

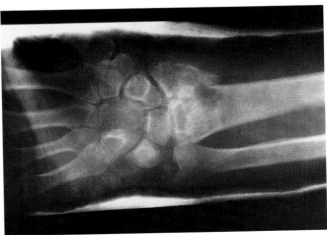

Fig. 5 An intra-articular fracture of the distal radius.

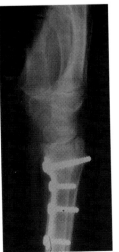
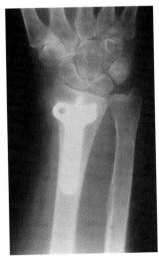

Fig. 6 A distal radius fracture following open reduction with internal fixation.

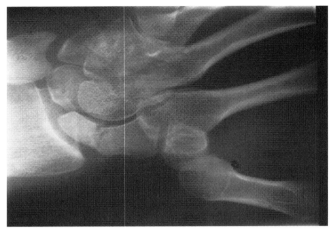

Fig. 7 A fractured scaphoid.

and the patient should be made aware of this fact from the time of initial presentation. The patient should be informed that the average time to union is 16 weeks and that only 50 per cent of scaphoid fractures are healed in 12 weeks. Of course, this means that a certain number of fractures takes a very long time to unite. Because such prolonged immobilization is unacceptable to many athletes (and workers), there may be some benefit in using early internal fixation of scaphoid fractures.[12] This allows short-term cast immobilization and hence earlier return to wrist motion and activity. This approach is currently under investigation in a number of centres, and may become more popular in subsequent years as methods of fixing the scaphoid internally are improved.

The difficulty in attaining union in such a seemingly minor fracture is directly related to the somewhat precarious blood supply to the scaphoid. Because the majority of the scaphoid consists of articular surface there are only a limited number of points where blood vessels enter this bone. In general, the blood supply is better in the distal portion of the bone and therefore fractures that occur proximally tend to be slower to heal. These fractures also have a higher incidence of non-union, but the exact incidence of this is not known.

The treatment of displaced scaphoid fractures is quite different from that for undisplaced fractures. Even apparently small amounts of displacement (1 mm) are considered to be significant. Such minor amounts of displacement are taken seriously because of the major ligamentous attachments to the scaphoid, as discussed in the section on anatomy. Displacement of fracture fragments by even 1 mm indicates that there is some form of ligamentous injury and therefore instability. This leads to difficulty in attaining union, but can also create long-term problems with carpal instability. Carpal instability is a very complex problem which requires an entire chapter of its own. It is sufficient to state that carpal instability occurs when there have been significant ligamentous injuries in the wrist which may lead to changes in the angular relationships between the carpal bones. Subsequently, this leads to abnormal wrist kinematics and secondary osteoarthritic change.

To avoid these difficulties, displaced fractures in the scaphoid are best treated with early open reduction and internal fixation to restore wrist anatomy as closely as possible to normal (Fig. 8). Obviously, depending on the amount of displacement of the fracture, the

associated ligamentous injury is variable. This will be discussed in more detail in the section on ligamentous injuries.

The major specific complication associated with fractures of the scaphoid is that of non-union. This is said to occur in only 1 per cent of cases if undisplaced fractures are treated from the time of injury. However, this number is based on very old data and may be too low. Proving that union has occurred is difficult, and there are many patients with scaphoid fractures said to have been united on the basis of plain radiographs when tomography reveals that the fracture line in the scaphoid is still clearly present and has not healed. Many of these patients are not symptomatic in the early stages.

The difficulty with non-union in the scaphoid is that, again, it may lead, to carpal instability. The scaphoid is a critical link between the proximal and distal rows of the carpus. With the link disrupted, wrist kinematics change and this leads to a specific pattern of degenerative arthritis in the wrist. Osteoarthritic change begins at the radioscaphoid joint and progresses through the scaphocapitate and capitolunate joints. Normally the radiolunate joint is spared and normal articular cartilage is present. All this degenerative change leads to a painful and stiff wrist. This specific form of degenerative arthritis is known as scapholunate advanced collapse (**SLAC**) or sometimes as a SLAC wrist. A salvage or reconstructive surgical procedure may be required to give these individuals relief from their pain. The exact frequency with which this complication occurs is not known. It has been suggested that it is the ultimate fate of all non-union scaphoids, but patients followed in all studies on this subject have been highly selected.[13] The incidence of asymptomatic non-union of long standing in the general population is not known. However, it does occur frequently, and therefore aggressive treatment for fresh scaphoid fractures and non-unions is probably justified in the young athlete.

Fractures of other carpal bones

Significant fractures of the other bones in the carpus are generally rare. Minor dorsal chip or capsular avulsion fractures are seen relatively frequently. After ascertaining that they are not associated with

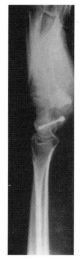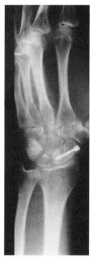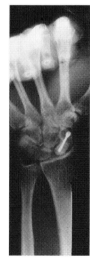

Fig. 8 A scaphoid fracture following open reduction with internal fixation and bone grafting.

major ligamentous disruptions in the carpus (discussed in detail in the section on ligament injuries), they can be treated with short-term immobilization for comfort, with an early return to motion and activity anticipated. Major fractures can be treated with casting alone if they are undisplaced; if they are displaced they will require open reduction and internal fixation to restore the joint surface to normal and produce a stable, normally functioning carpus.

One specific fracture that should be discussed here is that of the hook of the hamate. This rare injury is usually incurred by striking something solid with a club or a bat, and the force transmitted down the shaft results in fracture of the hook of the hamate. Patients will present with a typical history; frequently they are golfers who have struck a hidden tree root. They have pain and tenderness in the ulnar side of the palm. Symptoms of ulnar nerve irritation or compression may be present as this structure lies in close proximity within Guillon's canal. The diagnosis is confirmed with radiography, but the physician examining the patient must suspect this condition because a special radiographic view known as a carpal tunnel view is required to visualize the hook of the hamate adequately and see the fracture site.

If the diagnosis is made early and the fracture is undisplaced, a period of casting for 6 weeks, followed by repeat examination and radiography, is justified. If the presentation is late, the fracture is displaced, or union has not occurred following casting, surgical treatment is required. Treatment options consist of either excision of the fracture fragment or internal fixation of the fracture. Since no difference in the outcome of these two treatments has been shown, excision is favoured as internal fixation can be fraught with major complications such as ulnar nerve palsy.[14]

The major long-term complication of this fracture is rupture of the flexor digitorum profundus tendon to the little finger. This tendon, which passes directly across the fracture site as it moves through the carpal tunnel, becomes frayed and attenuated, and ultimately ruptures. It is for this reason that surgical treatment is justifiable, even if the patient is asymptomatic.

Ligamentous injuries

As discussed in the section on anatomy, a large number of functionally important ligaments support and maintain intercarpal relationships. It has recently been recognized that these ligaments are frequently injured. Unfortunately, these injuries are usually recognized late, either because the patient has assumed that the injury was minor or because the primary contact in the health care system makes the same assumption. Many of these patients have been told not to be concerned about the injury as it is only a sprained wrist. This information is partly correct in that the wrist is sprained; the problem lies in the fact that most of these so-called sprains are significant ligamentous tears that lead to long-term problems and complications. Consideration of each subtype of ligamentous injury and the various classifications available is beyond the scope of this chapter, but a discussion of the most common injuries is certainly warranted.

It is first necessary to understand that there are degrees of injuries that can occur. At one end of the spectrum is the 'sprained wrist', which follows a benign course, and at the other end is a carpal dislocation or a dislocation of the lunate. The spectrum of treatment will be as broad as the range of injuries. The major ligamentous

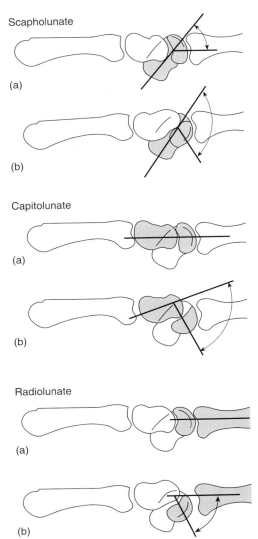

Fig. 9 A diagrammatic representation of various carpal angles as measured on the lateral radiographs (reproduced from Green DP. *Operative hand surgery*. New York: Churchill Livingstone, 1988: 891, with permission).

injuries are obviously dislocations of the wrist or of specific carpal bones (usually lunate, with all other dislocations being extremely rare).

These injuries are usually readily diagnosable as the patient presents with a swollen, often deformed, and very painful wrist associated with concomitant radiographic abnormalities. These injuries are devastating and are best treated with open reduction of the carpus, temporary pinning of the reduced carpus, repair of any ligaments that are reparable, and immobilization for 6 to 8 weeks. The aims of treatment are not to restore a normal wrist, but to attain a reasonable range of motion (60 to 80 per cent of normal) and perhaps 75 per cent of normal grip strength (Fig. 9). Attainment of normal carpal relationships on radiographs is very important. Other methods of treatment, such as closed reduction and casting, are outmoded because of the difficulties of maintaining normal carpal relationships. This inability to maintain critical relationships alters wrist kinematics irrevocably and leads to pain, stiffness, weakness, and in some instances degenerative arthritis, as has been discussed

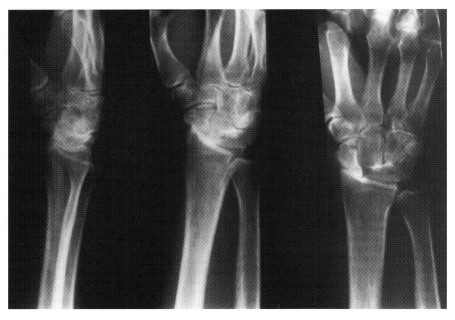

Fig. 10 A typical scapholunate advanced collapse (note advanced degenerative change at radioscaphoid and capitolunate joints).

previously. This phenomenon is known as carpal collapse and is easily diagnosed radiographically by those familiar with the normal carpal relationships and the measurement of specific carpal angles (e.g. the scapholunate, radiolunate, and capitolunate angles). Ultimately, the aim of the treatment of all ligamentous injuries about the wrist is the avoidance of significant carpal collapse.

The most common and more subtle ligamentous injury occurring in the wrist is scapholunate dissociation. This injury involves the ligaments of the scapholunate complex. Disruption of these ligaments allows the scaphoid to dissociate from the lunate. This means then that, in its most extreme form, the scaphoid rotates into an abnormal position of palmar fixation. These patients present with findings similar to those of a scaphoid fracture. Radiographs show no fractures, but radiographic abnormalities are often present. The fact that the scaphoid rotates into palmar flexion results in an abnormal gap between the scaphoid and the lunate on an anteroposterior plain radiograph of the wrist. This gap should be greater than 2 mm to be considered abnormal. In addition, the scaphoid appears to be foreshortened. On the lateral view of the wrist, specific angle changes occur which can be measured. (For further discussion, the reader is referred to more detailed works.[2,4]) These patients have an unstable scaphoid statically, as clearly the scaphoid is unstable even at rest with these abnormalities appearing on plain radiographs. In many instances, no radiographic abnormalities are identified on static films even though significant ligamentous injury has occurred.

The diagnosis of these injuries is often difficult even in experienced hands. The history is usually quite straightforward, with a fall on the outstretched hand being the mechanism of injury. Cineradiographs, an abnormal bone scan, and wrist arthroscopy may all be required to obtain an exact diagnosis and evaluation of scaphoid stability in these patients. Many of them have dynamic scaphoid instability, that is, at rest the scaphoid maintains its normal relationships to the remainder of the carpus, but when the wrist is loaded the attenuated ligaments do not maintain their position and the scaphoid becomes unstable. Arthroscopy shows obviously attenuated and disrupted ligaments, or disruption of one set of the three sets of ligaments that stabilize and support the scaphoid.

Treatment of scaphoid instability depends upon many factors, including the age and activity level of the patients and whether the diagnosis is made early or late. Early diagnosis is generally defined as within 3 weeks of the original injury. The degree of symptomatology and the wishes of the patient are also critical. The available treatments are varied and controversial and just one approach is presented here. The best treatment for an athlete with an acute scapholunate dissociation is to reduce the scaphoid to its normal position and K-wire it to the lunate and capitate temporarily. The reduction can be performed either closed or open. In addition, the patient is immobilized in a thumb spica case for 6 to 8 weeks. This allows time for some ligamentous healing to occur in the anatomical position. The patient is then generally mobilized and followed carefully with radiographs for signs of carpal collapse. Thumb spica immobilization with careful radiographic follow-up seems to be adequate treatment for those patients who may have an acute ligament injury but whose radiographs are normal. If radiographic abnormalities develop at any time in the early stages, more aggressive treatment can be applied.

There are significant differences in the individual presenting late with an unstable scaphoid. Ligamentous healing cannot occur, even if the scaphoid is reduced. Ligament reconstructions have been attempted in a number of centres, but without much success.

The first step in treating a patient with a late-presenting scapholunate dissociation is to have a detailed discussion with him or her about the magnitude of the symptoms. Treatment of the unrecognized unstable scaphoid involves significant surgical procedures, and many patients will want to leave well alone as they find their symptoms to be more of a nuisance than a major disability. However, if the patient's wrist is significantly disabled and he or she wishes something to be done, the next step should be a wrist arthroscopy (Fig. 10). This will allow diagnosis of the scapholunate ligament disruption to be confirmed, and will also allow the radioscaphoid joint to be assessed for degenerative change. Patients with scapholunate dissociation are at risk of the same long-term complications as those patients with a non-union of the scaphoid, that is, the specific form of degenerative arthritis known as scapholunate advanced collapse. The presence of degenerative change at the radioscaphoid joint will significantly alter the surgical management of these patients.

Given that no degenerative change is present and that the patient wishes some treatment to be applied, two choices are available.

The first, and certainly the most frequent, choice for most hand surgeons in North America is to attempt to stabilize the scaphoid in a good position by a limited carpal arthrodesis. Specifically, the most common procedure is an arthrodesis between the scaphoid, trapezium, and trapezoid, which is known as a triscaphe fusion or an STT arthodesis.[15] This is a significant surgical procedure producing reduction in wrist motion of approximately 35 per cent with a complication rate in published series approaching 52 per cent, including delayed union, non-union, infection, and neurological and vascular injury. At 10 year follow-up acceptable results were attained in approximately 80 per cent of cases.[16,17] It should be noted that these patients will develop excessive motion through other carpal joints and therefore are at high risk for the development of degenerative change elsewhere in the wrist following this procedure.

The other choice is an attempt to stabilize the scaphoid with a flap of the dorsal wrist capsule.[18] This is a much smaller operation in the sense that the reduction in wrist motion is far less, the time of immobilization is far shorter, and there are fewer complications. The problem with this particular procedure is that there are no large series available indicating how effective it is and what the results of long-term follow-up of the patients will be. Therefore patients must be told that the results of this procedure are basically unpredictable but that a certain number of them will benefit from the procedure. They should also be apprised of the fact that the downside risks of this operation are small, with a low complication rate, little restriction in wrist motion, and no risk of degenerative change elsewhere in the carpus as far as we are aware. For these reasons capsuldesis is the preferred first line of treatment in the very young patient or the very young athlete with scaphoid instability. Should this procedure fail, limited carpal arthrodesis can be considered as a second choice.

Other ligamentous injuries about the wrist are much less common than those of the scapholunate complex. In addition, the majority of other ligamentous injuries are not known to have major late sequelae such as degenerative arthritis. They tend to produce symptoms which are generally of a more minor nature than those associated with scapholunate instability. Given all this, the treatment of acutely injured ligaments can be short periods of immobilization for symptomatic relief. In the patient presenting with late ligamentous injuries, such as those with lunotriquetral instability, treatment can be predicted on the basis of the patient's symptoms. Specific instability can always be eliminated by some form of limited carpal arthrodesis, but with varying degrees of effectiveness in terms of symptomatic relief. For this reason these treatments are only embarked upon after careful discussion with the patient regarding the percentage of successful results, complications, and the amount of dysfunction produced by the surgical procedure.

These discussions are as important as, or more important than, the specific procedure carried out.

In summary, ligamentous injuries to the wrist represent a wide spectrum of injuries, many of which have been recognized with increasing frequency because of better awareness and improved diagnostic techniques such as wrist arthroscopy. Early recognition may lead to better treatment and the avoidance of long-term complications such as carpal collapse, degenerative arthritis, and the need for extensive surgical reconstruction.

The triangular fibrocartilage complex

The triangular fibrocartilage complex is another commonly injured structure in the wrist area. It is probably most frequently injured in association with fractures of the distal end of the radius. This injury may be represented by avulsion fracture of the ulnar styloid, as seen on plain radiographs in distal radius fractures. It can also be injured in isolation.

When injury to this structure is associated with distal radial fractures, it is obviously overshadowed by other symptoms and physical findings. In such cases adequate treatment of the fracture is all that is necessary, and these patients will rarely present with a fracture that has done well and a symptomatic tear of the triangular fibrocartilage complex. This does happen, but it is very uncommon. Patients presenting with an acute injury to the triangular fibrocartilage complex will have dorsal ulnar wrist pain and localized tenderness, and occasionally localized swelling. They may have symptoms of catching or locking with pronation and supination or with other wrist motions. Radiographs are normal, and it is often difficult to distinguish these patients from patients who have lunotriquetral tears and distal radio-ulnar joint pain.

One approach is to treat these individuals symptomatically, whereupon most will improve with time. Those that have persistent and aggravating symptoms can be considered as candidates for wrist arthroscopy, which is becoming the gold standard diagnostic tool for pathology in this region. During arthroscopy, the location and nature of the tear are evaluated. Classification systems for tears of the triangular fibrocartilage complex are available, but a significant number of patients will obtain symptomatic improvement from arthroscopic debridement of the tear. Other injuries, specifically avulsions from either the ulnar aspect or the radial aspect of the triangular fibrocartilage complex, will require reattachment to the radius or the ulna using either open or arthroscopic procedure for symptomatic relief to be obtained.

Distal radio-ulnar joint[19]

The distal radio-ulnar joint is also frequently injured, but the injuries are generally associated with more significant injuries such as distal radial fractures and tears of the triangular fibrocartilage complex. Isolated injuries are less common and frequently unrecognized. The patient will present acutely with pain and swelling, but generally little, if any, associated deformity. Initial physical examination will reveal tenderness well localized at the distal radio-ulnar joint. The pain is often exaggerated with full pronation and supination.

In the most dramatic cases, a frank dislocation of the joint occurs, and on a true lateral radiograph of the radius, the ulna is

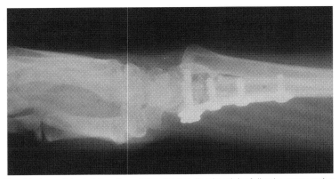

Fig. 11 A persistent dislocation of the distal radio-ulnar joint following open reduction with internal fixation of a distal radius fracture (note the dorsal location of the distal ulna on the lateral view).

identified most frequently dislocated dorsally and much less frequently dislocated volarly (Fig. 11). Acute injuries are easily treated with cast immobilization. Dorsally dislocated or unstable ulnas are treated with an above-elbow cast in full supination for 3 weeks, followed by 3 weeks of a below-elbow cast. Placing the arm in full supination reduces the dorsal dislocation and allows healing to occur in a reduced position. The opposite is true of the volarly unstable distal ulna where pronation is the position of stability for immobilization.

Most frequently, however, the patient will present late with vague symptoms of wrist pain with activity. Again, the late presentation is a result of the patient's lack of appreciation of the original injury or of failure to recognize this injury by the primary health care contact. Generally the only abnormal physical finding is well-localized tenderness to the distal radio-ulnar joint. Some patients will have an obvious prominence of the distal ulna. In others, the distal ulna can be excessively mobile in a palmar dorsal plane compared with the opposite wrist. Radiographic examination is generally unhelpful. A very small and highly selected number of patients may have a coronal CT scan performed to demonstrate that the affected wrist is asymmetrical through the distal radio-ulnar joint compared with the unaffected wrist. These patients are generally best treated non-surgically with physiotherapy and taping to try and aid stability and reduce their symptoms during activity.

A large number of surgical procedures which attempt to stabilize and reduce the distal radio-ulnar joint have been described. In general, these procedures do not achieve consistently reproducible results. Therefore these procedures are reserved as a final effort to try and stabilize the distal radio-ulnar joint in those patients with extremely disabling symptoms.

References

1. Linscheid RL, Dobyns JH. Athletic injuries of the wrist. *Clinical Orthopaedics and Related Research* 1985; **198**: 141–51.
2. Lichtman DM, ed. *The wrist and its disorders.* Philadelphia: WB Saunders, 1988.
3. Mayfield JK, Wrist ligamentous anatomy and pathogenesis of carpal instability. *Orthopedic Clinics of North America* 1984; **15**: 209–16.
4. Talesnik J, ed. *The wrist.* New York: Churchill Livingstone, 1985.
5. Palmer AK, Werner FW. The triangular fibrocartilage complex of the wrist—anatomy and function. *Journal of Hand Surgery* 1981; **6**: 153–62.
6. Rothjh, Haddad RG. Radiocarpal arthroscopy and arthrography in the diagnosis of ulner wrist pain. *Arthroscopy* 1986; **2**: 234–43.
7. Cooney WP, Evaluation of wrist pain by arthrogram, arthroscopy, and arthrotomy. *Journal of Hand Surgery* 1993; **18**: 815–22.
8. Cooney WP, Dobyns JH, Linscheid RL. Complications of Colles' fractures. *Journal of Bone and Joint Surgery* 1980; **62A**: 613–19.
9. Knirk JL, Jupiter JB. Intra-articular fractures of the distal radius in young adults. *Journal of Bone and Joint Surgery* 1986; **68A**: 657–9.
10. Axelrod TS, McMurtry RY. Open reduction and internal fixation of comminuted, intra-articular fractures of the distal radius. *Journal of Hand Surgery* 1990; **15A**: 1–11.
11. Cooney WP, Dobyns JH, Linscheid RL. Fractures of the scaphoid: a rational approach to management. *Clinical Orthopaedics and Related Research* 1980; **149**: 90–7.
12. Herbert TJ. Management of the fractured scaphoid using a new bone screw. *Orthopaedic Transactions* 1982; **6**: 464–5.
13. Kerloke L. McCabe SJ. Non-union of the scaphoid: a critical analysis of recent natural studies. *Journal of Hand Surgery* 1993: **18**: 1–3.
14. Watson HK, Rogers WD. Non-union of the hook of the hamate: an argument for bone grafting the non-union. *Journal of Hand Surgery* 1989; **14A**: 486–90.
15. Watson HK, Hempton RF. Limited wrist arthrodesis I. The triscaphoid joint. *Journal of Hand Surgery* 1980; **5**: 320–7.
16. Kleinman WB. Long term study of chronic scapholunate instability treated by scapho-trapezio-trapezoid arthrodesis. *Journal of Hand Surgery* 1989; **14A**: 425–8.
17. Kleinman WB, Carroll C IV. Scapho-trapezio-trapezoid arthrodesis for treatment of chronic, static and dynamic scapho-lunate instability: a 10-year perspective on pitfalls and complications. *Journal of Hand Surgery* 1990; **15A**: 408–14.
18. Green DP. Carpal dislocations and instabilities. In: Green DP, ed. *Operative hand surgery*, 2nd edn. New York: Churchill Livingstone, 1988: 875–938.
19. Bowers WH. The distal radioulnar joint. In: Green DP, ed. *Operative hand surgery*, 2nd edn. New York: Churchill Livingstone, 1988: 939–89.

Further reading

Green DP, ed. *Operative hand surgery*, 2nd edn. New York: Churchill Livingstone, 1988.
Rockwood CA Jr, Green DP, eds. *Fractures in adults*. Philadelphia: JB Lippincott.

7.8 Pain about the groin, hip, and pelvis

Harald P. Roos and Per A.F.H. Renström

Introduction

Pain syndromes in the hip and pelvis area are not uncommon in people involved in sports. The majority of the conditions are easy to diagnose and treat and will more or less disappear by themselves with rest. On the other hand, about 20 per cent[1] can be most challenging to diagnose and treat, and it requires experience to be able to recognize them. Many different conditions that involve other medical specialties can cause pain in the hip and pelvic area such as orthopaedics, urology/gynaecology, general surgery, and internal medicine. Therefore, it has been recommended that a multidisciplinary approach be taken for diagnosing and treating these injuries.[2] A complicating factor is that chronic groin, hip, and pelvic injuries are most often associated with diffuse and uncharacteristic symptoms. In addition, these are often difficult to detect because of secondary symptoms of overuse. In this situation, treating only the inflammatory overuse condition is not uncommon and thus the real mechanical problem may be overlooked, resulting in a poor treatment outcome. This is probably the most important explanation why many groin, hip, and pelvic injuries take a long time to resolve, with severe consequences for the injured athlete. However, with a well-planned diagnostic approach to the problem, this risk may be diminished (Fig. 1).

Although groin, hip, and pelvic injuries occur most commonly in sports such as soccer, team handball, ice hockey, they are also seen in individual sports such as fencing, speed skating, cross country skiing, hurdles, high jump, and horse riding.[3,4] In a prospective study of soccer injuries in Sweden in the 1970s, groin injuries accounted for 5 per cent of the total injuries (Fig. 2).[3] In a recent study in Swedish soccer players there was little change in the incidence of groin injuries: these comprised 7 per cent of the total injuries.[5] Approximately 2.5 per cent of all sports-related injuries are in the hip and pelvic area.[7]

Soft-tissue injuries are the most common cause of groin pain in athletes. A direct, blunt trauma, although not common, can cause these injuries as can an indirect strain to the muscle–tendon unit. Groin injuries are, however, usually subacute or chronic when first examined by the physician. The most commonly involved muscle–tendon units are the adductor complex (especially the adductor longus), the rectus femoris, rectus abdominis, and iliopsoas.[8] As

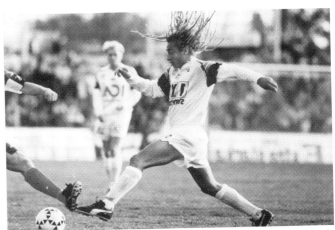

Fig. 1 An action in soccer that may cause groin problems (Bildbyrån, Hassleholm).

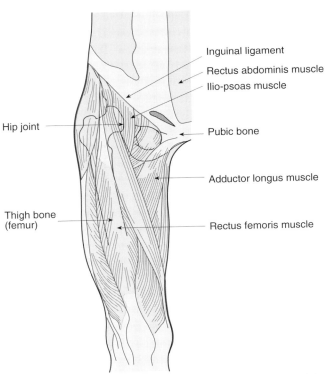

Fig. 2 Diagram of the muscles in the groin region. (Reproduced from ref. 6 with permission.)

mentioned above, pain in the groin area can have many other causes, especially hernias, and these will be discussed below. Pelvic and hip pain may involve fractures and degenerative joint disease.

Anatomy and basic biomechanics

The pelvic girdle consists of two paired innominate bones, the sacrum and the coccyx. Three fundamental parts make up the innominate bones—the ileum, the ischium, and the pubis, where one of each form a part of the hip socket (acetabulum). The fusion of vertebrae (five and three) form the sacrum and the coccyx, respectively. Movement across the joints in the pelvis is minimal and there is no muscle action at the joints. Anteriorly the pubic bones are joined at the symphysis pubis, where the bony surfaces are covered with hyaline cartilage and separated by a fibrocartilaginous disc. Strong ligaments stabilize the joint—superiorly by the suprapubic ligament, inferiorly by the arcuate portion of the pubic ligament, and additionally by the anterior interpubic ligament.

The sacroiliac joints form the connection posteriorly between the two ilia and proximal three vertebrae of the sacrum. The sacroiliac joints are covered with hyaline cartilage and are classified as diarthrodial joints. However, the presence of fibrous bands that sometimes obliterate the entire joint cavity makes them more or less semifused.[9] The strong posterior and dorsal sacroiliac ligaments reinforce the joints, as do the sacrotuberal and sacrospinous ligaments. The irregular joint shape itself also acts as a stabilizer.

Since there is little motion in the pelvic joint, the entire pelvis can thus be seen as a single link between the spinal column and the lower extremities. The most susceptible areas to traumatic injuries are the pubic symphysis, the pubic rami, and just lateral to the sacroiliac joints.[10] The pelvis is capable of two distinct movements: anteroposterior tilting and rotation.

Because of its ball and socket configuration the hip joint possesses a unique degree of internal stability.[9] Despite this there is a great mobility between the femoral head and the acetabulum. The motion in the hip joint is in three planes: sagittal, frontal, and transverse, with the greatest motion in the sagittal plane. Flexion of 120 degrees, abduction of 20 degrees, and rotation of 20 degrees are necessary for performing normal activities of daily living, and to participate in sport a significantly greater motion is often necessary.[11] During slow walking the maximum force transmitted across the hip joint is about 1.6 times bodyweight and in running the force increases to 5 times bodyweight during the stance phase.[12]

The most important muscles influencing the groin area are the adductor muscle complexes, which mainly consists of the adductor longus (Fig. 2), adductor brevis, pectineus, and gracilis muscles as well as the rectus abdominis, the rectus femoris, the sartorius, the iliopsoas; and the gluteus medius muscles. The close relationship between the different muscles makes the differentiation (by palpation) difficult. For example, the insertion of the rectus abdominis is very close to the origin of the adductor longus. Other muscles include muscles that abduct the hip joint, such as the anterior portion of the gluteus maximus, gluteus minimus, and the tensor fasciae latae. Those which externally rotate the hip, are the gluteus maximus and medius, the piriformis, the quadratus femoris, and the gemmelli muscles. The gluteus minimus, the adductor magnus, and the tensor faciae latae muscles produce internal rotation.

The peripheral nerves most commonly affected in the groin are the ilioinguinal, genitofemoral, and the lateral femoral cutaneous nerves. The ilioinguinal nerve is located proximal to the inguinal ligament and it supplies the area around the base of the penis, scrotum, and the labia majora. The genitofemoral nerve is located deeper and is divided into two parts: (1) ramus genitalia, (2) ramus femoralis. Through its first branch the nerve supplies the labia majora or scrotum and the second branch transmits signals from an area just distal to the inguinal ligament. The obturator nerve passes through the channel with the same name and innervates an area medially on the thigh, distal to that of the ilioinguinal nerve. The lateral femoral cutaneous nerve innervates the lateral border of the thigh almost down to the knee joint.

The inguinal channel is a 4-cm long tunnel. Its external orifice is located close to the pubic tubercle and the internal orifice between the tubercle and the anterior superior iliac spine. The ventral wall consists of the aponeurosis to the external oblique muscle and there is an opening just cranial to the ligamentum inguinale, which is the external inguinal annulus. The dorsal wall of the channel consists of the transversal fascia and its opening laterally forms the internal inguinal annulus. The internal oblique muscle and the transverse muscle provide the cranial cover. The inguinal ligament forms the caudal border of the inguinal channel

Diagnostic approach

History

Earlier problems
A history of congenital hip-joint disorders, which may contribute to an early onset of osteoarthritis, should be considered. Earlier histories of hip problems, such as transient synovitis or Legg–Calve–Perthes' disease, should be elicited. A history of a hip trauma combined with a period of restricted mobility may indicate a haemarthrosis of the hip joint with an increased risk for later segmental collapse.[13] Any kind of earlier surgery in the region such as appendectomy, laparoscopy, or hernioplasty will be recognized.

Onset of symptoms
The onset of symptoms can be a useful indicator to the primary cause of even very long-standing groin pain. A sudden onset during an activity indicates an injury to the muscle–tendon complex or a fracture. The former can be true even if the pain after the initial trauma subsides; this may not return until the activity gradually increases again, perhaps months later. Forgetting the very first occurrence of pain is easy and the condition will be interpreted as a typical overuse injury, when actually it had a true traumatic cause. A gradual onset of problems that may be associated with a change in physical activity, such as higher intensity of training, or changing methods, indicates an overuse injury most likely from the muscle–tendon complex. This may also signal a stress fracture. Sometimes there is no specific time of onset and no specific change in activities, but since the symptoms are most prominent in association with physical activity muscle–tendon units are most likely to be suspected as the source of pain. This may also be the case for groin pain, such as hernia, prostatitis, nerve entrapment, or osteoarthritis of the hip, typically caused by participating in sports.

Type of symptoms
The location of the pain or tenderness should be noted. Do the symptoms correspond to a specific tendon or are they more diffuse?

Radiation of pain into the abdomen, scrotum perineal area, buttock, or down to the leg will be important factors in the diagnosis. Functional impairment and swelling may be present. A feeling of fatigue in the area is not uncommon and changes in sensation may be present. Urogenital symptoms, such as dysuria, or discharge, and bowel symptoms should be asked for specifically, since these are easily missed.

Type of pain

A pain that is sharp, causes a catching sensation, and related to certain positions indicates a mechanical problem such as a loose body in the hip joint, an impingement of the acetabular labrum, or a snapping hip. A radiation of pain may be a sign of nerve entrapment or sciatica. If the pain is associated with sneezing or coughing and radiates to the scrotum the cause could be an inguinal hernia.

Probing for the relationship of the pain to physical activity is important. Pain and stiffness during the warm-up phases that gradually lessen or disappear, just to return with greater intensity after continued activity is a typical feature of subacute or chronic inflammatory conditions. If the patient tries to ignore this type of pain, he or she might be caught in the so-called vicious pain cycle with a risk for a chronic groin problem that is can be very difficult to manage.[3,8]

Pain can be mostly of skeletal origin, such as a stress fracture, but it may also be caused by joint disorders, for example hip osteoarthritis, sacroiliac disorders, or pain about the pubic symphysis—symphysitis (osteitis pubis).

The symptoms are generally more vague and diffuse in chronic cases of hip and pelvic disorders. The most common symptom is pain during exercise, but the symptoms can vary for the same diagnosis and in the same patient at different times.

Physical examination

The examination of a patient with long-lasting symptoms emanating from the groin must involve several different steps. It is recommended that a standardized procedure be followed when the patient is first examined. An examination of the spine may be considered logical, whereas a foot examination may be overlooked. However, if the patient is a long-distance runner and suffers from an overuse injury in the rotators of the hip or lateral hip bursa this could be associated with a hyperpronation of the foot.

Deciding whether there really is a muscle tendon injury involved is important, and isolating which muscle–tendon complex is vital. Functional muscular tests should be carefully performed. The condition may be labelled tendinitis only when the following three signs of tendinitis are fulfilled: (1) pain when the muscle contracts against resistance; (2) pain when the muscle is stretched; (3) tenderness over the insertion or origin.

It is not obvious what is normal as far as flexibility is concerned. Clearly there are differences in flexibility between males and females. It must also be kept in mind that differences occur between different types of athletes and in different playing positions, for example a soccer team.[14] What is normal for one category of athletes, for instance gymnasts, may not be normal for a track and field athlete. Side-to-side differences in the same patient may, however, indicate a pathological situation that should be treated.

Muscle strength is difficult to assess manually in a reproducible way, but functional tests, such as muscle resistive tests or standing on one leg, will indicate a decreased muscular function or muscle imbalance.

The following standardized clinical examination is divided into different sections depending on the position of the patient.

In standing position

- Inspection—for atrophies, scoliosis, asymmetries, knee and feet position;

- Leg-length discrepancy—if present, should be defined as being of a structural or functional origin;

- Movement in the spine;

- Trendelenburg sign;

- Functional tests—knee bending on one leg and toe-raising;

- Examination for inguinal hernia—is made through an invagination of the scrotum to the annulus inguinalis externus. The index finger of one hand is used while at the same time palpating over the inguinal channel with the other hand. This is performed first in the relaxed patient and then when the patient is asked to cough or to increase their abdominal pressure (Valsalva manoeuvre).

Prone position

- Palpation—of the spine and the sacroiliac joints;

- Flexibility testing—knee-extensors, hip flexors, and the hip abductors with the hip in extension;

- Resistive test for the hamstring muscles.

Supine position

- Range of movement of the hip joints;

- Straight-leg raising test;

- Flexibility testing—the hamstrings, the adductor muscles in 90 and 0 degrees of hip flexion, the abductor muscles, rotator muscles of the hip, and the triceps surae muscles;

- Resistive test—the adductor muscles, knee-extensors, abdominal muscles, hip rotators, and hip flexors;

- Sensitivity—test for blunt and sharp sensations in the groin region tracking the different peripheral nerves;

- Palpation—of the symphysis junction and other parts of the skeleton to note tenderness over tendinous insertions, lymphatic nodes, etc. Palpate the scrotum, the general abdomen, and check for hernias;

- Neurological examination—of the lower limb with testing of patellar and Achilles' reflexes, strength in toe-extensors and sensitivity. Palpation of the peripheral vessels—posterior tibial and dorsalis pedis arteries;

- Rectal examination—is mandatory in cases with a long history of pain emanating from the groin area. Note clinical signs of a prostatitis and also other palpable abnormalities. A rectovaginal examination is sometimes indicated in females.

Side position

- Hyperextension of the hip joints as a test for nerve entrapment;

- Palpation of the trochanteric region;

- Testing of segmental movement in the lumbar spine could be done in this position.

In certain cases, especially in long-distance runners, a more thorough biomechanical examination can be performed in an attempt to find malalignment.

Evaluation of clinical findings

In many cases of long-standing pain from the groin signs of tendinitis will be present in one or more locations. Whether this is the primary cause or a secondary phenomenon is difficult to establish. With a clear history of a training error the diagnosis is accepted and treatment given. On the other hand, where there is a clinical history of neither a training error nor a sudden onset of symptoms during activity it is important to be aware of the fact that the primary cause probably is not musculoskeletal in origin.

Further investigations

There are several diagnostic tools that can be used in the diagnosis of groin, hip, and pelvic pain. However, the various methods differ in importance based on the clinical findings in each patient. Although the clinical examination can be standardized this is not the case regarding the decision about requesting further investigations; instead, these must be strictly individualized.

Plain radiography

A plain radiograph of the pelvis is indicated in most cases of long-lasting symptoms arising from the groin and pelvis. After an acute injury, especially in teenagers, outlining an avulsion injury at the tendon insertion is important. Joint changes in the sacroiliac joint and in the pubic symphysis can be detected. If a hip-joint disorder, such as early osteoarthrosis is suspected, anteroposterior and lateral views of that joint should be taken. Preferably, these will be weight-bearing films, since these will detect osteoarthrosis at an earlier stage. Radiographs obtained in different positions of hip rotation seem to detect degenerative changes in the posterior aspects of the joint earlier, but they are not routinely performed.

Bone scan

This is the method of choice if a stress fracture must be outlined. Early osteoarthrosis of the hip joint can be detected by this method as well as disorders of the sacroiliac joint or the symphysis. A bone scan has been suggested to be a predictor for the later progression of osteoarthrosis.[15] Increased uptake can also indicate skeletal tumours with or without metastasis.

Ultrasonography

Fluid in the hip joint is best detected by ultrasonography, and this also makes the method useful in the diagnosis of arthritis. The method is valuable in a case of a child with suspected transient synovitis.[16] The amount of fluid in a joint can thus be determined, and this information will be helpful in deciding whether to aspirate the joint to lower the intra-articular pressure. Similarly, ultrasonography will be indicated in the case of a displaced hip fracture where a haemarthrosis might cause a high pressure. It has been shown that an increased intracapsular pressure in the hip compromises the blood supply to the femoral head, with a risk for a later segmental collapse.[13]

Kälebo et al. have recently demonstrated that an experienced radiologist is very capable of detecting partial and complete tendon tears, for example in the adductor longus tendon close to the origin on the pubic tubercle.[17] Thus, in cases of long-standing discomfort from the adductor muscle–tendon unit, ultrasonography of the tendon will be helpful in making the decision about further management, for example surgical intervention.

Computed tomography (CT)

Muscular disorders, for instance tears, may be visualized by this method, as well as hernias in the abdominal wall (Spigeli hernias). Skeletal disorders and loose bodies in the hip joint are well detected. The method can also be used to detect other disorders of the hip joint such as a torn acetabular labrum, especially in combination with arthrography (CT arthrography).

Magnetic resonance imaging (MRI)

MRI might be indicated for detecting and evaluating soft-tissue injuries, in particular the gadolinium-enhanced MRI technique.[18] Since an acetabular labral injury or chondral loose bodies are not well visualized by conventional radiography, Magnetic resonance arthrogram (MRA) is of considerable value in these cases as well as CT arthrography and arthroscopy. MRI has also become useful in the diagnosis of musculotendinous injuries, since it provides good soft-tissue contrast, multiplanar capability, and a high sensitivity to small injuries.[19,20] Theoretically, MRI should be a tool in the diagnosis of hernias, but for a hernia to be visualized it requires that the hernia is dislocated when the examination is performed.

Herniography

Clinical examination, even when performed by an experienced practitioner, is often insufficient to rule out the presence or absence of a hernia in the young athlete. Direct hernia may cause long-lasting groin pain in athletes, including soccer players.[21] This type of hernia is most often seen later in life ('old man's hernia'), but it seems as if the physical strain in sports provokes the development of these acquired hernias.

Positive-contrast peritoneography used for the diagnosis of hernia in the inguinal and pelvic region is called herniography. It is a very sensitive method for the demonstration of inguinal and femoral hernias. This method, developed by the Swedish radiologist Gullmo,[22] has become more common lately.[2,23,24] A contrast medium is injected intra-abdominally and films are taken at rest and when the patient is asked to increase the intra-abdominal pressure. Contrast medium that sinks down pathologically will be indicative of an existing hernia (Fig. 3(a,b,c)). This technique has been shown to be useful in the detection of hernias in athletes.[21] However, one must be careful since the specificity of the method can be questioned; because some of the hernias visualized may not be causative, the treatment will be unsuccessful.

The main indication for a herniography is obscure long-lasting groin pain, independent of whether a hernia is recognized by manual testing or not.[21,24] Thus, a patient with a subacute onset of symptoms, which initially are often unilateral (and where the preliminary diagnosis is not infrequently tendinitis and the treatment has been unsuccessful), is a candidate for herniography.

All hernias demonstrated by herniography need not necessarily be symptomatic. Thus, a demonstrated hernia is not always the explanation of the pain. All available data should be evaluated fully before a decision to operate is made. However, when a herniography is performed on the indications of long-lasting, one-sided groin

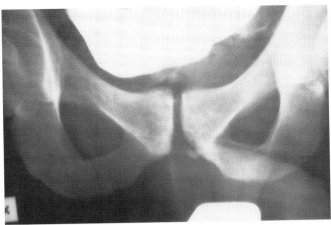

(a)

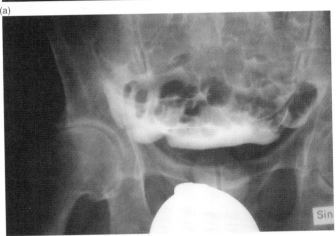

(b)

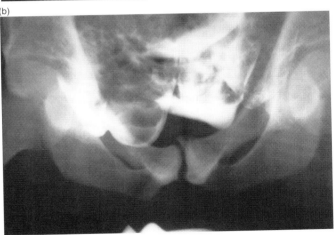

(c)

Fig. 3 Herniography (a) normal herniography, (b) small hernia changes on the left side. It should be pointed out that arthritis is also present in the hip that could cause problems. (c) Hernia on the right side.

pain, a demonstrated hernia on the symptomatic side is often the cause of the problem and surgery will be therapeutic.

Hernias in young adults, which otherwise are hardly noted by clinical examination because of the broad base of the hernia, are part of a condition described as an insufficient groin or sports hernia.[25] This condition is caused by a generalized weakness of the muscular and fascial apparatus of the groin. The bulging that is often seen is located medially and is caused by a weakness of the transversalis and soleus fasciae.

Arthroscopy

Hip arthroscopy is performed much less frequently than arthroscopies of other joints. The vulnerable blood supply to the femoral head, the close relationship of the neurovascular structures to the lower extremity, and the lack of well-designed instruments specific for hip arthroscopy account for this. However, once the technique has been mastered, the procedure provides an excellent visualization of the articular cartilage, labrum, and synovium that is superior to many radiographic methods.[18,26] An arthroscopy is of value in aiding the diagnosis of hip-joint disease, particularly in young athletes.[27,28] This technique allows synovial biopsies to be taken, chondral flap lesions and tears of the labrum to be resected, as well as the removal of loose bodies and resection of impinging synovial folds.

Laparoscopy

This may be the future method for detecting hernias with the obvious advantage of simultaneously treating the hernia endoscopically. However promising, there may still be difficulties in detecting medial defects (with the same limitation as with MRI), since it may be impossible to increase the intra-abdominal pressure enough to reproduce the defect in the abdominal wall. The lateral hernias will, on the other hand, be easily detected and could also be treated at the same time.

As yet, there is no clear consensus about which surgical technique should be used in young patients who have high demands of physical activity, for example soccer players (Smedberg, personal communication). Probably, the open, outside method of repair is to be preferred instead of a graft from the inside in these situations.

Laboratory tests

Erythrocyte sedimentation rate and white blood cell analysis will sometimes be of value in aiding the diagnosis of general inflammatory conditions. Blood analysis for rheumatoid diseases should be performed when inflammatory reactions in other joints, a synovitis of the hip, or radiological signs of a pelvospondylitis in the sacroiliac joints are present.

Examination of a discharge from the prostate, both microscopically and for the culture of micro-organisms, can be performed when there are clinical signs of a prostatitis or a symphysitis, or urogenital symptoms.

Specific injuries

Groin injuries

Muscle–tendon injuries

Adductor injuries

The hip–adductor complexes include the adductor longus, the adductor magnus, the adductor brevis, and the pectineus muscle. The gracilis and the inferior part of the gluteus maximus can also provide adduction in the hip joint. The adductor longus is the most frequently injured groin muscle–tendon unit in sports.[3,4] (Fig. 4). Noting the injury mechanism is important, as discussed earlier, since it could have major implications on the treatment; specifically if it is an acute muscle injury, tear, or an overuse injury caused by repetitive loading.

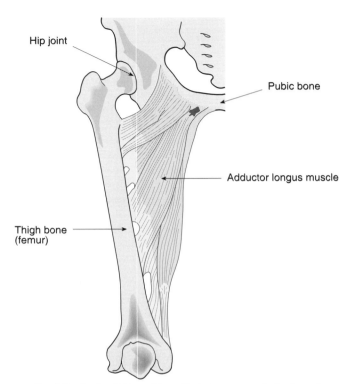

Fig. 4 Proximal partial tear of the adductor longus muscle–tendon unit.

An acute tear that occurs at the proximal musculotendinous junction of the adductor longus is most likely to be secondary to an increased collagen content in the tendon, and therefore reduced extensibility, as postulated by Noonan and Garrett.[29] Complete tears or grade III strains of the adductors are rare. They are mainly located in the distal part of the adductor longus at the femoral insertion site.[30]

The chronic pain condition in the adductor longus, mainly located in the proximal part of the muscle, could be caused by a partial tear that has not been recognized, and it is therefore most important to understand how the symptoms started. Resistant chronic pain that is very distinctly in the proximal part should be suspect for this diagnosis. Ultrasound examination[17] or an MRI scan[20] may be helpful in securing a proper diagnosis.

A strictly overuse-induced condition must be analysed for causative extrinsic factors such as equipment and training methods. Speed skating, cross-country skiing, and uphill running are all activities that provide repetitive loading to the adductor complex. However, intrinsic factors may also be important: malalignment, muscle strength and flexibility discrepancies, leg-length discrepancy, and also foot morphology must be looked for. Other predisposing factors are specific muscle weaknesses, especially of the muscles in the adductor group, and poor or asymmetrical muscular flexibility.[8]

Diagnosis Pain when the adductor muscles are passively stretched and pain at contraction against resistance, in combination with tenderness that is located to the insertion site, will give the location of the injury (Fig. 5). As mentioned above, these findings may not always be the real primary cause. It must be realized that the tendon injury response can be secondary to another condition

and, in this case, treatment of the tendinitis will not be curative. If the onset of symptoms does not fit well with a history of overuse, if the localization is inconstant from time to time (i.e. pain which moves around) or if there are positive findings at many sites then further diagnostic tests should be considered. This could also be true in cases where no positive findings, other than those from muscles or tendons, are present during the clinical examination.

Treatment The main treatment of an overuse injury in a tendon is usually by conservative or non-surgical means. The first rule is to avoid abuse and painful activities. Once the diagnosis is secured, the goal of the treatment of a muscle/tendon injury is to regain full range of motion and to restore muscle strength, endurance, balance, and coordination.

The non-surgical treatment is usually divided into three phases: (1) acute and early phases; (2) rehabilitation and strength-training phases; and (3) functional and return to activity phases.[4] Correction of a malalignment with orthotics, stretching and/or strengthening exercises in combination with symptomatic treatment can be successful. According to Thomeé and Karlsson, the latter could include different physiotherapeutic modalities in the three phases[4] as well as anti-inflammatory medications. If the treatment is unsuccessful after a proper rehabilitation of 2 to 4 months, then an injection with a local anaesthetic, with or without a corticosteroid, in the periosteal area at the insertion site of the tendon may be attempted. This treatment should be combined with resting the affected muscle for 1 to 2 weeks. The indications for corticosteroid injections in this area will be very strict and preferably administered by experienced personnel.[8] There is no indication for an injection of corticosteroids directly into the tendon itself.

In long-lasting cases surgery may be indicated. Several different methods for the treatment of these injuries have been described.[1,7,17,31,32] However, most studies report on just a small number of patients with a short- or medium-term, follow-up period. The causes of groin pain in some studies are not quite homogenous, which makes the results difficult to interpret. The postoperative rehabilitation period and the rest from physical activity may contribute to the promising results observed after surgical treatment.

The recent recommendation is that the tendon should be opened longitudinally, and in some, but not all, patients pathological granulation tissue can be found and removed. The pathological tissue

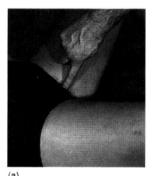
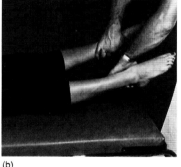

Fig. 5 (a) There may be tenderness on palpation over the muscle–tendon junction or at the insertion of the adductor longus muscle tendon on the left side. (b) Resistive adduction of the legs will elicit pain in the adductor longus muscle–tendon unit area.

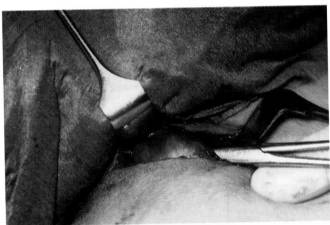

Fig. 6 Adductor longus muscle tendon in surgery.

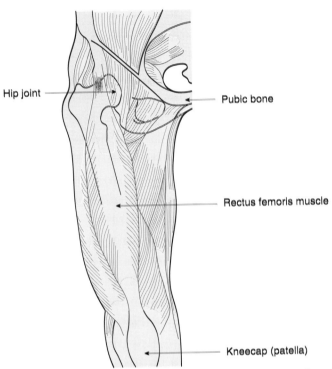

Fig. 7 Partial tear of the proximal muscle–tendon unit of the rectus femoris. (Reproduced from ref. 6 with permission.)

should be excised, in the direction of the fibre, until healthy tissue appears. The incision in the tendon should then be closed carefully with resorbable sutures.[4,8] In cases with no macroscopic findings in the tendon, a tenotomy at the origin can be performed[8] (Fig. 6). Good long-term results after tenotomy have been reported.[32] A somewhat different surgical approach has been described by Martens et al.,[31] who perform a tenotomy of the gracilis tendon and a partial tenotomy of the adductor brevis tendon. The authors strongly recommend leaving the adductor longus tendon intact, in contrast to others. Very limited information is available about surgery on tendons in this area. Surgery is seldom indicated for these problems.

A grade III strain or a complete rupture of the adductor longus can be sustained by a powerful eccentric contraction, such as when the muscle contracts during a simultaneous strong abduction force. A typical example is when two soccer players try to kick the ball at the same time. A complete disruption must be suspected if the ability to contract the muscle is totally lost. These tears are commonly located distally, towards the insertion point on the femur. Most often the complete disruptions are diagnosed after a long delay and are sometimes suspected of being a tumour.[30] The old complete disruptions can usually be treated conservatively after a soft-tissue tumour has been ruled out. In a fresh injury, surgical treatment may be considered in the athlete.

Management of injuries to the rectus femoris (Fig. 7), rectus abdominis, and the iliopsoas follow the same principles as the adductor longus.

Hernia

Inguinal and femoral hernias are not uncommon and may be symptomatic producing radiating pain diffusely in the groin. Typically, the pain radiates down to the scrotum and there is pain associated with sneezing and coughing. The pain is usually sudden and sharp and initially occurs in specific situations, but may be more constant chronically— probably due to the involvement of secondary structures. Inguinal and femoral hernias are usually easily recognized and treated successfully with surgery (Fig. 8). Return to sport is usually possible within 2 to 3 months.

In athletes with persistent pain, hernia should still be the working diagnosis to be looked for. Even if the clinical examination is negative, a hernia may be present and the cause of the pain. Hackney[25] has described a syndrome of a weakness in the posterior inguinal wall causing chronic groin pain, but without a clinically recognizable hernia. This condition has been named 'sports hernia', and is assumed to be caused by a congenital weakness of the posterior wall in the inguinal channel. Initially, it results in a symptomatic bulging in sports-active people, and probably later in life forms a fully developed hernia.[2] The pain from this injury is located

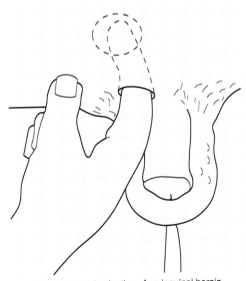

Fig. 8 Manual palpation of an inguinal hernia.

deeply. This pain progresses and the discomfort usually becomes more severe making it impossible to stride properly or turn quickly without a stab of pain. The pain is often worse on one side, but it may radiate laterally and across the midline down to the inside of the thigh into the adductor area and into the scrotum and testicle. About half the athletes give a history of pain when coughing. The examination reveals the main tenderness to be worse over the pubic tubercle of the affected side. The scrotum is then invaginated and the inguinal rings palpated from the inside. The area around the external ring is tender. Since the condition is difficult to detect by clinical examination a herniogram or a modified CT herniogram may be used for the diagnosis. Laparoscopy seems to have limitations in detecting this particular condition, as discussed earlier. The results of surgical repair to the posterior inguinal wall are described as excellent. Hackney[25] reported that 87 per cent of patients returned to full sporting activity within a couple of months and the remaining 13 per cent were improved.

Other type of hernias causing pain which also show a negative clinical examination for hernia have been called 'incipient hernias', which sometimes correspond to the sport hernias. These have been detected by herniography.[22,24] Herniography is a very sensitive method and the result must be carefully correlated to the presenting symptoms (Fig. 3(a,b,c)). Asymptomatic hernias will be found if the cohort of patients referred to herniography is inappropriate, which may result in unnecessary surgery, with a risk of an unsatisfactory outcome.

Bursitis

There are at least 13 permanent bursae in the hip region. Bursitis often occurs in parallel with tendon pathology and is usually difficult to differentiate from inflammatory conditions in the tendon insertions (tenoperiostitis). The bursa is often located in close association to a joint or over a bony prominence. The most commonly affected bursae in the pelvic region are the ischial, iliopectineal, and the trochanteric bursae.

Pathology in the bursa can be divided into traumatic and inflammatory bursitis.[3] The traumatic bursitis arises either after a direct blow to the bursa (such as a fall directly on to the bursa), or as an indirect trauma through a strain in a passing tendon resulting in a haemorrhage into the bursa. Small haematomas will usually be resorbed, but a major haematoma may result in scarring or calcifications. This can sometimes result in loose bodies inside the bursa that must be removed. An acute haemorrhagic bursitis should be treated by evacuation of the haematoma. The superficial trochanteric bursa is commonly affected by a direct trauma with a haemorrhage and bursitis as a result. The haematoma may be aspirated, using a thin needle, in the acute stage. In a chronic condition the treatment of choice will often be surgical excision. Sometimes a steroid injection gives good results.

The inflammatory bursitis is often divided into friction bursitis, chemical bursitis, and infection bursitis. A friction bursitis is caused by repeated movements of a tendon against a bursa. An example is the iliopectineal bursitis which is caused by the friction from the iliopsoas tendon (Fig. 9). The bursa is located anterior of the hip joint and dorsal to the iliopsoas tendon. It is the largest bursa in the body and it communicates with the hip joint in about 15 per cent of adults. An iliopectineal bursitis causes a feeling of swelling and ten-

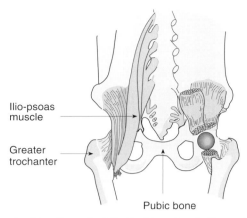

Fig. 9 Iliopectineal bursitis on the left side. (Reproduced with permission from ref. 6.)

derness, but rarely it can also give impingement with sudden position-related pain in the groin. This bursitis occurs with or without associated pathology of the iliopsoas.

Trochanteric bursitis will cause pain and tenderness just lateral to the greater trochanter or posterior to the prominence. Sometimes the pain radiates along the outside of the femur and might therefore be misinterpreted as a referred pain from a herniated lumbar disc. The pain is typically provoked by rotation of the hip joint. There are two lateral bursae. One superficial inside the iliotibial band and one deeper between the gluteus medius and the tensor fasciae latae muscles. The cause of a trochanteric bursitis may be a compensatory internal rotation of the extremity due to a hyperpronation of the foot. The causative factors for a possible hyperpronation should be analysed and corrected.

Ischial bursitis occurs after a blow to the ischial tuberosity with pain and tenderness in that region. The treatment is rest, ice, and compression and anti-inflammatory medication. In chronic pain, surgery may be indicated for removal of the bursae. Chemical or infectious bursitis in this region is not common.

Pain and haemorrhage over the iliac crest has been referred to as *hip pointer*.[33,34] This includes a variety of injuries, such as contusion, avulsion fracture, and periostitis. Consequently, the healing time is extremely variable according to Busconi and McCarthy,[18] which probably reflects the fact that the expression 'hip pointer' includes several different conditions with a variable outcome. It may be wise to use the term 'hip pointer' for a contusion injury to the iliac crest and for nothing else. Myositis ossificans has been described as a complication,[34] and corresponds to the site of contusion.

Nerve entrapment

Rarely, peripheral nerves will become entrapped in this region. Those that may be affected are the ilioinguinal, genitofemoral, and lateral cutaneous femoral nerves. Nerve entrapment most commonly occurs postoperatively after an appendectomy or hernioplasty. Another typical condition is the so-called meralgia paraesthetica, here the lateral cutaneous femoral nerve becomes entrapped after it has passed under the inguinal ligament just medially to the anterior superior iliac spine. The cause of this condition is commonly mechanical, such as tight pants (underwear) or weight gain. The ilioinguinal nerve may be affected after intensive training of the abdominal muscles. Hyperextension of the hip joint augments the pain. The most usual symptom or finding is hyperaesthesia in the area it supplies. Blocking the nerve with a local anaesthetic will confirm the diagnosis. The treatment initially is with non-steroidal anti-inflammatory medication, altered training methods, and alteration of clothing if necessary. Sometimes, but rarely, surgical treatment will be necessary. It has been debated whether release of the nerve or a resection is the preferable surgical method. Ekstrand[5] recommends routinely cutting the ilioinguinal nerve when a hernioplasty is performed, although this approach is controversial. The genitofemoral nerve may also be affected, following the same principles as for the ilioinguinal nerve. A report has shown that a long-lasting cure from entrapment of the ilioinguinal and genitofemoral nerves can be obtained from a nerve resection.[35]

Snapping hip syndrome

The snapping hip is a condition that is not very well defined. It can be confusing for the physician.[36,37] It may have intra-articular causes, for example loose bodies or labral tears, which may be diagnosed by MRI, CT, or arthroscopy. Superficial or external snapping is the way most people view this condition. The most common cause of the condition is either a thickened border of the iliotibial band or the anterior border gluteus maximus snapping over the greater trochanter producing a bursitis. Other causes of snapping are when the iliopsoas tendon passes over the iliopectineal eminence or the lesser trochanter, when the iliofemoral ligaments pass over the femoral head, or when the long head of the biceps passes the ischial tuberosity.

A snapping or even a popping noise associated with hip movements is most often the reason for complaint. The phenomenon is predominantly seen in females. If the snapping is only associated with a noise or a pop and no pain, it can be ignored and considered as a normal condition. Tenderness and pain in the area indicates the need for therapy. Superficial snapping is managed non-surgically, with the same principles of treatment as in the case of a bursitis due to other causes. Hyperpronation could be a cause of the condition in females and the triggering factor will need to be treated, sometimes in combination with local symptomatic treatment. Occasionally, surgical treatment is indicated in patients with continuous symptoms.

A deep snapping hip can be the result when the iliopsoas tendon snaps over the iliopectineal eminence, especially when the hip is abducted and externally rotated.[38] An iliopsoas bursography has been used to demonstrate that the sudden jerking movement of the iliopsoas tendon between the anterior/inferior iliac spine and iliopectineal eminence may be combined with pain and an audible snap.[39] Surgical treatment by exploring the iliopsoas tendon, its sheath, and the removal of hypertrophic nodules occasionally in combination with lengthening of the iliopsoas tendon can be tried if conservative measures fail to yield the desired effect. Surgery has been shown to reduce the snapping and the pain markedly.[39] Exploration and debridement of the iliopsoas bursa with arthroscopic assistance has recently been reported with promising results.[18]

Fractures

Fractures in this region are more common in the elderly population. However, femoral neck or trochanteric fractures may also be seen in younger athletes, mostly after traffic accidents or from overtraining. A femoral neck fracture in a young person will often require surgery, but the risk of future complications is high because of the vulnerable blood supply to the femoral head. Acetabular and pelvic fractures are usually caused by a direct trauma, such as falling on the ice or hard-packed snow when skating or skiing.

Avulsion fractures

Avulsion fractures can occur from any of the tendon insertions in the groin area, and is a condition mostly seen in adolescents. The most commonly involved locations are the anterior superior or inferior spine of the ileum, the ischial tuberosity, and the lesser trochanter. An avulsion fracture occurs during a heavy muscular activity, such as a sprint race or a soccer game, and is caused by the mechanical failure of bone due to the application of a tensile force through a musculotendinous unit or ligament.[40] The injury is usually generated by a sudden forceful concentric or eccentric contraction, or alternatively by an excessive passive lengthening.[41] There will be a loss of function in the affected muscle and localized tenderness. A plain radiography will establish the diagnosis. Surgery is recommended to restore the normal anatomy when the avulsed fragment is displaced significantly.

The most common locations are as follows:

1. Anterior/superior iliac spines seen with a traction injury of the sartorius muscle during jumping and running. The trauma occurs when the hip is extended and the knee is flexed, for example in a sprinting event. Active flexion or abduction of the affected side will cause pain. Significant displacement of the avulsed fragment is usually prevented by the tensor fascia lata and the inguinal ligament. Surgery has been recommended for severe displacement, rotation of large fragments, and for athletes who wish for a rapid return to sports.[34] Fortunately, functional disability after this kind of injury is not considered a significant problem.[8,18]

2. Avulsion of the anterior/inferior iliac spine occurs secondary to an excessive exertion of the straight head of the rectus femoris muscle. A common mechanism of injury is when the hip is hyperextended and the knee flexed, as in kicking the ball in soccer. Active flexion of the hip or extension of the knee will cause pain. The treatment in the majority of cases is non-surgical.

3. Avulsions of the ischial apophyses occur between the ages of 15 and 25 years (Fig. 10). Avulsion is caused by a maximum hamstring contraction with the pelvis fixed in flexion of the knee in extension. The injury is mainly seen in gymnasts, hurdlers, figure skaters, and water skiers.[42] The fusion of the apophyses may, as indicated, occur late, indicating that athletes can be susceptible to these injuries for a long time. A sudden onset of pain and tenderness at the ischial tuberosity are common and discomfort is increased with rising from the sitting position. Flexion of the hip against resistance will give pain. The treatment for this injury is controversial. Some authors recommend open reduction if the avulsed fragment is displaced more than 2 cm.[42,43]

Fatigue or stress fractures

These may occur in the femoral neck or shaft or on the inferior pubic bone. A stress fracture is an effect of repetitive loading which

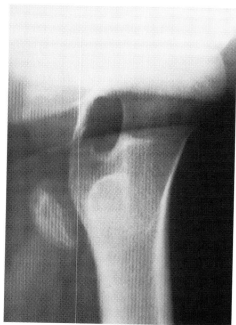

Fig. 10 Avulsion of the ischial tuberosity in combination with a hamstring tear.

will reach a point where the bone will break. The condition is seen mainly after excessive training, such as in track and field athletes, long-distance runners, and military recruits.[38,44] It can also be seen after a sudden change in training methods. Typically, a stress fracture occurs when the training is restarted after a period of rest, for example after an unrelated injury. Another important causative factor is a decreased strength in the bone itself, which has been noted in young female athletes who have an insufficient food intake and/or hormonal disturbances. They will become catabolic, and eventually osteoporosis will be established. Although stress fractures in female athletes might be common and thought to be associated with amenorrhoea, a presentation of unusual fracture sites necessitates a more thorough evaluation; causes such as Cushing's syndrome have been described.[45] Pain that is strictly related to exercise and provoked by movement in the hip joint may correspond to a stress fracture in the region. One negative radiographic examination will be insufficient to exclude the diagnosis of stress fracture and the radiographic examination must be repeated in 2 to 4 weeks if the diagnosis is suspected (Fig. 11). A bone scan verifies these fractures after 2 to 8 days.

The treatment of stress fractures is mainly conservative (rest), but a fracture of the cervical neck may displace with a risk for later vascular complications to the femoral head such as segmental collapse. Thus, these fractures might need surgical stabilization. Johansson *et al.* followed 23 athletes with stress fractures of the femoral neck for 6.5 years.[47] Of these, 16 were treated with internal fixation and the remaining 7 were conservatively treated. The seven patients treated conservatively developed major complications requiring surgery, of these five were displaced fractures. The authors concluded that the high incidence of displaced fractures might be caused by the delay between onset and diagnosis, and therefore a shortening of that delay would be advantageous for the outcome. It was mentioned earlier that displaced stress fractures of

the femoral neck seem to have a higher rate of complications and require a longer healing time than acute fractures.[46]

Pelvic stress fractures are also secondary to microtrauma, most often at the junction of the ischium and inferior pubic ramus. These fractures are mainly seen in female runners, and the treatment is always conservative with rest and alternative training regimes. It may be 3 to 5 months before the fractures are asymptomatic.

Hip-joint problems

According to Calliet,[48] there are four different structures about the hip joint that may cause pain:

(1) the fibrous capsule and the ligaments;

(2) the surrounding muscles;

(3) the bony periosteum;

(4) the synovium.

In the elderly, the most common cause of hip pain is degenerative disease. It has, however, been shown that former athletes, especially soccer players, and people with certain occupations have radiographic changes of osteoarthrosis in the hip joint earlier in life compared with controls.[49-54]

Lindberg *et al.*[52] showed in a group of 63 former, male soccer players with an average age of 43 years that about 7 per cent had hip-joint changes and that in 286 players with an average age of 53 years, the figure was 15 per cent. In non-soccer players the prevalence of hip osteoarthritis in these age groups was less than 1 and 3 per cent, respectively. The degenerative changes were especially found among those who had played at national or international level. This might indicate why athletes in their thirties may well have ongoing hip-joint degeneration (maybe not yet visible radiographically), as a cause of pain in the hip and pelvis. The condition can be detected with a bone scan or on MRI, or seen more easily with weight-bearing radiographs, preferably in different positions of rotation, where the posterior parts of the joint are more visible.

There is some controversy about the risk for runners developing hip osteoarthrosis. Most studies have not shown such a relationship,[55] except in extremely high-mileage runners or top-level athletes.[56,57]

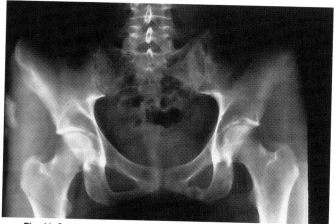

Fig. 11 Stress fracture of the inferior ramus in a long-distance runner.

Other causes of hip pain are osteochondritis dissecans and loose bodies. An avulsion of the labrum of the acetabulum can occur occasionally and will cause sharp and catching pain during exercise, sometimes with persistent pain afterwards. Sudden episodes of pain or catching sensations may occur as a sign of impingement into the hip joint. Theoretically, a capsular impingement may occur, but more probably it will be an impingement caused by the iliopectineal bursa, the acetabular labrum, or the lateral portion of the origin rectus femoris. Impingement can be diagnosed by MRI or CT scans combined with an arthrography. A diagnostic injection with local anaesthesia may also add information. Arthroscopy is sometimes indicated to evaluate the joint and to extract loose fragments. The treatment depends on the diagnosis. If there is any joint or cartilage damage, the athlete should avoid pounding activities and participate more in activities such as biking and swimming.

Hip-joint problems in children

Transient synovitis is the most common cause of hip joint complaints in children. This must be differentiated from Legg–Calvé–Perthes' disease, rheumatoid disorders, osteoid osteoma, and other rare conditions. However, secondary hip-joint degeneration can be seen early in life after Legg–Calvé–Perthes' disease. Segmental collapse may not only follow major traumas such as hip dislocation, but may also be seen after haemarthrosis of the joint a period of high intra-articular pressure.[16] Slipped capital epiphysis may occur in the age group 10 to 15 years, especially among boys. Hormonal, genetic, and mechanical factors have been discussed as aetiological factors. Males are affected twice as often as females, and black people have an unusually high incidence. The affected boys are usually obese and development of secondary sexual characteristics is delayed.[58] The treatment is surgical stabilization, if possible *in situ*, with threaded pins. The main complication with a slipped capital femoral epiphysis is osteonecrosis, reported to occur in as many as 15 per cent of the patients.[59] There is some controversy whether a prophylactic procedure should be performed on the asymptomatic side as well, because of the increased risk of sustaining the same injury, estimated to be 30 to 50 per cent. A prophylactic procedure with an atraumatic technique on the contralateral side is the treatment of choice in Sweden.[60]

Pelvis–buttock problems

Osteitis pubis

This condition was described in the German literature around 1950 as a benign condition, more or less as a radiographic finding without any clinical relevance. It is a well-recognized entity after surgery to the bladder or prostate and has also been reported to occur among athletes.[61] However, it is not uncommon; symptoms cause severe disability and sports participation is impossible because of pain from this area, most often symptoms are long-lasting. Typically, this condition occurs in soccer players, ice-hockey players, football players, long-distance runners, and weightlifters.[62,63] There is almost never a trauma, but instead a gradual onset with pain central in the groin, often radiating either up to the abdomen or down to the medial aspects of the thighs.[62,64] There is tenderness over the symphysis and painful passive abduction and active adduction and internal rotation of the hip. The insertion of the rectus abdominis muscles are often affected with pain associated with sit-ups. During the con-

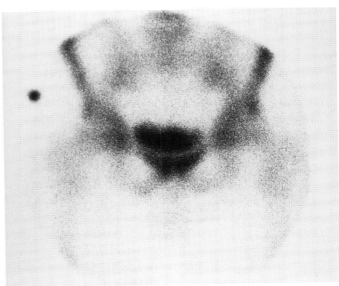

Fig. 12 Synovitis as seen on a bone scan.

dition, pain will move around to different tendons and it is common with pain at rest. A common complaint is pain in the morning after a training event, or pain when changing position in bed at night.

The precise aetiology is unclear, but muscle strain and stress fracture have been discussed. Ruling out any urogenital pathology is important. It has been speculated that prostatitis is a frequently overlooked differential diagnosis in patients with chronic groin pain, and these patients will have symptoms mimicking tendinitis of the adductor longus.[4,65] Symphyseal pain (symphysitis associated with prostatitis) especially caused by *Chlamydia trachomatis* has been suggested as a cause[65] (Fig. 12). The changes in the pubic symphysis are, however, often clearly not infectious and are probably not associated with an isolated traumatic episode. Pubic instability, secondary to adductor imbalance or trauma, may occur with an osteitis pubis.[8]

Early in the course of the disorder, a bone scan may show an increased uptake; after 2 to 3 weeks the typical radiographic findings will appear, such as erosion and/or sclerosis of the symphyseal junction (Fig. 13).[64] The condition is sometimes extremely long lasting and difficult to manage. The non-infectious osteitis pubis is self-limiting.[62] Proper management may reduce the time needed for a return to sport. If there is a prostatitis this will be treated with antibiotics according to existing recommendations, otherwise the treatment is, rest, non-steroidal agents, and physiotherapy. If the problems persist, a steroid injection may be given with the aid of a fluoroscope (Fig. 14). Some athletes can take part in all physical activities since they treat themselves with a fast-acting, non-steroidal anti-inflammatory drug (NSAID) before the start of the activity. Surgery is rarely indicated, but in extremely recalcitrant cases it has been tried with results described as successful.[66]

The return to sport is gradual and is possible within 4 to 8 months, although the average time for a return to competitive sports is approximately 8 to 9 months. Occasionally, the symptoms may last for 1 to 2 years.

Radiographic changes without tenderness corresponding to the symphyseal junction will not by itself be considered to be the reason

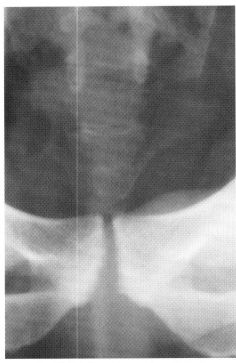

Fig. 13 Osteitis pubis on plain radiograph.

for the pelvic pain. The main differential diagnoses are osteomyelitis versus osteitis pubis, but the latter differs since it is usually bilateral to the symphysis, it has no sequestrum, and a negative culture. The condition will eventually heal, but the radiographic changes will, as indicated above, persist, however, with a negative bone scan. The long duration of the condition may sometimes ruin a promising athletic career.

Piriformis syndrome

Pain can sometimes be experienced when the piriform muscle is stretched. Compression on the sciatic nerve as it passes the piriformis muscle has been suggested to cause groin pain. A history of an earlier trauma is common and the patients will, in typical cases,

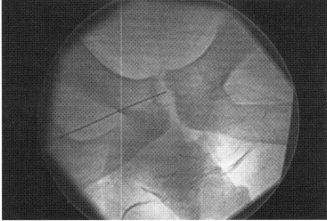

Fig. 14 Injection of corticosteroids with the aid of a fluoroscope.

have discomfort when sitting and in activities that cause hip flexion and internal rotation.[67] Pain is experienced when the examiner internally rotates and extends the thigh forcefully. This is called Pace's sign.[18] MRI may show a thickening of the inflamed nerve. The treatment is directed against the inflammatory reaction with NSAIDs or eventually a corticosteroid injection. Good results have been reported with physiotherapy eventually combined with NSAIDs. Sectioning of the piriform muscle has been reported to give acceptable results in long-lasting cases.[68]

Hamstring syndrome

A pain that is localized proximal on the back part of the thigh could be caused by a sciatic nerve irritation due to a compression provided by the hamstring muscles. This syndrome has been called hamstring syndrome,[69] and a characteristic complaint is that the pain appears when the patient is in the sitting position. The syndrome has been found among runners, especially sprinters and hurdlers; typically no pain is associated with slow-speed running.

The differential diagnosis is the piriformis syndrome, which also is an irritation of the sciatic nerve located more proximal in the buttock. Ischiogluteal bursitis causes a pain that is very similar to hamstring syndrome, but in this condition pain at rest is more common.

The clinical finding, when a hamstring syndrome is present, is a tenderness around the ischial tuberosity and pain when the leg is raised in the straight position. The treatment is initially conservative, but good results with nerve release have been described.[69]

Sacroiliac dysfunction

There is some controversy about how often this very solid articulation between the pelvis and sacrum may cause pain. O'Donoughue[70] reported that most injuries that are initially identified as sacroiliac sprains are found to be other entities. Clearly, some situations will generate forces to the sacroiliac joints that may cause pain at a later stage, for example a sudden violent contraction of the hamstrings or abdominal muscles, a severe direct blow to the buttocks, or forceful straightening from a crouched position. The main symptom is pain in the region and tenderness.

There are several tests for detecting sacroiliac joint pathology, one of which is the three-step test. Here the examiner's hand moves proximally to investigate first the hip and the iliopsoas muscle, then the sacroiliac joint, and finally the lumbar spine. The patient lies face down and the first step is to extend the hip joint, with a knee flexed, combined with pressure on the buttock; the second is when the examiner's hand is moved to the sacrum and further extension of the leg will affect the sacroiliac joint. The third step involves examining the lumbar spine, with the leg in the same position, while the other hand fixates on the thoracolumbar junction. Compression of the iliac wings or just an abduction in the hips when the patient is lying on his back can also detect pathology. Many different treatments have been tried, with a success rate depending on whether the diagnosis is accurate or not. Elastic support, NSAIDs, and, in some situations, steroid injections may help.

An inflammatory condition in these joints (sacroiliitis) is not uncommon, especially during winter in cross-country skiers. Pelvospondylitis can also affect the sacroiliac joint. The symptoms are often vague and diffuse, commonly with a pain in the lower lumbar spine radiating to the thighs. Acute septic osteomyelitis has also been described in the sacroiliac joint or the symphysis advancing through a haematogenous pathway.[71]

Referred pain

Pain from the spine may radiate out to the groin and down to the thigh. It may be caused by facet joint degradration or an arachnoiditis. Sciatic pain from a herniated lumbar disc, spinal stenosis, or spondylolisthesis can also be present in the groin region, especially when the L4 root is affected. Other causes of sciatic nerve compression have been discussed earlier, such as piriformis and hamstring syndrome. Visceral pain might also radiate down to the groin.

Coccyx pain

Coccygodynia arises mainly after a coccyx fracture. These fractures occur when there is a direct blow to the region, such as falling off a horse. The injury is extremely painful and recovery is usually slow. Eventually there will be a bony healing or a pain-free fibrous union. A doughnut-shaped pillow can give relief. Rarely, however, there will be persisting pain and disability, and a coccygectomy may be considered.

Tumours

The groin is not an uncommon site for tumours. Osteosarcomas, chondrosarcomas, schwannomas, and other tumours may appear in this region. Typically, the pain will be experienced initially in a sport such as soccer and it will be explained by a strain to a muscle or tendon. Persistent pain must thus be very carefully investigated to exclude a tumour. Radiography will always be included in the early stages of diffuse groin pain and MRI or CT scans will secure the diagnosis. A rectal examination at the first visit in the case of non-specific pain from the groin may help to shorten the delay to diagnosis.

Concluding remarks

As in many other situations in medicine the outcome of the treatment of a condition is dependent on a correct diagnosis. In the case of groin pain there is a significant problem because the symptoms are often vague and diffuse. Therefore it is important to have a multidisciplinary approach to the problem, each with expertise in different aspects of groin pain. Teamwork with an experienced physiotherapist will also be helpful.

A correct diagnosis at an early stage of groin pain will help to reduce the morbidity. Once the groin pain becomes chronic managing it may be difficult. There will be secondary symptoms that make a correct diagnosis more difficult to achieve. Groin injuries are some of the most challenging injuries in the field of sports medicine.

References

1. Muckle DS. Associated factors in recurrent groin and hamstring injuries. *British Journal of Sports Medicine* 1982; **16**: 37–9.
2. Ekberg O, Persson NH, Abrahamsson PA, Westlin N. Groin pain in athletes, a multidisciplinary approach. *Sports Medicine* 1988; **6**: 56–61.
3. Renström P, Peterson L. Groin injuries in athletes. *British Journal of Sports Medicine* 1980; **14**: 30–6.
4. Thomeé R, Karlsson J. Muscle and tendon injuries of the groin. *Critical Reviews in Rehabilitation Medicine* 1995; **7**: 299–313.
5. Ekstrand J. *Symposia of groin pain, 3rd Scandinavian Congress of Sports Medicine.* Linköping, Sweden, 1996.
6. Peterson L, Renström L. *Injuries in sports.* London: Dunitz, 1985.
7. Estanwik JJ, Sloane B, Rosenberg MA. Groin strain and other possible causes of groin pain. *Physician and Sportsmedicine* 1990; **18**: 59.
8. Renström PAHF. Tendon and muscle injuries in the groin area. *Clinics in Sports Medicine* 1992; **11**: 815–31.
9. Gross ML, Nasser S, Finerman GAM. Hip and pelvis. In: DeLee J, Drez D eds. *Orthopedic sports medicine.* Philadelphia: WB Saunders, 1994: 1068–85.
10. Kane WJ. Fractures of the pelvis. In: Rockwood CA Jr, Green DP, eds. *Fractures in adults.* Philadelphia: JB Lippincott, 1984: 1399–1479.
11. Johnson RC, Schmidt GL. Hip motion measurements for selected activities of daily living. *Clinical Orthopaedics* 1970; **72**: 205.
12. Morris JM. Biomechanical aspects of the hip joint. *Orthopedic Clinics of North America* 1970; **2**: 33.
13. Wingstrand H, Strömqvist B, Egund N, Gustavsson T, Nilsson LT, Thorngren KG. Hemarthrosis in undisplaced cervical fractures. Tamponade may cause reversible femoral head ischemia. *Acta Orthopaedica Scandinavica* 1986; **57**: 305–8.
14. Öberg B, Ekstarnd J, Möller M, *et al.* Muscle strength and flexiblty in different positions of soccer players. *International Journal of Sports Medicine* 1984; **5**: 213–16.
15. Dieppe P, Cusnaghan J, Young P, Kirwan J. Prediction of the progression of joint space narrowing in osteoarthritis of the knee by bone scintigraphy. *Annals of the Rheumatic Diseases* 1993; **52**: 557–63.
16. Wingstrand H, Egund N, Carlin NO, Forsberg L, Gustavsson T, Sundén G. Intracapsular pressure in transient synovitis of the hip. *Acta Orthopaedica Scandinavica* 1985; **56**: 204–10.
17. KŠlebo P, Karlsson J, SvŠrd L, *et al.* Ultrasonography of chronic tendon injuries in the groin. *American Journal of Sports Medicine* 1992; **20**: 634–9.
18. Busconi B, McCarthy J. Hip and pelvic injuries in the skeletally immature athlete. *Sport Medicine Arthroscopic Reviews* 1996; **4**: 132–58.
19. Beltran J, Noto A, Herman L, Lubbars L. Tendons: high-field strength surface coil imaging. *Radiology* 1987; **162**: 735.
20. Speer K, Lehnes J, Garett W. Radiographic imaging of muscle strain injury. *American Journal of Sports Medicine* 1993; **21**: 89.
21. Smedberg S, Broome A, Gullmo Å, Roos H. Herniography in athletes with groin pain. *American Journal of Sports Medicine* 1985; **149**: 378–82.
22. Gullmo Å. Herniography. The diagnosis of hernia in the groin and incompetence of the pouch of Douglas and pelvis floor. *Acta Radiologica Scandinavica* 1980; **361** (Suppl.): 1.
23. Ekberg O. Inguinal herniography in adults: technique, normal anatomy and diagnostic criteria for hernias. *Radiology* 1981; **138**: 31–6.
24. Ekberg O, Blomquist P, Olsson S. Positive contrast hernia in adult patients with obscure groin pain. *Surgery* 1981; **89**: 532.
25. Hackney RG. The sports hernia: a cause of chronic groin pain. *British Journal of Sports Medicine* 1993; **27**: 58–62.
26. McCarthy JC, Day B, Busconi B. Hip arthroscopy: application and technique. *Journal of the American Academy of Orthopedic Surgeons* 1995; **3**: 115.
27. McCarthy JC, Busconi B. The role of hip arthroscopy in the diagnosis and treatment of the hip disease. *Canadian Journal of Surgery* 1995; **38**: 13–17.

28. Ikeda T, Awaya G, Suzuki S, *et al*. Torn acetabular labrum in young patients: arthroscopic diagnosis and management. *Journal of Bone and Joint Surgery* (London) 1988; **70**: 13–16.

29. Noonan TJ, Garrett WE Jr. *Clinics in Sports Medicine* 1992; **11**: 783–806.

30. Peterson L, Stener B. Old total rupture of the adductor longus muscle. *Acta Orthopaedica Scandinavica* 1976; **47**: 653–7.

31. Martens MA, Hansen L, Mulier JC. Adductor tendinitis and musculus rectus abdominis tenopathy. *American Journal of Sports Medicine* 1987; **15**: 353–6.

32. Åkermark C, Johansson C. Tenotomy of the adductor longus tendon in the treatment of chronic groin pain in athletes. *American Journal of Sports Medicine* 1992; **20**: 640–3.

33. Paletta GA, Andrish JT. Injuries about the hip and pelvis in the young athlete. *Clinics in Sports Medicine* 1995; **14**: 591–628.

34. Canale ST, King RE. Pelvic and hip fractures. In: Rockwood CA Jr, Wilkins KE, King RE, eds. *Fractures in children*, 3rd edn. Philadelphia: JB Lipincott, 1991: 991–1120.

35. Westman M. Ilioinguinalis—och genitofemoralisneuralgi. *Lakartidningen* 1970; **67**: 5525–30. (In Swedish)

36. Schaberg JE, Harper MC, Allen WC. The snapping hip syndrome. *American Journal of Sports Medicine* 1984; **12**: 361.

37. Zoltan DJ, Clancy WG, Keene JS. A new operative approach to snapping hip and refractory trochanteric bursitis. *American Journal of Sports Medicine* 1996; **14**: 201.

38. Waters PM, Millis MB. Hip and pelvic injuries in the young athlete. *Clinics in Sports Medicine* 1988; **7**: 513–26.

39. Jacobsen T, Allen WC. Surgical treatment of snapping iliopsoas tendon. *American Journal of Sports Medicine* 1990; **18**: 470.

40. Fernbach SK, Wilkinsson RH. Avulsion fracture of pelvis and proximal femur. *American Journal of Roentgenology* 1981; **137**: 581–4.

41. Metzmaker JN, Pappas AM. Avulsion fractures of the pelvis. *American Journal of Sports Medicine* 1985; **13**: 349–58.

42. Wooton JR, Cross MJ, Holt KW. Avulsion of the ischial apophysis: the case for open reduction and internal fixation. *Journal of Bone and Joint Surgery* (London) 1990; **72**: 625–7.

43. Rosen LA, Micheli LJ, Treves S. Early scintigraphic diagnosis of bone stress and fracture in athletic adolescents. *Pediatrics* 1982; **70**: 11–15.

44. Devas MB. Stress fractures in the femoral neck. *Journal of Bone and Joint Surgery* 1965; **47B**: 728–31.

45. Licata AA. Stress fracture in young athletic women: case reports of unsuspected cortison-induced osteoporosis. *Journal of Medical Science and Sports Exercise* 1992; **24**: 955–7.

46. Blickenstaff LP, Morris JM. Fatigue fracture of the femoral neck. *Journal of Bone and Joint Surgery* (Am) 1966; **48**: 1031.

47. Johansson C, Ekenman I, Törnquist H, Eriksson E. Stress fractures of the femoral neck in athletes. The consequence of a delay in diagnosis. *American Journal of Sports Medicine* 1990; **18**: 524–8.

48. Calliet R. *Soft tissue pain and disability*. Philadelphia, FA Davis, 1978: 2–4.

49. Klünder K, Rud B, Hansen J. Osteoarthritis of the hip and knee in retired football players. *Acta Orthopaedica Scandinavica* 1980; **51**: 925–7.

50. Lindberg H, Danielsson LG. The relation between labor and coxarthrosis. *Clinical Orthopaedics* 1984; **191**: 159–61.

51. Axmacher B, Lindberg H. Coxarthrosis in farmers. *Clinical Orthopaedics* 1993; **287**: 82–6.

52. Lindberg H, Roos H, GŠrdsell P. Prevalence of coxarthrosis among former soccer players. *Acta Orthopaedica Scandinavica* 1992; **64**: 165–7.

53. Kujala UM, Kaprio J, Sarna S. Osteoarthritis of weightbearing joints of lower limbs in former elite male athletes. *British Medical Journal* 1994; **308**: 231–4.

54. Vingård E, Alfredsson, Goldie I, Hogstedt C. Sports and osteoarthrosis of the hip. An epidemiological study. *American Journal of Sports Medicine* 1993; **21**: 195–200.

55. Konradsen L, Berg Hansen E-M, Söndergaard L. Long distance running and osteoarthrosis. *American Journal of Sports Medicine* 1990; **18**: 379–81.

56. Marti B, Knobloch M, Tscopp A, Jucker A, Howald H. Is excessive running predictive of degenerative hip disease? Controlled study in former elite athletes. *British Medical Journal* 1989; **299**: 91–3.

57. Kujala UM, Kettunen J, Paananen H, *et al.* Knee osteoarthritis in former runners, soccer players and shooters. *Arthritis and Rheumatism* 1995; **38**: 539–46.

58. Hägglund G, Hansson LI, Hansson V, Karlberg J. Growth of children with physiolysis of the hip. *Acta Orthopaedica Scandinavica* 1987; **58**: 117–20.

59. Hartman J, Gates D. Recovery from cartilage necrosis following slipped capital femoral epiphysis. *Orthopedics Review* 1972; **1**: 33.

60. Hägglund G. The contralateral hip in slipped capital femoral epiphysis. *Journal of Pediatric Orthopedics* 1996; **5**: 158–61.

61. Wiley JJ. Traumatic osteitis pubis: The gracilis syndrome. *American Journal of Sports Medicine* 1983; **11**: 360.

62. Fricker PA, Taunton JE, Ammann W. Osteitis pubis in athletes: infection, inflammation or injury? *Sports Medicine* 1991; **12**: 266–79.

63. McMurty CT, Avioli LV. Osteitis pubis in an athlete. *Calcified Tissue International* 1986; **38**: 76–7.

64. Harris NH, Murray RO. Lesions of the symphysis in athletes. *British Medical Journal* 1974; **4**: 211–14.

65. Abrahamsson PA, Westlin N. Symphysitis and prostatitis in athletes. *Scandinavian Journal of Urology and Nephrology* 1985; **19** (Suppl. 93): 42.

66. Boland AL, Hosea TM. Hip and back pain in runners. *Postgraduate Advances in Sports Medicine* 1986; 3–15.

67. Barton PM. Piriformis syndrome: a rational approach to management. *Pain* 1991; **47**: 345–52.

68. Vandertop WP, Bosma NJ. The piriformis syndrome: a case report. *Journal of Bone and Joint Surgery* (Am) 1991; **73**: 1095–7.

69. Puranen J, Orava S. The hamstring syndrome. A new diagnosis of gluteal sciatic pain. *American Journal of Sports Medicine* 1988; **16**: 517–21.

70. O'Donoughue DH. *Treatment of injuries in athletes*. Philaldelphia: WB Saunders, 1970.

71. Hedström SÅ, Lidgren L. Acute hematogenous pelvic osteomyelitis in athletes. *American Journal of Sports Medicine* 1982; **10**: 44–6.

Index

Note: Since the subject of this book is sports medicine, index entries beginning "sport" have been kept to a minimum, and readers are advised to seek more specific references.

Page numbers in **bold** refer to principal discussions in the text. Page numbers in *italics* refer to tables. In disease-related entries "vs." refers to differential diagnosis.

The alphabetical order of the index is letter-by-letter.